VOLUME TWO

PATHOLOGY

VOLUME TWO

PATHOLOGY

Edited by

W. A. D. ANDERSON

M.A., M.D., F.A.C.P., F.C.A.P., F.R.C.P.A.(Hon.)

Emeritus Professor of Pathology and formerly Chairman
of the Department of Pathology, University
of Miami School of Medicine,
Miami, Florida

JOHN M. KISSANE, M.D.

Professor of Pathology and of Pathology in Pediatrics,
Washington University School of Medicine;
Associate Pathologist, Barnes and Affiliated Hospitals,
St. Louis Children's Hospital,
St. Louis, Missouri

SEVENTH EDITION

with 1728 figures and 6 color plates

THE C. V. MOSBY COMPANY

Saint Louis   1977

SEVENTH EDITION (two volumes)

Copyright © 1977 by The C. V. Mosby Company

Previous editions copyrighted 1948, 1953, 1957, 1961, 1966, 1971

Printed in the United States of America

Distributed in Great Britain by Henry Kimpton, London

The C. V. Mosby Company
11830 Westline Industrial Drive, St. Louis, Missouri 63141

Library of Congress Cataloging in Publication Data

Anderson, William Arnold Douglas, 1910-   ed.
  Pathology.

  Includes bibliographies and index.
  1. Pathology. I. Kissane, John M. II. Title.
[DNLM: 1. Pathology. QZ4 P2985]
RB111.A49   1977   616.07   77-1052
ISBN 0-8016-0186-X

CB/CB/B   9 8 7 6 5 4 3 2 1

CONTRIBUTORS

LESTER ADELSON, M.D.

Professor of Forensic Pathology, Department of Pathology, Case Western Reserve University School of Medicine, Cleveland; Chief Pathologist and Chief Deputy Coroner, Cuyahoga County Coroner's Office, Cleveland, Ohio

ARTHUR C. ALLEN, M.D.

Director of Laboratories, The Jewish Hospital and Medical Center of Brooklyn; Clinical Professor of Pathology, State University of New York Downstate Medical Center, Brooklyn, New York; Consultant, Hunterdon Medical Center, Flemington, New Jersey; Consultant, Fort Hamilton Veterans Administration Hospital, Brooklyn, New York

ROBERT E. ANDERSON, M.D.

Professor and Chairman, Department of Pathology, The University of New Mexico, Albuquerque; Consultant, Albuquerque Veterans Administration Hospital, Albuquerque; Consultant, Meson Physics Facility Policy Board, Los Alamos Scientific Laboratories, University of California, Los Alamos, New Mexico; Visiting Research Scientist, Radiation Effects Research Foundation, Hiroshima, Japan

W. A. D. ANDERSON, M.A., M.D., F.A.C.P., F.C.A.P., F.R.C.P.A.(Hon.)

Emeritus Professor of Pathology and formerly Chairman of the Department of Pathology, University of Miami School of Medicine, Miami, Florida

ROGER DENIO BAKER, M.D.

Professorial Lecturer, George Washington University School of Medicine and Health Sciences, Washington, D.C.

SAROJA BHARATI

Associate Director, Congenital Heart Disease Research and Training Center, Hektoen Institute for Medical Research; Research Associate Professor of Medicine, Abraham Lincoln School of Medicine, University of Illinois; Associate Professor of Pathology, Rush Medical School, Chicago, Illinois

CHAPMAN H. BINFORD, A.D., M.D.

Chief, Special Mycobacterial Diseases Branch, Geographic Pathology Division, Armed Forces Institute of Pathology, Washington, D.C.

JACOB L. CHASON, M.D.

Professor of Pathology (Neuropathology) and Chairman of the Department of Pathology, Wayne State University School of Medicine, Detroit, Michigan

MASAHIRO CHIGA, M.D.

Professor of Pathology, Department of Pathology and Oncology, University of Kansas Medical Center, Kansas City, Kansas

A. R. W. CLIMIE, M.D.

Associate Professor of Pathology, Wayne State University School of Medicine; Chief of Pathology, Harper-Grace Hospitals, Detroit, Michigan

SIR THEO CRAWFORD, B.Sc., M.D., F.R.C.P., F.R.C.Path.

Professor of Pathology, St. George's Hospital Medical School, University of London, London, England

GEORGE Th. DIAMANDOPOULOS, M.D.

Associate Professor of Pathology, Harvard Medical School, Boston, Massachusetts

HUGH A. EDMONDSON, M.D.

Professor of Pathology, University of Southern California School of Medicine, Los Angeles, California

GERALD FINE, M.D.

Staff Pathologist and Chief, Division of Anatomic Pathology, Department of Pathology, Henry Ford Hospital, Detroit, Michigan

L. M. FRANKS, M.D., F.C.A.P., F.R.C.Path.

Imperial Cancer Research Fund Laboratories, London, England

ROBERT J. GORLIN, D.D.S., M.S.

Professor and Chairman of the Division of Oral Pathology, University of Minnesota School of Dentistry, Minneapolis, Minnesota

JOE W. GRISHAM, M.D.

Professor and Chairman, Department of Pathology, University of North Carolina School of Medicine, Chapel Hill, North Carolina

PAUL GROSS, M.D.

Distinguished Research Professor, Department of Pathology, Medical University of South Carolina, Charleston, South Carolina

EMMERICH VON HAAM, M.D.

Professor Emeritus of Pathology, The Ohio State University College of Medicine, Columbus, Ohio

BÉLA HALPERT, M.D.

Emeritus Professor of Pathology, Baylor College of Medicine, Houston, Texas

GORDON R. HENNIGAR, M.D.

Professor of Pathology and Chairman of the Department of Pathology, Medical University of South Carolina, Charleston, South Carolina

CHARLES S. HIRSCH, M.D.

Associate Professor of Forensic Pathology, Department of Pathology, Case Western Reserve University School of Medicine, Cleveland; Associate Pathologist and Deputy Coroner, Cuyahoga County Coroner's Office, Cleveland, Ohio

HOWARD C. HOPPS, M.D., Ph.D.

Curators' Professor, Department of Pathology, University of Missouri Medical Center, Columbia, Missouri

†ROBERT C. HORN, Jr., M.D.

Late Chairman, Department of Pathology, Henry Ford Hospital, Detroit, Michigan

DAVID B. JONES, M.D.

Professor of Pathology, State University of New York Upstate Medical Center, Syracuse, New York

JOHN M. KISSANE, M.D.

Professor of Pathology and of Pathology in Pediatrics, Washington University School of Medicine; Pathologist, Barnes and Affiliated Hospitals, St. Louis Children's Hospital, St. Louis, Missouri

†Deceased.

FREDERICK T. KRAUS, M.D.

Director of Laboratory Medicine, St. John's Mercy Medical Center; Associate Professor of Pathology, Washington University School of Medicine, St. Louis, Missouri

JOSEPH F. KUZMA, B.S., M.D., M.S.

Clinical Professor of Pathology, Medical College of Wisconsin, Milwaukee, Wisconsin

PAUL E. LACY, M.D.

Mallinckrodt Professor and Chairman of the Department of Pathology, Washington University School of Medicine, St. Louis, Missouri

MAURICE LEV, M.D.

Director, Congenital Heart Disease Research and Training Center, Hektoen Institute for Medical Research; Professor of Pathology, Northwestern University Medical School; Professor of Pathology, Rush Medical School; Professorial Lecturer, Pritzker School of Medicine of the University of Chicago; Lecturer in the Department of Pathology, Abraham Lincoln School of Medicine, University of Illinois; Lecturer in the Department of Pathology, the Chicago Medical School, University of Health Sciences; Lecturer in the Department of Pathology, Loyola University, Stritch School of Medicine; Distinguished Professor in the Department of Pediatrics, Rush Medical College; and Career Investigator and Educator, Chicago Heart Association, Chicago, Illinois

VINCENT T. MARCHESI, M.D., Ph.D.

Anthony N. Brady Professor of Pathology and Chairman, Department of Pathology, Yale University School of Medicine, New Haven, Connecticut

RAÚL A. MARCIAL-ROJAS, M.D.

Professor of Pathology and Legal Medicine, University of Puerto Rico School of Medicine; Director, Institute of Legal Medicine, San Juan, Puerto Rico

WILLIAM A. MEISSNER, M.D.

Professor of Pathology at the New England Deaconess Hospital, Harvard Medical School, Boston, Massachusetts

JOHN B. MIALE, M.D.

Professor of Pathology, University of Miami School of Medicine, Miami, Florida

MAX MILLARD, M.A., M.B. (Dublin), F.R.C.P. (Ireland), F.R.C.Path. (England), D.C.P. (London)

Director of Pathology Laboratories, South Miami Hospital, Miami, Florida

FATHOLLAH K. MOSTOFI, A.B., B.Sc., M.D.

Associate Chairman, Center for Advanced Pathology; Chairman, Department of Genitourinary Pathology; Registrar, Urologic Registries; Head, World Health Organization International Reference Center on Tumors of Male Genitourinary Tract; Veterans Administration Special Reference Laboratory for Pathology at the Armed Forces Institute of Pathology; Clinical Professor of Pathology, Georgetown University Medical Center, Washington, D.C.; Professor of Pathology, University of Maryland School of Medicine; Associate Professor of Pathology, Johns Hopkins University Medical School, Baltimore, Maryland

WAYKIN NOPANITAYA, Ph.D.

Assistant Professor, Department of Pathology, University of North Carolina School of Medicine, Chapel Hill, North Carolina

JAMES E. OERTEL, M.D.

Chief of Endocrine Pathology, Armed Forces Institute of Pathology, Washington, D.C.

ROBERT L. PETERS, M.D.

Professor of Pathology, University of Southern California School of Medicine, Los Angeles; Director of Pathology and Laboratories, University of Southern California Liver Unit at Rancho Los Amigos Hospital, Downey, California

HENRY PINKERTON, B.S., M.D.

Emeritus Professor of Pathology, St. Louis University School of Medicine, St. Louis, Missouri

R. C. B. PUGH, M.D., F.R.C.Path.

Department of Pathology, St. Paul's Hospital, London, England

JUAN ROSAI, M.D.

Professor of Pathology and Director of Anatomic Pathology, University of Minnesota Medical School and University Hospitals, Minneapolis, Minnesota

ARKADI M. RYWLIN, M.D.

Professor of Pathology, University of Miami School of Medicine; Director, Department of Pathology and Laboratory Medicine, Mount Sinai Medical Center, Miami Beach, Florida

DANTE G. SCARPELLI, M.D., Ph.D.

Professor and Chairman, Department of Pathology, Northwestern University Medical School, Chicago, Illinois

THOMAS M. SCOTTI, A.B., M.D.

Formerly Professor of Pathology, University of Miami School of Medicine, Miami, Florida

STEWART SELL, M.D.

Professor of Pathology, School of Medicine, University of California at San Diego, La Jolla, California

†RICHARD SHUMAN, B.S., M.D.

Late Professor of Pathology, Medical College of Pennsylvania; Consultant in Pathology, Veterans Administration Hospital, Philadelphia, Pennsylvania; formerly Chief of Soft Tissue Section, Pathology Division, Armed Forces Institute of Pathology; formerly Head of International Center for Soft Tissue Tumors, World Health Organization, Washington, D.C.

RUTH SILBERBERG, M.D.

Professor of Pathology, Departments of Anatomy and Orthopedic Surgery, Hadassah Hebrew University, School of Medicine, Kiryat Hadassah, Jerusalem, Israel

STANLEY B. SMITH, M.D.

Pathologist, Variety Children's Hospital, Miami, Florida

SHELDON C. SOMMERS, M.D.

Director of Laboratories, Lenox Hill Hospital; Clinical Professor of Pathology, Columbia University College of Physicians and Surgeons, New York, New York; Clinical Professor of Pathology, University of Southern California School of Medicine, Los Angeles, California

STEVEN L. TEITELBAUM, M.D.

Associate Professor of Pathology, Washington University School of Medicine; Associate Professor of Oral Biology, Washington University School of Dental Medicine; Associate Pathologist, The Jewish Hospital of St. Louis; Pathologist, Shriners Hospital for Crippled Children, St. Louis, Missouri

ROBERT A. VICKERS, D.D.S., M.S.D.

Professor of Oral Pathology, University of Minnesota School of Dentistry, Minneapolis, Minnesota

NANCY E. WARNER, M.D.

Chairman, Department of Pathology, University of Southern California School of Medicine, Los Angeles, California

D. L. WILHELM, M.D., Ph.D.

Professor and Head of School of Pathology, University of New South Wales; Director of Pathology, The Prince Henry Hospital and The Prince of Wales Hospital, Sydney, Australia

LORENZ E. ZIMMERMAN, M.D.

Chief, Ophthalmic Pathology Branch, Armed Forces Institute of Pathology, and Clinical Professor of Ophthalmic Pathology, The George Washington University School of Medicine, Washington, D.C.

†Deceased.

PREFACE to seventh edition

The preface to the sixth edition of *Pathology* mentioned a merging between pathology and other so-called basic sciences that compelled a certain arbitrariness relating to inclusion or exclusion of many subjects in which recent advances had been made. In the preparation of this seventh edition, we have taken cognizance of some of those points of merging to which highly specific, not merely arbitrary, consideration must be given, that is, consideration regarding inclusion in the undergraduate medical curriculum. In planning for and executing this seventh edition, we recognized the fact that many schools now introduce pathology in the first year of the undergraduate medical curriculum. This fact compels teachers of pathology to place their contributions even more specifically in contextual relationship with the so-called "basic sciences" while maintaining relevant contemporariness in their applications to clinical medicine.

To these ends, several chapters have been rewritten by new contributors. We welcome them to this, our joint effort, at the same time that we thank those colleagues whom they have succeeded.

We hope that this revision will continue to entitle this work to the acceptance that preceding editions have enjoyed as a source for consideration by students during their preclinical years, no less than during their clinical years. A conscious effort has been made to continue the emphasis upon clinicopathologic correlations to the end that the work would continue to merit the confidence enjoyed by previous editions as a reliable, up-to-date source of information related to pathologic anatomy, important in the practice of the many defined areas of clinical medicine, including that of pathology itself.

W. A. D. Anderson
John M. Kissane

PREFACE to first edition

Pathology should form the basis of every physician's thinking about his patients. The study of the nature of disease, which constitutes pathology in the broad sense, has many facets. Any science or technique which contributes to our knowledge of the nature and constitution of disease belongs in the broad realm of pathology. Different aspects of a disease may be stressed by the geneticist, the cytologist, the biochemist, the clinical diagnostician, etc., and it is the difficult function of the pathologist to attempt to bring about a synthesis, and to present disease in as whole or as true an aspect as can be done with present knowledge. Pathologists often have been accused, and sometimes justly, of stressing the morphologic changes in disease to the neglect of functional effects. Nevertheless, pathologic anatomy and histology remain as an essential foundation of knowledge about disease, without which basis the concepts of many diseases are easily distorted.

In this volume is brought together the specialized knowledge of a number of pathologists in particular aspects or fields of pathology. A time-tested order of presentation is maintained, both because it has been found logical and effective in teaching medical students and because it facilitates study and reference by graduates. Although presented in an order and form to serve as a textbook, it is intended also to have sufficient comprehensiveness and completeness to be useful to the practicing or graduate physician. It is hoped that this book will be both a foundation and a useful tool for those who deal with the problems of disease.

For obvious reasons, the nature and effects of radiation have been given unusual relative prominence. The changing order of things, with increase of rapid, world-wide travel and communication, necessitates increased attention to certain viral, protozoal, parasitic, and other conditions often dismissed as "tropical," to bring them nearer their true relative importance. Also, given more than usual attention are diseases of the skin, of the organs of special senses, of the nervous system, and of the skeletal system. These are fields which often have not been given sufficient consideration in accordance with their true relative importance among diseases.

The Editor is highly appreciative of the spirit of the various contributors to this book. They are busy people, who, at the sacrifice of other duties and of leisure, freely cooperated in its production, uncomplainingly tolerated delays and difficulties, and were understanding in their willingness to work together for the good of the book as a whole. Particular thanks are due the directors of the Army Institute of Pathology and the American Registry of Pathology, for making available many illustrations. Dr. G. L. Duff, Strathcona Professor of Pathology, McGill University, Dr. H. A. Edmondson, Department of Pathology of the University of Southern California School of Medicine, Dr. J. S. Hirschboeck, Dean, and Dr. Harry Beckman, Professor of Pharmacology, Marquette University School of Medicine, all generously gave advice and assistance with certain parts.

To the members of the Department of Pathology and Bacteriology at Marquette University, the Editor wishes to express gratitude, both for tolerance and for assistance. Especially valuable has been the help of Dr. R. S. Haukohl, Dr. J. F. Kuzma, Dr. S. B. Pessin, and Dr. H. Everett. A large burden was assumed by the Editor's secretaries, Miss Charlotte Skacel and Miss Ann Cassady. Miss Patricia Blakeslee also assisted at various stages and with the index. To all of these the Editor's thanks, and also to the many others who at some time assisted by helpful and kindly acts, or by words of encouragement or interest.

W. A. D. Anderson

CONTENTS

xiv   Contents

COLOR PLATES

25/Testes, scrotum, and penis

FATHOLLAH K. MOSTOFI

TESTES
Anomalies

Excluding malposition of the testicle, other anomalies are very rare. Anorchidism (congenital absence) and monorchidism (one testicle) have been reported. Synorchidism (fusion of testicles) occurs intra-abdominally. Polyorchidism has been found at operation and necropsy.

Ectopic testis. Ectopic testis is a congenital malposition of the testicle outside of the normal channel of descent. This ectopia, according to its location, is classified as interstitial, pubopenile, femoral, crural, transverse, and perineal.

Cryptorchidism. When the congenital malposition results in retention of the testicle anywhere along the route of descent, it is known as cryptorchidism. The cause of cryptorchidism is not always evident. The various apparent causes are short spermatic vessels or vas deferens, adhesions to the peritoneum, poorly developed inguinal canal or superficial abdominal ring, maldevelopment of the scrotum or cremaster muscles, and hormonal influences. Incomplete descent is found quite frequently during the first few months of infancy. The incidence is about 4% in boys under 15 years of age and about 0.2% in adults. Histologically, the cryptorchid testis before puberty does not differ from the normally descended organ. After puberty, however, it is always smaller than normal. The capsule is somewhat thickened and wrinkled. The epididymis is separated from the mesorchium. There is progressive loss of germ cell elements. The tubules may be lined only with spermatogonia and spermatids, but occasionally there is spermatogenesis. In fact, foci of spermatogenesis are found in 10% of undescended testes. This condition has also been reported in abdominal testis. It is estimated that 10% of men with untreated cryptorchidism remain fertile. The basement membrane of the tubules thicken and hyalinize. In later stages spermatogenesis is rare or absent and the tubules are lined only with Sertoli cells. Tubules with completely occluded lumens are not uncommon. The collecting tubules and rete may be quite prominent, a condition that suggests hyperplasia and even adenoma. The intertubular tissue is sparsely cellular and becomes more dense with age. The interstitial cells of Leydig are conspicuous and vary in number. In some cases the Leydig cells are decreased in number, and in other cases they are increased both in size and in number. They are found singly, in small groups, and occasionally in large masses. In some cryptorchid testicles, most of the atrophied organ is composed of large groups of polyhedral Leydig cells between which may be found scanty fibrous tissue and a few fibrosed tubules. In rare instances, very few cellular elements are encountered and the entire testes become completely fibrosed.

The cause of atrophy of undescended and ectopic testes is not known. There is convincing evidence that an optimum temperature is necessary for spermatogenesis and that temperatures higher than that within the scrotum suppress spermatogenesis. When aspermia or hypospermia exists, the testicle atrophies. The chief function of the scrotum is to regulate the temperature for the testes. Ischemia caused by pressure, stressed by some authors, is definitely a minor factor in causing suppression of spermatogenesis in cryptorchidism. There is a high incidence of tumors of the testes in cryptorchidism.

Intersexuality. A *true hermaphrodite* or *ambisexual* is one who possesses an ovary and a testicle or two ovotestes with or without external genitalia of both sexes. A *pseudohermaphrodite* possesses gonads of one sex and genitalia of either both or opposite sexes. In the *male pseudohermaphrodite,* the testes are present, but the internal genitalia are of both sexes, and the penis and scrotum are poorly developed. In the *female pseudohermaphrodite,* the ovaries are present, usually in their normal position, the vagina is rudimentary and opens into the urethra, and the clitoris is hypertrophied.

Status of the testis in male infertility

About 15 out of every 100 marriages in the United States are barren, and male infertility accounts for about half of the cases. In all such patients quantitative determination of urinary 17-ketosteroids, estrogens, and gonadotropins; karyotyping; and testicular biopsy are essential to determine the specific cause of the male infertility and whether it is curable. Wong and his co-workers have proposed a simple classification of male infertility: pretesticular, testicular, and posttesticular.

Pretesticular causes of infertility are mainly hypopituitarism, endogenous or exogenous estrogen or androgen excess, hypothyroidism, diabetes mellitus, and glucocorticoid excess.

Hypopituitarism may be prepubertal or postpubertal. Prepubertal causes include lesions in or adjacent to the pituitary (e.g., craniopharyngiomas, trauma, and cysts). Such patients eventually manifest sexual infantilism, failure of somatic growth, and varying degrees of adrenal and thyroid hypofunction. Testicular biopsy shows small immature seminiferous tubules and immature Leydig cells similar to prepubertal testis.

Postpubertal hypopituitarism results from tumors, trauma, or infarction. Testicular biopsy shows maturation arrest, loss of germ cells, reduced diameter of tubules, and progressive thickening and hyalinization of tunica propria. The Leydig cells are small and shriveled.

Hypopituitarism may be the result of genetic defects in gonadotropin secretion. There are no demonstrable lesions of the pituitary and deficiencies of adrenal and thyroid function or growth. The patients may show deficiency of both follicle stimulating (FSH) and luteinizing hormones (LH), or the FSH may be normal but LH deficient. The patients are generally tall and eunuchoid. Testicular biopsy in the former shows small and immature seminiferous tubules resembling prepubertal testis. In the latter the seminiferous tubules show a greater degree of development than do the Leydig cells.

Estrogen excess may be endogenous (hepatic cirrhosis, adrenal tumor, Sertoli or Leydig cell tumor) or exogenous (administered to patients with cancer of prostate). Initially, the biopsy shows failure of maturation, progressive decrease of germinal elements, diminished diameter of seminiferous tubules, and thickening and hyalinization of tunica propria. Eventually there is complete sclerosis of tubules and atrophy of Leydig cells. The findings are identical to those of postpubertal hypopituitarism.

Androgen excess may be endogenous (adrenogenital syndrome, androgen-producing adrenal cortical or testicular tumors) or exogenous (oral administartion). Pathologic findings depend on whether the condition developed before or after puberty. If prepubertal, the result is virilism and failure of the testis to mature. If postpubertal, there is progressive loss of germ cells and, unless recognized and remedied, tubular sclerosis.

Glucocorticoid excess, whether endogenous (Cushing's syndrome) or exogenous (administered for treatment of ulcerative colitis, rheumatoid arthritis, or bronchial asthma) can result in oligospermia and maturation arrest or hypospermatogenesis.

Hypothyroidism and diabetes mellitus may result in decreased fertility. Hypospermatogenesis is followed by thickening of tunica propria. In uncontrolled diabetes autonomic neuropathy may result in impotence.

Testicular causes of infertility are agonadism, cryptorchidism, maturation arrest, hypospermatogenesis, absence of germ cells (Sertoli cell–only syndrome), Klinefelter's syndrome, mumps orchitis, and irradiation damage.

Agonadism

Congenital agonadism is extremely rare and consists of total absence of the testes. If this occurs in early embryonic life, the infant will be female. Occasionally in cryptorchid boys the epididymis ends blindly, but careful search fails to show any gonadal tissue (the "vanishing testis syndrome"). The chromosomal pattern is XY. Since testes must have been present in fetal life to initiate male development, they must have been resorbed after that period.

Bilateral anorchia may be associated with incomplete differentiation of male genitalia. The gonads and the internal genital structures may be absent or rudimentary. These findings suggest that the testes must have been present to initiate male sex development but vanished before maturity.

Jost showed that fetal testis played an important role in the early development of the wolffian structures and regression of müllerian elements. The development of wolffian structures was related to the local androgen production, whereas regression of müllerian elements seemed to be influenced by additional nonandrogenic factors. Federman's excellent discussion of the situation may be summarized as follows: If the male fetus begins life with dysgenetic testis, varying degrees of pseudohermaphroditism may ensue; if gonadal failure occurs before organization of the genital tract, female external genitalia will result; if gonadal failure occurs during the period of male sexual differentiation, ambiguous genitalia may result; if, however, testicular failure occurs after the sixteenth week of gestation, the male structures are established and the patient would develop as a male but without testes.

Cryptorchidism

The histology of cryptorchidism is described on p. 1013.

Maturation arrest

Maturation arrest is manifested in a testicular biopsy by the failure of normal spermatogenesis at some stage. Most commonly this is at the stage of primary spermatocytes. No secondary spermatocytes, spermatids, or spermatozoa are present. It may also be at the spermatid stage with few or no spermatozoa.

The Sertoli cells, testicular tunica propria, and Leydig cells are normal as is the diameter of the seminiferous tubules. There is oligospermia, or azoospermia. The urinary FSH, LH, and 7-ketosteroids are normal.

Hypospermatogenesis

Hypospermatogenesis is more difficult to detect. All cells of spermatogenic series are present in the same proportions as normal, but the number of each variety is decreased. The seminiferous tubules are of normal size. Sertoli and Leydig cells and the tunica of the tubules are normal. Patients have oligospermia with normal urinary FSH, LH, and 17-ketosteroids.

Absence of germ cells (Sertoli cell–only syndrome)

The characteristic feature of this group is the absence of germ cells with the seminiferous tubules lined solely by exuberant Sertoli cells. In a few tubules germ cells may persist. The diameter of seminiferous tubules is decreased; the tunica propria of the tubules is not thickened and the Leydig cells are normal. The secondary sex characteristics are well developed; the patients are potent but infertile. The urinary 17-ketosteroids are normal, but urinary FSH and LH are invariably high.

Klinefelter's syndrome

About 3% of male sterility is attributable to primary hypogonadism. This syndrome is characterized by testicular hypoplasia, azoospermia, gynecomastia, eunuchoid build, increase of urinary gonadotropin, and, not infrequently, subnormal intelligence. The diagnosis is seldom made before puberty. Chromosome studies reveal an XXY intersexuality caused by fertilization of an ovum whose divided X chromosome failed to separate. Such individuals have a sex-chromatin pattern similar to genetic females. However, other individuals with a similar or nearly similar syndrome are genetically males.

There is increased urinary excretion of pituitary gonadotropic hormones, but the reason is not that there are any abnormalities of the pituitary gland but is attributed to the absence of the controlling influence of some testicular hormones.

The tests are usually small (1.5×0.5 cm). The histology of the biopsy varies widely. It has been reported that the tubules are sclerosed and hyalinized and there is an apparent increase in the number of interstitial cells. Tubular fibrosis is progressive and is associated with retardation of spermatogenesis. Spermatogenic activity varies greatly. Careful examination of a biopsy may fail to show any activity whatsoever, but it may be found only on examination of the entire testis. Maturation as far as primary spermatogenesis, even to the stage of secondary spermatocytes and spermatids and, in rare instances, spermatozoa, has been reported. The release of sperm from the testis to the ejaculate is uncommon, but a few have been observed.

Mumps orchitis

The histology of mumps orchitis is described on p. 1017. Ten to 20 years after the initial infection, depending on the extent of testicular involvement, there may be oligospermia or azoospermia. The 17-ketosteroids and LH are normal, and the level of FSH is elevated.

Irradiation damage

Permanent germ cell destruction results from exposure to radiation so that in time the tubules are lined by Sertoli cells only. The diameter of seminiferous tubules is progressively smaller and the tunica is thicker, terminating in sclerosis. Leydig cells are preserved. The patient is azoospermic or oligospermic. Urinary FSH is elevated, but the 17-ketosteroids and LH are normal.

Posttesticular causes of infertility consist mainly of block, which may be congenital (absence or atresia of vas deferens or epididymis) or acquired. Acquired is more frequent and may be either on the basis of infection (gonorrhea, etc.) or surgical intervention (voluntary or iatrogenic). The clinical manifestation is azoospermia. The testicular biopsy in such patients shows active spermatogenesis. The seminiferous tubules may be dilated, and there may be hypospermatogenesis or cellular sloughing, or both.

Another cause of posttesticular infertility is impaired sperm mobility. Wong and his coworkers reserve this term specifically to those cases in which the sperm counts are adequate and the testicular biopsy specimens are normal, yet the mobility of spermatozoa in the semen is either greatly impaired or absent.

In all men with infertility, testicular biopsy is necessary for proper categorization and for prognosis.

Acquired atrophy

Excluding undescended testicles, acquired atrophy occurs in senility, prolonged hyperpyrexia, debility, avitaminosis, cirrhosis of the liver, hypothyroidism, schizophrenia, estrogen medication for carcinoma of the prostate, and diseases of the pituitary gland and hypothalamus. Faulty or suppressed spermatogenesis without other changes may questionably be considered as mild atrophy. The early findings in atrophy are degenerative changes of the spermatogonia cells. As atrophy progresses, the germinal epithelial cells disappear, leaving only Sertoli cells resting on a thickened basement membrane. The seminiferous tubules become small and farther apart, and the interstitial cells of Leydig appear prominent (Fig. 25-1).

Thrombosis and infarction

Hemorrhage, thrombosis, and infarction of the testicle occur in trauma, torsion, leukemias, bacterial endocarditis, and periarteritis nodosa (Fig. 25-2). Birth trauma may cause hemorrhage of the testicle. Many such hemorrhages are small hematomas that rapidly resorb.

Torsion

A sudden twisting of the spermatic cord results in strangulation of the blood vessels

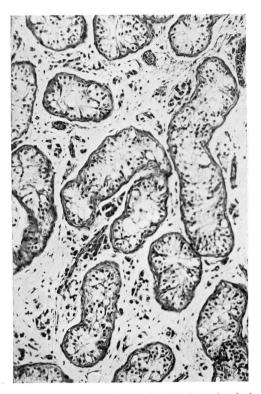

Fig. 25-1. Atrophy of testicle. Thickened tubular basement membranes lined with degenerated spermatogonia and Sertoli cells. Prominent Leydig cells in interstitial tissue.

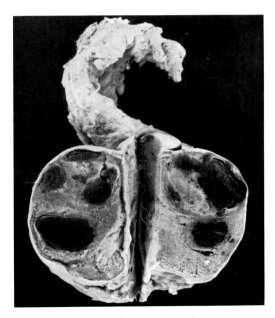

Fig. 25-2. Multiple infarcts of testicle in periarteritis nodosa.

serving the testicle and epididymis. The predisposing causes of torsion are free mobility and high attachment of the testicle. These anatomic features are found in such conditions as failure of the tunica vaginalis to close, large tunica vaginalis, absence of scrotal ligaments, gubernaculum testis or posterior mesorchium, or elongation of the globus minor. Abnormal attachment of the common mesentery and vessels to the globus minor and lower pole of the testicle provides attachment of the testicle by a narrow stalk instead of by a wide band. The exciting cause may be violent exercise or straining. The majority of the cases of torsion involve undescended testicles. Torsion may occur at any age. Cases have been reported in the newborn infant and in very elderly persons. The twist is commonly located in the free intravaginal portion of the cord. It may be a half turn to two full turns in either direction. The gross and microscopic findings depend on the degree of strangulation. Usually, the picture is that of congestion and hemorrhage followed by necrosis of the testicle. The interstitial tissue may or may not be infiltrated with leukocytes. The tubules suffer varying degrees of degeneration and necrosis. At times, the entire testicle is found to be necrotic and acellular, and "ghost" tubules remain as conspicuous components in the histologic picture.

Inflammation

Acute orchitis. Acute orchitis is (1) an infection via the vas deferens and epididymis, (2) a combination epididymo-orchitis, or (3) a metastatic lymphogenous or hematogenous infection. Epididymo-orchitis is predominantly secondary to urethritis, cystitis, and seminal vesiculitis. Acute orchitis may be a complication of mumps, smallpox, scarlet fever, diphtheria, typhoid fever, glanders, dengue fever, influenza, typhus fever, pneumonia, malaria, filariasis, and Mediterranean fever. Acute orchitis also has been encountered as a complication in focal infections such as sinusitis, osteomyelitis, cholecystitis, and appendicitis.

In acute orchitis, the testicle becomes firm, tense, and swollen. In gonorrheal orchitis, which is usually an extension from the epididymis, single or multiple abscesses develop, or the testicle may be diffusely infiltrated with neutrophilic leukocytes, lymphocytes, and plasma cells.

Chronic orchitis. Acute inflammation of the testicle may completely resolve, or the inflam-

mation may continue in a chronic form. The inflammation may be focal or diffuse, unilateral or bilateral. In some cases, fibrosis may be seen grossly. There is a varying degree of degeneration and disappearance of the tubular cells, and the basement membranes of the tubules become thickened and hyalinized. Many patients with testicular tumors give a history of some form of orchitis.

Mumps orchitis. The incidence of orchitis as a complication of parotitis is between 20% and 30%. This complication is rare in children, being seen mostly in adults. Grossly, the testicle is enlarged, and the tunica albuginea contains punctate hemorrhages. In the early stages, the parenchyma appears edematous. Microscopically, the acute inflammatory process is characterized by diffuse interstitial infiltration with polymorphonuclear neutrophils, lymphocytes, and histiocytes. Similar cellular elements fill the lumens and distend the tubules. Very few tubules suffer necrosis, but in severe cases the germinal epithelial cells and spermatogonia undergo degeneration, with subsequent loss of spermatogenesis. In subacute and chronic phases of mumps orchitis, the interstitial tissue is infiltrated with lymphocytes. When degeneration has been extensive, the testicle becomes smaller, and the thickened tubules are lined with a few Sertoli cells. The incidence of testicular atrophy and consequent sterility in this type of orchitis is not known.

Granulomatous orchitis. The etiology and pathogenesis of a rather characteristic type of nonspecific granulomatous orchitis that may be misinterpreted as tuberculosis have not been entirely clarified despite excellent research and studies of the lesion. It occurs predominantly among middle-aged men and frequently is associated with trauma. Grossly, the testis is enlarged, and the tunica albuginea may be normal or thickened. The tissue is usually grayish, white, tan, or brownish. Histologically, there is a striking tuberculoid pattern. The relatively circumscribed microscopic tubercles originate from and within the tubules. They are composed of epithelioid cells, lymphocytes, plasma cells, some polymorphoneuclear neutrophils, and multinucleated giant cells. The walls of the tubules are thickened by fibrous proliferation and, with the inflammatory cellular infiltrate, blend with the contiguous interstitial tissue. The interstitial tissue shows fibrosis and is predominantly infiltrated with lymphocytes and plasma cells. The origin of the epithelioid cells is from Sertoli cells lining the tubules. The transformation of the Sertoli cells to epithelioid or histiocytic cells is the result of the effect of a lipid fraction of spermatozoa. Berg[2] has produced granulomas in hamsters with an acid-fast staining lipid fraction of human spermatozoa.

Malakoplakia. One type of granulomatous orchitis, often with abscess formation, is characterized by infiltration with large histiocytes with small round or oval nuclei, and ground glass granular cytoplasm containing Michaelis-Gutmann bodies. The lesion is described on p. 985.

Tuberculosis of testicle and epididymis. Tuberculosis of the testicle without involvement of the epididymis is rare. Discrete tubercles in the testicle may be encountered in generalized miliary tuberculosis. Tuberculosis of the epididymis is usually unilateral, may occur at any age, and frequently is associated with tuberculosis of the lungs and genitourinary tract. The location of the primary focus of genital tuberculosis has stimulated considerable controversy among many investigators. Young's extensive surgical experience has convinced him that, in most of the cases of genital tuberculosis, the primary site is in the seminal vesicles. Walker[30] lends support to the advocates of the theory that the prostate gland or seminal vesicles harbor the primary focus.

The earliest lesions are seen as discrete or conglomerated, yellowish necrotic areas located in the globus minor. Microscopically, these reveal either characteristic tubercles or disorganized inflammatory cellular reaction consisting of polymorphonuclear leukocytes, plasma cells, desquamated epithelial cells, some large monocytes, occasional multinucleated giant cells, and many acid-fast bacilli. The early lesion may regress and become calcified. Usually, however, there is progressive invasion until the entire epididymis becomes involved. When the tunica vaginalis is invaded, a considerable amount of serofibrinous or purulent exudate develops. Usually, the tunica vaginalis serves as a barrier against extension into the testicle, and it is often surprising to find complete destruction of the epididymis with no invasion of the testicle.

Syphilis. The testicles are involved in almost every syphilitic patient. Syphilitic orchitis occurs either as a diffuse interstitial inflammation with fibrosis or as single or multiple gummas. Either of these types of lesions may be found in the acquired or congenital forms of syphilis. In contrast to tuberculosis, acquired syphilitic orchitis affects the testicle before the epididymis.

Grossly, in the diffuse interstitial type the testis is enlarged, the cut surface is bulging grayish to yellowish white, and there is loss of normal architecture. The gummatous testicle is enlarged, firm, globular, smooth, and, rarely, nodular. When sectioned, the yellowish white or grayish white gummas bulge from the surrounding parenchyma. Extension of the gumma into the tunica vaginalis causes adhesion to the scrotum, and secondary infection induces ulceration of the scrotum with herniation of the testicle. In fibrous syphilitic orchitis, the testicle is small and hard. When fibrosis is not pronounced, however, it is of normal size and somewhat indurated.

Microscopically, in secondary syphilis both the interstitial tissue and the seminiferous tubules are involved. The inflammatory reaction is similar to that as seen elsewhere in secondary syphilis. There is heavy infiltration with plasma cells, lymphocytes, and monocytes. The inflammatory reaction often surrounds small and large blood vessels that show hyperplasia of their walls. Angiitis of small arteries is characteristic. The involved seminiferous tubules resemble those of granulomatous orchitis with replacement of normal cell population with histiocytes, lipophages, and proliferating Sertoli cells. Spirochetes are readily demonstrable with Levaditi stains.

Microscopically, the gummas of the testicle are similar to those found elsewhere. The gumma is composed of a central area of necrosis surrounded by a zone of edematous fibrous tissue infiltrated with plasma cells, lymphocytes, and occasional multinucleated giant cells. There is decreased spermatogenesis and thickening of the basement membrane of the tubules. Spirochetes are readily demonstrable in this stage. In later stages, there is diffuse fibrosis, peritubular and basal hyalinization, with necrosis of the tubular cells, and shrinking of the tubules. The interstitial cells usually are well preserved and often may be hypertrophied. Spirochetes rarely are found in the fibrotic stage.

Chronic vaginalitis (chronic proliferative periorchitis, pseudofibromatous periorchitis). Chronic proliferative periorchitis frequently has been designated as multiple fibromas of the tunica vaginalis. The etiology of this peculiar inflammatory lesion is unknown. Some of the cases are definitely associated with trauma. The age incidence is between 20 and 40 years.

Grossly, the tunica vaginalis is found to be greatly thickened and nodular (Fig. 25-3).

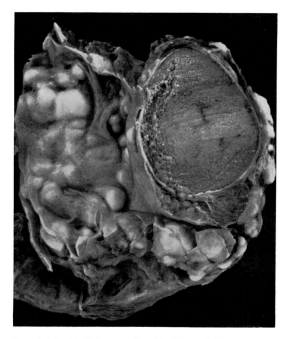

Fig. 25-3. Nodular vaginalitis (pseudofibromatous periorchitis). (Courtesy Dr. Robert S. Haukohl, Tampa, Fla.)

The surface is smooth and glistening. The nodules are multiple, scattered irregularly throughout the tunica vaginalis, and more numerous along the epididymis. The nodules range in size from 1 mm to 2 cm in diameter. On sectioning, some of the nodules are found to be circumscribed and resemble uterine fibroids, whereas others are ill defined or confluent. Occasionally, some nodules become calcified.

Microscopically, the sections reveal a scanty cellular collagenous fibrous tissue, often interlacing or having a whorling architecture, infiltrated with lymphocytes and plasma cells. In other cases, there is very little inflammatory cellular reaction.

Spermatic granuloma. Invasion of spermatozoa into the stroma of the epididymis provokes an inflammatory reaction designated as spermatic granuloma. The lesions are not uncommon, and similar lesions occur within the testes. Trauma or inflammation injures the wall of the tubule, and spermatozoa are spilled into the stroma. In some patients in whom vasectomy has been done, loss of ligature from the proximal (testicular) end of the vas allows extravasation of spermatozoa resulting in sperm granuloma. Such loss of ligature may also result in reestablishing communication between severed ends of the vas. The lesions

range from 3 mm to 3 cm in diameter. They are firm and white and may contain soft yellow or yellowish brown areas. They may be located in any part of the epididymis, but the majority occur in the upper pole.

Histologically, the early reaction is infiltration with neutrophilic leukocytes and phagocytes, followed by various mononuclear cells, among which are histiocytes and epithelioid cells. At this stage, the lesion is tuberculoid in character, with a center containing spermatozoa and debris. Lymphocytes appear among the epithelioid cells, and a mild fibroblastic proliferation replaces the epithelioid cells. The late lesions consist of hyalinized fibrous tissue, spermatozoa, granules of calcium, and very few inflammatory cells. Lipochrome pigment may be present in some lesions.

Tumors

The most important cell elements in the testis are the germ cells in various stages of maturation. These cells comprise the major population of adult normal seminiferous tubules, and their sole function is the production of spermatozoa. In addition to these cells, the seminiferous tubules also contain the sustentacular cells of Sertoli, which have three functions: they support the germ cells, produce estrogens, and form the basement membrane of the seminiferous tubules. The seminiferous tubules drain into collecting ducts, which join to form the rete testis, thence vasa efferentia, and finally the epididymis. These serve to transmit the spermatozoa out of the gonad. The seminiferous tubules are supported by a delicate fibrovascular stroma in which varying numbers of interstitial cells of Leydig are seen. The main functions of Leydig cells are that they constitute part of the supporting stroma of the gonad, and they produce hormones; they are the main source of testosterone and other androgenic hormones in man, and they produce estrogens and possibly progesterone and corticosteroids. Sertoli and Leydig cells are thus the hormone-producing cells of the male gonad and along with their homologs in the ovary (theca-granulosa cell) are designated the specialized stromal cells of the gonad to differentiate them from the usual fibrovascular stroma that the gonads have in common with all other organs. The entire structure is covered by tunica, which contains the smooth muscle layer of Dartos.

Symptomatically, there are no early symptoms of testicular tumors other than gradual enlargement of the testis, pain, and heavy or dragging sensation. Presence of a nodule or hardness with or without pain may be detected incidentally by a patient, patient's physician, or the wife or girl companion. Gynecomastia is seen in a number of patients. In all patients with gynecomastia the testicles should be carefully examined. In about 10% the symptoms are acute, simulating epididymitis, torsion, or infarction of the testis. A number of patients come in with generalized metastasis. The chorionic gonadotropins, follicle-stimulating hormones, and alpha fetoproteins are elevated in a number of patients, and the persistence of any of these after orchiectomy is most often indicative of metastasis.

There is no satisfactory clinical classification of testis tumors. They can be and are classified on a histologic basis only. In all patients suspected of testicular tumors, orchiectomy is mandatory, as biopsy is contraindicated because of frequency of local recurrence and metastasis in patients who have been biopsied.

The rarity of testicular tumors, the heterogeneity of their structure ranging from single cell tumors to complex neoplasms, and the absence of a readily available experimental model have resulted in considerable confusion about the origin, pathology, natural history, behavior of testicular tumors, and their effect on survival and mortality. The classic works of Friedman and Moore, and Dixon and Moore, who reported their observation on 1000 cases of testicular tumors collected at the Army Institute of Pathology (now the Armed Forces Institute of Pathology) in Washington, D.C., during World War II, followed by Mostofi's studies of an additional 6000 testicular tumors collected in the American Registry of Pathology housed at the Institute have clarified many of the problems. This account is based on these studies, the work of the W.H.O. Panel on Testicular Tumors, and the experimental research of Stevens and others.

The fibrovascular stroma may rarely develop various benign tumors (angiomas, fibromas, myomas) and more rarely, sarcomas. The majority of testicular tumors are derived either from the specialized gonadal stromal cells or from the germ cells.

Tumors derived from specialized gonadal stroma

To understand the hormonal and morphologic features of tumors derived from specialized gonadal stroma, one should remember that the primitive mesenchyme of the genital ridge forms the whole gonad of each sex except for the germ cells that migrate from their site of origin in the yolk sac entoderm. These primitive mesenchymal cells constitute the supporting stromal elements for the germ cells. In the female they give rise to theca, granulosa, and lutein cells and in the male, to the sustentacular cells of Sertoli and the interstitial cells of Leydig. The cells of origin of the testis and ovary are identical, and in neoplastic proliferation one might suppose that the strict control that directs the differentiation of these two dissimilar structures might be deranged so that structures reminiscent of either ovary or testis may develop. Thus Sertoli and Leydig cell tumors may be found in the ovary (in addition to granulosa cell, theca cell, and lutein cell tumors), and the latter three tumors may be seen in the testis (in addition to Sertoli cell and Leydig cell tumors).

Nodules consisting of Sertoli cell–lined tubules are not infrequent in the undescended testis, and although sometimes erroneously designated as adenomas, they are persistent or hyperplastic nodules. Unless there is a distinct, grossly visible tumor, the lesion should not be so designated.

Tumors of these cell types—Sertoli, granulosa, theca, or those showing admixtures—occur in all ages but more commonly in infants and children. They correspond to arrhenoblastoma and androblastomas of the ovary. About one third of adult patients show gynecomastia. Grossly, the tumors are usually fairly large, well circumscribed, round or oval, firm, and yellowish or yellowish gray. The cut surfaces are bulging and somewhat greasy.

Microscopically, three basic patterns may be recognized: tubular, stromal, or mixed. The tubular type presents tubules lined by high or low columnar Sertoli-like cells (Fig. 25-4), or cuboid cells resembling granulosa cells. The stromal type shows closely packed rounded or spindle-shaped cells with dark-staining nuclei and a small amount of cytoplasm, which resemble theca cells. The mixed type contains characteristics of both and even Leydig cells. These tumors have been designated as androblastoma by Teilum who reported three cases with gynecomastia. Mostofi has reported a series of 23 cases and suggested the designation "tumors of specialized gonadal stroma." These tumors are mostly benign—only about 10% are malignant and those that metastasize do so within 1 year.

The manifestations of Leydig cell tumors

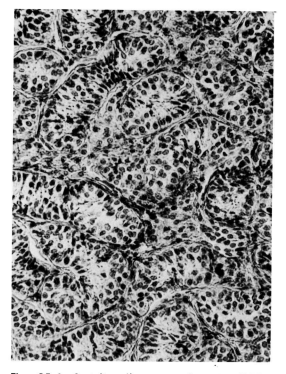

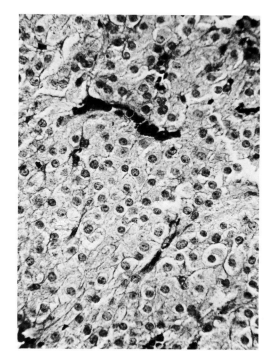

Fig. 25-4. Sertoli cell tumor of testis. (205×; AFIP 55-4720.)

Fig. 25-5. Interstitial cell tumor of testis. (250×; AFIP 989657.)

are extremely interesting. Normally, Leydig cells produce mostly testosterone but some estrogens and other hormones as well. They undergo morphologic and endocrine involutional changes beginning with fetal and newborn life, when they are stimulated by gonadotropins to appear as large epithelium-like cells; in infancy and childhood, they resemble fibroblastic cells; in adulthood, they are large and granular; and in old age, they are small and vacuolated, have a dark-staining nucleus, and are often again spindly.

Clinically, all the children with Leydig cell tumors manifest macrogenitosomia, with voice changes, enlargement of the penis, pubic and axillary hair, and precocious body development. In adult patients, no supermasculinizing features are observed, but about half show gynecomastia and other feminizing features. If the condition is not recognized and the tumor-bearing testis is not removed, premature closure of the epiphysis may occur, resulting in dwarfism. In others, gynecomastia develops as the child approaches adolescence. Gynecomastia may be attributable to the estrogen production or secondary to metabolism of increased or altered androgens. The tumors produce testosterone, estrogens, progesterone, and even corticosteroids.

Grossly, the testis usually is enlarged, although this may not be detected. About one half of the patients consult a physician because of gynecomastia, with the breasts about two times larger than normal. The testicular tumors are lobulated, well circumscribed, and homogeneously yellowish to mahogany brown. Areas of necrosis and hemorrhage are extremely rare, but calcification may be encountered.

Microscopically, the most common cell type consists of large polyhedral cells with vacuolated or eosinophilic cytoplasm with a round or oval vesicular nucleus and a single or double nucleolus (Fig. 25-5). Binuclear and trinuclear cells are not uncommon. In addition to lipids and brown pigment, the cytoplasm may contain crystals—Reinke's, which are characteristic for interstitial cells but seem to have no function. The tumors may recapitulate the various types of interstitial cells encountered in the normal testis in its involution. The cells are arranged in columns and cords separated by well-vascularized fibrous tissue, frequently giving the tumors an endocrine pattern.

Differentiation between hyperplasia and tumor (adenoma or carcinoma) is sometimes difficult, especially in children and in patients with adrenogenital syndrome. In tumors, there is a distinct mass, and there usually are no entrapped seminiferous tubules. Differentiation between a benign and a malignant interstitial cell tumor is difficult, if not impossible, on a histologic basis, but cellular anaplasia and vascular invasion are disturbing features. Fortunately, most of the tumors are benign. The only criteria for malignancy is metastasis, and this usually is late in development. It is important to do hormone assays in such patients, for a rise in or a persistently elevated androgen level after orchiectomy may alert the development of metastasis. Differentiation from a tumor derived from an adrenal rest is sometimes difficult, but adrenal rests occur almost entirely outside the tunica of the testis and tumors in the substances of the testis must be regarded as interstitial cell tumors. Histologically and endocrinologically, the two tumors frequently are indistinguishable.

Tumors derived from germ cells

Tumors derived from germ cells constitute the most common neoplasms of the testis comprising about 95% of tumors of this organ.

Incidence. The incidence of germ cell tumors is 3 per 100,000 male population, but in the age groups of 20 to 39 the annual morbidity is over 6. These tumors comprise 4% to 6% of all male genitourinary tumors; about 90% occur before the age of 45. Deaths from testicular tumors constitute the fourth most frequent cause of tumor deaths (after leukemias, Hodgkin's disease, and brain tumors) in the 18- to 34-year age group. A second peak incidence is seen in patients over 50. The histology and behavior of the tumors vary with different age groups. A doubling of mortality from testicular tumors has been reported between 1943-1947 and 1958-1962.

Etiology. The cause of testicular tumors is unknown. Several factors, however, are suspect. Genetic factors apparently play a role in the high incidence of testicular tumors reported in brothers, identical twins, monozygous twins, and members of the same family. Muller has reported a history of malignant disease of the testis in the next of kin in 16% of cases. Patients with one testis tumor have a high incidence of another tumor in the opposite testis. Many dysgenetic gonads develop tumors. There is a high incidence of testicular tumor in certain strains of mice, and this can be genetically manipulated.

Maldescent of the testis is associated with a high incidence of testicular tumors. In 2200 testis tumors we found 72 in undescended testis. Since cryptorchidism after 21 years of age affects only 1 in 250 men, this would indicate an incidence of 3.6% of maldescent in this group. Other studies have claimed that 1 in 80 inguinal testes and 1 in every 20 abdominal testes develop malignant tumors. The high incidence is attributed to the higher temperature that the undescended testis is subjected to in the groin or abdomen. Other possible factors are abnormal structure of the undescended testis and interference with blood supply. In man, there is a slightly higher incidence of tumors on the right side (52% versus 48%).

Many patients with testicular tumor give a history of mumps or other form of orchitis. Many patients give a history of trauma, but whether trauma initiates the process or simply brings to focus an abnormal testis has not been settled. In connection with trauma it may be mentioned that teratomas induced in fowl by intratesticular injection of zinc salts, alone or with pituitary gonadotropic hormones, are attributed to the necrotizing effects of the injection.

In recent years testicular tumors have been reported in two men after the use of lysergic acid diethylamide and in patients who have received certain drugs for long periods.

The high incidence of testicular tumors in a period of life when sexual activity is at its height, presence of elevated pituitary gonadotropins in some patients with testicular tumors, elevation of chorionic gonadotropins or estrogens or both in some patients with germ cell tumors of testis, the report of a seminoma in a patient who had received hormone treatment for sterility, and the fact that zinc-induced teratomas in the fowl occur only during the period of maximal pituitary gonadotropin secretion suggest that endocrines may play a role in induction of testicular tumors. In summary, maldescent, mumps orchitis, and trauma to the testis are at this writing three of the most important factors in the genesis of testicular tumors.

Histogenesis and classification. Willis[32] advocated two sites of origin of testicular tumors: cells in the seminiferous tubules and foci of plastic pleuropotential embryonic tissue that escaped the influence of the primary organizer during embryonic development. Based on this, he proposed a classification of these tumors into seminoma and teratoma. Since the latter category included tumors of different structure and behavior, the classifi-

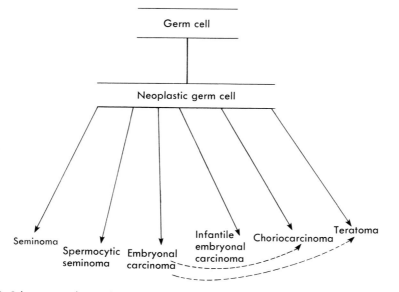

Fig. 25-6. Schematic relationship of T-testicular tumors. Individual histologic patterns probably arise directly from germ cells, but choriocarcinoma and teratoma may originate from embryonal carcinoma.

cation has not been accepted, even though it has been somewhat modified in recent years by English investigators. The American writers, on the other hand, have maintained that all of these tumors originate from the germ or sex cell. This position has now been conclusively confirmed by the experimental work of Stevens,[27] who demonstrated the origin of nonseminomatous tumors from the germ cells. Pierce and Beals[19] have shown that, ultrastructurally, embryonal carcinoma cells resemble the primitive germ cell.

Modern-day histologic classification of germ cell tumors is a modification of the Friedman and Moore classification proposed in 1943. We divide these tumors into *A*, those that are of single cell type (60%), and *B*, those that show more than one cell type (40%). In the first group there are six basic histologic patterns:

Tumors of one histologic type (Fig. 25-6)

1. Seminoma
2. Spermatocytic seminoma
3. Embryonal carcinoma
4. Yolk sac tumors or infantile embryonal carcinoma
5. Choriocarcinoma
6. Teratoma

Seminoma. Compared with the incidence of other teratoid tumors, seminoma is the most frequent, occurs in the older age group, and is relatively less malignant. Undescended testicles

harbor this tumor more frequently than other forms of teratoid tumors. The involved testicle may be only slightly enlarged or may be 10 times larger than normal, yet it usually maintains almost its normal contour. This gross feature is attributable to the fact that the tunica covering is rarely invaded. The neoplasm is opaque grayish white or yellowish white and not uncommonly contains yellowish and yellowish brown areas of necrosis (Fig. 25-7). Some tumors are homogeneous, whereas others are distinctly lobulated. The large tumors replace the entire testicle, whereas the small tumors are circumscribed but not encapsulated. Hemorrhagic necrosis is rare, and cysts are never found in pure seminomas.

Microscopically, seminomas are readily recognized because of their monocellularity. The cells are moderately large, round, cuboid, or polyhedral and quite uniform in size, and the majority reveal distinct cell borders. The cytoplasm usually is quite clear, containing glycogen, but occasionally it is slightly stained. The relatively large, round, centrally located nucleus may occupy one third to one half of the cell. The nucleolus is prominent and slightly eosinophilic, and some nuclei have two nucleoli (Fig. 25-8).

The cells are quite regular, and mitotic figures are infrequent. In about 10%, however, there is considerable anaplasia and increased mitotic activity (anaplastic seminoma) indica-

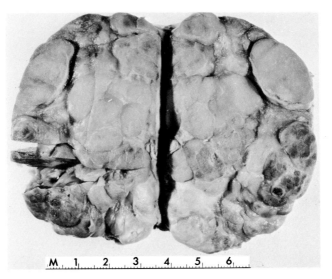

Fig. 25-7. Seminoma of testis. (AFIP 53-18346.)

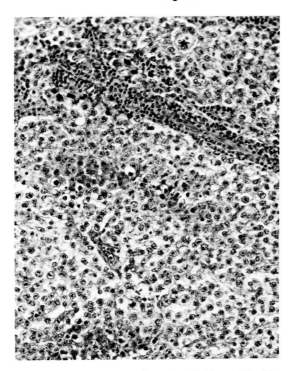

Fig. 25-8. Seminoma of testis. (145×; AFIP 69-6824.)

tive of a more aggressive tumor. The seminoma cells occur in cords, columns, or sheets; they may be infiltrating or intratubular. The stroma is usually delicate but almost invariably shows varying degrees of lymphocytic infiltration that may sometimes be quite prominent. In some the stroma may be granulomatous

and in a few, very fibrous. The stroma divides the tumor into lobules. This reaction of the stroma is interpreted as an immunologic response of the body to the tumor. The tumors are very radiosensitive, and the 5-year mortality is less than 5%.

Spermatocytic seminoma. Spermatocytic seminoma usually occurs in older patients. Grossly, it is more yellowish, softer, mucoid, with small or large spaces containing pinkish fluid than is seminoma. Microscopically, although the major cell population is of intermediate size similar to seminoma, there are a number of cells resembling secondary spermatocytes and huge mononucleate or multinucleate giant cells. The cytoplasm has no glycogen. The nuclei of the intermediate and large cells have a distinct chromatin distribution, which resembles the meiotic phase of normal primary spermatocytes and is described as filamentous or spireme.

Lymphocytic and granulomatous reactions are absent. The tumors may comprise up to 10% of seminomas, depending on the age of the patient population; the tumors are believed to be radiosensitive and the prognosis is quite good.

Embryonal carcinoma. Among germ cell tumors embryonal carcinoma ranks third in frequency. Grossly, the tumors are among the smallest. They distort the contour of the testicle more than the seminoma because of their invasion of the capsule and epididymis. The cut surfaces reveal a soft gray or grayish red tissue with areas of hemorrhage and necrosis (Fig. 25-9). The tumors are rarely cystic.

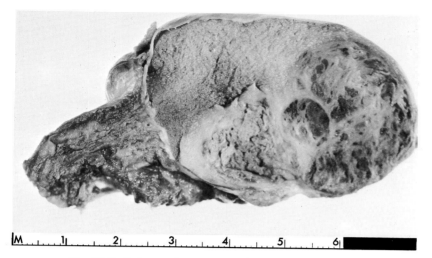

Fig. 25-9. Embryonal carcinoma of testis. (AFIP 53-21786.)

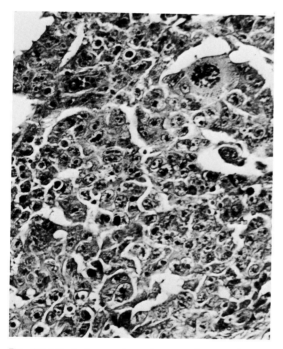

Fig. 25-10. Embryonal carcinoma of testis. (230×; AFIP 270230-3.)

Microscopically, the characteristic feature of these tumors is that they are made up of definitely carcinomatous cells—large, highly anaplastic with amphophilic cytoplasm, often with indistinct cell borders (Fig. 25-10). The nuclei are prominent and eosinophilic and may be quite large. Mitotic figures are always present and often numerous. The cells usually form glandular, tubular, papillary, or pseudocystic structures or rarely solid sheets. Hemorrhage and necrosis are not uncommon. The stroma does not have the distinct pattern of the seminoma. It may be imperceptible or abundant, fibrous, primitive, or even sarcomatous. The tumors are less sensitive to radiation than are seminomas, and the 5-year mortality is about 65%. Embryonal carcinoma also occurs in infants and has been designated as yolk sac tumor.

Yolk sac tumors (infantile embryonal carcinoma). These tumors have also been designated as endodermal sinus tumors because they resemble a yolk sac or an endodermal sinus. They are the most common testicular tumor in infants and children. Alpha fetoproteins are usually high. Grossly, the testicle is usually enlarged and the cut surface is yellowish gray, mucinous, and greasy. Microscopically, the tumor has a reticular pattern with epithelial cells that range from flattened to cuboid and even low columnar cells forming anastomosing tubular structure (Fig. 25-11). The 5-year mortality is about 33%.

Choriocarcinoma. Pure choriocarcinomas are the most malignant of germ cell tumors but, fortunately, are extremely rare (18 in 6000). They are usually small and always hemorrhagic and necrotic with a small rim of viable tissue at the periphery. Frequently, the patients, who are usually in their early twenties, come in with symptoms of metastasis. Sometimes, the primary lesion is completely missed until autopsy because of its small size. The level

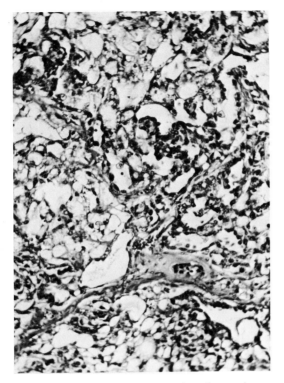

Fig. 25-11. Infantile pattern of embryonal carcinoma of testis. (130×; AFIP 69-6791.)

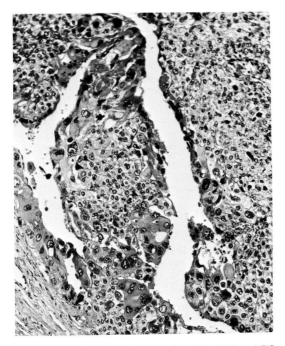

Fig. 25-12. Choriocarcinoma of testis. (100×; AFIP 70-2219.)

of chorionic gonadotropins is elevated and there is gynecomastia. To diagnose choriocarcinoma, one must recognize two types of cells, the cytotrophoblast and the syncytiotrophoblast (Fig. 25-12).

The cytotrophoblasts are polyhedral cells having a clear or pinkish cytoplasm with relatively large hyperchromatic nuclei. They lie in sheets or make up the major portion of the villuslike structures, which are usually bordered by syncytiotrophoblasts. The syncytiotrophoblasts are large, irregular, often huge, bizarre cells with pseudopodia extending between other cells. Their cell wall is indistinct. They possess a large amount of azurophilic cytoplasm, which frequently is vacuolated. Their deeply staining nuclei are large, irregular, and pyknotic. Some of the cells are multinucleated.

The syncytiotrophoblastic cells usually are located (as in choriocarcinoma of the uterus) in the advancing edge of the tumor, but distinct villous formation is very rare. All of our patients with pure choriocarcinoma of the testes were dead within 35 weeks of the diagnosis.

In contrast to the rarity of pure choriocarcinoma, it is not infrequent to see areas of choriocarcinoma in one of the other tumors—seminoma, embryonal carcinoma, and teratoma. The presence of choriocarcinoma in such cases affects the progress, but in contrast to the situation in pure choriocarcinoma, the prognosis is not hopeless. More frequently, syncytiotrophoblast-like cells also may be seen in many of the seminomas, embryonal carcinomas, and teratomas, but the evidence suggests that these probably do not have any prognostic significance. In a number of tumors where the primary has no demonstrable chorionic elements the metastasis will show choriocarcinoma.

Teratoma. Teratoma in the testis is defined as a complex tumor with recognizable elements of more than one germ layer. Grossly, the tumors are of moderate size, grayish white, cystic, and honeycombed with areas of cartilage and bone (Fig. 25-13). The cysts mostly contain keratohyaline matter but may contain mucin. In contrast to the ovaries, dermoid tumors are rare in the testes.

Microscopically, the testicular teratoma is a complex tumor revealing a disorderly arrangement of a great variety of fetal and adult structures originating from the three germ layers: ectoderm, mesoderm, and entoderm. The most common well-differentiated struc-

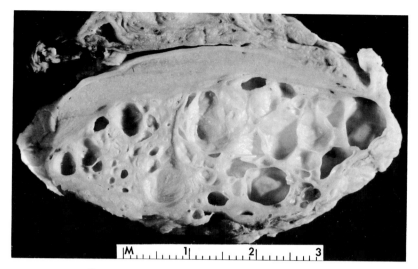

Fig. 25-13. Teratoma of testis. (AFIP 57-3396.)

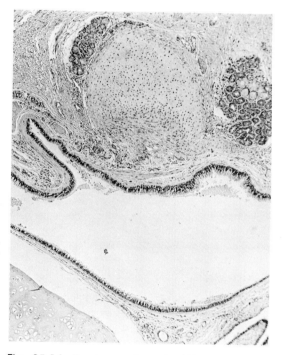

Fig. 25-14. Teratoma of testis. (48×; AFIP 154-883.)

tures are squamous cysts filled with keratohyaline substance, cartilage, smooth muscle, mucous glands, respiratory and gastrointestinal structures, and, in infants and children, nerve tissue (mature teratoma) (Fig. 25-14). Occasionally, the tumors are quite immature, showing primitive cartilage, mesenchyme, neuro-

ectodermal canals, and abortive intestinal and respiratory tubules (immature teratoma). Rarely a teratoma may show malignant transformation, e.g., squamous carcinoma. Although no malignant areas may be encountered, teratomas should not be regarded as benign, since about 29% show metastases and terminate fatally in 5 years. In infants and children the prognosis is much better.

Tumors of more than one histologic type

Forty percent of the tumors show more than one histologic type. Spermatocytic seminoma and yolk sac tumors tend to occur in pure forms, but other types may occur in any combination —either in the primary or the metastasis. The most frequent combination is that of teratoma and embryonal carcinoma commonly designated as teratocarcinoma, which constitutes 22% of testicular tumors. Many other combinations also occur.

Teratocarcinoma. By common usage "teratocarcinoma" is employed to designate tumors that contain both teratoma and embryonal carcinoma. Among germ cell tumors this is the second most common.

Grossly, teratocarcinomas are usually quite large and solid or contain a mixture of solid and cystic areas. They may have areas of necrosis and hemorrhage (Fig. 25-15). They are composed of a variety of teratomatous tissue intermingled with definite embryonal carcinoma. The 5-year mortality is about 50%.

Metastasis. Lymphogenous metastasis occurs much more frequently than hematogenous ex-

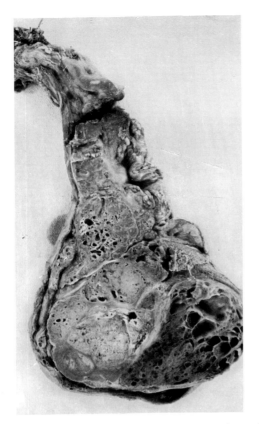

Fig. 25-15. Immature teratoma (teratocarcinoma) of testicle infiltrating spermatic cord.

cept in choriocarcinomas. The lymph nodes predominantly invaded are the iliac and peri-aortic and the mediastinal and supraclavicular groups. Sooner or later, hematogenous spread occurs, and the organs most frequently involved are the lungs, liver, and the kidneys, but no organ is immune. One of the most interesting features is that a primary lesion consisting of pure embryonal carcinoma, teratoma, or teratocarcinoma may metastasize individually as such, or as one of the other tumors, or as a choriocarcinoma. Seminomas may also do this, but rarely. Another interesting feature is that a primary lesion may consist of a small, benign-appearing teratoma, whereas the metastasis may be composed of embryonal carcinoma and choriocarcinoma. These observations have been explained by the fact that the primitive totipotential cell may develop into one cell type in the primary tumor and into another cell type in the metastasis. It is also possible that a small focus of the tumor cell type seen in the metastasis was missed in the primary lesion. Another unusual feature of these tumors is that oc-

casionally a small primary lesion may be burned out so that the testis shows only an area of scarring and calcific and hemosiderin deposition while there is widespread metastasis of embryonal carcinoma, choriocarcinoma, or teratoma.

Hormonal aspects. The blood and urine of some patients with germ cell tumors of the testicle contain chorionic gonadotropic hormone similar to that of pregnant women and, when injected in suitable animals, yields a positive pregnancy test. In addition, there may be a large amount of follicle-stimulating and other hormones and alpha fetoprotein. Biologic tests for gonadotropic hormones should be performed in every patient in whom a testicular tumor is suspected. In those patients in whom there are positive preoperative or persistent postoperative hormones, the prognosis is poorer. Postoperatively, a positive test for chorionic gonadotropins indicates metastasis. Negative results do not always indicate a good therapeutic response.

Tumors and tumorlike conditions containing both germ cell and gonadal stromal elements

These are usually seen in dysgenetic gonads, but rarely also in undescended and, more rarely, in normally located testis. The tumors designated as gonadoblastoma show large cells resembling seminoma and rarely embryonal carcinoma and small cells resembling immature Sertoli-granulosa cells and occasionally Leydig cells. The tumors are usually benign, but the germ cell element may metastasize.

EPIDIDYMIS

The epididymis should not be considered as a separate body. It is part of the testicle and, therefore, usually a partner with the testicle to the major diseases described in the preceding paragraphs. However, primary tumors may arise in the epididymis. Longo and others[40] collected 134 cases of primary tumors of the epididymis from the world literature. The ages of patients ranged from 21 to 78 years, with the average age about 41 years. Tumors occurred four times more often in the globus minor than in the globus major, and the left side was affected twice as often as the right. The tumors ranged from 1 to 5 cm in diameter.

The most common tumor of the epididymis is the *adenomatoid tumor* (Fig. 25-16). This tumor has been reported under a variety of headings such as mesothelioma, lymphangioma, and adenomyoma. Similar tumors are en-

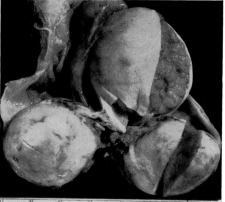

Fig. 25-16. Large adenomatoid tumor of lower pole of epididymis. Tumor bisected and almost as large as testis above. (Courtesy Dr. Paul C. Dietz, La Crosse, Wis.)

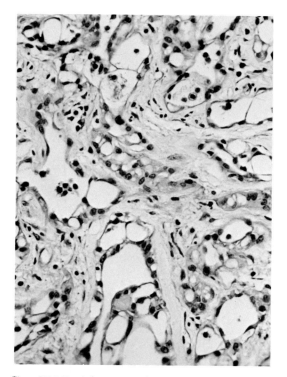

Fig. 25-17. Adenomatoid tumor of epididymis. (225×; AFIP 53-18326.)

countered in the tunica vaginalis, spermatic cord, posterior aspect of the uterus, fallopian tube, and ovary; thus such tumors develop along the course of the mesonephric duct.

Adenomatoid tumors are believed to originate from mesothelial cells. Most of the tumors occur in persons between 20 and 40 years of age. About 80% are attached to the epididymis, usually the globus minor, and the remaining are located on the tunica of the testes and in the cord. They are painless, single, firm, round, or ovoid nodules ranging in size from less than 1 cm to 5 cm in greatest diameter. The cut surfaces are homogeneous, grayish white, and fibrous, having a whorled appearance, and occasionally reveal yellow areas. Histologically, they reveal glandlike structures and irregular spaces and some contain cords of epithelium-like cells (Fig. 25-17). The stroma varies in amount and is composed of a loose or a dense fibrous connective tissue in which broad smooth muscle fibers are recognized. The glandlike structures may be lined with flat, cuboid, or low columnar cells. Many of the cells, particularly those arranged in cords, are vacuolated.

Leiomyoma is the second most common tumor of the epididymis and is frequently accompanied by a hydrocele. Other benign tumors reported in the literature are *angiomas, fibromas, lipomas, adrenal rests,* and *cholesteatomas.* The reported teratoid tumors and dermoid cysts are often associated with teratoid tumors of the testicle.

Carcinomas and sarcomas are extremely rare. Many patients with von Hippel–Lindau's disease show clear-cell adenomas and adenocarcinomas of the epididymis resembling similar lesions in the kidney.

SPERMATIC CORD

Anomalies. Anomalies of the spermatic cord consist of congenital absence or congenital atresia of the vas deferens. Sterility is present when either of these conditions is bilateral. Complete or incomplete duplication of the vas deferens has been reported.

Inflammation. Inflammation of the vas deferens is known as vasitis or deferentitis, whereas inflammation of the entire spermatic cord is termed funiculitis. Lymphangitis, phlebitis, and thromboangiitis may be attributed to a variety of causes. Vasitis may be caused by extension of epididymitis or lymphogenous transportation from urethritis and cystitis. The etiology of some cases of both vasitis and funiculitis is not definitely known, but trauma and focal and general infections are suspected. Tuberculosis of the spermatic cord is secondary to tuberculous epididymitis and seminal vesiculitis. Filarial funiculitis is associated with elephantiasis of the penis and scrotum. There is lymphangiectasia and fibrosis of the interstitial tissue. The walls of the lymph vessels become thickened and frequently reveal obliterative lymphangitis, with calcific and crystalline deposits. Calcified filariae may be found in whorls of hyalinized fibrous tissue. The various inflammatory cells encountered in filarial funiculitis are lymphocytes, plasma cells, eosinophils, and, in some cases, multinucleated giant cells.

Cysts. Cysts of the epididymis (spermatocele) or the testicular appendix (hydatid of Morgagni) or epididymal appendices are quite common. The most important are spermatoceles, which may be unilateral or bilateral, unilocular or multilocular. The epithelium is flattened or cuboid, or may be ciliated and surrounded by various amounts of hyalinized fibrovascular tissue and occasionally cholesterol crystals. The lumen is filled with fluid that is either neutral or slightly alkaline. The sediment contains lymphocytes, cellular debris, fat globules, and sometimes cholesterol. The presence of spermatozoa distinguishes these cysts from hydrocele.

Varicocele. Varicocele is a common condition in which the veins of the pampiniform plexus are dilated and elongated and their tortuosity increased. The cause of *primary* or *idiopathic varicocele* is not definitely known. Secondary or symptomatic varicocele is the result of pressure on the spermatic veins or its tributaries by an enlarged liver and spleen, pronounced hydronephrosis, muscle strain, and abdominal tumors. Primary varicocele usually involves the left spermatic cord and is predominant in young boys.

Tumors. Various tumors involving the spermatic cord have been observed. Benign tumors are lipomas, fibromas, myomas, angiomas, cystadenomas, teratomas, and dermoid cysts. Sarcomas (Fig. 25-18) and carcinomas are rare. Lipoma is the most common tumor involving the spermatic cord.

SCROTUM

Anomalies. Arrest of development may result in the formation of a separate pouch for each testicle. Half of the scrotum corresponding to undescended testicle may be rudimentary. A cleft scrotum resembling labia majora is encountered in pseudohermaphroditism. Partial cleft scrotum may accompany other congenital defects of the genitourinary system.

Dermatologic lesions. The common skin diseases of the scrotum are scabies (*Sarcoptes scabiei*), pediculosis, prurigo, eczema, erysipelas, psoriasis, and, not infrequently, syphilitic lesions. Sebaceous cysts are not uncommon. They may be multiple. They develop slowly and occasionally become calcified.

Gangrene. Gangrene of the scrotum may

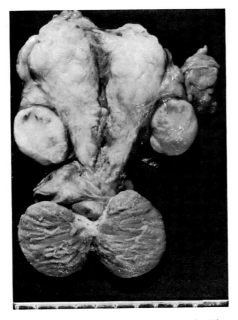

Fig. 28-18. Testis and spermatic cord. Fibrosarcoma of spermatic cord. (Courtesy Dr. Joseph L. Teresi, Brookfield, Wis.)

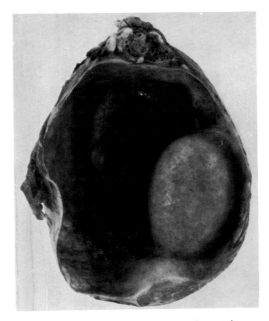

Fig. 25-19. Hydrocele. Normal testicle.

be caused by trauma or may be a complication of infectious diseases, phimosis, chancroid, balanitis, and periurethritis. The idiopathic or spontaneous gangrene is unassociated with trauma or infection. There is often associated gangrene of the penis.

Elephantiasis. Elephantiasis of the scrotum is characterized by diffuse increase and fibrosis of the subcutaneous tissue and obvious thickening of the skin resembling elephant's hide and resulting in enlargement of the scrotum. The disease is the result of lymph stasis either from blocking of the lymphatics by microfilaria *(Wuchereria bancrofti)* or from cicatricial closure of the lymph channels from chronic inflammation after trauma, excision of lymph nodes, or chronic lymphadenitis. In filariasis, the adult worm obstructs the lymph channels. Secondary infection, according to some investigators, is necessary to produce elephantiasis. The live worm apparently provokes little or no inflammation. The dead and disintegrating forms stimulate proliferation of the intima, followed by thrombosis and organization.

Hydrocele. A hydrocele is an abnormal accumulation of serous fluid in the sac of the tunica vaginalis (Fig. 25-19). Normally, there are a few drops of serous fluid between the visceral and parietal layers.

In the congenital type of hydrocele, there is a direct communication with the abdominal cavity as a result of failure of closure of the funicular process. In infantile hydrocele, there is an accumulation of fluid in the partly closed funicular process and the sac of the tunica vaginalis, but there is no communication with the abdominal cavity. Acute hydrocele may be a complication of gonorrhea, tuberculosis, syphilis, erysipelas, rheumatism, typhoid, or neoplasms. Between 25% and 50% of acute hydroceles are the result of trauma.

The fluid of the hydrocele is odorless, viscid, and straw colored to amber colored. The usual amount varies from 4 to 10 ounces. It has a neutral reaction, and its specific gravity varies from 1.020 to 1.026. It contains about 6% protein (serum albumin, serum globulin, and fibrinogen), alkaline carbonates, and sodium chloride. Occasionally, fibrous bodies coated with salts and fibrin are found floating in the fluid. The bodies originate from detached villous projections of the tunica vaginalis. If the hydrocele is infected, the fluid may be cloudy, or it may be brownish red if slight hemorrhage has occurred. Microscopic examination of comparatively clear hydrocele fluid reveals a few mesothelial cells, lymphocytes, cholesterin crystals, and lecithin bodies.

The sac of the hydrocele may be a single-chambered or multiple-chambered structure. The inner surface of the tunica vaginalis is usually smooth, but there may be adhesions and fibrous projections. The wall is variously thickened, composed of scanty cellular fibrous tissue infiltrated with lymphocytes and some plasma cells. Calcific deposits occasionally are encountered.

Hematoma. Hematoma of the scrotum is an effusion of blood within the tissue of the scrotal wall. The blood may collect beneath the tunica dartos, between the tunica vaginalis and the fibrous coat (paravaginal hematoma), or in the scrotal septum. Hematomas are usually of traumatic origin.

Hematocele. Hemorrhage in the sac of the tunica vaginalis is known as hematocele. Spontaneous hematocele is slow and insidious in its development, whereas a rapidly developing hematocele is invariably the result of trauma. The blood coagulates, fibrin settles out and organizes, and the wall becomes thick and rough. In long-standing hematocele, the tunica vaginalis becomes enormously thickened with dense fibrous tissue, which occasionally becomes partly calcified. Trauma may result in the formation of both hematoma and hematocele.

Tumors. Lipomas of the scrotum usually arise from the cord. They occur between the ages of 40 and 60 years and are seldom found in the adolescent or the aged. Sebaceous or epidermoid cysts are common. They are yellowish white, firm, and rounded and range from pinhead size to 3 cm in diameter. They occasionally become infected.

The most common malignant neoplasm of the scrotum is the squamous cell carcinoma. Etiologically, the well-known and almost legendary "chimney-sweeps' cancer" has been replaced by that arising among workers with tar, paraffin, and mineral oil, as well as by that arising in mule spinners in cotton mills.

Several types of sarcomas have been described but they are all rare.

PENIS
Anomalies

Phimosis. Phimosis is a condition in which the preputial orifice is too small to permit retraction of the prepuce behind the glans. It is independent of inflammation of the foreskin. An acquired phimosis may result from inflammation, trauma, or edema that narrows the preputial opening so that the prepuce cannot be retracted. *Congenital phimosis* predisposes to development of preputial calculi and squamous cell carcinoma. *Paraphimosis* is a condition in which the retracted prepuce cannot be reduced, with swelling of the prepuce and ulceration of the constricting tissue. It is usually a complication of gonorrhea, chancre, chancroid, balanitis, or trauma.

Hypospadias. Hypospadias is a developmental arrest in which the urethral meatus is present on the undersurface of the penis. It is probably attributable to disturbance of sex differentiation, causing imperfect closure of the urethral groove. The arrest may take place anywhere along the urethral groove, thus resulting in hypospadias with location from the glans penis to the perineum. Hypospadias is associated with a rather high incidence of genital anomalies such as cryptorchidism, enlarged prostatic utricle, and bifid scrotum. In about 25% of the cases, hypospadias is inherited as a recessive trait.

Epispadias is a rare form of congenital defect in which the urethral meatus is located at the upper surface of the penis. Its incidence in newborn infants is 1 in 50,000, and it frequently is associated with cryptorchidism, exstrophy of the urinary bladder, or absence of the prostate gland. In fact, it is a mild form of exstrophy.

Inflammation

Syphilis. The common site of a hard chancre is on the glans near the frenum or on the inner surface of the prepuce. It also may occur within or at the side of the urethral meatus or, rarely, on the shaft (see p. 437).

Chancroid. An acute venereal disease caused by *Haemophilus ducreyi* and usually transmitted by sexual intercourse, chancroid produces a painful ulcer on the corona, prepuce, or shaft of the penis. This ulcer is necrotic and suppurative and bleeds readily. It is not so indurated as the syphilitic chancre and is therefore termed "soft chancre" (see p. 430).

Herpes progenitalis. Herpes progenitalis is characterized by development of a group of vesicles on the glans or prepuce. The surrounding tissue is inflamed. The vesicles rupture, and small discrete or confluent ulcers develop that heal within a short time.

Granuloma inguinale. Granuloma inguinale usually begins in the inguinal region and spreads to the perineum, scrotum, and penis. Nodules and serpiginous ulcers develop on the

prepuce, and these spread to the glans and the shaft (see p. 431).

Lymphopathia venereum. Lymphopathia venereum is often confused with granuloma inguinale, but it is a specific venereal disease caused by a filtrable agent (see p. 434).

Fusospirochetosis. Erosive and gangrenous balanitis is a disease comparable to Vincent's angina and is caused by a fusiform bacillus (*Vibrio*) and a spirochete (see p. 449).

Plastic induration. Plastic induration (Peyronie's disease) is a fibrositis of the penis involving Buck's fascia and the sheath of one or both corpora cavernosa. The etiology is unknown. It resembles Dupuytren's contracture and keloids, and 25% of patients do show Dupuytren's contracture. The disease is more common than reports in the literature indicate. About 5% to 10% of cases reveal mild lesions. Two types are described: (1) thickening and contracture of the median septum and (2) localized nodules or indurated thickened areas involving the sides and underportion of the sheath of the corpus cavernosum. There is curvature of the penis on erection, pain on erection, and difficult or impossible intromission. Microscopically, there is a scanty cellular fibrous tissue in which there are few blood vessels and mild evidence of inflammation. The lesion often resembles scar tissue. Occasionally, the fibrous tissue undergoes ossification.

Tumors
Benign tumors

Squamous cell papillomas. Benign squamous cell papillomas reported under various names are common. Benign mesodermal tumors, however, are rare. Lipomas, fibromas, and angiomas have been reported.

Condyloma acuminatum. Incorrectly termed venereal wart, condyloma acuminatum is a raspberry-shaped or cauliflower-shaped tumor usually located on the sulcus. The tumor may be a single papilloma, or there may be multiple or conglomerated papillomas. These tumors frequently are associated with or occur after various inflammatory diseases of the penis. A viral etiology cannot be excluded. Microscopically, these are essentially squamous papillomas characterized by pronounced acanthosis and hyperplasia of the prickle cell layer. Parakeratosis is present but normal. The rete ridges are elongated and may be branching, but they all extend to about the same level. The growth is usually and characteristically upward toward the surface and not downward into the tissue. Sometimes, the tumor is quite extensive. One variety has received attention. This category, designated as giant condyloma or Buschke-Lowenstein tumor, forms grotesque cauliflower-like warty masses of large size with a strong tendency to extend, to perforate the prepuce, to destroy the underlying tissue, to ulcerate, to become infected, and to produce many fistulas. Clinically, they behave as cancer, and recurrence is the rule, but histologically they are benign. In contrast to the usual condylomas, the stratum corneum is thicker, parakeratosis is present, there is pronounced acanthosis and papillation and pronounced hyperplasia of the prickle cell layer. The papillae extend much deeper. Mitoses are limited to the basal layers, and stratification is normal. The tumors do not metastasize.

Verruca. Verruca is an ordinary squamous cell papilloma revealing hyperkeratosis and thus differing from a single condyloma, in which the epithelium is piled up in the middle layer (acanthosis).

Premalignant lesions

Erythroplasia of Queyrat. Erythroplasia of Queyrat is a pinkish, pagetoid lesion that usually involves the glans but occasionally may occur on the coronal sulcus or prepuce. It is shiny, pinkish red, flat, faintly elevated, and sharply marginated. The surface is smooth, slightly eroded, "velvety," more firm than the surrounding normal tissue, quite pliable, and with definite evidence of fixation to the underlying tissue. Histologically, erythroplasia of Queyrat shows an area of irregular acanthosis in which the keratin layer is decreased and there is parakeratosis. The epidermis is thickened and composed of atypical cells with loss of normal polarity and of normal maturation, many of the cells are vacuolated, and numerous mitotic figures are seen at all levels. The rete ridges are elongated and extend into the underlying stroma and sometimes are attached to each other. The subepithelial layer of dermis is edematous and shows infiltration that is predominantly plasmacytic.

Malignant tumors

Squamous cell carcinoma. In the United States, fewer than 2% of all cancers in men arise in the penis. The incidence in other parts of the world is as follows: China, 18.3%; continental Europe, 4.9%; Great Britain, 1.27%. In this country, it occurs about three or four times more frequently in blacks than in whites. The greatest incidence is between the ages of 45 and 60 years. Rare cases in childhood and early adult life have been reported.

It would not be an exaggeration to state that the presence of a foreskin is a predisposing cause for squamous cell carcinoma of the penis, since without this structure the incidence is insignificant. In India, the Muhammedans, who practice circumcision in infancy as a religious rite, rarely develop carcinoma of the penis, whereas the Hindus, who do not circumcise, have about a 10% incidence. Among Jews, who are also regularly circumcised in infancy, the disease is almost unknown. The exciting causes of this neoplasm are irritation by retained smegma, phimosis, and trauma. Smegma has been shown to be possibly carcinogenic (see p. 703). Many patients give a history of previous venereal disease.

The location of the neoplasm, in order of frequency, is the (1) frenum and prepuce, (2) glans, and (3) coronal sulcus. The tumors may be papillary or flat and ulcerating. They grow slowly. Histologically, they are of low-degree malignancy. Metastasis in the inguinal lymph nodes occurs in about 50% of the cases. Visceral metastasis is extremely rare.

Sarcoma. Fibrosarcoma, leiomyosarcoma, Kaposi's sarcoma, endothelioma, and malignant melanoma are seen rarely.

URETHRA
Mechanical disturbances

Diverticula. Urethral diverticula are fairly common in females but rare in males. They may be congenital or acquired. Congenital true diverticula, arising from the periurethral glands, always occur on the ventral wall of the anterior portion of the urethra, whereas acquired diverticula develop in the posterior portion. The acquired diverticula are caused by inflammation, trauma, or, in the male, obstruction of the urethra.

Prolapse. Prolapse of the urethra occurs almost exclusively in females. It usually involves the entire circumference, and the lumen is located in the center. Unless reduced promptly, pressure and infection produce vascular engorgement and acute inflammation.

Obstruction. Strictures of the urethra may be congenital or acquired. The former occurs usually in male infants either at the corona or the membranous urethra. Infant girls also may manifest congenital stricture of the distal portion of the urethra. Acquired strictures are the most common and most of them used to be complications of gonorrheal urethritis. This will probably be the case again with the recent increase in the incidence of venereal disease. About 10% are the result of trauma, but tuberculosis, other venereal diseases, periurethral abscesses, and caruncles also may cause urethral strictures. In the female, obstetric trauma is the chief cause. Whatever the cause, the urethra heals by proliferation of fibroblasts and scarring, resulting in contraction. If left untreated, sooner or later there is back pressure, dilatation of the urethra, hypertrophy of the vesical musculature, and eventually hydroureter and hydronephrosis.

Inflammation

Gonococcic urethritis. Acute urethritis may be attributed to a variety of bacteria. Gonococcic urethritis in the male, as a rule, involves the portion of urethra anterior to the triangular ligament (p. 429).

Nonspecific urethritis. Trauma, injection of chemical irritants, masturbation, coitus (in which female partner may suffer a nonspecific vaginitis), redundant foreskin, and "pinhole" meatus are causes of nonspecific urethritis. The same conditions that predispose to cystitis act similarly in the urethra. Various bacteria have been isolated, among which staphylococci, streptococci, and colon bacilli predominate.

Abscesses. Abscesses within and continuous to the urethra are infrequent. They are usually complications of gonorrhea, but they may be complications of nonspecific infections. These abscesses develop when the urethral glands are infected and their ducts occluded.

Reiter's disease. Urethritis, conjunctivitis, and arthritis form a clinical triad known as Reiter's disease. The etiology of this disease is not known, and tissue changes have not been investigated. Several workers have recovered viruslike agents by inoculating embryonated eggs with filtered urethral and conjunctival exudates. Spontaneous recovery is the rule, but relapses occur in about 25% and these may occur after a considerable silent period.

Urethrolithiasis

Calculi are rarely formed in the urethra. They either are dislodged bladder calculi or, when primary, originate in a urethral diverticulum.

Tumors
Benign tumors

The most common benign tumors of the urethra are caruncles, cysts, polyps, papillomas, adenomas, and angiomas. Fibromas and myomas are extremely rare.

Caruncles. Urethral caruncles are confined almost entirely to the female urethra. Their etiology is unknown. There are several theories: regional or circumscribed prolapse of urethral mucosa caused primarily by postmenopausal shrinkage of vaginal tissue with secondary trauma and infection, infection and chronic irritation resulting from lack of proper hygiene, and trauma consequent to coitus or childbirth.

Histologically, there are three somewhat arbitrary types:

The *papillomatous* type is frequently grossly lobulated as a result of clefts or crypts. The surface is covered by transitional and stratified squamous epithelium in various places. The epithelium continues along the crypts, from which sprouts extend deep into the stroma. Some of the epithelium-lined crypts on cross section appear as deep-seated nests of epithelial cells. Such areas may be confused with carcinoma. The stroma is usually infiltrated with inflammatory cellular elements.

The *telangiectatic* caruncle is highly vascular. The vessels are so numerous that the lesion has an appearance similar to the papillomatous type.

The *granulomatous* type lacks the epithelial hyperplasia and is almost entirely composed of granulation tissue.

There is an increasing opinion that the first two types of urethral caruncles represent precancerous lesions. Cases have been reported of carcinoma arising in a urethral caruncle.

Cysts. Cysts of the urethra may be congenital or acquired. Acquired cysts are most common and result from inflammatory occlusion of the urethral glands. The cysts of the posterior urethra arise from occlusion of the periurethral and subcervical ducts. Polyps are usually encountered in the folds of the urethra. Some of the polyps are difficult to differentiate from fibromas and papillomas. Papillomas occur in any part of the urethra, but the majority are encountered about the vesical neck at or near the meatus. Adenomas are small sessile or pedunculated tumors originating from the periurethral glands and usually encountered in the prostatic urethra. In the female, they arise from Skene's glands.

Malignant tumors

Malignant tumors of the urethra include squamous cell carcinoma, transitional cell carcinoma, and adenocarcinoma. Squamous cell carcinoma of either the male or female urethra is rare, but vulvourethral carcinoma is not infrequent. Transitional cell carcinomas resemble those of the bladder. Adenocarcinomas of the urethra are extremely rare. They originate from Littre's glands, lacunae of Morgagni, and Cowper's glands. Cowper's adenocarcinoma is characterized by extensive mucus production. In the female, adenocarcinoma usually develops from Skene's glands. In the male, adenocarcinomas of the posterior urethra are often extensions from prostatic carcinoma; however, in recent years an unusual papillary adenoma and adenocarcinoma of the utricle that resemble endometrial or endocervical tumors have been recognized.

REFERENCES
Testes

1 Atkin, N. B.: Br. J. Cancer 28:275-279, 1973 (testicular tumors).
2 Berg, J. W.: Arch. Pathol. (Chicago) 57:115-120, 1954 (granuloma).
3 Brown, R. C., and Smith, B. H.: Am. J. Clin. Pathol. 47:135-147, 1967 (malakoplakia).
4 Capers, T. H.: Am. J. Clin. Pathol. 34:139-145, 1960 (granulomatous orchitis).
5 Cohn, B. D.: Surgery 62:536-541, 1967 (histology of cryptorchidism).
6 Collins, D. H., and Pugh, R. C. B.: Br. J. Urol. 36 (suppl.):1-11, 1964 (testis tumors).
7 Dickinson, S. J.: J. Pediatr. Surg. 8:523-527, 1973 (structural abnormalities in undescended testis).
8 Dixon, F. J., and Moore, R. A.: In Atlas of tumor pathology, Sect. VIII, Fasc. 32, Washingston, D.C., 1952, Armed Forces Institute of Pathology.
9 Dow, J. A., and Mostofi, F. K.: South. Med. J. 60:193-195, 1967 (tumors and crypt).
10 Friedman, N. B., and Garske, G. L.: J. Urol. 62:363-374, 1949 (granulomatous orchitis).
11 Friedman, N. B., and Moore, R. A.: Milit. Surg. 99:573-593, 1943 (teratomatous tumors).
12 Givler, R. L.: Cancer 23:1290-1295, 1969 (leukemia).
13 Levin, H. S., and Mostofi, F. K.: Cancer 25:1193-1203, 1970 (plasmacytoma).
14 Maier, J., Van Buskirk, K. E., Sulak, M. H., Perry, R. H., and Shamber, D. T.: Trans. Am. Assoc. Genitourin. Surg. 60:71-74, 1962 (testis tumors).
15 Merrin, C., Sarcione, E., and Bohne, M., et al.: J. Surg. Res. 15:309-312, 1973 (alpha fetoprotein in testicular tumors).
16 Mostofi, F. K., and Price, E. B., Jr.: Tumors of male genital system. In Atlas of tumor pathology, Ser. 2, Fasc. 7, Washington, D.C., 1973, Armed Forces Institute of Pathology.
17 Mostofi, F. K., and Sobin, L. H.: International histological classification of tumors of testes, Geneva, 1977, World Health Organization.
18 Mostofi, F. K., Theiss, E. A., and Ashley, D. J. B.: Cancer 12:944-957, 1959 (gonadal stromal tumors).
19 Pierce, G. B., Jr., and Beals, T. F.: Cancer Res. 24:1533-1567, 1964 (testis tumors).
20 Price, E. B., Jr.: J. Urol. 102:708-713, 1969 (epidermoid cyst).
21 Price, E. B., Jr., and Mostofi, F. K.: Cancer 10:592-595, 1957 (secondary carcinoma of testis).
22 Reyes, F. I., and Faiman, C.: Can. Med. Assoc. J. 109:502-503, 1973 (development of testicular tumor during *cis*-clomiphene therapy).
23 Rosai, J., Khodadoust, K., and Silber, I.: Cancer 24:103-116, 1969 (spermatocytic seminoma).
24 Rosai, J., Silber, I., and Khodadoust, K.: Cancer 24:92-102, 1969 (spermatocytic seminoma).
25 Scorer, C. G.: Br. J. Surg. 49:357-367, 1962 (cryptorchidism).
26 Shiffman, M. A.: J. Urol. 98:493-496, 1967 (Sertoli cell tumor).
27 Stevens, L. C.: Dev. Biol. 2:285-297, 1960 (testis tumors).
28 Teilum, G.: Acta Endocrinol. (Kbn.) 4:43-62, 1950 (testis tumors).
29 Teoh, T. B., Stewart, J. K., and Willis, R. A.: J. Pathol. Bacteriol. 80:147-156, 1960 (infantile testis tumors).
30 Walker, K. M.: Lancet 1:435-440, 1913 (tuberculosis).
31 Westcott, J. W.: J. Urol. 96:243-246, 1966 (lymphoma).
32 Willis, R. A.: Pathology of tumors, ed. 4, London, 1967, Butterworth & Co. (Publishers) Ltd.
33 Young, H. H.: Arch. Surg. (Chicago) 4:334-419, 1922 (tuberculosis).

Epididymis, spermatic cord

34 Brosman, S. A., et al.: Urology 3:568-572, 1974 (rhabdomyosarcoma of testis and spermatic cord in children).
35 Broth, G., Bullock, W. K., and Morrow, J.: J. Urol. 100:530-536, 1968 (tumors of epididymis).
36 Glassy, F. J., and Mostofi, F. K.: Am. J. Clin. Pathol. 26:1303-1313, 1956 (sperm granuloma).
37 Jackson, J. R.: Cancer 11:337-350, 1958 (adenomatoid tumor).
38 Klingerman, J. J., and Nourse, M. H.: J.A.M.A. 200:673-675, 1967 (torsion).
39 Kyle, V. N.: J. Urol. 96:795-800, 1966 (leiomyosarcoma of cord).
40 Longo, V. J., McDonald, J. R., and Thompson, G. J.: J.A.M.A. 147:937-941, 1951 (neoplasms).
41 Lundblad, R. R., Mellinger, G. T., and Gleason, D. F.: J. Urol. 98:393-396, 1967 (malignant tumors).
42 Remzi, D.: South. Med. J. 66:1295-1297, 1973 (tunica vaginalis).
43 Silverblatt, J. M., et al.: Urology 3:235-237,

1974 (mesotheliomas of spermatic cord, epididymis, and tunica vaginalis).

44 Smith, B. A., Jr., Webb, E. A., and Price, W. E.: J. Urol. 98:743-750, 1967 (carcinoma, seminal vesicle).

45 Williams, G., and Banerjee, R.: Br. J. Urol. 41:332-339, 1969 (tumors).

Intersexuality, infertility, agonadism

46 Amelar, R. D.: Infertility in men. Philadelphia, 1966, F. A. Davis Co., pp. 13-14.

47 Ashley, D. J. B.: Human intersex, Edinburgh, 1962, E. & S. Livingstone, Ltd.

48 Charny, C. W.: In Behrman, S. J., and Kistner, R. W., editors: Progress in infertility, Boston, 1968, Little, Brown & Co., pp. 649-671 (male infertility).

49 Federman, D. D.: Abnormal sexual development: A generic and endocrine approach to differential diagnosis, Philadelphia, 1967, W. B. Saunders Co.

50 Goldberg, L. M., et al.: J. Urol. 11:84-85, 1974 (congenital absence of testis: anorchism and monorchism).

51 Inhorn, S. L., and Opitz, J. M.: In Bloodworth, J. M. B., editor: Endocrine pathology, Baltimore, 1968, The Williams & Wilkins Co.

52 Jirasek, J. E.: In Cohen, M. M., Jr., editor: Development of the genital system and male pseudohermaphroditism, Baltimore, 1971, The Johns Hopkins Press.

53 Jones, H. W., Jr., and Scott, W. W.: Hermaphroditism, genital anomalies, and related endocrine disorders, ed. 2, Baltimore, 1971, The Williams & Wilkins Co.

54 Jost, A.: Rec. Progr. Horm. Res. 8:379-418, 1953 (testicular biopsy).

55 Paulsen, C. A.: In Williams, R. H., editor: Text book of endocrinology, ed. 4, Philadelphia, 1968, W. B. Saunders Co., pp. 405-408 (testis).

56 Wong, T. W., Straus, F. H., and Warner, N. E.: Testicular biopsy in the study of male infertility: I. Testicular causes of infertility, Arch. Pathol. 95:151-159, 1973.

57 Wong, T. W., Straus, F. H., and Warner, N. E.: Testicular biopsy in the study of male infertility: II. Posttesticular causes of infertility, Arch. Pathol. 95:160-164, 1973.

58 Wong, T. W., Straus, F. H., and Warner, N. E.: Testicular biopsy in the study of male infertility: III. Pretesticular causes of infertility, Arch. Pathol. 98:1-8, 1974.

Scrotum

59 Borden, T. A., Rosen, R. T., and Schwartz, G. R.: Am. Surg. 40:193-194, 1974 (scrotal hematoma).

60 Burpee, J. F., and Edwards, P.: J. Urol. 107:812-814, 1972 (Fournier's gangrene).

61 Fardon, D. W., Wingo, C. W., Robinson, D. W., and Masters, F. W.: Plast. Reconstr. Surg. 40:482-488, 1967 (gangrene spider bite).

62 Exelby, P. R.: Cancer 24:163-168, 1974 (scrotal masses in children).

63 Himal, H. S., McLean, A. P., and Duff, J. H.: Surg. Gynecol. Obstet. 139:176-178, 1974 (gas gangrene of scrotum and perineum).

64 Keeler, L. L., and Harrer, W. V.: J. Med. Soc. N.J. 71:575-577, 1974 (lymphedema of scrotum and penis).

65 Kickham, C. J., and DuFresne, M.: J. Urol. 98:108-110, 1967 (carcinoma).

66 Lee, W. R., and McCann, J. K.: Br. J. Industr. Med. 24:149-151, 1967 (mule spinner carcinoma).

67 Smulewicz, J. J., and Donner, D.: J. Urol. 111:621-625, 1974 (gas gangrene of scrotum).

68 Vermillion, C. D., and Page, D. L.: J. Urol. 107:281-283, 1972 (Paget's disease of scrotum).

Penis

69 Bivens, C. H., Marecek, R. L., and Feldman, J. M.: New Eng. J. Med. 289:844-845, 1973 (Peyronie's disease).

70 Campbell, M.: J. Urol. 67:988-999, 1952 (epispadias).

71 Dehner, L. P., and Smith, B. H.: Cancer 25:1431-1447, 1970 (soft-tissue tumors of penis).

72 Editorial: Med. J. Aust. 2:1035-1036, 1973 (carcinoma of penis).

73 Frew, I. D. O., Jefferies, J. D., and Swinney, J.: Br. J. Urol. 39:398-404, 1967 (carcinoma).

74 Graham, J. H., and Helwig, E. B.: Cancer 32:1396-1414, 1973 (erythroplasia of Queyrat).

75 Grossberg, P., and Hardy, K. J.: Med. J. Aust. 2:1050-1051, 1973 (carcinoma of penis).

76 Gursel, E. O., Megall, M. R., and Veenema, R. J.: Urology 1:569-578, 1973 (penile cancer).

77 Hagerty, R. F., and Taber, E.: Am. Surg. 24:244-259, 1958 (hypospadias).

78 Horton, G. E., and Devine, C. J., Jr.: Plast. Reconstr. Surg. 52:503-510, 1973 (Peyronie's disease).

79 Johnson, D. E., Fuerst, D. E., and Ayala, A. G.: Urology 1:404-408, 1973 (carcinoma of penis).

80 Kaplan, C., and Katoh, A.: J. Surg. Oncol. 5:281-290, 1973 (erythroplasia of Queyrat [Bowens disease of glans penis]).

81 Masih, B. K., and Brosman, S. A.: J. Urol. 111:690-692, 1974 (webbed penis).

82 Melicow, M. M., and Ganem, E. J.: J. Urol. 55:486-514, 1946 (premalignant lesions).

83 Moulder, J. W.: The psittacosis group as bacteria (Ciba lectures in microbial biochemistry, 1963), New York, 1964, John Wiley & Sons, Inc. (lymphogranuloma venereum).

84 Najjar, S. S.: Clin. Pediatr. (Phila.) 13:377, 1974 (webbing of penis).

85 Ngai, S. K.: Am. J. Cancer 19:259-284, 1933 (cancer).

86 Poutasse, E. F.: J. Urol. 107:419-422, 1972 (Peyronie's disease).

87 Powley, J. M.: Br. J. Surg. 51:76-77, 1964 (condyloma—Buschke-Lowenstein tumor).

88 Rege, P. R., and Evans, A. T.: J. Urol. 111:784-785, 1974 (erythroplasia of Queyrat).

89 Smith, B. H.: Am. J. Clin. Pathol. 45:670-678, 1966 (Peyronie's disease).

90 Tan, R. E.: J. Urol. 92:508-510, 1964 (gangrene).

Urethra

91 Agusta, V. E., and Howards, S. S.: J. Urol. 112:280-284, 1974 (posterior urethral valves).

92 Bissada, N. K., Cole, A. T., and Fried, F. A.: J. Urol. **112:**201-203, 1974 (condylomata acuminata of male urethra and bladder).

93 Chambers, R. M.: Br. J. Urol. **46:**123, 1974 (anatomy of urethral stricture).

94 Cobb, B. G., Wolf, J. A., Jr., and Ansell, J. S.: J. Urol. **99:**629-631, 1968 (stricture, congenital).

95 Grewal, R. S., and Francis, J.: Int. Surg. **48:** 591-593, 1967 (foreign body).

96 Hill, B. H.: N.Z. Med. J. **69:**198-204, 1969 (nonspecific and gonorrheal urethritis).

97 Huvos, A. G., and Grabstald, H.: J. Urol. **110:** 688-692, 1973 (urethral meatal and parameatal tumors).

98 Kaplan, G. W., Buckley, G. J., and Grayhack, J. T.: J. Urol. **98:**365-371, 1967 (carcinoma of male urethra).

99 Klaus, H., and Stein, R. T.: Pediatrics **52:** 645-648, 1973 (urethral prolapse in young girls).

100 Knoblich, R.: Am. J. Obstet. Gynecol. **80:** 353-364, 1960 (adenocarcinoma of female urethra).

101 Malhoski, W. E., and Frank, I. N.: Urology **2:**382-384, 1973 (anterior urethral valves).

102 McEwen, C.: Trans. Coll. Physicians Phila. **34:**39-46, 1966 (Reiter's disease).

103 Marshall, F. C., Uson, A. C., and Melicow, M. M.: Surg. Gynecol. Obstet. **110:**723-733, 1960 (neoplasms and caruncles).

104 Meadows, J. A., Jr., and Quattlebaum, R. B.: J. Urol. **100:**317-320, 1968 (polyps).

105 Mitchell, J. P.: Br. J. Urol. **40:**649-670, 1968 (injuries).

106 Mogg, R. A.: Br. J. Urol. **40:**638-648, 1968 (anomalies).

107 Morrison, A. I.: Br. J. Vener. Dis. **43:**170-174, 1967 (nonspecific urethritis).

108 Williams, D. I., and Retik, A. B.: Br. J. Urol. **41:**228-234, 1969 (valves and diverticula).

26/Lung, pleura, and mediastinum

MAX MILLARD

Lung

PULMONARY STRUCTURE

The anatomy of pulmonary lobes and segments is left to specialized texts and the consideration here commences with the branching of the bronchi.

Bronchial branching occurs dichotomously up to 25 times, starting from the main bronchus at the hilus and ending with the terminal bronchiole near the periphery. Between these two points, the airways function as afferent and efferent air-conditioning tubes and play no active role in respiratory exchange. The latter role belongs to alveoli.

Walls of *bronchi* consist of mucosa, glands, muscle, and fibrous tissue with cartilage. The mucosa is mainly a pseudostratified ciliated columnar epithelium, with some intervening goblet cells and undifferentiated basal cells. From the latter, the other types are regenerated. The cilia beat rapidly against the undersurface of the covering mucus, moving it upward. The epithelium rests on a prominent continuous, thick, eosinophilic basement membrane, a feature easily seen in large bronchi, although still present in a much thinner form in the small ones. Beneath the mucosa are seromucinous glands, decreasing in number and becoming purely mucous as the bronchi branch. Glands disappear altogether at the level of the terminal bronchioles.

Bronchial muscle, surrounding the mucosa, is not circular but is in the form of a right and a left spiral of smooth muscle that extends up to the level of, and into, the alveolar ducts. This aids contraction and shortening, or dilatation and lengthening. A loose fibrous tissue sheath surrounds the muscle and allows the bronchial lengths and diameters to alter without affecting tensions in the neighboring alveoli. The hyaline cartilage plates extend, in diminishing size, into the small bronchi.

In large bronchi, the entire circumference is supported by cartilage, whereas in small bronchi this support is only partial, so that chance section may include no cartilage. Hence large bronchi have rigidity and can stay patent if there is massive collapse of the lung, in which condition small bronchi also will collapse.

Bronchioles, originally defined as those passages with a diameter of 1 mm or less, are now considered to be those airways distal to the last plate of cartilage and having no mucous glands and few goblet cells. Thus the mucosa, lined by cuboid epithelium with few or no cilia, is surrounded by smooth muscle and scanty fibrous tissue. It is important to realize how poor is their ability to drain themselves. There are no glands to secrete and wash away impurities and no cilia to move surface material, but only the few lymphatics and the macrophages of the alveoli and connective tissue.

The *terminal bronchioles* are the most peripheral bronchioles to have a complete epithelial lining. They come in a cluster of three to five from a final division, the preterminal bronchiole.

Terminal bronchioles give rise to *respiratory bronchioles* of similar caliber to their parent; the maintenance of the original diameter after branching serves to reduce the velocity of the air. Nevertheless, they differ in that a number of alveoli open directly into their muscular walls. Some respiratory bronchioles follow a recurrent path, bringing them back and parallel to their parent terminal bronchiole, with which their alveoli communicate by a narrow channel (Fig. 26-1). This bronchiolar-alveolar anastomosis becomes an important bypass in the event of bronchiolar obstruction. Between the openings of the alveoli, the respiratory bronchiole still has cuboid epithelium and smooth muscle, the latter surrounding the openings of the alveoli. A respiratory bronchi-

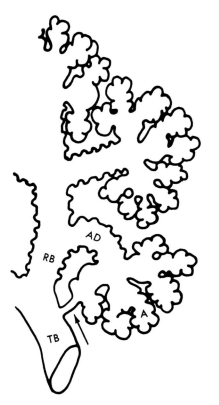

Fig. 26-1. Terminal branches of respiratory tree. **A,** Atrium with alveoli. **AD,** Alveolar duct. **RB,** First-order respiratory bronchiole. **TB,** Terminal bronchiole. *Arrow,* Bronchioloalveolar anastomosis.

ole will branch several times into further respiratory bronchioles.

The next division is into the *alveolar ducts.* These are elongated passageways that really do not have walls but only the framework of the continuous chain of alveoli opening from them. They therefore have no epithelial lining, but a ring of muscle surrounds the alveolar openings as in the respiratory bronchioles. The knobs of muscle are easily seen where the alveolar septa join the ducts.

Finally, from the alveolar ducts come about four air sacs or *atria*—structures in which muscle fibers end and the greatest number of *alveoli* are formed (Fig. 26-1).

Cellular components. Mention was made on the previous page of three long-recognized cells present in the epithelial lining of the airways. Ultrastructural studies in the mouse, rat, and pig have uncovered further cells, some of which are now known to occur in man.[11] The fourth cell is the *intermediate,* possibly a precursor of the ciliated cell. Fifth is the

brush cell, not yet confirmed in man. It is not ciliated, but has a brush border of microvilli; a function has not so far been attributed to it. Occurring centrally is the sixth, *serous cell,* like those in the submucosal glands. The seventh is also to be found centrally in man, an important cell with many confusing names. It lies basally and is the *Kulchitsky cell* (Feyrter cell, AFG [argyrophil-fluorescent granular] cell, a member of the APUD [amine precursor uptake and decarboxylation] family). This is the source of the pulmonary carcinoid (p. 1140) and it has an endocrine function. It appears to be the cell of the neuroepithelial body described by Lauweryns in babies that later seems to break up into its separate component cells. Finally comes the eighth cell, named after *Clara.* It is present in terminal bronchioles in man where it bulges into the lumen. Although it contains abundant rough endoplasmic reticulum rather than osmiophilic bodies, it appears to synthesize surfactant, which is extruded through the apex into the lumen (apocrine secretion).[20] There is a dispute as to the relative importance of the two sites of formation of this product, but some maintain that terminal bronchioles are themselves so narrow that they need surface tension–lowering activity. The view for the primacy of alveolar surfactant is stated by Meyrick and Reid.[15]

The electron microscope has settled the controversy about *alveolar structure* (Fig. 26-2). It shows a continuous alveolar surface (septal) epithelium, providing a covering to the septal capillary network, only 0.2 μm thick. This is the type I, or membranous pneumonocyte. It cannot be seen in ordinary sections, but occasional attenuated nuclei are visible (Fig. 26-27). These cells are extremely elastic to conform with respiration. Lying under the epithelium are the alveolar cells. Some drop off to be alveolar macrophages and are replaced by macrophages that have migrated from the bone marrow or by differentiation of alveolar septal fibroblasts.[5] Others, with large nucleus and granular cytoplasm, are believed to secrete pulmonary surfactant (dipalmitoyl lecithin).[9] These are the type II, or granular, pneumonocytes. Hardly recognizable under the light microscope, they are cuboid with, as seen under the electron microscope, characteristic osmiophilic lamellated bodies (Fig. 26-2), which, although associated with surfactant, have not been definitely proved to produce it. Some argue that these

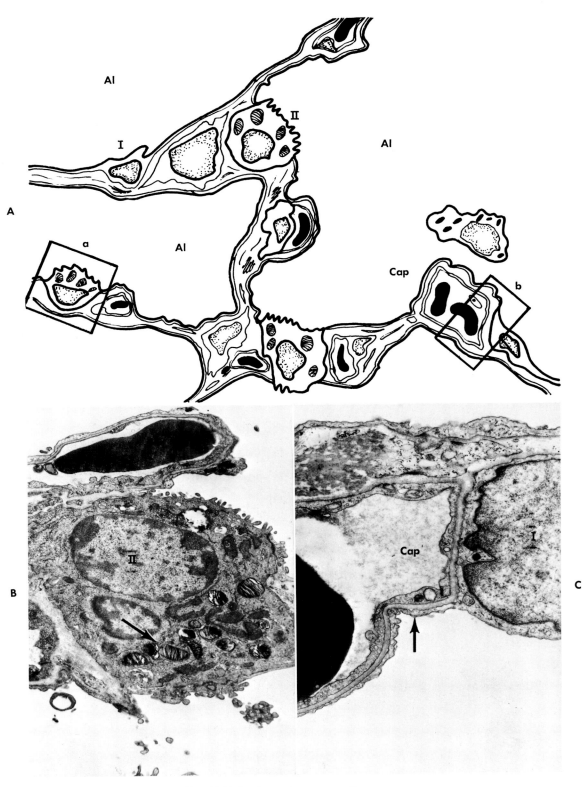

Fig. 26-2. For legend see opposite page.

cells are phagocytic and that the bronchiolar Clara cells are the source of surfactant.

A filmy surface layer of surfactant lipoprotein covers the alveoli. It helps the elastic recoil of the lung after expansion, and it maintains the alveoli open in expiration. Surfactant is needed throughout life and constantly needs to be replaced (it lasts about 3 days).[7] Morgan reviews the role played by loss of surfactant in many diseases, drowning, and surgery on the lung.[16]

The alveolar epithelium has its own basement membrane, continuous with that of the bronchioles, separated from that of the capillaries by an important tissue space containing reticulin and elastic fibers. A thickness of 0.5 to 2.5 μm of this blood-gas barrier has to be traversed by the respiratory gases.

Preparations of the alveolar septal capillary network indicate that the vessels branch so much that they almost touch each other. An elastic and reticular fiber network supports them, and pericytes are present ensheathed within the capillary basement membrane.[24] In the network are mesenchymal cells and phagocytes. The interalveolar septa have numerous pores of Kohn, 10 μm in diameter, which allow free intercommunication between alveoli—even those from different alveolar ducts or lobules. These are seen easily in organizing pneumonia, when young fibrous tissue grows through them, linking solidified alveoli (Fig. 23-30). Otherwise, the pores become an effective bypass if a bronchiole is blocked. However, Pump's investigations suggest that the pores are pathologic fenestrae produced by degeneration of the supporting elastic fibers.[17]

Functional units. Although the concept of the *lobule* as a functional unit is no longer favored, it will be defined so that the reader can understand older writings. The primary lobule, the respiratory tissue arising from one alveolar duct, has been abandoned as a unit because it is too small. "Lobule" is now synonymous with the secondary lobule. The latter is much larger and refers to the lung supplied by the three to five terminal bronchioles arising from a preterminal bronchiole.

Most practical of all is the concept of the *acinus,* the lung distal to one terminal bronchiole. It is a readily visible unit on the cut surface of a lung perfused with formalin. One lobule is composed of three to five acini. Acini are most easily recognized when black dust is deposited around their central bronchiole (Fig. 26-28). Near the sharp margins of the lungs, septa run a short way in from the pleura, often demarcating the sides of acini. These septa are inconstant and unreliable markers. Even where they are absent (which is the case deeper within the lung), a more trustworthy lateral boundary to the acinus can be found— a thin line, which is the acinar vein, a vessel that is always here, never in the center where the bronchiole and artery run.

One tends to assume that the whole lung is in uniform action at all times. Contrary evidence has been presented[22] that there are functional units that roughly correspond to present-day lobules, called "pneumons." Reserve pneumons are brought into use when needed by relaxation of bronchiolar and alveolar duct muscle.

Supporting structures. The lung remains expanded as atmospheric pressure stretches the supporting pulmonary framework of closely linked collagenous and elastic fibers.[12] Reticular fibers have a lesser function in this respect. When air enters the pleural cavity, the intrapulmonary and extrapulmonary pressures become equal, and the collagenous and elastic fibers pull the lung close to its root (collapse).

Collagenous and elastic fibers encircle and support the openings of all alveoli, just as they support the terminal air passages. They run from one alveolar duct to another, sending branch filaments to neighboring alveoli and vessels. Other fibers originate in vessel walls and then run out to alveoli. In this way, all the passages and vessels are linked to neigh-

---

Fig. 26-2. A, Normal alveolar wall with type I and type II pneumonocytes. Wall includes capillaries *(Cap)*, fibroblasts, collagen, and elastin. Macrophage may be seen free in alveolar space, *Al*, to right. **B,** Type II pneumonocyte as seen at **a** in **A.** Cell has few irregular processes on its free alveolar edge and lamellated bodies *(arrow)* in its cytoplasm. **C,** Blood-gas barrier, as seen at **b** in **A,** includes epithelial cell and endothelial cell. To right is nucleus of type I cell with thin cytoplasmic flange *(arrow)* covering capillary and separated from endothelial cell by respective basement membranes. Above, space between endothelium and epithelium is wider, since it includes collagen and elastin. (**B,** 7500×; **C,** 11,000×; **A** to **C,** courtesy Miss Barbara Meyrick, London, England.)

boring structures, allowing changing tensions to be spread evenly throughout. Elastic fibers are best demonstrated in the tips of the interalveolar septa, where alveoli open into air passages. When collagenous and elastic fibers are fragmented by disease, reticular fibers maintain the integrity of the alveolar capillary network.

Interlobular connective-tissue septa in the adult lung are mostly concentrated in the subpleural zone, particularly at the sharp edges and angles of the lungs.[18,19] They are relatively scarce over costal surfaces and absent over the fissural surface and deeper in the lung. It is fundamental to the operation of collateral air drift in the human lung that these septa are incomplete, not enclosing lobules. The mosaic pattern of subpleural lymphatics bears no constant relationship to the septa, although the two may overlap.[19]

Fetal and neonatal lung. In utero, the lung contains much fluid, but otherwise the alveolar surfaces are generally apposed. Intro-

duction of air by the first breath requires relatively great force to overcome the surface tension in the bronchioles and alveoli and also to move away the fluid.[4] Once the first airways open, their original surface tensions fall, and they tend to stay open. The next breath will open air spaces farther out in the lung and so on in a series (the "pop-pop-pop" mechanism).

From the beginning of their development, the lungs are covered by pleura. In the fetus at 26 to 28 days, the two main bronchi grow out from the trachea, which is, in turn, a bud off the foregut. They subdivide (Fig. 26-3) until, by the sixteenth week, all the airways down to the ends of the terminal bronchioles are created, and no more will be formed although cartilage will appear until the twenty-fourth week. Interlobar septa form very early and by 12 weeks the lobes are demarcated. A lung in this *"glandular"* or *"bronchial" phase* (fifth to sixteenth week) is recognized by the cuboid cells lining the airways, which

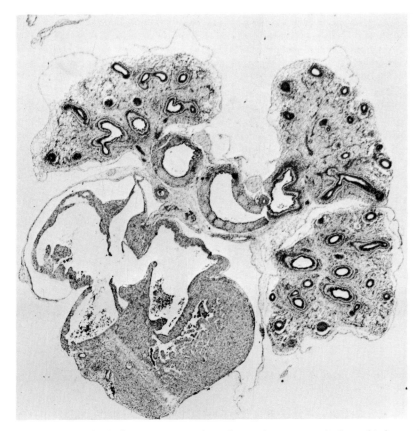

Fig. 26-3. Heart and both lungs in 8-week embryo showing early bronchial tree in undeveloped mesenchyme. (24×.)

are surrounded by mesenchyme. Pulmonary arteries are now in position. The *"canalicular" phase* occupies the sixteenth to twenty-fourth weeks. Rapid proliferation of capillaries between groups of epithelial cells of the air passages converts the epithelium into channels, on the surface of which lie networks of capillaries. A hasty glance at the lungs of a fetus of this age might lead one to believe that these are primitive vascular alveoli lined by cuboid cells. During this phase, the formation of surfactant commences, and attenuation of the epithelium of the channels begins, allowing the blood to approach closer to the alveolar lumen. Extrauterine life cannot be maintained prior to these events. While this vital opening of the distal airways is proceeding, the mesenchyme is contributing the bronchial cartilage and elastic and collagen fibers. Cilia and goblet cells have appeared by 13 to 14 weeks, and bronchial glands are in place 2 weeks later.

Not until the twenty-fourth[1] week (or twenty-eighth week[5]) does the *"alveolar" phase* begin. Fetal alveoli are very shallow evaginations of the primitive bronchiolar walls. Boyden's important wax reconstructions have shown that, from now on, functional lung tissue grows centripetally by the conversion of peripheral terminal bronchioles into respiratory bronchioles.[6] No further airways develop after the sixteenth week.

At birth the full-term infant has 20 million alveoli, which are so small that they barely resemble normal adult alveoli and are better termed "saccules."[6] True alveoli are formed only after birth. The number increases (with the growth of the thorax) to the adult total of 200 to 600 million by the eighth year, after which they further increase in size.[21] The original plump saccular lining cell of the saccular phase very slowly becomes attenuated. Even in an infant, many of them remain visible. Saccular septa of a newborn infant are thick-walled structures because of the prominent capillaries. Alveoli develop rapidly between the sixth and eighth postnatal week.

Throughout fetal life, the lower respiratory tract produces a highly complex lung fluid that is held under pressure during later fetal life by sphincterlike contraction of the laryngeal muscles. The resultant positive pressure is considered to be a factor in the expansion and growth of the lung. From time to time, the larynx relaxes and some fluid is released, to be promptly swallowed. Paralysis of the laryngeal muscles by damage to the vagus will be followed by atelectasis, a condition also found when there is a wide tracheoesophageal fistula.[22] The human fetus makes breathing movements in utero at a rate of 40 to 70 per minute for 70% of the time during the second half of gestation.[8]

As the fetus grows, the amount of phospholipid in lung fluid increases. The fluid in the upper trachea and larynx is mainly a highly viscous mucus, secreted locally by glands. It seems probable that this must be squeezed out of the infant (i.e., by vaginal delivery) rather than inspired. Absence of squeezing, as in cesarean section, may explain why babies delivered in this fashion are more prone to respiratory distress.[22] So it seems that fetal lung functions like an exocrine gland, secreting fluid and (from about the 900 gm stage) the surface tension–lowering lipoprotein, and that the bronchioles act as the excretory ducts. At birth, fluid is removed through pulmonary vascular and lymphatic channels.

The viable fetus (i.e., over 1000 gm) is able to remain alive without true alveoli because the bronchiolar capillaries are so well developed as to be able themselves to permit gaseous exchange.

Pulmonary blood and lymphatic vessels. The ultimate destination of the pulmonary arteries is the capillary network of the interalveolar septa. The return is into the *pulmonary venous system,* which also picks up blood from the bronchial arterial flow and from veins originating from larger bronchi. Other bronchial veins drain the pleural surfaces and the largest bronchi, entering the azygos vein on the right and the hemiazygos or innominate vein on the left.

In the adult, the ill-defined adventitia being omitted from the measurement, elastic *arteries* have been said to have an external diameter greater than 1 mm, smaller vessels being muscular arteries. In turn, the transition between these and arterioles was put at 0.1 mm.

Orthodox for many years, the foregoing concept is inaccurate because it is based on lungs in which the arteries have not been standardized by injection to their true size.[1]

Pulmonary arteries have an internal and an external elastic lamina, whereas in bronchial arteries only the internal elastica is well developed. Even more noticeable in bronchial arteries is an additional muscular layer in the intima, with its fibers appearing longitudinal, although most of them follow a spiral course.

It is difficult to tell an arteriole from a venule (unless the former can be traced to an artery), because neither vessel normally has any muscle. In other words, pulmonary arterioles are really precapillaries and do not resemble arterioles of other organs.[23]

At birth, the full-term infant has pulmonary arteries with thick-walled, muscular small branches. This narrow lumen reduces pulmonary blood flow, for which there is little need in utero. Within a few days, the walls become thin, and, before the end of a year, they are of adult type. Elastic arteries are recognized in the lung of the newborn infant by loose layers of connective tissue that surround them as well as by their predominantly elastic media.

Bronchial arteries exist to nourish bronchi, in whose walls they ramify as far as the terminal bronchioles. They do not have significant anastomoses with pulmonary arterial branches but can be an important source of collateral circulation when the pulmonary arterial circulation is blocked or in emphysema or diffuse fibrosis.

The *lymphatic vascular system* provides a pleural plexus of capillaries that may outline the lobules. This plexus drains to the hilar lymph nodes but also communicates with pulmonary lymph vessels, which begin at the respiratory bronchioles.[13] They drain the tissue spaces of the interalveolar septa and the bronchial and vascular trees into the hilar lymph nodes. From here, drainage is to tracheobronchial nodes and eventually to the right lymphatic duct and, on the left, to the thoracic duct. Some lymph also passes to scalene and retroperitoneal lymph nodes. As recently as 1974 Lauweryns demonstrated that there are no lymphatic vessels in interalveolar septa.[14] Their most distal representatives are the "juxta-alveolar lymphatics" situated in the space between alveoli and the outer border of interlobular, pleural, perivascular, or peribronchial connective-tissue sheets. Small lymphatics are easily seen in lungs of persons dying of drowning or hyaline membrane disease.

Lymphoid nodules occur at the bifurcation of bronchi, as far down as the respiratory bronchioles, so that collections of lymphocytes in the muscle coat are not necessarily proof of the presence of chronic inflammation.

CONGENITAL ANOMALIES

Total absence of lungs may occur in anencephalic monsters. Unilateral *atresia,* the absence of a lung, does not endanger life, but serious malformations often accompany it.[36] Usually, there is no trace of the missing lung's bronchus or vessels. Sometimes one lobe or a whole lung is *hypoplastic.* This may be primary or secondary to the pressure of a large tumor or cyst or to abdominal organs entering the thorax, as in congenital diaphragmatic hernia.[38a] *Potter's syndrome* is deformity of the ears, widely set eyes, prominent epicanthic fold, receding chin, and pulmonary hypoplasia, accompanying severe renal hypoplasia or cystic disease.

It is not uncommon to find an *excessive or diminished number of pulmonary lobes* in the absence of any functional effect. An *accessory lobe* (which may become infected) is an independent pulmonary structure, invested by its own pleura and supplied by an accessory bronchus. The *azygos lobe* is produced by a low-arching azygos vein pulling down into the right apex, rendering it bifid because the vein drags down with it a fold of pleura.

Bronchopulmonary sequestration

A sequestered pulmonary segment is one totally or partly separated from the normal lung, having developed from an accessory bronchopulmonary bud on the foregut. More often it is intralobar, meaning within a pulmonary lobe, but there is an extralobar variety. Mixed forms are beginning to be reported.[33]

Intralobar sequestration. Intralobar sequestration is observed in young adults in whom a large mass is found, generally in the left lower lobe. There is usually no communication with the bronchial tree, and blood is supplied from a large artery from the aorta, arising just above or below the diaphragm.[23] Venous return is pulmonary. The mass turns out to be a single large cyst, a cluster of small ones in firm fibrotic lung, or mainly solid lung tissue with abscesses.[28] In the cysts is pus or viscid material. Infection can be severe enough to spread to the pleura.

Extralobar sequestration. At first glance, extralobar sequestration is merely an accessory lobe but nearly always is basal and left-sided and shows no communication with the bronchial tree. It has a variable blood supply from the aorta, and its veins drain to the azygos system. Unlike the intralobar variety, it is covered by its own pleura and often is found in infancy.

Sequestration communicating with esophagus or stomach. On rare occasions, a sequestration of either type is served by a bronchus growing directly out of the midesophagus, lower esophagus, or gastric fundus.[31] This suggests that sequestrations are closely related to one another and to accessory bronchopulmonary tissues, all of which may be termed bronchopulmonary-foregut malformations.

Cystic disease

Pulmonary cysts in older children and adults frequently are so altered by inflammation and fibrosis that forms of bronchial distention distal to an occlusion, in bronchiectasis or in honeycomb lungs, cannot be distinguished from congenital cysts by any combination of clinical findings and microscopy. Findings in favor of cystic bronchiectasis are as follows:

1. Situation in a lower lobe
2. Earlier stages of bronchiectasis in other bronchi
3. Easy demonstration of a bronchus directly entering the cavity

Bronchial (bronchogenic) cyst. A tracheobronchial cyst is attached to the trachea near the bifurcation or to a main bronchus. This is really an accessory bronchial bud, although it rarely communicates with the lumen. It is a unilocular sphere containing watery fluid and having an attenuated wall of bronchial type, including surface epithelium, glands, muscle, and cartilage (which causes trabeculation of the lining). If detached from its parent bronchus, it appears as a mediastinal bronchogenic cyst. Other cysts, in exactly the same position, are found to be enterogenic—cysts of foregut origin lined by gastric or intestinal epithelium. Some bronchial cysts are paraesophageal or even within the esophageal wall.

A solitary bronchial cyst may be within the lung. Infection may convert it into an abscess.

Multiple cysts. Cysts up to 1 cm in diameter may be clustered in the periphery of one or more lobes. They are congenital anomalies of more distal bronchi, and hence their linings are simpler than those of central bronchial cysts. The lining is of columnar cells, sometimes ciliated, covering elastic and fibrous connective tissue with a little muscle. The cysts may or may not communicate with bronchi or with each other. Those entering a bronchus are originally filled with air. The blind ones contain fluid.

Some peripheral cysts are derivatives of the visceral pleura.[37] Folds of the latter may dip into clefts in the lung in the region of interlobular septa and, becoming separated, form into cysts. Possibly, too, pouches of mesothelium are nipped off between growing lung buds. In either case, the cyst lining resembles the structure of the pleura. There will be no muscle coat.

Multiple lung cysts may be present in patients with Marfan's syndrome or tuberous sclerosis.

Congenital cystic adenomatoid malformation. A rare diffuse hamartoma found in the newborn infant (especially the premature infant), congenital cystic adenomatoid malformation endangers life.[25] Generally confined to one lobe, it can be diagnosed radiograph-

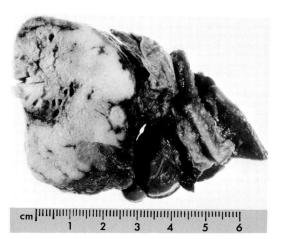

Fig. 26-4. Diffuse hamartoma (congenital cystic adenomatoid malformation of lung). Most of right lung replaced by firm white tissue containing tiny cysts. Left lung compressed and partly hidden by turned-down trachea.

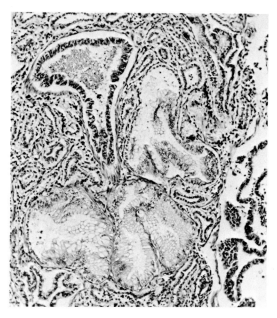

Fig. 26-5. Diffuse hamartoma. Mucinous and cuboid types of epithelium are present. (165×.)

ically by the presence of an enlarged lung with a mass containing cystic cavities. *Grossly,* the lobe, which requires surgical removal, displaces the mediastinum, partly compresses normal lung, and interferes with the hemodynamics of the heart (Fig. 26-4). Cysts of up to 3 cm bulge under the pleura and are found on the cut surface. They have one or more cavities containing air, since they communicate with the bronchial tree, but there is not a normal bronchial system. Around them is collapsed and indurated white lung.

Microscopically, the cysts and the remnants of the alveoli have two possible linings. One is a bronchial type (without underlying cartilage) sometimes thrown into a polypoid configuration, hence the name "adenomatoid." The second is a tall columnar cell with a small basal nucleus and a bounteous cytoplasm full of mucin. Around the epithelium is a thin layer of connective tissue and smooth muscle (Fig. 26-5). Inflammation may complicate the condition.

Congenital pulmonary lymphangiectasis. Congenital pulmonary lymphangiectasis is a bilateral, diffuse but irregular, dilatation of pulmonary lymphatic vessels and is found only in the newborn infant. These vessels, mainly under the pleura and in the interlobular septa, are distended with clear fluid to a diameter of several millimeters (Fig. 26-6). The cysts are lined by endothelium resting on a little fibrous tissue.[35]

The fully developed condition is incompatible with life. A number of the cases have been associated with malformations of the left side of the heart.[39]

Vascular anomalies

Arterial anomalies. The main pulmonary trunk or its right or left branch may be lacking, in which case the arterial supply is from a patent ductus, with contributions from bronchial arteries and accessory branches. Congenital stenosis of the pulmonary artery branches may be single or multiple, local or diffuse. There is right ventricular hypertrophy, and one can easily see dilatation distal to each arterial narrowing.[30]

Venous anomalies. In totally *anomalous venous drainage* of the lungs the four main veins converge behind the left atrium to form a chamber of their own (cor triatriatum). From it emerges a vein that runs into the left

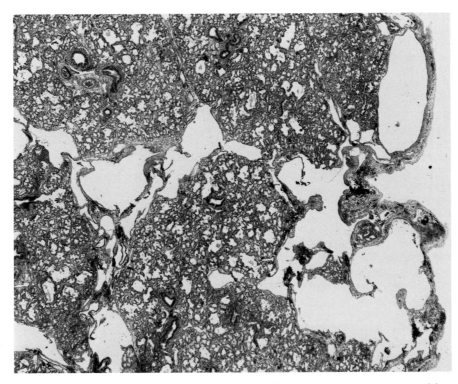

Fig. 26-6. Congenital pulmonary lymphangiectasis. Dilated spaces are not around bronchi and arteries; thus, condition is distinguished from interstitial emphysema. (21×.)

innominate vein, the coronary sinus, the right atrium, the inferior vena cava below the diaphragm, or the portal vein. Patients with such anomalies are cyanotic, but those in whom some of the veins drain normally can be quite asymptomatic. When drainage is totally anomalous, 75% of infants will die or require operation before their first birthday.[27]

An anomaly well known to radiologists is the "scimitar sign." A broad, curving paracardiac shadow is produced by abnormal right pulmonary venous drainage into the inferior vena cava at or below the diaphragm. Symptoms produced by this partial shunt from the left to the right side of the heart depend on the amount of blood involved. After this condition was first described, it was realized that two other abnormalities accompany it—a hyparterial right upper-lobe bronchus (the right tracheobronchial tree is a mirror image of the left) and systemic pulmonary arteries to the right lung. Accordingly, we now speak of the *scimitar syndrome*.[34] Conditions associated with this are bronchiectasis, anomalous right hemidiaphragm, atrial or ventricular septal defects, patent ductus arteriosus, aortic coarctation, and arteriovenous anomalies of the right lung.

One or more of the pulmonary veins may be *stenotic*.[32]

Arteriovenous fistula (aneurysm). Arteriovenous fistula is a tumorlike malformation that enlarges over the years. The usual site is immediately beneath the pleura (Fig. 26-7). Each lesion is an interweaving complex of arteries and very thin-walled veins, with one large vessel entering and one leaving. This abnormal communication is usually between a pulmonary arterial branch and a vein (occasionally a bronchial or an intercostal artery). If the shunt is large enough, the patient is polycythemic and cyanotic. Fatal rupture may occur into the lung or pleural space.

Among 63 cases at the Mayo Clinic, only three had a systemic blood supply and one third were multiple; 50 of the patients had hereditary hemorrhagic telangiectasia. In the presence of the last feature, there was an increased incidence of multiplicity and a greater rate of growth of the fistulas.[29]

ACQUIRED VASCULAR DISEASE
Acquired arteriovenous fistula

Some patients with cirrhosis (portal or caused by schistosomiasis) have decreased arterial oxygen saturation. A smaller number are cyanotic and have clubbed fingers. The

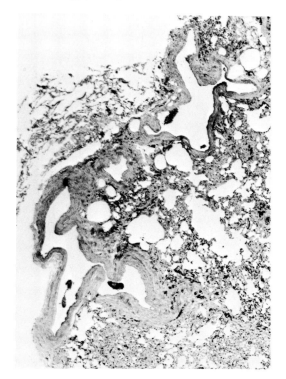

Fig. 26-7. Arteriovenous fistula. Large, misshapen, thick-walled vessels run aimlessly just below pleura. (24×.)

change in oxygen saturation is caused by the development of multiple, tiny, arteriovenous anastomoses in the lung.[43] If the pulmonary vessels are injected, many more such cases of pulmonary spider nevi will be uncovered. They may result from the same mechanism that produces them in the skin.

Hyperemia and congestion

Active hyperemia. Active hyperemia is the result of an acute infective condition of the lung or of the presence of a gaseous, liquid, or particulate irritant. The term implies active dilatation of pulmonary vessels, and hence edema is likely to appear soon after, characterized microscopically by the presence of fibrin strands and leukocytes.

Passive hyperemia. Passive hyperemia is usually called *congestion*, the result of left-sided heart failure, which interferes with pulmonary venous drainage. The lungs are dark blue and heavy, with diminished air content. Edema is frequent, evident from the bloody, frothy fluid pouring from the cut surface. This occurs because the alveolar capillaries are overdistended and because hypoxia and increased pressure promote escape of fluid across

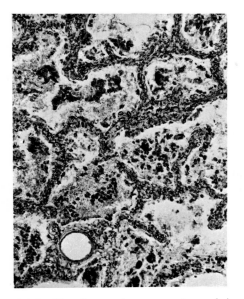

Fig. 26-8. Chronic passive congestion of lung. Alveolar septa are thickened because they are hypervascular. Alveoli contain pigment-laden macrophages and protein.

the vascular endothelium. The normal resorptive powers of the alveoli are overwhelmed.

Initially, a pale eosinophilic amorphous or granular material is seen in the alveoli, with erythrocytes and macrophages. Interalveolar septa are widened by prominent, hitherto inconspicuous, capillaries. Edematous thickening of interlobular septa is apparent, and the lymph channels within them and around vessels and bronchi are dilated. Veins in the walls of bronchi also are congested.

Chronic passive congestion. In chronic passive congestion, seen classically in mitral stenosis, the lungs are firmer and drier, with a faint brown tinge (brown induration). The alveoli contain many macrophages stuffed with brown hemosiderin granules (heart-failure cells) (Fig. 26-8). Tortuous alveolar capillaries are expanded to the width of several red cells, and the interalveolar septa undergo fibrosis. When this has developed, the alveolar surface cells become much more prominent. Fibrosis also thickens the interlobular septa and the perivascular and peribronchial tissues and ultimately may obliterate alveolar capillaries. In the most severe instances, the alveolar material becomes ossified, with neighboring areas combining to form particles of bone several millimeters in diameter, large enough to be recognized radiographically (Fig. 23-46).

The microscopic changes include medial and intimal thickening of the small muscular pulmonary arteries. Uncommonly, there is necrotizing arteritis.[47]

Iron in alveolar macrophages may not necessarily be the result of bleeding into the lung. The cells take up plasma protein in edema fluid, which includes acid mucopolysaccharide. The latter has the property of impregnating the mucin with iron, presumably from plasma transferrin.[44]

Simple brown induration should be differentiated from three conditions. The first is *idiopathic pulmonary hemosiderosis*. Nearly all the patients have been boys. Repeated sudden attacks of intra-alveolar bleeding cause severe anemia with dyspnea and jaundice. Death ensues after a few years. The changes resemble those of severe brown induration, and the hilar nodes also are brown. In the bleeding phase, alveoli are filled with fresh blood with a pronounced phagocytic reaction. Later, macrophages carry hemosiderin to the interalveolar septa, which become fibrotic, and to the interlobular, subpleural, peribronchial, and perivascular connective tissues. In all these sites, nodular fibrosis forms in reaction to hemosiderin. The elastic fibers in the alveolar septa, pulmonary stroma, and small and medium-sized pulmonary arteries are hemosiderin-encrusted. The vascular elastica may be degenerate. Alveolar surface cells are crowded, swollen, and occasionally multinucleated. Soergel and Sommers[46] have collected a total of about 100 reported cases. A total of nearly 50 cases in adults has been published.

The second disease to be distinguished from simple brown induration is *Goodpasture's syndrome*. This is an often lethal combination of an initial disease closely resembling (both clinically and pathologically) idiopathic pulmonary hemosiderosis but soon (although occasionally years later) followed by a severe proliferative glomerulonephritis. Most of the patients are in the third decade, and men predominate over women.[49] Immunofluorescence investigations indicate that the alveoli and glomeruli share antigens to which antibodies are formed, creating pulmonary and renal lesions in which immunoglobulins can be detected.[41] Attachment of antibody to alveolar and glomerular basement membranes causes activation of complement, which then leads to inflammation and necrosis of the related cells.

In patients having pulmonary signs of Goodpasture's syndrome but with normal urinalysis findings and normal light microscopic morphology in renal biopsy, newer studies have been surprising. When fluorescence microscopy is carried out on the renal tissue, some of the patients are found already to have positive linear glomerular immunofluorescence to anti-IgG and anti-C_3 antiserum; electron microscopic studies will show deposits in the glomerular basement membrane.[45] The importance of this is twofold. First, there can be extensive renal involvement before there is clinical renal abnormality; steroids have to be given at the earliest possible stage of the renal lesion, to prevent an inevitably fulminant course. Second, such cases would be falsely diagnosed as idiopathic pulmonary hemosiderosis. Ultrastructural differences between the lesions of the alveolar capillary basement membranes in these two diseases have now been demonstrated.[42]

A third, rare, condition to be distinguished from brown induration is *mechanical obstruction of the pulmonary veins,* in which an interstitial (septal) pulmonary fibrosis develops, with some deposition of hemosiderin.[40]

Hypostatic congestion. Hypostatic congestion is a gravitational congestion and edema of the lungs in persons with weakening cardiac and respiratory action. Such areas are ideal breeding grounds for bacteria, which bring about hypostatic bronchopneumonia in the immobile patient.

Massive pulmonary hemorrhage in newborn infants

Infants believed clinically to have died from hyaline membrane disease sometimes are found to have massive hemorrhage into the whole of two or more lobes. Most die by the end of their second postnatal day. Many resemblances are noted to hyaline membrane disease both in the patients at risk and in the course of the disease, but the condition also occurs in stillborn infants and may cause respiratory distress from the moment of birth. Massive hemorrhage and hyaline membrane disease often coexist.

The condition occurs in about 1 in 1000 live-born infants and causes acute collapse, accompanied by outpouring of bloody fluid from the trachea, mouth, and nose. It has been associated with severe birth asphyxia, hypothermia, hemolytic disease of the newborn, congenital heart disease and small-for-age development. The precipitating factor all of these have in common is acute left ventricular failure in a patient who is lying flat rather than sitting up. Numbers of investigators have analyzed the fluid and confirm that it is a form of severe hemorrhagic pulmonary edema, not pure blood.[48] One could say that this is a neonatal equivalent to adult shock lung. Nine percent of neonatal deaths show this as the cause of death when examined post mortem.

Edema and shock

Pulmonary edema, alone or with minimal congestion, is caused by administration of too much intravenous fluid, by conditions of increased intracranial pressure (by a reflex pathway), or by exposure to chemical or physical irritants (including irradiation, p. 356) or may occur in fulminating bacterial or viral infection, anaphylactic shock, and angioneurotic edema. Normally the lung's lymphatics actively pump excess fluid back to the systemic venous system. The rate of fluid flow through the lung's interstitial tissue can increase several times before there is a clinically measurable increase in the tissue's fluid contents (i.e., edema).[61] Theories of pulmonary edema are centered on considerations of factors affecting fluid filtration and clearance, and factors affecting microvascular membrane structure. Severe acute pulmonary edema may develop within 24 hours in unacclimatized young healthy persons who ascend to an altitude of 10,000 feet or more. Two young men who were natives of the mountains were reported to have died after returning from a visit of a month or two to lower altitudes.[50]

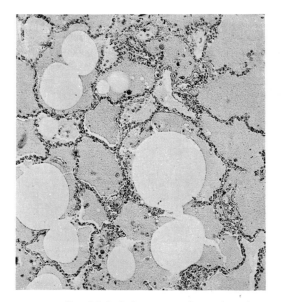

Fig. 26-9. Pulmonary edema.

In all types of pulmonary edema the lungs are large, pallid and wet, pit on finger pressure, and pour out copious frothy fluid when cut. When associated with fatal intracranial conditions, edema frequently is confined to one or both upper lobes.[52] Microscopically, the alveolar vessels are inconspicuous, and the interlobular septa, air spaces, and bronchi are filled by pale-staining, protein-containing fluid (Fig. 26-9).

Radiologists recognize edema by the appearance of Kerley's lines, which are produced by edema of various interlobular septa and distended lymphatics within them.

The two high-altitude victims mentioned previously also had hyaline membranes, thrombosis of the precapillaries, and wide dilatation of the pulmonary venous system, including the capillaries. Ultrastructural studies of rats in simulated high altitude have disclosed multiple vesicles protruding from the alveolar capillaries. These are considered to be edematous blebs, and they are so large and numerous as to cause considerable luminal narrowing. This, combined with vasoconstriction, appears to be the basis of mountain edema.[57]

Acute pulmonary edema. Acute pulmonary edema[52] has manifold causes. It is particularly likely to involve the pulmonary medulla.[53] As much as 2 or 3 liters of foamy fluid can appear within 1 to 2 hours, and a fulminating variety can be fatal in 10 to 20 minutes. Among the causes are myocardial infarction, pulmonary embolism, mitral stenosis, and disorders of cardiac rhythm. A cause of fulminating, often fatal and still unexplained, pulmonary edema is heroin overdosage.[58]

Shock lung. The "shock-lung syndrome" (hemorrhagic pulmonary edema, posttraumatic respiratory insufficiency, and congestive atelectasis are some of its synonyms) was first recognized in patients surviving major thoracic or nonthoracic injuries during World War II. Within hours or days of apparently successful treatment of a severe wound, there follows tachypnea, dyspnea, tachycardia, and cyanosis; mortality is high. A characteristic feature is labored rapid breathing with cyanosis, often resistant to oxygen therapy and assisted ventilation. Chest x-ray films demonstrate diffuse alveolar infiltrates that may progress to widespread consolidation.

Microscopically one finds severe interstitial edema of the peribronchial and pericapillary tissue, congestion, collapse of many alveoli, and focal bronchopneumonia. Less constant findings are alveolar edema, thromboemboli in the smallest pulmonary vessels, fat emboli, and hyaline membranes, plus intraalveolar and interstitial hemorrhage.[62] These cause petechiae to appear on the lungs' surfaces with focal congestion and collapse within, followed in later stages by widespread hemorrhagic consolidation in which the lungs resemble liver.

The effect on function is to increase capillary permeability, reduce the amount of surfactant, and damage the alveolar lining cells.[60a] The initiating event appears to be aggregation of platelets and leukocytes in the pulmonary microcirculation with release of vasoconstrictor and bronchoconstrictor agents from these cells.

Similar, but not identical, pathologic and clinical pictures are associated with the cardiopulmonary bypass procedure, burns, large transfusions of stored blood, and septic or endotoxic shock. The last condition has been shown experimentally to cause degranulation of neutrophils because of injury to their lysosomes by phagocytosed endotoxin.[51]

Fibrinous pulmonary edema. In the past, attempts have been made to distinguish at least two types of fibrinous pulmonary edema —that occurring in uremia ("uremic lung or pneumonitis") and that occurring in acute rheumatic fever ("rheumatic lung or pneumonitis"). For years, radiologists have recognized the butterfly or bat's wing hilar shadows produced by the protein-rich fluid that is concentrated around the roots (medullae) of both lungs. Uremia is one of the commonest causes and may produce the radiologic picture in a few days. Chronic left ventricular failure in essential hypertension is another important cause.[56]

The lung is dark purple, with a very soft, rubbery consistency. The edema fluid gives the lung around the hilum, particularly the lower lobes, an increase in consistency. Because it is so rich in fibrin, the cut surface is wet and glassy. "Solid edema" had been observed by pathologists for years prior to this distinction.

The fluid does not pour away easily because of the coagulation of the fibrin; firm pressure will release the fluid.

What damages the capillary walls so as to allow fibrinogen to pass through is not known. There is evidence that in conditions of anoxia or increased pulmonary venous pressure, the blood flow is much diminished in the outer parts of the lungs; thus the central distribution of the uremic change is encouraged. This is merely a manifestation of the division of the normal lung into two zones: (1) medulla,

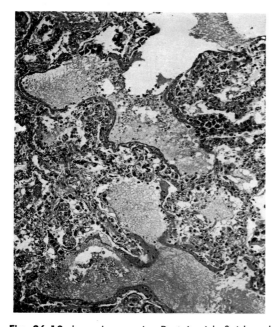

Fig. 26-10. Lung in uremia. Protein-rich fluid and erythrocytes fill alveoli, and hyaline membranes line septa, which are edematous and contain some macrophages. (115×.)

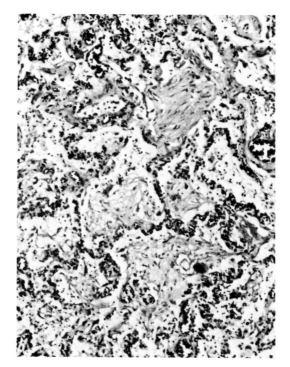

Fig. 26-11. Organizing pulmonary edema. Intra-alveolar fibrin with some erythrocytes is being organized into solid masses by young fibroblasts. No inflammatory reaction is present. Dark cells in alveolar capillaries are erythrocytes. (24×.)

comprising large bronchi and vessels and the lobules in the angles of their bifurcations and (2) cortex, the outer third, composed of most of the alveoli and of the small bronchi and vessels.[53]

Microscopically, the difference between the uremic lung and ordinary edema is the greater eosinophilia of the alveolar fluid in the former. Moreover, a hyaline membrane is very common. Fluid also will be found in the alveolar ducts, and edema of interlobular septa will be noticed. Any cellular infiltrate is scanty—mostly neutrophilic (Fig. 26-10). Given chronicity, it is possible for the fibrin to undergo organization in both alveoli and bronchioles (Fig. 26-11). These changes are not specific for uremia but can be seen in any case of high-protein edema, especially in left ventricular failure.[56] Undoubtedly in the past, the changes have been confused with organizing pneumonia. The young fibrous tissue contains hemosiderin macrophages and may be covered by proliferating alveolar epithelium, which also grows over alveolar septa.

A similar condition has been observed in patients given antihypertensive drugs such as hexamethonium, if the drugs prolong life, but the cause is cardiac failure, not the drug.

Lung in rheumatic fever. Grossly and microscopically, the lung in rheumatic fever has the nonspecific picture of pulmonary edema plus hemorrhagic areas. Added to this are many large mononuclear cells, both septal and intra-alveolar, which may compress the alveolar capillaries. Hemorrhage into alveoli is common, and rarely there is fibrinoid necrosis of the capillaries.[54] Small pulmonary arteries may contain thrombi and show fibrinoid mural changes. Aschoff bodies do not appear, but perivascular lymphocytes, histiocytes, and fibroblasts can be observed.

Finally, there is organization of alveolar exudate and septal fibrosis. Moolten[59] described 88 of 166 cases of rheumatic heart disease in which autopsy disclosed interstitial fibrosis of the lung. A number of these cases could be shown not to be attributable to chronic passive congestion but to "rheumatic pneumonia."

Thromboembolism and infarction

General remarks on the nature of thrombi, emboli, and pulmonary infarctions are found in Chapter 4.

Incidence. Pulmonary embolism has been

found in up to 25% of autopsies performed in general hospitals. Embolism is not synonymous with infarction, which is seen in about half the cases. Most of the patients are on medical (particularly cardiac) rather than surgical wards and are at least 40 years of age. Noncardiac medical patients are likely to have pleural effusions, pneumonia, or other lung disease. Pulmonary embolism may be a cause of unexpected death in supposedly normal persons.[63,65,70] Phlebothrombosis may be demonstrated in such patients. About 150 cases have been reported in children. There is also an association with childbirth, obesity, severe trauma, and thrombophlebitis (including that caused by intravenous therapy).

The risk of venous thrombosis is increased fourfold in women taking contraceptive pills. Persons with carcinoma (for some reason, most commonly of the stomach and pancreas) have an unexplained tendency to venous (even arterial) thrombosis.

Sites of origin. Thrombi form in the deep or superficial veins of the lower limb, the iliac, prostatic, or utero-ovarian veins, and the right side of the heart (atrial fibrillation, or endocardial damage by myocardial infarction). Frequently, search for the origin is in vain because the embolus is the whole thrombus. Less common sources are the mesenteric and portal veins and those of the neck and arms.

Gross appearance of embolus. A thrombus more than a few days old is readily distinguished from a postmortem clot. The latter is soft, moist, and red, with perhaps sedimentation into a dark lower layer of cells and an upper yellow layer of plasma. The typical thrombus is much drier and paler, is brittle, and has on its surface parallel wavy thin lines of Zahn. If it has been in situ for a few days or more, it may be partly adherent to the arterial intima. A thrombus only a day old on arriving in the lung may be indistinguishable from a postmortem clot. One should note whether it has the shape of a systemic vein or bears imprints of its valves. Otherwise one can never be sure. Present criteria for diagnosis of antemortem thrombus (i.e., embolus) may be too narrow. A newly formed thrombus at the advancing head of an older one is loosely attached and so can break free.

Obstructive effect. The largest emboli cannot pass the major pulmonary arteries unless they fragment, immediately or later. Smaller emboli also may block a major vessel or even the main bifurcation if they become coiled upon themselves. Obstruction of a main artery

can be relieved by a change in shape of a soft, loose embolus. Smaller emboli most commonly travel to the vessels of the lower lobes.

Massive emboli in the main pulmonary trunk or straddling the bifurcation commonly cause death instantly or in 10 to 15 minutes. This is too quick for infarction to supervene. The patients die in shock with acute right atrial dilatation that spreads to the right ventricle if the patient survives longer. Usually, bulging of the main pulmonary artery will be observed before it is opened. The lung may appear quite normal or may have suffered some collapse and edema. Often it will show several small older infarcts, since multiple infarctions are so common.

Effect of embolism. Why patients with embolism die is not known. Some patients with large emboli survive, with the vessels distended around almost completely occlusive thrombi.[68] The collateral circulation gives aid, and the patient may have few symptoms.[69] Possibly these were emboli that stimulated later thrombosis that extended retrogradely. Alternatively, they may simply be thrombi (p. 177).

Emboli that reach lobar or smaller arteries are those commonly causing infarction, but they may produce only "incipient infarction." In the latter condition, the territory of supply of the occluded vessel is congested by an inflow of blood from bronchial arteries in the surrounding lung. The area is red and microscopically is edematous, with greatly congested alveolar capillaries. The tissues are not necrotic and presumably can recover.

Embolization to small pulmonary arteries (miliary emboli) can have profound physiologic effects. Innocuous at first sight, they may be fatal or build up a cor pulmonale as new showers of emboli fall. Their effect is aggravated by superimposed thrombosis. Why a series of small infarcts in congestive heart failure brings about death is not known.[66] Pulmonary angiography has demonstrated that the affected area is well aerated but is not perfused with blood. Possibly oxygen desaturation brought about by thromboembolism leads to vasoconstriction and increasing pulmonary hypertension.[64] Release of serotonin, fibrinopeptides, and kinins also is suspected of playing a part.

Appearance of infarct. The classic sterile infarct is a wedge-shaped area up to 5 cm in greatest dimension. Some are irregular or quadrilateral. The base rests on the pleura, and often one can find the blocked vessel on cutting into the lung just proximal to the

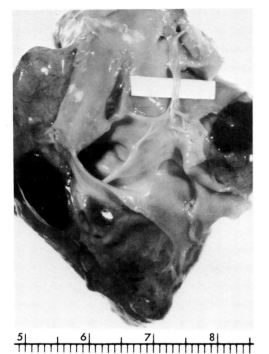

5| 6| 7| 8|

Fig. 26-12. Webs in major branch of pulmonary artery, which are residues of organized thrombi.

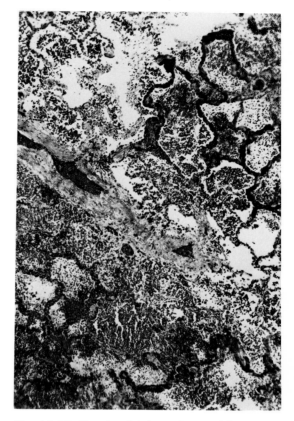

Fig. 26-13. Margin of infarct. *Bottom left,* Masses of erythrocytes and extensive necrosis of intra-alveolar septa. *Top right,* Earlier stage. *Top left,* Congestion only. (63×.)

apex of the infarct. After the first day, there is a covering fibrinous pleuritis, and the area bulges slightly. It is indurated and the cut surface is ill defined, moist and dark purple. One to 2 days later, the pleural surface is depressed, and the cut surface is dry, granular, and pale red, becoming brown; the margins are sharp. Organization and retraction leave a well-concealed thin scar at right angles to the pleura, which may have undergone local thickening. The thrombus is organized into a fibrous band or net[23] (Fig. 26-12).

Microscopically, intense alveolar capillary congestion and alveoli filled with blood are seen in the first 24 to 48 hours. After this stage, the interalveolar septa undergo coagulative necrosis (Fig. 26-13), nuclear detail is lost, and erythrocytes become pale discs. Their hemoglobin is converted into hemosiderin, taken up by phagocytes. During the second week, fibroblasts grow in from the periphery. Organization takes weeks or months, depending on how big the infarct is.

Septic emboli produce infarcts in which suppuration and abscess formation commence in the center. As the process spreads outward, the original similarity to a bland infarct is lost. Instead of a fibrinous pleurisy, there is a fibrinopurulent one.

Only earlier septic infarcts will be recognizable because of the peripheral tissue necrosis and central suppuration.

The emboli are small, coming as they do from brittle fragments released from veins or cerebral sinuses with purulent thrombophlebitis or from bacterial endocarditis on the right side of the heart. Consequently the infarcts are not massive.

Noninfected cavitation can occur as a rarity in pulmonary infarcts larger than 4 cm in diameter.[69]

Nonthrombotic embolism

Embolism by fat globules, air, etc. is discussed in Chapter 4.

Pulmonary arteriosclerosis

Pulmonary arteriosclerosis, no matter how advanced, is never so severe as that in the aorta. The plaques are smooth and only slightly raised. Heaped-up or ulcerated deposits rarely are seen, but secondary thrombosis does occur. The condition may be merely caused by old age, but it is also an accompaniment of pulmonary hypertension.

Primary (unexplained) pulmonary hypertension

Pulmonary arterial hypertension of unknown cause is an uncommon condition. After injection of radiopaque medium at hypertensive pressures into the pulmonary circulation of diseased and control lungs, it was decided that the essential lesion is obliterative cellular intimal thickening in the small, nonmuscular arteries and medial hypertrophy proximal to this.[71] Pulmonary vasoconstriction or thromboembolism may initiate the changes.

Most patients have been young women, although even children have been affected. The principal complaint is worsening exertional dyspnea. Syncopal attacks and chest pain are experienced by about half of the patients. Right ventricular hypertrophy is noticeable, and the pulmonary arteriogram resembles a pruned leafless shrub in autumn instead of the normal leafy bush of springtime.[74] Death comes in a few years from right-sided heart failure, sometimes quite suddenly or after cardiac catheterization or angiocardiography.

The vascular changes of primary and secondary pulmonary hypertension are similar. There are six stages[75a]:

1. Medial hypertrophy of small pulmonary arteries and arterioles (Fig. 26-14)
2. Added intimal and endothelial cell proliferation, often occluding the lumen
3. Progressive intimal fibrosis and massive medial muscular hyperplasia, often multilayered or longitudinal
4. Dilatation lesions[23]
   a. Dilatation causes thinning of some muscular arteries so that they resemble large veins.
   b. Dilated thin vessels surround a parent muscular artery in an angiomatous fashion (angiomatoid lesion) and then join alveolar capillaries (a revascularized thrombus?).
   c. A dilatation filled with narrow tortuous

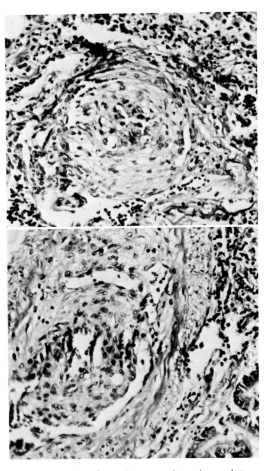

Fig. 26-15. Plexiform lesions. Complicated intertwining mass of tiny vessels with plump endothelial cells arises in relation to wall of larger pulmonary artery. (196×.)

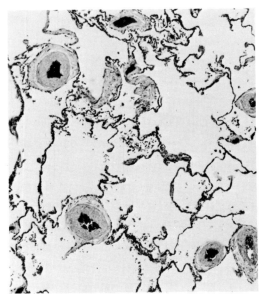

Fig. 26-14. Idiopathic pulmonary hypertension. Considerable muscular thickening of minor pulmonary arteries. (75×.)

vessels links its parent artery to thin wide vessels that join alveolar capillaries (plexiform lesion) (Fig. 26-15). Proximally, the parent small muscular pulmonary artery shows medial hypertrophy and intimal fibrosis. Then comes the dilated segment whose lumen is filled with the plexus of tortuous capillaries. Beyond this again, the blood enters the distal dilated artery. Plexiform lesions occur probably only in pulmonary hypertension from congenital heart disease with a shunt, in pulmonary schistosomiasis, and in primary pulmonary hypertension.[80]

5. Encrustation of the elastica with hemosiderin
6. Necrotizing arteritis (rare)

Secondary pulmonary hypertension

The following outline, based on Wood's simple approach,[82] lists the principal causes of secondary pulmonary hypertension. All of these must be excluded before the primary variety is diagnosed. There are four basic mechanisms, but, in general, the condition begins as pulmonary venous hypertension, which gives rise to vasoconstriction and induces pulmonary arterial hypertension.

1. Passive type—produced by diseases raising pulmonary venous pressure
   a. Mitral stenosis
   b. Chronic left ventricular failure (mostly in aortic stenosis, severe myocardial fibrosis, and essential hypertension)
   c. Myxoma of left atrium
   d. Ball valve thrombus, mitral orifice
   e. Totally anomalous pulmonary venous drainage
2. Reactive or hyperkinetic type—produced by congenital heart defects that cause increased blood flow through pulmonary vasculature
   a. Patent ductus arteriosus
   b. Atrial or ventricular septal defect
   c. Eisenmenger's complex
3. Vaso-occlusive type
   a. Obstructive
      (1) Multiple emboli or thrombosis
      (2) Sickle-cell disease
      (3) Miliary carcinomatosis
      (4) Polyarteritis nodosa
      (5) Amniotic fluid embolism
      (6) Schistosomiasis
      (7) Congenital pulmonary artery stenosis
   b. Vasoconstrictive—usually transient and related to hypoxia caused by alveolar hypoventilation; also high altitude
   c. Obliterative—caused by reduction of vascular bed by chronic parenchymal disease
      (1) Emphysema
      (2) Advanced fibrosis, all types
      (3) Pneumoconiosis
      (4) Granulomatosis

4. Kyphoscoliosis—chest deformity that leads to hypoventilation, pulmonary hypertension, and cor pulmonale with hypercapnea[75]

Vascular changes in secondary pulmonary hypertension are similar to those in the primary form, although muscular artery hyperplasia is not so advanced and plexiform dilatation lesions are seen only in certain types.

An intriguing, though unusual, cause of secondary pulmonary hypertension is that attributable to vasoconstriction secondary to airway obstruction by large tonsils and adenoids. All the 27 recorded cases have been in children. Two died, the rest were cured by surgical treatment, with complete disappearance of the hypertension.[73]

Wagenvoort has produced a schematic representation of the characteristic changes in five major groups of pulmonary vascular disease.[79]

Pulmonary artery thrombosis in the major arteries has been well authenticated.[77] It is fatal only when the cor pulmonale it produces becomes decompensated. Thrombosis of the smaller muscular branches alone is uncommon, seen mainly in pulmonary stenosis.[3] Ring and Bakke[76] have noted that:

1. 75% of the pulmonary-artery cross section may be occluded before systolic blood pressure falls.
2. 90% must be occluded before death occurs.
3. There is a reserve of readily distensible small vessels, and bronchial artery anastomosis will appear.
4. Much blood may still flow around the thrombus.

Rezek and Millard have discussed the difficulty of determining at autopsy whether an older thrombus originated from an earlier embolus or arose autochthonously.[2]

Most commonly pulmonary artery thrombosis is secondary to the impaction of multiple emboli. Microscopically, thrombi and emboli will be found in most of the small arteries and arterioles, in all stages from fresh to organizing and recanalizing thrombi.

Pulmonary veno-occlusive disease

The discussion above has emphasized arterial disease, but for the past 10 years there have been reports of children and young adults dying of progressive occlusion, by intimal thickening and fibrosis, of the smaller pulmonary veins and venules. Generally this is taken to be a consequence of thrombosis, of which the precipitating cause is unknown,[78] although

Wagenvoort suggests the possibility of a viral infection.[81]

ATELECTASIS AND COLLAPSE

It seems useful to maintain a distinction between the terms *atelectasis* and *collapse,* atelectasis meaning incomplete expansion of the newborn infant's lung and collapse meaning reduction in lung size due to loss of air.

Atelectasis

Atelectasis is a neonatal condition resulting from weak respiratory action. It tends to occur in premature infants and in infants with various forms of cerebral birth injury, central nervous system malformation, and intrauterine hypoxia. Total atelectasis is found in stillborn infants. In these infants, the lungs are dark blue and fleshy and devoid of crepitation. They are so small that they occupy only the posterocentral portions of the pleural cavities. No pleural lobular markings are visible. In microscopic slides, thick and vascular interalveolar septa and small alveolar spaces are seen. The spaces contain granular amniotic debris and nucleated squamous cells aspirated in utero under the stimulus of hypoxia (Fig. 26-16). Distended respiratory bronchioles also may be seen.

An infant who survives atelectasis for some hours must have some aerated lung. This will be mainly in the upper lobe, where scattered pinker areas are to be found. In these cases,

pneumothorax or interstitial emphysema is an indication of the infant's own violent efforts to breathe or of overstrenuous attempts at artificial respiration.

Frequently, it is not possible to say why an infant did not survive. To blame atelectasis is to beg the question of the cause of atelectasis in a healthy-looking child. One needs to examine the placenta and know the course of the pregnancy and labor.

Perinatal pneumonia and *intrauterine pneumonia* are grossly indistinguishable from atelectasis. There are three types[83]: (1) fetal, occurring near full term, (2) early perinatal, with death occurring on the first day, and (3) late perinatal, with death occuring in the first week but after the first day. The percentages of autopsies in which they were found were 10%, 25%, and 30%, respectively. The pneumonia sometimes is the result of inspiration of infected or irritant amniotic fluid. Neutrophils are found in the alveolar septa and the alveoli, which also contain recognizable amniotic fluid material. Often, the diagnosis is difficult to prove because, despite thickened septa, the inflammatory cells are scanty. Every effort must be made to obtain bacterial cultures. For further consideration of the significance of atelectasis and of the importance of pleural petechiae and of cultures, see the discussion by Rezek and Millard.[2] The presence of polymorphonuclear leukocytes is no proof of bacterial infection but may be a reaction to tissue degen-

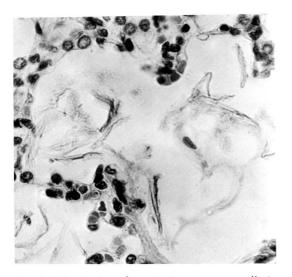

Fig. 26-16. Aspirated amniotic squamous cells in alveolus. One cell is nucleated. (564×.)

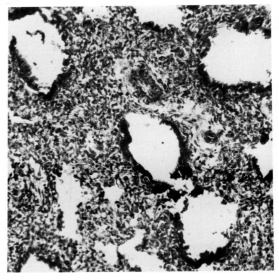

Fig. 26-17. Hyaline membrane disease. Homogeneous dark material lining air spaces is eosinophilic membrane. (152×.)

eration or, in the fetal lung, a reaction to hypoxia.[84]

Hyaline membrane disease. Hyaline membrane disease may be regarded as a special form of atelectasis or collapse occurring a few hours after birth and sometimes after apparently full expansion. The lungs become solid and airless, but there may be interstitial emphysema. Microscopically, interalveolar septa are apposed, but bronchioles are distended. Many of the terminal and respiratory bronchioles are internally coated with thick "hyaline membranes" of a homogeneous eosinophilic material (Fig. 26-17). The material has the staining characteristics of fibrin, a finding confirmed by the use of fluorescein-labeled fibrin antibody and by electron microscopy. The membranes take a little time to develop and are not found in infants who have never breathed.

Lauweryns[90] considers widespread distention of pulmonary lymphatics and impaired perfusion of small muscular pulmonary arteries and of pulmonary arterioles to be of pathogenetic importance. Membranes appear to form in situ after necrosis of the epithelial cells lining the affected bronchioles. Later, phagocytosis of the lining membrane and reformation of the epithelium are noted.

Those most susceptible to the disease are the premature infants (the greater the prematurity, the worse the disease) and full-term infants of mothers who have diabetes mellitus or who require cesarean section. Minutes or hours after birth, the infants progress to desperate anoxia, but if they survive the first 2 days, they seem to recover completely. Nevertheless there is reason to believe that what was considered to be *congenital pulmonary dysplasia* (Wilson-Mikity syndrome) is really residual oxygen damage in a premature infant treated and surviving. (Seventy infants were followed for 2 to 5 years after recovering from the disease; six had radiologic evidence suggestive of pulmonary fibrosis, confirmed by biopsy in two.[93])

The membranes are found in 20% to 40% of live-born infants dying in the first few days of life, or in up to 70% of infants dying in the early neonatal period in whom no other major abnormality is encountered. This amounts to 25,000 deaths annually in the United States. This should be reduced both by newer treatments such as continuous positive airway pressure and also by our ability to predict the occurrence of the disease while the child is still in utero, with the determination of the ratio of sphingomyelin to lecithin in the amniotic fluid. More recently it has been suggested that glucocorticoids be given to the mothers shortly before delivery since they stimulate lung maturation with respect to surfactant synthesis.[85,87] In correlation with this is the observation that adrenocortical size is reduced in these infants.[91]

The evidence is strong that these striking membranes do not cause the atelectasis and that atelectasis produces the membranes. Demonstration of the absence of the surface tension–lowering alveolar surface film does everything but explain its absence. The consequent inability of the infant to force open the alveoli (p. 1042) leads to congestive failure. Protein-containing fluid transudes from pulmonary capillaries into the alveoli. Under such circumstances, premature infants are forced to attempt respiration by means of the alveolar ducts, in which hyaline membranes then form (not in the alveoli).[82]

In recognition of the secondary role of the hyaline membrane, not present in every case, the alternative name of *respiratory distress syndrome* is employed, but this has also been confusingly applied to the adult shock-lung syndrome.

Commonly there are pressure ulcers on the true and false vocal cords.[92] These are considered to be caused by laryngeal dysfunction producing abnormal closure of the larynx.

There are *other causes of hyaline membrane* formation. It has been seen in children dying from kerosene poisoning and is common in adults with viral pneumonia, chemical pneumonitis, severe uremia, rheumatic involvement of the lung, severe pulmonary edema, bacterial pneumonia, and after irradiation. Of 156 adult patients at autopsy, seven had hyaline membranes. They also had a fibrinolytic defect.[88]

Massive pulmonary hemorrhage in newborn infants (p. 1049) has been confused with hyaline membrane disease. Another related disease is *chronic pulmonary insufficiency of prematurity.* This syndrome of delayed respiratory distress occurs in infants weighing less than 1250 gm at birth. It has a 10% to 20% mortality and seems to be caused by a lack of surfactant.[89]

Collapse

Two main types of collapse of the lung exist—compressive and obstructive, two important variants of the latter being acute massive collapse and middle lobe syndrome.

Compressive collapse. The mechanism in compressive collapse is external pressure, generally by pleural fluid and less often by air (pneumothorax), intrathoracic tumor (including a large heart), high diaphragm, or spinal deformity. The subpleural regions undergo greater collapse than do the central areas, and the lower lobes are affected most often. The effect tends to spread throughout the lung unless pleural fibrosis or adhesions help keep the lung expanded.

Collapsed lungs are dark red or blue, poorly crepitant, and smaller than normal, with slightly wrinkled pleura. For a long time, they remain capable of reexpansion, but, if this does not happen, low-grade inflammation will set in, to be followed by extensive fibrosis.

The microscopic view reflects the gross appearance. Alveolar septa are close together, and their vessels are prominent. The larger bronchi remain open. Later, the interlobular, perivascular, and peribronchial tissue increases, alveolar capillaries become increasingly bloodless, and arteriolar walls are thickened. Eventually, a condition resembling organizing pneumonia may be seen.

Obstructive (absorptive) collapse. The term *obstructive collapse* refers to the cutting off of air to a group of lobules or even a whole lobe by obstruction of many bronchioles or a large bronchus. Possible causes are pressure by enlarged lymph nodes, intrabronchial tumor, foreign body, or an especially viscid mucous secretion. The last results from acute bronchiolitis (especially in young children), suppression of the cough reflex (including neurologic diseases and anesthesia), severe bronchial asthma, cystic fibrosis of the pancreas, dehydration, and tracheotomy.

Obstructive collapse is less severe than the compressive variety because the absorbed air is largely replaced by edema fluid and bronchial secretion. The collapse is likely to be patchy, creating dark blue depressions in between apparently raised, normal pink areas over the lung surface (Fig. 26-18). If bronchial drainage is not restored, chronic or organizing pneumonia is likely, with areas of endogenous lipid pneumonia.

Acute massive collapse occurs occasionally in adults after surgery. Depressed cough reflex, immobile abdomen, and oversecretion of bronchial mucus combine to diminish the airway. Spencer[3] believes that the original injury is severe acute pulmonary edema, with severe secondary bronchospasm that attempts to overcome it. While air is slowly absorbed distal to blocked bronchi, oxygen and anesthetic gases disappear quickly, allowing prompt collapse.[95] The difference lies in the absence of nitrogen in anesthesia.

Middle lobe syndrome is a consequence of enlargement of the lymph nodes in the angle between the middle and lower lobar bronchi of the right lung. The middle bronchus is thereby kinked and obstructed, cutting off the air to the middle lobe and resulting in obstructive collapse. Just as in lobar emphysema of infants (p. 1060), exception has been taken to a purely mechanical explanation for middle lobe syndrome. In none of a series of nine patients was there obstruction of the lobar bronchus and its segmental bifurcation (as investigated by bronchoscopy or bronchography).[94]

EMPHYSEMA

Emphysema has passed beyond the simple concept of hyperinflation of alveoli called "diffuse vesicular emyphysema." Erroneous views were engendered by the examination of unfixed collapsed lungs. The inflation technique advocated by Laennec was ignored for over a century.

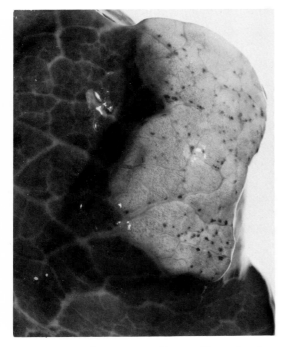

Fig. 26-18. Obstructive collapse. There is clear contrast between pale, still-aerated lung and dark depressed lung beside it. Normal pleural lymphatic network is easily seen.

Classification

Emphysema may mean something different to the pathologist, to the clinician, and to the radiologist. In the United States, it means an increase in size of air spaces distal to the terminal bronchioles, with destruction of their walls and minimal fibrosis. In Britain, the term is taken to include the combination of the effects of both chronic bronchitis (chronic productive cough and dyspnea) and emphysema and includes simple distention. Acceptance of these concepts permits four mechanisms of production of emphysema[1]:

1. *Atrophy* (emphysema of aging, coal miner's pneumoconiosis, bronchitis and bronchiolitis, and scar and paraseptal emphysema)
2. *Hypoplasia* during the postnatal phase of alveolar development (bronchitis and bronchiolitis of childhood and most cases of unilateral hyperlucent lung)
3. *Overinflation* (so-called compensatory emphysema, ball-valve obstruction, and infantile lobar emphysema)
4. *Destruction* (as when alveolar destruction is associated with chronic bronchitis or with scars)

A simple classification is as follows:
1. Localized
   a. Acute
   b. Chronic
   c. Paraseptal
   d. Lobar
   e. "Compensatory"
2. Generalized
   a. Centriacinar ("focal")
   b. Diffuse
      (1) Panacinar ("vesicular")
      (2) Acute obstructive
   c. Multiple focal
3. Aging lung ("senile")
4. Interstitial
5. "Bronchiolar"

More helpful to understanding is the classification shown in Fig. 26-19, in which the various mechanisms are displayed. Three concepts are vital to its understanding: (1) the alveoli are distended beyond the size normal in deep inspiration, (2) the unit involved in emphysema is the anatomic acinus (p. 1041), and (3) emphysema is either associated with airways obstruction (trapping) or it is not. When air is trapped, that lobe or lung will not deflate when removed from the body. Most clinically significant types of emphysema fall into the category of *irreversible airways obstruction*.

In this text, *emphysema is defined as* a condition of the lung characterized by permanent increase beyond normal in the size of the air spaces distal to the terminal bronchioles.

Localized emphysema
Acute localized emphysema

Acute localized emphysema is most often seen in association with bronchopneumonia or with bronchiolitis of children. Many lobules are affected by alternating areas of collapse and reversible overdistention *(hyperinflation)*.

Chronic localized emphysema

Chronic localized (irregular) emphysema is found in relation to chronic local inflammation and fibrosis, or to calcified foci, especially around apical scars. Frequently, the large empty spaces render the scar insignificant. Microscopically, in a central fibrous area, cuboid cells line residual terminal bronchioles and alveoli. Opening off these are fibrous, stretched-out septa that are poorly vascular, contain some dust, and enclose irregular giant air spaces.

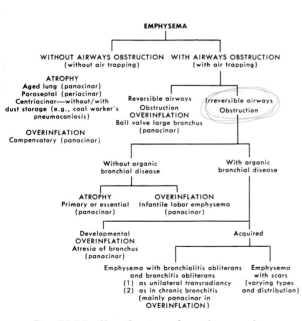

Fig. 26-19. Classification of emphysema by morphology and pathogenesis (see text). (Modified from Reid, L.: The pathology of emphysema, London, 1967, Lloyd-Luke [Medical Books] Ltd.)

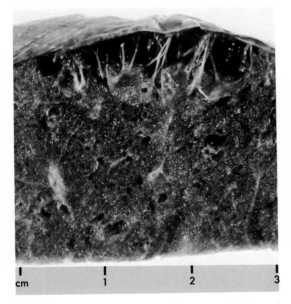

Fig. 26-20. Paraseptal emphysema. Subpleural distended air spaces are traversed by fibrotic strands of vessels, bronchioles, and septa.

Paraseptal emphysema

Paraseptal emphysema has a distribution all of its own, whether subpleural (Fig. 26-20) or within the lung. In the first instance, it is along the sharp edges of the lung or on the mediastinal or diaphragmatic surfaces. When internal, it is found against connective tissue septa, against larger vessels or bronchi (Fig. 26-21), or even within the angle of bronchial divisions. There is a beadlike row of uniform holes, each gently bending outward the apposed pleura. At first measured in millimeters, some eventually progress to be measured in centimeters. They are bounded by the subpleural connective tissue septa that eventually tear and allow confluence so that bullous emphysema is born (Figs. 26-22 and 26-26). The cavities of the internal variety do not attain great size.

Atrophy appears to be the cause of paraseptal emphysema. Remember two important facts: (1) it has nothing to do with centriacinar or panacinar emphysema (which could be present by coincidence), and (2) it rarely causes impaired respiratory function, unless a bulla ruptures (pneumothorax) or is big enough to compress neighboring lung.

Lobar emphysema of infants

In lobar emphysema of infants an upper or middle lobe of the lung is blown up with

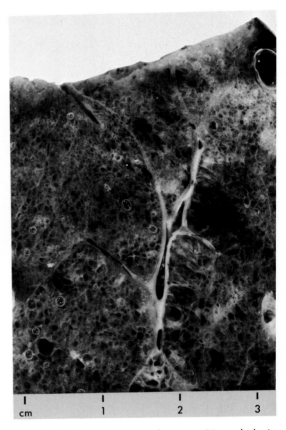

Fig. 26-21. Paraseptal emphysema. Distended air spaces are to right of vertically running blood vessel. Grade I panacinar emphysema also is present.

air so suddenly and severely that surrounding lung is collapsed and a serious mediastinal shift ensues. The diaphragm on that side is forced down. Without surgery the child may die quickly. Surgery also prevents permanent damage.

There are several causes: (1) partial intrabronchial obstruction by a congenital web, foreign body, or infection, (2) extrabronchial compression by an abnormally large or anomalous vessel, and (3) absence or hypoplasia of bronchial cartilages, permitting collapse of the walls during expiration. Nevertheless, most of the cases have no organic block and the obstruction is functional, probably within the alveoli.[1] The concept of an anomaly of cartilage has erroneously been seized upon because the variability of the state of development and maturity of bronchial cartilage in early life is not widely known, and neither is the fallacy of the random sectioning of a bronchus (p. 1038).

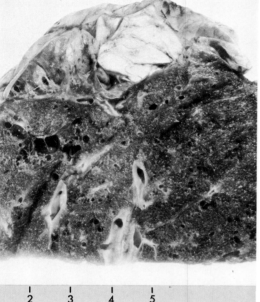

Fig. 26-22. Paraseptal emphysema in more advanced state than that shown in Fig. 26-21 displaying how condition can develop into bullous emphysema.

The disease is not to be confused with tension cyst (p. 1072).

The affected lobe is tense and hugely swollen. The alveoli give the cut surface a honeycomb pattern, and microscopically they have the look of large, unruptured, adult-sized air sacs.

Compensatory emphysema

Compensatory emphysema is a misleading term used for the expansion of remaining normal lung that occurs after another portion has been removed, or damaged by fibrosis or collapse. The lung is airy, and its alveoli are distended until they may give way, but there is no increase in functional activity—rather a decrease. The compensation is to fill the extra space that has been created.

Unilateral hyperlucent lung. A discussion of localized emphysema appears to be the appropriate place to mention unilateral hyperlucent lung. Named also the Swyer-James or the MacLeod syndrome, it refers to a lung with unilateral radiologic transradiancy, without collapse, with little ventilation, and with little pulmonary artery blood flowing through it. The lung is smaller than normal but airy. There is distortion or obliteration of many bronchi or bronchioles, hypoplasia of the pulmonary arteries, and emphysema.[111] The condition is the result of infective damage to the airways in childhood, with the small lung and its small arteries being secondary to this. Three children have been observed to begin with radiologically normal pulmonary vasculature and then develop secondary hypoplasia (retarded development) of alveoli and vessels after severe pneumonia.[111] Abnormally large alveoli in a small or normal-sized lung is a sign of pulmonary hypoplasia, since a lower than normal number of alveoli have to expand to fill the thorax.

Generalized emphysema

The discussion of generalized emphysema considers those varieties commonly implied by the word "emphysema."

Etiology. Theories that emphysema is related to primary vascular disease or destruction of alveolar elastic tissue have been abandoned. Suspicions of the danger of blowing wind instruments have been replaced by those of the dangers of coughing cigarette smoke. Emphysema is considered by McLean[106] to be the consequence of prolonged inflammation and obstruction of the respiratory bronchioles. Permanent damage leads to bronchiolar obliteration. Despite collateral ventilation via the pores of Kohn, the incomplete interlobular septa and the bronchioloalveolar anastomoses, air trapping is claimed to result. This may distend and even disrupt air passages distal to the obstructed bronchioles. If the pressure of the trapped air is high, as with coughing, so much the worse. Unfortunately, these inflammatory or obstructive bronchiolar lesions may not be seen, although it is inferred that the bronchioles have been destroyed from evidence of their numerical reduction.[106]

The view of Leopold and Gough[105] is that chronic inflammation damages the walls of the most distal respiratory bronchioles, which dilate more and more (centriacinar emphysema). Affected third-order respiratory bronchioles fuse into a dilatation (the "common pool") at the level of the second-order bronchiole. The process may come to involve the interalveolar septa also (panacinar emphysema) if there is inflammatory damage to alveolar ducts and the air sacs distal to these.

According to Spain and Kaufman,[115] the essence of emphysema is chronic inflammation in and around the terminal bronchioles. These become thickened, rigid, and narrowed, causing trapping of air in expiration, with distention of alveoli.

These three leading theories share a belief in the role of chronic bronchiolitis. It is a mistake to assume that there is only *one* cause of emphysema. Coal dust alone has been considered to cause centriacinar emphysema in miners.[101] The assumption that black particles in the lungs are necessarily carbon is false. Clinical and fine structural studies have demonstrated a mixture of inorganic silicates and aluminates, some trace metals, elemental carbon, and a highly soluble, probably organic pigment not yet identified.[108] Ferritin also is often present in patients with congestive heart failure.

What we are considering is not just coal dust (itself not pure carbon), not just tobacco derivatives, not just pollutants of our air. What we have done is to equate blackness with badness. We have assumed that the blackness of coal workers' lungs is to be equated with functional impairment. In fact, dust and centriacinar emphysema may co-exist and, equally, may exist independently (p. 1092). Gough[10] seems to add confusion by confining the term "focal dust emphysema" to the centriacinar emphysema of coal and other industrial workers and by regarding the morphologically similar condition of nonindustrial workers as having an inflammatory origin. More recently, he has reported on the findings in autopsies on 247 miners who had suffered from coal worker's pneumoconiosis.[112] This painstaking study, using a matching series of nonminers, showed that there was much more emphysema among miners and that it was of the focal dust type. Only a minority had what Gough would recognize as centriacinar or panacinar emphysema, and it was seen in areas with little or no dust.

The reader is referred also to the work of Reid,[109] who believes that the disease commences with inflammatory destruction of the walls in the junctional region between the terminal and respiratory bronchioles, and to a review by Thurlbeck.[116]

No basic discovery has been made as to the cause of disabling emphysema. We do not even know why air is trapped, but this is the key factor in causing functional impairment. The terminal bronchioles in the autopsy specimen are perfectly patent. Obstruction is created by premature collapse of these airways during expiration, because of loss of the normal elastic pull of surrounding alveoli.

Clinicians experience extraordinary difficulty in distinguishing chronic bronchitis from emphysema. The pathologist can describe the type of disease present but is too late to help the clinician. Consequently, the clinical literature concerning chronic bronchitis and emphysema cannot be otherwise than confusing. Emphysema is discussed and its manifestations described without authors' defining what emphysema means to them. This comment applies to some of the latest texts available in 1975. Refreshing frankness about the inaccuracy of the radiologist's opinion regarding the diagnosis of emphysema is disclosed by Felson who retails his frequent false-positive and false-negative reports and his inability to distinguish centriacinar from panacinar forms.[98] In fact, centriacinar emphysema cannot be seen in chest x-ray films unless it is in the rare "four plus" variety (see p. 1065). Many clinicians are unaware of the fallibility of the radiologic diagnosis of emphysema and are surprised when the eventual postmortem examination shows cor pulmonale and insignificant emphysema (i.e., chronic bronchitis was present).

Pathologists will be responsible for perpetuating misunderstanding if they do not perfuse lungs in potential emphysema cases, or if they simply report "emphysema" without stating the type and without quantitating it by degree of severity and percentage of cut lung surface involved. Until all concerned recognize the blandness of most cases of centriacinar emphysema as opposed to the seriousness of the higher grades of panacinar emphysema, statistics of clinical manifestations and survival will inevitably be false.

Finally, we must have sympathy with the clinical problems, which have led to introduction of terms such as "chronic obstructive pulmonary disease" and "obstructive airway disease." They do allow for the common coincidence of bronchitis and emphysema and for the difficulty in deciding which predominates.

A type of emphysema that has a specific causal relationship to an abnormality of a protein normally present in serum is that associated with alpha$_1$-antitrypsin (α_1-AT) deficiency. This is the predominantly lower lobe panacinar variety listed as "primary or essential" in Fig. 26-18. α_1-AT is a protease inhibitor (Pi) with a normal range of 180 to 280 mg per 100 ml.

In its absence or deficiency, leukocyte proteases may cause damage to the lung. It is the major component of serum alpha$_1$-globulin, and its production by the liver is governed by a single autosomal Pi locus, with multiple codominant alleles and over 20 phenotypes demonstrable by electrophoresis. The important homozygous phenotype producing very low levels of α_1-AT is Pi ZZ (see also pp. 1326, 1361, 1376, and 1391), estimated to occur in from 0.07% to 0.2% of the hospital population of the United States and Norway.[103,119] Such persons are vulnerable to the development of early childhood cirrhosis (because of accumulated α_1-AT in hepatocytes) and to dependent panacinar emphysema of early onset (third or fourth decade) with a higher proportion of women than is found in other types of emphysema.

Patients with Pi ZZ phenotype have only 10% of normal levels of alpha$_1$-globulin and hence can be detected by serum protein electrophoresis. It may be that as many as 88% of them will develop emphysema. The normal person is Pi MM, whereas 6% to 16% of the population are heterozygous Pi MZ with intermediate (40% to 80% of normal) serum levels of α_1-AT.

Familial cases have been uncovered (as many as 15 members in one family).[117] Some members of a family are Pi ZZ, others are Pi MM or Pi MZ. The risks of being Pi MZ are still being investigated, but Kueppers and Dönhardt are convinced that such persons are unusually prone to panacinar emphysema, but not necessarily at so early an age as the Pi ZZ population.[104]

The inhibitor acts against trypsin, thrombin, plasmin, and kallikrein as well as against elastase and collagenase from leukocytes. Leukocyte enzymes produce lysis of exudate in the distal respiratory tract and α_1-AT prevents their activity from going too far; unchecked they will destroy pulmonary tissue. The greater vascular perfusion at the bases of the pulmonary lobes allows more aging leukocytes to be sequestered there and discharge their enzymes.[100]

As to the origin of the deficiency, it lies in production of defective inhibitor by the liver, because of a lack of sialyl transferase, resulting

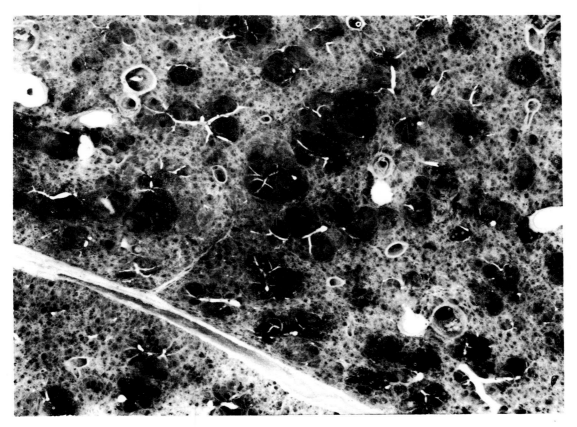

Fig. 26-23. Centriacinar emphysema. Lung fixed with formalin under pressure. Pulmonary arteries have been injected with barium-gelatin mixture. Dark spaces are centriacinar areas of atrophy. Around these, alveoli of normal size have been preserved. (3×; from Heard, B. E.: Thorax **13:**136-149, 1958.)

in accumulation of the faulty product in the liver, from which its release is diminished.[118]

Incidence. In the last decade study of the frequency of emphysema in the United States has revealed many more cases than were previously reported. In Great Britain, emphysema causes twice as many deaths in men as does carcinoma of the lung and is responsible for nine tenths of all cor pulmonale, which, in turn, accounts for 5% to 10% of all cases of cardiac disease.[97] In series of random autopsies, at least half of the patients have been found to have emphysema, not necessarily severe or symptomatic during life.

Centriacinar emphysema

Centriacinar emphysema refers to emphysema confined to the central portion of the acinus, its distribution being segmental, lobar, or generalized.

Lungs fixed by formalin perfusion. Simply by perfusing the bronchial tree for 3 days with formalin under gravitational pressure, one can recognize the condition of the cut surfaces. This allows one to see earlier phases, to grade severity of emphysema, and to recognize two important centriacinar types (atrophic and destructive[1]). In atrophy, the central hole in the acinus is composed of a group of widened air spaces crossed by tenuous strands of tissue (Fig. 26-23). Microscopically, the peripheral architecture is more or less preserved, although alveolar walls are flimsy. In the rarer destructive type, there is a completely empty central hole of 1 cm diameter or more. Its wall appears smooth and is composed of interrupted alveolar walls that have retracted and flattened. No evidence is available that atrophy progresses to destruction, and they are not usually found together. Even widespread and well-developed atrophic centriacinar emphysema gives no symptoms because great numbers of peripheral and perfect alveoli are available and because there is no air trapping. Nor is the condition a usual sequel of chronic bronchitis.

When centriacinar emphysema is so advanced that the periphery of the acinus is destroyed, the condition will be indistinguishable from panacinar emphysema of similar severity, and the degree of respiratory impairment will depend on the volume of lung destroyed. A few persisting normal alveoli at the periphery indicate centriacinar emphysema (Fig. 26-24).

One gets a better impression of emphysema from looking at the whole lung, perhaps with a hand lens, than from microscopic slides.

The detailed work of Snider et al.[114] and Reid,[1] has developed the concept of centriacinar emphysema as usually symptomless and as separate from deposits of dust. Therefore, when a mild to moderate degree of the condition is found at autopsy in a patient who had respiratory disability, chronic bronchitis is likely to have been responsible for these symptoms.

In London, centriacinar emphysema is found in one of five fluid-fixed lungs of persons with normal chest x-ray films and no clinical lung disease. We do not know if it contributes to disability when obstructive lung disease also is present. It is not a constant factor in disabled coal miners.

The lesions can expand or become confluent. They are more advanced in the upper lobes, particularly the upper parts of the lobes. Microscopically, pigment is concentrated along the course of the dilated bronchioles.[120] Their walls appear to have undergone fibrous thickening. An intramural and perimural infiltrate of lymphocytes is present. Damaged interalveolar septa are thinned and fractured.

Panacinar ("vesicular") emphysema

Panacinar emphysema is that form of the disease that comes to the average physician's mind when "emphysema" is mentioned. The disease is nearly as common as the centriacinar form. Mixed forms also occur.

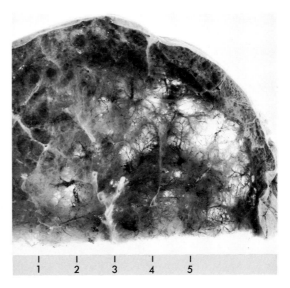

Fig. 26-24. Centriacinar emphysema—severe. Residues of normal lung tissue at periphery of acini situated beneath pleura are clue to naming this particular case centriacinar rather than severe panacinar.

"Panacinar" means that all alveoli of the acinus are uniformly distended. Localized forms occur in compensatory overinflation, in ball-valve obstruction of a large bronchus, in infantile lobar emphysema, and in unilateral hyperlucent lung. Involvement of most of both lungs will be seen in the aging lung, in association with chronic bronchitis or as idiopathic disease. Whereas centriacinar emphysema favors the upper two thirds of the lungs and is much commoner in men, the panacinar emphysema of the aging and idiopathic types involves all of the lungs and has an equal sex incidence. Panacinar emphysema occurring in alpha$_1$-antitrypsin deficiency is distinctive in that it preferentially damages the lower lobes.

Panacinar emphysema of lowest grade is seen in the perfused lung as innumerable 1 mm holes that are individual enlarged alveoli (Fig. 26-25). When of medium severity, the holes are several millimeters in size, and retraction of the damaged alveoli causes the vessels, bronchi, and septa to stand up. The most severe panacinar emphysema has confluent large holes occupying all of the acinus. It is to such advanced disease that the following description applies.

The patients have a barrel-shaped chest of increased anteroposterior diameter, with widened, nearly horizontal, intercostal spaces. There is moderate kyphosis, and the costal

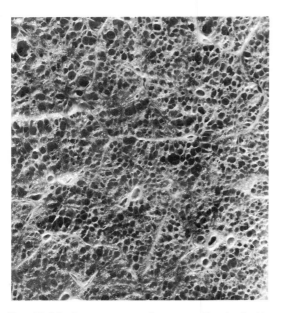

Fig. 26-25. Panacinar emphysema—Grade II. No part of acinus is spared.

cartilages may be calcified. Most of the patients are men 40 to 60 years of age.

The lungs are so full of air that they depress the diaphragm and hide the heart. The pleura is dry and smooth and the surface corrugated by indentations of the ribs, alternating with expansions representing the intercostal spaces. Pigment deposits tend to follow the rib markings. Finger pressure creates permanent depressions. Dryness is the outstanding feature of the airy, spongy, cut surface, which discloses innumerable empty spaces 1 to 2 mm in diameter. Normal alveoli in middle age are about 120 to 140 μm in diameter and thus cannot be appreciated by the unaided eye.

Formalin-perfused preparations reveal that alveoli are replaced by larger thick-walled empty spaces. These represent fused alveoli crossed by strands of obliterated vessels. Acini may communicate with one another, causing formation of bullae. The most advanced lesions are in the basal segments of the lower lobes and the lower part of the lingula and middle lobe.

In microscopic sections, alveoli appear enlarged or, their walls having ruptured, are fused into spaces of irregular size and shape into which the broken ends of the original septa project as spurs. All the septa are very thin, and their vessels are barely evident. An occasional dilated respiratory bronchiole may be recognized.

The great reduction of the number of alveolar capillaries is followed by muscular hypertrophy and hyperplasia of their parent vessels, which may have little lumen left. There is great expansion of the venous collateral circulation, whereby desaturated blood may be shunted from the systemic into the pulmonary veins when the right side of the heart fails. This will aggravate the anoxia and hypercapnia. In contrast, the bronchial arteries take on additional function. They enlarge and anastomose into the pulmonary arteriolar system. This is a demonstration of the uneven perfusion in such cases. Function is further impaired, in both bronchitis and emphysema, by greatly uneven ventilation brought about by the irregular distribution of airway obstruction. Consequently, one fourth of the lung spaces receive about nine tenths of the ventilation. Despite this inequality, the wasteful perfusion of these poorly ventilated areas is not proportionately reduced, so that blood gas disturbances ensue.[102]

Radiologic correlation. Even large air spaces in centriacinar emphysema do not produce radiologic changes of widespread emphysema. Such changes are produced only by the more severe grades of panacinar emphysema.[1] Hence, if clinical aspects are taken into consideration, a normal x-ray film will almost exclude gross widespread panacinar emphysema with air trapping.[113] Shadows seen in chest x-ray films of persons with heavy dust deposits are attributable to the dust alone, not to any disease caused by the deposits.

Clinical correlation. If one takes a group of adults suffering from dyspnea of pulmonary origin, there will be an association with idiopathic emphysema in 10% and with chronic bronchitis in the rest. Only 50% of patients with bronchitis who are short of breath have significant emphysema, 20% have normal lungs, 20% have panacinar emphysema of a degree expected at their age, and 10% have centriacinar emphysema (Reid[105]).

Idiopathic (primary) emphysema. Idiopathic emphysema is a form of panacinar emphysema that is not too common. When widespread it can be fatal. It occurs equally in both sexes. Bullae are common, and there is considerable air trapping. The emphysema is of a severe degree. Nothing is known of the cause except that the basic change is atrophy of the alveolar wall and capillary bed and that 10% to 20% of cases are associated with alpha$_1$-antitrypsin deficiency.

Emphysema with chronic bronchitis. Two circumstances have to be considered: (1) emphysema caused by chronic bronchitis, when infection damages and scars small airways and alveoli, and (2) emphysema associated with, but not caused by, chronic bronchitis, a circumstance in which the bronchitis is much more serious and the emphysema benign.

Chronic bronchitis causes destruction, overinflation, and atrophy, processes extending from bronchioli to alveoli. The emphysema is panacinar.

Bullous emphysema and blebs. Whereas bullae have been described as possible components of advanced panacinar emphysema, occasionally extremely large blebs are found (often in younger adults) in the absence of a history of chronic lung disease or emphysema. Blebs are the result of rupture of alveoli directly into the subpleural interstitial tissue plane. Such blebs cannot be demarcated laterally by interlobular septa and may compress much of a lobe. They are a common cause of spontaneous pneumothorax. A bulla is a manifestation of emphysema, whereby progressive dilatation and destruction of alve-

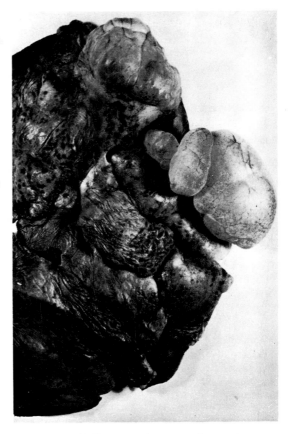

Fig. 26-26. Bullous emphysema of anterior margin of lung.

olar walls form a large subpleural air space, contained laterally by lobular septa. At the apices, along the anterior margin, and along free edges of the bases, distended alveoli often expand into bullae several centimeters in diameter (Fig. 26-26). Such large air cysts have smooth, tissue paper–thin walls, which are reticulated if there are clinging remnants of alveolar and tissue septa. The space may be crossed by strands of tissue, vessels, or bronchi. Bullae are found at the sites mentioned because here lobular septa are complete, and collateral air flow is therefore inadequate to dissipate the high pressure.

During life, a bulla cannot project from the lung as it so dramatically does in the pathologist's specimen. The thoracic cage is unyielding, and a bulla has to bulge into the lung. If large, it will compress a considerable volume of normal lung.

Various types of bullae occur.[1] Among them should be included "tension pneumatocele" or "vanishing lung" (p. 1072).

Complications of severe generalized emphysema

1. Right-sided heart failure (cor pulmonale)
2. Respiratory acidosis, causing fatal coma (from carbon dioxide retention, which depresses respiration; in addition, infection, sedatives, narcotics, and administration of pure oxygen cause further depression)
3. Acute and chronic peptic ulceration (found in up to 20% of emphysematous patients at autopsy)
4. Simulation of brain tumor in a small proportion of severe cases (hypercapnia appears to cause cerebral vasodilatation, which increases cerebrospinal fluid pressure[96])
5. Pneumothorax

Cor pulmonale is defined as right ventricular hypertrophy secondary to pulmonary disease (the term has been misused in many variants). The index of hypertrophy is a right ventricular thickness greater than 4 mm, a measurement reliable only when that ventricle is not dilated. Only by weighing the right ventricle can hypertrophy accurately be determined. Using Fulton's method, by which a weight of 80 gm is abnormal,[99] Millard showed that electrocardiography is not a reliable guide to the presence of right ventricular hypertrophy and that it is almost useless for quantitating the degree of hypertrophy.[107]

Diffuse acute obstructive emphysema

In diffuse acute obstructive emphysema, widespread obstruction is the result of severe acute bronchiolitis, asthma, pertussis, anaphylaxis, war gases, or suffocation. The condition is an acute overdistention. The lungs are so full of air that they cover the heart, yet they can be readily compressed manually. Such force probably overcomes many points of bronchial obstruction as a result of thick mucus, pus, or aspirated material.

Microscopic examination confirms that this is not a true emphysema, since the air spaces are overinflated without destructive changes.

Multiple focal emphysema

Multiple focal emphysema is seen in honeycomb lung and pneumoconiosis, in which interstitial fibrosis pulls on the surviving lung tissue, causing what has been called *paracicatricial emphysema* or, in pneumoconiosis, *focal dust emphysema*.[10]

Aging lung (so-called senile emphysema)

It used to be thought that "senile emphysema" was a lung disorder secondary to the development of a barrel chest. In fact, it is an aging atrophy of alveolar walls, unassociated with air trapping. In my experience it is the commonest type of emphysema to be seen, and it commences at about the age of 40 years. It is always a low-grade panacinar emphysema, inexplicably never known to progress to become clinically significant. The whole of each lung is affected.

The lungs are airy, fluffy, and small, for they lose air when the thorax is opened. Microscopically, although the alveoli are enlarged and their walls thin with reduced numbers of capillaries, the most telling changes are the reduction in number of alveoli and their simpler outline, as a result of the loss of some of the angles in their walls.

Interstitial emphysema

When air escapes into the connective tissue framework of the lung, it travels in the form of silvery bubbles 1 to 2 mm in diameter.

The bubbles will first be noted beneath the pleura, especially where it fuses with interlobular septa. They travel along perivascular sheaths to the hilum. From here, air can spread into the mediastinum, neck, and trunk.

The largest bubbles are at the hilum and may have compressed pulmonary vessels. Sometimes the pressure will tear a small vein, leading to air embolism. Rupture of a pleural bleb sets up a pneumothorax.

The condition is seen in newborn infants as a result of too powerful artificial respiration or positive pressure oxygenation. Other infants produce it themselves in a desperate effort to overcome bronchial obstruction by mucus or meconium or because of pneumonia, aspiration, atelectasis, intrapulmonary hemorrhage, or hyaline membrane disease.

In older patients, the cause is acute generalized emphysema, brought about by the raised intra-alveolar pressure of coughing in pertussis, penetrating trauma and rib fracture, air embolism, blast injury, intratracheal anesthesia, straining against a closed glottis, or introduction of the point of a needle through the chest wall into the lung.

Microscopically, there are distended alveoli (particularly noticeable in newborn infants), and alveoli may communicate with a pleural bleb. Clear spaces running outside the bronchi and blood vessels and in connective tissue septa are evidences of the passage of air. This is not true emphysema, for alveoli are not damaged.

"Bronchiolar" emphysema

"Bronchiolar" emphysema is a misconceived concept, named here to dispel the notion that it might have anything to do with emphysema. It is a form of honeycomb lung (p. 1099).

VIRAL AND RICKETTSIAL DISEASES

See Chapter 12.

FUNGAL DISEASES

See Chapter 13.

PROTOZOAL AND HELMINTHIC DISEASES

The effects of protozoal and helminthic diseases on the lung are discussed in Chapter 14. For *Pneumocystis carinii* pneumonia, see p. 1077.

PNEUMONIA
Bacterial pneumonia

Anthrax, pertussis, plague, glanders, melioidosis, *Klebsiella-Enterobacter* infection, and tularemia are discussed in Chapter 9. Leprosy is considered in Chapter 10, and spirochetal diseases in Chapter 11.

Lobar pneumonia

Pneumococcal pneumonia, the classic lobar variety, has become a rarity. Now it is seen mainly in persons who lie ill and unattended at home, those in whom chest injuries cause pulmonary congestion and edema, and those who recently have undergone general anesthesia or in alcoholics exposed to cold.

The route of infection is the bronchial tree. When the cocci reach the alveoli, there is a hyperemic response, with migration of macrophages and leukocytes to the area. The organisms multiply in the protein-containing fluid of the inflammatory reaction.

Phases. Untreated pneumococcal pneumonia follows a series of phases. The onset is in the hilar region, usually in a lower lobe, sometimes bilaterally. A whole lobe is not necessarily affected.

Initial phase. The initial phase (1 to 2 days) is one of acute congestion and edema, unlikely to be met with alone but commonly found as the advancing edge of a central consolidation. The region is gray-red, and frothy bloody fluid can be squeezed from it. Pneumococci are present in large numbers in smears made from the cut surface. Tiny fibrin plugs adhere to a knife edge scraped over the cut surface.

Microscopically, prominent alveolar capillaries can be seen. Nuclei of septal cells are prominent (Fig. 26-27), and neutrophils are migrating into the alveoli (Fig. 26-28, *A*). These are filled with eosinophilic fluid, and Gram stains will divulge the many cocci.

Early consolidation (red hepatization). In the phase of early consolidation (2 to 4 days), the oldest (central) area becomes voluminous and consolidated. Cellular exudation replaces edema. The cut surface is dry, very friable, dull red or pink, and granular (as a result of fibrin in the individual alveoli, the cut walls of which retract below the exudate). If the pleura has been reached, it has an easily removed coat of fibrin.

The main microscopic feature is replacement of alveolar fluid by densely packed neutrophils, thin strands of fibrin, and a few erythrocytes. Because engorgement is diminishing, alveolar septa are less prominent than in the first stage. (See Fig. 26-28, *B*.)

Late consolidation (gray hepatization). In the late consolidation phase (4 to 8 days), one lung may weigh 1500 gm. The cut surface is

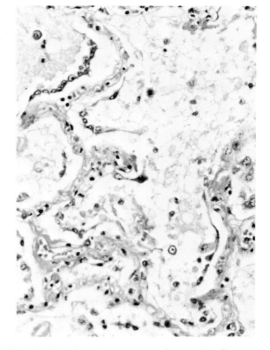

Fig. 26-27. Alveolar type I and type II cells stimulated in case of viral pneumonia. Only in such types of irritation are these cells seen clearly under light microscope. Elongated cytoplasm of type I cell readily apparent, whereas type II is cuboid. (215×.)

dry, granular, and gray (Fig. 26-29). The area is quite airless, with the consistency of liver, and slices of it retain straight, sharp edges. The lobe may have the marks of ribs and intercostal spaces. Fibrinous pleurisy is easily seen, and the bronchial mucosa is red.

During this stage, the fluid portion of the exudate has been removed, and a large amount of fibrin has been left behind. There are no organisms. Neutrophils in the exudate are reduced in number, and many are disintegrating, as their pyknotic nuclei indicate. Exudate is often separated from the septa by a thin clear space. (See Fig. 26-28, *C.*)

Resolution. In the resolution stage (8 days), exudate is liquefied by enzymatic action, and blood circulation becomes very active. The

tissue is friable. Some areas, generally the older central ones, are already softened. Resolution may start in such regions while consolidation is still spreading at the periphery. The cut surface is mottled and is gray, red, or dirty brown. It is smooth and moist. A large amount of frothy, yellow, creamy fluid can be squeezed out. (See Fig. 26-28, *D.*)

Microscopically, one sees large numbers of macrophages, some coming out of the septal walls into the shrunken fibrin masses and engulfing neutrophils and debris. Alveolar capillaries are congested.

Resolution and reaeration of the lung require 1 to 3 weeks. Antibiotic therapy induces resolution on about the third day.

Complications. The principal complications

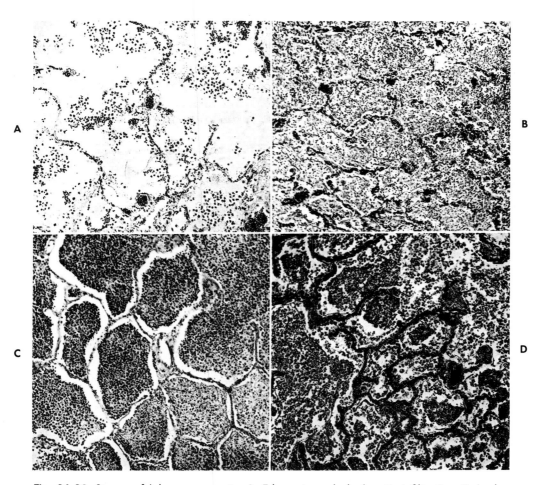

Fig. 26-28. Stages of lobar pneumonia. **A,** Edema in early leukocytic infiltration. **B,** Leukocytic stage. Engorgement persists. Fibrin is scanty. **C,** Late fibrinous stage. Beginning of contraction of alveolar exudate. Alveolar walls ischemic. **D,** Resolution. Macrophages predominate. Masses of fibrin free in alveolar spaces and alveolar capillaries engorged.

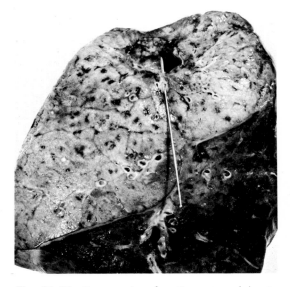

Fig. 26-29. Pneumonia of entire upper lobe in stage of gray hepatization. Disease stops sharply at interlobar septum and is in contrast with congested lower lobe. Abscess cavity has formed near apex and can be seen to drain into bronchus. (From Rezek, P. R., and Millard, M.: Autopsy pathology, Springfield, Ill., 1963, Charles C Thomas, Publisher.)

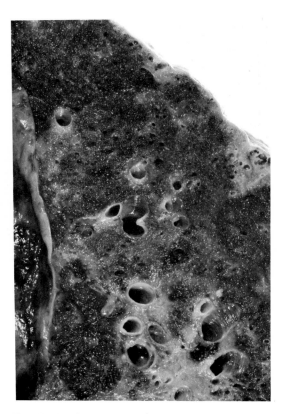

Fig. 26-30. Late stage of organizing pneumonia. Paler, solid areas are fibrous.

of pneumococcal pneumonia are as follows:

1. Organization of exudate (see following discussion)
2. Pleural effusion—5% of treated cases
3. Empyema—less than 1% of treated cases; pus is thick and green with clumps of fibrin; can either be free or be encysted in the pleural cavity or in an interlobar fissure; organization of such empyema creates a thick fibrous pleural casing in which fluid locules may be buried
4. Lung abscess—very rare complication that may actually indicate secondary infection by another organism
5. Mediastinitis
6. Cardiac complications—purulent pericarditis, acute bacterial endocarditis, and myocarditis
7. Meningitis
8. Acute otitis media and mastoiditis
9. Purulent arthritis—mainly in infants
10. Paralytic ileus

Organizing (nonresolving) pneumonia. Although resolution appears to depend on fibrinolysins, we do not know the full mechanism and cannot explain the few occasions when it does not work. The lobe is at first fleshy (carnification) and light brown–pink. Pleural

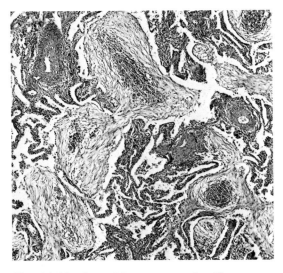

Fig. 26-31. Organizing pneumonia. Young connective tissue fills and distends alveoli and travels from one alveolus to another through pore of Kohn. (54×.)

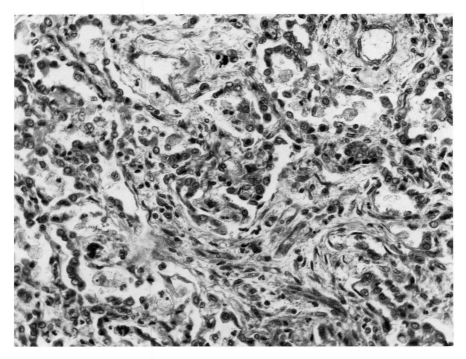

Fig. 26-32. Late stage of organizing pneumonia. Alveoli are contracted and lined by cuboid cells. (246×.)

adhesions form, and later the affected area becomes tough, airless, leathery, and gray (Fig. 26-30). At the margins, there may be focal emphysema. Bronchiectasis may follow. Seen microscopically, the fibrinous exudate undergoes organization. Interalveolar septa are preserved, but fibroblasts can easily be seen growing through the pores of Kohn, linking one solidified alveolus with its neighbor (Fig. 26-31). The fibrous tissue matures into poorly cellular scar tissue, and cuboid metaplasia coats the alveoli (Fig. 26-32).

Organizing pneumonia also is seen in the neighborhood of chronic suppuration, distal to bronchial obstruction or bronchiectasis, around a carcinoma, and in relation to granulomatous disease. There is an impression that organizing pneumonia has increased since the use of antibiotics. Possibly the drugs cut down the inflammatory response, thereby reducing the quantity of fibrinolysin.

Pneumococcus type III pneumonia

Pneumococci of type III have an abundant capsular mucopolysaccharide that imparts a slimy quality to the exudate and thus to the cut surface of the lung. Pneumococcal pneumonia with abscess formation is most likely to be caused by this organism.

Klebsiella pneumonia

Pneumonia caused by *Klebsiella pneumoniae* (Friedländer's bacillus) is particularly destructive. Older men, particularly alcoholics or those with diabetes or severe oral sepsis, most often are afflicted. Its preference for the posterior segment of the right upper lobe indicates an inhalational type of infection.[3] *Klebsiella pneumoniae* is a large gram-negative organism with plentiful capsular material recognized in the sticky mucoid exudate.

Infected lobules create red-gray consolidated nodules that, in confluence, become lobar. The infection is destructive, terminating by forming extensive abscesses, a point of distinction from pneumococcus type III pneumonia.

Microscopically, in the early stages the condition is distinguished by the bacteria in the alveolar exudate. Neutrophilic outpouring is accompanied by destruction of the interalveolar septa. Pronounced edema is seen in interlobular septa and around vessels and bronchi. Soon abscesses form, with breaking down of inflammatory cells and total loss of alveolar structure. A chronic state can supervene as granulation tissue turns to fibrosis and abscesses become simple cavities. The latter are fibrous walled, and the inflammatory cells are now lymphocytic.

Since the abscesses are usually apical, one's first impression is tuberculosis, although other bacteria, such as staphylococci, have to be considered. *Acinetobacter* can cause a pneumonia that is destructive and produces sticky pus (the organisms are encapsulated).[129] The important strains of the tribe are *Herellea vaginicola* and *Mima polymorpha* (both constitute *Acinetobacter calcoaceticus*). These are gram-negative pleomorphic aerobic rods and cocci, resistant to penicillin.

Staphylococcal pneumonia

Up to 5% of bacterial pneumonias are caused by *Staphylococcus pyogenes,* but the incidence rises during epidemics of influenza, pertussis, and measles. The mortality is around 20% and is even higher in young infants. A chronic state may precede death. The infection may terminate the course of leukemia or of cystic fibrosis of the pancreas.

A thick fibrinous or fibrinopurulent pleuritis coats the affected lung in nearly all cases. Infants, especially those infected in nursery epidemics, frequently develop empyema and bronchopleural fistula. They die in a few days. Those who die soonest appear to have only hemorrhagic consolidation or edema of the lungs, with little pleuritis. The bronchial mucosa is red if not covered by a shaggy yellow membrane. Under the microscope, the inflammatory element is not impressive in the beginning. Alveoli are filled with eosinophilic fluid, erythrocytes, a few neutrophils, and many cocci.

In older infants and adults, the condition tends to pass from this phase into one of multiple foci of gray-yellow consolidation. In a few days, these become irregular, small, yellow abscesses (Fig. 26-33). They tend to unite into a honeycomb or into a small number of large abscess cavities. In either case, bronchial communications are to be expected, and, if there is an empyema, it will turn into a pyopneumothorax. Infection can spill into other bronchi, setting up new infections.

In infants a check-valve obstruction at the junction of the bronchus and abscess can result in a rapidly expanding air-filled *tension cyst (tension pneumatocele)* because the surrounding inflammation interferes with the normal collateral ventilation. The cyst is spherical, can be centimeters in diameter, and has a thin wall. This is necrotic and ragged at first but later becomes fibrotic and smooth. Usually, the air is absorbed after infection is cured. A tension cyst may rupture and cause a simple

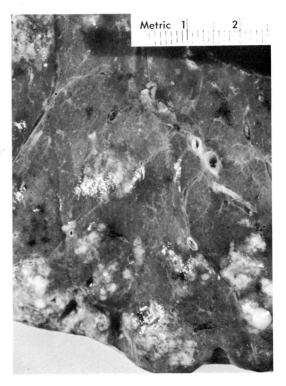

Fig. 26-33. Staphylococcal pneumonia. Numerous 1 to 2 mm areas are becoming confluent.

or tension pneumothorax, with or without empyema.

Tension cysts (so-called vanishing lung) also are seen in drug-treated tuberculosis.

Microscopically, abscess-forming staphylococcal pneumonia exhibits alveolar septa and air spaces packed with neutrophils. Often, the septa have been destroyed, and bronchioles are caught up in the same neutrophilic outpouring. There may be edema and neutrophilic filling of pulmonary septal lymphatics. The first pleural changes are congestion and fibrin exudation. Neutrophils pour into the fibrin, which rapidly thickens and, later on, fibroblasts grow into it. The wall of a pneumatocele is at first such inflamed and necrotic lung tissue, surrounded by a zone of compressed lung. Later, a thin wall of fibrous connective tissue forms.

Fulminating staphylococcal pneumonia of adults is fatal in 1 to 2 days. The lungs are heavy and watery but without consolidation. The patients are most likely to have had staphylococcal septicemia. The diagnosis will be missed if cultures are not taken from lung and blood, because only moderate neutrophilic activity is seen in the congested alveoli.

Streptococcal pneumonia

Most instances of streptococcal pneumonia (due to β-hemolytic *Streptococcus pyogenes*) are secondary to influenza, measles, or other childhood viral infections. Formerly, the disease comprised 3% to 5% of all childhood pneumonias, and 20% of the patients developed empyema. Others had abscesses, bronchopleural fistulas, or pericarditis, and the mortality was high. The organism was the main cause of death in the 1918-1919 influenza pandemic, with *Haemophilus influenzae* less frequently the causative organism.

Today the disease is rare, even as an accompaniment of influenza, but Welch et al.[135] have documented a small primary epidemic in previously healthy young men.

The heavy, blue-purple lungs are covered by fibrin. Streptococcal empyema is at first watery with fibrin flakes, turning thick and purulent with loculation of the fluid.

The mucosa of the respiratory tract is red and swollen and may be coated by a membrane. Ulcers may be found in the larynx, trachea, and bronchi, whose lumens are filled with bloody fluid. Streptococcal pneumonia is extensive, bilateral, interstitial, and bronchiolar. The most acute form resembles acute staphylococcal pneumonia. Later, the soggy lungs develop ill-defined, moist, consolidated areas that will become confluent or turn into abscesses. Smaller bronchi and the bronchioles are prominent because they are filled with pus and because their pale yellow walls are thickened by inflammation.

Microscopically, the airways are denuded of epithelium and are stuffed with neutrophils and debris. Neutrophils, fibrin, and some lymphocytes infiltrate the hyperemic walls of the airways and pour into alveoli. Lymphatic vessels are engorged with neutrophils. Pulmonary necrosis or abscess, bronchiectasis, mediastinitis, or pericarditis may be present. In nonfatal cases, the severe destruction can be repaired only by fibrosis.

Haemophilus influenzae pneumonia

Haemophilus influenzae was believed to cause influenza, but the great pandemic made clear the primary role of a virus. The combination of this organism and a virus produces a bronchopneumonia in which the walls of smaller bronchi and bronchioles are damaged or destroyed. Pure hemophilus pneumonia has complicated chronic lung disease in adults, with a gross appearance similar to that of streptococcal pneumonia.[133]

Mycoplasma pneumonia

Mycoplasma pneumoniae (formerly primary atypical pneumonia, Eaton agent pneumonia) is a common pathogen of the upper respiratory tract of children and young adults. Usually it produces only mild pharyngeal infections, but in 3% to 10% pneumonia develops. It has been reported that 8% to 39% of pneumonias in military recruits is caused by this agent, and in the civil population the percentage is similar. Although there is a response to antibiotics, the disease may spread to other areas of the lungs, and mixed infections are common. Moreover, there can be hemolytic anemia, purpura, gastroenteritis, hepatitis, arthritis, myocarditis, and dermatologic and neurologic complications.[130] Culture of the organism requires 10 days on special media.

Bronchopneumonia

Bronchopneumonia originates in bronchioles and extends into surrounding alveoli. The causes are as follows:
1. Inhalation of noxious gases and dusts
2. Aspiration of fluid and solid contents of the alimentary tract
3. Bacterial infection, either primary or complicating viral infections such as influenza or ornithosis, rickettsial diseases, congestive heart failure, bronchiectasis, bronchial obstruction, or pulmonary mycoses

Bacterial infection or aspiration tends to occur in weak individuals such as premature and full-term newborn infants and in bedridden or comatose patients.

The organisms commonly responsible are species of *Staphylococcus, Streptococcus, Klebsiella, Haemophilus, Pneumococcus,* and gramnegative bacilli.[132] In pseudomonal pneumonia there are well-demarcated, firm, necrotic nodules. These are composed of a necrotic coagulum, particularly situated around blood vessels and containing large numbers of the bacteria and a minimal inflammatory response of lymphocytes. Vascular thrombosis is inconstant. There is also a tuberculous bronchopneumonia (p. 1121).

Terminal or hypostatic bronchopneumonia is hard to recognize grossly, since it is hidden by the preexisting basal and posterior congestion and edema. The other types are classically patchy. Focal red or gray areas of consolidation (often centered on small bronchi) lie beside raised, pink, aerated normal areas and dark blue, sunken, collapsed areas (Fig. 26-34, *A*). This patchwork of 1 cm contrasting zones is,

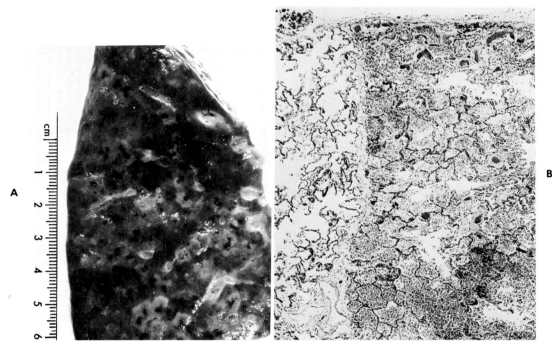

Fig. 26-34. A, Bronchopneumonia. Lighter small areas are groups of alveoli filled with inflammatory exudate. **B,** Bronchopneumonia. Inflammation is contained by vertically running septum. (**B,** 33×.)

however, not so common. It often takes the passage of the fingertips over the cut surface to pick up the areas of differing consistency. The bronchial mucosa is frequently bright red. Another variety is peribronchial pneumonia, in which infection picks out peribronchiolar alveoli only, and the consolidation parallels the bronchial tree. If progressive, bronchopneumonia will imitate lobar pneumonia. Careful inspection is likely to disclose a residual patchwork.

The complications of bronchopneumonia are generally those of lobar pneumonia, with a greater tendency for bronchopneumonia to cause permanent damage. Bronchiolar fibrosis and narrowing, with organization of exudate, may lead to bronchiectasis.

The microscopic lesions of bronchopneumonia are alveoli filled with neutrophils and fibrin, the septa being thickened by the congested capillaries, which contain leukocytes (Fig. 26-34, *B*). Acute bronchitis and bronchiolitis also will be seen.

Inhalation (aspiration) pneumonia

Inhalation pneumonia results from inhaling food, gastric contents, or a foreign body, which may occur when anesthesia has been induced

on a full stomach. Other predisposing conditions are drunkenness, convulsions, coma, and neurologic disorders interfering with the swallowing, coughing, and breathing mechanisms. Feeble infants or those with a tracheoesophageal fistula may aspirate food. Aspiration may occur in patients with necrotic oropharyngeal tumors and those vomiting copiously with intestinal obstruction.

Some die quickly from asphyxiation or laryngospasm, without pneumonia. The large airways are filled with the foreign material, and the mucosa may be reddened by irritation.

If smaller amounts are aspirated, the foreign material may trickle into narrower air passages, and often it is inhaled into alveoli; therefore, no foreign material may be visible to the naked eye.

Sterile foreign matter sets up a chemical pneumonitis. The lung undergoes severe congestion and edema, confirmed microscopically by alveoli filled with hemorrhagic fluid and neutrophils. Particles are found in bronchioles. Secondary bacterial infection is likely to occur. A few hours after aspiration, patients with chemical pneumonitis dramatically develop cyanosis, dyspnea, shock, and frothy, bloody sputum. They appear to be suffering from

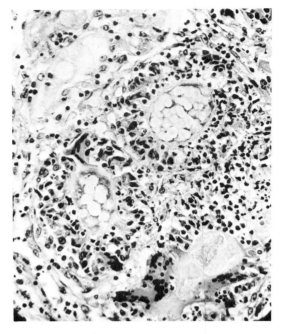

Fig. 26-35. Pulse pneumonia. Intense reaction around partly digested cotyledons of beans. (Approximately 300×.)

pulmonary edema and are likely to die of cardiac failure.

A nonsterile aspirate rapidly causes widespread bronchopneumonia, which forms confluent necrotic areas. These are yellow, green, or a dirty gray-green or brown, and they are poorly defined and foul smelling. Putrefactive anaerobes induce a friable gangrenous destruction of the lung, as opposed to the abscesses of pyogenic aerobes. Gangrenous cavities are more irregular and ragged.

The microscopic appearance is of tissue necrosis surrounded by alveoli filled with many erythrocytes and macrophages, a few neutrophils, and debris that may be recognizable as altered food or may be crystalline or amorphous. The starch-containing cotyledons of the pulses (lentils, peas, beans, and peanuts), cause local pneumonic infiltrates that may pass on to granulomas with giant cells (Fig. 26-35). Disintegration of the pulse may leave an apparently inexplicable giant cell pneumonia.

Very ill or postsurgical patients frequently aspirate food.[125] Barium introduced into the stomach immediately after death has been found in the lungs, sometimes even in the alveoli. Evidently moving the body and the force exerted in removing the lungs are responsible.[125] Therefore, gastric contents in bronchi or alveoli cannot be taken as evidence of antemortem aspiration unless the trachea is closed off immediately after death before the body has been moved. Microscopic signs of aspiration may be otherwise unexplained diffluent hemorrhage in dependent parts of the lungs. Some cellular response can be found even in patients dying quickly from aspiration. The cellular reaction continues in the lungs after clinical death.

Lipid pneumonia

Inflammatory and even fibrous reactions associated with the presence of intra-alveolar lipid have long been known.

Exogenous lipid pneumonia

The exogenous variety of lipid pneumonia is associated with the long-continued use of oily nosedrops or sprays taken for rhinitis or sinusitis. The base is mineral oil (liquid paraffin). This oil to taken regularly at bedtime and, during sleep, is quite easily aspirated in small amounts, which accumulate. There is a similar danger for young children who are forcibly given milk, oily vitamins, or other medicine. An enfeebled elderly person may not know that food has trickled into his bronchi. By no means does tube feeding protect against this accident, for there is regurgitation and the cardiac sphincter is lax.

A related condition is the occasional reaction to radiopaque contrast media instilled for bronchography. Practically all the patients eventually dispose of the medium by expectoration and phagocytosis, but in a few it remains as an irritant with a resulting lipid pneumonia.[122,124]

Nature of irritants. Least irritant are olive oil and the neutral vegetable oils used as contrast media. They stimulate slight fibrosis and can be slowly absorbed. Much more irritative is mineral oil, despite its being chemically inert. It is emulsified and engulfed by phagocytes, but the residue slowly induces fibrosis. Duration of action and amount of the oil are important factors. Animal oils (cod-liver, halibut, and milk) tend to decompose and are converted by human lipases into irritating fatty acids that stimulate a rather severe inflammation and more rapid fibrosis. The three types are distinguishable only histochemically (see following discussion).

Clinical picture. Lipid pneumonia often is unsuspected until revealed by radiographic examination or autopsy. It tends to be symptomless, unless a secondary bacterial infection ensues. Radiographic diagnosis of lipid pneumonia must be followed by lung biopsy. Neither presence nor absence of fat droplets in sputum is diagnostic.

Gross appearance. In more active patients, the lesions are mostly in the right middle and lower lobes and the left lower lobe. In those confined to bed, the lesions are found in the upper lobes. The commoner lesion is a diffuse process, commencing as scattered foci that subsequently fuse. Much or all of a lobe is indurated and noncrepitant, with a pale yellow, solid cut surface. Another finding is the oil granuloma, a well-localized rounded area, sometimes with scalloped margins. The firm mass can be mistaken for carcinoma. Neighboring lung may be slightly collapsed or show distinct inflammatory changes in the bronchi.

Microscopic appearance. The important characteristic of exogenous lipid is its existence, either free or in macrophages, as clear droplets. In the early stages, these are in the alveoli, accompanied by neutrophils. Macrophages become so numerous that the air spaces are filled. Alveolar phagocytes merge into giant cells, and rest on a fibrous framework. The

inflammatory reaction becomes lymphocytic (Fig. 26-36). Terminal bronchioles are dilated. Small arteries undergo obliteration by intimal proliferation and medial fibrosis. Fat droplets are released from the macrophages. Foreign-body giant cells and Langhans' giant cells, aided by the presence of epithelioid cells, create a resemblance to an infectious granuloma. The end stage is shown in Fig. 7-22. If some of the lipid is present as cholesterol, it gives the macrophages a foamy instead of a bubbly cytoplasm, but cholesterol needles are not seen. Within a few hours after cod-liver oil has entered alveoli, a hyaline membrane forms around the oil, and an obvious foreign-body giant cell reaction is stimulated. This oil can be resorbed with mineral fibrosis if the dose is small.

The Liebermann-Burchardt reaction demonstrates cholesterol in sections. Cod-liver oil is stained by scarlet red and Nile blue sulfate and forms a black precipitate with osmic acid. Mineral oil is stained by scarlet red and is nonreactive with osmic acid.

Endogenous lipid pneumonia

The endogenous variety of lipid pneumonia, of which cholesterol pneumonitis is an ex-

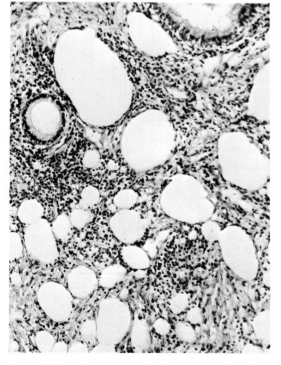

Fig. 26-36. Exogenous lipid pneumonia. Late stage with almost complete replacement of lung structure by fat and fibrous tissue. (105×.)

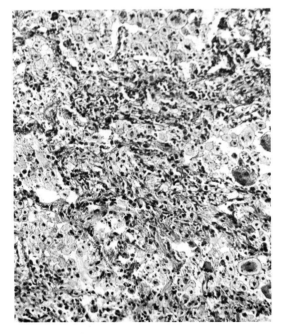

Fig. 26-37. Endogenous lipid pneumonia. Foamy macrophages fill alveoli. (109×.)

ample, is the result of metabolic, allergic, neoplastic, or inflammatory processes that release lipid by causing tissue breakdown. The commonest causes are nonresolving pneumonia, carcinoma, and abscesses (Fig. 26-86). Naked-eye differentiation from the exogenous form is impossible, unless the consolidation has the classic golden color seen in some cases. Of course, there is no gravitational distribution, but instead there is a relationship to the primary condition. The lipid tends to be finely dispersed in the cytoplasm of macrophages, changing them into foamy macrophages (Fig. 26-37), whereas large intracytoplasmic droplets (vacuoles) characterize exogenous lipid pneumonia. The interalveolar fibrosis and later replacement of lung tissue are the same as seen with exogenous lipid.

The lipid results from hyperactivity of type II pneumonocytes whose laminated cytosomes are extruded in excessive numbers into the alveolar spaces. Free in the alveoli, the type II inclusion bodies are taken into pulmonary macrophages, which feast on them until bloated and inactive. Lipid is released on the death of these cells and is sufficiently irritative to induce interstitial fibrosis.[123]

Pneumocystis carinii pneumonia

Also known as plasma cell pneumonia, *Pneumocystis carinii* pneumonia is rare in the United States but common in central Europe. Large numbers of the protozoon *Pneumocystis carinii* are present in the alveoli and are presumed to be responsible for the disease, the occurrence of which is mainly confined to the first few months of life. Infantile cases usually arise in epidemic form, but in some cases the children affected have been debilitated or have had abnormalities of gamma globulin. Many of the cases in adults and some in children are associated with leukemia, lymphoma, or cytomegalic inclusion disease.[134]

Up to 40% of the infants die and are found to have voluminous, gray-pink, firm, airless lungs. There is no pleuritis. The cut surface reveals confluent or completely homogeneous, firm, dry, gray tissue. The regional lymph nodes are unaltered, and the bronchi are empty.

Microscopically, the alveoli are filled with a foamy, pale, eosinophilic substance. In it are faintly staining dotlike bodies surrounded by a little clear space and a capsule, each no more than 1 μm in diameter (Fig. 26-38, *A*).

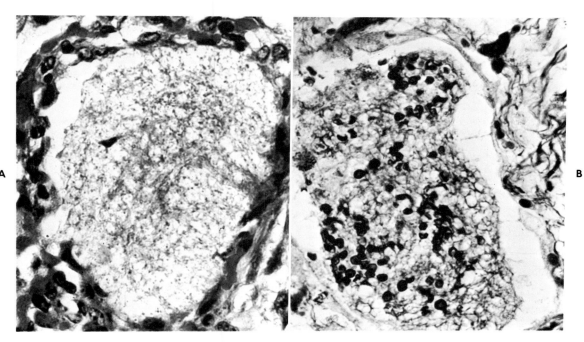

Fig. 26-38. *Pneumocystis carinii* pneumonia. **A,** Minute black dots are individual nuclei. **B,** Alveolus shown in **A** stained with methenamine silver. Dark spheres are capsules of individual organisms. (**A,** Hematoxylin and eosin; **A** and **B,** 600×.)

As many as eight of these may be gathered within a cyst 8 to 12 μm in diameter. Lymphocytes, monocytes, and plasma cells distend interalveolar septa in typical cases. Plasma cells are often predominant but in a number of reports have been absent, particularly in cases secondary to hematologic diseases. Hematoxylin does not always stain the organisms, which are seen better with the periodic acid–Schiff method. Gomori's silver methenamine staining brings out the cysts well (Fig. 26-38, B).

Variants of the disease are beginning to appear. Granulomas containing parasites have appeared in the lung, sometimes progressing to fibrosis and calcification. Some patients not only have pneumocystosis of the lung but also of the spleen, liver, lymph nodes, and bone marrow.[128]

Interstitial pneumonia

Although viral pneumonia is discussed in Chapter 12, it is necessary to mention the microscopic findings here to distinguish them from the pneumonias just described.[126,127] Some cases of organizing pneumonia are a combination of chronic interstitial pneumonia and superimposed acute pneumonia.[127] Many also may merge with diffuse interstitial pulmonary fibrosis.

In uncomplicated interstitial pneumonia, the exudate is in the interalveolar septa. These are greatly thickened by increased numbers of reticulin fibers and a gathering of lymphocytes, plasma cells, and histiocytes. Cuboid metaplasia may occur in the alveolar lining. Some alveoli are greatly reduced in size, while nearby there may be focal emphysema. Not only may connective tissue be laid down in the septa but also fibrosis may be initiated by alveolar cell proliferation on the alveolar surface.[126,127] Only in the latter case will the air space be compromised.

PULMONARY ABSCESS AND GANGRENE

Causes. The flood of antibiotics has barely dampened the fires of abscesses in the lungs. The most common cause is inhalation of foreign material. This may be food, decaying teeth, gastric contents, or necrotic tissue dislodged during surgery on the mouth, upper respiratory tract, or nasopharynx. Severely infected gingivae and teeth can be the source of pus draining into the lungs during sleep. When a bronchus has become obstructed, an abscess may form distally; this may be the first sign of a bronchial carcinoma or an impacted foreign body. Necrosis within a tumor, followed by bacterial infection, leads to an abscess. Severely infected cystic disease of the lung, or bronchiectasis, can develop into an abscess. Another important group of abscesses includes those arising during bacterial pneumonia. The organisms are most likely to be type III pneumococci, *Klebsiella pneumoniae,* staphylococci, and hemolytic streptococci. Only in a minority of cases is an abscess caused by septicemia or a septic infarct, as in acute osteomyelitis or bacterial endocarditis. Rare causes are trauma to the lung, and direct extension from a suppurating focus in the esophagus or mediastinum, subphrenic area, or vertebral column.

Distribution. Abscesses of inhalational origin are likely to be in the right upper lobe or in the apex of the right lower lobe. The more vertical course of the right bronchus puts it more in line with the trachea, thus rendering it more receptive to inhaled material. Suppuration beginning in a bronchus spreads distally in the air passages and is likely to destroy the bronchial wall and spread into the surrounding lung. Tiny foreign particles will set up inflammation in alveoli and are closer to the pleura. An abscess complicating pneumonia will have no primary relationship to a bronchus. Abscesses in septicemia are scattered throughout the lungs but are likely to be small and subpleural. Septic infarcts are described on p. 1053.

Appearance. Sympneumonic abscesses are described in the discussion of pneumonia under each organism. As to the other varieties, an early abscess is yellow or white and firm. Septicemic abscesses have a thin red rim. Soon the center undergoes liquefaction and cavity formation. The lining is ragged, yellow, and necrotic. Odor may be absent or extremely unpleasant, the latter indicating the need for anaerobic as well as aerobic cultures. With time, the pus is likely to become gray or green and to undergo complete liquefaction. Around it is a wall of granulation tissue, erroneously called a pyogenic membrane. An abscess in pneumonia is surrounded by a wide zone of consolidation. The chronic abscess has a thin, firm, fibrous wall and a greater amount of organizing pneumonia external to it. A communication with a bronchus may have persisted.

Course. Complete healing of a small abscess is possible. Resolution may leave a scar with a small central sterile cavity. An abscess close to the pleura induces fibrinous or purulent pleurisy, followed by empyema. An abscess can perforate into a bronchus (bronchopulmonary fistula) or into the mediastinum. The fistula promotes further spread through the lung, and a series of small intercommunicating abscesses may appear. Pulmonary septa form no barrier to inflammation, which can cross an interlobar fissure if the two surfaces have been united by adhesions. Serious bleeding will be produced by erosion of a vessel in the abscess wall. A distant complication of pulmonary abscess is dissemination to the brain, which occurs in 5% to 10% of cases. No antibiotics can repair the damage wrought by larger abscesses. However, the lining is converted into a smooth fibrous wall on which a single layer of squamous or columnar cells can be demonstrated microscopically. Tension pneumatocele is described on p. 1072.

Microscopic appearance. Destruction of alveoli or bronchial tissue is readily recognized, and masses of neutrophils fill the area. The center is likely to be necrotic and, peripherally, individual inflammatory cells are pyknotic. Hypervascularity will be observed at the edges, where plump young fibroblasts are proliferating to form a capsule. Bacterial colonies may be recognized without special stains. Around the abscess, alevoli are likely to be filled with organizing exudate.

Gangrene. The term "gangrene" is not accurately used with reference to the lung, since there is no massive ischemic necrosis followed by putrefaction. The lesion is a rather rapidly progressive abscess in which, in addition to aerobes, anaerobic organisms such as bacteroides, streptococci, clostridia, fusiform bacilli, and spirochetes play an active role. The abscess is not walled off, and destruction is extensive. Irregular cavities are surrounded by soft, airless, moist, green or black tissue. It is hardly possible to touch this tissue without its breaking, and strands of it float in the foul-smelling pus.

NONNEOPLASTIC ACQUIRED DISEASES OF BRONCHI
Acute bronchitis and bronchiolitis

In adults, acute bronchitis may be restricted to large and medium-sized bronchi. Infection may have descended from the upper respiratory tract or may be airborne. The mucosa is edematous and congested. It produces a plentiful mucin that may become purulent and yellow. More severe inflammation leads to mucosal ulceration. Diphtheria and severe pyogenic infection form a fibrinous membrane

covering the mucosa. Necrotizing and hemorrhagic bronchitis are the most severe forms, generally occurring in influenza with secondary infection.

This progression is mirrored microscopically. Increased secretion is observed in the glands and goblet cells. Then neutrophils appear in the bronchial wall and migrate into the lumen. Hypervascularity is apparent, and some mucosal cells are cast off, sometimes in strips. Once the wall is exposed, the inflammatory reaction is heightened. A membrane is recognized as a mesh of fibrin with entrapped necrotic leukocytes and epithelial cells.

Acute bronchitis in children[138] *and elderly persons*[137] is important because of accompanying bronchiolitis. In severe cases, there is a laryngotracheobronchitis, which may be associated with acute generalized or interstitial emphysema. Bronchioles are plugged with yellow, mucinous droplets. In acute inflammation, numerous goblet cells are rapidly formed by metaplasia in bronchioles that usually have none. Bronchopneumonia ensues around the terminal and respiratory bronchioles. The major danger is respiratory failure from blockage of so many bronchioles. There is the risk later of obliteration of the bronchioles by fibrous organization of the highly fibrinous exudate (bronchiolitis obliterans) (Fig. 26-39). Such a process is akin to what happens to alveolar exudate in organizing pneumonia. Most adult cases have occurred after exposure to poisonous gases. Bronchiolitis obliterans is otherwise rare as a widespread condition. Necrotizing bronchitis and bronchiolitis is seen in children dying from adenovirus infection, and in some there has also been bronchiolitis obliterans. Other agents causing necrotizing bronchitis are respiratory syncytial virus, parainfluenza virus, and mycoplasma.[136]

Chronic bronchitis

The only satisfactory definition of chronic bronchitis is a clinical one, that of the British Medical Research Council, accepted by the American Thoracic Society. It reads: "Chronic bronchitis is characterized by the production of sputum in the absence of cardiac or other pulmonary disease. The sputum must be produced on most days for at least three months of the year and for at least two years." Therefore, if one sees many lymphocytes in a bronchial wall, this condition cannot be called chronic bronchitis. I suggest "lymphocytic bronchitis," which describes a true inflammatory reaction. In fact, "chronic bronchitis" is

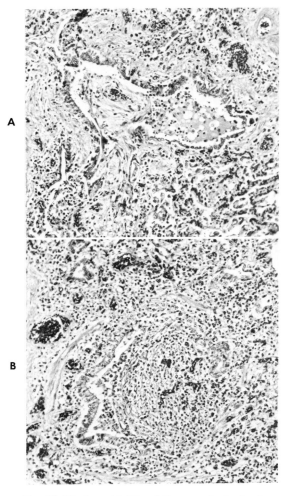

Fig. 26-39. Bronchiolitis obliterans. **A,** Early stage. **B,** Later stage. Young vascular fibrous tissue is growing into lumen of bronchus, organizing exudate and obliterating lumen. (**A** and **B,** 165×.)

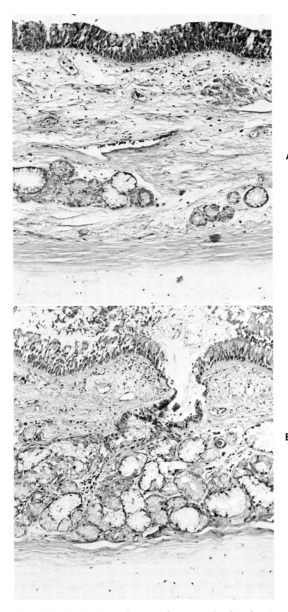

Fig. 26-40. A, Bronchus with normal glands. **B,** Pronounced hypertrophy and hyperplasia of bronchial glands in chronic bronchitis (gland/wall ratio, about 0.6). (**A** and **B,** 145×.)

a most unsuitable name for the disease we are discussing.

The sputum is produced by an increased number of mucous cells throughout the bronchial tree. The fact that the glands are hypertrophied can be seen (and measured). The Reid index is the ratio of the depth of the glands to the thickness of the mucosa (the gland/wall ratio—0.14 to 0.36 normally but 0.41 to 0.79 in chronic bronchitis)[1] (Fig. 26-40). In bronchioles, where glands are not present, goblet cells in large numbers replace the ciliated epithelium. Changes in the proportion of different cell types of the bronchial glands result in a change in the components of the bronchial secretion.[1]

The disease has its highest incidence and is most severe in Great Britain, where it causes nearly 10% of all deaths. Its incidence in the United States is much underrated, mainly because of its being confused with emphysema, an error made even by some workers in the field of respiratory disease.[139,140]

Chronic bronchitis often is provoked by nasal sinusitis, is perpetuated by repeated respiratory infections, and often leads to emphysema and cor pulmonale. Chronic passive congestion of the lungs in heart failure is a common precursor of chronic bronchitis. Climate, air pollution, and cigarette smoking are important external factors, but why it commences and becomes a long-continuing disease is unknown. *Haemophilus influenzae* and pneumococci are the most common pathogens in chronic bronchitis.

At first, there is mucosal edema with hypersecretion. Later, bacterial infection creates a purulent fluid. This is believed to be the most important factor in causing permanent destruction of the bronchi and bronchioles. Later, the mucosa of larger bronchi is purple, velvety or granular (hypertrophic), or thin, pale, and smooth, with longitudinal and transverse gray ridges (atrophic). In either case, the wall is thickened, and eventually inflammation spreads into peribronchial tissues, causing patchy pneumonia and a thin investment of fibrous tissue. Here, too, from involvement of terminal bronchioles, lies the origin of some cases of emphysema. Chronic suppuration can cause bronchiectasis. In the bronchioles and alveoli there is ulceration, fibrosis and stenosis, all secondary to infection.

Microscopically, hyperplasia of the mucous glands and goblet cells of the bronchi occurs at the expense of serous cells and of cilia, so that the increased secretion is removed poorly or not at all, with a consequent risk of bacterial infection. Only during attacks of acute infection is there infiltration by inflammatory cells, with damage to the epithelium. Many patients undergo squamous metaplasia of the mucosa. Large numbers of goblet cells make their appearance in the bronchiolar epithelium and create mucous plugs.

Clinical correlation. Chronic bronchitis should be considered in conjunction with the discussion of emphysema (p. 1058), where it is stressed that in life the airway obstruction that both diseases can cause may make them indistinguishable. The degree of hypersecretion has little correlation with the patient's disability. The disability is caused by obstruction of small airways, which may be blocked by pus or mucopus and damaged by fibrosis. Bronchographic study in severe chronic bronchitis often will disclose a variety of structural and obstructive abnormalities in the peripheral bronchial tree.[148]

It is extremely difficult to recognize wherein lies the airway obstruction that is so serious in chronic bronchitis. In normal persons the resistance to air flow in distal airways is only 25% of the total, with the other 75% being provided by the proximal airways.[145] In bronchitis, bronchiectasis, and emphysema, this peripheral resistance is increased at least four times. This is caused by mucous plugging and narrowing and obliteration of the small airways, without a check valve (Laennec's original theory). Accordingly, some investigators now use the term "chronic obstructive disease of small airways."[147]

Disability can be present in patients who deny habitual expectoration but who have "morning catarrh" or "throat clearing." Most of the excess secretion comes from the glands, but it is the hypersecretion in the peripheral small airways that is mainly responsible for the disturbance of respiratory function.

Infection has not been demonstrated to be a prime cause of the damage, and prospective studies have cast further doubt upon the role of infection.[143,144] Trials of prophylactic chemotherapy have not reduced the number of exacerbations but have lessened the severity and duration of each episode. Retained secretions are the key factor in the onset of respiratory failure.

Since cigarette smoke and air pollutants are potent factors in aggravating the symptoms, it has been suggested that the role of antibiotics in the management of chronic bronchitis be reassessed.[149]

"Blue bloaters and pink puffers" is the colorful phrase crystallizing the opposite mechanisms at work in the relatively uncommon pure forms of chronic bronchitis and emphysema. The typical case of chronic bronchitis has no overinflation (hence normal total lung capacity) but has increased residual volume (from air trapping) and reduced maximal expiratory flow rate. This contrasts with emphysema, which is characterized by increased functional residual capacity (overinflation), increased residual volume, reduced maximal expiratory flow rate, and loss of elastic recoil.[141] Because of these factors and the impaired ventilation and perfusion (p. 1068), the patient who has predominant emphysema (type A, pink puffer) is dyspneic but maintains normal blood gases by hyperventilation. He has a low diffusing capacity probably because of loss of blood vessels in the poorly ventilated area. His condition is grave, but it is safe to give oxygen. The person who has mainly chronic bronchitis (type B, blue bloater) has abnormal blood gases (raised P_{CO_2}) with cyanosis, little dyspnea, but a

nearly normal diffusing capacity.[102] He suffers recurrent episodes of carbon dioxide retention with cyanosis and edema. Oxygen therapy must be carefully controlled to avoid carbon dioxide narcosis.

Bronchiectasis

Bronchiectasis is the persistent dilatation of, and fibrosis around, bronchi resulting from inflammatory damage to their walls. About one half of the patients give a history of previous pneumonia or bronchopneumonia, particularly during infectious diseases of childhood. Infection during the course of tuberculosis and cystic fibrosis of the pancreas also belongs in this group. Bronchial obstruction is the other important cause and may be attributable to bronchial tumor, inhaled foreign body, or bronchial compression by diseased hilar nodes or aortic aneurysm. A third group of cases is associated with pulmonary fibrosis, such as the pneumoconioses. *Congenital bronchiectasis* of children and young adults usually is confined to one lobe. It is probably a form of congenital cystic disease in which normal alveolar tissue does not form, and the proximal bronchial tree develops chronic inflammation.

Patients with bronchiectasis cough up great volumes of foul sputum. In some, this is blood stained, and a minority suffer massive hemoptysis. Finger clubbing, chest pain, and exertional dyspnea are fairly common.

Bronchial inflammation leads to hypersecretion of mucus, which becomes infected and viscous. Infection advances into the wall, and its destruction begins. When obstruction comes first, it is followed by hypersecretion and then by infection. In either case, the lung adjoining the involved bronchus participates in the inflammation. The normal expansile forces in the lung can pull on the damaged bronchi, causing them to be widened. There is sufficient cartilage in the first four divisions of lobar bronchi to protect them from dilatation.

Bronchiectasis involves bronchi running more or less vertically, usually in the lower lobes. In an upper lobe, it is likely to be secondary to destructive tuberculous lesions. A single site of bronchiectasis is most likely to be the result of a relatively large obstruction.

The dilatation is most often cylindrical, a uniform widening of considerable length. Bronchi of a diameter of several millimeters travel right down to the pleura where no scissors will normally reach. Sometimes the widening is fusiform. A common variant is varicose bronchiectasis, in which numerous constrictions break the dilated bronchi into segments. In the saccular variety, in which the bronchiectasis has changed into a spherical abscess, there are beadlike bulges along the course of the bronchi. These remain even if the inflammatory process is cured.

The early mucosal change is a soft, hyperemic, velvety thickening. Later, there is ulceration and, with mucosal atrophy, a rope-ladder pattern is produced in which the mucosa is folded over prominent bands of circular muscle. The normal longitudinal mucosal folds provide the vertical lines. In the presence of suppuration, the lining is necrotic with underlying granulation tissue. Small bronchi or bronchioles distal to these areas may have suffered fibrous obliteration. Lung tissue close by the affected bronchi undergoes pneumonitis. Widening of the bronchial arteries and an increase in their communications with the pulmonary arteries are demonstrable. Eventually, the pleura is involved with chronic inflammation and fibrosis. In the end stages, affected bronchi are thickened by mural and peribronchial fibrosis, a reaction diminished by adequate antibiotic therapy (Fig. 26-41, *A*).

Microscopically, the mucosa becomes edematous, ulcerated, and converted into granulation tissue. Loss of epithelium, or conversion of ciliated cells to goblet cells or metaplastic stratified squamous epithelium, is important in nonobstructive cases, for it causes retention of secretion. The wall is extensively infiltrated by lymphocytes and plasma cells. Sometimes, these are collected into submucous lymphoid nodules large enough to raise the mucosa (Fig. 26-41, *B*).

Later, all components of the normal wall are replaced, allowing dilatation. The lining is now very similar to an abscess wall. The end result is a fibrous wall lined by a single atrophic epithelial layer or stratified squamous epithelium.

Complications of bronchiectasis are localized pleurisy, empyema, bronchopleural fistula, lung abscess, acute and chronic pneumonia, cerebral abscess, meningitis, and right ventricular hypertrophy. Some bronchiectatic cavities give rise to squamous cell carcinoma and tumorlets.

Foreign bodies in bronchi

Most of the patients who inhale foreign bodies into the bronchi are children. In adults, aspiration under anesthesia or a sudden gasp while holding something in the mouth is the usual cause. The object tends to enter the

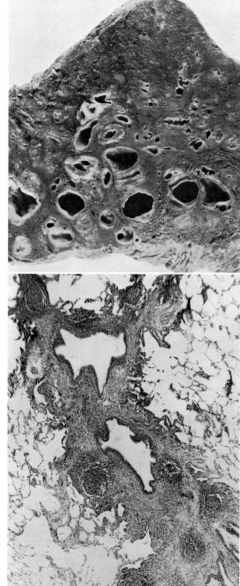

Fig. 26-41. Bronchiectasis. **A,** Lower lobe of child's lung removed surgically. At lower left is bronchiectatic abscess. **B,** Dilatation and fibrous thickening of wall of bronchiole. Mucosal lining is preserved. Nodular and diffuse lymphocytic infiltration. (**B,** 40×.)

more vertical right main bronchus. It causes edema and inflammation, which impact it more tightly. Complete obstruction, or a ball-valve action, lets air out only, so that the supplied segment collapses. A check-valve ef-

fect, letting air in only, causes hyperinflation. Mucosal pressure is followed by inflammation, ulceration, and suppuration. From this can result bronchial stenosis, bronchiectasis, pneumonia, lung abscesses, or gangrene. In addition, the foreign body may act as a chemical irritant.

Broncholithiasis. Broncholithiasis is the presence of stony bodies in the bronchial lumen. These are portions of calcified hilar lymph nodes that have eroded into the air passage. Rarely they come from an intrapulmonary granuloma. The usual site is the left middle lobe bronchus, because a node lies in the acute angle between it and the lower lobe bronchus.

Mucoid impaction. In some patients with chronic bronchitis, but also in those with asthma, cystic fibrosis, or bronchopulmonary aspergillosis (p. 514), segmental bronchi may become stuffed with putty-like plugs. These are firmer than simple mucus and tend to be in the upper lobes and to recur even if they are treated or are coughed up. They widen the bronchus and may cause suppuration distal to the obstruction. Some present radiologically as solitary nodules; the majority can be recognized as densities in the shape of a V, Y, or cluster of grapes, which represent the bronchial branching. The cause is unknown.[146]

Such plugs are laminated structures with layers of mucin and fibrin continually being added. In them are numerous eosinophils and bronchial epithelial cells. If unrelieved, the condition will cause localized bronchiectasis.

Bronchial fistulas

Three types of abnormal tracts originate in bronchi: bronchopleural, bronchoesophageal, and bronchodiaphragmatic fistulas.

Bronchopleural fistula is the commonest and is a complication of tuberculosis, pneumonia caused by staphylococci, streptococci, and *Klebsiella,* bronchiectasis, lung abscess, and pulmonary mycosis. Complications are tension pneumothorax and empyema.

Bronchoesophageal fistula is less common and is most often the result of an esophageal carcinoma, perforation by foreign bodies, and trauma. Food is inhaled into the lungs.

Bronchodiaphragmatic fistula is least common. Subphrenic and hepatic abscesses, whether pyogenic, amebic, or echinococcal, may cause obliteration of the pleura. The abscess can then penetrate the diaphragm and break into the lung, with eventual communication with a bronchus.

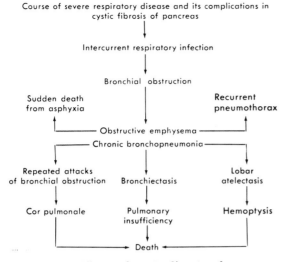

Course of severe respiratory disease and its complications in cystic fibrosis of pancreas

↓

Intercurrent respiratory infection

↓

Bronchial obstruction

↓

Sudden death from asphyxia ——— Obstructive emphysema ——— Recurrent pneumothorax

——— Chronic bronchopneumonia ———

Repeated attacks of bronchial obstruction   Bronchiectasis   Lobar atelectasis

Cor pulmonale   Pulmonary insufficiency   Hemoptysis

→ Death ←

Fig. 26-42. Effects of cystic fibrosis of pancreas on lung. (Slightly modified from di Sant'Agnese, P. A.: *Am. J. Med.* **21**:406-422, 1956.)

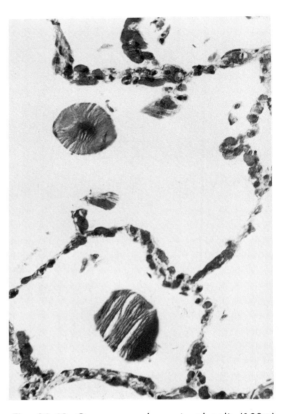

Fig. 26-43. Corpora amylacea in alveoli. (108×.)

CYSTIC FIBROSIS OF PANCREAS

Cystic fibrosis of the pancreas causes the majority of cases of chronic nontuberculous pulmonary disease in children in the United States. The cause is the abnormal and inspissated mucin secreted by the bronchial glands. See Fig. 26-42.

Respiratory complications are often fatal. Originally there was only a 1% survival at 10 years of age, but this has changed to 72% at age 12 and 45% at age 20; half of these have no or minimal respiratory symptoms. The reasons for this improvement are debated.[129] The disease is described in full on pp. 1459 to 1461.

UNUSUAL CAUSES OF PULMONARY CONSOLIDATION
Pulmonary alveolar microlithiasis

Pulmonary alveolar microlithiasis is a diffuse bilateral filling of the majority of alveoli by calcific concretions called "calcospherites." Radiologically they mimic miliary tuberculosis, yet the disease is asymptomatic for many years. Eventually, there is pulmonary insufficiency and right ventricular hypertrophy. Sex incidence is about equal, and most patients have been middle-aged. Familial cases are known, but the cause of the disease is a mystery except for rare cases of the milk-alkali syndrome (p. 272).

The lungs together weigh 2 to 4 kg. Except for some adhesions, the pleura is not affected.

Beneath it, gritty particles can be felt, and the lungs are solid, especially the basal regions. If it is possible to cut the lungs with a knife, a grittiness creates much resistance; a saw may be needed. The concretions on the dry, bloodless cut surface glisten in reflected light and may be picked out with the fingernails. Other tissues are not involved.

Microscopic examination shows concentrically laminated calcified bodies in one fourth to three fourths of the alveoli. Their size ranges between 50 and 200 μm. The centers stain more darkly, and they resemble the noncalcified eosinophilic corpora amylacea commonly found in the alveoli of aged individuals[150] (Fig. 26-43). Ossification is sometimes seen around the calcospherites, but this is not to be confused with the ossified nodules of mitral stenosis (Fig. 26-44). Alveolar walls may be unaltered, but many areas have undergone considerable fibrous thickening.

Metastatic and dystrophic calcification bear no relationship to alveolar microlithiasis. Metastatic calcification is by far the commoner in the lung, where it appears in routine stains

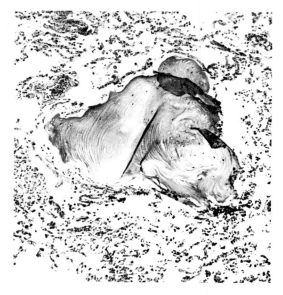

Fig. 26-44. Ossified nodule in mitral stenosis. (66×.)

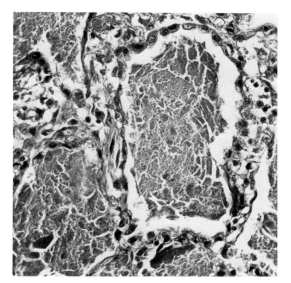

Fig. 26-46. Pulmonary alveolar proteinosis. Prominent type II cells. (Hematoxylin and eosin; 330×.)

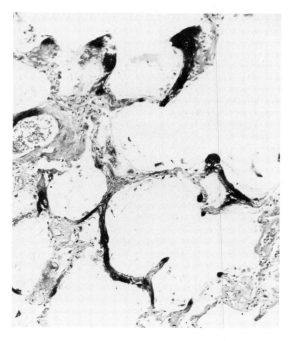

Fig. 26-45. Metastatic calcification. (105×.)

as a blue line marking the alveolar and bronchiolar basement membranes (Fig. 26-45).

An important, sometimes forgotten, cause of dystrophic calcification is varicella pneumonia. Necrosis in the acute phase is followed 2 to 7 years later by widespread pulmonary calcification, readily diagnosed in chest x-ray films.[151]

Pulmonary alveolar proteinosis

The first published report, citing 27 cases, appeared in 1958.[156] The total reported number now is over 150 cases.

The disease affects adults, preponderantly men, and is manifested by dyspnea, cough (often with yellow sputum), increasing fatigue, and loss of weight. About one third of the patients have died after a chronic course. Over the years, cor pulmonale builds up. Approximately 10% of the cases reported also have had nocardiosis (not always pulmonary).

Only the lungs are involved. Confluent gray 2 cm nodules of consolidation appear under the pleura. The intervening lung is likely to be affected. In the late stages, no normal lung is recognizable. Each lung weighs between 1 and 2 kg.

The microscopic feature is a filling of many alveoli with finely and coarsely granular eosinophilic material. Within it are fine needle-shaped spaces, deeper eosinophilic, rounded, structureless bodies, desquamated and degenerating septal cells, and other rounded laminated bodies the size of large cells. The alveolar septal cells proliferate in great number and project into the alveoli (Fig. 26-46). They may be multinucleated. Their cytoplasm is plentiful and gives the same staining reactions (periodic acid–Schiff positive and alcian blue negative), as does the material in the alveoli. Vacuolated cytoplasm indicates the presence of lipid. It is possible to see septal cells becoming detached, the nuclei being fragmented or pyknotic, and the cytoplasm becoming granular like the alveolar material. As the cells degenerate further, the nucleus disappears and the cytoplasm is transformed into the laminated or round bodies already mentioned.

The alveolar septa are devoid of inflammation or abnormal deposits, and their capillaries appear normal. The proteinaceous content of the alveoli is also to be found in bronchioles. It is sometimes possible to diagnose the disease by recognizing the peculiar eosinophilic content of the sputum, and the diagnosis can be confirmed during life by the demonstration of lamellar bodies in bronchial washings.[153]

The alveolar material appears to be palmityl lecithin devoid of surface tension–lowering activity in the patient, although it still has activity when tested after removal from the lung. Since it is not foreign to the alveolus, this explains the lack of cellular reaction to it.[155]

We can postulate that surfactant accumulates in excess because of overload of the normal clearance mechanism or decreased degradation of alveolar lipid. Alveolar macrophages in which it is stored appear defective, releasing the substance into the alveolar spaces.[153]

It is likely that there is more than one pathway to proteinosis. One of my patients was a young man who died after a lifetime of repeated pulmonary and dermal infections. A chest x-ray film of good quality, taken a week before death, was normal, yet at autopsy there was extensive bilateral proteinosis. Corrin and King have produced an identical condition by exposing rats to cristobalite, quartz, aluminum, and other dusts. They showed that the alveolar material originated from type II pneumonocytes.[123] Four young sandblasters had a rapidly fatal illness characteristic of acute silicosis but were found to have a combination of interstitial fibrosis and alveolar proteinosis.[152] In 13 fatal cases of thymic alymphoplasia in infancy, six were found to have a condition microscopically indistinguishable from pulmonary alveolar proteinosis. It is not yet possible to say whether the latter condition is related to hypogammaglobulinemia.[154]

ALLERGIC GRANULOMAS AND RELATED CONDITIONS

To be considered in this discussion are bronchial asthma, Löffler's syndrome, tropical eosinophilia, eosinophilic pneumonias, drug reactions, hypersensitivity pneumonitis, Wegener's granulomatosis, lethal midline granuloma, allergic granulomatosis, and angiitis.

Bronchial asthma

Asthma is defined as obstructive narrowing of the bronchi that changes in severity over short periods of time, either spontaneously or in response to treatment. It is not caused by cardiovascular disease and appears to be a hypersensitivity reaction related either to allergy or infection, particularly bronchitis. The allergen may be extrinsic or intrinsic and the antibody is IgE.

Recent work has disclosed additional antigens causing asthma. Among them in atopic subjects in Britain and the United States are the spores of *Aspergillus fumigatus*, which grow within their lungs, although not causing the disease aspergillosis.[161] This demonstrates type I of the four different types of allergic reaction in man.[160] The reaction is in the bronchi, whereas in nonatopic subjects the invasive and destructive form of aspergillosis occurs. Dutch workers have uncovered the role of acarine mites of species of the genus *Dermatophagoides* as the antigen of house dust, bedding, and human dander.[159]

Few people die directly from asthma. Among 68 fatal cases, asthma was primary in 52 and secondary to bronchitis in 16. Infection and psychologic factors were most important in precipitating attacks, often of the status asthmaticus variety.[157] Anaphylactic accidents also were important.

Impacted viscid mucous plugs are a significant factor in causing death, but right ventricular failure sometimes plays a role. Bronchospasm is not considered to be a major factor. Estimates have been made of a mortality of 1.5 per 1000 asthmatic patients per year.

The lungs are pale and distended, but not emphysematous. The cut surface reveals thick-walled large and small bronchi. Those of medium and small size are plugged by thick, viscid mucus (Fig. 26-47).

Microscopically, the lumens of all bronchi contain mucin, in which are many eosinophils and shed epithelial cells. The glands are enlarged and hyperactive, their wide ducts filled with mucin. Many goblet cells are present in the mucosa, the basement membrane of which is thickened many times over into a broad, homogeneous, bright pink, wavy band. The mucosa is thrown into folds by contraction of the hypertrophied muscle coat. This does not necessarily reflect the degree of spasm during life (Fig. 26-48). Shedding of the ciliated cells is prominent and is attributed to transudation of edema fluid from the submucosa.[158] This will greatly impair clearance of the bronchi. Bronchial epithelium in some areas displays

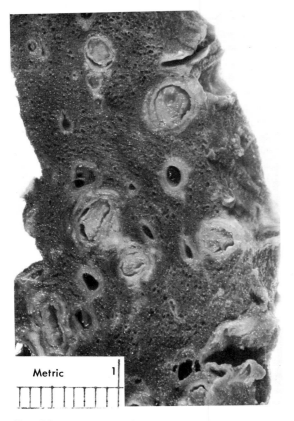

Metric 1

Fig. 26-47. Portion of formalin-fixed lung from patient dying in status asthmaticus. (From Rezek, P. R., and Millard, M.: Autopsy pathology, Springfield, Ill., 1963, Charles C Thomas, Publisher.)

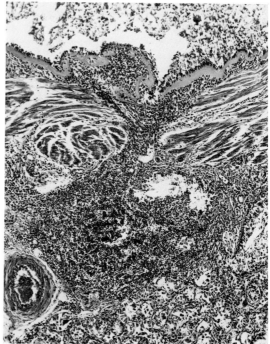

Fig. 26-48. Asthma. From top to bottom: desquamated epithelium, thickened basement membrane, muscular hyperplasia, dense infiltration by eosinophils, and glandular hyperplasia. (75×.)

regenerative activity, including mitoses. There is no satisfactory explanation for the thickening of the basement membrane.

Löffler's syndrome; tropical eosinophilia

In 1932, Löffler described a group of patients seen radiologically to have transient, irregular, small opacities throughout the lung. Many of the patients appear to have asthma, and all have respiratory symptoms. There is a peripheral blood eosinophilia of up to 50% or 60%. No specific infecting or infesting agent has even been demonstrated, and the condition is benign.

The salient features are massive filling of alveoli with eosinophils, some macrophages and giant cells, and eosinophilic infiltration of bronchial walls, which have thick hyaline basement membranes.[163]

An allied condition is *tropical eosinophilia*, seen widely in India, Malaysia, China, the Philippines, Polynesia, Africa, and the Caribbean. The roentgenographic findings resemble those in Löffler's syndrome. The patients are sicker, with fever, severe, persistent coughing, and a prolonged illness with blood eosinophilia. In many the condition is a hypersensitivity reaction to circulating microfilariae.[164] These are still unidentified and are considered to be of a type infecting animals and incapable of a complete cycle in human beings. This work does not exclude alternative causes such as ascariasis, fungi, mites, and molds.

The lung is covered by a fibrotic pleura. Its cut surface is a blend of small hemorrhages and gray-white nodules up to 1 cm in size. Microscopically, many eosinophils are found in the alveoli and interstitium, with smaller numbers of lymphocytes and plasma cells. Eosinophils also are present in the secretion filling the bronchi. Foreign body type of granulomas are present in the inflammatory foci. Elsewhere there is interstitial fibrosis.

Eosinophilic pneumonias

Liebow and Carrington[165] discuss all the varieties of pulmonary disease with eosinophilia. They then present a number of cases of eosinophilic pneumonia, a chronic severe illness with fever, night sweats, weight loss, and dyspnea. Only some of the patients had asthma. X-ray films showed rapidly progressive, dense, peripheral infiltrates. In biopsy material, alveoli are filled with eosinophils and vacuolated mononuclear cells. The former may be so packed as to resemble abscesses with necrotic centers and granulomatous response. Eosinophils, with a smaller number of plasma cells and lymphocytes, infiltrate the interstitial tissues and the walls of small bronchi and bronchioles. Although the cause is unknown, the prognosis is generally good, particularly if the patient responds to steroids.

This disease bears some resemblance to infection by *Aspergillus fumigatus* in which growth in the medium-sized bronchi of atopic individuals causes a mixed type I and type III reaction. It is more severe because the reaction is around, as well as in, the bronchi, with alveolitis in addition. Superimposed on asthma are repeated, transient pulmonary infiltrations, eosinophilic pneumonia, and thick bronchial mucous plugs at the site of which there is an irregular bronchiectasis, possibly the result of a type III reaction focally in the wall.[162] (See mucoid impaction, p. 1083.)

Drug reactions

Detailed consideration of the allergic types of drug-induced lung disease is not possible here. Davies has presented an extensive review.[166] Some examples are asthma induced by many antibiotics, radiopaque organic iodides, antisera, vaccines, pituitary snuff (see below); pulmonary eosinophilia caused by nitrofurantoin; and hydralazine-induced systemic lupus erythematosus. What appears to be allergic lung disease in drug addicts is cumulative pulmonary vascular obstruction attributable to insoluble particulate contaminants in the intravenously administered drugs (see Chapter 7).

Hypersensitivity pneumonitis caused by inhaled organic antigens (extrinsic allergic alveolitis)

Certain conditions can be gathered under the heading "hypersensitivity pneumonitis caused by inhaled organic antigens." Their symptoms and pathologic manifestations are similar but their origins are diverse.[171]

Group I—Antigenic molds (thermophilic actinomycetes, genus *Micropolyspora* and *Thermoactinomyces*)

Moldy hay
  Farmer's lung (*M. faeni, M. vulgaris*) (p. 1098)
Moldy residue of sugar cane
  Bagassosis (*M. vulgaris*) (p. 1097)
Compost for growing mushrooms
  Mushroom worker's disease (*M. faeni, M. vulgaris*)
Contamination of air-conditioning and heating systems[169] (thermophilic actinomycetes)

Group II—Antigenic bird droppings
  Bird-breeder's lung (pigeons; budgerigars)

Group III—Antigenic fungus in dead wood
  Maple bark–stripper's disease (*Cryptostroma corticale*, which may persist in the human lesion and be mistaken for *Histoplasma*)[168]
  Sequoiosis (redwood sawdust; *Graphium* and *Pullularia*)
  Suberosis (oak and cork dust; organic dust)
  Malt-worker's lung (*Aspergillus clavatus*)

Group IV—Antigen in wheat flour (*Sitophilus granarius*; wheat weevil)

Group V—Antigen is porcine and bovine posterior pituitary
  Pituitary snuff-taker's disease

Bird-breeder's (fancier's) lung. All the foregoing groups of conditions represent a type III (Arthus) allergic response to the avian serum protein in droppings. Antigen-antibody reactions form immune complexes that activate complement, so causing tissue damage. Intermittent exposure results in attacks that come on acutely after 5 or 6 hours, with the patient having fever, malaise, and muscle pains followed by cough and dyspnea. Regular, frequent exposure results in the insidious development of the disease, concealing the causal relationship. The morphologic responses are mainly in the alveolar tissues, and x-ray films show miliary infiltrations either basally or widespread. There is weight loss.

In biopsy material from bird-breeder's lung, alveolar septa are thickened by an infiltrate of lymphocytes, plasma cells, and histiocytes. Many large foamy macrophages are seen in the alveolar septa and lumens, intermingled with the other inflammatory cells or massed together. Foci of lymphocytes, without germinal centers, are common, especially beside bronchioles. Foreign body giant cells and sarcoid-like granulomas are common (Fig. 26-49). Eosinophils, vasculitis, and necrosis are not found.

When the disease becomes chronic, the foam cells of the early phase are diminished but, as shown in Fig. 26-50, obliterative and fibrotic changes ensue, and the basic lesion becomes chronic interstitial pneumonia with fibrosis.[170]

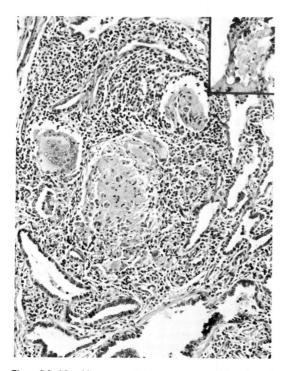

Fig. 26-49. Hypersensitivity pneumonitis. Small granulomas resembling those of sarcoidosis have formed in relation to several bronchioles and are accompanied by leukocytic and plasmacellular reaction. *Inset,* Foam cells that were found in another part of same slide. Allergen was not identified in this case. (177×.)

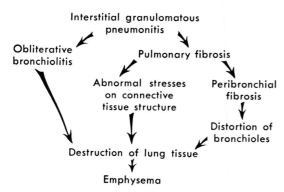

Fig. 26-50. Diagram showing how interstitial hypersensitivity (granulomatous) pneumonitis can lead to permanent pulmonary damage. (From Schlueter, D. P., Fink, J. N., and Sosman, A. J.: Ann. Intern. Med. **70:**457-470, 1969.)

In a recent fatal case there was diffuse fibrosis with honeycomb change.[167]

One must remember the following maxim when evaluating lung biopsies—if a dyspneic nontubercular patient has widespread miliary or nodular opacities on radiologic examination, consider first hypersensitivity pneumonitis. The most severe is farmer's lung (p. 1098), but there must be many as yet unrecognized causes of interstitial inflammation with sarcoidlike granulomas. New sources of environmental contamination are constantly being found (in cheese washers, furriers, coffee workers), often allergenic fungal spores.[169a]

Wegener's granulomatosis

The disease is a pathologic triad consisting of (1) necrotizing granulomas in the nose, paranasal sinuses, and lung, (2) vasculitis of small arteries and veins, and (3) glomerulitis. Clinically, there is a corresponding triad of intractable rhinitis and sinusitis, nodular pulmonary lesions with cough and hemoptysis, and terminal uremia.

As of 1969, at least 150 cases have been reported. All have been fatal, usually within 6 months, with a few patients lingering up to 4½ years. More recently, with the hypothesis that this is an immune complex–induced disease, treatment with cyclophosphamide and renal dialysis has been successful.[175] Some fulminating cases appear to have responded to immunosuppressive drugs, followed by renal transplantation.[180]

It is important to me to preserve the "sanctity of the syndrome." Unless an error by earler writers can be demonstrated or new information added that must modify earlier opinion, one cannot include cases satisfying only two of the three criteria. Carrington and Liebow have recognized this in reporting cases of necrotizing pulmonary granulomatosis under the title "limited forms of angiitis and granulomatosis of Wegener type."[174] Some of these patients have had multiple, bilateral, round masses in the lungs which have been classified microscopically as a lymphomatoid variant of "limited Wegener." On the other hand, some patients with the triad have additional evidence of vasculitis in the spleen, synovia, central nervous system,[173,178] orbit, breast, and skin, so that the patient may be first in the care of a dermatologist, a neurologist, an ear, nose, and throat specialist, or a general physician.

The changes in the paranasal sinuses are described on p. 1215 and the kidneys are described on p. 956.

Our present interest is in the lungs. In advanced cases, these are large and nodular. Over such nodules is a fibrinous pleuritis. When the lung is cut, several well-circumscribed firm areas are disclosed. Their centers tend to be softer than the rubbery periphery and are yellow or red-brown compared with the gray of the edges. There may be central cavitation. Some reach a diameter of 5 cm, but 3 cm is average. Infarcts of various sizes also are present. Small ulcers of the bronchial mucosa are common.

The key to the diagnosis is the microscopic demonstration of arteritis and phlebitis away from large areas of necrosis. Unlike polyarteritis nodosa and hypersensitivity angiitis, fibrinoid necrosis and eosinophilic infiltration of vascular walls are almost never seen. Most of the involved vessels are 2 mm or less in diameter. All their layers are infiltrated by lymphocytes and plasma cells, with some histiocytes and rare giant cells. A simple (nonfibrinoid) necrosis and abundant granulation tissue replaces much of the wall and narrows the lumen. Similar changes are seen in nearby small bronchi and bronchioles. Initial lung biopsies have been mistakenly diagnosed as rheumatoid granulomas.

It can be difficult to prove the diagnosis microscopically because necrosis may destroy the evidence of vasculitis (Fig. 26-51). Necrotic areas tend to be confluent. They may show no residue of structure or have a hazy stromal pattern in which there is cellular debris. Beyond the necrosis is a zone of granulation tissue with lymphocytes, plasma cells, and neutrophils. Giant cells of foreign body type and Langhans' type are numerous. At the periphery is a well-formed zone of fibroblasts.

From the category of "limited Wegener" a smaller group has been separated. Known as *lymphomatoid granulomatosis,* it is described as an angiocentric and angiodestructive lymphoreticular proliferative and granulomatous disease involving predominantly the lungs.[182] Usually the lymph nodes, spleen, and bone marrow are spared, but generalized atypical lymphoid hyperplasia may precede the lesions in the lung. Eventual cutaneous, renal, and central nervous system involvement is common; 26 of the first 40 patients have died, some with atypical lymphoma. The cellular infiltrations are variegated, with atypical and plasmacytoid forms; angiitis involves both pulmonary arteries and veins.

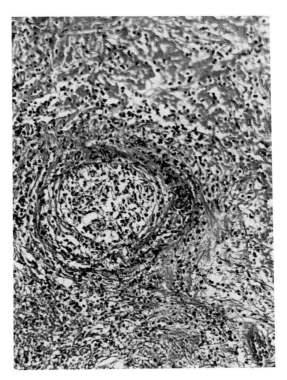

Fig. 26-51. Wegener's granulomatosis. Remnants of artery destroyed by vasculitis and surrounded by inflammatory and necrotic tissue. (150×.)

Liebow has described two more pulmonary granulomatoses. *Necrotizing "sarcoid" angiitis and granulomatosis* is relatively benign and confined to the lungs.[181] *Bronchocentric granulomatosis* appears to be a form of allergic bronchopulmonary aspergillosis.[179a]

Lethal midline granuloma

The term "lethal midline granuloma" fits the pathologic findings in a small group of patients suffering from a mutilating, progressive, ulcerating condition of the nose, sinuses, face, palate, and upper respiratory tract, including neighboring bone. The disease has been considered by some to be just one form of vasculitis and by others to be related to Wegener's granulomatosis.[172] (See p. 1089.)

Allergic granulomatosis

Patients with allergic granulomatosis resemble those with Wegener's granulomatosis. They differ in having a definite allergic history, asthma, and blood eosinophilia. There is no upper respiratory tract necrosis, and there is a Löffler type of pneumonia.[183] It is suggested that the condition belongs in the pulmonary-infiltrate-with-eosinophilia (PIE) syndrome

(p. 1087) as a subtype accompanied by pulmonary arteritis.[176]

Angiitis

The several conditions mentioned here are discussed in detail in Chapter 21.

The variety of *hypersensitivity angiitis* that is rapidly fatal after the administration of a drug is a necrotizing process very similar to polyarteritis nodosa but, unlike the latter, is prone to affect the lungs, where small infarcts are the result. Heart and kidney are also subject to damage.

Polyarteritis nodosa is uncommon in the lungs.

Unifying remarks

Most pathologists accept the concept of "lymphoma" as referring to definite histologic types having corresponding clinical courses. They also recognize that one type may convert into another or terminate as leukemia. To me, the just-described granulomas of the respiratory tract are analogous to the lymphomas. Certain pathologic types are associated with a certain course, but transformation and borderline cases are known to occur. An attempt to demonstrate this point is shown in Fig. 26-52.

PNEUMOCONIOSIS

A century ago Zenker coined the etymologically correct term "pneumonokoniosis," meaning "dust retained in the lungs." Modern definitions stating that the dust must stimulate fibrosis are incorrect. Pneumoconiosis is the focal desposition in the lungs of dusts that may be inert or may be fibrogenic. "Massive fibrosis" is induced in any pneumoconiosis by an infection, usually tuberculous. The *inert dusts* are gypsum, cement, and the oxides of tin, iron, and barium. Pure coal dust is almost inert. The *harmful dusts* are silica, asbestos, bauxite, and beryllium (see also p. 314).

Anthracosis and simple coal worker's pneumoconiosis

Anthracosis is the deposition in the lungs of coal, soot, and dust particles inhaled from the open air. Much of the material will be expectorated, but some is taken by macrophages from the alveoli into the pulmonary lymphatic vessels, ending up as fixed cells beneath the pleura, in septa, around vessels and bronchioles, and in the periphery of scars of the lung. This is the well-known blackening seen in virtually every adult lung.

Simple coal worker's pneumoconiosis (closely

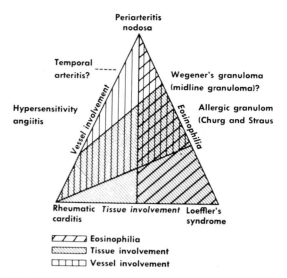

Fig. 26-52. Interplay between various types of vasculitis and granulomatosis in lung. At base are two conditions in which tissue involvement predominates and vascular involvement is negligible. Löffler's syndrome is a benign, transitory eosinophilic infiltration. Proceeding along right side of triangle, there is increasing vascular involvement as we reach allergic granuloma, which combines vasculitis and eosinophilia. Wegener's granulomatosis is closer to periarteritis nodosa, in which eosinophilia is a minor finding; tissue granulomas and vasculitis are prominent. Periarteritis nodosa is antithesis of Löffler's syndrome in that vasculitis is major feature and tissue involvement negligible. Passing down left side of triangle, we encounter conditions with vasculitis and no eosinophilia. In temporal arteritis; tissue involvement is not a feature, nor is it in hypersensitivity angiitis. Finally, we reach rheumatic carditis with its high incidence of tissue changes (Aschoff bodes). (From Sokolov, R. A., Rachmaninoff, N., and Kaine, H. D.: Am. J. Med. **32:**131-141, 1962.)

related to anthracosis) is seen in those who handle soft bituminous coal—either in the mines or by shoveling it in large quantities. No silicosis is involved, and the focal centriacinar emphysema found in miners may be coincidental. There is no impairment of health.

Simple coal worker's pneumoconiosis can only be diagnosed in life by radiographic changes induced by radiopaque components of the dusts (dust reticulation). Cigarette smoking probably potentiates the effects of the dust, but wives of miners have a higher prevalence of respiratory symptoms than do wives of nonminers. This suggests that other environmental factors must be at work.[196]

The first modern survey of coal worker's pneumoconiosis in the United States, based on new radiologic criteria and endeavoring to exclude sampling and observer errors was issued in 1973.[210] It showed a 30% incidence of pneumoconiosis in bituminous coal miners (22% had coal worker's pneumoconiosis of the lower (simple) grade, 6% had higher grades, and there was progressive massive fibrosis in 2%). In anthracite miners these figures are higher—60% had pneumoconiosis (22% with coal worker's pneumoconiosis of the higher grade and 14% with progressive massive fibrosis). A second review followed in 1976.[211] That all grades of simple coal worker's pneumoconiosis are associated with little respiratory impairment and disability is also demonstrated, a view coinciding with that of the British Industrial Injuries Advisory Council. A strongly contrary view is held by Davies.[206]

The gross lesion is the *coal macule,* which surrounds a respiratory bronchiole. It is 1.5 to 10 mm in diameter and can range from a limited distribution to wide dissemination in the whole of the lungs. Firm but not fibrous, it is seen as a black nodule. Dilatation of the related bronchiole and of neighboring alveoli gives rise to the focal emphysema of miners that cannot be distinguished from the centriacinar variety (p. 1061).

The dust penetrates the epithelium of the respiratory bronchioles and may enter the lymphatic vessels as free particles, some traveling to the hilar nodes and other farther, particularly to abdominal lymph nodes. Still others enter the bloodstream and are carried to the liver and spleen.

Some of the dust-filled macrophages collect in alveoli in such relatively fixed areas as the septa and subpleura and around arteries and bronchioles. Because alveoli in such situations have a limited ventilatory excursion, clearance of dust from them is limited.

Coal particles that reach the alveoli are no larger than 5 μm in diameter. They reach all parts of the lungs, but their concentration is greatest in the upper lobes. Some dust is carried not to the hilar nodes but to the normal small lymphoid collections. Here, the macrophages are held up indefinitely, and some die, releasing the dust. Coal macules are the result. Connective tissue response to the particles is irregularly arranged bundles of fibers but not a functionally significant fibrosis (see also p. 313).

Silicosis and coal worker's pneumoconiosis

Simple coal worker's pneumoconiosis and coal worker's pneumoconiosis sound so similar yet refer to a bland and a serious condition, respectively. The effects of silica-contaminated coal dust can be (1) simple coal worker's pneumoconiosis, (2) nodular silicosis, or (3) progressive massive fibrosis. The last two conditions comprise coal worker's pneumoconiosis.

Silica (silicon dioxide) and silicates occur all over the world. Wherever rock is to be cut, whether to gain granite, coal, gold, copper, or tin, silica dust is likely to fill the air. In the case of coal, it is the hard or anthracite variety that is accompanied by large amounts of silica. Other workers face the hazard—particularly stonemasons, sandblasters, boiler scalers, and those preparing clay for the manufacture of pottery (see also p. 314).

Role of silica. It has long been believed that were silica totally insoluble, it would not cause serious disease. It is poorly and weakly soluble, but the products of its solution are not the direct cause of disease. Only those particles less than 5 μm in diameter are significant. The apparent importance of particles less than 1 μm and even of ultramicroscopic size (less than 0.2 μm) is being studied. The nature of the reactive surface area and the total weight of dust present are vital factors. Many more factors are discussed in the publication of the American Medical Association's Council on Occupational Health.[184] Current opinion is that silica particles, in conjunction with or coated by the patient's plasma proteins, form an antigen the response to which leads to fibrosis.

Some inhaled silica particles will never get past an alveolar lumen. Others will adhere to the alveolar wall, damage the membranous pneumonocyte, and enter the interalveolar space, where they will be taken up by macrophages. A macrophage dies because the ingested particle damages the wall of the phagosome in which it lies, releasing lysosomal enzymes. Chemical substances released from the dead cell are fibrogenic, not the silica itself, and the greater the extent of destruction of macrophages, the greater the fibrosis.[3]

Still more silica particles penetrate the alveolar wall in the free state and can pass in this way to the hilar nodes, where at last they are trapped. When the particles are fine, some will enter the bloodstream, to be taken up by the liver and spleen.

It takes 10 to 15 years for the disease to develop except in the acute or rapid variety. The earliest symptoms are dyspnea and dry cough. Chest pain, night sweats, and hemoptysis occur later.

Gross appearance. The particles in lymphatic vessels are carried to the pulmonary lymphoid nodules at the bifurcations of major vessels and airways. Dying macrophages begin their irritative reaction in these sites, and the earliest lesions are only 1 to 2 mm in width, mostly in the upper lobes. It is nodularity that gives silicosis its unique appearance among the pneumoconioses. The nodules are fibrous and slowly increase in size until they can be recognized on roentgenographic examination. As nodules reach the surface of the lung, pleural adhesions are formed. Whatever anthracotic pigment is inhaled tends to be caught in the nodules, blackening them. By the time the patient dies of the disease, all parts of the lung are affected, the pleural cavities may be obliterated, and the nodules are readily palpated. They are black or gray-white and hard, and grate when cut. In an advanced case, the lungs may be almost completely solid. The hilar nodes are much enlarged, and their cut surface resembles the nodules. Important complications are emphysema, bronchiectasis, and cor pulmonale. Any cavities found should be considered to be a complicating tuberculosis until proved otherwise (see following discussion).

Microscopic appearance. The silica indirectly provokes connective tissue proliferation, and this becomes collagenous and densely hyalinized. The fibers are arranged in concentric bands that may interweave—a pattern seen much better with a reticulin stain (Fig. 26-53). No inflammatory reaction is present, but there may be some central necrosis. The periphery usually is quite sharply demarcated, although strands may weave into the neighboring interstitium of alveolar septa. Most of the trapped carbon will be at the periphery, where the silica mainly lies. Silica crystals can be seen only with polarized light. The nodule may obliterate perivascular lymphatic vessels or destroy an arterial or bronchial wall.

Variants of silicosis

Silicosis with tuberculosis. In some countries, two thirds of men with silicosis also have pulmonary tuberculosis. According to other reports, it occurs in 10%—still a high incidence. Large nontuberculous cavities occur in a minority of patients with silicosis as a result of ischemia and necrosis. There appears to be a synergism between silica and tubercle bacilli. In a number of patients, the disease advances fast and is fatal. The bacilli reproduce more rapidly in tissues in the presence of silica and strains not normally virulent lead to progressive tuberculosis in guinea pigs made to inhale quartz dust.

This type of tuberculosis is a central caseation of silicotic nodules with a peripheral reaction of tuberculous inflammation. The usual tubercles will be found in the nonsilicotic areas of the lung.

Progressive massive fibrosis. Progressive mas-

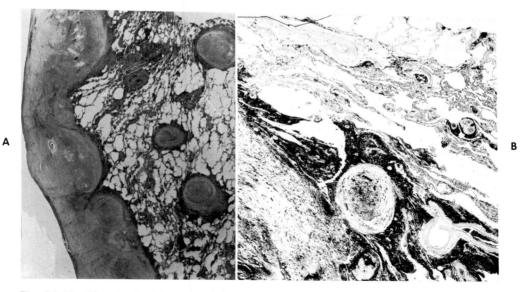

Fig. 26-53. Silicosis. **A,** Silicotic nodules in lung and pleura. **B,** Dense fibrosis with entrapped carbon. In center, silicotic nodule with concentric collagenous fibers. Normal lung above. (**A,** Low power; **B,** 22×.)

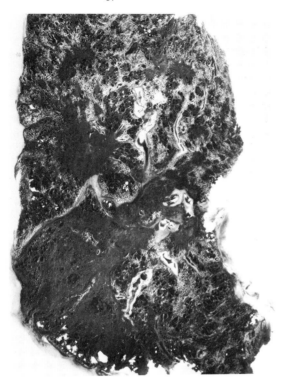

Fig. 26-54. Progressive massive fibrosis. Black areas were almost stony hard, attributed not to calcification, but to dense collagenization. Small dark areas are nodular lesions of silicosis.

sive fibrosis (tuberculosilicosis; conglomeration) also is known as complicated pneumoconiosis. After the onset of tuberculosis or a nonspecific infection in a patient with preexisting silicosis, conglomerate areas of fibrosis will develop (Fig. 26-54). These masses are irregular and slowly enlarge. There is occasionally central cavitation attributable either to caseation or to ischemia. Ischemic cavities tend to be small and slitlike and contain nonpurulent black fluid. They are caused by vascular obliteration induced by the fibrosis. Small pulmonary arteries are compressed and often totally fibrosed. The disease is not typical of tuberculosis in a nonsilicotic lung, and tubercles may not be seen. Mycobacteria may be hard to isolate, and in some patients there is no demonstrable cause of massive fibrosis.

Bronchitis and emphysema become superimposed upon the pneumoconiosis. Emphysema and cor pulmonale are now the most important causes of death in silicosis.

A black lung with the features of silicosis is found in *graphite* miners and those who work with the dust. Once again, silica is the fibrogenic agent.

Diatomite fibrosis. Diatomaceous earth contains fossil diatoms of almost pure silica less than 1 μm in diameter. The disease produced by it appears in 1 to 3 years. It causes not a nodular but a linear fibrosis of the pulmonary stroma. This is similar to the effects of pneumoconiosis from fuller's earth, a complex silicate.[198]

Rapid silicosis. Rarely, in men suffering heavy exposure to silica, typical silicosis will appear in 2 years. One reported case is that of a sandblaster who developed silicosis in 17 months and died 2 years after starting his occupation.[193] The authors who reported the case quote the estimate that this would require exposure to 100 million particles of pure silica per cubic foot of air. The patient's lungs weighed 3750 gm, and the right ventricular myocardium was 1 cm thick.

Rheumatoid pneumoconiosis. A modification in the pattern of silicosis has been observed in coal miners who develop rheumatoid arthritis.[185] It is a superimposition of the typical rheumatoid nodule upon silicotic lesions of a rather massive and extensive nature (Caplan's syndrome). This may occur quite early in the disease. Calcification, rare in progressive massive fibrosis, is seen in rheumatoid pneumoconiosis. The disease has been seen not only in coal workers, but also in sandblasters, potters, persons working with asbestos, and those working in foundries. Not all patients with pneumoconiosis and extrapulmonary rheumatoid disease develop rheumatoid lung lesions.[197]

Asbestosis

Asbestosis differs from other dust diseases in that the particles are relatively large fibers up to 50 μm by 0.5 μm. These are derived by crushing of the rock in which the fibers are up to 2 cm long. There is danger to the miners but more to the crushers and to workers in the many industries employing asbestos (fire-resistant materials, paper, plastics, brake linings, acoustical tiles). The products are ubiquitous. Usually, the disease develops about 15 years after exposure commenced, but occasionally this time is very much shorter. Breathlessness and cough appear relatively early, even when radiologic changes are minimal or absent.

Evolution of asbestosis. Pathogenesis is discussed on p. 315. The flexible, sharp-pointed fibers at first lie in the respiratory bronchioles, where they act as physical rather than chemical irritants. Nearly all of them are in the lower lobes. In time, a number pass into alveolar ducts and alveoli. The response is proliferation of connective tissue (later to be hyalinized) around the respiratory bronchioles and in the interalveolar septa, interlobular septa, and visceral pleura. British workers noted an increased incidence of tuberculosis in these patients in the 1940s, when the level of dust exposure was far greater than it is now; concomitant tuberculosis has virtually disappeared. Those who have had lengthy industrial exposure (20 years or so) have at least a tenfold risk of developing lung carcinoma in the affected lobe.[188] Furthermore, there is a heightened susceptibility to pleural mesothelioma (p. 316) or, through the diaphragm, peritoneal mesothelioma.[187,199] Although the risk of carcinoma is greatest in those exposed to asbestos for more than 20 years (whether or not they develop fibrosis), mesothelioma can arise earlier and from smaller doses.[191,201] A patient seen by me developed mesothelioma 30 years after 6 months of exposure to asbestos. Asbestos could still be found in the lung sections.

Gross appearance. An immediately noticeable change is great pleural fibrosis, frequently sufficient to obliterate the pleural space around the lower lobes. The pleura is so thick that it becomes rigid. Such a change is most characteristically seen as wide hyaline plaques of a cartilaginous consistency. They are composed of dense laminated acellular collagen, presumed to be a reaction to asbestos. In advanced disease, the lung is firm and small, with the lower lobe being more severely damaged. The cut surface of the lung is a sponge of alveoli and bronchioles surrounded by a fibrous network. Eventually, the fibrosis obliterates much lung tissue. Cor pulmonale and bronchiectasis are common. Because the asbestos fibers are too large to enter lymphatic vessels, there is no significant change in the hilar nodes.

Microscopic appearance. Interstitial fibrosis begins around bronchioles, slowly extending into and obliterating alveoli. Many alveolar cells have undergone cuboid metaplasia. Later, alveolar lumens are filled by fibrous tissue, although special stains will reveal an intact elastic framework. Fibrosis will envelop and destroy many lymphatic vessels, bronchioles, and small vessels. It is erroneous to regard the well-known asbestos bodies as pathognomonic. First, lungs commonly contain asbestos bodies without the disease asbestosis being present. Second, patients with talc pneumoconiosis have in their lesions material very similar to

asbestos bodies. Third, formation of bodies resembling asbestos bodies is not to be confused with pathogenicity. Although apparently identical, the central fiber may not be asbestos, a fact leading Gross to propose the term "ferruginous body." He was able to produce them in hamsters given fibrous aluminum silicate, silicon carbide whiskers, cosmetic talc, and glass fibers.[190]

An asbestos body is a simple fiber hidden beneath a yellow or golden-brown encrustation of iron salts and protein. Uneven deposition of this coat is responsible for the beaded shape with drumstick ends. By this stage of the disease, it is probable that the bodies cannot move. They lie where alveolar spaces used to be and are enveloped in fibrous tissue. Sometimes foreign body giant cells are close by (Fig. 26-55). Greenberg discusses the diagnostic importance of demonstrating ferruginous bodies in sputum.[189]

Finally, work in Britain and New York has demonstrated submicroscopic asbestos fibers (chrysotile) with or without asbestos bodies, in the lungs of workers exposed to these fibers. One patient suffered from what was morphologically fibrosing alveolitis.[194] We are thus left with the questions of how much asbestosis we

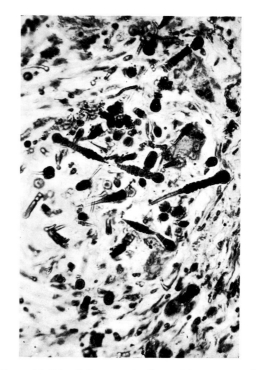

Fig. 26-55. Asbestos bodies. (Approximately 400×.)

miss by not using the electron microscope and how many cases of fibrosing alveolitis may be attributed to dust particles.

Berylliosis

Miners and handlers of crude beryl and related ores do not suffer from berylliosis. This affects those who extract beryllium from the ores or who handle it in industry, as in the making of alloys (see also p. 317).

Acute berylliosis is a chemical broncho-alveolitis induced by breathing fumes of beryllium oxide during the extraction process. Some patients die in 2 weeks. Others recover and appear to be well, although their chest x-ray films are abnormal. A third group of patients develop the chronic pulmonary form.

In the acute phase, the lungs are extremely heavy because of great edema. Alveoli are filled with fluid in which are macrophages, erythrocytes, fibrin, and some neutrophils.

To diagnose *chronic berylliosis,* one must know the risk of exposure because of the close resemblance to sarcoidosis. There is also similarity to farmer's lung. It is possible to demonstrate minute amounts of beryllium in tissue sections by use of microemission spectrography.[213]

Chronic berylliosis is of insidious onset, with lassitude, shortness of breath, loss of weight, and bilateral pulmonary infiltration shown in x-ray films.

There is pleural fibrosis, and the cut surface discloses streaks and nodules of fibrous tissue. The intra-alveolar granulomatous reaction of the early stage spreads to interstitial tissue. Initial lesions coalesce, forming focal, small, gray-white fibrous areas. Small cystic spaces with fibrous walls are also present. The fibrosis increases irregularly, and small nodular fibrotic areas are present in the pleura and hilar nodes. All parts of the lungs are affected. Granulomas also will be found in the skin, liver, kidney, skeletal muscle, and extrathoracic lymph nodes.

Microscopically, the basic lesion is the non-caseating granuloma, formed in vast numbers in the interstitial tissue beneath the pleura, in the septa, and around vessels and bronchi.[202] The earliest lesion is a loose collection of epithelioid cells surrounded by an ill-defined zone of lymphocytes, plasma cells, and Langhans' giant cells. In the latter, and sometimes lying free, may be seen any of three types of foreign body, which also are to be found in sarcoidosis. First is a sharp-edged birefringent, 3 to 10 μm crystal, occurring singly or in clumps. It

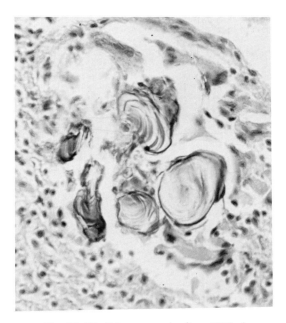

Fig. 26-56. Schaumann bodies. (390×.)

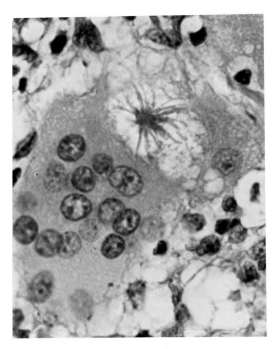

Fig. 26-57. Asteroid. (1026×.)

is calcium carbonate in the form of calcite, and it forms the nidus of the second type. Next is the conchoidal (Schaumann) body, so called because of its scalloped margin (Fig. 26-56). It may be as large as 50 μm, it has a concentric, laminated, deeply basophilic structure, and in the very center there may be a refrac-

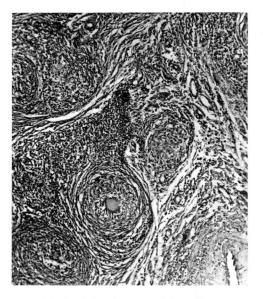

Fig. 26-58. Nodular lesions of beryllium granuloma in subcutaneous tissue. There is lamination of collagenous fibers around central giant cell.

tile crystal. The laminations appear to be successive depositions of calcium and iron upon a beryllium–plasma protein compound.[192] Further investigations suggest that they originate from aggregation of residual bodies (end products of activated lysosomes).[203] The third foreign body is the asteroid, which has a delicate, acidophilic, star-shaped cytoplasmic structure (Fig. 26-57). Its occurrence is quite infrequent compared with the 46% incidence of birefringent crystals and 42% incidence of conchoidal bodies in Williams' series.[202] Histochemical methods have failed to establish the composition of asteroids.

The granuloma ultimately undergoes fibrosis and hyalinization (Fig. 26-58). Meanwhile, lymphocytes and plasma cells advance into the interalveolar septa, which also become fibrotic. Damage to the alveolar septa results in the cyst formation seen grossly. Granulomas similar to those in the lung are to be found in the hilar nodes and follow the same changes.

Siderosilicosis

Iron oxide appears to be almost innocuous, but frequently silica accompanies it. The result is a modified silicosis, seen in hematite miners, welders, boiler scalers and other iron workers, and silver polishers.

The lungs of a miner of pure hematite may be the color of brick but free of fibrosis. When silica also has been present, changes similar to those of coal worker's nodular silicosis or progressive massive fibrosis are produced. Some patients have small fibrous nodules in the upper lobes, centrally red and whorled and peripherally dark red-brown. This is silicosis with a hematite hue, and the microscopy need not be repeated. Hematite is orange in polarized light, in contrast to the white of silica, and tissue reactions around the nodules liberate iron from hematite, so that a Prussian blue stain is positive.

The lungs of *silver polishers and arc welders* may be blackened by iron oxide dust and fumes, respectively. It is deposited in vessel walls and alveolar septa and fills some alveolar spaces. Once within macrophages, it can give a Prussian blue reaction. Accompanying silica may induce fibrosis in some arc welders.

Talcosis

Workers who prepare hydrated magnesium silicate (talc) or use it in factories may succumb to the fibrogenic impurities that accompany it. Among these is tremolite, which is one mineral form of asbestos. It causes a disease characterized by small fibrous nodules in the lower lobes. The nodes are gray and may coalesce to produce larger fibrous areas that are likely to undergo central cavitation. The absence of carbon distinguishes talcosis from coal miner's pneumoconiosis. Talc particles are taken into macrophages in alveolar septa, around small, but not large, vessels, and under the pleura. They are doubly refractile, irregular, and 1 to 2 μm in size. Tremolite fibers will form asbestos-like bodies and will induce further interstitial fibrosis.

Synthetic fibers

As the manufacture of synthetic fibers has multiplied, fears have been expressed that their inevitable inhalation by factory workers would prove harmful. This has not been the case for fiber glass, but textile workers manipulating and using acrylic and polyester fibers are now reported as suffering from fibrosing respiratory disease.[212]

OCCUPATIONAL LUNG DISEASES

In this section are discussed those inhalational lung diseases in which the noxious agents are molds or fumes.

Bagassosis

Bagasse (from an old word referring to the waste skin left after the oil is pressed out of olives) is the fibrous cellulose part of sugar cane, the residue after the juice has been crushed out. Bagasse is used in the manufacture of insulating materials. When men take it in a dry state from storage, they develop symptoms of hypersensitivity pneumonia, particularly in the upper lobes. This condition results only after several weeks or months of exposure. In some patients, it progresses to interstitial fibrosis with bronchiectasis and emphysema.

The cause is thermophilic actinomycetes. The disease was believed to be peculiar to New Orleans, but it has been seen in countries in which sugar cane is grown and in those to which bagasse is exported (see also p. 1088).[209]

Farmer's lung

Persons who work continuously with grain or hay in silage or spoiled by dampness may suddenly become very ill, with dry cough, severe dyspnea, and fever. This disease, known as farmer's lung, is attributable to sensitization to *Thermopolyspora polyspora* (p. 1088) in the moldy grain. In the United States, Wisconsin has had the most cases. Patients require several months to recover, and, if they return to the same work, their illness will recur more severely. The microscopic picture is the standard reaction of hypersensitivity pneumonitis (p. 1088 and Fig. 26-49).

Farmer's lung is recognized in Britain as an occupational disease. By 1968, in a chest clinic serving a population of 90,000 in a rural area of Wales, 245 cases of the disease had been registered.[215] It is most incapacitating when chronic, rather than when acute, and is then productive of airways obstruction. Five autopsies in the Welsh series have shown diffuse interstitial pulmonary fibrosis, honeycombing, histologic changes of pulmonary hypertension, and cor pulmonale. From a neighboring area in England comes an account of the first fatal acute case, a farmer's son who died after a few weeks of illness.[204]

Byssinosis

A nonfatal but disabling disease, byssinosis (Greek *bussos,* 'fine flax, fine linen') occurs in persons who work with cotton, flax, and hemp. It is characterized by its asthma-like symptoms, with severe chronic bronchitis that is never present on Sunday and worse on return to work on Monday. Byssinosis is a nonfibrogenic disease. Round or oval dust bodies are present in the lungs. They may be as large as 10 μm, with a black center surrounded by yellow. Apparently cotton dust contains a substance that releases endogenous histamine from lung tissue, causing bronchiolar contraction. The source is the bract rather than the fibers.

Byssinosis is an interesting disease because it gives the false impression of being caused by antigens released in textile dust or from cotton, hemp, or flax and because its existence is so often denied or its eradication falsely claimed.[207]

Diseases caused by industrial fumes

Mention already has been made of arc welder's disease and acute berylliosis. The fumes of cadmium and bauxite also are dangerous.

The risk from *cadmium* arises in atomic reactors, electroplating, and the production of alloys. About one in five men exposed to the fumes of cadmium oxide dies. Within the day, the affected person develops dyspnea, cough, and fever—an acute chemical pneumonitis (see Fig. 26-59 and p. 293 and Fig. 7-34).

Abrasives are manufactured from calcined *bauxite* at a high temperature, which releases fumes of submicron-sized silica and alumina (corundum). Although the lungs of those who work with these chemicals contain much silica, they do not have silicotic nodules, and the responsible component of bauxite fumes is not known. Aluminium is suspected, for it is no

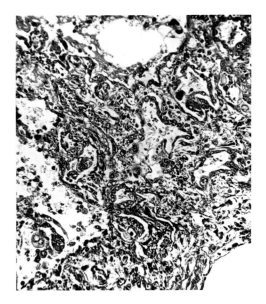

Fig. 26-59. Cadmium pneumonitis, example of chemical pneumonitis. Deformed alveoli lined by hyperplastic septal cells. Air spaces largely occupied by masses of similar cells, including bizarre giant cells.

longer considered harmless. Dust of aluminum metal has caused lung disease.

The chemical pneumonitis leads to a diffuse interstitial fibrosis that is followed by pronounced peripheral emphysema with bullae. Spontaneous pneumothorax is extremely common. The hilar nodes undergo a simple enlargement.

Silo filler's disease may be confused with farmer's lung because of the relationship to grain and farmers. A silo is a large, airtight chamber in which green crops are pressed and kept for fodder. In it, nitrogen dioxide is released by fermentation. The gas is present in greatest amount in the first 7 to 10 days after the silo is filled. Anyone entering may become unconscious in minutes and never recover. Other patients have a latent period of several days or weeks.

The oxides of nitrogen are readily soluble in water, forming nitrous and nitric acids. *Nitrous fumes* are a potential hazard in many industries and cause a disease identical to that suffered by silo fillers.[3,214] Those most severely affected die in a few days (p. 312).

PULMONARY FIBROSIS

Although the various occupational diseases cause pulmonary fibrosis, that term tends to be used in reference to diseases such as organizing pneumonia (p. 1070), lipid pneumonia (p. 1075), and brown induration (p. 1048). In the section that follows are discussed pulmonary fibrosis as found in connective tissue diseases, sarcoidosis, eosinophilic granuloma, diffuse interstitial fibrosis, and fibrosis from drugs.

First, some general information about alveolocapillary block and honeycomb lung is pertinent. *Alveolocapillary block* is a term coined to encompass certain clinical, physiologic, and pathologic changes. There is progressive dyspnea, tachypnea at rest, cyanosis (eventually even at rest), basal rales, and absence of wheezing or evidence of bronchial obstruction. Later, there is right-sided heart failure, and there may be clubbing of digits. There is reduction of diffusing capacity of the lung and reduced lung volume. The pathologic process is a diffuse widespread fibrosis of the interalveolar septa, or septal thickening by fluid, collagen, and proliferated cells of other than connective tissue origin. The causes include sarcoidosis, irradiation, the pneumoconioses, carcinomatous lymphangiosis, miliary tuberculosis, eosinophilic granuloma, progressive systemic sclerosis, rheumatoid lung, fibrosing alveolitis, and other granulomas and fibroses of uncertain cause.

Honeycomb lung is an excellent description of widespread disease in which large numbers of small cysts are formed in fibrotic lungs (Fig. 26-60), the causes being those of alveolocapillary block. There is obliteration, by fibrosis

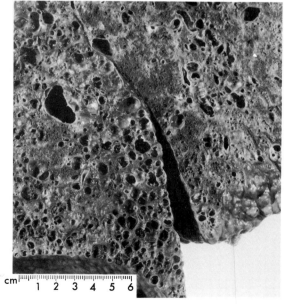

Fig. 26-60. Honeycomb lung showing at bottom right nodularity of pleural surface that has misled some to call condition "muscular cirrhosis."

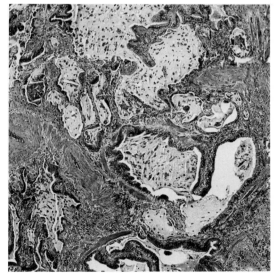

Fig. 26-61. Adenomatous proliferation of terminal bronchiolar cells in fibrous area of lung. (67×.)

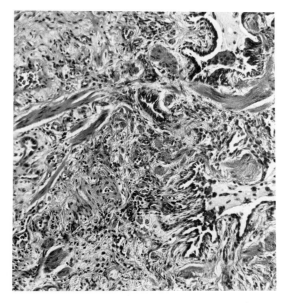

Fig. 26-62. Smooth muscle hyperplasia in fibrotic area of lung. (102×.)

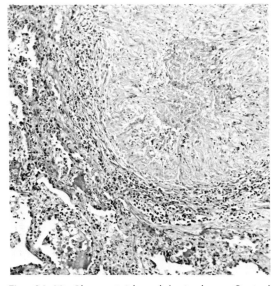

Fig. 26-63. Rheumatoid nodule in lung. Central necrosis with peripheral palisading of reactive cells and outer inflammatory exudate. (165×.)

or granuloma, of some of the bronchioles and their subdivisions.[218] Neighboring unaffected bronchioles undergo dilatation, forming cysts next to consolidated or fibrotic areas. Associated with this is alveolar septal fibrosis, often abetted by chronic pneumonitis or the specific pathologic process in the particular case. Some cysts become lined by flat or cuboid epithelium, which may be ciliated and mucin secreting (Fig. 26-61). Squamous metaplasia is common, and there is a risk of scar carcinoma (p. 1127). The interstitial and pericystic tissue is composed of young fibroblasts, with lymphocytes, plasma cells, histiocytes, some giant cells, elastic tissue, and smooth muscle.

Considerable masses of smooth muscle may proliferate from bronchi, bronchioles, arteries, veins, and lymphatic vessels[219] (Fig. 26-62). The muscle bundles run in various directions in relation to the channels from which they originated. Since these channels tend to become obliterated, muscle seems to arise directly out of interstitial fibrous tissue, the pulmonary septa, or the visceral pleura (Fig. 26-60).

Connective tissue diseases
Rheumatoid lung

The recognition of extra-articular manifestations of rheumatoid diseases has been especially centered on the cardiovascular system, central nervous system, and lungs. The

pulmonary lesions differ in that there is male instead of female preponderance.

In some patients, pleurisy with effusion accompanies exacerbations of rheumatoid arthritis. In others, it precedes joint disease by several years. A constantly noted characteristic of the pleural fluid is a very low glucose level (less than 10 mg to 15 mg per 100 ml). The common findings in the pleura are nonspecific adhesions and dense fibrosis. Only in a minority of patients have pleural biopsies revealed granulomas similar to those in the subcutaneous tissue.

In addition, there can be interstitial pneumonia, fibrosis, or honeycombing. The earliest change is a nonspecific interstitial pneumonia that can resolve. This is seen as edema and congestion of interalveolar septa. Lymphocytes infiltrate the septa and the area around vessels and bronchioles. Fibrin and some macrophages are in the alveoli.[216]

Should this condition persist, alveolar septa undergo progressive fibrosis. Germinal centers appear in some of the collections of lymphocysts, an important clue to the possibility of rheumatoid disease. Nodules form and may be 1 cm in diameter (Fig. 26-63). These are areas of fibrosing interstitial pneumonia, rarely containing small granulomas of the rheumatoid type (central necrosis with infiltrating neutrophils and a wavy palisade of radially arranged macrophages and, beyond this, scanty giant cells and a zone of lymphocytes and plasma cells). Sometimes there may just be inflammatory cells with small collections of macrophages and areas of fibrosis. Rheumatoid nodules are much commoner in miners with rheumatoid arthritis than in other persons with that disease.

The next stage is bronchiolectasis, consequent upon fibrosis. Many small and medium-sized arteries undergo fibrosis, beginning in the intima, extending into the media, and causing great luminal narrowing. The dilated bronchioles retain a muscle coat. Their epithelial lining is a single layer of flat or cuboid cells. Dilatation is eventually great enough to lead to a honeycomb appearance apparent to the naked eye, bronchioles now being surrounded by thick fibrous tissue containing many lymphocytes and plasma cells with occasional macrophages. Septal fibrosis is still apparent, and some alveoli are dilated.

Caplan's syndrome, or rheumatoid pneumoconiosis, is discussed on p. 1094. Rheumatoid lung bears a relationship to some cases of fibrosing alveolitis (p. 1104) although Scadding[220] is more cautious about accepting it than is Spencer.[3]

Systemic lupus erythematosus

In systemic lupus erythematosus, pleurisy (with or without effusion) is common and may cause the first symptoms. The patient frequently appears to have nonspecific patchy bronchopneumonia or interstitial pneumonia, with repeated attacks in different areas of the lungs. No diagnostic microscopic features are known, there being eventual fibrosis. In a few lungs, there is arteritis with fibrinoid degeneration.[216a]

Progressive systemic sclerosis (scleroderma)

Patients with pulmonary involvement by scleroderma are likely to be women in later life. Localizing symptoms are a dry or productive cough and increasing dsypnea. These may precede the cutaneous findings, and a pulmonary component is rather common. There is an increased collagen-like deposition in the basement membranes of small pulmonary vessels. In turn, there is fibrosis of alveolar septa and interstitial tissue (Fig. 26-64). As arteriolar lumens become narrowed, alveolar tissues become necrotic, and microcysts are formed. Fibrosis is progressive, and the lung loses its elasticity. In the end, even the bronchi undergo fibrosis, with areas of constriction and sacculation.

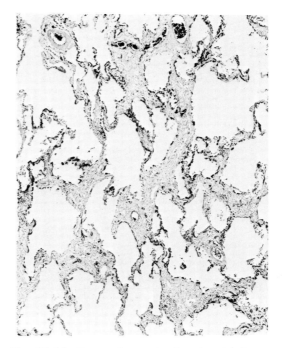

Fig. 26-64. Progressive systemic sclerosis. Severe interstitial fibrosis. (52×.)

Grossly, the lower lobes suffer most. The pleura is fibrotic. On the cut surface, a network of interstitial fibrosis encloses cystic spaces no bigger than 1 cm in diameter. There are also fibrous nodules of 1 to 15 mm in diameter. The cysts are frequently peripheral, and the dense, fibrous, airless areas are central.[217] In the latter, the vascular and alveolar structures are replaced. Bronchiectasis is common. As might be expected, in such far-advanced cases there is pulmonary hypertension and right ventricular hypertrophy.

Microscopically, in the earlier stage the alveolar septa are thickened by cellular proliferation and prominent capillaries. As they are smothered by ever-increasing collagen deposition, the septa undergo disruption and now surround spaces larger than alveoli. Lymphocytes in moderate numbers infiltrate this tissue, and the alveolar lining cells proliferate. Arterioles are obliterated, and slowly, over some years, the fibrosis progresses until in many areas alveoli cannot be recognized. Meanwhile, the inflammatory reaction has abated.

Sarcoidosis

Sarcoidosis (sarcoid, 'fleshlike') remains a mystery. Its characteristic lesion closely resembles that of any granuloma in a nonnecrotic or noncaseous stage, whether fungal or tuberculous, and it is indistinguishable from beryl-liosis and from certain lesions of leprosy and histoplasmosis. Histologic reactions identical to it are well known in the regional lymph nodes draining a carcinoma.[228] I have seen such lesions develop within a couple of months in a wound resulting when a child fell against a stone step. Such lesions are silicon granu-lomas, identical to the sarcoid lesion except for the presence of doubly refractile crystals, usually in the foreign body giant cells.[230] Users of deodorant containing zirconium sometimes develop local reactions like that of sarcoidosis. Many patients with sarcoidosis-like lesions live in pine forest regions; pine pollen is acid-fast and produces sarcoidosis-like lesions when in-jected into ginuea pigs. However, the incidence of sarcoidosis is higher in nonpiny rather than in piny areas of the countries concerned.

British investigators believe, in part because of the persistent teachings of Scadding,[231] that sarcoidosis is a manifestation of tuberculosis. In his series of 230 cases, tubercle bacilli were isolated from 18 patients in the sarcoid phase, from 11 during overt caseating tuberculosis that preceded sarcoidosis, and from five when sarcoidosis was followed by caseating tuber-culosis. Bacilli were of the human strain and were virulent for guinea pigs, and the orga-nisms were sometimes first isolated when the disease passed from the clinical picture of sarcoidosis to one of caseating tuberculosis. This coincided with a change from the state of tuberculin negativity to that of positivity. In a study[222] similar to Scadding's, there were 14 black adults, five of whom developed sar-coidosis after well-documented tuberculosis. Six started with sarcoidosis, developed tuber-culosis, and then reverted to the sarcoid state. In three patients, the two diseases coexisted.

Scadding suggests that an immunologic ab-normality precedes the sarcoidosis and that this results in tuberculosis infection being associ-ated with sarcoidosis instead of tuberculosis. Whether this explains the failure of sarcoidosis to respond to antituberculous drugs is doubt-ful. The lesions are modified by steroids.

Further evidence of a relationship to tu-berculosis is as follows:

1. The prevalence of sarcoidosis changes in the same direction as tuberculosis in sev-eral ethnic groups.[232]
2. A prospective study of 360 sarcoidosis patients in Philadelphia disclosed the sub-sequent development of tuberculosis in 13 (3.6%).[226]
3. A joint study from Cincinnati and

Czechoslovakia has demonstrated acid-fast bacilli in 100 patients with sarcoido-sis.[236]
4. A more speculative argument is based on the demonstration that, although pa-tients with tuberculosis or sarcoidosis often also are infected with mycobac-teriophages, only in those with sarcoidosis is there an absence of antibody to the phage; perhaps this makes the difference between their developing tuberculosis or sarcoidosis.[229] Phage-infected mycobac-teria lose their acid-fastness and hence are difficult to identify. Lack of phage-neutralizing antibodies may acount for the lack of caseation in sarcoidosis and the relative anergy to tuberculin. It may be that patients who already have sar-coidosis have increased vulnerability to mycobacterial infection.[234]

The Kveim test (p. 1103) is nearly always negative in tuberculosis and leprosy. There are well-documented cases of sarcoidosis-like lesions after BCG vaccination, and even clin-ical sarcoidosis has occurred.[223] Others merely become Kveim-positive. These findings accen-tuate the complex interrelationship of sar-coidosis, tuberculosis, and Kveim antigen.

Many have suggested that the worldwide sarcoidosis with identical clinical, radiologic, and pathologic findings is a syndrome of many causes, so that one might speak of tuberculous sarcoidosis, beryllium sarcoidosis, or, in the case of the injuries mentioned previously, quartz or silica sarcoidosis. What we are now discussing may be "idiopathic sarcoidosis." Waksman's hypothesis is attractive: "that all lesions of sarcoid type are immunologic re-actions to more or less widely disseminated antigens which are either of low solubility or unmetabolisable."[237] Scadding's admittedly fanciful conclusion is that, if most sarcoidosis is mycobacterial and since tuberculosis is de-clining, the controversy around the etiology of sarcoidosis may not be resolved before the disease disappears![232]

Clinical picture and diagnosis. Sarcoidosis spares practically no organ. Epithelial and endothelial surfaces and the adrenal glands are strange exceptions to this. Although its manifestations are protean, its course may be so silent that only a routine chest x-ray ex-amination discloses its presence. A joint study from London and New York indicates that symptomatic sarcoidosis (respiratory, dermato-logic, and lymph node) is balanced by an equal amount of silent disease.[225] Many cases have been unexpected findings at autopsy, and many others undergo spontaneous regression. There is a significant female predominance, and the highest incidence of the disease is among blacks and Scandinavians. The majority of the blacks are young women. Most childhood cases in the United States have been in blacks. The lung is a common site of involvement, usually with initial hilar lymphadenopathy. Rarely, this may incite a middle lobe syndrome by bronchial compression. Otherwise, the complaints are vague and slight—persistent cough, sometimes loss of weight, and occasionally fever and sweating. Pulmonary insufficiency is rare and indicates extensive fibrosis. Few persons die from sarcoidosis; the commonest cause of death is heart failure associated with severe pulmonary damage. Others succumb to direct cardiac or cerebral involvement.

Dyspnea worsens with increasing pulmonary function changes and advancing radiologic staging of sarcoidosis.[221] Dyspnea is most frequently associated with expiratory slowing, to which both pulmonary restriction and intrinsic bronchial obstruction contributed. In 107 patients with bronchopulmonary sarcoidosis it was shown that dyspnea is associated with irreversible disease, inasmuch as it could rarely be relieved by corticosteroids.

A worldwide survey indicates a mortality risk of 5% in patients with this disease.[235]

Serum protein levels often are abnormal, with reduced albumin and with globulin of 3.5 or more grams per 100 ml. In 10% to 20% of patients, there is a serum calcium of 11 to 15 mg per 100 ml, with normal phosphorus levels.

The *Kveim test* involves the use of a saline extract of known human sarcoid tissue that, when injected intradermally into persons with sarcoidosis, will slowly produce a local sarcoid granuloma in 60% to 90% of cases. This must be identified by biopsy 4 to 7 weeks later. The reaction is weaker or negative in quiescent stages and becomes positive again with recurrences. The Kveim test is positive in 84% of those with histologic sarcoidosis and in many without it who later develop such lesions.[233] The rate of false positivity is 1% to 2%.[233]

The reliability of the Kveim test has been questioned. It has been found to be positive in many patients with Crohn's disease, and in a recent study of patients with sarcoidosis, it was positive only when there was pronounced lymphadenopathy. Furthermore, it was positive in patients with chronic lymphocytic leukemia, tuberculosis, infectious mononucleosis, and nonspecific cervical adenitis.[224] This appears to be the result of defects in the antigen used. The debate giving the opposing views of Israel and Siltzbach on the reliability of the test should be read.[225]

A valuable differential point for clinical diagnosis is a biopsy from the gastrocnemius, which is not likely to be affected by tuberculosis but may reveal sarcoid granulomas. Scalene node and liver biopsies are also fruitful.

About 10% of 227 patients with sarcoidosis had pleural fibrosis or effusion; granulomas could be found when pleural biopsies were taken.[238] During thoracotomy, granulomas are sometimes noted projecting from the surface of the visceral pleura. Pleural involvement is an important sign of progression of the disease.

Gross appearance. The hilar and mediastinal lymph node enlargement is sometimes so great that the designation "potato nodes" has been applied. This is only in the early stages, because later on there is healing that ranges from restoration of the normal state to fibrosis without calcification. In the lung, there are disseminated miliary or nodular fibrous foci with diffuse linear infiltrations. They extend out from the hila in a bilaterally symmetric fashion, tending to become broader and more extensive. Interstitial fibrosis and transformation of alveoli into enlarging cysts create the rare examples of sarcoid honeycomb lung. The nodular variety of sarcoidosis produces lesions measured in a few millimeters, but they may reach 2 cm in diameter. Cavitation is very rare.

Microscopic appearance. The characteristic appearance has been mentioned in the discussion of berylliosis (p. 1096). There is a small, sharply delimited collection of epithelioid cells. Among them are foreign body giant cells, Langhans' giant cells, and the Schaumann and asteroid bodies, which have little value in diagnosis since they are nonspecific. Peripherally, there is a small zone of lymphocytes and plasma cells (Fig. 26-65, *A*). These discrete nodules appear in clusters and, by partial coalescence, form larger complexes (Fig. 26-65, *B*).

It is incorrect to believe that central coagulative necrosis, or even apparent caseation, rules out the diagnosis of sarcoidosis. Small zones of eosinophilic granular necrosis may occur (but with intact reticulin), and acid-fast stains will be negative. If regression is

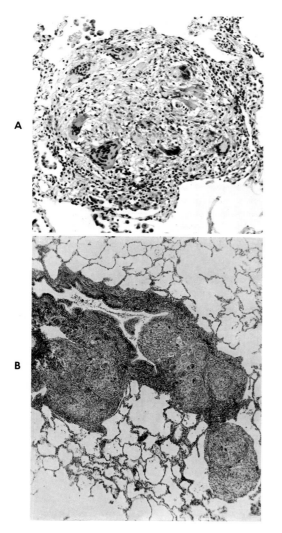

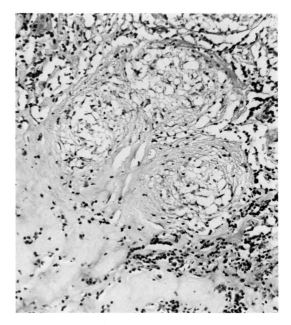

Fig. 26-66. Collagenization of sarcoid lesion. (165×.)

Fig. 26-65. Sarcoidosis. **A,** Single noncaseating granuloma. **B,** Nodular granulomas surround bronchiole and small vein. (**A,** 153×; **B,** 40×.)

taking place, fibroblasts grow in and lay down a dense collagen between the epithelioid cells (Fig. 26-66). This is the tissue that produces pulmonary fibrosis. The lesions are in alveolar walls but are also perivascular and peribronchial. Sarcoidosis can often be diagnosed by random biopsy of bronchial mucosa. Fibrosis in such situations can lead to stenosis of bronchi or bronchioles.

In conclusion, I must say that microscopic evidence does not prove a diagnosis of sarcoidosis. The report must be in such terms as "tuberculoid granuloma compatible with sarcoidosis" if such is the clinical impression.

Diffuse interstitial pulmonary fibrosis (fibrosing alveolitis)

Many diseases fulfill the descriptive designation "diffuse interstitial pulmonary fibrosis." Hamman and Rich believed that they were describing a new and relatively acute entity. We now recognize an acute disease that becomes chronic, "characterized by an inflammatory process in the lung beyond the terminal bronchiole having as its essential features (1) cellular thickening of the alveolar walls showing a tendency to fibrosis, and (2) the presence of large mononuclear cells, presumably of alveolar origin, within the alveolar spaces."[249] This is a broad general category of disease and inflammation. In the first cases described, the patients survived 6 weeks to 6 months. We now know that most patients live for a number of years. A survey of 96 patients disclosed that only 16% had a worthwhile response to corticosteroids, and the 5-year-survival of this group was 67%. Only 20% of the nonresponding patients lived for 5 years. In all, there were 59 deaths.[250]

Liebow and associates[241,242] call the disease under discussion "usual interstitial pneumonia" to distinguish it from "desquamative interstitial pneumonia" and from "lymphoid interstitial pneumonia." Scadding finds that term confusing because there is no pneumonia in the usual sense of the term and "interstitial" is not synonymous with "interalveolar." Hence "alveolitis" is preferable, and it is of a "fibrosing" type.[248]

Most patients have been adults 30 to 50 years of age, but six cases have been recorded in infancy.[240] They have progressive dyspnea, unproductive cough, cyanosis, and weight loss. Tachypnea, fever, and cyanosis at rest are common in the later stages.

Grossly, the lungs in earlier cases have increased consistency. Microscopic changes are already well under way. Eventually, the lung becomes rather solid, often with pleural fibrosis. Typically, there is the widespread bilateral, but not uniform, appearance of honeycomb lung. In some lungs, the surface is nodular, since the raised areas are up to 1 cm and correspond to projecting cysts. The depressions between them are of fibrous tissue. Such changes are greatest in the lower and outer zones and resemble the exterior of a hobnailed liver.

Microscopically, the initial changes are edema and increased vascularity of the interalveolar septa. Then mononuclear and histiocytic infiltration of the septa appears with fibrous exudate in the alveoli. Reticulin fibers are being laid down. Alveolar lining cells become cuboid, and relatively few erythrocytes and leukocytes are seen in the alveolar space. A hyaline membrane is sometimes seen. Reticulin becomes collagen, and alveolar capillaries gradually are replaced, whereas in other places they undergo a remarkable hyperplasia in the midst of young fibrous tissue. The disease is also active around terminal bronchioles and alveolar ducts. As interstitial fibrosis advances, many alveoli and bronchioles are converted by metaplasia of their lining into a pseudoglandular pattern (Fig. 26-61). The small pulmonary arteries undergo intimal thickening. Intra-alveolar fibrosis follows, and alveoli are squeezed out of existence. Smooth muscle hyperplasia is apparent in the fibrous tissue (Fig. 26-62). Small cysts are created.[220] The normal tiny lymph follicles of the lungs become hyperplastic. Even in a late stage of the disease, coexisting early lesions can be found nearby.

With the knowledge from the roentgenogram that the condition is diffuse and bilateral, that the known causes of honeycomb lung have been excluded, and that the patient suffered a (usually) chronic course, the pathologist can diagnose fibrosing alveolitis. This means the exclusion of late stages of hypersensitivity pneumonias, sarcoidosis, berylliosis, connective tissue disorders, silo filler's disease, mercury vapor inhalation, irradiation damage, and rheumatoid diease. Fifteen families are now known in which many members (starting sometimes in early childhood) have fibrosing alveolitis, transmitted as an autosomal dominant.[251] In 27% of one series of cases, rheumatoid factor was present in the patients' sera. In another series, 14% of the patients had rheumatoid arthritis. Deposits of IgM and rheumatoid factor have been demonstrated along the alveolar walls.[220]

Desquamative interstitial pneumonia

Desquamative interstitial pneumonia causes dyspnea, dry cough, fatigue, and weight loss without fever. About 50 cases have been reported. Radiologic changes include a ground glass opacity in the base of each lobe. This corresponds to patchy, firm, airless, yellow-gray areas. Striking microscopic findings are the uniform diffuse masses of intact desquamated granular pneumonocytes and macrophages filling many alveoli. They are large, with plentiful PAS-positive, brown, granular cytoplasm that is free of lipid and contains little iron. Lined up along the alveolar septa, they continue to divide after desquamation. Hyperplastic lymphoid follicles are prominent. Despite the name of the disease, interstitial inflammatory activity is slight and fibrosis usually insignificant. Consequently, the patients do quite well and are helped by steroids. Nevertheless, after a long follow-up of 13 cases of the disease, one third either died or were showing progressive disability despite immunosuppressive and steroid therapy.[246]

Probably the disease is a densely cellular, lightly fibrous variant of fibrosing alveolitis,[249] and several more cases are reported suggesting this.[245] Further, some patients have microscopic features of both types.[248]

Giant cell interstitial pneumonia is a very rare disease, possibly related to desquamative interstitial pneumonia. Bilaterally, there is a lymphocytic interstitial infiltrate, and bizarre multinucleated giant cells fill the alveoli.[247]

Lymphoid interstitial pneumonia

Lymphoid interstitial pneumonia appears to be an immunoproliferative disorder not related to fibrosing alveolitis. Many of the patients have hypergammaglobulinemia without a monoclonal peak,[239] but the latter also is recorded.[244] This is a slowly progressing disease with increasing dyspnea. In sections, one sees alveolar septa distended by masses of mature lymphocytes with some intermingled large monocytes and plasma cells. The infiltrate extends into interlobular septa and encloses bronchioles and vessels.[243] Differentiation from lymphoma can be difficult and relies on the mixture of mature cells and the absence of lymph node involvement.

Eosinophilic granuloma and related conditions

All members of the histiocytosis X triad, when disseminated, also may affect the lung,[252] but *eosinophilic granuloma* may be solely pulmonary. Hand-Schüller-Christian disease and Letterer-Siwe disease are discussed elsewhere (p. 1510). Eosinophilic granuloma is a chronic inflammatory disease of unknown etiology characterized primarily by the presence of histiocytes, eosinophils, and fibroblasts. Many cases confined to the lung have been described. To date, electron microscopic studies have failed to elucidate the nature of the disease in the lung.[253]

Most of the patients have been young men. A number are discovered by routine chest x-ray examination, which discloses increasing diffuse, bilateral reticulonodular densities. Some patients remain well for as long as 15 years. Others suffer progressively worsening cough and dyspnea, which may be totally disabling as the disease advances. Corticosteroids have aided these patients. Because of the formation of bullae, pneumothorax is a common complication.

The few open thoracotomies performed have allowed observation of many nodules up to 1 cm in diameter. In advanced cases, there is extensive fibrosis and honeycomb lung, more pronounced in the upper lobes.

Pulmonary biopsies reveal fairly well-demarcated, nodular, interstitial lesions composed of eosinophils and histiocytes, with some lymphocytes and plasma cells. Alveoli are filled with histiocytes, and the septa are thickened by proliferation of fibroblasts. Some histiocytes contain hemosiderin. Later, eosinophils become scanty, interstitial fibrosis is predominant, and many distal air spaces are lined by cuboid or low columnar epithelium. Diagnosis at this stage is difficult, and one should look for the iron-containing histiocytes and make multiple sections, for one of the characteristics of eosinophilic granuloma is its variability of development from one area to

another. A helpful point is that the elastic fibrils and laminae of alveolar septa, bronchioles, and vessels become progressively more disrupted and scanty and finally they disappear. Although this also is observed in sarcoidosis and viral pneumonia, it is not seen in fibrosing alveolitis.

They are not primarily pulmonary diseases. Another condition of more generalized nature is *chronic granulomatous disease*. This syndrome consists of chronic suppurative lymphadenitis, hepatosplenomegaly, eczematoid dermatitis, and pulmonary infiltrations associated with hypergammaglobulinemia. These lesions resemble those of cat-scratch disease, with numerous pigmented histiocytes. In the classic form, confined to boys, death comes in the first decade. The basic anomaly is the failure of the patient's neutrophils to kill bacteria after ingesting them, because of delay in release of lysosomal enzymes. There are other familial and nonfamilial variants, some in girls, some with defective immunoglobulins.[254]

Fibrosis caused by drugs

A number of drugs have been reported to cause interstitial pulmonary fibrosis. Among them are busulfan (Myleran), nitrofurantoin (Furadantin), hexamethonium, methysergide, and oxygen. It is always difficult to prove that a particular drug is responsible, but at least there is an association.[258] Heard and Cooke[255] have shown that the alleged interstitial fibrosis of busulfan and hexamethonium is intraalveolar because of organization of fibrinous edema presumably caused by the drugs. Busulfan also stimulates epithelial cells in various parts of the body to enlarge, including the alveolar lining cells, which reach up to 40 μm by 20 μm in size (Fig. 7-15). Ingestion of the herbicide Paraquat can cause fatal interstitial fibrosis.

That *oxygen* in high concentration is poisonous to animals has been known for many years. Not until 1967, when Nash et al.[257] reported on 70 cases, was there wide acceptance of the danger of mechanical respirators. Damage is related to the concentration of oxygen and the duration of exposure. It begins to appear in about 4 days, and concentrations greater than 80% are the most damaging (see also p. 260).

Experiments on monkeys show that the alveolar lining epithelium is almost completely destroyed in 4 days and that the type I cells are replaced by type II cells, which, with interstitial fibers and cells, greatly thicken the alveolar septa. Initially the injury is to the alveolar capillary endothelial cells. In these experiments, complete return to normal function was possible.[256]

The damage caused by oxygen has complicated interpretation of manifestations of a number of diseases, especially hyaline membrane disease and postperfusion lung.

The lungs are heavy, relatively dry, and beefy. In the early phases, there is congestion, edema, and hemorrhage in the alveoli. A fibrin exudate is turned into a hyaline membrane. No inflammation is seen. Later, edema is pronounced in the alveolar and interlobular septa. Alveolar lining cells are prominent and hyperplastic, and beneath them fibroblasts begin to proliferate (Fig. 26-67). By now damage is severe and alveolocapillary block has started. The dilemma is there—oxygen is needed and "the brain softens before the lung hardens."

TUBERCULOSIS

Tuberculosis is the infectious disease caused by several different species of mycobacteria. Originally only *Mycobacterium tuberculosis* var. *hominis* and *M. tuberculosis* var. *bovis* were identified as pathogenic for man. In recent years, the unclassified (anonymous, atypical) mycobacteria have become important.

Prevalence

The high infectivity of pulmonary tuberculosis and the extent of disease in cows have caused this to be one of the most common and lethal infectious diseases throughout the world. In North America and Western Europe, improved hygiene and living standards have greatly diminished the prevalence of tuberculosis, with pasteurization of milk and control of herds playing an important role. Earlier diagnosis and more effective treatment also play their part. In the United States in 1965, about 52,000 new cases of pulmonary tuberculosis were reported. This dropped to 44,000 in 1967, still an enormous number of cases of a largely preventable disease. In England and Wales in 1971 there were 11,700 cases of tuberculosis and 1460 deaths. The infection rate in Indian immigrants is 12 times and in Pakistanis 26 times that of British natives. Most of them contract the disease after arriving in Britain. In the United States in 1970 there were 37,000 new cases of tuberculosis and 5560 deaths (an increased mortality of 4.1% over the previous year). The 1970 case

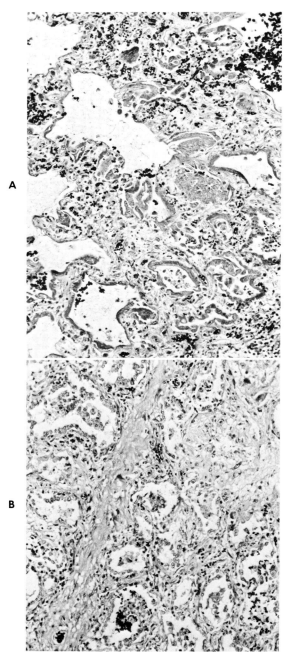

Fig. 26-67. Oxygen toxicity. **A,** Early stage—about sixth day. Hyaline membrane, reactive alveolar cells, and pronounced interstitial edema and congestion without inflammatory reaction. **B,** Later stage—about fourteenth day. Progression to early interstitial fibrosis, still without significant inflammation. (**A** and **B,** 165×.)

rate for whites was 12.4 per 100,000 and for nonwhites 59 per 100,000, although in some cities the rates were two times greater than these figures.

Wide differences between death and case rates are shown by the 1959 figures from Japan—death rate, 35.4; case rate, 537.7. Moreover, these data represent the prevalence of *tuberculous disease,* whereas if the entire population was given skin tests, there would be a third, even higher figure—the prevalence of *tuberculous infection.* This includes active disease and disease overcome in the past, but with skin allergy persisting. Even in the Western world, the sharp decline in the death rate has not been accompanied by a proportionate fall in the number of new cases. The death rate in Africa and Asia stands at about 300 per 100,000. The lowest incidence rates are in Holland, Denmark, New Zealand, and Australia (in order of increasing figures). The total of world deaths from the disease per year is 5 million.

Organism

Mycobacterium tuberculosis is a slender, straight, or slightly curved rod. Its length varies from 1 to 4 μm, with occasional longer filamentous forms. It is either homogeneous or beaded in the Ziehl-Neelsen stain. There is no way of identifying microscopically which species of *Mycobacterium* has caused the disease.

The organism is aerophilic but can multiply slowly at fairly low oxygen tensions, as would be found near the center of a caseous lesion or when a lung is collapsed or the blood supply to the center of a lesion is cut off. Bacilli do not proliferate in the center of closed caseous areas, yet often multiply at an enormous rate if aeration is reestablished, as by a bronchus or blood vessel opening into the lesion. It is also likely that this will alter the pH of the region in favor of more rapid growth. Fatty acids released in caseous areas inhibit their growth. A single organism is potentially infective, but there must be 1 million bacilli or clumps of bacilli per milliliter of bacterial suspension before microscopic examination reveals more than one organism per 10 oil-immersion fields. Therefore, the report of "absent or scanty organisms" can be extraordinarily misleading.

Chemistry of tubercle bacillus

The tubercle bacillus does not have exotoxins or endotoxins to explain its virulence, but there are important chemical components in its body that produce far-reaching effects in the human being. Fifty percent of the organism is a lipid that, although no longer believed to form a waxy coat, is in some way responsible for acid-fastness. The more virulent the organism, the more lipid it contains. Lipids also seem to stimulate monocytes and macrophages to become epithelioid cells or to divide into multinucleated Langhans' cells.

The protein fraction, "tuberculoprotein," is principally important for inducing sensitization in the patient, but it also stimulates formation of Langhans' and epithelioid cells. The carbohydrate, in the form of polysaccharides, provokes a neutrophilic reaction locally and an outpouring of young neutrophils from the bone marrow.

Tuberculin test

Products derived from tuberculoprotein can be injected intracutaneously for the Mantoux test. These include old tuberculin (OT) and purified protein derivative (PPD). A positive test indicates that a person now has, or had in the past, active tuberculosis. Thus it is mainly of exclusionary value except in "conversion"—when a patient previously known to be negative becomes positive to a later test.

Unclassified (atypical) mycobacteria

A possible relationship between saprophytic acid-fast bacilli and human disease was first considered in 1935. About 1948, infections by what were called "yellow" or "atypical" acid-fast bacilli were being reported. Today, in the United States, subject to regional variations, 1% to 10% of persons believed to have tuberculosis have *mycobacterial pseudotuberculosis* (nontuberculous mycobacteriosis) caused by what are now called anonymous or unclassified mycobacteria. They differ vastly from *M. tuberculosis* in that their cultural characteristics are distinct, they do not cause progressive disease in guinea pigs but sometimes do so in mice, and they are resistant to streptomycin, isoniazid, and para-aminosalicylic acid. Some newer drugs have been effective, and the group II organisms have been found particularly susceptible to chemotherapy. These organisms are not mutants produced by drugs.

The term "unclassified" means that characteristics are not yet sufficiently established to allow designation of species. The grouping that follows is not classification in the biologic sense.

Four groupings of these organisms have

been made.[276] Group I, the photochromogens, includes *M. kansasii*. About two thirds of mycobacterial infections in Britain are attributable to group I. In the United States, organisms of this group cause mainly pulmonary disease in older white males, particularly in Kansas, Illinois, and Texas. The group was found to be the cause of 9% of mycobacterial disease in Dallas.[279] These organisms cause cervical lymph node infection in children.[293] Among 99 patients in Dallas having *M. kansasii* infection of the lungs, there were 85 with cavitary disease. Thirty-eight of the whole group previously had normal lungs, the rest having had signs or symptoms of "chronic pulmonary disease."[274]

Group II, the scotochromogens *(M. scrofulaceum)*, is an important cause of acute or subacute lymphadenitis in children.[300] Members of this group very rarely cause pulmonary disease. The organisms can be isolated from the sputum and saliva of many healthy people. Group III, the nonphotochromogens, includes the important Battey type, the chief cause of pulmonary mycobacteriosis of white men in Georgia, Alabama, and Florida.[265] Cervical lymphadenitis in children also is caused by organisms of group III. The Battey organism has been named *M. intracellulare*. Nine cases of disseminated tuberculosis caused by this organism are now on record.[278] A minor member of the group is *M. avium,* which causes less than 0.1% of mycobacterial infections.[268] Group IV, the rapid growers, includes *M. fortuitum,* a rare cause of pulmonary disease, sometimes fatal. Also in group IV is *M. balnei (marinum)* found in the slime of freshwater and saltwater swimming pools. They grow in skin scraped by the rough pool walls, causing "swimming pool granulomas." The organism also grows in fish tanks.[264]

Some unusual mycobacteria are *classified,* because even though they are photochromogens, they have clearly defined characteristics. One is *M. ulcerans,* the cause of the extensive superficial ulcers of the skin of children and young adults in the Buruli district of Uganda. An associated fat necrosis can extend down to muscle or bone, producing gigantic "Buruli ulcers," never causing systemic tuberculosis.

Tendon sheaths, joints, and bursae or soft tissues may be infected by unclassified mycobacteria.[277] Osteomyelitis has been caused by a nonphotochromogen. Such cases indicate hematogenous infection.

Nontuberculous mycobacteriosis of lymph nodes tends to be more suppurative than tuberculosis, but in the lungs the two are considered to be indistinguishable pathologically. Among a group of 36 children with atypical mycobacterial lymphadenitis, seven had suppurative and granulomatous inflammation, alone or with typical tuberculous reaction, and four had a nonspecific diffuse granulomatous or chronic inflammatory reaction.[289] This was not considered characteristic enough to be diagnostic. Others have commented on finding longer, wider, and more heavily beaded acid-fast organisms in mycobacteriosis.

Therefore, only the bacteriologist or special skin tests can demonstrate the difference between the two types of mycobacterial disease. Patients suffering from pulmonary mycobacteriosis mistakenly treated in tuberculosis sanatoriums are in danger of a superinfection by tuberculosis. The primary disease in such patients will not respond to standard antituberculous chemotherapy, so that surgery may be the only cure.

Special purified protein derivatives (PPD) have been prepared for each important group, and their use has demonstrated widespread reactivity (e.g., 70% with PPD-Battey in some

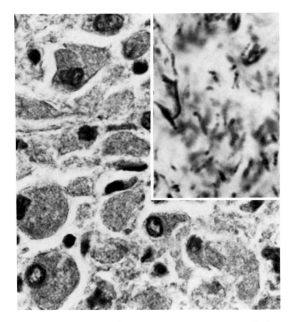

Fig. 26-68. Large histiocytes were main cellular reaction in fatal case of widely disseminated mycobacterial pseudotuberculosis. Cytoplasmic granularity is caused by large numbers of organisms. *Inset,* Ziehl-Neelsen stain of these cells. (837×; inset, 1620×.)

southeastern areas). More blacks than whites react, whereas most of the patients with actual disease are white. Only about half of the patients react to standard PPD.

The noncontagious nature of pulmonary mycobacteriosis has been demonstrated.[265] Not one case was discovered among 500 contacts (including 151 spouses) of 158 patients infected by nonphotochromogens. Isolation is therefore unnecessary. The organisms are opportunists capable of producing serious respiratory disease only after resistance has been lowered by other disease. Most patients are from rural areas and of low social and economic status.[288] We do not know how these persons become infected or where the organisms reside. Soil is considered a possibility.

An uncommon variant deserves comment. Occasionally a child presents with enlargement of spleen and lymph nodes. Bone marrow smears contain numerous cells of the Gaucher type. They are also in the spleen and lymph nodes and are found to be histiocytes packed with acid-fast bacilli that create the foamy appearance (Fig. 26-68). Caseating granulomas do not appear, but there are "hard" tubercles among the histiocytes.

Transmission of tuberculosis

The main routes of tuberculous infection are (1) pulmonary, (2) intestinal, (3) tonsillar, (4) cutaneous, and (5) placental (congenital). The disease usually is spread by droplets from a patient with a cavitary lesion that opens into a bronchus. Coughing, sneezing, and spitting emit a potent spray to which members of the family frequently are exposed. Infection in a child is too often the first indication that grandpa's cough is not caused by smoking. The organisms are quite resistant to drying and persist as infective agents in dust. According to one illustrative report,[286] infected dust particles in crew's quarters lingered after four sailors with pulmonary tuberculosis were removed from a ship. The particles appeared to be responsible for a high rate of tuberculin conversion among the remaining members of the crew for a period of several months.

Occupational hazards exist for all hospital personnel, and the risk for British laboratory workers is two to nine times the national rate.

In some parts of the world, infected milk causes up to 10% of cases of tuberculosis, whereas in countries with a well-supervised dairy industry, this is unknown. Organisms swallowed from outside the body (usually the bovine variety) may infect the tonsils and cervical lymph nodes. The tonsillar disease may pass unnoticed, whereas the cervical node enlargement is prominent. Similarly, the first intestinal lesion is mucosal ulceration, which tends to heal readily, leaving the impression that disease commenced in the mesenteric lymph nodes. After the catastrophe at Lübeck resulting from accidental oral administration of BCG contaminated by living tubercle bacilli to 251 newborn infants, advanced pulmonary lesions of progressive primary type were found in 15 of the 72 who died. These were attributed to direct aspiration of bacilli. Primary lesions were found in the alimentary tract in every case.

Inoculation of tubercle bacilli into the skin is among the lesser dangers faced by pathologists and rarely leads to infection of the internal organs. Butchers may be infected by handling contaminated meat.

Congenital tuberculosis is rare, there being only 158 cases accepted by one group of investigators[266] up until 1960. For this diagnosis to be accepted, lesions must have been present at birth or must have appeared within a few days, with the child having been immediately separated from all infectious persons. The primary complex is found in the liver and portal lymph nodes, since infection has been blood borne through the placenta. Less often, infection is from swallowing tuberculous amniotic fluid (leading to intestinal and mesenteric disease) or inhalation (causing pulmonary lesions).

New variants of clinical tuberculosis

Variant types of disease have appeared. In England one sees patients with multiple tuberculous ulcers and strictures of the intestine. None are in the late stages of pulmonary tuberculosis, are on steroids, or have access to unpasteurized milk; they do not even have a quiescent pulmonary disease or abnormal chest x-ray films. Some are native born, others are immigrants from the Indian subcontinent who have been in Britain for years. Usually they are surgical cases, rarely diagnosed until microscopic slides are examined.[296] Osseous, renal, and testicular tuberculosis occur in adult Londoners with no pulmonary disease.

A rise in the incidence of tuberculous cervical lymphadenitis has been noted in Chicago. Twenty-two cases of all ages were treated; none was caused by atypical mycobacteria and none had a history or clinical evidence of pulmonary tuberculosis.[287] It was accepted that the disease was part of a generalized lymphohematogenous dissemination, a view also held by those reporting a similar series from London.[272]

To explain these variants requires knowledge of the behavior of early tuberculosis. The mycobacteria multiply at the site of entry and in the nodes draining it. Leukocytes disseminate the organisms in the blood and lymphatic vessels. Usually the primary and metastatic sites heal, but infection may lie dormant in either. If local defences break down in the future, an extrapulmonary focus will arise in a person with no lung disease or no apparent source of fresh external infection.

Factors determining course of infection

Native resistance. Native resistance occurs among the different species. Rats are highly resistant to tuberculosis, although the organisms readily multiply within their bodies. Rabbits are susceptible to the bovine organism, but, by virtue of developing an acquired resistance to infection by human mycobacteria, they appear to have native resistance. Lurie has observed that "the natural resistance of human beings to tuberculosis bears a certain relationship to the resistance of the rabbit to the human tubercle bacillus. The vast majority of civilized mankind completely recovers from its primary infection just like the rabbit. There is no race of human beings which is completely immune to tuberculosis."[281] The guinea pig has virtually no resistance to tuberculosis. Studies from the United States Army, where whites and blacks are housed and fed together, indicate that black soldiers have a somewhat higher incidence of the disease and a four times greater mortality than do white soldiers. Tuberculosis in American blacks follows a course intermediate between generalized rapidly progressive primary disease and the localized (pulmonary) chronic ulcerative disease of white adults. It is believed that black adults react to tuberculous infection strikingly differently from white adults.[290] When influences such as dosage, previous infection, and environment are equalized, blacks are found to have a lower degree of racial resistance.

Age and sex. Age and sex have an influence on the incidence of the disease. There are considerably more male than female patients after 25 years of age. Tuberculosis is at its lowest incidence during infancy but has a high death rate. Many healthy persons pick up resistance from subclinical infection. At the beginning of this century, probably the entire population up to 20 years of age was

tuberculin positive. Now, less than 20% of young American adults have a positive reaction, confirming the statistics that show that, in countries with low case rates, tuberculosis is a disease of older people.

Economic status. It is difficult to assess the importance of racial differences when poverty alone can explain much of the higher incidence. The increase in numbers of cases of tuberculosis during famine and war points to the importance of diet and housing conditions. Debilitating diseases may predispose a person to tuberculosis, and the combination aggravates the tuberculosis, increasing the death rate.

Hormonal influences. Whether diabetes has a direct effect on tuberculosis has not been decided. Hyperthyroidism exerts a favorable effect on the course of tuberculosis, and hypothyroidism acts in the opposite way. Cortisone and ACTH will worsen active disease and rekindle the inactive, unless antituberculous drugs are given at the same time. It is not certain that pregnancy (as a hormonal effect) has a deleterious effect on the tuberculous mother. Any worsening of the disease could be merely caused by defective nutrition, inadequate rest, and excessive physical work.[290]

Tissue susceptibility. In children, the lymph nodes are particularly heavily attacked, and the meninges, lungs, and spleen often are involved. Among adults, the lungs bear most of the disease. Second place is shared roughly by the adrenal glands, kidneys, fallopian tubes, epididymides, meninges, and serous membranes. The liver, spleen, bone, red bone marrow, and lymphoid tissue come next. The mucosae of the upper respiratory tract and intestine of adults are rather resistant unless the dose is massive. Rarely infected are cardiac and skeletal muscle, stomach, thyroid gland, pancreas, testis, and breast.

Reactions of tissues to infection

After introduction of tubercle bacilli into animals, the more virulent the strain and the more vulnerable the organ, the greater the extent of the immediate reaction: edema, hyperemia, and neutrophilic infiltration.[281] Having taken up bacilli, the neutrophils die and are ingested by phagocytes. At first the bacilli multiply within the cells. More mononuclear phagocytes collect at the periphery of the nodule that is being formed. What happens at the very beginning is unknown. We cannot explain why tubercle bacilli inspired throughout the lungs usually produce a lesion in only one area.

Infection is by very small clumps of bacilli or even by single ones. In a special search among 1000 persons who died suddenly, not a single prenecrotic focus of macroscopic size attributable to airborne infection could be found, although there was evidence of tuberculosis in three fourths of the bodies examined.[283]

With equal infecting doses, the quantity of exudate in the early lesions is greater in hypersensitive tissues than in nonsensitized. From this observation has come the concept of the exudative and the proliferative lesions.

Exudative reaction. The exudative reaction is an expression of poorer host resistance than is met with in the proliferative reaction and is most often seen in the lungs in rapidly progressive tuberculosis. There is exudation of fibrinous fluid into the alveoli, with outpouring of neutrophils. It may progress to massive caseation that is poorly localized. Numerous organisms are present in acute exudative tuberculosis. However, if the lesion becomes caseous, few organisms can be found in the cheesy matter. If it later softens further so as to become semiliquid, the organisms usually multiply at a great rate.[261] Different reticulin patterns are present in the proliferative, softening, and healing phases.[295]

Proliferative reaction. The end of the proliferative reaction is the hard tubercle, a nonspecific granuloma also seen in sarcoidosis, deep mycoses, syphilis, and berylliosis and in some forms of leprosy. The term "hard" signifies merely that there is no necrosis. Tubercle bacilli are much fewer than in the exudative phase.

The *hard tubercle* is a compact collection of a score or so of a special form of mononuclear phagocyte. This has plentiful, pale eosinophilic cytoplasm and an oval vesicular nucleus. Although the cells have only the faintest resemblance to epithelial cells, they were long ago called "epithelioid." Their peculiarity is the bacterial lipoprotein in the cytoplasm. Among the cells, or at their periphery, there is often a cell with plentiful pink cytoplasm and as many as 20 to 40 round or oval nuclei (Fig. 26-69). When the nuclei are arranged in a complete or partial marginal ring, the cell is described as a Langhans' giant cell. If the nuclei are uniformly scattered, the cell resembles a common foreign body giant cell. Both types of giant cell originate from phagocytes,

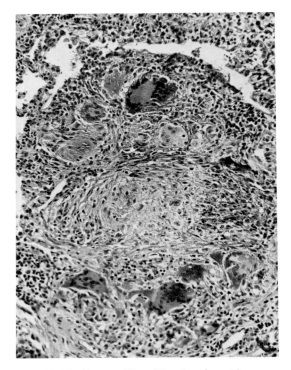

Fig. 26-69. Young ("hard") tubercle with prominent epithelioid cells. (120×.)

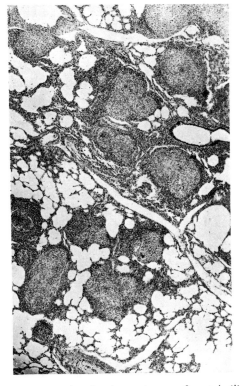

Fig. 26-70. Tubercles becoming confluent (miliary tuberculosis).

and neither is important in making the diagnosis of tuberculosis. An acid-fast bacillus must be seen to identify the hard tubercle as mycobacterial. It is very unusual to find organisms in Langhans' cells. The few that are demonstrable are free or in epithelioid cells.

The tubercle enlarges by migration of more macrophages from blood and tissues, and its periphery is cuffed by a zone of lymphocytes. Tubercles exist side by side and may fuse with one another (Fig. 26-70). This will render them grossly visible for the first time.

The next stage is the conversion to the *soft tubercle*. Starting in its center the epithelioid cells become necrotic and are replaced by an eosinophilic substance at first coarsely granular and dotted with nuclear remnants (Fig. 26-71). Once it becomes homogeneous and quite structureless, it is termed caseous (cheesy), having the naked-eye appearance of a thick, pasty, pale yellow-white substance in the 1 to 2 mm miliary tubercle. In turn, "miliary" implies a resemblance to the millet seed, an object seen by few occidental pathologists. This total obliteration of structure (Fig. 26-72) is what distinguishes caseation from coagulation necrosis because even the interstitial fibrous tissue has gone. The dead tissue is rich in

lipids, and it may persist for a very long time, apparently because the lipids inhibit proteolytic enzymes.

Bacilli are variable in distribution in necrotic tissue.[283] They range from numerous to totally absent. They may be found only in the center in some cases, even in colony formation, whereas in other lesions they are near the periphery of the area of necrosis. A known long-standing necrotic lesion with a peripheral fibrous zone can never be assumed to be innocuous.

Chemotherapy affects the presence of tubercle bacilli in the tissues. In a proportion of treated patients, resected lung specimens may show readily stainable nonculturable bacilli whose significance is uncertain.[299] The assumption that the bacilli are dead is questionable, although varied techniques fail to "revive" them.[298] Nevertheless, their visible persistence may be an indication for surgery. The lowest yield of positive cultures from resected lungs is obtained in those patients whose sputum has become negative within 3 months of chemotherapy or has been negative for more than 6 months before surgery.[280]

There is much evidence that caseation does not occur before hypersensitivity has been es-

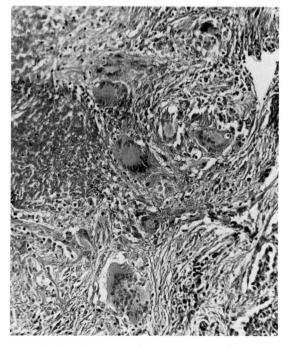

Fig. 26-71. Granular necrotic material appearing in center of tubercle. (168×.)

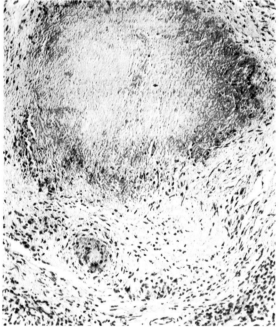

Fig. 26-72. Soft tubercle. Caseous center and early formation of fibrous capsule.

tablished. It begins to appear about 2 weeks after injection of large doses of virulent bacilli into relatively resistant animals. Caseation is progressive as long as tubercle bacilli can proliferate in the tissues, allowing the process to extend. When the macrophages can destroy bacilli as rapidly as they are reproduced, effective fibrous encapsulation can occur. Capsules can protect against progressive caseation only if they are complete. The danger is survival of a minority of organisms that lie dormant almost as if they were spores. They can immediately be reactivated by oxygen brought in by rupture of the capsule or bleeding into the caseous center. Fresh tuberculoprotein now released may induce further caseation and obliteration of the fibrous barrier. Even on reaching this stage, the tubercle is not histologically diagnostic. It is a "caseating tuberculoid granuloma," awaiting a positive Ziehl-Neelsen stain or successful culture.

What happens next is either further spread or healing, depending on the host-bacillus relationship. "Healing" as used in pathology lacks the connotation of restitution to normal. In tuberculosis it refers to increasing fibrosis creeping into the diseased area, creating a scar. Very common also is calcification, in no sense a protective process. Calcium carried in blood plasma to caseous areas is deposited as relatively insoluble compounds, possibly influenced by the high concentration of lipids.

Among the infants in the Lübeck series, calcification was first seen at 58 days. Calcification can appear in primary lesions after 2 months, whereas in postprimary infection 6 months are required.[269] Calcium must accumulate for about a year to be seen radiologically. After about 3 years, the lesion attains a chalky character. Stony foci are at least 5 years old and may be ossified. At first, calcium is seen in routine sections as irregular pale blue clouds. With time, the color intensifies, particularly at the periphery. Viable bacilli may still be present in noncalcified areas.

Calcification in tuberculosis, therefore, merely indicates that caseous necrosis has taken place but is not evidence of cure or sterilization. Identical pulmonary calcification can be produced by histoplasmosis.

Pathogenicity of tubercle bacilli

To be infectious, tubercle bacilli must be inhaled with particles no larger than 15 μm in order to reach the aveoli. Bigger clumps will be returned by cilia to the sputum.

Tubercle bacilli are readily phagocytosed.

It is believed that within these phagocytes the most effective processes of immunity take place. The overcoming of infection probably depends on the power of the host's monocytes to kill the engulfed bacilli. For some days they multiply freely as if harmless cellular parasites. Similar multiplication is seen in lepromatous leprosy and Johne's disease of cattle. It also occurs in human infection by anonymous mycobacteria. At about 15 days, the peaceful relationship between mycobacteria and host cells is suddenly altered by the appearance of sensitization to tuberculoprotein. Tubercle bacilli begin to act with virulence. During the relatively slow disintegration of the organisms within the phagocytes, complex antigens are released. This happens only in vivo.

Nature of hypersensitivity and immunity

Around tuberculoprotein and the nature of Koch's phenomenon appears to revolve the complicated reaction to tuberculous infection. The nature of *Koch's phenomenon* is this. When a healthy guinea pig is injected with live tubercle bacilli, a nodule appears at this site in 10 to 14 days. It enlarges and becomes an ulcer that persists until the animal dies of generalized tuberculosis. The regional lymph nodes also become tuberculous. Living tubercle bacilli or their breakdown products injected into already tuberculous guinea pigs immediately elicit, at the new site of injection, an acute exudative response that, within 2 to 4 days, advances to shallow ulceration that heals. Regional lymph nodes do not react. This is the simplest expression of the complex hypersensitivity to tuberculoprotein. The animal has reacted hypersensitively but has localized the infection and disposed of it.

It has been much disputed whether this hypersensitivity or allergy is also the mechanism of the patient's *acquired immunity*. It is more likely that they are responses to different antigenic agents. Tuberculin sensitivity cannot be induced by the injection of tuberculin. Injection of tuberculoprotein may sensitize normal animals to tuberculoprotein but not to tuberculin. Heat-killed tubercle bacilli produce typical tuberculous lesions, but these regress. Only tuberculoprotein associated with tubercle bacilli induces sensitivity to tuberculin. Animals have been successfully desensitized to tuberculoprotein and then have been shown still to have greater immunity than a normal animal. The chief mechanism of immunity is the increased capacity of mononuclear phagocytes to inhibit the growth of tubercle bacilli.

Nevertheless, under certain conditions hypersensitivity may aid in protection.[281] Although various antibodies are found in sera of tuberculous patients, they confer no immunity on susceptible animals. Sera of highly immunized animals have no in vitro bactericidal effect on tubercle bacilli.

As hypersensitivity appears, the macrophages become epithelioid cells, and all but the most virulent organisms are killed. The more epithelioid cells, the more quickly this phase progresses. The change in the appearance of the cells is attributable to the fine, intracytoplasmic dispersion of lipid from the bacilli. Thus the appearance of epithelioid cells is associated with death of the bacilli. In reinfection tuberculosis, the bacilli cannot multiply as they can in primary infection, and formation of nodules and epithelioid cells is accelerated. Under these conditions, the mononuclear cells have a directly augmented activity independent of any contribution from the patient's serum. They are not only phagocytic, but also bacteriostatic.

Silk bags containing collodion and tubercle bacilli were placed in the peritoneal cavities of normal and immune rabbits. These bags allow body fluids to enter but bar the animals' cells. The fluids of immune animals inhibited growth of the bacilli in vivo.[281] Hence, there must be a humoral component of acquired resistance.

All these sequences in animals apply equally to man. Whether or not hypersensitivity can be equated with immunity, the inflammatory process in the reinfected patient develops more quickly and in the more destructive form of caseation. Yet, these lesions are more effectively localized by fibrous tissue, and regional lymph node inflammation is not so prominent a feature as it is in primary disease. In this sense, hypersensitivity is associated with better defenses. Therefore, hypersensitivity may be said to work with the increased monocytic function that is the major activity of immunity. On the other hand, hypersensitivity has an unfavorable action in that it is responsible for serious tissue destruction, even though this will also decrease the local multiplication of tubercle bacilli.

A few organisms usually survive in the primary site and years later can start a new bout of progressive disease (p. 1118). Under these circumstances, the host-parasite relationship is an unstable equilibrium. Over a long time, the ascendancy can pass to either one in a cycle of progressive and quiescent disease. In the same organ, there can simultaneously be healing and progressing lesions.

There is no immunity without hypersensitivity. Patients with either primary or reinfection tuberculosis are hypersensitive, the state being more pronounced in children than in adults. It is not known why this difference exists. The *bacille Calmette-Guérin (BCG)* is a permanently attenuated living bovine organism that almost invariably causes harmless infection. Blattner has reviewed a dozen instances of death in children from disseminated "BCG tuberculosis" within some months of vaccination.[260] Many had hypogammaglobulinemia, and others suffered repeated infections or were debilitated prior to vaccination. These conditions, therefore, are contraindications to giving BCG, as is a positive tuberculin reaction. BCG is injected to immunize human beings, but there is no way to measure the immunizing potency of any particular batch. Considerable variation occurs. Vaccination is offered to tuberculin-negative persons in areas with a high risk of infection.

The Medical Research Council in England has conducted follow-up studies of over 50,000 tuberculin-negative children for 7 to 10 years. They were vaccinated with BCG or another nonpathogenic organism, the vole bacillus *(M. tuberculosis* var. *muris)*. The incidence of tuberculosis in the vaccinated group was only one fifth that of a similar but unvaccinated group, and the protection appeared to be long-lasting.[267,282]

In regard to the histopathology of BCG vaccination, of particular interest is the frequent occurrence of Schaumann bodies in the tuberculoid granulomas. They are probably formed from fatty acids. It has been speculated that the bodies are part of the morphologic expression of the development of the antigenic response to the bacilli.[297]

Populations with a low rate of tuberculosis are not vaccinated because other methods of control of the disease have been successful. In these people, tuberculin conversion is a valuable sign to disclose a new case. BCG vaccination can always be given if a high incidence of tuberculin positivity appears in a group exposed to a special risk.

Tuberculosis of lung
Primary tuberculosis and primary complex

When tuberculosis was a very common disease in the Western world, "primary" tuberculosis and "childhood" tuberculosis were synonymous. Now, a person may be unexposed to the risk until adult life, so the term "primary" is used. Most often, primary tuberculous infection is overcome without signs or symptoms or with only slight fever, cough, or chest pain. Only skin testing discloses that it has occurred.

The *primary complex* is a focal lung lesion with a beady chain of miliary tubercles running in the lymphatic vessels to the third component, the enlarged hilar lymph nodes (Fig. 26-73).

The *pulmonary component* is the primary (Ghon) focus. It occurs with equal frequency on either side and tends to be subpleural, in the midportion of a lobe rather than apical. Rare multiple primary complexes may be the result of exposure to a source of heavy infection. One lesion can be in the lung and the other extrapulmonary.

The true early lesion rarely is seen. It resembles nontuberculous bronchopneumonia, passing through red and gray stages of consolidation. Around it is an extremely wide, red, less firm perifocal reaction. The latter is an alveolar filling with serum, phagocytes, and

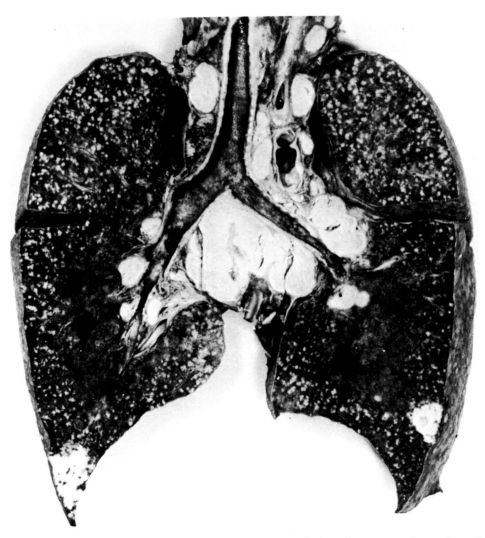

Fig. 26-73. Bilateral tuberculous primary complexes. Subpleural caseous primary focus in each lower lobe. Hilar and tracheobronchial nodes have undergone massive enlargement and caseation. In addition, advanced miliary dissemination can be seen. (From Giese, W.: In Kaufmann, E., and Staemmler, M., editors: Lehrbuch der speziellen pathologischen Anatomie, vol. II, Berlin, 1959-1960, Walter De Gruyter & Co.)

erythrocytes but without inflammatory cells. This is rapidly converted into a quite well-demarcated area of consolidation 1 to 2 cm in diameter. Its cut surface is a rather dry or crumbling, gray or white caseous tissue surrounded, during the most active phase, by a red zone of tuberculous granulation tissue. Rarely does it undergo complete resolution. More often, the area becomes caseous, encapsulated by fibrous tissue (which has formed from the granulation tissue), and it is sometimes calcified. Such a calcified (even ossified) residue may be only a few millimeters in diameter. In other patients, the remnant is a small, puckered, pleural scar.

The early histologic response has been described on p. 1112. This passes on to caseation and, in patients with good resistance, to creation of a fibrous capsule.

The *lymphatic vessel component* may not be seen at all in a random slice made into the lung. It heals with complete resolution.

The *lymph node component* is a massive enlargement of hilar and tracheobronchial nodes that in children is much greater than the area drained. In some adults, the reverse is the case. Generally, all the nodes in the group are necrotic and matted into a yellow-white conglomeration with spots of calcification. The greatest enlargement and most caseation occur in the hilar nodes. Encapsulation and extensive calcification follow, but not

before the anterior mediastinal, and sometimes even cervical and abdominal, lymph nodes have been involved. Nodal lesions take longer to regress than those in the lung, often years, and they remain a potential source of reinfection. Much later, these lymph nodes shrink to normal size but are largely calcified. Microscopic examination of the lymph nodes discloses the extensive caseation, with peripheral tubercles and fibrosis.

Progressive primary infection

There is progression of the primary complex in a small number of persons—especially in those subjected to very heavy infection. Most often affected are black infants or children.

The process is tuberculous bronchopneumonia with caseation (Fig. 26-74). It spreads in three ways: (1) by direct extension, (2) into bronchi, and (3) into the bloodstream. The periphery is irregular and poorly defined, and there is no limiting zone of granulation tissue.

Bronchial dissemination arises by one of two methods. First, caseous matter erodes into the lumen of a small bronchus and is distributed along the ramifications of the bronchus into previously healthy lung. This creates a pyramid with its base on the pleura. Second is a similar infection of a much larger bronchus by caseous material from a hilar node. The resultant

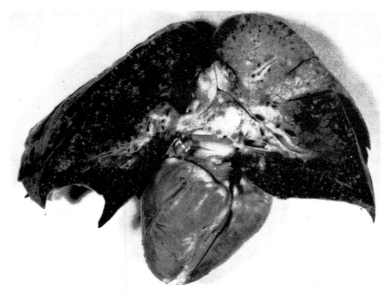

Fig. 26-74. Progressive primary tuberculosis (posterior view) in 18-month-old infant. Coalescent tuberculous bronchopneumonia of right upper and middle lobes. Acinar-nodose tuberculosis in remainder of lungs. Caseation of hilar nodes.

bronchopneumonia can be extensive and fatal. If a cavity forms, its wall is shaggy and its outer wall is ill defined, without a capsule.

Rupture of the tuberculous lesion into a blood vessel may result in hematogenous dissemination, i.e., generalized miliary tuberculosis (see following discussion).

Progressive primary tuberculosis may be arrested at any stage. Exudative lesions can be resolved, and caseous areas can be encapsulated and calcified. Eventually, the lung will have multiple, relatively large calcified and fibrous areas. The microscopic appearance of these lesions has been described previously. Tuberculous caseous pneumonia is described on p. 1121.

Miliary tuberculosis

Tubercle bacilli may spill into the blood, directly or through the lymphatic vessels. Penetration of a pulmonary vein is likely to infect all of the body, whereas entrance of bacilli into a pulmonary artery is likely to restrict them to its territory within the lung. Mycobacteria entering a major lymphatic vessel will be returned by the right ventricle to both lungs. Cells of the reticuloendothelial system destroy many of them, often by forming small noncaseating tubercles that disappear after they have performed their task. A harmless infection leaves a residue of tiny calcified dots in the liver, spleen, apices of the lungs, meninges, or skeletal system. For a while, it is possible for one of these to flare up as active disease. If so, the condition of miliary tuberculosis is set up. However, there is reason to believe that organisms, despite their lodging in susceptible tissues, can be promptly killed. This is more likely in adults than in infants.

Infection may come from a primary focus or from a later stage of tuberculosis, in which the miliary disease may be merely a terminal event. In the adult, miliary tuberculosis is more likely to be of extrapulmonary origin, even though the lung is seen to be infected the most heavily and even though it contains chronic lesions that initiated extrapulmonary disease. More and more cases of miliary tuberculosis are being reported in elderly persons, with half of the cases in those past the age 60 years being "cryptic." This means that the usual clinical and radiologic features are absent. A typical patient is an elderly woman with pyrexia, pancytopenia, or leukemoid reaction. Many such patients have been fruitlessly investigated for blood dyscrasia, and sometimes lymphocytic leukemia has

been erroneously diagnosed. Therapeutic trial has been advocated as a method of diagnosis.[292]

In children, miliary tuberculosis may be more or less confined to the lungs. More often, in addition, liver, spleen, and kidneys bear a great number of tubercles, followed by meninges, bone marrow, lymph nodes, and thyroid gland. Only muscle tissue is spared.

The pleura generally shows little reaction. The cut surface of the lung is studded with firm white tubercles 1 mm in diameter or caseating tubercles several millimeters in diameter (Fig. 26-73). Tubercles in the upper lobes are the largest, but the distribution of tubercles is even throughout. The heavier the infection, the closer and more numerous they will be. Tubercles grow smaller as the infection is resisted. Specific chemotherapy will allow scar formation and disappearance of the lesions after only a few weeks, as opposed to several months in untreated patients. The latter may develop fibrosis or scar emphysema. Childhood miliary tuberculosis can heal without trace, but the adult variety rarely does.

The tubercles are chiefly within alveolar septa where the bacterial emboli lodge. They are of the hard variety at first but enlarge and caseate. Fibrous capsules are formed in those patients who survive a longer time.

Chronic and recurrent types of pulmonary miliary tuberculosis occasionally are found in adults. Giese[269] refers to Gujer's 176 cases of miliary tuberculosis, 54 of which were subacute or chronic. The lungs are heavy, and the pleura is fibrotic. On the cut surface, tubercles are seen to have coalesced into small nodules with central caseation and eventual cavitation. In other patients, there is extensive fibrosis around the nodules. Chronic disseminated tuberculosis involving several organs also has been described.[262]

Reactivation (reinfection) tuberculosis

Reinfection can be endogenous, resulting from reactivation of a primary focus, or exogenous, caused by organisms received from an external source. Numerous authorities in many countries believe that endogenous reactivation is by far the commoner mechanism. Stead[294] presents persuasive evidence that exogenous reinfection is uncommon and that nearly all chronic pulmonary tuberculosis develops from reactivation of dormant foci implanted during primary infection. In Medlar's series,[283] 91% of the progressive pulmonary lesions in patients under 40 years of age were the result of continuation and endogenous reactivation of primary disease.

Reactivation favors the subapical region of any lobe, especially the right, some 2 to 4 cm below the apex. The reason for this characteristic site is not known. The lesion is a small area of dry, confluent, tuberculous bronchopneumonia that tends to fan out to the pleura. Regional lymph node involvement is minor.

Healing leaves a small scar around which dust tends to collect in blocked lymphatic vessels. Such scars are restricted almost entirely to the pleura, which is thick, hyalinized, calcified or, rarely, ossified. The pleural surface is uneven, often puckered, and slaty blue or black, and pleural adhesion is common. Often, the scar has an area of several square centimeters but little depth. Sometimes one finds a 5 mm calcified nodule or a zone no more than 1 cm deep in which the lung is black and airless or contains a tiny cavity with a smooth inner lining. Focal emphysema may surround the scar. The entire process is spoken of as *arrested tuberculosis.*

The microscopic lesions begin with an exudative reaction that passes into tubercle formation, caseation, and peripheral fibrosis. Further caseation and tissue destruction produce the gross lesion. "Arrest" is recognized by the reduced amount of caseous matter, with a strong fibrocalcific reaction. The lesions of arrested tuberculosis lack Langhans' cells and stainable acid-fast bacilli, but may still be infectious for the guinea pig.

Progressive reactivation (reinfection) tuberculosis. An advancing lesion occupies much of the upper lobe, undergoes massive central caseation, and, if it breaks into a bronchus, will form a cavity. The latter type is *chronic ulcerative tuberculosis,* and the noncavitary

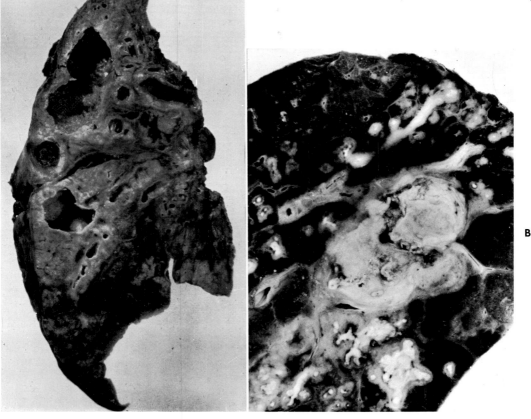

Fig. 26-75. Fibrocaseous tuberculosis. **A,** Advanced lesion with cavitation. Cavities have thick walls and communicate with larger bronchi by wide openings. **B,** Large areas of caseation with attempts at fibrous encapsulation. There is also extensive tuberculous bronchitis. (From Giese, W.: In Kaufmann, E., and Staemmler, M., editors: Lehrbuch der speziellen pathologischen Anatomie, vol. II, Berlin, 1959-1960, Walter De Gruyter & Co.)

variety is *chronic fibrocaseous tuberculosis.* No matter how soft the center, a cavity cannot form without drainage into a bronchus or bronchiole.

Some patients develop *acute cavities,* usually during caseous pneumonia. The outline of such a lesion is irregular or branching, corresponding to the fusion of lobular areas. The lining is shaggy and necrotic and may contain remnants of septa, vessels, and bronchi. It may break through the pleura, setting up a tuberculous pyopneumothorax. Other specimens disclose tubular cavities, which indicate a destructive caseous bronchitis. Progression of the cavity is rapid, with little likelihood of its becoming chronic.

A newly formed *chronic cavity* has necrotic, ragged walls, with adherent, pale yellow, cheesy material. No odor is present. Active cavities have three definite linings. Innermost is the caseous tissue with debris, many bacilli, and, in places, epithelioid cells and some fibroblasts. Beyond this is a red zone of tuberculous granulation tissue composed of many dilated capillaries, epithelioid and Langhans' cells, and fibroblasts. The external layer is a thin gray zone of loose connective tissue, which has arisen from organization of the perifocal zone. This merges indefinitely into consolidated or normal lung. The opening into the bronchus may be very small.

Chronicity is indicated by a fibrous outer wall, which forms from organization of the perifocal reaction and is 1 to 2 mm thick. The outline tends to be irregular because of uneven breakdown of the tissues. Several cavities may intercommunicate, and the bronchus of each may be identified (Fig. 26-75, *A*).

The lining of older cavities is gray or pink and shaggy. A smooth fibrous lining replaces this granulation tissue as infection is overcome. Around it are foci of tuberculous bronchopneumonia, caseation, fibrosis, and bronchiectasis. Overlying pleura is fibrotic. The pleural space may develop empyema or be totally obliterated by adhesions. The pleural fibrosis is protective against bronchopleural fistula, empyema, and transpleural dissemination of infection into neighboring lung. It cannot prevent the cavity from enlarging, and new fibrous tissue is laid down as the older is destroyed from within. Little change is to be found in the regional nodes.

All these changes, except cavitation, occur in fibrocaseous tuberculosis (Fig. 26-75, *B*).

Cavities of 5 cm or more may be crossed by strands of connective tissue, blood vessels,

or bronchi. The vessels usually have been obliterated by thrombosis. If not, the tuberculous process may weaken their walls, permitting aneurysm formation or massive, often fatal, bleeding. Bleeding is more likely to come from a vessel in the cavity wall. The incidence of fatal hemoptysis has not been decreased by chemotherapy.

Cavities enlarge either by constant destruction of their lining or by neighboring areas of caseation breaking into the cavity. The oldest lesions are in the upper posterior portion of the lung. Usually, the anterior portion of the lung is spared. Most of a lobe may be converted into large coalescing cavities surrounded by solid lung tissue altered by tuberculosis in different stages. Fibrosis may obliterate many vessels and induce pulmonary hypertension.

In closed healing of cavities, the bronchus is obliterated at its entry to the cavity. This may be mediated by collapse of the lung, endobronchitis, a caseous plug in the bronchial lumen, or a gradual pinching off of the bronchus by contraction of surrounding granulation tissue. The cavity fills with necrotic material, air and fluid are absorbed, calcification follows, and either nothing is left but a radial scar or, in the case of larger cavities, there is considerable contraction and walling off.[259] Closing occurs more readily in the smaller, more pliable and collapsible bronchi of children. Children suffer less frequently than adults from chronic cavities.

Early, emptied small cavities have walls thin and pliable enough to become apposed and adherent. Healing will leave only a minimal scar. The effects of chemotherapy are discussed on p. 1123.

Complications of reinfective tuberculosis. Cavitation, pleurisy, and empyema have just been discussed. From cavities comes the danger of bronchial dissemination of bacilli. An upper lobe cavity tends to infect other parts of that lobe and the apex of the lower lobe, less often its posterobasal region. Infection can spread to the opposite lung, usually its lower lobe. Bacilli in sputum may set up ulcerative tracheal or laryngeal tuberculosis or, in late stages, infect the tongue and mucosal lymphoid tissue of the small and large intestines. Apart from hematogenous miliary dissemination, there is danger of active disease in a single site, particularly meninges, kidney, bone, epididymis, and fallopian tube. Infection of mediastinal lymph nodes is usually not significant. Patients with extensive chronic tuberculosis may develop amyloidosis.

Tuberculous caseous pneumonia

Tuberculous caseous pneumonia is rapidly progressive. It occurs in children when a caseous hilar node erodes a bronchial wall, and in unusually hypersensitive adults when there is perforation of a tuberculous cavity into a bronchus. A great amount of infected material is spilled over, and the condition is analogous to Koch's phenomenon in guinea pigs. The affected area at first includes one or two lobules, which are solid, dry, gray, and granular. Enough lung tissue remains to cause confusion with diffusely infiltrating bronchial carcinoma, adenocarcinoma, or gray hepatization.

Large quantities of tuberculoprotein reach uninfected tissue of an already hypersensitive individual, provoking a vigorous exudative response in the alveoli, with many bacilli. Tissue necrosis follows rapidly, and adjacent foci enlarge and coalesce. Microscopic tubercles are uncommon. Soon the gray turns to yellow or gray-red, and the whole lobe is firm. A whole lung, or most of both lungs, can be affected, and those parts not massively consolidated may show patchy bronchopneumonia centered around caseous bronchi. The peripheral zones may be moist, translucent, shiny, smooth, and somewhat gelatinous (gelatinous pneumonia, a term that should not be applied to the entire tuberculous lesion). Gelatinous pneumonia is seen microscopically as filling of intact thick-walled alveoli by much fluid and by fibrin with many macrophages. Inflammatory cells are scanty.

The larger the diseased areas, the more likely it is that caseation and cavitation will occur in older areas, beginning around bronchi. The cut surface is firm, dry, opaque, and yellow-white. Tubercles are found in and around the bronchi, which are ulcerated and may be destroyed. Tuberculous pleurisy and caseous hilar nodes are frequently present. Eventually, an opening will be forced into a large bronchus. Miliary dissemination is common. The most severe cases used to be called "galloping consumption."

If such widespread disease can be arrested, fibrosis is most extensive. Resolution of exudate is possible only before necrosis occurs.

Nonreactive tuberculosis

Since 1882, persons have been reported with severe hypersensitivity and low resistance and who have developed widespread pulmonary tuberculosis lacking the characteristic histologic response.[284] Disease of the hematopoietic system often is present (primary or secondary). Should tuberculosis be unsuspected and the patient be given steroids, the disease may advance rapidly. Some such lungs have contained a number of yellow miliary to nodular areas, but in others the lesion resembles an ill-defined bacterial pneumonia, sometimes with abscess cavities. Nodular areas are seen under the microscope to be fairly well-defined eosinophilic necroses with some nuclear debris, mostly from inflammatory cells. Caseation is not common and is early and limited. Granulation tissue, epithelioid cells, and Langhans' cells are lacking. In lungs that appear pneumonic, there is widespread hyperemia, hemorrhagic alveolitis with edema, or widespread necrosis like that of an ischemic infarct. Whichever type is present, there will be an enormous number of tubercle bacilli (Fig. 26-76). Regional nodes, liver, spleen, and bone marrow may contain similar lesions.

Acinar (acinonodose) tuberculosis

In both cavitary and fibrocaseous tuberculosis, an entire lobe or lung may be riddled by

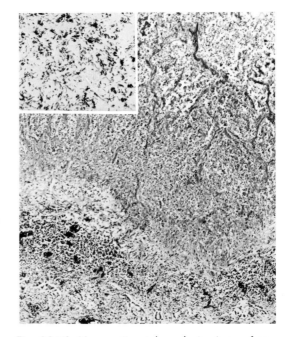

Fig. 26-76. Nonreactive tuberculosis. Area of central cavitary necrosis (top right), vascular zone with cellular necrosis (middle), and hypervascular and early fibrous area (bottom). No cellular reaction typical of tuberculosis. *Inset,* Masses of tubercle bacilli found in vascular zone. (75×; *inset,* 460×.)

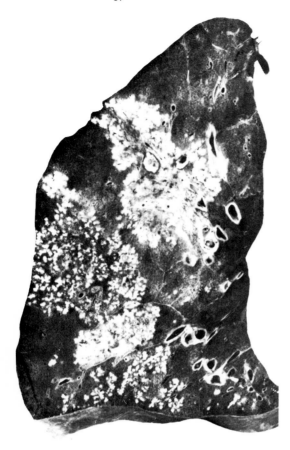

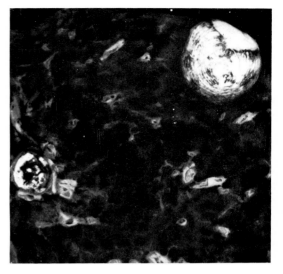

Fig. 26-78. Lamellated tuberculoma formed from Ghon tubercle in adult.

Fig. 26-77. In upper lobe is large, chronic, fibrocaseous area with small central cavity. Condition is spreading peripherally. In lower lobe is typical, partly confluent, acinar tuberculosis. (From Giese, W.: In Kaufmann, E., and Staemmler, M., editors: Lehrbuch der speziellen pathologischen Anatomie, vol. II, Berlin, 1959-1960, Walter De Gruyter & Co.)

what appears to be magnified miliary disease. This is acinar tuberculosis, caused by infection of acini by aspiration from chronic tuberculosis higher up in the lung. These units undergo caseation with a cloverleaf pattern, followed later by fibrosis. Close inspection always discloses a small, central, thick-walled bronchus in each area. Cavitation does not occur. Individual areas may fuse and reach a size of 1 to 2 cm (Fig. 26-77).

Acinar lesions are a hallmark of reinfection tuberculosis when resistance is good. Healing by fibrosis is possible, leaving only gray-black bands of connective tissue. Should the lesions progress, lobular pneumonia is the result. Microscopically, there is an initial alveolar exudation of fibrin and neutrophils, rapidly overshadowed by tubercle formation.

Tuberculous bronchitis

Tuberculous bronchitis is commoner with lower lobe disease and with cavitation. Its incidence increases with the severity of the pulmonary disease.[275] A search among 197 autopsies in a mental hospital disclosed scars of large bronchi in 27%,[270] a figure similar to those in a number of European reports. The scars form depressed troughs and rings covered by mucosa.

The earliest lesion is the submucosal tubercle. As caseation appears, the mucosa becomes ulcerated. Finally, segments of the bronchus are lined by tuberculous granulation tissue. The latter tends to heal with fibrosis, a complication compounded by fibrous tissue laid down in concomitant inflammatory processes around the bronchus. The lumen is narrowed or may even be closed, either by fibrosis or by caseous material. Distal to this there may be bronchiectasis. Patchy collapse of the lung follows bronchial obliteration.

Dissemination of tuberculosis within peribronchial lymphatic vessels eventually infects bronchial walls. Affected bronchi fan out from the hilum. They look like thick-walled white tubes from which caseous material can be squeezed. Normal lung lies between the bronchi.

In young children in whom primary tuberculosis has led to pulmonary collapse, bronchiectasis frequently develops.[271] Less often, bronchial strictures occur, and only one third of such children have normal bronchi.

Tuberculoma

A tuberculoma is a nodular, conglomerate area of caseous necrosis with a well-formed fibrous capsule. It occurs in adults with reactivation tuberculosis. Tuberculomas vary in size from 0.5 to 4 cm. Most are solitary and in an upper lobe. The cut surface shows uniform or lamellated, dry, caseous matter with areas of calcification (Fig. 26-78) or a cavity. The capsule is 1 to 3 mm thick, and the surrounding lung is normal or has minimal tuberculosis. Although tuberculomas are considered as inactive, they may break down and discharge their contents into a bronchus, indicating reactivation.[291]

Pathology of treated pulmonary tuberculosis

Surgical procedures that aim at physical collapse of the diseased lung are followed by pronounced fibrosis of the pleura and the tuberculous foci of the lung. "Closed healing" of small cavities is described on p. 1120. Large cavities leave a residum of inspissated necrotic tissue within a thick capsule surrounded by looser fibrous tissue.

Specific chemotherapy accelerates healing. Cavities undergo "open healing." They are converted to spherical cysts filled with air under tension, with a fibrous wall 1 to 2 mm thick. The cyst may be 10 to 15 cm across. An active cavity is distinguished by its irregular and frankly tuberculous inner surface.

The cyst, also called a tension cavity, has a smooth or slightly wrinkled gray or graypink glistening lining, on which a small amount of pink granulation tissue may rest. In some surgically removed specimens, small foci of caseation remain at the periphery. A bronchus will nearly always be found entering the cyst, which probably exists because of patency of the bronchocavitary junction.

The cyst is bigger than the original cavity because of a check-valve action at the bronchocavitary junction by tuberculous granulation tissue in the early stages. During the response to treatment, the valve effect is lost and the cavity diminishes. Any fluid remaining becomes inspissated and calcified.

The outstanding feature of drug therapy in tuberculosis is regression of perifocal lesions and healing of tuberculous ulcers with regeneration of epithelium, which may be flat or stratified squamous.[259] This permits drainage and inactivation of the infection of the wall, and hence only a thin, fibrous, outer zone appears. Usually, no tubercle bacilli can

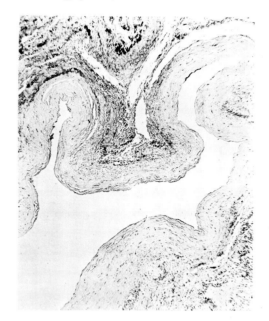

Fig. 26-79. Thin, fibrous cavity wall in lobe removed after 1 year of chemotherapy.

be isolated. A patient so "healed" is still in danger of aspergilloma, perforation, suppuration, bleeding, or reactivation. Therefore, surgical removal often is performed.

Reported incidence of open healing varies from 6%[263] to 10%. In the days before chemotherapy, open healing was very uncommon.[259]

Microscopically, the healed part of the wall is hyalinized connective tissue, with scanty capillaries and a few lymphocytes. Scattered calcium deposits are present (Fig. 26-79). There is a sharp demarcation from adjacent lung. On the inner surface, there are flattened connective tissue cells, not an epithelium, although cells may grow in from the entering bronchus for a short way. Granulation tissue in any active areas can be so vascular as to form a source of bleeding.

Chemotherapeutic agents also can cause closed healing, a hyalinization and calcification brought about in a few months instead of 1 to 2 years. Healing is always more rapid if the necrotic tissue has not undergone liquefaction.

Noncavitary caseous disease responds to chemotherapy by rapid disappearance of the peripheral lesions and by forming a thin fibrous capsule. There is a much lower incidence of fibrosis in the lung.

Causes of death from tuberculosis

Murasawa and Altmann[285] analyzed in 1958 the causes of death in 570 autopsies performed at a hospital for tuberculosis. In 52%, pulmonary tuberculosis was considered the main cause. After this came arteriosclerotic heart disease, malignancy, and surgery on the lung. A 1963 report[273] reviews 295 autopsies performed on tuberculous patients in the period from 1950 to 1960. In 1950, progressive tuberculosis was listed as the principal cause of death in 74% of cases. In 1959 and 1960, this was the cause of death in only 15%. Conditions unrelated to tuberculosis, such as carcinoma, myocardial infarction, and cerebral hemorrhage, rose from 6% to 64% as causes of death. Conditions related to tuberculosis, but not necessarily associated with active disease, increased from 20% in 1950 to 31% in 1959 and 1960. These were pulmonary hemorrhage, pulmonary insufficiency, spontaneous pneumothorax, death during thoracic surgery, cor pulmonale, and amyloid disease. One third of the autopsied patients were considered to have healed tuberculosis.

CARCINOMA

The commonest tumor of the lung is *metastatic carcinoma,* with the lungs being involved in 20% to 45% of all cases of carcinoma. Most often, the tumor cells arrive in the pulmonary arteries. Less often, they come retrogradely in lymphatics, by direct invasion, or in the bronchial arteries. Some tumors metastasize to a bronchus, sometimes simulating a bronchial primary.[311a]

No fixed pattern is observed. There may be one or innumerable secondary tumors, ranging in size from a millimeter to many centimeters. They are nearly always spherical, often with a finely or deeply scalloped edge. Metastatic renal carcinoma, seminoma, and sarcoma are particularly well rounded, producing the radiologic "cannonball lesions." It is not often possible even to guess at the source of a metastasis, although the brown of melanoma and the pink and red of chorioepithelioma are characteristic, as is the moist fish-flesh appearance of many sarcomas.

Primary carcinoma

The overwhelming number of primary tumors of the lung are carcinomas.

Classification

Many pathologists have not followed the World Health Organization's classification of lung tumors. Both Spencer[3] and Melamed[332] have found need to modify it. A major objection is its largely artificial separation of adeno-

carcinoma from alveolobronchiolar carcinoma (p. 1136). In this discussion are considered most of the following tumors, classified by their origin:

Bronchial epithelium
  Squamous cell (epidermoid) carcinoma (with variants spindled and papillary)
  Oat (small) cell carcinoma
  Undifferentiated large cell carcinoma
  Melanoma

Bronchial epithelium and glands
  Adenocarcinoma (with variant giant cell carcinoma)
  Carcinoid
  Adenoid cystic carcinoma
  Mucoepidermoid carcinoma
  Clear cell carcinoma
  True adenoma
  Benign clear cell tumor (origin mesenchymal?)

Bronchiolar and alveolar epithelium
  Peripheral adenocarcinoma (bronchioloalveolar carcinoma)
  Scar carcinoma (glandular or squamous)
  Tumorlet
  Peripheral carcinoid

Mesenchymal
  Connective tissue tumors (benign and malignant)
  Granular cell myoblastoma of bronchus
  Chemodectoma
  Lymphoma

Mixed
  Hamartoma
  Blastoma
  Teratoma

Pleural
  Mesothelioma

Pseudotumor
  Plasma cell granuloma
  Sclerosing angioma
  Pseudolymphoma

Incidence

The increased incidence of carcinoma of the lung is too great to explain by blaming errors in diagnosis in earlier years. By 1970, the lung cancer death rate for males in England and Wales was 72 per 100,000 population, and in the United States it was 52.1. The figures for females were 11.6 and 10.3, respectively. The number of deaths from carcinoma of the lung in the United States rose from 27,000 in 1955 to 55,000 in 1968, with an estimate of 81,000 in 1975. Over the preceding 35 years in the United States, male deaths from lung cancer have increased 15 times and female deaths have been roughly doubled. At the beginning of this century (before cigarettes became popular), the sex incidence was roughly equal. About

85% of patients are men. In Britain, the disease accounts for more than 10% of all deaths in persons between 45 and 64 years of age (see also p. 719).

Etiology

The close relationship between certain types of lung carcinoma and *cigarette smoking* has been made well known, as has the lesser relationship to cigar and pipe smoking. Whether or not a cause-and-effect relationship has been proved is a blend of logical, statistical, and emotional argument. It is impossible adequately to summarize the issue here. Opinion prevails in Britain that cigarettes are an etiologic factor, based particularly on Doll and Hill's study of over 40,000 doctors.[317] The 1964 United States Surgeon General's Advisory Committee report concluded that cigarette smoking is causally related to lung carcinoma in men and that its effect far outweighs all other factors. Risk increases with the duration of smoking and the amount smoked daily. A heavy cigarette smoker has at least a 20 times greater risk of having lung carcinoma than a nonsmoker. Data for women point to the same conclusion.[339] A study has been made of 163 cases of lung cancer in women compared with 1192 cases in men attending the same hospital during the same period.[347] In the women, the ratio of cigarette-associated carcinoma (squamous and oat cell) to the other varieties was 0.34:1, compared to 3.05 : 1 in the men. When lung cancer was surveyed during a 3-year period at Memorial Hospital, 8 nonsmokers out of 401 (2%) men and 26 nonsmokers out of 64 (41%) women were found. Adenocarcinoma was present in 5 of the men and most of the women.

The carcinogen has not been identified, nor is it known whether this agent might be only one link in a chain of causality, having an effect, for example, on an enzyme or oxidation-reduction reaction. Various hydrocarbons have been extracted from burning cigarettes and polluted atmosphere. Most carcinogenic to the skin of mice and rats are the benzopyrenes, but one cannot accurately assess their significance in relation to the mucosa of human lungs. Carcinoma of the lung has not been reproduced in animals by products extracted from burning tobacco. Anderson reviews experiments that succeeded in producing carcinoma in animals exposed for long periods to nitro-olefins—products that are possibly found in automobile engine exhausts.[301]

In mining and textile manufacturing areas of England and Wales, an inverse ratio has been discovered between the incidence of chronic bronchitis and of lung cancer. Coal miners have less lung cancer than expected statistically if they have chronic bronchitis.[302] Yet in Manchester smokers have a greater risk of developing chronic bronchitis than do nonsmokers and those who do develop chronic bronchitis are more likely to have lung cancer.[340]

Associated factors may be of importance— atmospheric pollution, the cigarette paper, different tobaccos favored in different countries, simultaneous pulmonary disease such as chronic bronchitis and emphysema, contaminants, length of the discarded butt (filter action), etc.

Atmospheric pollution from industrial and automobile exhausts has long been considered a significant factor in lung carcinoma.

Although the place with the world's highest per caput consumption of cigarettes (the Channel Islands) has the highest incidence of lung carcinoma, one is puzzled by the much lower incidence in heavy smokers in the rural areas of any country as compared with their urban counterparts. It may be because the countryman's carcinogens are received only from cigarettes—not from the air as well. This is also suggested by the fall in lung cancer deaths in Greater London. The city has achieved a dramatic drop in air pollution, greater and sooner than anywhere else, while Londoners' smoking habits have not been altered.[325]

Several occupational lung cancers occur. In uranium mines at Jachymov (Joachimstal), Czechoslovakia, half of all miners' deaths were caused by lung carcinoma. In cobalt mines at Schneeberg, Saxony, three fourths of deaths were caused by carcinoma of the lung. The common factor was radioactive ore and radon gas. Many hundreds of men died before safety measures were employed. Mortality from lung carcinoma in uranium miners in Colorado is four times greater than expected.[348]

Increased risk is recognized among those working in the preparation of asbestos (p. 316), chromates, nickel, arsenic, and iron dust, ore, or fumes.[311]

Changes in the mucosa of large bronchi are commonly found away from the region of the tumor. They range from basal cell hyperplasia with or without atypism, to stratification (flattening of the superficial cells), to squamous metaplasia, and, finally, to carcinoma in situ (Fig. 26-80). These changes have been found

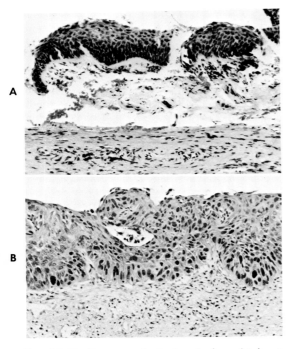

Fig. 26-80. Degrees of atypism in bronchial epithelium. **A,** Moderate dysplasia. **B,** Squamous cell carcinoma in situ. (**A** and **B,** 300×.)

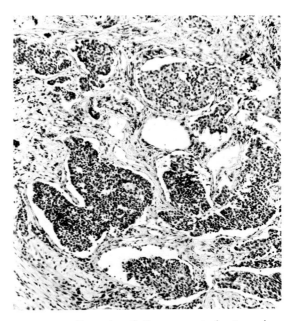

Fig. 26-81. Tumorlet. Cells appear to be in endothelium-lined spaces. (109×.)

in 98.8% of multiple sections of the tracheobronchial tree of men who died with pulmonary carcinoma.[305] Almost as many sections from smokers who died with other diseases had the changes. Only 16.8% of the sections from nonsmokers exhibited mucosal abnormality, which rarely exceeded basal cell hyperplasia. In children, the changes were found in 16.6% of sections, chiefly squamous metaplasia and stratification (14.6%) and basal cell hyperplasia (2.4%).[304] In children, there is a frequent association between the epithelial lesion and healing of mucosal ulcers.

Chronic inflammation progressing to fibrosis is associated with lung tumors of two varieties, the *tumorlet* and the *scar carcinoma*. The initial stage is *atypical bronchiolar proliferation*. When fibrous tissue surrounds and replaces alveoli, the surviving alveoli are lined by uniform small cuboid cells with dark regular nuclei (cuboid metaplasia from alveolar epithelium). This may be seen in tuberculosis, nonresolving pneumonia, chronic pneumonitis, bronchiectasis, lipid pneumonia, chronic abscess, in and around infarcts, anthracosis, and in honeycomb lungs.[333]

In other cases, adenomatous proliferation of cells of the terminal bronchioles is apparent. Dilated spaces are lined by a single layer of uniform low or tall columnar cells with small basal nuclei and pale cytoplasm (Fig. 26-61). When such areas are large, the problem of adenomatosis versus carcinoma arises (p. 1136).

Tumorlet is the name chosen for the next stage, which has areas up to 3 mm in diameter. In one or more fibrous areas of the lung, in the mucosa or walls of bronchi or bronchioles, or in the wall of a chronic abscess, there are isolated groups of small hyperchromatic cells of spindled or oat cell appearance (Fig. 26-81). Often, there is a suggestion of a palisade layer. Cytoplasm is scanty, and the nuclei are quite uniform, with very rare mitoses. In some slides, the cell clusters are observed directly arising from metaplastic cuboid epithelium or alveoli or bronchioles. The more pulmonary scars are examined microscopically, the more tumorlets will be found. Confusion with the rather similar small peripheral carcinoids (p. 1140) and chemodectomas (p. 1144) may be hard to avoid. In 1976 electron microscopic studies showed neurosecretory granules in 14 of 15 tumorlets, a ratio suggesting that there are minute carcinoid tumors.[312a]

Tumorlets are often within spaces resembling lymphatic vessels. In one published report of 90 tumorlets,[334] lymph nodes contained metastases of the cells in five cases. Survival

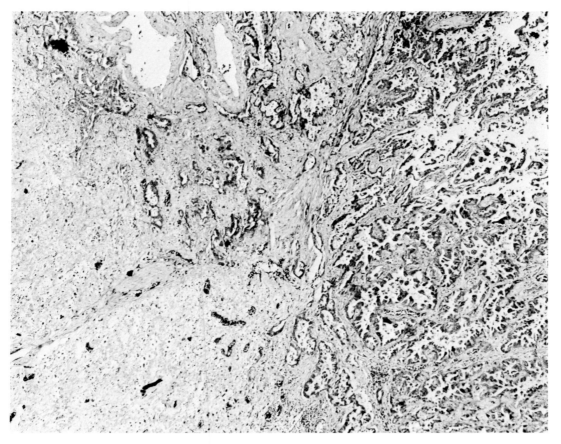

Fig. 26-82. Scar adenocarcinoma. Proliferating atypical glands trapped in scar on left, progressing to rather poorly differentiated adenocarcinoma on right. (52×.)

in perfect health is recorded as long as 12 years after removal of many tumorlets.[331] Tumorlets appear to be nearly always benign, whereas lung carcinomas of the same tiny size often are associated with fatal metastases.

Lung scar carcinoma was brought into prominence about 1940 by Friedrich and by Rössle. Tumorlets do not appear to turn into scar cancers, which, as the name implies, are always malignant. Because pathologists prior to the 1960s often did not recognize the nature of scar adenocarcinoma, a review of the literature is pointless. The true incidence of these tumors is higher than recorded. About two thirds of the tumors are less than 3 cm in diameter. Most are subpleural and appear as puckered scars. The cell type is usually adeno-carcinomatous[309] (Fig. 26-82) but is sometimes squamous or undifferentiated.[352]

These small tumors can set up massive, early metastases in lymphatic vessels and in nodes around large bronchi, creating the false impression that the hilar mass is the site of origin.

A change in the radiologic appearance of a long-stable pulmonary scar should promptly raise the suspicion of carcinoma. There is also an increased incidence of all cell types of lung carcinoma in patients with long-standing fibrosing alveolitis.[319]

Types of carcinoma

If "bronchial carcinoma" is considered to refer to tumors arising from mucosa, this group comprises squamous cell carcinoma, oat cell carcinoma, pleomorphic and giant cell types, and undifferentiated carcinoma. To these could be added bronchial adenocarcinoma. Arising from the mucosa or glands are carcinoid, adenoid cystic carcinoma, and mucoepidermoid carcinoma. Epithelium of the respiratory bronchioles possibly gives rise to bronchiolar carcinoma.

Variation in diagnostic criteria renders numerous series of cases incapable of comparison. Some carcinoids have been misdiagnosed oat cell or poorly differentiated squamous cell

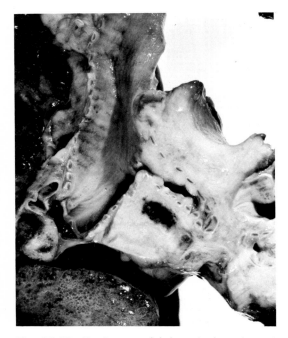

Fig. 26-83. Carcinoma of left main bronchus almost completely occluding its lumen and growing along bronchial tree. Note preservation of cartilage in main bronchus. (From Rezek, P. R., and Millard, M.: Autopsy pathology, Springfield, Ill., 1963, Charles C Thomas, Publisher.)

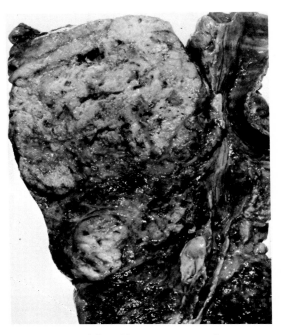

Fig. 26-84. Widely infiltrating variety of squamous cell carcinoma simulating lobar pneumonia or tuberculosis. (From Rezek, P. R., and Millard, M.: Autopsy pathology, Springfield, Ill., 1963, Charles C Thomas, Publisher.)

carcinomas. Some will diagnose squamous cell carcinoma only if intercellular bridges, epithelial pearls, or keratinization is present. Other tumors will be called undifferentiated. In the absence of these findings, other pathologists, using their experience of squamous cell carcinoma elsewhere, feel justified in diagnosing poorly differentiated squamous cell carcinoma. Different opinions about adenocarcinoma and bronchiolar carcinoma create further difficulties. Finally, there is the common experience that the more sections one cuts, the likelier one is to observe a combination of cellular patterns, such as squamous and glandular. The incidence of mixed glandular, oat cell, and squamous carcinoma of the lung in the literature ranges from 3% to 19%, with a figure of about 7% being common.

Bronchial carcinoma

In this section is discussed squamous cell, oat cell, and undifferentiated large cell carcinomas. This group has its peak incidence between the ages of 40 and 65 years. Only a few dozen cases are reported before 20 years of age.[314]

Gross appearance

About 60% to 75% of carcinomas involve a main bronchus (Fig. 26-83) or its bifurcation or even extend to the carina. Two thirds of tumors in resected specimens are peripheral. About one third of squamous cell carcinomas, three fourths of adenocarcinomas, and one fifth of oat cell carcinomas arise in the periphery of the lung.[3] Hence, a hilar tumor is likely to be squamous or oat cell. Of the two, the oat cell variety is smaller, has less chance of central necrosis, and is particularly likely to metastasize early.

Beginning as a roughening of the mucosa that becomes warty, growth continues into the lumen, filling it with white tissue that becomes yellow, soft, and friable. Growth also occurs through the bronchial wall into contiguous lung, initially sparing cartilages. Later, the neoplasm may become fused with its metastases in the hilar nodes. Although any large tumor will be necrotic, yellow, granular, cheesy material usually is associated with squamous cell carcinoma and it closely resembles caseating tuberculosis (Fig. 26-84). Otherwise, gross morphology does not assist much

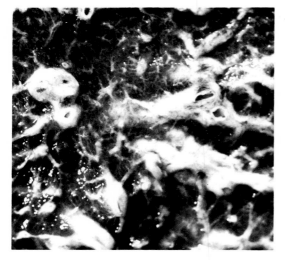

Fig. 26-85. Bronchial carcinoma with widespread peribronchial dissemination. (From Rezek, P. R., and Millard, M.: Autopsy pathology, Springfield, Ill., 1963, Charles C Thomas, Publisher.)

in the recognition of the type of tumor present.

Given time, the tumor will grow along the branches of the stem bronchus, removing any chance of deciding the point of origin. The tumor may even cross the carina. In an investigation of the bronchial stump in 100 surgical cases, there was direct extension of tumor in the bronchus, proximally in 12, submucosal lymphatis spread in six, and significant epithelial metaplasia in 15.[315] One must examine the stump microscopically in every case in order to evaluate the chance of recurrence.

A more limited spread is along a medium-sized bronchus and its smaller branches (Fig. 26-85). Their walls are thickened by white tumor tissue. A similar "pipestem" pattern may be seen in metastatic tumors, especially from the breast and stomach. Carcinoma arising some distance from the hilum is inclined to invade the lung so as to create a fairly well-demarcated, peripherally firm, and centrally friable gray-white sphere (Fig. 26-86). It is often difficult to demonstrate its bronchial origin.

An uncommon type of tumor is shown in Fig. 26-87. This has been called exophytic endobronchial carcinoma.[343] The carcinoma is polypoid or papillomatous, with superficial invasion of the bronchial wall. The prognosis appears to be much better than for more invasive types, perhaps because symptoms of bronchial obstruction arise early.

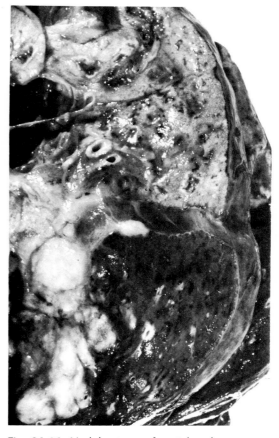

Fig. 26-86. Nodular type of peripheral squamous cell carcinoma. In upper portion of lung is paler area of endogenous lipid pneumonia (see Fig. 26-84).

Multiple primary bronchial carcinomas

Painstaking studies have been made of the tracheobronchial trees of 255 patients who died of bronchial carcinoma. Nine patients (3.5%) had two or more bronchial primary lesions. With less rigid criteria, such multiplicity could be found in up to 12.5%.[306] There is a later report of 55 patients with a second bronchial primary carcinoma.[344a]

Local effects

Obstruction of the lumen is caused either by intraluminal growth or by a stenosing tumor encircling the wall. If the lumen is partly blocked, a valve effect may induce obstructive overinflation in the distribution of the bronchus. Usually obstruction will later become complete, and the air is then absorbed. The collapsed area is usually the site of organizing pneumonia. Obstruction also can lead to infection of retained secretions, bronchiectasis,

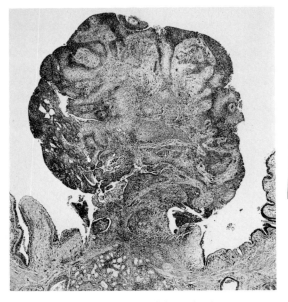

Fig. 26-87. Exophytic endobronchial squamous cell carcinoma with superficial submucosal invasion. (19×.)

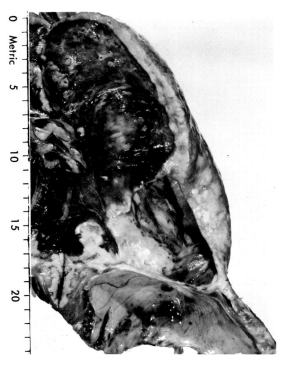

Fig. 26-88. Metastatic squamous cell carcinoma encasing entire lung. Without demonstrating primary lung tumor, this appearance also would be compatible with mesothelioma or sometimes even with fibrous end stage of pyogenic or tuberculous empyema.

abscess, or gangrene. Chronic pneumonitis or an abscess is a common first sign of carcinoma and may even cause death. The cavity is lined by necrotic tumor and does not have the dirty gray or pink lining of an uncomplicated lung abscess.

The primary tumor or its metastases can compress a pulmonary artery or vein or grow around and into the superior vena cava. The latter happens most often when the tumor is in the right main bronchus. The effect is great venous distention of the head, neck, and upper arms, with edema and cyanosis of these areas. Erosion of a large vessel in the wall of a bronchus or cavitated carcinoma can cause fatal bleeding. Hilar tumor may destroy the recurrent laryngeal and phrenic nerves as they run along the trachea. It may extend into the pericardium. If the tumor reaches the pleura, it sets up serous or sanguinous effusion and, if cavitated, its rupture may be responsible for empyema. Seeding of the pleura can thickly coat the entire lung like a mesothelioma (Fig. 26-88). Growth can continue into the chest wall or into a neighboring lobe. An apical tumor can destroy the neighboring ribs and brachial plexus. Invasion of the cervical sympathetic trunk brings about Horner's syndrome (ptosis of the upper eyelid, constricted pupil, and decreased sweating on the same side of the face). All primary neoplasms of the lung and practically all metastases are fed by systemic arteries.

Microscopic appearance

The largest series in which a realistic classification of lung carcinomas was used is the 5000 cases from Memorial Hospital.[332] It should form the basis of comparison for future series from other large centers. The series was divided as follows: squamous, 40%; large cell anaplastic, 33%; combined adenocarcinoma and bronchiolar, 16%; oat cell, 11%. Do understand that these figures will be different in a surgical series (biased toward resectable and peripheral tumors) and an autopsy series (including hopelessly inoperable central tumors).

Squamous cell carcinoma. A well-differentiated keratinizing tumor of the squamous cell variety is uncommon in the lung. More often, one can recognize epithelial pearl formation, intracellular bridges, or a whorling of cells within true pearls. There may be only an occasional deeply eosinophilic, individually keratinized cell.

The cells are in sheets, cords, and bundles

separated by varying amounts of vascular connective tissue. Cellular pleomorphism usually is pronounced, but mitoses are not necessarily numerous. Often, the outer cell layer has a palisade effect, and this, when cut at a particular angle, can give a pseudoglandular appearance. At times, some of the larger tumor cells are of the signet type (Fig. 26-89), but mucin stains will be negative. This imitation of adenocarcinoma is seen in tissues where

there is no possibility of two cell types being present, particularly in cervical metastases from carcinoma of the oral cavity.

One variety of endobronchial squamous carcinoma (Fig. 26-90) is the *papillary carcinoma*, sometimes multiple and sometimes built up of neoplastic transitional type of epithelium rather than squamous.

Oat cell carcinoma (small cell carcinoma). The name "oat cell carcinoma" applies to a

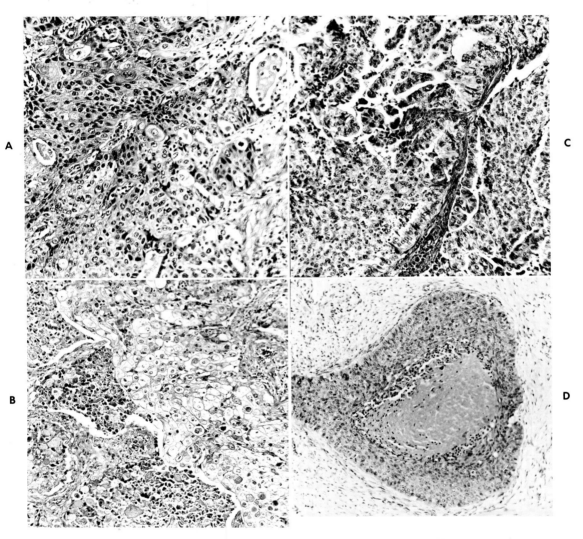

Fig. 26-89. Squamous cell carcinoma. **A,** Lesion in upper left corner readily recognized as squamous cell carcinoma. In remainder of photomicrograph, tumor is poorly differentiated and forms pseudoglands, which appear to contain secretion that is actually degenerating material. **B,** Formation of large clear cells that look as though they might contain mucin but do not react with mucin stains. This clarity of cytoplasm is probably attributable to hydropic degeneration. Same tumor as shown in **A. C,** Area with mixture of undifferentiated and tall columnar glandular cells. **D,** Necrotic form of squamous cell carcinoma, form more often seen in upper respiratory tract but also resembling comedocarcinoma of breast. (**A,** 150×; **B,** 109×; **C,** 132×; **D,** 141×.)

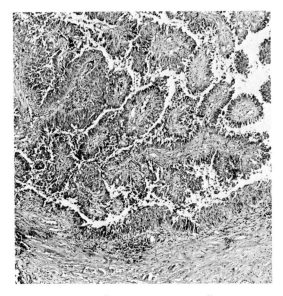

Fig. 26-90. Papillary squamous cell carcinoma of bronchus, type sometimes called transitional carcinoma. (90×.)

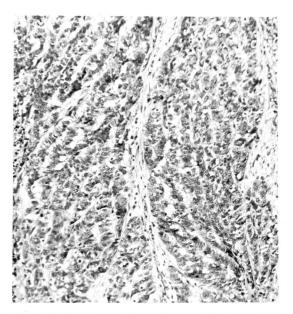

Fig. 26-92. Oat cell carcinoma. Variant with cells arranged in ribbons. (152×.)

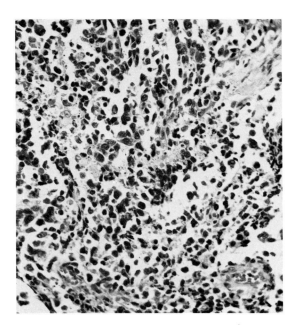

Fig. 26-91. Oat cell carcinoma, "usual" type. (234×.)

specific tumor that appears to develop beneath the columnar mucosal layer. Mitoses are common, and, in lighter-staining nuclei, prominent nucleoli are present. The tumor usually is characterized by diffuse sheets of closely packed cells about 8 μm in diameter, somewhat larger than a lymphocyte in formalin-fixed tissue.

There is little or no cytoplasm—merely very hyperchromatic round, oval, or spindle-shaped nuclei in which little structural detail is visible (Fig. 26-91). Metastases of these cells in lymph nodes often can only be appreciated initially because they replace normal structure. Careful search will always disclose the elongated forms and set aside the diagnosis of lymphosarcoma. In 84% of one series of cases,[350] the nuclei of lymph node metastases were larger and paler, and there was more cytoplasm, resembling cells of anaplastic squamous cell carcinoma. Some definite structural pattern has been noted.[307] The cells may be arranged in "streams" (i.e., clumps of cells with a parallel orientation of their long axes). Another variant is the "ribbon," one to several cells in width, often running in festoons (Fig. 26-92). Pseudo-rosettes, rosettes, tubules, and ductules also can be seen. Ductules sometimes contain epithelial mucin, but there is no resemblance to poorly differentiated adenocarcinoma.

Serious misconceptions have been held for many years about the nature of oat cell carcinoma. For a long time it was believed to be a mediastinal lymphosarcoma and then, till recently, an anaplastic (possibly epidermoid) carcinoma. The fallacy of the latter was demolished in three stages: (1) Azzopardi's demonstration of the structural pattern,[307] (2) the recognition of endocrine activity in some of these tumors (p. 1134), and (3) the electron microscopic delineation of the close relationship of oat cell carcinoma to carcinoid.

Rarely in pathology is orthodoxy so profoundly demolished and reconstructed as in the work of Bensch et al.[310] They have confirmed that in normal bronchial epithelium (especially in the first year of life) occasional argyrophilic Kulchitsky[329] cells are present (p. 1039). Electron microscopy disclosed neurosecretory granules in their cytoplasm. Similar granules are present in the cytoplasm of oat cell carcinomas and of bronchial carcinoids. Here lies the explanation of the difficulty we sometimes experience in deciding whether we are looking at an oat cell carcinoma or a carcinoid. Perhaps this is a clue as to why most endocrine syndromes caused by lung cancer are associated with the oat cell variety.

Undifferentiated large cell carcinoma. Undifferentiated large cell carcinomas have cells of varying types. The diagnosis begins by exclusion of recognizable features of squamous cells, oat cells, or glandular cells. With differing criteria, this group swells and diminishes in various studies. The cells are close together in a medullary or solid alveolar arrangement. Invasion of small blood vessels and lymphatic vessels is common. Individual cells are oval, spindled, angular, or polyhedral. Results of nuclear and cytoplasmic staining are very variable, but the nuclei tend to be large, with prominent nucleoli.

The variant known as *giant cell carcinoma* is uncommon, invades blood vessels, is more widely metastasizing, and is the most rapidly fatal of all lung carcinomas. The cells are loosely set in a stroma, scanty even when subjected to reticulin stains. Cells are nearly all of the multinucleated giant cell type, frequently extremely bizarre and hyperchromatic (Fig. 26-93). Occasionally, one tumor cell is seen ingesting another. Smaller single-nucleated pleomorphic cells are present, and there are areas with spindled and strap cells, suggesting rhabdomyosarcoma but without cross striations.[338] Tissue culture shows that the cells are epithelial. Melamed[332] considers that this is just one form of undifferentiated large cell carcinoma. There is reason for believing that most, if not all, giant cell carcinomas may be anaplastic adenocarcinoma.[322]

Spindle cell carcinoma. Spindle cell carcinoma frequently has been mistaken for carcinosarcoma, which accounts for the excessive number of case reports of the latter. In sites such as the esophagus, urinary bladder, and oral mucosa, squamous cell carcinoma is well

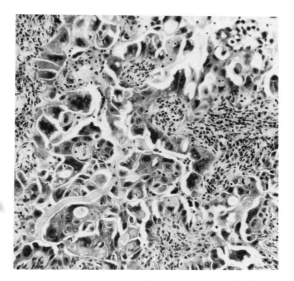

Fig. 26-93. Giant cell carcinoma. (168×.)

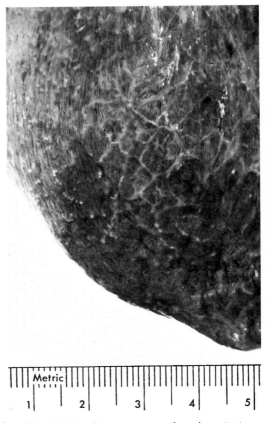

Metric

1   2   3   4   5

Fig. 26-94. Carcinomatous lymphangiosis.

known to undergo transition to a spindled form, as can malignant melanoma. In breast carcinoma, cartilaginous and osseous metaplasia is recognized. Therefore, the diagnosis of carcinosarcoma of the bronchus is difficult to uphold as opposed to carcinosarcoma of lung (p. 1144).

Pattern of metastases

Lymphatic spread. Spread to hilar lymph nodes is seen in the majority of cases, particularly when the tumor is in a large bronchus. Extension then occurs to the mediastinal and paratracheal groups. When the hilar lymph nodes have been destroyed, retrograde flow in the pulmonary lymphatic vessels reaches the subpleural plexus. The condition of carcinomatous lymphangiosis is the delicate white lacework produced when vessels of the plexus are totally permeated (Fig. 26-94). This condition is often also secondary to numerous small arterial emboli of tumor cells. Tumor cells may travel into the chest wall through lymphatic vessels in pleural adhesions. By retrograde extension through the diaphragm, lymph nodes along the abdominal aorta are colonized. Of great prognostic importance is the group of small nodes on the scalenus anterior muscle. These nodes are frequently biopsied, for their involvement renders the disease incurable. Invasion and obstruction of the thoracic duct cause chylothorax.

Hematogenous spread. Carcinoma of the lung can spread in the blood to any part of the body. Collier et al.[313] examined resected lungs for blood vessel invasion. They found that in patients with such invasion the 5-year survival rate was 6%, whereas 72% of the few patients without vascular invasion lived for 5 years.

Extrathoracic metastases are usual, partly because the pulmonary veins are so often invaded. In one large series of autopsied cases, no metastases were present in 10.5%, most of which were squamous cell tumors.[346] Studies of other large groups of cases indicate that metastases are found in the liver in about one third, in the adrenal glands in 20% to 33%, in the skeletal system in 15% to 21%, in the brain in about 18%, in the kidneys in 14% to 17%, and in the spleen in about 5%.[3] Involvement of the liver can be massive at an early stage and may cause both jaundice and seeding back to the lungs. Frequently, metastases from carcinoma of the lung present clinically as primary brain tumors. Extensive meningeal involvement can simulate meningitis or encephalitis.

Skin, pancreas, myocardium, and intestine occasionally are invaded. The pituitary gland, particularly the posterior lobe, often has metastases, and these rarely cause deficiency syndromes.

Extrapulmonary manifestations of bronchial carcinoma

Some bronchial carcinomas produce hormones or effects on the neuromuscular system. To date, the following have been recorded: adrenocorticotropin, glucagon, serotonin or related substances, antidiuretic hormones, parathormone-like and insulin-like substances, and gonadotropin.

The clue to *gonadotropin* is the appearance of gynecomastia, seen in four men, who had large anaplastic carcinomas of the bronchus.[356] Nearly all the endocrine syndromes are associated with oat cell carcinoma, and the commonest is *Cushing's syndrome,* 115 examples of which had been collected by 1965.[353] (Islet cell carcinomas and thymomas sometimes also have this association). Cushing's syndrome secondary to lung carcinoma comes on rapidly and may be fulminant. The tumor either produces ACTH or a corticotropin-like substance that stimulates the adrenal glands and depresses ACTH secretion by the pituitary gland. Sixteen of 20 patients with oat cell carcinoma (and without Cushing's syndrome) had increased numbers of pituitary hyaline basophils (Crooke's cells).[358] This is the hallmark of increased circulating cortisone type of hormones. In the Cushing cases, the adrenal glands are hyperplastic (two to three times normal weight) but, even without the syndrome, autopsies on patients who had oat cell carcinoma frequently disclose lesser degrees of adrenocortical hyperplasia. The latter is taken to indicate that there are two types of adrenocorticopin, one relating to adrenal weight and the other (in Cushing's syndrome) to steroid production. Cushing's syndrome may be associated with bronchial carcinoid.[362] Again, we see a relationship between the latter and oat cell carcinoma.

Inappropriate antidiuretic hormone activity has been reported about 26 times, with nearly all the tumors being oat cell carcinoma, with occasional adenocarcinoma.[353] The hormone may be produced directly by the tumor. The clinical effects include hyponatremia and urinary sodium wastage, absence of edema, and renal and adrenal malfunction—these leading to lethargy, confusion, and coma. The last three are the symptoms of hypercalcemia of malignancy and of *parathormone-like activity.* Hypercalcemia was found in 25 of 200 patients with unresectable bronchial carcinoma, 14 of whom had no osseous metastases. There were 12 with squamous cell carcinoma and 2 with large cell anaplastic carcinoma.[308] A number of authors have confirmed that even with bone secondaries, hypercalcemia is rare in adeno-carcinoma and does not occur in oat cell carcinoma.

Another mysterious combination, and the commonest, is the group of neuromuscular abnormalities that may be associated with carcinoma of the lung.[354] *Cortical cerebellar degeneration* produces loss of cerebellar function. *Peripheral neuropathy,* usually purely sensory, is associated with degeneration of neurons in the posterior root ganglia. In some patients, *mental changes* are prominent. They are considered a metabolic effect of the tumor, since they occur in the absence of metastases. The effects range from impaired mental acuity to severe dementia. All three neuromuscular disorders may be combined. A fourth abnormality, a muscle weakness termed *carcinomatous myopathy,* is recognized. There are degenerative changes in the muscles of the limb girdle and trunk. These variants were found in 16% of the 250 patients examined in one study.[355] By 1966 a review had collected 165 cases, and oat cell carcinoma comprised 54% of the lung tumors in the patients.[360] Some

patients with oat cell carcinoma developed a myasthenic syndrome with a relatively poor response to neostigmine.[357] This may be seen in as many as 6% of cases.[359]

Prognosis

A computer analysis of survival of 2155 patients with lung cancer surveyed the significance of 28 factors, such as size of tumor, site, and presence of metastases. A major finding was that squamous cell carcinoma had the best prognosis and that there was virtually no survival with oat cell carcinoma.[336]

Discussion of the value of early diagnosis of lung cancer remains pessimistic, particularly because a lesion visible in chest x-ray films is already a late one. Six-monthly examinations of large numbers of men in London and Philadelphia have not improved survival in those who developed lung cancer[341] while under surveillance. In the Philadelphia study 121 of 6136 men developed lung cancer during a 10-year period; 67 of them did so within 6 months of a chest x-ray film being read as negative. When their films were reviewed, the tumor was seen in 30% to 42% of all the cases, the figure varying with the reviewer.[351] By contrast, when occult carcinoma has been diagnosed by selective bronchial washing, only 2 (3%) of 61 patients have died of the disease.[346a]

Analysis of the results of surgical therapy

Table 26-1. T, N, and M categories for carcinoma of the lung*

T	Primary tumors
T0	No evidence of primary tumor
TX	Tumor proved by the presence of malignant cells in bronchopulmonary secretions but not visualized roentgenographically or bronchoscopically
T1	A tumor that is 3 cm or less in greatest diameter, surrounded by lung or visceral pleura and without evidence of invasion proximal to a lobar bronchus at bronchoscopy
T2	A tumor more than 3 cm in greatest diameter, or a tumor of any size that, with its associated atelectasis or obstructive pneumonitis, extends to the hilar region. At bronchoscopy the proximal extent of demonstrable tumor must be at least 2 cm distal to the carina. Any associated atelectasis or obstructive pneumonitis must involve less than an entire lung, and there must be no pleural effusion
T3	A tumor of any size with direct extension into an adjacent structure such as the chest wall, the diaphragm, or the mediastinum and its contents; or demonstrable bronchoscopically to be less than 2 cm distal to the carina; any tumor associated with atelectasis or obstructive pneumonitis of an entire lung or pleural effusion
N	**Regional lymph nodes**
N0	No demonstrable metastasis to regional lymph nodes
N1	Metastasis to lymph nodes in the ipsilateral hilar region (including direct extension)
N2	Metastasis to lymph nodes in the mediastinum
M	**Distant metastasis**
M0	No distant metastasis
M1	Distant metastasis such as in scalene, cervical, or contralateral hilar lymph nodes, brain, bones, lung, liver, etc.

*Each case must be assigned the highest category of T, N, and M that describes the full extent of disease in that case.

Table 26-2. Stage grouping in carcinoma of the lung

Occult carcinoma	
TX N0 M0	An occult carcinoma with bronchopulmonary secretions containing malignant cells but without other evidence of the primary tumor or evidence of metastasis to the regional lymph nodes or distant metastasis.
Invasive carcinoma stage I	
T1 N0 M0	A tumor that can be classified T1 without any metastasis or with metastasis
T1 N1 M0	to the lymph nodes in the ipsilateral hilar region only, or a tumor that
T2 N0 M0	can be classified T2 without any metastasis to nodes are distant metastasis. Note: TX N1 M0 and T0 N1 M0 are also theoretically possible, but such a clinical diagnosis would be difficult if not impossible to make. If such a diagnosis is made, it should be included in stage 1.
Stage II	
T2 N1 M0	A tumor classified as T2 with metastasis to the lymph nodes in the ipsilateral hilar region only.
Stage III	
T3 with any N or M	Any tumor more extensive than T2, or any tumor with metastasis to the lymph
N2 with any T or M	nodes in the mediastinum, or with distant metastasis.
M1 with any T or N	

in 2156 patients suffering from bronchial carcinoma has revealed that in only 464 was resection possible, and 347 of these survived the operative phase. The 5-year survival of the 347 patients was 28%, or slightly under 5% for the whole group.[320]

A better prognosis can be expected in cases of solitary nodular carcinomas of lung. When these are no bigger than 4 cm in diameter, the resection-for-cure rate is as high as 94%, and in persons surviving the operation for curative resection, the 5-year survival is 51%. In a series of 193 such tumors, 58% were adenocarcinoma and alveolar cell carcinoma, 39% squamous and large cell carcinoma, and 3% oat cell carcinoma.[327]

A review[337] of 51 patients living 5 years after surgical therapy disclosed no special factors, such as early diagnosis, that would explain this survival. Of 2540 patients, 56 survived 10 years, but some still developed recurrences or new primary tumors. In one series, of those patients who survived surgery, the 5-year survival in those with oat cell carcinoma was 9%; large anaplastic carcinoma, 30%; squamous cell carcinoma, 42%; and adenocarcinoma, 54%.[328] There were 767 patients, of whom only 184 could be offered surgery with a hope of cure (24%). Out of the 767, only 8% lived 5 years.

The American Joint Committee for Cancer Staging and End Results Reporting has developed a clinical stage classification for carcinoma of the lung, using the TNM System.[300a] Applicable separately to the different histologic types, it has been accepted by the International Union Against Cancer. The categorization is outlined in the following Tables 26-1 and 26-2.

The *causes of death* from bronchial carcinoma are various combinations of pneumonia, lung abscess, bronchiectasis, asphyxia, bleeding, fistulas to the pleura or eosphagus, and the effects of the various metastases. Adrenocortical insufficiency is rare, even when the glands are extensively replaced.

Pulmonary adenomatosis, bronchioloalveolar carcinoma, and adenocarcinoma

Clear distinctions between pulmonary adenomatosis, bronchioloalveolar carcinoma, and some cases of adenocarcinoma of the lung often are difficult and perhaps unnecessary. *Adenomatosis* was referred to in the discussion of scar tumors and of changes in areas of chronic inflammation and fibrosis (p. 1126). Another variety is seen in the absence of fibrosis, when a single layer of well-differentiated tall columnar cells lines the alveoli in one or more areas (Fig. 26-94). The cells have basal nuclei and copious pale cytoplasma that sometimes contains mucin. Cilia are rare. Sometimes, the cells are separated slightly from one another, creating a peglike appearance. Although usual, histologic criteria of malignancy are lacking, the description may be the same in many cases of metastasizing *bronchioloalveolar carcinoma*.

Several cases have been described in which carcinoma of the pancreas and a few from the stomach, ovary, or breast metastasized to the lung, exactly imitating bronchioloalveolar carcinoma microscopically.[324]

The only way to recognize *adenocarcinoma* is to see it arising grossly as a roughening of the mucosa of a bronchus, with microscopic origin from the mucosa or submucosal glands.

The preceding discussion gives reasons leading some to the view that all three lesions are only variants of one type of neoplasm. Shinton[344] considers bronchioloalveolar carcinoma to be "a form of spread" of adenocarcinoma "rather than a histologic type." Liebow has not been able to distinguish the two unless by noting origin of a poorly differentiated adenocarcinoma from a small bronchus and by being aware of its rapid growth and early bloodborne metastases.[330]

It seems best to consider that these tumors, which nearly always are peripheral, can be well differentiated (bronchioloalveolar carcinoma and the very rare adenomatosis) or poorly differentiated (adenocarcinoma). They can be gathered under the title *peripheral adenocarcinoma* with qualifying titles if necessary, such as "well-differentiated" or "poorly differentiated" or "scar adenocarcinoma." Half of one series of 100 cases arose in scars.[309] True adenocarcinoma of bronchial glands or mucosa is seen only occasionally.

Further light has been shed in 1975 by a study of five cases in which the true tumor cell was considered to be either a metaplastic bronchiolar mucous cell (the typical tall columnar cell of bronchiolar carcinoma) or a bronchiolar stem cell with ultrastructural features of both the ciliated and nonciliated (Clara) cell of the bronchus. In the light microscope the latter two tumor cells are low columnar or cuboid with big hyperchromatic nuclei. It is postulated that the type II cells believed by a number of observers to be neoplastic are merely hyperplastic, stimulated by the proximity of the tumor cells.[321] The conclusion is that true alveolar cell carcinoma is rare. Some of the cases have admixed areas of oat cell or squamous cell carcinoma.[316]

Nature of peripheral adenocarcinoma

Peripheral adenocarcinoma occurs with equal frequency in men and women. However, it is proportionately a more frequent carcinoma of the lung in women because they have only one sixth the number of bronchial carcinomas suffered by men. The incidence of the tumor appears to be increasing. Cases have been noted arising in pulmonary scars, in honeycomb lung, in fibrosing alveolitis,[319,333] and in progressive systemic sclerosis.[318] Three cases were complications of chronic mineral oil pneumonia.[312] Although an infectious disease of similar microscopic appearance is quite common in sheep *(jagsiekte)* and in horses, guinea pigs, and rats, this does not unravel the mystery. Discord arises as to whether multiple lesions in the lung indicate multicentricity. The majority view is that there is one origin with prolific airborne dissemination along alveolar septa and the bronchial tree.[323]

Gross appearance

In the unusual instance of *adenocarcinoma arising from bronchial mucosa,* the lesion will be close to the hilum and will resemble other hilar tumors. Microscopically, there are small, well-formed but irregular glands lying in a connective tissue stroma and lined by a single or pseudostratified layer of tall columnar cells. These have large hyperchromatic nuclei and pale cytoplasm and may be ciliated.

Adenocarcinoma and *bronchioloalveolar carcinoma* cannot be distinguished grossly even by those who regard them as separate conditions. Multiple cuts should be made through the tumor in search of a scar that may be central or off-center. About half the cases are of nodular type, one third diffuse (lobular or

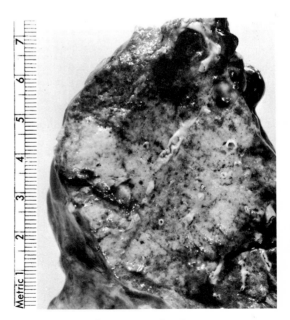

Fig. 26-95. Diffuse type of adenocarcinoma resembling diffuse type of squamous cell carcinoma (see Fig. 26-84).

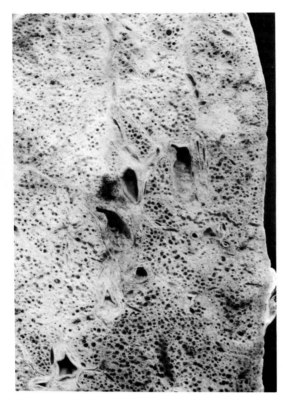

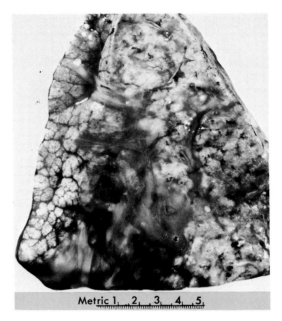

Fig. 26-97. Mucoid adenocarcinoma. Most of lung replaced by white soft tumor. Lower two thirds of cut surface covered by tenacious mucin, so that specimen resembles that of very mucinous pneumococcal or *Klebsiella* pneumonia.

Fig. 26-96. Adenocarcinoma. Patient had no nodules of tumor, but most alveoli in both lungs were lined by single layer of well-differentiated cells like those shown in Fig. 26-98, *A*. Patient died of alveolocapillary block without metastases, and by some this would be regarded as an example of pulmonary adenomatosis.

nodes were affected in 26%, liver in 13%, and the following sites (listed in descending order) each involved in less than 10%: abdominal nodes, bones, adrenal glands, brain, pleura, kidneys, pericardium, cervical nodes, spleen, heart, and diaphragm.[345]

Microscopic appearance

In the best-differentiated adenocarcinoma, a layer of tall columnar cells lines alveolar septa (Fig. 26-98, *A*). Nuclei are small, basal, hyperchromatic, and fairly uniform, and the cytoplasm is pale or full of mucin. Mucin may distend some alveoli and even flatten the tumor cells lining them. Slender papillae of the cells may project into the alveoli. When respiratory bronchioles are recognized, tumor cells will be seen growing along the mucosal surface, and, proximally, a transition to the more cuboid normal respiratory lining cells may be seen. Because cells line a fine membrane and enclose spaces the size and shape of alveoli, it does not mean that they are alveoli. Very likely, the membranes are often just fine stromal strands. Characteristically, at the periphery of the lesions it is easy to find tumor cells along some alveolar septa. Many cells, apparently viable, are free in the alveoli. A few cells lining septa are ciliated, a feature

lobar) (Fig. 26-95), and the remainder mixed. In about two thirds, both lungs are ultimately affected to a significant degree, in striking contrast to bronchial carcinoma.

The nodules are gray-white consolidated areas averaging 3 to 5 cm and are fairly well demarcated. Very often they are multiple and present in some or all lobes. The diffuse variety is so extensive that it mimics a gray area of pneumonia (Fig. 26-96) or the yellow-white of organizing or lipid pneumonia. Central necrosis is common. Often, mucin secreted by the tumor cells makes the cut surface resemble that of *Klebsiella* or *Pneumococcus* type III pneumonia (Fig. 26-97). Efforts to demonstrate an origin from a bronchus will nearly always fail.

In a report on 205 cases of bronchioloalveolar carcinoma, metastases were found to be present in 54% (19% local only, 16% distant only, and 20% local and distant). Mediastinal

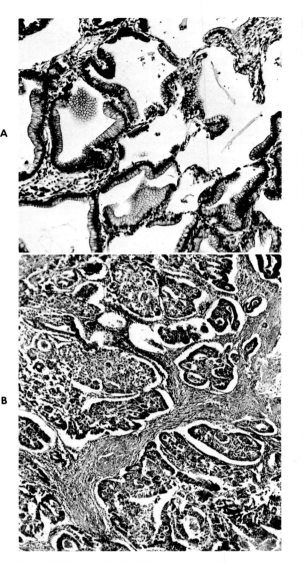

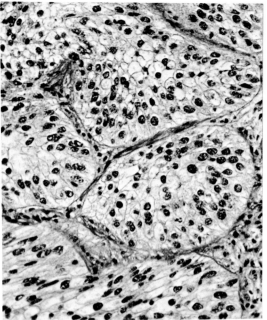

Fig. 26-99. Clear-cell carcinoma. (189×.)

Fig. 26-98. A, Well-differentiated adenocarcinoma growing along interalveolar septa. **B,** Poorly differentiated adenocarcinoma with little resemblance to alveolar pattern. (**A,** 124×; **B,** 111×.)

not seen in any other tumor of the lung. In less-differentiated forms, nuclear characteristics of malignancy appear—hyperchromasia, irregularity and pleomorphism, and mitoses. Origin from a scar may be recognized (Fig. 26-82). There is a sclerotic form in which the tumorous "acini" are separated from one another by connective tissue. Of still lower differentiation are the varieties with irregular glands no longer the shape and size of aveoli (Fig. 26-98, *B*) or with a cribriform pattern as if a duct were crossed by interlacing strands of tumor cells.

Clear-cell carcinoma (Fig. 26-99) has been considered by some as a poorly differentiated adenocarcinoma.[335] There are sheets and alveolar clumps of large rounded cells with clear nonstaining cytoplasm that often reacts with mucin stains. Others have identified glycogen in some of the cells. Some examples appear to be variants of squamous cell carcinoma with hydropic cytoplasm. One must exclude the presence of a primary carcinoma in the kidney.

"Bronchial adenoma"

The term "bronchial adenoma" should mean a benign glandlike proliferation of bronchial mucosa, but only 11 cases had been collected by 1967, all apparently in larger bronchi.[369] Seven years later only one more case could be added. Even rarer are benign mixed tumors of the bronchi.

In practice, the term "bronchial adenoma" is used to designate a group of malignant or potentially malignant tumors: carcinoid, adenoid cystic carcinoma, and mucoepidermoid carcinoma. In a collection of 162 of these tumors, 89.5% were carcinoids, 8% were adenoid cystic carcinoma, and 2.5% (four cases) were mucoepidermoid carcinoma.[371] By 1973 there were 50 recorded cases of mucoepidermoid lung tumors.[364]

"Bronchial adenomas" appear some years

earlier than do carcinomas of the lung, and the sex distribution is equal. The types cannot be distinguished grossly, although adenoid cystic carcinoma tends to be closer to the carina and may be in the trachea. The tumors are polypoid or sessile, but although they extend into the lumen, they are likely to grow into the bronchial wall and expand into neighboring lung as a dumbbell shape, so that removal by bronchoscope is impossible. The surface of the endobronchial part is covered by intact mucosa and is smooth or lobulated. Gross examination gives no clue as to malignancy.

The microscopic appearance is the same as described for these tumors in the salivary gland and gastrointestinal tract (Fig. 26-100). *Carcinoids* of the lung have a number of microscopic variants. Osseous metaplasia may occur between the tumor cells (Fig. 26-101). A few carcinoids have pink granular cells of the oncocytic type. Glandular differentiation and mucin secretion are quite common in carcinoids and in no way rule out that diagnosis.[368] A carcinoid is quite often poorly differentiated and can have a hardly recognizable organized pattern with extreme nuclear irregularity, which may be mistaken for undifferentiated bronchial carcinoma. A distorted bronchial biopsy specimen makes this an even

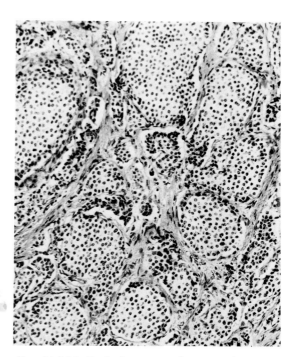

Fig. 26-100. Typical pattern of carcinoid. (153×.)

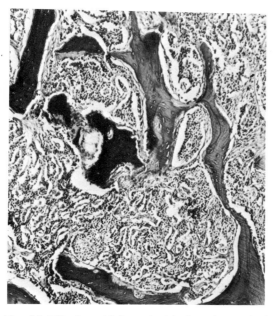

Fig. 26-101. Bronchial carcinoid. Greatly ossified stroma. (96×.)

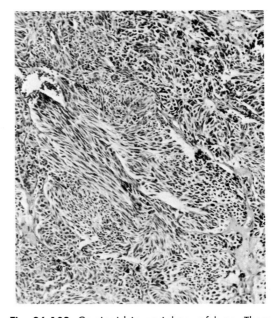

Fig. 26-102. Carcinoid in periphery of lung. There is pronounced spindled pattern. This tumor was malignant, although cellular pattern is not indicative of this. (165×.)

more difficult decision. Spindle-celled carcinoids also have to be recognized (Fig. 26-102). They are especially to be found peripherally, where carcinoids with granular cytoplasm also occur. Both types tend to be small, probably arising from small bronchi or bronchioles.[366] The presence of bronchial mucosa to one side of the poorly defined tumor and the absence of a scar would point to a peripheral carcinoid. The relationship of tumorlets to carcinoids is discussed on p. 1126.

In difficult cases, one cannot rely on argyrophilic or argentaffin stains for cytoplasmic granules, since these are hard to see in any bronchial carcinoid. One may demonstrate the granules in electron microscopic studies of formalin-fixed tumor tissue.

Malignancy of carcinoids in the lung can be as difficult to determine as it is in the intestine.[373] Five percent of 203 bronchial carcinoids excised at the Mayo Clinic metastasized.[370] With the recognition of the relationship to oat cell carcinoma (p. 1133), some tumors that might in the past have been wrongly classed as oat cell carcinoma will now be recognized as malignant carcinoids.

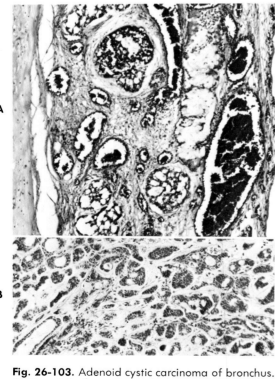

Fig. 26-103. Adenoid cystic carcinoma of bronchus. **A,** Its origin from mucosal glands. **B,** Deeper infiltrating portion. (**A,** 84×; **B,** 119×.)

About 12 examples of carcinoid syndrome in association with a metastasizing bronchial carcinoid are on record.[367] Carcinoids of different embryonic parts of the gut have differing carcinoid syndromes. That of the bronchi (foregut) is remarkable for severe and prolonged episodes of flushing, apparently because carcinoids have produced histamine and 5-OH-tryptophan instead of serotonin. Such variation is characterized ultrastructurally by recognizable differences in the morphology of carcinoids in different sites.[365] Bronchial carcinoids are argyrophilic but not argentaffin.

As of 1968, there were 21 cases of "bronchial adenoma" in children under the age of 16 years. Of those that were microscopically identified, nine were carcinoids, three adenoid cystic, and two mucoepidermoid.[375] A handful of cases of mediastinal carcinoids has been seen. Their origin is believed to be mediastinal remnants of bronchial anlagen.

These tumors also may arise in the *trachea* as is noted in a report of 16 cases that could be resected.[372] Of these, seven invaded the thyroid and four the esophagus. Hematogenous metaseases were found in the lung in five patients and the brain in one. Only one patient had regional lymph node metastases.

Prognosis

In one reported series, only 57% of 21 patients with bronchial *carcinoid* survived 5 years, and 44% of 27 patients with such tumors had metastases.[368] In another series, *adenoid cystic carcinoma* was a slowly growing, infiltrating malignancy, invading adjacent structures, destroying cartilage, and eventually producing distant metastases[371] (Fig. 26-103). Most of the two dozen or so reported cases of *mucoepidermoid carcinoma* of the bronchus have been low grade (Fig. 26-104), and the three metastasizing cases cited in one study are unusual.

RARE PULMONARY TUMORS
Bronchial chondroma

Bronchial chondroma is a smooth-surfaced but lobulated, pedunculated, or sessile tumor projecting into the lumen. Grossly, its cartilaginous nature is recognized on the cut surface, and it is seen microscopically to be well-formed hyaline cartilage. It is not to be confused with hamartoma (below).

Bronchial papillomatosis

The commoner laryngeal papillomatosis rarely extends down the trachea into the bron-

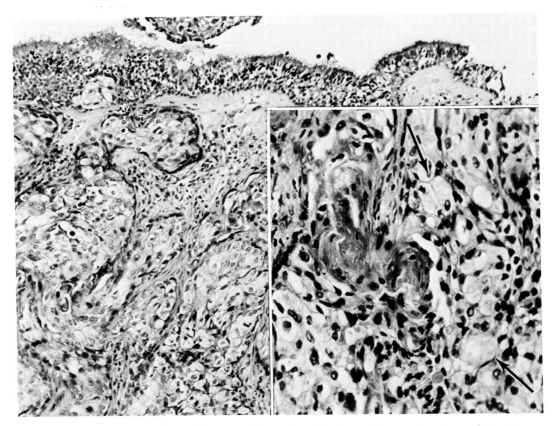

Fig. 26-104. Mucoepidermoid tumor of bronchus showing submucosal nature of tumor. *Arrows in inset,* Mucin-containing cells, to left of which is well-developed keratinization of other cells. (177×; inset, 330×.)

chial tree. Most of the patients are children, but occasionally adults are affected. Death in such cases is from obstruction, aspiration, and pulmonary infection. The innumerable bronchial lesions are warty, with a microscopic structure of acanthotic stratified squamous epithelium covering the papillary and branching connective tissue core. There may be epithelial atypism or even malignant change.

Lipoma

One fifth of pulmonary lipomas arise in fat normally present beneath the pleura. The remaining tumors are in the normal fat of the bronchial submucosa. When symptomatic, they mimic carcinoma. Histologically, they resemble lipomas seen in any part of the body.[388] By 1968, only 33 bronchial lipomas had been recorded.[379]

Bronchial hamartoma

Albrecht's original definition of hamartomas is "tumorlike malformations in which occur only an abnormal mixture of the normal constituents of the organ in which they are found. These malformations may consist of a change in the quantity, arrangement, degree of differentiation, or any combination of these."*

Bateson believes that this is a tumor of undifferentiated mesenchyme in the bronchial submucosa and that it may grow into or away from the lumen.[377] This relieves us of trying to explain why no cases have been seen in childhood.

Most of the tumors are close to the pleura. They are 1 to 4 cm in diameter and spherical or ovoid, with lobulation. They shell out easily

---

*Translated from Albrecht, E.: Verh. Dtsch. Pathol. Ges. 7:153-157, 1904.

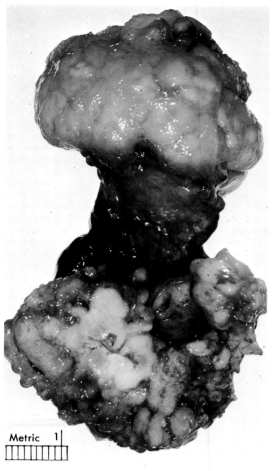

Metric 1

Fig. 26-105. Surgically removed hamartoma of lung. Some of cut surface can be seen in lower portion.

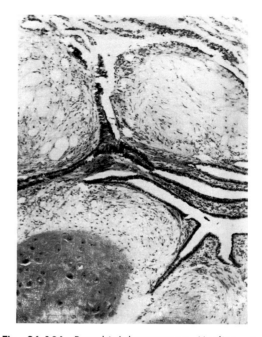

Fig. 26-106. Bronchial hamartoma. Hyaline cartilage, lower left, surrounded by loose connective tissue and fat and covered in turn by bronchial epithelium. Beneath this in places are smooth muscle fibers.

and have a cartilaginous appearance, often with foci of calcification (Figs. 17-1 and 26-105). Those with much fat are yellow. Usually, the principal microscopic component is hyaline cartilage, but some have elastic cartilage. In the typical cases, between the masses of cartilage are clefts lined by bronchial epithelium, beneath which are fat and smooth muscle fibers (Fig. 26-106). Sometimes, cartilage is replaced by fibromyxomatous tissue. About 1% of pulmonary hamartomas are endobronchial. Up to 1965, only 53 cases of the latter were recorded in the English literature.[384]

Lymphoma and leukemia

Lymphoma frequently is found to have spread to the lungs. Primary lymphoma in the lungs is difficult to prove once the disease has become disseminated,[392] whereas many cases labeled lymphosarcoma are undoubtedly "pseudolymphoma" (p. 1146). Over 90 cases of primary lymphoma of the lung, most of which were lymphosarcoma, were collected by Saltzstein.[389] Pulmonary involvement in leukemia is commonest in the pleura and subpleura, but leukemic infiltration also is found in the interalveolar septa and around vessels and bronchi.[380] It may cause symptoms of alveolocapillary block, especially in lymphocytic leukemia.

Diffuse hamartoma
See p. 1045 for discussion.

Pulmonary blastoma and carcinosarcoma

A *blastoma* is a tumor arising from a pluripotential cell of one germ layer that can undergo progressive and unlimited expansion. In the lung, it has appeared at any age between adolescence and late adult life, manifested as a well-demarcated white mass. Microscopically, there are solid tubelike cords of epithelial cells and irregular glandlike structures resting in an immature stroma of spindled or stellate cells (Fig. 26-107). Some consider this to be a replication of fetal lung. Metastases of such tumors occur.[379a,383]

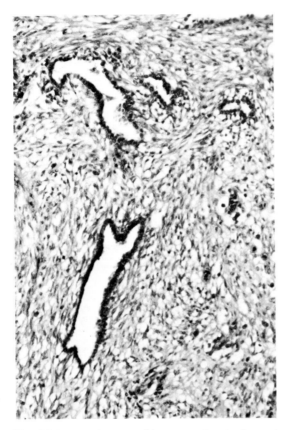

Fig. 26-107. Pulmonary blastoma. Poorly formed tubular pattern in abundant mesenchymal stroma. (165×.)

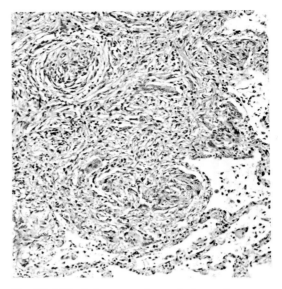

Fig. 26-108. Pulmonary chemodectoma from case with pulmonary hypertension. (147×.)

Carcinosarcoma may be related to, or even be, a more malignant form of blastoma. It is grossly similar, has a similar age incidence, metastasizes more often, and may be either multiple or endobronchial.[391] Microscopically, there are various types of adenocarcinoma intermingled with fibrosarcoma, sometimes with osteosarcoma or chondrosarcoma.

No explanation has been made that is satisfactory to all authorities. Spencer[3] believes that it is a counterpart of Wilms' tumor (a mesoblastic tumor) and does not explain the absence of childhood cases. Barson et al.[376] are convinced that the similarity to fetal lung is fortuitous and that all the tumors must be carcinosarcomas of varying degrees of malignancy. Adult mesenchymal tissue may contain undifferentiated cells that could revert to their pluripotential embryonic state. I incline to the carcinosarcoma theory, keeping in mind the analogy not of Wilms' tumor but of cystosarcoma phyllodes of the breast.

Other tumors

Chemodectoma, benign clear cell tumor, fibroma, leiomyoma, neurofibroma, granular cell myoblastoma, and sarcoma of the lower respiratory tract are great rarities.[3] Reviews have lately appeared on leiomyosarcoma,[381] lymphangiomyomatosis,[390] and hemangiopericytoma.[387]

Of this group, *sarcomas* of muscle are among the least rare. Over 40 leiomyosarcomas have been reported.[386] They should not be confused with spindle cell carcinoma (p. 1133) and fibrous histiocytoma (p. 1145). Many are bronchial rather than pulmonary.[3] Only nine rhabdomyosarcomas are known to have occurred in the lung.[378]

Chemodectoma may be a functional hyperplasia of normal nonchromaffin paraganglionic tissue in relation to pulmonary venules (Fig. 26-108). Perhaps the cells "sample" the blood before it returns to the heart. This concept has been contradicted by ultrastructural studies showing similarity to the cells of meningioma.[377a] The lesion is infrequent and usually multiple.

Benign clear cell tumor is rare but important, since it may be confused with metastatic renal cell carcinoma and sclerosing hemangioma. It appears as a coin lesion chiefly in middle-aged persons. Microscopically, it is composed of uniform, large, pale clear cells, rich in cytoplasmic glycogen, and has a sinusoid blood supply.[385] It appears to arise from pericytes or smooth muscle cells.[382]

SOLITARY PULMONARY NODULES

One of the most important clinical problems is evidence of a single radiopaque nodule, often discovered by chance. In one study[394] of resected solitary pulmonary nodules from 887 men, in 316 cases the nodules were malignant (280 primary, 26 metastatic, seven "adenoma," and three miscellaneous). There were 65 cases of hamartoma and 474 of granuloma. Most of the latter were histoplasmosis (164), tuberculosis (122), and coccidioidomycosis (98). A miscellaneous group of 23 comprised entities such as infarct, bronchial cyst, pneumonitis, and vascular disorder. There were nine cases of tumor of pleura or chest wall. In patients over 50 years of age, 56% of the nodules were malignant. A study of 1134 patients showed that the solitary nodule in 392 of them was a bronchial carcinoma.[393]

These represent the findings in surgical series of cases. In public health surveys, the yield of primary malignancies is 5% or less of persons found to have solitary nodules by x-ray examination.[393a] One important lesson is that calcification does not necessarily exclude the diagnosis of malignancy.

PSEUDOTUMORS
Histiocytoma

In the soft tissues of the body, we have become aware of the large family of *fibrous histiocytomas* (fibrous xanthomas), some members of which are malignant, and which takes its protean nature from the ability of the tissue histiocyte to convert into a fibroblast. Two members of the family seem to have settled in the lung, sclerosing hemangioma and plasma cell granuloma. Excision is curative.

Sclerosing hemangioma

Sclerosing hemangioma takes the form of a benign solitary nodule in the lung, sometimes involving a bronchus. It is oval or spherical and well encapsulated, usually ranging in diameter from 1.5 to 8 cm.[401] Most have been in the lower lobes and in women. The cut surface is gray-pink and fleshy, with yellow and hemorrhagic areas. Microscopically, there are closely packed papillary processes separated by branching epithelial spaces (Fig. 26-109). Intervening stroma varies from clusters of large pale or clear cells to acellular hyalinized areas. Vessels and vascular spaces are not

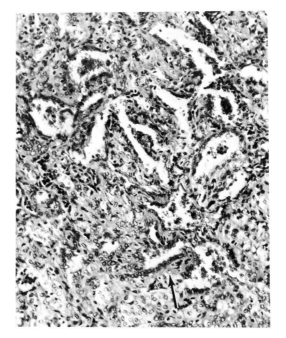

Fig. 26-109. Sclerosing hemangioma. Pale or clear cells among dilated small vessels. *Arrow,* Cuboid change in trapped alveoli. (195×.)

prominent; lipid is demonstrable in the stroma and around some smaller vessels or in relation to small hemorrhages.[395,406]

Spencer[3] does not believe that this is primarily a proliferation of vessels, and he is supported by Kennedy's ultrastructural studies.[399] These lay stress on the epithelial papillary pattern. It appears that these cells and many of the stromal cells are type II pneumonocytes. There is confusion in the literature created by authors not distinguishing plasma cell granuloma from sclerosing hemangioma.[402] Kennedy suggests that "papillary pneumonocytoma" would be a better term.

Plasma cell granuloma

Plasma cell granuloma is another rare cause of a large solitary nodule, especially in younger persons. The alternative name, *inflammatory pseudotumor,* hints at the possible etiology. Grossly, some have been well-demarcated nodules of 2 to 4 cm, but larger ones, occupying much of a lobe, have been seen, and they may obstruct bronchi or the trachea. When hard, they have a streaky gray-white cut surface. Softer forms are yellow. Microscopically, there are masses of plasma cells, both mature and immature. Lymphocytes and even lymphoid follicles may be present.[396]

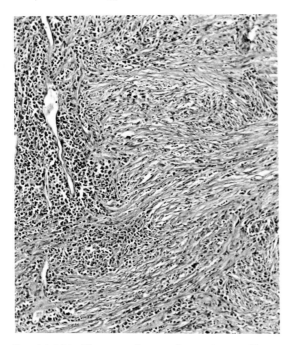

Fig. 26-110. Plasma cell granuloma. Strong fibroblastic reaction (fibers arranged in parallel bundles) is heavily infiltrated by plasma cells. (165×.)

Often, parallel bands of cellular fibrous tissue make up the bulk of the mass (Fig. 26-110), sometimes with foamy histiocytes in the interstices. This mass is no form of myeloma or plasmacytoma, although true myeloma of the lung does occur (6.9% of the Mayo Clinic cases of myeloma, in which admittedly nearly all the cases were examples of direct invasion of the lung from ribs or vertebrae).[398] Plasma cell granuloma is an infectious process with a massive immunologic component.[396] It is not likely that *tumoral amyloidosis* of the lung[397] is a later stage in which masses of amyloid are laid down. Some patients with pulmonary amyloidosis have it in the form of multiple nodules and their prognosis is good.[400] Others have it as a diffuse alveolar septal process, with greater disability.[403]

Pseudolymphoma

Sometimes, unexplained accumulations of lymphoid tissue are found in the lung. Although unencapsulated and frequently very large, the lesions do not become disseminated and have histologic features that further distinguish them from lymphomas. An individual pseudolymphoma may be several centimeters in diameter or may replace most of a lobe.

The cut surface is gray-white and homogeneous. Microscopically, the important finding is a mixed cellular infiltrate, predominantly of mature lymphocytes, with some reticulum cells, plasma cells, and neutrophils. Of great significance is the presence of true germinal centers, not found in lymphomas, and the noninvolvement of the hilar lymph nodes. Sometimes, these distinctive features are lacking, and only time will tell if a true lymphoma is present.[389, 404] The condition is similar to that seen in the mediastinum (p. 1150) and must bear a close relationship to lymphoid interstitial pneumonia[405] (p. 1105).

Pleura
PNEUMOTHORAX

Air or gas may enter the pleural cavity in the following conditions, usually as a result of "spontaneous" rupture: trauma, emphysema, cystic disease of lung, tuberculosis, bronchopleural fistula, abscess, septic infarct, pneumonia, bronchiectasis, perforation of the esophagus or stomach, honeycomb lung, berylliosis, diffuse interstitial fibrosis, influenza, and without demonstrable cause.

In most cases, pneumothorax is not dangerous, but sometimes the air collects under pressure because of valve action. The lung on the involved side will be totally collapsed, and the mediastinal structures will be displaced to the opposite side. The air usually is slowly resorbed. Complications are effusion, hemorrhage, infection, interstitial emphysema, and rapid death.

PLEURAL FLUID

Three classes of pleural fluid can be present: transudates, exudates, and a miscellaneous group.

A *transudate* or hydrothorax is the result of passage of fluid brought about by increased hydrodynamic pressure or decreased colloid-osmotic pressure of the blood or lymph in the vascular bed of the visceral or parietal pleura. Most commonly, this is the circulatory disturbance of cardiac failure. It also may be attributable to mechanical obstruction, as when a hilar tumor blocks lymphatic drainage or when the superior vena cava or azygos vein is obstructed. Changes in plasma osmotic pressure occurring in hypoproteinemia or sodium retention also will allow fluid to escape into the pleural cavity. The cause of the hydrothorax accompanying ovarian fibroma (Meig's syndrome) is unknown.

An *exudate* is the result of pleural inflammation—either primary or secondary to bacterial infection in the underlying lung, viral and rickettsial disease, fungal infection, or parasitic infestation (amebiasis, trichinosis, paragonimiasis). Noninfective irritant causes include tumors of the lung and pleura, pulmonary infarction, rheumatic fever, collagen disease, and pneumothorax.

Transudates are watery, straw-colored fluids of low specific gravity and low protein content, none of which features are constant enough to be reliable.[2] Exudates, apart from their possible cellular or microbial content, have more protein. It is usual to classify transudates as serofibrinous, purulent, or sanguineous. The serofibrinous fluid of early tuberculosis is pale yellow and either contains small rounded fibrin balls when removed or clots in vitro. Shaggy fibrin coats the pleural surfaces to varying degrees and may organize into a fibrous mantle or obliterate the pleural cavity. Most chest physicians believe that the term "idiopathic pleural effusion" should not be used and that the condition should be assumed to be tuberculosis until efforts have been made to exclude this diagnosis (roentgenography, culture of the fluid, skin testing, and pleural biopsy).

Polyserositis (Concato's disease) is characterized by effusions in pleural, pericardial, and peritoneal cavities, terminating in constrictive pericarditis, "sugar icing" of the liver and spleen, and fibrous thickening of the linings of all these cavities.

Hemorrhagic exudates raise the suspicion of tuberculosis, cancer, or pulmonary infarction.

The collection of purulent exudate in the pleural space is called *empyema*, or pyothorax. It is the result of pyogenic or tuberculous inflammation of the lung, necrotic infected tumor, lung abscess, fistula, infection introduced at surgery, systemic mycosis. bloodborne infection, subdiaphragmatic abscess, bronchopleural fistula, trauma, or mediastinitis. The three commonest organisms are pneumococci, staphylococci, and hemolytic streptococci. At first, a thick shaggy fibrin layer covers the pleurae, with the surfaces being separated by pus. Commonly, the empyema becomes walled off or encysted, either in the main pleural cavity, at the base of the lung, against the mediastinum, or in an interlobar fissure. In the final stage, organization of this material so encases the lung that it cannot expand. The effect is even worse in childhood because there is retarded growth of the thoracic cage on the affected side. At any age, the organized tissue may become calcified.

Tuberculous empyema varies between a thin, watery, yellow-white fluid and a thick, creamy, or caseous yellow fluid. Either variety may be blood stained.

The chief member of the *miscellaneous group* of fluids is *chylothorax*. This means the presence of chyle in the pleural cavity because of obstruction of, or injury to, the thoracic duct or its tributaries. Obstruction is most often the result of pressure by enlarged mediastinal lymph nodes, though the trauma can be either accidental or a complication of intrathoracic surgery. There is a rare congenital chylothorax, which may be fatal. The fluid is an emulsion of fat globules that give it an opalescent creamy appearance, and it separates into an upper fatty layer on standing. It is odorless and alkaline and can be cleared by adding fat solvents, or stained with dyes such as scarlet red. This distinguishes chylothorax from a *pseudochylous effusion,* a fluid that is turbid or milky from cholesterol and lecithin or albuminous particles in fine suspension. There are no fat droplets. Lipoid nephrosis, subacute glomerulonephritis, and tuberculous pleurisy are the causes. *Chyliform effusion* appears creamy because of its content of breaking-down inflammatory or neoplastic cells.

PLEURAL TUMORS

Pleural plaques are not neoplasms, and their relationship to asbestosis and mesothelioma has been overstressed (see p. 1095). Most of the patients are elderly men. There are discrete thickenings (up to 5 mm) of the parietal pleura of the tendinous portion of the diaphragm or lower half of the thoracic wall. Often they are bilaterally symmetric, have a smooth ivory surface, irregular but sharp outlines, and may be 10 cm across. Microscopically they are composed of poorly cellular laminated hyalinized collagen; there may be foci of calcification. The etiology is unknown.[409]

Very rarely, there are benign or malignant tumors of the subpleural connective tissues. Except for these, and subpleural tumors of the lung, the only pleural tumor to consider is the *mesothelioma.* A firm diagnosis of mesothelioma cannot be made without proof that there is no carcinoma in the body, for metastases of adenocarcinoma of the stomach, colon, pancreas, ovary, or adrenal gland with pronounced desmoplasia can mimic mesothelioma. The relationship to asbestosis[407] is discussed on p. 316. A survey of 52 cases of pleural mesothelioma revealed a history of industrial association with asbestos in 80% of the series.[411] Mesothelial cells can form phagocytes, fibroblasts, and epithelial cells. Recognition of this fact removes intellectual qualms about the varied pictures of these tumors, and tissue cultures appear to have proved the mesothelial origin of the tumor. Valuable confirmation of this fact comes from an electron microscopic study that showed characteristics of mesothelial cells in epithelial cells of diffuse mesothelioma.[410] There are two kinds—localized mesothelioma and diffuse spreading mesothelioma.

Localized mesothelioma occurs in late middle age in either sex and is rarely malignant. It creates an encapsulated, pedunculated, or sessile firm mass on the surface of the lung, in a fissure, or buried within the lung. Size ranges from a few to many centimeters. The cut surface is yellow or gray-white, sometimes with a pink tinge or with cystic areas containing pale yellow fluid. The microscopic picture is of a fibroma, with interweaving bundles of fibroblasts lying in a collagenous tissue. In this may be small clefts lined by a single layer of flat or cuboid cells (Fig. 26-111). Other varieties have a predominantly papillary pattern, with or without tubular structures. The fibrous component may be very cellular or may, in places, be hyalinized.

Blood-stained pleural fluid is common even in benign varieties, and mitoses can be found in the connective tissue component of even clinically benign solitary mesotheliomas. Only recurrence with intrathoracic spread or invasion of the chest wall indicates malignancy, for metastasis of this variety is not reported.[408]

Diffuse spreading mesothelioma is always malignant. A thick white or pink tissue ensheathes part or all of a lung, particularly the basal portion. It may involve the visceral pleura, and the pleural space contains watery or bloody fluid until the tumor becomes so thick that the space is obliterated. Underlying lung is collapsed but not otherwise involved. The tumors spread by direct extension, invasion of neighboring tissues and organs, pleural implantation, and lymphatic and hematogenous metastases. Microscopically, both epithelial and connective tissue elements resemble those of the solitary form, although the degree of atypism may be greater. The epithelial cells may be in a cordlike, tubular, glandular, or papillary carcinomatous pattern. The connective tissue ranges from quite well-differentiated to fibrosarcomatous types.

Mediastinum

The mediastinum is the median connective tissue in which are slung the heart and the hila of the lungs, while posteriorly the aorta, thoracic duct, and esophagus run through it. The *superior mediastinum* lies above the pericardium and contains the aortic arch, great vessels, thymus, trachea, esophagus, and thoracic duct. The *inferior mediastinum* has three compartments: anterior, middle, and posterior. The *anterior mediastinum* is the shallow space between the pericardium and body of the sternum, containing some lymph nodes. The *middle mediastinum* contains the heart and pericardium, the tracheal bifurcation, and the pulmonary arteries and veins. The *posterior mediastinum* is behind the trachea, pericardium, and posterior surface of the diaphragm. It is the space in front of the vertebral column containing the thoracic aorta, azygos and hemiazygos veins, esophagus, and thoracic duct.

INFLAMMATORY DISEASES

Mediastinal emphysema. Mediastinal emphysema is the escape of air into the interstitial tissue. It usually comes from the lungs

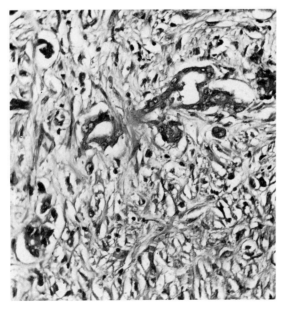

Fig. 26-111. Mesothelioma. (228×.)

but sometimes escapes from the esophagus in certain kinds of trauma.

Mediastinitis. Mediastinitis is a serious acute inflammation most often caused by trauma, external or internal. The latter includes rupture of the esophagus by swallowed foreign bodies or incoordinated vomiting. Perforation of the trachea or esophagus by carcinoma is an important cause. Mediastinal infection can be set up from the local lymph nodes, pleural cavity, pericardium, subdiaphragmatic abscess, and osteomyelitis of the thoracic cage. In some patients, there is widespread mediastinal cellulitis, whereas others develop an abscess.

Chronic fibrous mediastinitis. Chronic fibrous mediastinitis is a manifestation of granulomatous disease such as histoplasmosis and tuberculosis. Sometimes, patients have fibrocaseous granulomatous disease from which organisms cannot be cultured.[412,430] The commonest effect is constriction of the superior vena cava, but obstruction may be apparent in the tracheobronchial tree, pulmonary veins, and esophagus. Cases without granulomas may be variants of idiopathic mediastinal fibrosis (below) more often than is suspected.[426]

Idiopathic mediastinal fibrosis. Idiopathic mediastinal fibrosis is a proliferation of fibrous tissue in the superior mediastinum. It surrounds the great veins at the formation of the superior vena cava and thus sets up venous hypertension in its catchment area. The patient is saved from serious consequences by a slowly developing collateral circulation. This disease resembles idiopathic retroperitoneal fibrosis.[423] In a reported series of 20 cases,[419] there was partial or complete caval obstruction in 12, involvement of the tracheobronchial tree in four, esophageal obstruction in two, and one death from stenosis of the pulmonary vein.

TUMORS AND CYSTS

Diseases of the thymus are considered in Chapter 35. There remain the following categories: (1) enlargement of lymph nodes, (2) mesenchymal tumors, (3) nerve tissue tumors, (4) intrathoracic thyroid and parathyroid glands, (5) cysts, and (6) teratomas. These are arranged in order of incidence and site of relative frequency in the following list*:

Superior mediastinum
  Goiter
  Bronchogenic cyst

*Modified from Schlumberger, H. C.: Tumors of the mediastinum. In Atlas of tumor pathology, Sect. V, Fasc. 18, Armed Forces Institute of Pathology.

  Parathyroid adenoma
  Myxoma
  Lymphoma
Anterior mediastinum
  Thymoma
  Teratoma
  Goiter
  Parathyroid adenoma
  Lymphoma
  Lipoma
  Fibroma
  Lymphangioma
  Hemangioma
  Chondroma
  Giant cell node hyperplasia
  Thymic cyst
  Rhabdomyosarcoma
Middle mediastinum
  Bronchogenic cyst
  Lymphoma
  Pericardial cyst
  Plasma cell myeloma
Posterior mediastinum
  Neurilemoma
  Neurofibroma
  Ganglioneuroblastoma
  Malignant schwannoma
  Fibrosarcoma
  Lymphoma
  Goiter
  Xanthofibroma
  Gastroenteric cyst
  Chondroma
  Myxoma
  Heterotopia of bone marrow
  Meningocele
  Paraganglioma

An example of the incidence of mediastinal tumors in a large hospital is to be found in the 215 cases at the Cleveland Clinic.[413] Of these 89 (41%) were malignant and 20 of them were asymptomatic. Altogether 94 asymptomatic tumors (44%) were found in routine chest x-ray films. The major types were thymic, 20%; lymphoid, 17%; neurogenic, 23%; teratomatous, 12%; thyroid, 11%; developmental cysts, 7%; vascular, 6%; and mesenchymal, 4%.

Infants and children have a greater proportion of malignant mediastinal tumors than do adults. Among 105 patients at the Mayo Clinic under the age of 16 years, the commonest lesions were neurogenic, 34%; teratoma, 20%; developmental cysts, 12%; and lymphoma, 8.5%.[433]

Enlargement of lymph nodes

In this group are the lymphomas and leukemias, metastases, infections, and granulomas. They may press upon the trachea, esophagus, large veins, hilar structures, or thoracic duct. Two additional entities require discussion.

Mediastinal lymph node hyperplasia produces single or multinodular masses 5 to 15 cm in diameter, mainly in the posterior mediastinum. The cut surface is soft and homogeneously gray-red. The masses are considered to be hamartomas, since the lesions have occurred in regions in which lymph nodes are not found, including soft tissues of the neck and shoulder and within skeletal muscle.[423] Later authors have drawn attention to a distinctive, large systemic arterial supply to the mass. No longer is there the normal vascular supply to a lymph node but proliferation (with endothelial cell mitoses) of stromal vessels originating from the capsular region. If the lesion is a vascular hamartoma modifying lymphoid tissue, then the alternative term *angiomatous lymphoid hamartoma* is preferable.[432]

Microscopically, the tissue does not have the structure of true lymph nodes, because there is no corticomedullary pattern, medullary cords, hilum, or subcapsular sinuses.[421]

A clinicopathologic analysis has been made of 81 cases of giant lymph node hyperplasia, 70 of which were intrathoracic; the remainder were cervical, intrapulmonary, axillary, retroperitoneal, and pelvic.[422] Two histologic varieties are distinguished. In the commoner (91% of these cases) the follicle centers are small and transfixed by radially penetrating capillaries, many of which are ensheathed by collagenous hyalinization *(hyaline vascular type)*. These structures can resemble Hassall's corpuscles (Fig. 26-112) because the cells become concentrically layered and flattened. Between the follicles, proliferated capillaries with plump endothelial cells replace lymphoid sinuses; these capillaries also may be encased in hyaline. The second variety is one with reactive follicle centers that are normal sized or larger and that have mitoses and many histiocytes. Between such follicles are sheets of plasma cells, among which some remnants of normal sinuses and follicles are to be found *(plasma cell type)*. This second type is distinguished clinically by a tendency for the patient to have fever, anemia, and hyperglobulinemia.

Such manifestations are believed to indicate an infectious or inflammatory etiology. All the lesions are benign and are cured by excision.

Massive intrathoracic hematopoiesis appears in some persons with chronic hemolytic anemia or hereditary spherocytosis. Single or multiple masses of bone marrow, up to 7 cm in diameter, are found paraspinally in the posterior mediastinum.[414]

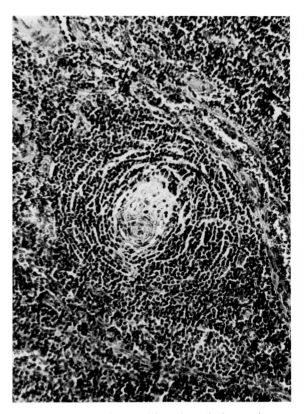

Fig. 26-112. Mediastinal lymph node hyperplasia (hyaline vascular type) with pseudo-Hassall's corpuscles. (150×.)

Mesenchymal tumors

Of the mesenchymal tumors, lipoma is the commonest, but it is in itself a rarity.[427]

Nerve tissue tumors

The commonest tumors of the mediastinum are nerve tissue tumors, with teratoma and thymoma coming next. They are found in the paravertebral region, since they arise from sympathetic nerve trunks or intercostal nerves. They occur at all ages, but the more malignant ones appear in the young, who are more likely to have tumors arising from ganglion cells. The tumors of nerve sheaths, in descending order of frequency, are neurilemoma, neurofibroma, and malignant schwannoma (neurofibrosarcoma). Tumors of ganglion cells are ganglioneuroma, ganglioneuroblastoma, and neuroblastoma (sympathicoblastoma).

The benign tumors may reach 20 cm in diameter and are generally firm and well encapsulated.[428] They are rounded, lobulated, or, if growing intraspinally into the mediastinum, dumbbell shaped. Neurilemoma is encapsulated and often centrally necrotic. Neurofibroma may be mistaken for a malignant tumor because it has no capsule. Ganglioneuroma can form the largest of all mediastinal tumors. Attachment to the sympathetic trunk or an intercostal nerve is frequently demonstrable.

Intrathoracic thyroid and parathyroid glands

When thyroid and parathyroid glands are displaced into the mediastinum, they are subject to their usual diseases. A large mediastinal goiter can compress the trachea. Parathyroid glands enjoy a variety of positions, including the anterior mediastinum, behind the esophagus, or within the thymus.

Cysts

All mediastinal cysts are rare. The most frequent are bronchogenic, pericardial, lymphatic, gastric and enterogenous, and nonspecific cysts.[420,425] *Bronchial cysts* are described on p. 1045. When mediastinal, they may cause obstruction of the tracheobronchial tree of children.[418]

Pericardial cysts lie in one of the cardiophrenic angles. They rarely communicate with the pericardial cavity but are attached to the anterior pericardium directly or by a pedicle. Microscopically, there is a thin connective tissue wall lined by one layer of flat or cuboid cells.

Lymphatic cysts vary from unilocular through multilocular to cavernous lymphangioma. Sometimes, they undertake an infiltrative character and are then called *cystic hygroma*. Large lymphangiomas often are associated with chylothorax and apparent obliteration of the thoracic duct. It may be that the ductal changes are primary and the "lymphangioma" secondary.[415]

Gastroenterogenic cysts are most likely to be found posteriorly near the hila on either side of the midline and are, in infants, the commonest cause, after neuroblastoma, of a posterior mediastinal mass. They arise from a diverticulum of the developing foregut that becomes adherent to the notochord. This explains their close attachment or relationship to the vertebrae and the frequency of accompanying vertebral malformations. The cyst may be lined by gastric epithelium or small or large intestinal epithelium. A related cyst is the *esophageal cyst,* attached to the esophagus and lined by noncornifying stratified squamous epithelium and sometimes by ciliated cells. About 100 cases of esophageal and gastroenterogenic cysts have been recorded.

Nonspecific cysts are considered to be the result of inflammation and hemorrhage in the various types just described.[425]

To this group of mediastinal cysts can be added the *intrathoracic meningocele,* which arises by extension of dura and subarachnoid through a spinal nerve foramen, creating a large cystic dilatation beneath the pleura. The wall is of delicate vascular connective tissue resembling arachnoid.

Teratomas

The anterior mediastinum is the third commonest site of teratoma after the ovary and testis. How these tumors start in the mediastinum is caught up in the mystery of the nature of all teratomas. The *benign cystic teratoma* (dermoid cyst) is as described in the ovary and is two or three times commoner than the malignant variety.

Malignant teratoma is predominantly solid and may have recognizable bone or cartilage. There may be extension into the pericardium or lung. Nineteen of the 20 recorded[431] cases occurred in men, and survival after diagnosis is usually less than 1 year.[429] The malignant component is squamous or glandular carcinoma, rarely sarcoma.

Chorioepithelioma is a highly malignant teratoma that is friable and very hemorrhagic. When it is found in men, a primary tumor in the testis should be excluded. Some authorities will not accept a case as arising extratesticularly if there is even a scar or cyst in the testis.

Seminoma of the mediastinum is a very rare tumor, probably a variant of teratoma. Thirty-one cases of seminoma were collected in a 1968 review,[417] but the total recorded is over 100.

A collection of 30 cases of primary mediastinal germ cell tumors[424] comprises 10 pure seminomas and 20 embryonal carcinomas (mostly with seminomatous or teratoid elements). The ages of the patients were 15 to 35 years, and 22 patients were men. The prognosis was found to be worse than for tumors of similar types in the testis or ovary.

REFERENCES
General

1 Reid, L.: The pathology of emphysema, London, 1967, Lloyd-Luke (Medical Books) Ltd.
2 Rezek, P. R., and Millard, M.: Autopsy pathology, Springfield, Ill., 1963, Charles C Thomas, Publisher.
3 Spencer, H.: Pathology of the lung (excluding

pulmonary tuberculosis), ed. 2, New York, 1968, Pergamon Press, Inc.

Pulmonary structure

4 Avery, M. E., and Fletcher, B. D.: The lung and its disorders in the newborn infant, ed. 3, Philadelphia, 1974, W. B. Saunders Co.
5 Bertalanffy, F. D.: Am. Rev. Resp. Dis. **91:** 605-609, 1965.
6 Boyden, E. A.: Am. J. Anat. **121:**749-761, 1967.
7 Clements, J. A.: In Liebow, A. A., and Smith, D. E., editors: The lung, Baltimore, 1968, The Williams & Wilkins Co. (surface-active materials in lungs).
8 Dawes, G. S.: New Eng. J. Med. **290:**557-559, 1974.
9 Divertie, M. B., and Brown, A. L., Jr.: Med. Clin. North Am. **48:**1049-1054, 1964.
10 Gough, J.: Postgrad. Med. J. **41:**392-400, 1965.
11 Jeffery, P. K., and Reid, L.: J. Anat. **120**(2): 295-320, 1975.
12 Krahl, V. E.: Am. Rev. Resp. Dis. **80**(July suppl.):24-44, 1959.
13 Lauweryns, J. M.: Am. Rev. Resp. Dis. **102:** 877-855, 1970.
14 Lauweryns, J. M., and Baert, J. H.: Ann. N.Y. Acad. Sci. **221:**244-275, 1974.
15 Meyrick, B., and Reid, L.: Proc. Roy. Soc. Med. **66:**386-387, 1973.
16 Morgan, T. E.: New Eng. J. Med. **284:**1185-1193, 1971.
17 Pump, K. K.: Chest **65:**431-436, 1974.
18 Reid, L.: Thorax **13:**110-115, 1958.
19 Reid, L.: Thorax **14:**138-145, 1959.
20 Smith, P., Heath, D., and Moosavi, H.: Thorax **29:**147-163, 1974.
21 Thurlbeck, W. M., and Angus, G. E.: Chest **67**(suppl.):3S-7S, 1975.
22 Towers, B.: In Assali, N., editor: Biology of gestation, New York, 1969, Academic Press, Inc. (fetal and neonatal lung).
23 Wagenvoort, C. A., Heath, D., and Edwards, J. E.: The pathology of the pulmonary vasculature, Springfield, Ill., 1964, Charles C Thomas, Publisher.
24 Weibel, E. R.: Microvasc. Res. **8:**218-235, 1974.

Congenital anomalies

25 Belanger, R., LaFlèche, L. R., and Picard, J.-L.: Thorax **19:**1-11, 1964.
26 Bessolo, R. J., and Maddison, F. E.: Am. J. Roentgenol. **103:**572-576, 1968.
27 Bonham Carter, R. E., Capriles, M., and Noe, Y.: Br. Heart J. **31:**45-51, 1969.
28 Borrie, J., Lichter, I., and Rodda, R. A.: Br. J. Surg. **50:**623-633, 1963.
29 Dines, D. E., Arms, R. A., Bernatz, P. E., and Gomes, M. R.: Mayo Clin. Proc. **49:**460-465, 1974.
30 Franch, R. H., and Gay, B. B.: Am. J. Med. **35:**512-529, 1963.
31 Gerle, R. D., Jaretzki, A., III, Ashley, C. A., and Berrie, A. S.: New Eng. J. Med. **278:** 1413-1419, 1968.
32 Good, C. A.: Am. J. Roentgenol. **85:**1009-1024, 1961.

33 Iwai, K., Shindo, G., Hajikano, H., Tajima, H., Morimoto, M., Kosuda T., and Yoneuda, R.: Am. Rev. Resp. Dis. **107:**911-920, 1973.
34 Kittle, C. F., and Crockett, J. E.: Ann. Surg. **156:**222-233, 1962.
35 Laurence, K. M.: J. Clin. Pathol. **12:**62-69, 1959.
36 Maltz, D. L., and Nadas, A. S.: Pediatrics **42:** 175-188, 1968.
37 Moffat, A. D.: J. Pathol. Bacteriol. **70:**361-372, 1960.
38 Moncrieff, M. W., Cameron, A. H., Astley, R., Roberts, K. D., Abrams, L. D., and Mann, J. R.: Thorax **24:**476-487, 1969.
38a Reale, F. R., and Easterly, J. R.: Pediatrics **51:** 91-96, 1973.
39 Rywlin, A. M., and Fojaco, R. M.: Pediatrics **41:**931-934, 1968.
39a Takahashi, M., Ohno, M., Mihara, K., Matsu-ura, K., and Sumiyoshi, A.: Radiology **114:**543-549, 1975.

Acquired vascular disease
Hyperemia and congestion

40 Andrews, E. C., Jr.: Bull. Johns Hopkins Hosp. **100:**28-42, 1957.
41 Beirne, G. J., Octaviano, G. N., Kopp, W. L., and Burns, R. O.: Ann. Intern. Med. **69:** 1207-1212, 1968.
42 Donald, K. J., Edwards, R. L., and McEvoy, J. D. S.: Am. J. Med. **59:**642-649, 1975.
43 Hutchinson, D. C. S., Sapru, R. P., Sumerling, M. D., Donaldson, G. W. K., and Richmond, J.: Am. J. Med. **45:**139-151, 1968.
44 McCarthy, C., Reid, L., and Gibbons, R. A.: J. Pathol. Bacteriol. **87:**39-47, 1964.
45 Mathew, T. H., Hobbs, J. B., Kalowski, S., Sutherland, P. W., and Kincaid-Smith, P.: Ann. Intern. Med. **82:**215-218, 1975.
46 Soergel, K. H., and Sommers, S. C.: Am. Rev. Resp. Dis. **85:**540-552, 1962.
47 Spain, D. M.: Arch. Pathol. (Chicago) **62:** 489-493, 1956.
48 Trompeter, R., Yu, V. Y. H., Aynsley-Green, A., and Robertson, N. R. C.: Arch. Dis. Child. **50:**123-127, 1975.
49 Whitworth, J. A., Lawrence, J. R., and Meadows, R.: Aust. N.Z. J. Med. **4:**167-177, 1974.

Edema and shock

50 Arias-Stella, J., and Kruger, H.: Arch. Pathol. (Chicago) **76:**147-157, 1963.
51 Balis, J. U., Gerber, L. I., Rappaport, E. S., and Neville, W. E.: Exp. Mol. Pathol. **21:**123-137, 1974.
52 Dalldorf, F. G., Carney, C. N., Rackley, C. E., and Raney, R. B., Jr.: J.A.M.A. **206:**583-586, 1968.
53 Fleischner, F. G.: Am. J. Cardiol. **20:**39-46, 1967.
54 Grunow, W. A., and Esterly, J. R.: Chest **61:** 298-301, 1972.
55 Hardaway, R. M., James, P. M., Jr., Anderson, R. W., Bredenberg, C. E., and West, R. L.: J.A.M.A. **199:**779-790, 1967.
56 Heard, B. E., Steiner, R. E., Herdan, A., and Gleason, D.: Br. J. Radiol. **41:**161-171, 1968.

57 Heath, D., Moosavi, H., and Smith, P.: Thorax **28:**694-700, 1973.
58 Karliner, J. S., Steinberg, A. D., and Williams, M. H., Jr.: Arch. Intern. Med. (Chicago) **124:**350-353, 1969.
59 Moolten, S. E.: Am. J. Med. **33:**421-441, 1962.
60 Pietra, G. G.: Hum. Pathol. **5:**121-122, 1974.
60a Solliday, N. H., Shapiro, B. A., and Gracey, D. G.: Chest **69:**207-213, 1976.
61 Staub, N. C.: Am. Rev. Resp. Dis. **109:**358-372, 1974.
62 Wardle, E. N.: J. Roy. Coll. Phys. Lond. **8:** 251-265, 1974.

Thromboembolism and infarction

63 Breckenridge, R. T., and Ratnoff, O. D.: New Eng. J. Med. **270:**298-299, 1964.
64 Editorial: Lancet **1:**91-92, 1964.
65 Fleming, H. A., and Bailey, S. M.: Br. Med. J. **1:**1322-1327, 1966.
66 Gorham, L.W.: Arch. Intern. Med. (Chicago) **108:**8-22, 189-207, 418-426, 1961.
67 Grieco, M H., and Ryan, S. F.: Am. J. Med. **45:**811-816, 1968.
68 Hampton, A. O., and Castleman, B.: Am. J. Roentgenol. **43:**305-326, 1940.
69 Leinassar, J. M., and Niles, N. R.: Circulation **17:**60-64, 1958.
70 Zimmerman, T. S., Adelson, L., and Ratnoff, O. D.: New Eng. J. Med. **283:**1504-1505, 1970.

Pulmonary hypertension

71 Anderson, E. G., Simon, G., and Reid, L.: J. Pathol. **110:**273-293, 1973.
72 Braun, A., Greenberg, S. D., Malik, S., and Jenkins, D. E.: Arch. Pathol. **95:**67-70, 1973.
73 Djalilian, M., Kern, E. B., Brown, H. A., et al.: Mayo Clin. Proc. **50:**11-14, 1975.
74 Evans, W., Short, D. S., and Bedford, D. E.: Br. Heart J. **19:**93-116, 1957.
75 Fishman, A. P.: In Zorab, P. A., editor: Proceedings of a symposium on scoliosis, London, 1965, National Fund for Research into Poliomyelitis and other Crippling Diseases.
75a Heath, D., and Edwards, J. E.: Circulation **18:** 533-547, 1958.
76 Ring, A., and Bakke, J. R.: Ann. Intern. Med. **43:**781-806, 1955.
77 Schein, C. J., Rifkin, H., Hurwitt, E. S., and Lebendiger, A.: Arch. Intern. Med. (Chicago) **101:**592-605, 1958.
78 Thadani, U., Burrow, C., Whitaker, W., and Heath, D.: Q. J. Med. **44:**133-159, 1975.
79 Wagenvoort, C. A.: Chest **64:**503-504, 1973.
80 Wagenvoort, C. A., and Wagenvoort, N.: Circulation **42:**1163-1184, 1970.
81 Wagenvoort, C. A.: Chest **69:**82-86, 1976.
82 Wood, P.: Mod. Conc. Cardiovasc. Dis. **28:** 513-518, 1959.

Atelectasis and collapse
Atelectasis

83 Langley, F. A., and Smith, J. A. M.: J. Obstet. Gynaecol. Br. Emp. **66:**12-25, 1959.
84 Osborn, G. R.: Lancet **1:**275, 1962.
    Hyaline membrane disease
85 Avery, M. E.: New Eng. J. Med. **292:**157-158, 1975.

86 Barter, R. A., Byrne, M. J., and Carter, R. F.: Arch. Dis. Child. **41:**489-495, 1966.
87 Brown, B. J., Gabert, H. A., and Stenchever, M. A.: Obstet. Gynecol. Survey **30:**71-90, 1975.
88 Capers, T. H., and Minden, B.: Am. J. Med. **36:**377-381, 1964.
89 Krauss, A. N., Klain, D. B., and Auld, P. A. M.: Pediatrics **55:**55-58, 1975.
90 Lauweryns, J. M.: Hum. Pathol. **1:**175-204, 1970.
91 Naeye, R. L., Harcke, H. T., and Blanc, W. A.: Pediatrics **47:**650-657, 1971.
92 Osborn, G. R., and Flett, R. L.: J. Clin. Pathol. **15:**527-541, 1962.
93 Shepard, F. M., Johnston, R. B., Jr., Klatte, E. C., Burko, H., and Stahlman, M.: New Eng. J. Med. **279:**1063-1071, 1968.

Collapse

94 Culiner, M. M.: Dis. Chest **50:**57-66, 1966.
95 Raffensperger, J. G., Diffenbaugh, W. G., and Strohl, E. L.: J.A.M.A. **174:**1386-1388, 1960.

Emphysema

96 Editorial: Br. Med. J. **1:**272-273, 1958.
97 Editorial: Br. Med. J. **2:**229-231, 1959.
98 Felson, B.: Postgrad. Med. **54:**76-82, 1973.
99 Fulton, R. M.: Q. J. Med. **22:**43-58, 1953.
100 Greenberg, S. D., Jenkins, D. E., Stevens, P. M., and Schweppe, H. I.: Am. J. Clin. Pathol. **60:**581-592, 1973.
101 Hepplestone, A. G., and Leopold, J. G.: Am. J. Med. **31:**279-291, 1961.
102 King, J. K. C., and Briscoe, W. A.: Postgrad. Med. **54:**101-108, 1973.
103 Kueppers, F., and Black, L. F.: Am. Rev. Resp. Dis. **110:**176-194, 1974.
104 Kueppers, F., and Dönhardt, A.: Ann. Intern. Med. **80:**209-212, 1974.
105 Leopold, J. G., and Gough, J.: Thorax **12:** 219-235, 1957.
106 McLean, K. H.: Am. J. Med. **25:**62-74, 1958.
107 Millard, F. J. C.: Br. Heart J. **29:**43-50, 1967.
108 Newman, J. K., Vatter, A. E., and Reiss, O. K.: Arch. Environ. Health (Chicago) **15:** 420-429, 1967.
109 Reid, L.: Br. J. Radiol. **32:**294-295, 1959.
110 Reid, L.: Personal communication, 1968.
111 Reid, L., Simon, G., Zorab, P. A., and Seidelin, R.: Br. J. Dis. Chest **61:**190-192, 1967.
112 Ryder, R., Lyons, J. P., Campbell, H., and Gough, J.: Br. Med. J. **3:**481-487, 1970.
113 Simon, G.: Clin. Radiol. **15:**293-306, 1964.
114 Snider, G. L., Brody, J. S., and Doctor, L.: Am. Rev. Resp. Dis. **85:**666-683, 1962.
115 Spain, D. M., and Kaufman, G.: Am. Rev. Tuberc. **68:**24-30, 1953.
116 Thurlbeck, W. M.: Am. J. Med. Sci. **246:**332-353, 1963.
117 Townley, R. G., Ryning, F., Lynch, H., and Brody, A. W.: J.A.M.A. **214:**325-331, 1970.
118 Weiser, M. A., Lamont, J. T., and Walker, W. A.: New Eng. J. Med. **292:**205-206, 1975.
119 Williams, W. D., and Fajardo, L. F.: Am. J. Clin. Pathol. **61:**311-320, 1974.
120 Wyatt, J. P., Fischer, V. W., and Sweet, H. C.: Lab. Invest. **10:**159-177, 1961.

121 Wyatt, J. P., Fischer, V. W., and Sweet, H. C.: Dis. Chest **41**:239-259, 1962.

PNEUMONIA

122 Cabrera, A., Pickren, J. W., and Sheehan, R.: Am. J. Clin. Pathol. **47**:154-159, 1967.
123 Corrin, B., and King, E.: Thorax **25**:230-236, 1970.
124 Friedell, G. H., Kaufman, S. A., Laforet, E. G., and Strieder, J. W.: Am. J. Roentgenol. **87**:847-852, 1962.
125 Gardner, A. F. N.: Q. J. Med. **27**:227-242, 1958.
126 Gross, P.: Arch. Pathol. (Chicago) **69**:706-715, 1960.
127 Gross, P.: Arch. Pathol. (Chicago) **72**:607-619, 1961.
128 Henderon, D. W., Humeniuk, V., Meadows, R., and Forbes, I. J.: Pathology **6**:235-241, 1974.
129 Mearns, M. B.: Br. J. Hosp. Med. **12**:497-506, 1974.
130 Murray, H. W., Masur, H., Senterfit, L. B., and Roberts, R. B.: Am. J. Med. **58**:229-242, 1975.
131 Robinson, R. G., Garrison, R. G., and Brown, R. W.: Ann. Intern. Med. **60**:19-27, 1964.
132 Tillotson, J. R., and Lerner, A. M.: Medicine (Baltimore) **45**:65-76, 1966.
133 Tillotson, J. R., and Lerner, A. M.: Arch. Intern. Med. (Chicago) **121**:428-432, 1968.
134 Walzer, P. D., Perl, D. P., Krogstad, D. J., Rawson, P. G., and Schultz, M. G.: Ann. Intern. Med. **80**:83-93, 1974.
135 Welch, C. C., Tombridge, T. L., Baker, W. J., and Kinney, R. J.: Am. J. Med. Sci. **242**:157-165, 1961.

Nonneoplastic acquired diseases of bronchi
Acute bronchitis and bronchiolitis

136 Case 12-1975, Case Records of Massachusetts General Hospital, New Eng. J. Med. **292**:634-640, 1975.
137 Ham, J. C.: Ann. Intern. Med. **60**:47-60, 1964 (adults).
138 Wittig, H. J., and Chang, C. H.: Pediatr. Clin. North Am. **16**:55-66, 1969 (children).

Chronic bronchitis

139 Bates, D. V.: New Eng. J. Med. **278**:546-551, 600-605, 1968.
140 Fletcher, C. M., Jones, N. L., Burrows, B., and Niden, A. H.: Am. Rev. Resp. Dis. **90**:1-13, 1964.
141 Fraser, R. G.: Am. J. Roentgenol. **120**:737-775, 1974.
142 Garston, B.: Dis. Chest **40**:530-538, 1961.
143 Gregg, I.: Respiration **26**(suppl.):123-130, 1969.
144 Gregg, I.: Aspen emphysema conference **11**:235-248, 1968.
145 Hogg, J. C., Macklem, P. T., and Thurlbeck, W. M.: New Eng. J. Med. **278**:1335-1360, 1968.
146 Irwin, R. S., and Thomas, H. M.: Am. Rev. Resp. Dis. **108**:955-959, 1973.
147 Macklem, P. T., Thurlbeck, W. M., and

Fraser, R. G.: Ann. Intern. Med. **74**:167-177, 1971.
148 Simon, G. Br. J. Radiol. **32**:292-294, 1959.
149 Tager, I., and Speizer, F. E.: New Eng. J. Med. **292**:563-571, 1975.

Unusual causes of pulmonary consolidation
Pulmonary alveolar microlithiasis, calcification

150 Baar, H. S., and Ferguson, F. F.: Arch. Pathol. (Chicago) **76**:659-666, 1963.
151 Raider, L.: Chest **60**:504-507, 1971.

Pulmonary alveolar proteinosis

152 Buechner, H. A., and Ansari, A.: Dis. Chest **55**:274-278, 1969.
153 Gold, D. W., Territo, M., Finley, T. N., and Cline, M. J.: Ann. Intern. Med. **85**:304-309, 1976.
154 Haworth, J. C., Hoogstraten, J., and Taylor, H.: Arch. Dis. Child. **42**:40-54, 1967.
155 Ramirez, J., and Harlan, W. R., Jr.: Am. J. Med. **45**:502-512, 1968.
156 Rosen, S. H., Castleman, B., and Liebow, A. A.: New Eng. J. Med. **258**:1123-1142, 1958.

Allergic granulomas and related conditions
Bronchial asthma

157 Cardell, B. S., and Pearson, R. S. B.: Thorax **14**:341-352, 1959.
158 Dunnil, M. S.: J. Clin. Pathol. **13**:27-33, 1960.
159 Editorial: Lancet **1**:1295-1296, 1968.
160 Gell, P. G. H., and Coombs, R. R. A.: Clinical aspects of immunology, ed. 3, Oxford, 1975, Blackwell Scientific Publications.
161 Pepys, J., and Simon, G.: Med. Clin. North Am. **57**:573-591, 1973.
162 Scadding, J. G.: J. Roy. Coll. Physicians London **2**:35-41, 1967.

Eosinophilia

163 Bedrossian, C. W. M., Greenberg, S. D., and Williams, L. J.: Am. J. Med. **58**:438-443, 1975.
164 Danaraj, T. J.: Arch. Pathol. (Chicago) **67**:515-524, 1959.
165 Liebow, A. A., and Carrington, C. B.: Medicine (Baltimore) **48**:251-285, 1969.

Drug reactions

166 Davies, P. D. B.: Br. J. Dis. Chest **63**:59-70, 1969.

Hypersensitivity pneumonitis caused by inhaled organic antigens (extrinsic fibrosing alveolitis)

167 Edwards, C., and Luntz, G.: Br. J. Dis. Chest **68**:57-64, 1974.
168 Emanuel, D. A., Wenzel, F. J., and Lawton, B. R.: New Eng. J. Med. **274**:1413-1418, 1966.
169 Fink, J. N., et al.: Ann. Intern. Med. **84**:406-413, 1976.
169a Fraser, R. G., and Paré, J. A. P.: Sem. Roentgenol. **10**:31-42, 1975.
170 Hensley, G. T., Garancis, J. C., Cherayil, G. D., and Fink, J. N.: Arch. Pathol. (Chicago) **87**:572-579, 1969.
171 Schlueter, D. P.: Am. J. Med. **57**:476-491, 1974.

Lethal midline granuloma

172 DeRemee, R. A., McDonald, T. J., Harrison, E. G., and Coles, D. T.: Mayo Clin. Proc. **51**:777-781, 1976.

Allergic granulomatosis, angiitis, Wegener's granulomatosis

173 Åström, K. E., and Lidholm, S. O.: J. Clin. Pathol. **16**:137-143, 1963.
174 Carrington, C. B., and Liebow, A. A.: Am. J. Med. **41**:497-527, 1966.
175 Case 29-1974, Case records of Massachusetts General Hospital, New Eng. J. Med. **291**:195-202, 1974.
176 Clausen, K. P., and Bronstein, H.: Am. J. Clin. Pathol. **62**:82-87, 1974.
177 Divertie, M. B., and Olsen, A. M.: Dis. Chest **37**:340-349, 1960.
178 Drachman, D. A.: Arch. Neurol. (Chicago) **8**:145-155, 1963.
179 Fienberg, R.: Am. J. Med. **19**:829-831, 1955.
179a Katzenstein, A., Liebow, A. A., and Friedman, P. J.: Am. Rev. Resp. Dis. **111**:497-537, 1975.
180 Kjellstrand, C. M., Simmons, R. L., Uranga, V. M., Buselheimer, T. J., and Najarian, J. S.: Arch. Intern. Med. **134**:40-43, 1974.
181 Liebow, A. A.: Am. Rev. Resp. Dis. **108**:1-18, 1973.
182 Liebow, A. A., Carrington, C. R. B., and Friedman, P. J.: Hum. Pathol. **3**:457-558, 1972.
183 Sokolov, R. A., Rachmaninoff, N., and Kaine, H. D.: Am. J. Med. **32**:131-141, 1962.

Pneumoconiosis

184 American Medical Association Council on Occupational Health: Arch. Environ. Health (Chicago) **7**:130-171, 1963.
185 Caplan, A., Payne, R. B., and Withey, G. L.: Thorax **17**:205-212, 1962.
186 Elmes, P. C.: Postgrad. Med. J. **42**:623-635, 1966.
187 Enticknap, J. B., and Smither, W. J.: Br. J. Industr. Med. **21**:20-31, 1964.
188 Gilson, J. C.: Proc. Roy. Soc. Med. **66**:395-403, 1973.
189 Greenberg, S. D., Hurst, G. A., Mattage, W. T., Miller, J. M., Hurst, I. J., and Mabry, L. C.: Ann. N.Y. Acad. Sci. **271**:353-364, 1976.
190 Gross, P., deTreville, R. T. P., Cralley, L. J., and Davis, J. M. G.: Arch. Pathol. (Chicago) **85**:539-546, 1968.
191 Knox, J. F., Holmes, S., Doll, R., and Hill, I. D.: Br. J. Industr. Med. **25**:293-303, 1968.
192 McCallum, R. I., Rannie, E., and Verity, C.: Br. J. Industr. Med. **18**:133-142, 1961.
193 Michel, R. D., and Norris, J. F.: Arch. Intern. Med. (Chicago) **113**:850-855, 1964.
194 Miller, A., Langer, A. M., Tierstein, A. S., and Selikoff, I. J.: New Eng. J. Med. **292**:91-93, 1975.
195 Miller, A. A., and Ramsden, F.: Br. J. Industr. Med. **18**:103-113, 1961.
196 Ortmeyer, C. E., Costello, J., Morgan, J. W. C., Swecker, S., and Peterson, M.: Arch Environ. Health **29**:67-72, 1974.
197 Rickards, A. G., and Barrett, G. M.: Thorax **13**:185-193, 1958.
198 Sakula, A.: Thorax **16**:176-179, 1961.

199 Selikoff, I. J., Churg, J., and Hammond, E. C.: J.A.M.A. **188**:22-26, 1964.
200 Thomson, J. G., and Graves, W. M., Jr.: Arch. Pathol. (Chicago) **81**:458-464, 1966.
201 W.H.O. Advisory Committee on Asbestos Cancers: Ann. Occup. Hyg. **16**:9-18, 1973.
202 Williams, W. J.: Br. J. Industr. Med. **15**:84-91, 1958.
203 Williams, W. J., and Williams, D.: J. Pathol. Bacteriol. **96**:491-496, 1968.

Occupational lung diseases

204 Barrowcliff, D. F., and Arblaster, P. G.: Thorax **23**:490-500, 1968.
205 Bouhuys, A., Barbero, A., Lindell, S.-E., Roach, S. A., and Schilling, R. S. F.: Arch. Environ. Health (Chicago) **14**:533-544, 1967.
206 Davies, D.: Br. Med. J. **2**:652-655, 1974.
207 Editorial: New Eng. J. Med. **277**:209-210, 1967.
208 Hapke, E. J., Seal, R. M. E., and Thomas, G. O.: Thorax **23**:451-468, 1968.
209 Hearn, C. E. D., and Holford-Strevens, V.: Br. J. Industr. Med. **25**:267-282, 283-292, 1968.
210 Morgan, W. K. C., Burgess, D. B., Jacobson, G., et al.: Arch. Environ. Health **27**:221-226, 1973.
211 Morgan, W. K. C., and Lapp, N. L.: Am. Rev. Resp. Dis. **113**:531-559, 1976.
212 Pimentel, J. C.: Thorax **30**:204-219, 1975.
213 Prine, J. R., Brokeshoulder, S. F., McVean, D. E., and Robinson, F. R.: Am. J. Clin. Pathol. **45**:448-454, 1966.
214 Rafii, S., and Godwin, M. C.: Arch. Pathol. (Chicago) **72**:424-433, 1961.
215 Seal, R. M. E., Hapke, E. J., and Thomas, G. O.: Thorax **23**:469-489, 1968.

Pulmonary fibrosis

216 Cruickshank, B.: J. Dis. Chest **53**:226-236, 1959.
216a Fayemi, A. O.: Mt. Sinai J. Med. **42**:110-118, 1975.
217 Getzowa, S.: Arch. Pathol. (Chicago) **40**:99-106, 1945.
218 Heppleston, A. G.: Thorax **11**:77-93, 1956.
219 Liebow, A. A., Loring, W. E., and Felton, W. L., II: Am. J. Pathol. **29**:885-911, 1953.
220 Scadding, J. G.: Proc. Roy. Soc. Med. **62**:227-238, 1969.

Sarcoidosis

221 DeRemee, R. A., and Andersen, H. A.: Mayo Clin. Proc. **49**:742-745, 1974.
222 Haroutunian, L. M., Fisher, A. M., and Smith, E. W.: Bull. Johns Hopkins Hosp. **115**:1-28, 1964.
223 Hart, P. D., Mitchell, D. N., and Sutherland, I.: Br. Med. J. **1**:795-804, 1964.
224 Israel, H. L., and Goldstein, R. A.: New Eng. J. Med. **284**:345-349, 1971.
225 Israel, H. L., and Siltzbach, L. E.: In Ingelfinger, F. J., editor: Controversy in internal medicine, II, Philadelphia, 1974, W. B. Saunders Co., pp. 339-360.
226 Israel, H. L., and Sones, M.: Am. Rev. Resp. Dis. **94**:887-895, 1966.

227 James, D. G., Siltzbach, L. E., Sharma, O. P., and Carstairs, L. S.: Arch. Intern. Med. (Chicago) **123:**187-191, 1969.
228 Lennert, K.: Virchows Arch. (Pathol. Anat.) **358:**241-247, 1973.
229 Mankiewicz, E.: Acta Med. Scand., suppl. 425, pp. 68-73, 1964.
230 Millard, D. R., and Maisels, D. O.: Am. J. Surg. **12:**119-123, 1966.
231 Scadding, J. G.: Br. Med. J. **2:**1617-1623, 1960.
232 Scadding, J. G.: Sarcoidosis, London, 1967, Eyre & Spottiswoode (Publishers) Ltd.
233 Siltzbach, L. E.: J.A.M.A. **178:**476-482, 1961.
234 Siltzbach, L. E.: Practitioner **202:**613-618, 1969.
235 Siltzbach, L. E., et al.: Am. J. Med. **57:**847-852, 1974.
236 Vaněk, J., and Schwarz, J.: Am. Rev. Resp. Dis. **101:**395-400, 1970.
237 Waksman, B. H.: Medicine (Baltimore) **41:**93-141, 1962.
238 Wilen, S. B., Rabinowitz, J. G., Ulreich, S., and Lyons, H. A.: Am. J. Med. **57:**200-209, 1974.

Diffuse interstitial pulmonary fibrosis (fibrosing alveolitis) and variants

239 Greenberg, S. D., Haley, M. D., Jenkins, D. E., and Fischer, S. P.: Arch. Pathol. **96:**73-80, 1973.
240 Hewitt, C. J., Hull, D., and Keeling, J. W.: Arch. Dis. Child. **52:**22-37, 1977.
241 Liebow, A. A.: In Liebow, A. A., and Smith, D. E., editors: The lung, Baltimore, 1968, The Williams & Wilkins Co.
242 Liebow, A. A., and Carrington, C. B.: In Simon, M., editor: Frontiers of pulmonary radiology, New York, 1969, Grune & Stratton, Inc.
243 Macfarlane, A., and Davies, D.: Thorax **28:**768-776, 1973.
244 Montes, M., Tomasi, T. B., Jr., Noehren, T. H., and Culver, G. J.: Am. Rev. Resp. Dis. **98:**277-280, 1968.
245 Patchefsky, A. S., Banner, M., and Freundlich, L. M.: Ann. Intern. Med. **74:**322-327, 1971.
246 Patchefsky, A. S., Fraimow, W., and Hoch, W. S.: Arch. Intern. Med. **132:**222-225, 1973.
247 Reddy, P. A., Gorelick, D. F., and Christianson, C. S.: Chest **58:**319-325, 1970.
248 Scadding, J. G.: Thorax **29:**271-281, 1974.
249 Scadding, J. G., and Hinson, K. F. W.: Thorax **22:**291-304, 1967.
250 Stack, B. H. R., Choo-Kang, Y. P. J., and Heard, B. E.: Thorax **27:**535-542, 1972.
251 Swaye, P., Van Ordstrand, H. S., McCormack, L. J., and Wolpaw, S. E.: Dis. Chest **55:**7-12, 1969.

Eosinophilic granuloma and related conditions

252 Carlson, R. A., Hattery, R. R., O'Connell, E. J., and Fontana, R. S.: Mayo Clin. Proc. **51:**542-547, 1976.
253 Gracey, D. R., Divertie, M. B., and Brown, A. L.: Chest **59:**5-8, 1971.

Chronic granulomatous disease

254 Schlegel, R. J.: J.A.M.A. **231:**615-617, 1975.

Fibrosis caused by drugs

255 Heard, B. E., and Cooke, R. A.: Thorax **23:**187-193, 1968.
256 Kapanci, Y., Weibel, E. R., Kaplan, H. P., and Robinson, F. R.: Lab. Invest. **20:**101-118, 1969.
257 Nash, G., Blennerhassett, J. B., and Pontoppidan, H.: New Eng. J. Med. **276:**368-374, 1967.
258 Rosenow, E. C., III, DeRemee, R. A., and Dines, D. E.: New Eng. J. Med. **279:**1258-1262, 1968.

Tuberculosis

259 Auerbach, O.: Am. J. Surg. **89:**627-636, 1955.
260 Blattner, R. J.: J. Pediatr. **65:**311-314, 1964.
261 Canetti, G.: The tubercle bacillus in the pulmonary lesion of man, New York, 1955, Springer Publishing Co., Inc.
262 Cleve, E. A., Young, R. V., and Vicente-Mastellari, A.: Dis. Chest **32:**671-677, 1957.
263 Corpe, R. F., and Stergus, I.: Am. Rev. Tuberc. **75:**223-241, 1957.
264 Cortez, L. M., and Pankey, G. A.: J. Bone Joint Surg. **55-A:**363-370, 1973.
265 Crow, H. E., Corpe, R. F., and Smith, C. E.: Dis. Chest **39:**372-381, 1961.
266 Davis, S. F., Finley, S. C., and Hare, W. K.: J. Pediatr. **57:**221-224, 1960.
267 Editorial: Br. Med. J. **1:**966-967, 1963.
268 Falk, G. A., Hadley, S. J., Sharkey, F. E., Liss, M., and Muchenheim, C.: Am. J. Med. **54:**801-810, 1973.
269 Giese, W.: In Kaufmann, E., and Staemmler, M., editors; Lehrbuch der speziellen pathologischen Anatomie, vol. II, Berlin, 1959-1960, Walter de Gruyter & Co.
270 Grosz, H. J.: Dis. Chest **36:**514-520, 1959.
271 Hill, L. E., and Pearson, J. E. G.: Br. J. Dis. Chest **53:**278-295, 1959.
272 Iles, P. B., and Emerson, P. A.: Br. Med. J. **1:**143-145, 1974.
273 Jenney, F. S., and Cohen, A. C.: Dis. Chest **43:**62-67, 1963.
274 Johanson, W. G., Jr., and Nicholson, D. P.: Am. Rev. Resp. Dis. **99:**73-85, 1969.
275 Jones, R. S., and Alley, F. H.: Am. Rev. Tuberc. **63:**381-398, 1951.
276 Karlson, A. G.: Surg. Clin. North Am. **53:**905-912, 1973.
277 Kelly, P. J., Weed, L. A., and Lipscomb, P. R.: J. Bone Joint Surg. **45-A:**327-336, 1963.
278 Koenig, M. G., Collins, R. D., and Heyssel, R. M.: Ann. Intern. Med. **64:**145-154, 1966.
279 LeMaistre, C.: Ann. N.Y. Acad. Sci. **106:**62-66, 1963.
280 Lester, W., Colton, R., and Kent, G.: Am. Rev. Resp. Dis. **85:**847-857, 1962.
281 Lurie, M. B.: Am. J. Med. **9:**591-610, 1950.
282 Medical Research Council: Br. Med. J. **1:**973-987, 1963.
283 Medler, E. M.: Am. J. Med. **9:**611-622, 1950.
284 Montes, M., and Phillips, C.: Am. Rev. Tuberc. **79:**362-370, 1959.

285 Nurasawa, K., and Altmann, V.: Sea View Hosp. Bull. **17:**85-94, 1958-1959.
286 Ochs, C. W.: J.A.M.A. **179:**247-252, 1962.
287 Ord, R. J., and Matz, G. J.: Arch. Otolaryngol. **99:**327-329, 1974.
288 Prather, E. C., Bond, J. O., Hartwig, E. C., and Dunbar, F. P.: Dis. Chest **39:**129-139, 1961.
289 Reid, J. D., and Wolinsky, E.: Am. Rev. Resp. Dis. **99:**8-12, 1969.
290 Rich, A. R.: The pathogenesis of tuberculosis, ed. 2, Springfield, Ill., 1950, Charles C Thomas, Publisher.
291 Rüttimann, A., and Suter, F.: Schweiz. Med. Wochenschr. **83:**591-600, 1953.
292 Sahn, S. A., and Neff, T. A.: Am. J. Med. **56:**495-505, 1974.
293 Salyer, K. E., Votteler, T. P., and Dorman, G. W.: J.A.M.A. **204:**1037-1040, 1968.
294 Stead, W. M.: Am. Rev. Resp. Dis. **95:**729-745, 1967.
295 Steer, A.: Am. Rev. Resp. Dis. **95:**200-208, 1967.
296 Stott, R. B., and Mallinson, C. N.: Guy's Hosp. Rep. **122:**259-267, 1973.
297 Vortel, V.: Am. Rev. Resp. Dis. **86:**336-349, 1962.
298 Wayne, L. G.: Am. Rev. Resp. Dis. **82:**370-377, 1960.
299 Wayne, L. G., and Salkin, D.: Am. Rev. Tuberc. **74:**376-387, 1956.
300 Wolinsky, E.: Ann. N.Y. Acad. Sci. **106:**67-71, 1963.

Carcinoma

300a American Joint Committee for Cancer Staging and End Results Reporting: Clinical staging system for carcinoma of the lung, Chicago, 1973, the Committee.
301 Anderson, W. A. D.: Am. J. Clin. Pathol. **46:**1-26, 1966.
302 Ashley, D. J. B.: Br. J. Cancer **21:**243-259, 1967.
303 Ashley, D. J. B., and Davies, H. D.: Thorax **22:**431-436, 1967.
304 Auerbach, O., Stout, A. P., Hammond, E. C., and Garfinkel, L.: Am. Rev. Resp. Dis. **82:**640-648, 1960.
305 Auerbach, O., Stout, A. P., Hammond, E. C., and Garfinkel, L.: New Eng. J. Med. **265:**253-267, 1961.
306 Auerbach, O., Stout, A. P., Hammond, E. C., and Garfinkel, L.: Cancer **20:**699-705, 1967.
307 Azzopardi, J. G.: J. Pathol. Bacteriol. **78:**513-519, 1959.
308 Bender, R. A., and Hansen, H.: Ann. Intern. Med. **80:**205-208, 1974.
309 Bennett, D. E., Sasser, W. F., and Ferguson, T. B.: Cancer **23:**431-439, 1969.
310 Bensch, K. G., Corrin, B., Pariente, R., and Spencer, H.: Cancer **22:**1163-1172, 1968.
311 Boyd, J. T., Doll, R., Faulds, J. S., and Leiper, J.: Br. J. Industr. Med. **27:**97-105, 1970.
311a Braman, S. S., and Whitcomb, M. E.: Arch. Intern. Med. **135:**543-547, 1975.
312 Bryan, C. S., and Boitnott, J. K.: Am. Rev. Resp. Dis. **99:**272-274, 1969.
312a Churg, A., and Warnock, M. L.: Cancer **37:**1469-1477, 1976.
313 Collier, F. C., Enterline, H. T., Kyle, R. H., Tristan, T. T., and Greening, R.: Arch. Pathol. (Chicago) **66:**594-603, 1958.
314 Compton, H. L., and Kittle, C. F.: Am. Surg. **29:**26-32, 1963.
315 Cotton, R. E.: Br. J. Dis. Chest **53:**142-150, 1959.
316 Delarue, N. C., Anderson, W., Sanders, D., and Starr, J.: Cancer **29:**90-97, 1972.
317 Doll, R., and Hill, A. B.: Br. Med. J. **2:**1071-1081, 1956.
318 Fox, B., and Risdon, R. A.: J. Clin. Pathol. **21:**486-491, 1968.
319 Fraire, A. E., and Greenberg, S. D.: Cancer **31:**1078-1086, 1973.
320 Gifford, J. H., and Waddington, J. K. B.: Br. Med. J. **1:**723-730, 1957.
321 Greenberg, S. D., Smith, M. A., and Spjut, H. J.: Am. J. Clin. Pathol. **63:**153-167, 1975.
322 Hathaway, B. M., Copeland, K., and Gurley, J.: Arch. Surg. (Chicago) **98:**24-30, 1969.
323 Hawkins, J. A., Hansen, J. E., and Howbert, J.: Am. Rev. Resp. Dis. **88:**1-5, 1963.
324 Hewer, T. F.: J. Pathol. Bacteriol. **81:**323-330, 1961.
325 Higgins, I. T. T.: Arch. Environ. Health **28:**121-129, 1974.
326 Hukill, P. B., and Stern, H.: Cancer **15:**504-514, 1962.
327 Jackman, R. J., Good, C. A., Clagett, O. T., and Woolner, L. B.: J. Thorac. Cardiovasc. Surg. **57:**1-8, 1969.
328 Kirklin, J. W., McDonald, J. R., Clagett, O. T., Moersch, H. J., and Gage, R. P.: Surg. Gynecol. Obstet. **100:**429-438, 1955.
329 Lauweryns, J. M., and Peuskens, J. C.: Life Sci. **8:**577-585, 1969.
330 Liebow, A. A.: Adv. Intern. Med. **10:**329-358, 1960.
331 MacMahon, H. E., Werch, J., and Sorger, K.: Arch. Pathol. (Chicago) **83:**359-363, 1967.
332 Melamed, M. R.: In Watson, W. L., editor: Lung cancer, St. Louis, 1968, The C. V. Mosby Co.
333 Meyer, E. C., and Liebow, A. A.: Cancer **18:**322-351, 1965.
334 Mikail, M., and Sender, B.: Am. J. Clin. Pathol. **37:**515-520, 1962.
335 Morgan, A. D., and Mackenzie, D. H.: J. Pathol. Bacteriol. **87:**25-27, 1964.
336 Mountain, C. F., Carr, D. T., and Anderson, W. A. D.: Am. J. Radiol. **120:**130-138, 1974.
337 Overholt, R. H., and Bougas, J. A.: J.A.M.A. **161:**961-963, 1956.
338 Ozzello, L., and Stout, A. P.: Cancer **14:**1052-1056, 1961.
339 Report of Advisory Committee to Surgeon General: Smoking and health, Washington, D.C., 1964, U.S. Government Printing Office.
340 Rimington, J.: Br. Med. J. **2:**373-375, 1971.
341 Rhodes, M. L.: Chest **64:**741-746, 1973.
342 Rosenblatt, M. B., Lisa, J. R., and Trinidad, S.: Dis. Chest **49:**396-404, 1966 (metastases to bronchi).
343 Sherwin, R. P., Laforet, J. W., and Streider, E. G.: J. Thorac. Cardiovasc. Surg. **43:**716-730, 1962.
344 Shinton, N. K.: Br. J. Cancer **17:**213-221, 1963.

344a Smith, R. A., Nigam, B. K., and Thompson, J. M.: Thorax 31:507-516, 1976.

345 Storey, C. F. S., Knudtson, K. P. K., and Lawrence, B. J. L.: J. Thorac. Surg. 26:331-406, 1953.

346 Strauss, B., and Weller, C. V.: Arch. Pathol. (Chicago) 63:602-611, 1957.

346a Tyers, G. F. D., and McGavran, M. H.: Chest 69:33-38, 1976.

347 Vincent, T. N., Satterfield, J. V., and Ackerman, L. V.: Cancer 18:559-570, 1965.

348 Wagoner, J. K., Archer, V. E., Lundin, F. E., Jr., Holaday, D. A., and Lloyd, J. W.: New Eng. J. Med. 273:181-188, 1965.

349 Watson, W. L.: Cancer 18:133-135, 1965.

350 Watson, W. L., and Berg, J. W.: Cancer 15:759-768, 1962.

351 Weiss, W., and Boucot, K. R.: Arch. Intern. Med. 134:306-311, 1974.

352 Yokoo, H., and Suckow, E. E.: Cancer 14:1205-1215, 1961.

Bronchial carcinoma

Extrapulmonary manifestations of bronchial carcinoma

353 Bower, B. F., and Gordan, G. S.: Annu. Rev. Med. 16:83-118, 1965.

354 Brain, Lord: Lancet 1:179-184, 1963.

355 Croft, P. B., and Wilkinson, M.: Lancet 1:184-188, 1963.

356 Fusco, F. D., and Rosen, S. W.: New Eng. J. Med. 275:507-515, 1966.

357 Greene, J. G., Divertie, M. B., Brown, A. L., and Lambert, E. H.: Arch. Intern. Med. (Chicago) 122:333-339, 1968.

358 Kennedy, J. H., Williams, M. J., and Sommers, S. C.: Ann. Surg. 160:90-94, 1964.

359 Kennedy, W. R., and Jimenez-Pabon, E.: Neurology (Minneap.) 18:757-766, 1968.

360 Morton, D. L., Itabashi, H. H., and Grimes, O. F.: J. Thorac. Cardiovasc. Surg. 51:14-29, 1966.

361 Nichols, J., and Gourley, W.: J.A.M.A. 185:696-698, 1963.

362 Riley, C. J., and Lécutier, M. A.: Br. Med. J. 2:291-292, 1969.

"Bronchial adenoma"

363 Allen, M. S., Marsh, W. L., and Geissinger, W. T.: J. Thorac. Cardiovasc. Surg. 67:966-968, 1974.

364 Axelsson, L., Burcharth, F., and Johansen, A.: J. Thorac. Cardiovasc. Surg. 65:902-908, 1973.

365 Black, W. C., III: Lab. Invest. 19:473-486, 1968.

366 Felton, W. L., Liebow, A. A., and Lindskog, G. E.: Cancer 6:555-567, 1953.

367 Frank, H. D., and Lieberthal, M. M.: Arch. Intern. Med. (Chicago) 111:791-798, 1963.

368 Goodner, J. T., Berg, J. W., and Watson, W. L.: Cancer 14:539-546, 1961.

369 Kroe, D. J., and Pitcock, J. A.: Arch. Pathol. (Chicago) 84:539-542, 1967 (true adenoma).

370 Okike, N., Bernatz, P. E., and Woolner, L. B.: Ann. Thorac. Surg. 22:270-277, 1976.

371 Payne, W. S., Ellis, F. H., Woolner, L. B., and Moersch, H. J.: J. Thorac. Cardiovasc. Surg. 38:709-726, 1959.

372 Pearson, F. G., Thompson, D. W., Weissberg, D., Simpson, W. J. K., and Kargin, F. G.: Ann. Thorac. Surg. 18:16-29, 1974.

373 Smith, R. A.: Thorax 24:43-50, 1969.

374 Tauxe, W. N., McDonald, J. R., and Devine, K. D.: Arch. Otolaryngol. (Chicago) 75:364-376, 1962.

375 Verska, J. J., and Connolly, J. E.: J. Thorac. Cardiovasc. Surg. 55:411-417, 1968.

Rare pulmonary tumors

376 Barson, A. J., Jones, A. W., and Lodge, K. V.: J. Clin. Pathol. 21:480-485, 1968.

377 Bateson, E. M.: Cancer 31:1458-1467, 1973.

377a Churg, A. M., and Warnock, M. L.: Cancer 37:1759-1769, 1976.

378 Conquest, H. F., Thornton, J. L., Massie, J. R., and Coxe, J. W., III: Ann. Surg. 161:688-692, 1965.

379 Crutcher, R. R., Waltuch, T. L., and Ghosh, A. K.: J. Thorac. Cardiovasc. Surg. 55:422-425, 1968.

379a Fung, C. H., Lo, J. W., Yonan, T. N., Milloy, F. J., Hakami, M. M., and Changus, G. W.: Cancer 39:153-163, 1977.

380 Green, R. A., and Nichols, N. J.: Am. Rev. Resp. Dis. 80:833-844, 1959.

381 Guccion, J. G., and Rosen, S. H.: Cancer 30:836-847, 1972.

382 Hoch, W. S., Patchefsky, A. S., Takeda, M., and Gordon, G.: Cancer 33:1328-1336, 1974.

383 Karcioglu, Z. A., and Someren, A. O.: Am. J. Clin. Pathol. 61:287-295, 1974.

384 Kurrus, F. D., and Conn, J. H.: J. Thorac. Cardiovasc. Surg. 50:138-140, 1965.

385 Liebow, A. A., and Castleman, B.: Yale J. Biol. Med. 43:213-222, 1971.

386 McNamara, J. J., Paulson, D. L., Kingsley, W. B., Salinas-Izaquirre, S. F., and Urschel, H. C., Jr.: J. Thorac. Cardiovasc. Surg. 57:635-641, 1969.

387 Meade, J. B., Whitwell, F., Bickford, B. J., and Waddington, J. K. B.: Thorax 29:1-15, 1974.

388 Plachta, A., and Hershey, H.: Am. Rev. Resp. Dis. 86:912-916, 1962.

389 Saltzstein, S. L.: Cancer 16:928-955, 1963.

390 Silverstein, E. F., Ellis, K., Wolff, M., and Jaretzki, A.: Am. J. Roentgenol. 120:832-850, 1974.

391 Stackhouse, E. M., Harrison, E. G., Jr., and Ellis, F. H.: J. Thorac. Cardiovasc. Surg. 57:385-399, 1969.

392 Sternberg, W. H., Sidransky, H., and Ochsner, S.: Cancer 12:806-819, 1959.

Solitary pulmonary nodules

393 Higgins, G. A., Shields, T. W., and Keehn, R. J.: Arch. Surg. 110:570-575, 1975.

393a McClure, C. D., Boucot, K. R., Shipman, G. A., Gilliam, A. G., Milmore, B. K., and Lloyd, J. W.: Arch. Environ. Health (Chicago) 3:127-139, 1961.

394 Steele, J. D.: Thorac. Cardiovasc. Surg. 46:21-39, 1963.

Pseudotumors

395 Arean, V. M., and Wheat, M. W., Jr.: Am. Rev. Resp. Dis. 85:261-271, 1962.
396 Bahadori, M., and Liebow, A. A.: Cancer **31:** 191-208, 1973.
397 Duke, M.: Arch. Pathol. (Chicago) 67:110-117, 1959.
398 Herskovic, T., Andersen, H. A., and Bayrd, E. D.: Dis. Chest 47:1-6, 1965.
399 Kennedy, A.: J. Clin. Pathol. 26:792-799, 1973.
400 Lee, S. C.: Thorax 30:178-185, 1975.
401 Liebow, A. A., and Hubbell, D. S.: Cancer 9: 53-75, 1956.
402 Nair, S., Nair, K., and Weisbrot, I. M.: Chest 65:465-468, 1974.
403 Poh, S. C.: Thorax 30:186-191, 1975.
404 Reich, N. E., McCormack, L. J., and van Ordstrand, H. S.: Chest 65:424-427, 1974.
405 al-Saleem, T., and Peale, A. R.: Am. Rev. Resp. Dis. 99:767-772, 1969.
406 Titus, J. L., Harrison, E. G., Clagget, O. T., Anderson, M. W., and Knaff, L. J.: Cancer 15:522-538, 1962.

Pleural tumors

407 Borow, M., Conston, A., Livomese, L., and Schalet, N.: Chest 64:641-646, 1973.
408 Manguikian, B., and Prior, J. T.: Arch. Pathol. (Chicago) 75:236-249, 1963.
409 Robinson, J. J.: Arch. Pathol. 93:118-122, 1972.
410 Wang, N.: Cancer 31:1046-1054, 1973.
411 Whitwell, F., and Rawcliffe, R. M.: Thorax 26:6-22, 1971.

Mediastinum

412 Aronstam, E. M., and Thomas, P. A., Jr.: Dis. Chest 41:547-552, 1962.
413 Benjamin, S. P., McCormack, L. J., Effler, D. B., and Groves, L. K.: Chest 62:297-303, 1972.

414 Coventry, W. D., and LaBree, R. H.: Ann. Intern. Med. 53:1042-1052, 1960.
415 Dische, M. R.: Am. J. Clin. Pathol. 49:392-397, 1968.
416 Editorial: Br. Med. J. 2:135-136, 1969.
417 El-Domeiri, A. A., Hutter, R. V. P., Pool, J. L., and Foote, F. W., Jr.: Ann. Thorac. Surg. 6:513-521, 1968.
418 Grafe, W. R., Goldsmith, E. I., and Redo, S. F.: J. Pediatr. Surg. 1:384-393, 1966.
419 Hache, L., Woolner, L. B., and Bernatz, P. E.: Dis. Chest 41:9-25, 1962.
420 Herlitzka, A. J., and Gale, J. W.: Arch. Surg. (Chicago) 76:697-706, 1958.
421 Krasznai, G., and Juhász, I.: J. Pathol. 97: 148-151, 1969.
422 Keller, A. R., Hochholzer, L., and Castleman, B.: Cancer 29:670-683, 1972.
423 Lattes, R., and Pachter, M. R.: Cancer 15:197-214, 1962.
424 Martini, N., Golbey, R. B., Hajdu, S. I., Whitmore, W. F., and Beattie, E. J.: Cancer 33: 763-769, 1974.
425 Morrison, I. M.: Thorax 13:294-307, 1958.
426 Nelson, W. P., Lundberg, G. D., and Dickerson, R. B.: Am. J. Med. 38:279-285, 1965.
427 Pachter, M. R., and Lattes, R.: Cancer 16:74-117, 1963.
428 Pachter, M. R., and Lattes, R.: Dis. Chest 44: 79-87, 1963.
429 Pachter, M. R., and Lattes, R.: Dis. Chest 45: 301-310, 1964.
430 Silver, C. P., and Steel, S. J.: Lancet 1:1254-1256, 1961.
431 Spock, A., Schneider, S., and Baylin, G. J.: Am. Rev. Resp. Dis. 94:97-103, 1966.
432 Tung, K. S. K., and McCormack, L. J.: Cancer 20:525-536, 1967.
433 Whittaker, L. D., and Lynn, H. B.: Surg. Clin. North Am. 53:893-904, 1973.

27/Ophthalmic pathology

LORENZ E. ZIMMERMAN

This chapter is concerned not only with pathologic processes affecting the eyeball, but also with alterations in the eyelids, conjunctiva, and orbital tissues.

EYELIDS

The eyelids are covered externally by epidermis and internally by the palpebral conjunctiva (Fig. 27-1), between which are the corium, subcutaneous tissues, layer of skeletal and smooth muscles, and the tarsal plate with its contained meibomian glands. In general, pathologic processes affecting the eyelids are not sufficiently different from those observed elsewhere to warrant separate discussion, even though the eyelids are sites of predilection for many dermatologic entities such as basal cell carcinoma, nevi, the melanotic freckle of Hutchinson, extrasacral mongolian spots, cavernous hemangioma, neurofibroma, senile and sebaceous keratosis, xeroderma pigmentosum, verruca filiformis, xanthomas (xanthelasma and juvenile xanthogranuloma), lipid proteinosis, molluscum contagiosum, keratoacanthoma, pseudoepitheliomatous hyperplasia, trichoepithelioma, and syringoma. These are described in the chapter on the skin. A few conditions, however, should be considered here.

Dermoid and epidermoid cysts

Dermoid cyst is a developmental anomaly usually encountered in the upper eyelid, most often temporally, and sometimes involving the orbit as well as the eyelid. Its wall is composed of epidermal and dermal tissues, including such adnexal structures as hair follicles, sebaceous glands, and sweat glands, all of which typically contribute their products to the contents of the cyst, the principal ingredient of which is desquamated keratin (Fig. 27-2).

Epidermoid cysts also are encountered in the eyelids. These differ from dermoid cysts in that they are lined by epidermal tissue

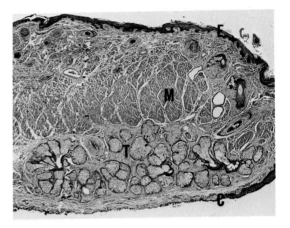

Fig. 27-1. Normal eyelid. **E,** Epidermal surface. **C,** Conjunctival surface. **M,** Muscular plane. **T,** Tarsal plate with meibomian glands. (19×; AFIP 61-3230; from Boniuk, M.: Int. Ophthalmol. Clin. 2:239-317, 1962; Little, Brown & Co.)

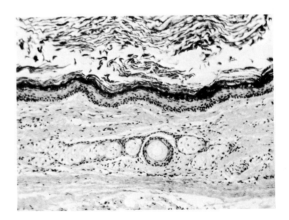

Fig. 27-2. Dermoid cyst. Lumen (top of field) filled with desquamated keratin and lined by epidermis. Hair follicles and sebaceous glands present in its wall. (125×; AFIP 72852-24102; from Hogan, M. J., and Zimmerman, L. E.: Ophthalmic pathology, ed. 2, Philadelphia, 1962, W. B. Saunders Co.)

without adnexal structures and the lumen contains only keratin.

After trauma, the contents of dermoid and epidermoid cysts may escape into the adjacent tissues, provoking a severe foreign body granulomatous reaction and presenting a clinical picture suggestive of a rapidly growing malignant neoplasm.

Sty

Sty, or external hordeolum, is an acute suppurative inflammation of one of the specialized glandular structures associated with the eyelash follicles. Frequently a complication of a staphylococcal blepharitis, the infection involves the sebaceous glands of Zeis, the apocrine glands of Moll, and the eyelash follicles.

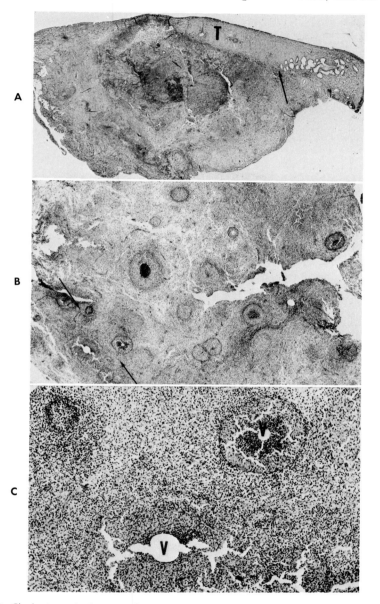

Fig. 27-3. Chalazion. **A,** Large inflammatory mass continuous with scarred tarsus, *T*, occupies most of eyelid. *Arrow,* Juncture of chalazion with residual meibomian gland. **B,** Biopsy specimen revealing multiple discrete granulomatous lesions and abscesses. Area between *arrows* shown at greater magnification in **C. C,** Lipoidal vacuoles, *V,* in center of two granulomas. (**A,** 9×; AFIP 56-10004; **B,** 15×; AFIP 56-22051; **C,** 63×; AFIP 56-22049; **B** and **C,** from Hogan, M. J., and Zimmerman, L. E.: Ophthalmic pathology, ed. 2, Philadelphia, 1962, W. B. Saunders Co.)

Much less frequently encountered is an acute suppurative inflammation of the meibomian gland called an internal hordeolum.

Chalazion

Chalazion is the name given to a chronic inflammatory process involving the meibomian glands. Pathogenetically, it is believed to develop as a consequence of obstruction to the drainage of secretions. It is, therefore, often seen as a complication of various tumors and other disease processes at the eyelid margin. In the course of its slowly progressive evolution, the inflammatory process leads to a destruction of the walls of some of the meibomian glands and ducts and a consequent escape of secretions and inflammatory products into the tarsal plate. The process may then spread within the tarsus to involve adjacent glands, or it may perforate through to either the conjunctival surface posteriorly or the muscular plane and subcutaneous tissues anteriorly. Clinically, the resultant indurated mass may be mistaken for a deeply situated neoplasm. An important problem in clinical diagnosis here is differentiating a chalazion from a carcinoma of the meibomian glands, because both develop within the tarsus and because a tumor of the meibomian glands actually may produce a chalazion.

Microscopically, the chalazion is a great imitator, for the resultant histopathologic picture may resemble that of tuberculosis, sarcoidosis, cat-scratch disease, lipogranulomas, foreign body granulomas, or even plasmacytomas (Fig. 27-3). Although there is nothing highly specific about the microscopic picture, the diagnosis is based on two main features: (1) location in the tarsus and (2) presence of globules of fat in the center of some of the granulomas and abscesses. The lipid deposits, of course, appear as empty spaces in paraffin sections, but their histochemical characteristics can be demonstrated with frozen sections and stains for fat.

Sebaceous carcinoma

Sebaceous carcinoma is an exceedingly rare tumor elsewhere in the body, but in the eyelids it is second in frequency among malignant tumors only to basal cell carcinoma. In my experience, it is observed more frequently than either squamous cell carcinoma or malignant melanoma. Although basal cell carcinomas have a predilection for the lower eyelid, sebaceous carcinomas arise more frequently in the upper eyelid, perhaps because the mei-

bomian glands are larger and more numerous in the upper than in the lower lids. Although sebaceous carcinomas are generally believed to arise mainly from the meibomian glands within the tarsal plate, we have observed a number of cases in which the sebaceous glands of Zeis, which are associated with the lash follicles, were either solely responsible or participated along with the meibomian glands in giving rise to the tumor. Clinically, these tumors may produce a localized or a diffuse thickening of the tarsus, an ulcerated or a papillomatous tumor at the eyelid margin, or the picture of an inflammatory process variously resembling a chalazion, a chronic blepharitis, or a keratoconjunctivitis.

Microscopically, most sebaceous carcinomas show sufficient maturation to permit easy differentiation from basal cell carcinoma and squamous carcinoma. Areas usually can be found in which the tumor produces lobules showing progressive sebaceous differentiation of the constituent cells as they pass from the basaloid reserve cells peripherally toward the large sebaceous cells with abundant foamy cytopalsm centrally (Fig. 27-4). The ducts of the meibomian glands normally produce some

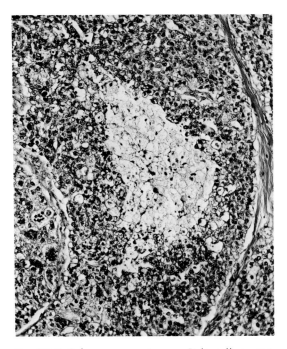

Fig. 27-4. Sebaceous carcinoma. Pale cells in center of lobule are swollen with cytoplasmic lipid. (130×; AFIP 58-13416; from Hogan, M. J., and Zimmerman, L. E.: Ophthalmic pathology, ed. 2, Philadelphia, 1962, W. B. Saunders Co.)

keratin as they approach the eyelid margin, and one should therefore not be surprised if some production of keratin is occasionally observed. Diagnosis may be difficult when one has only small biopsy fragments to examine, but if the possibility of sebaceous carcinoma has been considered, frozen sections and stains for fat should be used to help establish the correct diagnosis. When one has, in addition to the tumor itself, enough of the adjacent normal eyelid to permit orientation, demonstration that the tumor has arisen within the tarsal glands or in the vicinity of the eyelash follicles where the glands of Zeis are located will greatly facilitate correct histopathologic interpretation. These points are emphasized because it has been my impression that in the past many pathologists have mistakenly interpreted sebaceous carcinomas of the eyelid as either basal cell or squamous cell carcinoma. Correct diagnosis is not merely of academic interest, for sebaceous carcinomas are among tumors of the eyelid second only to malignant melanoma in their capacity to metastasize.

Extramammary Paget's disease

Extramammary Paget's disease has been observed rather frequently in association with sebaceous carcinoma of the eyelids. This is the only important exception to the usual experience that mucus-secreting, apocrine type of carcinomas are those that are typically responsible for the invasion of the overlying epidermis by individual neoplastic cells and the consequent development of a chronic eczematoid inflammatory process that often accounts for long delays in arriving at a correct diagnosis.

In the eyelids, we have often observed this phenomenon secondary to carcinomas arising in the meibomian and Zeis glands. Individual neoplastic cells containing sebaceous secretions in their cytoplasm may be observed in both the epidermal and conjunctival surfaces along the eyelid margin (Fig. 27-5). Sometimes, these cells also may be observed at a remarkable distance away from the underlying tumor in the tarsal glands. We have seen several cases in which even the bulbar conjunctiva and cornea were so affected. In such cases, the patients had presented clinically with the picture of a chronic unilateral keratoconjunctivitis that was unresponsive to all forms of medical therapy. Whether the neoplastic cells observed in the cornea and bulbar conjunctiva have actually migrated there from the eyelid margin or have undergone a peculiar neoplastic metaplasia in situ remains to be determined.

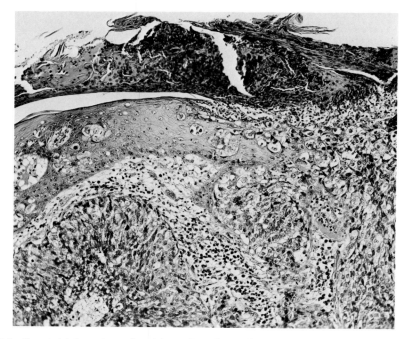

Fig. 27-5. Pagetoid invasion of epidermal surface of eyelid by sebaceous carcinoma of meibomian gland derivation. (115×; AFIP 58-13414; from Hogan, M. J., and Zimmerman, L. E.: Ophthalmic pathology, ed. 2, Philadelphia, 1962, W. B. Saunders Co.)

The affected epidermal and conjunctival tissues are typically acanthotic and exhibit varying degrees of hyperkeratosis and parakeratosis as well as subacute inflammation.

CONJUNCTIVA AND CORNEA

The conjunctiva and cornea are discussed together here because so many of the more common pathologic processes affect them together, either concurrently or sequentially.

The conjunctiva covers the inner surface of the eyelids, where it is firmly attached to the tarsal plates. This portion is called the tarsal or palpebral conjunctiva. At the upper end of the upper eyelid and at the lower end of the lower eyelid, the conjunctiva is redundant and loosely attached to the underlying tissues as it is reflected onto the surface of the globe, where it is called the bulbar conjunctiva. Most of the bulbar conjunctiva is rather loosely attached to the underlying sclera, but it becomes more firmly attached as it merges with the cornea (Fig. 27-6).

The transitional zone between the bulbar conjunctiva and the cornea is called the limbus. The corneal margin of the limbus is easily defined and recognized by the fact that the stratified squamous epithelium of the cornea and its basement membrane are very intimately and firmly adherent to Bowman's membrane, the most superficial portion of the corneal stroma. Bowman's membrane termi-

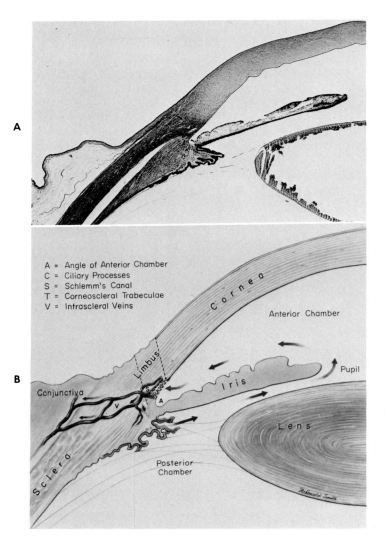

Fig. 27-6. Normal eye. **A,** Actual section. **B,** Artist's drawing. (**A,** 11×; AFIP 56-11490; **B,** AFIP 57-18073; from Zimmerman, L. E.: In Saphir, O., editor: A text on systemic pathology, New York, 1958-1959, Grune & Stratton, Inc.; by permission.)

nates abruptly at the limbus, where a loose connective tissue (the substantia propria) containing capillaries begins to make its appearance between the epithelium and the sclera. In the limbal area, the conjunctival epithelium is nonkeratinizing stratified squamous with very few goblet cells. Peripherally goblet cells become more numerous, and the conjunctival epithelium becomes progressively more stratified columnar in type.

Dermoid tumors

Dermoid tumors are solid choristomatous malformations that are seen most frequently in the limbal area temporally. They are typically covered with keratinized epidermal tissue beneath which are masses of dermal collagen and adipose tissue containing various adnexal structures, including hair follicles (Fig. 27-7). A related choristoma, the **dermolipoma,** is typically devoid of skin appendages and contains more adipose tissue. It usually is encountered in the bulbar conjunctiva near the outer canthus.

Conjunctivitis and keratoconjunctivitis

Conjunctivitis and keratoconjunctivitis are very common, for the conjunctiva and cornea

are exposed to a broad range of chemical, physical, microbial, and allergenic stimuli capable of evoking the full gamut of humoral, cellular, and tissue responses that are observed in acute, subacute, and chronic forms of inflammation. In addition to the general aspects of inflammation that are important wherever the processes develop, there are certain special aspects of ocular inflammations.

The eye is an exceptionally sensitive organ in many ways, including hypersensitivity to pain and light. Thus the acutely inflamed eye is typically very painful and photophobic. Relatively trivial lesions that affect the cornea may not only be exquisitely painful but also may cause a sharp reduction in vision by affecting corneal transparency in a variety of ways. In the acute stages of inflammation, corneal edema and infiltration by inflammatory cells may have a profound effect on corneal transparency. In more chronic forms of inflammation, blood vessels invade the normally avascular cornea. In the late stages of the interstitial keratitis of congenital syphilis, for example, the main clinical and histopathologic alteration is the deep stromal vascularization.

Pannus formation is another important corneal complication of keratoconjunctivitis. The inflammatory pannus is a wedge of vascularized connective tissue infiltrated by lymphocytes and plasma cells that invades the superficial layers of the cornea from the limbus, after destroying portions of Bowman's membrane and some of the most superficial stromal lamellae (Fig. 27-8).

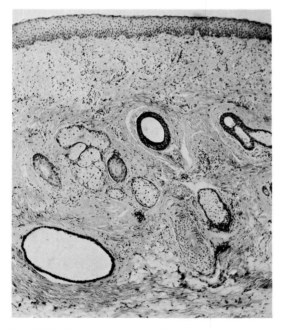

Fig. 27-7. Dermoid tumor of limbus consisting of choristomatous mass of cutaneous and adnexal tissues. (75×; AFIP 203027-24101; from Hogan, M. J., and Zimmerman, L. E.: Ophthalmic pathology, ed. 2, Philadelphia, 1962, W. B. Saunders Co.)

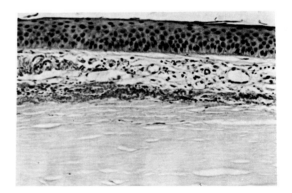

Fig. 27-8. Inflammatory pannus. Thick layer of vascularized connective tissue infiltrated by inflammatory cells has replaced Bowman's membrane and some superficial lamellae of corneal stroma. (AFIP 47564; from Hogan, M. J., and Zimmerman, L. E.: Ophthalmic pathology, ed. 2, Philadelphia, 1962, W. B. Saunders Co.)

Among the tissue responses that characterize the conjunctival reaction to chronic inflammation, two deserve special comment: **follicular hyperplasia** and **papillary hypertrophy**. Although the conjunctiva does not normally contain lymph nodes, it does have an amazing capacity to respond to chronic irritation, especially to such chronic infections as trachoma, by the proliferation of an abundance of lymphoid tissue with the formation of lymph follicles that contain prominent germinal centers (Fig. 27-9). The follicular hyperplasia of lymphoid tissue may become so prominent that it is readily recognizable by the clinician, especially on slit-lamp examination. The lymph follicles produce avascular grayish white granular elevations in the normally smooth transparent conjunctiva. Papillary hypertrophy is the result of a proliferation of blood vessels and connective tissue elements in the substantia propria in multiple foci, causing irregular elevations of the overlying epithelium (Fig. 27-10). Between the papillae, cryptlike proliferations of mucus-secreting conjunctival epithelium are formed. Since the papillae contain a prominent core of blood vessels and the lymph follicles in follicular hyperplasia are avascular, the ophthalmologist usually has no difficulty in distinguishing these two types of tissue response.

Infectious causes of conjunctivitis and keratitis include bacteria (e.g., the gonococcus, pneumococcus, streptococcus, staphylococcus, Koch-Weeks bacillus, diplobacillus of Morax-Axenfeld, tubercle bacilli, leprosy bacilli, *Francisella tularensis,* etc.), fungi (opportunistic pathogens such as various species of *Aspergillus, Cephalosporium,* and *Fusarium* as well as

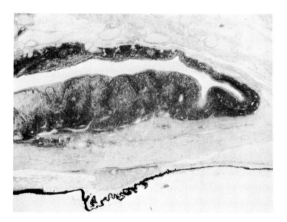

Fig. 27-9. Massive lymphoid hyperplasia of bulbar and fornical conjunctiva in trachoma, with formation of lymph follicles. (39×; AFIP 67237; from Hogan, M. J., and Zimmerman, L. E.: Ophthalmic pathology, ed. 2, Philadelphia, 1962, W. B. Saunders Co.)

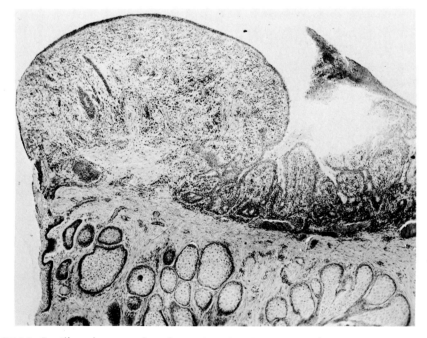

Fig. 27-10. Papillary hypertrophy of tarsal conjunctiva in vernal conjunctivitis. (50×; AFIP 60-5084; from Hogan, M. J., and Zimmerman, L. E.: Ophthalmic pathology, ed. 2, Philadelphia, 1962, W. B. Saunders Co.)

some of the better known pathogens such as *Coccidioides immitis, Nocardia asteroides, Sporothrix schenkii,* and *Rhinosporidium seeberi*), parasites (one of which, *Oncocerca volvulus,* is responsible for a great deal of blindness in Africa and in Central America), and several groups of viruses (especially the adenoviruses, *Chlamydia,** herpesviruses, and poxviruses). Viral infections are especially important because of their prevalence and high degree of contagiousness and, in some cases, because of their chronicity (e.g., trachoma) or tendency to recur (e.g., herpes simplex) coupled with their potential for producing severe corneal opacification leading to blindness.

Trachoma and **inclusion conjunctivitis** are caused by very closely related agents that have been placed in the genus *Chlamydia: Chlamydia trachomatis* and *Chlamydia oculogenitalis,* respectively. Collectively, they are commonly called the TRIC agents. The agent causing trachoma under natural conditions appears to be infectious only for the conjunctival epithelium of man. The disease is extremely prevalent in many countries in which poverty and poor personal hygiene are widespread. It is estimated that about 400 million people are infected and that about 1 in 20 have been blinded by the disease.

Early in the course of infection, the trachoma agent proliferates in the conjunctival epithelium, where it can be recognized in the form of basophilic cytoplasmic inclusion bodies (of Halberstaedter and Prowazek). The conjunctival epithelium becomes hyperplastic and infiltrated by mononuclear inflammatory cells. Lymph follicles develop in the substantia propria (Fig. 27-9). As the disease progresses, degeneration and necrosis of epithelial cells stimulate a more intense inflammatory reaction. Macrophages containing phagocytosed cellular debris (Leber cells) appear and papillary hypertrophy becomes pronounced. The stroma is greatly thickened and heavily infiltrated by plasma cells as well as lymphocytes. An inflammatory pannus invades the cornea. Scarring and vascularization of the cornea account for the blindness that is so common a complication of trachoma.

Inclusion conjunctivitis, although caused by an agent that is morphologically indistinguishable from that causing trachoma, is a much less severe disease. Two main forms of infection are recognized, both attributable to a genital reservoir. Inclusion blennorrhea is an acute, purulent conjunctivitis of the newborn infant resembling gonorrhea neonatorum epidemiologically in that the infection is acquired from the mother's genital tract during birth. Inclusion conjunctivitis in the adult is a less acute follicular conjunctivitis that may occur in epidemic form when large numbers of people are exposed as, for example, when swimming in nonchlorinated pools—hence the name "swimming pool conjunctivitis." Both in infants and in adults, the disease tends to be self-limiting and the cornea is spared.

Vernal conjunctivitis is a chronic recurring type of inflammation involving mainly the upper tarsal conjunctivas of boys in the spring. Noticeable papillary hypertrophy dominates the picture (Fig. 27-10). The large papillae, which develop broad flat tops, contain a stroma that is heavily infiltrated by chronic inflammatory cells and eosinophils.

Metabolic disorders

Metabolic disorders may affect the cornea or conjunctiva, sometimes producing lesions that are very helpful in clinical diagnosis.

In **Wilson's hepatolenticular degeneration,** for example, there is a curious deposit of a copper compound in Descemet's membrane of the peripheral cornea (Fig. 27-11). This gives rise to a peculiar ruby red to greenish brown opacification, the Kayser-Fleischer ring, that is pathognomonic of the disease (see p. 1376).

In **cystinosis,** fine scintillating polychromatic cystine crystals are deposited in the substantia propria of the conjunctiva and in the corneal stroma, where they can be readily observed with the slit lamp and obtained for microscopic examination by biopsy.

In **ochronosis,** brownish discoloration occurs in the outermost scleral and episcleral connective tissues (Fig. 27-12) and in the peripheral cornea of the interpalpebral zone, where these tissues are exposed to air and light.

In **hypercalcemia,** regardless of the specific cause, calcium salts may be deposited in Bowman's membrane.

In **familial hypercholesterolemia** and in certain other forms of **disturbed lipid metabolism,** arcus senilis becomes prominent at an early

---

*Although it is still common practice as well as convenient to consider the *Chlamydia* that cause trachoma, inclusion conjunctivitis, psittacosis, and lymphogranuloma venereum as viruses because they pass through Berkefeld filters, are obligate intracellular parasites, and produce inclusion bodies resembling those of poxviruses, they have now been placed in a separate taxonomic family, the *Chlamydiaceae.*

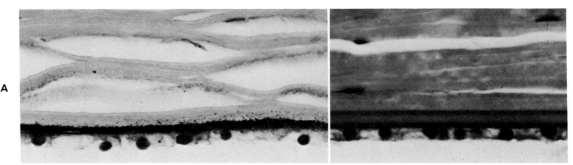

A

B

Fig. 27-11. A, Kayser-Fleischer ring. Dark band is copper compound that has been deposited in Descemet's membrane close to endothelium. **B,** Normal cornea for comparison. (**A,** 600×; AFIP 264768; **B,** 600×; AFIP 64-1883; **A,** from Hogan, M. J., and Zimmerman, L. E.: Ophthalmic pathology, ed. 2, Philadelphia, 1962, W. B. Saunders Co.)

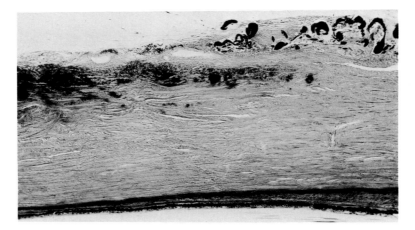

Fig. 27-12. Ochronosis. Strong pigmentation in degenerated elastic and collagenous tissues of sclera and episclera. (70×; AFIP 59-699; from Rones, B.: Am. J. Ophthalmol. **49:**440-446, 1960.)

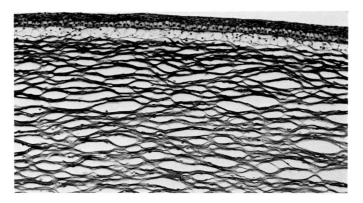

Fig. 27-13. Hurler's disease. Collection of histiocytic cells, cytoplasm of which is filled with acid mucopolysaccharide, is present in superficial layers of corneal stroma. (90×; AFIP 68-4418.)

age, and the corneal disturbance is appropriately called arcus juvenilis. Clinically, this is a milky opacification of the corneal stroma in a ring-shaped band peripherally, with a thin clear zone between it and the limbus. In ordinary paraffin sections of the cornea, no abnormalities are noted, even though clinically the arcus may have been very pronounced. Frozen sections and stains for fat are required to demonstrate the large amount of lipid present in Bowman's and Descemet's membranes and in the corneal stroma.

In **Hurler's disease** (gargoylism), there is a definite clouding of the cornea that may be present at birth but often begins near the end of the first year and severely interferes with vision. It is the result of an accumulation of abnormal mucopolysaccharides in the stromal and endothelial cells of the cornea and in histiocytic cells that may accumulate in large numbers, replacing Bowman's membrane (Fig. 27-13). Similar changes are observed in the Morquio, Scheie, and Maroteaux-Lamy syndromes, which are also the result of disturbances in mucopolysaccharide metabolism. Highly characteristic changes also are found in **Fabry's disease.** There is a diffuse haziness in the corneal epithelium and denser opacities that radiate out toward the periphery in wavy lines and bands from a focus near the center. Histologically, the basal cell layer of the corneal epithelium is swollen by an accumulation of glycolipids.

Pinguecula

Pinguecula is a common degenerative process believed to be a consequence of excessive actinic damage to the collagen in the substantia propria of the bulbar conjunctiva. It occurs most frequently in the interpalpebral region, where the tissues are most exposed, and appears clinically as a yellowish thickened area. Histologically, it is characterized by senile elastosis between the often atrophic overlying epithelium and the unaffected underlying sclera (Fig. 27-14). When a pinguecula becomes large, it may become secondarily irritated and inflamed. As a result, pseudoepitheliomatous hyperplasia of the overlying epithelium may develop and give rise to concern about cancer (Fig. 27-15). In some individuals, the actinic stimulation affects the epithelium as well as the substantia propria, giving rise to dyskeratotic lesions similar to those of the epidermis in senile keratosis. Only rarely, however, do these acanthotic lesions progress to squamous carcinoma. When they do, however, they are typically very low grade, well-differentiated, nonmetastasizing tumors.

Pterygium

Pterygium is believed to be a lesion very closely related to the pinguecula. The essential difference is that the pterygium arises at the limbus and typically progresses into the cornea, forming a wedge of vascularized connective tissue that dissects the epithelium away from Bowman's membrane. It is a more important lesion than the pinguecula because it is potentially sight-impairing as it progresses toward the center of the cornea, diminishing the transparency of the latter, because it is cosmetically much more objectionable and because it is more difficult to excise permanently since it has a greater tendency to recur. Secondary epithelial changes (pseudoepitheliomatous hyperplasia and dyskeratotic processes) may complicate the picture just as with the pinguecula.

Epidermidalization

Epidermidalization is a nonspecific descriptive term used to designated metaplasia of the

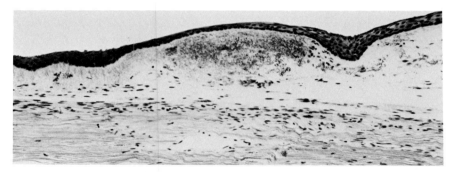

Fig. 27-14. Pinguecula. Noticeable elastosis of collagen in substantia propria. (120×; AFIP 86530; from Hogan, M. J., and Zimmerman, L. E.: Ophthalmic pathology, ed. 2, Philadelphia, 1962, W. B. Saunders Co.)

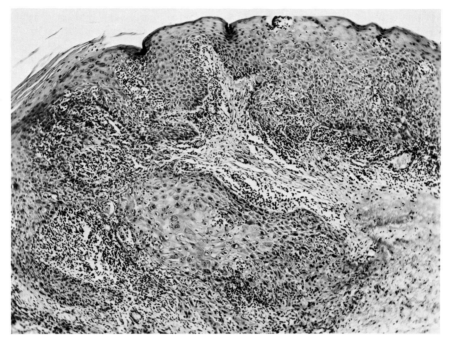

Fig. 27-15. Pseudoepitheliomatous hyperplasia of bulbar conjunctiva complicating inflammation of pinguecula. (75×; AFIP 55-16489.)

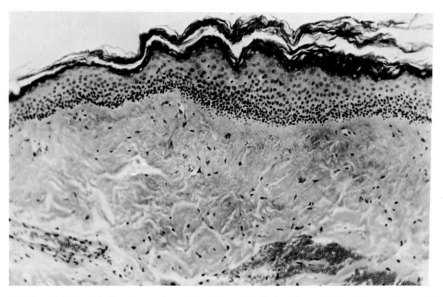

Fig. 27-16. Epidermidalization of conjunctiva. Well-developed keratin and prominent granular layer are present. These are not normally seen in conjunctiva. (125×; AFIP 338247-13081; from Hogan, M. J., and Zimmerman, L. E.: Ophthalmic pathology, ed. 2, Philadelphia, 1962, W. B. Saunders Co.)

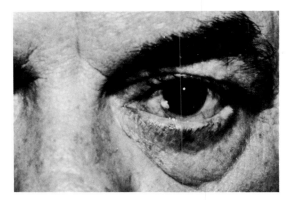

Fig. 27-17. Leukoplakia of limbus. (AFIP 60-5604; from Zimmerman, L. E.: In Boniuk, M., editor: Ocular and adnexal tumors, St. Louis, 1964, The C. V. Mosby Co.)

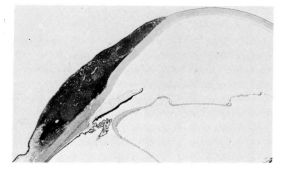

Fig. 27-18. Malignant melanoma of limbus that arose in compound nevus of conjunctiva. (7×; AFIP 57-16759; from Hogan, M. J., and Zimmerman, L. E.: Ophthalmic pathology, ed. 2, Philadelphia, 1962, W. B. Saunders Co.)

normally thin, transparent, nonkeratinized conjunctiva into a thicker, acanthotic, keratinizing squamous epithelium that may have a striking resemblance microscopically to epidermis (Fig. 27-16). Clinically, the affected tissue appears pearly white, and when localized to a placoid area, the descriptive term "leukoplakia" is appropriate (Fig. 27-17). This term, however, implies nothing etiologically or prognostically, nor does it indicate what the histopathologic picture might be, for other processes besides epidermidalization can produce leukoplakic lesions. Leukoplakia should, therefore, be used only for clinical description. A variety of factors may lead to epidermidalization, including an insufficiency of tears, excessive drying when the eyeball is chronically exposed as a result of neuroparalytic disorders or pathologic processes affecting closure of the eyelids (e.g., severe exophthalmos), vitamin A deficiency, etc. Bitot's spots are foci of keratinization in which xerosis bacilli proliferate saprophytically in the keratin layer, producing a foamy substance that can be wiped away.

Tumors
Benign tumors

Benign tumors of the conjunctiva include papillomas, nevi, angiomatous malformations, neurofibromas, and lymphomas. All others are too rare to mention, and only the so-called *lymphoma* requires comment here.

Most of the massive proliferations of lymphoid tissue that present clinically as epibulbar tumors prove to be benign, both on histopathologic examination and upon long-term follow-up study. When follicle formation is

evident and when a significant admixture of other inflammatory cells besides the lymphocytes can be seen, the lesion can rather easily be recognized as a reactive lymphoid hyperplasia. However, when lymphocytes without formation of follicles are seen almost exclusively, then the possibility of a well-differentiated lymphosarcoma or a lymphocytic leukemia must be given serious consideration and appropriate clinical and hematologic studies undertaken. It is only very rarely, however, that an epibulbar tumor is the initial clinical manifestation of a malignant lymphoma or leukemia.

Malignant tumors

Malignant tumors of the conjunctiva are rare and only two, malignant melanoma and squamous cell carcinoma, will be considered here. Both arise much more frequently on the bulbar conjunctiva than on the palpebral conjunctiva or in the fornices, and both are observed most frequently in the limbal area of the interpalpebral zone.

Malignant melanomas. Malignant melanomas of the conjunctiva may arise from preexisting nevi, within an area of acquired melanosis, or anew in apparently normal conjunctiva. Malignant melanomas arising in conjunctival nevi are very similar histopathologically to those of the skin (Fig. 27-18).

Clinically, the patient, who is often a young or middle-aged adult, usually is able to give a very meaningful history. A pigmented spot is known to have been present in the exposed part of the bulbar conjunctiva since early childhood. For years, it did not change in appearance and then began to grow larger, typically as an exophytic epibulbar mass. Patients with malignant melanomas arising in areas of acquired melanosis give a different history. They tend to be older and deny the presence of any conjunctival lesion during childhood or during the early adult years. During middle age, they become aware of a slowly progressive brownish discoloration of the conjunctival epithelium of one eye. There is a great deal of variability in the degree and extent of this acquired melanosis. In some patients almost the entire conjunctiva and much of the corneal epithelium may be affected, whereas in others only a relatively small area may be involved. After a period of years, during which time the pigmentary disturbance may have progressed steadily, waxed and waned, or remained stationary, about one fifth of the patients develop one or more nodules within the area of melanosis. These may or may not be pigmented. Such a change is always a cause for alarm, because it usually is an indication that a malignant melanoma has arisen and calls for excision or biopsy.

When feasible, the entire area of pigmentary disturbance should be excised for histopathologic study, but when considered too extensive, one or more of the nodules alone may be excised for microscopic examination. With only the malignant melanoma itself available for histopathologic study, the pathologist usually cannot determine whether the tumor arose from a nevus, in acquired melanosis, or started again. This distinction is best made by the clinician, but if the pathologist has a sufficiently generous sample of the surrounding conjunctiva available for examination, as is the case when the orbital contents have been exenterated, he often can make the differential diagnosis microscopically. When the adjacent tissues contain clusters of benign nevoid cells and cystic inclusions of conjunctival epithelium in the substantia propria, these are features typical of a preexisting compound nevus. If, on the other hand, no nevoid clusters are present in the substantia propria but the conjunctival epithelium exhibits intense melanotic pigmentation, activated clear cells, and intraepithelial nests of large atypical melanocytes, these features are characteristic of acquired melanosis (Fig. 27-19).

Acquired melanosis often has been called "precancerous" melanosis in the ophthalmic literature, but because the development of a malignant melanoma in the affected tissues is the exception rather than the rule, occurring

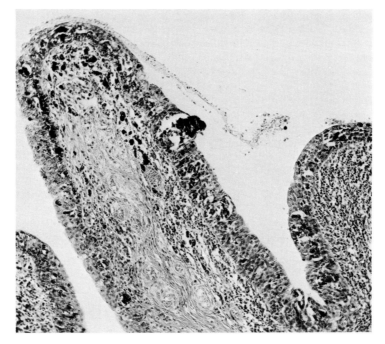

Fig. 27-19. Acquired melanosis of conjunctiva. Heavily pigmented conjunctival epithelium contains many large prominent nests of nevoid cells, and there is dense infiltrate of chronic inflammatory cells in substantia propria. (115×; AFIP 897677; from Smith, M. E.: In Ackerman, L. V., and Rosai, J.: Surgical pathology, ed. 5, St. Louis, 1974, The C. V. Mosby Co.)

in only 15% to 20% of cases, this term gives a false impression as to the neoplastic potential of the pigmentary disturbance. The condition is believed to be the conjunctival equivalent of the melanotic freckle of Hutchinson.

Malignant melanomas of the conjunctiva, regardless of their histogenetic derivation, carry a guarded prognosis. Although less frequently lethal than melanomas of the skin, they do have the capacity for invasion of lymphatic and vascular channels. Those that are still quite localized and confined to the limbal zone often can be controlled by simple excision, whereas those that involve the conjunctiva more diffusely with spread onto the eyelids, caruncle, or canthi usually must be treated by a more radical procedure such as exenteration of the orbital contents.

Squamous cell carcinoma. Squamous cell carcinoma of the conjunctiva presents most often as a very well defferentiated exophytic mass at the limbus on the nasal or temporal side (Fig. 27-20). It is rather rare in the United States and in Europe, but there is evidence that it is encountered more frequently in the Middle East, Africa, and India. Most squamous cell carcinomas seem to arise at sites of actinic keratosis. This fact, coupled with the unavailability of adequate medical care to permit removal of all cosmetic blemishes on the conjunctiva, probably offers the best explanation for the apparent geographic variation in the occurrence of these tumors. Other factors, such as racial susceptibility and tribal customs also may play a role.

Although actinic keratosis is probably the most important precursor lesion responsible for the development of squamous cell carcinomas, there is another group of epithelial changes that seem to play a role. They seem to be analogous to the spectrum of intraepithelial changes observed in such other mucous membranes as the uterine cervix, ranging from dysplasia through carcinoma in situ to invasive carcinoma (Fig. 27-21). In the ophthalmic literature, these intraepithelial lesions have often been called collectively "Bowen's disease." Although convenient, this is an inappropriate designation because there is only a superficial similarity of these conjunctival lesions to the distinctive cutaneous tumor that Bowen described.

Clinically, the dysplasia–carcinoma in situ group often can be differentiated from the actinic keratosis group. The latter almost always is confined to the exposed conjunctival and limbal tissues in the interpalpebral area and have a leukoplakic appearance because of the tendency of the acanthotic epithelium to develop a keratotic crust over its surface. Dysplasia and carcinoma in situ develop in portions of the conjunctiva covered by the eyelids as well as in the exposed areas, spread more frequently into the cornea, and are characterized by a grayish opalescent or gelatinous appearance of the affected epithelium that is less acanthotic and seldom covered by a keratotic crust.

Regardless of their histogenesis, squamous cell carcinomas of the conjunctiva carry a

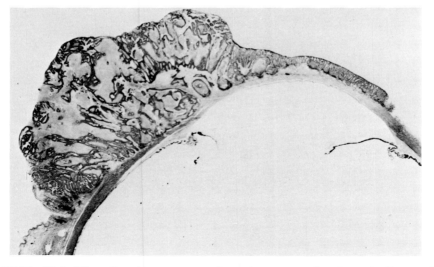

Fig. 27-20. Well-differentiated squamous cell carcinoma growing in typically exophytic manner from bulbar conjunctiva. (10×; AFIP 72108; from Hogan, M. J., and Zimmerman, L. E.: Ophthalmic pathology, ed. 2, Philadelphia, 1962, W. B. Saunders Co.)

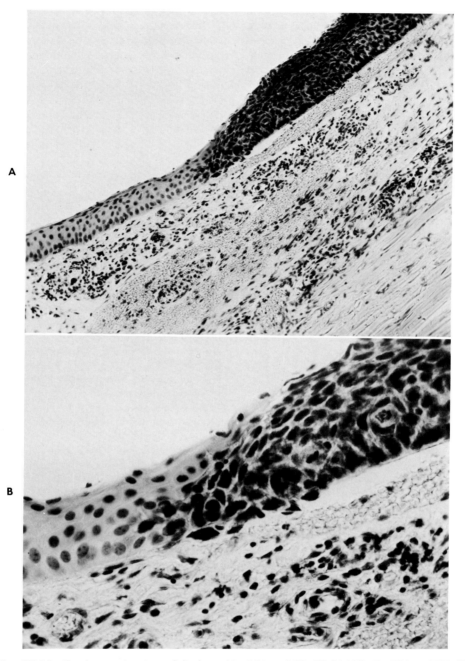

Fig. 27-21. Carcinoma in situ of limbus. (**A,** 160×; AFIP 53-21692; **B,** 570×; AFIP 53-21693; **B,** from Hogan, M. J., and Zimmerman, L. E.: Ophthalmic pathology, ed. 2, Philadedphia, 1962, W. B. Saunders Co.)

very favorable prognosis and should be treated by the most conservative excisional methods feasible. If permitted to grow large, they may invade the eye or the orbit, but metastasis is very rare.

ORBIT

In addition to the eyeball and optic nerve, the orbit contains the extraocular muscles, many blood vessels and peripheral nerves, and one important epithelial structure, the lacrimal gland—all embedded in a matrix of adipose tissue. Although these orbital tissues may be involved in a broad range of systemic as well as localized disease processes, the single most important aspect of orbital pathologic abnormalities is the formation of a space-occupying mass that displaces the eyeball, usually with protrusion forward (proptosis or exophthalmos). These orbital tumors include benign and malignant neoplasms, hamartomatous and choristomatous growths, and inflammatory masses that are commonly (although inap-

propriately!) called inflammatory pseudotumors. In addition, the orbital tissues may become diffusely involved in pathologic processes related to systemic diseases.

Endocrinopathic exophthalmos

Endocrinopathic exophthalmos is a convenient term under which the main ophthalmic manifestations of Graves' disease can be grouped collectively. Graves' disease usually is divided into two types: mild, often referred to as thyrotoxic or benign exophthalmos, and severe, also called thyrotropic, malignant, or infiltrative exophthalmos.

Although eyelid retraction and an apparent exophthalmos are characteristic features of Graves' disease, in its classic form one rarely sees evidence of more than a minimal effect on the orbital tissues, and severe secondary damage to the eyeball is not observed. In thyrotropic exophthalmos, on the other hand, the orbital tissues and extraocular muscles may become so massively involved that an extreme

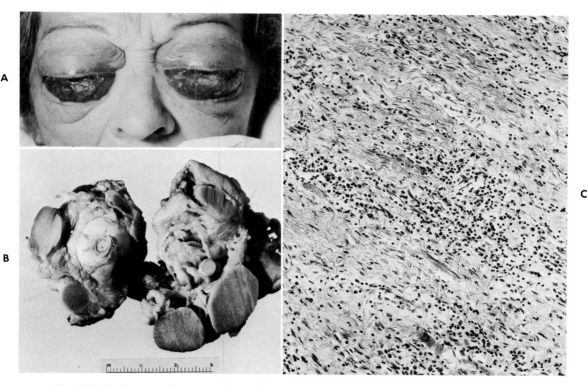

Fig. 27-22. Graves' disease with malignant exophthalmos. **A,** Severe periorbital edema and chemosis as well as proptosis. **B,** Massively enlarged extraocular muscles. **C,** Greatly degenerated extraocular muscles scarred and infiltrated by mononuclear inflammatory cells. (**A,** AFIP 55-3860; **B,** AFIP 55-10706; **C,** 145×; AFIP 58-13128; from Zimmerman, L. E.: In Ackerman, L. V., in collaboration with Butcher, H. R., Jr.: Surgical pathology, ed. 3, St. Louis, 1964, The C. V. Mosby Co.)

degree of rapidly progressive exophthalmos develops (Fig. 27-22, *A*). This may so seriously threaten the eye that the eyelids must be sutured together to prevent exposure keratitis. This form of endocrinopathic exophthalmos often is called "malignant exophthalmos" because of its severity, difficulty to control, and damaging sequelae. It is typically a bilateral disorder, but unilateral involvement occurs with sufficient frequency that it is considered by many ophthalmologists to be the leading cause of unilateral proptosis in adults. The pathologic changes include an accumulation of water-binding mucopolysaccharides throughout the orbital tissues, severe degeneration of ex-

traocular muscles that may become massively enlarged (Fig. 27-22, *B*) and eventually scarred (Fig. 27-22, *C*), and diffuse lymphocytic infiltration.

Anderson[21] has recently reviewed a large amount of the very abundant current literature on the mechanisms involved in the pathogenesis of Graves' disease and endocrine exophthalmos and has prepared an admirable summary. Because the old terms "thyrotoxic" and "thyrotropic" exophthalmos give an erroneous oversimplified concept of the pathologic physiology involved and because the many descriptive terms that have been used for various clinical manifestations of Graves' dis-

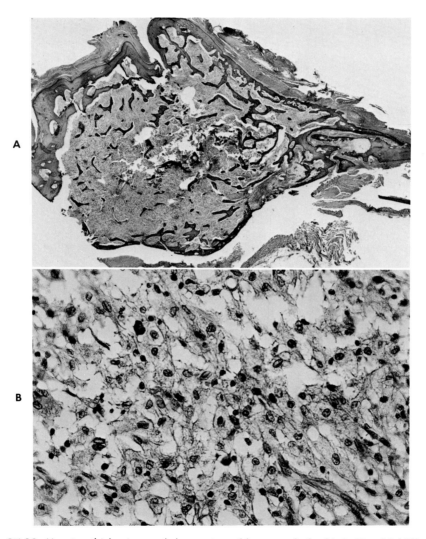

Fig. 27-23. Massive thickening and destruction of bony roof of orbit in Hand-Schüller-Christian disease. (**A**, 6×; AFIP 58-5349; **B**, 305×; AFIP 58-4501; **A** and **B**, from Hogan, M. J., and Zimmerman, L. E.: Ophthalmic pathology, ed. 2, Philadelphia, 1962, W. B. Saunders Co.)

ease are equally objectionable. Werner[33] has recently proposed a new objective classification: *class 0*, no signs or symptoms; *class 1*, only signs, no symptoms; *class 2*, symptoms and signs; *class 3*, proptosis; *class 4*, extraocular muscle involvement; *class 5*, corneal involvement; *class 6*, optic nerve involvement with loss of sight.

Histiocytosis X

Histiocytosis X, a group of related disorders that includes Hand-Schüller-Christian disease, eosinophilic granuloma of bone, and Letterer-Siwe disease, may have unilateral or bilateral proptosis as an important, sometimes presenting, clinical manifestation.

In Hand-Schüller-Christian disease, massive thickening and destruction of the bony walls of the orbit by the xanthogranulomatous process, with infiltration also into the soft tissues, occur so frequently that proptosis is considered one of the cardinal signs of the disease (Fig. 27-23). In eosinophilic granuloma of bone, there is often only a single focus of bone destruction, but this may be located in the orbit, most often in the upper temporal region, where thickening of the soft tissues of the eyebrow and eyelid may be a prominent clinical sign. Orbital involvement is rare in Letterer-Siwe disease.

Phycomycosis

Phycomycosis (often called mucormycosis) is described here because it is typically encountered as a most impressive complication of uncontrolled acidosis, especially in diabetic patients. It is a mycotic infection that is described more fully in Chapter 13, but because of its frequently devastating ocular and orbital complications, it must be mentioned here.

Pathogenetically, it has been shown that some of the saprophytic fungi belonging to the Phycomycetes become extremely virulent when the host is acidotic. Clinically insignificant infections involving the nose and paranasal sinuses may then lead to rapidly spreading orbital cellulitis with frequent vascular complications (occlusive arteritis as well as thrombophlebitis). Gangrenous areas rapidly appear about the orbit, nose, and palate, and ischemic infarction involving the optic nerve and retina produce a rapidly progressive blindness. If not recognized early in its development and if the underlying disorder (diabetic acidosis, etc.) is not corrected promptly, the infection and its vascular complications spread back into the brain, resulting in a fatal outcome, often within a week of onset of symptoms.

Leukemia and malignant lymphoma

Leukemia and malignant lymphoma may involve any of the orbital tissues, but only rarely is the orbital lesion the initial manifestation of the disease. In some patients (especially in children) destined to develop acute granulocytic leukemia, a mass of very immature cells of the granulocytic series, often resembling the cells of reticulum cell sarcoma, may appear in the orbit long before any hematologic evidence of leukemia is found. Primary reticulum cell sarcomas of the orbit are extremely rare. Whenever a tumor suggestive of a reticulum cell sarcoma is encountered in the orbit, the pathologist should investigate the possibility that the lesion is, in actuality, a granulocytic sarcoma (also called chloroma), an undifferentiated or transitional carcinoma that has spread into the orbit from an asymptomatic primary lesion in the nasopharynx or paranasal sinuses, or an inflammatory pseudotumor in which an exuberant reactive hyperplasia of reticulum cells has dominated the picture.

There is only one form of malignant lymphoma that involves the orbital tissues frequently—*Burkitt's African lymphoma*. This peculiar, highly undifferentiated malignant lymphoma has a curious predilection for the bones of the face and jaws. There is often bilateral involvement of the maxillae with spread into the soft tissues of the orbit. Consequently, proptosis with upward displace-

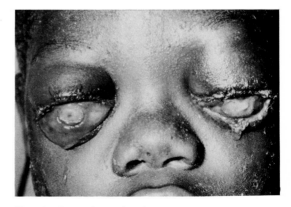

Fig. 27-24. Bilateral orbital involvement in Burkitt's African lymphoma. (AFIP 68-7157-5; from Karp, L. A., Zimmerman, L. E., and Payne, T.: Arch. Ophthalmol. [Chicago] **85:**295-298, 1971.)

ment of the eyeball is not an unusual presenting manifestation (Fig. 27-24).

Macroglobulinemia and other dysproteinemias

Macroglobulinemia and other dysproteinemias may be accompanied by massive proliferation of lymphoid tissue in extra–lymph
nodal sites. We have seen several cases in
which a mass in the orbit, with or without
lacrimal gland involvement, was the initial
clinical manifestation.

Microscopic examination typically shows a
mixed population of cells, including lymphocytes, plasma cells, and reticulum cells, but
particularly impressive are those that seem to
represent intermediate stages of plasmacytoid
differentiation. The demonstration of plasmacytoid cells in which eosinophilic intranuclear
inclusions staining positively with periodic
acid–Schiff are conspicuously present (Fig.
27-25) should always suggest the possibility
of a dysproteinemia and call for appropriate
studies of the serum proteins.

Sjögren's syndrome

Sjögren's syndrome, characterized ophthal-
mologically by the occurrence of keratoconjunctivitis sicca in middle-aged arthritic wom-
en, may lead to either shinkage or enlargement of the lacrimal and salivary glands.

Microscopically, the changes observed include nonspecific atrophy with disappearance
of variable amounts of the glandular parenchyma and replacement by an infiltrate of
lymphocytes, plasma cells, and reticulum cells
with or without fibrosis. In some cases, Godwin's benign lymphoepithelial lesion is strikingly obvious. Whenever this alteration is observed in an enlarged lacrimal or salivary
gland, the pathologist should investigate the
possibility that the patient may have clinical
manifestations of Sjögren's syndrome. The
benign lymphoepithelial lesion is characterized
by a peculiar proliferation of both the epithelial and the myoepithelial cells of the larger
ducts of the lacrimal or salivary glands and
a virtually complete disappearance of all other
glandular structures in the immediately adjacent areas. Thus one sees the epimyoepithelial islands in a sea of lymphoid cells (Fig.
27-26). Frequently, the lumens of the affected
ducts are obliterated and some lymphocytes
also are observed among the proliferated epimyoepithelial cells. In some cases of Sjögren's
syndrome, the affected glands show a striking
plasmacytoid reaction, and the PAS-positive
inclusions that are always so suggestive of a
dysproteinemia may be conspicuously present.

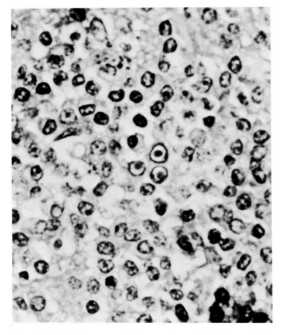

Fig. 27-25. Three cells in center of field contain intranuclear inclusions that stain positively with periodic acid–Schiff reaction in lymphoid pseudo-tumor in patient with macroglobulinemia. (Periodic acid–Schiff; 750×; AFIP 69-4960.)

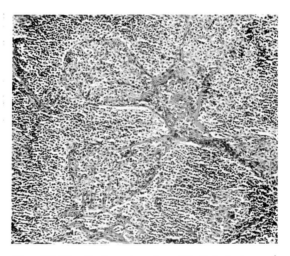

Fig. 27-26. Benign lymphoepithelial lesion of lacrimal gland. Epimyoepithelial islands such as one shown are all that remain of lacrimal gland, which is massively replaced by lymphoid cells. (115×; AFIP 63-1260.)

Mikulicz's syndrome

Mikulicz's syndrome is characterized by enlargement of multiple lacrimal and salivary glands. It may be observed in patients with Sjögren's syndrome, but it also may be observed in those with various other conditions (e.g., sarcoidosis, macroglobulinemia, leukemia, malignant lymphoma, etc.).

The term "Mikulicz's disease" always has been confusing because nobody really knows what disease process Mikulicz's patient had. Most writers today seem to be in agreement that this term therefore should be dropped and that the term "Mikulicz's syndrome" should be used only clinically for descriptive purposes.

Recklinghausen's neurofibromatosis

Recklinghausen's neurofibromatosis is another example of a very different type of systemic disease in which the orbit often is involved. In addition to having localized plexiform neurofibromas in the orbit or eyelids, patients with neurofibromatosis may exhibit gross disfigurement of the orbit (usually unilaterally) as a consequence of severe maldevelopment of both the osseous and soft tissues of the orbit. The eye also is often involved, and it may become either grossly enlarged, usually from an associated glaucoma, or shrunken from complications leading to phthisis bulbi.

Tumors

The following is a practical classification of tumors of the orbit.

Primary orbital tumors

1. Choristomatous (examples, dermoid cysts and teratomas)
2. Hamartomatous (examples, hemangiomas and lymphangiomas)
3. Mesenchymal
   a. Adipose
   b. Fibrous
   c. Myomatous
   d. Cartilaginous
   e. Osseous
   f. Vascular
4. Neural
   a. Peripheral nerves
   b. Optic nerves
5. Melanomatous (in association with nevus of Ota)
   a. Cellular blue nevus
   b. Malignant melanoma
6. Epithelial
   a. Lacrimal gland
   b. Ectopic lacrimal gland
7. Inflammatory "pseudotumors"
   a. Lymphoid
   b. Plasmacytoid

c. Sclerosing nongranulomatous
d. Granulomatous
e. Lipogranulomatous

Secondary orbital tumors—from primary sites in adjacent tissues

1. Intraocular
   a. Malignant melanoma
   b. Retinoblastoma
2. Epibulbar
   a. Carcinoma
   b. Malignant melanoma
3. Eyelids and skin of face
   a. Basal cell carcinoma
   b. Sebaceous carcinoma
   c. Malignant melanoma
   d. Squamous cell carcinoma
4. Upper respiratory tract
   a. Carcinoma of various types
   b. Malignant melanoma
   c. Mucocele
5. Intracranial
   a. Meningioma
   b. Pituitary adenoma

Metastatic

1. Carcinoma
2. Malignant melanoma
3. Sarcoma
4. Neuroblastoma

As with all classifications, there are lesions that would seem to fit into more than one category and there are others that do not seem to fit well into any. In the orbit, a good example is the fibrous xanthoma, a lesion that we are recognizing with increasing frequency. Is it a neoplasm or a peculiar form of inflammatory pseudotumor? If it is a neoplasm, is it basically fibrous, vascular, or histiocytic? At the present time, these questions cannot be answered satisfactorily.

It is difficult to comment on the relative frequency of orbital tumors because there is so much variation depending on the nature of one's particular experience. The pathologist who practices in a pediatric hospital will see many examples of orbital involvement late in the course of such conditions as neuroblastoma, leukemia, and Hand-Schüller-Christian disease, but the ophthalmic pathologist rarely sees such cases. He and the clinical opthalmologist, who deal primarily with those conditions whose initial manifestations are ocular or orbital, are much more likely to see hemangiomas, rhabdomyosarcomas, and gliomas of the optic nerve in their pediatric patients. One of the most common orbital tumors in the experience of radiologists is the mucocele of the paranasal sinuses, yet the ophthalmic pathologist rarely sees these lesions. In geriatric practice, one sees secondary and metastatic

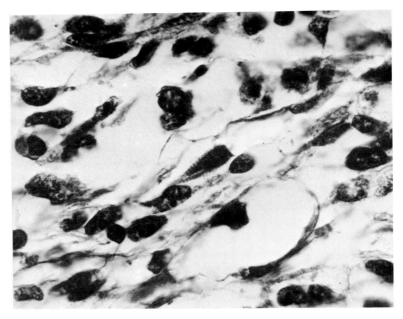

Fig. 27-27. Embryonal rhabdomyosarcoma of orbit. One cell in center of field has well-formed cross striations, whereas all others appear to be undifferentiated mesenchymal cells. (720×; AFIP 65-3236.)

tumors of the orbit much more frequently than primary tumors. In equatorial Africa, primary malignant lymphoma involving the orbital bones is relatively common, whereas this is a very rare orbital neoplasm everywhere else in the world.

Although the foregoing comments indicate that it is difficult to generalize about orbital tumors, there does seem to be general agreement that endocrinopathic endophthalmos, hemangiomas, and inflammatory pseudotumors are the most frequent causes of proptosis in adults. Hemangiomas also are frequent in childhood. Of especial importance in childhood are rhabdomyosarcomas, gliomas of the optic nerve, leukemia, and lymphoma.

Rhabdomyosarcomas. Rhabdomyosarcomas of the orbit are usually of the embryonal type (Fig. 27-27) and are seen almost exclusively in the first 15 years of life. They arise diffusely in the orbital tissues (only rarely in the substance of one of the extraocular muscles) and have a predilection for the upper inner portion, producing a downward and temporal displacement of the globe.

Typically sudden in appearance, the tumor often grows with alarming rapidity and frequently has spread diffusely by the time the orbit is explored. It is not only highly invasive, with a distinct tendency to invade the cranium, but it is also capable of metastasizing widely by the bloodstream. Its prognosis is very poor, although the treatment of orbital rhabdomyosarcomas has been more successful than has that of other embryonal rhabdomyosarcomas. This tumor does not generally affect visual acuity, although the displacement of the globe may cause diplopia. With severe proptosis, exposure keratitis eventually may complicate the picture.

Glioma of optic nerve. Glioma of the optic nerve is another orbital tumor encountered almost exclusively in the pediatric age group, with about half of the cases being recognized by the age of 5 years. It is typically a very low grade, well-differentiated, fibrillary type of astrocytoma that grows slowly within the parenchyma of the nerve (Fig. 27-28), gradually destroying the latter's axons as it displaces the eye forward. Those tumors that arise anteriorly in the nerve, close to the globe where the central retinal artery and vein pass through the nerve to enter the eye, are likely to compress and occlude these vessels. Thus the child with a glioma of the optic nerve often shows a number of important ocular complications not often seen in patients with rhabdomyosarcomas of the orbit, including severe loss of vision, optic atrophy, papilledema, retinal hemorrhages and exudates, and even infarction of the retina.

Although prognosis for vision in the affected

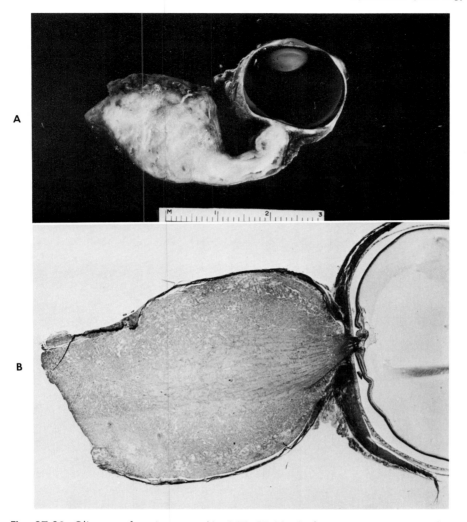

Fig. 27-28. Gliomas of optic nerve. (**A,** AFIP 57-890-3; from Hogan, M. J., and Zimmerman, L. E.: Ophthalmic pathology, ed. 2, Philadelphia, 1962, W. B. Saunders Co.; **B,** AFIP 55-17314; from Zimmerman, L. E.: In Saphir, O., editor: A text on systemic pathology, New York, 1958-1959, Grune & Stratton, Inc.; by permission.)

eye is very poor, prognosis for life is good. After a period of growth during childhood, the tumors seem to become quiescent. Spread from the optic nerve back into the brain is unusual, orbital recurrence is very rare, and hematogenous spread unknown, even though the tumor may have been untreated or incompletely resected.

Gliomas of the optic nerve occur more frequently in patients with Recklinghausen's neurofibromatosis than in otherwise normal individuals, and in such patients they may be bilateral, but less than 15% of patients with these tumors show evidence of neurofibromatosis.

Meningiomas. Meningiomas, in contrast with gliomas, occur more frequently in adults than in children. There are three possible histogenetic explanations for the occurrence of orbital meningiomas.

One group arises from the leptomeningeal coverings of the optic nerve (Fig. 27-29). This type is almost always of the meningothelial variety, and psammoma bodies are usually demonstrable. The tumor often compresses or infiltrates the parenchyma of the optic nerve, producing optic atrophy and visual loss as well as proptosis.

Meningiomas of the second major group have an intracranial site of origin that clin-

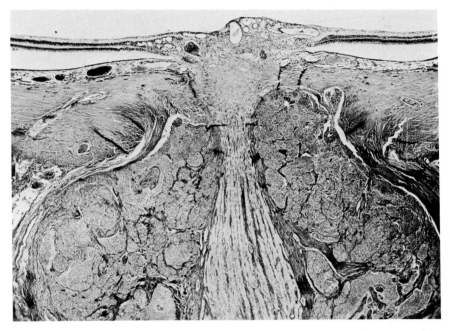

Fig. 27-29. Meningioma of optic nerve. (22×; AFIP 55939; from Smith, M. E.: In Ackerman, L. V., and Rosai, J.: Surgical pathology, ed. 5, St. Louis, 1974, The C. V. Mosby Co.)

ically may be silent and difficult to detect. These tumors reach the orbit by infiltrating directly into the orbital bones or along the vessels and nerves that pass through the various foramina. They usually do not affect the optic nerve itself, and visual loss is therefore not characteristic.

The third group of meningiomas is mainly of theoretic interest. It is postulated that meningiomas may arise from meningeal rests in the orbit. We know that ectopic neuroglial and meningeal tissue may be encountered in the orbit, giving rise to space-occupying choristomatous cysts and tumors (encephaloceles and meningoceles), but proof of the origin of meningiomas from such rests is most difficult to establish. It is possible that some of the fibroblastic and fibroxanthomatous tumors encountered in the orbit may have taken origin from such ectopic meningeal tissue, but the majority of unequivocal meningothelial and psammomatous meningiomas in the orbit either are of optic nerve origin or are secondary from an intracranial site of origin.

Leukemia and lymphoma. Leukemia and lymphoma have been mentioned earlier in this chapter (p. 1177). As an initial manifestation of a previously undetected leukemia, the child more likely than the adult may be seen with an apparently isolated tumor in the orbit, eyelids, or periorbital tissues. Thus, in the differential diagnosis of any undifferentiated neoplasm encountered in the orbital tissues of a child, leukemia must be considered and appropriate hematologic investigations may be undertaken. Burkitt's African lymphoma is the most important malignant lymphoma that affects the orbit (p. 1177).

Postirradiation sarcomas and carcinomas. Postirradiation sarcomas and carcinomas were once of great importance in children who had received intensive radiation therapy for retinoblastoma. There was a period when 7500 to 10,000 rads were being delivered through one or two portals in an effort to save at least one eye in selected patients with bilateral retinoblastoma. This treatment was frequently successful in controlling the retinoblastoma, but intraocular complications leading to eventual enucleation of the eye were common, and occasionally a second tumor appeared in the irradiated tissues 5 to 20 years later. Most of these were sarcomas and, of these, osteogenic and chondromatous sarcomas were seen most often. This is of pathogenetic significance because in nonirradiated orbital tissues malignant bone tumors are exceedingly rare neoplasms (except in adults who have Paget's disease of bone).

In recent years, with the availability of bet-

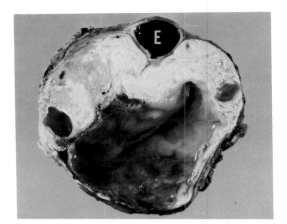

Fig. 27-30. Teratoma that massively enlarged orbit of newborn infant. Note size of eye, **E**, for comparison. (From Casanovas, R.: Arch. Ophthalmol. [Chicago] **77**:795-797, 1967; AFIP 66-7224.)

ter methods of radiation therapy, it has been learned that much smaller doses of radiation in selected patients can control the retinoblastoma without adversely affecting the eye or adjacent orbital tissues, and it is hoped that postradiation cancers will no longer be encountered in this area.

Other primary malignant orbital tumors in children. Other primary malignant tumors of the orbit in children such as embryonal carcinoma, meningeal sarcoma, and alveolar soft-part sarcoma are encountered too rarely to warrant further comment here.

Metastatic neuroblastoma. Metastatic neuroblastoma is the only important metastatic tumor of the orbit in children. It generally is encountered late in the clinical course, long after the child has been recognized as having a malignant retroperitoneal tumor. Thus it rarely presents a diagnostic problem for either the ophthalmologist or the ophthalmic pathologist. Typically, the orbits are affected bilaterally, and there is often a hemorrhagic appearance to the affected eyelids and orbital tissues.

Benign orbital tumors. Benign orbital tumors in children are numerous. They include the relatively common dermoid cysts, the rare teratomas, which often are already huge at birth (Fig. 27-30), ectopic masses of neurogenic and meningeal tissues (encephaloceles and meningoencephaloceles), hemangiomas, lymphangiomas, and neurofibromas, and even such lesions that are more typically seen in adults such as meningiomas, lacrimal glands tumors, and inflammatory pseudotumors.

Lacrimal gland tumors. Lacrimal gland tumors include, in addition to the primary epithelial neoplasms, enlargements resulting from a variety of other pathologic processes. When a patient is seen with a mass in the position of the lacrimal gland, there is about a 50-50 chance that the cause will be found to be an epithelial neoplasm.

Enlargements not the result of epithelial neoplasms are most frequently caused by nonspecific inflammatory processes ("pseudotumors"), but they also may be observed when the gland is involved in such specific granulomatous diseases as sarcoidosis, tuberculosis, and leprosy or when it is invaded by neoplasms that have arisen elsewhere. As was indicated in the discussion of Mikulicz's syndrome, the lacrimal glands may be enlarged along with one or more salivary glands in leukemia, malignant lymphoma, macroglobulinemia, Sjögren's syndrome, and a variety of other conditions. If both lacrimal glands are enlarged, one can be relatively certain that the cause is not an epithelial neoplasm because these are, almost without exception, always unilateral.

Epithelial neoplasms. Epithelial neoplasms of the lacrimal gland are very similar to those of the salivary glands, but one does not see such a great variety of tumor types in the lacrimal gland, and certain tumors (e.g., Warthin's tumor) that are relatively common in the salivary glands are either very rare or nonexistent in the lacrimal gland. For practical purposes, a very simple classification may be used. There are two major groups: the mixed tumors and carcinomas that are unrelated to mixed tumors.

The mixed tumors of the lacrimal gland are virtually identical to those of the salivary glands (p. 1262). Most of the mixed tumors are benign, but about one third are malignant. The median age of patients with benign mixed tumors is 35 years, whereas patients with malignant mixed tumors tend to be about 15 years older. The malignant mixed tumor by definition is one that contains areas of benign mixed tumor but, in addition, areas exhibiting histologic features of malignancy. The latter are usually adenocarcinomatous, sometimes squamous, and very rarely sarcomatous. The malignant change may be evident when the tumor is first removed, or it may be observed only some years after a benign mixed tumor has been incompletely removed and then allowed to recur.

Adenocarcinomas that are unrelated to

mixed tumors exhibit considerable architectural variation microscopically, but one type is of particular importance. This is the adenoid cystic or cylindromatous variety, which is comparatively more frequent in the lacrimal than in the major salivary glands. It is a tumor that in the past often has been confused with benign mixed tumors (and vice versa). Benign mixed tumors carry a favorable prognosis, whereas adenoid cystic carcinomas are extremely infiltrative, with a remarkable tendency to spread into and along nerves and through the bony wall of the orbit. Although the cure rate for benign mixed tumors is high, it is most unusual to be able to save a patient who has an adenoid cystic carcinoma of the lacrimal gland. Thus the histopathologic delineation of adenoid cystic carcinoma from benign mixed tumor has been a major contribution to the study and prognosis of lacrimal gland tumors.

Pseudotumor. Pseudotumor is a term that has variable connotations. It is perhaps most precisely used when surgical exploration of the orbit fails to reveal any evidence of a mass in a patient who clinically was believed to have an orbital tumor. It is most frequently used, however, together with the adjective "inflammatory," to designate a mass composed of inflammatory tissue that clinically had been suspected of being a neoplasm. Microscopically, some of these can be placed in well-established categoric groups (e.g., sarcoidosis, tuberculosis, echinococcosis, foreign body granulomas, and sclerosing lipogranulomas), but the majority are very nonspecific in their histopathologic appearance. They tend to be characterized by the production of variable proportions of dense fibrous connective tissue and lymphoid aggregates, the latter often exhibiting prominent reactive centers. In other instances, one may see a conspicuous vasculitis with eosinophilia, suggesting the possibility of an allergic process. In still other cases, the mass involves mainly skeletal muscle, suggesting a primary myositis of obscure cause.

Collectively, these inflammatory pseudotumors constitute a large and important segment of the orbital tumor problem in adults because of their relative frequency, their obscure etiology, and their ineffectual therapy.

INFLAMMATIONS

Inflammations of the eye are named after the tissues that are principally affected. Since the uveal tract is the most highly vascular tissue of the eye, it tends to be the site of the major inflammatory response in most cases, and the term "uveitis" often is used in ophthalmology as an all-inclusive synonym for the more appropriate designation ocular inflammation. Both the clinician and the pathologist, however, should try to identify the main sites of involvement and use more appropriate terminology:

Sites of inflammation	Term
Entire uveal tract	Panuveitis
Iris	Iritis
Ciliary body	Cyclitis
Choroid	Choroiditis
Retina	Retinitis
Retina and choroid	Chorioretinitis or retinochoroiditis
Sclera	Scleritis
Sclera and uvea	Sclerouveitis
Cornea	Keratitis
Cornea and sclera	Sclerokeratitis
Exudate in anterior chamber	Hypopyon
Interior of eye	Endophthalmitis
Interior plus all tunics	Panophthalmitis
Optic nerve	Optic neuritis
Optic nerve head	Papillitis
Retina and optic nerve	Neuroretinitis

The terms provide no information as to specific cause or pathogenesis, nor do they indicate the type of pathologic process that is involved. For descriptive purposes and to facilitate a consideration of pathogenesis, it is convenient to classify intraocular inflammations as follows:

> Acute suppurative
> > Exogenous
> > Endogenous
>
> Chronic nongranulomatous
> > Exogenous
> > Endogenous
>
> Chronic granulomatous
> > Exogenous
> > Endogenous

Acute suppurative inflammations

Acute suppurative inflammations are most often exogenous, after penetrating or perforating wounds of the globe with or without the introduction of foreign bodies. Bacteria, fungi, certain chemicals, including acids and alkalis, and all sorts of organic matter are potent irritants. When introduced into the eye, they tend to provoke a massive polymorphonuclear response leading to endophthalmitis or panophthalmitis. Much less frequently, acute suppurative inflammation develops after intraocular surgery, after perforation of a corneal ulcer (Fig. 27-31), or as a result of spread from an orbital cellulitis.

Endogenous suppurative inflammation is

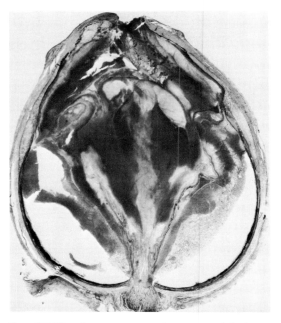

Fig. 27-31. Acute suppurative panophthalmitis secondary to perforation of corneal ulcer. (AFIP 28817; from Hogan, M. J., and Zimmerman, L. E.: Ophthalmic pathology, ed. 2, Philadelphia, 1962, W. B. Saunders Co.)

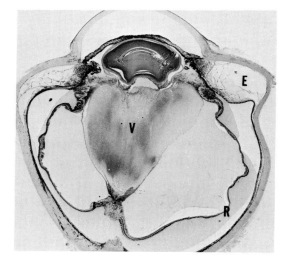

Fig. 27-32. Endogenous acute suppurative endophthalmitis, complication of meningococcemia in patient who also had meningitis. Purulent exudate in vitreous body, **V,** which has become detached from retina, **R,** which also is detached. Serous exudate present in preretinal, subretinal, and epichoroidal spaces, **E.** (5.5×; AFIP 56-9989; from Zimmerman, L. E.: In Saphir, O., editor: A text on systemic pathology, New York, 1958-1959, Grune & Stratton, Inc.; by permission.)

much less common. It is almost always the result of hematogenous infection of the eye from a primary bacterial or mycotic focus elsewhere in the body (Fig. 27-32), but extension to the eye through the optic nerve or subarachnoid fluid from an intracranial infection is also possible. Demonstration of the causative bacteria or fungi in cases of suppurative endophthalmitis or panophthalmitis usually requires a careful search of sections that have been appropriately stained for these organisms.

Mycotic infections deserve special comment not because they are more frequent or more devastating than the bacterial but because the eye is vulnerable to many organisms that are so lowly virulent that they are generally regarded as nonpathogenic saprophytes. The cornea and vitreous, being without an intrinsic blood supply and much slower to react to inflammatory stimuli, seem to permit saprophytic organisms to proliferate and establish themselves before an effective suppurative response can be developed to eradicate them. These fungi may be introduced from the soil or from vegetation when the cornea is scratched or the vitreous body penetrated. Prophylactic antibiotic therapy used in the

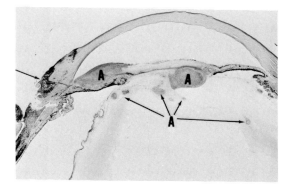

Fig. 27-33. Nocardial endophthalmitis that developed after cataract extraction. *Arrows,* Surgical wound. Multiple abscesses, **A,** present in iris, posterior chamber, and vitreous. (6×; AFIP 68-2841; slightly modified from Meyer, S. L., Font, R. L., and Shaver, R. P.: Arch. Ophthalmol. [Chicago] 83:536-541, 1970.)

management of ocular injuries has greatly reduced the frequency of serious bacterial infection, but at present no satisfactory drugs are available to protect the eye against infection by species of *Aspergillus, Cephalosporium, Fusarium,* and other fungi that may be introduced at the time of injury or surgery (Fig. 27-33).

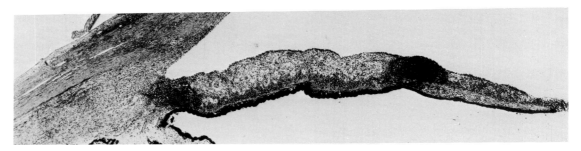

Fig. 27-34. Chronic nongranulomatous iridocyclitis. (40×; AFIP 60392.)

Chronic nongranulomatous inflammations

Chronic nongranulomatous inflammations stand in contrast to the acute suppurative inflammations. They are seldom exogenous and rarely are attributable to a specific infectious agent. The inflammatory reaction is most frequently restricted to the uvea, often to the iris and ciliary body (Fig. 27-34).

Because the tissues are infiltrated by lymphocytes and plasma cells, often with many Russell bodies being present, it is generally assumed that an immunopathologic mechanism is involved. Neither the clinician nor the histopathologist has enjoyed much success in the etiologic classification of nongranulomatous uveitis, although certain systemic diseases such as ankylosing spondylitis and Still's disease often are complicated by this type of uveitis.

Chronic granulomatous inflammations

Granulomatous inflammations are of special interest to the pathologist because they frequently present patterns of tissue reaction that fall into meaningful pathogenetic groups, even though a specific causative agent is not demonstrable in the tissue. Important examples of both posttraumatic and purely endogenous granulomatous inflammation must be considered. In the first category are sympathetic ophthalmia, phacoanaphylaxis (described in the discussion on cataracts), and foreign body granulomas. Of these, however, only the latter can be considered entirely exogenous because systemic autosensitivity is believed to play an important role in the pathogenesis of the other two.

Sympathetic ophthalmia. Sympathetic ophthalmia is a diffuse granulomatous uveitis that affects both eyes after a penetrating injury to one eye. It is fortunately a rare complication because it often leads to very severe visual loss in both eyes, but it does occur periodically after intraocular surgery as well

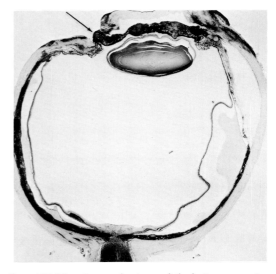

Fig. 27-35. Sympathetic ophthalmia occurring after penetrating wound of limbus with prolapse of iris and ciliary body (arrow). Almost all of uvea thickened by infiltrate of lymphocytes and epithelioid cells. (4×; AFIP 53904-17111; from Friedenwald, J. S., Wilder, H. C., Maumenee, A. E., Sanders, T. E., Keyes, J. E., Hogan, M. J., Owens, W. C., and Owens, E. U.: Ophthalmic pathology, Philadelphia, 1952, W. B. Saunders Co.)

as after accidental wounds. A prolapse or loss of uveal tissue seems to be an important predisposing factor.

The condition is believed to develop as a result of an autosensitivity reaction to uveal tissue that has become altered in some mysterious way after the injury. The entire uveal tract becomes thickened by an infiltrate of lymphocytes and epithelioid cells (Fig. 27-35). There is no necrosis, and virtually no polymorphonuclear leukocytes or plasma cells are observed.

Endogenous granulomatous inflammation. Endogenous granulomatous inflammation includes a large infectious group and a miscellaneous group of unknown cause. Many of the important systemic infectious diseases that characteristically produce a granulomatous response may involve the eye. Examples are tuberculosis, leprosy, syphilis, blastomycosis, cryptococcosis, coccidioidomycosis, sporotrichosis, cysticerosis, toxoplasmosis, visceral larva migrans, and cytomegalovirus infection. Since the ocular complications of most of these infections and their histopathologic characteristics are not particularly noteworthy, only the two especially important examples will be described here—toxoplasmosis and toxocariasis.

Toxoplasma chorioretinitis occurs in two main forms: congenital and acquired. In those cases in which congenital toxoplasmosis results in a stillborn baby or a neonatal death, there is a very high incidence of severe chorioretinitis. Less overwhelming congenital infections may be characterized by nonfatal damage to the brain and areas of chorioretinitis. There is also evidence that unilateral or bilateral chorioretinitis may be the only recognizable clinical manifestation of congenital toxoplasmosis. The intraocular inflammation in such cases often leads to chorioretinal scarring, but the infection may or may not be eradicated.

The causative protozoan parasite may remain viable in an encysted form for long periods, giving rise periodically to bouts of renewed activity. The other form of the disease is acquired toxoplasmosis occurring in adults, usually without any other associated clinical manifestations of systemic disease such as fever,

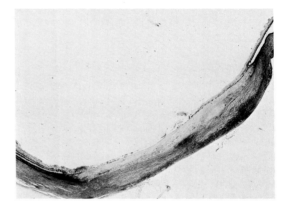

Fig. 27-36. Chorioretinitis caused by toxoplasmosis. (7×; AFIP 754058; from Smith, M. E.: In Ackerman, L. V., and Rosai, J.: Surgical pathology, ed. 5, St. Louis, 1974, The C. V. Mosby Co.)

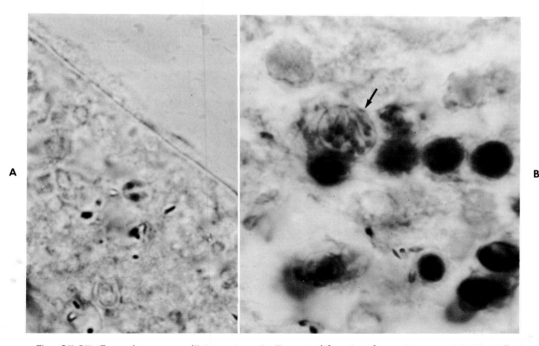

Fig. 27-37. *Toxoplasma gondii* in retina. **A,** Two proliferative forms in necrotic retina. **B,** *Arrow,* Encysted forms in necrotic retina. (**A,** 1800×; AFIP 211318-21011; from Wilder, H. C.: Arch. Ophthalmol. [Chicago] **48:**127-136, 1952; **B,** 1920×; AFIP 754058; from Zimmerman, L. E.: In Ackerman, L. V. [in collaboration with Butcher, H. R., Jr.]: Surgical pathology, ed. 4, St. Louis, 1968, The C. V. Mosby Co.)

malaise, skin rash, or lymphadenopathy. In these cases, the retina seems to be particularly vulnerable to infection by *Toxoplasma gondii*, providing the only focus where the parasite establishes itself in a pathogenetically significant manner.

What one sees microscopically in both the congenital and the acquired forms is a discrete area of coagulative necrosis in the retina (Fig. 27-36). Usually, the pigment epithelium and occasionally variable amounts of the adjacent choroid and sclera also exhibit coagulative necrosis. Surrounding the areas of coagulative necrosis, there is a diffuse granulomatous reaction affecting the choroid, sclera, and episclera. Away from this discrete focus of chorioretinitis, the picture is more variable and nondiagnostic. Often, there is a panuveitis that may be purely nongranulomatous or distinctly granulomatous. Usually, it is only in the area of coagulative necrosis that the free bow-shaped protozoans or their encysted forms can be seen (Fig. 27-37), although sometimes the encysted forms can be identified in the adjacent viable retina.

Ocular larva migrans is a nematodal endophthalmitis caused by larvae of *Toxocara canis* that wander into the eye through the uveal or retinal circulation. This, then, is the ocular equivalent of visceral larva migrans. *Toxocara canis* is a common inhabitant of the dog's intestinal tract, and its eggs contaminate the soil everywhere dogs are present. Young children who put dirty objects in their mouths or who actually eat soil (pica) are the ones who are most likely to become infected.

In the eye, the nematode larvae seem to have a predilection for the retina and vitreous body, producing a chronic, sclerosing inflammatory reaction in the vitreous and retina, usually without external signs and symptoms of ocular inflammation. Eosinophils often are present in large numbers in the vitreous. Eosinophilic abscesses and small granulomas often develop about the disintegrating larvae (Fig. 27-38). The vitreal reaction eventually produces a massive retinal detachment and a leukokoria that often leads to a clinical diagnosis of retinoblastoma.

Less frequently, the parasite may become localized in the choroid or between the choroid and retina, producing a focal chorioretinal mass in the vicinity of the macula or optic disc. Ocular larva migrans is almost always a unilateral condition that is not accompanied by systemic manifestations, except perhaps for a mild eosinophilia. Why children with visceral manifestations of larva migrans should not have ocular complications and why those with ocular larva migrans should not have systemic manifestations are unexplained.

Noninfectious granulomatous disease. Non-

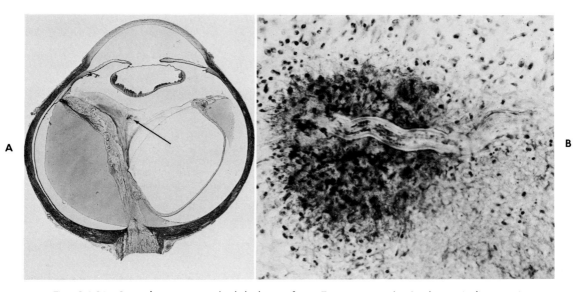

Fig. 27-38. Granulomatous endophthalmitis from *Toxocara canis*. **A,** *Arrow* indicates site of granuloma containing larva shown in **B.** Preretinal inflammatory membrane has led to total detachment of retina. **B,** Nematode larva in granuloma in vitreous. (**A,** 3×; **B,** 400×; **A** and **B,** from Wilder, H. C.: Trans. Am. Acad. Ophthalmol. Otolaryngol. **55:**99-109, 1950; AFIP 198761.)

infectious granulomatous disease of various types may affect the eye. Three examples that are particularly striking will be discussed: sarcoidosis, rheumatoid sclerouveitis, and juvenile xanthogranuloma.

Sarcoidosis frequently is complicated by the development of a granulomatous iridocyclitis (Fig. 27-39) and less often by a retinitis or chorioretinitis. The intraocular lesions, like those of other affected tissues, are typically noncaseating epithelioid tubercles. The gran-

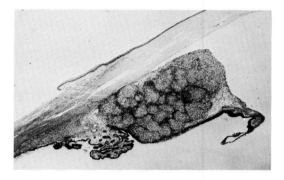

Fig. 27-39. Granulomatous iridocyclitis in sarcoidosis. (20×; AFIP 71412-08121; from Hogan, M. J., and Zimmerman, L. E.: Ophthalmic pathology, ed. 2, Philadelphia, 1962, W. B. Saunders Co.)

ulomatous lesions of the iris and ciliary body often erupt into the anterior or posterior chambers, producing various complications (e.g., cataract, glaucoma, hypotony, and corneal damage) that seriously affect vision and may lead to blindness. The retinal lesions are usually much less massive than those occurring in the anterior segment and tend to be distributed along the major vessels (Fig. 27-40), producing an ophthalmoscopic picture that has been described as resembling drippings of candle wax. Involvement of the central nervous system is said to occur with great frequency among those patients who are found to have this curious retinal form of sarcoidosis.

Rheumatoid sclerouveitis is characterized by the formation of patchy areas of coagulative necrosis of collagen in the sclera, usually anteriorly between the limbus and the equator of the globe. These areas are surrounded by a palisade of epithelioid cells, so that the lesions are reminiscent of the rheumatoid nodules that develop in the subcutaneous tissues, tendons, or other collagenous structures such as the dura mater in patients who have rheumatoid arthritis. When only a discrete focus of involvement is present, the lesion often is called a "rheumatoid nodule" of the sclera.

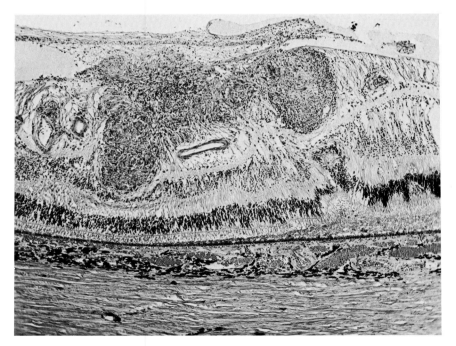

Fig. 27-40. Perivascular distribution of tubercles in patient with sarcoidosis who died as consequence of involvement of central nervous system. (50×; AFIP 63-1450.)

Often, however, there are extensive areas of diffuse thickening and induration resulting from a massive infiltration by lymphocytes, plasma cells, and histiocytes (Fig. 27-41). Clinically, this gives rise to a picture that has usually been called "brawny scleritis." In some patients, the same basic disorder seems to

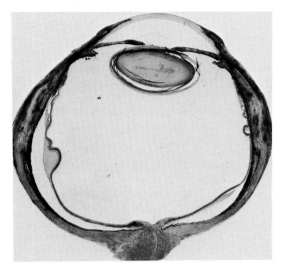

Fig. 27-41. Brawny scleritis. Sclera anteriorly is massively thickened by chronic granulomatous inflammatory reaction. (5×; AFIP 67159; from DeCoursey, E., and Ash, J. E.: Atlas of ophthalmic pathology, Rochester, Minn., 1942, American Academy of Ophthalmology and Otolaryngology.)

lead to a sharp dissolution of the sclera with minimal inflammatory thickening. In such cases, the uvea may herniate through defects in the sclera, and the globe becomes vulnerable to rupture from minimal trauma. This form of the disease is called "scleromalacia perforans." In only about half of the patients who present with these various forms of sclerouveitis is there a well-established clinical history of rheumatoid arthritis or some other related systemic disease.

Juvenile xanthogranuloma is typically a benign, spontaneously regressing, granulomatous dermatosis of infants and young children who have no important visceral lesions. The only important exception to this generalization is observed in the rare child who develops lesions in the iris and ciliary body (Fig. 27-42). This uveal involvement frequently leads to one or both of two serious complications: spontaneous hemorrhage into the anterior chamber and secondary glaucoma resulting from an accumulation of histiocytic cells in the anterior chamber angle. The iris and ciliary body are infiltrated by lipid-laden histiocytes similar to those found in the skin lesions, and Touton giant cells are often present. Ocular involvement is virtually always unilateral.

Complications

Complications of ocular inflammation may be very serious, leading to blindness. In the

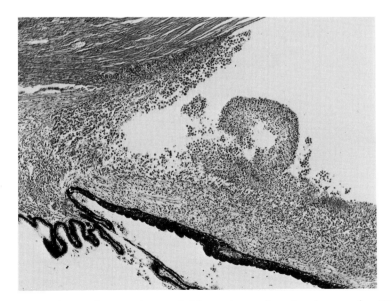

Fig. 27-42. Juvenile xanthogranuloma of iris and anterior chamber angle. (50×; AFIP 60-2778; from Hogan, M. J., and Zimmerman, L. E.: Ophthalmic pathology, ed. 2, Philadelphia, 1962, W. B. Saunders Co.)

acute suppurative and granulomatous forms, necrosis of the retina and choroid leads to permanent scarring and loss of function of these tissues. If the macula or all of the retina is affected, severe visual loss is inevitable. When there has been more widespread destruction of intraocular tissues, severe scarring and gliosis are observed and the internal architecture of the globe becomes disorganized. The production of aqueous humor may be so greatly reduced that the eye becomes soft, atrophic, and shrunken. This state of advanced degeneration and disorganization of the entire eyeball is called phthisis bulbi (Fig. 27-43). Phthisical eyes present not only a cosmetic problem but are often irritable. Malignant melanoma may arise in such blind, phthisical

eyes, and, because it is invisible, as a result of opacification of the ocular media, the tumor often spreads out of the eye before it is detected (Fig. 27-44). For all these reasons, phthisical eyes often are enucleated.

More limited inflammatory processes, including those of the chronic nongranulomatous variety, also may produce a variety of significant complications, including leakage of plas-

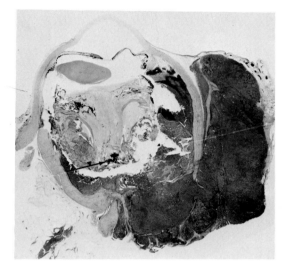

Fig. 27-44. Malignant melanoma of choroid that arose in phthisic eye that had been blind for 22 years after missile injury. *Arrow,* Retained metallic foreign body in scarred vitreous body. Note massive extraocular extension of tumor. (2×; AFIP 57-14185; from Hogan, M. J., and Zimmerman, L. E.: Ophthalmic pathology, ed. 2, Philadelphia, 1962, W. B. Saunders Co.)

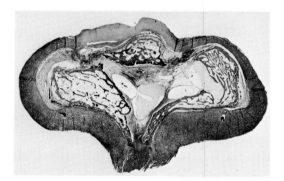

Fig. 27-43. Phthisis bulbi. (3×; AFIP 112917-07091; from Friedenwald, J. S., Wilder, H. C., Maumenee, A. E., Sanders, T. E., Keyes, J. E., Hogan, M. J., Owens, W. C., and Owens, E. U.: Ophthalmic pathology, Philadelphia, 1952, W. B. Saunders Co.)

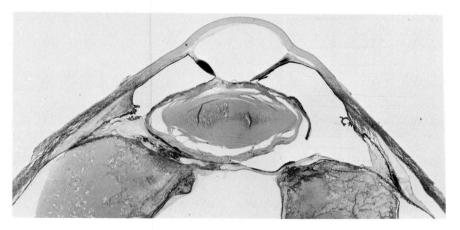

Fig. 27-45. Several complications of chronic iridocyclitis are present: broad peripheral anterior synechias, seclusion of pupil by posterior synechias, occlusion of pupil by fibrovascular membrane, iris bombé, and formation of cataract. (5×; AFIP 66-13055.)

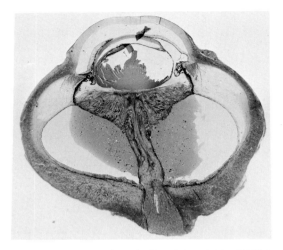

Fig. 27-46. Atrophia bulbi. (4×; AFIP 54885-07091; from Friedenwald, J. S., Wilder, H. C., Maumenee, A. E., Sanders, T. E., Keyes, J. E., Hogan, M. J., Owens, W. C., and Owens, E. U.: Ophthalmic pathology, Philadelphia, 1952, W. B. Saunders Co.)

ma proteins and an accumulation of inflammatory cells in the aqueous humor and vitreous, adherence of the iris to the lens (posterior synechias) or to the cornea (anterior synechias), formation of a pupillary membrane that occludes the pupil and obstructs the flow of aqueous humor (Fig. 27-45), opacification of the cornea, formation of cataracts, diminution of aqueous production, chorioretinal degeneration, and optic atrophy. As a consequence of these complications, the eye may become glaucomatous or hypotonic, or it may first become glaucomatous and then later hypotonic when damage to the ciliary body becomes sufficiently severe. In cases of long-standing severe hypotony, one often sees a detachment of the retina and uvea, papilledema, and shrinkage of the globe or atrophia bulbi (Fig. 27-46).

GLAUCOMA

Glaucoma is the name given to a large group of ocular disorders that have in common a rise in intraocular pressure sufficient to damage various tissues, especially optic nerve fibers. Theoretically, such an increase in intraocular pressure could arise from an excessively rapid production of aqueous humor by the ciliary body or from a great increase in episcleral venous pressure with consequent impairment of aqueous flow out of the globe, but for all practical purposes the cause is almost always found to be an obstruction to aqueous flow within the eyeball.

There are three main sites at which the flow of aqueous humor most often is obstructed: at the pupil, in the angle of the anterior chamber, and within the outflow pathways that lie between the anterior chamber angle and the episcleral veins (Fig. 27-6). When the anatomic obstruction is the result of a developmental malformation, the glaucoma is classified as congenital. All other glaucomas are acquired and traditionally are subdivided into secondary and primary forms. The secondary glaucomas are those that develop as a complication of some other primary disease process (e.g., uveitis, trauma, intraocular hemorrhage, and neoplasms) and are usually unilateral. The primary glaucomas are typically bilateral, occurring in eyes that are not obviously affected by some other condition.

Secondary glaucoma

Secondary glaucoma is produced by one or more of four main types of obstruction:
1. Posterior synechias
2. Anterior synechias
3. Accumulation of cells or cellular debris in the anterior chamber angle
4. Damage to the outflow channels in the trabecular meshwork, canal of Schlemm, ciliary body, scleral spur, etc.

Posterior synechias are adhesions between the pupillary margin of the iris and the anterior surface of the lens that usually develop as a result of inflammation of the iris (iritis). These adhesions may bind the iris to the lens completely, a condition called "seclusion of the pupil" (Fig. 27-45). One often sees accompanying the formation of posterior synechias the outgrowth of a fibrovascular membrane from the pupillary margin of the iris across the pupil. Obstruction of the pupil by such a membrane is called "occlusion of the pupil." Either seclusion of the pupil or occlusion of the pupil will prevent the flow of aqueous humor from the posterior chamber through the pupil into the anterior chamber. This leads to an increase in pressure within the posterior chamber and a forward ballooning of the iris (iris bombé).

Adhesions between the anterior surface of the iris at its periphery and the trabecular meshwork and cornea are called peripheral anterior synechias. Inflammation of the iris and ciliary body (Fig. 27-34), neovascularization of the iris (called rubeosis iridis—Fig. 27-47), and organization of hemorrhages and exudates in the anterior chamber angle are the most frequent causes for the development of peripheral anterior synechias.

Particulate matter in the aqueous humor often gets caught in the trabecular meshwork as the aqueous humor drains through this structure into the canal of Schlemm and other related outflow channels (Fig. 27-48). Grossly (and clinically), the angle of the anterior chamber may appear to be completely normal, although careful biomicroscopic examination may reveal evidence of the accumulation of cellular debris in the angle. These, then, are cases of secondary open-angle glaucoma in contrast with the angle-closure secondary glau-

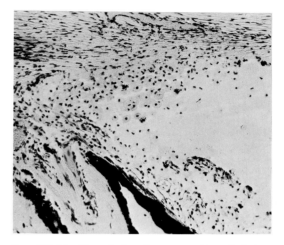

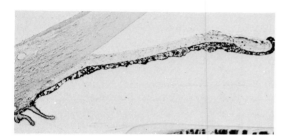

Fig. 27-47. Peripheral anterior synechia resulting in neovascularization of iris in patient with diabetes mellitus (diabetic rubeosis iridis). Thickened and vacuolated pigment epithelium is characteristic of iris in diabetic patients. (24×; AFIP 55-8505.)

Fig. 27-48. Phacolytic glaucoma. Liquefied lens cortex and macrophages have accumulated in angle of anterior chamber in eye that had hypermature senile cataract. (150×; AFIP 54-25767; from Zimmerman, L. E.: In Maumenee, A. E., and Silverstein, A. M., editors: Immunopathology of uveitis, Baltimore, 1964, copyrighted by The Williams & Wilkins Co.)

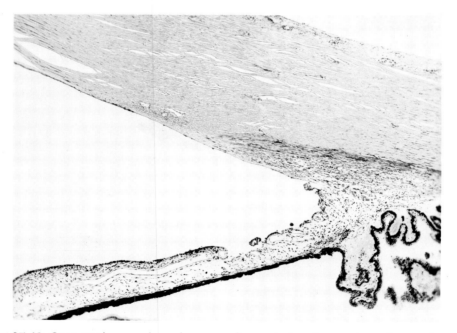

Fig. 27-49. Open-angle secondary glaucoma after contusion damage to outflow pathways. Injury produced tear into face of ciliary body with consequent deepening of angle of chamber. (50×; AFIP 58-5478; from Hogan, M. J., and Zimmerman, L. E.: Ophthalmic pathology, ed. 2, Philadelphia, 1962, W. B. Saunders Co.)

comas resulting from the formation of peripheral anterior synechias. Many different pathologic processes may lead to the accumulation of cells and debris in the outflow pathways: hemorrhage into the anterior chamber or the vitreous, uveitis, liquefaction and escape of lens protein in hypermature cataracts, tumor cells shed from uveal melanomas or retinoblastomas, pigmented cells from the iris (in pigmentary glaucoma and pseudoexfoliation of the lens capsule), etc.

Finally, the trabecular meshwork and other tissues containing outflow passages may become thickened and their passages narrowed as a result of tissue damage accompanying any of the foregoing conditions that permit cellular debris to become trapped in these tissues. They may become similarly affected after contusions to the eye (Fig. 27-49) or from chemical damage such as in siderosis bulbi resulting from a retained intraocular ferrous foreign body.

Primary glaucoma

Primary glaucoma is of two main types: chronic open-angle (often called chronic simple) glaucoma and acute angle-closure (often called acute congestive) glaucoma.

Chronic open-angle glaucoma appears to be a genetically determined disease that becomes evident with aging. It is characterized by a very insidious onset and slowly progressive rise in intraocular pressure, resulting from an increased resistance to aqueous outflow of undetermined cause and at an undetermined site. Early in the course of the disease, the eyes may seem to be perfectly normal except for the elevated intraocular pressure. Gradually, the increasing rise in intraocular pressure leads to a typically painless loss of vision and eventually to complete blindness.

Acute angle-closure glaucoma is an entirely different form of primary glaucoma occurring most often in individuals who typically have small hyperopic eyes with relatively shallow anterior chambers and very narrow anterior chamber angles. These peculiar anatomic features, which can be readily recognized by ophthalmic examination, predispose the eye to bouts of angle-closure glaucoma, especially as the lens grows larger with aging or with the development of a cataract. Normally in such eyes there is a closer than normal approximation of the iris to the lens so that a relatively small increase in the anteroposterior diameter of the lens may impair the flow of aqueous humor between the lens and the iris at the pupil, even without the formation of synechias (a physiologic block). When this situation develops, the pressure rises in the posterior chamber, the iris becomes bowed forward, and the already very shallow anterior chamber angle becomes obliterated by the apposition of iris to the trabecular meshwork. If this situation is permitted to remain uncorrected by medical or surgical therapy, adhesions between the iris and cornea lead to permanent occlusion of the angle of the anterior chamber. Bouts of angle-closure glaucoma tend to develop very suddenly, and the intraocular pressure rises to very high levels in a relatively short time. Consequently, the affected eye becomes very red and painful. Often, the patient complains of headache, nausea, and vomiting. The sudden rise in pressure to the very high levels (three to four times normal) produces severe corneal edema and, if unrelieved for more than a few hours, severe damage to the nerve fibers in the optic nerve head. The creation of a new passage for aqueous flow from the posterior chamber into the anterior chamber by peripheral iridectomy or iridotomy overcomes the pupillary block and is therefore a procedure that is used both in the treatment and prevention of attacks of acute angle-closure glaucoma.

Effects

Effects of glaucoma on the eye vary with the type of glaucoma, but common to all is the eventual damage to optic nerve fibers and consequent blindness. When glaucoma develops congenitally or very early in infancy, it typically causes an opacification and enlargement of the cornea (Fig. 27-50) even though the elevation of intraocular pressure may not be very great. Thus the corneal findings are of great significance in the clinical recognition of congenital and infantile glaucoma.

The optic nerve tolerates pronounced elevation in intraocular pressure very poorly and, regardless of cause, a sudden rise of pressure into the range of 50 to 90 mm Hg, if unrelieved for more than a day or two, may produce such ischemic necrosis of the optic nerve head that all vision is destroyed. Corneal edema, but without enlargement of the cornea, is a characteristic feature of acute glaucoma, regardless of its specific cause. Pronounced elevations in intraocular pressure also often produce areas of ischemic necrosis in the iris and foci of opacification in the superficial lens cortex.

On the other hand, the eye often tolerates

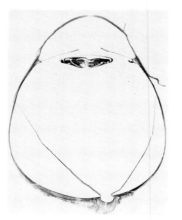

Fig. 27-50. Congenital glaucoma has led to noticeable enlargement of cornea and deep cupping of optic nerve head. (AFIP 38269; from Friedenwald, J. S., Wilder, H. C., Maumenee, A. E., Sanders, T. E., Keyes, J. E., Hogan, M. J., Owens, W. C., and Owens, E. U.: Ophthalmic pathology, Philadelphia, 1952, W. B. Saunders Co.)

small or moderate rises of pressure remarkably well, particularly when the elevation in pressure has developed very slowly, as it does in the chronic forms of primary and secondary glaucomas. Eventually, however, chronic glaucoma leads to an atrophy of optic nerve fibers, usually, however, sparing those from the macula until very late, so that the patient who has lost most of his peripheral field of vision may still retain good visual acuity. This fact accounts for the not unusual experience that a patient with chronic glaucoma may suffer optic nerve damage and be unaware of his visual loss as long as his macular function remains reasonably good. This is why a routine check of intraocular pressure and of the peripheral field of vision is recommended as part of the annual physical examination of all adults.

After glaucoma has produced atrophy of the optic nerve fibers, the physiologic cup that is normally observable in the optic nerve head gradually becomes larger and deeper. The elevated intraocular pressure tends to bow the lamina cribrosa backward, accentuating the enlargement of the cup. This is called glaucomatous cupping (Fig. 27-50). It is a late complication of glaucoma.

Other late complications include atrophy of all ocular tissues and chronic corneal edema leading to bullous keratopathy. Atrophy of the ciliary body eventually will lead to a diminution of aqueous formation, compensating

somewhat for the impaired outflow of aqueous humor. Although this tends to relieve the elevated intraocular pressure, it is not without sequelae, for the normal production and circulation of aqueous humor are necessary for the nutrition of such avascular tissues as the lens, vitreous, and cornea. Advanced glaucoma, therefore, often is complicated by cataract formation, severe degenerative keratopathy, and alterations in the vitreous body.

CATARACT

Opacification of the lens, regardless of its cause, is termed a cataract. Some cataracts are present at birth. These congenital cataracts may be genetically determined, the result of rubella acquired in utero, or associated with other malformations produced by chromosomal abnormalities (e.g., trisomy 13-15) or they may be sporadic and idiopathic. Opacification of the lens acquired after birth may be the result of ocular trauma (traumatic cataracts), a complication of some other primary ocular or systemic disease such as uveitis, malignant melanoma of the uvea, or diabetes mellitus (complicating cataracts), a consequence of chemical intoxication as occurred when dinitrophenol was used for weight reduction and MER-29 was employed for the reduction of blood cholesterol levels, or simply a manifestation of aging (senile cataracts).

The lens is one of the most unusual tissues of the body. Derived from the surface ectoderm, it is a mass of modified epithelial cells that become sequestered in the posterior chamber very early in embryologic development. Devoid of stroma and containing no blood supply, the lens depends on the circulating aqueous humor for its nutrition, oxygenation, and removal of catabolites. It is also a unique epithelial tissue in that it has no way of desquamating its oldest cells. These merely get compressed into the central (nuclear) part of the lens as new lenticular cells (cortical fibers, as they are generally called) are formed at the equator from the epithelial layer. The mystery, therefore, is not why the lens sometimes becomes opaque but rather how it generally remains optically clear for so many years in most individuals.

Microscopically, the changes observed in cataractous lenses are not specifically related to the cause of the cataract. Very minimal variations in the size, shape, and water content of cortical cells may cause opacification readily detectable by the ophthalmologist on slit-lamp examination, yet the pathologist may find it

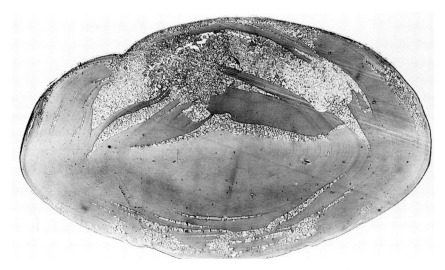

Fig. 27-51. Mature cortical and nuclear cataract. There is advanced degeneration of lens fibers which are considerably fragmented. (27×; AFIP 66872; from DeCoursey, E., and Ash, J. E.: Atlas of ophthalmic pathology, Rochester, Minn., 1942, American Academy of Ophthalmology and Otolaryngology.)

impossible to be certain whether he sees any abnormalities. With more advanced cortical degeneration, the integrity of the cells breaks down. Fragmentation and dissolution of the tissue become very obvious (Fig. 27-51).

With the breakdown of lens protein and because of associated alterations in the lens epithelium, movement of water into the lens may become increased and the lens swells (intumescent cataract), leading to an increase mainly in its anteroposterior diameter. This is one factor that may produce a block of aqueous flow through the pupil and provoke an attack of acute congestive glaucoma.

With more complete breakdown of lens protein, total liquefaction of the cortex may be observed. In such cases, the hard yellowish nucleus may be observed to float about within the milky liquefied cortex. This type of hypermature senile cataract is called a morgagnian cataract (Fig. 27-52). Often, the lens epithelium becomes completely necrotic in these morgagnian cataracts, and as the lens protein breaks down into smaller molecules, the latter diffuse out through the lens capsule, carrying water along. This leads to a shrinkage of the lens, and in advanced states only the nucleus remains within the capsule. Only rarely does the entire lens substance become absorbed in this fashion, but it accounts for some of the rare spontaneous cures of blindness caused by cataract. Posterior dislocation of a cataractous lens provides another explanation of such "cures."

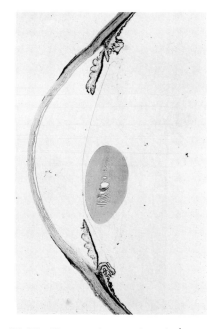

Fig. 27-52. Hypermature cataract (morgagnian type). Lens cortex has become completely liquefied and dense nuclear portion has settled downward (vertical plane of section). (7×; AFIP 54-25766; from Flocks, M., Littwin, C. S., and Zimmerman, L. E.: Arch. Ophthalmol. [Chicago] **54**:37-45, 1955.)

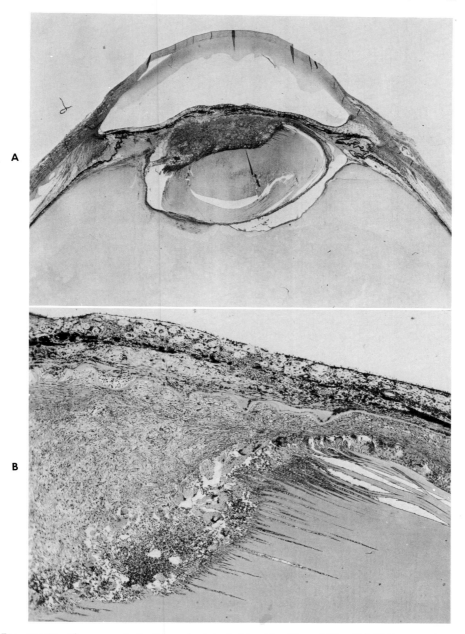

Fig. 27-53. Phacoanaphylactic endophthalmitis. (**A**, 10×; AFIP 55-22260; **B**, 53×; AFIP 55-22261; from Zimmerman, L. E.: In Ackerman, L. V. [in collaboration with Butcher, H. R., Jr.]: Surgical pathology, ed. 2, St. Louis, 1959, The C. V. Mosby Co.)

The passage of liquefied cortex of a hypermature cataract through the lens capsule into the aqueous humor often provokes an outpouring of macrophages, which then phagocytize the escaped lens matter. These macrophages, together with the remaining liquefied lens cortex in the aqueous humor, often obstruct the outflow of aqueous humor in the anterior chamber angle (Fig. 27-48). Typi-cally, this produces a rapidly developing form of open-angle acute congestive glaucoma that is called "phacolytic glaucoma" because pathogenetically it is the result of lysis of the lens (phacolysis). Cataract extraction and ir-rigation of the anterior chamber may control the glaucoma and restore vision if performed soon after the onset of glaucoma.

Because the lens does become sequestered

and encapsulated by a remarkably thick basement membrane (called the lens capsule) so early embryologically, the body's immunologic system for recognizing its own unique proteins never gets the opportunity to recognize those of the lens. Thus, later on in life, when as a result of accidental trauma or a surgical procedure the lens capsule is ruptured, lens protein escapes into the aqueous humor, from which it can be absorbed into the bloodstream. The reticuloendothelial system then gets its first opportunity to encounter these proteins. Autosensitization may ensue, but, fortunately, lens proteins seem to be very weakly antigenic, even when injected in a different species, and it is believed that some other factor acting as an adjuvant is necessary to permit significant autosensitization to develop. There is one condition believed to be at least partially dependent on autosensitization to lens protein for its occurrence—*phacoanaphylaxis*. This is almost always a complication of some injury that ruptures the lens capsule. In the days when extracapsular cataract extraction was the standard operation for senile cataracts, phacoanaphylactic endophthalmitis was relatively more important because if the operation performed on the first eye sensitized the patient, then when the operation was subsequently performed on the second eye, the stage was set for a severe immunopathologic reaction when the aqueous became flooded with antigen released from the lens.

The histopathologic picture of phacoanaphylactic endophthalmitis is very characteristic (Fig. 27-53). An intense inflammatory reaction is seen centered about the lens. In those cases that occur after a penetrating wound, one sees a massive invasion of the lens by inflammatory cells at the site where the lens capsule is ruptured. A typically granulomatous reaction develops in the lens. Necrotic lens tissue infiltrated by polymorphonuclear leukocytes becomes surrounded by a zone of epithelioid cells and giant cells about which there develops an even broader zone of granulation tissue heavily infiltrated by lymphocytes and plasma cells. The iris becomes firmly adherent to the inflammatory mass that surrounds the lens and it, too, is diffusely infiltrated by lymphocytes and plasma cells. The inflammatory reaction spreads into the vitreous and, as a result, retinal detachment often complicates the situation.

DISLOCATION OF LENS

The lens is held in place by the bundles of collagenous filaments passing from the ciliary epithelium to the lens capsule (the zonular ligament). These zonular fibers may be ruptured as a result of trauma, and the lens may lose all or a part of its support. If only a part of the zonular ligament is ruptured, the lens becomes only partially dislocated or subluxated to one side. When all of the support has been lost, the lens may become completely dislocated posteriorly or anteriorly. When dislocated into the anterior chamber, there is often obstruction to aqueous outflow and an acute secondary glaucoma develops. Thus surgical removal is usually undertaken when anterior dislocation is observed. If the lens capsule has not been broken, the eye usually tolerates posterior dislocation quite well. If the lens is ruptured, however, phacoanaphylactic endophthalmitis may develop. Dislocated lenses usually become cataractous and also may give rise to a phacolytic glaucoma.

Dislocation or subluxation of the lens also may develop spontaneously as a result of damage to the zonular ligament in certain ocular or systemic diseases. Two notorious examples are Marfan's syndrome and homocystinuria (Fig. 27-54). Patients with late syphilis also are believed to be prone to develop spontaneous dislocation of the lens.

INTRAOCULAR NEOPLASMS

There are only two important primary intraocular malignant neoplasms, malignant melanoma of the uvea and retinoblastoma. All others are so rare that no mention of them need be made here. In addition, there is the

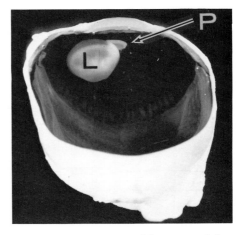

Fig. 27-54. Spontaneous subluxation of lens, **L,** in homocystinuria. Note that lens is dislocated to left of its normal position behind pupil, **P.** (AFIP 64-3737.)

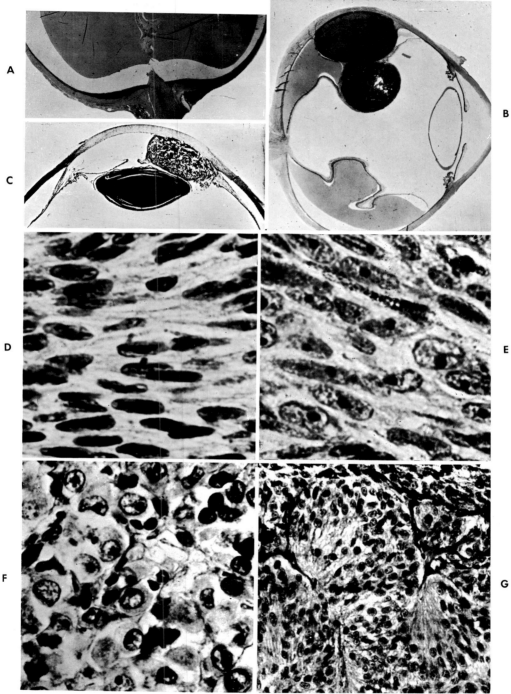

Fig. 27-55. Melanoma of uvea. **A,** Flat diffuse type. **B,** Collar-button type, extension through break in Bruch's membrane. **C,** Tumor in ciliary body and iris. **D** to **F,** Callender cell types. **D,** Spindle cell A. **E,** Spindle cell B. **F,** Epithelioid cell. **G,** Fascicular type. (AFIP; **A, B, D, E,** and **G,** from DeCoursey, E., and Ash, J. E.: Atlas of ophthalmic pathology, Rochester, Minn., 1942, American Academy of Ophthalmology and Otolaryngology.)

problem of metastatic tumors that must be considered.

Malignant melanoma

Malignant melanoma of the uvea is observed almost exclusively in white adults. Because of its selective occurrence in whites, it rarely is encountered in Africa, the Orient, and in those parts of Central and South America where there has been a large degree of intermarriage among Indians, blacks, and whites. In North America and in Europe, it is the most common of all intraocular tumors (primary or secondary, benign or malignant).

Uveal melanomas usually are slow growing and late in metastasizing. They have a much better prognosis than malignant melanoma of the skin (60% 10-year survival after enucleation of the eye). Two main cell types are observed: spindle and epithelioid (Fig. 27-55). Melanomas composed entirely of slender spindle-shaped cells with thin, elongated nuclei and no nucleoli (spindle cell A type) have the most favorable prognosis (85% 10-year survival). Those composed of larger, plumper spindle-shaped cells containing more ovoid nuclei with nucleoli (spindle cell B type) have a slightly less favorable prognosis (80% 10-year survival). Those composed entirely of large, pleomorphic cells with hyperchromatic nuclei and large, prominent nucleoli (epithelioid cells) carry the worst prognosis (35% 10-year survival). When there is a mixture of spindle and epithelioid cells, the tumors are said to be of the "mixed cell type." The 10-year survival for this group is 45%. Regardless of cell type, uveal melanomas show great variations in the production of melanin. Some are totally devoid of pigment, whereas others are jet black, and between these extremes are all shades of gray.

Melanomas arising in the choroid and ciliary body generally attain a fairly large size (10 to 20 mm in diameter) before they are detected, whereas those arising in the iris, where they can be seen by the patient and his family, are usually very much smaller. For this reason and because they are more accessible for surgical excision, iris tumors rarely have to be treated by enucleation of the eye, which operation must be done for most melanomas of the choroid and ciliary body. Since most iris tumors are not only small but also are frequently composed of the most favorable cell type (spindle cell A), which grows in a compact cohesive manner, they generally can be removed by iridectomy or iridocyclectomy

without tumor cells being disseminated throughout the anterior chamber. Thus recurrence is usually not a problem, and metastasis is very rare. The overall mortality from iris melanomas is less than 5%.

Melanomas of the choroid and ciliary body typically grow inward, toward the vitreous body, producing first an elevation and then a detachment of the retina. This causes visual disturbance for which the patient seeks ophthalmologic examination. Other complications of uveal melanomas include intraocular hemorrhage, inflammation (especially when the tumor develops areas of necrosis), cataract formation, and glaucoma. Thus the possibility of an intraocular melanoma often must be considered in the differential diagnosis of many ocular disorders.

Retinoblastoma

Retinoblastoma, in sharp contrast with uveal melanomas, is observed almost exclusively in very young children, and no racial group is spared. For this reason, it is encountered in all parts of the world. Often, if not always, it is present at birth, although it may take 2 to 3 years or more before it is discovered. Some cases are genetically determined, and in these patients there is a very high incidence of multicentricity and bilaterality. Survivors of bilateral retinoblastoma are very likely to transmit the disease to about one half of their progeny. Sporadic unilateral retinoblastomas are believed to be the result of a somatic mutation, in which case the survivor would not be capable of transmitting the disease to his offspring. Unfortunately, however, one can never be certain that a unilateral sporadic retinoblastoma appearing in a family in which there is no known history of retinoblastoma will not turn out to be the result of a genetic mutation that has expressed itself in only one eye.

Retinoblastoma, as the name implies, is a retinal neoplasm composed of anaplastic, poorly differentiated retinal cells (Fig. 27-56). These cells tend to grow in all directions—into the vitreous, beneath the retina, and along the retina. By each of these routes the tumor tends to invade the optic nerve head, through which it spreads back into the optic nerve and meninges. The extent of invasion of the optic nerve is important in prognosis, particularly if the tumor extends to the point of transection. The amount of choroidal invasion is also related to prognosis. A fatal outcome often is attributable to intracranial

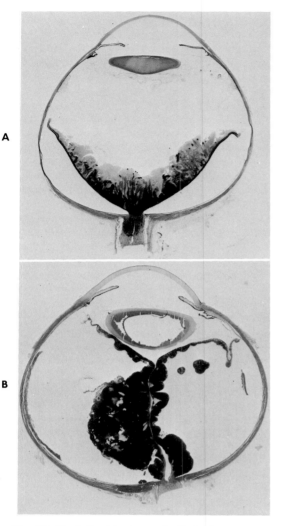

A

B

Fig. 27-56. Retinoblastoma. **A,** Endophytic pattern of growth with invasion of optic nerve. **B,** Exophytic growth with total detachment of retina. (**A,** AFIP 211405; **B,** AFIP 183030; from Friedenwald, J. S., Wilder, H. C., Maumenee, A. E., Sanders, T. E., Keyes, J. E., Hogan, M. J., Owens, W. C., and Owens, E. U.: Ophthalmic pathology, Philadelphia, 1952, W. B. Saunders Co.)

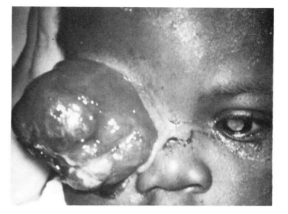

Fig. 27-57. Massive orbital invasion by retinoblastoma of right eye. Left eye also affected, as evident from leukokoria. (Courtesy Dr. V. T. Curtin; from Zimmerman, L. E.: Med. Ann. D.C. **38:**366-374, 1969.)

The majority of cases are detected when a parent first notices something peculiar about the child's eye. Usually, this is a change in the appearance of the normally jet black pupil. The white mass in the retina tends to reflect light rays entering the eye, producing a white, yellow, or grayish discoloration of the pupil (a sign called leukokoria—Fig. 27-57). Other pathologic processes in the retina or vitreous body may produce similar pupillary changes and thus lead to enucleation in the mistaken belief that the eye contains a malignant neoplasm. Congenital malformations, endophthalmitis produced by wandering larvae of *Toxocara canis*, exudative retinopathies (e.g., Coats' disease), traumatic or idiopathic retinal detachment, and the retinopathy of prematurity are some of the more important causes for leukokoria, leading to confusion with retinoblastoma. Besides leukokoria, other manifestations of retinoblastoma include strabismus, inflammation, glaucoma, and intraocular hemorrhage.

Metastatic tumors

Metastatic tumors of many different types have been encountered in the eye, but metastasis from two sources are notorious. In women, metastasis from carcinoma of the breast is by far more frequent than from all other sources combined. Usually, metastasis to the eye occurs after mastectomy has been performed, although rarely the ocular tumor may be the initial clinical manifestation. If the ocular metastasis occurs long after mastectomy at a time when the patient appears to

spread via the optic nerve and subarachnoid fluid. The tumor also has the capability for vascular invasion and hematogenous dissemination. It also can spread back into the orbit, and in neglected cases the child may present with a large fungating mass that fills the orbit (Fig. 27-57). Before the turn of the century, this was the typical picture of retinoblastoma. Fortunately, today—at least in our more highly civilized countries, where the public as well as physicians are better educated—such advanced stages rarely are seen.

be in good general health, the possibility of metastatic carcinoma may not be suspected by either the patient or ophthalmologist. In such cases, enucleation may be performed in the mistaken belief that the eye contains a malignant melanoma.

In men, bronchogenic carcinoma is the most frequent source of metastasis to the eye. This tumor is more likely than breast cancer to remain undetected until after enucleation has been carried out because of a suspected uveal melanoma. Thus in the differential diagnosis of malignant melanoma of the uvea, one must always be alert to the possibility of metastatic carcinoma, and appropriate studies should be undertaken before enucleation is recommended. Some ophthalmologists still seem to want to rush a patient suspected of having an intraocular melanoma to surgery for enucleation, afraid that any delay might jeopardize the patient's chances for a cure. Melanomas, however, are slow growing and generally have been present for a very long time before they have been discovered, so that taking the additional time for a thorough clinical, laboratory, and radiologic work-up would be time well spent.

Metastatic tumors in the eye almost always selectively involve the uvea rather than the retina, optic nerve, or any other tissue. The choroid is by far the part of the uvea most frequently involved (Fig. 27-58), and the iris is the least frequently affected. In the iris, however, the metastatic carcinoma very char-

acteristically produces clinical signs and symptoms of a uveitis, whereas the metastatic tumor in the choroid rarely is accompanied by such manifestations. The reason for this difference is unknown.

Benign tumors

Benign tumors include nevi of the uveal tract, melanocytomas of the optic disc, hemangiomas of the choroid, and other hamartomatous lesions of the phakomatoses (Sturge-Weber syndrome, von Hippel–Lindau disease, Recklinghausen's disease, and Bourneville's disease). It should be noted that the various ocular lesions typical of the phakomatoses also may be observed as isolated lesions in individuals who seem to have no systemic manifestations.

In the Sturge-Weber syndrome, there is a cavernous hemangioma of the choroid (Fig. 27-59) and often an ipsilateral congenital glaucoma associated with an extensive cavernous hemangioma (nevus flammeus) of the face, involving the eyelids. In von Hippel–Lindau disease, the characteristic ocular lesion is angiomatosis retinae (Fig. 27-60). Huge, tortuous vessels course to a vascular tumor of the retina that microscopically resembles closely a hemangiopericytoma. In Recklinghausen's neurofibromatosis, the eye may show any one or more of many different lesions, including discrete nevi and neurofibromas, diffuse neurofibromatous thickening of the uvea with or without hyperpigmentation, plexiform neurofibromas of the ciliary nerves, juvenile astrocytoma of the optic nerve, congenital glaucoma, congenital enlargement of the globe, atrophia bulbi, etc. In Bourneville's disease,

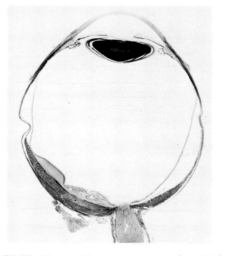

Fig. 27-58. Metastatic carcinoma in choroid from breast cancer. (AFIP 37637; from DeCoursey, E., and Ash, J. E.: Atlas of ophthalmic pathology, Rochester, Minn., 1942, American Academy of Ophthalmology and Otolaryngology.)

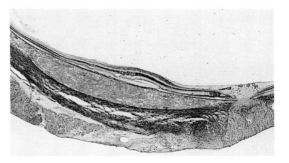

Fig. 27-59. Cavernous hemangioma of choroid. (8×; AFIP 171647-26081; from Friedenwald, J. S., Wilder, H. C., Maumenee, A. E., Sanders, T. E., Keyes, J. E., Hogan, M. J., Owens, W. C., and Owens, E. U.: Ophthalmic pathology, Philadelphia, 1952, W. B. Saunders Co.)

the characteristic lesion is the astrocytic hamartoma that involves the optic nerve head or the retina, or both. These benign astrocytic tumors tend to undergo calcification, giving rise to the giant drusen that are seen most frequently protruding from the nerve head.

RETINAL DISEASES

Retinal diseases are extremely important not only because the retina is the single most important ocular tissue but also because it often is affected by a very broad range of systemic as well as ocular disease processes, far too many to be considered here. Only a few of the most important will be considered.

Retinopathy of prematurity

Retinopathy of prematurity, also called retrolental fibroplasia, is a curious condition that first made its appearance early in the 1940s when modern incubators fed by pure oxygen became available for the routine treatment of premature babies. Soon the disease became a leading cause of blindness in children. After much intensive research, it was shown that the incompletely vascularized retina of the premature baby is exquisitely sensitive to hyperoxia. The proliferating retinal capil-laries under the influence of continuous high-oxygen tension not only cease their normal growth to the retinal periphery but also may become permanently obliterated. After oxygen therapy is discontinued, abnormal vasoproliferative changes occur proximal to the points where the retinal vessels are permanently obliterated. These proliferating new vessels often penetrate the internal limiting membrane of the retina and grow into the vitreous (Fig. 27-61). There they leak fluid and blood, which may subsequently lead to organization, produce traction on the retina, and cause retinal detachment and blindness. After the cause of this retinopathy of premature babies was discovered, appropriate control measures were instituted, and the disease virtually disappeared.

Diabetic retinopathy

Diabetic retinopathy is the second leading cause of new adult blindness in the United States, and it is one of the most dreaded of all the vascular complications that await the diabetic patient. It is particularly among those who developed diabetes in childhood and who have had the disease for 15 to 20 years that retinopathy is most frequently observed and

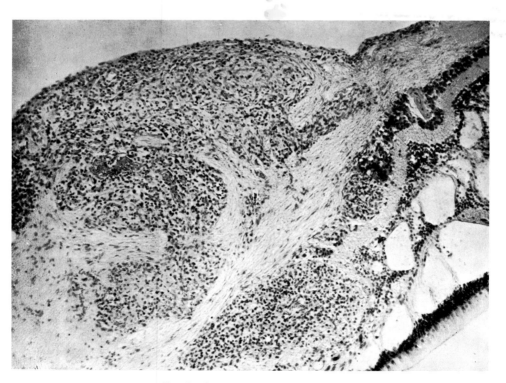

Fig. 27-60. Angiomatosis retinae.

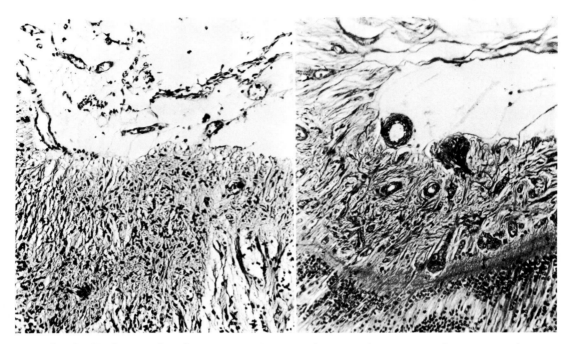

Fig. 27-61. Retinopathy of prematurity. Intraretinal neovascularization can be seen on right and proliferation of vessels in vitreous on left. (From Friedenwald, J. S., Owens, W. C., and Owens, E. U.: Trans. Am. Ophthalmol. Soc. **49:**207-234, 1951.)

is most disabling, just when the patient is in what should be his most productive years. The duration of diabetes rather than the adequacy of its control seems to be the most significant pathogenetic factor, for diabetic retinopathy was not a significant problem in the preinsulin era when young diabetic patients rarely survived more than a few years.

The selective retinal capillary microangiopathy of diabetes seems to begin with a degeneration of the mural cells or pericytes, but in patchy areas one also observes capillaries that appear to be totally ischemic, showing a loss of endothelial cells as well as pericytes (Fig. 27-62). Immediately adjacent to these ischemic foci are focal saclike aneurysmal dilatations of the capillaries. Most of these microaneurysms are too small to be visible by ordinary ophthalmoscopy, but some of the larger ones do become visible, especially when associated with a diapedesis of erythrocytes, producing the small dot hemorrhages. At about the same time that microaneurysms and dot hemorrhages make their appearance, "soft exudates" in the superficial layers of the retina also are seen. These are believed to be microinfarcts involving the nerve fiber layer, similar to those responsible for the cotton wool spots of hypertensive retinopathy (see

below). Venous dilatation and irregularity are typically present. The microangiopathy includes a loss of permeability with the formation of hard exudates in the deeper layers of the retina (Fig. 27-63). These are rich in proteins and lipids and have a yellowish appearance. Histiocytes swollen with ingested lipids often are present in large numbers in these deeply situated exudates.

Midway in the course of diabetic retinopathy, new capillaries proliferate, often at the optic disc or along one of the major veins. These erupt through the internal limiting membrane of the retina into the vitreous. These also leak, and an accumulation of connective tissue develops along the preretinal vessels. Hemorrhage from these intravitreal vessels and contraction of connective tissue eventually lead to traction on the retina and its detachment (Fig. 27-64).

It is clear, therefore, that visual loss from diabetic retinopathy may be ascribed to a number of pathologic processes—retinal ischemia, formation of hemorrhages and exudation in the retina, presence of microinfarcts, proliferation of new vessels and connective tissue on the retinal surface, hemorrhages into the vitreous, and retinal detachment.

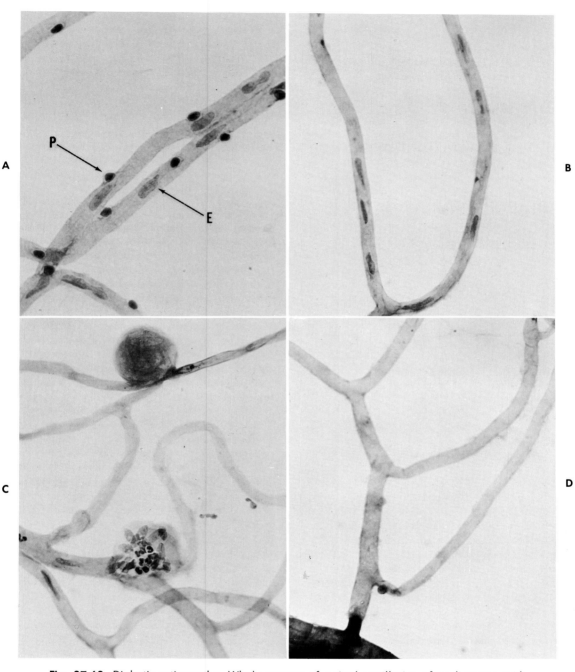

Fig. 27-62. Diabetic retinopathy. Whole mounts of retinal capillaries after digestion with trypsin. **A,** Nuclei of endothelial cells, *E,* and of pericytes or mural cells, *P,* are normally observed in about 1:1 ratio. **B,** Selective loss of mural pericytes, one of earliest changes in diabetes. **C,** Saccular microaneurysms characteristic of diabetic retinopathy. One in upper part of field is hyalinized, whereas one in lower part shows endothelial proliferation and adherent leukocytes. **D,** Many of ischemic vessels showing loss of all nuclei in advanced diabetic retinopathy. (**A,** AFIP 64-7004; **B,** AFIP 64-7010; **C,** AFIP 64-7009; **D,** AFIP 64-7008.)

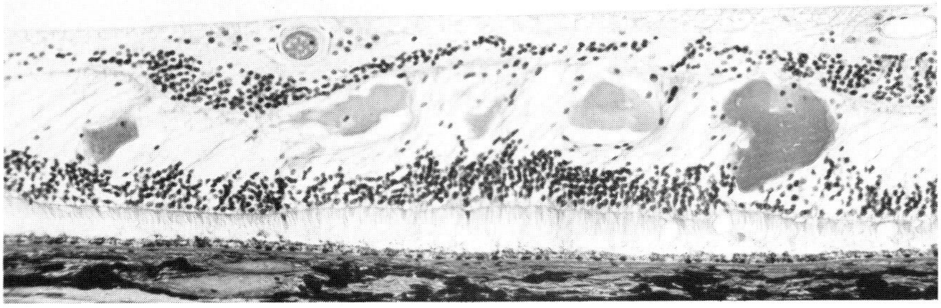

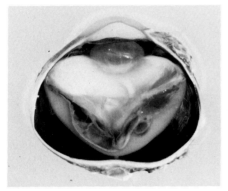

Fig. 27-63. Diabetic retinopathy. Ischemic degeneration of inner layers and exudates in outer plexiform layer. (205×; AFIP 84800; from Friedenwald, J. S., Wilder, H. C., Maumenee, A. E., Sanders, T. E., Keyes, J. E., Hogan, M. J., Owens, W. C, and Owens, E. U.: Ophthalmic pathology, Philadelphia, 1952, W. B. Saunders Co.)

Fig. 27-64. Diabetic retinopathy has led to retinitis proliferans, intravitreal hemorrhage, and retinal detachment. (AFIP 57-5060.)

Hypertensive retinopathy

Hypertensive retinopathy is observed most frequently and in its most severe form in the acutely progressive type of malignant hypertension. There is a generalized narrowing of retinal arterioles leading to retinal ischemia. Microinfarcts are commonly present. Clinically, these appear as soft, fluffy, superficial exudates (called cotton-wool spots) protruding forward from the retina. Microscopically, however, these are not exudates but focal areas of ischemic infarction, typically involving only the nerve fiber and ganglion cell layers of the retina (Fig. 27-65). The lesion is associated with edematous swelling and a disappearance of nuclei. Within the swollen nerve fiber layer one sees peculiar cell-like structures (cytoid bodies), which are tremendously swollen necrotic axons (end bulbs of Cajal). In hypertensive retinopathy, flame-shaped superficial hemorrhages and watery exudates in the deeper retinal layers frequently are present. Often, the retina is diffusely edematous, and there may be considerable papilledema. The accumulation of protein-rich exudate and lipid-laden macrophages in the outer plexiform layer of the macula leads to the formation of a series of linear hard exudates radiating out from the foveal area (macular star figure). Retinal changes similar to those observed in malignant hypertension also may be observed in other conditions such as eclampsia, periarteritis nodosa, lupus erythematosus, etc.

Vascular occlusive disease

Vascular occlusive disease may affect either the arterial or the venous side and may develop suddenly or slowly. Sudden total occlusion of the central retinal artery is usually the result of atherosclerosis leading to hemorrhage or thrombosis in the vicinity of a subintimal plaque that has already greatly narrowed the lumen. This vascular accident produces complete ischemic infarction of those retinal layers that are totally dependent on the central retinal artery, and the patient experiences a sudden loss of vision (Fig. 27-66).

The same clinical and histopathologic picture may be observed when an embolus obstructs the central retinal artery. Endocardial vegetations, mural thrombi after myocardial infarction, and the cardiac myxoma are sources of large emboli. Smaller emboli from atherosclerotic plaques in the great vessels of the neck more frequently lodge in branches of the central retinal artery, producing smaller areas of retinal infarction. Microscopically, the retinal infarct is characterized by an early edematous thickening of the inner half of the

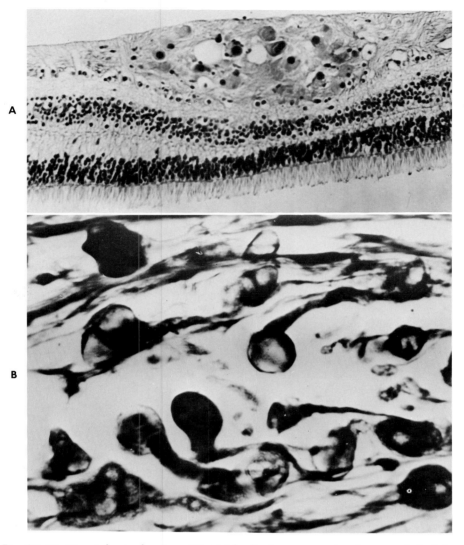

Fig. 27-65. Microinfarct of retina. "Cytoid bodies" are axonal enlargements in infarcted nerve fiber layer. **A,** Paraffin section. **B,** Frozen section stained by Hortega's method. (**A,** 210×; AFIP 69808; from Friedenwald, J. S., Wilder, H. C., Maumenee, A. E., Sanders, T. E., Keyes, J. E., Hogan, M. J., Owens, W. C., and Owens, E. U.: Ophthalmic pathology, Philadelphia, 1952, W. B. Saunders Co.; **B,** from Wolter, J. R.: Am. J. Ophthalmol. **48:**473-485, 1959.)

retina and a dissolution of nuclei in the ganglion cell and inner nuclear layers. Clinically, the edematous retina appears gray, and only in the fovea where the inner layers of the retina are normally absent does the choroidal circulation give the fundus its normal pink hue. Later on, as the edema subsides, the retina regains its transparency, and microscopically one sees only a thinning of the inner retinal layers from which the nerve fibers, ganglion cells, and almost all of the cells in the inner nuclear layer have disappeared.

Thrombosis of the central retinal vein leads to hemorrhagic infarction of the entire retina (Fig. 27-67). All of the retinal veins and capillaries are engorged. Rupture of the latter leads to bleeding into all retinal layers. Bleeding into the vitreous or beneath the retina may also be observed. An important complication of thrombosis of the central retinal vein is hemorrhagic glaucoma, which typically makes its appearance after about 3 months. This is the result of a proliferation of capillaries in the anterior chamber angle from the root of

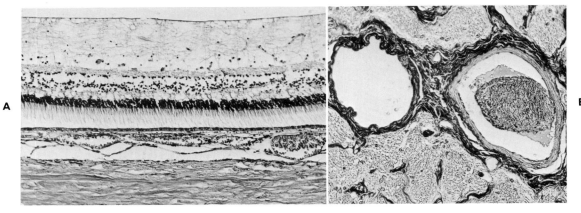

A

B

Fig. 27-66. Acute ischemic infarction of retina, **A,** produced by embolus in central retinal artery, **B,** from mural thrombus in left ventricle of patient who had sustained myocardial infarction. (AFIP 951983; **B,** from Zimmerman, L. E.: Arch. Ophthalmol. [Chicago] **73:**822-826, 1965.)

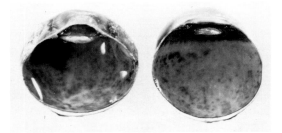

Fig. 27-67. Hemorrhagic infarction of retina. (AFIP 64-2232.)

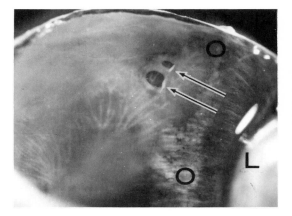

Fig. 27-68. Two holes are present in peripheral retina. Dense white retinal tissue at anterior border of each hole *(arrows)* is retracted operculum torn away in formation of holes. **O—O,** Ora serrata. **L,** Posterior surface of lens. (AFIP 65-3203-1.)

the iris and face of the ciliary body, obstructing the outflow of aqueous humor and leading to hemorrhage into the anterior chamber. Similar anterior segment changes may be observed after occlusion of the central retinal artery, but much less frequently. They also may be seen with other retinopathies, especially diabetic retinopathy, and it is suspected that the cause is a vasostimulatory factor liberated from the hypoxic retina.

Slowly progressive vascular insufficiency most often affects not just the retinal circulation but also the uveal blood supply, because it is observed mainly in those occlusive vascular diseases that affect the aortic arch and the great vessels of the head and neck (e.g., atherosclerosis of the carotid arteries, cranial arteritis, and pulseless disease).

Retinal detachment

Retinal detachment is a separation of the sensory retina from its normally tenuous juxtaposition to the retinal pigment epithe-

lium. The tips of the rods and cones normally are interdigitated with villous projections from the retinal pigment epithelium, but they are not attached by any specialized structures such as desmosomes. Thus these two tissues separate very readily—artifactitiously when a normal eye is opened in the laboratory without prior fixation or in vivo as a result of many pathologic processes. In general, retinal detachment can be expected to occur as a consequence of any of the following three pathogenetic mechanisms: (1) traction on the retina resulting from pathologic processes developing in the vitreous or in the anterior segment of the eye, including abscesses and hemorrhages in the vitreous, complications of intraocular surgery, or accidental trauma, etc., (2) exudation of fluid from the choroid opening up the potential subretinal space, as often occurs when there is an inflammatory process or tumor in the choroid, or (3) passage of liquefied vitreous or aqueous humor through a hole or tear in the retina. (See Fig. 27-68.)

It is the latter type that generally is treated by various surgical procedures designed to drain off the subretinal fluid and then to seal off the hole or tear by creating permanent adhesions between the adjacent retina and the pigment epithelium.

Since the outer layers of the retina are dependent on the choroidal circulation for nutrition and oxygenation, retinal detachment leads to a spatial separation of the retina from the choroid and a consequent ischemic loss of function. The aim of surgical reattachment of the retina is to get the retina back in place before irreparable damage has occurred in the retinal rods and cones.

REFERENCES
General

1 Boniuk, M., editor: Ocular and adnexal tumors; new and controversial aspects, St. Louis, 1964, The C. V. Mosby Co.
2 Hogan, M. J., and Zimmerman, L. E.: Ophthalmic pathology; an atlas and textbook, Philadelphia, 1962, W. B. Saunders Co.
3 New Orleans Academy of Ophthalmology: Industrial and traumatic ophthalmology, St. Louis, 1964, The C. V. Mosby Co.
4 New Orleans Academy of Ophthalmology: Symposium on surgical and medical management of congenital anomalies of the eye, St. Louis, 1968, The C. V. Mosby Co.
5 Reese, A. B.: Tumors of the eye, ed. 2, New York, 1963, Paul B. Hoeber Medical Division, Harper & Row, Publishers.
6 Zimmerman, L. E., editor: Int. Ophthalmol. Clin. **2:**237-557, 1962 (tumors of eye and adnexa).

Eyelids

7 Boniuk, M.: In Zimmerman, L. E., editor: Int. Ophthalmol. Clin. **2:**239-317, 1962 (tumors of eyelids).
8 Boniuk, M. In Boniuk, M., editor: Ocular and adnexal tumors; new and controversial aspects, St. Louis, 1964, The C. V. Mosby Co., pp. 75-100 (differentiation of squamous cell carcinoma from other epithelial tumors of eyelid).
9 Boniuk, M., and Zimmerman, L. E.: Trans. Am. Acad. Ophthalmol. Otolaryngol. **72:**619-642, 1968 (sebaceous carcinomas).

Conjunctiva and cornea

10 Ashton, N., Kirker, J. G., and Lavery, F. S.: Br. J. Ophthalmol. **48:**405-415, 1964 (ochronosis).
11 Cogan, D. G., and Kuwabara, T.: Arch. Ophthalmol. (Chicago) **61:**553-560, 1959 (arcus senilis).
12 Cogan, D. G., and Kuwabara, T.: Arch. Ophthalmol. (Chicago) **63:**51-57, 1960 (cystinosis).
13 Cogan, D. G., Albright, F., and Bartter, F. C.: Arch. Ophthalmol. (Chicago) **40:**624-638, 1948 (hypercalcemia).
14 Finley, J. K., Berkowitz, D., and Croll, M. N.: Arch. Ophthalmol. (Chicago) **66:**211-213, 1961 (arcus senilis).
14a Goldberg, M. F., Maumenee, A. E., and McKusick, V. A.: Arch. Ophthalmol. (Chicago) **74:**516-520, 1965 (mucopolysaccharidoses).
14b McKusick, V. A.: Am. J. Med. **47:**730-747, 1969 (mucopolysaccharidoses).
15 Newell, F. W., and Koistinen, A.: Arch. Ophthalmol. (Chicago) **53:**45-62, 1955 (gargoylism).
16 Reese, A. B.: Am. J. Ophthalmol. **61:**1272-1277, 1966 (acquired melanosis).
17 Spaeth, G. L., and Frost, P.: Arch. Ophthalmol. (Chicago) **74:**760-769, 1965 (Fabry's disease).
18 Witschel, H., and Mathyl, J.: Klin. Monatsbl. Augenheilkd. **154:**599-605, 1969 (Fabry's disease).
19 Zimmerman, L. E.: Arch. Ophthalmol. (Chicago) **76:**307-308, 1966 (acquired melanosis).
20 Zimmerman, L. E.: In Rycroft, P. V., editor: Corneo-plastic surgery, New York, 1969, Pergamon Press, Inc., pp. 547-555 (cancerous, precancerous, and pseudocancerous lesions).

Orbit

21 Anderson, D. R.: Am. J. Ophthalmol. **68:**46-57, 1969 (endocrinopathic exophthalmos).
22 Ashton, N., and Morgan, G.: J. Clin. Pathol. **18:**699-714, 1965 (rhabdomyosarcoma).
23 Dutcher, T. F., and Fahey, J. L.: J. Natl. Cancer Inst. **22:**887-917, 1959 (macroglobulinemia).
24 Font, R. L., Yanoff, M., and Zimmerman, L. E.: Am. J. Clin. Pathol. **48:**365-376, 1967 (benign lymphoepithelial lesion of lacrimal gland and Sjögren's syndrome).
25 Forrest, A. W.: In Zimmerman, L. E., editor: Int. Ophthalmol. Clin. **2:**543-553, 1962 (tumors after radiation about eye).
26 Godwin, J. T.: Cancer **5:**1089-1103, 1952 (benign lymphoepithelial lesion of salivary gland).
27 Hoyt, W. F., and Baghdassarian, S. A.: Br. J. Ophthalmol. **53:**793-798, 1969 (natural history of optic gliomas).
28 Jones, I. S., Reese, A. B., and Krout, J.: Trans. Am. Ophthalmol. Soc. **63:**223-255, 1965 (rhabdomyosarcoma).
29 Kroll, A. J., and Kuwabara, T.: Arch. Ophthalmol. (Chicago) **76:**244-247, 1966 (endocrinopathic exophthalmos).
30 Little, J. M.: Trans. Am. Acad. Ophthalmol. Otolaryngol. **71:**875-879, 1967 (macroglobulinemia).
31 Porterfield, J. F., and Zimmerman, L. E.: Virchows Arch. (Pathol. Anat.) **335:**329-344, 1962 (rhabdomyosarcoma).
32 Straatsma, B. R., Zimmerman, L. E., and Gass, J. D. M.: Lab. Invest. **11:**963-985, 1962 (phycomycosis).

33 Werner, S. C.: Am. J. Ophthalmol. **68:**646-648, 1969 (endocrinopathic exophthalmos).

34 Zimmerman, L. E., Sanders, T. E., and Ackerman, L. V. In Zimmerman, L. E., editor: Int. Ophthalmol. Clin. **2:**337-367, 1962 (epithelial tumors of lacrimal gland).

Inflammations

35 Ashton, N.: In Rycroft, P. V., editor: Corneoplastic surgery, New York, 1969, Pergamon Press, Inc., pp. 579-591 (*Toxocara canis* and the eye).

36 Fine, B. S. Lab. Invest. **11:**1161-1171, 1962 (intraocular mycotic infections).

37 Gould, H. L., and Kaufman, H. E.: Arch. Ophthalmol. (Chicago) **65:**453-456, 1961 (sarcoidosis).

38 Wilder, H. C.: Trans. Am. Acad. Ophthalmol. Otolaryngol. **55:**99-109, 1950 (ocular larva migrans).

39 Wilder, H. C.: Arch. Ophthalmol. (Chicago) **48:**127-136, 1952 (*Toxoplasma* chorioretinitis).

40 Zimmerman, L. E.: Lab. Invest. **11:**1151-1160, 1962 (mycotic keratitis).

41 Zimmerman, L. E.: Am. J. Ophthalmol. **60:** 1011-1035, 1965 (juvenile xanthogranuloma).

42 Zimmerman, L. E., and Maumenee, A. E.: Am. Rev. Resp. Dis. **84**(Nov. suppl.):38-44, 1961 (sarcoidosis).

Glaucoma; cataract

43 Flocks, M., Littwin, C. S., and Zimmerman, L. E.: Arch. Ophthalmol. (Chicago) **54:**37-45, 1955 (phacolytic glaucoma).

44 Kolker, A. E., and Hetherington, J., Jr.: Becker-Shaffer's Diagnosis and therapy of the glaucomas, ed. 3, St. Louis, 1970, The C. V. Mosby Co.

45 Wolff, S. M., and Zimmerman, L. E.: Am. J. Ophthalmol. **54:**547-563, 1962 (postcontusion glaucoma).

46 Zimmerman, L. E.: In Maumenee, A. E., and Silverstein, A. M., editors: Immunopathology of uveitis, Baltimore, 1964, The Williams & Wilkins Co., pp. 221-242 (lens-induced inflammation in human eyes).

47 Zimmerman, L. E.: In New Orleans Academy of Ophthalmology: Symposium on glaucoma, St. Louis, 1967, The C. V. Mosby Co., pp. 1-30 (histology and pathology of outflow channels).

48 Zimmerman, L. E. Am. J. Ophthalmol. **65:**837-862, 1968 (congenital rubella syndrome).

49 Zimmerman, L. E., and Font, R. L.: J.A.M.A. **196:**684-692, 1966 (congenital malformations).

Retinal diseases

50 Cant, J. S., editor: The William Mackenzie centenary symposium on the ocular circulation in health and disease, St. Louis, 1969, The C. V. Mosby Co.

51 François, J., et al.: Ophthalmologica **170:**405-425, 1975 (genetics of retinoblastoma).

52 Goldberg, M. F., and Fine, S. L., editors: Symposium on the treatment of diabetic retinopathy, Washington, D. C., 1968, U. S. Government Printing Office, United States Public Health Service Publ. no. 1890.

53 McPherson, A., editor: New and controversial aspects of retinal detachment, New York, 1968, Paul B. Hoeber Medical Division, Harper & Row, Publishers.

54 Redler, L. D., and Ellsworth, R. M.: Arch. Ophthalmol. **90:**294, 1973 (prognostic factors in retinoblastoma).

55 Schepens, C. L., and Regan, C. D. J., editors: Controversial aspects of the management of retinal detachment, 1965, Boston, Little, Brown & Co.

56 Wolter, J. R.: Am. J. Ophthalmol. **48:**473-485, 1959 (pathology of cotton wool spot).

57 Wolter, J. R.: Trans. Am. Ophthalmol. Soc. **65:** 106-127, 1967 (cytoid bodies).

58 Wolter, J. R., Philips, R. L., and Butler, R. G.: Arch. Ophthalmol. (Chicago) **60:**49-59, 1958 (macular star figure and hypertensive retinopathy).

59 Zimmerman, L. E.: Discussion of Wolter, J. R.: Trans. Am. Ophthalmol Soc. **65:**106-127, 1967 (historical review of cytoid bodies as axonal enlargements).

28/Upper respiratory tract and ear

JOHN M. KISSANE*

UPPER RESPIRATORY TRACT

Gross and microscopic features of the upper respiratory tract influence both the pathology and the clinical course of lesions that develop in this area. The thin walls of the perinasal sinuses allow inflammatory processes or neoplasms to spread from one area to another. A tumor originating in a maxillary sinus may remain clinically silent until it produces symptoms of pressure by filling the sinus, at which time the lesion may be difficult to eradicate. Otherwise inconsequential inflammatory or proliferative lesions may prove life threatening if located on a vocal chord or elsewhere in the airway. Proximity of components of the upper airway to the central nervous system has important clinical consequences. Inflammatory or neoplastic lesions, primary in the upper respiratory tract, may give rise to clinical manifestations by involving the central nervous system. The failure of therapeutic measures directed against the primary process may be followed relatively promptly by neurologic complications.

Morphologic features of inflammatory and neoplastic lesions of the upper respiratory tract depend on the structure of the epithelial surfaces of specific regions. The nares are lined by stratified squamous epithelium endowed with pilosebaceous elements. At birth the entire upper respiratory tract except the surfaces of the true vocal chords is lined by respiratory (simple or pseudostratified columnar) epithelium, which overlies mucous glands and a stroma containing erectile blood vessels. Soon after birth, many components of the upper respiratory tract come to be lined by nonkeratinized stratified squamous epithelium. In the adult, only the laryngeal ventricles and the infraglottic chamber of the larynx are consistently lined by respiratory epithelium. The submucosa of the upper respiratory tract contains relatively uniformly distributed mucous glands, which discharge upon the epithelial surface. In the nasopharynx, the submucosa contains discrete aggregates of lymphoid tissue that collectively constitute Waldeyer's ring, which consists of the palatine tonsil posterosuperiorly, the pharyngeal tonsils laterally, and the submucosal aggregates of lymphoid tissue at the base of the tongue anteroinferiorly (Fig. 28-1).

Conventional topographic anatomy distinguishes the external nose from the internal nasal cavity and paranasal sinuses. All three components serve functionally as antechambers of the upper respiratory tract whose diseases they share. The pharynx, an arbitrarily defined delta-like common conduit shared by upper respiratory and alimentary tracts, is subdivided into nasal pharynx, oropharynx, and laryngeal (hypo)pharynx. The first and third of these participate in disease processes of the upper respiratory tract and are considered here. The oropharynx participates in diseases of the upper alimentary tract and is considered in Chapter 30.

Nose, nasal cavity, paranasal sinuses, and nasopharynx
Malformations

The external nose is always malformed in cases of alobar holoprosencephaly, congenital aberrations in lateralization of the forebrain that are associated with abnormal assignment of olfactory lobes. In the most basic abnormality, a tubular proboscis presents rostral to variably fused optic vesicles. More commonly, the nose in the normal position possesses a single, often imperforate nostril.

Although uncommon, *choanal atresia* and *stenosis* are important congenital malformations. In this situation, either an epithelial membrane or an osteocartilaginous septum occludes the posterior nasopharynx. In choanal stenosis the obstructive membrane bears a minute orifice. Newborn infants reflexly

*Much of the original text and illustrations in this chapter was retained after revision of an earlier version by Dr. J. Daniel Wilkes.

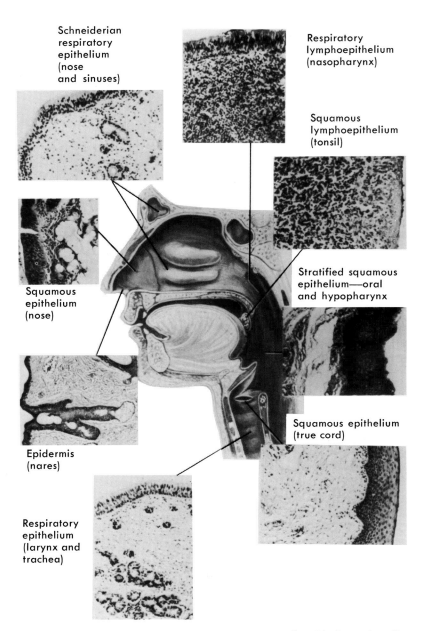

Schneiderian
respiratory
epithelium
(nose
and sinuses)

Respiratory
lymphoepithelium
(nasopharynx)

Squamous
lymphoepithelium
(tonsil)

Stratified squamous
epithelium—oral
and hypopharynx

Squamous
epithelium
(nose)

Squamous epithelium
(true cord)

Epidermis
(nares)

Respiratory
epithelium
(larynx and
trachea)

Fig. 28-1. Hemisection of head showing various types of epithelium that line specific anatomic sites of upper respiratory tract. (From Ash, J. E., Beck, M. R., and Wilkes, J. D.: Tumors of the upper respiratory tract and ear. In Atlas of tumor pathology, Sect. IV, Fasc. 12 and 13, Washington, D.C., 1964, Armed Forces Institute of Pathology; AFIP 70-1150-3.)

breathe through the nose and must learn oral breathing. Infants with choanal atresia or stenosis, therefore, experience respiratory distress while nursing and may be asphyxiated. Surgical perforation of the choanal septum constitutes a neonatal emergency.

Acquired lesions

Cutaneous lesions. The external nose is subject to disorders of the skin generally or to those disease processes to which special considerations such as exposure to solar radiation or pronounced investment of sebaceous glands render it particularly susceptible. The cutaneous investment of the nose is therefore particularly subject to lesions of lupus vulgaris, lupus erythematosus, or actinic keratosis. *Rhinophyma* is a sequela of extreme acneiform hypertrophy of sebaceous glands of the alae of the nose and adjacent regions of the face. Eventually fibrosis of the dermis produces nodular enlargement of the nose. Microscopic features include hypertrophy and hyperplasia of the sebaceous glands, dilatation and keratinous plugging of ducts, a chronic dermal inflammatory infiltrate, and progressive fibrosis.

Inflammation

Acute rhinitis. The most common etiologic agents responsible for acute rhinitis are viruses. Many viruses may cause acute catarrhal rhinitis, characterized by hyperemia of the nasal mucosa, edema, and exudation of serous and mucinous fluid. In performing its function of cleansing, warming or cooling, and humidifying the inspired air, the nasal mucosa is constantly challenged by antigens from the environment. Allergic rhinitis, characterized by a gray, mucinous discharge containing numerous eosinophils, is a common consequence of such exposure.

Histologically, there is edema of the submucosa and a cellular infiltrate composed of eosinophils, lymphocytes, and plasma cells. In chronic forms of rhinitis, squamous metaplasia may occur with fibroblastic proliferation of the stroma. Eventually, the subepithelial basement membrane shows characteristic thickening and hyalinization.

Atrophic rhinitis (ozena). Atrophic rhinitis affects predominantly the inferior turbinate. It is characterized clinically by pronounced crusting of the nasal mucosa and the characteristic offensive odor. The histologic appearance varies with the stage of the condition. Early, there is abundant lymphocytic and plasmacytic infiltration with desquamation of epithelium and squamous metaplasia. Atrophy of mucosal glands and stromal fibrosis occur later. The condition occurs most frequently in young females.

Rhinitis caseosa. A rare disease, rhinitis caseosa is characterized by accumulation in the nose of an extremely malodorous cheesy mass accompanied by a seropurulent discharge. The disorder is usually unilateral and may give rise to polypoid excrescences or eventually nasal deformities. Pathologic changes are not specific but reflect a chronic inflammatory process, the cause of which is not clear. The disease is comparable to cholesteatoma of the ear.

Sinusitis. Sinusitis usually accompanies rhinitis and may be acute or chronic, infectious, irritative, or allergic. Anatomically, perinatal sinuses drain poorly. Their ostia are easily occluded by edema and acute inflammation. Histologic features of sinusitis resemble those of rhinitis. Important complications of sinusitis relate to their nearness to other structures. Purulent ethmoiditis may give rise to orbital cellulitis and subsequent intracranial infection. Frontal sinusitis may be followed by osteomyelitis of the frontal bone and meningitis. Thrombophlebitis may arise in facial structures and propagate retrogradely into the cranial cavity. Retrobulbar neuritis may result from sphenoiditis.

Specific chronic infections

Syphilis. Primary syphilis rarely occurs at the mucocutaneous border of the nose. Chronic coryza and bony destruction with saddle-nose deformity are characteristic of congenital syphilis. Tuberculosis and leprosy also may involve the nasal cavity.

Rhinoscleroma. The chronic granulomatous inflammation, rhinoscleroma, involves the nose and nasopharynx and may extend into the oral cavity, larynx, and trachea. Deforming nodular masses eventually result in partial obstruction of the nose, nasal cavity, and the nasopharynx. This disease is rare in the United States, although over 100 cases have been reported. It is seen more frequently in Mediterranean areas, especially Egypt. A gram-negative diplobacillus, *Klebsiella rhinoscleromatis,* is always found in the lesion, usually in foamy, mononuclear cells (Mikulicz's cells); however, the organism may also be found in the nasopharynx and throat of otherwise healthy individuals. The disease has never been produced in experimental animals. The etiologic role of the organism remains obscure.

The inflammatory process confines itself to soft tissue; cartilage and bones are not involved. Rhinoscleroma is characterized by submucosal accumulation of plasma cells and foamy histiocytes and later by proliferation of fibrous tissue with formation of dark red nodular masses in the nasal mucosa that give rise to subsequent scarring and contractions with resulting deformities. Ulceration is not a constant feature.

Rhinosporidiosis. Rhinosporidiosis is attributed to infection by the morphologically defined organism *Rinosporidium seeberi.* The organism has not been cultivated on artificial media. The disease is relatively common in tropical areas, infrequent in medically advanced countries. Rhinosporidiosis usually presents as a bleeding nasal polyp. A similar process may rarely involve the conjunctiva, nasopharynx, or larynx. The polyps have a rough hemorrhagic surface in contrast to the smooth appearance of conventional allergic or inflammatory polyps.

Microscopically, organisms in all stages of development are distributed throughout the vascular myxomatous connective tissue of the inflammatory polypoid lesion. The earliest stage is a small, round cell about the size of an erythrocyte and containing clear, vacuolated cytoplasm and a distinct membrane. This spore enlarges to form mature cysts approximately 200 μm in diameter, which contain thousands of spores. The entire structure may ultimately rupture to disseminate spores in the submucosa and onto the surface of the mucosa of the involved region (Fig. 28-2).

Phycomycosis. Phycomycosis is a generic designation of infections by filamentous fungi of the class Phycomycetes. Many such infections are appropriately encompassed by the designation *mucormycosis,* but the role of members of the genus *Aspergillus* in such infections is insufficiently appreciated. Phycomycetes are ubiquitous opportunistic molds. Great caution must be exercised, therefore, in evaluating the significance of identification of one or another species in cultures from body fluids or exudates. The syndrome of phycomycosis consists of nasal, paranasal sinus, orbital, and central nervous system involvement. It is almost confined to severely acidotic patients, most commonly those with uncontrolled diabetes mellitus. Clinical detection of an acute necrotizing inflammatory process in the nasal or orbital area in a debilitated, acidotic patient demands

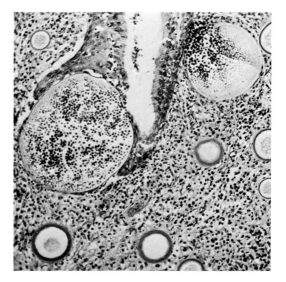

Fig. 28-2. Rhinosporidiosis. Mature cyst has ruptured and small spores are disseminating onto mucosa. (AFIP 70-1150-1.)

immediate consideration of phycomycosis. Smears, cultures, and biopsy specimens assist in establishing the diagnosis.

Histologic features are characteristic in that these fungi have a greater affinity for hematoxylin than most other organisms. Broad, irregular hyphi of variable diameter and branching dichotomously in a haphazard fashion are characteristic. They grow profusely in tissues. Infiltration of the walls of blood vessels is particularly characteristic (Fig. 28-3).

Lethal midline granuloma. An aggressive, necrotizing inflammatory process, lethal midline granuloma consists of an ulcerative destructive process involving midline structures of the face—the nose, paranasal sinuses, soft palate, and pharynx. From this clinically characterized melange three processes, definable in terms of their histopathologic features and natural history, have partially emerged. Malignant lymphoma of varying histologic features may produce a chronic destructive ulcerative process in the upper respiratory tract. Wegener's granulomatosis may produce predominant lesions in the upper respiratory tract or even the surface structures of the midline of the face. Other cases that lack the visceral lesions of Wegener's granulomatosis remain and are not readily classifiable as resembling any described form of malignant lymphoma except perhaps mycosis fungoides. These cases have recently been characterized as midline malignant reticulosis.[32]

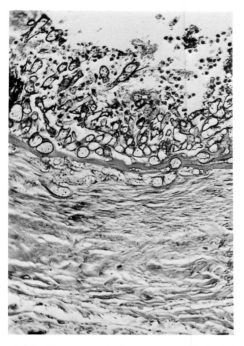

Fig. 28-3. Phycomycosis (mucormycosis). Twisting, branching, large nonseptate hyphae have peculiar tendency to invade vessels. (AFIP 58-7380.)

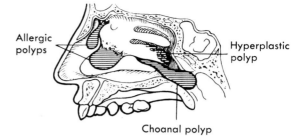

Fig. 28-4. Location of nasal polyps. Allergic polyps occur more commonly in upper area of lateral nasal wall, involving anterior middle turbinate especially. Choanal polyps have long pedicle and present in nasopharynx. Hyperplastic or neoplastic polyps and epithelial papilloma are not so pedunculated and involve posterior aspect of middle turbinate. (AFIP 70-1150-2.)

Wegener's granulomatosis. A syndrome of unknown etiology, Wegener's granulomatosis is characterized by necrotizing granulomatous lesions, usually including a vasculitis, involving the respiratory tract and often other organ systems, and a necrotizing glomerulonephritis. Partial expressions of the syndrome have recently been recognized. The disorder is generally believed to involve immune mechanisms. Patients often have histories of protracted rhinitis, sinusitis, or otitis. Nodular or diffuse pulmonary infiltrations sometimes with cavitation may occur. Necrotizing granulomatous lesions occur in both the upper and lower respiratory tracts. A vasculitis involving arteries and veins may be recognized microscopically. In cases with visceral involvement, a necrotizing glomerulitis is characteristic. Immunosuppressive chemotherapy has produced prolonged remissions.[32]

Relapsing polychondritis. Relapsing polychondritis most frequently involves the cartilages of the ears but may involve cartilages of the nose, larynx, trachea, joints, or the sclera of the eye. The disease is believed to be a disorder in chondromucin metabolism and has been associated with immunologic processes that include rheumatoid arthritis, systemic lupus erythematosus, and Hashimoto's thyroiditis.

Tumors and tumorlike conditions

The upper respiratory tract is exposed to a variety of infectious, chemically irritating, antigenically stimulating, mechanically traumatic, and undoubtedly many other influences. Consequences of these multifaceted deleterious exposures include the formation of tumorlike and truly neoplastic conditions that involve the upper respiratory tract. A variety of non-neoplastic but tumorlike conditions involve the upper airway, which is also subject to a considerable variety of true neoplasms.

Polyps. Nasal polyps are tumorlike, essentially nonneoplastic tumefactions that arise from the mucosa of the nasal cavity. Allergic and inflammatory factors underlie the pathogenesis of nasal polyps. *Choanal polyps* are a clinically defined category of inflammatory polyps that extend by an elongated pedicle from the nasal cavity through the choanae to present in the nasopharynx (Fig. 28-4).

Nasal polyps present in adolescence or early adulthood as usually multiple opalescent myxoid excrescences protruding into the nasal cavity from the lateral nasal wall. Obstructive symptoms predominate; the lesions rarely bleed. The occurrence of nasal polyps has recently emerged as an uncommon manifestation of cystic fibrosis.

Microscopically, nasal polyps consist of an edematous myxoid stroma overlaid by a hypersecretory respiratory epithelium in which patches of squamous metaplasia may occur. The stroma is infiltrated by inflammatory cells in which eosinophils may be conspicuous. The subepithelial basement membrane may become thickened. Polyps associated with chronic nasal allergy (allergic polyps) differ quantitatively

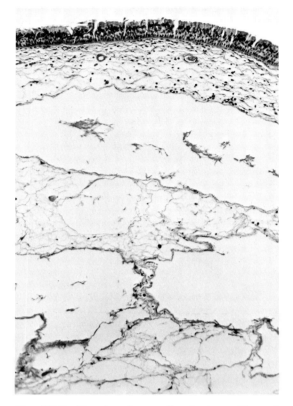

Fig. 28-5. Nasal polyps, allergic type. Stromal edema with pseudocyst formation.

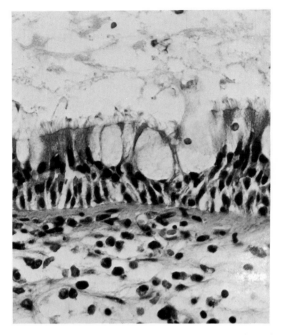

Fig. 28-6. Nasal polyp, allergic type. Ciliated pseudostratified columnar respiratory epithelium shows increased mucin production. Thickened basement membrane is evident. Inflammatory infiltrate is predominantly plasma cell.

from those attributable to chronic nasosinusoidal infection (inflammatory polyps) (Fig. 28-5). Eosinophils are more prominent in the cellular infiltrate of "allergic" than "inflammatory" polyps and the basement membrane is more frequently thickened (Fig. 28-6). "Allergic polyps" are more likely to recur after excision and are more often bilateral and multiple than are "inflammatory polyps."

Benign tumors

Juvenile nasopharyngeal angiofibroma. Juvenile nasopharyngeal angiofibroma is a rare tumor that occurs predominantly in adolescent and young adult males. The striking male preponderance, accelerated growth of the tumor at puberty, and stability or spontaneous regression thereafter all suggest hormonal factors in pathogenesis, no mechanism of which has been established. Most of these lesions originate from the roof of the nasal cavity, from which location they may secondarily erode into orbit, maxillary sinus, or external nose.

Grossly, nasopharyngeal angiofibroma is a bulky, gray-white rubbery lesion that may be

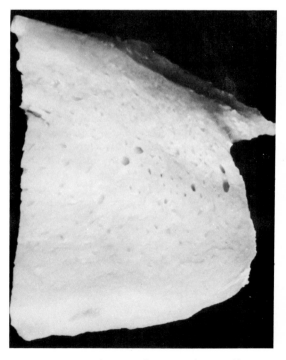

Fig. 28-7. Juvenile nasopharyngeal angiofibroma. Large blood vessels apparent on cut surface of portion of large tumor. (AFIP 56-18303-2.)

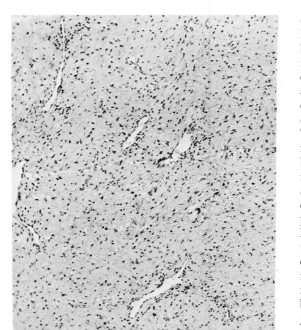

Fig. 28-8. Juvenile nasopharyngeal angiofibroma. Stroma consists of vascular spaces and dense cellular fibrous tissue. (AFIP 56-9683.)

distorted by contact with surrounding structures and is usually covered by an intact mucosa. Major vascular supply is usually grossly recognizable as dilated channels in the base of the lesion (Fig. 28-7). Microscopically, the lesion consists of a stroma of stellate and fusiform cells sparsely arrayed among myxoid intracellular material (Fig. 28-8). Dilated vascular channels are conspicuous. Overlying mucosa is usually of respiratory type. The vascular component of the tumor is distinguished by lacking a tunica elastica and by discontinuity of its tunica muscularis. Ultrastructural studies have confirmed these lesions and verify that the stromal cell is a fibroblast. Stromal fibroblasts often contain peculiar electron-dense nuclear inclusions.[12] Mast cells, smooth muscle cells, and various types of inflammatory cells may be found in the edematous myxoid interstitium.

A major factor in the natural history of nasopharyngeal angiofibroma is the tendency to bleed upon surgical manipulation. That at least some such lesions stabilize or even regress in young adulthood must be taken into account in assessment of the risks of therapy. Malignant transformation is very rare.

Epithelial papilloma. Epithelial papillomas occur predominantly in adult males with about

one twenty-fifth the frequency of nasal polyps. Most such lesions arise from the middle turbinate, but entirely analogous tumors arise from the septum, elsewhere in the nasal cavity, or in paranasal sinuses. They may be multiple and tend to recur after excision. The nomenclature of epithelial papillomas of the nasal cavity has become bewilderingly complex. The designation "cylindrical cell papilloma" reflects the origin of all epithelial papillomas basically from respiratory epithelium indigenous to the upper respiratory tract. *Transitional cell papilloma* is a purely morphologic designation reflecting a similarity of some papillary lesions of the nasal cavity to nonkeratinizing lesions, e.g., of the lower urinary tract. Although most epithelial papillomas are exophytic, i.e., they proliferate external to the mucosal surface, some undermine contiguous mucosal surfaces. This topographic feature has been endowed with the designation *inverted papilloma* (Fig. 28-9, *A*). The inverting epithelium may be squamous or respiratory in character (Fig. 28-9, *B*). We tend to subscribe to the nomenclature of Ringertz[15] in designating such lesions as cylindrical cell papillomas, since that designation assigns a cell of origin, but not excluding, however, the capacity of that cell to undergo a variety of metaplasias.

Malignant tumors

Carcinomas of nasal mucosa. Carcinomas of nasal mucosa occur predominantly in adult life. A slight female preponderance is evident in Western countries. Epistaxis and nasal obstruction are prominent symptoms. Grossly, the lesions consist of locally ulcerative and proliferative lesions. Nonkeratinizing epidermoid carcinoma is the most common histologic pattern. A nonkeratinizing epidermoid carcinoma infiltrated by lymphocytes constitutes *lymphoepithelioma,* a pattern of nasopharyngeal carcinoma, particularly common in males, particularly common in Chinese, and particularly prone to present clinically with early metastases to cervical lymph nodes.

Benign and malignant connective tissue neoplasms of the nasopharynx are uncommon.[8-11]

Synovial tumors of hypopharynx. Synovial tumors of the hypopharynx resemble synovial sarcomas of the joints. There are ample normal synovial tissues in the neck to provide a source for the tumor, including the bursae associated with the hyoid bone and the cricoarytenoid joints and those in the upper posterior portion of the neck. The mesothelial

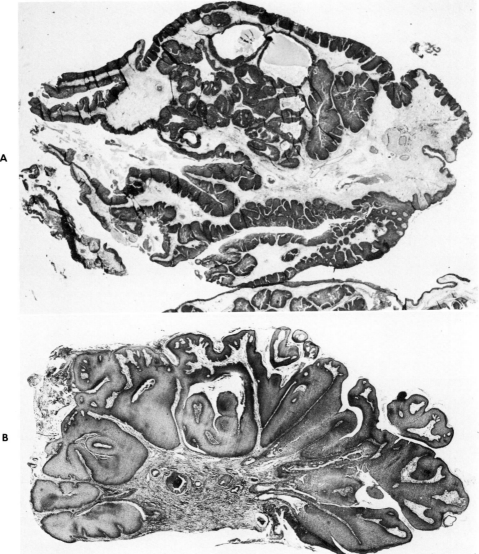

Fig. 28-9. Epithelial papillomas of nasal cavity. **A,** Inverted papilloma **B,** Squamous cell papilloma. (**A** from Norris, H. J.: Laryngoscope **72:**1784, 1962; **B, 73:**1, 1963.)

portion of the pharyngeal tumor usually is more differentiated than in the joint tumor.

Extramedullary plasmacytoma. Extramedullary plasmacytoma occurs most commonly in the nasal cavity and nasopharynx. Diagnosis usually is based on histologic features which include orientation of plasma cells in broad sheets on a delicate stroma and replacement of other tissue by such plasma cell sheets (Fig. 28-10). Since there is a definite relationship between extramedullary plasmacytoma and multiple myeloma, appropriate diagnostic studies to detect the latter are necessary.

These include immunoelectrophoresis, bone x-ray studies, and bone marrow examination.

Neurogenic tumors. A review of neurogenic tumors in the upper respiratory tract indicates that the majority of fibrillar tumors are of neural origin and often are confused with fibrous mesenchymal tissue (Fig. 28-11).

The sources of origin of the neurogenous tumors may be divided into three categories:
1. Peripheral neural elements
2. Central neural elements
3. Extrusions of brain tissue through defects

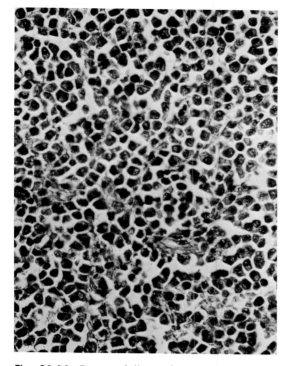

Fig. 28-10. Extramedullary plasmacytoma, which occurs predominantly in nasal cavity. Pleomorphic plasma cells completely replace stroma. (AFIP 870263.)

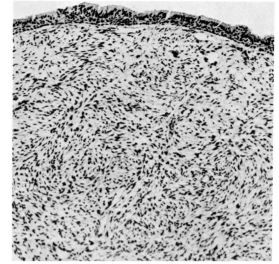

Fig. 28-11. Fibrosarcoma of nasal cavity. Interlacing fascicles of neoplastic fibrous cells evident. (AFIP 831866.)

in the cribriform plate and glabellar and occipital sutures

Tumors originating from peripheral nerve elements include the neuroma, neurofibroma, neurilemoma (schwannoma), malignant schwannoma (Fig. 28-12), ganglioma, and gangliofibroma. Central neural crest elements that have migrated simultaneously with cranial nerve are the source of origin of the ganglioglioma, neuroblastoma (esthesioneuroepithelioma), and medulloblastoma. Sympathetic neural elements that are derived from central neural elements give rise to the ganglioneuroma, sympathicoblastoma, and paraganglioma. Secondary neurogenous tumors include the meningioma, ependymoma, and retinoblastoma.

The olfactory neuroblastoma is a neoplasm that originates in the olfactory placode. It is presumed that the tumor arises from a stem cell, termed "esthesioneuroblast," because the usual location is in the olfactory area of the nasal cavity. The architecture varies, especially the proportion and arrangement of the cellular and fibrillar elements. Small, round or oval, primitive neural epithelial cells that are slightly pointed at one end grow in clusters that are

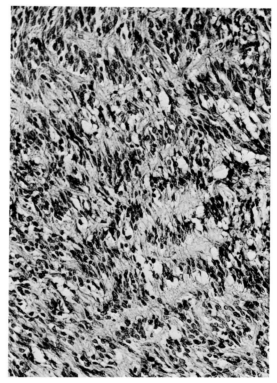

Fig. 28-12. Malignant schwannoma of nasal cavity, which originally was interpreted as fibrosarcoma. Palisading of nuclei became apparent when tumor recurred. Nuclear palisading characteristic of neurogenic tumors but not of fibrosarcomas. (AFIP 304290.)

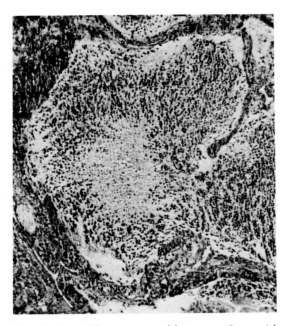

Fig. 28-13. Olfactory neuroblastoma. Organoid masses of neurocytoblasts associated with delicate neural fibrils pathognomonic for this lesion. (AFIP 64-8034-1.)

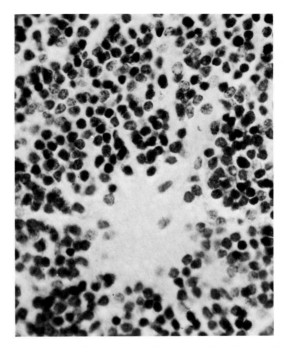

Fig. 28-14. Olfactory neuroblastoma. Small, round or oval, primitive neuroepithelial cells grow in rosette clusters around bundle of fine fibrillar neural stroma. (AFIP 64-8034-2.)

closely associated with bundles of fine neural fibrils (Figs. 28-13 and 28-14). Although rosette formation among the cells occurs, it is not so prominent a feature as in sympathicoblastoma and retinoblastoma. Olfactory neuroblastoma is apparently the most sensitive neurogenous tumor to irradiation therapy.

The **nasal glioma (congenital ganglioglioma)** occurs in the newborn infant, in whom the presence of an intranasal polypoid mass is almost pathognomonic of brain extrusion. Wide separation of the infant's eyes usually is associated with this condition. The lesion results from a congenital herniation of the cerebral vesicle through the skull, most commonly in the occipital and nasal frontal areas.

A nasal glioma may present as a smooth, nonulcerated, subcutaneous mass in the nasofrontal area attached by a fibrous stalk to the brain through the glabellar sutures. Intranasally, the mass may seem to arise from a turbinate, but its attachment to the cribriform plate is usually obvious. When the lesion is an encephalocele that communicates with the cerebral ventricles, it will enlarge when the patient cries or strains. Most nasal gliomas present a monotonous pattern of brainlike adult glial tissue interspersed with fine fibrous septae (Fig. 28-15). Meningitis may occur if an encephalocele is removed intranasally through a communicating ependyma-lined sinus.

Sarcoma botryoides (malignant mesenchymoma). Sarcoma botryoides is a recognized entity of the urogenital tract in children (p. 996). Recently, it has also become recognized as an equally specialized entity in the upper respiratory tract. The lesion occurs in the nasopharynx, palate, and ear. Although usually classified as a form of rhabdomyosarcoma, we have seen some congenital mesenchymal tumors containing no recognizable striated muscle elements. They are composed of neoplastic fibrous tissue, bone, or cartilage.

Since embryonal mesenchyme is the tissue of origin, the histologic appearance is varied because many of the tissues that normally are derived from embryonal mesenchyme are represented in the neoplastic growth. Fibromatous and myomatous elements usually are present in varying proportion. The large strap cell is characteristic of the primitive muscle component (Fig. 28-16). Neoplastic bone and cartilage may be present. Typically, the tumor metastasizes early and death rapidly ensues.

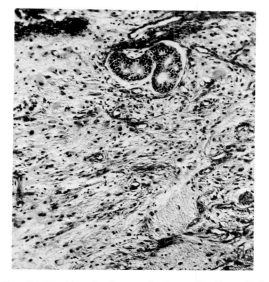

Fig. 28-15. Nasal glioma. Delicate fibrillar glial tissue with plump gemistocytic astrocytes extends to level of sweat gland in skin of glabellar region.

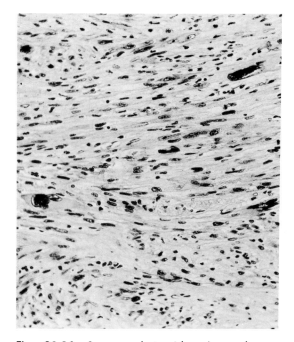

Fig. 28-16. Sarcoma botryoides. Large hyperchromatic nuclei in cells with abundant cytoplasm characteristic of primitive striated muscle components.

Larynx
Malformations

The commonest malformations of the larynx of clinical importance are laryngeal webs, delicate fibromembranous septa that fuse a variable extent of the true vocal chords and produce stridor and occasionally respiratory distress in the newborn infant. Usually they can be handled conservatively by dilatation.

Posterior cleft larynx is a malformation reflecting incomplete separation of respiratory and alimentary components of the embryonic foregut related to the more common tracheoesophageal fistula (p. 1280). Some cases are familial.

Laryngeal atresia produced either by a delicate fibrous septum that traverses the entire larynx or a thick, knobby fibrocartilaginous mass produces immediate respiratory distress after birth and perinatal death unless dealt with by emergency tracheostomy.

Inflammations

Inflammatory lesions of the larynx are rarely subjected to pathologic examination for diagnostic purposes. The larynx, of course, participates in many infectious processes that involve the upper respiratory tract whether viral, bacterial, or fungal. Diphtheria has become much less common in recent decades, although epidemics continue to occur even in medically advanced countries. Other infectious forms of croup have assumed greater diagnostic importance. Acute epiglottitis, often attributable to infection by *Haemophilus influenzae* may be life threatening and require prompt clinical recognition and the institution of appropriate antibiotic therapy. The disease is most common in infants and young children but may occur even in adults.

Tumors and tumorlike conditions

Nodules. Laryngeal nodules are acquired lesions that usually occur on the anterior third of one or both vocal cords, often as consequences of vocal abuse. This concept of pathogenesis is reflected in a variety of synonyms, e.g., singer's nodes, screamer's nodes, preacher's nodes, etc. The lesion is believed to originate at sites of local trauma along the course of the cords and to progress through stages characterized as *fibrous, polypoid, varicose,* and *fibrinoid* (Fig. 28-17). Unless the patient is reeducated in utilization of the voice, recurrence after excision is likely.

Papilloma. Multiple epithelial papillomas occur in the upper respiratory tract, chiefly the larynx but occasionally also in the trachea and major bronchi. Papillomas that occur in adolescence are possibly viral in etiology. The

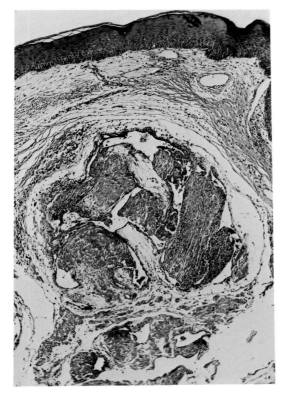

Fig. 28-17. Laryngeal nodule—fibrinoid stage. Darker staining material in edematous stroma characteristic of this stage.

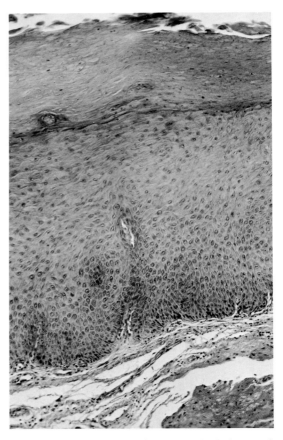

Fig. 28-18. Pachyderma laryngis. Thick layer of keratin not normally present on true vocal cords. Squamous epithelium thickened.

lesions present grossly as multiple warty excrescences that microscopically consist of focal proliferations of well-differentiated squamous epithelium. Recurrences after local excisions are the rule. Malignant transformation has occurred after irradiation therapy. In adults, papillomas occur as so-called hyperkeratotic papillomas, usually solitary lesions that respond to local excision. Rarely, papillomatous material may be aspirated into lower air passages where it appears to be capable of reimplantation and growth.

Hyperkeratosis. Hyperkeratosis of squamous epithelium of the true vocal cords constitutes the lesion designated in the older literature "pachyderma laryngis." The lesion produces focal or diffuse epithelial thickening along the true cords by the formation of a layer of true keratin (Fig. 28-18). The lesion occurs most commonly in men subject to external pollutants, particularly cigarette smoke. The correlation with epidermoid carcinoma is not great.[66]

Carcinoma. Conventional classifications divide carcinoma of the larynx into *extrinsic*

forms, originating in the hypopharynx or arytenoid folds, epiglottis, piriform fossa, false cords, or laryngeal ventricles, and the *intrinsic* type involving the mucosa of the true cords or infraglottic larynx, the former being by far the most common. Clinical courses of these two categories differ widely although the pathologic features may not be strikingly different. Most lesions are nonkeratinizing, relatively well-differentiated epidermoid carcinomas. Well-differentiated exophytic (verrucous carcinoma) occurs in the larynx as in the oral pharynx.[77]

Nonepithelial tumors of larynx. Nonepithelial tumors of the larynx are uncommon neural (neurilemoma and nonchromaffin periganglioma) and vascular (hemangiopericytoma) tumors (hemangiotomas) are probably the most common of these.

Carcinoma. The older classification divided carcinoma of the larynx into (1) an extrinsic type originating in the hypopharynx, arytenoid

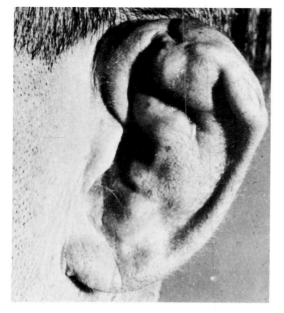

Fig. 28-19. Keloids of ear (cauliflower ear).

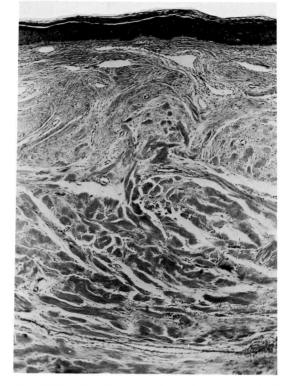

Fig. 28-20. Keloid of ear. Dense bands of keloid collagen in subcutaneous tissue.

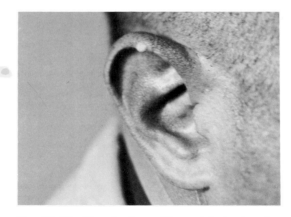

Fig. 28-21. Chondrodermatitis nodularis chronica helicis. Location and clinical appearance characteristic of this painful nodule. (From Shuman, R., and Helwig, E. B.: Am. J. Clin. Pathol. **24:**126-144, 1954; AFIP 165134.)

folds, epiglottis, and piriform fossae and (2) an intrinsic type involving the mucosa lining the larynx. The clinical course of these two categories differs widely, although the pathologic may not be strikingly different.

Extrinsic laryngeal carcinoma grows more rapidly than intrinsic. Diffuse extension of extrinsic carcinoma renders it less amenable to treatment. Intrinsic carcinoma of the larynx is overwhelmingly squamous and usually is a well-differentiated tumor. It occurs predominantly in older men. The majority of the tumors arise on the vocal cords. They grow relatively slowly and remain superficial for prolonged periods. When they infiltrate, however, the extension is rapid.

EAR
External ear

The external ear is subject to a variety of disease processes. Congenital deficiencies or malformations of auricular cartilages occur often in association with renal malformations. Rare inflammatory processes such as onchocerciasis, leprosy, blastomycosis, and coccidioidomycoses may involve the external ear. Keloids developed on the external ear (as *cauliflower ear*) after repeated trauma such as is experienced by boxers and wrestlers (Figs. 28-19 and 28-20). Epidermoid carcinoma and basal cell carcinoma occur on the ear as on the skin elsewhere. Chondrodermatitis nodularis chronica helicis specifically involves the external ear, where it presents as a painful tumorlike nodule on the superior concave surface of the helix (Figs. 28-21 and 28-22). At this site the skin is in direct contact with cartilage without a protective vascular sub-

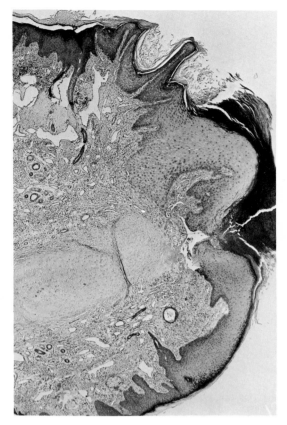

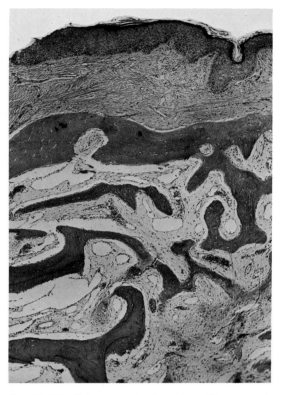

Fig 28-23. Osteoma of external auditory canal. Spicules of hypertrophic bone apparent.

Fig. 28-22. Chondrodermatitis nodularis chronica helicis. Superficial parakeratotic plaque with acanthotic squamous epithelium overlying cartilage showing fibrinoid degeneration.

cutaneous layer. The pathogenesis of the lesion is unknown. Compromise of the blood supply is suggested. The lesion is benign.

External auditory canal, middle ear, temporal bone
Tumors and tumorlike lesions

Tumors of the external auditory canal are rare. The majority of them arise in the skin that lines the canal. These tumors include the junctional nevus, an occasional malignant melanoma, and the squamous cell papilloma that has histologic characteristics similar to those of the lesion arising in the mucosa of the upper respiratory tract. Special entities of this area are osteoma and exostosis, ceruminal adenoma, and otic polyp.

Osteoma. Osteomas appear most often in adolescent boys and young men, arising most commonly at the chondro-osseous junction of the external auditory canal (Fig. 28-23). These lesions of bone occur more frequently in persons who habitually swim in cold water. Experimental support for this observation was furnished when overgrowths of bone were produced in the otic canals of guinea pigs by injecting cold water into the canals at intervals for long periods. The lesions are benign and do not recur after excision.

Ceruminal adenoma. Although ceruminal adenoma occurs in man, it is more common in lower animals, especially dogs and cats (Fig. 28-24). The ceruminal glands are modified sweat glands of the apocrine type, normally situated deep in the dermis near the cartilage of the canal. The tumor is particularly pleomorphic histologically. Squamous metaplasia is not uncommon, although its basic epithelial cell retains similarity to the apocrine type of the parent gland (Fig. 28-25). Although frequently interpreted as an adenocarcinoma, we have no record of an authentic ceruminal gland tumor that has metastasized.

Polyps. Polyps arise in the middle ear as a complication of chronic otitis media and protrude into the external canal through a perforated tympanic membrane. They are com-

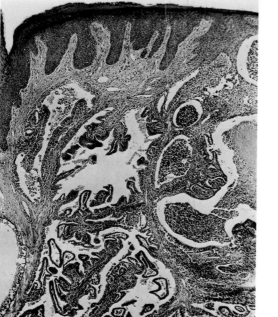

Fig. 28-24. Ceruminal adenoma of external auditory canal in cat. Papillary character seen more frequently in lesions in dogs and cats than in those in human beings.

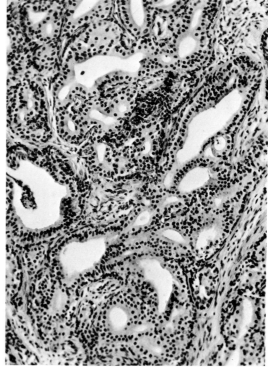

Fig. 28-25. Ceruminal adenoma of external auditory canal. Glandular pattern retained.

posed chiefly of granulation tissue and chronic exudate, but wide variations are also possible in the proportion of their other constituents—epithelium, blood vessels, and fibrous tissue (Fig. 28-26). The lesion most often is covered by squamous epithelium that has resulted from metaplasia of the normally modified respiratory epithelium of the middle ear.

Cholesteatoma. Cholesteatoma is most frequently a postinflammatory pseudotumor and is classified as a primary lesion when it arises from an embryonal inclusion of squamous epithelium in the temporal bone, especially in the petrous portion. The lesion is almost always a consequence of chronic otitis media in which there is marginal perforation of the external tympanic membrane. Through this opening, squamous epithelium from the external canal gains access to the middle ear and either reepithelializes the denuded surface or burrows under the epithelium normally present and replaces it (Fig. 28-27). From this epithelium, flaky keratin is constantly being shed, the accumulation of which eventually causes pressure erosion of bone. The term

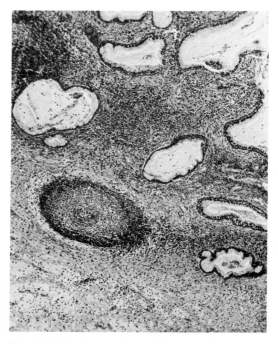

Fig. 28-26. Otic polyp. Chronic inflammation, pseudogland formation, and lymphoid follicle present.

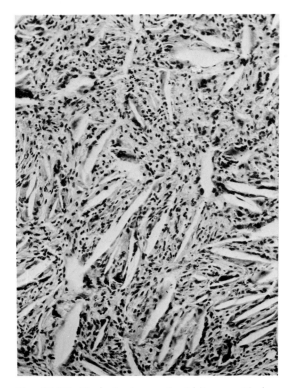

Fig. 28-27. Cholesteatoma of middle ear. Cholesterol-slit spaces, foreign body giant cells, and chronic inflammatory changes evident. (AFIP 56-2028-2.)

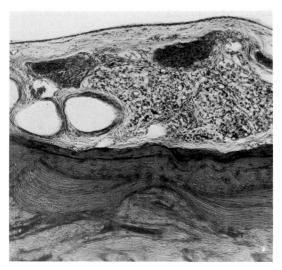

Fig. 28-28. Glomus jugularis with floor of middle ear below.

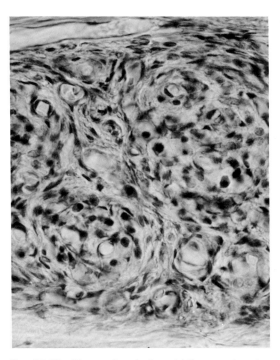

Fig. 28-29. Glomus jugularis, middle ear, showing characteristic histologic details of glomus body (high power).

cholesteatoma is an unsatisfactory one in that the occasional cholesterol deposits are the result of hemorrhage or chemical degradation of the keratin lipid. However, this nomenclature is universally accepted and would be difficult to change.

Nonchromaffin paraganglioma (glomus jugulare tumor). Nonchromaffin paraganglioma arises from structures in the human temporal bone similar to the carotid bodies, the glomus jugularis. In the middle ear, more than 90% of the tumors arise from the glomus jugularis that lies in the jugular canal immediately under the floor of the middle ear (Figs. 28-28 and 28-29). Additional foci of chemoreceptor glomera in the temporal bone region are located along the tympanic branch of the glossopharyngeal nerve along the auricular branch of the vagus nerve and in the jugular ganglion of the vagus nerve.

For many years, chemoreceptor structures have been classified as nonchromaffin paraganglionic tissue to differentiate them from the catecholamine-containing, chromaffin-reacting paraganglonic tissue such as the adrenal medulla and autonomic nervous system. However, recent observations suggest that the normal paraganglionic structures of the neck and temporal bone, and the tumors of these structures, contain and may secrete physiologically active catecholamines. Until the true fre-

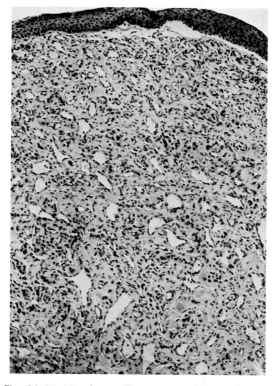

Fig. 28-30. Nonchromaffin paraganglioma (glomus tumor) of middle ear originally diagnosed as hemangioma because of prominent vascular component. However, nests of epithelioid cells with hyperchromatic oval nuclei can be noted protruding into vascular spaces.

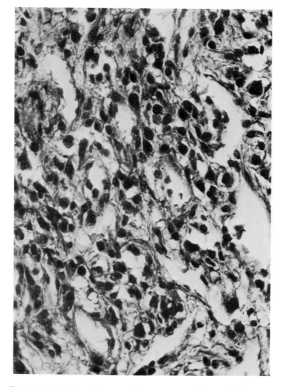

Fig. 28-31. Nonchromaffin paraganglioma (glomus tumor) of middle ear. Organoid nests of epithelioid cells in proximity to capillary spaces. Note that nests tend to protrude into vascular spaces, retaining characteristic pattern of chemoreceptor organs.

quency of functioning tumors is known, all patients with suspected paragangliomas or chemodectomas arising in the glomus jugularis complex should have routine preoperative determinations of urinary catecholamines and their metabolites. If these are found to be elevated before operation, the management is similar to that of pheochromocytoma.

These tumors may be misdiagnosed as hemangioendotheliomas. However, the structure of the glomus is readily recognized in that the lesion tends to retain the characteristic pattern and cell type (Fig. 28-30). The tumor cells are arranged in organoid intercapillary clumps, which sometimes assume an acinar pattern around small capillaries (Fig. 28-31). Since the tumor is difficult to excise, it usually recurs locally. Instances of metastasis have been reported.

Sarcoma botryoides. Sarcoma botryoides occurs most commonly between the ages of 1 and 6 years. It usually presents as a swelling situated either in the temporal bone posterior to the auricle or in the external auditory

canal. The histologic characteristics of this tumor are similar to those of sarcoma botryoides in other sites. Occasionally, a large protoplasmic strap cell is noted (see p. 1220).

Only a few cases of primary squamous cell carcinoma and adenocarcinoma of the temporal bone have been reported.

Otosclerosis

Otosclerosis generally is considered a primary, often symmetric, dystrophic disease involving the labyrinth of the temporal bone adjacent to membranous inner ear structures. There is replacement of the altered bone by localized foci of abnormal weblike bone exhibiting prominent cement lines, irregularly shaped and distributed osteocytes, and prominent vascular connective tissue marrow spaces (Fig. 28-32). This process can, over many years, replace extensive adjacent areas of temporal bone surrounding inner ear structures, or the disease may become inactive or quiescent in whole or in part at any time, with the formation of a histologically more

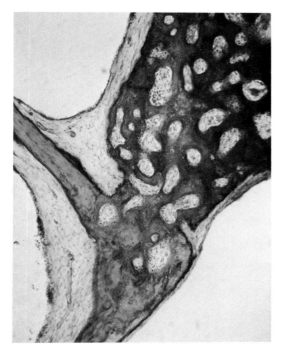

Fig. 28-32. Otosclerosis. Hypertrophic bone.

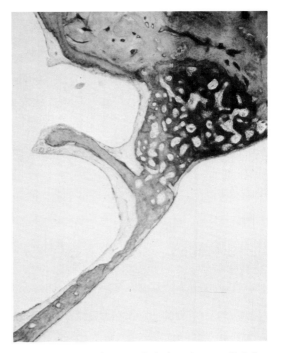

Fig. 28-33. Otosclerosis. Ankylosed stapedial foot plate.

sclerotic, mosaic type of bone. A definite etiology has not been established. Certain peculiarities have been confirmed such as occurrence only in human beings, a prominent familial predisposition, a predominance in males over females in a ratio of 2:1, and its rarity in blacks and Orientals as compared to whites. A high incidence of otosclerosis has been established in association with osteogenesis imperfecta. The onset of clinical otosclerosis varies from midchildhood to late middle adult life, with the majority of patients noting hearing loss soon after puberty.

The primary foci of otosclerotic bone most frequently are found in an area of the temporal bone just anterior to the oval window, with other primary sites, listed in order of frequency, being the bone surrounding the round window, the internal auditory canal, and the semicircular canals. Extension of the foci usually is found to involve the bony wall adjacent to the membranous cochlear structures. The auditory ossicles, with the exception of the footplate of the stapes, have not been clearly determined as primary foci of the disease.

Otosclerosis found in the majority of routinely examined temporal bones produces no appreciable clinical symptoms, being referred to in such cases as histologic otosclerosis. When the disease process advances to either impact or ankylose the stapedial footplate (Fig. 28-33), a conduction type of deafness results. It is then that surgical intervention may ensue, with an attempt to mobilize the fixed footplate or complete removal of the stapes with replacement by various types of prostheses. The pathologist should be reminded that the surgeon must submit the stapedial footplate if a histologic diagnosis of otosclerosis is likely to be made, for seldom will the disease be found to involve the crura or head of the stapes. A sensorineural type of deafness has been described in clinical otosclerosis and is believed to be in some way attributable to involvement by the disease of the bone adjacent to the membranous cochlear structures.

REFERENCES
Miscellaneous

1 Ash, J. E., and Raum, M.: Atlas of otolaryngic pathology, Washington, D. C., 1956, American Academy of Ophthalmology and Otolaryngology, American Registry of Pathology, and Armed Forces Institute of Pathology (general).

2 Holdcraft, J., and Gallagher, J. C.: Ann. Otol. Rhinol. Laryngol. 78:5-20, 1969 (malignant melanomas).

3 Kraus, F. T., and Perez-Mesa, C.: Cancer 19: 26-38, 1966 (verrucous carcinoma).

4 Masson, J. K., and Soule, E. H.: Am. J. Surg. 110:585-591, 1965 (embryonal rhabdomyosarcoma).

5 Pang, L. Q.: Arch. Otolaryngol. (Chicago) **82**: 622-628, 1965 (carcinoma of nasopharynx).

6 Prior, J. T., and Stoner, L. R.: Cancer **10**:957-963, 1957 (sarcoma botryoides).

7 Al-Saleem, T., Harwick, R., Robbins, R., and Blady, J. V.: Cancer **26**:1383-1387, 1970 (malignant lymphomas of pharynx).

Upper respiratory tract
  Nose, nasal cavity, paranasal sinuses,
  and nasopharynx

8 Fu, Y. S., and Perzin, K. H.: Non-epithelial tumors of the nasal cavity, paranasal sinuses and nasopharynx: A clinicopathologic study. I. General features and vascular tumors, Cancer **33**:1275, 1974.

9 Fu, Y. S., and Perzin, K. H.: Non-epithelial tumors of the nasal cavity, paranasal sinuses and nasopharynx: A clinicopathologic study. II. Osseous and fibro-osseous lesions including osteoma, fibrous dysplasia, ossifying fibroma, osteoblastoma, giant cell tumor and osteosarcoma, Cancer **34**:1289, 1974.

10 Fu, Y. S., and Perzin, K. H.: Non-epithelial tumors of the nasal cavity, paranasal sinuses and nasopharynx: A clinicopathologic study. III. Cartilaginous tumors (chondroma, chondrosarcoma), Cancer **34**:453, 1974.

11 Fu, Y. S., and Perzin, K. H.: Non-epithelial tumors of the nasal cavity, paranasal sinuses and nasopharynx: A clinicopathologic study. IV. Smooth muscle tumors (leiomyoma, leiomyosarcoma), Cancer **35**:1300, 1975.

12 McGavran, M. H., Sessions, D. G., Dorfman, R. F., Davis, D. O., and Ogura J. H.: Nasopharyngeal angiofibroma, Arch. Otolaryngol. **90**:68, 1969.

13 Norris, H. J.: Papillary lesions of the nasal cavity and paranasal sinuses. Part I. Exophytic (squamous) papillomas. A study of 28 cases, Laryngoscope **72**:1784, 1962.

14 Norris, H. J.: Papillary lesions of the nasal cavity and paranasal sinuses. Part II. Inverting papillomas. A study of 29 cases, Laryngoscope **73**:1, 1963.

15 Ringertz, N.: Pathology of malignant tumors arising in the nasal and paranasal cavities and maxilla, Acta Otolaryngol. **27**(suppl.):31, 1938.

16 Snyder, R. N., and Perzin, K. H.: Papillomatosis of nasal cavity and paranasal sinuses (inverted papilloma, squamous papilloma). A clinicopathologic study), Cancer **30**:668, 1972.

Phycomycosis

17 Battock, D. J., Grausz, H., Bobrowsky, M., and Littman, M. L.: Ann. Intern. Med. **68**:122-137, 1968.

18 Bergstrom, L., Hemenway, W. G., and Barnhart, R. A.: Ann. Otol. Rhinol. Laryngol. **79**:70-81, 1970 (mucormycosis).

19 Berk, M., Fink, G. I., and Uyeda, C. T.: J.A.M.A. **177**:511-513, 1961.

20 Hoagland, R. J., Sube, J., Bishop, R. H., Jr., and Holding B. F. Jr.: Am. J. Med. Sci. **242**:415-422, 1961.

21 McBride, R. A., Corson, J. M., and Dammin, G. J.: Am. J. Med. **28**:832-846, 1960.

22 Straatsma, B. R., Zimmerman, L. E., and Gass, J. M. Lab. Invest. **11**:963-985, 1962.

Lethal midline granuloma, Wegener's granulomatosis

23 Alarcón-Segovia, D., and Brown, A. L., Jr.: Proc. Mayo Clin. **39**:205-222, 1964.

24 Berman, D. A., Rydell, R. E., and Eichenholz, A.: Ann. Intern. Med. **59**:521-530, 1963.

25 Byrd, L. J., Shearn, M. A., and Tu, W. H.: Arthritis Rheum. **12**:247-253, 1969 (Wegener's granulomatosis).

26 Cassan, S. M., Divertie, M. B., Hollenhorst, R. W., and Harrison, E. G. Jr.: Ann. Intern. Med. **72**:687-693, 1970 (orbital pseudotumor and Wegener's granulomatosis).

27 Edgerton, M. T., and Desprez, J. D.: Br. J. Plast. Surg. **9**:200-211, 1956.

28 Elsner, B., and Harper, F. B.: Arch. Pathol. (Chicago) **87**:544-547, 1969 (Wegener's granulomatosis).

29 Feldman, F., Fink, H., and Gruezo, Z.: Am. J. Dis. Child. **112**:587-592, 1966 (Wegener's granulomatosis).

30 Fisher, J. H.: Can. Med. Assoc. J. **90**:10-14, 1964 (Wegener's granulomatosis).

31 Greenspan, E. M.: J.A.M.A. **193**:74-76, 1965 (therapy).

32 Kassel, S. H., Echevarria, R. A., and Guzzo, F. P. Malignant reticulosis, Cancer **23**:920, 1969.

33 Kunkel, G., Hüttemann, U., and Nickling, H. G.: Dtsch. Med. Wochenschr. **94**:959-965, 1969 (Wegener's granulomatosis).

34 McIlvanie, S. K.: J.A.M.A. **197**:130-132, 1966 (therapy).

35 Novack, S. N., and Pearson, C. M.: New Eng. J. Med. **284**:938-942, 1971 (therapy—Wegener's granulomatosis).

Relapsing polychondritis

36 Dolan, D. L., Lemmon, G. B., Jr., and Teitelbaum, S. L.: Am. J. Med. **41**:285-299, 1966.

37 Kaye, R. L., and Sones, S. A.: Ann. Intern. Med. **60**:653-664, 1964.

38 Spritzer, H. W., Weaver, A. L., Diamond, H. S., and Overholdt E. L.: J.A.M.A. **208**:355-357, 1969.

Juvenile nasopharyngeal angiofibroma

39 Apostol, J. V., and Frazell, E. L.: Cancer **18**:869-878, 1965.

40 Furstenberg, A. C., and Boles, R.: Trans. Am. Acad. Ophthalmol. Otolaryngol. **67**:518-523, 1963.

41 Schiff, M.: Laryngoscope **69**:981-1016, 1959.

Synovial tumors of hypopharynx

42 Cadman, N. L., Soule, E. H., and Kelly, P. J.: Cancer **18**:613-627, 1965.

43 Harrison E. G., Jr., Black, B. M., and Devine, K. D. Arch. Pathol. (Chicago) **71**:137-141, 1961.

44 Jernstrom, P.: Am. J. Clin. Pathol. **24**:957-961, 1954.

45 McCormack, L. J., and Parker, W.: Cleve. Clin. Q. **23**:260-264, 1956.

46 Mackenzie, D. H.: Cancer **19:**169-180, 1966.

47 Martens, V. E.: J.A.M.A. **157:**888-890, 1955.

Extramedullary plasmacytoma

48 Rawson, A. J., Eyler, P. W., and Horn, R. C., Jr.: Am. J. Pathol. **26:**445-461, 1950.

49 Stout, A. P., and Kenney, F. R.: Cancer **2:**261-278, 1949.

50 Webb, H. E., Hoover, N. W., Nichols, D. R., and Weed, L. A.: Cancer **15:**1142-1155, 1962.

Neurogenic tumors

51 Berger, L., and Coutard, H.: Bull. Assoc. Franc. Cancer **15:**404-414, 1926.

52 Cummings, C. W., Montgomery, W. W., and Balogh, K., Jr.: Ann. Otol. Rhinol. Laryngol. **78:**76-95, 1969 (neurogenic tumors of larynx).

53 Fisher, E. R.: Arch. Pathol. (Chicago) **60:**435-439, 1955.

54 Fruhling, L., and Wild, C.: Arch. Otolaryngol. (Chicago) **60:**37-48, 1954.

55 Lewis, J. S., Hutter, R. V. P., Tollefsen, H. R., and Foote, F. W.: Arch. Otolaryngol. (Chicago) **81:**169-174, 1965.

56 McCormack, L. J., and Harris, H. E.: J.A.M.A. **157:**318-321, 1955.

57 Mendeloff, J.: Cancer **10:**944-956, 1957.

58 Oberman, H. A., and Sullenger, G.: Cancer **20:**1992-2001, 1967.

59 Schall, L. A., and Lineback, M.: Ann. Otol. Rhinol. Laryngol. **60:**221-229, 1951.

60 Seaman, W. B.: Radiology **57:**541-546, 1951.

61 Thaler, S. U., and Smith, H. W.: Arch. Otolaryngol. (Chicago) **83:**233-236, 1966.

Larynx

62 Addy, M. G., Ellis, P. D. M., and Turk, D. C.: *Haemophilus* epiglottitis: nine recent cases in Oxford, Br. Med. J. **1:**40, 1972.

63 Batsakis, J. G., and Fox, J. E.: Rhabdomyosarcoma of the larynx, Arch. Otolaryngol. **91:**136-140, 1970.

64 Batsakis, J. G., and Fox, J. E.: Supporting tissue neoplasms of the larynx, Surg. Gynecol. Obstet. **131:**989-997, 1970.

65 Bauer, W. C., Edwards, D. L., and McGavran, M. H.: A critical analysis of laryngectomy in the treatment of epidermoid carcinoma of the larynx, Cancer **15:**263-270, 1962.

66 Bauer, W. C., and McGavran, M. H.: Carcinoma-in-situ and evaluation of epithelial changes in laryngo-pharyngeal biopsies, J.A.M.A. **221:**72-75, 1972.

67 Booth, J. B., and Osborn, D. A.: Granular cell myoblastoma of the larynx, Acta Otolaryngol. (Stockh.) **70:**279-293, 1970.

68 Burroughs, N., and Leape, L. L.: Laryngotracheoesophageal cleft: Report of a case successfully treated and review of the literature, Pediatrics **53:**516, 1974.

69 Holinger, P. H., and Brown, W. T.: Congenital webs, cysts, laryngoceles, and other anomalies of the larynx, Ann. Otol. Rhinol. Laryngol. **76:**744, 1967.

70 Holinger, P. H., Schild, J. A., and Maurizi, D. G.: Laryngeal papilloma; review of etiology and therapy, Laryngoscope **78:**1462-1474, 1968.

71 McGavran, M. H., Bauer, W. C., and Ogura, J. H.: Isolated laryngeal keratosis; its relation to carcinoma of the larynx based on a clinicopathologic study of 87 consecutive cases with long-term follow-up, Laryngoscope **70:**932-951, 1960.

72 Meesen, J., and Schultz, H.: Electron microscope demonstration of a virus in human laryngeal papilloma, Klin. Wochenschr. **35:**771-773, 1957.

73 Moore, R. L., and Lattes, R.: Papillomatosis of the larynx and bronchi, Cancer **12:**117-126, 1959.

74 Rabbett, W. F.: Juvenile laryngeal papillomatosis. The relation of irradiation to malignant degeneration in this disease, Trans. Am. Bronchoesoph. Assoc. **45:**115-129, 1965.

75 Tefft, M.: The radiotherapeutic management of subglottic hemangioma in children, Radiology **85:**207-214, 1966.

76 Vetters, J. M., and Toner, P. G.: Chemodectoma of the larynx, J. Pathol. **101:**259-265, 1970.

77 VanNostrand, A. W. P., and Olafsson, J.: Verrucous carcinoma of the larynx. A clinical and pathologic study of 10 cases, Cancer **30:**691, 1972.

78 Witzleben, C. L.: Aplasia of the trachea, Pediatrics **32:**31, 1963.

Ear

79 Batsakis, J. G., Hardy, G. C., and Hishiyama, R. H.: Arch. Otolaryngol. (Chicago) **86:**66-69, 1967 (ceruminal gland tumors).

80 Cankar, V., and Crowley, H.: Cancer **17:**67-75, 1964 (ceruminal gland tumors).

81 Kingery, A. J.: J.A.M.A. **197:**137, 1966 (chondrodermatitis helicis).

82 Levit, S. A., Sheps, S. G., Espinosa, R. E., Remine, W. H., and Harrison, E. G., Jr.: New Eng. J. Med. **281:**805, 1969 (glomus tumors).

83 Rosenwasser, H.: Arch. Otolaryngol. (Chicago) **88:**1-40, 1968 (glomus tumors).

84 Schermer, K. L., Pontius, E. E., Dziabis, M. D., and McQuiston, R. J.: Cancer **19:**1273-1280, 1966 (glomus tumors).

85 Shuman, R., and Helwig, E. B.: Am. J. Clin. Pathol. **24:**126-144, 1954 (chondrodermatitis helicis).

86 Simonton, K. M.: J.A.M.A. **206:**1531-1534, 1968 (glomus tumors).

Otosclerosis

87 Altman, F.: Henry Ford Hospital International Symposium on Otosclerosis, Boston, 1960, Little, Brown & Co.

88 Guild, S. R.: Ann. Otol. Rhinol. Laryngol. **53:**246-266, 1944.

89 Gussen, R.: Acta Otolaryngol. (Stockh.) suppl. 248, pp. 1-38, 1969.

90 Shambaugh, G. E., Jr.: Surgery of the ear, ed. 2, Philadelphia, 1967, W. B. Saunders Co., p. 475.

91 Transactions of the American Otological Society, Inc., vol. LIV, (Ninety-ninth annual meeting, April 18 and 19, 1966), St. Louis, 1966, American Otological Society, Inc. (Z-P Graphic Arts Service, Inc.).

29/Face, lips, teeth, mouth, jaws, salivary glands, and neck

ROBERT A. VICKERS
ROBERT J. GORLIN

FACE AND LIPS
Developmental anomalies including minor variations from normal

Facial clefts. Facial cleft, occurring in approximately 1 of every 800 white births, may exist as an isolated anomaly or in combination with other developmental disturbances (about 15% of clefts are so associated). Clefts have a racial predilection. They are most frequent in Amerindians and least common in Afro-Americans.[1,11] Clefts in combination with other developmental disturbances may be so well known as to constitute a syndrome. These symptom complexes are numerous and only a few may be considered here. Similarly, details of lateral facial clefts, pseudoclefts, cleft uvula, and microforms are left for comprehensive discussions.[2,11]

Facial clefts arise from the failure of the ectomesenchyme to cross the junction of fusion of facial processes about the sixth or seventh week in utero. Thus *cleft upper lip (harelip),* the most common facial cleft, results from failure of fusion of the lower part of the median nasal (globular) process with the maxillary process. Unilateral cleft is about eight times more common than bilateral involvement. It is more common in males (about 60%) and on the left side (about 2 : 1). The degree of cleavage may vary from a slight notch at the lateral border of the philtrum to a complete separation extending into the nostril.[1,2]

Commonly (in about 50% of cases), cleft lip (cheiloschisis) is associated with *cleft palate* (palatoschisis). When the cleft extends through the line of fusion between the premaxilla and the maxilla, the area subsequently to be occupied by the developing lateral incisor frequently is disturbed. Supernumerary, impacted, or (most commonly) missing maxillary lateral incisors often are observed.

Cleft palate also may exist to varying degrees, ranging from fissure of the azygos or tip of the uvula (uvula fissa) to complete cleft. Not uncommonly, a submucous palatal cleft may remain undetected. Cleft palate unassociated with cleft lip (about 25%) is seen more commonly in females. Associated with abnormally small mandible (micrognathia) and tongue (microglossia) and posterior displacement of the tongue (glossoptosis), it is known as *Robin anomaly.* Cleft lip and cleft palate may be associated with chromosomal abnormalities; e.g., cleft lip with cleft palate is seen in trisomy 13, cleft palate occurs in about 5% of the cases of the XXXXY syndrome (a poly-X variant of Klinefelter's syndrome), and cleft lip or cleft palate, or both, occur in about 15% of the cases of trisomy 18.[11]

The tongue is cleft into two to four lobes in association with asymmetric cleft palate, pseudocleft of the upper lip, and digital anomalies in the *orofaciodigital syndromes.*[2]

Congenital lip pits. Congenital paramedian pits of the lower lip vary in size from small bilateral dimples on the vermilion border to large snoutlike structures in the midline (Fig. 29-1). Resulting fistulas are lined by stratified squamous epithelium and are connected at the base with the mucous glands of the lip by means of communicating ducts. Mucus may be observed exuding from the openings.

The pits may occur alone or in combination with cleft palate or cleft lip as part of a syndrome (66%). Inheritance is autosomal dominant with variable expressivity.[8] An unrelated condition, *commissural lip pits,* is observed on one or both sides in frequencies up to 15% of those examined.

Median rhomboid "glossitis." Median rhomboid "glossitis" is manifest as a roughly diamond-shaped reddish pattern on the dorsum of the tongue, immediately anterior to the

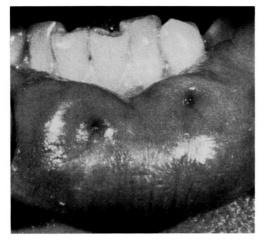

Fig. 29-1. Congenital lip pits (fistulas). Usually bilateral, frequently associated with facial clefts, and symmetrically situated on vermilion border of lower lip, fistulas represent failure of closure of evanescent sulci that appear in 10 to 14 mm embryo.

circumvallate papillae. Occurring in somewhat less than 1% of individuals, it reportedly represents developmental failure of coverage of the tuberculum impar by the lateral tubercles of the tongue. *Candida albicans* infection has also been etiologically implicated. It may arouse suspicion of malignant neoplasm in the minds of clinicians unaware of the nature of this condition.[1,5]

Fissured tongue. Fissured tongue occurs in about 5% of the population, with the frequency increasing with age. It is noted more commonly in Down's syndrome, being present in about 30% of affected individuals, and is also part of the Melkersson-Rosenthal syndrome (upper facial edema, facial palsy, cheilitis granulomatosa).[1,5]

Fordyce's granules. Fordyce's granules are collections of sebaceous glands symmetrically located on the lateral vermilion part of the upper lip and on the buccal mucosa of approximately 65% of adults. The most common oral mucosal sites are lateral to the angle of the mouth about Stensen's papilla, and lateral to the anterior pillar of the fauces.[1,5]

TEETH
Developmental anomalies of teeth

Anomalies of number. Rarely is there complete absence of teeth (anodontia) or noticeable suppression in tooth formation (oligodontia). More commonly, a mild reduction in number (hypodontia) is observed.[4,24] The

third molars, less commonly the maxillary lateral incisors and second premolars, are the teeth most likely to be missing. Radiation to the jaws may injure or inhibit developing tooth buds. Supernumerary teeth occasionally are observed—most commonly mesiodens in the midline of the maxilla and extra molars, posterior to the third molars.[4,24]

Anomalies of size. Rarely are all the teeth too large or too small. More frequently, a single tooth is reduced in size (microdontia) or disproportionately enlarged (macrodontia).

Anomalies of shape. An anomaly called "dens invaginatus (dens in dente)" is manifest most commonly in the maxillary lateral incisor. A similar anomaly may occur in premolars.[4,24]

Anomalies of eruption. Rarely (1 in 2000 white infants, but more common among Amerindians) are teeth present at birth (natal teeth). This condition may occur idiopathically or, occasionally, in association with other anomalies (chondroectodermal dysplasia, pachyonychia congenita, oculomandibulodyscephaly) in the neonatal period. Delay in eruption may be related to physical obstruction (impaction), endocrine disturbances (cretinism), or a multitude of other causes (cleidocranial dysplasia, fibromatosis gingivae, etc.).[1,2,4]

Anomalies of dental pigmentation. The teeth may be discolored as a result of exogenous (usually chromogenic bacteria) or endogenous (usually altered blood pigments) factors—internal hemorrhage from trauma, congenital porphyria, erythroblastosis fetalis, etc.[1,4,25] Tetracyclines administered to the mother during the last trimester of pregnancy or to the infant are also incorporated in developing teeth, producing a yellow to gray color. Their presence may be demonstrated by a noticeable yellow fluorescence under ultraviolet light.[25]

Premature loss of teeth. Premature loss of a tooth or teeth may be attributable to trauma, mercury poisoning, hypophosphatasia, cyclic or chronic neutropenia, premature periodontoclasia with hyperkeratosis of palms and soles (Papillon-Lefèvre syndrome), or histiocytosis X.[1,4,5]

Hereditary enamel defects. These occur in about 1 in 16,000 children, affecting both dentitions. According to Witkop and Rao[25] there appear to be at least 10 distinct types.

In the hereditary enamel dysplasias, the teeth are frequently brown and the enamel has a tendency to flake off, but the enamel

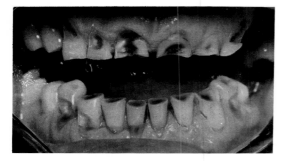

Fig. 29-2. Dental erosion. Characterized by smooth surface dissolution of enamel, especially at cervical portion, condition is of unknown etiology.

varies in hardness and thickness according to the specific type. The underlying dentin and the root formation are entirely normal, in contrast to dentinogenesis imperfecta and dentin dysplasia.

Hereditary dentin defects. Only two dentin defects may be considered here: dentinogenesis imperfecta (hereditary opalescent dentin) and dentin dysplasia. Both are transmitted as autosomal dominant traits.[4,5a,25]

Dentinogenesis imperfecta usually occurs as an isolated phenomenon (1 in 8000 individuals). A somewhat similar condition may occur as a component of osteogenesis imperfecta, blue scleras, otosclerosis, laxity of ligaments, etc. Both deciduous and permanent teeth have an opalescent blue to brown color. Because of poor attachment at or near the dentinoenamel junction, the enamel fractures off. The roots are frequently thin and short and the canals obliterated. Microscopically, irregularly arranged dentinal tubules and defective matrix formation are noted.[4,24,25]

Dentin dysplasia is characterized by rootless malaligned teeth, generally exhibiting an absence of pulp chambers and canals but normal-appearing crowns.[25] Many teeth exhibit large periapical radiolucencies, and a pathognomonic half moon–shaped pulp chamber may be seen on roentgenographic examination.

Other enamel disturbances. Nonhereditary enamel disturbances may affect either dentition, and they may be widespread or involve but a single tooth. The disturbance may be severe, causing deep pitted grooves, or so mild as to be manifest by only a small chalky spot. Defective enamel may result from injury to the enamel organ at any time from the earliest period of matrix formation to the last stage when calcification is taking place or result from acquired abnormalities such as in dental erosion (Fig. 29-2).

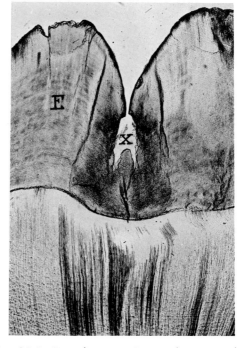

Fig. 29-3. Dental caries. Fissure lesion resulted in establishment of cavity, **X**, in enamel, **E**. Ground section of molar.·

Nutritional deficiencies (calcium, phosphorus, vitamin D), endocrine and related disorders (hypoparathyroidism, pseudohypoparathyroidism, hypophosphatasia, rickets), congenital syphilis, infection of the deciduous precursor *(Turner's tooth)*, ingestion of excessive fluoride (in excess of 1.5 ppm), and many miscellaneous conditions can injure the developing ameloblast, producing enamel hypoplasia.[1]

Other dentin disturbances. The rate of dentin formation is less than normal in scurvy. In rickets, the developing dentin is hypocalcified, with a wide margin of predentin analogous to the wide osteoid seams in forming bone.

Vitamin D–resistant rickets, an X-linked dominant trait, is associated with defective dentin formation and resultant periapical abscess development. Similar changes have been reported in a variety of related metabolic disorders.[1,4,5a]

Diseases of teeth

Dental caries. Dental caries is a disease of the enamel, dentin, and cementum that produces progressive demineralization of the calcified component and destruction of the organic component, with the formation of a cavity in the tooth (Fig. 29-3). Microorganisms are present at all stages of the disease and, from the results of animal experiments, appear to be essential etiologic factors.[1,4,17,17a,19] Specific strains of streptococci have been shown to induce dental caries in rats and in hamsters. Destruction of tooth structure by caries is easily differentiated from dental erosion and abrasion.

Tooth decay occurs or has occurred in the majority of individuals living in the United States, Canada, and Europe. Once a carious cavity has formed, the defect is permanent. The designation DMF (decayed, missing, filled) has proved useful in comparative studies of the frequency of dental caries, particularly in children and young adults. After the introduction of fluoride to the drinking water (1 ppm)—the more practical method—the DMF rate has generally decreased over a period of years by more than 50%.[16,16a,21,22]

Studies throughout the world have given striking evidence of the efficiency of fluoridation of communal water supplies in reducing the rate of tooth decay in children.[23a] Partial control of tooth decay by this method constitutes an important public health achievement. Topical applications of fluoride solutions to tooth surfaces and brushing the teeth with dentifrices containing fluoride appear to be effective in further reducing susceptibility to dental caries.

Excessive amounts of fluoride cause a condition called mottled enamel. It occurs in children who have consumed drinking water containing 1.5 ppm fluoride or more during the time when tooth enamel is being deposited in the developing, unerupted teeth.

Caries occurs in areas on tooth surfaces where saliva, food debris, and bacterial plaques accumulate. These areas are chiefly the pits and fissures, cervical part of the tooth, and interproximal surfaces. Surfaces that are cleansed by the excursion of food and the action of the tongue and cheeks are usually free of caries. If this process is interfered with (e.g., by prosthetic appliances or lack of saliva), caries may develop rapidly.

The formation of bacterial plaques in areas of stagnation precedes cavity formation in, especially, smooth dental surfaces. Acidogenic and aciduric bacteria, together with filamentous forms, are present in such plaques[4,17] (Fig. 29-4).

Pulp and periapical periodontal disease. The tooth, projecting into the oral cavity through the mucous membrane and extending deep into the jawbone, affords a surprisingly direct pathway for infection after exposure and infection of the dental pulp and after ulceration or breakdown of the epithelial attachments.

Carious destruction of dental hard tissues frequently produces pulpitis or inflammation of dental soft tissue, including, by way of extension, those surrounding the end or apex of the tooth. An alternative, yet equally dentally threatening pathway exists through the gin-

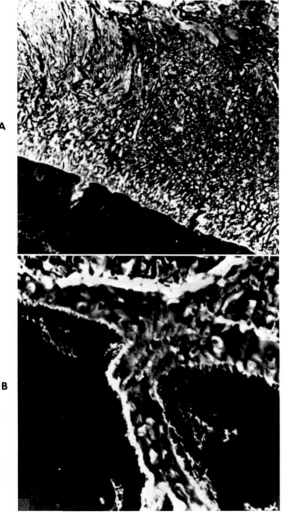

A

B

Fig. 29-4. Bacterial plaque isolated by acid flotation from clinically noncarious enamel. **B,** Mass of bacteria at enamel surface extending from plaque into lamella. (**A,** 2000×; **B,** 6000×; **A** and **B,** from Scott, D. B., and Albright, J. T.: Oral Surg. **7:**64-78, 1954.)

gival attachment (see following discussion concerning periodontal disease).

Inflammation of the dental pulp may be noninfected. Trauma to the tooth from a blow, which may or may not fracture the tooth, from dental operations, or from excessive thermal changes may also induce inflammation. This may be minimal with recovery, particularly in teeth with incompletely formed roots, or it may be severe leading to necrosis.

Pulpitis, regardless of the etiologic agent, may be acute or chronic. In acute pulpitis, pain is usually severe and increased by heat or cold. Pulpitis, acute or chronic, may be asymptomatic or accompanied by a mild fever and leukocytosis. Periapical tissues become involved by extension.

Acute alveolar or periapical abscess is usually the result of spread of suppurative infection from the tooth pulp through the root canals to the periodontal ligament about the

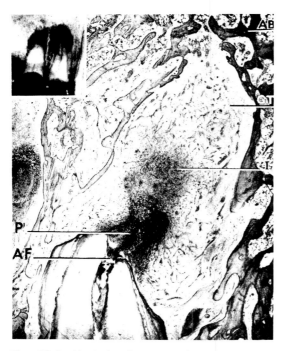

Fig. 29-5. Mesiodistal section through apex of maxillary first premolar with granuloma. *Inset,* Roentgenogram of specimen shows large areas of bone destruction around root ends of both maxillary premolars. **AB,** Alveolar bone. **AF,** Apical foramen. **GT,** Granulation tissue. **I,** Dense cellular infiltration next to foramen. **P,** Breaking down of tissue and formation of pus at foramen. (From Boyle, P. E., editor: Kronfeld's Histopathology of the teeth and their surrounding structures, Philadelphia, 1955, Lea & Febiger.)

tooth root ends. Drainage to the surface of adjacent skin of the face or neck may follow.

A more common sequela to dental pulp infection is the dental granuloma. Clinically, this may be completely symptomless. Radiographic examination frequently discloses an area of bone rarefaction about a tooth root apex, with a chronically infected or partially obliterated root canal. This area is usually spherical and well demarcated. Histologically, the tissue consists of fibrous connective tissue, often heavily infiltrated by lymphocytes and plasma cells, surrounding necrotic tissue at the apex of the root canal foramen or within the pulp canal. Peripherally, loose and dense connective tissue merges into the surrounding bone, which may develop a definite cortical layer (Fig. 29-5).

Remnants of epithelium (rests of Malassez) are found in the periodontal ligament, surrounding the teeth. In granulomas, this epithelium may proliferate. The root end may become surrounded by fluid with epithelium lining the surface, thus forming a cyst. The cyst may enlarge to a considerable size. Although epithelium is present in practically all granulomas and often proliferates to line small cystic cavities, the development of large cysts is relatively uncommon. (See also section on odontogenic cysts.)

Periodontal disease. The inflammatory and degenerative processes that develop at the gingival margin and progress until the tooth-supporting structures are lost have much in common with periapical periodontal disease. In both instances, chronic asymptomatic infection by the common oral pathogens is usual, although episodes of acute suppuration may occur. The reactions in both are a walling-off process with a pronounced chronic inflammatory cell infiltration. The proliferation of epithelium is always present in the marginal form of periodontal disease. It represents an attempt to cover the surface of the chronic ulcer that develops about the involved tooth root area (Figs. 29-6 and 29-7).

The disease commonly begins as a gingivitis. Deposits of plaque and calculus upon the tooth surfaces, impaction of food, decayed teeth, overhanging margins of dental restorations, and ill-fitting dental appliances are among the local causes.[23] Once this "pocket" has been established below the gingival margin, calcified deposits form on the tooth root surfaces and act as an infected foreign body, thus prolonging and promoting the inflammatory process, with progressive resorption of tooth-sup-

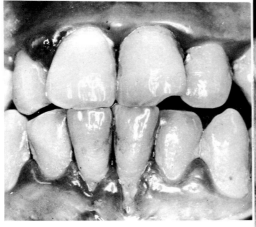

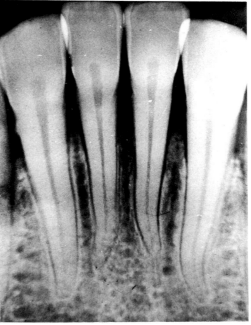

Fig. 29-6. Periodontitis. Edema, periodontal abscess, hemorrhage upon slight pressure, tissue recession with retraction of gingival margin, color change from light pink to deep red, loss of tissue in interdental area, horizontal bone loss, and widening of periodontal space. See Fig. 29-7.

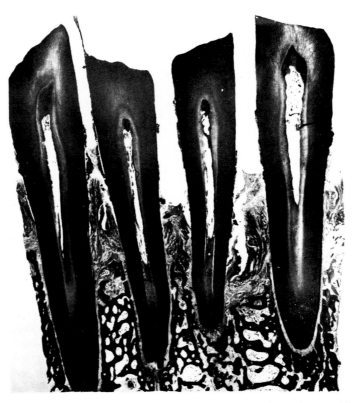

Fig. 29-7. Periodontitis (advanced). Mesiodistal section through mandibular incisors. Chronic inflammation of gingiva followed by proliferation of epithelium of gingival attachment along cementum, excessive osteoclastic resorption of interdental bone, and deep periodontal pocket formation between gingiva and surface of roots.

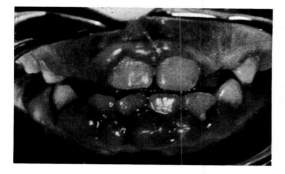

Fig. 29-8. Hyperplasia of gingiva associated with diphenylhydantoin (Dilantin).

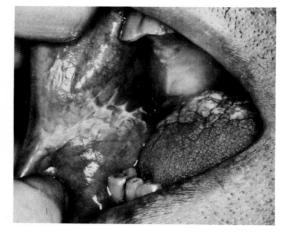

Fig. 29-9. Lichen planus of buccal mucosa. Dorsum of tongue also involved. (Courtesy Dr. Jens O. Andreasen, Copenhagen.)

porting structures. Proliferation of epithelium to line the pocket occurs concomitantly with the loss of tissue. A purulent discharge from periodontal pockets can usually be elicited by digital pressure in many adult patients and even may occur in adolescents. Some individuals may show great resistance to the development of periodontal pockets despite adverse local factors, just as others have an extraordinary resistance to dental caries. Periodontal disease is more common in older individuals, and after middle age it becomes the chief cause of tooth loss.[23]

Pregnancy with its change in endocrine balance frequently is accompanied by gingivitis and hyperplastic inflammatory responses. Gingivitis may be somewhat more frequent during puberty.[70]

Drug action may cause gingival response. The hyperplasia associated with the use of diphenylhydantoin (Dilantin) sodium may be so extensive that the teeth are almost completely covered by gingival enlargement[18,23, 27,70] (Fig. 29-8).

MOUTH
Mucocutaneous diseases

Although mucocutaneous disorders constitute a heterogeneous group, they are conveniently discussed together.

Lichen planus. Lichen planus usually appears as an irregular, lacelike whitening of the buccal mucosa (Fig. 29-9), but other oral areas (gingiva, tongue, palate, etc.) also may be involved and the clinical appearance also may be bullous or erosive. Approximately one third of affected patients have only oral lesions. The other two thirds have only cutaneous or skin and oral manifestations. Mucosal surfaces of other body sites are much less frequently involved. The diagnosis may be suspected when the lacelike whitening of the surface of the

buccal mucosa (Wickham's striae) is seen. Biopsies of nonulcerated whitenings may be used in the diagnosis.[26,63]

The cause of lichen planus is not known. Patients are most frequently between 40 and 60 years of age. Oral lesions of lichen planus do not itch. Symptoms may not be present, but pain and discomfort have been observed, especially with bullous or atrophic types of the disease. Approximately one half of the patients observe concurrent "nervous stress" and express anxiety or fear of having oral cancer.

Pemphigus. Pemphigus, especially pemphigus vulgaris, characteristically involves the oral mucosa during its course and may appear initially in this location. The oral tissues are very red, friable, and pebbly (Fig. 29-10). Vesicle and bulla formation is observed, but the blisters do not remain intact for long periods in the mouth. Smear preparations, biopsies of oral sites, and immunofluorescence are most useful in establishing a diagnosis (Fig. 29-11).

Benign mucous membrane pemphigoid. Benign mucous membrane pemphigoid is a vesicular or bullous disease involving the oral mucosa. Conjunctival tissues are frequently affected also, and the associated inflammation and scarring of this site are most serious sequelae.[39] Microscopically, vesicle formation occurs immediately below the epithelium, and biopsy specimens of the short-lived vesicles are helpful in establishing the diagnosis, as are immunofluorescence studies.[50]

Erythema multiforme. Erythema multiforme is characterized by large, erosive, frequently hemorrhagic lesions of the lips, buccal mucosa, and tongue. Oral and facial tissues are in-

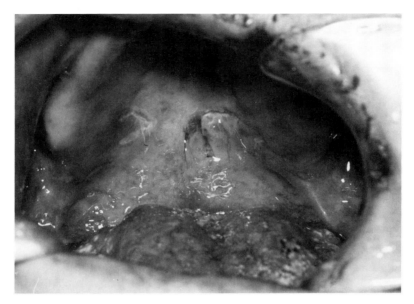

Fig. 29-10. Pemphigus involving palatal mucosa.

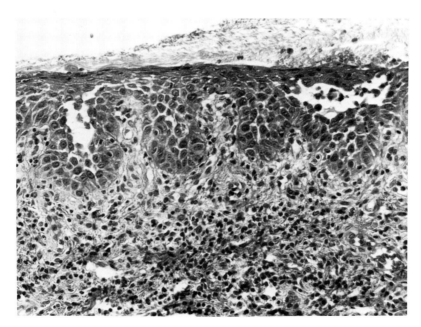

Fig. 29-11. Biopsy of oral mucosa in pemphigus showing intraepithelial acantholysis.

volved in approximately 25% of the patients.

Stevens-Johnson syndrome is a term applied to clinically severe examples of erythema multiforme, especially when the conjunctiva, genitalia, and, often, lungs are involved. Further, many consider these conditions closely related to Reiter's syndrome, Behçet syndrome, and Sutton's disease.[1]

Epidermolysis bullosa. Oral tissues are involved in clinical and genetic types of epidermolysis bullosa (see p. 1814). Microstomia, after the scarring of buccal mucosa, and dental abnormalities are complications of the dystrophic forms of this disease.[44]

Others. *Keratosis follicularis* (Darier's disease),[1] *lupus erythematosus,* and *herpes zoster* are additional examples of so-called mucocutaneous conditions with oral manifestations.

Lipoid proteinosis (Urbach-Wiethe syndrome) causes extreme induration of the oral mucosa, especially that of the lips and the tongue, which becomes atrophic and bound down to the oral floor. In *primary amyloidosis,* infiltration of the tongue may be associated with *macroglossia.* Enlargement of the tongue also may be seen in an unusual form of glycogen-storage disease of muscle. Deposits of secondary amyloid in the gingiva are not clinically manifested. *Scleroderma* and *acrosclerosis* occasionally (about 7%) are associated with a widening of the periodontal ligament of the teeth.

Hairy tongue is associated with proliferation of saprophytic organisms that cause extrinsic staining of elongated filiform papillae. Although the eiology is unknown, hairy tongue may follow therapeutic use of antibiotics or radiation. *Benign migratory glossitis* (geographic tongue), also of unknown etiology, is characterized by irregular superficial areas devoid of filiform papillae. It is more common in females and is seen in about 2% of the population.[1]

Oral and labial *papillomatosis* may be associated with both the juvenile (benign) and adult (malignant) forms of *acanthosis nigricans.*[1] The oral lesions, in contrast to the cutaneous, are not pigmented.

Inflammatory diseases

Acute herpetic gingivostomatitis. Acute herpetic gingivostomatitis is the most common manifestation of primary infection with the herpes simplex virus, type 1. It is frequently misdiagnosed as necrotizing ulcerative gingivitis or Vincent's stomatitis. Occurring in less than 1% of the population, it is rarely, if ever,

seen in a child under 1 year of age. It reaches its peak between the ages of 1 and 3 years, although it also is observed in older children and in young adults. The incubation period is 4 to 6 days. The gingiva is red and swollen, is exquisitely tender, and bleeds easily. Numerous vesicles and bullae are present on the labial, lingual, and buccal mucosae.[1,5,40a,53]

Microscopically, the herpes simplex vesicle shows multinucleated giant cells having two to 15 nuclei per cell, and eosinophilic "inclusion bodies" are seen within the nuclei. Intraepithelial edema (ballooning degeneration) and intracellular edema are especially pronounced.

The herpes simplex virus may be identified by determination of neutralizing antibody titer, complement fixation, or specific skin test taken after the infection. There is a high incidence (70% to 90%) of neutralizing antibody in the adult population.[40a]

Recurrent herpes (cold sore, fever blister). Recurrent herpes simplex infections occur most frequently about the face and lips and tends to recur at the same site. The condition is characterized by groups of small, clear vesicles on an erythematous base. The recurrent lesions seem to be induced by such agents as sunshine, fever, mechanical trauma, menses, and allergy. Intraoral involvement is rare but may involve the hard palate and gingiva with pinhead-sized, grouped ulcers.[40a,45a]

Recurrent aphthae (canker sores). Although resembling the lesions of recurrent herpes, recurrent aphthae are not caused by the herpes simplex virus. Somewhat similar lesions are seen on the oral mucosa in *Reiter's syndrome* (arthritis, conjunctivitis, and urethritis) and Behçet's syndrome (orogenital ulcerations and iridocyclitis).[1,38,56,62a]

Infectious mononucleosis. Infectious mononucleosis may present pronounced oral signs. In addition to inflammation of the oral pharynx and lymphadenopathy, about one third of patients will exhibit a grayish or grayish green membrane resembling that of diphtheria or Vincent's angina over the throat or posterior buccal mucosa. The gingiva bleeds easily and becomes enlarged, resembling that in leukemia or scurvy.[30]

Hand-foot-and-mouth disease. Generally unrecognized, hand-foot-and-mouth disease is a self-limited, febrile disease caused by group A coxsackieviruses, principally type 16, less often types 5 and 10. It is manifest by many small vesicles or punched-out ulcers of the lips and buccal mucosa. The gingiva characteristically is spared, in contrast to herpetic stomatitis.

Those affected are principally children under 10 years of age. Cutaneous involvement is usually limited to the palms, soles, and ventral surfaces and sides of fingers and toes.[1,5]

Agranulocytosis. Agranulocytosis often is manifest by ragged necrotic ulcers of the gingiva, palate, tonsils, or oropharynx.[1] Sialorrhea may be profuse. Drug sensitivity, especially to the barbiturates, amidopyrine, and the sulfonamides, is the best-known cause. Similar lesions are seen in *cyclic neutropenia,* a heritable disorder in which the neutrophils are decreased every 21 days.[1,5] Various *cytotoxic agents* employed in cancer chemotherapy produce severe oral ulceration.

Lethal granuloma (midline lethal granuloma). Probably a form of malignant reticulosis, lethal granuloma involves the palate, sinuses, and nasopharynx in a severe, progressive, ulcerative, destructive process.[1,5,61]

Wegener's granulomatosis. Considered to be a form of hypersensitivity, Wegener's granulomatosis, a possible variant of polyarteritis nodosa, may be heralded by "multiple pyogenic granulomas" of the interdental papillae of the gingiva.[61]

Acute necrotizing gingivitis (Vincent's disease, fusospirochetosis). Acute necrotizing gingivitis is far less common than supposed.[23] Often the term "trench mouth" is used as a catchall to include primary herpetic gingivostomatitis, herpangina, infectious mononucleosis, etc. This is especially true in children, for fusospirochetosis is extremely uncommon in childhood (except in Africa), afflicting instead young and middle-aged adults. The disease is almost exclusively limited to the interdental papillae and the free gingival margin, rarely extending to the faucial area *(Vincent's angina).* Necrosis and ulceration of one or more interdental gingival papillae, mild fever, fetid breath, malaise, and local discomfort characterize the condition. Predisposing conditions seem to allow penetration of the oral tissues by several symbiotic organisms normally inhabiting the mouth, among these a fusiform bacillus and an oral spirochete, *Borrelia vincentii.*

Noma (cancrum oris, gangrenous stomatitis). Noma may occur as a complication of acute necrotizing gingivitis in children or, rarely, in adults debilitated by infectious disease or possibly malnourishment. It is rare other than in the Far East and Africa. The process usually begins in a gingival ulceration and rapidly spreads to involve the cheeks, lips, and jawbones. The tissues become blackened and necrotic. Pneumonia and toxemia are common sequelae.[1,4,65]

Syphilis. In both the prenatal and the acquired forms, syphilis may be manifest about the mouth.[1,4,5] In the acquired form, the primary lesion or *chancre* may appear on the lips or tongue, simulating a squamous cell carcinoma.[53a] The secondary stage is characterized by the mucous patch (a milky white, focal, superficial ulcer of the oral mucosa), sore throat, and occasionally condyloma at the corner of the mouth (split papule). The hard palate may be perforated in the tertiary stage as a result of gumma formation. The tongue may be involved with a diffuse inflammatory process *(syphilitic glossitis)* that may predispose to the development of squamous cell carcinoma. Prenatal syphilis may be demonstrated by rhagades or radiating scars about the mouth and characteristic alteration in the form of the permanent teeth *(Hutchinson's incisors* and *mulberry molars),* in addition to the changes seen in the secondary and tertiary stages of acquired syphilis.[4,60a]

Gonorrhea. The variable, clinical conditions associated with oral, tonsillar or pharyngeal infection by the gram-negative intracellular diplococcus *Neisseria gonorrhoeae* are perhaps too poorly appreciated and diagnosed. Its identification, though rare, has been documented.[36a] Generally acute, erythematous, and ulcerative with associated systemic symptoms, it may also be pseudomembranous or even vesicular in its manifestations. Burning and itching have been early subjective symptoms.

Yaws. Yaws presents lesions somewhat similar to those of syphilis. The secondary papular lesions are commonly perioral. Tertiary lesions *(gangosa)* result in extensive destruction of the soft palate, hard palate, and nose.[1]

Granuloma inguinale. Oral lesions of granuloma inguinale occur and are the most common extragenital (about 5% to 6%) manifestations of the disease.[1]

Actinomycosis. Actinomycosis of the cervicofacial type arises through invasion of oral mucous membranes or a tooth socket, spreading to involve the jawbones, musculature, and salivary glands. Multiple foci of suppuration lead into sinus tracts that drain to the cutaneous surface or oral mucosa, liberating pus containing the typical and diagnostic "sulfur granules" of *Actinomyces israelii.*[134]

Other granulomatous infections

Histoplasmosis. Oral lesions of histoplasmosis appear most frequently as nodular or ulcerated areas on the tongue or palate.[32] *Tuberculosis* of the oral tissues is rare and usually is associated with advanced pulmonary disease. The typical lesion is an irregular, slowly enlarging, painful ulcer of the base of the tongue or palate.[48]

Many other fungal and tropical diseases have oral lesions—among them tropical sprue, leishmaniasis, scleroma, leprosy, and South American blastomycosis.[1]

Candidosis (thrush). Candidosis is a fungal disease occurring most often in debilitated persons, infants, or especially individuals who have been taking oral antibiotics. It also may be associated in the form of a syndrome with hypoparathyroidism, keratoconjunctivitis, and Addison's disease. A chronic hyperplastic candidosis is often present. It is characterized by a pseudoepitheliomatous hyperplasia, with fungal invasion and a noticeable chronic inflammatory reaction. The fungus may invade the oral mucosa, skin, female genitalia, or urinary tract. Since the fungus *Candida albicans* is a normal oral inhabitant, the diagnosis cannot be made by smear alone. The presence of hyphae is more significant diagnostically. The clinical appearance is that of numerous milk-white plaques—occasionally covering the entire oral mucosa—that are easily stripped off, leaving a bleeding surface because of penetration of the mycelia. Overclosure of the jaws in the edentulous patient or in the patient with poorly constructed dentures commonly results in low-grade chronic infection at the corners of the mouth, attributable at least in part to candidal organisms. This is called *perlèche,* or *angular cheilitis.* Cheilosis caused by deficiency of one or more of the B complex vitamins is rare.

Childhood exanthematous diseases. The childhood exanthematous diseases frequently manifest oral lesions. *Koplik's spots,* one of the prodromal signs of measles, are pinhead-sized, bluish white spots surrounded by erythematous halos. They appear in the buccal or labial mucosa about 18 hours prior to the skin rash. *Warthin-Finkeldy* giant cells may be histologically observed in the tonsils or other oral lymphatic lesions.

Disturbances of pigmentation

Melanotic pigmentation. Melanin may occur in the oral mucosa and about the lips under both normal and pathologic conditions.[1,2,40] Racial pigmentation, especially of the gingiva, is the most common type and appears to be directly related to skin color. It is present not only in nearly all blacks but also in Oriental peoples and those of Mediterranean background. Little melanin is present at birth. It is deposited largely during the first decade.

Chronic adrenocortical insufficiency (Addison's disease), hemochromatosis, and Albright's syndrome (polyostotic fibrous dysplasia and precocious puberty)[33] may be associated with pigmentation of the oral mucosa as well as of the skin. Pigmentation also is seen in chronic steatorrhea and in the Peutz-Jeghers syndrome. The latter is characterized by gastrointestinal polyposis, mucocutaneous pigmentation, and autosomal dominant inheritance.[2] Palatal melanotic pigmentation may be seen after extensive use of various antimalarial drugs, such as amodiaquin (Camoquin) or chloroquine.[73] It also may be seen in patients with oral lichen planus ("melasmic" staining).

All types of melanotic nevi have been reported in oral surroundings, as has malignant melanoma.[64]

Nonmelanotic pigmentation. Nonmelanotic pigmentation usually is caused by heavy metals. Amalgam tattoo results from implantation of particles of filling material under the mucosa at the time of dental procedures. Lead, bismuth, arsenic, and mercury intoxications may be associated with a deposit of the metallic sulfide in the inflamed gingival margin.

Tumors and tumorlike lesions
Benign tumors and tumorlike lesions of the oral soft tissues

Generalized or localized enlargement of the gingiva should arouse clinical suspicion of neoplastic disease.

Enlarged gingival papillae, with bleeding upon slight pressure, are found in vitamin C deficiency (scorbutic gingivitis). Clinically similar appearances may indicate the local infiltration of the gingiva with immature leukocytes characteristic of one variety or another of leukemia.

In contrast, the gingiva may show localized or generalized enlargements that are dense and firm and that show little or no tendency to hemorrhage upon pressure. These may be associated with chronic local irritation and represent a formation of scar tissue. Diphenylhydantoin sodium (Dilantin) frequently causes a striking enlargement of the gingiva associated with a dense overgrowth of fibrous tissue (Fig. 29-8).

All gingival enlargements become traumatized during mastication, toothbrushing, etc. Plasma cells, characteristically present in the

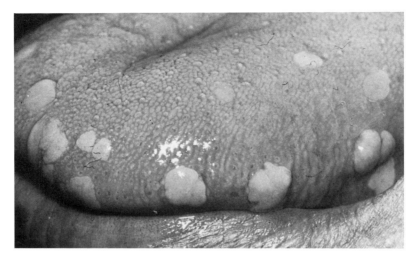

Fig. 29-12. Multiple lesions of focal epithelial hyperplasia on tongue. (From Praetorius-Clausen, F.: Pathol. Microbiol. **39:**204-213, 1973.)

gingiva in small numbers, may increase under inflammatory stimuli to simulate plasma cell myeloma or solitary plasmacytoma, but the presence of other inflammatory cells suggests plasma cell granuloma.

Fibromatosis gingivae. Fibromatosis gingivae represents a proliferation of the entire gingiva. Inflammation is characteristically absent, since the gingiva is of normal color and hard texture. The normal eruption of teeth is prevented. Fibromatosis gingivae may rarely be associated with hypertrichosis, seizures, and mental retardation. An autosomal dominant genetic pattern is common.[2] There are other varieties.[71a]

Papilloma. Papilloma is an arborescent growth consisting of numerous squamous epithelial fingerlike projections, each of which contains a well-vascularized, fibrous connective tissue core. Although it may be seen throughout the mouth, the tongue and periuvular area are common sites.[1]

Focal epithelial hyperplasia. This condition was first described by Heck as occurring on oral mucosal tissue of Navajo children and has since been observed in others, most prominently Greenlandic Eskimos.[60] It is usually a soft, nonulcerated white or reddish papule approximately 0.5 cm. in diameter (Fig. 29-12). The lesions are frequently multiple, of likely viral etiology, and have now been observed in the United States and other countries.

Fibroma. The most common benign oral mucous membrane mass is "fibroma" that occurs as a discrete superficial pedunculated mass. Such lesions appear to be nonneoplastic

in nature, arising as an exuberant response to physical trauma or other inflammatory agents. An example of this type of reaction is the so-called denture-injury tumor. Microscopically, these fibromas are composed of collagenic fibrous connective tissue covered by keratinized or parakeratinized stratified squamous epithelium. Myxomatous degeneration, metaplastic bone formation, or fatty infiltration is noted in the connective tissue.[70]

Lipoma and "amputation neuroma." Although uncommon, lipoma and "amputation neuroma" may occur, particularly in the mandibular gingivobuccal sulcus. The amputation neuroma is a pseudotumor consisting of congeries of peripheral nerve bundles that have proliferated into a knotlike mass, usually subsequent to trauma in the region of the mental foramen.[70]

Neurilemoma and neurofibroma. Neurilemoma and neurofibroma are also observed in oral environs, especially the tongue. Neurofibroma may occur as an isolated lesion or as part of Reckinghausen's *neurofibromatosis*. The lesions of the latter condition may be of at least three types: discrete, diffuse, or plexiform.[70] Both *osteoma* and *chondroma* have also been reported in the tongue.

Granular cell tumor or granular cell myoblastoma. First described by Abrikossoff in 1926 and assumed initially to be of striated muscle origin, granular cell tumor has, in recent years, been the subject of considerable controversy. Many investigators believe it to be of neural origin, whereas others suggest that it represents not a true neoplasm but

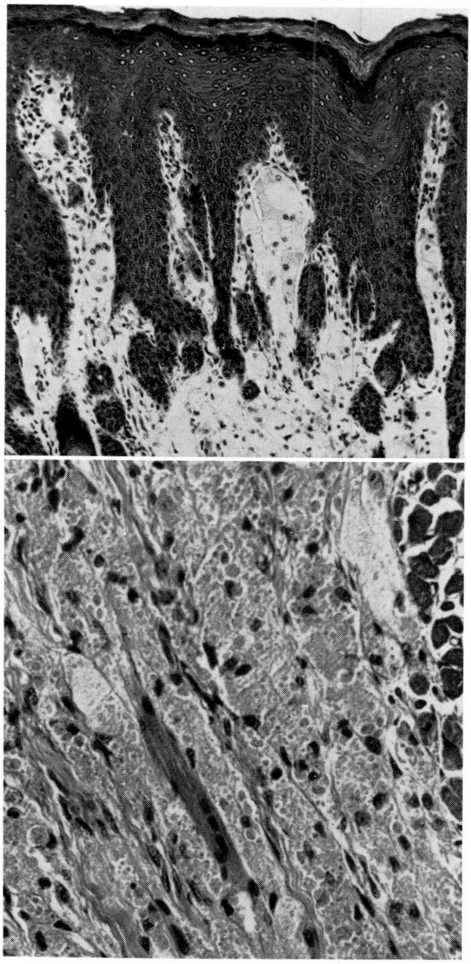

Fig. 29-13. Granular cell tumor (granular cell myoblastoma). Tongue and skin are two most frequent sites. **A,** Pseudoepitheliomatous proliferation may be pronounced, simulating squamous cell carcinoma. **B,** Tumor consists of sheet of large cells with granular eosinophilic cytoplasm and small hyperchromatic nuclei.

a special type of muscle degeneration. Histochemical and electron microscopic investigations have added support to the neural theory of origin.[28,70,72]

Granular cell myoblastoma is usually benign. Although having its origin in many tissues, especially the skin, about 40% arise in the tongue. There appears to be no age preference except for a possible variant that occurs at birth on the anterior alveolar ridges and has been called *congenital epulis of the newborn.* It is seen almost exclusively in female infants.[82a]

Microscopically, the tumor consists of large polyhedral cells with an acidophilic granular cytoplasm. Ultrastructural studies have demonstrated that the "granules" are lysosomal structures. The nucleus is small, somewhat pyknotic, and eccentrically placed. Pseudoepitheliomatous hyperplasia, characteristically absent in the congenital epulis, may be so pronounced in the tongue lesion that a diagnosis of squamous cell carcinoma is made (Fig. 29-13). Although the histology of this lesion is clear, its histogenesis is not. Other benign muscle tumors, *leiomyoma* and *rhabdomyoma,* have been reported in the tongue, lip, and uvula but are rare.[70]

Hemangioma. Hemangioma of the oral mucous membranes is essentially similar to that of the skin and may occur in any area of the mouth with many appearances. Although it is most commonly of the capillary type, cavernous and mixed types also are seen. These often congenital lesions should not be confused with the exuberant overgrowth of granulation tissue designated as *granuloma pyogenicum,* which apparently arises as the result of trauma and nonspecific infection. The granuloma pyogenicum is indistinguishable, microscopically, from the so-called *pregnancy tumor* that arises on the gingiva during the second trimester of gestation in approximately 10% of gravid females. Consisting of new capillaries, fibroblasts, and polymorphonuclear neutrophils, these lesions frequently last long after termination of pregnancy, eventuating in a fibroma-like lesion.[70]

Hereditary hemorrhagic telangiectasia (Osler-Rendu-Weber disease). Hereditary hemorrhagic telangiectasia is manifest by numerous spiderlike angiomatoses of the lips and tongue. Nasal mucosal involvement results in frequent epistaxis. Usually noted at puberty, the condition is inherited as an autosomal dominant characteristic. Microscopically, the individual lesion is a superficial blood vessel surrounded by abnormal elastic fibers that permit dilatation.[2]

Encephalofacial angiomatosis (Sturge-Weber syndrome). Encephalofacial angiomatosis consists of superficial and deep-seated hemangiomas, usually of the upper two thirds or half of the face, associated with leptomeningeal angiomas, cerebral calcifications, seizures, glaucoma, and mental retardation. There are many clinical variations.[2,70]

Lymphangioma. The majority of lymphangiomas are found at birth in the head and neck region and may cause enlargement of the tongue (macroglossia) and the lip (macrochelia). *Cystic hygroma* is a special type of lymphangioma occurring in the cervical region in the newborn infant.

Solitary plasmacytoma. Solitary plasmacytoma of the mouth occurs as a soft-tissue lesion without bone involvement (especially about the tonsillar area and antrum) or as part of a generalized myeloma. About one third of the cases of solitary plasmacytoma eventuate in multiple myeloma. There is a definite predilection for males (about 2 : 1). Rarely are they seen in individuals under 30 years of age. Grossly, they are smooth, soft, and somewhat rubbery tumors. Microscopically, they are indistinguishable from plasma cell myeloma. Differential diagnosis includes *plasma cell granuloma.*[59]

White lesions of oral mucosa

A change in color of the normally reddish oral mucosa to white constitutes one of the most frequently encountered oral abnormalities. Failure to recognize and identify the cause of this alteration can be a serious omission, since early squamous cell carcinoma may appear white.[70b]

The term "leukoplakia" has been used so differently by so many that it has come to signify only a 'white patch' that does not rub away.[58,67]

Hyperkeratoses. An increased retention and production of keratin by mucosal stratified squamous epithelium is the most frequent cause of white patches of the oral cavity. This is termed hyperkeratosis and may be associated with chronic mechanical irritation and other factors. Biopsies of oral white patches may demonstrate cytologic and histologic alterations of a degree to warrant consideration as dysplasia. Specific alterations of dysplastic or "premalignant" character include those of dyskeratosis, abnormal nuclear shapes and size, and increased numbers of mitotic figures. Most pathologists term such alterations *epithelial dysplasia.* Microscopic examination of oral white patches that do not resolve with conservative management within a short time (e.g., 1 to 2 weeks) is indicated. *Leukoedema* is a slight whitening of oral mucosa without dysplasia or abnormalities of keratinization.[29]

"*Snuffbox granuloma*" is a term denoting the white, leathery, oral patches seen in patients using snuff or intraoral tobacco. Patients using snuff have an increased incidence of oral carcinoma. The microscopy is characteristic.[64a,69]

Other white lesions. The *white oral lesions of lichen planus* were discussed previously (p. 1237 and Fig. 29-9). Wickham's striae or lace-like patterns in this condition are characteristic. Several hereditary conditions feature whitenings of the oral cavity. *Hereditary benign intraepithelial dyskeratosis, white sponge nevus (leukokeratosis heredita), pachyonychia congenita, Darier's disease,* and *dyskeratosis congenita (Zinsser-Engman-Cole syndrome)* are examples.[1,2]

Aspirin burns resulting from the unprescribed use of tablets as dental topical anesthetics or troches frequently are seen. Soft, focal, oral whitenings that peel away easily, leaving a raw, bleeding surface, are seen in *candidosis.*

Malignant tumors of oral cavity
Squamous cell carcinoma

Squamous cell carcinoma (epidermoid carcinoma) is the most common oral malignant neoplasm, and approximately 7 per 100,000 deaths in the United States are currently attributed to it annually. Further, investigations in Minnesota indicated that among adults 45 years of age or older, 1 in every 1000 examined had this lesion of the lip or other oral structure.[71] Tobacco, syphilis, and alcohol have been etiologically implicated for many years, although they are not considered primary causes.[70a] Chronic inflammations caused by poorly fitting prostheses, poor oral hygiene, or inadequate dental restorations probably is not an important etiologic factor. Approximately 10% of patients having or having had oral carcinoma have or will have another.[62] Oral white patches are observed in association with squamous cell carcinoma in up to 75% of instances, and it is considered likely that many superficial malignancies evolve in this fashion.[58]

The clinical appearance of small or early examples of the malignancy may vary from white, thickened, or verrucous to soft, red, velvety or ulcerative. Induration is also clinically suggestive of oral malignancy.

Squamous cell carcinomas of the lip or oral cavity are, generally, histologically well differentiated and occur in males 40 years of age and older. The oral cavity offers epithelial neoplasms with as great a clinicopathologic diversity as any body part; however, metastasis most frequently occurs first in ipsilateral, submandibular, or cervical lymph nodes. The presence or absence of lymph node metastasis is an important index of the clinical stage of the disease. A sarcoid reaction may be seen in regional cervical lymph nodes in perhaps 6%

of cases of carcinoma of the tongue, parotid gland, and oral cavity, especially after radiation therapy, probably as a result of the necrotic products of the tumor.

Squamous cell carcinoma of lip. Squamous cell carcinoma of the lip is almost exclusively a male disease, with less than 3% of the cases occurring in women. Originating most frequently in the sixth to eighth decades, approximately 90% arise on the vermilion border of the lower lip, usually on one side of the midline. It presents as a painless, characteristically indurated, ulcerated or exophytic lesion. Usually, lip carcinoma is well differentiated (about 60%) and slow to metastasize to the submental and submandibular nodes. Prognosis is good[70a] whether the lesion is treated by radiation or by surgery, 5-year cure rates being about equal (80%). Carcinoma of the lip is more common in individuals of light complexion, especially in those who, because of their occupation, receive an unusual amount of actinic radiation, such as farmers, sailors, and policemen. About 6% have multiple lip carcinomas, either simultaneously or at intervals. Over 10% have at least one cancer of the skin, and over 3% have an oral, pharyngeal, laryngeal, or esophageal carcinoma.

Early or premalignant alterations of lip epithelium appear as localized keratotic plaques that may resolve, only to reappear. Alternately, malignant degeneration is indicated by diffuse, thin whitening of superficial portions of the vermilion border of the lip.

Squamous cell carcinoma of tongue. Squamous cell carcinoma of the tongue is the most frequent intraoral malignant lesion, comprising about one half of the cases. It is less exclusively a male disease (about 75% in males) than is carcinoma of the lip. Approximately 80% of the cases arise in the sixth to eighth decades.[70a] In Scandinavia, however, the disease is not rare in women and commonly is associated with *Plummer-Vinson syndrome* (atrophy of mucous membrane, iron deficiency anemia, and dysphagia). There appears to be a positive correlation between carcinoma of the tongue, especially of the dorsal surface, and syphilitic glossitis, the incidence of carcinoma of the tongue being about four times more common in individuals with syphilis (Fig. 29-14) than in those without syphilis.

The lateral border and ventral surfaces of the tongue are frequent sites of carcinoma (about 65%). Metastases, frequently bilateral (about 20%), are present in about 35% of

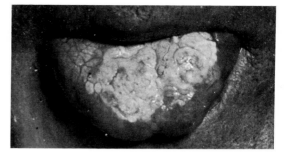

Fig. 29-14. Leathery and warty whitening ("leukoplakia") of tongue associated with carcinoma of low-grade malignancy.

the patients at the time of hospital admission. Contralateral metastasis occurs in less than 3%.

Survival figures indicate that the prognosis for patients with squamous cell carcinoma of the tongue is dependent on several factors. The small, early lesion of low-grade malignancy without evidence of metastasis or conspicuous local invasion may be successfully managed by surgery or radiation therapy. Approximately 60% of such patients live 5 years or more. This figure is reduced to 30% in instances where the tumor is anaplastic or has metastasized.[70a]

Squamous cell carcinoma of floor of mouth. Squamous cell carcinoma of the floor of the mouth (about 15% of oral cases) is typically manifest as an indurated ulcer in the anterior portion about the openings of the sublingual and submandibular glands, with over 80% occurring in males. The carcinoma invades rapidly, spreading to the submandibular lymph nodes (about 50%) and to the submandibular and sublingual salivary glands, tongue, and mandibular gingiva. Treatment, usually radiation, yields a survival rate similar to that for carcinoma of the tongue. Although white patches are observed throughout the oral cavity in a variety of clinical circumstances, the white patch on the mouth floor, however subtle, should be thoroughly investigated. Early squamous cell carcinoma of the area frequently will be overlooked if this is not done.

Squamous cell carcinoma of buccal mucosa. Squamous cell carcinoma of the buccal mucosa constitutes from one fourth to one third of all oral carcinomas and varies in frequency in different geographic areas. In India and other countries in which betel nut and tobacco chewing are commonplace, buccal carcinomas are the major cancer. Abnormal keratinization is especially common in this group. *Oral submucous fibrosis* may be another premalignant mucosal alteration.[57] Progressive infiltrative growth, local recurrence after treatment, and local lymph node metastasis characterize squamous cell carcinoma originating in the cheeks. Five-year survival figures vary, but approximately 50% of affected patients survive this period after diagnosis and adequate surgical or radiation therapy. Patients rarely succumb to the disease from complications associated with distant metastasis. Rather, malnutrition, asphyxia, pneumonia, etc. complicate local tumor growth and lead to death.

An unusual form of epidermoid carcinoma most frequently involving the buccal mucosa and mandibular gingiva is *verrucous carcinoma*.[43] In the United States, in the mid-south, it is commonly associated with the prolonged use of snuff placed in the gingivobuccal sulcus. It is characteristically associated with leukoplakia, growing into large, fungating, soft, papillary masses. Microscopic diagnosis may be difficult and delayed, for the tumor presents an unusually well-differentiated pattern. Although destruction may be extensive and recurrence frequent (about 75%), metastasis is unusual. Patients are especially prone to develop additional, sometimes less differentiated oral carcinomas.

Squamous cell carcinoma of gingiva. Squamous cell carcinoma of the gingiva constitutes about 10% of oral malignancy and is more common in men than women (about 4 : 1). It has been more frequent on the mandibular gingiva, and its early, clinical resemblance to more common inflammatory conditions in this location may lead to delayed diagnosis. Tobacco and syphilis are less clearly related etiologically to gingival carcinoma than to carcinomas of the tongue or cheek. Early involvement of contiguous structures, such as bone and lymph nodes, characterizes the tumor.[36,70a]

Squamous cell carcinoma of palate. Squamous cell carcinoma of the palate may be ulcerative or tumorous or both. The tumors are more often of high-grade malignancy and occur about four times more frequently in men than in women. Although the lesions often are symptomless, patients may complain of a dental prosthesis that has become ill fitting. Pain may be a late clinical feature. Early involvement of underlying bone is a common feature. The soft palate is the more frequent site.

Pseudosarcoma (carcinosarcoma)

Pseudosarcoma (carcinosarcoma) occasionally is associated with an intramucosal or in situ squamous cell carcinoma of the mouth or oral pharynx. Bizarre, sarcoma-like proliferation of neoplastic cells results in bulky polypoid masses that may only faintly resemble carcinoma.[70a]

Carcinoma in situ

An occasional oral carcinoma, regardless of location, may demonstrate all cytologic features of malignant neoplasia yet fail to show any histologic evidence of invasion. The term *carcinoma in situ* has been used in this case. Considerable variability in the clinical appearance of carcinoma in situ has been experienced. The terms bowenoid (see Bowen's disease of skin, p. 1843), erythroplastic (see erythroplasia of Queyrat, p. 1844), and leukoplakia-like are used to describe the variable clinical appearance.

Lymphoepithelial carcinoma

Lymphoepithelial carcinoma may be found in the faucial area and base of the tongue, as well as in the nasopharynx and nasal cavity. Since the primary lesion is frequently small and undiscovered, the first clinical sign is often regional adenopathy and dysphagia. The "lymphoepithelioma" consists of syncytial masses of large polyhedral cells with eosinophilic cytoplasm, a large nucleus, large eosinophilic nucleoli, and a stroma infiltrated by numerous small lymphocytes (Regaud type of lymphoepithelial carcinoma). The cells of the "transitional cell carcinoma" are large, poorly differentiated, and anaplastic (Schmincke type of lymphoepithelial carcinoma). Radiation therapy is employed for both neoplasms, with the survival rate approaching 30%.

Other tumors

Kaposi's sarcoma, liposarcoma, rhabdomyosarcoma, embryonal rhabdomyosarcoma, alveolar soft-part sarcoma, etc. have been reported but are uncommon. Leukemic infiltration of the gingiva is seen frequently in affected patients.[52,55,70]

Primary malignant melanoma

Primary malignant melanoma of the oral cavity is relatively rare. About twice as common in males as in females, the peak incidence is in the sixth decade. Seldom has a case been reported in anyone under 20 years of age. Approximately 80% arise in the hard palate, alveolar ridge, or soft palate. Metastatic spread is exceedingly common. The 5-year survival rate appears to be about 5%.[64]

JAWS
Developmental lesions

Exostoses (tori). Exostoses or bony protuberances are not uncommon about the mouth. The most frequent is *torus palatinus,* which occurs in the midline of the hard palate in about 20% of the population. *Torus mandibularis* is less frequent (about 7% of the population), generally bilateral (80%), and is found on the lingual surface of the mandible, usually opposite the premolars. It is inherited as an autosomal dominant trait. *Multiple exostoses* are still less common and occur as small nodular outgrowths on the buccal surface of the maxilla and mandible, opposite the premolars and molars.

Osteomatosis. Osteomatosis may be associated with polyposis and adenocarcinoma of the colon and multiple cutaneous and mesenteric fibromas and lipomas (Gardner's syndrome). Epidermoid inclusion cysts are scattered over the body. The syndrome is transmitted as an autosomal dominant trait.[2,102]

Microscopically, the bony growths consist of dense, irregular bone with well-marked haversian systems and fibrous medullary portions. Cartilage is never observed. Blood calcium, phosphorus, and alkaline phosphatase levels are within normal limits.

Melanotic neuroectodermal tumor of infancy (retinal anlage tumor, melanoameloblastoma, melanotic progonoma). A tumor of the jaws, the melanotic neuroectodermal tumor, is a rare benign lesion of neural crest origin, largely restricted to the maxilla of infants.[74,77] At time of discovery of the tumor, the infant is nearly always under 6 months of age. A few similar tumors have been reported in the shoulder, epididymis, mandible, calvaria, brain, and mediastinum. There is little evidence of odontogenic origin and insufficient evidence to imply origin in the retinal anlage. Borello and Gorlin[77] have demonstrated that a tumor elaborated vanilmandelic acid, and neural crest origin appeared likely. Ultrastructural evidence supports this view.[86a]

Grossly, the tumor is often pigmented and well circumscribed, although no well-defined capsule is present. Microscopically, the tumor consists of a fibrous connective tissue stroma in which tubules or spaces are present in large numbers (Fig. 29-15). The spaces are lined

by a single layer of large cuboid cells with abundant cytoplasm in which are found numerous melanin granules. The spaces frequently are filled with many deeply staining cells that are smaller than the duct cells and contain much less cytoplasm. They appear to be neuroblasts.

Inflammatory and metabolic lesions

Acute suppurative osteomyelitis. Acute suppurative osteomyelitis of the jaws has become a relatively rare disease with the advent of antibiotics.[1,5] Usually because of infection of the marrow cavity with *Staphylococcus aureus* subsequent to jaw fracture or severe periapical disease, the process spreads, especially in the lower jaw, causing severe pain and facial cellulitis. When the resistance of the host is high or the virulence of the organism low, a chronic focal sclerosing osteomyelitis or condensing osteitis is seen.

Osteomyelitis of jaw of newborn infants. A distinct clinical entity, osteomyelitis of the jaw of the newborn infant almost exclusively involves the upper jaw.[90]

Garré's chronic sclerosing osteomyelitis with proliferative periosteitis. Garré's chronic sclerosing osteomyelitis with proliferative peri-

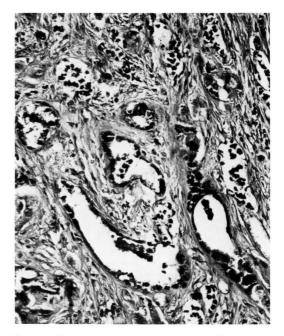

Fig. 29-15. Pigmented neuroectodermal tumor of infancy. This choristomatous lesion is composed of numerous tubules in fibrous connective tissue stroma. Tubules lined by large cuboid cells containing melanin. Within lumens are cells resembling neuroblasts.

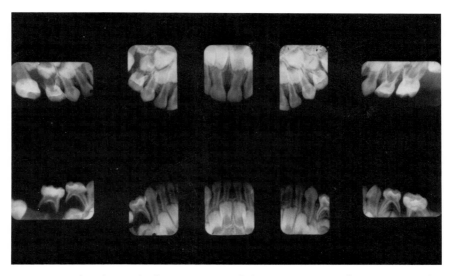

Fig. 29-16. Dental radiographs from patient with histiocytosis X. Molars appear to float in areas of bone loss.

osteitis is a nonsuppurating type seen most often in the lower jaw in children and young adults.[1]

Infantile cortical hyperostosis (Caffey's disease). Infantile cortical hyperostosis appears in infants, usually within the first 3 months of life, as a bilateral cortical thickening of the mandible, being inherited as an autosomal dominant trait.[2]

Osteoradionecrosis of the jaws. Osteoradionecrosis of the jaws, principally affecting the mandible, occurs after extensive therapeutic radiation in about 5% of patients. The severity seems to be proportional to the radiation dose, the presence of peridental sepsis, the degree of trauma to the tissue by ill-fitting dentures, and the susceptibility of the host.

Osteitis deformans (Paget's disease of bone). Osteitis deformans may involve the jaws, especially the maxilla, with progressive enlargement and displacement of teeth as part of the generalized disease. This becomes especially apparent if the patient wears dentures.

Histiocytosis X (Letterer-Siwe disease, Hand-Schüller-Christian disease, eosinophilic granuloma). In histiocytosis X, the jaws are sites of deposits of foamy histiocytes. It has been reported that 93% of patients had sore, swollen necrotic gingivae and 78% had loose, sore teeth that rapidly exfoliated (Fig. 29-16). The premolar-molar region of the mandible more frequently than the maxilla is the common area of involvement. Loss of trabeculae, pseudocyst formation, and dental root resorption are typical roentgenographic findings.[94]

Giant cell granuloma. Giant cell "reparative" granuloma is a nonneoplastic lesion of unknown etiology that appears to be limited to the jaws.[70] Treatment consists of simple excision and curettage. Although resembling true giant cell tumor of bone, it has certain properties and microscopic characteristics that separate it as a distinct entity. It constitutes about 3% of benign jaw tumors. It is found either centrally or peripherally, being about equally distributed. It is somewhat more common in the mandible and in females. The roentgenographic appearance is not pathognomonic, being solitary, radiolucent, and sharply delineated. The lamina dura may be displaced. Grossly, the tissue is usually reddish brown or black, depending on the amount of hemorrhage. Not uncommonly, the surface is eroded or ulcerated.

Microscopically, the giant cell granuloma consists of an admixture of multinucleated giant cells scattered in a very cellular stroma from which the giant cells probably are derived (Fig. 29-17). The stromal cell has a round or oval nucleus, small nucleolus, prominent nuclear membrane, and poorly delineated cytoplasmic boundaries. Nuclear pleomorphism, hyperchromatism, and increased mitotic activity are characteristically absent. Hemosiderin pigment, evidence of old hemorrhage, often is seen lying free or ingested by mononuclear phagocytes. Collagen production is quite common, whereas osteoid is present less often, and both are nearly always absent from the true giant cell tumor.

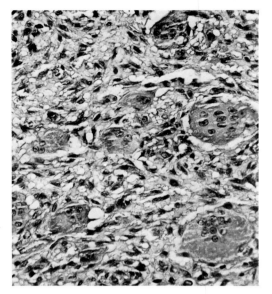

Fig. 29-17. Giant cell granuloma. Lesion characterized by numerous multinucleated giant cells in fibrous cellular stroma from which giant cells are derived. Collagen, osteoid, or bone are formed.

Microscopic differentiation should include true giant cell tumor (extremely rare in the jaws), cherubism, fibrous dysplasia, and aneurysmal bone cyst. The lesions of *hyperparathyroidism* cannot be differentiated on a microscopic basis from central giant cell granuloma, and in the case of recurrence or multiple or satellite lesions, blood and urinary calcium levels always should be determined. Also suggestive of hyperparathyroidism is disappearance of the lamina dura about the teeth, but this is less common than is generally believed.

Tumors and tumorlike lesions

Fibrous dysplasia. The jaws may be involved in fibrous dysplasia of the monostotic or polyostotic types.[101,106] The monostotic form is the more common and seems to be more frequent in children and young adults. Clinically, it is manifest by a painless swelling of the bone. Displacement of teeth may be present. Polyostotic fibrous dysplasia, in addition to manifestation in several or many bones, may be accompanied by melanotic pigmentation of the skin and oral mucosa and endocrine disturbances, including precocious puberty in females *(Albright's syndrome)*.

Cherubism. Cherubism is an autosomal dominantly inherited disease essentially limited to the jawbones. It has been imprecisely referred to as familial fibrous dysplasia.[65] This condition is characterized by enlargement of the jaws usually during the second or third year of life, especially in the mandibular molar area. Bony expansion increases for a few years and then tapers off, usually regressing by puberty. Associated with the jaw anomaly are upturning of the eyes, revealing a rim of sclera, and nonspecific submandibular lymphadenopathy.

Microscopically, the bony lesion consists of vascular and usually collagenic fibrous connective tissue, having an abundant admixture of perivascular osteoclastic giant cells. Not uncommonly, fibrin is deposited around small capillaries.

Malignant tumors metastatic to jaws. Malignant tumors metastatic to the jaws are uncommon, spread probably taking place through the vertebral system of veins. In an extensive survey, there was an indication of the following order of frequency: carcinoma of breast, lung, large intestine, prostate and kidney, thyroid gland, and testis.[82]

The tooth-bearing area of the body and the molar regions of the mandible are the most frequent sites, possibly because of greater arterial blood supply in these regions. In about one half of the cases, the oral metastasis is the first sign of the generalized cancer. Swelling, pain, and anesthesia are the most common symptoms (Fig. 29-18).

Osteosarcoma (osteogenic sarcoma). Approximately 10% of osteosarcomas occur in the jaws. Accessibility, a feature leading to early treatment, and greater histopathologic differentiation likely contribute to the relatively more favorable prognosis appreciated by this malignant tumor when observed in oral sites.[76]

Chondrosarcoma. Less frequently encountered in the jaws than osteosarcoma, chondrosarcoma has been less successfully managed and may be more biologically malignant than chondrosarcoma of long bones. Microscopically, chondrosarcoma and osteosarcoma may appear benign early in their development. Although both these entities may contain bone and cartilage, only the neoplastic cells of the latter, osteosarcoma, produce osteoid.[80]

Fibrosarcoma. Fibrosarcomas of jaws also have been observed. They may originate in periosteal or central locations. Histopathologic interpretation and diagnosis are complicated by the numerous other fibrous or spindle cell neoplasms observed in the jawbones.

Multiple myeloma and Ewing's sarcoma. Rarely multiple myeloma and Ewing's sar-

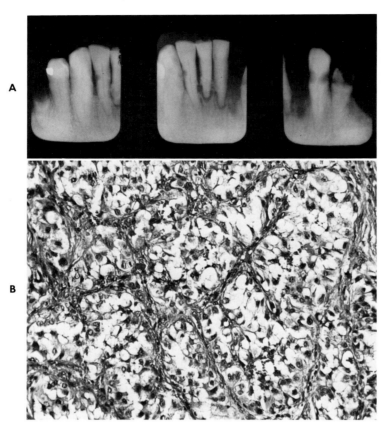

Fig. 29-18. Clinical radiographic, **A,** and histologic, **B,** appearance of metastatic adeno-carcinoma of kidney. Similarity to inflammatory conditions of dental tissue in radiograph may be striking.

coma may be initially manifest as a lesion of the jaws. Usually, jaw involvement is merely a part of the generalized disease.[2]

Malignant lymphoma. In contrast to most other primary malignancies of the jawbones, malignant lymphomas of the jaws occur more frequently in the maxilla.[2]

Burkitt's lymphoma. An undifferentiated lymphosarcoma, Burkitt's lymphoma, has been described in the jaws and abdominal viscera of equatorial African children from 3 to 8 years of age, constituting about 50% of all malignant tumors in this age group. Arising most often in the maxillary alveolar process, it is destructive, effecting loss of deciduous molars. The process extends to involve the parotid gland, antrum, nasopharynx, and orbit. Usually, there is no associated lymphadenopathy.[79]

Evidence suggests that the Epstein-Barr virus is immunologically associated with Burkitt's tumor and infectious mononucleosis (see also p. 718).

Cysts

Cysts of the jaws and mouth usually are classified according to their odontogenic or nonodontogenic origin. However, a number of oral lesions called "cysts" on clinical or roentgenographic evidence alone do not fall within the definition of a pathologic, epithelium-lined cavity containing fluid or debris. The salivary gland retention cyst (mucocele), ameloblastoma, traumatic bone cyst, static bone cyst, and the lesions of hyperparathyroidism all fall within this category.[1]

Odontogenic cysts

Periodontal cyst. The most common odontogenic cyst is the periodontal cyst. Most often it is observed at the apex of an erupted tooth *(radicular type)*. The origin of this cyst appears to be in the cystic degeneration of epithelialized granulomas that have resulted most frequently as sequelae to dental caries and pulpitis. The origin of the stratified squamous epithelium lining these cysts is the epithelial

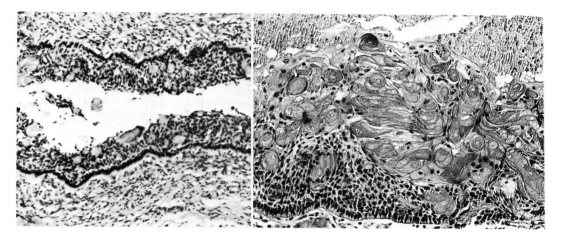

Fig. 29-19. Calcifying odontogenic cyst. Note pronounced basal layer with palisaded cells and large masses of partially keratinized "ghost" cells.

rests of Malassez, which lie in the periodontal ligament. They are derived from Hertwig's root sheath. The walls of smaller cysts usually are infiltrated with chronic inflammatory cells.[78b]

Gingival cyst. The gingival cyst, multiple as a rule, occurs in the anterior jaws of infants and children.[1,86] This type becomes uncommon with increasing age. Those situated on the lateral surface of the root of erupted teeth have been called *lateral periodontal cysts*.

Dentigerous cyst. Cyst formation may be associated with unerupted teeth and originates from epithelium of the dental lamina or dental organ. The mandibular third molars and maxillary canines are most often involved. This cyst has significance because of the occasional massive resorption of involved jawbone that results from its unhampered expansion. Whereas the incidence of ameloblastomatous transformation within dentigerous cysts has not been precisely determined, the fact that such transformation does occur, the fact that ameloblastomas may appear cystic, and, finally, that histopathologic examination is required for these determinations render pathologic examination of such material prudent.[105] Carcinoma arising in dentigerous cysts has also been observed.[1]

Eruption cyst. A special type, occasionally bilateral, that does not involve bone, the eruption cyst, is seen rarely in the gingiva overlying erupting deciduous canines or molars.

Multiple cysts (odontogenic keratocysts). Multiple cysts of the jaws are associated in a syndrome with multiple nevoid basal cell carcinomas and skeletal anomalies, especially bifid rib and kyphoscoliosis.[85] The syndrome has autosomal dominant inheritance. Lamellar calcification of the dura is common. Medulloblastoma and bilateral calcified ovarian fibromas also may be part of the syndrome. Odontogenic keratocyts are observed without the syndrome.[78a]

Calcifying odontogenic cyst. The calcifying odontogenic cyst (Fig. 29-19) is characterized by masses of "ghost" or aberrantly keratinized epithelium intermixed with the cells lining the cystic cavity. About one third of these cysts occur extraosseously.

Nonodontogenic cysts

As the name implies, nonodontogenic cysts are not derived from the tissues of the developing tooth. Many have been classified as *fissural* or *inclusion cysts*, since they are believed to have their origin in epithelial rests in bone resulting from fusion of two or more embryologic processes.

Median anterior maxillary cyst (nasopalatine duct cyst, incisive canal cyst, cyst of palatine papilla). The most common nonodontogenic cyst is the median maxillary cyst, which arises from the epithelial remnants of the nasopalatine duct. It often is discovered in routine dental roentgenograms. It lies above and midway between the roots of the maxillary central incisors.

Globulomaxillary cyst. The globulomaxillary cyst is intraosseous and is located between the maxillary lateral incisor and canine at the embryologic junction of the globular process with the palatine process of the maxilla.

Nasoalveolar (nasolabial) and dermoid cysts. In contrast to the intraosseous cysts just mentioned, the nasoalveolar cyst and dermoid cyst are formed within soft tissue. The nasoalveolar cyst is formed at the junction of the globular, lateral nasal, and maxillary processes, being located at the ala of the nose and frequently extending into the nostril. The dermoid cyst is especially common in the head and neck, with the floor of the mouth being the principal site. Dermoid cysts probably are derived from enclaving of epithelial debris in the midline during closure of mandibular and other branchial arches.

• • •

From the practical standpoint, few cysts of the jaws can be differentiated from each other on microscopic basis alone. Generally, roentgenographic evidence and further information such as history, clinical appearance, and evidence derived from tooth vitality tests are necessary to establish a definite diagnosis. However, the following hints may help. Gingival, periodontal, dentigerous, primordial, and fissural (globulomaxillary, median anterior maxillary, nasoalveolar, etc.) cysts usually are lined by nonkeratinizing, stratified squamous epithelium overlying dense fibrous connective tissue. The dermoid cyst, on the other hand, is lined by a keratinized stratified squamous epithelium plus skin appendages. The radicular, periodontal, and fissural cysts commonly show secondary chronic inflammatory infiltrate especially rich in plasma cells. Far less frequently is this seen in dentigerous or gingival cysts. Fissural cysts of the maxilla not uncommonly are lined by ciliated columnar epithelium, at least in their superior part. The odontogenic keratocyst is lined by a thin layer of keratinized or parakeratinized epithelium. Mucous glands and congeries of blood vessels and nerves frequently are noted in the connective tissue wall of the median anterior maxillary cyst. The mandibular dentigerous cyst occasionally may be lined in part by goblet cells or have lymphoid follicles or epithelial cell rests beneath the lining in the cyst wall. These proliferated rests of Malassez are responsible occasionally for an incorrect diagnosis of ameloblastoma.

Traumatic bone cyst (solitary or unicameral bone cyst). The traumatic bone cyst is not a true cyst. It is not lined by epithelium but by a thin membrane of connective tissue. Usually, no content is found other than a small amount of blood, serum, or granulation tissue laden with hemosiderin, macrophages, and a few foreign body giant cells.[75a]

Static or latent bone cyst (Stafne's cyst). The static or latent bone cyst is not a cyst but is a developmental defect usually containing salivary gland tissue. It is located on the inferior surface of the mandible just in front of the angle.

Gastric or intestinal epithelium–lined cyst. The gastric or intestinal epithelium–lined cyst is rare. It has been observed almost exclusively in males. The most common location is in the anterior portion of the oral floor or body of the tongue. It corresponds to developmental abnormalities ("duplications") seen elsewhere in the gastrointestinal tract.

Odontogenic tumors

Odontogenic tumors of the jaws arising from tooth-forming tissues are uncommon. There has been an interest in them, however, and classifications have been relatively numerous dating from that of Broca in 1867. Goldman and Thoma classified odontogenic tumors according to their tissue origin as epithelial, mesodermal, and mixed. Pindborg and Clausen, in 1958,[93] presented a classification that stressed the phenomenon or phenomena of induction in addition to histogenesis. Subsequent authors have expanded on this slightly.

Since there is a certain necessary complexity, the World Health Organization adopted a classification that allows for evaluation of the numerous transition forms. The interested reader is referred to this work[3] and that of Gorlin[1] for a comprehensive discussion of the subject.

The classification that follows presents odontogenic tumors in a fashion that attempts simplification without sacrifice of histogenetic considerations. Moreover, it emphasizes clinical behavior in the traditional manner.

Benign
1. Ameloblastoma
2. Adenomatoid odontogenic tumor
3. Calcifying epithelial odontogenic tumor
4. Ameloblastic fibroma
5. Odontomas
6. Cementomas
7. Myxoma/myxofibroma

Malignant
1. Ameloblastic carcinoma (malignant ameloblastoma)
2. Ameloblastic fibrosarcoma

Ameloblastoma. Ameloblastoma is the most common of epithelial odontogenic tumors. It is comparatively uncommon, reportedly comprising about 1% of tumors and cysts arising in the jaws. It may arise from the epithelial lining of a dentigerous cyst, the remnants of dental lamina and enamel organ, or from the basal layer of the oral mucosa.

Analysis of over 1000 cases reveals that ameloblastoma appears most commonly in the third to fifth decades.[95] No sex or racial preference is noted. Over 80% occur in the mandible, and 70% of these arise in the molar-

ramus area. Rarely, an extraosseous example is discovered.

Because of its invasive property and tendency to recur, the ameloblastoma has been usually considered "locally malignant" but is benign. Distant metastases,[87] especially to the lungs, have been reported in rare instances, but factors such as aspiration and transplantation are considered significant in most.[1] Frankly carcinomatous neoplasms resembling dental organ epithelium are best considered *amelo-*

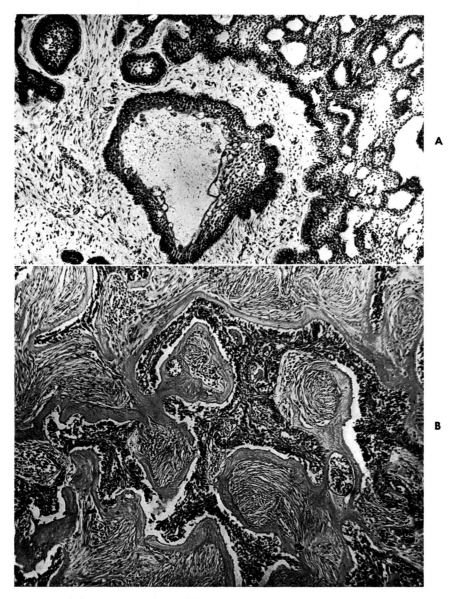

Fig. 29-20. Ameloblastoma. **A,** Amebloblastoma of mandible showing solid strands of enamel organs with formation of cystic spaces. Fibrous stroma. **B,** Atypical solid ameloblastoma of mandible. Cords of irregularly shaped epithelial cells surrounded by hyaline zone of very dense fibrous stroma.

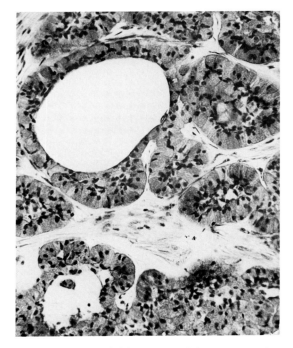

Fig. 29-21. Ameloblastoma exhibiting granular cell pattern. Occasionally, whole tumor may be composed of large granular cells with eosinophilic granular cytoplasm.

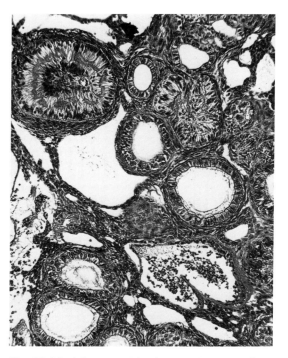

Fig. 29-22. Adenomatoid odontogenic tumor. Consists of congeries of tubules. Possibly arises from preameloblast.

blastic carcinoma. Traditionally, ameloblastoma has been divided into solid and cystic types, but nearly all ameloblastomas demonstrate some cystic degeneration. Microscopically, many subtypes or patterns have been suggested: follicular, plexiform, acanthomatous, granular cell (Figs. 29-20 and 29-21), and vascular varieties. However, two or more types may occur within the same tumor, and there is no evidence that any subtype is more aggressive than any other.

The majority of ameloblastomas demonstrate one of the two predominant patterns, follicular or plexiform, the former being the more common. In the follicular type there is an attempt to mimic the dental organ epithelium. The outermost cells resemble those of the inner dental epithelium of the developing tooth follicle, i.e., the ameloblastic layer. The cells are tall columnar, with polarization of the nuclei away from the basement membrane.[105] The central portion of the epithelial island is composed of a loose network of cells resembling stellate reticulum. Squamous metaplasia within the stellate reticulum gives rise to the acanthomatous type. The epithelial islands demonstrate no inductive influence upon the collagenized connective tissue stroma.

Enamel and dentin are never formed by the ameloblastoma. The plexiform pattern demonstrates irregular masses and interdigitating cords of epithelial cells with a minimum of stroma.[3]

Adenomatoid odontogenic tumor (ameloblastic adenomatoid tumor). A benign lesion, the adenomatoid odontogenic tumor probably arises from the preameloblast or inner enamel epithelium.[1,3,91] It appears to be more common in females, arises somewhat more often in the anterior region of the upper jaw, and occurs most frequently in the second decade of life. Frequently it is associated with an unerupted canine. Although the tumor expands, it is not invasive and does not recur even after extremely conservative surgical therapy.

Microscopically, the lesion consists of congeries of ductlike structures, lined by medium to tall columnar epithelium, in an extremely scant fibrous connective tissue stroma (Fig. 29-22). Small calcified deposits are often seen scattered throughout the epithelial tissue.

Calcifying epithelial odontogenic tumor. The calcifying epithelial odontogenic tumor is a rare lesion. The tumor has been invasive and may be locally recurrent. It seems to occur more commonly in the fourth and

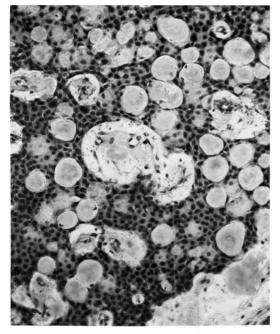

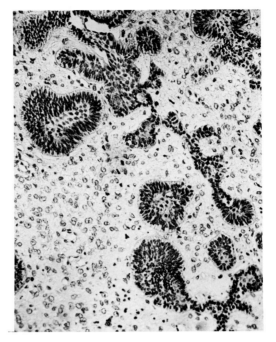

Fig. 29-23. Calcifying epithelial odontogenic tumor. Very rare, somewhat aggressive tumor arising from reduced enamel epithelium. Droplets of calcified amyloid material frequently exhibit Liesegang rings.

Fig. 29-24. Ameloblastic fibroma. Consists of numerous islands of odontogenic epithelium in cellular mesenchymal matrix. This tumor is nonaggressive and must be differentiated from ameloblastomas, which lack mesenchymal matrix.

fifth decades. There is no sex predilection. Several of the reported cases have arisen in the mandibular premolar-molar area in association with an embedded tooth.[1,3,5,89]

Microscopically, the tumor is composed of polyhedral epithelial cells with scanty stroma. The closely packed cells frequently demonstrate nuclear pleomorphism. Intracellular degeneration results in numerous spheric spaces filled with eosinophilic homogeneous material that in time becomes calcified. This has been shown to be amyloid or a similar substance[104] (Fig. 29-23).

Ameloblastic fibroma. The ameloblastic fibroma is characterized by proliferation of both epithelial and mesenchymal elements in the absence of hard tooth structure, i.e., enamel or dentin. In contrast to ameloblastoma, the tumor for which it is most commonly mistaken, the ameloblastic fibroma usually occurs in a young age group, rarely being seen in individuals over 21 years of age. Clinical behavior is entirely benign.[1,3,5,81]

Microscopically, the ameloblastic fibroma is composed of strands and buds of epithelial cells in a very cellular connective tissue stroma (Fig. 29-24). The presence of this mesenchymal portion clearly differentiates this lesion

from ameloblastoma. For the most part, the cells composing the strands of epithelial cells are cuboid and are two cell layers thick. Only occasionally a stellate reticulum is present. In contrast to ameloblastoma, simple curettage of the ameloblastic fibroma is usually adequate treatment.

Odontomas. Three subtypes or varieties of odontogenic tumors featuring production of calcified parts of teeth are usually considered: *complex odontoma,* in which enamel, dentin, cementum, etc., have not differentiated to the point where an actual tooth can be recognized; *compound odontoma,* in which a tooth or teeth, regardless of size or fine form, can be discerned; and *ameloblastic odontoma,* in which an additional component resembling dental organ epithelium (ameloblastomatous) is observed in addition to enamel, dentin, etc.[1]

Complex odontoma has been most frequently encountered in molar areas of the mandible and more often observed in female patients. Differentiation is poor, and a variety of calcified patterns is observed. The enamel, dentin, and cementum may be virtually unidentifiable. Although the tumors occasionally achieve considerable proportions, they are entirely benign. Growth and symptomatology are

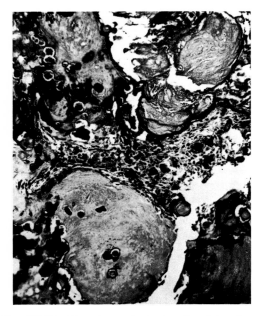

Fig. 29-25. Complex odontoma. Consists of un-organized mass of dentin, enamel, cementum, and pulpal tissue and occasional areas of enamel epithelium.

slight. They are frequently diagnosed after routine radiographic examinations (Fig. 29-25).

Compound odontoma presents a higher degree of differentiation than does complex odontoma, and the individual lesion characteristically consists of masses of small, misshapen teeth. Some may have as few as three teeth, whereas the exception has been reported containing 2000 denticles. These odontomas behave in an entirely benign fashion. They are more commonly encountered in anterior regions of the jaws and in the maxilla more often than in the mandible.

Ameloblastic odontoma is much less frequent than either complex or compound odontoma. Although dental hard tissues such as enamel and dentin in the odontomas under discussion necessarily form through action of ameloblasts and odontoblasts, certain odontomas are encountered that possess a striking epithelial component. In these instances, the term *ameloblastic odontoma* has been employed. They are considered benign but may, on occasion, behave more aggressively and recur locally after conservative surgical removal.[1,3,5]

Cementomas. Three, possibly four, apparently unrelated lesions of the jaws can be identified within this group characterized by benign neoplastic formation of cementum or cementum-like hard tissue within a cellular fibrous connective tissue.[1,3,5,88]

Cementoma or periapical fibrous dysplasia (periapical cemental dysplasia) has been the most frequently encountered, and estimates place the prevalence at 2 to 3 per 1000 individuals. Females are principally affected. Multiple mandibular teeth are usually involved by asymptomatic, small radiolucencies or, later, radiopacities that may be confused with dental inflammations. Treatment is not required.

Familial multiple cementomas, much less frequently encountered, have been reported with varying terminology in middle-aged black females. There is swelling and deformity, and multiple areas of both jaws appear to be affected.[1]

Diagnosis of the several fibrous, ossifying, or "cementifying" jaw lesions, such as the so-called true cementomas, cementoblastomas, cementifying fibromas, fibrous dysplasias, etc., represents a most consuming exercise of pathology. In such instances, the clinical history, radiographic examination, histopathology, and, occasionally, blood chemistry are required.

Myxoma and myxofibroma, odontogenic fibroma. Myxoma of bone does not occur outside of the jaws.[1,3,75] Most investigators believe that this lesion is of tooth germ origin (dental papilla) and have called it **odontogenic myxoma.** Some examples are associated with the proliferation of large numbers of small epithelial rests of Malassez. The **odontogenic fibroma** differs microscopically from the myxoma only by the presence of collagenic fibrous connective tissue and greater numbers of odontogenic epithelial rests.

About 60% of odontogenic myxomas and fibromas occur during the second and third decades. The maxilla and mandible are equally affected. The tumors are slow growing. Bony expansion may be great, however, producing obvious facial deformity. Microscopically, the myxoma consists of loose stellate cells with long, anastomosing cytoplasmic processes (Fig. 29-26). Occasionally, an inactive strand of odontogenic epithelium is noted around the edge of the tumor.

Malignant ameloblastoma (ameloblastic carcinoma). We have encountered four neoplasms, three maxillary and one mandibular, that besides possessing histologic criteria of ameloblastoma manifest malignant cytologic features such as numerous mitotic figures and clinical aggressiveness. Although one is struck

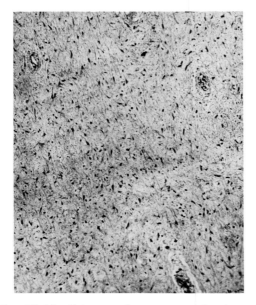

Fig. 29-26. Odontogenic myxoma. Consists of loose, embryonal connective tissue. Occasionally, strands of odontogenic epithelium are present.

by the relative rarity of malignant odontogenic neoplasms, this possibility may not at the present time be excluded.[1,3,5]

Ameloblastic fibrosarcoma. Ameloblastic fibrosarcomas have also been rarely observed. Initially, these pathologic "curiosities" presented histopathologic features of ameloblastic fibroma. Recurrences were characterized by an increasingly malignant-appearing connective tissue portion, diminution or absence of the epithelial component, and malignant behavior. Pain has preceded the nine instances available for analysis, a feature differing from other odontogenic tumors. In no case yet studied has metastasis occurred. Death follows extensive local recurrence and extension.

SALIVARY GLANDS
Development

Both the major and the minor salivary glands develop as buds of oral ectoderm, arising in much the same manner as teeth. The epithelial bud proliferates into the adjacent mesenchyme, enlarging at its most distal end to form alveoli, with the epithelial cords becoming hollow to form ducts. The parotid and submandibular gland anlagen first become apparent by the sixth fetal week (13 to 15 mm embryo), although acini are not developed until the fifth month in utero. During the eighth week (19 to 25 mm embryo), the buds of the sublingual gland become apparent. The minor salivary glands are initiated by the tenth week.

Labial glands arise as epithelial buds of the vestibular epithelial plate prior to the opening of the alveolabial sulcus. Buccal and molar glands arise at the same time, associated with the terminal portion of Stensen's duct. Retromolar glands develop in the fifth fetal month.

The major salivary glands are subject to many developmental anomalies. One or more lobes (rarely, whole glands) may be congenitally absent or aplastic. Total absence of all major glands also has been reported. Accessory glands and glands ectopically placed within the body of the mandible have been noted. Major salivary ducts may be congenitally atretic or, rarely, imperforate.

Structure and types

The salivary glands, both major and minor, are tubuloalveolar structures. Both the parotid and submandibular glands are well encapsulated, although the sublingual is not. The adult parotid gland is serous in type, whereas the submandibular and sublingual glands are mixed, the former being predominantly serous and the latter mucous. Minor salivary glands are widespread, being scattered over the lips, buccal mucosa, palate, and tongue. Pure serous glands are seen about the circumvallate papillae (glands of von Ebner); pure mucous glands, in the palate and base of the tongue (Weber's glands). All others are of the mixed type.

Function

Saliva, the product largely of the major salivary glands, varies in quantity from 150 to 1300 ml per day (mean, 345 ml). The amount and the degree of viscosity depend on many factors (mechanical, chemical, and psychologic) but ultimately upon the type of nerve stimulus received by the glands.

The secretory nerve fibers to the salivary glands are under both parasympathetic and sympathetic control. Sympathetic stimulation of the submandibular gland via the superior cervical ganglion, for example, evokes a secretion of thick viscous mucus, whereas parasympathetic stimulation via the chorda tympani elicits a copious, thin watery flow.

The saliva performs several known functions, the most important being lubrication for deglutition and speech. Both mucin, a glycoprotein elaborated by mucous glands, and the voluminous watery secretion of the parotid glands aid in this process. In cases of diminished flow (xerostomia), poor oral hygiene and increased dental decay are observed. Taste is altered greatly. Saliva has antibacterial properties and a high buffering capacity. It probably contributes little toward digestion, although it contains a salivary amylase (ptyalin) capable of transforming starch to maltose and of splitting glycogen.

Disturbances of salivary flow

Increased salivary flow, sialorrhea (ptyalism), can result from many causes. It most commonly is associated with acute inflammation of the oral cavity, such as herpetic or aphthous stomatitis, and with "teething." It often is seen in mentally retarded individuals, in deteriorated schizophrenics, and in patients with neurologic disturbances with lenticular involvement. Mercury poisoning, acrodynia, pemphigus, pregnancy, rabies, epilepsy, nausea, and ill-fitting dentures all may be accompanied by an increased degree of salivation. Also, increased gastric secretion is accompanied by increased salivary flow. These may be pronounced sialorrhea in familial autonomic dysfunction and in one of the periodic diseases, periodic sialorrhea.

Recurrent sialadenitis and periodic sialorrhea. Recurrent sialadenitis and periodic sialorrhea are similar to other periodic diseases in their regular recurrence at short intervals, chronic course, resistance to therapy, and generally benign behavior.

Single pairs or all glands, most commonly the parotid, enlarge at regular intervals of weeks or months. Periodic sialorrhea is more common in women and may be an autosomal dominant trait. It not uncommonly accompanies other recurrent periodic diseases such as periodic abdominalgia or periodic neutropenia.

Familial autonomic dysautonomia (Riley-Day syndrome). Familial autonomic dysautonomia is characterized by excessive perspiration, sialorrhea, erythematous blotching of the skin, defective lacrimation, wide blood pressure fluctuation, emotional instability, cold hands and feet, and hyporeflexia. It is first manifest in infancy by impaired sucking and swallowing and an absence of tears. Growth is retarded, and the ability to sit, walk, and speak is delayed. The sialorrhea is especially noticeable during excitement.[160] The disorder is inherited as an autosomal recessive trait. It occurs almost exclusively in Jews of Ashkenazi extraction.

Xerostomia. Decreased salivary flow, xerostomia, is also associated with many conditions. Rarely, there is congenital absence of one or more major glands or ducts.[1] Epidemic parotitis (mumps) and sarcoidosis (uveoparotitis) are associated with reduced flow. Sjögren's syndrome[1,116,123] (keratoconjunctivitis sicca, rhinitis sicca, polyarthritis) and the other so-called "autoimmunization" syndromes and diseases (Mikulicz's, Felty's, Waldenström's, lupus erythematosus, etc.) also exhibit xerostomia. Therapeutic radiation to the lateral cervical area commonly produces fibrotic changes after acinar destruction of the parotid glands. Megaloblastic anemias (pernicious anemia, anemia of pregnancy) are not uncommonly associated with decreased salivary output. The majority of cases of xerostomia appear to be idiopathic. Many of these are associated with a smooth atrophic tongue.

Enlargements

Enlargement of one or more salivary glands may be associated with sialorrhea, xerostomia, or normal salivary secretion. A single glandular enlargement may denote localized inflammation, cyst, or neoplasm. Bilateral enlargement may signify an inflammatory process, such as mumps or sarcoid, or a diffuse neoplastic infiltrate (leukemia or lymphoma), or it may be attributable to unknown factors related to malnutrition, alcoholic cirrhosis, or hormonal disturbance.

Cysts

Cysts of salivary gland origin fall under three categories: true cysts, ranula, and mucocele or superficial retention cyst.

True cyst. The true cyst is usually small, 1 cm or less in diameter, and located within the body of the parotid or submandibular gland. It is lined by stratified squamous epithelium.[1,148]

Ranula. Ranula is a term used rather loosely to indicate a thin-walled, cystic lesion located on the floor of the mouth, and it includes sublingual gland mucoceles and a deep burrowing lesion that frequently extends through the mylohyoid muscle.[1,120]

Mucocele (retention cyst). The mucocele is a cavity lined by granulation tissue containing an eosinophilic hyaline material (mucus) composed of a variable number of mucus-laden macrophages (Fig. 29-27). Trauma, chiefly mechanical, appears to be responsible for damage to the ducts of minor salivary glands, resulting in the spillage of mucus into the lamina propria and submucous tissue.[165]

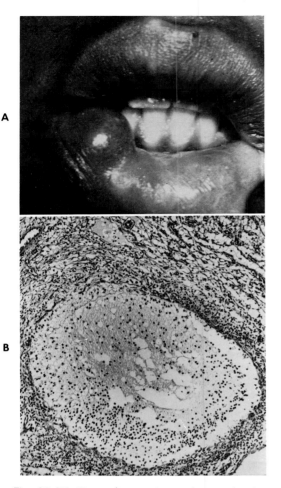

Fig. 29-27. Mucocele or minor salivary gland retention "cyst." **A,** Most commonly observed on lower lip, mucoceles are observed throughout oral cavity. They arise from spillage of mucus into surrounding connective tissue. **B,** Low-power photomicrograph illustrating extraductal mucus surrounded by inflammation. Note absence of epithelium.

This mucous pool may be localized and surrounded by a wall of granulation tissue. Mucocele of the glands near the ventral tip of the tongue is called cyst of Blandin-Nuhn.

Enlargements related to malnutrition

The relationship of parotid gland enlargement to malnutrition has been pointed out by many investigators. Hypertrophy also has been noted in cases of alcoholism and cirrhosis. Enlargement of the submandibular glands also has been noted occasionally in these cases. It is well known that both restricted dietary intake and alcohol contribute toward hepatic cirrhosis. The enlargement may be associated with excessive salivation. Experimentally, parotid enlargement can be produced in rats on a protein-free diet or by feeding proteolytic enzymes.

Parotid enlargement has also been reported in mental patients and in Amerindian hospital patients who were assumed to be receiving adequate diets. Past dietary history was not known, however. Cases also have been cited in association with diabetes mellitus, pregnancy and lactation, thyroid disease, cardiospasm, and menopause. In association with diabetes, the parotid swelling may precede the elevation in blood glucose by many months.

Microscopic changes consist of acinar hypertrophy, swelling of cells, and fatty infiltration. No inflammatory changes are observed. The pathogenesis is unknown, although reference is often made to morphologic and functional similarities between the parotid gland and the pancreas.[191]

Inflammatory diseases

Acute parotitis (secondary suppurative type). Acute parotitis is caused by ascent of microorganisms, usually *Staphylococcus aureus,* up Stensen's duct when salivary flow is reduced by inadequate fluid balance from fever, diuretics, starvation, etc. This may become recurrent, leading to scarring and chronic parotitis. Experimental production of secondary parotitis has confirmed clinical evidence. Experimental obstruction alone does not produce the classic microscopic change.

Microscopically, there is widespread destruction of acini and replacement with fibrous connective tissue. Plasma cell and lymphocytic infiltration usually is considerable. Ducts and acini frequently are dilated.

Chronic submandibular adenitis. Chronic submandibular adenitis is almost always attributable to blockage by stricture or calculi (sialoliths). This, in turn, renders the gland susceptible to retrograde bacterial invasion.

Sjögren's syndrome. Sjögren, in 1933, first described a syndrome consisting of conjunctivitis sicca, pharyngolaryngitis sicca, rhinitis sicca, polyarthritis, parotid (occasionally submandibular enlargement, and xerostomia.[1, 116, 119, 173] This syndrome subsequently was shown to have a relationship to other disorders such as Felty's syndrome, polyarteritis, lupus erythematosus, purpura and hypergammaglobulinemia of Waldenström, scleroderma, and Hashimoto's thyroiditis. Patients with Sjögren's syndrome reportedly have a higher incidence of lymphomas[173] (see also p. 1178).

The patient, usually a postmenopausal female, clinically presents red, burning eyes, photophobia, and lack of tears. Dysphagia and dysphonia may be pronounced, and the oral mucosa, especially that of the tongue, is atrophic and shiny. Dental caries is usually widespread.

Sjögren's syndrome has been designated by many authors as an autoimmune disorder. It has been suggested that an antigen released from damaged acini coming into contact with lymphatic tissue (normally present with parotid gland) would result in the production of antibodies that, in turn, would damage more acinar epithelium, continuing the cycle. Arguing for the autoimmune nature of the disease are the following:

1. Associated rheumatoid arthritic changes in over 50%
2. Hypergammaglobulinemia
3. Rheumatoid factor found in over 75%
4. Antithyroglobulin antibodies (about 35%) and antinuclear factors (about 65%)
5. Autoantibody reaction with salivary duct cytoplasm noted in over 50%

It has been suggested that there is impaired IgG autoantibody production. A model for the syndrome has been described in NZB mice.[146]

Microscopically, the changes were long recognized under the name of either *Mikulicz's disease* or *benign lymphoepithelial lesion*. Initially, there is a periductal mononuclear cell infiltrate consisting predominantly of small lymphocytes. Later, large lymphocytes and reticular cells appear. The acinar tissue is eventually totally replaced (Fig. 29-28). Epimyoepithelial islands arising from ductal proliferation are scattered throughout the tissue. Similar changes have been described in the lacrimal glands[133] and the minor salivary glands of the lip and palate.[109,122]

Sialolithiasis. Sialolithiasis, the occurrence of salivary stone or calculus, is found most commonly in the submandibular gland or especially its duct. Involvement of the parotid gland is relatively unusual (estimates ranging from 4% to 21%). Calculus in the sublingual and minor salivary glands, although not unknown, is rare.[1]

Although the etiology is unknown, theories have been advanced that salivary retention, with resultant precipitation of calcium salts, is the significant factor. Whether the retention is preceded by inflammation of the duct because of a foreign body, bacteria, or other factor is debatable.

Because of the intermittent obstruction of

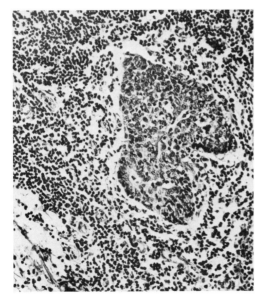

Fig. 29-28. Sjögren's syndrome (benign lymphoepithelial lesion). Acini replaced by pronounced lymphocytic infiltrate. Differentiation from lymphosarcoma made with difficulty.

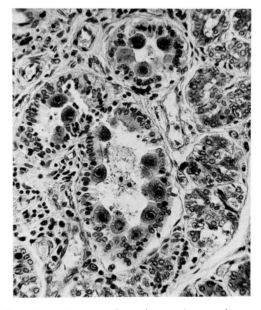

Fig. 29-29. Cytomegalic inclusion disease illustrating numerous, large, doubly contoured inclusion bodies within cytoplasm of duct cells of parotid gland. (Courtesy Dr. R. Marcial-Rojas, San Juan, Puerto Rico.)

the duct system, inflammation of the proximal portion of the gland occurs. Contrast media may be employed to demonstrate tortuous dilatation of the principal ducts and the presence of strictures. There is atrophy of the acinar cells, with replacement by scar tissue and fat cells if the obstructive process continues.

Cytomegalic inclusion disease. Cytomegalic inclusion disease is a widespread viral disease that becomes clinically manifest in only a small percentage of the population. It appears to be largely harmless outside infancy but remains a risk to the fetus if first contracted by the mother during pregnancy (see p. 481).

Described in 1932 by Farber and Wolbach as coincidental findings in intact salivary and lacrimal gland epithelium in more than 10% of all infant autopsies, the disease was proved to have viral etiology in 1956.

Although initially believed to be limited to salivary and lacrimal glands, it was subsequently shown to be generalized, producing a clinical picture resembling erythroblastosis or hepatitis in neonates and characterized by a train of events: mild jaundice, hepatosplenomegaly, bruising, and, finally, purpura. Interstitial pneumonitis, Addison's disease, or interstitial nephritis with hematuria also may eventuate. A high proportion of fatal cases have exhibited a peculiar laminar necrosis immediately beneath the ependyma of the brain. These areas become calcified and simulate congenital toxoplasmosis.

Microscopically, the inclusions may be seen in the salivary glands, lacrimal glands, liver, kidney, lung, etc. In the salivary gland, the inclusions are seen as round, highly refractile, homogeneous, eosinophilic bodies within the cytoplasm or nucleus of ductal cells (Fig. 29-29). These cells also may be seen with standard Wright's stain in gastric washings, subdural fluid, or sediment from freshly voided urine.

Epidemic parotitis (mumps). Epidemic parotitis is an acute, highly contagious viral disease. Despite the name, it is systemic, affecting many organs other than the parotid gland. It is probable that some degree of pancreatitis (and orchitis in male adults) occurs in nearly every case, but severe complication is rather uncommon. Oophoritis also may occur but is quite rare.[1]

There is diffuse tender enlargement of one or both parotid glands, accompanied by mild fever. Less commonly, the submandibular and sublingual glands are involved and, very rarely, the lacrimal glands. Examination of the buccal mucosa during the active state usually will reveal an erythematous halo about the opening of Stensen's duct.

In adolescents and adult males, clinical orchitis (usually unilateral) is present in about 25%. Only rarely is sterility produced, however. Pancreatitis, manifested by epigastric pain and nausea, although not very common as a severe complication, is probably a constant factor, causing elevated serum amylase and lipase levels.

Microscopically, in the parotid glands there are degenerative changes of the ductal epithelium, with infiltration of lymphocytes and macrophages about the ducts. The acini may undergo pressure atrophy.

Uveoparotid fever (Heerfordt syndrome). Uveoparotid fever is a form of sarcoidosis originally described by Heerfordt in 1909. The syndrome consists of a triad of signs: parotid enlargement, uveitis, and facial paralysis. It usually is seen in the second and third decades and is decidedly more common in black females. It represents about 10% of the cases of sarcoidosis.

The parotid swelling, which is bilateral in over half of the cases, often is preceded by mild fever, lassitude, and anorexia. The swell-

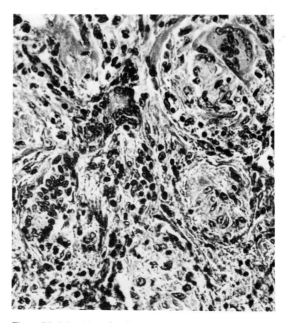

Fig. 29-30. Heerfordt's syndrome (uveoparotid fever) or sarcoidosis. Acini replaced by multiple, usually discrete, sarcoidal granulomas. Lacrimal glands, as well as major salivary glands, enlarged and associated with facial nerve paralysis.

Table 29-1. Tumors of major and minor salivary glands

Tumor type	Major	Minor
Benign		
Pleomorphic adenoma (mixed tumor)	55-65%	45-55%
Papillary cystadenoma lymphomatosum	5-6%	—
Oxyphil granular cell adenoma (oncocytoma)	Rare	Rare
Papillary cystadenoma	Rare	2-3%
Benign hemangioendothelioma	Rare, except in infants	—
Miscellaneous (adenoma, lipoma, neurilemoma, neurofibroma, sebaceous adenoma, etc.)	Rare	Rare
Malignant		
Carcinoma in pleomorphic adenoma	3-5%	2-3%
Adenocarcinoma (includes "classic," trabecular, etc.)	4-5%	10-18%
Cylindroma (adenocystic carcinoma)	4-5%	16-20%
Mucoepidermoid carcinoma	12-15%	10-12%
Acinic cell adenocarcinoma	2-3%	Rare
Squamous cell carcinoma	3-4%	?
Undifferentiated carcinoma	Rare	Rare
Miscellaneous (unclassified, oxyphil adenocarcinoma, melanoma, lymphoma, etc.)	Rare	1-2%

ing, in contrast to mumps, is not painful and is firm and nodular. The lacrimal glands occasionally are involved (Fig. 29-30). Ocular involvement, usually bilateral, may be severe and prolonged. Uveitis, iridocyclitis, and optic neuritis are not uncommon complications. Paralysis of the facial nerve is common in about 25% of the patients in uveoparotid fever.[1]

Necrotizing sialometaplasia. The condition is one microscopically confused with malignancy, especially squamous cell carcinoma of the palate.[108a]

Tumors (Table 29-1)

Benign hemangioendothelioma. The benign hemangioendothelioma is the most common tumor of the parotid gland during the first year of life, usually appearing within the first 3 months (Fig. 29-31). It occasionally is noted at birth. It also may arise in the submandibular gland. Skin hemangiomas may overlie the salivary gland hemangioendothelioma.

Histologically, the benign hemangioendothelioma is composed of capillary vessels lined by two or more layers of endothelial cells. The vessel lumens often are obscured as a result of the strong cellularity. It is never encapsulated, infiltrating the gland, replacing the acini, and leaving only the ductal elements.

Pleomorphic adenoma or mixed tumor. The benign pleomorphic adenoma is the most common tumor of the major (about 60%) and minor (about 50%) salivary glands.[1,121,132,135]

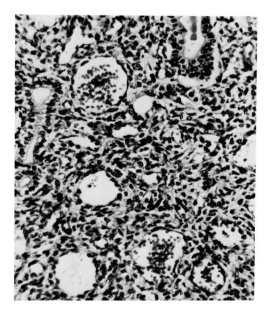

Fig. 29-31. Hemangioendothelioma of parotid gland—most common tumor of parotid gland in children under 1 year of age. Usually of capillary type, with few well-defined lumens.

It occurs most frequently in the parotid gland and less commonly in the submandibular gland—in the ratio of about 9:1.[130] Only rarely does it occur in the sublingual gland.

It arises most frequently in the fourth to sixth decades and is found somewhat more commonly in women. It is extremely rare in children. The primary growth occurs as a single nodule or mass in contrast to the recurrence, which is usually multilobulated. Although usually single, multiple mixed tumors[152] have been reported, arising either in two independent sites within the same gland, bilaterally, or within the homolateral parotid and submandibular glands.

Numerous theories of origin have been postulated: mesenchymal, branchiogenic, embryonal gland anlagen, and adult epithelial or myoepithelial tissue. Of special interest are the histochemical studies,[111,137] which support a theory of histogenesis from intercalated ducts. Two types of mucus have been demonstrated: an epithelial type elaborated by glandular structures and a "mesenchymal" type found in myxomatous areas, apparently the product of myoepithelial cells.[147]

Grossly, the pleomorphic adenoma is not truly encapsulated, a condition that was responsible for its high rate of recurrence in the past. Most tumors are from 2 cm to 5 cm in size, although some have attained gigantic proportions. The cut surface is grayish white

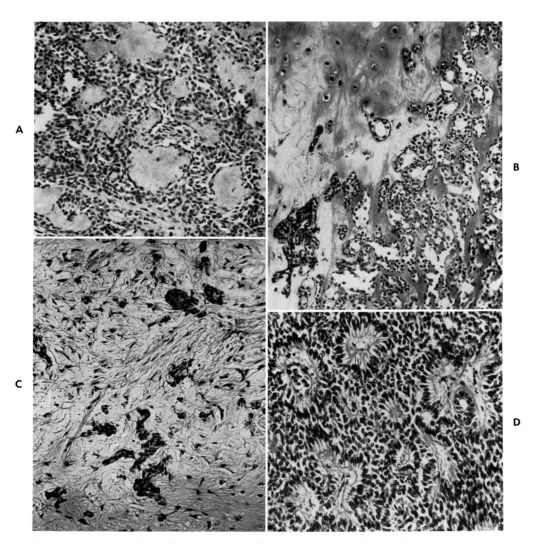

Fig. 29-32. Pleomorphic adenoma or mixed tumor Considerable variability of microscopic picture. **A,** Some tumors are exceedingly cellular, consisting of masses or sheets of small oval or rounded cells exhibiting little tendency to form ducts. **B,** Some tumors exhibit large masses of cartilage-like tissue. True cartilage occasionally produced by metaplasia of fibrous connective tissue stroma. Numerous ductlike structures manifest in this tumor. **C,** Certain tumors contain only few islands of epithelial cells in sea of loose mucoid matrix. **D,** Unusual variant of pleomorphic adenoma, so-called adenomyoepithelioma.

or yellowish and translucent. Areas containing cartilage appear bluish. Secondary cyst formation or hemorrhage is rare.

Microscopically, a wide variety of patterns may be found, both within the same tumor and in different tumors (Fig. 29-32). Myxoid areas occur in possibly 90%, whereas over one-third exhibit such an area as a dominant feature. One half will contain pseudocartilage. Squamous epithelial masses are seen in about 25%, and a pseudoadenoid arrangement of epithelial cells resembling cylindroma (adenoid cystic carcinoma) is manifest in about 10% of the cases.

A histologic feature in many pleomorphic adenomas is the presence of well-differentiated ductlike structures. Some tumors are composed entirely of these structures, having well-defined lumens with no admixture of mucoid material. These have been called *adenomas.* Other pleomorphic adenomas are composed almost entirely of mucoid pools, with only scant evidence of epithelial elements.

The epithelial cells vary in appearance from single-layered or double-layered high columnar to low cuboid. Material found in the ductlike lumens in some cases resembles colloid and in others, mucin. The former has been called epithelial mucin, whereas the latter has been characterized as being of mesenchymal origin. This mesenchymal product may simulate cartilage. True cartilage and even bone are observed in a small percentage of these tumors. In some, islands of acidophilic granular cells (oncocytes) are noted. Cylindromatous areas may cause considerable difficulty in diagnosis, especially if the biopsy specimen is small. Fortunately, cylindroma rarely, if ever, arises in mixed tumor.

Although several investigators have attempted to classify the mixed tumor into numerous subtypes on the basis of histologic pattern, clinical behavior is probably similar. The local recurrence rate is low. Various investigators have estimated this to be in the range of 0 to 5%. Because there is seldom any change in histologic pattern with recurrence, poor encapsulation or pseudoencapsulation has been suggested by many as the responsible factor.

Papillary cystadenoma lymphomatosum. (Warthin's tumor, adenolymphoma). Papillary cystadenoma lymphomatosum is a benign tumor of the parotid gland, arising most commonly in the lower portion of the gland overlying the angle of the mandible. It comprises from 2% to 6% of all parotid neoplasms. It chiefly affects males (5:1) from 40 to 70 years of age.[175] About 7% of the tumors occur bilaterally. The tumor may be superficial or deep to parotid fascia, within the substance of the gland or occasionally posterior to it. Rarely, an extraparotid lesion is encountered. A malignant variant has been described.[166]

There have been numerous theories of the histogenesis of papillary cystadenoma lymphomatosum.[175] The most plausible theory is that proposed by Albrecht and Arzt in 1910 and supported by numerous investigators. According to this concept, the tumor represents neoplastic proliferation of heterotopic salivary gland rests entrapped during growth and development in lymph nodes adjacent to or within the parotid gland.

Grossly, this well-encapsulated tumor is round or oval or often flattened. Its surface is usually smooth, occasionally lobulated, and commonly pinkish gray in color. The cut surface is studded with whitish nodules that correspond to the germinal centers. Irregular cystic spaces filled with serous or milky fluid and containing papillary projections are observed.

Microscopically, the essential components of the neoplasm are epithelial parenchyma and lymphoid stroma. The parenchymatous tissue is composed of tubules and dilated cystic spaces into the lumens of which project slender, fingerlike, papillary processes, giving the neoplasm its characteristic appearance (Fig. 29-33). The lining epithelium is composed of two rows of cells, the inner row of tall nonciliated columnar cells with oxyphilic granular cytoplasm and the outer layer of cuboid, polygonal, or rounded cells. The cell nuclei of the inner layer tend to be deeply stained and are evenly arranged toward the luminal end. The nuclei of the basal layer are round or vesicular, with a distinct nuclear membrane and one or two nucleoli. Occasionally a mucous or goblet cell is observed. Within the tubular and cystic spaces, a pink, granular or, more often, homogeneous substance is seen, probably a product of the lining epithelial cells. A thin basement membrane separates the epithelium from the lymphoid stroma. When present in abundant quantities, the lymphoid stroma contains numerous germinal centers.

Electron microscopic studies have demonstrated that the epithelial cells are oncocytic (i.e., essentially bags of mitochondria).[154,179] The mitochondria are of two types, the usual form and the giant form, which is two to three

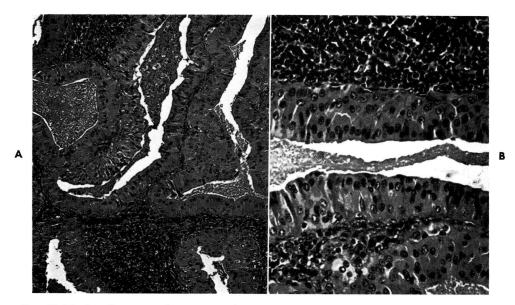

Fig. 29-33. Papillary cystadenoma lymphomatosum of parotid gland. **A,** Papillae extending into cavity contain lymphoid core covered by columnar epithelium. **B,** High magnification of area of **A** showing layer of columnar epithelium and lymphoid tissue.

times the size of the former. The cristae of the giant form are in the shape of closely packed lamellae. Preoperative diagnosis has been aided by scanning with technetium.[126]

Oxyphil granular cell adenoma (oncocytoma). A rare, benign neoplasm of glandular origin, oxyphil granular cell adenoma is composed of large epithelial cells containing oxyphil granular cytoplasm. Although cases have been reported in other major and minor salivary glands, it occurs almost exclusively in the parotid gland. Similar tumors may occur in the thyroid gland (Hürthle cell adenoma), parathyroid glands, kidney, adrenal glands, and pancreas. The tumor apparently arises from oxyphil granular cells (oncocytes), which have been reported to be present in a large number of organs (thyroid gland, parathyroid glands, pituitary gland, testicles, pancreas, liver, etc.) as well as in normal salivary glands. Hamperl[140,141] has suggested that the oncocyte is derived by a special degenerative metaplasia that does not prevent the cell from dividing.

Clinically, the tumor is indistinguishable from pleomorphic adenoma. It is usually firm, well demarcated, and freely movable. The facial nerve is almost never involved. Grossly, the tumor is round or oval, solid, and well encapsulated. The cut surface is usually grayish red and is divided into lobules by thin strands of fibrous connective tissue.

Microscopically, the oxyphil granular cell adenoma is composed of large cells of different sizes and shapes, sharply delineated from one another, somewhat resembling hepatic or adrenocortical cells (Fig. 29-34). The abundant eosinophilic cytoplasm contains numerous small, uniform granules. The nuclei are usually single and small, with one or more prominent nucleoli. The cells are commonly arranged in columns or cords, occasionally in tubular or acinar fashion. Rarely, an occasional focus of cartilage is found. Rarely also, diffuse collections of oncocytes or even focal oncocytomas are seen in typical pleomorphic adenomas.

Electron microscopic studies have shown a mitochondrion-rich cytoplasm.[112] This is borne out by the histochemical demonstration of an abundance of oxidative enzymes and adenosine triphosphatase. A strong metachromasia is noted with thionine or cresyl violet.[112]

Oxyphil granular cell carcinoma (malignant oncocytoma). The oxyphil granular cell carcinoma has been described in the salivary, thyroid, and adrenal glands.[140,141]

Sebaceous lymphadenoma. Sebaceous lymphadenoma is a rare benign lesion of the parotid gland. Microscopically, it is composed of a well-demarcated mass of lymphoid tissue in which there are numbers of islands of ductlike structures exhibiting sebaceous cell differentiation.[110,125]

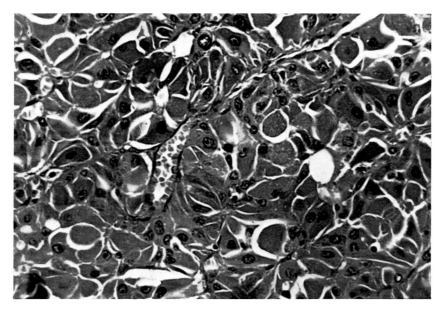

Fig. 29-34. Oxyphil granular cell adenoma (oncocytoma) of parotid gland. Sheets and glandular formations of tall columnar cells with eosinophilic granular cytoplasm.

Mucoepidermoid carcinoma. Of ductal origin, mucoepidermoid carcinoma exhibits cells of various ranges of activity, from the mucus-secreting cell to those that are quite squamous in character.

Although originally considered to be of two types, benign and malignant, further observation has indicated that occasionally the most benign-appearing ones have metastasized. All are now classified as carcinoma, and the degree of malignancy is estimated as low or high. One should understand that this is purely an arbitrary microscopic classification and not a hard-and-fast clinical evaluation.

Clinically, mucoepidermoid carcinoma of low-grade malignancy usually resembles the pleomorphic adenoma. It presents itself as a painless swelling, usually of the parotid gland. The appearance depends on the stage of differentiation, with the mature tumor being smaller, less firm, more movable, and more prone to mucous cyst formation than is the more malignant type. Encapsulation, although not uncommon in the better-differentiated tumor, is quite rare in the more anaplastic type. The low-grade tumor is more commonly found in females in the fourth to fifth decades. Involvement of the facial nerve in patients not operated upon is exceedingly rare.[144,169]

In contrast, the high-grade (more malignant) mucoepidermoid tumor not uncommonly manifests pain or facial nerve paralysis, or both, as an initial symptom. Sex predilection is not observed. Metastases to lung, brain, and bone frequently occur early in the course. The 5-year survival rate is about 25%.

The tumor also may occur within the body of the jaws, principally the mandible, in the retromolar area, where it makes its presence known early.[170] The prognosis of the tumor in this location is good.

Microscopically, the appearance is quite variable and depends on the degree of differentiation of the tumor, with those of low-grade malignancy having an abundance of mucous cells, whereas the more anaplastic have few to no mucous cells and may be mistaken for squamous cell carcinomas (Fig. 29-35). A mucin stain such as Meyer's muci-carmine or Schiff stain should be employed in all doubtful cases. There are three cell types evident: those that are frankly mucoid, others that are evidently epidermoid, and an intermediate type that is neither but has the capacity of maturing in either direction. Not uncommonly, the squamous epithelial cell nests of low-grade malignant tumors become hydropic. The presence of small cysts is very common in these well-differentiated tumors. The cysts become filled with mucus and commonly rupture. Cystic arrangement is uncommonly seen in the more malignant variety. Here, the pattern is more nestlike or sheetlike, with mucous cells being uncommon in the

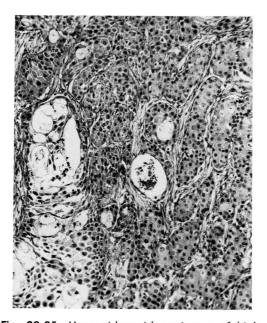

Fig. 29-35. Mucoepidermoid carcinoma of high-grade malignancy, strongly resembling squamous cell carcinoma. Careful search usually will reveal few cells that are producing mucus. Periodic acid–Schiff stain may aid in diagnosis.

primary tumor. However, metastases from these tumors not rarely manifest mucous cells.

Cylindroma (adenocystic carcinoma, cylindromatous adenocarcinoma). Cylindroma constitutes about 5% to 10% of parotid gland tumors, 18% submandibular gland tumors, 25% malignant oral salivary gland tumors, and over 50% of the glandular tumors of the tongue. Its origin appears to be the intercalated duct.[171] The same tumor occurs in the nasopharynx, paranasal sinuses, and lower respiratory system. It is most commonly observed in the sixth decade. The tumor is slow growing and of a moderate to low-grade malignancy but is widely infiltrative. It is poorly encapsulated. Facial nerve involvement is common, invasion of perineural lymphatics usually being readily demonstrated in section. The tumor is usually small (2 to 4 cm), firm, homogeneous, and grayish white in cross section. Multiple recurrence is common, with regional and finally generalized metastasis. The 5-year survival rate is about 35%. Prognosis for the palatal cylindroma is far better than that for cylindromas in the major salivary glands.[121,135]

Microscopically, the tumor demonstrates a striking pattern of anastomosing cords of small, darkly staining cells with scant cytoplasm (Fig.

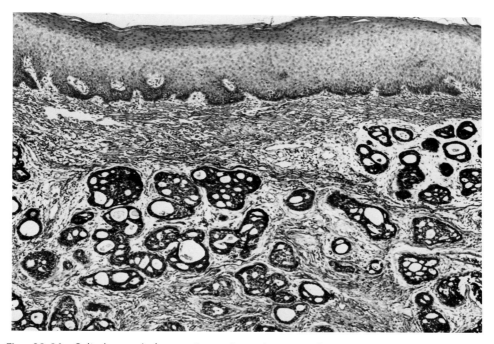

Fig. 29-36. Cylindroma (adenocystic carcinoma) arising from minor salivary glands of palate.

29-36). These cords are separated by acellular areas containing hyalin or mucicarmine-positive material. The cells have regular, rounded, rather vesicular nuclei. Chromatin clumping, mitotic figures, and prominent nucleoli are characteristically absent. There are two principal patterns: cribriform and solid. There appears to be a better prognosis if the pattern is cribriform rather than solid. Frequently, centripetal perineural extension can be demonstrated.[131,156]

Although the tumor is moderately radiosensitive, recurrence after radiation therapy is rather common despite an initially favorable response.

Acinic cell adenocarcinoma (clear cell carcinoma, serous cell adenocarcinoma). Acinic cell adenocarcinoma appears to arise from the intercalated duct cells of normal glands, chiefly the parotid gland. It is uncommon, constituting about 2.3% of major salivary gland tumors.[107] It occurs about twice as frequently in women as in men.

The tumor is usually rounded and is well encapsulated in about one half of the cases. It is slow growing but has a tendency to recur, especially when poorly encapsulated. The recurrent lesion is usually multiple. Characteristically, metastasis occurs to the lungs, bones, and brain. Regional spread is rather uncommon. The tumor occurs most commonly in the third and fourth decades. On cut section, it is gray to reddish tan, soft, friable, and, occasionally, somewhat cystic.

Histologically, acinic cell adenocarcinoma occurs in two distinct forms—the granular cell, which is the more common, and the clear cell. Some tumors are admixtures of the two types. The granular cell type is composed of large polyhedral or rounded cells with small, dark, eccentrically placed nuclei. The cytoplasm is abundant, granular, and somewhat basophilic. PAS-positive material may be present, especially in microcystic areas. Occasionally, a lymphoid stroma is present. In over 10% of the tumors, the principal cell is clear, at times exhibiting a pseudoglandular papillary or cystic arrangement, greatly resembling adenocarcinoma (hypernephroma) of the kidney (Fig. 29-37). Ultrastructural studies have demonstrated that the granular cell variety is composed of cells that resemble the serous acinar cells of normal glands; i.e., they contain secretory granules and histochemically are identical with serous cells.[107,128,134,143]

Cells of the clear-cell variety, as the name implies, do not stain with hematoxylin and eosin and do not react with stains for glycogen or mucin. Electron microscopic studies have demonstrated a large number of free ribosomes and few mitochondria and other organelles. The clear appearance is attributable to the clumping and margination of the free ribosomes after formalin fixation. Presumably, the clear cell variety arises from the striated ducts.

Carcinoma in pleomorphic adenoma. Confusion exists regarding the "malignant mixed tumor," and two separate views regarding it are available. One ascribes the term to those salivary gland neoplasms that are histologically similar to pleomorphic adenoma but, because of cellular activity (mitotic index), nuclear pleomorphism, and growth characteristics, are felt more likely to recur or metastasize. On the other hand, if serial sections are made on examples of all proved salivary gland malignancies, a focus of "typical" mixed tumor may be found, allowing the diagnosis. Obviously, divergent clinicopathologic data ensue from these two tumor groups.[159]

Squamous cell carcinoma. Squamous cell carcinoma comprises about 4% of major salivary gland tumors, arising predominantly in males in the sixth or seventh decade. The high degree of malignancy indicated by its histologic appearance is confirmed by its ag-

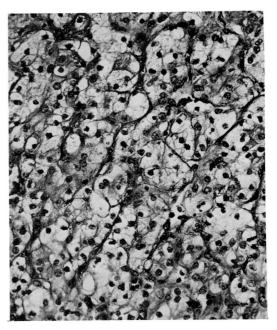

Fig. 29-37. Acinic cell adenocarcinoma. Note hypernephroid appearance.

gressive clinical behavior. Completely replacing salivary gland acini, the tumor infiltrates the skin and involves the facial nerve early in its clinical course. Pain may be severe. Metastatic spread is common. Care must be exercised to differentiate the squamous cell carcinoma from the poorly differentiated malignant mucoepidermoid carcinoma.

Papillary cystadenoma and cystadenocarcinoma. Papillary cystadenoma and cystadenocarcinoma occur most frequently in the parotid gland, less commonly in the submandibular and minor salivary glands. The majority of the adenocarcinomas are slow growing, somewhat invasive, and slow to metastasize. Microscopically, the tumor consists of glandlike spaces lined with tall columnar epithelium having eosinophilic cytoplasm. Mucin is commonly produced and may fill the glandlike spaces. Metastasis usually occurs to the regional lymph nodes and vertebrae (Figs. 29-38 and 29-39).

Undifferentiated carcinoma. Undifferentiated carcinoma consists of sheets or cords of anaplastic epithelial cells surrounded by varying amounts of fibrous stroma. Pleomorphism usually is noticeable, and mitotic figures are abundant. At times, some degree of differentiation into glandlike structures is noted, but this does not seem to have any effect upon

prognosis. Invasion of adjacent structures such as auditory canal, paranasal sinuses, and mandible is common, as well as local and widespread metastasis. Prognosis is poor—only radical surgery being of any value, for the tumor is characteristically radioresistant. It appears to run a more malignant course in children than in adults.

Other tumors of salivary glands. Several other tumors having their origin in the stromal tissues of salivary glands have been described: lipoma, rhabdomyosarcoma, leiomyoma, neurofibroma, neurilemoma, leiomyosarcoma, xanthoma, lymphangioma, malignant hemangioendothelioma, and fibromatosis.

Tumors of minor salivary glands. Tumors of the minor salivary glands include all those that occur in the major glands (parotid, submandibular, sublingual), with the exception of sebaceous cell adenoma and hemangioendothelioma.[121,135]

Pleomorphic adenoma appears to be the most common tumor arising from the intraoral minor salivary glands. Next in order of frequency are cylindromatous adenocarcinoma, mucoepidermoid tumor, and adenocarcinoma. Benign tumors occur most frequently in the fourth and fifth decades. The malignant tumors are most common in the sixth decade. The palate is the site of greatest predilection,

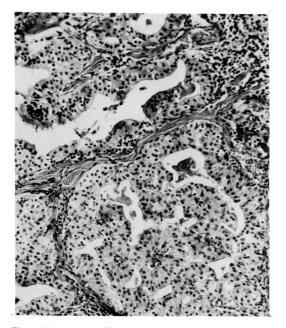

Fig. 29-38. Papillary cystadenoma. This tumor arises from neoplastic proliferation of ducts, being essentially a Warthin tumor without lymphoid stroma.

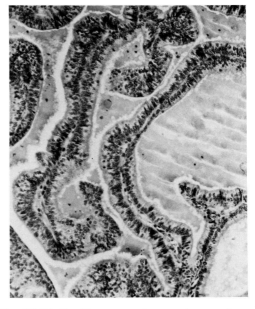

Fig. 29-39. Papillary cystadenocarcinoma. A most uncommon tumor, it occurs in both major and minor salivary glands.

followed by the upper lip, buccal mucosa, tongue, oral floor, and retromolar region. Cylindroma occurs about twice as frequently in women and in a slightly older age group. Minor salivary gland tumors rarely may occur entirely within the mandible.

NECK
Tumors

Carotid body tumor. Carotid body tumor (nonchromaffin paraganglioma, chemodectoma) arises in the carotid bodies, small ovoid nodules situated on the medial aspect of the bifurcation of the common carotid arteries. Histologically identical tumors are found in the aortic bodies, the glomus jugulare (paraganglion tympanicum), and the ganglion nodosum of the vagus nerve. All of these structures are apparently derived from neuroepithelial elements of the cranial nerves. They subsequently migrate to areas of mesodermal concentration about the vessels of the embryonic branchial arches.[136]

The tumor may become manifest at any age but rarely before puberty. There is a slight female predilection. About 5% are bilateral.

Microscopically, the tumor is lobulated and thinly encapsulated or embedded in loose connective tissue. It consists of nests of rather large polyhedral cells grouped together in an alveolar or organoid pattern (Fig. 29-40). The cell nests are separated by loose connective

tissue and a vascular stroma. The individual epithelial cells present rounded vesicular nuclei with pronounced nucleoli. Their cytoplasm is pale, eosinophilic, and frequently vacuolated, with indistinct cell boundaries. Rarely, bizarre, hyperchromatic cells, active mitoses, and capsular invasion may be observed. Spread to regional nodes or even distant dissemination has been noted but does not seem to adversely affect the patient.

Fibromatosis colli

Fibromatosis colli (torticollis, wryneck) occurs both as a primary and as a secondary disease.[138] Primary or congenital torticollis is manifest by a firm, fusiform swelling of the sternocleidomastoid muscle either at birth or within the first few weeks of life. The swelling usually increases for several weeks and then regresses, occasionally disappearing between the sixth and eighth month.

Grossly, the muscle is shortened, contracted, and fibrous. Clinically, the chin becomes tilted upward and toward the unaffected side. If untreated, facial asymmetry results, with adaptive scoliosis of the lower cervical and upper thoracic spine, foreshortening of the skull, and flattening of the facial bones on the involved side. Etiology is unknown, but theories have implicated birth trauma or, especially, uterine malposition. Often (35% to 50%) it is associated with breech delivery.

Microscopically, the muscle fibers are widely separated by dense, scarlike fibrous connective tissue (Fig. 29-41). Secondary torticollis is usually caused by a myositis that is attributed to a "chill." Occasionally it occurs after a

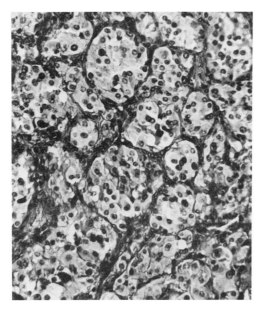

Fig. 29-40. Carotid body tumor.

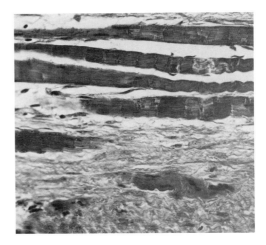

Fig. 29-41. Torticollis. Fibrous connective tissue replaces striated muscle fibers.

tumor of the cervical cord, or it may be a hysterical manifestation.

Cysts

Thyroglossal duct cysts. The thyroid gland arises as an anlage in the region of the foramen cecum of the tongue and descends into the anterior neck. If it persists in its embryonal position, it is spoken of as lingual thyroid.[126,127] Rarely, a strand of epithelium persists and connects the base of the tongue with the normally positioned thyroid gland. The thyroglossal duct cyst results from cystic degeneration of this tract. It is situated in the midline of the neck in the region of the hyoid bone, through which the tract usually passes. The cyst is lined by respiratory or stratified squamous epithelium, or by both types. The cyst may become infected and drain, becoming a thyroglossal duct fistula.[117]

Lymphoepithelial cyst. The lateral cervical cyst (branchial cyst) is located anterior to the sternocleidomastoid muscle near the angle of the mandible. The alleged association of these cysts or sinuses with squamous carcinoma appears unwarranted. Microscopically, the cyst is lined by either stratified squamous or pseudostratified ciliated columnar epithelium. Beneath the epithelium is abundant lymphoid tissue with germinal centers. The cysts are believed to arise from cystic degeneration of epithelium enclaved in cervical lymph nodes. The cyst usually becomes apparent during the third decade. Similar lesions may occur in the parotid gland or on the oral floor.

Parathyroid cyst. Microscopic cysts of the parathyroid glands are seen in at least 50% of normal specimens. Nevertheless, cysts large enough to produce clinical symptoms are rare.[139,177] (See also p. 1656.)

The parathyroid cyst is solitary and slow growing and may cause dysphagia and displacement of the trachea to the contralateral side, producing hoarseness by pressure on the recurrent laryngeal nerve. In several instances, this symptom has led to a preoperative diagnosis of thyroid carcinoma. It is found anywhere in the lateral neck from the angle of the mandible deep to the sternocleidomastoid muscle to the mediastinum. Most of the patients have been over 30 years of age, and a 2 : 1 female and left-sided predilection is evident.

The cyst is usually very thin and filled with a clear, watery fluid. Microscopically, it is lined by a somewhat flattened cuboid to low columnar epithelium. Within the collagenic connective tissue wall, one usually notes several types of parathyroid cells: water-clear cells, chief cells, and, occasionally, oxyphil cells. Not all three types are always present.

Cervical thymic cyst. Occasionally, remnants of thymus primordium are left in the neck, where they may remain undisturbed or, rarely, may undergo cystic alteration and subsequent enlargement. The cysts probably arise from degeneration of Hassall's corpuscles.[113] They present clinically most often at about the age of 3 to 6 years, and there appears to be a 2:1 male sex predilection. The cysts are usually elongated and may assume quite large proportions. They usually are located in the lateral neck at the angle of the mandible just anterior to the sternocleidomastoid muscle.

Microscopically, the cysts are lined by stratified squamous epithelium and often contain a thick reddish brown fluid. Rarely, cuboid epithelium is found. In the walls, thymic structures (i.e., Hassall's corpuscles) may be identified. The cyst is well encapsulated and often exhibits cholesterol crystals among the connective tissue fibers. (See also p. 1594.)

Cystic hygroma colli. The cystic hygroma or diffuse lymphangioma is manifest as a rather poorly defined soft-tissue mass in the neck. It is present at birth. Usually located behind the sternocleidomastoid muscle, it may extend to involve the shoulder or mediastinum.[118]

Microscopically, it consists of large endothelium-lined lymphatic spaces in a loose connective tissue stroma (Fig. 29-42).

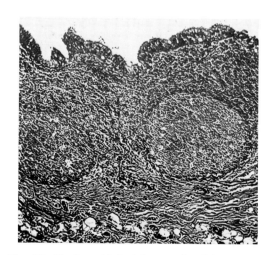

Fig. 29-42. Branchial cleft cyst lined by respiratory epithelium with lymphoid tissue in connective tissue wall.

Inflammatory disease

Ludwig's angina. Ludwig's angina is a severe, boardlike cellulitis of the neck involving all of the submandibular spaces. Prior to the advent of antibiotics, this was a rare complication of periapical infection of the mandibular molars or extension from an acute osteomyelitis occurring after compound fracture of the mandible. Drainage of a mixed infection through the lingual plate of the mandible into one or more spaces and subsequent extension with pronounced edema of the glottis commonly resulted in death through severe toxemia and asphyxiation.[142]

REFERENCES
General

1 Gorlin, R. J., and Goldman, H.: Thoma's Oral pathology, ed. 6, St. Louis, 1970, The C. V. Mosby Co.
2 Gorlin, R. J., Pindborg, J. J., and Cohen, M. M., Jr.: Syndromes of the head and neck, ed. 2, New York, 1976, McGraw-Hill Book Co.
3 International histological classification of tumours. No. 5. Histological typing of odontogenic tumours, jaw cysts and allied lesions, Geneva, 1971, World Health Organization.
4 Pindborg, J. J.: Pathology of the dental hard tissues, Philadelphia, 1970, W. B. Saunders Co.
5 Shafer, W. G., Hine, M. K., and Levy, B. M.: Oral pathology, ed. 3, Philadelphia, 1974, W. B. Saunders Co.
5a Stewart, R. E., and Prescott, G. H., editors: Oral facial genetics, St. Louis, 1976, The C. V. Mosby Co.

Face and lips

6 Beckwith, B.: Birth Defects 5(2):188-196, 1969 (macroglossia-omphalocele syndrome).
7 Boughman, R. A.: Oral Surg. 34:781-799, 1972 (lingual thyroid).
8 Cervenka, J., Gorlin, R. J., and Anderson, V. E.: Am. J. Hum. Genet. 19:416-432, 1967 (congenital lip fistulas).
9 Fogh-Andersen, P.: Acta Chir. Scand. 129:275-281, 1965 (macrostomia).
10 Glass, D.: Br. J. Oral Surg. 1:194-199, 1964 (hemifacial atrophy).
11 Gorlin, R. J., Cervenka, J., and Pruzansky, S.: Birth Defects 7(7):3-49, 1971 (facial clefting and clefting syndromes).
12 Halperin, V., Kolas, S., Jeffries, K. R., Huddleston, S. O., and Robinson, H. B. G.: Oral Surg. 6:1072-1077, 1953 (developmental oral anomalies).
13 Monroe, C. W.: Plast. Reconstr. Surg. 38:312-319, 1966 (median cleft of mandible).
14 Nevin, N. C., Dodge, J. A., and Kerhohan, D. C.: Oral Surg. 29:443-446, 1970 (aglossia).
15 Gorlin, R. J., Old, T., and Anderson, V. E.: Z. Kinderheilkd. 108:1-11, 1970 (hypohidrotic ectodermal dysplasia—genetic heterogeneity).

Teeth

16 Ast, D. B., Kantwell, K. T., Wachs, B., and Smith, D. J.: J. Am. Dent. Assoc. 53:314-325, 1956 (study of fluorine on caries in Newburgh and Kingston).
16a Backer-Dirks, O.: Int. Dent. J. 17:582-605, 1967 (dental caries).
17 Darling, A. I.: In Gorlin, R. J., and Goldman, H. M., editors: Thoma's Oral pathology, ed. 6, St. Louis, 1970, The C. V. Mosby Co. (dental caries).
17a Edwardson, E.: Arch. Oral Biol. 13:637-646, 1968 (Streptococcus mutans).
18 Goldman, H. M., and Cohen, D. W.: Periodontal therapy, ed. 4, St. Louis, 1968, The C. V. Mosby Co. (experimental periodontal disease).
19 Keyes, P. H.: Arch. Oral Biol. 1:304-320, 1960 (infectious nature of caries).
20 Keyes, P. H.: J. Am. Dent. Assoc. 76:1357-1373, 1968 (research in dental caries).
21 Murray, J.: Br. Dent. J. 126:352-354, 1969 (fluoride and caries).
22 Naylor, M. N.: Proc. Roy. Soc. Med. 62:839-844, 1969 (caries research).
23 Ruben, M. P., Goldman, H. M., and Schulman, S. M.: In Gorlin, R. J., and Goldman, H. M., editors: Thoma's Oral pathology, ed. 6, St. Louis, 1970, The C. V. Mosby Co. (periodontal disease).
23a Scherp, H. W.: Science 173:1199-1205, 1971 (dental caries: prospects for prevention).
24 Schulze, C.: In Gorlin, R. J., and Goldman, H. M., editors: Thoma's Oral pathology, ed. 6, St. Louis, 1970, The C. V. Mosby Co. (developmental abnormalities of teeth).
25 Witkop, C. J., Jr., and Rao, S.: Birth Defects 7(7):153-184, 1971 (inherited defects in tooth structure).

Mouth

26 Andreasen, J. O.: Oral Surg. 25:31-42, 158-166, 1968 (lichen planus).
27 Angelopoulos, A., and Goaz, P. W.: Oral Surg. 34:888-906, 1972 (Dilantin gingival hyperplasia).
28 Aparacio, S. R., and Lumsden, C. E.: J. Pathol. 97:339-355, 1969 (granular cell tumor—ultrastructure).
29 Archard, H. O., Carlson, K. P., and Stanley, H. R.: Oral Surg. 25:717-728, 1968 (leukoedema).
30 Banks, P.: Br. J. Oral Surg. 4:227-234, 1967 (infectious mononucleosis—oral lesions).
31 Barron, S. L., Roddick, J. W., Jr., Greenlaw, R. H., Rush, B., and Tweeddale, D. N.: Cancer 21:672-681, 1968 (multiple primary cancers).
32 Bennett, D. E.: Arch. Intern. Med. (Chicago) 120:417-427, 1967 (histoplasmosis).
33 Bowerman, J. E.: Br. J. Oral Surg. 6:188-191, 1969 (oral pigmentation—Albright's syndrome).
34 Bronner, M., and Bronner, M., editors: Actinomycosis, London, 1969, John Wright & Sons, Ltd.
35 Browne, W. G., Izatt, M. M., and Renwick, J. H.: Ann. Hum. Genet. 32:271-281, 1969 (white sponge nevus).
36 Cady, B., and Catlin, D.: Cancer 23:551-569, 1969 (gingival carcinoma).
36a Chue, P. W. Y., J. Am. Dent. Assoc. 90:1297-1301, 1975 (oral gonorrhea).
37 Clausen, F. P., Mogeltoft, M., Roed-Petersen,

B., and Pindborg, J. J.: Scand. J. Dent. Res. 78:287-294, 1970 (focal epithelial hyperplasia).

38 Cook, B. E. D.: Br. Dent. J. 109:83-96, 1960 (recurrent aphthae).

39 Cook, B. E. D.: Br. Dent. J. 109:83-96, 131-138, 1960 (oral bullous lesions).

40 Dummett, C. O., and Barens, G.: J. Periodont. 38:369-378, 1967 (oral pigmentation—review).

40a Eilard, U., and Hellgren, L.: Dermatologica (Basel) 130:101-106, 1965 (herpes).

41 Einhorn, J., and Wersäll, J.: Cancer 20:2189-2193, 1967 (oral cancer and oral leukoplakia).

42 Forman, G.: Br. Dent. J. 119:83-84, 1965 (occupational oral keratosis).

43 Goethals, P. L., Harrison, E. G., Jr., and Devine, K. D.: Am. J. Surg. 106:845-851, 1963 (verrucous oral carcinoma).

44 Gorlin, R. J.: Oral Surg. 32:760-767, 1971 (epidermolysis bullosa).

45 Green, D.: Oral Surg. 15:1312-1324, 1962 (scleroderma—oral changes).

45a Greenberg, M. S., et al.: J. Dent. Res. 48:385-391, 1969 (intraoral herpes).

46 Himalstein, M. R., and Humphrey, T. R.: Arch. Otolaryngol. (Chicago) 87:389-395, 1968 (pseudosarcoma).

47 Jepsen, A., and Winther, J. E.: Acta Odontol. Scand. 23:239-256, 1965 ("speckled leukoplakia").

48. Komet, H., Schaefer, R. F., and Mahoney, P. L.: Arch. Otolaryngol. (Chicago) 82:649-651, 1965 (tuberculosis—oral manifestations).

49 Lehner, T., and Sagebiel, R. W.: Br. Dent. J. 121:454-456, 1966 (aphthae—electron microscopic changes).

50 Lever, W. F.: Pemphigus and pemphigoid, Springfield, Ill., 1965, Charles C Thomas, Publisher (pemphigus and pemphigoid).

51 Martin, J. L., and Crump, E. P.: Oral Surg. 34:49-58, 1972.

52 Masson, J. K., and Soule, E. H.: Am. J. Surg. 110:585-591, 1965 (rhabdomyosarcoma).

53 Muller, S. A.: Oral Surg. 32:752-759, 1971 (oral viral infections).

53a Meyer, I., and Shklar, G.: Oral Surg. 23:45-57, 1967 (acquired oral syphilis).

54 Nally, F. F., and Ross, I. H.: Oral Surg. 32:221-234, 1971 (herpes zoster).

55 O'Day, R. A., Soule, E. H., and Gores, R. J.: Oral Surg. 20:85-93, 1965 (oral embryonal rhabdomyosarcoma).

56 Pindborg, J. J., Gorlin, R. J., and Asboe-Hansen, G.: Oral Surg. 16:551-560, 1963 (Reiter's syndrome—oral lesion).

57 Pindborg, J. J., and Sirsat, S. M.: Oral Surg. 22:764-779, 1966 (oral submucous fibrosis).

58 Pindborg, J. J., Renstrup, G., Silverman, S., Jr., and Poulsen, H. E.: Acta Odontol. Scand. 21:407-414, 1963 (clinical and histologic signs of malignancy—leukoplakias).

59 Poole, A. G., and Marchetta, F. C.: Cancer 22:14-21, 1968 (plasmacytoma).

60 Pretorius-Clausen, F.: Pathol. Microbiol. (Basel) 39:204-213, 1973 (focal epithelial hyperplasia).

60a Putkonen, T.: Acta Dermat. Vener. (Stockholm) 42:44-62, 1962 (congenital syphilis—dental changes).

61 Scott, J., and Finch, L. D.: Oral Surg. 34:920-933, 1972 (Wegener's granulomatosis).

62 Sharp, G. S., Bullock, W. K., and Helsper, J. T.: Cancer 14:512-516, 1961 (multiple oral carcinoma).

62a Ship, I. I.: Oral Surg. 33:400-406, 1972 (recurrent aphthae).

63 Silverman, S., Jr., and Griffith, M.: Oral Surg. 37:705-710, 1974 (lichen planus).

64 Simons, J. N.: Am. J. Surg. 116:494-498, 1968 (oral malignant melanoma).

64a Smith, J. F.: Arch. Otolaryngol. 101:276-277, 1975 (snuff granuloma).

65 Snijman, P. C.: Br. J. Oral Surg. 4:106-110, 1967 (gangrenous stomatitis).

66 Soderquist, N. A., and Reed, W. B.: Arch. Dermatol. (Chicago) 97:31-33, 1968 (pachyonychia congenita).

66a Southam, J. C., Colley, I. T., and Clarke, N. G.: Br. J. Dermatol. 80:248-256, 1968 (herpetic gingivostomatitis).

67 Sprague, W. G.: Oral Surg. 16:1067-1074, 1963 (terminology of "leukoplakia").

68 Thoma, K. H.: In Gorlin, R. J., and Goldman, H. M., editors: Thoma's Oral pathology, ed. 6, 1970, The C. V. Mosby Co., St. Louis.

69 Van Wyk, C. W.: Med. Proc. (Johannesb.) 11:531-537, 1965 (oral lesion caused by snuff).

70 Vickers, R. A.: In Gorlin, R. J., and Goldman, H. M., editors: Thoma's Oral pathology, ed. 6, St. Louis, 1970, The C. V. Mosby Co. (oral soft-tissue neoplasms).

70a Waldron, C. A.: In Gorlin, R. J., and Goldman, H. M., editors: Thoma's Oral pathology, ed. 6, St. Louis, 1970, The C. V. Mosby Co. (oral epithelial tumors).

70b Waldron, C. A., and Shafer, W. G.: Cancer 36:1386-1392, 1975 (oral leukoplakia).

71 Vickers, R. A., Gorlin, R. J., and Lovestedt, S. A.: Northwest Dent. 44:339-342, 1965 (oral cancer—mass screening).

71a Witkop, C. J., Jr.: Birth Defects: Original Article Series. Part XI. Orofacial structures, VII (7):210-221, 1971 (heterogeneity in gingival fibromatosis).

72 Whitten, J. B.: Oral Surg. 26:202-213, 1968 (granular cell tumor—ultrastructure).

72a Wyk, C. W. van: J. Oral Pathol. 6:1-24, 1977 (focal epithelial hyperplasia).

73 Zachariae, H.: Acta Derm. Venereol. (Stockholm) 43:149-153, 1963 (palatal pigmentation—antimalarial drugs).

Jaws

74 Allen, M. S., Jr., et al.: Am. J. Clin. Pathol. 51:309-314, 1969 (melanotic neuroectodermal tumor).

75 Barros, R. E., Dominguez, F. V., and Cabrini, R. L.: Oral Surg. 27:225-236, 1969 (odontogenic myxoma).

75a Beasley, J. D., III: J. Am. Dent. Assoc. 92:145-152, 1976 (traumatic cysts of jaws). 206, 1966 (melanotic neuroectodermal tumor)

76 Bennett, J. E., Tignor, S. P., and Shafer, W. G.: Am. J. Surg. 116:538-541, 1968 (osteosarcoma of jaws).

77 Borello, E., and Gorlin, R. J.: Cancer 19:196-206, 1966 (melanotic neuroectodermal tumor of infancy).

78 Brady, R. O., and King, F. M.: In Hers, H. G., and Van Hoff, F., editors: Lysosomes and storage diseases, New York, 1973, Academic Press, Inc. (Gaucher's disease).

78a Brannon, R. B.: Oral Surg. 43:233-255, 1977 (odontogenic keratocyst).

78b Browne, R. M.: J. Oral Pathol. 4:31-46, 1975 (odontogenic cysts—review).

79 Burkitt, D.: Cancer 20:756-759, 1967 (Burkitt's lymphoma—review).

80 Chaudhry, A. P., Robinovitch, M. R., Mitchell, D. F., and Vickers, R. A.: Am. J. Surg. 102: 403-411, 1961 (chondrosarcoma in jaws).

81 Cina, M. T., Dahlin, D. C., and Gores, R. J.: Mayo Clin. Proc. 36:664-678, 1961 (ameloblastic fibroma).

82 Clausen, F., and Poulsen, H.: Acta Pathol. Microbiol. Scand. 57:361-374, 1963 (carcinoma metastatic to jaws).

82a Fuhr, A. H., and Krogh, H. J.: J. Oral Surg. 30:30-35, 1972 (congenital epulis of the newborn).

83 Gardner, D. G., Michaels, L., and Liepa, E.: Oral Surg. 26:812-823, 1968 (calcifying odontogenic tumor).

84 Gorlin, R. J., Chaudhry, A. P., and Pindborg, J. J.: Cancer 14:73-101, 1961 (odontogenic tumors—review).

85 Gorlin, R. J., and Sedano, H. O.: Birth Defects 7(8):140-151, 1971 (nevoid basal cell carcinoma syndrome).

86 Harless, C. F., Jr.: Oral Surg. 20:684-689, 1965 (gingival cysts).

86a Hayward, A. F., Fickling, B. W., and Lucas, R. B.: Br. J. Cancer 23:702-708, 1969 (melanotic neuroectodermal tumor of infants—ultrastructure).

87 Hoke, H. F., and Harrelson, A. B.: Cancer 20: 991-999, 1967 (metastatic ameloblastoma).

88 Jacobsohn, P. H., and Quinn, J. H.: Oral Surg. 26:829-836, 1968 (ameloblastic odontoma).

89 Krols, S., and Pindborg, J. J.: Arch. Pathol. 98:206-210, 1974 (calcifying epithelial odontogenic tumor).

90 Norgaard, B., and Pindborg, J. J.: Acta Ophthalmol. (Kbh.) 37:52-58, 1959 (osteomyelitis of jaw in infants).

91 Philipsen, H. P., and Birn, H.: Acta Pathol. Microbiol. Scand. 75:375-398, 1969 (adenomatoid odontogenic tumor).

92 Pincock, L. D., and Bruce, K. W.: Oral Surg. 7:307-311, 1954 (odontogenic fibroma).

93 Pindborg, J. J., and Clausen, F.: Acta Odontol. Scand. 16:293-301, 1958 (odontogenic tumors —classification).

94 Sedano, H. O., Cernea, P., Hosxe, G., and Gorlin, R. J.: Oral Surg. 27:760-771, 1969 (histiocytosis X—oral changes).

95 Small, I. A., and Waldron, C. A.: Oral Surg. 8:281-297, 1955 (ameloblastoma).

96 Smith, J. F., Blankenship, J., Drake, J., and Robbins, M.: Oral Surg. 17:618-627, 1964 (ameloblastoma—granular cell variety).

97 Spouge, J. D.: Oral Surg. 24:392-403, 1967 (odontogenic tumors).

98 Spouge, J. D., and Spruyt, C. L.: Oral Surg. 25:447-457, 1968 (odontogenic tumors).

99 Steg, R. F., Dahlin, D. C., and Gores, R. J.: Oral Surg. 12:128-141, 1959 (malignant lymphoma).

100 Topazian, R. G., and Costich, E. R.: J. Oral Surg. 23:559-568, 1965 (cherubism).

101 Waldron, C. A.: J. Oral Surg. 28:58-64, 1970 (fibrous lesions of jaws).

102 Weary, P. E., Linthicum, A., Cawley, E. P., Coleman, C. C., Jr., and Graham, G. F.: Arch. Dermatol. (Chicago) 90:20-30, 1964 (osteomatosis-polyposis or Gardner's syndrome).

103 Wright, D. H.: Br. J. Surg. 51:245-251, 1964 (Burkitt's lymphoma in jaws).

104 Vickers, R. A., Dahlin, D. C., and Gorlin, R. J.: Oral Surg. 20:476-480, 1965 (amyloid-containing odontogenic tumors).

105 Vickers, R. A., and Gorlin, R. J.: Cancer 26: 699-710, 1970 (histopathologic criteria of ameloblastoma).

106 Zegarelli, E. V., Kutscher, A. H., Napoli, N., Iurono, F., and Hoffman, P.: Oral Surg. 17: 219-224, 1964 (cementoma, periapical fibrous dysplasia).

Salivary glands and neck

107 Abrams, A. M., Cornyn, J., Scofield, H. H., and Hansen, L. S.: Cancer 18:1145-1162, 1965 (acinic cell carcinoma).

108 Abrams, A. M., and Finck, F. M.: Cancer 24: 1057-1063, 1969 (sialadenoma papilliferum).

108a Abrams, A. M., and Melrose, R. J.: Cancer 32: 130-135, 1973 (necrotizing sialometaplasia).

109 Abramson, A. L., Goodman, M., and Kolodny, H.: Arch. Otolaryngol. (Chicago) 88:91-94, 1968 (Sjögren's syndrome—palatal salivary glands).

110 Assor, D.: Am. J. Clin. Pathol. 53:100-103, 1970 (sebaceous lymphadenoma).

111 Azzopardi, J. G., and Smith, O. D.: J. Pathol. Bacteriol. 77:131-140, 1959 (histochemistry of mucins in salivary gland tumors).

112 Balogh, K., and Roth, S. I.: Lab. Invest. 14: 310-320, 1965 (electron microscopy of oncocytoma).

113 Barrick, B., and O'Kell, R. T.: J. Pediatr. Surg. 4:355-358, 1969 (thymic cysts).

114 Bazaz-Malik, G., and Gupta, D. N.: Z. Krebsforsch. 70:193-197, 1968 (malignant oncocytoma).

115 Bergman, F.: Cancer 23:538-543, 1969 (minor salivary gland tumors).

116 Bloch, K. J., Buchanan, W. W., Wohl, M. J., and Bunim, J. J.: Medicine (Balt.) 44:187-231, 1965 (Sjögren's syndrome—review).

117 Brintnall, E. S., Davies, J., Huffman, W. C., and Lierle, D. M.: Arch. Otolaryngol. (Chicago) 59:282-289, 1954 (thyroglossal duct cysts).

118 Broomhead, I. W.: Br. J. Plast. Surg. 17:225-244, 1964 (cystic hygroma).

119 Bunim, J. J., Buchanan, W. W., Wertlake, P. T., Sokoloff, L., Bloch, K. J., Beck, J. S., and Alepa, F. P.: Ann. Intern. Med. 61:609-630, 1964 (Sjögren's syndrome—review).

120 Catone, G. A., Merrill, R. G., and Henny, F. A.: J. Oral Surg. 27:774-786, 1969 (ranula).

121 Chaudhry, A. P., Vickers, R. A., and Gorlin,

R. J.: Oral Surg. **14**:1194-1226, 1961 (minor salivary gland tumors—review).

122 Chisholm, D. M., and Mason, D. K.: J. Clin. Pathol. **21**:656-660, 1968 (Sjögren's syndrome —labial salivary glands).

123 Davidson, D., Leibel, B. S., and Berrie, B.: Ann. Intern. Med. **70**:31-38, 1969 (Sjögren's syndrome).

124 Deppisch, L. M., and Toker, C.: Cancer **24**: 174-184, 1969 (ultrastructure of mixed tumor).

125 Deysine, M., and Mann, B. F., Jr.: Ann. Surg. **169**:437-443, 1969 (sebaceous lymphadenoma).

126 Dodds, W. J., and Powell, M. R.: Am. J. Roentgenol. **100**:786-791, 1967 (lingual thyroid scanning with technetium).

127 Downton, D., and O'Riordan, B. C.: Br. J. Oral Surg. **1**:29-32, 1963 (lingual thyroid).

128 Echevarria, R. A.: Cancer **20**:563-571, 1967 (acinic cell carcinoma, clear cell carcinoma—ultrastructure).

129 Eneroth, C. M., Blanck, C., and Jakobsson, P. A.: Acta Otolaryngol. (Stockholm) **66**:477-492, 1968 ("malignant mixed tumor").

130 Eneroth, C. M., Hjertman, L., and Moberger, G.: Acta Otolaryngol. (Stockholm) **64**:514-536, 1967 (submandibular gland tumors).

131 Eneroth, C. M., Hjertman, L., and Moberger, G.: Acta Otolaryngol. (Stockholm) **66**:248-260, 1968 (cylindroma).

132 Eneroth, C. M.: Cancer **27**:1415-1418, 1971 (salivary gland tumors).

133 Font, R. L., Yanoff, M., and Zimmerman, L. E.: Am. J. Clin. Pathol. **48**:365-376, 1967 (Sjögren's syndrome—lacrimal glands).

134 Fox, N. M., ReMine, W. H., and Woolner, L. B.: Am. J. Surg. **106**:860-867, 1963 (acinic cell carcinoma).

135 Frable, W. J., and Elzay, R. P.: Cancer **25**: 932-941, 1970 (minor salivary gland tumors).

136 Glennier, G. G., and Grimley, P. M.: In: Atlas of tumor pathology, Ser. 2, Fasc. 9, Washington, D.C., 1973, Armed Forces Institute of Pathology (extra-adrenal paraganglion system tumors).

137 Grishman, E.: Cancer **5**:700-707, 1952 (histochemistry of mixed tumors).

138 Gruhn, J., and Hurwitt, E. S.: Pediatrics **8**: 522-526, 1951 (fibroblastic sternomastoid tumor of infancy).

139 Haid, S. P.: Arch. Surg. (Chicago) **94**:421-426, 1967 (parathyroid cysts).

140 Hamperl, H.: Cancer **15**:1019-1927, 1962 (oncocytoma, benign and malignant).

141 Hamperl, H.: Virchows Arch. (Pathol. Anat.) **335**:452-483, 1962 (oncocytoma).

142 Herd, R. M., and Hall, J. F.: Oral Surg. **4**: 1523-1527, 1951 (Ludwig's angina).

143 Hübner, G., Klein, J., and Kleinsasser, O.: Virchows Arch. (Pathol. Anat.) **345**:1-14, 1968 (ultrastructure of acinic cell carcinoma).

144 Jakobsson, P. A., Blanck, C., and Eneroth, C. M.: Cancer **22**:111-124, 1968 (mucoepidermoid carcinoma).

145 Kauffman, S., and Stout, A. P.: Cancer **16**: 1317-1331, 1963 (salivary gland tumors in children).

146 Kessler, H. S.: Am. J. Pathol. **52**:671-685, 1968 (Sjögren's syndrome—animal model).

147 Kierszenbaum, A. L.: Lab. Invest. **18**:391-396, 1968 (ultrastructure of mixed tumor).

148 Kini, M. G.: Br. Med. J. **2**:415, 1940 (parotid cyst).

149 Kleinsasser, O., and Klein, H. J.: Arch. Klin. Exp. Ohren Nasen Kehlkopfheilkd. **190**:272-285, 1968 (malignant mixed tumor).

150 Kleinsasser, O., Klein, H. J., and Hübner, G.: Arch. Klin. Exp. Ohren Nasen Kehlkopfheilkd. **192**:100-105, 1968 (salivary duct carcinoma).

151 Leake, D., and Leake, R.: Pediatrics **46**:203-207, 1970 (neonatal parotitis).

152 Lenson, N., and Strong, M. S.: New Eng. J. Med. **254**:1231-1233, 1956 (multiple mixed tumors—review).

153 Luna, M. A., Stimson, P. G., and Bardwil, J. M.: Oral Surg. **25**:71-86, 1968 (minor salivary gland tumors).

154 McGavran, M. H. P.: Virchows Arch. (Pathol. Anat.) **338**:195-202, 1965 (papillary cystadenoma lymphomatosum—electron microscopy).

155 Macsween, R. N., Goudie, R. B., Anderson, J. R., Armstrong, E., Murray, M. A., Mason, D. K., Jasani, M. K., Boyle, J. A., Buchanan, W. W., and Williamson, J.: Ann. Rheum. Dis. **26**:402-411, 1967 (Sjögren's syndrome—autoimmune studies).

156 Market, J.: Arch. Klin. Exp. Ohren Nasen Kehlkopfheilkd. **184**:496-500, 1965 (ultrastructure of cylindroma).

157 Marsden, A. T. H.: Br. J. Cancer **5**:375-381, 1951 (salivary gland tumors in Malaya).

158 Masson, J. K., and Soule, E. H.: Am. J. Surg. **112**:615-622, 1966 (head and neck desmoid tumors).

159 Moberger, J. G., and Eneroth, C. J.: Cancer **21**:1198-1211, 1968 (malignant mixed tumor).

160 Moses, S. W., Rotem, Y., Jagoda, N., Talmor, N., Eichhorn, F., and Levin, S.: Isr. J. Med. Sci. **3**:358-371, 1967 (familial dysautonomia).

161 Myerson, M., Crelin, E. S., and Smith, H. W.: Arch. Otolaryngol. (Chicago) **83**:488-490, 1966 (salivary gland duct duplication).

162 Reimann, H. A., and Lindquist, J. N.: J.A.M.A. **149**:1465-1467, 1952 (periodic sialorrhea).

163 Reynolds, C. T., McAuley, R. L., and Rogers, W. P., Jr.: Am. J. Surg. **111**:168-174, 1966 (minor salivary gland tumors).

164 Richard, E. L., and Ziskind, J.: Oral Surg. **10**: 1086-1090, 1957 (ectopic salivary glands).

165 Robinson, L., and Hjørting-Hansen, E.: Oral Surg. **18**:191-205, 1964 (mucocele).

166 Ruebner, B., and Bramhall, J. L.: Arch. Pathol. (Chicago) **69**:110-117, 1960 (malignant papillary cystadenoma lymphomatosum).

167 Sandstead, H. R., Koehn, C. J., and Sessions, S. M.: Am. J. Clin. Nutr. **3**:198-214, 1955 (parotid enlargement in malnutrition).

168 Scher, I., and Scher, L. B.: Br. Dent. J. **98**: 324-325, 1955 (imperforate salivary ducts).

169 Schwartz, I. S., and Feldman, M.: Cancer **23**: 636-640, 1969 (mucoepidermoid tumors).

170 Silverglade, L. B., Alvares, O. F., and Olech,

E.: Cancer **22:**650-653, 1968 (central muco-epidermoid tumors in jaws).

171 Smith, L. C., Lane, N., and Rankow, R. M.: Am. J. Surg. **110:**519-526, 1965 (cylindroma).

172 Stebner, F. C., Eyler, W. R., DuSault, L. A., and Block, M. A.: Am. J. Surg. **116:**513-517, 1968 (papillary cystadenoma lymphomatosum and technetium).

173 Talal, N., Sokoloff, L., and Barth, W. F.: Am. J. Med. **43:**50-65, 1967 (Sjögren's syndrome—lymphoma).

174 Thackray, A. C., and Lucas, R. B.: Atlas of tumor pathology, Ser. 2, Fasc. 10, Washington, D.C., 1974, Armed Forces Institute of Pathology (salivary gland tumors).

175 Thompson, A. S., and Bryant, H. C., Jr.: Am. J. Pathol. **26:**807-849, 1950 (histogenesis of papillary cystadenoma lymphomatosum).

176 Welsh, R. A., and Meyer, A. T.: Arch. Pathol. (Chicago) **85:**433-447, 1968 (histogenesis of mixed tumors).

177 Wood, J. W.: Arch. Surg. (Chicago) **92:**785-790, 1966 (parathyroid cysts).

178 Wukl, M. J., and Bloch, K. J.: Postgrad. Med. **45:**108-116, 1969 (Sjögren's syndrome).

179 Yarington, C. T., Jr., and Zagibe, F. T.: J. Laryngol. **83:**361-365, 1969 (ultrastructure of papillary cystadenoma lymphomatosum).

30/Alimentary tract

ROBERT C. HORN, Jr.
GERALD FINE

CONGENITAL ANOMALIES
Atresia

Most malformations of the alimentary tract are congenital and are related to the formation of the bowel lumen or bowel rotation. Interruption in the continuity of the bowel lumen, which may be partial (stenosis) or complete (atresia), manifests itself in early infancy and is incompatible with life without prompt surgical correction. The common sites involved are the esophagus, small intestine, and anus. Esophageal atresia is frequently associated with tracheoesophageal fistulas. Webs of vascularized fibrous tissue covered by mucosa may be the cause of narrowing of the upper or lower portion of the esophagus (Fig. 30-1). Those in the former site are more often seen in women and frequently are associated with atrophic glossitis, iron-deficiency anemia, and dysphagia (Plummer-Vinson syndrome). Intestinal atresia may be associated with *meconium ileus* (see discussion of cystic fibrosis, p. 1459), which has been considered by some to be the cause of the atresia. Faulty development of the hindgut, which is intimately related to the development of the cloacal septum, is frequently associated with fistulas between the rectum and urinary or genital tract or the perineum. Failure of the proctodeum to invaginate or of the anal plate to be absorbed results in *imperforate rectum* or *anus*.

Heterotopia

Gastric mucous membrane may be found in the cervical esophagus or associated with other malformations such as Meckel's diverticulum, duplications, or enteric cysts. *Pancreatic tissue,* in the form of discrete nodules of acinar and ductal tissue and occasionally islets of Langerhans, are most common in the stomach and duodenum and less frequently in the jejunum, Meckel's diverticulum, and appendix. The *adenomyoma,* an admixture of ducts and smooth muscle, is encountered in the stomach and gallbladder.

Duplications and enteric cysts

These are segments of gastrointestinal tube in apposition to any portion of the alimentary canal that may be completely independent of the adjacent normal intestine or share its lumen and mesentery and muscle coats. They develop in one of two ways—multicentric recanalization of the proliferated luminal gut epithelium or persistence, growth, and sequestration of diverticular buds of the developing intestine. The two are similar in makeup, but the cysts are more or less spheric and usually lack communication with the gut lumen. Duplications are commonest in the region of the terminal ileum, whereas cysts are most

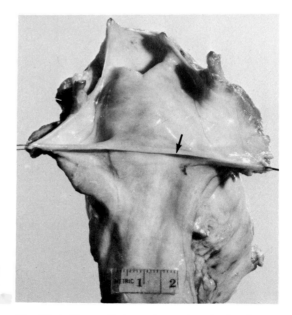

Fig. 30-1. Congenital esophageal web. Esophagus has been opened posteriorly.

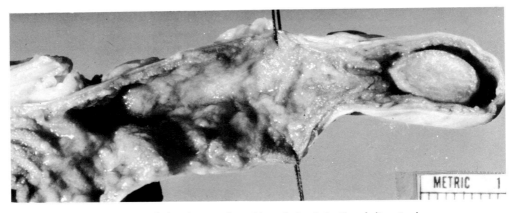

Fig. 30-2. Meckel's diverticulum. Note fruit pit in tip of diverticulum.

often intrathoracic and related to the esophagus. They may be lined by small intestinal, gastric, or even bronchial mucous membrane; if gastric, peptic ulceration with concomitant hemorrhage or perforation may occur.

Meckel's diverticulum

Meckel's diverticulum is a diverticulum on the antimesenteric aspect of the terminal ileum, 1 inch to 6 feet proximal to the ileocecal valve, and possesses all the layers of small bowel (Fig. 30-2). It represents the commonest of many possible residua of the omphalomesenteric-duct; others are umbilical sinus, cyst between the ileum and umbilicus, and ileoumbilical fistula. Its mucosa is usually that of the small intestine, but in 25% of the cases gastric mucosa with or without pancreatic tissue may be present. It may make itself clinically known as a result of peptic ulceration and hemorrhage, obstruction of its lumen, intussusception, or diverticulitis.

Aganglionic megacolon (Hirschsprung's disease)

Aganglionic megacolon is characterized by symptoms of partial or complete intestinal obstruction usually from birth or very early in life with great dilatation and hypertrophy of the colon. The underlying anatomic defect is a lack of ganglion cells in Auerbach's (myenteric) plexus and Meissner's (submucous) plexus in a narrowed, nonhypertrophied segment of intestine distal to the extremely dilated and hypertrophied colon, which is innervated normally (Plate 2, *A*). The aganglionic area usually does not extend higher than the sigmoid colon, but instances of involvement of the entire colon and even the small intestine occur. The diagnosis can be made on the failure to find ganglion cells on adequate rectal biopsy. Surgical resection of the aganglionic segment relieves the condition.

Pyloric stenosis

Gross narrowing of the pylorus secondary to an unexplained hypertrophy of the pyloric muscle manifests itself, usually in male infants, by vomiting with attendant dehydration and malnutrition in *congenital pyloric stenosis*. Surgical relief is obtained by incision of the hypertrophied muscle. A similar condition is occasionally seen in adults, but only rarely is it unassociated with a gastric or duodenal ulcer.

Plate 2
A, Congenital aganglionic megacolon (Hirschsprung's disease).
B, Multifocal epidermoid carcinoma of esophagus. Photograph of gross specimen superimposed upon roentgenogram demonstrating lesion with aid of contrast medium.
C, Familial multiple polyposis of colon.
D, Multiple chronic gastric (peptic) ulcers. Pylorus is just to left of ulcer on left.
E, Carcinomatous ulcer of stomach. Lesion presumed to have been malignant from its inception. *Lower left,* Focus of carcinoma.
F, Carcinoma of stomach, linitis plastica type. Surgically resected specimen.
G, Multiple carcinoid tumors of ileum. Patient had lymph node and liver metastases and demonstrated carcinoid syndrome.

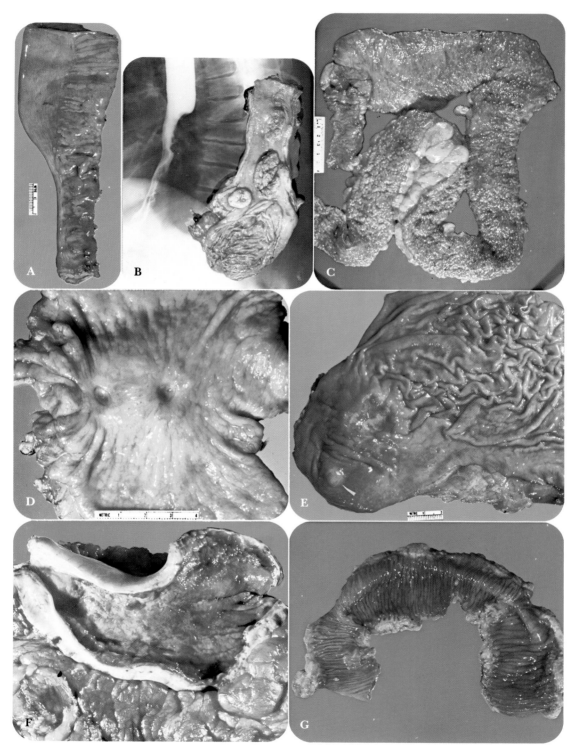

Plate 2
For legend see opposite page.

Achalasia of esophagus

Achalasia of the esophagus predominates in women, usually becomes manifest in adult life, and is associated with pronounced dilatation and hypertrophy of the entire esophagus, except the distal spastic segment.

Various changes in the ganglia of the spastic segment have been reported—partial or complete absence or degeneration. Vagus nerve degeneration has also been implicated in the pathogenesis of this condition.[18]

Miscellaneous

A variety of anomalies of position may involve the gastrointestinal tract—the presence of portions of the tract in internal or external or diaphragmatic hernial sacs, malrotation or failure of descent of the intestine, transposition associated with transposition of other viscera, and variations in development or attachment of the mesentery. Any or all of these anomalies may be responsible for volvulus and intestinal obstruction.

Abnormal peritoneal bands also may produce obstruction. A *congenitally short esophagus* may be associated with herniation of a portion of gastric cardia into the thoracic cavity, so-called *hiatus hernia* (p. 1281).

Multilocular rectal cysts with variable epithelial lining—squamous, columnar with mucin, or transitional—presumably having their origin from the neurenteric canal or postanal gut, may be responsible for intestinal obstruction, abscesses or fistulas. Association of the cysts with a dimple of the anal mucous membrane in its posterior midline has been reported.

ACQUIRED MALFORMATIONS
Diverticula

Acquired diverticula of the gastrointestinal tract are for the most part "false" (pulsion diverticula), representing herniations of the mucous membrane and muscularis mucosae through weakened areas or defects in the muscularis propria. Their walls do not have

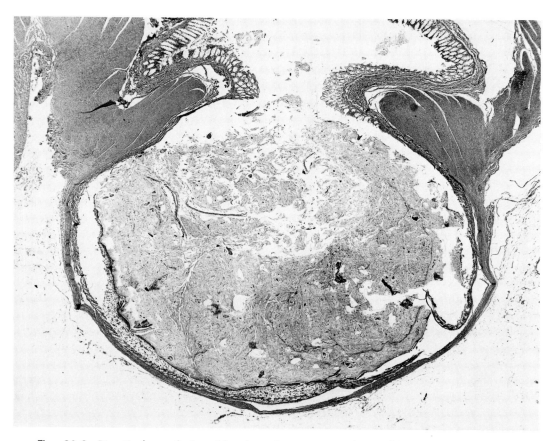

Fig. 30-3. Diverticulum of sigmoid colon, demonstrating hernia-like nature. Note fecal content. (17×.)

all the layers of the segment of alimentary tract from which they arise but are composed of mucous membrane, muscularis mucosae and areolar tissue (Fig. 30-3). They occur at the junction of the esophagus and hypopharynx (Zenker's diverticulum), in the second portion of the duodenum, in the small intestine, and in the appendix, but they are most frequent and clinically significant in the colon. In the last site, they are frequently multiple and most prevalent in the descending and sigmoid colon. They ocur on the convexity of the intestine opposite the mesenteric attachment and between the long muscle bands (taenias). Although numerous, they may be difficult to discern, being hidden externally by epiploic appendages and internally by muscle contraction, which diminishes their luminal orifice. Clinical manifestations may be acute or chronic or related to one of a number of factors or combination of factors, e.g., bowel spasm, occlusion of diverticula by fecalith and diverticulitis with and without perforation.

The less commonly acquired diverticula, "true" (traction) diverticula, occur in the esophagus and first portion of the duodenum just distal to the pylorus. In both sites, they are the result of inflammation and scarring; those in the esophagus are related to hilar and mediastinal lymph node disease, whereas those in the pylorus are secondary to duodenal or pyloric ulcers.

Pneumatosis cystoides intestinalis

In pneumatosis intestinalis, gas-filled cysts are found in the submucosa or wall of the small intestine, less frequently in the colon, and rarely in the stomach and esophagus at necropsy (Fig. 30-4). The process is associated with gastric or duodenal ulcers, enterocolitis, or respiratory disease, notably asthma. It now appears that the condition can be explained on a mechanical basis in association with (1) obstruction with ulceration, (2) trauma from biopsy, sigmoidoscopic examination, etc., or (3) respiratory disease with severe cough. In the last case, it is postulated that pneumo-mediastinum occurs after pulmonary alveolar rupture, since the air then dissects retroperitoneally and reaches the intestine along the path of the mesenteric blood vessels. The gas cysts range in diameter from a few millimeters to a centimeter or more and may be lined by flattened endothelium-like cells resembling lymphatic spaces or multinucleated giant cells, or they may have no visible lining. The cysts do not communicate with the intestinal lumen

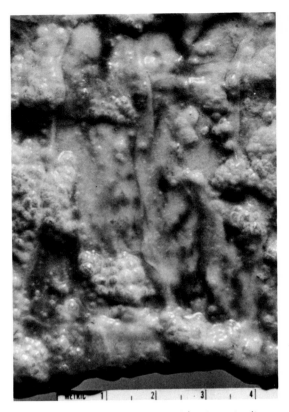

Fig. 30-4. Pneumatosis cystoides intestinalis.

or with each other. The symptoms of pneumatosis are generally nonspecific. Spontaneous resolution with radiographic clearing can and does occur.

Melanosis of colon

The mucous membrane of the colon and appendix may acquire a brown color because of the accumulation of brown granular pigment in phagocytes in the lamina propria. Although the pigment is referred to as melanin, its exact nature is unknown. The condition is not of clinical significance. One suggestion is that it is related to colonic stasis and the habitual use of anthracene laxatives.

Endometriosis

Foci of endometrial glands and endometrial stroma may involve the colon, usually the sigmoid or rectum, appendix, or small bowel. It may be responsible for obstructive symptoms, colic, and diarrhea, or even rectal bleeding. Obstruction is the result of fibrosis or muscle spasm, and cancer can be simulated both radiographically and at operation. Less commonly a *decidual reaction* associated with pregnancy may be found involving the serosa of the bowel.

Miscellaneous

Many of the malformations more commonly seen as congenital lesions also may be acquired. For example, *esophagotracheobronchial fistulas* may result from infection, trauma, or neoplasm, and *acquired megacolon* in the adult may result from a destructive lesion of the myenteric plexus.

MECHANICAL DISTURBANCES
Obstruction

The relative incidence of the various causes of *intestinal obstruction* varies, but hernias, adhesions, and neoplasms are the common causes. Other causes are volvulus, foreign objects, inflammatory disease, stricture, and external compression by tumors, cysts, enlarged viscera, etc., as well as such congenital lesions as annular pancreas, meconium ileus, and the atresias, bands, etc., previously noted.

Hernia

Hernia is the protrusion of tissue, organ, or part of an organ through an abnormal opening in the wall of the body cavity in which it is normally confined. The majority of hernias are abdominal, resulting from herniation of abdominal contents through the internal or external inguinal rings, femoral ring, or defects in the abdominal wall resulting from trauma or improper healing after a surgical procedure. Less common are internal hernias, wherein loops of intestine penetrate normally small peritoneal recesses, such as the fossa at the junction of the duodenum and jejunum. Diaphragmatic hernias are not a significant cause of intestinal obstruction. Herniation of abdominal viscera through congenital defects in the diaphragm is infrequent compared to *hiatus hernia,* which is the protrusion, often intermittent ("sliding" hernia), of a portion of the stomach and abdominal esophagus through the esophageal hiatus of the diaphragm into the thoracic cavity. Symptoms in the latter—a disease of obese, middle-aged individuals—are related to the reflux of gastric secretions into the esophagus, with resultant so-called peptic esophagitis, ulceration, and hemorrhage. Herniation of the gastric cardia through the esophageal hiatus also may occur alongside the esophagus, called paraesophageal hernia.

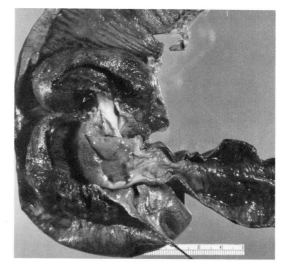

Fig. 30-5. Ileocecal intussusception with infarction.

Adhesions

In addition to congenital bands, peritoneal adhesions secondary to inflammation and after laparotomy may be responsible for intestinal obstruction, usually the small intestine.

Neoplasms

Intestinal obstruction may result from primary or secondary bowel involvement by neoplasm. The more common obstructing primary tumors are the encircling carcinomas that occur in the left half of the colon where the intestinal content is semisolid.

Intussusception

This is the invagination of a segment of intestinal tract (the intussusceptum) into the immediately adjacent (almost always distal) intestine (the intussuscipiens). It is primarily a disease of infants and young children, but it does occur in adults, in whom it may be initiated by a pedunculated benign or malignant primary tumor or a metastatic growth. In children it is more common in the ileocecal region, with the ileum telescoping into the colon and the ileocecal valve retaining its normal position (Fig. 30-5). Less common are ileoileal and colocolonic intussusception. Masses of lymphoid tissue, polyps, or the ileocecal valve itself may form the advancing head of the intussusception, or the lesion may be the result of uncoordinated muscle contractions of the bowel. Bowel obstruction or compromise of blood supply to the involved intestine requires surgical intervention if spontaneous correction does not occur. Multiple foci of intussusception, unassociated with any reaction, are seen occasionally at necropsy and are believed to be agonal.

Volvulus

Volvulus is the twisting of a loop (or loops) of intestine upon itself through 180 degrees or more that produces obstruction of both the intestine and the blood supply of the affected loop. Causative factors are usually long mesenteric attachment, redundant intestine, abnormal bands, congenital or acquired, or abnormal attachments of the intestine. The lesion is most common in the sigmoid colon and predominates in men. Because strangulation occurs almost simultaneously with obstruction, operative treatment must be prompt to avoid death of the patient.

Obturation obstruction

A foreign body, exogenous or endogenous, large or small, may obstruct the intestinal lumen by inducing bowel spasm or becoming entrapped in areas of anatomic or pathologic narrowing of the intestinal lumen. Gallstone obstruction of the small intestine complicating cholecystogastric or cholecystoduodenal fistula, large-bowel obstruction by enteroliths and appendiceal obstruction by fecaliths are examples of common endogenous obstruction. Almost any conceivable ingested foreign body may produce bowel obstruction. Fruit pits and bezoars—masses of ingested hair (trichobezoars) or vegetable residues (phytobezoars), most notably persimmons—are worthy of mention. Parasites, particularly *Ascaris lumbricoides,* are also causes of intestinal obstruction.

Stricture

Intrinsic narrowing of the intestinal lumen may be the result of scarring in one or more of its layers as a result of chemical injury (e.g., lye in the esophagus), peptic ulceration of the esophagus or duodenum, x-ray irradiation, scarring at the sites of surgical anastomosis or intestinal resection, or scleroderma.

Adynamic (paralytic) ileus

The clinical picture of acute intestinal obstruction may occur in the absence of mechanical or organic obstruction as a result of paralysis of the musculature of a portion or all of the intestinal tract. Abdominal distention and accumulation of gas and fluid in the intestine may be extreme, producing the same effects as mechanical obstruction. It frequently occurs after laparotomy, usually in a mild

form. It may be associated with intra-abdominal infection, trauma, or other disease (e.g., ureteral stone) or systemic infection (e.g., pneumonia in children). Peritonitis secondary to acute appendicitis with perforation, perforated peptic ulcer, etc., is probably the most important single underlying cause. A related condition is *acute dilatation of the stomach,* which occasionally complicates surgery, usually abdominal.

Effects of intestinal obstruction

The systemic effects of bowel obstruction are variable in their severity, being dependent on the site involved and the degree of obstruction. They are related to fluid and electrolyte loss, distention with fluid and gas, and damage to the bowel wall and resulting permeability to bacteria and, potentially, peritonitis. One or more of the following may be associated with the obstruction—dehydration, acidosis, alkalosis, hemoconcentration, decrease in intracellular fluid, and finally renal suppression. The bowel proximal to the obstruction shows varying degrees of dilatation and hypertrophy depending on the location and the completeness of the obstruction, as well as the duration.

Mallory-Weiss syndrome

Any action that increases intra-abdominal pressure, but particularly bouts of repeated and forceful vomiting, may produce one or more lacerations of the gastric cardia that may be the source of gastrointestinal hemorrhage, sometimes massive. This syndrome, known eponymically by those who first described it, frequently occurs in alcoholics or is associated with atrophic gastritis. The tears occur in the long axis of the stomach and esophagus, occasionally crossing the esophagogastric junction.

VASCULAR DISTURBANCES
Esophageal varices

Elevated pressure in the portal venous system, most often the result of cirrhosis of the liver but, at times, caused by such other lesions as portal vein thrombosis, commonly results in esophageal varices. The esophageal venous plexus receives blood from the gastric and coronary veins of the stomach, forming part of one of the routes by which portal venous blood may bypass the liver to reach the right atrium. As a result, the submucosal veins of the lower part of the esophagus, and sometimes of the upper part of the stomach as well, become greatly dilated, tortuous, and engorged. They are covered by a thin mucous membrane. The increased venous pressure, with or without inflammation or ulceration, often results in massive and frequently fatal hemorrhage.

Infarction of intestine

Compromise of the blood supply to the intestine may result in its necrosis (gangrene). Excluding strangulation, as discussed previously, the causes of infarction in order of decreasing frequency are sclerosis of the mesenteric arteries with or without associated thrombosis; embolism; venous thrombosis; vascular diseases such as arteriolar sclerosis, thromboangiitis obliterans, and periarteritis nodosa; and hypotension in association with non-occlusive atheromatous disease, which by itself has compromised the blood supply short of producing infarction. Emboli may be vegetations or thrombi in the diseased left side of the heart or atheromatous material dislodged from aortic plaques. The superior mesenteric vessels and consequently the jejunum and proximal part of the ileum are involved most frequently, although any part or all of the gastrointestinal tract may be affected.

Infarction from arterial occlusion is usually anemic initially but with time becomes hemorrhagic. Venous occlusion preceding arterial blockage causes infarction that is hemorrhagic from its inception. The bowel becomes dusky and purple red because of hemorrhage into the bowel wall and lumen and subsequent necrosis and inflammatory cell infiltration. The resulting paralysis of the bowel muscle produces an intestinal obstruction with its attendant physiologic alterations.

Ischemic enteritis

Reduction in blood flow to the intestine insufficient to produce a full-thickness infarct may result in a variety of nonspecific lesions—ulceration, inflammation, cicatrization with stricture formation and "intestinal angina." The distinction between such lesions and those believed to be related to potassium ingestion is not always clear.

Hemorrhoids

Hemorrhoids are varicosities of the hemorrhoidal vein—"internal" and covered by mucous membrane if of the superior hemorrhoidal plexus and "external" and covered by skin if of the inferior hemorrhoidal plexus. The former are the more important and the more troublesome. They result from increased venous pressure related to such causes as portal hypertension, cardiac failure, carcinoma of the rectum, or myomatous or pregnant uterus, but chronic constipation appears to be far more important in their pathogenesis.

The coincidence of hemorrhoids and rectal carcinoma is sufficiently great to make search for the latter mandatory in every patient with hemorrhoids.

Complications of hemorrhoids are thrombosis with associated inflammation, scarring, pain, and hemorrhage in the form of bright red blood passed by rectum. Organization of a thrombus may produce a histologic picture that may mimic the malignant hemangioendothelioma.

Gastrointestinal hemorrhage

Bleeding into the gastrointestinal tract may be the result of a wide variety of lesions and may be minimal, producing anemia, or massive and life threatening. If the blood is eliminated orally or rectally soon after escaping from the vascular system, it is bright red, but if it is confined to the alimentary tract for a period of time before being eliminated, it is brown or black (coffee-ground vomitus and tarry stools —melena). The most important sources of massive hematemesis (vomiting of blood) are esophageal varices, gastric or duodenal (peptic) ulcer, and leiomyoma. Other tumors (benign or malignant), hiatus hernia, gastritis, etc. usually produce bleeding of lesser degree. Massive bleeding from the rectum or anus is less common than massive hematemesis. Hemorrhoids, diverticular disease, or the polyps of the Peutz-Jeghers syndrome may cause it. However, these lesions also may be associated with bleeding of small amount, as is commonly found in carcinoma of the large intestine and, less often, with other tumors, regional enteritis, ulcerative colitis, and anal fissure. The lesions causing hematemesis are also associated with blood in the stool, which may be occult (i.e., detectable only by chemical means. Other conditions that should be considered as potential causes of any type of gastrointestinal bleeding include hereditary telangiectasis (Rendu-Osler-Weber disease), other vascular malformations, any of the blood dyscrasias, and anticoagulant therapy.

INFLAMMATIONS
Esophagitis

Inflammation of the esophagus is most commonly the result of reflux of gastric secretion associated with hiatus hernia, achalasia, and scleroderma and less commonly caused by the ingestion of corrosive substances such as lye and viral infections—herpes simplex and chicken pox. Scarring with degrees of stricture are most frequently associated with the ingestion of lye and long-standing reflux of gastric secretions.

Esophageal pseudodiverticulosis is a condi-

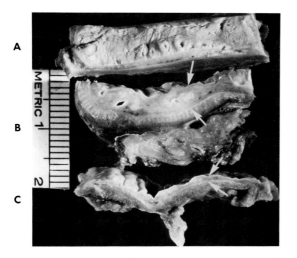

Fig. 30-6. A and **B,** Pseudodiverticulosis of esophagus. **C,** Normal esophagus. Ducts of esophageal glands are prominent in thickened submucosa *(arrows)* in pseudodiverticulosis, and their openings on mucosal surface are accentuated, **A.** (Courtesy Dr. Aaron Lupovitch, Detroit, Mich.)

tion that radiographically mimics diverticula but that pathologically is dissimilar. The x-ray changes are attributable to dilatation and tortuosity of the esophageal glands and their ducts, but there is no abnormal extension of mucosa beyond the confines of the esophageal submucosa. The process appears to be the result of inflammation and obstruction of the increased number of esophageal glands (Fig. 30-6).

Gastritis and gastroenteritis

The gastritis and gastroenteritis that are such common clinical complaints rarely come to the attention of the pathologist. They are the result of exogenous agents, e.g., alcohol, therapeutic drugs (salicylate, etc.), irradiation, and corrosive agents, or endogenous agents, e.g., bacterial and viral agents involving the bowel or other organs and allergy. *Phlegmonous gastritis,* usually of streptococcal origin, is secondary to inflammation elsewhere in the body, e.g., osteomyelitis.

Eosinophilic granuloma and eosinophilic gastroenteritis

These manifest themselves, either as a localized, fibrotic, polypoid, tumorlike mass (inflammatory fibroid polyp,[60] Fig. 30-7) or as a diffuse infiltration throughout all coats of the gut wall. Eosinophils make up a prominent part of the histopathologic picture in

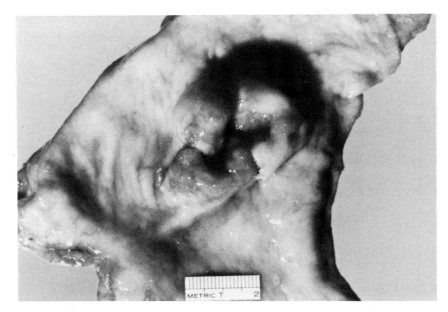

Fig. 30-7. Eosinophilic granuloma (inflammatory fibroid polyp) of stomach.

both lesions, but blood eosinophilia and a history of allergy are associated only with the diffuse lesion. Sites of involvement in order of frequency include the stomach, jejunum, ileum, and cecum. The colon and rectum are rarely involved.

Ulcers of stomach and duodenum

Ulcers, usually small and multiple and not penetrating the muscularis mucosae (erosions), are frequently encountered in the stomach as a terminal event in a variety of conditions. Acute ulcers of the stomach or duodenum may be associated with extensive burns (Curling's ulcers, Fig. 30-8), Cushing's disease, hypothalamic lesions, stress or trauma; they may also be iatrogenic (corticosteroid therapy, gastric tubes). They may be fatal as a result of uncontrolled hemorrhage or spontaneous perforation and peritonitis.

Nonspecific ulcers in the small intestine have been encountered with increasing frequency. They may be complicated by scarring and partial intestinal obstruction. Vascular changes and potassium, a known tissue irritant therapeutically employed in enteric coated tablets, have been implicated in their pathogenesis.

Peptic ulcer

Incidence and etiology. Chronic ulcers having certain similarities and distinct differences occur in the stomach and duodenum. Duodenal ulcers are more common and more often found in young and middle-aged men, whereas gastric ulcers are more frequent in women. Duodenal ulcer has been associated with tension, stress, and anxiety, but this is by no means always the case and there is no agreement on the importance of stress in its pathogenesis. Peptic ulcers occur only in the environment of acid gastric secretions: the stomach, duodenum, lower esophagus, jejunum just distal to the site of surgical gastroenteric anastomosis, and malformations containing gastric mucosa. The mucous membrane not accustomed to the acid-pepsin environment is the site involved. Thus gastric ulcers occur in the antrum, infrequently in the cardia, whereas the acid secretion is usually limited to the fundus.

Hypersecretion of gastric juice and emotional factors have been considered to be important in the pathogenesis of peptic ulcers. The gastroduodenal mucous membrane is protected against digestion by normal gastric secretions not only by its mucous coating but also by dilution and neutralization with swallowed food, saliva, and regurgitated duodenal fluids. Hypersecretion of hydrochloric acid into the fasting stomach at night is regarded by Dragstedt as the cause of duodenal ulcer. This is considered to be the result of vagal stimulation and can be abolished by section of the vagus nerve. He regards the gastric ulcer also to be the result of increased hydrochloric acid secretion attributable to a humoral (gastrin) stimulation brought about by stasis of ingested food in an atonic stomach.

Emotional factors responsible for vagal stimulation through the hypothalamus–anterior pituitary–adrenal cortex stress mechanism have been shown by Wolf to affect gastric function. Cortisone, which may be the cause of ulcers, usually gastric, may also activate a preexisting ulcer and be responsible for perforation or hemorrhage.

Morbid anatomy and histology. Gastric ulcers most commonly occur on or near the lesser curvature of the stomach, usually within about 5 cm of the pylorus. They are more numerous on the posterior than the anterior wall. A few occur in the cardia, and a few seemingly straddle the pylorus, making it difficult to assign them definitely to either stomach or duodenum. Duodenal ulcers usually occur in the first centimeter or two distal to the pylorus on the anterior or posterior wall rather than laterally.

Although some gastric ulcers are large and irregular, the typical peptic ulcer is small (± 1 cm in the duodenum; 1 to 2.5 cm in the stomach). It is characteristically "punched

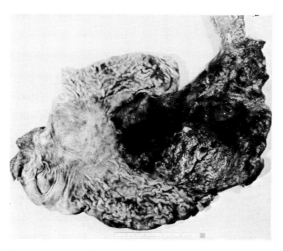

Fig. 30-8. Curling's ulcer of proximal part of stomach.

out," with sharply defined margins, sometimes sloping distally. The ulcer penetrates deeply. Its edges are neither raised nor overhanging (Plate 2, *D*). The mucosal folds converging upon the ulcer are distinct to the edge of the lesion. In the case of *gastric ulcer*, it is important, although often difficult and sometimes impossible, to differentiate the lesion from a *malignant ulcer*. The latter is usually a bowl-shaped lesion, and the entire ulcer tends to be raised above the surface of the rest of the stomach (Plate 2, *E*). Penetration is not usually deep, and the progress of the mucosal folds toward the crater is interrupted by nodular mucosal or submucosal thickening.

Microscopically, the bed of the ulcer is seen to be covered by fibrinous exudate containing fragmented leukocytes. Separating this from the scar tissue base is fibrotic granulation tissue with a plasma cell and lymphocytic infiltrate. Occasionally, eosinophils are prominent. The scar tissue is dense and avascular and occupies a full-thickness defect in the muscularis. Hypertrophic nerve bundles may be conspicuous, and at times a large artery, often thrombosed or sclerotic, may be seen. In some bleeding ulcers, such a vessel may be recognized on gross examination.

Many ulcers heal, and epithelium grows over the defect in a single layer. In time, glandlike structures may develop, but a completely normal mucous membrane is not regenerated. Because of the dense scar, the muscle does not regenerate, and evidence of the ulcer will remain indefinitely.

Complications. The principal complications of peptic ulcer are hemorrhage, perforation, and obstruction. Which, if any, occurs is dependent in part on the location of the ulcer. Both gastric and duodenal ulcers are subject to massive hemorrhage. Duodenal ulcers are especially prone to perforation. Any ulcer, but especially those located posteriorly, may bleed in smaller amounts, producing melena or evidence of occult blood in the stool.

Anterior duodenal ulcers may perforate into the free peritoneal cavity, with resultant generalized peritonitis. Perforating posterior ulcers more often penetrate into the pancreas, producing intractable pain. Posterior perforation also may occur into the lesser peritoneal sac, leading to localized peritonitis. The omentum or adhesions to adjacent organs also may serve to localize peritoneal inflammation. The peritonitis from perforated peptic ulcer is initially a chemical inflammation, but bacterial contamination soon follows.

Pyloric obstruction may be a complication of an ulcer, gastric or duodenal, situated near the pylorus. It usually results from a combination of cicatricial narrowing and spasm. The stomach becomes greatly dilated and hypertrophied.

The development of carcinoma has been referred to as one of the complications of peptic ulcer. It seems probable that carcinoma can develop in a preexisting ulcer, but it is equally probable that it is a rare event. It is extremely difficult to establish the fact of such a sequence of events in any particular case.

A complication of surgical treatment of ulcer is the development of a *marginal (stomal) ulcer*—peptic ulceration of the jejunum just distal to the site of anastomosis with the stomach after gastroenterostomy or gastric resection with gastrojejunostomy. Such ulcers may perforate. If perforation into the transverse colon takes place, gastrojejunocolic fistula is the result.

Regional enteritis

Regional enteritis (Crohn's disease) is a chronic inflammatory disease of unknown etiology affecting a portion of the intestinal tract, occurring in young adults, and frequently producing partial intestinal obstruction. The disease most commonly involves the terminal ileum, often with extension into the cecum and sometimes into the ascending colon as well. It is usually in the terminal ileum that narrowing produces partial obstruction. In more than half the cases, multiple areas of both small and large intestine are involved in segmental fashion, i.e., lengths of normal intestine separate areas of disease (so-called skip areas). Changes may be limited to the colon, segmentally or involving the whole organ. Crohn's disease of the colon (or granulomatous colitis) is being recognized with infrequency (Fig. 30-9).

The inflammatory changes are nonspecific and more or less granulomatous. The mucosal surface has a reddened, nodular, cobblestone-like appearance, with multiple, linear ulcerations. All coats of the diseased intestine are thickened—the mucosa by inflammatory infiltrate, chiefly of lymphocytes and plasma cells, the submucosa and subserosa by fibrosis, and the muscularis by hypertrophy (Fig. 30-10). The fibrosis and infiltrate extend into the mesentery.

Histologically, irregular ulceration with a neutrophilic leukocytic reaction is seen. In the

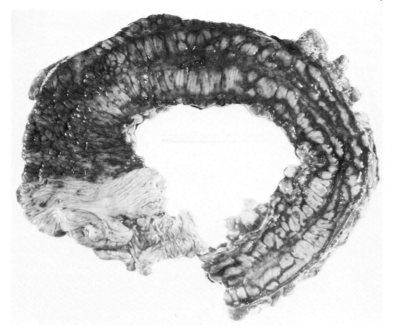

Fig. 30-9. Granulomatous colitis (Crohn's disease of colon) involving almost entire large bowel.

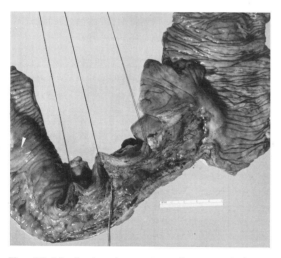

Fig. 30-10. Regional enteritis of terminal ileum. Note abrupt cessation of pathologic change at ileocecal valve.

preserved mucous membrane, the glands are dilated, goblet cells are absent or decreased in number, and Paneth cells are more prominent than usual. Peculiar glands resembling Brunner's glands of the duodenum or pyloric glands frequently are seen. The muscularis mucosae is hypertrophied, and nerves in the involved segment are increased in number, size, and prominence. Lymphoid nodules are conspicuous in the submucosa, and often in the subserosa as well. Tubercles composed of epithelioid cells, with occasional multinucleated giant cells but without necrosis, are conspicuous in some cases. They have given rise to the speculation of etiologic identity with Boeck's sarcoid, an idea that has been abandoned. Deep ulcers may give rise to sinus tracts and perforations, which usually are walled off by omentum or adhesions. Fistulas may complicate long-standing cases. The fistulas may be internal, involving other organs or other segments of intestine, or external, opening on the skin of the abdomen, after surgical procedures. The regional lymph nodes are enlarged. They usually show nonspecific inflammatory changes but may contain granulomas like those in the intestine.

Lymphatic obstruction is believed to play a primary role in the pathogenesis of regional enteritis, giving rise to submucosal edema. This, in turn, is followed by fibrosis, lymphoreticular hyperplasia, and, ultimately, secondary mucosal ulceration, inflammation, and the other changes described. Ammann and Bockus[71] suggest that ulceration results from shortening and distortion of Kerkring's folds, in turn the result of shortening of the muscularis mucosae early in the development of the disease.

Appendicitis

Acute appendicitis is uncommon at the extremes of age and is most frequently seen in older children and young adults. The most important factor in its pathogenesis is obstruction of the lumen—the most frequent cause being a fecalith—a molded mass of inspissated fecal material that may develop rock-hard consistency. Fecaliths are found in at least three fourths of acutely inflamed appendices and in virtually all that are gangrenous. In youth, the lymphoid tissue of the mucous membrane may become sufficiently hyperplastic, at times in association with systemic infection, to produce obstruction leading to appendicitis or to cause symptoms and signs indistinguishable from those of mild acute appendiceal inflammation. Other causes of obstruction are scars representing a residual of previous attacks of appendicitis, tumors, external bands, adhesions, rarely masses of parasites (especially pinworms), foreign bodies, and possibly spasm of the muscle at the base of the appendix. The immediate cause of acute appendicitis is bacterial infection from the intestinal lumen although bacterial invasion from the bloodstream in systemic disease is possible. All species of bacteria common to the intestinal tract can be identified, and usually multiple organisms can be isolated from an individual case.

Inflammation of limited extent may manifest itself grossly only by mild hyperemia. Microscopic examination may show only small amounts of purulent exudate in the lumen although careful study may reveal one or more foci of inflammation with ulceration of the mucosa. Many examples of *focal appendicitis* are not merely an early phase of diffuse inflammation but a milder form of the disease, perhaps dependent on temporary or incomplete obstruction by such mechanisms as lymphoid hyperplasia or muscle spasm. The inflammation may appear to be limited to the muscle coat or subserosa, or both, but careful search usually shows mucosal involvement.

Hyperemia and margination of leukocytes in the peripheral blood vessels of the appendix, or even infiltration of polymorphonuclear leukocytes into the subserosal tissues may occur as a result of trauma during a surgical procedure, particularly if appendectomy is performed incidentally after a complex operation. Inflammatory change in the serosa and subserosa (periappendicitis) may be associated with disease primarily outside the appendix (e.g., salpingitis). At times a few neutrophilic leukocytes may be found in the lumen of an incidentally removed appendix without there being any evidence of inflammation of the appendiceal wall.

Diffuse acute appendicitis almost always occurs in an obstructed appendix. Increased intraluminal pressure compromises the blood supply and thus the effects of ischemia and bacterial infection contribute to an anatomic picture that is dependent on the time when the appendix is removed. Degrees of ulceration of the mucous membrane, infiltration of leukocytes, and hemorrhagic necrosis result in a distended appendix whose vessels are engorged and whose surface is dulled by a fibrinopurulent exudate. Perforation or sloughing of part or all of the appendix may result in *peritonitis*, which may be generalized, or walled off to form an *appendiceal abscess*. Infrequently encountered complications are pylephlebitis and liver abscess.

Not every instance of appendicitis follows this course. If tissue destruction is minimal, resolution follows or there may be cicatrization. Occasionally, true chronic inflammation of the appendix occurs, usually associated with fistula formation or a foreign body (intestinal content) after acute appendicitis with perforation. Otherwise true chronic appendicitis as a distinct entity does not exist.

Obliteration of part or all of the appendiceal lumen by a mixture of fibrous tissue, lymphocytes, lymphoid follicles, and nerve bundles is a common finding. Although frequently referred to as "obliterative appendicitis," there is no evidence that it is the result of inflammatory disease.

The appendix may be involved in diseases primarily affecting other portions of the gastrointestinal tract, such as regional enteritis, typhoid fever, and amebiasis and in certain systemic diseases (e.g., measles). In the prodromal stage of measles, characteristic Warthin-Finkeldy giant cells may be seen in the lymphoid tissue of the appendix, as well as in the lymphoid tissues of the rest of the body.

Many parasites may be found in the appendix. *Enterobius vermicularis* is the parasite most often encountered and may be noted on gross and histologic examination. Ordinarily they merely inhabit the appendix and have no relationship to appendiceal disease. On occasion, however, they may penetrate the wall and become the center of granulomatous inflammatory reaction.

Chronic ulcerative colitis

Chronic (idiopathic) ulcerative colitis is usually a disease of young adults, although its onset may be at any age. It runs a very protracted course. It frequently has been suggested that ulcerative colitis and regional enteritis might represent expression in different sites of an identical or related fundamental disease process. However, there are many differences, and although some features are common to both conditions, each generally forms a distinctive total pathologic picture. Although there are instances difficult to assign to one or the other category, it is now generally accepted that the distinction usually can be made between Crohn's disease involving the colon (granulomatous colitis) and chronic ulcerative colitis.

In many respects, ulcerative colitis appears to be a systemic disease rather than a condition affecting only the colon. It is generally believed that psychogenic factors are frequently of etiologic importance. Evidence has been accumulating recently to implicate hypersensitivity as a factor in causation, very likely secondary, since an immune basis for the disease has not been demonstrated. In patients with ulcerative colitis, the occurrence of drug and transfusion reactions, erythema nodosum, iritis, arthritis, hemolytic anemia, and elevated serum gamma globulin support this concept. In 1960, Priest et al.[89] demonstrated, in "skin windows" in patients with ulcerative colitis, the exudation of an unusually large number of basophilic leukocytes in response to a nonspecific injury. This was followed by the demonstration of increased numbers of mast cells in the exudate in the lesions of at least some cases of ulcerative colitis.

It frequently is stated that ulcerative colitis begins in the rectum or sigmoid and progresses proximally to involve the left side of the colon or the whole colon. This is not universally accepted, and it is possible that the theory is based upon the relative ease of establishing the diagnosis by proctoscopic examination. When the whole colon is examined, all or almost all of it is affected in the majority of cases. When a limited segment is involved, it is usually in the left half. It is probable that some of the instances of segmental distribution really represent regional enteritis (or enterocolitis). The terminal ileum is involved in approximately one fourth of cases, almost always in direct continuity with colonic disease.

The pathologic appearance of the colon varies greatly in different stages of the disease. Invariably, there is hyperemia, and the mucosa is dark red or purplish red and velvety (Fig. 30-11). At first, tiny erosions appear, later becoming deeper and coalescing to form linear ulcers, which have the appearance of

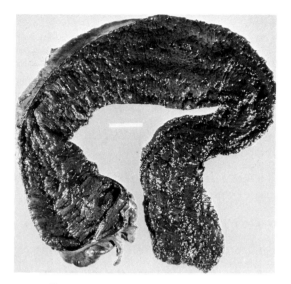

Fig. 30-11. Chronic ulcerative colitis.

longitudinal furrows distributed in the long axis of the colon. The ulcers are often undermining, partially freeing ragged remnants of mucous membrane. In occasional acutely progressing cases, the entire colon may be extremely friable and bleed freely. The muscle is thickened, apparently by contraction, and rigid, having lost, in whole or in part, its distensibility. This produces shortening as well as narrowing, and as the disease progresses, the colon comes more and more to resemble the garden hose to which it has been compared. Inasmuch as chronic ulcerative colitis is a disease of remissions and exacerbations, periods of relative quiescence and healing alternate with periods of activity.

The earliest histologic lesion in most cases is a crypt abscess—the accumulation of polymorphonuclear leukocytes in the crypts of Lieberkühn, with breakdown of the crypt wall. The crypt abscesses tend to coalesce to form enlarging, shallow ulcers. Along with the neutrophilic exudate are noted the other usual changes of inflammation, i.e., hyperemia, edema, hemorrhage, and, more deeply, accumulation of lymphocytes and plasma cells. Frequently, eosinophils as well as basophils are present in impressive numbers. The former are readily seen in routine histologic preparations, but special techniques are necessary to demonstrate basophils. Some authors have emphasized vasculitis as an early feature, but this is striking only in occasional cases. Ulcerative colitis is primarily a mucosal disease, with infrequent and usually limited involvement of the other layers, whereas regional enteritis is a disease of the submucosa and deeper tissues. Also, the inflammation of ulcerative colitis is not characteristically productive of abundant fibrous scar tissue. Granulomas with giant cells, like those of regional enteritis, are only an occasional finding in ulcerative colitis. When the ulcers heal, they are covered by a single layer of epithelium. Although there is an attempt to reform crypts, regeneration is not complete, and structural abnormalities persist. In quiescent chronic disease, the mucosa remains red and granular. As noted in the discussion of regional enteritis, chronic ulcerative colitis is to be distinguished from granulomatous colitis.

Pseudopolyps are a frequent and striking finding in ulcerative colitis. They consist of polypoid masses of granulation tissue that include distorted, inflamed crypts, often with hyperplastic epithelium. In contrast to adenomatous polyps, they vary greatly in size and shape, may be long and pendulous, and show no clear distinction between stalk and main body of the polyp. True adenomatous polyps do occur, however, in association with these inflammatory pseudopolyps.

There is a distinctly increased incidence of carcinoma of the colon in patients with ulcerative colitis of very long standing, particularly when the onset has been in childhood or adolescence. There may be multiple carcinomas. Whether or not this complication represents progression from pseudopolyp to adenomatous polyp to carcinoma is debated. Another important complication is acute dilatation of the colon in fulminant disease—so-called toxic megacolon. It constitutes an emergency and may progress to perforation.

Pseudomembranous enterocolitis

Pseudomembranous (staphylococcal) enterocolitis is an occasional complication of a major surgical procedure (usually on the intestinal tract) and is highly lethal. It almost invariably occurs in patients who have had antibiotic therapy, and it results from disturbance of the normal balance of the intestinal flora and infection by *Staphylococcus aureus (Micrococcus pyogenes)*, which elaborates a potent enterotoxin. The condition occurs more rarely as a terminal phenomenon in diverse other diseases, among them treated leukemia and lymphoma.

Pseudomembranous enterocolitis may involve any portion of the gastrointestinal tract from the lower esophagus to the rectum, most often the ileum. The lesion is an acute in-

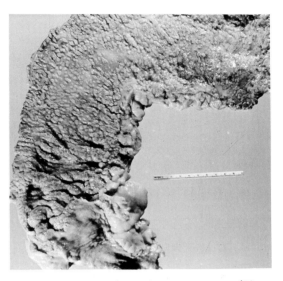

Fig. 30-12. Pseudomembranous enterocolitis.

flammation with necrosis, initially patchy, of the mucous membrane, producing focal erosions leading to diffuse ulceration. There is intense hyperemia, edema, and neutrophilic infiltration, often with perivascular hemorrhages. Characteristically, the ulcerated surface is covered by a pseudomembrane consisting of a fibrin mesh and mucus with entrapped inflammatory and blood cells and bacteria (Fig. 30-12). Large amounts of fluid distend the intestine. The disease usually develops between the third and seventh postoperative days and is attended by profuse watery diarrhea, dehydration, and profound shock.

Tuberculosis

Primary intestinal tuberculosis, ordinarily the result of ingestion of foods (especially dairy products) infected with the bovine tubercle bacillus, has become rare in the United States. Tuberculosis of the gastrointestinal tract is almost invariably associated with advanced open pulmonary disease with discharge from the lung lesions, and subsequent swallowing, of large numbers of bacilli. In fatal pulmonary tuberculosis, gastrointestinal involvement is quite common, and in disseminated disease, gastrointestinal lesions may be widespread.

The usual isolated gastrointestinal lesion involves the ileocecal or anal region. Rarely the esophagus, stomach, or intestine may be involved. Differentiation must be made from other infrequently encountered granuloma-producing conditions—Boeck's sarcoid, syphilis, and fungal and parasitic infections—and the granulomas of talc and barium.

Necrotizing enterocolitis

Necrotizing enterocolitis is an inflammatory process that involves primarily the mucosa and submucosa or the entire wall of the terminal ileum and varying lengths of the colon, principally of premature infants within the first few days of life and less commonly full-term infants or children in the first 2 months of life. Air, either superficial in the bowel wall or in the peritoneum, is not an infrequent accompaniment and in the latter site may be an aid in recognizing the condition by x-ray examination. Factors considered important in the etiology of the condition are ischemia resulting from a Shwartzman-like reaction, shunting of blood from the involved areas such as might occur with hypoxia and anoxia that is commonly seen in these infants, bacterial infections, and endotoxins. The disease is rapidly progressive and requires aggressive supportive therapy and surgical intervention in some instances if a cure is to be affected.

Fungal infections

Involvement of the gastrointestinal tract, in particular the esophagus and stomach, by fungi of the genus *Candida* is not an uncommon finding at necropsy in patients with chronic debilitating diseases or who have received prolonged intensive antibiotic therapy. Other fungi, e.g., *Mucor* and *Cryptococcus,* are rarely seen.

Intestinal histoplasmosis may mimic tuberculosis in histopathologic detail, and its differentiation is made by demonstration of the causative organism either in microscopic sections or in cultures. It is most common in the ileocecal region, but widespread gastrointestinal lesions may be present as part of a generalized histoplasmosis.

When *actinomycosis* involves the gastrointestinal tract, it too shows predilection for the ileocecal region or appendix.

Lymphopathia venereum

Lymphopathia (lymphogranuloma) venereum involving the anorectal region is a disease of male or female homosexuals. Initially the perirectal fat is involved by chronic inflammatory change and fibrosis, rendering it very firm. The lymphatic lesions may suppurate and inflammation spreads to involve the rectal wall proper. Characteristically, stricture formation follows.

Parasitic infestations

Amebiasis. *Entamoeba histolytica* most frequently involves the cecal or rectal region and less commonly extensive segments of the large intestine. In the earliest lesions, there is a minimal mononuclear and eosinophilic leukocytic infiltration associated with the trophozoites penetrating the colonic epithelium. This produces tiny, small, yellow nodular elevations that eventuate in flask-shaped ulcerations. Organisms may be variable in number and difficult to identify without special staining procedures (Fig. 30-13). In the advanced case, the mucosa may have a shaggy appearance with shreds of fibrin and tags of underlying mucous membrane attached to the margins of the ulcers. The colon may be greatly thickened and there may be many adhesions to adjacent loops of intestine or to the mesentery. Amebic granulomas may develop.

Schistosomiasis. Ova of the parasite *Schistosoma mansoni* or *S. japonicum* in the mucosa and submucosa may excite a tubercle-like reaction and a polypoid adenomatoid hyperplasia of the mucous membrane of the colon or rectum. Less often, adult worms may be found in the submucosal veins. Various other parasites that inhabit the intestinal tract are considered in Chapter 14.

Malakoplakia

A disease of unknown etiology generally affecting the urinary tract has been reported in the appendix and colon. The histopathologic condition is identical to that seen in the urinary tract—macrophages harboring calcium-containing Michaelis-Gutmann bodies and periodic acid–Schiff–positive granules.

Other forms of gastrointestinal inflammation

Iatrogenic. *Ionizing irradiation* given for treatment of cancer, usually of the female generative organs may be responsible for inflammation in one or more focal areas of the small intestine or colon. More intense tissue damage leads to ulceration, the healing of which commonly leads to stricture formation. The changes are not specific although vascular changes (fibrous intimal thickening of medium-sized and small arteries and hyalinization of arterioles) are often conspicuous. Irradiation ulcers in the rectum may be associated with considerable scarring.

Drugs used in therapy (aminopterin, 5-fluorouracil, lincomycin, clindamycin, etc.) have been associated with changes in the intestinal tract. Inflammation, usually mucosal

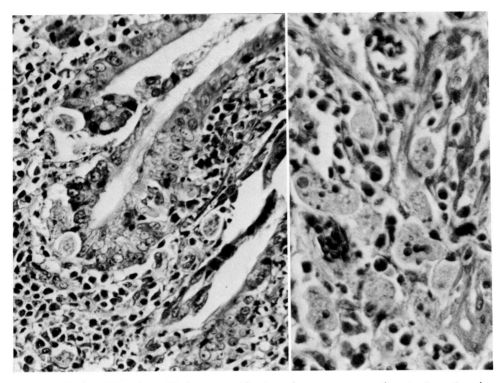

Fig. 30-13. Amebic colitis. Higher magnification demonstrates erythocyte ingestion by trophozoites.

and submucosal and accompanied by ulceration of the mucous membrane is responsible for a variety of gastrointestinal symptoms that subside after cessation of the drug.

Poisons. *Mercury and arsenic* may be responsible for nonspecific inflammation or necrosis in the colon, with the changes being less apparent and less extensive with arsenic. In addition, consumption of inorganic arsenical compounds such as Paris green may produce similar changes in the stomach and small intestine.

Metabolites. Accumulation of metabolic products such as occurs in patients dying with uremia may be responsible for changes ranging from minimal nonspecific inflammation to extensive necrotizing colitis. Some of the lesions may represent pseudomembranous enterocolitis or other specific infection.

Virus infections. Intestinal changes associated with viruses responsible for brief bouts of gastroenteritis are not encountered by the pathologist. Rarely, one sees at necropsy inclusion bodies of chicken pox and herpes simplex in the esophageal epithelium and inclusions of the cytomegalic virus in the mucosa and granulation tissue of ulcers of the intestine.

Granuloma. Granulomatous inflammation characterized by tubercle formation is uncommon in the intestinal tract with the exception of that seen in Crohn's disease. It may occur anywhere in the gut but is more common in the ileocecal region. Diagnostic considerations include sarcoidosis, tuberculosis, Crohn's disease, syphilis, foreign body (food, barium, etc.), leprosy, fungi, and parasitic infestations. Since the histology is not diagnostic unless a causative agent is identified, one must often rely heavily on clinical information and gross findings for their distinction. Even then, the various granulomas cannot always be differentiated.

Anorectal lesions

Stercoraceous (stercoral) ulcers are irregular and involve the mucous membrane of the rectum and less often of the colon resulting from trauma caused by impacted, inspissated fecal masses. They may be associated with perforation and peritonitis or with hemorrhage.

Colitis cystica profunda may be diffuse and involve extensive areas of the large intestine, but it usually is confined to the rectum. It is characterized by mucous cysts and glands lined by goblet cells in the submucosa. They are often

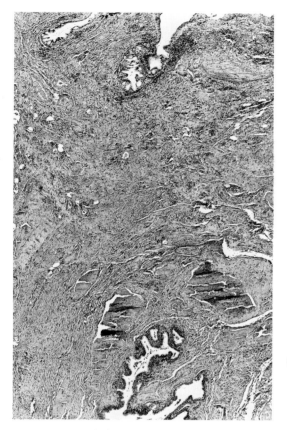

Fig. 30-14. Anal ducts. Small portion of epithelial lining of anal canal visible above, and anal ducts present both superficially and deep within muscle. (55×.)

associated with chronic inflammatory change and extraglandular accumulation of mucin. The condition may result from extension of surface epithelium along granulation tissue tracts after deep ulceration. Lesions with a similar appearance are infrequently encountered in the stomach.

The crypts of Morgagni have traditionally been implicated in the causation of most anorectal inflammatory disease, specifically perirectal *abscesses* and *anorectal fistulas*. Corresponding to the columns in the sinuses of Morgagni is a circular band, 0.3 to 1.1 cm wide, of "transitional" or "cloacogenic" epithelium interposed between rectal and anal mucous membrane. This transitional epithelium, often including mucus-secreting cells, lines the sinuses of Morgagni and the anal ducts or glands that communicate with them. The distribution of the ducts and glands varies greatly. They may extend caudally penetrating the internal anal sphincter or cephalad beneath the rectal mucosa and may branch in complex fashion (Fig. 30-14). It is infection in the crypts of Morgagni and of these anal ducts that is responsible for the very troublesome perianal and ischiorectal abscesses, which in turn are responsible for anal fistulas which may open internally in the region of the anorectal junction or externally on the perianal skin. Histologically, inflammation in this area is nonspecific often with a foreign body reaction, no doubt because of contamination with fecal matter.

Anal fissures are acute or chronic ulcers situated posteriorly in the anal canal just distal to the anorectal junction. These various anal, perianal, and anorectal lesions are insignificant in themselves, but they may be the source of great discomfort and disability.

PERITONEUM, OMENTUM, RETROPERITONEUM, AND MESENTERY
Peritonitis

Inflammation of the peritoneum is an acute or chronic response, diffuse or localized, to a variety of agents—bacterial, chemical, viral, or foreign material. The acute variety is most frequently encountered and is usually associated with inflammation of abdominal organs with or without perforation, e.g., appendicitis, cholecystitis, intestinal infarction, diverticulitis, perforated peptic ulcer, and hemorrhage attributed to ruptured ectopic pregnancy. Less commonly encountered is the "primary" form caused by the pneumococcus or hemolytic streptococcus. The organisms causing acute peritonitis are numerous and most commonly include one or more of the normal flora of the gastrointestinal tract, most commonly *Escherichia coli, Proteus,* and *Enterococcus,* but *Bacteroides* and *Clostridium* are also important. Initially, there is hyperemia, edema, and extravasation of red cells followed by exudation of leukocytes and fibrin, all of which account for the loss of the serous membrane's normal glistening sheen. To a limited extent, the character of the peritoneal exudate depends on a particular dominant organism. Although it may be thin, watery, and only slightly turbid, it usually is frankly purulent or fibrinopurulent.

As the process progresses, the plastic exudate may cause adhesions between loops of intestine, omentum, and abdominal parietes forming abscesses in localized areas, rather than permitting general spread of the process. Such abscesses are prone to develop in the lumbar gutters, the subphrenic space between the liver and diaphragm, the subhepatic area and the pelvic cul-de-sac. After widespread peritonitis subsides, such focal accumulations of exudate may persist and necessitate surgical drainage. Complications of acute peritonitis are adynamic or paralytic ileus and fibrous peritoneal adhesions.

Adhesions associated with inflammatory disease of the female pelvic organs, most importantly the fallopian tubes, are especially noteworthy. The causative infections are usually primarily of gonococcal etiology, but secondary superinfection is common. The disease is usually characterized by recurring episodes of acute but low-grade inflammation, and the resulting adhesions may become very dense and complicated, although generally limited to the pelvis.

Tuberculous peritonitis may occur as a manifestation of disseminated tuberculosis, miliary or otherwise, or in association with intestinal involvement. It also may be secondary to disease of the female generative organs. The disease process is the same as that in other parts of the body. It may be productive of widespread, dense adhesions.

A variety of irritants may be responsible for peritonitis—bile, hydrochloric acid and other intestinal contents that gain access to the peritoneum as a result of rupture of a viscus (gallbladder, bile duct, duodenum, etc.), hemorrhage from an ectopic pregnancy or corpus luteum, and other foreign material such as *Lycopodium* spores and talc.

Bile may produce a profound initial systemic reaction in the host, but the nature of the resulting pathologic process is dependent on the source of the contaminating bile and the type and number of associated bacteria.

Foreign body granulomas may result from *Lycopodium spores* and *talc crystals*—material used as dusting powders for surgical rubber gloves in the past. The use of absorbable starch has eliminated such granulomas but the starch does not appear to be completely innocuous. Instances of peritonitis and foreign body granuloma have been reported, presumably developing on the basis of hypersensitivity to the starch.

Infrequently *oily materials* used in salpingography, *parasites* or their ova, *barium sulfate* administered for diagnostic radiographic study and escaping into the peritoneum as a result of perforation, and sclerosing agents used in the treatment of hernia may be incitants of a foreign body reaction.

Periodic disease (familial Mediterranean fever, familial recurring polyserositis)

Periodic bouts of pain occur particularly in the abdomen, but they may also be noted in the chest and joints. During intervals between attacks, the patients are in excellent health. The disease is a genetic disorder of unknown etiology and pathogenesis affecting patients of Armenian, Arab, or Jewish ethnic origin, the last being predominantly the non-Ashkenazi Jews—the Sephardi and Iraqi ethnic groups. Sterile exudates in the involved serous surfaces are minimal, consisting of focal collections of neutrophils, fibrin stands, and ecchymoses, and only rarely are fibrinous adhesions and scars produced despite the many attacks. Amyloid of the perireticular type described in the kidneys, spleen, adrenals, pulmonary alveolar capillaries, and hepatic sinusoids but not in other organs, may result in the patient's death. Otherwise the course is a protracted one.

Ascites

Ascites is the condition of transudation of clear, low-specific gravity fluid into the peritoneal cavity. The protein content is less than 3%. It is most commonly seen with portal cirrhosis of the liver but may result from other causes of hypertension in the portal venous system, such as thrombosis or cardiac decompensation, or from hypoalbuminemia. Chylous ascites, in which the fluid appears milky and has a high fat content, is related to obstruction of the thoracic duct, usually neoplastic.

Retroperitoneal lesions

The retroperitoneum is an ill-defined area that may share in the complications of diseases of the many organs that lie within it or impinge upon it. Hemorrhage, infections, and extensions of neoplasms are the important complications and may be related to the urinary tract, adrenal glands, pancreas, gastrointestinal tract, retroperitoneal lymph nodes, and blood vessels, including the aorta and vena cava, etc.

A number of possibly related conditions involve the mesenteric and retroperitoneal adipose tissue. At one end of the spectrum is a self-limited, chronic, productive inflammation of the mesentery, usually of the small intestine. This has been variously termed "mesenteric panniculitis," "lipogranuloma," and "isolated lipodystrophy" and likened to Weber-Christian disease. It may produce a significant mass and may or may not be symptomatic. Retractile mesenteritis is a similar condition, distinguished by fibrosis and hyaline scarring and retraction of the mesentery, with distortion of intestinal loops productive of episodes of pain, constipation, and obstruction.

Idiopathic retroperitoneal fibrosis is a lesion characterized by dense fibrosis and a limited, nonspecific inflammatory reaction that frequently presents with ureteral obstruction. The disease also occurs in the mediastinum. A similar lesion has been observed in association with methysergide therapy. It usually regresses after withdrawal of the drug.

Torsion of omentum

Omental torsion, secondary to adhesions, tumors, etc. or, at times, of unknown cause, may result in infarction and give rise to signs and symptoms simulating those of acute appendicitis but usually without vomiting. Similarly, epiploic appendages may become in-

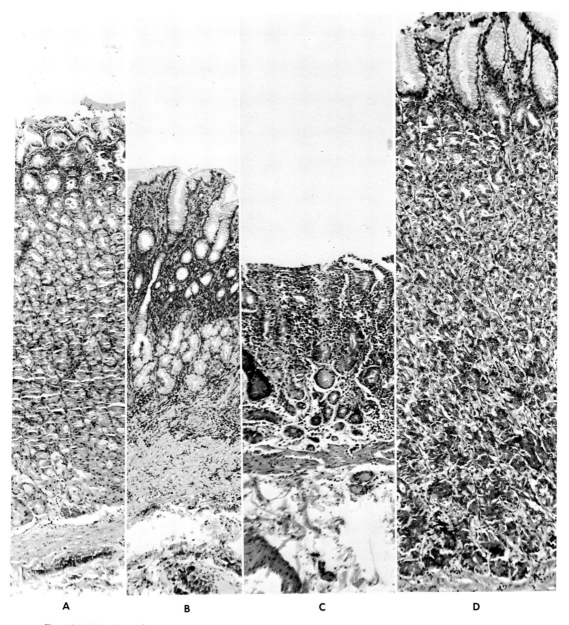

A	B	C	D

Fig. 30-15. A and **B**, Normal stomach. **A,** Fundus. **B,** Antrum. **C,** Atrophic gastritis. **D,** Gastric rugal hypertrophy. (**A** to **D,** 90×.)

farcted. Fat necrosis of an appendage, presumably a late result, is not uncommon.

FUNCTIONAL STATES
Gastric atrophy (atrophic gastritis)

So-called atrophic gastritis is not properly classified as an inflammatory condition. The term is used by some as a synonym for gastric atrophy. Others consider the two as different stages of the same pathologic process.

In atrophic gastritis, the mucous membrane is greatly thinned, and the gastric glands are correspondingly shortened and also widely separated. On naked-eye inspection, the mucosa in advanced atrophy is smooth, is patently thinned, and has a waxy cast. The striking cellular changes in the gastric glands are two: (1) a decrease in number or, in the fully developed case, complete absence of parietal cells and (2) the occurrence, usually in the deeper part of the mucosa, of glands identical with those of the small intestine (Fig. 30-15, *C*). All cell types normally found in the glands of the small intestine may be represented. This change has been regarded as "intestinal metaplasia" by some and as heterotopia by others. The decrease or absence of parietal cells, which has been demonstrated to be associated with an autoantibody in a high percentage of patients with atrophic gastritis, accounts for

deficient hydrochloric acid secretion or complete achlorhydria. Large numbers of lymphocytes and plasma cells are present in the lamina propria, but the increase may be more apparent than real. The changes described occur focally in many stomachs without overt disease. They are seen more often and in more widespread and advanced degree with increased age.

Atrophic gastritis commonly is associated with gastric carcinoma, but a postulated predisposing role has not been demonstrated. Advanced atrophy regularly accompanies polypoid carcinoma and adenomatous polyp. Indeed, the appearance of many of the latter and of some polypoid carcinomas strongly suggests origin from glands typical of the small intestine. Gastric atrophy also regularly accompanies pernicious anemia, a disease associated with achlorhydria and a high incidence of gastric carcinoma. An antibody to parietal cells has been demonstrated in a proportion of patients with atrophic gastritis. These patients are predisposed to develop pernicious anemia, in contrast to those in whom the antibody cannot be demonstrated.[124] However, in general, it has been difficult to correlate the pathologic findings of atrophic gastritis with clinical disease or with radiologic or gastroscopic findings.

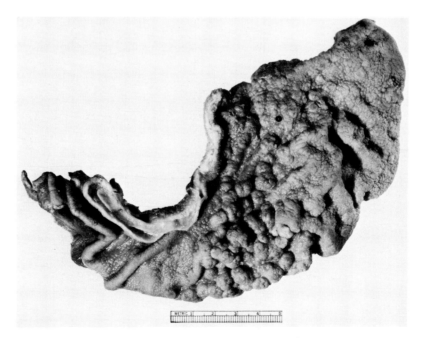

Fig. 30-16. Gastric rugal hypertrophy.

Gastric rugal hypertrophy

Gastric rugal hypertrophy (called hypertrophic gastritis by some) is characterized by enlargement of the gastric mucosal folds in both length and breadth, producing thickening and convolution of the mucous membrane reminiscent of the appearance of the cerebral convolutions (Fig. 30-16). Histologically, it appears to be a true thickening, and there is an apparent striking increase in the depth of the glands and in the number of parietal cells. At times, glands penetrate the muscularis mucosae (Fig. 30-15, *D*). The changes may be diffuse and pronounced or localized and of limited degree. It seems likely that pathologists have failed to recognize localized instances or minor degrees of the condition, accounting, perhaps, for the difficulty they have had in supporting clinical and radiologic diagnoses of "hypertrophic gastritis."

Gastric rugal hypertrophy has been associated with hyperchlorhydria (in some instances with extreme gastric hypersecretion), hypoproteinemia, and *tumors or hyperplasias of multiple endocrine glands*. It is postulated that gastric rugal hypertrophy is one manifestation of a syndrome consisting additionally of islet cell tumor, primary chief cell hyperplasia of the parathyroid glands, and, at times, abnormalities of other endocrine glands, especially the adrenal cortex and pituitary, and having several different modes of clinical expression.

The principal ones are as follows:

1. The *Zollinger-Ellison syndrome,* with intractable peptic ulcer, often in an unusual location
2. The *Verner-Morrison syndrome,* with intractable watery diarrhea, the result of incomplete neutralization in the intestine of the very large amounts of highly acid gastric juice
3. Hyperparathyroidism

These syndromes are familial in some instances. In the Zollinger-Ellison syndrome, the islet cell tumor is often malignant, often in the duodenum instead of the pancreas, and characteristically composed of alpha cells that secrete gastrin, which, in turn, stimulates gastric secretion. However, insulin-secreting beta cell tumors also occur.

Malabsorption syndrome

The malabsorption syndrome is characterized by impaired intestinal absorption, especially of fats, and is manifested by diarrhea with bulky, foul stools, abdominal distention, and malnutrition with attendant vitamin deficiencies, all in varying degree. The clinical picture may be associated with a wide variety of underlying diseases, and the cases may be conveniently subdivided into primary and secondary groups. Among the numerous causes of secondary malabsorption are the following: cystic fibrosis of the pancreas, chronic incom-

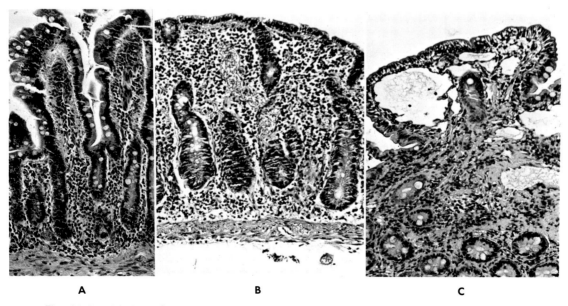

Fig. 30-17. A, Normal jejunum. **B,** Jejunum in nontropical sprue. **C,** Lymphangiectases of jejunum in protein-losing enteropathy. (**A** to **C,** 150×.)

plete intestinal obstruction, surgical resection of significant segments of the gastrointestinal tract, infections (especially enteric), antibiotics, biliary tract disease, scleroderma, Whipple's disease, parasitic infestations, regional enteritis, diabetes, neoplasms (notably lymphoma), possibly allergy, etc.

Celiac disease and sprue. The names given to primary malabsorption or steatorrhea are *celiac disease* in infants and children, *nontropical sprue* in the adult, and *tropical sprue*.

In the first two conditions there seems to be an identical, genetically controlled, enzymatic or metabolic defect that is converted to overt clinical disease by a number of possible triggering mechanisms, the most important and most frequently occurring of which is sensitivity to, or intolerance of, gluten. In this case, the elimination of gluten from the diet usually relieves the symptoms and permits normal development, although it does not cure the underlying defect. The small intestine in this state has a flat surface, partially or completely lacking villi. The mucosal crypts appear elongated, dilated, and more widely spaced than normal. The surface epithelial cells are cuboid or low columnar with irregular nuclei (Fig. 30-17, *B*). When a gluten-free diet produces clinical remission, the anatomic lesion can be reversed to some degree, although usually not completely. The change is most conspicuous in the upper part of the jejunum, becoming less so in the ileum and duodenum. This pathologic picture is not specific for nontropical sprue or celiac disease, but when full-blown is very nearly so. A variant not responding to the elimination of gluten and characterized additionally by the deposition of eosinophilic hyaline material in the lamina propria of the small intestine has been described.[131]

Tropical sprue is very similar to nontropical sprue in its clinical and morphologic expressions. The pathologic changes usually are not so noticeable and are reversible with folic acid therapy, but they are unaffected by elimination of gluten from the diet. Macrocytic anemia is usually a feature.

Protein-losing enteropathy (exudative enteropathy)

In protein-losing enteropathy, which also may be associated with steatorrhea, large amounts of serum protein are lost in the intestine, and serum levels (of both globulin and albumin) are abnormally low. Like the malabsorption state, it may be secondary to some specific gastroenteric disease state or congestive heart failure, or it may be idiopathic.

Some of the gastrointestinal diseases that may be associated with considerable protein loss are gastric rugal hypertrophy, sprue, regional enteritis, and ulcerative colitis. Constrictive pericarditis is the most important underlying cardiac lesion. In some patients with "idiopathic" protein-losing enteropathy, dilatation of lymphatic channels (lymphangiectasia) in the intestinal mucosa and mesentery has been demonstrated (Fig. 30-17, *C*). Some of these latter patients have had systemic lymphatic abnormalities, but in others no cause of lymphatic obstruction is found.

GASTROINTESTINAL MANIFESTATIONS OF SYSTEMIC DISEASE

The gastrointestinal tract may be the site of involvement in a number of diseases involving multiple organs. Such involvement may produce symptoms, which are the first manifestations of the disease, or it may be occult. In both situations biopsy of the intestinal tract may be helpful and an easily accessible means of establishing the diagnosis. Symptoms that may be present—diarrhea, steatorrhea, and those of malabsorption—may be unassociated with histologic changes in the gut or there may be degrees of villous mucosal atrophy. Gastrointestinal manifestations may be seen in a variety of endocrine diseases (diabetes, thyrotoxicosis, hyperparathyroidism, and hypoparathyroidism), skin diseases (dermatitis herpetiformis), pseudoxanthoma elasticum, Ehlers-Danlos syndrome, mastocytosis, etc.

Cystic fibrosis

The most important gastrointestinal manifestation is malabsorption with steatorrhea and azotorrhea, secondary to pancreatic achylia, and deficient secretion of the intestinal glands. Approximately 10% of patients have intestinal obstruction in the newborn period as the result of *meconium ileus*. The abnormal accumulations of meconium distend the loops of intestine, which in one third of the cases rotate upon themselves producing a volvulus. Another complication is intestinal perforation in utero with the development of sterile peritonitis, so-called *meconium peritonitis*. The escaping of epithelial cells, mucus, and cellular debris usually stimulate a foreign body reaction, and calcification, visible radiographically, frequently takes place. (See also p. 1459.)

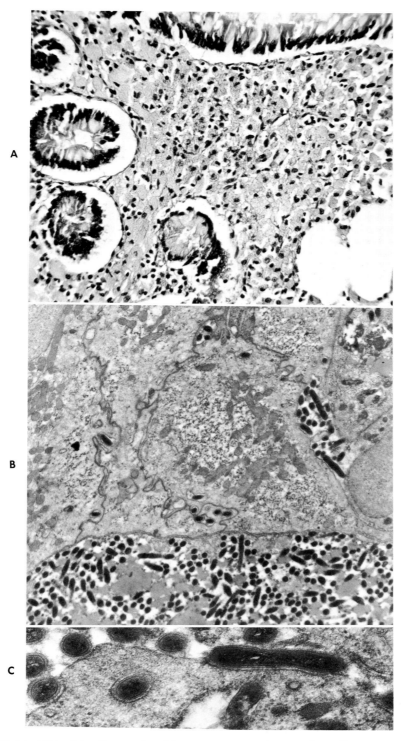

Fig. 30-18. Whipple's disease involving mucous membrane of small intestine. **A,** Pale macrophages in mucosa. **B,** Bacilliform bodies are extracellular. **C,** Encapsulated bodies are seen both intracellularly and extracellulary. (**A,** 300×; **B,** 8100×; **C,** 45,000×.)

Progressive systemic sclerosis (scleroderma)

Although any portion of the intestinal tract may be involved, the esophagus is the most frequent site. There is hyaline sclerosis of the submucosa with lymphocytic infiltration, and atrophy and fibrosis of the muscularis. The overlying mucous membrane may be thin and become ulcerated. In the esophagus, the rigidity of the wall may predispose to regurgitation of acidic gastric juice from which there may be further complications.

Other collagen diseases, *dermatomyositis* and *lupus erythematosus,* may also involve the gastrointestinal tract affecting the musculature in the former condition and blood vessels in both instances.

Whipple's disease (intestinal lipodystrophy)

Originally considered to be a disorder of intestinal function involving lipid metabolism, Whipple's disease has been generally recognized more recently as a systemic disease. Aggregates of large, pale macrophages bearing intracytoplasmic sickle-shaped inclusions in the intestinal mucous membrane and mesenteric lymph nodes that react strongly with the periodic acid–Schiff staining procedure dominate the anatomic picture, but similar deposits have also been described in virtually every organ of the body. Lipid deposits are striking in lymph nodes, especially those of the mesentery.

It is generally a condition of adult males that may be familial. The manifestations are diarrhea, gradual wasting, and migratory polyarthritis. An infectious etiology has replaced the concept of a disorder of lipid metabolism. This is based largely on the belief, generated from electron microscopic studies, that the "inclusions" are in fact bacilliform microorganisms (Fig. 30-18). Thus far, it has not been possible to identify or culture organisms from material from patients with Whipple's disease. Previously considered a progressive and usually fatal disease, it has been found to respond favorably to antibiotic therapy.

Storage disease

Deposits of one of a number of substances seen in a variety of diseases—Tay-Sachs, Niemann-Pick, Fabry's, Hurler's, Gaucher's glycogen storage, and metachromatic leukoencephalopathy—may be found in ganglion cells, histiocytes, or nerve fibers in the gut.

Tangier disease is an autosomal recessive inherited disease in which there is deposition of cholesterol esters in the reticuloendothelial system as well as in histiocytes of the mucous membrane of the pharynx and intestine. The disorder is benign except for a possible predisposition to atherosclerosis.

Wolman's disease is also inherited as an autosomal recessive disease in which cholesterol esters may be found deposited in histiocytes in the lamina propria of the intestine as well as in the reticuloendothelial system of the liver, spleen, lymph nodes, and bone marrow. Calcification of the adrenal glands is a common accompaniment. The central nervous system appears not to be involved. The reported patients have died before attaining 6 months of age.

Congenital beta-lipoprotein deficiency, an autosomal recessive disease, manifests itself in the intestinal tract by deposition of lipid droplets in the mucosal epithelial cells with practically no fat droplets in the lamina propria and submucosa. It usually manifests itself within the first 2 years of life a mild steatorrhea and neurologic symptoms resembling Friedreich's ataxia.

The frequent involvement of the intestinal tract in these storage diseases has made biopsy of the gut an easy approach to diagnosis.

Rectal biopsy has also proved useful in a large number of other disease entities for obtaining diagnostic information—schistosomiasis, amyloidosis, amebiasis, Crohn's disease, Hirschsprung's disease, melanosis coli, ulcerative colitis, pneumatosis, hemochromatosis, and the changes produced by chemotherapeutic agents and antibiotics. The finding of *colonic macrophages* (muciphages) however must be carefully evaluated. The variation in interpretation given to them by different authors—early phase of Whipple's disease, ceroid-containing phages, etc.—appears to be in part the result of nonuniformity in the histochemical methods employed in their study. Recent investigations carried out on surgical and necropsy material indicate their frequent occurrence and lack of clinical significance. It appears that they are unrelated to the many storage diseases cited previously and that they are the result of phagocytosis of mucin released from the goblet cells of the colonic mucous membrane.

NEOPLASMS
Adenomatous polyps, papillary adenomas, and miscellaneous polyps

Benign polypoid glandular neoplasms occur throughout the gastrointestinal tract, from the stomach to the rectum, occurring in greatest

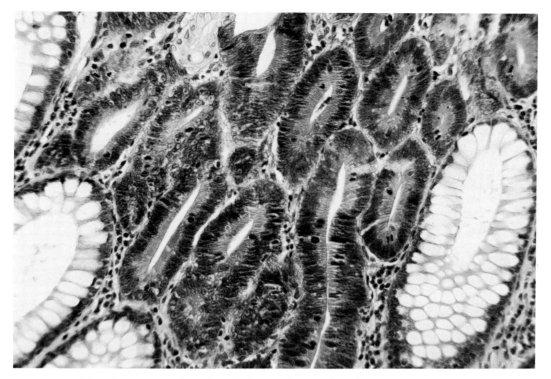

Fig. 30-19. Adenomatous (neoplastic) change in glands of colon in contrast to normal glands at left and in right lower corner. (300×.)

number in the colon and rectum. Estimates of their incidence range as high as 25% to 50% in an autopsy population of the older age groups (60 to 80 years). Their incidence increases after 30 years with advancing age. In one fourth or more of cases, they are multiple, frequently but not regularly limited to one part of the intestine. Approximately 75% of adenomatous polyps occur in the rectum and sigmoid colon, although their exact incidence in various segments of the large intestine varies from one reported series to another.

The earliest adenomatous change that can be recognized is the replacement of some of the lining cells of the crypts, beginning at the base, by cells that are generally taller, more slender, and more deeply stained than the normal. They have hyperchromatic nuclei and lack vacuoles indicative of mucin secretion (Fig. 30-19). Mitotic figures may be numerous. Proliferation progresses with the formation of a focal nodule that is generally lobulated and berry-like, usually less than 2 cm in diameter and attached to the intestinal wall by a pedicle of varying length, composed of normal mucous membrane (Fig. 30-20). A number of polypoid epithelial lesions of the colon bear a

resemblance to the adenomatous polyp and are commonly confused with it. At times, *abnormal folds* or minute elevations of the mucous membrane are mistaken for adenomas on proctoscopic or sigmoidoscopic examination. Rather frequently occurring polyps, best termed *hyperplastic* or *metaplastic,* are lesions composed of enlarged, regular glands with scalloped luminal borders showing excessive mucin secretion but lacking the neoplastic change of the adenomatous polyp described previously (Fig. 30-21). Another lesion that must be distinguished from the adenomatous polyp and that does not have any relationship to cancer is the *juvenile polyp.* Also referred to as a retention polyp, it is usually single—a smooth, rounded nodule, 1 to 3 cm in diameter, composed of large, hyperplastic or cystic glands with a very abundant, well-vascularized fibrous stroma infiltrated by inflammatory cells (Fig. 30-22). It is supported on a stalk of normal mucous membrane. The most frequent clinical manifestation is bleeding. It is a lesion of children, although similar polyps occasionally occur in adults. Polypoid inflammatory or nonspecific granuloma-like nodules—inflammatory polyps—are occasionally seen as soli-

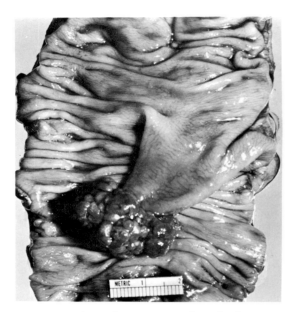

Fig. 30-20. Adenomatous polyp of colon.

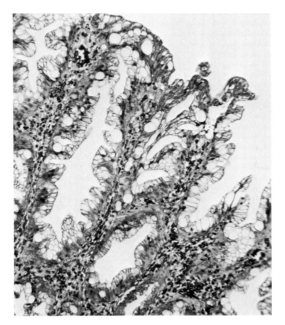

Fig. 30-21. Hyperplastic polyp of colon. (175×.)

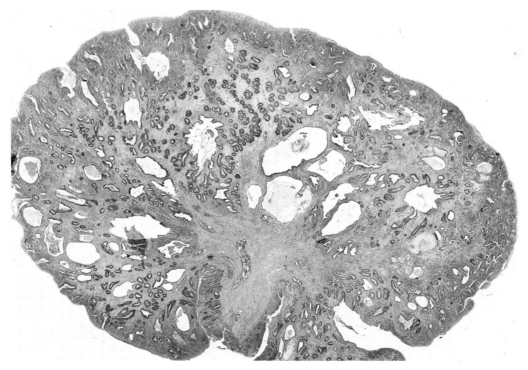

Fig. 30-22. Juvenile polyp of rectum. Cystic dilatation of glands and abundant stroma. (13×.)

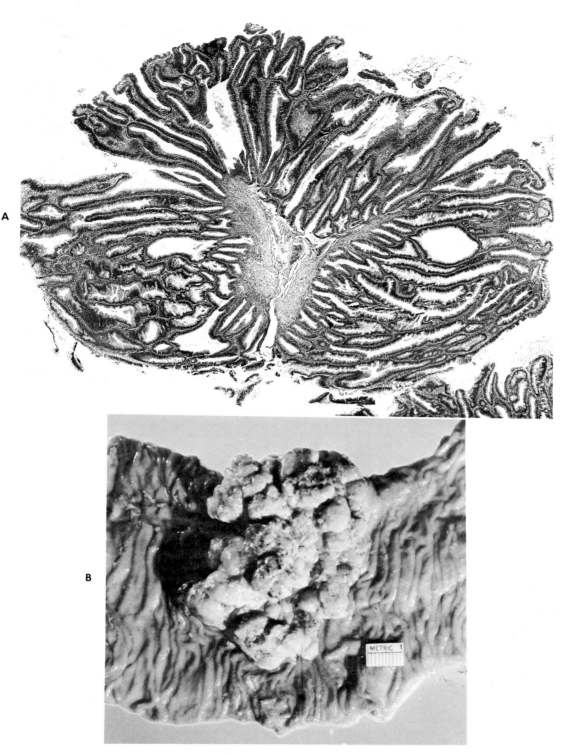

Fig. 30-23. A, Papillary (villous) adenoma of rectum. Papillary configuration readily apparent. **B,** Papillary adenoma of colon. (**A,** 25×.)

tary lesions, but the typical inflammatory polyp or pseudopolyp is that seen in long-standing chronic ulcerative colitis.

The *papillary adenoma* (known also as *villous adenoma* and *villous papilloma*) is a neoplasm related to, but much less common than, the adenomatous polyp. It is encountered more often in the rectum than in other parts of the large intestine. It is characterized by neoplastic proliferation from the mucosal surface into the lumen and develops a gross papillary configuration (Fig. 30-23, *A*), as opposed to the lobulated, berry-like nodule of the polyp. Characteristic examples are large and sessile (Fig. 30-23, *B*). Large papillary adenomas have been recognized as the occasional cause of severe fluid and electrolyte loss, especially of potassium, producing electrolyte imbalance, which may threaten life.

Papillary adenomas and adenomatous polyps may coexist, and many lesions have morphologic characteristics of both. The distinction is particularly difficult in small lesions and especially when study is limited to small fragments of biopsy material. Both papillary adenomas and adenomatous polyps occur rarely in the small intestine.

In *familial multiple polyposis* (Plate 2, *C*), the entire colon is studded with polyps, usually tiny and sessile. The disease is transmitted as an autosomal dominant trait and usually makes its existence known in childhood or adolescence. The incidence of carcinoma in this disease is so high and the cancers occur so often in young adults (or even adolescents) that total colectomy is generally regarded as the treatment of choice once the diagnosis has been established.

Polyps may be associated with other abnormalities. In *Gardner's syndrome* polyposis of the colon is associated with neoplasms of both bone and soft tissues elsewhere in the body—epidermoid cyst, fibroma, and osteomas (in the mandible and maxilla)—and sometimes with polyps in other portions of the gastrointestinal tract. Colorectal carcinomas develop in a large number of these patients.

In *Peutz-Jeghers syndrome,* one finds melanin spots on the buccal mucosa, lips, and digits associated with polyps occurring most anywhere in the gastrointestinal tract. The disease is transmitted as a simple mendelian dominant trait. The polyps differ from those generally found in the intestinal tract in that they are hamartomatous (i.e., composed of normal-looking, but irregularly arranged glands of any of the types normally occurring in the mucous

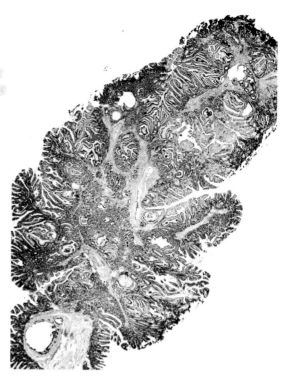

Fig. 30-24. Polyp of ileum from patient with Peutz-Jeghers syndrome. Note irregularities and variegated appearance. (16×; from Horn, R. C., Jr., Payne, W. A., and Fine, G.: Arch. Pathol. [Chicago] **76:**29-37, 1963.)

membrane of origin and may include bands of smooth muscle; Fig. 30-24). Thus parietal cells may be present in gastric polyps, Brunner's glands in duodenal lesions, etc. The polyps of the large intestine are not always readily distinguishable from adenomatous polyps. The principal clinical manifestations of the Peutz-Jeghers syndrome are hemorrhage and intussusception. Instances of development of gastrointestinal carcinoma in patients with this syndrome have been documented, but progression of the Peutz-Jeghers polyps to genuine cancer must be rare. Cytologic atypia is frequent, but it is apparently not of significance, nor is the pseudoinvasive appearance suggested by the smooth muscle within the polyps. Rarely encountered are isolated polyps resembling the Peutz-Jeghers polyp, but without the other manifestations of the syndrome.

In the *Cronkhite-Canada syndrome* one finds multiple polyposis of the colon associated with ectodermal changes—alopecia, nail atrophy, and hyperpigmentation—as well as polyps in the stomach and small intestine. The polyps morphologically have the features of retention polyps.

In the *Turcot syndrome* polyps of the colon are found combined with brain tumors.

Relationship of adenomatous polyps and papillary adenomas to carcinoma of colon

It has been usual to regard the benign epithelial proliferations of the large intestine as precursors of cancer, but in recent years this point of view has been seriously challenged. Taking all the facts into consideration, one may observe that carcinomas of the large intestine can, and do, take origin in adenomatous polyps. However, in all probability, carcinomas arising on this basis are infrequent, and colonic carcinomas are malignant neoplasms from their inception. This statement may not be true for the papillary adenoma, concerning which the consensus continues to be that the danger of cancer is great. This is based upon the frequent finding, by study of numerous blocks and sections, of associated foci of invasive growth and of lymph node metastasis, as well as upon the frequency of locally recurrent growth occurring after excision, and upon recurrence as frank invasive cancer.

Gastric polyps

The epithelium of gastric polyps more closely resembles the epithelium of the small intestine and retention polyps of the colon than true adenomas. The belief that adenomatous polyps of the stomach offer the threat of transformation into cancer is held by many, although the seriousness of the threat is not a matter of general agreement.

In the stomach, polyps are commonly associated with carcinomas, and when polyps are multiple as is the case in one third to one half of instances, there is almost always an associated carcinoma. In addition, atypical cytologic changes, consistent with interpretation as carcinoma in situ, are not uncommonly present in parts of gastric polyps. Nevertheless despite the fact that some gastric cancers may arise in pre-existing polyps, not all polyps will become invasive cancers, and relatively few cancers can be traced to polyps as precursors. Gastric polyps have an incidence of less than 10% of that of gastric cancer.

Carcinoma of colon and rectum

Incidence. Carcinoma in these sites accounts for the highest incidence of cancer in the body. Roughly three fourths of carcinomas of the large intestine occur in the rectum and sig-

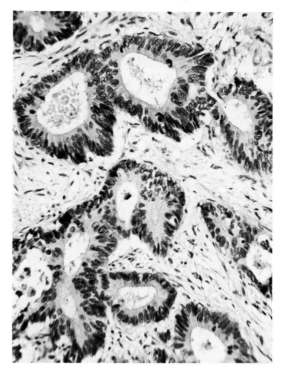

Fig. 30-25. Typical well-differentiated adenocarcinoma of colon. (300×.)

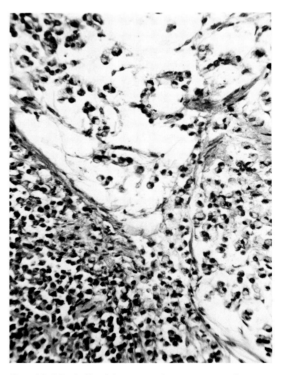

Fig. 30-26. Colloid (mucinous) carcinoma of cecum. Both patterns of pools of mucin and of sheets of individual signet-ring cells are seen. (300×.)

moid colon. Of the remainder, a majority arise in the cecum and ascending and descending colon, with the flexures and transverse colon being least often affected.

Histology and morbid anatomy. Generally they are well-differentiated tumors reproducing the appearance of normal colonic glands, more or less faithfully (Fig. 30-25). The usual cellular aberrations of neoplasia are generally obvious. Mucin production by the tumor is variable, but not infrequently one encounters tumors capable of secreting very large amounts

of mucin. Signet-ring cells (cells in which a large vacuole of mucin pushes the nucleus off to one side) may be conspicuous in some of these tumors (Fig. 30-26). In others, signet-ring cells may grow within the colonic wall without any readily apparent mucosal lesion, thus producing a linitis plastica type of growth.

Distinct differences between the growth patterns of carcinoma of the right and left half of the colon can be observed. Those in the right colon are usually bulky and may show extensive necrosis because they outgrow their

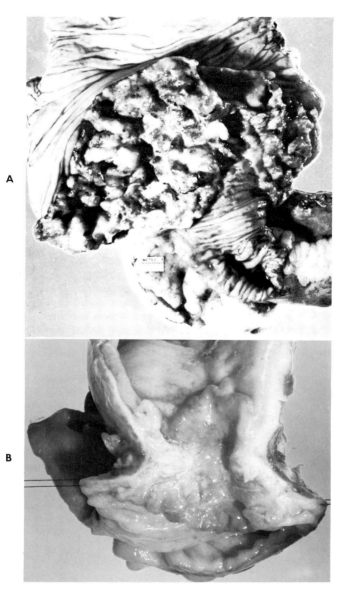

Fig. 30-27. A, Characteristic bulky, ulcerated carcinoma of right side of colon. Lesion in cecum. **B,** Characteristic constricting, "napkin-ring" carcinoma of left side of colon. Tumor does not quite involve full circumference. Hypertrophied proximal bowel above.

blood supply (Fig. 30-27, *A*). Occult bleeding is common, and the presenting symptoms may be generalized weakness and anemia. In the more distal portions of the colon, the tumor frequently has a napkin-ring configuration (Fig. 30-27, *B*). Considerable fibrous-tissue stroma accompanies the tumor and accounts for contraction and narrowing of the bowel lumen and thus a higher incidence of obstruction than carcinoma in the right colon. Carcinomas of the rectum do not have a characteristic gross anatomic pattern. Bleeding is a common symptom. Many are discovered on routine proctoscopic or digital examination. Not uncommon in the rectum is the bulky "colloid" carcinoma presenting as a vari-colored mass with extensive ulceration. The smaller, more or less flat carcinomas that occur in the rectum and sigmoid colon commonly undermine the peripheral normal mucous membrane as they grow centrifugally. It is thus possible to obtain only overlying normal mucosa by a proctoscopic or a sigmoidoscopic biopsy, if the forceps bite is not deep enough.

Spread. By the time the lesion is first observed penetration of the muscular wall with involvement of the serosa and subserosa have usually occurred. Of greatest significance to the patient's longevity is spread via the lymphatics. Extension is generally to anatomically predictable lymph nodes proximal to the growth. Knowledge of the anatomy of the lymphatic circulation and associated lymph nodes is the basis for properly planned surgical treatment of carcinoma in general, as well as specifically of carcinoma of the colon and rectum. Metastatic spread bypasses uninvolved nodes infrequently. In the laboratory the isolation of lymph nodes and demonstration of lymph node metastases are facilitated by clearing techniques.

Blood vascular spread of colonic cancer is also highly significant. Cancer cells have been found circulating in the bloodstream, but their significance remains incompletely understood. The finding of cancer cells in the circulating blood and the establishment of metastatic foci are not synonymous. In general, when venous invasion and blood-borne metastases are present, local growth and lymphatic spread are also extensive. However, striking examples are encountered of extensive venous dissemination of otherwise localized carcinomas and of locally far-advanced, highly invasive tumors without significant lymphatic or venous spread.

The bulky tumors producing large amounts of mucin are prone to spread widely over the peritoneal surface and are in contrast to the usual carcinomas of the large intestine. This type of spread may result in the formation of a metastatic tumor mass palpable on rectal examination in the rectovesical or rectouterine space, the so-called rectal shelf. Implantation of cancer cells at the suture line of intestinal anastomosis or in the peritoneum is another mode of tumor spread.

A number of classifications of colonic and rectal carcinoma, the most important of which are based on degree of differentiation and on the extent of spread both directly through the intestinal wall and via the lymphatics following a proposal of Dukes, correlate reasonably well with the end results of surgical treatment. The 5-year survival rates after intestinal resection vary from 15% to 20% to better than 60%, depending on the parts of the intestine involved and the extent of the disease at the time of diagnosis and treatment. The foregoing figures take into account only those tumors not so far advanced as to be considered inoperable.

Carcinoma of stomach

Incidence. The incidence varies greatly in various parts of the world and among various peoples. It is known to be particularly frequent in Japan, very rare among the Malay population of Java, but by no means rare among the Chinese inhabitants of Java. In Iceland it accounts for 35% to 45% of all fatal cancers in males. This high incidence has been attributed to the consumption of considerable amounts of smoked fish and meat, particularly the former. It thus appears that the geographic variation in the incidence of gastric carcinoma may depend, at least in part, upon the dietary customs and resultant exposure to carcinogens. The incidence in women is about half that in men. For other geographic factors see p. 719.

Classification. Most carcinomas of the stomach arise from the mucus-secreting cells. Differentiation is variable as to the extent and regularity of gland formation, mucus secretion, cytologic features, etc., but in general they tend to be less well differentiated and less characteristic than the carcinomas of the colon and rectum (Fig. 30-28). The commonest site of involvement is the antrum on or near the greater curvature. Ulcerative cancers in particular have a predilection for location in proximity to the greater curvature or to the pylorus.

Of the many classifications of gastric carcinoma, a large proportion lack the merit of

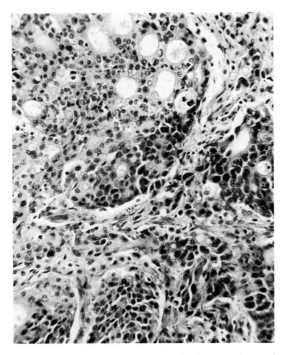

Fig. 30-28. Carcinoma of stomach showing limited degree of glandular differentiation. (300×.)

clinical significance. An exception is that of Borrman.[175] It is based upon the extensiveness of the lesion as judged by gross examination, showing a gradual gradation between the less malignant tumors that grow mainly within the lumen of the stomach and those prognostically less favorable, which are deeply invasive and penetrate the gastric wall. Stout's classification is somewhat similar, being based upon direction of growth and the resultant gross configuration of the tumor. He recognized (1) a fungating or polypoid type, (2) an ulcerating type (ulcer-cancer), (3) a superficial spreading type, and (4) a diffusely spreading type (linitis plastica).[183]

Polypoid or fungating gastric carcinomas have a particularly favorable prognosis. An exception is the fungating carcinoma of the cardioesophageal junction, which is prone to become very extensive, both locally and in terms of lymph node spread before giving rise to symptoms. Superficial spreading is also a relatively favorable type. Unfortunately these two forms of gastric carcinoma are relatively infrequent varieties. Linitis plastica type, equally or more rare, is hopeless in its outlook.

The various classifications and their clinical correlations support the concept that tumor growth by frank infiltration offers a greater and more immediate threat to the life of the host than does the gastric cancer that grows expansively, essentially pushing aside the host tissue. Defects in the classification of gastric carcinomas arise in the fact that they often cannot be assigned to any of the categories, either because they are too far advanced to yield a clue to their initial gross configuration or because they show features of tumors of two or more growth types.

Morbid anatomy. *Polypoid gastric carcinomas* resemble adenomatous polyps except that they are usually larger and have a less delicate and often less distinct pedicle because of carcinomatous invasion. Benign polyps are commonly seen, and atrophic gastritis is always present in stomachs that are the site of polypoid carcinomas. Pernicious anemia may be associated. They usually show good glandular differentiation, and the neoplastic glands very often resemble those of the small intestine.

The macroscopic differences between ulcer cancers and peptic ulcers have been described in the discussion of peptic ulcer (Plate 2, *D* and *E*). The old controversy over how many gastric cancers have their origin in peptic ulcers seems to have been largely resolved. Current opinion is that a small number of gastric carcinomas may arise in preexisting ulcers. Conviction of such an occurrence must rest upon demonstration of a characteristic peptic ulcer with cancer limited to one portion of its base or margin. Caution must be exercised not to misinterpret cytologically atypical, proliferative epithelial changes in the mucous membrane at the edge of an ulcer as malignant. A majority of ulcer cancers are malignant lesions from their inception, either because of primarily deeply penetrating growth or because of early peptic ulcerations of a small cancer. Ulcerative cancer has no specific histologic features.

Superficial spreading type. This is a distinctive variety of gastric carcinoma that spreads superficially in the mucosa or submucosa of the stomach forming a serpiginous lesion that may cover a large portion of the mucosal surface. Even without deeper penetration, lymph node metastases may take place. This type of tumor may be multicentric.

In the *linitis plastica or diffusely spreading* type of carcinoma, the wall of the entire stomach is thickened, more or less uniformly, by neoplastic infiltration and new fibrous tissue production. The shrunken stomach with its relatively rigid wall has earned the descriptive term "leather-bottle stomach" (Plate 2, *F*).

Characteristically, the mucosa displays no focal lesion, although it may show thickening and irregularities, with flattening and distortion of its folds. Tumor infiltration involves all layers, but the submucosa and subserosa are chiefly affected. Lymphatic permeation is usual within the gastric wall proper, as well as into the adjacent omentum. Extension into the duodenum is generally sharply limited, although the subserosa may be involved to some extent. Histologically, carcinomas of the linitis plastica type tend to be undifferentiated, and at times distinction from malignant lymphoma is difficult or impossible. If a tumor secretes mucin, this may be a helpful diagnostic feature. At times, mucin secretion may be abundant, and signet-ring cells may be the predominant cells. Desmoplasia often is pronounced and dominates the histologic picture, making recognition of cancer cells difficult. The prognosis is essentially hopeless in this variety of gastric cancer because of the extent of the disease by the time it is clinically recognized. Occasionally, focal fibrotic thickening of the antrum, apparently of inflammatory nature, may simulate cancer clinically and on naked-eye inspection of the specimen.

The majority of gastric carcinomas, which do not meet the criteria of any one of these groups, are extremely variable in gross appearance and histologic pattern. Again, because they are usually far advanced before an opportunity for treatment is offered, the outlook is poor.

Spread. Direct spread and spread by way of the lymphatics are of foremost importance in dictating principles of surgical treatment and in assessing the individual patient's prognosis. Metastasis to lymph nodes along the greater and lesser curvatures of the stomach is frequent. Extension to the para-aortic and celiac lymph nodes is also often seen. Metastasis to the left supraclavicular lymph nodes by way of the thoracic duct may be a presenting sign of gastric carcinoma, so-called Virchow's (Ewald's) node. Spread into the esophagus, especially submucosal, and to the mediastinal lymph nodes may be a feature. In occasional cases, there may be permeation of pulmonary lymphatics and the bone marrow (with clinically unexplained anemia) as early manifestations of the disease.

Liver metastasis, common even in cases believed to be "early," results from invasion of the tributaries of the portal venous system. Peritoneal spread and carcinomatosis occur, and gastric cancer is an important diagnostic consideration when a rectal shelf is demonstrated clinically. Carcinoma of the stomach, as well as other parts of the gastrointestinal tract, may metastasize early to the ovaries so that the ovarian tumor dominates the clinical picture, the so-called *Krükenberg tumors*. The typical Krükenberg tumor is characterized by signet-ring cancer cells with abundant fibrous-tissue stroma.

Carcinoma of esophagus

Among gastrointestinal cancers, *epidermoid carcinoma of the esophagus* ranks behind only carcinoma of the colon and rectum and carcinoma of the stomach in frequency. It is a disease of older age groups, affecting men more often than women. Geographic features are discussed on p. 715. Half of the cancers arise in the mid-third of the esophagus, the remainder being approximately equally distributed between the upper and lower thirds. It is generally an ovoid growth with its long axis parallel to the long axis of the esophagus (Plate 2, *B*). Central ulceration of the elevated plaque-like growth undermines the peripheral mucous membrane. It may extend to involve the full circumference of the esophagus and commonly infiltrates the full thickness of the esophageal wall. Lymphatic spread and mediastinal invasion are frequent. As a result, carcinoma of the esophagus is generally well established when recognized, and the results of treatment, as measured in terms of 5-year survivals, are, as might be expected, quite poor.

Although epidermoid carcinomas are by far the most common in the esophagus, glandular carcinomas are occasionally seen. Although most of the adenocarcinomas are primary tumors of the gastric cardia with the extension into the esophagus, occasionally they take origin in esophageal glands and may grow in an adenoid cystic pattern.

Carcinoma of small intestine

This is an infrequent primary malignant tumor and when it occurs in the duodenum, one may have difficulty in distinguishing it from pancreatic carcinoma or carcinoma of the common bile duct secondarily infiltrating the duodenum. With the exception of some of the periampullary carcinomas, many of which resemble the biliary duct system tumors morphologically, carcinomas of the small intestine are similar in appearance and behavior to those of the large intestine, although their clinical diagnosis may be more difficult and their evolutionary stage more advanced when they are diagnosed. An occasional carcinoma of the small intestine may take origin in a papillary adenoma.

Carcinoma of anal region

A number of different epithelial tumors take origin in the vicinity of the anus and anorectal junction. The *epidermoid carcinoma* arising from the squamous epithelium of the anal mucous membrane appears and behaves similarly to epidermoid carcinomas of other squamous epithelial mucous membranes. They spread freely by way of the rich perianal lymphatic plexuses to the lymph nodes of the groin.

The so-called *basoloid tumors* having histologic resemblance to the common basal cell epitheliomas of the skin, presumably arise from the mucosa of the transitional or cloacogenic zone separating the rectal and anal mucous membranes. Although they may spread as the epidermoid carcinomas of the anus do, studies indicate a more favorable prognosis than that of the anal epidermoid carcinomas.

Occasional epidermoid tumors in this area include some glandular elements or individual cells with mucin secretions—*mucoepidermoid carcinomas.*

Anal duct carcinoma is an infrequent tumor, usually glandular and mucin-secreting, that occurs in the anorectal area without apparent involvement of the anal skin or anal or rectal mucous membrane. It arises from anal glands or ducts and usually is not recognized as being malignant until some time has elapsed, often while treatment has been directed toward such conditions as fistula in ano.

Rarely, *epidermoid carcinomas* arise in the rectum without anatomic continuity with the anus. They also occur, but even more rarely, in the stomach as do mixed glandular and epidermoid tumors—adenoacanthomas.

Malignant melanoma

Malignant melanomas have been encountered in many parts of the gastrointestinal tract, and with the exception of those primary in the anus and esophagus, they are considered to be metastatic. Unlike the metastases from carcinoma, they are infrequently accompanied by peritoneal spread. The appearance and behavior of the primary tumors do not differ from those of the corresponding skin lesions. Anal malignant melanomas may present primarily as rectal lesions because anal sphincteric action may cause them to grow cephalad initially.

Establishment of the primary nature of gastrointestinal malignant melanomas rests upon demonstration of junctional change, with the recognition of neoplastic proliferation in the area of the junction of epithelium and subepithelial stroma.

Carcinoid tumor

Carcinoid (argentaffin) tumors are relatively uncommon neoplasms whose endocrine secretion may produce systemic effects. They are found throughout the gastrointestinal tract, from the stomach to the rectum, as well as in the gallbladder and in teratoid ovarian tumors. Morphologically and functionally identical tumors arise in the bronchial and tracheal mucous membranes. The cell of origin is believed to be the Kulchitsky cell, one of the cell types occurring in the crypts of Leiberkühn, characterized morphologically by the presence of cytoplasmic granules capable of reducing ammoniacal silver nitrate (argentaffin granules). It has been suggested that more than one cell type may be involved, since argentaffin granules are found frequently in the midgut carcinoids and rarely, if at all, in tumors of the bronchi, stomach, and hindgut. Argyrophil granules, which stain with metallic silver after the addition of exogenous reducing agent, have a similar distribution pattern as do the argentaffin granules but are seen with greater frequency in tumors of the bronchi, stomach, and hindgut than are the argentaffin granules. The argentaffin cells secrete serotonin (5-hydroxytryptamine), a hormone also found in blood platelets and concerned with blood coagulation, probably through a vasoconstrictive action. Serotonin has also been shown to have a normal central nervous system function, and these facts, together with its pathologic role in the development of cardiovascular lesions and the "carcinoid syndrome," accounts for the widespread interest it has generated. Some carcinoids are grossly indistinguishable from carcinomas, but generally the lesions are small submucosal nodules or merely focal areas of submucosal thickening. Their yellow color has been emphasized, but many are actually gray or gray-white. Muscle hypertrophy is often considerable in the involved area, and this, together with the characteristic fibrosis and perhaps peritoneal adhesions, may produce kinking and partial obstruction (Plate 2, *G*).

Two histologic types of carcinoid tumors are recognized. The "classic" variety, composed of solid nests of uniform small cells with round or oval nuclei that are usually regular,

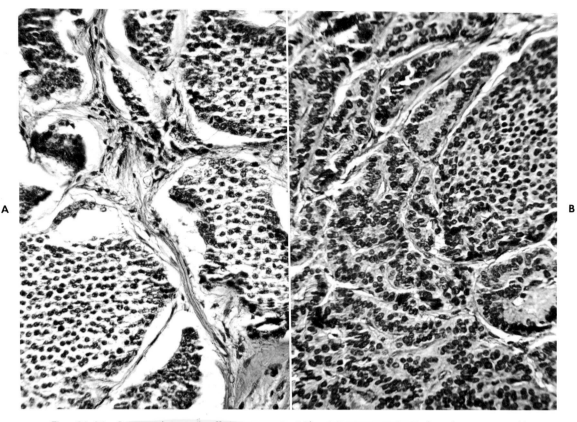

Fig. 30-29. Carcinoid (argentaffin) tumor. **A,** "Classic" pattern. **B,** Trabecular pattern. (**A** and **B,** 300×.)

is more commonly encountered. The less common histologic pattern is that of trabeculae of interanastomosing bands or ribbons of tumor cells. Rosette-like formation may occur with either type of tumor and both patterns may be seen in some tumors (Fig. 30-29). Mucus-secreting cells may be found in either variety of tumor, and in some instances when they are in great numbers, the diagnosis of mucus-producing carcinoma may be suggested. The argentaffin granules when present appear to be concentrated at the periphery of the cell about one pole of the nucleus. The tumors tend to grow invasively and do have the potential for metastasizing by way of lymphatics and bloodstream. However, even when metastases occur, it is not uncommon for a patient to live an essentially asymptomatic life for many years.

Carcinoid tumors occur more frequently in the appendix and rectum than elsewhere and they are usually asymptomatic, being found during the course of proctoscopic examination or in the appendix removed surgically for acute inflammation or other reasons. However,

roughly 10% to 15% of rectal carcinoid tumors, usually those more than 2 cm in diameter invade the muscularis propria and behave like rectal carcinomas, although perhaps progressing more slowly. Occasionally, very small tumors may be associated with distant, even widespread, metastases. Carcinoid tumors that metastasize and prove fatal, as well as those associated with the "carcinoid syndrome," most often are encountered in the ileum and commonly are multiple. The "carcinoid syndrome" consists of diarrhea, a peculiar cyanotic flushing of the skin, and right-sided heart failure, the last being based on organic disease of the tricuspid or pulmonic valves. Almost invariably, extensive liver metastases are present in patients with the syndrome. In the usual functioning carcinoid tumor, 5-hydroxyindoleacetic acid (5-HIAA), a degradation product of 5-hydroxytryptamine (5-HT), can be demonstrated in the urine. The cardiac lesion consists of dense, fibrous endocardial thickening, the fibrous tissue apparently being deposited upon the surface of the endocardium of the pulmonic valve, tricuspid valve, or endocardium of the auricle. Less commonly other chambers of the heart, the great vessels and coronary sinus may be involved. As the result of these changes, functional pulmonary stenosis and tricuspid insufficiency may result. Normally, serotonin is destroyed in the lungs by monamine oxidase, accounting for the preponderance of right-sided cardiac disease.

The fibrosis seen in the heart and in the vicinity of the primary carcinoid tumor has been considered to be the result of release of histamine and mucopolysaccharides from mast cells, which in turn produce local edema, and fibrin deposition with organization of the latter resulting in fibrosis.

Williams and Sandler[201] have subdivided carcinoid tumors into three groups: (1) those of the bronchus and stomach, arising from the foregut; (2) those of the jejunum, ileum, and cecum, arising from the midgut; and (3) those of the rectum developing from the hindgut. They point out that those from the foregut are often of trabecular pattern and sometimes secrete 5-hydroxytryptophan, a precursor of serotonin, and store the latter poorly; those of midgut origin are the classic lesions, both morphologically and tinctorially (positive argentaffin reaction) and in the ability to store large amounts of serotonin; those of the hindgut are usually of trabecular pattern and lack secretory function. The syndrome, as well as 5-HIAA excretion, is more frequent with midgut tumors than those from the foregut and hindgut.

Neoplasms of smooth muscle

With the exception of the uterus, the muscle of gastrointestinal tract gives rise to more tumors of smooth muscle than any other organ or organ system of the body. As is true also of the uterus, *leiomyomas* far outnumber *leiomyosarcomas*. They arise in any portion of the alimentary tract, from the esophagus to the rectum but are more common in the stomach than elsewhere. The small intestine is next most frequently involved. They may grow primarily into the gut lumen (Fig. 30-30), and in that part of the intestine supported on a mesentery, they may become pedunculated and form the head of an intussusception. They also may project primarily from the serosa and grow to a large size without producing gastrointestinal symptoms. Some tumors are dumbbell-shaped lesions, projecting in both directions. It is common for gastrointestinal muscle tumors to ulcerate and undergo extensive central necrosis, thus accounting for the frequency

of hematemesis (or melena). A small leiomyoma of the intestine may be the cryptic source of massive, even exsanguinating, hemorrhage.

These neoplasms are most frequently composed of interlacing bundles of fusiform cells with long processes and nuclei with blunted ends, often bearing a striking resemblance to normal smooth muscle. Less commonly, they feature round or polygonal cells that are frequently vacuolated and sometimes associated with spindle cells more characteristic of smooth muscle. This pattern is now generally considered to represent an atypical growth pattern of smooth muscle tumors and is referred to as bizarre leiomyoma, leiomyoblastoma, and round cell leiomyoma. Although they appear well delineated grossly, under the microscope no capsule is seen, and tumor muscle fibers usually can be seen to interdigitate with those of the muscularis propria or, occasionally, the muscularis mucosae. The histologic distinction between leiomyoma and leiomyosarcoma may be difficult in whichever microscopic pattern the tumor presents; the atypical appearance of the leiomyoblastoma by itself is not indicative of malignancy. Occasional sarcomas appear very orderly and well differentiated, giving no hint of malignancy until metastasis occurs. More often, however, completely benign tumors show great cellularity and nuclear pleomorphism, even to the presence of bizarre giant cells. The presence of mitotic figures in appreciable numbers is generally a reliable indication of malignancy.

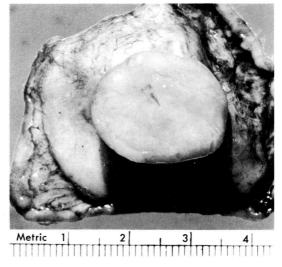

Fig. 30-30. Leiomyoma of stomach. Growth essentially endogastric.

Distant metastasis of leiomyosarcomas are usually blood borne, but some display a tendency to spread over the peritoneal surface and some are only locally invasive. Capacity for local invasion only is particularly true of those arising in the retroperitoneum, most of which are classified as sarcomas, largely because of the impossibility of removing them

completely and thus affecting cure, although they metastasize infrequently.

Lymphoma

A benign lesion, often referred to as *lymphoma of the rectum,* but also known as *lymphoid polyp* or *rectal tonsil,* is occasionally encountered on proctoscopic examination and

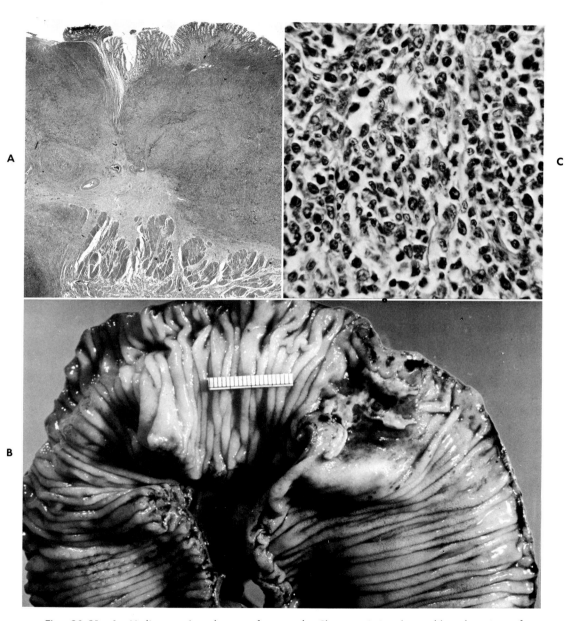

Fig. 30-31. A, Malignant lymphoma of stomach. Characteristic plateaulike elevation of mucosa and pronounced thickening of submucosa well demonstrated. At left, muscle has been freely invaded. **B,** Malignant lymphoma of small intestine, with multiple sites of involvement. Note similarity to gross appearance of carcinoid tumor illustrated in Plate 2, G. **C,** Malignant lymphoma of stomach showing considerable pleomorphism. (**A,** 13×; **C,** 625×.)

removed as a "polyp." It is usually only a few millimeters in diameter but may reach a dimension as great as 1.5 cm. It can be recognized microscopically as benign by its excellent organization with "germinal centers" and its usual limitation to the mucosa and submucosa without invasion of the muscle coat. It is of significance only in differential diagnosis. With this exception, the lymphomas of the gastrointestinal tract are malignant. Such malignant lymphomas may arise as primary, or apparently primary, gastrointestinal tumors or may be but one manifestation of generalized disease. The latter situation is more common, and all varieties of malignant lymphoma encountered in the lymphoid tissue of the body generally, may involve the alimentary tract. The same varieties also occur as "primary" lesions, but some (e.g., Hodgkin's disease and plasmacytoma) are very rare, whereas lymphosarcoma and reticulum cell sarcoma are relatively more frequent. Gastrointestinal lesions in generalized malignant lymphoma (including the leukemias) are of importance in and of themselves, and they may demand treatment when they are responsible for problems relative to gastrointestinal hemorrhage or obstruction. Malignant lymphomas readily perforate, occasionally at multiple sites, especially after irradiation therapy.

"Primary" malignant lymphoma of the gastrointestinal tract is most often seen in the stomach, less commonly in the rectum, cecum, and ascending colon and infrequently elsewhere. Gastric malignant lymphomas usually simulate carcinoma in their clinical manifestations, and they may do so as far as their gross pathologic appearance is concerned as well. However, many characteristically appear as flat, disclike or plateaulike elevations with rather sharply defined borders (Fig. 30-31, *A*). They are raised a few millimeters or a centimeter or so above the surrounding mucous membrane, and if they involve the antrum, their pyloric margin is abrupt. Frequently involvement is multifocal, and ulceration is usual, producing shallow saucerlike lesions. In the intestine, involvement of submucosa, as opposed to mucosa, is a prominent feature, and again multicentric origin is frequent. As with carcinoid tumors, kinking and incomplete obstruction may bring the disease to the patient's attention (Fig. 30-31, *B*).

Lymphomas may be difficult to distinguish histologically from carcinoma, and at times they can be distinguished from inflammatory hyperplasia only with great difficulty (Fig. 30-31, *C*). In some cases, the distinction from the latter requires observation of the clinical course over a period of years.

Although malignant lymphomas of the gastrointestinal tract have their greatest incidence in the same age range as carcinoma, they have a greater incidence during early ages, including childhood. Primary malignant lymphoma of the stomach, the most common malignant gastric tumor next to carcinoma, offers a distinctly better prognosis than does carcioma in terms of 5-year survival after surgical treatment. On the other hand, so-called primary malignant lymphomas of the colon and rectum in the majority of instances prove to be manifestations of systemic disease, although the extraintestinal involvement may not be apparent at the time of recognition of the colonic or rectal lesion.

Occasional cases of multiple, polypoid, relatively well-differentiated and organized lymphoid lesions of the gastrointestinal tract (so-called gastrointestinal pseudolymphomas) are encountered. They are extremely difficult to differentiate from malignant lymphoma and in some instances observation of the clinical course over a period of years is necessary for their distinction.

Miscellaneous rare tumors

Although *mucocele of the appendix* is not a true neoplasm, it will be considered here. It is a cystic dilatation of the appendix distal to a complete obstruction, usually the result of cicatricial stricture after inflammation. The mucocele is distended with thick, glairy mucus, its wall is thin, and the normal mucous membrane is replaced by glands resembling those of the colon or by a single layer of mucus-secreting cells. In a number of cases, there are associated pseudomucinous ovarian cysts. Rupture of a mucocele (or of a pseudomucinous cyst) results in the lesion known as *pseudomyxoma peritonei*—spread of mucus-secreting cells over the peritoneal surfaces, with accumulation of mucoid material in the peritoneal cavity. A difference of opinion exists as to whether pseudomyxoma represents actual neoplastic epithelial proliferation or a nonneoplastic proliferation of serosal cells under the stimulus of irritation. It seems likely that either or both mechanisms may be operative in individual cases. The behavior of pseudomyxoma peritonei is one of a locally infiltrating surface growth that generally cannot be eradicated.

Lipomas occasionally are encountered in

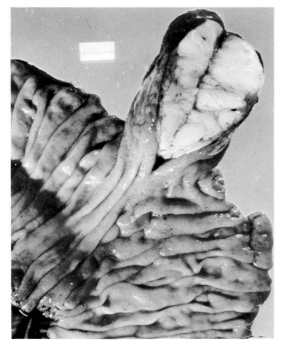

Fig. 30-32. Lipoma of jejunum.

various parts of the gastrointestinal tract, most often in the colon and rectum, and particularly in the vicinity of the ileocecal valve, where appreciable submucosal adipose tissue is usually present. They are submucosal, often superficially ulcerated, and may lead to an intussusception (Fig. 30-32). In instances of incipient intussusception, there may be puckering of the overlying serosa, and this, coupled with induration as the result of inflammation, accounts for their occasionally being mistaken for carcinoma at operation.

Vascular tumors, especially *cavernous hemangiomas,* have been reported as occuring in various parts of the gastrointestinal tract. Multiple hemangiomas may be seen as part of *Osler-Weber-Rendu* disease. *Lymphangiomas* occur less frequently. Characteristic *glomus tumors* may form polypoid, sometimes painful, gastric tumors. Rarely gastrointestinal lesions occur in *Kaposi's sarcoma.*

The gastrointestinal tract and mesentery may be involved by tumors of *nerve origin*—neurofibroma, neuroblastoma, ganglioneuroma and paraganglioma, *teratoma,* and *choriocarcinoma. Adenomas,* or papillary cystadenomas, arise from the apocrine sweat glands in the region of the anus and may give rise to Paget's disease. *Granular cell myoblastomas* have been encountered in the stomach, rectum, and esophagus.

Carcinosarcoma is a rare but spectacular tumor of the esophagus incorporating both epithelial growth (usually epidermoid) and a sarcomatous or sarcoma-like stroma, which may dominate the picture. Many such tumors are polypoid. There is no agreement as to the nature of the stromal change—whether it is genuinely malignant or pseudosarcomatous. The carcinosarcomas are distinctly less malignant than the much more common epidermoid carcinomas. Although they may be grossly simulated by the *polypoid fibrovascular tumors* occurring most commonly in the upper one third of the esophagus, their malignant histologic features should serve adequately to distinguish the two growths. Metastases, which are relatively infrequent, may be carcinomatous, sarcomatous, or mixed.

Mesothelial cysts are encountered rarely in the mesentery or retroperitoneum. Of greater importance and slightly greater frequency are tumors arising from the serosal lining cells—mesotheliomas. They may be solitary and fibrous, in which case they may be amenable to surgical removal, but more often the peritoneal mesotheliomas, in contrast to most of those of the pleura, are diffuse and result in widespread adhesions. They have a tubular pattern, forming multiple small spaces lined by mesothelium, and may secrete mucin. The histologic picture may simulate carcinoma very faithfully. Rare peritoneal mesotheliomas may present as multiple small papillary growths whose first discovery may be in a hernial sac. They may be difficult, if not impossible, to distinguish from mesothelial cell hyperplasia and metastatic carcinoma.

Metastatic tumors

Metastatic tumors, especially carcinoma, are common in the peritoneal cavity. Spread over the serosal surfaces to involve multiple organs and produce widespread adhesions is a frequent autopsy finding in disseminated cancer. The primary tumor may not be readily apparent without complete autopsy study; thus the distinction of metastatic carcinoma from diffuse mesothelioma is made difficult, if not impossible.

REFERENCES
Congenital anomalies
General

1 Estrada, R. L.: Anomalies of intestinal rotation and fixation, Springfield, Ill., 1958, Charles C Thomas, Publisher.
2 Kissane, J. M.: Pathology of infancy and childhood, ed. 2, St. Louis, 1975, The C. V. Mosby Co.

Atresias

3 Bernstein, J., et al.: Am. J. Dis. Child. **99:** 804-818, 1960.
4 DeLorimer, A. A., Fonkalsrud, E. W., and Hays, D. M.: Surgery **65:**819-827, 1969.

Esophageal webs

5 Shamma'a, M. H., and Benedict, E. B.: New Eng. J. Med. **259:**378-384, 1958.

Imperforate anus

6 Kiesewetter, W. B., Turner, C. R., and Sieber, W. K.: Am. J. Surg. **107:**412-421, 1964.

Heterotopia
Heterotopic gastric mucous membrane

7 Bosher, L. H., Jr., and Taylor, F. H.: J. Thorac. Surg. **21:**306-312, 1951.
8 Rector, L. E., and Connerley, M. L.: Arch. Pathol. (Chicago) **31:**285-294, 1941.

Heterotopic pancreatic tissue

9 Martinez, N. S., Morlock, C. G., Dockerty, M. B., Waugh, J. M., and Weber, H. M.: Ann. Surg. **147:**1-12, 1958.
10 Tonkin, R. D., Field, T. E., and Wykes, P. R.: Gut **3:**135-139, 1962.

Heterotopic pulmonary tissue

11 Marsden, H. B., and Gilchrist, W.: J. Pathol. Bacteriol. **86:**532-534, 1963.

Duplications and cysts

12 Bremer, J. L.: Arch. Pathol. (Chicago) **38:** 132-140, 1944.

Meckel's diverticulum

13 Johns, T. N. P., Wheeler, J. R., and Johns, F. S.: Ann. Surg. **150:**241-256, 1959.
14 Weinstein, E. C., Cain, J. C., and ReMine, W. H.: J.A.M.A. **182:**251-253, 1962.

Aganglionic megacolon (Hirschsprung's disease)

15 Gherardi, G. J.: Arch. Pathol. (Chicago) **69:** 520-523, 1960.

Pyloric stenosis

16 Benson, C. D., and Lloyd, J. R.: Am. J. Surg. **107:**429-433, 1964.
17 Cassella, R. R., Brown, A. L., Jr., Sayre, G. P., and Ellis, F. H., Jr.: Ann. Surg. **160:**474-487, 1964.

Achalasia of esophagus

18 Seagram, C. G. F., Louch, R. E., Stephens, C. A., and Wentworth, P.: Can. J. Surg. **11:** 369-373, 1968.

Multilocular rectal cysts

19 Edwards, M.: Dis. Colon Rectum **4:**103-110, 1961.

Acquired malformations
Diverticula

20 Borow, M., Smith, M., Jr., and Soto, D., Jr.: Am. Surg. **33:**373-377, 1967 (duodenum).
21 Edwards, H. C.: Ann. Surg. **103:**230-254, 1936 (jejunum).

22 King, B. T.: Surg. Gynecol. Obstet. **85:**93-97, 1947 (esophagus).
23 Morson, B. C.: Br. J. Radiol. **36:**385-392, 1963 (colon).
24 Reichman, H. R., and Watkins, J. B.: J.A.M.A. **182:**1023-1028, 1962 (colon).

Pneumatosis intestinalis

25 Culver, G. J.: J.A.M.A. **186:**160-162, 1963.
26 Doub, H. P., and Shea, J. J.: J.A.M.A. **172:** 1238-1242, 1960.
27 Keyting, W. S., McCarver, R. R., Kovarik, J. L., and Daywitt, A. L.: Radiology **76:**733-741, 1961.
28 Skendzel, L. P.: Arch. Pathol. (Chicago) **67:** 333-338, 1959.
29 Smith, B. H., and Welter, E. H.: Am. J. Clin. Pathol. **48:**455-465, 1967.

Melanosis of colon

30 Ecker, J. A., and Dickson, D. R.: Am. J. Gastroenterol. **39:**362-370, 1963.

Endometriosis

31 Tagart, R. E. B.: Br. J. Surg. **47:**27-34, 1959.

Esophagotracheobronchial fistula

32 Wychulis, A. R., Ellis, F. H., Jr., and Andersen, H. A.: J.A.M.A. **196:**117-122, 1966.

Mechanical disturbances
Obstruction
Hernia
Inguinal hernia

33 Mayo, C. W., Stalker, L. K., and Miller, J. M.: Ann. Surg. **114:**875-885, 1941.

Hiatus hernia

34 Barrett, N. R.: Br. J. Surg. **42:**231-243, 1954.
35 Grimes, O. F., and Stephens, B. H.: Ann. Surg. **152:**743-766, 1960.
36 Marchand, P.: J. Thorac. Surg. **37:**81-92, 1959.

Intussusception

37 Benson, C. D., Lloyd, J. R., and Fischer, H.: Arch. Surg. (Chicago) **86:**745-751, 1963.

Obturation obstruction

38 Norberg, P. B.: Am. J. Surg. **104:**444-447, 1962.

Stricture

39 Fabrikant, J. I., Anlyan, W. G., and Credick, R. N.: South. Med. J. **52:**1136-1191, 1959 (irradiation).
40 Norton, J. H., Jr., Rev-Kury, H., and White, H. J.: Gastroenterology **46:**471-473, 1964.
41 Perkins, D. E., and Spjut, H. J.: Am. J. Roentgenol. **88:**953-966, 1962 (irradiation).

Effects of intestinal obstruction

42 Storck, A., Rothschild, J. E., and Ochsner, A.: Ann. Surg. **109:**844-861, 1939.
43 Tumen, H. J.: In Bockus, H. L.: Gastroenterology, ed. 2, Philadelphia, 1964, W. B. Saunders Co.

Adynamic (paralytic) ileus

44 Ochsner, A., and Gage, I. M.: Am. J. Surg. **20:**378-404, 1933.

Mallory-Weiss syndrome

45 Baue, A. E.: J.A.M.A. **184**:325-328, 1963.
46 Dagradi, A. E., Broderick, J. T., Juler, G., Wolinsky, S., and Stempien, S. J.: Am. J. Dig. Dis. **11**:710-721, 1966.
47 Dobbins, W. O., III: Gastroenterology **44**:689-695, 1963.

Vascular disturbances
Esophageal varices

48 Baker, L. A., Smith, C., and Lieberman, G.: Am. J. Med. **26**:228-237, 1959.
49 Liebowitz, H. R.: J.A.M.A. **175**:874-879, 1961.

Infarction of intestine

50 Glotzer, D. J., and Shaw, R. S.: New Eng. J. Med. **260**:162-167, 1959.
51 Marston, A.: Lancet **2**:365-370, 1962.

Ischemic enteritis

52 Frengley, J. D., and Reid, J. D.: New Zeal. Med. J. **63**:212-218, 1964.

Gastrointestinal hemorrhage

53 Brief, D. K., and Botsford, T. W.: J.A.M.A. **184**:18-22, 1963.
54 Ecker, J. A., Doane, W. A., Dickson, D. R., and Gebhardt, W. F.: Am. J. Gastroenterol. **33**:411-421, 1960.
55 Smith, C. R., Jr., Bartholomew, L. G., and Cain, J. C.: Gastroenterology **44**:1-6, 1963 (hereditary hemorrhagic telangiectasia).
56 Thompson, H. L., and McGuffin, D. W.: J.A.M.A. **141**:1208-1213, 1949.

Inflammations
Esophagitis

57 Lupovitch, A., and Tippins, R.: Radiology **113**:271-272, 1974 (pseudodiverticulosis).
58 Moses, H. L., and Cheatham, W. J.: Lab. Invest. **12**:663-669, 1963 (herpetic).

Gastritis and gastroenteritis
Phlegmonous gastritis

59 Cutler, E. C., and Harrison, J. H.: Surg. Gynecol. Obstet. **70**:234-240, 1940.

Eosinophilic granuloma and eosinophilic gastroenteritis

60 Helwig, E. B., and Ranier, A.: Surg. Gynecol. Obstet. **96**:355-367, 1953.
61 Ureles, A. L., Alschibaja, T., Lodico, D., and Stabins, S. J.: Am. J. Med. **30**:899-909, 1961.
62 Boley, S. J., Allen, A. C., Schultz, L., and Schwartz, S.: J.A.M.A. **193**:997-1000, 1965.

Ulceration of stomach and duodenum
Nonspecific ulceration

63 Czaja, A. J., McAlhany, J. C., and Pruitt, B. A., Jr.: J.A.M.A. **232**:621-624, 1975 (duodenal disease in burns).
64 Goldman, H., and Rosoff, C. B.: Am. J. Pathol. **52**:227-244, 1968.
65 Pruitt, B. A., Jr., Foley, F. D., and Moncrief, J. A.: Ann. Surg. **172**:523-539, 1970 (Curling's ulcer).
66 Wayte, D. M., and Helwig, E. B.: Am. J. Clin. Pathol. **49**:26-40, 1968.

Peptic ulcer

67 Dragstedt, L. R.: J.A.M.A. **169**:203-209, 1959.
68 Illingworth, C. F. W.: Peptic ulcer, Edinburgh, 1953, E. & S. Livingstone, Ltd.
69 Kirsner, J. B., Kassriel, R. S., and Palmer, W. L.: Adv. Intern. Med. **8**:41-124, 1956.
70 Wolf, S.: Ann. Intern. Med. **31**:637-649, 1949.

Regional enteritis*

71 Ammann, R. W., and Bockus, H. L.: Arch. Intern. Med. (Chicago) **107**:504-513, 1961.
72 Lockhart-Mummery, H. E., and Morson, B. C.: Gut **1**:87-105, 1960 (and ulcerative colitis).
73 Meadows, T. R., and Batsakis, J. G.: Arch. Surg. (Chicago) **87**:976-982, 1963.
74 Saltzstein, S. L., and Rosenberg, B. F.: Am. J. Clin. Pathol. **40**:610-623, 1963 (and ulcerative colitis).

Appendicitis

75 Altemeier, W. A.: Ann. Surg. **107**:517-528, 1938 (bacteriology).
76 Collins, D. C.: Surg. Gynecol. Obstet. **101**:437-455, 1955.
77 Davidsohn, I., and Mora, J. M.: Arch. Pathol. (Chicago) **14**:757-765, 1932 (measles).
78 Fitz, R. H.: Am. J. Med. Sci. **92**:321-346, 1886.
79 Schenken, J. R., and Moss, E. S.: Am. J. Clin. Pathol. **12**:509-517, 1942 (parasites).
80 Tashiro, S., and Zinninger, M. M.: Arch. Surg. (Chicago) **53**:545-563, 1946.
81 Therkelsen, F.: Acta Chir. Scand. **94**(suppl. 108):1-48, 1946.
82 Wangensteen, O. H., and Dennis, C.: Ann. Surg. **110**:629-647, 1939.

Chronic ulcerative colitis†

83 Glotzer, et al: New Eng. J. Med. **282**:582-587, 1970 (ulcerative and granulomatous colitis).
84 Hawk, W. A., Turnbull, R. B., Jr., and Farmer, R. G.: J.A.M.A. **201**:738-746, 1967.
85 Kent, T. H., Ammon, R. K., and DenBesten, L.: Arch. Pathol. (Chicago) **89**:20-29, 1970.
86 Kirsner, J. B.: J.A.M.A. **191**:809-814, 1965.
87 Lewin, K., and Swales, J. D.: Gastroenterology **50**:211-223, 1966.
88 Lumb, G.: Gastroenterology **40**:290-298, 1961.
89 Priest, R. J., Rebuck, J. W., and Havey, G. P.: Gastroenterology **38**:715-720, 1960.

Pseudomembranous enterocolitis

90 Prohaska, J. V., Mock, F., Baker, W., and Collins, R.: Int. Abstr. Surg. **112**:103-115, 1961.
91 Torma, M. J., DeLemos, R. A., Rogers, J. R., Jr., and Diserens, H. W.: Am. J. Surg. **126**:758-761, 1973 (necrotizing).

Tuberculosis

92 Abrams, J. S., and Holden, W. D.: Arch. Surg. (Chicago) **89**:282-293, 1964.
93 Cullen, J. H.: Q. Bull. Sea View Hosp. **5**:143-160, 1940.

---

*See also references 83 to 89.
†See also references 71 to 74.

Fungal infections

94 Putnam, H. C., Jr., Dockerty, M. B., and Waugh, J. M.: Surgery 28:781-800, 1950.

95 Rubin, H., Furcolow, M. L., Yates, J. L., and Brasher, C. A.: Am. J. Med. 27:278-288, 1959 (histoplasmosis).

Lymphopathia venereum

96 Grace, A. W.: J.A.M.A. 122:74-78, 1943.

Parasitic infestations*

97 Dimmette, R. M., Elwi, A. M., and Sproat, H. F.: Am. J. Clin. Pathol. 26:266-276, 1956 (schistosomiasis).

98 Frye, W W.: J.A.M.A. 183:368-370, 1963 (small intestine).

99 Juniper, K., Jr.: Am. J. Med. 33:377-386, 1962 (amebiasis).

100 Kean, B. H., Gilmore, H. R., Jr., and Van Stone, W. W.: Ann. Intern. Med. 44:831-843, 1956 (amebiasis).

101 Koppisch, E.: J.A.M.A. 121:936-942, 1943 (schistosomiasis).

102 Prathap, K., and Gilman, R.: Am. J. Pathol. 60:229-245, 1970 (amebiasis).

Malakoplakia

103 Rywlin, A. M., Ravel, R., and Hurwitz, A.: Am. J. Dig. Dis. 14:491-499, 1969.

Other forms of enteritis and colitis†

104 Abrahamson, R. H.: Arch. Surg. (Chicago) 81:553-557, 1960 (radiation).

105 Gonzales, T. A., Vance, M., Helpern, M., and Umberger, C. J.: Legal medicine, pathology and toxicology, ed. 2, New York, 1954, Appleton-Century-Crofts (chemicals).

106 Tedesco, F. J., Stanley, R. J., and Alpers, D. H.: New Eng. J. Med. 290:841-843, 1974 (clindamycin).

Anorectal lesions

107 Grinvalsky, H. T., and Bowerman, C. I.: J.A.M.A. 171:1941-1946, 1959 (stercoraceous ulcers).

108 Grinvalsky, H. T., and Helwig, E. B.: Cancer 9:480-488, 1956.

109 McGovern, V. J.: In Sommers, S. C., editor: Pathology annual, New York, 1969, Appleton-Century-Crofts, vol. 4, pp. 127-158.

110 Parks, A. G.: Br. Med. J. 1:463-469, 1961.

111 Wayte, D. M., and Helwig, E. B.: Am. J. Clin. Pathol. 48:159-169, 1967.

Peritoneum, omentum, retroperitoneum, and mesentery

112 Altemeier, W. A., and Holzer, C. E.: Surgery 20:810-819, 1946 (torsion of omentum).

113 Eiseman, B., Seelig, M. G., and Womack, N. A.: Ann. Surg. 126:820-832, 1947 (talc).

114 Horsley, J. S.: Arch. Surg. (Chicago) 36:190-224, 1938 (peritonitis).

115 Means, R. L.: Am. Surg. 30:583-588, 1964 (bile peritonitis).

116 Mitchison, M. J.: J. Clin. Pathol. 23:681-689, 1970 (idiopathic retroperitoneal fibrosis).

117 Rogers, C. E., Demetrakopoulos, M. S., and Hyamns, V.: Ann. Surg. 153:277-282, 1961 (mesenteric lipodystrophy).

118 Schwartz, F. D., Dunea, G., and Kark, R. M.: Am. Heart J. 72:843-844, 1966 (methysergide and retroperitoneal fibrosis).

119 Sobel, H. J., Schiffman, R. J., Schwarz, R., and Albert, W. S.: Arch. Pathol. (Chicago) 91:559-568, 1971 (starch granulomas).

120 Sohar, E., Gafni, J., Pras, M., and Heller, H.: Am. J. Med. 43:227-253, 1967 (familial Mediterranean fever).

121 Tedeschi, C. G., and Botta, G. C.: New Eng. J. Med. 266:1035-1040, 1962 (retractile mesenteritis).

Functional states
Gastric atrophy (atrophic gastritis)

122 Bernhardt, H., Burkett, L. L., Fields, M. L., and Killian, J.: Ann. Intern. Med. 63:635-641, 1965.

123 Magnus, H. A.: J. Clin. Pathol. 11:289-295, 1958.

124 Strickland, R. J., and Mackay, I. R.: Am. J. Dig. Dis. 18:426-440, 1973.

Gastric rugal hypertrophy

125 Moldawer, M.: Metabolism 11:153-156, 1962.

126 Morrison, A. B., Rawson, A. J., and Fitts, W. T., Jr.: Am. J. Med. 32:119-127, 1962.

127 Murphy, R. T., Goodsitt, E., Morales, H., and Bilton, J. L.: Am. J. Surg. 100:764-778, 1960.

Malabsorption syndrome

128 Rubin, C. E., Brandborg, L. L., Phelps, P. C., and Taylor, H. C., Jr.: Gastroenterology 38:28-49, 1960.

129 Shiner, M.: J.A.M.A. 188:45-48, 1964.

130 Shiner, M., and Doniach, I.: Gastroenterology 38:419-440, 1960.

131 Weinstein, W. M., Saunders, D. R., Tytgat, G. N., and Rubin, C. E.: New Eng. J. Med. 283:1297-1301, 1970.

Protein-losing enteropathy (exudative enteropathy)

132 Davidson, J. D., Waldmann, T. A., Goodman, D. S., and Gordon, R. S., Jr.: Lancet 1:899-902, 1961.

133 Pomerantz, M., and Waldmann, T. A.: Gastroenterology 45:703-711, 1963.

134 Waldmann, T. A., Steinfield, J. L., Dutcher, T. F., Davidson, J. D., and Gordon, R. S., Jr.: Gastroenterology 41:197-207, 1961.

Gastrointestinal manifestations of systemic disease
Cystic fibrosis

135 di Sant'Agnese, P. A., and Lepore, M. J.: Gastroenterology 40:64-74, 1961.

136 Donnison, A. B., Schwachman, H., and Gross, R. E.: Pediatrics 37:833-850, 1966.

Progressive systemic sclerosis (scleroderma)

137 Goldgraber, M. B., and Kirsner, J. B.: Arch. Pathol. (Chicago) 64:255-265, 1957.

138 Hoskins, L. C., Norris, H. T., Gottlieb, L. S.,

---

*See also reference 79.

†See also references 39 and 41.

and Zamcheck, N.: Am. J. Med. **33**:459-470, 1962.

Whipple's disease (intestinal lipodystrophy)

139 Maizel, H., Ruffin, J. M., and Dobbins, W. O., III: Medicine (Balt.) **49**:175-205, 1970.
140 Ruffin, J. M., Kurtz, S. M., and Roufail, W. M.: J.A.M.A. **195**:476-478, 1966.
141 Sieracki, J. C., and Fine, G.: Arch. Pathol. (Chicago) **67**:81-93, 1959.
142 Watson, J. H. L., and Haubrich, W. S.: Lab. Invest. **21**:347-357, 1969.

Storage disease

143 Azzopardi, J. G., and Evans, D. J.: J. Clin. Pathol. **19**:368-374, 1968 (muciphages).
144 Bale, P. M., Clifton-Bright, P., Benjamin, B. N. P., et al.: J. Clin. Pathol. **24**:609-616, 1971 (Tangier disease).
145 Brett, E. M., and Berry, C. L.: Br. Med. J. **3**: 400-403, 1967 (rectal biopsy).
146 Dobbins, W. O., III: Gastroenterology **50**: 195-210, 1966 (beta-lipoprotein deficiency).
147 Lou, T. Y., Teplitz, C., and Thayer, W. R.: Hum. Pathol. **2**:421-439, 1971 (histiocytosis).
148 Lough, J., Fawcett, J., Wiegensberg, B., et al.: Arch. Pathol. **89**:103-110, 1970 (Wolman's disease).

Neoplasms
Adenomatous polyps, papillary adenomas, and miscellaneous polyps

149 Dukes, C. E.: Proc. Roy. Soc. Med. **40**:829-830, 1947 (difference between adenomatous polyp and papillary adenoma).
150 Dukes, C. E.: Can. Med. Assoc. J. **90**:630-635, 1964 (familial polyposis).
151 Helwig, E. B.: Dis. Colon Rectum **2**:5-17, 1959.
152 Horn, R. C., Jr., Payne, W. A., and Fine, G.: Arch. Pathol. (Chicago) **76**:29-37, 1963 (Peutz-Jeghers syndrome).
153 Klepinger, C. A., and Pontius, E. E.: Am. J. Clin. Pathol. **42**:371-380, 1964 (inflammatory polyp).
154 Lane, N., and Lev, R.: Cancer **16**:751-764, 1963.
155 McKusick, V. A.: J.A.M.A. **182**:271-277, 1962 (genetic factors).
156 Roth, S. I., and Helwig, E. B.: Cancer **16**: 468-479, 1963 (juvenile).
157 Sunderland, D. A., and Binkley, G. E.: Cancer **1**:184-207, 1948.
158 Turcot, J., Despres, M. P., and St. Pierre, F.: Dis. Colon Rectum **2**:465-468, 1959 (familial polyposis and tumors of the central nervous system).
159 Wells, C. L., Moran, T. J., and Cooper, W. M.: Am. J. Clin. Pathol. **37**:507-514, 1962 (electrolyte imbalance).
160 Wheat, M. W., Jr., and Ackerman, L. V.: Ann. Surg. **147**:476-487, 1958.

Relationship of adenomatous polyps and papillary adenomas to carcinoma of colon

161 Enterline, H. T., Evans, G. W., Mercudo-Lugo, R., Miller, L., and Fitts, W. T., Jr.: J.A.M.A. **179**:322-330, 1962.

162 Horn, R. C., Jr.: Cancer **28**:146-152, 1971 (malignant potential of polypoid lesions).
163 Spratt, J. S., Jr., Ackerman, L. V., and Moyer, C. A.: Ann. Surg. **148**:682-698, 1958.

Gastric polyps

164 Eklof, O.: Acta Radiol. (Stockholm) **57**:177-198, 1962 (also duodenum).
165 Ming, S. C., and Goldman, H.: Cancer **18**: 721-726, 1965.
166 Monaco, A. P., Roth, S. I., Castleman, B., and Welch, C. E.: Cancer **15**:456-467, 1962.
167 Tomasulo, J.: Cancer **27**:1346-1355, 1971.

Carcinoma of colon and rectum

168 Dukes, C. E.: J. Pathol. Bacteriol. **35**:323-332, 1932.
169 Dukes, C. E.: J. Pathol. Bacteriol. **50**:527-539, 1940.
170 Gilchrist, R. K.: Dis. Colon Rectum **2**:69-76, 1959.
171 Grinnell, R. S.: Cancer **3**:641-652, 1950.
172 Laufman, H., and Saphir, O.: Arch. Surg. (Chicago) **62**:79-91, 1951.
173 Moore, G. E., and Sako, K.: Dis. Colon Rectum **2**:92-97, 1959.
174 Southwick, H. W., Harridge, W. H., and Cole, W. H.: Am. J. Surg. **103**:86-89, 1962.

Carcinoma of stomach

175 Borrman, R.: In Henke, F., and Lubarsch, O., editors: Handbuch der speziellen pathologischen Anatomie und Histologie, Berlin, 1926, Julius Springer Verlag.
176 Boswell, J. T., and Helwig, E. B.: Cancer **18**: 181-192, 1965 (squamous cell carcinoma and adenoacanthoma).
177 Dungal, N., and Sigurjonsson, J.: Br. J. Cancer **21**:270-276, 1967.
178 Friesen, G., Dockerty, M. B., and ReMine, W. H.: Surgery **51**:300-312, 1962.
179 Golden, R., and Stout, A. P.: Am. J. Roentgenol. **59**:157-167, 1948.
180 Horn, R. C., Jr.: Gastroenterology **29**:515-525, 1955.
181 Monafo, W. W., Jr., Krause, G. L., Jr., and Medina, J. G.: Arch. Surg. (Chicago) **85**:754-763 1962.
182 Saphir, O., and Parker, M. L.: Surg. Gynecol. Obstet. **76**:206-213, 1943.
183 Stout, A. P.: Arch. Surg. (Chicago) **46**:807-822, 1943.

Carcinoma of esophagus

184 Block, G. E., and Lancaster, J. R.: Arch. Surg. (Chicago) **88**:852-859, 1964 (cardioesophageal adenocarcinoma).
185 Burgess, H. M., Baggenstoss, A. H., Moersch, H. J., and Clagett, O. T.: Surg. Clin. North Am. **31**:965-976, 1951.
186 Kay, S.: Surg. Gynecol. Obstet. **117**:167-171, 1963.

Carcinoma of small intestine

187 Benson, R. E.: Ann. Surg. **157**:204-211, 1963.
188 Darling, R. C., and Welch, C. E.: New Eng. J. Med. **260**:397-408, 1959 (tumors of small intestine).

189 Wiancko, K. B., and MacKenzie, W. C.: Can. Med. Assoc. J. 88:1225-1230, 1963.

Carcinoma of appendix

190 Sieracki, J. C., and Tesluk, H.: Cancer 9:997-1011, 1956.

Carcinoma of anal region*

191 Helwig, E. B., and Graham, J. H.: Cancer 16:387-403, 1963.
192 Kline, R. J., Spencer, R. J., and Harrison, E. G., Jr.: Arch. Surg. (Chicago) 89:989-994, 1964.
193 Lone, F., Berg, J. W., and Stearns, M. W., Jr.: Cancer 13:907-913, 1960.
194 Zimberg, Y. H., and Kay, S.: Ann. Surg. 145:344-354, 1957.

Malignant melanoma

195 Quan, S. H. Q., White, J. E., and Deddish, M. R.: Dis. Colon Rectum 2:275-283, 1959.

Carcinoid tumor

196 Bates, H. R., Jr., and Clark, R. F.: Am. J. Clin. Pathol. 39:46-53, 1963.
197 Black, W. C., III: Lab. Invest. 19:473-486, 1968.
198 Hernandez, F. J., and Reid, J. D.: Arch. Pathol. (Chicago) 88:489-496, 1969.
199 Horn, R. C., Jr.: Cancer 2:819-837, 1949.
200 Moertel, C. G., Sauer, W. G., Dockerty, M. B., and Baggenstoss, A. H.: Cancer 14:901-912, 1961.
201 Williams, E. D., and Sandler, M.: Lancet 1:238-239, 1963.

Neoplasms of smooth muscle

202 Berg, J., and McNeer, G.: Cancer 13:25-33, 1960.
203 Bogedain, W., Carpathios, J., and Najib, A.: Dis. Chest 44:391-399, 1963.
204 Camishion, R. C., Gibbon, J. H., Jr., and Templeton, J. Y., III: Ann. Surg. 153:951-956, 1961.
205 Skandalakis, J. E., Gray, S. W., and Shepard, D.: Int. Abst. Surg. 110:209-226, 1960.
206 Starr, G. F., and Dockerty, M. B.: Cancer 8:101-111, 1955.
207 Tallquist, A., Salmela, H., and Lindstrom, B. L.: Acta Pathol. Microbiol. Scand. 71:194-202, 1967 (leiomyoblastoma).

Lymphoma

208 Azzopardi, J. G., and Menzies, T.: Br. J. Surg. 47:358-366, 1960.
209 Cornes, J. S.: Cancer 14:249-257, 1961.
210 Cornes, J. S., Wallace, M. H., and Morson, B. C.: J. Pathol. Bacteriol. 82:371-382, 1961 (benign lymphoma of rectum).
211 Dawson, I. M. P., Cornes, J. S., and Morson, B. C.: Br. J. Surg. 49:80-89, 1961.
212 Jacobs, D. S.: Am. J. Clin. Pathol. 40:379-394, 1963 (malignant lymphoma and pseudolymphoma).
213 Joseph, J. I., and Lattes, R.: Am. J. Clin. Pathol. 45:653-669, 1966.

Miscellaneous rare tumors

214 Ackerman, L. V.: In Atlas of tumor pathology, Sect. VI, Fascs. 23 and 24, Washington, D.C., 1954, Armed Forces Institute of Pathology (tumors of the retroperitoneum, mesentery, and peritoneum).
215 Cohen, R. S., and Cramm, R. E.: Dis. Colon Rectum 12:120-124, 1969 (myoblastoma).
216 Hughes, J.: Ann. Surg. 165:73-76, 1967 (mucocele and pseudomyxoma).
217 Hyun, B. H., Palumbo, V. N., and Null, R. H.: J.A.M.A. 208:1903-1905, 1969 (hemangioma).
218 Jang, G. C., Clouse, M. E., and Fleischner, F. G.: Radiology 92:1196-1200, 1969 (fibrovascular polyp).
219 Kay, S., Callahan, W. P., Jr., Murray, M. R., Randall, H. T., and Stout, A. P.: Cancer 4:726-736, 1951 (glomus tumor).
220 Kepes, J. J., and Zacharias, D. L.: Cancer 27:61-70, 1971 (paraganglioma).
221 Lane, N.: Cancer 10:19-41, 1957 (carcinosarcoma).
222 Perea, V. D., and Gregory, L. J., Jr.: J.A.M.A. 182:259-263, 1962 (neurofibromatosis).
223 Regan, J. F., and Cremin, J. H.: Am. J. Surg. 100:224-233, 1960 (chorioepithelioma).
224 Sahai, D. B., Palmer, J. D., and Hampson, L. G.: Can. J. Surg. 11:23-26, 1968 (lipoma).
225 Stout, A. P.: J. Tenn. Med. Assoc. 44:409-411, 1951 (mesothelioma).
226 Stout, A. P., Hendry, J., and Purdie, F. J.: Cancer 16:231-243, 1963 (omentum).
227 Winslow, D. J., and Taylor, H. B.: Cancer 13:127-136, 1960 (mesothelioma).
228 Yannopoulos, K., and Stout, A. P.: Cancer 16:914-927, 1963 (mesentery).

*See also reference 108.

31/Liver

HUGH A. EDMONDSON
ROBERT L. PETERS

Liver disease has steadily gained recognition as a major health problem principally because of the worldwide distribution of virus hepatitis and the ubiquity of cirrhosis of the liver. The symptoms of liver disease, such as jaundice, fever, abdominal enlargement, and encephalopathy, are striking phenomena that bring the patient to the physician. The interpretation of the increasing number of laboratory and radiologic tests plus needle biopsy of the liver makes it imperative that the physician have a sound knowledge of the pathology of this most interesting organ and its multitudinous functions.

STRUCTURE AND CIRCULATION
Structure and embryology

The liver arises from the hepatic diverticulum in the 20- to 25-somite embryo. The primitive hepatic cells grow into the septum transversum, where the entodermal cells proliferate rapidly, while at the same time rapid growth of the mesoderm produces angioblasts and sinusoids.[14] Glycogen granules are noted at 8 weeks. The development of intrahepatic bile ducts is completed at 3 months[7] at which time bile secretion is said to begin. In the third month, the liver begins to store iron, and concurrently becomes the chief blood-forming organ of the embryo. The site of hematopoiesis is the extravascular component of the lobule.[6,17,18] This function is gradually transferred to the bone marrow as the latter develops, so that by time of birth, only an occasional focus of hematopoiesis remains. In premature infants, areas of hematopoiesis are abundant. At birth, the liver weighs about 300 gm and projects well below the costal margin. The left lobe is relatively large in the newborn infant. During fetal life, this lobe receives well-oxygenated blood from the umbilical vein. The latter structure atrophies and becomes the round ligament. The omphalomes-

enteric veins drain into the larger right lobe of the liver, and from these develops the portal vein.

The liver grows at a relatively slower rate than the rest of the body, so that in an adult it weighs approximately 1350 gm. At maturity, the liver is located most commonly at or above the costal margin. However, it is not unusual for the lower edge to be 1 to 3 cm below the costal margin.[12] The right lobe has become much larger than the left, and the organ is held firmly in the right hypochondrium and epigastrium by the falciform and triangular ligaments. Anatomically, the dividing line between the right and left lobe is 1 to 1.5 cm to the right of the falciform ligament, approximating the gallbladder-caval line. The division of the liver into various segments, each with its separate blood supply makes a study of surgical anatomy worthy of emphasis.[9]

A firm, smooth layer of connective tissue (Glisson's capsule) encloses the liver and is continuous with the connective tissue of the porta hepatis, the latter forming a sheath around the portal vein, hepatic artery, and bile ducts that enter the hilum of the liver. This connective tissue surrounds all subdivisions of the blood vessels and ducts to the finest radicles, where it joins the inner aspect of Glisson's capsule. The portal vein, hepatic artery, and common hepatic duct divide in the porta hepatis into right and left branches that supply the two lobes of the liver. In their subsequent ramification through the liver, the branches of the artery, vein, and hepatic duct are always together in the portal canals. Injection and corrosion methods have shown that, among the structures of the portal triad, the portal vein is the largest. The hepatic artery, being much smaller, tends to twine about it like a vine over the trunk of a tree. The size of the branches of the hepatic duct is about the same as that of the hepatic artery. The latter is subject to many gross anatomic variations.[10]

The hepatic parenchyma, as may be seen with the naked eye, or more clearly with the microscope, is composed of innumerable small lobules, each with a diameter of 0.5 to 2 mm and the shape of an irregular and somewhat pyramidal hexahedron. At the center of each lobule is the intralobular or central efferent vein, while around the periphery are four or five portal spaces arranged at regular intervals. This is the classic lobule of the liver.[5] Rappaport[13] has described the functioning lobule or liver acinus that has at its center a portal triad and around its periphery portions of several classic lobules. The liver acinus probably represents the true functioning unit of the liver, but because it is difficult to recognize, grossly and microscopically, pathologists in their descriptions of gross and microscopic specimens use the term *lobule* in its classic sense.

The lobules are composed of hepatocytes so arranged between sinusoids that at least two cells at their poles opposite the sinusoids may form bile canaliculi.[5] Depending on the angle at which the cells are sectioned for histologic preparations, one may see cell groups of variable thickness. It is important from the functional standpoint that a hepatocyte-sinusoidal system does exist, so that every hepatic cell abuts upon a sinusoid through which blood passes from the portal vessels to the central veins and that the cell has access to the bile canalicular system. Liver cell membranes form the lining of the canaliculi and are seen to be arranged as microvilli when viewed with the electron microscope.[15] The canaliculi form an interlacing network that impinges upon at least one side of every hepatic cell. These lead into larger channels that finally join the bile ductules at the margin of the lobule. At the junction, biliary duct epithelium and liver cells join in an uneven

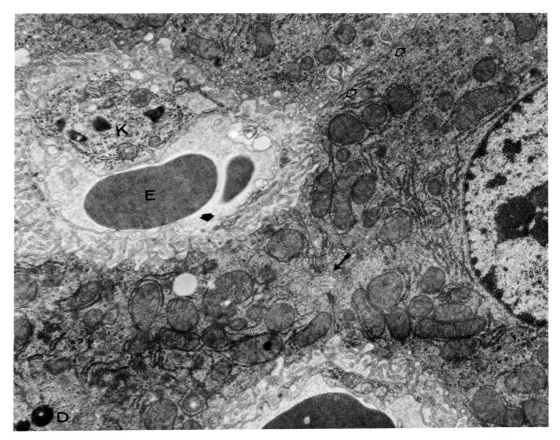

Fig. 31-1. Interlocking of liver cells is furnished by studlike projections of intercellular membrane *(open arrowheads)*. Erythrocyte, **E,** in sinusoid. Kupffer cell, **K.** Dense body, **D.** *Arrow,* Bile canaliculus. *Black arrowhead,* Pore in endothelium lining.

manner over a short distance.[15] Just before the passage is surrounded by a rosette of biliary epithelium, it has been termed *duct of Hering* or *bile preductule*.[15] The sinusoids form a radial network that allows the blood to come into contact with every parenchymal cell as it flows to the central veins. The lining cells of the sinusoidal system are best known as Kupffer cells. They apparently are held in place by interdigitations of their microvilli with the microvilli of the parenchymal cells. The Kupffer cells form an incomplete lining of the sinusoidal system, so that blood plasma may circulate freely in the space between the Kupffer cells and the parenchyma (Fig. 31-1). This space is known as Disse's space. It is not large enough to accommodate erythrocytes or leukocytes but averages about 0.33 μm or 300 to 400 nm in width. The cytoplasm of the Kupffer cells usually contains many lysosomes and vacuoles. The rough endoplasmic reticulum and mitochondria are abundant.[11] Kupffer cells are actively phagocytic, taking up many kinds of particulate matter.

The liver cells have a polyhedral shape, a round nucleus, and a fairly prominent nucleolus. The fine structure of liver cells has been extensively investigated in recent years.[8] The surface of the liver cell is in contact with (1) its neighbors, from whom it is separated by narrow intercellular spaces, (2) Disse's space, and (3) the bile canaliculus (Fig. 31-1). Along the lateral surface desmosomes are present. Near the canaliculus, tight junctions are formed by the fusion of the external leaflets of the neighboring plasma membranes. The bile canaliculi are lined by rather short microvilli of adjoining liver cells. A large portion of the surface of the parenchymal cell is exposed to Disse's space. Combined cytochemical and electron microscopic studies have shown that the plasma membrane along the sinusoidal surface has strong alkaline phosphatase and nucleoside monophosphatase activities whereas nucleoside triphosphatase is most active on the bile canaliculus side. The hepatocytes contain many mitochondria, more in the periportal than in the centrilobular zones. The endoplasmic cisternae are considered to be the distribution system that transports nutrients to all parts of the cell.[8] The Golgi apparatus has a convex and concave surface and is located between the nucleus and the bile canaliculus. It is considered to be the "packaging plant" of the liver cell. For example, very low density lipoproteins (VLDL) and glycoproteins are present. The bilirubin-conjugating enzyme is present in the smooth endoplasmic reticulum, but the transport mechanism for bilirubin is not known. Normally, glycogen is abundant throughout the cytoplasm. Lysosomes are numerous and, in the functioning liver, vesicles and vacuoles of variable size are present near Disse's space. Vesicular invaginations of the plasma membrane are noted to occur between the bases of the microvilli that project into Disse's space. Bile canaliculi form a polygonal network throughout the lobule, so that a small portion of every liver cell contributes to the canalicular system.[4] The central veins course through the centers of the lobules in a longitudinal fashion and empty into sublobular veins. The sublobular veins have specialized connective tissue walls and are distinguished from branches of the portal vein by the fact that they are not associated with arteries and bile ducts. The sublobular veins unite to form the hepatic veins. The latter combine to form two large trunks and several smaller ones that open into the inferior vena cava where it passes through a groove on the posterior surface of the liver. Large trunks of the hepatic vein form a simple branching system that is not nearly so angulated and tortuous as are the large branches of the portal vein.

Circulation

The liver receives into its sinusoidal system about 1500 ml of blood per minute. It is estimated that about 600 ml comes from the hepatic artery and 900 ml from the portal vein. Some 50% to 60% of the oxygen is supplied by the portal vein.[16] The latter system differs from the systemic venous system in that the blood is under a pressure of 8 to 10 mm Hg and has a relatively high oxygen content, usually about 80% saturated. The mixture of blood from a high-pressure arterial system (90 mm Hg) and a low-pressure venous system (8 to 10 mm Hg) is accomplished by a drop in arterial pressure consequent to the fine subdivisions of the hepatic arterioles that form a periductular plexus before the blood enters the peripheral sinusoids. Some small branches from the hepatic artery flow directly into the peripheral sinusoids, where it has a siphoning effect on the sinusoidal system as blood with a faster velocity flows to the central veins.[13] An intermittent type of flow has been observed that is no doubt regulated by the tonus of the hepatic arteriolar system and precapillary sphincters.

FUNCTION AND LABORATORY DIAGNOSIS

In health the hepatocytes perform a multitude of functions that are concerned with the following[76]:

1. Secretion of bile and other substances
2. Intermediate metabolism of proteins, lipids, and carbohydrates
3. Storage of certain foodstuffs and minerals
4. Detoxification of various compounds as well as metabolism of hormones and drugs
5. Elaboration of proteins with specific activities or functions

In disease one or more of these vital functions may be disturbed and can be measured by laboratory tests or the cause can be diagnosed by tissue examination. Furthermore, enzyme and electron microscopic studies have elucidated many aspects of malfunction in liver disease. It is important in the evaluation of each laboratory test that the physician have an understanding of the normal physiologic mechanisms involved as well as the various diseases that cause the abnormal findings. In the following discussion of hepatic tests that are most commonly used to detect disease, an attempt is made to relate some of these to disturbance of normal physiology and to fine structural change.

Among the laboratory tests used in the evaluation of liver disease are those that are related to the liver functions as outlined above, plus either those that measure soluble enzymes that enter the blood when the liver cells are injured by disease or those tests that measure abnormal substances, proteins or otherwise, that are elaborated by diseased liver cells. Tests that measure specific antibodies produced by the reticuloendothelial system against infective agents or organ-specific tissues are widely used.

Hepatic tests

Serum bilirubin and sulfobromophthalein (BSP). One of the most common findings in liver disease is the accumulation of bilirubin in serum and tissue fluids. Approximately 300 mg per day of bilirubin are formed in the reticuloendothelial system from the catabolism of heme, 80% to 90% of which is a component of hemoglobin released from senescent erythrocytes. The remainder arises from certain hepatic enzymes such as cytochromes and catalases or from precursors of hemoglobin in the marrow.[23,49,53] This early labeled bilirubin is derived from two sources, one related to erythropoiesis and the other is non-erythropoietic. The latter is apparently synthesized mostly in the liver, from "free" heme and heme proteins.[68] The erythrocyte component probably comes from the bone marrow, but its source is yet to be determined.[80] Arriving in Disse's space as an albumin-linked, lipid-soluble nonpolar susbstance, bilirubin is freed of albumin and enters the liver cell, where it is accepted by two specific binding proteins, Y and Z.[22] These same proteins also bind BSP. In the smooth endoplasmic reticulum, the bilirubin is converted to an excretable, water-soluble form by conjugation to 2 molecules of glucuronide per bilirubin molecule.[67] In this process, glucuronide is transferred from uridine pyrophosphate glucuronate by means of the enzyme glucuronyl transferase. Conjugated bilirubin leaves the liver cell by what must be an active-transport mechanism to enter the canaliculus, the flow being partially dependent on bile salt excretion.[44] From the canaliculi, bile passes into the small bile ducts and finally enters the gut by way of the biliary duct system. Bilirubin levels will rise in the serum and tissues, producing jaundice:

1. If a greatly increased load of bilirubin must be removed from the blood for conjugation and excretion
2. If abnormal liver cell function either prevents removal of "unconjugated" bilirubin from serum or inhibits the conjugation of the bilirubin with glucuronide in the liver cell, or both
3. If the excretion of bile via the duct system is impeded

The adult liver has sufficient reserve to handle much more than the normal quantity of bilirubin formed by the breakdown of erythrocytes, but the liver of the newborn infant or of the patient with parenchymal cell disease is often unable to cope with an increased pigment load that results from hemolysis. Hyperbilirubinemia is a common early sign of liver disease, but its detection and fractionation is usually of little help in the differential diagnosis. The "direct-reacting" bilirubin, which is a rough quantitation of the polarized water-soluble or conjugated bilirubin, will rise in about equal proportions to the indirect-reacting bilirubin in most jaundice disorders except those that are associated with an increase in pigment load (hemolysis) or in the hereditary hyperbilirubinemias (specific enzymic deficiency disorders). Unconjugated bilirubin, because of its lipid solubility, may pass in small amounts through the intestinal mucosa into the gut.[66,84,85] The unconjugated bilirubin rarely rises above 5 mg per 100 ml in uncomplicated hemolytic diseases.[32] Conjugated bilirubin is water soluble and is excreted by the kidney. It is probable that serum levels become elevated because conjugated bilirubin becomes loosely associated with albumin. In biliary tract obstruction, bilirubin levels generally do not rise above 25 mg per 100 ml because of the excretion of bilirubin through the kidney. However, in the presence of kidney disease, the hyperbilirubinemia may exceed this level.

The most commonly used dye for diagnostic purposes is sulfobromophthalein (BSP). It quickly binds to plasma proteins after intravenous injection. From 70% to 80% is removed by the liver and the remainder by muscle, kidney, and other organs.[65] BSP is conjugated by the liver cell to glucuronide and excreted by way of the biliary passages in a fashion similiar to that in which bilirubin is secreted. The disappearance rate is measured as an indication of the removal and excretory ability of the liver cell. The test is sensitive to minimal liver disease of almost any type, but is most valuable in the diagnosis of mass lesions, infiltrative disease, and some of the hereditary hyperbilirubinemias. However, the test is subject to interpretative errors because for any given body weight there can be considerable variation in plasma volume. Secondly, the removal of the dye depends on the hepatic blood flow; this may be altered by heart failure or by shock.[32] It is probable that much of the BSP retention observed in cirrhotic patients is the result of inadequate exposure of liver cells to sinusoidal blood. Furthermore, some blood may not enter the sinusoids because of intrahepatic shunts. Obviously, either liver cell damage or biliary tract obstruction will produce BSP retention in serum. In biliary obstruction, much of the serum BSP is conjugated to BSP-glucuronide.

Cerebrospinal fluid glutamine levels. The severely damaged or malfunctioning liver fails to appropriately dispose of circulating ammonia absorbed from the intestinal tract. The level of ammonia is closely related to nervous system dysfunction known as hepatic encephalopathy. The mechanism whereby encephalopathy is produced is apparently by the action of ammonia on Krebs cycle intermediate, α-ketoglutaric acid, to form glutamic acid. Glutamic acid reacts with another ammonia molecule to form glutamine. The depletion of important α-ketoglutarate rather than the direct effect of ammonia is considered to be the cause of the encephalopathy.[26,27] Since blood ammonia levels may drop but the central nervous system Krebs intermediaries remain depleted, there is better correlation between coma and CSF glutamine levels than between hepatic coma and blood ammonia levels. Blood ammonia analysis is also fraught with technical problems whereas CSF glutamine levels are reproducibly determined.[25,55]

Serum proteins. The major fractions of serum proteins, the albumin and the globulins, usually are measured simultaneously. The albumin level is a measure of liver cell function, but globulins are derived from many sources. Hypoalbuminemia is most often caused by one of the following:

1. Building blocks are inadequate. Hypoalbuminemia may be seen in starvation or in conditions in which the amino acid components are used preferentially in production of other proteins.
2. The liver cell in advanced chronic disease or in severe acute damage is incapable of sustaining normal levels of albumin. The serum albumin level often is closely monitored in order to judge the course of disease.
3. Excessive loss of albumin from the gastrointestinal system or the kidneys produces a low serum level.

About 12 gm of albumin is synthesized daily by the ribosomes of the rough endoplasmic reticulum. The albumin is apparently then transported to the plasma membrane for release into the bloodstream.

The serum globulin level may become elevated in the course of any chronic inflammatory disease. Usually, it is the gamma fraction that increases. In the United States, where the incidence of parasitic and mycotic disease is small, chronic liver disease is one of the more common causes of prolonged hyperglobulinemia.

The numerous flocculation and turbidity tests used in the past were based on a poorly understood insolubility of gamma globulin in certain reagents when the quantity of albumin was reduced or its quality was altered. There seems to be little use for such tests in a modern laboratory.

Prothrombin. Of the known coagulation factors, prothrombin (factor II), labile factor (factor VII), fibrinogen (factor I), and plasma thromboplastin component (PTC, factor IX), as well as plasma thromboplastin antecedent (PTA, factor XI) and Stuart factor (factor X), are produced by rough endoplasmic reticulum in hepatocytes.[79] All these components may be partially depleted in advanced chronic or severe acute liver disease, and their quantitation may be used in prognosis. The coagulation test used most commonly in assessment of liver disease is the prothrombin time. Because of its shorter half-life,[28] however, factor VII is theoretically superior, for the serum level reflects the parenchymal cell status more closely.

It has been shown that prothrombin synthesis by hepatocytes is cyclic. Usually only 10% to 30% of the cells are active at any one moment. The rate depends on the level of prothrombin in the blood,[24] and the synthesis of prothrombin factors V and VII is dependent on the availability of vitamin K. This vitamin is stored in the liver. The warfarin (Coumadin) anticoagulants all act by blocking vitamin K utilization. It is uncommon for dietary deficiency of vitamin K to occur, but impaired absorption of lipids from the gut will include inadequate assimilation of vitamin K. Those conditions that inhibit the absorption of lipid-soluble vitamin K from the gastrointestinal system include the spruelike diseases, pancreatic insufficiency, impaired bile flow, and chronic use of mineral oil. Sterilization of the gut by antibiotics will reduce available vitamin K made by bacteria.

A normal flow of bile into the intestine allows emulsification of lipids, including vitamin K. This emulsification is necessary for esterification and absorption. Thus either chronic biliary obstructive disease or liver cell disease may be associated with a low prothrombin activity. If vitamin K is administered parenterally, the reduction of prothrombin activity associated with chronic obstructive biliary tract disease is quickly reversed, whereas that related to parenchymal cell disease is not.

α_1-Antitrypsin (α_1-AT). α_1-Antitrypsin, also known as protease inhibitor (Pi), is a glycoprotein[63] with a molecular weight of 54,000[34] produced by the hepatocyte. Pi normally acts to inhibit certain proteolytic enzymes including trypsin, chymotrypsin, elastase, collagenase, thrombin, fibrinolysin, and some granulocytic proteases.[63,89] Levels of Pi are inconsistently reduced in serum of patients with massive hepatocellular necrosis[35] and are generally increased in sera of patients with inflammatory diseases and in most patients with cirrhosis. The quantitative determination of Pi has little reliability in evaluation of hepatic function, but one genotype, homozygous ZZ, is associated with

high incidence of a liver disease that usually appears transiently in infancy and later reappears as a fatal cirrhotic disorder in the juvenile (see pp. 1063 and 1376). Pi ZZ occurs in 0.07 to 0.2% of the population. Not all patients with Pi ZZ develop a hepatic disorder. Of the phenotypes described, only Pi ZZ is *definitely* related to disease. Pi SZ[36,38] or FZ[38] may rarely be associated with an adult variety of cirrhosis.

Alkaline phosphatase activity. The phosphomonoesterases with optimal activity in the alkaline pH range are grouped together and called *serum alkaline phosphatase*.[59] Alkaline phosphatases are present in endothelium, surface epithelia of many mucosal surfaces, neutrophils, placenta, bone, renal tubules, and to some extent, liver canaliculi.[37] Despite its uncertain source and largely undetermined function, serum alkaline phosphatase activity is a valuable and sensitive liver test. For practical purposes, only liver diseases, bone abnormalities, bone growth, and late pregnancy are associated with elevations in activity. Although the serum alkaline phosphatase activity may rise in the presence of any liver disease, the greatest elevations occur in biliary tract obstruction. This increase, plus BSP retention, may be the only laboratory alterations detected in a patient with a space-occupying mass in the liver.

Electrophoretic studies of elevated alkaline phosphatase in the serum suggest that one band, L, is the isoenzyme derived from the liver. The isoenzymes from the intestine and bone are indicated as band I and band B. Increase in "liver" alkaline phosphatase may be associated with liver disease but is elevated in some patients with bone disorders and others with no hepatic disease.[33] Thus it appears that isoenzyme quantitation still lacks good clinical correlation.

Leucine aminopeptidase (LAP, leucine arylamidase) and 5′-nucleotidase (5-Nase). These enzymes have widespread distribution in body tissues, but serum activity levels are rarely elevated except in obstructive diseases of the biliary tract. Either test is helpful in patients who have elevated alkaline phosphatase activity without evidence of liver disease. Since bone disease is not associated with elevated serum activities of LAP or 5-Nase, an increase in LAP and 5-Nase levels indicates that the elevation of alkaline phosphatase activity is related to hepatobiliary disease.[82]

α-**Glutamyl-transpeptidase (GGTP).** Although this enzyme is abundant in the kidney and somewhat less so in the pancreas, the liver is apaparently the source of the enzyme found in serum. The normal function of the enzyme is to catalyze a reaction between glutathione and an amino acid. Serum levels of GGTP are erratic and quantitatively unrelated to the extent of hepatocellular necrosis. However, the test is useful in detecting some additional abnormality in patients with quiescent liver disease. Alcoholic patients who have regained a stable pattern of laboratory test values develop elevated GGTP levels if they start drinking again. The GGTP may be the only test that shows abnormal results in sera of patients who have resumed alcoholism.

Transaminases. SGOT and SGPT are the two parenchymal cell enzymes that are most frequently quantitated in the evaluation of liver cell necrosis. Hepatocellular damage brings about the release of many cytoplasmic components. Some are unstable, and others that may also originate in extrahepatic tissues are unsuitable for diagnosis. GPT is fairly restricted to liver tissue. It is unbound to ultrastructures and is quite soluble,[81] and it apparently leaks through damaged but viable cell membranes. GOT is present in other tissues but in smaller quantities than in the liver.[71] In hepatocytes, the GOT is found in the soluble fraction (GOT I) and in mitochondria (GOT II) in a ratio of 1:4.[29] The different electrophoretic activities, pH optima, and substrate affinities[30,31,46] have prompted some investigators to attempt to separate the types or extent of cell necrosis by differential analysis of transaminase isoenzymes, but the technique awaits thorough clinical trials. The GOT not only is tissue-bound and less soluble than GPT, but also is cleared more rapidly from blood. GOT II is cleared more rapidly than GOT I.[45] Thus SGPT is a more satisfactory indicator of liver cell damage.

Lactic acid dehydrogenase fraction, isocitric dehydrogenase, sorbital dehydrogenase, glutamate dehydrogenase, ornithine carbamyl transferase, alcohol dehydrogenase, and guanase. These enzymes are present in liver in much higher quantities than in other tissues. They are released as a result of hepatocellular damage. The determination of levels in sera seems to have no diagnostic advantage over assessing the SGOT & SGPT levels.

Hepatitis B surface antigen (HBsAg). This lipoprotein, 20 nm particulate material, is a product of hepatitis B virus apparently noninfective of itself. The hepatitis virus, which proliferates in the hepatocytes, produces its surface coating in great excess to be released into the serum as HBsAg. HBsAg can be demonstrated histologically in the liver tissue in some patients with chronic varieties of hepatitis B.[42,50-52] Demonstration is by immunoperoxidase reaction specifically toward HBsAg[19,56] or by orcein stain,[86] which apparently demonstrates the disulfide bonding of HBsAg. Recently HBsAg has been demonstrated in tissue of some patients with chronic liver disease when serum levels of the antigen were undetectable.[19]

A confirmed positive test for HBsAg is definitive proof of infectivity (either acute or chronic) by hepatitis B.

Anti–hepatitis B core (anti-HBc). Anti–hepatitis B core is an antibody to the protected core of the hepatitis B virus. It becomes positive in essentially all patients who develop hepatitis B at about the time of maximal elevation of serum transaminase activity and remains elevated to a lesser extent for a long period of time, apparently years. Patients who retain the hepatitis B virus in their liver maintain a high titer of anti-HBc. Performance of the test is restricted by the difficulty of obtaining sufficient quantities of hepatitis B core (HBc). Testing for anti-HBc is undertaken by complement fixation,[54] immune adherence hemagglutination, or radioimmunoassay.

Another antigen-antibody system associated with hepatitis B is the *e* system (HBeAg and anti-HBe); *e* antigenemia is closely associated with viral DNA polymerase, the presence of Dane particles, and infectivity of the serum. Anti-HBe is a marker of low or no infectivity. HBe is present early in acute hepatitis B, and either HBe or anti-HBe can be detected in the sera of about 60% of patients with chronic varieties of hepatitis B. As of 1977, only the relatively insensitive technique of agar gel immunodiffusion is available for detection of HBeAg or anti-HBe.

Lymphocyte transformation. Lymphocyte transformation may be applied to test the cellular immune response to specific drugs or infective agents. Cellular immunity may persist after humoral immune responses have subsided or may be present when the latter have failed to develop. The test may be applied to investigations of diseases of organs other than liver, but it has been applied to identification of cellular immunity to hepatitis B and to some hepatotoxic drugs.[41,64,88] Lymphocyte transformation involves incubating the patient's lymphocytes with the suspected antigen, followed by incubation of the same lymphocytes in a tritiated precursor to DNA, usually thymidine. If the T lymphocyte has been previously exposed to the antigen and is normal in its response, it will "transform" to the immunoblast form, incorporating the labeled DNA precursor into its nucleus. The extent of the incorporation, and thus the percentage of transformation, is calculated. If the patient has not been previously sensitized to the antigen or has been exposed but has deficient or functionally abnormal T lymphocytes, little tritiated DNA-precursor will be incorporated.

Ameba antibodies. Antibodies to *Entamoeba histolytica* usually develop in patients with tissue invasion by the organism, which usually means a hepatic amebic abscess. The antibody levels are usually elevated at the time the patient enters the hospital with symptoms.

The antigen used in testing is the extract of a mutant strain of *E. histolytica* that can be grown on artificial cell-free culture media. Testing may be done by complement fixation or by hemagglutination after coating tannic acid–treated erythrocytes with semipurified amebic antigenic material.[39,61] The antibody levels considered significant for an amebic abscess must be established at each laboratory performing the test, but usually positive hemagglutination levels are in dilutions of 1:512 or greater. The level of the antibody is not directly related with the clinical severity of the disease.

Smooth muscle antibody. In many diseases associated with hepatic necrosis an antibody develops to components of muscle, apparently actin.[48] Apparently the hepatocyte has a protein that is immunologically similar to actomyosin.[47] Most often the antibody is IgM type and detection of nonselective smooth muscle antibody has little diagnostic value. However, in sera of patients with chronic active lupoid hepatitis and in some with cryptogenic cirrhosis, an IgG class of antibodies to smooth muscle is detectable in high titer.

Mitochondrial antibody. For inexplicable reasons, patients with primary biliary cirrhosis develop an antibody against mitochondrial membranes, particularly those in renal tubules. The antibody is IgG type and is demonstrated in a fashion similar to that for smooth muscle antibody. About 84% of patients with primary biliary cirrhosis have mitochondrial antibodies. In a properly controlled laboratory, there are few false positives.[62]

Liver-kidney microsomal antibodies (LKM antibodies). A rare antibody to microsomal membranes distinct from but easily confused with mitochondrial antibodies has been demonstrated by immunofluorescence in a fashion similar to that for smooth muscle and mitochondrial antibodies. Localization is in hepatocytes and renal proximal convoluted tubules in a very fine particulate distribution. The antibody has been detected in a very small percentage of patients with liver disease, about 75% of those with LKM antibody have chronic liver disease. Most but not all of the patients lack smooth muscle antibodies, mitochondrial antibodies, or hepatitis B surface antigen.[77,78,87]

Alpha fetoprotein (AFP). The fetal hepatocyte normally produces an alpha$_1$ globulin of unknown function that drops to inconsequential serum levels shortly after birth. Later in life some diseases, especially hepatocellular carcinoma (HCC), are associated with serum AFP levels of over 1000 nanograms per milliliter.[21] The AFP is produced by the tumor cells and can be demonstrated by immunofluorescent techniques.[74] Approximately 70% of patients with HCC have AFP levels over 800 ng in their sera, but AFP of 800 to 2000 ng/ml appears in sera of patients with fulminant hepatitis who are still in coma but have a good chance to recover.[60] It is also in maternal sera during fetal distress and in most hepatic disorders of infancy. It appears in higher levels in sera of infants with neonatal giant cell transformation than in those with biliary atresia.[90] Most patients with testicular or ovarian teratocarcinomas have AFP in their sera, as do children with ataxia-telangiectasia, hereditary tyrosinosis, and (Asian) Indian childhood cirrhosis.[21] The nonneoplastic conditions in which serum levels of AFP are elevated are usually readily distinguished on clinical grounds from hepatocellular carcinoma. Normal serum levels are 2.3 to 30 ng/ml, in viral hepatitis 50 to 1000 ng/ml, and in patients with chronic active hepatitis, usually less than 500 ng/ml.[21] The cellular mechanisms responsible for production of AFP are unknown. The elevated levels are not simply a result of increase in hepatocyte replication; the high elevation of AFP levels in sera of patients who ultimately survive fulminant viral hepatitis is not duplicated in patients who survive fulminant hepatic necrosis resulting from a hepatotoxic agent, even though the clinical and laboratory features may be otherwise indistinguishable and the morphologic extent of necrosis similar. Neither does it rise to levels over 800 ng/ml in sera of patients who have undergone subtotal hepatic resection.

Bile salts. Normally, the serum bile acids are low, ranging from 2 to 4 μmoles per liter[73] and are present in a conjugated form. However, in some diseases, such as the blind loop syndrome, they may be elevated and are present as free acids.[40] Differences in serum levels have been noted between chenodeoxycholic acid and cholate in certain diseases.[70] The total levels as well as levels of certain conjugates are sensitive although they are nonspecific indicators of early or minimal liver disease.

Needle biopsy

A needle biopsy of the liver is frequently obtained for study by means of both light and electron microscopy. These studies have added immeasurably to the knowledge of liver disease. Morphologic details unobtainable in autopsy material are seen and are useful in the diagnosis, prognosis, and treatment of hepatic disease.[43,57,83]

The clinician is careful not to perform a biopsy on a patient with common bile duct obstruction because of the danger of bile leakage. A prothrombin value below 40% of normal also is a contraindication because of the possibility of hemorrhage. Portions of the biopsy often are used for bacterial cultures, for analysis of iron or copper, and for other analyses heretofore impossible. Study with the electron microscope is most valuable in research, but this instrument is not yet used in the routine surgical pathology laboratory.

Angiography and scintiscans

Hepatic angiography and scintiscans have become important aids in the diagnosis of liver disease. Angiograms of a liver that contains a space-occupying lesion discloses its size and location and often is helpful in differentiating neoplasms from other diseases.[20] Scintiscans are now being used extensively in the diagnosis of focal intrahepatic lesions.[58,69,72,75]

CLASSIFICATION OF LIVER DISEASES

The discussion of liver disease in this chapter will generally follow the clinicopathologic concept shown in Table 31-1. Acute disorders of the liver may be subdivided into those in which there is primarily necrosis and those in which there is predominantly cholestasis. Chronic liver disease includes the many stages of precirrhosis and cirrhosis as well as other disorders. There may be episodes of jaundice or other indications of acute liver disease. The onset of chronic liver disease is often insidious.

Sooner or later, however, the clinical and laboratory evidence of cirrhosis becomes manifest in most patients. A heterogeneous group includes those acute and chronic liver diseases in which the principal finding is hepatomegaly. Although the chronic form may be attributable to some relatively acute disease like amebic abscess, most often it is long standing and the patient has few or no symptoms.

NECROSIS

Liver cells may be injured sufficiently to undergo necrosis by any one of many agents of infectious, chemical, metabolic, or nutritional origin, as well as by ischemia. The microscopic recognition of liver cell necrosis is dependent on irreversible pathobiologic changes of several hours' duration. The point of irreversibility is not distinguishable by present histotechniques. From a diagnostic standpoint, the limited forms that the necrotic liver cell may assume are expanded by differences in distribution and extent of necrosis and by the variable inflammatory responses that occur in diseases of diversified etiology. The different patterns of necrosis that are observed must reflect distinct pathways of molecular pathology, but there is little understanding of the pathogenesis of necrosis at the ultrastructural level.

Necrosis of liver cells is most frequently of a *lytic* type, as though early lysosomal release had caused self-destruction. Experimentally,[102] other changes occur before lysosomal destruction. Lytic necrosis usually involves only parenchymal cells, sparing the stroma. After lysis, the necrotic cell or cells are not visualized—only the area of dropout or hepatocytolysis.

Coagulative necrosis, on the contrary, is a mummified change of cells in which an eosinophilic granular cytoplasm develops, the nucleus disappears, and the shadow of the cell persists. Such cells are only slowly removed. Coagulative necrosis is a characteristic feature of anoxia and suggests that aerobic conditions are necessary for lytic necrosis. *Caseous and gummatous necrosis,* as well as *liquefactive necrosis,* may be observed in the liver.

Acidophilic necrosis is a singular type of unicellular death in which the cell becomes globular and small and it loses its pyknotic nucleus by extrusion. Other names for this type of necrosis include Councilman bodies and shrinkage necrosis.[97] Among the many conditions in which this type of necrosis is found

Table 31-1. Laboratory findings in acute and chronic liver disease*

Normal values	Transaminases SGPT, 5-35 units; SGOT, 8-40 units	Bilirubin (1.2 mg per 100 ml or less)	Urine urobilinogen (positive in 1:4 dilution)	Alkaline phosphatase (depends on methods†)	Prothrombin		Serum proteins Albumin, 3.5-4.5 gm; Globulin, 3-4 gm
					% of normal level (100%)	Response to vitamin K	
Acute liver disease							
1. Necrosis							
a. Viral hepatitis	High elevation (500-4000) early; SGPT usually > SGOT	Mild to sharp increase (2-40)	Increased early and late but may be absent during phase of deepest jaundice	Normal or mild increase	Moderate to sharp decrease (10%-80%)	Poor	Normal except in a prolonged course or in elderly patients
b. Infectious mononucleosis	Moderate elevation (100-500)	Normal or mild increase (2-5)	Mild or moderate increase	Normal or mild increase	Normal or mild decrease	Poor	Normal
c. Chemical (CCl₄, methyldopa, halothane, isoniazid, paracetamol)	High elevation (500-5000); SGPT usually > SGOT	Mild to sharp increase (2-40)	Usually increased but may be decreased during period of deepest jaundice	Normal or mild increase	Moderate to sharp decrease (5%-80%)	Poor	Normal
d. Acute alcoholic liver disease	SGOT, 75-300; SGPT, 50	Usually moderately elevated	Mild to moderate increase	Slight elevation	Normal to sharp decrease	Poor	Albumin acutely decreased; globulin normal in early stage
2. Cholestasis							
a. Drug-induced	Mild to moderate elevation (usually <300); SGOT and SGPT approximately equal	Mild to moderate increase (3-15)	Variable—mild decrease to mild increase	Moderate to sharp increase	Normal or mild decrease (50%-100%)	Good	Normal
b. Extrahepatic obstruction (1) Stone	Mild to moderate increase (100-300); SGOT and SGPT equal	Mild to moderate increased; fluctuations (2-15)	Variable—may be absent but occasionally increased	Moderate to sharp increase	Normal or moderate decrease (40%-100%)	Good	Normal

(2) Cancer with duct occlusion	Same as for stone	Moderate elevation without fluctuation (10-20)	Absent	Moderate to sharp increase	Variable decrease, mild to sharp (20%-80%)	Good	Normal except for possible decrease in albumin because of malnutrition
Chronic liver disease							
1. Biliary cirrhosis							
a. Secondary	Mild to moderate increase (100-300); SGOT often >SGPT	Mild to moderate increase (3-15)	Variable—decreased to increased	Moderate to sharp increase	Mild to moderate decrease	Variable, poor to good	Albumin decreased; globulin increased
b. Primary	Same as for secondary	Same as for secondary	Same as for secondary	Sharp increase	Mild to moderate decrease	Variable, poor to good	Albumin decreased; globulin increased
2. Alcoholic cirrhosis	Same as for biliary cirrhosis	Anicteric to episodes of jaundice (2-40)	Usually increased	Normal or mild increase	Moderate to sharp decrease	Poor	Albumin decreased; globulin increased
3. "Lupoid" cirrhosis or chronic active hepatitis	Sharp increase during jaundice episodes (500-1500); SGOT often > SGPT	Mild to moderate increase (2-20)	Usually increased	Variable—normal to sharp increase	Moderate to sharp decrease	Poor	Albumin decreased; globulin increased (often sharply)
Other lesions							
1. Abscess	Mild increase (< 200)	Normal or slightly elevated	Normal	Normal to moderate increase	Normal		Albumin may be decreased if chronic
2. Cancer, primary or metastatic	Mild increase (< 200)	Normal unless major bile ducts involved	Normal	Usually a moderate to sharp increase	Normal		Usually normal, but albumin may be decreased
3. Granulomas	Mild increase (< 200)	Normal	Normal	Same as for cancer	Normal		Normal

*Many tests are necessarily omitted; e.g., the BSP retention test is valuable but is used only for anicteric patients.

†May be measured in King-Armstrong units, Bodansky units, or Bessey-Lowry units.

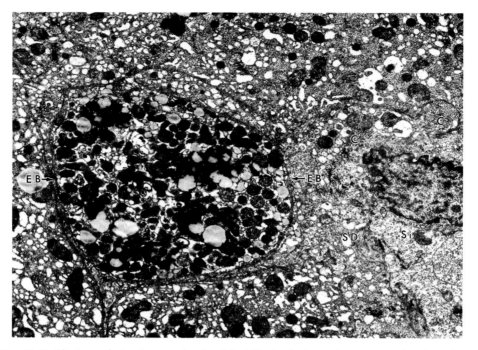

Fig. 31-2. Electron photomicrograph of acidophilic body just prior to extrusion into sinusoid. Note collagen in Disse's space not generally detectable on light microscopy. **C,** Collagen. **EB,** Eosinophilic (acidophilic) body. **SD,** Disse's space. **Si,** Sinusoid. (Courtesy Dr. Hisando Kobayashi, Nagoya, Japan.)

are viral hepatitis, yellow fever, and partial loss of blood supply.[97] On ultrastructural examination, the cytoplasm seems to have become dehydrated and the organelles compressed (Fig. 31-2). The acidophilic body is expelled into the sinusoid, where it may be ingested by a Kupffer cell.

Hyaline necrosis is another type of single cell necrosis that often follows hydropic degeneration of the liver cell. The hyaline bodies are relatively insoluble, are deeply eosinophilic, and are most frequently seen in alcoholic liver disease. They are called either "alcoholic hyaline body" or "Mallory body" after the investigator who originally described it. Hyaline necrosis also is observed in Wilson's disease, in infantile cirrhosis in India, and, rarely, in primary biliary cirrhosis, jejunoileal bypass, and α_1-antitrypsin deficiency.[103]

Liver cell necrosis, depending on its distribution, has been divided into *focal, zonal,* and *diffuse* types. Further definition is achieved by grading the severity as focal, submassive, and massive necrosis. There is a lack of uniformity, however, among pathologists as to the use of these descriptive terms. Nevertheless, *the distribution* of cell necrosis

and the particular kind of necrosis are important features in microscopic diagnosis.

Focal necrosis

Focal necrosis has no zonal pattern. Generally, single cells or small clusters of cells undergo lytic necrosis and are immediately replaced by swollen macrophages, Kupffer cells, and lymphocytes. Often, rapidly dividing adjacent liver cells will quickly heal the defect. Focal necrosis usually is related to an infective agent; viral hepatitis is the prototype. Rare foci of unicellular necrosis may be found in the liver of patients who have extrahepatic infections. In tuberculosis, sarcoidosis, and other granulomatous disorders, both hepatocellular focal necrosis and granulomas may occur. Focal necrosis is seen in typhoid fever, tularemia, and certain cases of rapidly progressive Hodgkin's disease. Biliary obstruction also may lead to focal necrosis and "bile lake" formation.

Zonal necrosis

Zonal necrosis is the usual reaction to toxins. Apparently, liver cells in corresponding lobular areas have a similar sensitivity. Depending on the noxious agent, necrosis may be centrilobular, midzonal, or peripheral (periportal).

Centrilobular necrosis is the commonest type of zonal necrosis. It most often is caused by ischemia and may be seen in patients with congestive failure or shock from any cause. Most necrotizing hepatotoxins have a centrilobular effect. The best known of these, because it is used so frequently in experimental pathology, is carbon tetrachloride (Fig. 7-41). It is postulated that this compound is split by microsomal enzymes into —CCl_3 and —Cl free radicals. These attack methylene bonds of the unsaturated fatty acids of microsome membranes, producing lipoperoxidases that cause severe membrane alterations.[98,99] The free radicals also damage microsomal proteins and P_{450}. Cysteine protects the liver cell from necrosis, possibly by reducing the binding of the free radical to the microsomal proteins.[92] Compounds such as chloroform and trinitrotoluene also cause centrilobular necrosis. Centrilobular necrosis in the fatty liver of alcoholic patients is discussed on p. 1366.

Midzonal necrosis is characteristic of yellow fever but may be seen in other infective conditions. The midzonal lesions are sharply delineated (Fig. 12-24) and are characterized by fatty change, eosinophilic necrosis, ballooning of liver cells and the formation of eosinophilic or Councilman bodies from the third to the seventh day.[94] The sequence of nuclear and cytoplasmic changes has been studied in yellow fever–injected rhesus monkeys.[91]

Peripheral necrosis has been described in phosphorus poisoning and in eclampsia. Yellow phosphorus in sufficient doses leads to peripheral fatty change and necrosis of liver cells.[93] In addition, centrilobular necrosis has been described after phosphorus poisoning.[100]

Diffuse necrosis

Viral hepatitis is by far the most common cause of diffuse, submassive, or massive necrosis of the liver that has previously been called *acute yellow atrophy*. Furthermore, massive or submassive hepatic necrosis may be seen after therapy with monoamine oxidase inhibitors,[95] zoxazolamine, iproniazid, ethionamide, diphenylhydantoin,[96] and others.[101]

Although the mechanisms of liver cell damage undoubtedly differ for many agents, certain features of pathogenesis are common. The initial molecular pathophysiologic change is generally unknown but is often specific for the liver cell, since many of the toxic agents enter other cells without ill effect.

VIRAL HEPATITIS

Viral hepatitis is a necrotizing inflammatory lesion of the liver produced by any one of at least three infecting agents, two of which have been isolated and partially characterized as viruses. The one or ones remaining are assumed to be viral. Acute viral hepatitis (AcVH) is the most common acute liver disease of children and of young adults, occasionally assuming epidemic proportions when hygienic conditions are suboptimal. The majority of infections are apparently subclinical, although occasionally a rapidly fatal course ensues. Hepatitis results in chronic liver disease in a relatively small number of patients; such chronic disorders almost invariably follow clinically inapparent or mild acute disease.

History

Although it has been known for more than a century that hepatitis was often associated with fecally contaminated material and that percutaneous injection could result in another form of hepatitis, it was not until 1942 that "serum hepatitis" gained widespread recognition. Some 24,664 United States troops contracted hepatitis after receiving injections from nine of the lots of yellow fever vaccine made with pooled human sera, an incidence of 56.64 cases per 1000 doses.[208]

In 1951, MacCallum showed, by means of series of feeding and inoculation experiments, that there were at least two viral agents producing similar diseases but that there was no cross immunity between the two. The two agents produced their diseases after different incubation periods; one had maximal infectivity by mouth, the other by percutaneous injection.[180] MacCallum suggested that the orally transmitted shorter incubation agent be called *hepatitis A virus* (HAV) and the parenterally transmitted longer incubation one *hepatitis B* (HBV), a proposal that has only recently been widely accepted.[130]

During the 1960s and 1970s knowledge continued to expand,[169,171,173] but a major breakthrough occurred in 1965 when Blumberg[115] discovered a serum factor that subsequently proved to be an identifiable antigenic component of HBV, thus allowing investigators to specifically identify that disease.[130] Meanwhile Deinhart and Holmes had shown that the short incubation, orally infective HAV could be transmitted to marmosets whereas HBV could not.[137,158] On the other hand, HBV was shown to be transmissible to chimpanzees,[110] and occasionally a non-B type of hepatitis has been transmitted to man from chimpanzee.[145] By 1974, immunoelectron microscopy had been employed by Feinstone and colleagues to identify HAV particles in stools of infected individuals; conversely the technique also allowed identification of antibody to the fecal HAV particles,[142] the antibody appearing fairly early in the patient's disease.

After the above means of identification were used, it became apparent that some patients with hepatitis were infected with an agent that seemed to be neither A nor B.[143,186] These are now tentatively called hepatitis non-A non-B (NAB) virus.

Hepatitis A

Etiologic agent. Viral hepatitis A (VH-A, epidemic hepatitis, infectious hepatitis, infective hepatitis, Botkin's disease, and, older yet, catarrhal jaundice) is caused by an orally acquired, fecally excreted virus that is 27 nm in diameter.[119] Apparently the virus is of RNA type and is believed to proliferate in hepatocyte cytoplasm. Hepatitis A virus (HAV) infectivity is totally destroyed by heating to 100° C for 5 minutes, reduced by heating to 60° C for 1 hour, almost completely inactivated by ultraviolet irradiation, and destroyed after 3 days of incubation at 37° C in 1:4000 formalin.[200] Infectivity is neutralized by addition of convalescent serum. Hepatitis A particles have not been demonstrated in sera of infected individuals, but their brief presence in serum is presumed by inference since serum taken from a patient in the prodrome of VH-A is infective for a second susceptible human. Although HAV can be transmitted by percutaneous routes, it apparently is rarely the agent of posttransfusion hepatitis.[143,198] Hepatitis A particles are demonstrable for a brief period in the stool of infected patients by the technique of immune electron microscopy[142] whereby the viral particles in ultracentrifugal fractions of the stool are agglutinated by convalescent sera, allowing the electron microscopic visualization of not only the clusters of the 27 nm round structures but also of the halo of antibodies attached to the viral bodies (Fig. 31-3). The particles appear in the stool about 2 weeks prior to symptoms and 5 days before development of abnormal transaminase levels and can be found until near the time of peak transaminase elevation.[137,171] The site of the viral

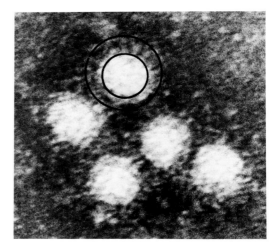

Fig. 31-3. Hepatitis A particles from stool of infected patient, agglutinated by anti-HA. Note fuzzy halo around particles representing antibodies. (One particle and halo *encircled.*) (Courtesy Dr. Jorge Rakela, Santiago, Chile.)

replication during the entire 15- to 45-day incubation period is unsettled.

Marmosets can be infected with HAV producing a hepatitis[137,158] so mild that any comparison with the pathogenesis of the disorder in man is tenuous.

Although past epidemics of hepatitis were apparently caused by HAV, much less is known about it than the virus for hepatitis B. Similarly uncertain is the pathogenesis of the disease produced by HAV and the sequelae, if any, of the infection. The term VH-A should be confined to the disease in which the viral particle can be specifically agglutinated from stool, or in which the patient develops a titer of antibody to VH-A or, presumptively, to a disease that can be related to a foodborne or waterborne epidemic with a high percentage of secondary cases in a family.

Clinical and immunologic aspect. Hepatitis A is highly infective by the fecal-oral route and is thus predominantly an epidemic disease in children, but the disease also occurs where there is poor sanitation or overcrowding. Although the usual route of entry of HAV is oral, it can be transmitted parenterally.[169,171,173] In children from poor hygienic environments the disease is probably common but usually overlooked as a mild influenza-like illness.

Toward the end of the prodrome, fatigue increases, nausea, vomiting and anorexia are frequent, and a distaste for cigarettes often develops. Patients with acute viral hepatitis type A (AcVH-A) also usually have fever, lymphadenopathy, and tender hepatomegaly. Biliuria is followed by icterus; the highest serum bilirubin level is usually reached 1 to 2 weeks after onset of jaundice, at which time the patient usually becomes subjectively improved. The patient is usually free of signs and symptoms of the disease 6 weeks after onset of jaundice.

Patients who develop AcVH-A rapidly develop an antibody that appears 8 or more days after infection, often rising to immune adherence titers between 1:1280 and 1:100,000 and slowly decreasing after convalescence to lower levels.[157] One infection with HAV seems to confer lifelong immunity; passive transfer of small amounts of convalescent serum to a patient at risk protects from clinically evident infection for about 6 months. Commercially available "hyperimmune" gamma globulin contains antibody to HAV of titers between 1:2000 and 1:8000 by immune adherence technique.

Epidemiology. Type A hepatitis has a worldwide distribution and is apparently a disease of man; other primates are only occasional secondary hosts, deriving the disease from man.[152] In 1960 it was found that certain mollusks harvested from polluted seawater concentrated the virus, and ingestion of raw or partially cooked mollusks was associated with an occasional epidemic.[139] It is usually considered that asymptomatic carriers of HAV are rare if they exist at all. Because of its high infectivity, its mode of transmission, the apparent rarity of either animal vectors or chronic carrier state, and the conferred immunity, VH-A tends to occur in epidemics only as a new susceptible population reaches an age where there is intimate contact with older children. The continual entry of new susceptible individuals is necessary for the maintenance of the virus. For unknown reasons, incidence figures for VH-A disease also show seasonal variation. In most countries of the world, the incidence of AcVH-A is decreasing.[186,188]

Hepatitis B

Etiologic agent. Viral hepatitis B (VH-B, syringe jaundice, homologous serum jaundice, serum hepatitis) is caused by a percutaneously transmitted virus that has a complicated morphology. The complete virion is a 40 nm double-shelled structure, called the "Dane particle" (after the investigator who first described the form), sparsely distributed in serum of infected individuals.[133] The outer shell of the Dane particle is a lipoprotein with the anti-

genic specificity identified as *hepatitis B surface antigen* (HBsAg). Beneath the HBsAg of the Dane particle is a 28 nm hexagonal core that is antigenically dissimilar to HBsAg; the antigen characteristic of the core is called *hepatitis B core antigen* (HBcAg).[130] DNA is apparently associated with the core. It has been claimed that a DNA polymerase is sandwiched between the outer HBsAg shell and the inner HBcAg of the Dane particle. Dane particles are very sparse in serum, which contains large amounts of material that is antigenically identical to the outer surface of the Dane particle but without core, DNA, or DNA polymerase. This "excess" surface material is in the form of 20 nm spheres or 20 nm diameter tubular structures of variable lengths. The abundant HBsAg is detectable in the patients' sera and is the basis of tests for hepatitis B infection. The excess material is apparently an aberrant noninfective by-product of viral replication. There are antigenic subtypes of HBsAg,[165,176] a universal type *a,* and sets of alleles (*d* and *y, w* and *r* as well as several other less well characterized), which have interestingly different geographic distributions.[177] The subtypes are characteristics of the virus, not the host. The manner in which the virus infects the hepatocyte is unclear. After infection, however, the "core" apparently replicates in the nucleus of the infected hepatocyte, whereas the HBsAg originates in cytoplasm, probably in the endoplasmic reticulum as a thin filamentous material that undergoes additional morphologic rearrangement before release from the hepatocyte, either as the protective coating of the Dane particle, as 20 nm spheres, or as the tubular structures (Fig. 31-4).

An additional antigenic substance in sera of about 10% of patients with acute viral hepatitis B has been recognized. This antigen, *e* (HBeAg), or its antibody, anti-e (anti-HBe), is found in about 60% of patients with chronic varieties of hepatitis B.[184,185,190] The full significance of e and anti-e awaits further clarification, but the presence of e in serum is related to infectiveness and is a feature of the virion rather than HBsAg. Serum of HBsAg-positive patients seems relatively noninfective if it contains anti-HBe.

Clinical and immunologic aspects. Hepatitis B attacks adults more frequently than does VH-A and is more often associated with serious liver disease. Whether the diseases differ in severity in age-matched individuals is unclear, but many clinicians believe that even in age-matched patients VH-B is still a more severe

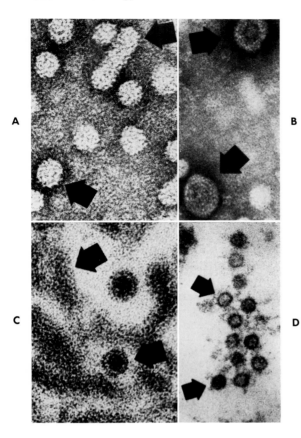

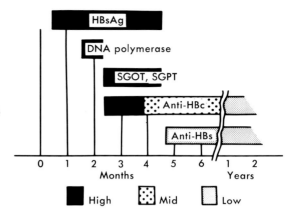

Fig. 31-5. Chart showing the laboratory changes associated with acute hepatitis B infection.

100 nm

Fig. 31-4. Electron microscopic appearance of components of hepatitis B virus. HBsAg is found in serum, **A,** as 20 nm spheres *(left arrow)* or tubular structures *(right arrow)* but is also found sparsely in serum, **B,** as the Dane particle *(arrow),* apparently the complete virion. In hepatocyte cytoplasm, **C,** HBsAg is form of long filamentous structures; rarely a spherical shell surrounds a hexagonal core, apparently the complete virus *(arrow).* Liver cell nuclei contain core, which is inner part of Dane particle without HBsAg envelope, **D.** (Courtesy Alfred E. G. Dunn, Los Angeles.)

illness. Chronic liver disease apparently is more frequently a sequela of AcVH-B than of AcVH-A; in fact it is unlikely that chronic liver disease ever follows VH-A.

Prodromal influenza-like symptoms, joint swelling, and effusion, all possibly a manifestation of acute immune-complex disease, are apparently more common in the prodrome of AcVH-B than in AcVH-A or AcVH-NAB. Prodromal skin rashes and pruritus occur in about equal frequency in AcVH-B and in AcVH-NAB. Some patients develop no pro-

dome with AcVH-B. Patients with AcVH-B may have fewer gastrointestinal symptoms than do patients with AcVH-A, but nausea, vomiting, and fatigue are the principal symptoms.

The serologic manifestations of VH-B infection are indicated in Fig. 31-5. Note that HBsAg may be detectable in less than 1 month after percutaneous inoculation with hepatitis B, but only at 1½ to 6 months after inoculation do clinical symptoms develop. The rise of bilirubin levels lags behind the rise in SGPT and SGOT activities.[54]

The average patient convalescing from AcVH-B develops evidence of T-cell response to HBsAg usually between 4 and 12 weeks after onset of illness. This response can be measured by lymphocyte transformation. According to preliminary studies, the accelerated capacity of the lymphocytes to transform when presented with HBsAg is retained for years if not forever.[88] The duration of time that anti-HBs remains in serum after convalescence is highly variable. Most patients who have had VH-B lose the anti-HBs, apparently in a matter of months[88] unless there has been repeated exposure or inoculation.

Epidemiology. Viral hepatitis type B has a worldwide distribution, but in contrast to VH-A, a large reservoir of asymptomatic carriers exist. Although transmission of overt disease in the United States is usually by inoculation of human blood products, it is not dependent on such artificial techniques for its propagation. Since HBsAg has been encountered in saliva,[121,194,227] tears, ascitic fluid, sneeze droplets,[227] blood-sucking insects,[199,232] menstrual fluid,[134] and, rarely, urine[227] many mechanisms of person-to-person transmission that have in-

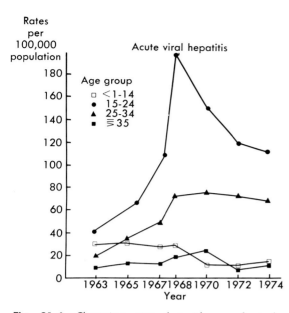

Fig. 31-6. Changing annual incidence of viral hepatitis in different age groups in California. Note that despite increased incidence in 15 to 24 year olds, the age group with hepatitis most often related to transfusion has no change of incidence over 10-year period.

volved kissing,[157,227] biting,[183] sharing of razors and toothbrushes,[186] and sexual[154,155] and transplacental transmission[210,216] have been described or suggested.

Hepatitis B incidence increased at alarming rates until 1970 in large cities, mostly because of the practice of needle sharing by parenteral drug users (see hepatitis in intravenous drug users, p. 1340). It is uncertain whether a recent decrease has resulted from diminished percutaneous drug abuse of the creation of a majority of immune individuals among the drug users.

The sale of blood by indigents to commercial blood banks had resulted in increased infectivity to those who received commercially prepared blood products (Fig. 31-6) although donor selectivity at some donor centers was sufficient to maintain a low-risk product.[109] In some cities, the incidence of clinical hepatitis acquired from a blood transfusion had been as high as 20 per 1000 units of blood although two thirds of the patients contracting hepatitis had developed subclinical disease only.[108,150,221] Screening for HBsAg reduced the total incidence of posttransfusion hepatitis about 25%. Despite sensitive screening of donor blood, a few cases of posttransfusion hepatitis are still

type B. Pooling of blood products obviously increases the risk of transmitting the agent. It has been shown that storage of plasma for 6 months at room temperature is not effective in completely inactivating the agent,[203] contrary to the belief in the 1950s and 1960s.[106] Blood fibrinogen carries a particularly high risk of transmitting hepatitis B,[116] a risk reduced but not eliminated by HBsAg screening of donors. However, heat-treated serum albumin and Cohn-fractionated gamma globulin are free of infectivity.[187] Reports of removal of the risk of posttransfusion hepatitis by reconstituting washed, frozen erythrocytes are encouraging.[124] Passive protection against HBV has been achieved by inoculation of high-titer anti-HBs,[172,219] and recent human and chimpanzee experimental data indicate that inoculation of heated HBsAg confers active immunization against hepatitis B.[156,170] Protection is apparently related to the immune response to HBsAg. Any protection by immune response to HBcAg is unknown.

Hepatitis non-A non-B (VH-NAB)

Little information is available about viral hepatitis that is neither type A nor type B. However several studies have confirmed an earlier observation of Allen and Saymon[105] that a distribution curve of incubation times for patients developing posttransfusion hepatitis was not a bimodal composite curve of a short and a long incubation period but was a unimodal curve with a peak at 45 to 49 days. One would expect a trough in the distribution curve at that point if only HAV and HBV were involved.

Further evidence for VH-NAB is given by reports of patients who had more than two separate bouts of VH with intervening complete recovery.[151,162,178,209] All patients with multiple bouts have been intravenous drug users. In recent studies, such patients have been shown to have VH-B on only one occasion, VH-A on only one, and one or more bouts of hepatitis with absence of serologic evidence of VH-A or VH-B.[186] Other investigators have shown that the patients who develop posttransfusion hepatitis with serum negative for HBsAg rarely develop antibodies to HAV.[143,198] Such patients are considered to have hepatitis NAB. The clinical illness and the epidemiology are not distinguishable from VH-B, and neither a universally acceptable viral antigen nor corresponding antibody response is demonstrable at this time (Table 31-2).

Table 31-2. Viral hepatitis

Clinical disease	Abbreviation	Older names	Agent	Infective material	Transmission methods	Incubation	Antigen and antibody	Course
1. Acute viral hepatitis type A	AcVH-A	Infectious hepatitis Catarrhal jaundice Epidemic hepatitis MS-1	HAV	Stool 4+ Urine 3+ Blood 1+	Fecal-oral	15-45 days	Blood anti-HA Stool HAV	Recovery
2. Viral hepatitis type B* a. Acute (1) Acute viral hepatitis type B	AcVH-B	Serum hepatitis Homologous serum jaundice MS-2	HBV	Blood 4+ Body fluid 1 to 3+ Stool 0	Percutaneous, unknown	45-180 days	Early: HBsAg Recovery: anti-HBs anti-HBc	Recovery 85% Fulminant 1% Subacute (impaired regeneration) fatal < 0.2% Persistent viral hepatitis 10%-12% Chronic active viral hepatitis type B < 3%
(2) Fulminant viral hepatitis type B	FVH-B	Acute red atrophy Acute yellow atrophy Subacute yellow atrophy	HBV	(As above)	Percutaneous, unknown	45-180 days	Early: HBsAg Late: not applicable	Death in days 75% Complete recovery 25% (age related)
(3) Viral hepatitis type B impaired regeneration syndrome	VH-B-IRS	Subacute yellow atrophy Subacute hepatic necrosis Chronic aggressive hepatitis? Protracted hepatitis	HBV	(As above)	Percutaneous, unknown	45-180 days	Early: HBsAg Recovery: anti-HBs anti-HBc	Slow recovery in elderly Fatal in 50%
b. Chronic (1) Persistent viral hepatitis type B	PVH-B	Transaminitis Chronic hepatitis Unresolved viral hepatitis B Chronic persistent hepatitis	HBV	(As above)	Transplacental, percutaneous, unknown	45-180 days	Anti-HBc HBsAg	Continued antigenemia nonprogressive 90% Recovery 10%
(2) Chronic active viral hepatitis	AVH-B	Chronic hepatitis Subacute aggressive Chronic aggressive hepatitis	HBV	(As above)	Transplacental, percutaneous, unknown	45-180 days	Anti-HBc HBsAg	Progression to cirrhosis probably 100%
(3) Active (or) inactive viral cirrhosis, type B		Postnecrotic cirrhosis Posthepatitis cirrhosis Macronodular cirrhosis	HBV	(As above)	Transplacental, percutaneous, unknown	45-180 days	Anti-HBc HBsAg	Death from complication of cirrhosis
3. Acute viral hepatitis non-A non-B	AcVH-NAB	Infectious hepatitis Serum hepatitis	Not identified	Body fluid?	Percutaneous, unknown	Peak at 45 days	Unknown	Recovery 85%

Pathology

Acute viral hepatitis A, B, and NAB produce microscopic lesions indistinguishable from one another by present methods. The changes do vary considerably, however, depending on the temporal stage of the disease, severity of the process, and individualized cellular and reparative response.

In a liver biopsy taken *prior to the onset of symptoms* and before there is biochemical evidence of cell necrosis, the hepatocytes have slightly enlarged nuclei and sharp nuclear membranes. The size and number of Kupffer cells, as well as the number of lymphocytes in the sinusoids, are increased. Sparse areas of cell dropout or *hepatocytolysis* may be seen, but generalized liver cell damage develops just prior to the onset of symptoms and simultaneously with serum biochemical abnormalities.

Three nearly concurrent independently variable morphologic changes characterize viral hepatitis at the *height of clinical disease:* (1) hepatocyte damage, (2) hepatocyte regeneration, and (3) lymphoid and reticuloendothelial reaction.

The *hepatocyte damage* is generalized. All the cells become swollen with a watery-appearing cytoplasm; this change is most severe in the centrilobular regions where the hydropic change at the sinusoidal margin contrasts sharply with the perinuclear and pericanalicular condensation of cytoplasm. In the early stage, the hepatocyte cord arrangement becomes disrupted because of the cytoplasmic swelling and onset of hepatocyte regeneration (Fig. 31-7). The nuclei are slightly but uniformly enlarged with a finely divided, granular nuclear chromatin, a prominent nucleolus, and a sharp nuclear membrane. Hepatocytolysis is randomly distributed throughout, but prominent in the centrilobular regions, where the intercellular membranes often become indistinct and structures that resemble syncytial giant cells are seen. Severe cell destruction leaves only a spongy stromal network in the centrilobular area. The lysis of dying cells must be rapid, since dead liver cells as such usually are not identifiable on biopsy. An exception is the type of cell death that results in the acidophilic body (see discussion of necrosis, Fig. 31-2, and Plate 3, *A*).

The *lymphoid and reticuloendothelial response* often produces the most obvious change. Kupffer cell activity is greatly increased, and unicellular foci of hepatocytolysis usually are replaced by macrophages and Kupffer cells that have phagocytosed lipo-

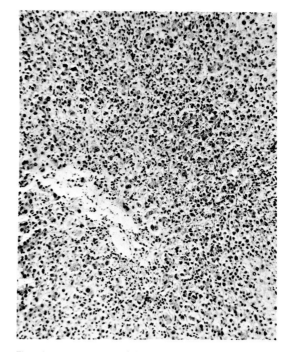

Fig. 31-7. Acute viral hepatitis. Appearance generally seen on needle biopsy. Note swollen liver cells, lack of cord pattern, and focal necrosis.

chrome pigment. These foci are further marked by numerous lymphocytes and a few plasma cells. In the portal areas, proliferative cholangiolar epithelium and poorly formed duct structures are found, and lymphocytes, plasma cells, and mononuclear cells often traverse the limiting plates of portal areas producing a saw-toothed effect.

Concurrently with acute damage and necrosis, *regeneration* without nodularity occurs with frequent mitotic figures. Regeneration is manifest by zones of massed hepatocytes, without the regular relationship of hepatocyte to sinusoids. The periportal cells particularly have a solid pavement appearance early in the disease.

Centrilobular canalicular cholestasis is variable, but even when extensive, there are no clinical features that distinguish cholestatic from ordinary viral hepatitis. Conversely, patients who have unusually high elevations of alkaline phosphatase activity in association with AcVH do not have unusual cholestasis on biopsy. If jaundice is prolonged, the Kupffer cells also contain bile pigment, but there is usually little bile staining of the cytoplasm of the swollen hepatocytes.

Late histologic changes. After clinical recovery, the serum transaminase levels are normal, but pigmented Kupffer cells are in scattered foci of previous cell necrosis, and hepatic parenchymal cells develop a cobblestone configuration. A slow reestablishment of the sinusoidal and cord pattern often requires a year. The cytoplasmic condensation and centrilobular accentuation of cell damage disappear, and the portal lymphoid hyperplasia often remains prominent for months.

Electron microscopic studies. Electron microscopic studies disclose that viral particles are extremely sparse during acute VH, but the opposite is true of the liver of the patient who is a chronic carrier or who has HBsAg-positive chronic liver disease.

Other changes observed in liver cells and Kupffer cells are nonspecific.[222] Early, the endoplasmic reticulum becomes irregularly dilated and vesicular and often is separated or destroyed by ballooning of the cytosol. The nuclei enlarge and nucleoli are prominent. Free ribosomes increase in the cytoplasm, and glycogen deposition is irregular. The intercellular membranes, instead of being destroyed as one would anticipate from light microscopy, actually develop microvilli, and the space between adjacent cells is widened. Fine strands of collagen often are found in Disse's space and in the intercellular space (Fig. 31-2).

The acidophilic, or Councilman-like, body is observed most often in viral hepatitis, although it may be seen in many other diseases in man and animals. Councilman described the bodies in yellow fever.[132] Some doubt has been expressed as to whether the bodies are the same as those seen in viral hepatitis. Most hepatopathologists use the term "acidophilic body" and "Councilman's body" interchangeably. The acidophilic body is composed of condensed cytoplasm from which ribosomes have largely disappeared but in which the shadowy, electron-dense remains of many cell organelles are still visible.[114,126,167]

Several histologic variants of AcVH may occur, but these are based on host response and not on differences of viral strains nor expression of antigenic subgroups. The immunologic reaction and parenchymal reparative properties of the host may be affected by external environmental factors.

The pathogenesis of viral hepatitis (A, B, or NAB) is unsettled. The older concept that hepatocyte death results from a viral cytopathic effect has not been disproved but seems inadequate to explain the variations in course. It has been proposed that viral components incorporated into hepatocyte cell membranes act as the target for an immune response (perhaps T-cell mediated).[141] An immunocytopathic basis for cell destruction can be expanded to explain many of the variations in the course of patients with viral hepatitis, as defects in immune responsiveness of the patient can often be correlated with the disease pattern that develops.[141,224]

Hepatitis in intravenous drug users

Although it appears that acute VH-B is on the decrease, and perhaps also the illicit use of intravenous drugs, a relatively increased frequency of serum hepatitis among drug addicts has been recognized for many years.[178,196] The development of the "hippie" culture with its philosophy of greater sharing of earthly goods, including needles and a wide variety of intravenous mixtures, expanded the hepatitis problem enormously. In Los Angeles County, the frequency of hepatitis associated with common needle use jumped from 19% of all reported cases of hepatitis in 1964 to 56% in 1968. Among patients with AcVH-B, 78% to 88% were associated with common needle use. At a large drug rehabilitation center in Los Angeles, 21.6% of patients had a history of jaundice during the time they were using drugs.[202] Since prospective transfusion studies indicate that for every patient with icteric serum hepatitis there are three who have anicteric disease, it would appear that nearly all intravenous drug users develop hepatitis on one or more occasions.

The exact relationship between the decreasing rate of AcVH-B and level of intravenous drug use is unclear. Since most drug users have acquired immunity to hepatitis B, the numbers of new cases of AcVH-B in that group reflects the entry of new susceptibles into the drug-using pool. In that respect the situation is analogous to other infectious diseases in which a high endemic rate follows an epidemic.

Twenty-seven percent of drug users admit having sold blood. The anticipated development of icteric serum hepatitis in a recipient who receives blood obtained from an addict is 70 times greater than the incidence of hepatitis in recipients of blood from highly selected donors.[129] Peculiarly, however, even at the height of the epidemic of hepatitis in drug users the predominant subtype of hepatitis B acquired from blood transfusions was *ad*, differing from the predominant subtype of the drug abuser, which was *ay*.[187] At the time of

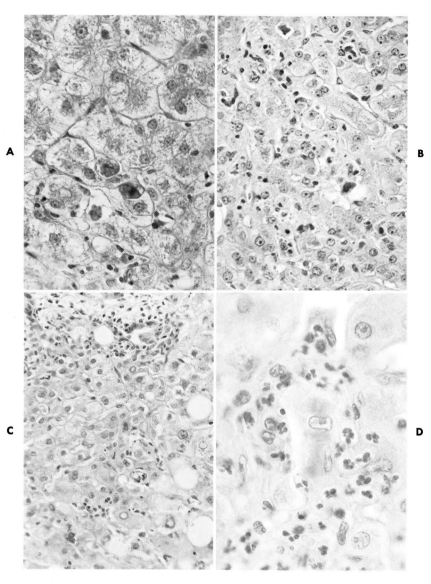

Plate 3
A, Needle biopsy in epidemic hepatitis. Two acidophilic bodies present near bottom. Cytoplasm swollen and granular and cell membranes indistinct.
B, Centrilobular bile stasis in patient taking oral contraceptive.
C, Acute pericholangitis and cholestasis in needle biopsy. Later at surgery, stone removed from common bile duct.
D, Hyaline necrosis in alcoholic. Many neutrophils in sinusoids.

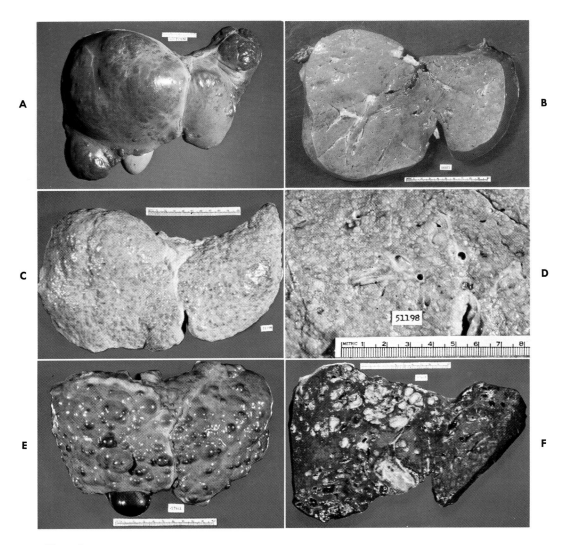

Plate 4

A, Submassive hepatic necrosis from viral hepatitis, with bulging areas of residual liver and much shrinkage and collapse of left lobe. Patient lived 24 days after onset of clinical symptoms.

B, Hypertrophic, firm, smooth alcoholic fatty liver.

C, Eutrophic, hard, finely pseudolobular alcoholic cirrhosis in 65-year-old man.

D, Cut surface of alcoholic cirrhosis showing pseudolobular pattern.

E, Atrophic, firm, megalonodular lupoid cirrhosis, quiescent in 20-year-old woman.

F, Suppurative cholangitis with multiple abscesses secondary to carcinomatous obstruction of common duct.

the increased incidence of hepatitis in the age group 15 to 24, there was no increase in rate of those over 55, that age group probably receiving the most transfusions (Fig. 31-6). Unquestionably, however, the illicit drug user, by increasing the incidence of AcVH-B, resulting in the usual 10% to 12% development of PVH, has increased the numbers of carriers of VH-B in the United States with consequences that will undoubtedly be long standing.

Singularly, the addict may develop icteric serum hepatitis on more than one occasion; some have had four and five episodes; several have had three. Multiple bouts of icteric viral hepatitis in other patients, including those who receive hundreds of units of blood or blood products, is rare. Immunoglobulin levels of addicts who develop multiple bouts of hepatitis are not depressed.[193]

On biopsy the needle user with hepatitis often has more lymphoid proliferation in the portal areas, even to the degree that lymph follicles form. Similarly, the patients often have lymph node hyperplasia that may be related to the repeatedly inoculated foreign material. After multiple bouts of hepatitis, the portal areas may become widened, but nodular regeneration does not develop. In a new recurrent episode of AcVH, the hepatocytes do not become hydropic, and a cord arrangement is maintained more often than in ordinary viral hepatitis. At one time in the Los Angeles area, heroin and other opiates were often adulterated or "cut" with substances that included talc-like particles. The repeated intravenous injection of these talc-containing drugs resulted in a recognizable lesion in which the polarizable crystals are present in the portal areas and in Kupffer cells. The crystals do not cause true granulomas but there may be an associated mild increase of connective tissue. In the past, crystals were noted in the biopsies of 20% of patients with hepatitis at the Los Angeles County–University of Southern California Medical Center and the John Wesley Hospital, but more recently the percentage is much less, apparently reflecting a different agent for "cutting" of heroin and other illicit drugs.

Fatal viral hepatitis
Fulminant viral hepatitis

Fulminant viral hepatitis is the clinical designation for the abrupt onset of liver failure with coma that always results from acute massive hepatic necrosis and usually occurs after

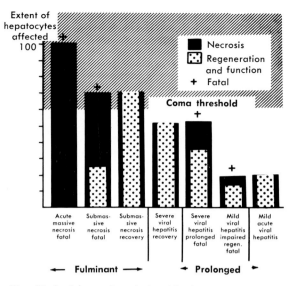

Fig. 31-8. Schematic relationship between extent of necrosis, regeneration and function, and survival. First three bars reflect extensive necrosis to extent that coma develops (fulminant). First bar depicts total destruction (thus no regeneration or function). Second bar has regeneration and function inadequate to regain original mass. Third bar reflects recovery because of greater regeneration, despite amount of necrosis similar to that of second bar. Remaining bars indicate that, with less necrosis, fatality may still occur if regeneration and function are impaired.

severe submassive hepatic necrosis resulting from viral hepatitis. One percent of patients hospitalized with viral hepatitis develop such abrupt and complete liver cell necrosis that hepatic insufficiency ensues (Fig. 31-8, bars *1*, *2*, and *3*). In such patients coma develops after less than 4 weeks of hepatitis, and death follows in 24 hours to a few days. The liver morphology is determined by the extent of necrosis, amount of regeneration, and duration of survival of the patient after onset of fulminant disease.

Recovery of patients with acute viral hepatitis is based on a balance of four semi-independent factors: (1) extent of hepatocellular loss, (2) extent and rapidity of regeneration of residual hepatocytes, (3) adequacy of functional activity of residual hepatocytes, and (4) adequacy of mechanisms of defense against continued viral replication and activity. The relationship of the clinical course to the sum effects of extent of necrosis, adequacy of regeneration, and function of residual liver are charted in Table 31-2.

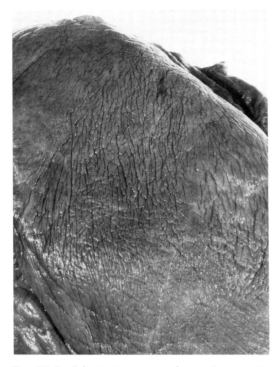

Fig. 31-9. Fulminating serum hepatitis occurring after blood transfusions given 140 days before onset of jaundice. Note typical wrinkling of capsule of liver when flexed.

In *acute massive necrosis,* morphologically the most severe and clinically the most rapidly progressive, the liver weighs from 1 to 1.2 kg, only modestly less than normal. Its capsule is smooth, but the liver is limp. On sectioning, the centrilobular areas are deeply reddened and retracted and may closely resemble severe acute passive congestion or even simulate the appearance of spleen, a pattern once referred to as *acute red atrophy* (Fig. 31-9). With complete necrosis there has not been sufficient time for bile pigments to accumulate; thus neither the patient nor the liver is deeply icteric.

Microscopically, the hepatocytes are destroyed, the Kupffer cells are large and numerous, and there is a variable amount of lymphocytic infiltrate and hyperplasia. The liver stroma is intact and little collapse is noted. The bile ducts show little hyperplasia. Since all hepatocytes are destroyed, the factors of regeneration, function, and continued viral activity are not operative (Fig. 31-8, bar *1*).

A patient with *submassive necrosis* (Fig. 31-8, bars *2* and *3*) of the liver may die in less than 1 week but may live for 2 or 3 weeks

when there is enough surviving liver parenchyma or greater regenerative and functional capacity. The deeply icteric swollen parenchymal cells remaining in periportal areas impart a golden yellow color that caused Rokitansky in 1842 to use the term *acute yellow atrophy* to describe the liver of those who survived only a few days. After more than a week of survival in coma from submassive necrosis, all of the parenchymal cells disappear in large zones but periportal remnants remain in other areas. The stroma is collapsed where there was previous necrosis, and the liver is shrunken to about 800 to 900 gm. It is wrinkled and deeply icteric (Fig. 31-9), particularly in the areas of less collapse. In those who survive 3 weeks or more, the collapse that follows continued destruction of all cells in some areas contrasts sharply with the irregular bulging yellow residual liver that has only undergone regeneration (Plate 4, *A,* and Fig. 31-10). In the past this stage was called *subacute yellow atrophy.* However, the necrosis is acute, even though the patient may have a prolonged survival when there is enough functionally active residual liver. If the patient lives for several weeks after submassive hepatic necrosis, the blood channels in the collapsed stroma of the liver may sclerose, areas of collapse become pale, and lose the congested "splenic" appearance. The morphologic features of the liver after submassive necrosis may range from (1) a flabby, mottled yellow and red organ, (2) one with large plaque-like islands of regenerating tissue in a background of red collapsed stroma, or (3) even a misshapen liver with scattered bulging yellow tumorlike masses in a bloodless collapsed stroma. These patterns, often misinterpreted as cirrhosis, are called (1) early, (2) middle, and (3) late stages of submassive necrosis respectively. Microscopically, in late submassive necrosis there are striking numbers of bile plugs and microconcretions of bile in periportal canaliculi.

In both massive or submassive necrosis, changes such as minimal ascites, pleural effusion, and peripheral edema may be present. The regional lymph nodes and spleen are generally enlarged at autopsy. Hemorrhagic phenomena may be seen in various tissues because of deficiency of coagulation factors normally produced by the liver. Hemorrhages are often present in the intestine, lungs, and mesentery, and gastrointestinal bleeding may contribute to death. Acute pancreatitis occasionally is noted at autopsy.

At the University of Southern California

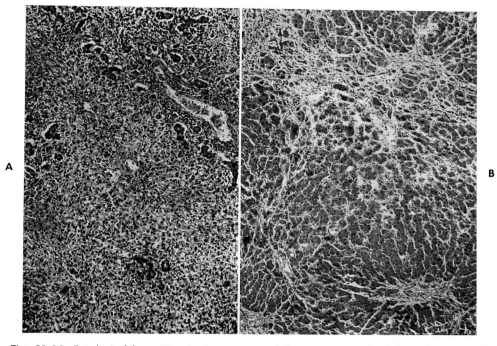

Fig. 31-10. Fatal viral hepatitis. **A,** Appearance of liver on ninety-third day, showing collapsed areas. **B,** Residual liver. (From Lucké, B.: Am. J. Pathol. **20:**595-619, 1944.)

Liver Center from 1960 to 1975, the average age of patients with clinically fulminant hepatitis who succumbed with acute massive necrosis was 25.1 whereas those with submassive necrosis was 37.7.[192] Younger patients who apparently have hepatocellular regenerative capacity completely recover if they do not expire in the initial fulminant phase. Some of the older patients may have enough residual liver to allow survival for a short period of time, but regeneration is apparently inadequate to permit recovery.[122]

Mortality. Estimates of the survival rates after fulminant viral hepatitis have ranged around 10%, an occasional study reflected survival rates of 35%.[135] In recent years in the United States, the overall survival rate has been 25%.[204,226] The more favorable survival figures noted during the years from 1965 to 1972 probably reflect the striking increase in drug-associated viral hepatitis in younger individuals (Fig. 31-6) with a correspondingly larger proportion of fulminant hepatitis in the same group. Chance of survival in younger individuals is greater; of 81 patients with fulminant hepatitis admitted to University of Southern California–John Wesley Hospital from 1965 to 1972, there was a 47.3% survival of the 11 to 20 age group, 25% survival in the

21 to 40 age group, and none in those over 40 years old.[204] All but one of 22 survivors of fulminant hepatitis at the University of Southern California–John Wesley Hospital Liver Unit since 1965 have been under 30 years of age. Consequently survival statistics for patients with fulminant hepatitis will differ, depending in part on whether the statistics were derived from areas where there is a heavy illicit drug use or from regions with a minimal drug problem, since the average age of the patients with fulminant hepatic necrosis will differ in the two environments. None of 22 survivors of the 81 cases of clinically fulminant hepatitis has developed cirrhosis or any other hepatic sequela.[164]

Viral hepatitis with impaired regeneration syndrome (VH-IRS)
Protracted viral hepatitis, subacute hepatic necrosis

As depicted in Fig. 31-8, even if necrosis is not severe enough to cause coma, the disease may still be protracted or even fatal if regeneration is inadequate. The patients with VH-IRS are older than those recovering in a normal fashion from viral hepatitis, since capacity for regeneration of hepatocytes apparently decreases with increasing age. The average age of the patients who die is 63.3. More than half are over 75 years old, whereas the average age of patients who die of fulminant hepatitis is much younger.[192] Viral hepatitis with impaired regeneration and a nonfulminant course accounts for 18% of fatal cases of hepatitis in our hospital. Death in patients under 30 with viral hepatitis IRS rarely occurs unless necrosis is severe enough for coma to develop.

Biopsies of the liver from nonfatal cases show regular, straight liver cords that are frequently somewhat shrunken, apparently a reflection of the failure of those cells to proliferate at an accelerated rate. Otherwise, in initial aspects of the disease, the histologic appearance is like that of AcVH. However, when the necrosis is more severe, areas of confluent hepatocellular destruction are not replaced by regenerating hepatocytes but are marked by collapsed stroma. When this stroma produces "bridging" bands that connect adjacent portal areas or central regions throughout the biopsy specimen, the pattern has been referred to as *subacute hepatic necrosis* (SHN).[118] "Bridging" can be seen when there has been either severe acute necrosis or an ordinary degree of necrosis with impaired regeneration. The liver of the patient who succumbs is shrunken and slightly toughened but limp. The surface is bumpy or irregular with few regenerative areas. On microscopic examination, the liver cells are shrunken and there is little exudate in the parenchyma, but hyperplasia of the lymphoid and reticuloendothelial system within widened portal areas simulates that of ordinary viral hepatitis. There is considerable collapse within each lobule, and thin fingers of collapsed stroma and collagen extend from both the portal and the central areas. Regeneration is minimal; thus the hepatic cords are straight and obvious.

Relapse of viral hepatitis

Two percent of patients have a relapse of viral hepatitis within 3 months after recovery. The symptoms are indistinguishable from the initial episode, although it is usually somewhat milder. Occasionally, the relapse may be more severe but rarely fatal. The biopsy changes in the liver are similar to those of the initial attack. Recovery occurs after the relapse.

Chronic varieties of hepatitis
Inadequacy of defense mechanisms against continued viral replication

The foregoing discussion has dealt with the relationship between the (1) extent of necro-

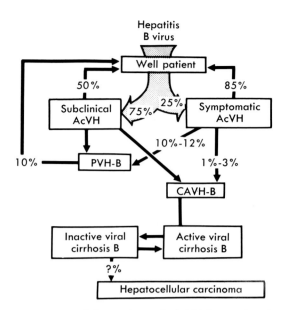

Fig. 31-11. Relationship of AcVH-B to chronic forms of disorder.

sis, (2) regenerative capacity, and (3) adequacy of hepatocellular functional activity. The fourth variable deals with the ability or inability of the patient to get rid of the virus. This introduces chronic viral disease (Fig. 31-11).

Persistent viral hepatitis (PVH) (unresolved viral hepatitis, transaminitis, asymptomatic carrier state, chronic persistent hepatitis)

Ten percent of adults who ostensibly recover from icteric viral hepatitis[201] and 50% of pediatric patients who recover from anicteric viral hepatitis[170] maintain asymptomatic smoldering or episodic elevations of SGPT activity. HBsAg remains in their sera if the original disease was VH-B. This condition is called *persistent viral hepatitis*.[161,192,201] The percentage of patients who develop PVH after AcVH-B and those who develop PVH after AcVH-NAB seems to be the same (10% to 12% in adults), but it is generally believed that AcVH-A is rarely if ever followed by PVH. PVH-B has been studied more than PVH-NAB, since HBsAg remains in the sera and in the liver. In a large population, between 0.1% and 15% of people (depending on the country) will asymptomatically have HBsAg in their sera, most of whom will have no history of acute viral hepatitis. It is presumed that the initial disease was subclinical. A small percentage of these asymptomatic carriers will have chronic

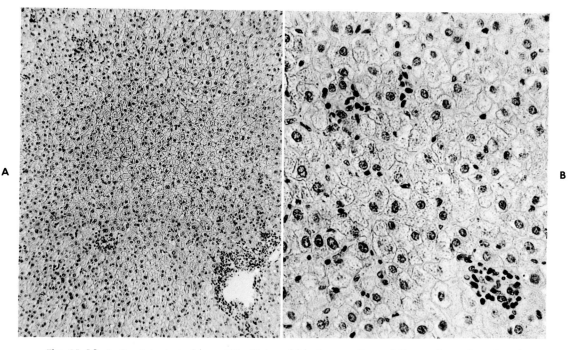

Fig. 31-12. A, Persistent viral hepatitis. Note cobblestone pattern of liver cells and scattered areas of focal necrosis. **B,** Higher magnification, emphasizing focal necrosis.

active hepatitis (see p. 1347), but most have the clinical and histologic features of PVH. Many investigators have demonstrated HBsAg in hepatocytes of such carriers.[50,51,140,146,160,168,217]

Microscopically, the hepatocytes in patients with PVH are hydropic and are of uniform size throughout the lobule. In livers of 88% of patients with PVH, the cord pattern is replaced by a cobblestone-like arrangement of regular, polygonal hepatocytes, there are occasional small foci of hepatocytolysis in which there are clusters of lymphocytes in livers of over 90% (Fig. 31-12). The Kupffer cells may be slightly hypoplastic, and there is a variable amount of portal lymphoid hyperplasia in two thirds of the patients. The changes closely simulate those that persist for several months after acute viral hepatitis.

In addition to the 10% to 12% incidence of development of PVH in otherwise normal individuals as sequela to AcVH, patients with acquired impairment of immune response have a much higher frequency of PVH after a bout of AcVH-B. Often the initial acute disease in such patients is associated with minimal symptoms. Thus patients with lymphomas,[115] those on chronic renal dialysis programs,[179,224] mongoloids who have spent their early child-

hood in institutions,[218] lepromatous leprosy patients,[115] and individuals receiving immunosuppressant therapy develop PVH readily. In addition, asymptomatic HBsAg positivity develops at about 2 months of age in over half of the children of mothers who acquire AcVH-B in the third trimester of pregnancy. Such infants continue to have PVH-B thereafter.[211] Ultrastructurally, the infant livers have nuclear viruslike particles that probably represent the core of the developing HB virion. For reasons that are unclear, only 5% or 6% of pregnant women with PVH-B in the United States transmit a demonstrable infection to their offspring in contrast to the 50% who transmit the disease when they develop acute VH-B in late pregnancy. Yet in Taiwan where the HBsAg-positive carrier make up 15% of the population, about half of the pregnant women with PVH-B transmit the virus to their offspring.[216] Almost invariably maternal patients with HBeAg in their sera transmit HBV to their offspring; patients with anti-HBe do not. Those with neither HBeAg nor anti-HBe demonstrable only occasionally transmit the disease. Oriental patients with PVH-B have HBeAg much more frequently than do patients with PVH-B in the U.S.A.

Biopsies from about 25% of the patients

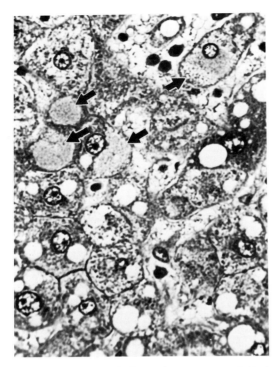

Fig. 31-13. "Ground-glass" hepatocytes of Hadziyannis *(arrows)* may be found either in persistent viral hepatitis B or chronic active viral hepatitis B.

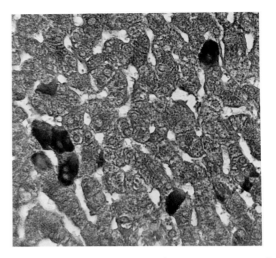

Fig. 31-14. Immunoperoxidase stains reveal HBsAg in "ground-glass" cells of Hadziyannis. (Courtesy Dr. Angelos Afroudakis, Athens, Greece.)

with PVH-B contain scattered hepatocytes with all or a discrete part of the cytoplasm replaced by a uniform granular change referred to as ground-glass cells of Hadziyannis[51] (Fig. 31-13). The ground-glass cells stain intensely for HBsAg by immunofluorescence,[50] immunoperoxidase methods[146] (Fig. 31-14), or by a stain that demonstrates the disulfide link of HBsAg, the Shikata-orcein stain.[212] Some hepatocytes other than ground-glass cells stain less intensively, an indication that many parenchymal cells other than ground-glass cells contain HBsAg. Electron microscopically, the ground-glass hepatocytes contain filamentous material (Fig. 31-4, *C*) that localizes immunoperoxidase directed to HBsAg.[146] However, peroxidase-labeled antibody to HBsAg also localizes in surrounding endoplasmic reticular membranes,[146,213] an indication that the antigenic components are present before the filaments that eventually appear within the cisternae. Cytoplasmic filamentous structures have been demonstrated in livers of patients with PVH by many investigators,[19,50,51,160,212,215,217] but demonstration of any component of viral structures in AcVH is generally unsuccessful. Some investigators describe a distinct nuclear or cytoplasmic distribution pattern of the virus that relates to whether the disease is PVH, CAVH, or PVH in an immunorepressed patient.[50,140,159,168]

Persistent viral hepatitis is not a progressive disorder; none of the patients develop cirrhosis. The incidence of PVH in the general population differs in various parts of the world from less than 0.1%[166] in some parts of the United States to 15% in Taiwan.[225] In the larger cities of the United States, such as Los Angeles where intravenous drug usage has been a problem in the 1960s and early 1970s, the incidence of persistent viral hepatitis-B in the "normal" population was about 0.4%.[109] The incidence of PVH-NAB is not known but must be higher since elimination of the HBsAg-positive blood donor has resulted in only a 25% reduction of posttransfusion hepatitis.[107,148]

Population studies in Korea[128] and Taiwan[131] reveal that a higher percentage of asymptomatic carriers of HBsAg have histologic features of subtle chronic active hepatitis than is the case with asymptomatic carriers in the United States where most of them have PVH. Many of the carriers from Korea and Taiwan have been said to ultimately develop cirrhosis.

The term *chronic persistent hepatitis* was recommended in 1968 by an international committee[136] for a histologic pattern in which there was portal lymphoid "infiltration" and little else. This was prior to the recognition of the relationship between HBsAg and hepatitis

B. The committee did not suggest that "chronic persistent hepatitis" might or might not be related to viral hepatitis but were attempting to assign terms to different histologic patterns; the nonspecificity of the lesion was not denied. It is unfortunate that the term "hepatitis" was used for a nonspecific hyperplasia of the normal lymphoid component of the portal area, which is a physiologic response, not a disease of the liver. After the asymptomatic carrier state for hepatitis B became more widely recognized (just described as *persistent viral hepatitis*) many clinicians adopted the term "chronic persistent hepatitis" for that condition without regard to the histologic pattern. We recommend discarding the term "chronic persistent hepatitis," not only because of the redundancy of *chronic* and *persistent,* but also because the term implies a disease rather than a reaction and is used widely to describe a clinicopathologic entity that the committee did not consider. It is also confusing that most intravenous drug users, after repeated injections of infectious and foreign materials, have striking lymphoid and reticuloendothelial proliferation unrelated to the viral hepatitis that such patients almost always contract sooner or later. We refer to the condition as "nonspecific lymphoid hyperplasia." Two microscopic features are helpful in distinguishing PVH from nonspecific lymphoid hyperplasia: (1) There is a lack of a regular sinusoidal-cord pattern in the former, imparting a cobblestone appearance to liver. The cobblestone appearance is uniform from central to periportal areas and from one lobule to the next. This is present in 88% of patients with PVH. (2) There is a diminution of Kupffer cell activity in PVH in contrast to the hyperplasia usually seen in the nonspecific reaction described by the European pathologists.[192] Portal lymphoid "infiltrate," the principal criterion for the condition described by the international committee, is found in only half of the patients with PVH.

Chronic active hepatitis

Chronic active hepatitis (CAH) (active chronic hepatitis, chronic aggressive hepatitis) is characterized by recurrent episodes of disease that simulate mild viral hepatitis, yet most patients eventually develop cirrhosis, usually a coarsely nodular type. Previously under dispute as to whether it represented nonhealing viral hepatitis,[223] an autoimmune disease,[181,230] or an autoimmune reaction precipitated by a viral infection,[182] investigators now

generally believe that multiple etiologies produce the same or a similar morphologic lesion and similar clinical patterns.

Most patients with CAH develop portal hypertension, including esophageal varices and ascites. Some have borderline encephalopathy for years. Only a few patients who have recurrent symptoms survive for 10 years or more; however, there has been increasing realization that some patients, particularly those who are identified through HBsAg screening techniques, may lead an entirely asymptomatic life for 30 years or so. Although rare, a patient may die a few weeks after the diagnosis is made.

Since at least one drug can produce all the features of chronic active lupoid hepatitis, including the positive lupus erythematosus preparation and histologic pattern, it is necessary to consider exogenous agents in the etiology of a disease that has been considered autoimmune in type.

Biopsies taken at the onset of symptoms usually disclose features of both acute and chronic liver disease. Cirrhosis may be present, but there are also changes that resemble those

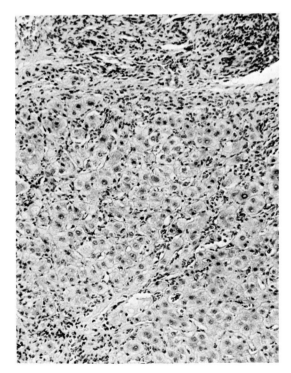

Fig. 31-15. Diffuse inflammation and liver cell necrosis in regenerative nodule from liver in chronic active hepatitis.

of viral hepatitis, with unicellular cytolytic foci surrounded by lymphocytes or plasma cells and Kupffer cell hyperplasia. The residual parenchymal cells are hydropic with large nuclei that are often vesicular. The normal cord pattern is absent. There is usually portal widening with increased collagen and both lymphoid and plasmacellular exudate, as well as focal destruction of the limiting plate ("piecemeal necrosis"). Although the hydropic swelling and occasionally the stratification of duct epithelium have been emphasized,[127,197] we have not found these features characteristic nor diagnostically useful (Fig. 31-15).

Many of these changes are also found in the liver of patients who have atypical varieties of acute viral hepatitis. Unfortunately, the morphologic criteria described for *chronic aggressive hepatitis* deal almost exclusively with portal changes.[136] Many pathologists have drawn their criteria from that description, which was inadequate, to exclude many other inflammatory reactions.

The following features distinguish chronic active hepatitis from atypical acute viral hepatitis:

1. The centrilobular areas do not have the most severe degenerative and necrotizing changes, as the entire lobule is more or less uniformly involved, or a zone of severe periportal damage may be recognized.
2. There is a lack of uniformity of lobular involvement in CAH. One lobule may have changes that resemble acute viral hepatitis, the next appears quiescent, and yet another has the cobblestone arrangement of hydropic hepatocytes, often bulging into adjacent parts of the lobule where the cells may appear somewhat more orderly.
3. In acute viral hepatitis there is uniformity of nuclear size and staining, whereas in CAH there are often considerable differences in nuclear size and staining, with some parts of a lobule having large numbers of polyploid nuclei or dysplastic cells.

Conditions that must be distinguished from chronic active hepatitis are as follows:

1. Viral hepatitis with severe necrosis such as that in patients recovering from fulminant viral hepatitis, or those who have had ordinary AcVH except for a prothrombin activity level of about 20% to 25%. Such livers show recent confluent necrosis in each lobule—an un-

likely development in CAH. Each lobule is similar in severity and stage; there is little continuing focal necrosis or exudate because regeneration dominates the histologic pattern.
2. Impaired regeneration (subacute hepatic necrosis. It usually occurs in those over 50 years old who develop severe acute viral hepatitis and who have reduced capacity for regeneration resulting in bridging collapse between adjacent portal areas or between portal and central areas. This type of viral hepatitis may be at times most difficult to distinguish from CAH, but the regularity of involvement from one lobule to another in subacute hepatic necrosis and the presence of "bridging" at each portal area have been emphasized.[118] In addition, in VH-IRS, the liver cords are usually straight, the cells are slightly shrunken, continuing necrosis is meager, and there is usually a narrow zone of nearly confluent cell loss around the central vein.
3. Patients with unusually exuberant inflammatory response to their viral hepatitis. As one finds in lymphoid tissue elsewhere, some individuals in response to a stimulus develop an inflammatory hyperplasia much more striking than that in others, which is ostensibly the same. Patients who have continually stimulated their reticuloendothelial system by challenge with injected foreign material may have an extremely hyperplastic and exudative reaction in the portal areas of each lobule upon which the changes of viral hepatitis become engrafted. The drug user with hepatitis, because of the widened portal areas infiltrated with unusual numbers of plasma cells, is probably the type of patient most frequently overdiagnosed as having chronic active hepatitis. In our experience such patients recover from viral hepatitis in a normal fashion.
4. Livers with preexisting increased portal collagen and superimposed viral hepatitis. Patients with alcoholic liver disease or fibrosis from prior gallstone disease, or the patient who has been an intravenous drug user for many years before acquiring AcVH, all have an increase in collagen density and in size of portal areas. The microscopic diagnosis of superimposed AcVH may be difficult. Since such patients are usually older than the average patient with AcVH, recovery is often

delayed. The prognosis is better than that of CAH, but patients with alcoholic cirrhosis may not recover.

During periods of clinical quiescence, the acute changes of CAH disappear but regenerative activity continues and progresses toward a coarsely nodular cirrhosis (Plate 4, *E*). The regenerative nodules may become large, and the cells may reassume a cord arrangement. The intervening regions of collapse may contain small islands of liver cells. They are heavily infiltrated by lymphocytes and plasma cells. The collagen in the areas of collapse is loose and permits the ready growth of large nodules. Recrudescence of necrosis usually does not affect all nodules to the same extent or severity.

Although serum albumin is moderately depressed, during active stages of the disease the serum globulin levels become greatly elevated, usually over 6 gm per 100 ml, occasionally over 8 gm per 100 ml. Most patients have elevations of IgG and IgM, and some have elevation of IgA.[144] Serum transaminase activities are elevated, often in the range of 1000 units. The SGOT level is usually elevated to a greater degree than the SGPT, just the opposite of ordinary AcVH. During the periods when the patient becomes anicteric and asymptomatic, the serum globulin levels may drop to normal or near normal ranges, and the transaminase activities either remain in the range of 100 to 200 units or reach normal levels.[205]

It is convenient to separate chronic active hepatitis into four groups based on presumed differences in etiology and a few subtle differences in clinical pattern.[123,149,206] The names used are chronic active *viral* hepatitis (CAVH), chronic active *lupoid* hepatitis (CALH), chronic active *toxic* hepatitis (CATH), and *cryptogenic* chronic active hepatitis (CCAH).

Chronic active viral hepatitis

Since discovery of HBsAg, it has been recognized that a large percentage of patients with chronic active hepatitis who have negative LE cell preparations and who lack smooth muscle antibodies, do have circulating HBsAg in their sera.[147,231] About 1% to 3% of patients with viral hepatitis who are ill enough for hospitalization will develop chronic active viral hepatitis that leads to cirrhosis. About four to five times as many patients will develop the disease without a clinically apparent acute attack. In contrast to the preponderance of females with chronic active lupoid hepatitis, there is a slight

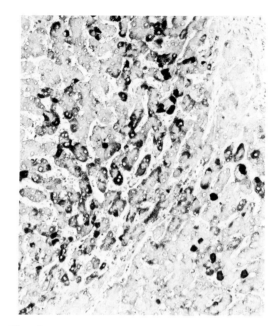

Fig. 31-16. Immunoperoxidase demonstration of HBsAg in CAVH-B. (Courtesy Dr. Angelos Afroudakis, Athens, Greece.)

preponderance of men with chronic active viral hepatitis. Systemic symptoms, such as amenorrhea, skin rashes, and joint pains, or psychiatric problems are much fewer in CAVH than in CALH, and the serologic changes of autoimmune disease are absent. Except for the occasional occurrence of "ground-glass" cells of Hadziyannis or hepatocytes stainable for HBsAg in CAVH-B, microscopic and gross findings in the liver in CAVH are indistinguishable from those of CALH (Fig. 31-16).

The pathogenesis of chronic active viral hepatitis remains unknown. It has been proposed that the patient with CAVH-B has a partially impaired immune response that allows the virion to replicate in some cells but to be destroyed or inactivated in certain other cells that undergo an immunocytopathic type of destruction. In support of this hypothesis, patients with CAVH-B have an impairment of immune responsiveness of cellular immune response specifically to HBsAg although response to other antigens is not diminished. The impairment is not so complete as is found in patients with PVH-B.[88]

The clinical course of chronic active viral hepatitis and the corresponding histologic pattern fall into three somewhat variable patterns: (1) classic CAVH, (2) subclinical CAVH, and (3) CAVH developing subclinically after a single bout of hepatitis.

Classic CAVH. The course of the disease is characterized by remission and exacerbations. There is a high incidence of chronic active viral hepatitis B among patients with hepatocellular carcinoma,[74,191,214,225,228] but rarely do they have symptoms of CAVH. It would appear that either most patients with CAVH who have repeated bouts of illness succumb to some aspect of the disease before reaching the stage of neoplasia, or the more quiescent insidious varieties of CAVH have a greater propensity to progress to malignancy than do those with repeated episodic necrosis.

Subclinical CAVH. The majority of patients found to have cirrhosis with HBsAg in their sera or in their hepatocytes (see viral cirrhosis type B, p. 1371) have no history of clinically recognizable hepatitis. Most have been ostensibly in good health until complications of cirrhosis appear. Consequently, studies of the liver during the development of disease have been either fortuitous or have resulted from the discovery of HBsAg in serum. The liver of such a patient has very little inflammatory component, either in portal areas or in parenchyma. However, usually a few foci of hepatocytolysis can be found with cuffs of mononuclear cells. Whatever inflammatory foci are found are irregularly distributed and unrelated to lobular architecture. However, there are faint, ill-defined areas of bulging "cobblestone" hepatocytes compressing adjacent parenchyma that has a cord pattern. Some hepatocytes have polyploid nuclei or dysplastic nuclei, and usually some zones where Kupffer cells are hyperplastic can be identified. If "ground-glass" or stainable antigen-positive cells are found, they tend to be in clusters rather than evenly distributed as they typically are when found in persistent viral hepatitis. The changes are sufficiently subtle that often the biopsies of such patients have been interpreted as *persistent hepatitis*. Only detailed prospective study will establish with certainty whether or not a consistently accurate distinction can be made between PVH and subclinical CAVH.

CAVH after a single bout of viral hepatitis. Occasionally a patient with a previously normal liver may have a fairly mild attack of hepatitis that progresses to cirrhosis within a year. The patient may be clinically asymptomatic after recovering from the acute disease until complications of cirrhosis develop.

The HBsAg can be demonstrated within hepatocytes of the liver affected with CAVH-B, especially when the disease is quiescent. In contrast to PVH where the HBsAg is in scattered hepatocytes but involves the cytoplasm of those cells quite heavily, the HBsAg distribution in CAVH-B is variable. It may be membrane bound, may have scattered solidly involved cells, and may have many cells with faint diffuse involvement, all in proximity.[104] HBcAg is abundant in hepatocellular nuclei in livers with CAVH-B.

Rarely, posttransfusion VH-non-B progresses to CAH and cirrhosis.

Chronic active lupoid hepatitis (CALH)

Cirrhosis is usually present when the patients are first studied, and the disease generally progresses over a period of years to death by hepatic failure, bleeding esophageal varices, or other complications of chronic liver disease. Early reports[111,174] indicated a preponderance in women, with findings of recurrent fever, menstrual irregularities, arthralgia, and hyperglobulinemia. Some patients with the same symptom complexes were found to have positive lupus erythematosus (LE) cell tests[111,113,153,163] and the term *lupoid hepatitis* was used. Although originally described in young women,[111] CALH may affect anyone from childhood to senility[205] but remains preponderantly a disease of women.

Most hepatologists accept the differences between CAVH and CALH as significant, admitting that the prognostic and therapeutic importance of establishing the type into which specific cases fit remains to be established. The characteristic features of CALH differing from other varieties of chronic active hepatitis are as follows:

1. Ninety percent of patients with CALH are women in contrast to those with CAVH-B, which is a disease more common in men.

2. The elevation of serum gamma globulin levels in lupoid hepatitis are usually much more striking than that found in other varieties of CAH.

3. It is rare for patients with CALH to have HBsAg-positive sera.

4. Chronic active lupoid hepatitis with all serologic markers may be produced by the drug oxyphenisatin in susceptible individuals, a finding that shows that viral infection may not be necessary to produce the disease.

5. In contrast to CAVH-B, CALH rarely if ever forms the basis for hepatocellular carcinoma (HCC). In a recent study at

Los Angeles County and John Wesley Hospitals, 71% of the hepatocellular carcinomas arising in nonalcoholic cirrhotic livers were in patients with CAVH-B; none of over 100 patients with HCC on whom LE preparations and smooth muscle antibodies of IgG type were studied had either autoimmune marker.

6. Patients with CALH usually have amenorrhea and are infertile. Many of the women with CAVH-B have become pregnant, carrying their infants to term.

Biologic false-positive reactions to serologic tests for syphilis occur in 25% or less of patients with chronic active lupoid hepatitis[182,205]; 50% have a positive latex fixative reaction for rheumatoid arthritis; 75% have antinuclear antibodies[182]; and 90% or more have a positive reaction for smooth muscle IgG antibodies.[230]

Chronic active toxic hepatitis

At least one drug, a formerly popular laxative containing oxyphenisatin, when used habitually did produce chronic active hepatitis. Some patients developed positive LE cell preparations and smooth muscle antibodies. Progression of the disease disappears with discontinuance of the laxative, but all features reappear with challenge.[206] Most other drugs that produce a lesion resembling CAH actually induce severe necrosis with collapse that may be very difficult to distinguish from CAH. Such drugs include methyldopa and isoniazid. Methyldopa is important to consider because the LE phenomenon often develops in a patient with or without a hepatic lesion when the patient is taking methyldopa. Interestingly, methyldopa liver necrosis is a disease predominantly of women (10:1). The fact that a drug may precipitate a disease previously believed to be autoimmune makes it mandatory that an exogenous sensitization be considered as possibly etiologic in any case of chronic active lupoid hepatitis.

Cryptogenic chronic active hepatitis

Many patients with the clinical, laboratory, and hepatic lesions of chronic active hepatitis have no evidence of exogenous sensitization. They do not have the LE factor, antinuclear antibody, smooth muscle antibody, or HAA. Cryptogenic chronic active hepatitis could have the same etiology as one of the types previously described, with the patient ultimately lacking demonstrable quantities of the serum factors that would allow classification as lupoid or viral or toxic types of disease. Alternatively, an etiologic agent not yet recognized may be at fault, or hepatitis NAB may occasionally give rise to chronic active hepatitis. No evidence has been forthcoming to indicate that VH-A progresses to cirrhosis.

Hemodialysis

In renal hemodialysis and organ transplant centers a major problem concerning viral hepatitis and certain other infections has arisen. Although the patients may develop mild or subclinical hepatitis,[175,179,195,220] the medical staff and the spouses of infected patients are at considerable risk for development of disease that may be severe.[125,207] The increase in hepatitis among patients seems to be related to the problems of sterilization of equipment that is used in common, or by the blood transfusions given to the anemic patients continually needing hemodialysis. The high incidence of HBsAg carrier state, far above that for hemophiliac patients, is probably a result of an impaired immune response. Work by Tong has shown that both the T and B lymphocytes are reduced in patients with chronic renal failure and that the number of null cells is increased.[224]

Type B hepatitis has received more study in hemodialysis centers than has non-B hepatitis or cytomegalovirus (CMV) infection. Within any one hemodialysis unit, the HBV subtype has been uniform. In most hemodialysis centers, the subtype has been *ad* but in a few it has been *ay*. This is supportive evidence of a common source of infection. Control efforts include isolation of HBsAg carriers and passive immunization[117,138]; both methods show promise.

The histologic changes of hepatitis in a patient undergoing renal dialysis differ somewhat from those seen in patients with ordinary acute viral hepatitis. Because of the difference in immune response, the sequelae also differ from those ordinarily seen. There is lymphoid hyperplasia in the portal areas, occasionally with germinal centers that produce a prominent widening of the portal areas. Occasionally thin collagen strands extend from the portal areas. Usually the Kupffer cells contain hemosiderin because of numerous transfusions, and, if there is chronic anemia, the hepatocytes contain hemosiderin. Usually the viral hepatitis is mild, although fulminant cases have been described.[120] Complete recovery from AcVH is erratic; instead of subsidence of disease as in

85% of "average" individuals who develop AcVH, or the development of the uniform cobblestone pattern of hepatocytes seen in PVH, the liver biopsy of the patient requiring hemodialysis tends to have a prolonged process of what histologically resembles acute viral hepatitis. The centrilobular hepatocytes are swollen and hydropic, Kupffer cells are modestly hyperplastic, and there is focal hepatocytolysis. These changes involve every lobule; in contrast to CAH, however, because of the widened, hyperplastic portal areas, the liver biopsy is often interpreted as "chronic active hepatitis." The clinical course suggests that the disorder is more a retardation of recovery than a progressive liver disease. Some patients lose HBsAg in their sera 1 or 2 years after they acquire it, an event that seems to be more common than it is in the patients with PVH-B or CAVH-B. Significant numbers of patients on chronic hemodialysis develop ascites that is unrelated to hepatic disease and unassociated with portal hypertension.

Many patients do develop persistent viral hepatitis with the unusual portal lymphoid hyperplasia and portal widening. In our dialysis center, true chronic active hepatitis seems to be seen much less than is diagnosed elsewhere.[229]

Some patients with microscopic alterations and elevation of serum transaminase activity that do not have HBsAg in their sera have been categorized as "nonviral hepatitis."[112] Obviously it is difficult to exclude a non-B viral agent in the pathogenesis of such hepatic changes.

Laboratory diagnosis

Tests that indicate cell necrosis or damage, such as SGPT, SGOT, isocitric dehydrogenase (ICD), lactic acid dehydrogenase (LDH), and LDH isoenzymes, are the most helpful in the diagnosis of viral hepatitis (Table 31-1). The transaminases are more stable than the others under laboratory conditions. Glutamic pyruvic transaminase is more selectively a liver parenchymal cell enzyme than is GOT. Serum GPT and SGOT activities rise above normal about 1 week prior to symptoms and continue to rise to levels usually above 1000 units, occasionally to 3000 units and rarely to 5000 units. The SGPT is higher than the SGOT in 85% of patients with viral hepatitis.

Serum bilirubin levels do not indicate the severity of disease, although anicteric viral hepatitis is usually a milder disease and never

fatal. The direct and indirect fractions are about equally divided. In younger patients, the serum albumin remains within normal range, but in older patients or severely ill younger patients, it may decrease. The change in albumin level is probably a reflection of functioning capacity of liver cells. The prothrombin activity is of little help in making the diagnosis of viral hepatitis, but it is of considerable prognostic value. A fall in prothrombin activity is of serious consequence, although death rarely occurs when the prothrombin activity (by Owren-Ware technique) remains above 5%.[135] The hepatitis-B antigen (HBsAg) in sera is strong evidence for hepatitis B. Serum alkaline phosphatase activity usually is slightly elevated (5 to 10 Bessey-Lowry units). Although patients who have considerable cholestasis on liver biopsy are often histologically classified as having cholestatic viral hepatitis, such patients usually have only a slight elevation of alkaline phosphatase activity. Conversely, the occasional patient with a fivefold to sevenfold increase in alkaline phosphatase activity rarely has cholestasis on liver biopsy.

In hepatic coma, most of the clinical and laboratory data are of little help in determining the amount of liver destruction in contrast to that which is viable but temporarily nonfunctional. However, good regenerative capacity and a better prognosis are suggested if alpha fetoprotein is detected. The best prognostic sign is a rise in prothrombin activity or of factor VII levels.

ENCEPHALOPATHY

The chief manifestation of hepatic failure is encephalopathy. This occurs in both acute and chronic liver disease. In fulminant hepatitis, the onset is sudden and the mortality high.[135] In chronic liver disease, the symptoms of hepatic encephalopathy are more likely to be mild and the onset gradual. The symptoms are of a neuropsychiatric nature, varying from minor disturbances of consciousness and behavior to drowsiness, confusion, and coma. Often, a flapping tremor of the extremities is evident. Despite the severe neurologic features that may develop, histopathologic changes are minimal, apparently limited to enlargement and increased numbers of protoplasmic astrocytes.[233] One of the surprising aspects of hepatic coma is the rapid and complete recovery that may occur if hepatic failure is ameliorated.

The etiology of hepatic encephalopathy is

related to the absorption of toxic products, primarily ammonia, from the intestine.[236] However, not all patients with encephalopathy have increased ammonia levels in the blood. Other substances, such as amino acids and short-chain fatty acids that might not be cleared by the diseased liver presumably could be partially responsible for encephalopathy. It has been proposed that the liver produces substances that are important for brain function and the lack of these might contribute to encephalopathy.[236] The control of blood ammonia levels is still the key concern of the clinicians.[234]

Ammonia, formed by the kidney and by urea-splitting organisms in the gut, is removed from portal blood by the intact liver to form urea. Patients on diuretic therapy or who have potassium depletion have a greater renal production of ammonia. The relative amounts of NH_3 and NH_4 in blood are critical, since only NH_3 passes through the cell membrane. The ratio follows the Henderson-Hasselbalch equation of $pH = 9.15 + \log\dfrac{[NH_3]}{[NH_4]}$. Thus alkalosis will increase the amount of diffusible NH_3. In the central nervous system, NH_3 is believed to produce its deleterious effects by diverting α-ketoglutarate from the tricarboxylic cycle with consequent loss of high-energy phosphate bond formation and reduction of aerobic metabolism.

Encephalopathy often increases as a result of spontaneous or surgical vascular bypass of the liver. In the latter group, patients past 60 are more severely incapacitated.[237] A close correlation has been demonstrated between the inability to synthesize urea and the development of encephalopathy.[238,239]

OTHER ACUTE INFECTIONS

There are other acute diseases of the liver of infectious origin that occur less frequently than viral hepatitis. Among these are yellow fever (pp. 487 and 1333), typhoid fever, Weil's disease, and infectious mononucleosis. Although rarely accompanied by jaundice, a classic example of focal necrosis of the liver is that produced by typhoid fever. Jaundice, high fever, and sore muscles always should bring to mind Weil's disease (p. 446). Infectious mononucleosis, a disease produced by the Ebstein-Barr (E-B) virus, may be accompanied by hepatomegaly, jaundice, and focal necrosis of the liver.[240] The portal tracts are heavily infiltrated with mononuclear cells; there is sinusoidal lymphocytosis, Kupffer cell hyperplasia, and

occasional punched-out areas of necrosis, but hepatocytes are not swollen. The disease is rarely fatal, but in autopsy material herpeslike particles have been noted on electron microscopic examination.[241] Cytomegalovirus disease, when transmitted by transfusion of fresh whole blood, closely resembles infectious mononucleosis in histologic appearance.[242,244] Rarely, a highly fatal liver disease may be caused by herpes simplex infection.[243] Livers involved have irregular serpiginous areas of coagulative necrosis with deeply eosinophilic intranuclear inclusions at the margins of the necrotic areas. Formerly common only in infants with kwashiorkor, herpetic liver necrosis has been described in patients with induced or acquired immune deficiency, and occasionally in pregnancy. In the past, focal necrosis of the liver attributable to some of the pyogenic organisms was known to complicate the course of septicemia, but the jaundice that was occasionally seen was possibly secondary to hemolysis caused by the organisms. In fatal chickenpox, irregular areas of necrosis often involve both the triads and portions of the lobules. The blood vessels of the triads usually are included in the necrotizing process.

CHEMICAL AND DRUG INJURY

Among the many functions of the smooth endoplasmic reticulum (SER) is the hydroxylation of many normally occurring lipid-soluble compounds, such as the steroids and bile salts, after which they may be combined with glucuronic acid, sulfate, or other anions, to make them water soluble. In the latter form they can be excreted in the urine or bile. Many chemicals, noxious susbstances, and drugs are metabolized by the same enzyme system in the SER. This system is an electron-carrier chain composed of NADPH–cytochrome P_{450} reductase and cytochrome P_{450}. Reduced nicotinamide adenine dinucleotide phosphate (NADPH) and molecular oxygen are necessary for its function.[253,261] The drug-metabolizing enzymes are inducible[267]; e.g., repeated doses of phenobarbital or ethanol are powerful stimulants. The increased SER is easily seen with the electron microscope. The metabolic pathway is nonspecific, however, and any one of many drugs or chemicals can be detoxified at an increased rate.

The location of the detoxifying enzymes in the liver has made the hepatocyte a target for many types of chemical and drug-related injury. These vary from mild disease that is diagnosed only by a rise in serum enzymes to instances of massive necrosis and death. Some reactions are relatively innocuous even though the patient is jaundiced. Many reactions occur after exposure to or ingestion of an injurious agent that is not related to therapy. However, by far the largest group does occur after the use of drugs. In the first group there is a direct toxic reaction on the liver of man and experimental animals that is dose-related and fairly prompt. The morphologic expression, commonly known as *toxic hepatitis,* is usually uniform and predictable. Among these hepatotoxins are carbon tetrachloride, chloroform,[270] chlorinated naphthalenes, phosphorus, and the toxin of *Amanita phalloides.* They usually produce a zonal type of necrosis accompanied by fatty change. Other body organs may be affected and, if death does not occur, recovery is complete. In mushroom poisoning, there is damage to both nuclei and cytoplasm at the ultrastructural level, particularly in the periportal zones.[263] Fatty change is seen in fatal cases but not in nonfatal cases.[274] The latter is characterized by centrilobular necrosis and collapse. The ultrastructural changes in carbon tetrachloride injury include the dislocation of ribosomes and dilatation of cisternae[245,269] (see p. 302).

Among the drugs used for therapeutic purposes there are innumerable examples of liver damage. This type of damage has been termed *drug-induced jaundice* or *drug-induced liver disease.* Recently, the term *toxic reaction* has been given to the cases with more severe injury.[262] The problem of drug-induced liver disease has assumed such proportions that it is now essential to question every jaundiced patient about drug usage. This is especially true when the jaundice is of the obstructive type, i.e., with a high alkaline phosphatase level and normal or slightly elevated transaminase levels; otherwise the condition may be misdiagnosed and the patient subjected to unnecessary surgery.

Several drugs that cause hepatic necrosis in humans as well as in animals, such as acetaminophen and furosemide, are apparently metabolized to intermediates that form a covalent linkage to macromolecules that are necessary for vital function of the cell. When this occurs, cell necrosis often results. In animals, glutathione prevents the covalent linkage with the macromolecules. It is of interest that pretreatment of the animals with enzyme inducers causes an increased severity of the hepatic necrosis, presumably because of the SER forming more of the toxic intermedi-

ates.[250] The protection of the liver against carbon tetrachloride–induced necrosis by protein deficiency is abolished if phenobarbital is given prior to exposure to carbon tetrachloride. Extensive studies with isoniazid suggests that a similar enzyme mechanism is involved, especially in those patients in whom the liver rapidly acetylates the drug. These individuals form an intermediate metabolite, acetylhydrazine.[261,262]

Liver disease based on allergy is usually assumed when a drug causes injury in only a small percentage of patients, is not dose-related, and is accompanied by allergic manifestations, such as skin rash, fever, and eosinophilia.[261]

A useful clinicopathologic classification of drug-induced liver disease is given in Table 31-3. The list of drugs given that are capable of causing liver injury is by no means complete. In the first group, there is usually simple cholestasis without cell necrosis or inflammation, although the effect of drugs or of any single drug can vary considerably, and an occasional necrotic liver cell as well as minimal inflammation is sometimes seen. Rarely, severe necrosis may ensue. As a group, these cholestatic drugs produce reversible injury to the secretory mechanism that prevents bilirubin glucuronide from entering the canaliculi normally. The bilirubin that does enter the canaliculi tends to accumulate and form bile plugs that are obvious on microscopic examination, especially in the centrilobular zone (Plate 3, *B*). There is usually some swelling or hydropic change of the hepatocytes. The electron microscope discloses a distortion and disappearance of the canalicular microvilli and widening of the canalicular ectoplasm.[265] After the drug is discontinued, the liver returns to normal.

It is of interest that women who have had benign jaundice of pregnancy, presumably because of excess production of sex hormones, will often have a recurrence of jaundice when they take one of the oral contraceptives.[251] The estrogens appear to be responsible for the rare instances of jaundice that follows the use of oral contraceptives.[268] The 17α-alkyl-19-norsteroids cause the most difficulty with bile secretion.[260] Although thrombosis of the hepatic veins, Budd-Chiari syndrome, has been reported as a rare complication from oral contraceptive use,[254] patients with Budd-Chiari syndrome at the University of Southern California Liver Unit have no greater incidence of oral contraceptive use than does the remainder of the hospital population.

In the second and largest group of patients, there is liver cell injury as well as cholestasis, so that the laboratory findings occasionally include a rise in the serum transaminases. The number of drugs that cause this type of injury seems endless. The phenothiazine drugs, and other commonly used drugs, such as nicotinamide[275] and aspirin[256] may cause liver injury. On microscopic examination, the findings are variable, but cell ballooning, focal necrosis of hepatocytes, cholestasis, and inflammation along the portal tracts usually are present. The reaction of the triads vary greatly. In some biopsies there is an increase of connective tissue and an inflammatory exudate in which round cells, neutrophils, or eosinophils may predominate. Ductular proliferation may also be seen. Granulomas with eosinophilic infiltrate may result from sensitivity to one of the sulfonamide drugs. Most patients in this second group recover when the offending drug is discontinued. A few have a long illness with the laboratory findings of biliary cirrhosis,[272] but most of these patients eventually get well.

In the third group of patients, liver cell necrosis with a minimal to moderate inflammatory response occurs, accompanied by hyperbilirubinemia and high serum transaminase activity. Although mild centrilobular necrosis that heals rapidly is occasionally noted after the use of isoniazid, this drug may cause massive necrosis and death. Elevated serum transaminase levels have been reported in about 20% of adults given isoniazid for tuberculosis prophylaxis.[257,258] Halothane and similar compounds—methoxyflurane (Penthrane)—occasionally are associated with liver necrosis.[264] The exact path of biotransformation of the inhalation anesthetics is not yet known, but it has been proposed that it is the same as that of fixed drugs and involves the same enzyme system in the SER. None of the known metabolic products are toxic to man.[247,266] The possibility of an allergic reaction has to be considered.[248] Halothane-associated liver damage in most instances occurs after more than one exposure, usually in a patient who has had an unexplained fever after the first halothane-induced anesthesia.

In fatal massive necrosis after halothane anesthesia, three stages can be recognized: necrotic, absorptive, and regenerative. In the *necrotic* stage, dead liver cells are still recognizable and occur in the first 5 days after onset of jaundice (Fig. 31-17). In the *absorptive*

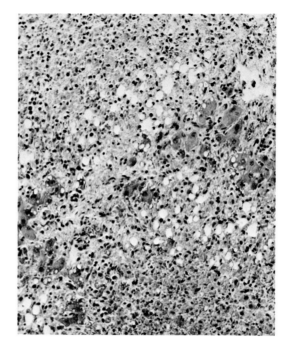

Fig. 31-17. Massive hepatocellular necrosis after halothane anesthesia. (From Peters, R. L., Edmondson, H. A., Reynolds, T. B., Meister, J. C., and Curphey, T. J.: Am. J. Med. **47**:748-764, 1969.)

stage, the liver cells have disappeared, leaving areas of collapse. This is the period in which most of the patients die, usually 1 to 2 weeks after the onset of jaundice. In the *regenerative* stage, submassive necrosis has occurred, and in this stage the patients live from 2 weeks to a month. These subjects are older and have insufficient regenerative capacity to restore the liver parenchyma. Individuals under 30 years of age who survive for 3 weeks after the onset of jaundice may be expected to recover.

In a small miscellaneous group (*4* in Table 31-3), the abnormalities produced are distinctive for each drug.[252] There are no common findings in the liver. A characteristic foamy type of fatty change occurs in the liver after the use of large amounts of intravenous tetracycline (Fig. 31-18).[246] The tetracycline interferes with the production of protein by RNA. Thus formation of lipoprotein necessary for the transfer of fat from the liver is blocked. Novobiocin inhibits the action of glucuronyl transferase, in this way producing an unconjugated hyperbilirubinemia.

Both an acute liver cell damage resembling mild viral hepatitis and a disorder indistinguishable from chronic active hepatitis have been described after the use of laxatives that

Table 31-3. Drug-induced liver disease*

Action of drug	Incidence	Pathologic condition— liver and other	Symptoms	Serum bilirubin	Transaminases	Alkaline phosphatase	Prothrombin activity	BUN
1. Cholestatic								
a. Anabolic steroids with a 17-alkyl group† / Methyl testosterone	High	Centrilobular cholestasis	Uncomplicated jaundice	Elevated, usually < 15 mg	Normal	Elevated often above 20 BL units	Normal	Normal
b. Oral contraceptives	1/10,000	Centrilobular cholestasis	Itching and jaundice	Mild elevation	Mild increase	Elevation mild to moderate		
2. Cholestatic, plus variable degree of necrosis								
Phenothiazine drugs / Sulfonamides / Thiouracil / Tolbutamide‡ / TAO / Mercaptopurine	< 1% / 0.6% / / High / / < 5%	Centrilobular bile stasis and focal necrosis; inflammation of triads in many instances	In addition to jaundice, may be fever, rash, and eosinophilia	Elevated, usually < 15	Mild rise, < 500; occasionally 1000 or more	Elevated	Normal	Normal
3. Necrosis, zonal or massive								
Halothane / Isoniazid / Ethionamide / PAS / Phenurone / Phenylbutazone / Acetaminophen / Methyldopa	1-10,000 / Very rare / Low / High / 2% / Rare / Suicide / variable F:M::9:1	Liver cell injury, massive necrosis or zonal necrosis	Severe jaundice usually; may proceed to hepatic coma and death	Moderate to high	> 500 to 1000	Elevation normal to mild	Decreased	May rise
(Acetaminophen)			Jaundice	Not elevated	1000 to 2000	0	Often decreased	Normal
4. Other								
Tetracycline, especially in pregnancy	Unknown	Fine, foamy fatty change; cholestasis; pancreas, brain, and kidney also involved	Jaundice; coma	Elevated	< 500	Elevated	Moderate decrease	High often renal failure
Novobiocin	Unknown		Newborn infants more susceptive	Elevated unconjugated bilirubin	Normal	Normal	Normal	Normal
Oxyphenisatin	Uncommon	Acute cell injury or chronic active hepatitis	Malaise	Mild elevation	> 500	Normal or elevated	Decrease	Normal

*Data in part from Zimmerman, H. J.: Am. J. Gastroenterol. **49:**39-56, 1968.

†Rarely, cases of liver necrosis have been reported.

‡Data from Pannekoek, J. H.: In Meyler, L., and Herxheimer, A., editors: Side effects of drugs, vol. 6, Baltimore, 1968, The Williams & Wilkins Co.

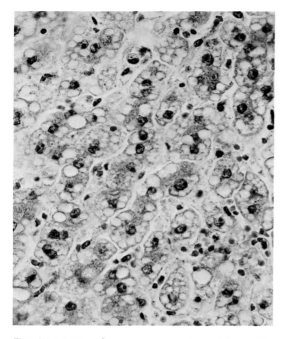

Fig. 31-18. Fine foamy vacuolization of liver after large amounts of intravenously administered tetracycline. (From Peters, R. L., Edmondson, H. A. Mikkelsen, W. P., and Tatter, D.: Am. J. Surg. 113:622-632, 1967.)

contain the agent oxyphenisatin (acetphenolisatin).[206] Methyldopa produces a similar type of liver damage that is quickly reversible when the drug is discontinued. Massive necrosis may also occur after the use of methyldopa.[259,271] Patients who chronically ingest large doses of vitamin A may develop symptoms of hypervitaminosis that may include hepatomegaly and ascites. The principal changes in the liver are perisinusoidal fibrosis and the accumulation of lipid-storage cells (Ito cells).[255] An unusual form of chronic liver disease has been reported in patients with psoriasis who have taken methotrexate.[249] Diffuse fibrosis along the sinusoidal walls and the presence of megalohepatocytes is characteristic. The disease may proceed to cirrhosis, almost silently.[273] Liver damage seems to be related to frequent small doses.[249]

RADIATION INJURY

Heavy irradiation of the liver, 3000 to 5900 rads, produces centrilobular necrosis, intense hyperemia, and damage to the small hepatic veins that resembles veno-occlusive disease.[278] The microscopic changes in a needle biopsy specimen taken in the acute stage of irradiation damage are most difficult to distinguish from the Budd-Chiari syndrome. In the chronic stage, after several months, there is a shrunken atrophied liver with lobular collapse and portal tract fibrosis. Vascular damage is still present. The presence of both acute and chronic changes may be looked upon as an intermediate stage of damage.[277] Experimentally, irradiation produces a fine structural change in the rough endoplasmic reticulum, characterized by the formation of dense membranes.[276]

BILIARY OBSTRUCTION
AND LIVER ABSCESS
Obstruction

A most important form of acute liver disease is that caused by obstruction of the extrahepatic biliary tract, sometimes called *surgical jaundice*. The obstruction may occur at any point between the hilus of the liver and the papilla of Vater. The most common causes are carcinoma, stone, or stricture. Carcinoma of the bile ducts or the head of the pancreas usually produces complete obstruction with pronounced dilatation of the biliary tree, for which the term *hydrohepatosis* has been used. There is jaundice accompanied by little or no pain. In calculous obstruction, or choledocholithiasis, there is often a history of gallbladder disease, and jaundice is accompanied by pain. Although calculus impacted in the papilla of Vater may produce complete obstruction, stones in the common duct are usually mobile and the jaundice tends to fluctuate or even disappear for varying periods of time. Obstruction of the common duct attributable to carcinoma causes a prompt rise in the serum alkaline phosphatase that precedes the rise in serum bilirubin, which with complete obstruction can go to levels of 20 to 30 mg per 100 ml, and higher if there is renal failure (Table 31-1). The blood prothrombin decreases but responds to parenterally administered vitamin K. Bile appears in the urine, and there is an absence of stercobilin in the stool. In choledocholithiasis the serum bilirubin level usually does not go so high and tends to fluctuate. The alkaline phosphatase level likewise does not show the constant rise usually seen in cancerous obstruction. An increase in bile acids in the serum is held responsible for the pruritus that is so common in patients with biliary obstruction.[293]

The sequence of events that follows obstruction of the bile duct depends to some extent on the severity of obstruction and infection that so often occurs in the stagnant column of bile present in the dilated ducts behind the obstructing lesion. The microscopic changes seen soon after obstruction include dilatation of the small ducts and particularly the prominence of the ductules where they penetrate the limiting plate to join the canaliculi. The dilated ductules are usually outlined by neutrophils just beneath their basement membranes. Bile accumulates in the centrilobular canaliculi, forming green-yellow to brown plugs (Plate 3, *C*). Later, in unrelieved obstruction, the ducts enlarge further and may proliferate. The bile canaliculi become more distended with plugs. In this stage, clinical acute cholangitis may supervene, characterized by chills and fever in addition to the jaundice. The periductal neutrophils become more numerous and penetrate the lumen of the ducts. The cholangitis is of bacterial origin. Organisms often are found in stagnant bile when obstruction is attributable to stone or stricture but are only rarely present in surgical specimens when the obstruction is caused by tumor.[294] In obstruction, electron microscopic studies show flattening of the canalicular microvilli and condensation of the pericanalicular ectoplasm.[279] The liver cells often contain intracytoplasmic bile, and Kupffer cells are enlarged by easily discernible masses of bile pigment. Foci of necrosis may appear within the lobules, accompanied by bile lakes and a rise in the serum transaminase levels. Often a feathery type of degeneration of liver cells is noted.[285] Increased connective tissue around the bile ducts may assume a lamellar arrangement, and small prolongations enter the periphery of the lobules. Occasionally, the infection of the stagnant bile is more severe and *suppurative cholangitis* occurs, resulting in a surgical emergency as the patient has a high fever, often with a positive blood culture, and may go into shock. The borderline between suppurative cholangitis and multiple liver abscesses, particularly microabscesses, is indistinct, as both may be present. Percutaneous transhepatic cholangiography and drainage has been used successfully in diagnosis and treatment at this stage of the disease.[296] Thus the spectrum of changes that follow obstruction begins with a mild pericholangitis and includes the various stages of infectious cholangitis, multiple liver abscesses and even biliary cirrhosis. For all of the above conditions, the authors use the term *obstructive biliopathy*. The severity of infection and abscess formation may vary considerably from one part of the liver to another.

Many clinicopathologic features are important. The finding of cholangitis or pericholangitis on needle biopsy does not necessarily correlate with clinical symptoms of cholangitis. The clinical entity was described in 1877 by Charcot[282] as intermittent hepatic fever, usually in patients with a stone in the common duct.

Because fatal cholangitis may quickly occur after obstruction by a stone in the diabetic patient, the screening of all diabetics past 40 years of age for cholelithiasis by oral cholecystograms should be a clinical consideration. In a small percentage of patients with choledocholithiasis, clinical features of acute cholangitis occur in the absence of jaundice.

Abscess

Pyogenic liver abscesses (Table 31-4) have been classified on the basis of the mode of entry, i.e. (1) ascension of the biliary tract (cholangitis), (2) by means of the hepatic artery (septicemia), (3) through the portal vein (pylephlebitis), (4) by direct extension (subphrenic abscess), (5) secondary to trauma, and (6) from unknown sources. The pathologic changes may result in multiple microscopic lesions or in single or multiple macroscopic abscesses.[291]

Although acute cholangitis consequent to obstruction of the common duct is the most common cause of multiple abscesses (Plate 4, *F*), septicemia and pylephlebitis must also be considered. Septicemias may produce multiple liver abscesses of variable size as well as abscesses of other organs in adults, infants, and children. In children, they usually occur before the age of 5 years, particularly in patients with acute blastic leukemia.[283] In the neonate, liver abscesses may complicate umbilical infections. Compared with the past, pylephlebitis is now rarely seen but does occur as an extension from suppurative appendicitis or other suppurative disease in areas drained by the portal vein. The emboli or bacteria are carried to the liver where they tend to form either multiple or solitary abscesses. These most often occur in the right lobe when the suppurative disorder is drained by the superior mesenteric vein, whereas disease on the left side of the abdomen may cause suppuration in one or both lobes.[288] Thrombosis of intrahepatic branches of the portal vein may accompany carcinomas of the biliary tract or the head of the pancreas and produce multiple infarcts. If obstructive cholangitis is present, some of the infarcts may suppurate, forming

Table 31-4. Suppurative disease of liver

	Bilirubin	Alkaline phosphatase	White blood cell count	Blood culture	Scan
1. Suppurative cholangitis with or without multiple abscesses	Usually 15	Greatly elevated	High: 15,000	Often positive	Filling defects not usually seen
2. Multiple abscesses from septicemia	Normal or slightly increased	Moderately elevated	High: 15,000	Positive	Filling defects not usually seen
3. Multiple abscesses from pylephlebitis	Normal or slightly increased	Moderately elevated	High: 15,000	Often positive	Filling defects not usually seen
4. Solitary abscesses	Normal	Moderately elevated	Varies	Negative	Positive
5. Amebic abscesses	Normal	Moderately elevated	High: 15,000	Negative	Positive
6. Actinomycosis	Normal	—	—	Negative	Positive

septic infarcts (an entity apparently not recognized in the literature).

Solitary abscesses may occur after both penetrating and nonpenetrating injuries to the liver, contiguous infections, and intra-abdominal suppuration.[291] In many patients with solitary abscesses, no recognizable sources can be found. Such abscesses have been reported in diabetic patients.[286] In livers of patients with a solitary abscess who do not have jaundice, the scintiscan shows a filling defect far more often than in patients with multiple small hepatic abscesses.

Pyogenic abscesses occur with equal frequency in men and women usually past 50 years of age, producing fever and a large liver accompanied by pain and tenderness in the right upper quadrant. Laboratory examination reveals a leukocytosis, elevated alkaline phosphatase level, and often a positive blood culture. Chest roentgenograms often disclose basilar atelectasis or pneumonitis, an elevated right diaphragm, and a pleural effusion. A hepatic scintiscan is an important diagnostic aid as it shows the filling defect in most patients.[291]

The most common organisms found in liver abscesses are *Escherichia coli* and *Staphylococcus aureus,* although many other organisms have been identified. Anaerobic organisms have been cultured, alone or in combination with aerobes.[287,292] *Bacteroides fragilis* as the cause of liver abscesses should be suspected at operation when there is a particularly foul odor to the abscess material.[284]

Liver abscesses vary from microscopic size to a diameter of several centimeters and, by coalescence, can form large cavities. Necrosis,

cellular disintegration, and leukocyte accumulation are found in the areas of abscess. Occasionally, there is the complication of rupture or spread of the infection to adjacent tissues. In a few cases endocarditis and other more distinct complications occur. Septicemia may occur after needle biopsy in patients with acute cholangitis and microabscesses.

Pyogenic infection may complicate any one of several congenital diseases of the liver. In polycystic disease infection may convert the cysts to innumerable abscesses.[281] Congenital hepatic fibrosis may be complicated by an acute and chronic cholangitis that resists treatment and may cause death.[290]

Differential diagnosis. Abscesses of the liver may also be of amebic or actinomycotic origin (discussed on pp. 518 and 523). These are much less common than pyogenic abscesses but have similar clinical and x-ray findings. Amebic abscess is caused by spread of *Entamoeba histolytica* from intestinal lesions by way of the portal vein. It is predominantly a disease of men, about 4:1, occurs before the age of 50 years, and is one of the serious diseases noted among travelers exposed to the organism. It is extremely rare in individuals who have not been outside the United States. Children are also susceptible to abscess formation.[289] A history of diarrhea weeks or months before onset of symptoms is given in approximately 50% of patients. However, trophozoites are not always demonstrable in the stools. Fever, leukocytosis, pain in the right upper quadrant, and a tender enlarged liver are common findings. An antibody to partially purified extract of cultured amebas forms the basis for a hemagglutination test in titers oc-

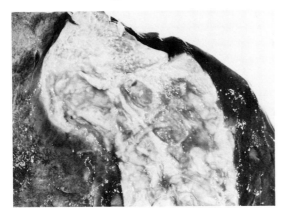

Fig. 31-19. Amebic liver abscess with rough, irregular lining of necrotic tissue.

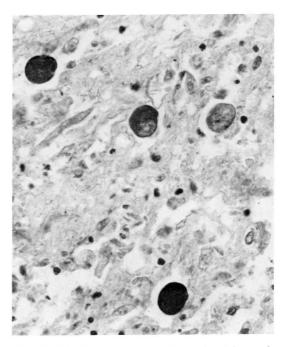

Fig. 31-20. Amebas in necrotic wall of liver abscess. (PAS stain.)

casionally as high as 1:30,000. Many patients will have a visible bulge of the rib margin and even edema over the right lower anterior portion of the chest. Roentgenograms and a liver scan usually will disclose the location of the abscess. Antiamebic therapy usually leads to rapid recovery. Scintiscans show that healing takes 2 to 4 months in most patients.[295]

The abscesses may vary greatly in size but are usually solitary and located in the superoposterior portion of the right lobe (Fig. 31-19). The contents of the abscess varies, depending on its age. Early, the purulent material may be gray-white and thick; later it takes on the classical "anchovy sauce" appearance or is more light colored and watery. The lining of the abscess is usually gray-white and rough, and small necrotic penetrations into the surrounding liver are seen. A striking "foam rubber" lining has been noted in much of our material. The abscess wall has an irregular lining composed of exudate and necrotic liver tissue. The contents usually stain deeply with hematoxylin, in contrast to pyogenic abscess. Amebas are most easily found in the marginal liver tissue, often in colonies with a clear zone about each ameba. A PAS stain accentuates the contrast between ameba and body cells (Fig. 31-20). The amebic infection may involve the branches of the portal and hepatic veins, producing an amebic phlebitis and thrombosis, thus accentuating the necrotic process.

Actinomycotic abscesses of the liver usually have a pathogenesis similar to the pyogenic pylephlebitic abscesses. Spread to the liver from intestinal lesions is by the portal venous channels. Multiple, small ragged abscess cavities are produced, in which the actinomycotic colonies can be found.[280] A honeycomb type of calcification sometimes is seen on roentgenograms (see also p. 518 and Fig. 13-26).

CIRRHOSIS

Cirrhosis results from a series of alterations that lead to a quantitative increase of dense fibrous connective tissue that subdivides the liver into nodules (pseudolobules) of variable size. Most often the fibrosis includes both the portal tissue and the venous outflow tract, but either may be almost exclusively involved. The nodular regeneration further distorts the portal and central relationship. Episodes of necrosis and regeneration of the liver parenchyma may occur continuously or intermittently from the inception of the disease.

Although the term "cirrhosis" (derived from the Greek word *kirrhos,* meaning 'tawny' or 'orange-colored') was applied originally because of color changes, fibrosis and nodular regeneration of liver cells, with distortion of vascular and architectural relationships, rather than any distinctive color now constitute the definition of cirrhosis.[312]

Many conditions are etiologically associated with cirrhosis, but in only a few of these is the full cause-and-effect relationship clear.

Thus it is difficult to classify cirrhosis by etiology. Earlier classifications based on morphology ignored the dynamic, changing character of the cirrhotic liver and often only a single feature, nodular size, was used to designate the various types. Although an etiologic classification correlates best with clinical disease, an ideal description should also include the following:

1. A morphologic term
2. Indication of cirrhotic or precirrhotic condition
3. An appropriate designation for the functional state of the liver

The suggested classification for cirrhosis is based on the etiology or, if not established, the major associated condition and includes the following:

1. Alcoholic cirrhosis or fibrosis—associated with chronic alcoholism
2. Cryptogenic active (or inactive) cirrhosis—follows cryptogenic chronic active hepatitis
3. Active (or inactive) viral cirrhosis, type B—the cirrhotic stage of chronic active hepatitis, type B
4. Active (or inactive) viral cirrhosis, type NAB—the cirrhotic stage of chronic active viral hepatitis, non-A non-B. Such classification, pending a laboratory method of identification, requires knowledge of inoculation and incubation times
5. Active (or inactive) lupoid cirrhosis—cirrhotic stage of chronic active lupoid hepatitis
6. Active (or inactive) toxic cirrhosis—the cirrhotic stage of chronic active toxic hepatitis
7. Hemochromatotic cirrhosis-ferrocirrhosis—consequent to excess storage of iron within the liver
8. Wilson's disease cirrhosis (W-D cirrhosis)—cirrhosis associated with Wilson's disease
9. Pi ZZ juvenile cirrhosis or fibrosis—cirrhosis associated with aberrant protease inhibitor (α_1-antitrypsin) type ZZ
10. JI bypass cirrhosis or fibrosis—cirrhosis associated with jejunoileal bypass surgery
11. Primary biliary cirrhosis or precirrhosis associated with idiopathic destruction of interlobular bile ducts
12. Secondary biliary cirrhosis or fibrosis—chronic liver disease occurring after mechanical obstruction, acquired or congenital
13. Miscellaneous, including syphilitic, parasitic, and cardiac fibroses and cirrhoses that complicate other diseases

Although the proposed classification leaves unsettled many aspects such as whether a particular feature is directly etiologic, indirectly etiologic, or simply associated, it sets up a framework within which there may be considerable leeway. It allows a clinician to characterize cirrhosis while there is yet ignorance of the morphologic type, and it saves the pathologist the problem of trying to choose a term that may not have any clinical credence.

Morphologic characterization

The dual requirements of simplicity and accuracy that would satisfy both gross and microscopic descriptions are not easily met; however certain gross features that characterize cirrhosis include (1) liver size, (2) extent of fibrosis, (3) size of functional unit (lobule or nodule), and (4) integrity (distinctness) of functional unit. The final diagnosis requires gross and microscopic study. Each category has one of several grades of change.

Size is a crude measure of degree of advancement of chronic liver disease. In early stages of all types of cirrhosis the organ is enlarged, apparently reflecting the response of hepatocytes to impaired function of the total organ. As cirrhosis progresses, reparative effort fails to compensate for dysfunction or ultimately to even maintain a stable amount of parenchyma because of continual destruction or attrition. Such an atrophic liver may be nonpalpable and may weigh less than half normal. Hepatic size is usually independent of the other morphologic features. The histologic features noted in a small sample do not allow the pathologist to predict whether 700 gm or 2000 gm of liver are present. The quantity of liver present is an integral part of its functional capacity.

The size categories are divided into (1) *hypertrophic*—over 1800 gm, (2) *eutrophic*—1200 to 1800 gm, and (3) *atrophic*—under 1200 gm.

Fibrosis. Some types of cirrhosis, particularly those related to alcoholism, are characterized by dense collagen that forms hard, white septa and scars, and fine collagen filaments in the interstices about individual hepatocytes within the nodule. The collagen restricts nodular size and obscures their margins. It is uncommon for certain kinds of nonalcoholic cirrhosis to be densely sclerotic. The density of the scars seems to be partly revers-

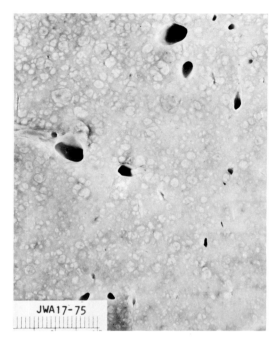

JWA17-75

Fig. 31-21. Cut surface of liver of alcoholic cirrhotic patient with atrophic, sclerotic, finely insular alcoholic cirrhosis. Note denser scarring to *right* of photograph.

ible, since they often become revascularized by numerous vessels that are tortuous and even cavernous. In the process pliability is restored to the liver.

The fibrosis in the liver may be graded depending on the amount, flexibility, and firmness of the connective tissue: (1) In *sclerotic* livers collagen is deposited in hard white bands 0.1 cm or greater in width, resulting in relatively nonpliable, unyielding liver that contains hard, ill-defined scars 1 cm or more wide (Fig. 31-21). (2) *Hard* cirrhotic livers are quite dense and stiff but without broad, hard scars (Plate 4, *C*). Sclerotic and hard livers are most characteristic of alcoholic cirrhosis. (3) *Firm* cirrhotic livers are compact and resistant, but their nodularity is more prominent than the fibrous tissue. (4) *Loose* describes the inactive cirrhotic liver with broad, loose connective tissue separating soft regenerative nodules, from which a slice of cirrhotic liver can be folded over onto itself.

Functional unit size. The functional unit refers to the cirrhotic regenerative nodule or to the lobule in the precirrhotic liver. In early cirrhosis these nodules are always small and ill defined. Large nodules may arise with progression of disease; their size is determined by (1) the density of the surrounding connective tissue, (2) the amount of continuing destruction and collagen deposition within the nodules, and last (3) the stimulus to regeneration.

Since the terminology for chronic liver disease includes precirrhotic as well as cirrhotic livers, (1) *normolobular* describes the livers with the least distortion and smooth capsular surfaces, prior to development of cirrhosis (Plate 4, *B*); (2) *granular* describes those in which there is early, regular fibrosis in either or both central and portal areas resulting in a hepatic surface that resembles sandstone, also precirrhotic (Fig. 31-25). Cirrhotic liver nodules are (3) *fine*—nodules under 0.3 cm (Plate 4, *D*), (4) *coarse*—nodules 0.3 to 0.8 cm, or (5) *megalonodular,* if over 0.8 cm (Plate 4, *E*).

Integrity of regenerative or lobular units. The integrity of the regenerative nodules is better correlated with etiology than is nodular size. The regenerative units are characterized as (1) nodular, if they bulge greatly on the capsular and cut surfaces, (2) insular, if they appear as slightly raised discs embedded in dense collagen on cut surface (Fig. 31-21), (3) pseudolobular, if the margins are ill defined by fibrosis and the cut surface of the liver resembles pancreas or salivary gland (Plate 4, *E*). In the past the term *pseudolobule* has been used interchangeably with *nodule.* However the truly *nodular* liver does not have the appearance of the cut surface of a lobulated organ, but the cut surface of some cirrhotic livers with poorly defined regenerative units does. This is particularly true of alcoholic cirrhosis. The poorly defined margin indicates the amount of collagen invading the substance of the nodule.

Disease. The definition of cirrhosis as proposed in 1956, required the presence of nodules. However, many patients who have only severe fibrosis exhibit the clinical and hemodynamic features of cirrhosis. Examples include many stages of alcoholic liver disease, the early stages of primary biliary cirrhosis, and the earlier stage of Banti's disease. Thus livers may be classified as "cirrhotic" when there is architectural distortion by regenerative units, "precirrhotic" when there is fibrosis only, and "liver disease" when there has been no morphologic study. The precirrhotic stage may be more specifically characterized. Thus a diagnosis may be "alcoholic *fatty liver and fibrosis* with hepatic failure."

Function

The functional status of the liver as measured by the clinical laboratory and morphologic parameters may be included in the pathologic evaluation as "with hepatic failure," "with cholestasis," "with focal alcoholic hyalin," "with activity," "quiescent," or other appropriate terms.

Alcoholic liver disease

On a worldwide basis, the most common type of cirrhosis that has been described has had a multitude of names. Among these are alcoholic cirrhosis, portal cirrhosis, diffuse cirrhosis, nutritional cirrhosis, septal cirrhosis, and hobnail cirrhosis. One term that has had particularly widespread usage is "Laennec's cirrhosis." It is impossible for any author to know exactly how the last term is used in various geographic regions. There may be considerable variation, depending on the morphologic criteria used by individual pathologists in various countries. Whereas most references in the past to "Laennec's cirrhosis" have applied to cirrhosis in the alcoholic, many pathologists in using the designation "Laennec's cirrhosis" have been referring to an ill-defined morphologic pattern since the description of the liver mentioned by Laennec was extremely meager. The most common type of cirrhosis seen in the United States occurs in the alcoholic patient; we have come to use the term *alcoholic cirrhosis* to indicate this background. This is not to imply that alcohol is the sole etiologic agent in the production of the cirrhosis in the alcoholic but that it is the most consistent single factor yet identified.

Alcoholism, incidence, and disease

The reported autopsy incidence of cirrhosis varies between 1% and 10% throughout most of the world. In various centers in the United States, it has varied from 1.6% to 11%. The age range of patients with alcoholic cirrhosis varies from 12 years to senility, but the peak incidence is in middle life (50 to 55 years), with most patients between 40 and 65 years of age. Alcoholic cirrhosis affects men more frequently than women. In women the peak age incidence is about a decade earlier than in men. In the Los Angeles County–University of Southern California Medical Center in 1970, at a time that 25% of underlying causes of death were from alcoholism, the frequency of cirrhosis at autopsy was 11%, principally of the alcoholic type. The highest frequency was among Mexican-American and other white

men over 20 years old, 25% and 18%, respectively.

Alcoholic cirrhosis follows the long-continued consumption of ethanol. The epidemiologic evidence indicates that the mortality from cirrhosis is directly related to the per capita consumption of ethanol from wine and spirits.[430] In India, Africa, and certain other parts of the world in which cirrhosis is common, alcoholism is not etiologically important. A relationship between alcoholism and cirrhosis is unquestionable, but the exact mechanism of its injurious effect is not known. It would appear that the development of cirrhosis in the alcoholic patient has some relationship to three factors at least:

1. Susceptibility to hepatic injury, which varies among alcoholics, with the often-quoted figure of 8% of all alcoholics developing cirrhosis being probably too low[353,359]
2. Amount of ethanol consumed daily and the duration of excessive consumption
3. Degree and duration of malnutrition, particularly of protein containing the essential amino acids

It is difficult to define chronic alcoholism other than to say that the individual drinks to such excess that he is incapable of leading a normal existence, primarily from the social and economic standpoints. The basis for this is the individual's loss of control for ethanol consumption. Among patients with cirrhosis, a history of excessive use of alcohol has been found in 30% to 92% in various series in the United States. At the Los Angeles County–University of Southern California Medical Center, more than 900 new patients with cirrhosis are seen annually. About 90% of these have a history of 5 to 15 years of heavy consumption of alcohol. Many consume as much as a quart of whiskey or a gallon of wine per day. In addition to steady drinking, most patients will periodically drink excessively for 1 or 2 weeks, during which time they eat little or no food. These bouts often terminate in an attack of jaundice, pneumonia, pancreatitis, or delirium tremens.

Ethanol metabolism

After ingestion and absorption, ethanol is distributed in the water space of the body. The rate of metabolism is constant and is decreased by fasting and increased by fructose, chronic ethanol ingestion, and certain drugs. Various parameters have been examined for their influence on the rate of metabolism; however the

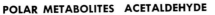

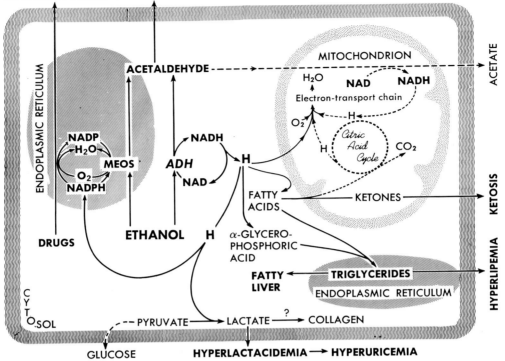

Fig. 31-22. Effects of oxidation of ethanol on intermediary metabolism in liver. *Broken lines,* Pathways inhibited by ethanol. Coupling of oxidation of ethanol with reduction of oxalo-acetate is hypothetical. (From Lieber, C. S.: J.A.M.A. **233:**1080, 1975.)

rate of metabolism is higher in small animals. Therefore experimental studies of the pathway and rates of ethanol metabolism must be compared cautiously with the proposed pathways in humans. Within 24 hours, 90% of the ingested ethanol is oxidized to carbon dioxide and a small amount (5% to 10%) is excreted unchanged by the lungs and kidneys. More than 90% of the ethanol metabolism occurs in the liver where it is oxidized to acetate, and up to 75% of the splanchnic oxygen supply is required for the conversion of ethanol to acetate. Studies in humans indicate that 50% to 100% of the ethanol entering the liver may appear in the hepatic venous outflow as acetate.[373]

The major pathway for hepatic ethanol oxidization is shown in Fig. 31-22 (of Lieber). The enzyme alcohol dehydrogenase (ADH) is present in sufficient activity to account for the maximal rate of ethanol metabolism. Because the enzyme ADH has a wide range of substrates, the physiologic role of the enzyme has been debated. The finding of measurable levels of ethanol in the portal blood of non-

drinking rats supported the concept that the primary function of ADH was for ethanol oxidation.[362] As ethanol is oxidized to acetaldehyde by ADH, the cofactor NAD is reduced to NADH. The same cofactor is reduced in the second step where it is catalyzed by the enzyme acetaldehyde dehydrogenase (AcDH). The sharp change in the NAD/NADH ratio is the fundamental biochemical alteration that may be related to many of the metabolic changes during ethanol metabolism. The rate-limiting step in ethanol metabolism by ADH is the regeneration of NAD, and the faster metabolic rate in certain situations is related to increased regeneration of NAD. Alternate pathways for ethanol oxidation are the "microsomal ethanol-oxidizing system" (MEOS), which is associated with the microsomes, and the coupled catalase system, which is associated with the peroxisomes.[369] The oxidation of ethanol by a microsomal system has been controversial for several years and the purification of the enzyme system may be confirmed in several laboratories in the near future. The microsomal system is attractive theoretically because it provides a biochemical mechanism to explain the enhanced rate of ethanol oxidization in subjects on long-term enthanol ingestion. Furthermore, ultrastructural studies of the hepatocytes from chronic alcoholics show hypertrophy of the smooth endoplasmic reticulum. However, other investigators with elaborate ultrastructural morphologic evaluations dispute this finding of increased smooth endoplasmic reticulum.[324] The physiologic role of MEOS seems small in the normal nondrinking person, but it may play some role in the metabolic adaptation seen in the chronic alcoholic person.

The site of ethanol metabolism may be important in the understanding of ethanol hepatotoxicity. Alcohol dehydrogenase does not have a uniform distribution within the hepatic lobule. Studies based on microdissection indicate that the predominant activity of ADH is in the central vein area, whereas other techniques indicate the larger amount to be in the periportal regions. Alcohol dehydrogenase and acetaldehyde dehydrogenase have several isoenzyme forms, which vary with age, species, and drug treatments, and these factors may also influence hepatotoxicity.

The molecular mechanism for ethanol toxicity may be related to (1) inhibition of the Na/K ATPase by ethanol producing the hydropic change, (2) immunologic injury with production of antibody to alcoholic hyalin, (3) increased fibrogenesis induced by the direct stimulation of fibroblasts by ethanol, (4) membrane damage from lipoperoxidation by· the free radicals that may be formed during ethanol metabolism. There is evidence for all of these mechanisms. Fatty change may occur with very mild social drinking, but functional impairment associated with mild fatty liver is rarely apparent. Whereas several mechanisms for ethanol-induced fatty liver have been proposed, recent analysis challenges several of these interpretations.[344] A major advance in the study of ethanol hepatotoxicity was the production of the morphologic lesion of acute and chronic alcoholic liver disease in baboons on an alcoholic diet supplemented with adequate nutritional factors.[414] Therefore ethanol and its metabolites may produce cellular damage, but deficient diet is not required for liver injury in the chronic alcoholic. It still remains possible that the effect of alcohol at the cellular level may be nutritional. This possibility is raised by the observation that hepatic disease that occasionally occurs after jejunoileal bypass is indistinguishable from alcoholic liver disease.[395]

Pathogenesis

The chronic use of ethanol may produce morphologic changes in the liver that are characteristic and allow a presumptive diagnosis to be made on these grounds alone. The study of a large number of biopsies, many of them taken serially, in conjunction with the study of autopsy material has disclosed a number of microscopic features of liver disease in the alcoholic that are helpful in explaining the clinical findings as well as the histogenesis of cirrhosis. In recent years, the term *alcoholic liver disease* has been used for all of the changes that occur, beginning with the earliest seen on needle biopsy and continuing to the end stage of cirrhosis.

Although, broadly speaking, three stages may be recognized—presymptomatic, acute liver disease or "alcoholic hepatitis," and chronic liver disease, which is usually cirrhosis—these may merge one into the other. Furthermore, acute changes sometimes are superimposed upon chronic liver disease. Biopsies and autopsies disclose that the disease often progresses through each of the first two stages before cirrhosis occurs. However, some alcoholic patients are symptomless until the advanced stage of cirrhosis is reached. In this latter group, the various steps leading to cirrhosis are unknown, but are presumed to be similar but less severe than those below, allowing the patient to live to a more advanced stage without occurrence of the clinical features of acute alcoholic liver disease.

Presymptomatic stage. In the presymptomatic stage before liver disease is manifest, the first discernible alterations may appear after a few years of heavy drinking. The patient may be seen by the physician or be hospitalized for any one of several conditions often seen in the alcoholic. These include delirium tremens, nausea and vomiting, trauma, acute infection, and alcoholic pancreatitis. The liver in presymptomatic disease often is enlarged but not to an unusual degree. Hepatic abnormalities include a mild rise in SGOT levels and BSP retention. In a biopsy study of this group,[330] it was noted that fatty vacuolization and hydropic change are the most common abnormalities, having been noted in 95% of biopsies. In addition, a mild but definite increase of connective tissue often thickens the walls of the central veins and centrilobular sinusoids. In an occasional patient, minute foci of hyaline necrosis and sinusoidal sclerosis occur. Most patients entered the hospital because of delirium tremens or nausea and vomiting. They had been drinking excessively for many years, and many had eaten poorly or not at all for short periods before entry.

The time interval between the onset of heavy drinking and microscopic abnormalities in the liver is not known. Alcohol given to young nonalcoholic volunteers produced fatty vacuolation in two days.[413] However, the fat was uniformly distributed throughout the lobule, and droplets were relatively small (usually from 5 to 15 μm) and different from the fat deposition of symptomatic stages of alcoholic liver disease.

Acute alcoholic liver disease. It is difficult to predict when the disease in an alcoholic whose biopsy shows the early changes just described will progress to the point at which symptoms of acute liver disease develop. These symptoms differ somewhat, depending on the morphologic abnormalities in the liver. Most commonly, however, the patient has a more or less sudden onset of jaundice that often is accompanied by fever. In the literature, these patients have been described as having "alcoholic hepatitis." A liver biopsy usually discloses one of three structural changes, each of which may be rather complex: (1) fatty liver with cholestasis, (2) fatty liver that undergoes a lytic type of necrosis, and (3) liver that undergoes sclerosing hyaline necrosis. There may be some overlap between the three types.

The simplest microscopic change is a fatty liver with cholestasis. A mild thickening of sinusoidal and central vein walls is common, but little or no increase of portal connective tissue is seen. Upon hospitalization, the patients usually recover in a period of a few weeks. It is remarkable how rapidly a large fatty liver shrinks when the patient partakes of an adequate diet and abstains from alcohol. In addition to hyperbilirubinemia, the hepatic tests usually show a moderate rise in alkaline phosphatase levels.

The second microscopic change in acute alcoholic liver disease is a fatty liver that undergoes a lytic type of necrosis. The lytic foci are usually centrilobular and devoid of inflammatory exudate. Cholestasis, bile staining of cytoplasm, and bile in Kupffer cells are uniformly present. Some of the patients become critically ill and may die in hepatic coma. At autopsy, the liver is hypertrophic, weighing as much as 5000 gm, and the capsule is smooth and usually tautly stretched about bulging fatty icteric parenchyma although, if lytic necrosis is sufficiently severe, the liver will be limp and soft as in other conditions in which there has been hepatocellular destruction. In such instances of severe necrosis, there is centrilobular depression and deep bile staining. Microscopically, the bloated hydropic centrilobular hepatocytes appear autolyzed; they are usually foamy. Those toward the periphery are filled with a large single fat globule. Upon the patient's admission to the hospital, the laboratory findings are similar to those in the patients with fatty liver with cholestasis except that the SGOT level may reach 300 units and the SGPT remains normal. The prothrombin activity may be decreased to the range of 20%.

For the third type of microscopic change in acute alcoholic liver disease, we use the term *sclerosing hyaline necrosis.*[330,403] In sclerosing hyaline necrosis, the centrilobular cells undergo hydropic and hyaline change that precedes necrosis. This change is most striking in a liver with few fat vacuoles, although fatty livers are not spared. The hyalin first appears as clumps in the cytoplasm and then as large masses that often have an eccentric location in the cell (Plate 3, *D*). Often, there are many neutrophils in the sinusoids around the necrotic cells. They may even penetrate the cytoplasm of the cell and possibly assist in its liquefaction. The latter appears to be a slow process. Various stages in the progression of hyaline necrosis are seen in the liver at any one time. A remarkable increase of collagen occurs in the centrilobular areas (Fig. 31-23). This is associated with increased numbers of cells that appear to be derived from Kupffer cells and function as fibroblasts. The increased connective tissue leads to obliteration of many of the central sinusoids and veins. The changes in sclerosing hyaline necrosis may be so severe that death ensues, but many patients recover. The necrotic cells finally disappear, the connective tissue condenses, and, although the regenerative response is poor, the remaining cells in the altered lobules resume their functions. In the acute phase, the patients often have jaundice, ascites, abdominal pain, and an exceptional neutrophilic leukocytosis.[331] Hyaline bodies when studied ultrastructurally do not have a limiting membrane and contain many filaments having an appearance of "twisted rope."[388] Branching and tubular microfilaments have been recognized. Electrophoretic studies of the isolated and homog-

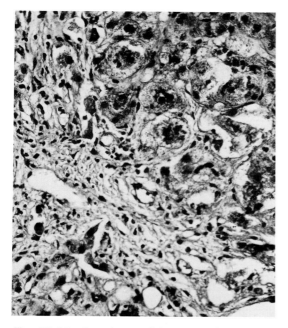

Fig. 31-23. Cytoplasm of hepatic cells contains eosinophilic granular material, so-called alcoholic hyalin. Cells appear swollen, and cell borders are indistinguishable. Sclerosis of vascular walls has begun. Needle biopsy of liver of 42-year-old Indian, chronic alcoholic who had been on long drinking spree before entering hospital.

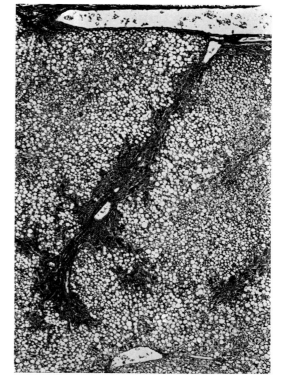

Fig. 31-24. Early stage of cirrhosis in fatty liver of alcoholic. Fibrosis and bile duct proliferation can be seen along terminal branch of portal tree. Irregular manner in which connective tissue invades periphery of lobules clearly shown. Little change around sublobular and central vein at bottom.

enized hyaline bodies show several bands identical with protein bands in normal liver.

Precirrhotic chronic alcoholic liver disease. As the *early changes of alcoholic liver disease* evolve toward cirrhosis, three different patterns are recognizable. In the first pattern, the fatty liver still has its lobular pattern, there is little or no centrilobular injury, but the portal tracts may have an increase in amount and density of connective tissue and bile duct proliferation. The widened portal area assumes an arachnoid configuration as the limiting plate disappears. Irregular prolongation of the portal connective tissue encroaches upon the periphery of the lobules and may extend directly along the sinusoids (Fig. 31-24). This may result in a pure portal fibrosis, with little or no necrosis, nor necessarily any regenerative nodules. In early cirrhosis some features are similar to fatty change alone. The liver is always hypertrophic, sometimes weighing as much as 2000 to 5000 gm. The capsule has finely granular regular areas of retraction and is unthickened but taut. The liver is yellow with fat or is yellow green with bile and fat. Even before true cirrhosis is present, there is slightly to moderately in-

creased resistance upon cutting to a degree that would be characterized as *firm*. The bulging parenchyma is greasy, and thin sections of the liver float in water. The lobules are enlarged, and the central veins may be indistinct.

In the second type, centrilobular fibrosis is the major hepatic change. Portal fibrosis is minor. We call the lesion *chronic sclerosing hyaline disease*. This disorder usually represents a sequela of acute sclerosing hyaline necrosis in which the necrosis and inflammatory reaction has subsided, but the fibrous tissue obstructing the venous outflow tract at the level of the central veins and sublobular veins becomes condensed (Fig. 31-25, *A*). Patients with the chronic sclerosing disease have an indolent clinical course characterized by muscle wasting and resistant ascites and frequently by functional renal failure. Wedged hepatic vein pressure is nearly always elevated.[407] At autopsy, the liver may be *eutrophic*

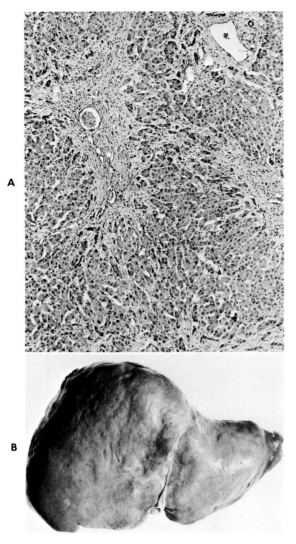

Fig. 31-25. Chronic sclerosing hyaline disease with eutrophic, hard, granular precirrhotic pattern. **A,** Fibrous destruction of centrilobular areas and slight widening of portal areas. **B,** Surface has sandstone appearance.

or atrophic but has a smooth or fine sandstone-like thickened capsule that encloses a tough hard liver parenchyma (Fig. 31-25).

In a third pattern found in most patients with alcoholic liver disease, there is both a centrilobular and a portal component, and both fatty change and centrilobular sclerosis are observed. The lobular pattern is altered, small regenerative nodules are seen, and communicating septa may connect centrilobular and portal areas. This stage is called *alcoholic fatty liver with central and portal fibrosis.* Should the patient discontinue alcohol consumption,

the fat will disappear in about 3 months but the fibrosis will remain.

Cirrhosis. Although there are all degrees of severity in the cirrhotic process, the next step in progression may be called *cirrhosis.* The morphologic pattern that develops in the alcoholic is a result of the continual encroachment of collagen fibers into regenerating nodules that proliferate most exuberantly during periods of improved nutrition and cessation of alcoholic intake. The outcome is a cirrhotic liver usually made up of poorly defined irregularly sized nodules with thin collagen fibers insinuated between the hepatocytes. In this early stage, the liver is hypertrophic, weighs 2000 to 4000 gm, and has a firm rubbery quality. It is more resistant to cutting, and the fibrous septa delineate fairly uniform-sized nodules 1 to 2 mm in diameter. As the cirrhosis progresses to the moderate stage, one or more areas of dense scarring may develop. The scars are irregular in configuration and are usually about 1.5 cm in greatest dimension. At the margin of the scars, the pseudolobules are smaller than those in liver remote from the scar. Near the center of the scar the pseudolobules are absent. The pathogenesis of these scars is unknown; the area most frequently involved is in a line between the gallbladder bed and the hepatic vein orifices, a less vascular area in that the line drawn between these structures represents the boundary separating the true median portion of left lobe from the true right lobe. Often the scarring results in a U-shaped area of retraction of the capsule over the dome of the liver. In alcoholic cirrhosis severe obliterative change along the hepatic venous outflow tract is noted in nearly all cases. The central veins have disappeared or are in the process of obliteration (Fig. 31-26). The small hepatic veins (sublobular veins) are severely damaged, and even larger veins are sclerosed in some areas, particularly where there is gross scarring. The vascular sclerosis probably occurs after earlier subclinical attacks of sclerosing hyaline necrosis, although a milder degree of connective tissue proliferation about hepatic venous tributaries does occur in fatty livers in which there has been no demonstrable sclerosing hyaline necrosis. There are no lobules with a normal pattern. Instead, arachnoid connective tissue septa now surround and invade pseudolobules of variable size. Regeneration occurs in some portions of the liver, and this further distorts the normal architecture so that the hepatic and portal veins may come to occupy positions near one another in

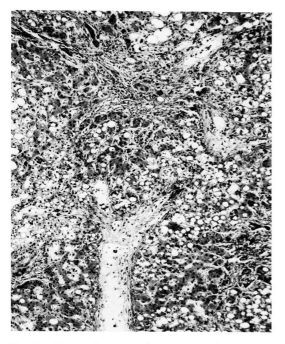

Fig. 31-26. Moderate cirrhosis. Fatty change and early obliteration of central and subhepatic veins. Granular fatty liver of 25-year-old male Mexican with history of chronic alcoholism.

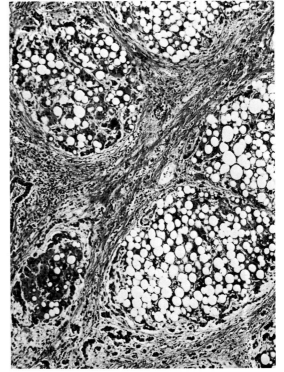

Fig. 31-27. Advanced stage of cirrhosis in 49-year-old white woman, known alcoholic for many years. Increase of connective tissue forms septa that subdivide liver into many small pseudolobules. Patient died in hepatic coma. Portacaval shunt done 1 year before death, but patient continued to drink excessively.

the fibrous septa. Infiltration with round cells and, occasionally, neutrophils may occur in the septa. Fatty change is usually found in the early stages of alcoholic cirrhosis; however if alcoholism is discontinued at any stage, the fat is diminished and parenchymal regeneration becomes prominent, resulting in the formation of larger, more discrete regenerative nodules.

In the histogenesis of moderately advanced stages of cirrhosis, there is both portal and centrilobular sclerosis. Attacks of necrosis may result in subdivision of preexisting nodules. The necrosis in turn acts as a stimulus to further regeneration and larger nodules form, particularly if there is cessation of alcoholic intake for awhile. The patients who die in this stage of cirrhosis die most often in hepatic coma but may also succumb to bleeding or intercurrent infection, especially pneumonia.

In the advanced stage of alcoholic cirrhosis, the liver is *atrophic,* usually being between 800 and 1200 gm. The nodules are usually more well defined (nodular or insular) and are often between 1 and 4 mm in diameter (finely or coarsely), but occasionally individual nodules may be as large as 1 cm. The capsular surface is deformed by the projecting nodules (Plate

4, *C*). The liver is resistant to cutting, and, after sectioning, the characteristic yellow mahogany-brown nodules are sharply outlined and appear as though they have been embedded in the pale gray bands of connective tissue (Plate 4, *D*). In some irregular areas, there may be complete absence of parenchymal tissue. On microscopic examination, the liver is composed entirely of pseudolobules and wide bands of connective tissue (Fig. 31-27). Much of the outflow tract is obliterated, especially its smaller radicles. The larger and thick-walled hepatic veins that remain may be near some of the larger portal triads, the two being separated only by the connective tissue bands. Most often the cirrhosis would be characterized as *atrophic sclerotic finely insular alcoholic cirrhosis.*

There is usually diminution or absence of fat in the atrophic stage. The collagenous connective tissue is dense, but there may be small foci of hyaline necrosis, usually without inflammatory exudate or sclerosis of sinusoids. Focal areas of cholestasis secondary to loss of communication between the regenerative nodules and functioning bile ducts may be observed. Often the liver cells in the hyperplastic nodules have abnormally large hyperchromic nuclei or even two nuclei. The cells in areas of recent regeneration lack any lipochromic pigment. In the atrophic stage, the cord pattern usually becomes reestablished and regular within the nodules; apparently the stimulus for or the response to regeneration has abated. Occasionally, in quiescent alcoholic cirrhosis, adenomatous hyperplasia occurs, and the scattered adenomatous nodules are two or three times larger than their neighbors and are dark brown. Since such nodules are more common in those patients who have a hepatocellular carcinoma elsewhere, it is possible that the adenomatous nodules are preneoplastic.

After surgery for a portacaval anastomosis, many patients will abstain from further use of ethanol, and a biopsy taken at the time of surgery may be compared with autopsy material many years later. There is usually considerable improvement or at least an increase in regenerative activity at the expense of the connective tissue septa, which, after revascularization, have become thinner and less cellular. The liver is often atrophic, hard, and coarsely nodular. The portal lymphatics are less prominent, and the liver cells in the pseudolobules often are normal in appearance, and liver cords become reestablished.

In some alcoholic patients, the first symptoms may not develop until the advanced stage of atrophic cirrhosis. There may be nothing in the history to indicate that the patient ever had a large fatty liver with an attack of jaundice that would indicate necrosis of liver cells. It would seem that in some such individuals, the cirrhotic process many progress through various stages of severity to the atrophic and coarsely nodular liver with little or no fat demonstrable on biopsy. The quantitative aspects of alcohol consumption and malnutrition may well determine whether fibrosis and pseudolobules occur with or without fatty changes. Certainly in the presence of severe fatty change, the sequence of necrosis of hepatic cells, jaundice, and coma is more likely to develop. Also alcoholic patients who develop fatal infections, pancreatitis, and delirium tremens seem to have fatty liver more often than not.

It has been shown by injection-corrosion casts of normal and cirrhotic livers that in cirrhosis there is an enlargement of the hepatic arteries and the arterial bed, with an increased number of communications between the hepatic arteries and portal veins.[345] The portal and hepatic venous systems are reduced in size, the change being much more severe on the hepatic vein side. The reduction of venous systems often is associated with fibrosis. Anastomotic channels occasionally are seen between portal and hepatic veins, but no significant differences were observed in the vascular pattern of alcoholic liver disease when compared with that of coarsely nodular cryptogenic cirrhosis.

In the advanced stages of alcoholic cirrhosis, portal hypertension with variceal bleeding, hepatic failure with encephalopathy, and functional renal failure are the most common causes of death. An increased frequency of peptic ulcer also occurs in these patients, and bleeding from this source must always be considered. In some patients, ascites may become chronic and resistant to treatment, whereas in others the ascites is easily controlled or spontaneously disappears. Hepatic encephalopathy is easily precipitated by hemorrhage, infection, or further insults to the liver.

Viral, lupoid, toxic, and cryptogenic cirrhosis

Viral, lupoid, toxic, and cryptogenic cirrhosis may be considered together because of similarity in morphology and pathogenesis, despite probable differences in etiology. All appear to have their genesis in chronic active hepatitis, often so mild that symptoms of repeated attacks are absent. Occasional patients remain well during life, but cirrhosis is unexpectedly found at autopsy. The cirrhosis arises in response to intermittent bouts of hepatocellular destruction, usually followed by a period in which destruction becomes relatively quiescent and hepatocellular regeneration takes place. In contrast to alcoholic liver disease, deposition of dense, hard collagen is not the rule, instead the fibrous septa are composed of loosely arranged stroma. Although a former term for this type of cirrhosis was "postnecrotic" cirrhosis, there is no evidence that a single episode of submassive necrosis ever leads to cirrhosis.[164] Conversely, only occasionally is there a history of viral hepatitis prior to signs of chronic liver disease, and submassive or severe clinical disease as an antecedent event is nonexistent in our experience. The liver at the advanced stage is atrophic (500 to 1000 gm), often limp and distorted by coarsely nodular

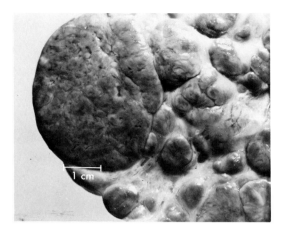

Fig. 31-28. Cut surface of atrophic, firm, megalo-nodular B-viral cirrhosis.

or megalonodular cirrhosis (Fig. 31-28 and Plate 4, *E*). In the early stages when the patient is asymptomatic, the liver may be *eutrophic, firm, finely granular, and precirrhotic.* Microscopically, there may be considerable variation in the amount of chronic inflammation, continuing necrosis, and the rate at which cirrhosis develops (Fig. 31-29).

Viral cirrhosis type B. Chronic active viral hepatitis type B leads inexorably to a soft coarsely nodular or megalonodular cirrhosis. When viewed by peritoneoscopy in the early stages, the liver may appear firm, granular, and normolobular. Viral cirrhosis type B accounts for 41% of the patients who died of soft macronodular or megalonodular nonalcoholic cirrhosis at the University of Southern California Liver Unit since 1969 (see p. 1335). It appears that a firm megalonodular cirrhosis viral type B is the leading type of cirrhosis in Africa and in the Orient. (In the United States alcoholic cirrhosis is much more common.) Widespread HBsAg testing should lead to statistical data that will give some measure of the temporal relationship between events that might have disseminated HBV compared with peaks of occurrences of B-viral cirrhosis as well as hepatocellular carcinoma (e.g., widespread use of pooled plasma, drug use in the 1960s and 1970s). B-viral cirrhosis appears to be one of the most common precursors of hepatocellular carcinoma.

Viral cirrhosis, NAB. Little information is available regarding cirrhosis that occurs after non-A non-B hepatitis, but occasionally a patient develops NAB hepatitis after a blood transfusion that progresses rapidly to cirrhosis. How frequently this occurs is uncertain. The

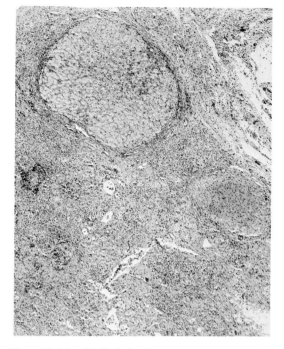

Fig. 31-29. Well-defined regenerative nodule amid collapsed inflamed stroma in coarsely nodular cryptogenic cirrhosis.

diagnosis can only be made when the disease has been traced from the inoculation through an intermediate incubation (about 45 days) to development of hepatitis to cirrhosis.

Lupoid cirrhosis. Lupoid cirrhosis is morphologically indistinguishable from B-viral cirrhosis. However, the disease usually occurs in women who have unusually high globulin levels, amenorrhea, and several serologic abnormalities such as positive lupus erythematosus preparations, smooth muscle antibodies, and, less consistently, false-positive serologic tests for syphilis and antinuclear antibodies. Hepatocellular carcinoma has not been reported as a complication of lupoid cirrhosis.

Toxic cirrhosis. Most drugs and toxins that adversely affect the liver do so by producing cholestasis, hepatocellular necrosis, or a combination of both. Those drugs producing submassive necrosis may result in lesions that, at certain stages, microscopically resemble cirrhosis but that are not truly nodular. Thus it seems a requirement that there be continual or repeated exposure to a drug that produces a minimal type of hepatocellular necrosis similar in extent to that seen in chronic active viral hepatitis. The drug oxyphenisatin may produce chronic active hepatitis that results in cirrhosis. It is uncertain whether the necrosis that occurs occasionally with methyldopa and with isoniazid and halothane may be minimal enough to allow prolonged continual use of the drug and development of true cirrhosis, but cases of chronic active hepatitis are reported after each.[271,381] Discontinuance of the affending drug stops the progression of the liver disease. How much reversal of the cirrhotic process can occur is uncertain.

Cryptogenic cirrhosis. The category of *cryptogenic cirrhosis* includes hepatic disorders of diverse causes, many of which are similar to the foregoing group. Some livers that ordinarily would be included in this group have been shown to have HBsAg demonstrable in hepatocyte cytoplasm by immunoperoxidase staining, whereas repeated serum testing for HBsAg by radioimmunoassay has been negative.[19] It is possible that excess HBsAg is not always produced in HBV infection. Thus many cirrhoses could be viral type B without serologic confirmation. Since CAVH-B patients have some tissue immunity to HBV, it is possible although not yet proved that some patients may recover from their HBV infection but retain residual inactive cirrhosis.

There is evidence that posttransfusion VH-NAB may occasionally result in cirrhosis. Thus viral hepatitis other than VH-B may be to blame for many cases of "cryptogenic cirrhosis." There is little or no evidence to suggest the development of cirrhosis after either clinically evident or subclinical hepatitis A, but no detailed serologic studies for anti-HAV have been undertaken on a significant number of patients with cryptogenic cirrhosis.

Patients with *alcoholic liver disease* who discontinue their alcoholic consumption will revascularize the dense hepatic collagen, allowing the pseudolobules to enlarge into well-demarcated bulging nodules. Such livers have been classified as "postnecrotic" in the past.[412] The reticence of many patients to admit alcoholism is well known and the disease in these patients is often erroneously classified as cryptogenic cirrhosis.

The possibility that cryptogenic cirrhosis may be attributable to drugs is important, since the prognosis of the liver disease is more favorable than in other kinds of cirrhosis if the offending agent is discontinued. In countries such as Africa the importance of fungal and plant toxoids in the production of the coarsely nodular and megalonodular cryptogenic cirrhosis is still unsettled. There may be other types of chronic liver disease that terminate with coarse nodules, but without a prior biopsy the antecedent disease cannot be identified.

Hemochromatotic cirrhosis

The liver is a major participant in the metabolism of iron as it stores the metal and also synthesizes transferrin, an iron-binding protein necessary for the transport of iron. Normally, the body contains 3 to 4.5 gm of iron, most of which is present in hemoglobin. The amount of iron absorbed daily is regulated through the intestinal mucosa so that in general increased blood loss results in increased absorption. The absorption is a stepwise process in which the rate-limiting step is the transfer of iron from the mucosal cell to plasma. This transfer is apparently controlled by luminal, humoral, and storage factors and requires oxidation of ferrous to ferric stage, a step catalyzed by ceruloplasmin.[341] Increased absorption follows an increase in iron presented to the mucosal surface and, also, by adding appropriate saccharides to make the iron more available. However, normal gastric secretions contain a substance that binds iron, reducing its absorption.[323] Absorption may also be diminished by increasing the amount of combining or chelating substances in the intestine. Pancreatic secretions reduce iron absorption.[322] A high-protein diet diminishes iron absorption if iron is administered with the protein.[318] After absorption, iron is transported by transferrin, an iron-binding protein synthesized by hepatocytes. The latter cells also have a limited capacity to store iron as ferritin. When this capacity is exceeded, the iron is stored in lysosomes in the form of large aggregates of hemosiderin. The iron leaves the liver cells when needed for hemoglobin synthesis, again attached to transferrin. Iron also may leave the liver by another avenue, for it has been shown that it can be excreted in the bile.[314] In addition to the role of the hepatocyte in iron metabolism, the sinusoidal lining cells, being part of the reticuloendothelial system, break down senescent erythrocytes, thus preserving the iron for reuse by the bone marrow.

Iron absorbed in excess of capacity for utilization by heme-forming tissue is deposited primarily in the hepatocyte, whereas iron in excess of need derived from destruction of erythrocytes or iron-containing cells is deposited in the reticuloendothelial system. In conditions such as a chronic hemolytic anemia, there is both parenchymal iron from increased iron absorption and reticuloendothelial iron from hemolysis.

Hemochromatosis is a condition whereby great quantities of hemosiderin in hepatocytes is associated with tissue fibrosis and cirrhosis. When there is no recognizable cause for in-

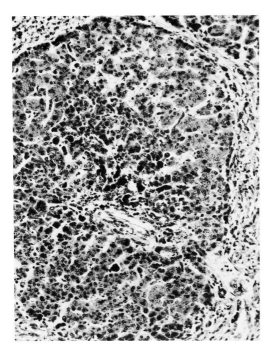

Fig. 31-30. Idiopathic hemochromatosis with pigmentary cirrhosis (54-year-old white man who died of primary carcinoma of liver). Liver cells and Kupffer cells contain fine granules of hemosiderin. In area of recent necrosis near center, histiocytes are filled with hemosiderin.

crease in iron absorption, the condition is referred to as *idiopathic hemochromatosis* (Fig. 31-30). When a cause, such as chronic anemia or prolonged ingestion of iron compounds can be identified, the condition is called *secondary* hemochromatosis. The deposition of hemosiderin in parenchymal or Kupffer cells in the absence of tissue fibrosis is called parenchymal or reticuloendothelial *hemosiderosis* respectively.

Idiopathic hemochromatosis is an inheritable disorder characterized by excessive iron absorption and deposition in certain organs, associated with damage and malfunction of the involved organs. The liver is cirrhotic, and pancreatic deposition results in diabetes. Other tissues that frequently have striking iron deposits and associated dysfunction include myocardial fibers, gastric mucosa, endocrine epithelium, and testes. The classical clinical triad is hepatomegaly, diabetes, and skin pigmentation, but often the patient may complain of impotence, easy fatigability, or signs of heart failure. Signs or symptoms of hepatic failure or portal hypertension are not the usual presenting features.

The reasons for the increased absorption that results in idiopathic hemochromatosis are not known although many hypotheses have been advanced.[341] These vary from abnormal luminal secretions and mucosal cell function to aberrant reticuloendothelial system function. Studies of families with the disease indicate two modes of inheritance. In the first of these, where there is evidence of an autosomal dominant type of inheritance, the males outnumber females 10 to 1 and the onset of symptoms is usually between 40 and 50 years of age. In the second, or presumed, autosomal recessive type, the distribution of males to females is equal. The parents show no evidence of disease and the onset of disease is usually seen in the late teens or early twenties.[410]

In one study of the relatives of patients with idiopathic hemochromatosis, it was found that many of them had excess hepatic iron, whereas the families of those with alcoholic cirrhosis did not have such findings.[397]

Ionic iron does not appear in the serum. Instead, 2 molecules of ferric iron are bound to 1 molecule of a carrier protein, transferrin. Normally, excess transferrin is present. Only one third is combined with iron. The remainder is unbound. In hemochromatosis, the transferrin levels may be unchanged, but the degree of saturation or binding is usually nearly 100%.

Patients with chronic anemia also may have increased iron absorption and saturated iron-binding capacity. Recently serum ferritin levels have been found to be greatly increased in untreated patients with idiopathic hemochromatosis.[400] Isoferritins in the heart, pancreas, and kidney are different from those in normal controls.[398]

A number of cases of fairly rapid storage of iron in the liver have been observed after portacaval shunts in patients with cirrhosis of the liver.[341,342] A similar increase has been demonstrated in experimental animals after shunt surgery.[325]

Pathology

Grossly, early in idiopathic hemochromatosis the external surface of the liver may be smooth, but as cirrhosis develops it becomes granular, less often nodular. The weight varies from 1 to 3 kg. On sectioning, the liver has a dark rusty brown appearance. At necropsy, it is rewarding to use the Prussian blue test on all livers that are excessively brown. On analysis, the liver in hemochromatosis contains between 1 and 10 gm of iron per 100 gm of liver, dry weight. This is compared with a normal figure of 0.188 gm or less.[316] A quantitative determination of iron may be done on a biopsy specimen of the liver.[304] This test uniformly discloses far more iron than is found in alcoholic cirrhosis. In addition to iron, excess quantities of lead, molybdenum, and copper are present.[315]

Microscopically, early in the disease there may be a uniform distribution of hemosiderin (iron-containing pigment) within the liver cells and Kupffer cells without fibrosis. Ordinarily, however, there is a variable degree of proliferation of fibrous tracts, leading to well-defined cirrhosis (Fig. 31-30). Although there is some correlation between the amount of iron present and the severity of cirrhosis, it is not invariable, as some livers with advanced cirrhosis will not have as much stainable iron as will those with poorly developed fibrous septa. The hemosiderin appears to have some predilection for the peripheral portion of the lobules. As the iron increases, the aggregates become larger and cellular detail may be obscured. Masses of hemosiderin are also seen within Kupffer cells, although this does not usually parallel the amount of hemosiderin within the hepatic cells. Focal areas of necrosis may occur, and after healing, such areas are marked by closely packed macrophages whose cytoplasm contains dense accumulations of hemosiderin. After necrosis, regenerative nodules develop that have little or no stainable iron within their cells. Fibrous tissue septa connecting the portal spaces are similar to those in alcoholic cirrhosis except for iron-filled macrophages and, occasionally, iron-encrusted connective tissue fibers. An iron-free pigment, hemofuscin, may accumulate within both the fibrous tracts and the hepatic cells. Fatty change is seen in a small proportion of patients but is most prevalent in those who have diabetes mellitus. The latter, when present, is usually mild. The presence of increased iron or melanin in the skin may give the patient a blue-gray or bronzed appearance, hence the name *bronze diabetes* for this complication of hemochromatosis. In many patients with pigmentary cirrhosis, there is a long course (10 years or more) that exceeds the duration in most other types of cirrhosis. Portal hypertension and ascites are not common complications, but primary carcinoma of the liver occurs more often than in any other type of cirrhosis,[313,316] up to 25% of patients in some series.[399]

The question of whether iron produces fibrous scarring is unanswered. There is clinical evidence suggesting that iron is involved in the pathogenesis of hemochromatosis.[341] In our experience there does seem to be an association between the density of iron deposition and the degree of fibrosis in both liver and pancreas. The Bantu who stores large amounts of iron absorbed from his diet, however, develops a meager degree of fibrosis. Experimental iron-loading experiments have usually failed to produce significant fibrosis with notable exceptions.[372]

The mechanism by which iron may damage the liver and pancreas, producing necrosis and fibrosis, is not known. Studies with the electron microscope show that iron is deposited within the lysosomes of the liver cell and, to a lesser extent, in some of the mitochondria. The latter may then degenerate. It is likely that a point is reached where some of the liver cells populating the lobules are unable to survive with so much of their cytoplasm occupied by iron.[431]

Secondary hemochromatosis

Hepatic iron stores may become greatly increased secondary to other disorders. When cirrhosis is also a part of the primary disease, distinction from idiopathic hemochromatosis may become impossible on histologic grounds alone. Quantitative analysis generally reveals that this deposition is much less in secondary hemochromatosis; liver iron usually is calculated to be less than 2 gm per 100 gm dry weight of liver when the iron loading is secondary to another disorder. Patients other than those with idiopathic hemochromatosis in whom iron is found in hepatocytes in excessive amounts include the following:

1. A small percentage of patients with any type of cirrhosis
2. A small percentage of patients who have undergone a portacaval shunt for portal hypertension
3. Any chronically anemic patient except one having iron deficiency
4. Some patients with porphyria cutanea tarda
5. Patients who have excessive dietary intake of iron salts

Patients in group 5 are seen principally in South Africa, where the Bantus often ingest large quantities of iron in food or drink prepared in iron utensils. This condition has been known as *Bantu siderosis*. It may lead to increased iron absorption and storage within the reticuloendothelial system and liver.[313] When the iron content of the liver is over 2% of the dry weight, classical signs of hemochromatosis may develop. In refractory anemias, especially those characterized by accelerated erythropoiesis and defects in normoblast maturation, secondary hemochromatosis and cirrhosis eventually may develop.[357,358] How important the additional iron loading from multiple transfusions is remains uncertain.[389] In an autopsy series of patients who had thalassemia with and without transfusions, a definite relationship of fibrosis to quantity of iron and age of patient was observed.[409]

The most common form of excess iron storage associated with liver disease occurs in alcoholism. The excessive deposition may be seen in any stage of alcoholic liver disease, from fatty liver to advanced cirrhosis. It has been stated that ethanol increases the absorption of iron once cirrhosis is present.[349] The reasons for increased iron absorption in alcoholic patients are not entirely clear. The daily intake of iron, 15 mg or more, by those who drink cheap wine may be of such magnitude that increased absorption results.[374] Both a low-protein diet and chronic anemia favor iron absorption. The effects of the alcoholic beverage itself, pancreatic dysfunction,[322] hepatocellular regeneration,[380] and portal hypertension are unsettled. Gastric atrophy is common in the alcoholic, possibly resulting in decrease of secretion of iron-binding protein in gastric juices leaving more iron available to absorb.[323] We have observed excess iron in livers of those patients who presumably drank only distilled liquor. In our biopsies from patients with alcoholic liver disease, about 5% have some degree of siderosis. Ordinarily, the iron in alcoholic liver disease is minimal or moderate when compared with the degree of cirrhosis. There are rare instances in which the amount of secondary iron loading in a cirrhotic liver is such that it is impossible on biopsy to distinguish alcoholic liver disease with excess iron storage from idiopathic hemochromatosis.

Wilson's disease (hepatolenticular degeneration)

Wilson's disease (hepatolenticular degeneration) is an inheritable disorder characterized by the abnormal metabolism of copper[434] in which the patient is in positive copper balance and excess quantities of copper are stored first in the liver and eventually in other tissues, especially the brain, cornea, and kidney. The disease is inherited in an autosomal recessive manner. Both homozygotes and heterozygotes occur in the same families.[427] In the homozy-

gote there is a defect in the excretion of the copper by the liver that appears to be responsible for the accumulation of copper in the body.[337]

Studies with radioactive copper have shown that slightly over 50% is absorbed in the normal person,[427] most of which is quickly stored in the liver, attached to hepatic proteins, but some circulates for a short time loosely bound to serum albumin. A small amount is probably bound to amino acids and can pass through a semipermeable membrane. This portion is probably responsible for the normal excretion of copper in the urine. The radioactive copper soon disappears from the blood and a secondary rise in the plasma occurs after its incorporation into ceruloplasmin (blue protein) by the hepatocytes and secretion of this alpha globulin into the blood.

In Wilson's disease it has been shown that radioactive copper is absorbed in a normal fashion, but in the symptomatic patient where the liver is saturated with copper the excess spills over into other tissues and into the urine. No secondary rise in plasma copper bound to ceruloplasmin is noted. This failure is probably the best diagnostic test for Wilson's disease.

The failure to excrete absorbed copper leads to its accumulation in the liver. The liver has the capacity to store copper far in excess of that needed in the normal person or in the heterozygote. It has been termed the "copper pot."[429] In the presymptomatic homozygote, the "pot" is not full. Only after it is full does the copper spill over into the blood and other tissues and into the urine in large quantities. Because the copper cannot be stored in the symptomatic patient with liver disease, it is stored in other tissues, especially the brain and kidney, and is excreted in the urine. Storage in the liver is achieved by combination with a protein, copperthionein. In patients with Wilson's disease, this metalloprotein has a copper-binding constant four times greater than that in control subjects.[334] The hepatocytic copper increase appears to occur first in the cytoplasm,[340] where the copper ion is capable of causing episodes of necrosis. These may produce attacks of jaundice and a rise in serum transaminase levels. All the stages in the progression from hepatocellular necrosis to cirrhosis in Wilson's disease have not been documented. However, hyaline necrosis[366] (Fig. 31-31) and chronic hepatitis[425] probably play a part. Other changes include fatty vacuolization, increase of lipochrome pigment, and glycogen-filled nuclei. Electron micro-

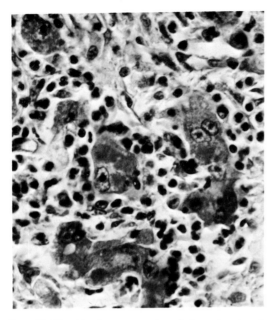

Fig. 31-31. Hyaline necrosis of hepatocytes in Wilson's disease. Abundant neutrophilic and round cell infiltrate in sinusoids.

scopic studies have disclosed striking abnormalities of the mitochondria that may be related to the fatty change.[424] Further studies suggest that a defect in lysosomes may account for the low biliary copper excretion.[426] In the advanced stage, the septa are usually thin, the regenerative nodules are large, and areas of collapse may be present.

The laboratory findings in Wilson's disease usually include a low-serum copper, low-serum ceruloplasmin, increased copper in the urine, and decreased copper in the stool. A sharp increase in urine copper occurs after the administration of penicillamine. A needle biopsy of the liver, when analyzed for copper with the emission spectrograph, shows a sharp increase of the metal. An amount above 25 mg per 100 gm dry weight of liver is characteristic. The abnormal retention of ^{64}Cu 72 hours after intravenous injection allows the clinician to distinguish between the normal patient and heterozygote carrier. There is some overlap, however, between heterozygotes and homozygotes.[346]

The hepatic form of Wilson's disease begins at a younger age (usually before 20) than that of the central nervous system.[427] The disease should always be suspected in a child or young person with symptoms of liver disease. The symptoms include abdominal pain, jaundice, ascites, and anemia, especially hemolytic ane-

mia. The presence of brown pigmentation of Descemet's membrane at the limbus of the cornea, the Kayser-Fleischer ring (Plate 5, *C*, and Fig. 24-11) is pathognomonic of Wilson's disease. When the disease is recognized in a family, all of its members should be examined for evidence of presymptomatic disease. It is important that the diagnosis of Wilson's disease be made in its early stages because treatment with penicillamine may restore the patient to health.

Cirrhosis and protease inhibitor ZZ

A deficiency of alpha$_1$ globulin noted in 1963 in adult patients with pulmonary emphysema resulted in the characterization of certain genetic determinants for this globulin[365] now known as α_1-antitrypsin (α_1-AT) or protease inhibitor (Pi). In 1968 the recognition of the same deficiency in serum of a juvenile cirrhotic identified a major type of juvenile liver disease.[416]

Protease inhibitor is a 54,000–molecular weight glycoprotein formed in the hepatocytes and normally released into serum.[34,363] Its electrophoretic rate in acid starch, but not its antigenic characteristics, is genetically determined by 23 different codominant alleles. The different genetic types of protease inhibitor are named according to the rate of migration in acid electrophoresis. MM is the common type of protease inhibitor and moves at medium speed in electrophoresis; those faster are designated by letters in the first part of the alphabet, those slower are named by letters in the last part. One type, Pi ZZ, is definitely related to liver disease, and Pi type SZ may also be occasionally found in patients with cirrhosis. Pi ZZ occurs in 0.07 to 0.1% of the population. In patients with Pi ZZ, the α_1-AT produced is deficient in sialic acid, either because there are low levels of sialic acid transferase in hepatocytes of Pi ZZ patients[333] or because of anomalous biosynthesis of the Pi peptide to the extent that normal glycosylation does not occur.[352] When the liver of a ZZ patient was replaced by an organ from a donor who was MM, the recipient thereafter produced Pi MM.[396]

The liver disease often associated with Pi ZZ typically has its onset in the first few weeks. If a biopsy is taken, it is usually interpreted as "neonatal hepatitis" although there are histologic changes in bile duct structures (see diseases of infants and children, p. 1391). Although the infant typically recovers from the initial jaundice and ostensibly im-

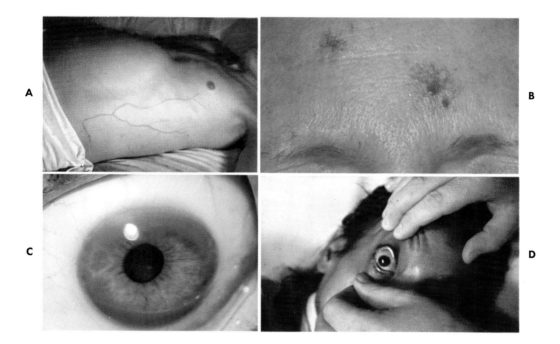

Plate 5
A, Hepatic cirrhosis. Ascites, congested veins, pigmented male nipple, axillary alopecia, and absence of striae.
B, Arteriovenous fistulas (vascular spiders) in diabetic cirrhosis. Arterial blood supply in center of lesion.
C, Kayser-Fleischer ring in Wilson's disease.
D, Jaundice and biliary cirrhosis after ligation of common bile duct.
(**A** and **D,** From Wiener, K.: Skin manifestations of internal disorders, St. Louis, 1947, The C. V. Mosby Co.)

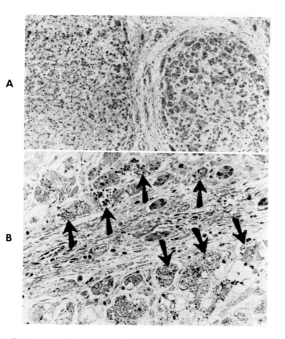

Fig. 31-32. Juvenile cirrhosis in alpha$_1$-antitrypsin deficiency (Pi ZZ). Note **A,** lamellar fibrosis and duct deficiency, and **B,** marginal hepatocytes filled with glycoprotein droplets *(arrows).*

proves, signs of chronic liver disease appear about 6 years to 10 years later, leading to death. Microscopically, the bile ducts are sharply numerically diminished, and fibrosis extends from portal areas in parallel bundles, surrounding small nodules of liver tissue that have a feathery margin. These resemble primary biliary cirrhosis or the late changes from biliary atresia. The peripheral hepatocytes are hydropic and often foamy but contain small hyaline eosinophilic bodies ranging from submicroscopic size to about 15 μm, most being 2 to 4 μm. The bodies are quite variable in numbers from one nodule to another (Fig. 31-32). The bodies are the protease inhibitor, apparently lacking the sialic acid component. The Pi bodies stain with diastase PAS, alcian blue, specifically by immunofluorescence or by immunoperoxidase techniques for α_1-antitrypsin. The protease inhibitor can also be demonstrated in hepatocytes of some patients with MZ or SZ Pi types. The protease inhibitor is located within cisternae of the rough endoplasmic reticulum (RER) and, to a lesser extent, the smooth endoplasmic reticulum (SER). As the bodies seem to be submicroscopic when viewed with the electron microscope, it is possible that the large bodies may be artifacts caused by coalescence.[321]

A deficiency in formation of biliary ductules in cirrhosis associated with Pi ZZ may be responsible for an increase in copper storage in the presence of normal ceruloplasmin levels.[351] A similar increase in copper storage has been noted in primary and prolonged secondary biliary cirrhosis.

Most individuals with Pi ZZ do not develop liver disease but instead acquire pulmonary emphysema in midadult life. The glycoprotein is demonstrable in the noncirrhotic liver. Few patients in the United States but several in Scandinavian countries[309,338] have had Pi ZZ reported with Pi ZZ cirrhosis recognized in adulthood. Rarely, adult patients with atrophic, firm, coarsely nodular cirrhosis of unknown causes have been found to have anomalous heterozygous Pi types.

A relationship of the cirrhosis in adults with Pi ZZ to hepatocellular carcinoma (HCC) has been suggested.[308,338] If there is a relation, it must account for a very small proportion of patients with HCC. Serum testing at our unit of 80 patients with HCC showed no significant differences in pattern from normal blood donors and only one patient with Pi ZZ.[74]

Biliary cirrhosis

Obstruction of the biliary tract (either extrahepatic or intrahepatic) may, if prolonged, lead to cirrhosis of the liver.[394] The causes of biliary obstruction have already been discussed (p. 1357). The appearance of the liver in extrahepatic obstruction depends on the degree of blockage and the time factor. Neoplastic obstruction is usually complete, and the patient dies before a true cirrhosis develops. The biliary tree proximal to the neoplasm is greatly dilated. The liver is green to greenish brown and finely granular. An increase of connective tissue along the large bile ducts near the hilum of the liver usually is noted. The organ is usually increased in size and palpable before death, although there is little increase in weight. Occasionally, a carcinoma obstructing the ducts grows very slowly and the increase in connective tissue is such that the liver cuts with increased resistance, and the diagnosis of early biliary cirrhosis is justified. Obstruction of the common duct caused by a calculus or a benign stricture is usually incomplete. Therefore the distention of the ducts and bile stasis in the liver are not so extreme as with cancerous obstruction. On occasion, a stone or a stricture may obstruct the common duct for years and lead to true biliary cirrhosis. The liver has a granular appearance or may

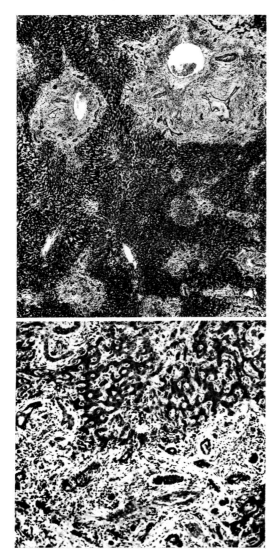

Fig. 31-33. Biliary cirrhosis.

even be nodular. It cuts with increased resistance, and fibrosis is as pronounced as it is in alcoholic cirrhosis. In neglected patients, biliary cirrhosis of this type may, on rare occasions, cause portal hypertension, splenomegaly, and hemorrhage from esophageal varices. A portacaval shunt may become necessary.[297]

In the early stage of extrahepatic obstruction, microscopic examination reveals that dilatation of the large ducts near the hilum is constant, whereas the size of the smaller ducts is variable. Some increase of fibroblastic activity with the formation of spurs is seen within 30 to 50 days.[420] Bile stasis is predominantly centrilobular. In the intermediate stage, between 60 and 100 days, connective tissue is more abundant and often has a concentric configuration around the bile ducts. Both at this stage and in the later cirrhotic phase, the arrangement of the connective tissue may give a "pipestem" effect (Fig. 31-33). Bile duct proliferation is present in only a small percentage of the total. The mononuclear type of exudate may be increased. Focal necrosis of hepatic cells, of either the lytic or the eosinophilic type, is frequent. Consequent to necrosis, particularly of cells in the peripheries of the lobules, bile lakes may form. The central veins are present and a normal lobular architecture can be seen throughout most of the liver. A few abnormal hyperplastic nodules may make their appearance at this stage. Later, especially in patients with calculus obstruction or stricture, a well-developed cirrhosis is noted, with connective tissue septa outlining pseudolobules. Intralobular bile stasis is irregular but is now both central and peripheral. There is usually no bile stasis within the interlobular ducts, probably because it is absorbed within the lobule. Occasionally, a liver may exhibit wide connective tissue septa, with abundant bile duct proliferation. Fatty changes, extensive necrosis of parenchyma, and even abscesses may complicate the disease.

Primary biliary cirrhosis

Primary biliary cirrhosis is a chronic disease of unknown etiology that occurs most frequently in middle-aged women. It primarily affects the interlobular bile ducts, although the clinical features are similar to those of prolonged partial obstruction of the extrahepatic bile ducts. The name is somewhat of a misnomer since cirrhosis is a late development although it is progressive and fatal.[298]

Primary biliary cirrhosis was not recognized until Hanot wrote his thesis "Hypertrophic Cirrhosis with Jaundice" in 1876.[410] He described the initial lesion as a catarrhal inflammation of the small bile ducts that he believed originated from a toxic or possibly an infective process.

Primary biliary cirrhosis is a disease that affects women in the ratio of about 9:1 over men. The onset is generally insidious, beginning with pruritus that may be present for several months to a year before the onset of dark urine or icterus. After jaundice has been present for months, the patient notices foul fatty stools, and slowly the skin manifestations of hyperlipemia become noticeable as xanthomas or fine yellowish deposits in the creases

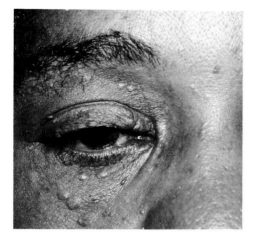

Fig. 31-34. Xanthomas of eyelid in primary biliary cirrhosis.

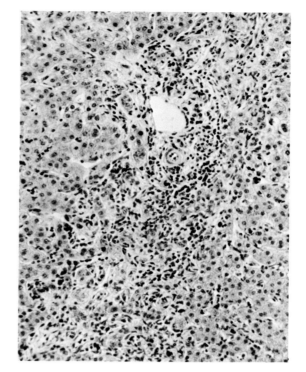

Fig. 31-35. Destruction of bile ducts and limiting plate in primary biliary cirrhosis.

of the palms of the hands, antecubital spaces, and elsewhere (Fig. 31-34).

From the onset, there is hepatomegaly, and about one half of the patients have splenomegaly. The impaired flow of bile into the intestine causes a deficiency of the absorption of vitamin D and calcium that results in osteomalacia, often with bone pain and even compression fractures of the vertebrae. Weight loss occurs as greater amounts of the ingested fat are excreted in the stool. The course is slowly downhill, with the duration of life after the diagnosis is established being from 5 to 15 years.

In a liver biopsy taken early in the disease, the interlobular ducts and the limiting plate are destroyed[302,329] (Fig. 31-35). Lymphocytes, sometimes accompanied by plasma cells, infiltrate and widen the portal areas and often completely surround the larger bile ducts. The arterioles usually are thickened. The liver cords are regular, but the cells generally are shrunken. Alcoholic hyaline is seen in many instances, especially in the periportal hepatocytes.[375] The Kupffer cells are hyperplastic, and occasional foci of lymphocytes or plasma cells are seen. Bile stasis is more frequently periportal than central. Primary biliary cirrhosis is the only disease in which periportal cholestasis predominates. Bile lakes, an occasional autopsy finding in the liver of patients with extrahepatic biliary tract obstruction, are not a feature of primary biliary cirrhosis.[302] Although epithelioid granulomas in the portal areas have been reported in as many as one third of the patients, they are much less frequent in our material. Ultrastructural studies have disclosed certain distinctive features in primary biliary cirrhosis. The bile duct epithelium shows intracytoplasmic filamentous structures as well as numerous other changes.[319]

Mallory bodies (alcoholic hyaline bodies) may be found in periportal hepatocytes in a significant percentage of patients with primary biliary cirrhosis.[375] It is indistinguishable by light and electron microscopy from that of the liver of the alcoholic patient.[385] The alcoholic hyaline bodies are sparsely distributed in a narrow zone of periportal hydropic hepatocytes, although typically hydropic hepatocytes do not occur in primary biliary cirrhosis except when there are degenerative changes that include alcoholic hyaline bodies. This change may be episodic but is a helpful diagnostic feature when present. Only rarely are alcoholic hyaline bodies found in periportal hepatocytes of patients with mechanical duct obstruction.

It has been maintained that envelopment of the septal and larger bile ducts by a nodular arrangement of lymphocytes, histiocytes with epithelioid change, plasma cells, and eosinophils is the earliest change in primary biliary cirrhosis. We find this change suggestive in the context of other changes, but not pathognomonic. In our material the large lymphoid aggregates are found somewhat later in the disease than is small duct dissolution. The abnormal bile duct epithelium described in livers of patients with primary biliary cirrhosis and with chronic active hepatitis has not been a prominent feature in our material.[127]

As the disease progresses, the portal areas widen and may unite. Pseudoductules proliferate considerably throughout the later stages of the disease and may be mistaken for ductules. Pseudoductules consist of paired columns of cells rather than round ductular structures with lumens. Regenerative nodules may occur late in the disease, but at autopsy true regenerative nodules are not usually present. Instead, portal areas have united to produce a finely granular liver. Rarely, 3 to 5 mm nodules will replace the lobular architecture. Signs of portal hypertension are a late occurrence. Only an occasional patient will have esophageal varices.

Among the diseases associated with primary biliary cirrhosis is ulcerative colitis. Usually when the bile ducts are affected in ulcerative colitis, the larger ducts are involved and not the ductules. However, in rare instances, classic primary biliary cirrhosis does follow ulcerative colitis.[384]

The laboratory findings in primary biliary cirrhosis resemble those of prolonged obstruction of the extrahepatic bile duct. Total bilirubin levels are usually in the range of 2 to 15 mg per 100 ml. The serum alkaline phosphatase activity is elevated, usually to 25 times the normal range, levels far greater than those seen in most other obstructive diseases of the biliary tract. The serum cholesterol, triglycerides, and particularly phospholipid levels all are greatly elevated. The serum is not lactescent, apparently because of the high levels of phospholipid. If the serum is frozen, the lipids are deemulsified and form a creamy layer at the meniscus. However, prolonged extrahepatic biliary obstruction or, rarely, prolonged cholestatic reactions to drugs[367] may produce similarly elevated serum lipid levels. Serum albumin levels may drop when the disease progresses. Serum globulin elevations are attributable to increases in low-density beta lipoproteins. The IgG component contains the mitochondrial antibody that acts upon the inner membrane of mitochondria from any one of the mammalian species.[311] The test has proved helpful in the diagnosis of primary biliary cirrhosis.[361] Serum transaminase activities generally are elevated in the 200 to 400 unit range. This elevation has led many clinicians to misdiagnose the disease as chronic active hepatitis.

An impaired T-cell response has been demonstrated in patients with primary biliary cirrhosis,[336,376] but etiologic relationships of autoimmune or toxic conditions are unclear. Although there is no abnormality in the level of serum ceruloplasmin in primary biliary cirrhosis, the levels of copper in the liver may be increased as much as twenty-five-fold.[335] Apparently the elevated levels reflect the impaired ability to excrete copper in bile, its usual route of disposal.

Several disorders of connective tissue may be associated with primary biliary cirrhosis. One combination is with Osler-Weber-Rendu syndrome (hereditary hemorrhagic telangiectasia), or with calcinosis, Raynaud's phenomenon, scleroderma, telangiectasia (CRST).[406] A small percentage of patients with rheumatoid arthritis may have primary biliary cirrhosis, sometimes accompanied by Sjögren's syndrome.[437] This syndrome, which consists of keratoconjunctivitis sicca (dry eyes) and xerostomia (dry mouth), may be partially or wholly expressed clinically. It is an immunologic disorder of the secreting tear and salivary glands. Some clinical, laboratory, or radiologic evidence of this syndrome has been reported in nearly all patients with primary biliary cirrhosis.[299] Chronic active hepatitis may also be complicated by Sjögren's syndrome. Conversely, patients who have a generalized connective tissue disorder, such as rheumatoid arthritis, disseminated lupus erythematosus, progressive systemic sclerosis, and others may eventually have chronic liver disease, particularly primary biliary cirrhosis.

The differential diagnosis between primary biliary cirrhosis and sarcoidosis may be difficult when granulomas are present in biopsy material.[423] Distinguishing features include a positive serum mitochondrial antibody test in primary biliary cirrhosis and a positive Kveim-Siltzback test that is present in about 75% of patients with sarcoidosis. Lack of jaundice and pruritus in patients with sarcoidosis is helpful. However, patients with sarcoidosis may have extensive involvement of the liver and occasionally cirrhosis, and in rare instances a patient with primary biliary cirrhosis may have multisystem involvement with noncaseating granulomas. Primary biliary cirrhosis has been reported with primary cutaneous amyloidosis.[423]

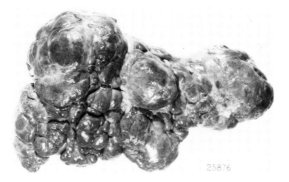

Fig. 31-36. Deeply scarred liver (hepar lobatum syphiliticum) that weighed only 710 gm (79-year-old white woman, known syphilitic, who had received some antisyphilitic therapy 3 years before death). Several large hyperplastic nodules present. Stringy adhesions bridge some deep transverse fissures.

Syphilitic cirrhosis

In congenital syphilis of the liver, now a rare entity, there is an overgrowth of mesenchymal tissue along the sinusoids that causes wide separation of the hepatic cells. Small gummas or even large soft ones occasionally are seen. Usually, spirochetes are easily demonstrable. Syphilitic cirrhosis rarely eventuates. In the tertiary stage of acquired syphilis, it is stated that about one sixth of all patients will develop gummas of the liver.[427] Gummas may be solitary or multiple and confluent, sometimes forming a large mass. On sectioning, they have a dull gray-yellow area of central necrosis, an irregular outline, and a marginal zone of gray-white, glassy-appearing granulation tissue. They often are widespread and, in healing, the scar tissue replacing them contracts to form deep scars that may incompletely divide the liver into masses of irregular size—hepar lobatum syphiliticum. In other instances, the crevices are not so deep, but stringy adhesions may bridge the indentations (Fig. 31-36). More rarely, the liver is deformed by linear depressions. This occurs alone or in combination with the deeply scarred organ. Beneath these linear deformities are bands of connective tissue that do not have the appearance of healed gummas. In hepar lobatum syphiliticum, there may be little more than the normal amount of connective tissue, or, on the contrary, the connective tissue may be diffusely increased.

Microscopically, in the gummatous stage there are isolated areas of necrosis surrounded

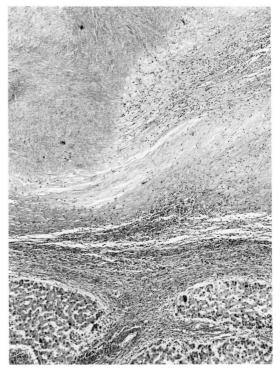

Fig. 31-37. Margin of gumma showing irregular outline, sparsity of epithelioid cells, and zone of granulation tissue (41-year-old woman who died of massive gastrointestinal hemorrhage; syphilis not diagnosed ante mortem).

by granulation tissue relatively poor in fibroblasts and usually sparse in epithelioid cells (Fig. 31-37). The granulation tissue impinges upon the liver parenchyma, and necrosis of the latter appears to occur at this junction. Lymphocytes and plasma cells are common, both around the areas of gummatous necrosis and along the portal tracts. Later, wide bands of scar tissue are irregularly distributed throughout the liver, sometimes in combination with unhealed gummas. In some areas, it appears that connective tissue septa may form without an intervening gummatous stage. The plasma cell infiltrate is helpful in distinguishing gummas from tuberculosis of the liver. Occasionally, a patient with advanced syphilis of the liver is a chronic alcoholic, and in this case the liver will be fatty.

Parasitic cirrhosis

Fibrosis in the liver may result from infection with the liver fluke, *Clonorchis sinensis,* or with schistosomes.

Clonorchis sinensis, prevalent in the Far East and in India, lodges in the biliary system, where it may, at times, cause sufficient obstruction to result in a cholangitic biliary cirrhosis (p. 1378).

Schistosomiasis causes hepatic fibrosis and cirrhosis attributable to the lodgment of ova in the portal vein branches.[435] Cirrhosis occurs particularly with *Schistosoma mansoni* and less frequently with *S. japonicum* and *S. haematobium.* The liver is nodular and firm and shows pale gray fibrotic areas on the cut surface. The fibrosis outlines the portal tracts, and it has been called Symmers' fibrosis or pipestem fibrosis.[300] The fibrosis causes narrowing and obliteration of much of the intrahepatic portal venous system. A fine network of thin-walled vessels develops around the portal veins.[348] The hepatic artery tends to enlarge and a presinusoidal hypertension develops. The hepatic veins are unchanged. Ova or remnants of ova may be seen along the portal tracts. In later stages, clinical manifestations may be similar to those of portal cirrhosis, with ascites, splenomegaly, anemia, and esophageal varices (Fig. 14-20).

Congestive or cardiac cirrhosis

The condition known as congestive or cardiac cirrhosis is a fibrosis and alteration of architecture of the liver associated with severe and prolonged passive hyperemia of the type that occurs most often in patients with rheumatic heart disease, hypertensive heart disease, arteriosclerotic heart disease, or in the rare patient with constrictive pericarditis. The serum bilirubin may be elevated and often there is sulfobromophthalein (BSP) retention.[326,418] Repeated bouts of decompensation appear to favor development of fibrosis. Because it is the end result of prolonged passive congestion, it is discussed with this disorder on pp. 157 and 1403. In myxedema a centrilobular congestive fibrosis has been described in a few cases.[303]

Miscellaneous types of cirrhosis

Cirrhosis may complicate the course of any one of many serious diseases that are systemic or that primarily involve other organs in the body. Liver abnormalities are common in ulcerative colitis. Among these are fatty change, portal inflammation and fibrosis, pericholangitis, chronic active hepatitis, granulomas, amyloidosis, cirrhosis, bile duct carcinoma, and sclerosing cholangitis.[327,384] In Crohn's disease, the liver changes may be similar to those in ulcerative colitis.[328] The liver disease in both ulcerative colitis and Crohn's colitis has been reported to improve after colectomy. Pericholangitis and fibrosis may lead to protracted jaundice and finally a biliary type of cirrhosis. Young women with ulcerative colitis may have "lupoid hepatitis" or "chronic active hepatitis" that eventuates in cirrhosis.

In diabetes mellitus, fatty changes[436] and even cirrhosis may occur, especially in patients whose disease is poorly controlled. Cirrhosis in nonalcoholic diabetic patients is rare. It has been observed that patients with alcoholic cirrhosis may secondarily become diabetic.[339] Rheumatoid arthritis,[355] regional enteritis,[320] scleroderma,[305] rheumatic fever, hyperthyroidism,[301] and various bacterial infections[360] occasionally may be complicated by cirrhosis. A mild degree of cirrhosis is not infrequently noted in the liver of elderly persons. This seems to be a slow progressive disease that occurs in patients in whom there are no etiologically demonstrable factors except possibly poor eating habits. In Boeck's sarcoidosis, the lesions in the liver may progress to cirrhosis.[387] In sickle-cell anemia, a coarsely nodular type of cirrhosis may be seen. Presumably, this is caused by anoxic necrosis from stagnation of the sickled red blood cells in the sinusoids.[422] There is also the possibility that patients who receive many transfusions may develop serum hepatitis followed by cirrhosis.

Thorotrast

It is well known that Thorotrast after a number of years may give rise to malignant tumors in the liver. However, it is also a cause of cirrhosis. Apparently the intense fibrosis is produced by irradiation.[433]

PATHOPHYSIOLOGY OF CHRONIC LIVER DISEASE

Many pathophysiologic phenomena are associated with chronic liver disease. Although some of these are the direct result of hepatic disease, others are unexplained. The concept that hepatic failure or insufficiency may occur to a variable degree is important. The most severe form of hepatic failure that results in coma is discussed on p. 1352. Only occasionally does the cirrhotic patient die in deep coma without some complication. The patient with cirrhosis, however, may from time to time have episodes of encephalopathy that are reversible. Some of these mild forms of encephalopathy are indicated by an inability to perform simple mental tests. More severe forms include flapping tremor, agitation, and disorientation.

Among the most common complications of chronic liver disease that progresses to cirrhosis are portal hypertension, esophageal varices, and ascites.

Portal hypertension

Resistance to the flow of blood within the liver in chronic liver disease is the most common cause of portal hypertension. This is the intrahepatic type, in contrast to the posthepatic type caused by lesions of the hepatic veins and the prehepatic type in which the obstruction is the result of disease of the portal vein.

Any form of cirrhosis may be associated with *intrahepatic portal hypertension.* The mechanism of obstruction has been attributed to compression by regenerative nodules.[356] However, at least in the alcoholic patient, significant portal hypertension develops in response to centrilobular intrasinusoidal collagen deposition before the development of regenerative nodules.[407] The normal pressure in the portal vein is 6 to 10 mm Hg.[405] In cirrhosis, it may rise to 20 or 30 mm Hg. The rise in pressure is directly related to the resistance to blood flow within the liver.

In about 15% of patients in whom portacaval shunt has been performed, the pressure on the hepatic side of a clamp placed on the vein is higher than it is on the splanchnic side, indicating that there is a reversal of portal vein blood flow in these patients.[383] The pressure within the portal system also may be measured with a fair degree of accuracy by introducing a catheter, via an antecubital vein, the superior vena cava, and the inferior vena cava, into a small branch of the hepatic venous system. The catheter, when wedged into the vein, gives a pressure reading similar to the pressure within the portal vein system.[408] The so-called wedged hepatic vein pressure is quite helpful in determination of whether the point of obstruction is within the liver or is extrahepatic. In the latter, normal wedged pressures are observed.

The portal vein averages 7 cm in length and is formed by the confluence of the superior mesenteric and splenic veins. The inferior mesenteric vein joins the latter about 3 cm from its junction point. Thus the portal blood is received from the gastrointestinal tract, mesentery, spleen, gallbladder, and pancreas. Obstruction to the flow of blood through the portal trunk results in hypertension throughout the system. In cirrhosis, this develops slowly but finally results in chronic passive hyperemia of the tissues drained by the portal vein. The intestines and peritoneum appear congested and edematous. The spleen is enlarged, firm, and dark red, and it may weigh between 300 and 1000 gm. There is poor correlation between the size of the spleen and increased pressure in the portal system.

Posthepatic portal hypertension is rare. It results from impaired entry of hepatic vein blood into the vena cava. Neoplastic obstruction, thrombosis of the hepatic veins or of the inferior vena cava, and prolonged congestive heart failure may transmit elevated pressure through the hepatic vascular bed to the portal vein.

Prehepatic portal hypertension is an uncommon condition in which the liver is presumed not to be involved. Banti's disease (idiopathic portal hypertension) is the principal example (p. 1405). Extrahepatic portal vein thrombosis has been considered a cause of portal hypertension.[415,417] However, neoplastic occlusion of the extrahepatic portal vein produces neither portal hypertension nor splenomegaly. In thrombosis of the portal vein associated with portal hypertension, it is likely that sludged blood already under increased pressure caused the thrombus to form.[382] Congenital absence of the portal vein has been reported.[390]

Rarely, myelofibrosis will produce portal hypertension. The elevated pressure probably results from the fibrous involvement of all of the intrahepatic portal structures rather than increased blood flow through the enlarged spleen.

Esophageal varices

As a result of the increase in pressure within the portal system, the blood tends to bypass the liver and return to the heart by various collaterals (Fig. 31-38). These develop more prominently cephalad than caudad. Although hemorrhoids are common, they do not cause serious complications. More important are the large varices susceptible to erosion and fatal bleeding that arise in the mucosa at the lower end of the esophagus (Fig. 31-39). The blood entering these veins is short-circuited from the portal system via the coronary veins of the stomach and also the left gastroepiploic and vasa brevia. In the lower third of the esophagus, the submucosal veins are poorly supported and are subjected to trauma by the

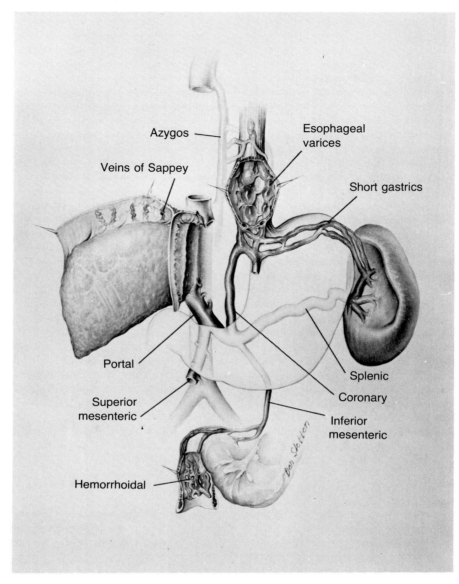

Fig. 31-38. Portal vein and its major tributaries showing most important routes of collateral circulation between portal and caval systems.

passage of food and also may be eroded by regurgitation of gastric juice. In patients with cirrhosis, both esophagoscopy and roentgenograms are used to demonstrate the presence of these varices. The exsanguination that follows rupture of the esophageal varices is a precipitating cause of death in 15% of cirrhotic patients. An additional 35% die of liver failure after esophageal hemorrhage.[392] *Other anastomoses* between the portal circulation and systemic veins may develop between the hilum of the liver and the umbilicus along the para-

umbilical plexus of veins. These may cause enlargement of the umbilicus (caput medusae). When greatly enlarged paraumbilical veins are present, the term "Cruveilhier-Baumgarten syndrome" sometimes is applied, especially when a murmur is heard. The cutaneous vessels over the upper abdomen may be enlarged. Other communications may be established through the veins of Retzius in the posterior mesentery and directly through the diaphragm via the veins of Sappey. It has been demonstrated that blood may even find

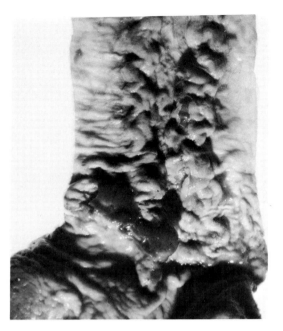

Fig. 31-39. Large esophageal varices on mucosal surface of opened esophagus.

its way through the periesophageal veins directly to the pulmonary veins and the left atrium.[317]

In patients who have esophageal varices demonstrable by esophagoscopy or by roentgenograms and who may or may not have had an episode of hemorrhage, the construction of a portal-systemic shunt[377] is performed in order to decompress the portal system. This is usually of the portacaval type.[378] If an end-to-side anastomosis is used, it prevents any possible retrograde flow in the portal vein through anastomoses with branches of the hepatic artery within the liver. It has been proposed that a side-to-side anastomosis may help the nutrition of the liver by allowing more hepatic artery blood to circulate through the parenchyma and then out through the portal vein (reversed flow). Following either procedure, the varices tend to decrease in size, as does the spleen in about one half of the patients. Further variceal hemorrhage is rare. The status of the fibrotic process in the liver is unaffected by surgery. Proper diet and abstinence from ethanol are of most value in allaying the progress of the disease. In extrahepatic obstruction, a portacaval shunt is usually impossible and a splenorenal shunt may be done.

Ascites

Ascites often accompanies portal hypertension, especially in the advanced stages of cirrhosis (Plate 5, *A*). The fluid within the abdomen is in the nature of a transudate, having a specific gravity of around 1.010. The mechanism of formation is complex and many factors are involved.

1. Portal hypertension and increased capillary filtration pressure
2. Postsinusoidal block
3. Hypoalbuminemia
4. Impaired renal function
5. Inferior vena cava hypertension
6. Hyperaldosteronism

The simple *elevation of portal pressure and increased capillary filtration pressure* may produce a soft-tissue transudate from the entire splanchnic bed and liver surface. *Postsinusoidal block* is believed to be the fundamental mechanism of ascites formation. Not only does increased lymph form, but the liver surface tends to "weep considerable amounts of fluid." *Hypoalbuminemia* may contribute to ascites by reduction of osmotic pressure in plasma, but its importance is believed to be minimal.

Impaired renal function in cirrhosis may be caused by pooling of splanchnic blood that results in a diminution of *effective* blood volume, reduced glomerular filtration rate, and sodium retention. There is also evidence that renal dysfunction is more directly related to hepatic disease. It has been suggested that in some unexplained fashion the liver may have a direct effect on the kidney's ability to excrete sodium. The failure to excrete sodium would be responsible for increased blood volume and partially responsible for ascites.[370]

Inferior vena cava hypertension has been proposed as a contributing feature in the formation of ascites.[386] Frequently in cirrhosis, an enlarged caudate lobe will compress the inferior vena cava into an elliptical shape that may cause a pressure differential between the abdominal and thoracic inferior vena cavae. It has been suggested that such narrowing may impair both hepatic venous and renal venous return, thus accentuating hepatic postsinusoidal portal hypertension and renal sodium clearance.

Aldosterone has strong sodium-retaining properties and is frequently found in increased amounts in the plasma and urine of cirrhotic patients, particularly those with ascites.[371,391] Whether the elevated levels are a primary or secondary feature in relation to ascites is unknown. Certainly *hyperaldosteronism* is not a prerequisite for ascites.

Other changes

Arteriovenous fistulas of skin. Arteriovenous fistulas of the skin, also called vascular spiders, are often observed in chronic liver disease (Plate 5, *B*). Recently, similar lesions in the lung have been described and recognized as a possible cause of finger clubbing and cyanosis that is common in patients with alcoholic cirrhosis.[310] Other findings in the cirrhotic patient may include palmar erythema,[306] pallor of the fingernails, enlargement of the salivary glands, and Dupuytren's contractures of the palmar fascia. In women with cirrhosis, a decrease in menstruation or amenorrhea is frequent.

Testicular atrophy. Testicular atrophy is a common accompaniment of cirrhosis.[307] This is often accompanied by signs of feminization in those with alcoholic liver disease.[432] These include a decrease in beard, development of gynecomastia, and impotence. The plasma levels of testosterone are decreased, and those of estradiol are normal or reduced. The plasma gonadotropins are normal or elevated, which presumably rules out hypothalmic-pituitary failure. The possibility exists that nonsteroidal estrogens are involved.[432]

Functional renal failure. Functional renal failure is a common cause of death in cirrhotic patients. Those who develop ascites tend to develop elevated creatinine levels, followed by a less striking rise of serum urea. Although it is well established that functional renal failure occurs after reduced renal plasma flow and an even more pronounced decrease in glomerular filtration rate, the pathogenesis is unknown. The total plasma volume actually is increased, although it is possible that splanchnic pooling of blood secondary to portal hypertension may reduce *effective* plasma volume.[332,393] Recent research indicates that the liver disease is linked somehow with the impaired renal capacity to excrete sodium and with consequent fluid retention.[370] Functional renal failure is not associated with any recognized pathologic changes in the kidneys.

Cirrhotic glomerulosclerosis. Cirrhotic glomerulosclerosis, a diffuse thickening of the glomerular basement membrane, occurs in up to 28% of cirrhotic patients.[354] There is disagreement as to functional importance of the lesion. In our experience, it is not associated with impaired renal function. It may represent an agonal edematous thickening of the basement membrane.

Proximal convoluted tubular epithelial proliferation. In patients who die of hepatic failure, the parietal layer of Bowman's capsule may be involved by a peculiar proliferation of swollen eosinophilic cuboid epithelium like that in the proximal convoluted tubules. Only scattered glomeruli may be involved. The cause of hepatic failure seems unimportant.

Burr cell hemolytic anemia and cirrhosis. Patients with cirrhosis and those with other liver diseases associated with absence of the spleen may develop a hemolytic process with large numbers of circulating erythrocytes that have spurlike projections from their surface producing distortion. The syndrome is associated with anemia and hyperbilirubinemia, predominantly in the indirect fraction. Conflicting experimental results have been reported regarding whether or not the defect is in the erythrocytic cell membrane[421] or in a plasma fraction.[343] The prognosis is poor. Occasionally, *hypersplenism* is associated with portal hypertension. The pancytopenia may be a major concern in Banti's disease.

Folate deficiency. Folate deficiency is relatively common in alcoholic liver disease, producing anemia, although rarely to the extent that megaloblastosis is prominent. Usually, folate deficiency is blamed on inadequate dietary intake,[347] but it is possible that the damaged liver may be incapable of adequate storage.

Hemorrhagic phenomena. Hemorrhagic phenomena are common in patients with hepatic disease. A number of defects in the clotting mechanism have been studied.[402] Fibrinogen, prothrombin, and factors VII, IX, X, and V all are produced by the liver parenchymal cell, and the platelet count may be reduced by hypersplenism.

Immunologic defects. It is well known that patients with cirrhosis, particularly the alcoholic type, often die of severe and often fulminating bacterial infection. A severe leukotactic defect attributable to the presence of abnormally high levels of a chemotactic factor inactivator has been reported.[379] An increase in the number of T cells and a failure to develop delayed hypersensitivity have been noted.[308,438] Hyperglobulinemia is commonly observed. It has been suggested that this may be caused by the failure of the liver to sequestrate antigens absorbed from the intestine, since these circulate through the rest of the body because of the collateral circulation in cirrhosis.

DIFFERENTIAL DIAGNOSIS OF JAUNDICE

A rise in either the indirect-reacting or direct-reacting bilirubin fraction in the blood results in yellow pigmentation of the skin, or jaundice. More than 97.5% of normal patients have serum bilirubin levels between 0.1 and 1 mg per 100 ml. Although a serum bilirubin above 1.2 mg per 100 ml is abnormal, jaundice does not become manifest until a level of 2 mg per 100 ml or more is reached. Since jaundice is dependent on bilirubin in tissue fluids, there may be a lag between the rise of the serum bilirubin level and evident jaundice. Minimal jaundice is best detected by examination of the scleras. Bilirubin has an affinity for elastic connective tissue, so that these structures are more deeply pigmented (Plate 5, *D*). However, in severe jaundice, the skin, interstitial fluids, and most of the body tissue (with the exception of the central nervous system) become bile stained. In chronic jaundice, the skin may appear a deep green-yellow and, in a few instances, an increase in melanin may result in a dark brown to black skin.

Pigments other than bilirubin may cause a yellow skin. Patients who ingest large quantities of carrots or carrot juice may have carotenemia. This pigment is best seen in the palms of the hands but not in the scleras. Atabrine, an antimalarial drug, also is capable of causing a yellow skin, as is dinitrophenol.

When confronted with a jaundiced patient, the physician has the responsibility for making an etiologic diagnosis as quickly as possible. The use of the terms "medical" and "surgical" jaundice emphasizes the importance of etiology. The most common causes of jaundice are viral hepatitis, cirrhosis, extrahepatic biliary obstruction, and drug-induced liver disease. In patients under 40 years of age, jaundice frequently is caused by viral hepatitis and drug sensitivity. In those over the age of 40 years, extrahepatic biliary obstruction is more common. Cirrhosis is a common cause of jaundice both before and after 40 years of age.

A careful history and physical examination followed by the performance of essential hepatic tests and, on occasion, by a needle biopsy of the liver usually will lead to a correct diagnosis. The patient should be questioned about exposure to other jaundiced individuals, transfusions, and needle sharing, all related to viral hepatitis. Further questioning about ingestion of hepatotoxic drugs or exposure to hepatotoxic chemicals is necessary.

A family history of jaundice may suggest an inheritable disease or a common infective, toxic, or dietary disorder. Questions regarding alcohol intake are important but often are ignored in the private hospital. Travel outside the United States may point to hepatitis A. If pain is present, its location, type, severity, and radiation are important. The patient should be questioned about pruritus and a change in stool color. The presence or absence of previous attacks of jaundice should be ascertained. Neoplasms usually cause an unremitting jaundice, whereas calculus obstruction, cirrhosis, and chronic active hepatitis are usually intermittent.

On physical examination, the size and consistency of the liver and the presence or absence of tenderness, nodules, or masses should be determined. A normal liver may extend below the costal margin but is too soft to palpate. The cirrhotic liver has a firm palpable edge. Even in advanced cirrhosis, when the liver is contracted, the lower margin may be felt on deep inspiration. In early to moderate cirrhosis, the liver is enlarged as a rule and the edge may be as low as the umbilicus. A small liver rarely is associated with biliary tract obstruction but often develops after liver cell necrosis. Careful palpation for an enlarged gallbladder, splenomegaly, and minimal ascites is likewise helpful in diagnosis. Splenomegaly, ascites, and many vascular spiders suggest chronic liver disease in the jaundiced patient. Primary carcinoma of the gallbladder may produce a hard palpable organ that is associated with jaundice as the initial symptom. A tense distended gallbladder favors neoplastic obstruction rather than choledocholithiasis. In cholelithiasis, the gallbladder usually becomes too fibrotic to undergo distention when the common bile duct is obstructed by a stone.

Usually no single laboratory test is relied upon to diagnose the cause of jaundice, but certain combinations of abnormal tests (Table 31-1) help to delineate various subgroups that narrow the possibilities to be considered by the clinician. The total serum bilirubin, as well as the direct-reacting and indirect-reacting fractions, always is determined. The test is usually performed at frequent intervals, for it gives valuable information as to the course of the disease.

Jaundice may be associated with an elevation of the indirect-reacting fraction of the serum bilirubin or, as is far more common, an elevation of both the direct-reacting and indirect-reacting fractions. The van den Bergh reactions shows that only a few diseases cause an excess of indirect-reacting bilirubin in the adult. Among these is the excess production of bilirubin that follows severe hemolysis. Congenital hemolytic anemia, mismatched blood transfusions, and severe hemorrhage into tissues or body cavities are examples. A different etiology is noted in Gilbert's disease, in which there is a failure to remove a normal quantity of unconjugated bilirubin from the blood. Jaundice caused by a lack of UDP-glucuronyl transferase in the infant, Crigler-Najjar disease, is discussed on p. 1401. A similar disease in the adult has been reported. The drug novobiocin may inhibit glucuronyl transferase and thus cause an unconjugated hyperbilirubinemia. Occasionally, patients with alcoholic cirrhosis may have a predominance of indirect-reacting bilirubin that is often associated with spur cell anemia or hypersplenism. The unconjugated bilirubin does not filter through the glomerulus; so there is no bilirubinuria, as is seen in jaundice caused by conjugated hyperbilirubinemia.

In most cases of jaundice (i.e., those caused by viral hepatitis, cirrhosis, biliary tract obstruction, and drugs), there is an increase of both direct-reacting and indirect-reacting bilirubin. Accompanying the rise in direct-reacting bilirubin there is also an increase in indirect-reacting bilirubin, often to as much as 50% in some disorders. The level of the total bilirubin may bear some relationship to the severity of disease in patients with liver cell necrosis and obstruction of the bile ducts but is more useful in following the course of the disorder. Declining levels of the serum bilirubin reflect the healing phase of hepatitis, drug jaundice, and other disorders. The height of the serum bilirubin is regulated not only by degree of hepatic dysfunction and red cell destruction, but also by rate of excretion of the water-soluble conjugated fraction in the urine. This fraction binds to albumin and is not freely excreted. The direct-reacting bilirubin may rise to higher levels in parenchymal cell disease than in obstructive disease for unknown reasons. Although biliuria is prominent early in viral hepatitis, biliuria decreases as jaundice deepens even though the direct-reacting bilirubin in serum rises.

Patients with hyperbilirubinemia who have greatly elevated serum transaminase levels and little or no rise in the alkaline phosphatase are considered to have liver cell necrosis or hepatocellular jaundice. Viral hepatitis, chemicals, poisons, and certain drugs must be con-

sidered in differential diagnosis. In some instances, a rise in alkaline phosphatase occurs in viral hepatitis and may, in older patients, be difficult to differentiate from obstructive biliary tract disease, particularly if the patient is at the stage where serum transaminase levels have dropped to a range of 500 units or less. Patients in shock or severe heart failure may have anoxic centrilobular necrosis associated with high serum transaminases and jaundice, but usually the bilirubin levels are in the range of 5 mg or less.

An increase in serum bilirubin levels accompanied by a high alkaline phosphatase usually is associated with intrahepatic or extrahepatic biliary obstruction. Although extrahepatic biliary obstruction caused by stone, cancer, or stricture is a well-known cause of jaundice with a high alkaline phosphatase, the possibility of drug-induced liver disease must always be ruled out. On occasion, obstructive disease may be accompanied by a moderate rise in serum transaminase (Table 31-1). The prothrombin activity may be reduced in either hepatocellular or prolonged obstructive disease. Administration of parenteral vitamin K will correct prothrombin deficiency induced by biliary tract obstruction but will have little effect on the impairment caused by liver cell necrosis.

Primary biliary cirrhosis in its early stage is often impossible to differentiate from extrahepatic obstruction on the basis of history and the physical and laboratory examinations. A needle biopsy is sometimes performed, but this may be hazardous if the jaundice is really caused by common bile duct obstruction, for bile leakage or hemorrhage may ensue. As a consequence, the diagnosis of obstructive biliary tract disease usually is made by clinical and laboratory means. Patients with choledocholithiasis tend to have a painful disorder that is often associated with cholangitis that produces bed-shaking chills, fever, and a high incidence of gram-negative bacteremia. Similar episodes of cholangitis may develop in the patient with a bile duct stricture. Cholangitis is uncommon in a patient with a malignant obstruction.

Unless the patient is quite ill from duct obstruction, with signs and symptoms of cholangitis not responding to antibiotics, or has diabetes, conservative treatment is the rule for a period of time in the hope that improvement will follow. A drop in bilirubin level or alkaline phosphatase is evidence against a malignant obstruction, except for carcinoma of the papilla of Vater, parts of which may slough periodically. A return of the bilirubin level to normal indicates a benign lesion and a cholecystogram often is performed. In the absence of gallstones, normal concentration by the gallbladder suggests that drug cholestasis is the cause of jaundice.

If jaundice does not abate, and doubt remains as to whether the disease is medical or surgical, one of two methods may be used for the radiologic visualization of the biliary tree.[404] One is by endoscopic retrograde cannulation of the papilla of Vater, and the other is by a recent modification of transhepatic opacification of the biliary tree. In the latter method, the needle is inserted into the liver toward the bifurcation of the common hepatic duct and contrast media is slowly injected under fluoroscopy as the needle is withdrawn. The contrast media entering the duct system will usually outline any obstructive lesion.

In patients suspected of having primary biliary cirrhosis, the results of needle biopsies, the serum mitochondrial antibody test, and the percutaneous angiogram may be definitive enough so that surgery is not considered for diagnostic purposes. Occasionally, the diagnosis may still be in doubt and surgery is performed.

The presence of underlying chronic liver disease in the jaundiced patient usually is manifested by a low serum albumin and a high serum globulin. An enlarged, firm liver, splenomegaly, vascular spiders, and ascites are nearly conclusive evidence of chronicity. The first symptom of chronic active hepatitis and alcoholic liver disease may be jaundice, even though chronic liver disease already is present. The jaundice that occurs in the patient with chronic liver disease is usually of limited duration, but more than one episode is not uncommon.

Occasionally more than one etiologic factor is responsible for the presence of jaundice. An example is *postoperative jaundice,* which is usually a benign condition[364] and may be caused by one or more of the following: (1) increased pigment load, (2) impaired hepatocellular function, and (3) extrahepatic obstruction. In some patients with hypotension and hypoxemia the jaundice has been called *benign postoperative intrahepatic cholestasis* and has to be distinguished from bile duct injury. Among the rare causes of postoperative jaundice is fat embolism.[401]

The diagnosis, care, and management of the jaundiced patient remain a challenge to the clinical acuity of the physician. This has been true for over 100 years, since the pioneers in the study of liver disease first published their observations.

DISEASE IN INFANTS AND CHILDREN

Neonates, infants, and children all are subject to liver disease. In the neonate, acute liver disease predominates. In infants and children, both acute and chronic disease occur. Normally an acholuric, nonhemolytic type of jaundice (so-called physiologic jaundice) is noted in most infants from the second to the fourth day of life. This may be attributable to a lack of a normal amount of glucuronyl transferase necessary to form bilirubin glucuronide, or to a lack of the intracellular acceptor of bilirubin, protein Y.[478] This protein along with protein Z are the organic anion–binding proteins that facilitate the transfer of both bilirubin and sulfobromophthalein. In the premature infant, however, the jaundice may be more severe and prolonged, leading to higher levels of unconjugated bilirubin in the plasma. When the serum bilirubin rises above 20 mg per 100 ml, irreversible damage to the central nervous system, called kernicterus, may be caused by unconjugated bilirubin entering nerve cells, particularly those in the basal ganglia. Inasmuch as unconjugated bilirubin circulates bound to albumin, a low serum albumin or drug therapy that replaces the bilirubin bound to albumin will allow central nervous system damage at levels lower than 20 mg per 100 ml. Ethnic differences in the frequency of neonatal jaundice have been observed in the frequency of high levels of unconjugated bilirubin in Orientals.[468]

The hyperbilirubinemias of the neonate have been classified as unconjugated and conjugated.[473] However, regardless of etiology, this separation does not become too evident before the liver has enough glucuronyl transferase to conjugate bilirubin. This occurs by the fifth to the seventh day of life. The etiology of mild hyperbilirubinemia in the neonate often is not established. In the Los Angeles County–University of Southern California Medical Center, this includes approximately 50% of all neonates with hyperbilirubinemia.

In the premature infant with hyaline membrane disease, jaundice may occur on the third day, and eventually the bilirubin rises to levels that produce kernicterus.

In *hemolytic disease of the newborn,* jaundice is apparent within the first 24 hours. When caused by ABO incompatibility, the disease is usually mild, although kernicterus can occur if the serum bilirubin level rises excessively. A far more serious disorder occurs when the Rh factor is involved. In the past, this disease was known as *erythroblastosis fetalis* or *icterus gravis neonatorum.* Usually, the liver is unable to secrete the large amount of unconjugated bilirubin that results from the hemolysis of erythrocytes. In fatal instances, there is an even distribution of bile in canaliculi and also in the hepatic cells. Liver cell necrosis of variable degree may occur and probably accounts for an increase in conjugated bilirubin that is sometimes seen in hemolytic disease of the newborn infant. Extramedullary erythropoiesis is common and may be extensive not only in the liver, but also in other organs. Because of the danger of kernicterus, severe hyperbilirubinemia often is treated by exchange transfusions. More recently, other methods of treating hyperbilirubinemia have been attempted. The mother may be treated with phenobarbital in the last weeks of pregnancy, and the drug is also given to the newborn infant. Phenobarbital is capable of increasing the smooth endoplasmic reticulum of hepatocytes, which is associated with the formation of glucuronyl transferase necessary for the conjugation of bilirubin and glucuronide.[455,491] It also has been shown that exposure of the newborn infant to blue light will cause a breakdown of the unconjugated bilirubin in the blood.[477] Fortunately, the practice of administration of anti-D to Rh-negative mothers of newborns who have the sensitizing D antigen in their erythrocytes has sharply reduced the incidence of serious erythroblastosis.

Other causes of unconjugated hyperbilirubinemia in the neonate include septicemia, especially that caused by gram-negative organisms, hematomas, and maternal diabetes mellitus. In the latter, the infant is usually large and hypotonic and has hypoglycemia. Congenital syphilis still occurs and may be manifested by hepatosplenomegaly and unconjugated hyperbilirubinemia.[510] Fibrosis, cellular injury, and cholestasis are the usual microscopic findings. It has been noted that serologic tests on the neonate who has congenital syphilis of the liver may be negative, whereas the tests on the mother will be positive.[495] A newly recognized disease, *fatal neonatal hepatic steatosis,* occurring in siblings, has been reported.[494]

Although any one of several diseases may cause an increase in conjugated bilirubin,[449] it may not become manifest until after the first week of life, for the liver is incapable of conjugating a large amount of bilirubin. The diseases most often responsible are either *infections* or *biliary atresia.*[511] It has been estimated that as many as 90% of infants with an obstructive type of jaundice have either neonatal hepatitis or biliary atresia.[504] It is important to differentiate between these, because surgical exploration is necessary in biliary atresia. Two tests may be of help: first, quantitative differences in the bile acid content of the serum and the response to cholestyramine therapy has been observed;[70] second, the serum level of lipoprotein X differs in the two diseases as to amount and also the response to the administration of cholestyramine.[451] There are many morphologic variations in atresia of the extrahepatic bile ducts.[497] When only a segment of the more distal portion of the extrahepatic bile duct system is affected, surgical correction is often possible. When the proximal portion or all of the system is atretic, an anastomosis is impossible. In these patients, liver transplantation has been attempted.[499] On microscopic examination of the liver, there is cholestasis that is predominantly centrilobular (but sometimes also peripheral and within the bile ducts), bile duct proliferation,[449] and periductular fibrosis that is often lamellar (Fig. 31-40). In some instances, foci of necrosis may surround pools of bile in the periphery of the lobules—the so-called bile lakes. Fibrosis along the biliary tracts usually leads to biliary cirrhosis, so that at autopsy one third or more of the liver is composed of fibrous tissue. However, there is considerable variation in severity not related to the duration of the obstruction. Furthermore, when the obstruction is relieved by surgery, the biliary cirrhosis may regress.[503] Children with unrelieved atresia who survive several years may develop portal hypertension and die of bleeding esophageal varices. A hepatoma has also been reported.[485]

Neonatal hepatitis is a term applied by clinicians and pathologists alike to nonobstructive jaundice conditions in the newborn.[442] Originally the term was used for a disorder characterized by transformation of hepatocytes to gigantic multinucleated syncytial cells (Fig. 31-41) that may have eight to 40 nuclei. The latter is often called *giant cell hepatitis.* In the absence of an inflammatory process or evidence of an infective agent that would justify the designation *"hepatitis,"* more proper ter-

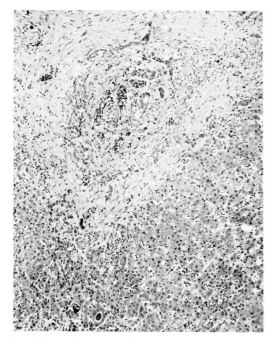

Fig. 31-40. Concentric bands of periportal connective tissue and bile stasis characteristic of biliary cirrhosis (5-month-old infant with atresia of common bile duct).

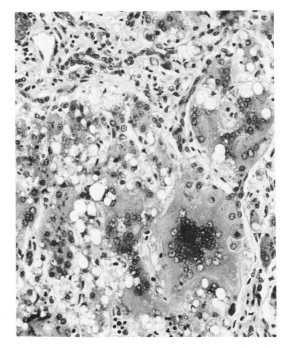

Fig. 31-41. Neonatal hepatitis (3-week-old male infant). Multinucleated giant cells compose most of parenchyma. Increased connective tissue can be seen along sinusoids and in periportal space. Intracanalicular bile stasis at upper right and lower left.

minology would be *idiopathic neonatal jaundice* or *neonatal giant cell transformation*. In addition to the giant cells, which are most prominent, the cells usually are hydropic and contain bile pigment. With progression of the disease, the giant multinucleated cells become more numerous, bile stasis is more prominent, and often there are intralobular tubules filled with bile. Rather characteristic is the diffuse formation of intralobular connective tissue that tends to sharply surround the circumscribed giant cells. Excess hepatic hematopoiesis is nearly always present. A majority of patients have an increased amount of iron in the liver cells and usually excess iron in the spleen.[493] There is ordinarily some increase of connective tissue in the periportal spaces, but the bile ducts are usually not so prominent as they are in biliary atresia.

Between 18%[490] and 40%[440] of infants with neonatal "hepatitis" have α_1-antitrypsin anomalous type ZZ (protease inhibitor, or Pi ZZ) (see pp. 1063 and 1361). The infants usually become asymptomatic after a period of jaundice in the first few months of life and later develop cirrhosis in the juvenile or adolescent period[481] (see discussion on cirrhosis, p. 1376).

Rarely do Pi ZZ infants with neonatal jaundice progress rapidly to death in the neonatal period.[450] The histologic changes in the liver of infants with Pi ZZ who develop neonatal jaundice are reported to fall into one of three histologic patterns: (1) cholestasis with some increase in portal fibrosis but ostensibly normal ducts, (2) extensive portal fibrosis with ductular regeneration and proliferation with little cholestasis, and (3) great reduction of interlobular bile ducts. All groups have one common feature: a demonstrable protease inhibitor glycoprotein in periportal hepatocytes. The glycoprotein that accumulates may be difficult to identify on routine hematoxylin and eosin preparations during the neonatal period, but it can be demonstrated by use of PAS stains, by electron microscopy, or by use of specific immunofluorescent techniques. One third of the third group, none of the second, and one half of the first group are reported to show giant cell transformation.[462a]

The precise relationship of Pi ZZ to biliary dysgenesis (Fig. 31-42), neonatal jaundice, and juvenile cirrhosis is unclear, because not all infants with Pi ZZ develop neonatal jaundice or subsequent liver disease. The two dis-

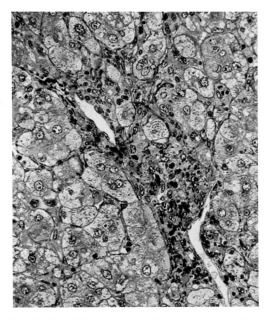

Fig. 31-42. Biliary dysgenesis associated with Pi ZZ. Note poorly defined portal area with deficient duct structures.

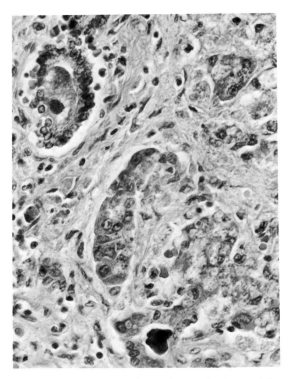

Fig. 31-43. Cytomegalic inclusion body in bile duct epithelial cell at upper left. Cholestasis and liver cell necrosis evident. Patient had jaundice since birth and died at 2½ months of age.

orders, often concurrent, may have a closely linked genetic background. Although HBsAg has been reported in a few infants with neonatal jaundice,[490] such relationship seems fortuitous.

When neonatal jaundice with giant cell transformation is noted on needle biopsy or at autopsy, every effort should be made to establish its etiology. The rubella syndrome, cytomegalic inclusion disease, galactosemia, toxoplasmosis, and biliary atresia may cause similar microscopic findings. However, there remains a sizable group of patients in whom no etiologic factor is recognized. The majority of the patients recover with no sequelae. Some die in the acute stage, and in a few (probably those with Pi ZZ but perhaps others) the liver involvement progresses to cirrhosis. (See discussion on cirrhosis, p. 1376, and Pi ZZ, p. 1326.)

A number of specific infections characterized by liver cell injury are rare causes of neonatal jaundice. *Viral hepatitis* is rarely recognized in infancy. The disease has been reported occurring after both intrauterine transfusion and transfusions given to newborns. More commonly, positive laboratory findings are noted on an infant when the mother has had acute viral hepatitis during the third trimester of pregnancy. More than one half of such infants become HBsAg positive. Infants who acquire

the hepatitis B agent during this period of immune paralysis retain the agent in their sera and their livers indefinitely.[140,210] In the United States, transmission of hepatitis B from a mother who has persistent viral hepatitis (PVH) to the infant is rare,[211] but in Taiwan where some 15% of the patients are asymptomatic carriers of HBsAg, 90% of mothers transmit the infection to offspring that are asymptomatic.[216] The benign clinical features of viral hepatitis, occurring during infancy, add support to the concept that tissue-immune responses augment the severity of the disease in later life. In *cytomegalic inclusion disease,* bile stasis is prominent. Some multinucleated giant cells may be seen, but necrosis of liver cells is variable. When present, the giant intranuclear inclusions are diagnostic (Fig. 31-43). As a rule, they are more easily found in the kidney. Cytomegalovirus hepatitis may produce jaundice in the adult.[509] In *herpes simplex,* the transmission of the disease is probably through the placenta, and the death rate is high.[460] There is hepatomegaly and a rise in SGOT but no jaundice as a rule.[445,483] An extensive coagulation necrosis is seen in the liver. The individual virus particles and the method of their exodus from the nucleus have been studied by electron microscopy.[487] In *coxsackie viremia*, there may be extensive necrosis of the liver and jaundice.[476] Massive necrosis may also occur after *echovirus 14* infection.[470]

Severe hepatitis with cholestasis and giant cell change has been observed in the rubella syndrome.[456] Coagulative necrosis also has been reported.[501] Many infants with trisomy of number 18 chromosome (E trisomy) have neonatal hepatitis and also may have biliary atresia.[443,492]

Extensive necrosis of the liver in the neonate that is associated with excessive iron has been observed.[492] Recently a disease characterized by hereditary recurrent cholestasis with lymphoedema has been described in Norway.[439]

In the first 2 to 3 weeks of life, if an infant with galactosemia is given cow's milk, the liver may enlarge and jaundice supervene. The diagnosis of this condition is highly important, because the removal of galactose from the diet relieves the symptoms.[452] The newborn infant with galactosemia may present with severe infection and septicemia. Recognition of the disease may be delayed for a few months, depending on the symptomatology. Various screening methods have been used for its detection.[462,466] The toxic effects of galactose accumulation is noted in the liver, in the eye where lenticular opacities may develop quickly, and in the brain where degeneration and mental retardation may result.[457,506] The pathology and inheritance of the disease have been studied extensively.[446,453]

The liver is enlarged and fatty and may become cirrhotic. Microscopically, the lobules are large, a moderate to severe degree of fatty change is present, and bile stasis is the rule. The bile plugs are contained within large acini. Often numerous bile ducts entering the periphery of the lobules are likewise filled with bile (Fig. 31-44). An irregular increase of connective tissue widens and lengthens the periportal spaces, sometimes connecting adjacent ones, so that cirrhosis can be diagnosed. The combination of large liver lobules, fatty change, and bile stasis seems to be characteristic of galactosemia. More rarely in galactosemia, the liver contains an excess of glycogen, with the cytoplasm of the cells being almost water clear, and rather delicate septa connect the periportal spaces, resulting in a different type of cirrhosis. In both of the foregoing

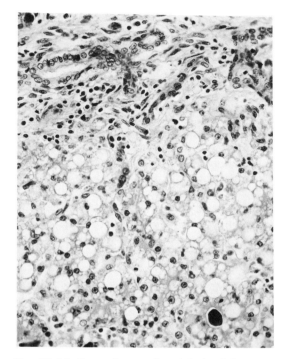

Fig. 31-44. Fatty change, intralobular bile stasis, and some increase of periportal connective tissue characteristic of galactosemia (3-week-old white male infant).

types, the central veins are visible and regenerative change seems to be minimal. It is of interest that in children with proved cirrhosis and ascites, proper treatment results in an apparent cessation of the disease process.

Neonatal cirrhosis has been described, predominantly in males 5:1.[502] During the period of infancy (up to 2 years of age), *infantile cirrhosis* may follow some of the conditions just described, such as atresia of the common bile duct and galactosemia, or it may occur occasionally as a complication of congenital syphilis. In instances of neonatal hepatitis in which the infant survives for a year or more, fibrosis may be of such severity that the liver could be classified as cirrhotic.

Other rare inheritable disorders of infancy include *tyrosinosis*, in which the liver may become cirrhotic and death is attributable to liver failure.[471] There is tyrosinemia, multiple renal tubular defects,[459] and increased urinary excretion of phenolic acids. Apparently the disease is caused by a lack of the enzyme *p*-hydroxyphenylpyruvic acid oxidase. On microscopic examination, regeneration, fatty change, and fibrosis are noted. Liver cell carcinoma may arise late in the disease.[463] In a child with features of tyrosinosis, recovery after dietary treatment has been reported.[464] At times it is difficult to distinguish tyrosinemia from galactosemia[472] and hereditary fructosemia.[479] *In fructose intolerance,* hepatomegaly and jaundice occur. This disorder is attributable to deficiency of the enzyme fructose phosphate-1-aldolase. In the liver there is fatty change, fibrosis, and cirrhosis.[489] *GM₁ gangliosidosis* is a genetically determined deficiency of β-galactosidase. Light and electron microscopy discloses many vacuoles in the hepatocytes and Kupffer cells. These have a characteristic ultrastructural appearance.[488]

Hypoglycemia in the neonate as well as in infancy and childhood may be caused by one of the hepatic enzyme deficiencies.[486] These include glycogen-storage disease, galactosemia, and fructose intolerance. Reye's syndrome also may cause hypoglycemia. In this disorder there is severe encephalopathy associated with fatty degeneration of the viscera. Most often it

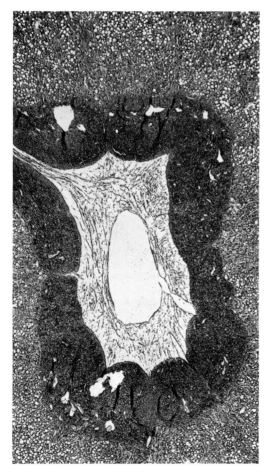

Fig. 31-45. Veno-occlusive disease of liver. (Slide courtesy Dr. G. Bras.)

occurs after an upper respiratory infection, usually viral. There is vomiting, delirium, and coma that is followed by death or recovery in a few days. The children are not jaundiced, but at necropsy the liver is yellow and the hepatocytes contain innumerable fine fat vacuoles. The disease has been associated with epidemics of influenza type B[467,480] and with the ingestion of aflatoxin.[447] An elevation of short-chain fatty acids has been observed in this disease.[507]

Niemann-Pick disease usually runs its course before the age of 4. Hepatomegaly, severe liver changes, and persistent jaundice may be noted in type D.[454] In the West Indies, both children and adults who have ingested "bush tea" made from boiling the leaves of *Crotalaria fulva* and *Senecio discolor* may develop occlusive disease of the central and sublobular veins, with resultant hepatomegaly, ascites, and often jaundice[448,496,500] (Fig. 31-45). The disease has also been reported in South America.[461] The venous lesion is first characterized by edema and later by collagenization. The large hepatic veins usually are unaffected. The sinusoids are remarkably congested, and the centrilobular hepatic cells atrophy. Later, in chronic cases, a nonportal type of cirrhosis may develop. A similar disease apparently occurs after the use of flour contaminated with *Senecio* in Africa.[496] Egyptian children also suffer from a disease involving the hepatic veins.[465]

In India, a disease known as *Indian childhood cirrhosis* (ICC) has been studied extensively.[441] This disease may be seen in patients from 6 months to 14 years of age. Five different histologic types have been recognized. The largest number of patients were in group II, which is predominantly a degenerative disease characterized by ballooning of liver cells, hyaline necrosis, neutrophilic exudate, and giant cell transformation. There is also fibrosis and loss of lobular architecture. It seems that only children in India are affected by the group II type of change. The other four types are not distinctive. In the limited material available for study, we have had difficulty in distinguishing the changes in group II from sclerosing hyaline necrosis seen in alcoholism.

Several of the inborn errors of metabolism may be responsible for cirrhosis in the juvenile patient. *Glycogenosis* has been defined as any condition in which the glycogen concentration of a tissue is increased.[482] Normally, the glycogen concentration in the liver should not exceed 6% of the wet weight. *Glycogen-storage disease* of the liver is now divided into types

I to X, each with its specific enzyme defect. Septa only have been observed in types III, VI, IX, and X. Only type IV may progress to cirrhosis that is fatal.[469,482] Many features of glycogen-storage disease are noted on electron microscopic studies. Among these is the storage of glycogen in abnormal lysosomes called "lysosomal bags." In this disorder, *Pompe's disease,* there is an absence of α-1,4-glucosidase.[498] Although clinical, laboratory, and morphologic studies are helpful, the final diagnosis rests on quantitative biochemical analysis of the tissue.[482] Fibrosis associated with *Gaucher's cells* may lead to scarring and finally a nodular liver. Liver changes may be observed in several of the mucopolysaccharidoses.[454] In *Hurler's syndrome* (gargoylism), the liver may be greatly enlarged, but cirrhosis rarely develops.[444] In this disorder there is an excess of dermatan sulfate and heparan sulfate in the urine and tissues, along with a decrease of β-galactosidase in the tissues.[454] The hepatocytes are highly vacuolated. When studied with the electron microscope, these vacuoles have a single membrane and contain both granular material and poorly staining areas. In *Hunter's syndrome,* hepatic changes are similar.[454] Liver changes have also been observed in *alpha-fucosidosis.*[454]

In children and infants with cystic *fibrosis of the pancreas,* the liver may contain focal areas of fibrosis associated with dilated bile ducts containing eosinophilic casts. Prolonged jaundice with cholestasis may be observed in the neonate.[508] In more advanced states of liver disease, a true cirrhosis may develop, with formation of nodules of variable size. A liver scan is important in diagnosis.[459]

Congenital hepatic fibrosis is a variant of polycystic disease,[474] for microcysts are present in the dense fibrous tissue that surrounds the lobules. These may be associated with polycystic disease of the liver, kidney, and pancreas. The disease was first described in children[475] but may become symptomatic in adults.[484] Portal hypertension is the predominating symptom in patients who have normal liver function tests. It is characterized by an excessive amount of dense connective tissue that is laid down around small bile ducts.[505] The histologic findings are characteristic in that portal fibrosis surrounds lobules that have intact central veins. Intrahepatic saccular dilatation of the biliary ductal system (Caroli's disease) is often associated with congenital hepatic fibrosis but rarely produces symptoms in childhood. (See also p. 1393.)

The term *juvenile cirrhosis* is sometimes used for patients in this particular age group. With careful study, most of these cases can be put in one or the other of the various etiologic types of cirrhosis outlined in the classification, particularly α_1-antitrypsin deficiency, Wilson's disease, or chronic active hepatitis of unknown etiology.

DISEASE IN PREGNANCY

The frequency of jaundice in pregnancy is about 1 in 1500 patients.[521] Some liver diseases occur almost exclusively in pregnancy, but consideration also must be given to more common illnesses, such as viral hepatitis, stones, and drug jaundice.[519] Viral hepatitis occurring during pregnancy seems to be no different from that seen in nonpregnant women. In our series of cases of fulminant hepatitis from 1918 to 1970, none of the patients were pregnant.

Among the disorders peculiar to pregnancy is obstetric cholestasis or recurrent jaundice of pregnancy, a familial disorder that has its onset in the third trimester. It is accompanied by pruritus and tends to recur with succeeding pregnancies. Pruritus of pregnancy without jaundice is a variant. It is likely that the disorder is caused by an increased level of hormones in susceptible patients, especially since investigators have shown that the same patients who develop recurrent jaundice of pregnancy, develop similar cholestasis and symptoms after the use of estrogens, progesterone, or both as in oral contraceptives.[251,518] A biopsy discloses centrilobular cholestasis without necrosis. Laboratory findings include a serum bilirubin level of less than 10 mg per 100 ml, a sharp elevation of serum alkaline phosphatase, and only a mild rise in SGOT levels. An associated rise in plasma bile acids is probably responsible for the pruritus.

Idiopathic *fatty liver of pregnancy,* initially described in 1940,[525] is a rare, highly fatal disorder that occurs in the third trimester. During the early 1960s, many cases of fatty liver of pregnancy were reported, but most of them occurred after the intravenous administration of tetracycline given for the treatment of pyelonephritis. It became apparent that tetracycline hepatotoxicity in pregnancy produced a fatty liver indistinguishable from the idiopathic type. Both are characterized by epigastric pain, vomiting, jaundice, and symptoms of hepatic and renal failure. The laboratory findings usually consist of hyperbilirubinemia, lactic acidosis, azotemia, hyperamylasemia, and depressed prothrombin activity. The transaminase levels are usually under 500 units. Those who survive an attack of idiopathic fatty liver of pregnancy may subsequently have an uncomplicated pregnancy.[514] At autopsy, the liver is moderately decreased in size and is soft. Fatty change of a foamy type is present, the fat being most prominent on the sinusoidal border of the liver cell with the displacement of the granular portion of the cytoplasm to the area around the bile canaliculus. Cholestasis is not prominent. Necrosis is hardly visible, but syncytial change of hepatocytes is prominent in centrilobular foamy cells. Pathologic changes also are seen in the renal tubules, pancreas, and brain. It is probable that tetracycline inhibits the synthesis of the proteins essential to the formation of lipoproteins, the principal form by which fat leaves the liver, thus leading to fatty liver.[324,522,523] Disseminated intravascular coagulation may complicate acute fatty liver of pregnancy.[516]

Eclampsia only rarely produces hepatic symptoms or clinical liver disease. Only one instance of fatal hepatic failure associated with the liver lesion of eclampsia was found at the Los Angeles County–University of Southern California medical complexes from 1918 to 1970. How-

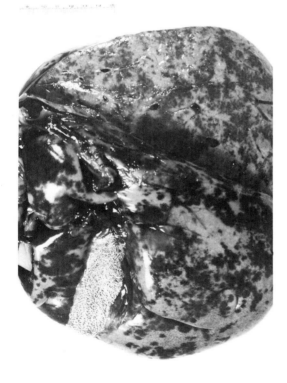

Fig. 31-46. Liver in eclampsia showing hemorrhagic appearance.

ever, patients who die from eclampsia generally have a mottled discoloration of the liver with hemorrhagic areas alternating with zones of pale ischemic necrosis and intact liver (Fig. 31-46). The periportal regions often have fibrin in the sinusoids and are often necrotic. The small branches of the portal vein may be thrombosed. Zones of infarction may cover several lobules. Occasionally, patients develop such hepatic alterations without the convulsions of eclampsia.[517,524] Rarely, diffuse coagulative necrosis occurs as a terminal event. Spontaneous rupture of the liver is a rare complication, usually in the third trimester of a multipara who has toxemia with or without eclampsia.[515] The rupture nearly always occurs in the right lobe as a complication of subcapsular hematoma.[512] It is of interest that rupture of the liver may occur in women taking contraceptive drugs.[520]

Most chronic diseases of liver preclude pregnancy, although rarely a cirrhotic patient may become pregnant.[513] Liver disease is often difficult to evaluate because of alterations of laboratory values that are associated with pregnancy. The serum albumin level is ordinarily depressed to a range of 2.8 to 3.7 gm per 100 ml (normal is 3.5 to 4.8 gm per 100 ml), and the alkaline phosphatase activity often is elevated to as much as twice the upper limits of normal.

In the differential diagnosis of liver disease in pregnancy, in addition to the liver diseases occurring almost exclusively in pregnancy, consideration also must be given to more common illnesses, such as stones, toxins, and viral hepatitis, which may occur in a pregnant woman.

DISEASES OF INTRAHEPATIC BILE DUCTS

The most common disease of the intrahepatic bile ducts (i.e., acute cholangitis) is discussed on p. 1358. However the ducts are subject to other disease, both primary and secondary. Among conditions unique to the ducts alone are sclerosing cholangitis, aneurysmal dilatation of the ducts, intrahepatic calculi, and pneumobilia.

Sclerosing cholangitis is a disease of the common bile duct that may extend into the liver, causing severe deformity of the intrahepatic ducts with characteristic "beading." In autopsy material, primary sclerosing cholangitis is a rare disorder.[536] The cause of the disease is unknown, but the possibility of its being an autoimmune reaction has been considered. A similar cholangitis is sometimes associated with one of the following: ulcerative colitis, retroperitoneal fibrosis, or fibrous mediastinitis.[531] The association of sclerosing cholangitis with ulcerative colitis is not unusual. The patient may be jaundiced for a variable period but often becomes asymptomatic. A few cases will go on to biliary cirrhosis or be complicated by a carcinoma of the ducts.[533,535]

Congenital dilatation of the *intrahepatic bile ducts,* or *Caroli's disease,* is a rare disorder. The cystic dilatations are easily seen on cholangiograms and may involve many of the intrahepatic bile ducts. The dilatations are filled with bile and have a characteristic gross and microscopic appearance.[528] The disease may be associated with choledochal cysts as well as with congenital hepatic fibrosis and is occasionally complicated by carcinoma.[527] *Intrahepatic calculi* most often occur as a complication of a chronic obstruction of the extrahepatic biliary tract but may, on occasion, be primary in the liver. An unusual disease seen in Chinese immigrants as well as in East Asia has been called *cholangiohepatitis* (Hong Kong disease). The patients may have calculi in the bile ducts, much sludge, and often remnants of *Clonorchis sinensis.*[532] Air in the intrahepatic biliary tract, or *pneumobilia,* is most often attributable to a cholecystoduodenal fistula.[530] The diagnosis is usually made on roentgenograms. The clinical entity of hemobilia, or hemorrhage into the biliary tract, is characterized by biliary colic, gastrointestinal hemorrhage, and often bilirubinuria and clinical jaundice. Both melena and hematemesis may be present. Unrecognized hemobilia has a high mortality. Among the causes of hemobilia are trauma (p. 1399), needle biopsy of the liver[526] and neoplasms of the intrahepatic bile ducts or of the hepatic parenchyma, and aneurysms (hemocholecyst)[534] of the hepatic artery. Diseases of the gallbladder and extrahepatic ducts may also give rise to hemobilia. Superior mesenteric angiography is considered the best diagnostic procedure for the diagnosis of hemobilia.[529]

REGENERATION

The liver has a great capacity for regeneration after resection, injury, or destruction of its cells. After removal of 30% to 70% of the liver in experimental animals, there is rapid liver cell hypertrophy followed by cell division.[541] The mitoses are concentrated at the periphery of the liver unit during the first 24 hours of the response.[540] Deoxyribonucleic acid (DNA) synthesis during regeneration shows values reaching 50 times normal. In the rat the peak of DNA synthesis occurs 21 to 23 hours after resection in most animals. Mitotic activity is limited after 48 hours but the liver returns to normal size.[542] The factor or factors that control regeneration have been extensively studied.[541] Much evidence has accumulated that one factor responsible is contained in portal vein blood, especially in that part of the blood that comes from the splenic vein and presumably from pancreas. Pancreatic insulin and glucagon appear to provide some advantage to the regenerating liver according to some experiments,[548] whereas others indicate that this is not true.[545,547] Furthermore it appears that blood circulated through a regenerating liver contains a factor that initiates a regenerative response in a normal liver.[543] Angiographic studies show that during regeneration the arteries probably hypertrophy and appear stretched, but no new vessels are observed.[537]

A major portion of the liver may be extirpated in the treatment of severe traumatic injury and neoplastic disease. After this, the patient may have hypoglycemia, hypoalbuminemia, and a bleeding diathesis. The last is caused by decreased levels of prothrombin and fibrinogen but usually is not severe. All of these complications are of short duration.[9]

TRANSPLANTATION

Many orthotopic liver transplants have now been attempted, usually in patients who have a primary carcinoma of the liver or congenital biliary atresia.[538,544,546,549] Several patients have survived for more than 2 years, but graft failure is common.[539] Most important is sepsis that is related to immunosuppression. Other complications have been encountered, among which are leakage from the biliary anastomosis, and breakdown and bleeding from the vascular anastomoses. Thrombosis of the hepatic artery or portal vein and hemorrhage unrelated to vascular anastomosis may also cause graft failure. Rejection alone is not one of the common causes of death. In autopsy material, the changes in the liver that are attributable to rejection alone are difficult to evaluate. These include a dense mononuclear cell infiltrate in the triads and sinusoids with prominent immunoblasts. Centrilobular necrosis and cholestasis are present. Immunoblastic and lymphocytic infiltration about portal and, later, central vein branches seems to be a characteristic feature. After recovery from apparent rejection, collagen fibers may be seen in the space of Disse. The vascular changes consist of a thickened arterial intima, many lipophages, and disruption of the internal elastic lamina. The results of transplantation of 27 cases in England have been published.[538,550]

DEGENERATIONS

Degenerative changes that affect the liver, such as cloudy swelling and glycogen infiltration, are adequately discussed elsewhere in the text (p. 112).

Atrophy. Generalized atrophy may occur in old age and in starvation states such as anorexia nervosa. The atrophy may or may not be accompanied by an increase of lipochrome that gives the liver a deep brown appearance. In the atrophic state the liver often weighs less than 1000 gm and the hepatocytes appear shrunken. Segmental and lobar atrophy of the liver may occur after certain disease states of the liver, such as vascular or biliary obstruction, hepatocellular damage, or a combination of factors.[556] It is important when such changes are seen at surgery to remedy any correctable cause.

Amyloidosis. Hepatic involvement is seen with almost equal frequency in primary and secondary amyloidosis.[558] Hepatomegaly, splenomegaly, and ascites are common; the last is usually caused by cardiac or renal amyloidosis. The liver is enlarged, firm, and has a dense capsule. The edges are rounded and the organ has a pale color. The cut surface is abnormally translucent in the areas of amyloid accumulation. Amyloidosis is predominantly portal in distribution, but in those patients where it is predominantly intralobular, there is usually massive hepatomegaly, cardiac and renal involvement, and ascites. The amyloid appears as a hyaline material between the lining cells of the sinusoids and the liver cells. Its continued accumulation causes compression, atrophy, and disappearance of the liver cells. Amyloidosis of vessel walls exclusively is more likely to be present in the primary form of the disease. The course is variable, and the diagnosis often is established by needle biopsy.

Calcification. When differential diagnosis becomes of clinical importance, calcifications in the liver may be observed on roentgenograms.[557] The most common cause is metastatic mucinous adenocarcinoma from the colon and stomach. Calcifications in other metastatic lesions, such as osteogenic sarcoma, carcinoid, neuroblastoma, lymphoma, and Zollinger-Ellison syndrome,[552] are rare occurrences. Several primary tumors of the liver, including liver cell carcinoma (especially in infants), hemangioendothelioma, and hemangioma, as well as the granulomatous lesions (tuberculosis and histoplasmosis), may cause calcifications. Simple cysts, hydatid cysts, actinomycosis, and pyogenic abscesses are other rare causes.[560]

Fatty change. Fatty change in the liver is common, perhaps more frequent than in any other organ, and it may be of severe degree. Because of the rapid transport of free fatty acids from the peripheral adipose tissue to the liver and the formation of triglyceride, phospholipid, and cholesterol esters that must be secreted into the blood as lipoprotein, anything that interferes with the intracellular metabolism of the lipids can quickly result in recognizable fatty change. Excess mobilization of fat also may result in the accumulation in the liver. The fat usually accumulates in the center of the lobules, where, when abundant, it forms large globules that distend the hepatic cells. Nearer the peripheries of the lobules, the globules tend to be smaller and only partially fill the hepatic cells. In chronic ulcerative pulmonary tuberculosis, a peripheral type of fatty change predominates. In prolonged passive congestion, the fatty change may be most noticeable at the centers of the lobules. With gross fatty accumulation, the liver is increased in size and has a tense capsule and rounded margins. The cut surface bulges slightly and is pale yellow to yellow (Plate 4, *B*). The lobular markings are obscured.

By far the most common cause of severe fatty change is chronic alcoholism (p. 1367). Fatty livers also are found in association with obesity, malnutrition, and wasting diseases (e.g., tuberculosis and malignant tumors) and in some cases of diabetes mellitus. Certain poisons, such as phlorhizin, carbon tetrachloride, chloroform, and ether, may cause fatty change. In kwashiorkor, a common disease in the tropical regions that is associated with protein malnutrition, the fatty change may be extreme.[562] The fat accumulates in large vacuoles, sometimes forming fatty cysts.[563] The changes seen with the electron microscope are rather mild. The patients may be lethargic or in coma. Hypoglycemia is common.

In experimental animals, a pronounced centrilobular fatty change may be produced by deficiency of choline, and peripheral fatty changes are produced by certain amino acid deficiencies that must be accompanied by a sufficient intake of carbohydrate.[561]

Fatty change resulting from ethionine administration is apparently caused by a lack of adenosine triphosphate (ATP) in the liver cells.[554]

In some cases of sudden death in young adults, pronounced fatty change in the liver has been the only finding.[555] A peculiar fatty change seen in late pregnancy is described on p. 1395.

Severe fatty change has been noted in obese patients who have had a jejunoileal or jejunocolic bypass for the treatment of obesity. Death has been reported in such cases.[551,553,559]

CONGENITAL AND ACQUIRED ABNORMALITIES OF FORM AND POSITION

Congenital abnormalities of the liver are not common. Reidel's lobe is a downward projection of the right lobe, which may be mistaken for a tumor or believed to be a displaced kidney. The liver may be displaced in position in association with a congenital diaphragmatic hernia. Severe abnormalities that require surgery are seen rarely.[564] Atrophy of the left lobe of the liver may be caused by some interference with the left branch of the portal vein.

Acquired abnormalities of position are mainly downward or upward displacement by some extrahepatic cause, such as a subdiaphragmatic abscess or an abdominal tumor. Abnormalities of form may be the result of contraction of scar tissue (e.g., hepar lobatum) or nodularity from irregular regenerative hyperplasia or neoplastic growth. Transverse, oblique, or sagittal grooves on the upper or anterior surface of the liver are common. They have been attributed to pressure of the ribs, folds of the diaphragm, and tight clothing. They often are associated with chronic cough, emphysema, and bronchitis caused by pressure from hypertrophied diaphragmatic muscle bundles. The capsule is thickened at the depths of the folds, and adjacent hepatic parenchyma may show slight atrophic changes. Such grooving does not appear to be of any functional significance.

TRAUMA

The liver, because of its size, weight, and soft consistency, is susceptible to blunt injury, especially in vehicular accidents at high speed. Collision with the steering wheel is particularly harmful. Blunt injuries most often affect the right lobe, producing lacerations of variable configuration and severity that require surgery. Severe injury without laceration of the capsule may cause continued bleeding that results in a subcapsular hematoma and delayed

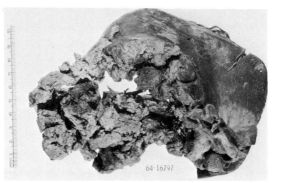

Fig. 31-47. Shattered right lobe of liver after bullet wound. Specimen surgically resected.

rupture into the abdominal cavity 24 hours or more after the accident. A peritoneal tap may aid in the diagnosis of intrahepatic hemorrhage.[569] In some instances an intrahepatic hematoma ruptures into the biliary tract with resultant hemobilia,[568] in which the patient has gastrointestinal bleeding, often with hematemesis.

Stabbings and gunshot wounds are common causes of injury to the liver.[569] Gunshot wounds may destroy much of the liver (Fig. 31-47). The treatment of traumatic injury may require special surgical techniques,[9,569] especially when the hepatic veins and inferior vena cava are injured; the former may be actually torn from the vena cava. In some instances the hepatic artery must be ligated to control hemorrhage.[567] The highest mortality is from gunshot blasts and blunt trauma. Injury to other organs also increases the mortality.[596] In traumatized liver removed at surgery, there is a variable amount of hemorrhage and necrosis of the injured parenchyma, often with a neutrophilic exudate. On rare occasions, an arteriovenous fistula has been known to occur after liver injury.[566] These are often present for many years before they are diagnosed and lead to portal hypertension and ascites. They are curable by surgery.

Subcapsular hematomas, of small or large size, occur occasionally in newborn infants, especially those born prematurely, and require surgery, or prove fatal.[565] These hematomas may be caused by trauma during birth or may accompany blood dyscrasias, such as erythroblastosis fetalis.

PIGMENTATION

Anthracotic pigment may be carried to the liver by the bloodstream after rupture into

Table 31-5. Hereditary hyperbilirubinemias

Syndrome	Age of onset of jaundice	Symptoms and course	Serum bilirubin			BSP excretion	Cholecysto-gram	Gallstones	Pathologic condition
			Range	Conjugated	Unconjugated				
Crigler-Najjar 1.	Neonate	Jaundice at birth with or without kernicterus; death in first year of life	>20 mg per 100 ml	—	Increased	Normal	Visualization	—	Few bile thrombi
2.		May be past 50	<20 mg per 100 ml	—	Increased	Normal	—	—	Few bile thrombi
Gilbert's constitutional hyperbilirubinemia	Birth to middle age (average, 18 years)	Jaundice may be precipitated by fatigue, intermittent infections, alcohol, and stress; nausea, anorexia, and vague abdominal distress may occur	<5 mg per 100 ml	Normal	Increased	Normal	Visualization	Increased frequency	Hypertrophy of smooth endoplasmic reticulum
Dubin-Johnson 1. Classic	Most often 15 to 25 years	Pain over liver and hepatomegaly, especially during attacks of jaundice; dyspepsia; problem exists throughout life with fluctuations of jaundice	N to 6 mg per 100 ml	Increased	Increased	Retention with late rise after 90 minutes	No visualization	Occur in approximately 10%	Pigment in liver, probably melanins
2. Variants in family members	Mild elevation of serum bilirubin after 10 years	None	>1 mg in 20% of family	Normal or increased	Normal or increased	Normal	Normal		Pigment in many but not related to increased serum bilirubin
Rotor	Early in life, usually before 20 years	Jaundice fluctuates	N to 6 mg per 100 ml	Increased	Increased	Retention with no late rise	Visualization		None

the pulmonary veins of a thoracic lymph node containing carbon pigment. The carbon particles are phagocytized by the Kupffer cells and tend to be carried to portal spaces, where they accumulate.

Silver pigment may be found under the sinusoidal endothelial cells of the liver in argyria. After the injection of Thorotrast, macrophages in the periportal areas and Kupffer cells may store thorium for decades.

Hemosiderin accumulation in the liver is common. In hemolytic anemias, the hemosiderin tends to be distributed diffusely. The pigment is found in both the hepatic cells and the phagocytic Kupffer cells of the sinusoids. In hemochromatosis, the pigment is largely hemosiderin, but hemofuscin is present as well.

In malaria, hematin pigment may accumulate in large amount, mainly in the Kupffer cells of the sinusoids. It may be sufficient to give the liver a dark grayish brown color. A similar pigment may be found in the liver in schistosomiasis.

Bile pigmentation of the liver is seen in any variety of jaundice. When seen fresh, the liver is yellowish but soon changes to green as a result of oxidation of the bilirubin to biliverdin. Masses of pigment may be seen distending the bile capillaries and small ducts and also within the hepatic cells.

The differential diagnosis of increased lipochrome in the liver as seen on biopsies is discussed on p. 1419.

HEREDITARY HYPERBILIRUBINEMIA

Several syndromes that are caused by inborn errors in the metabolism of bilirubin have been described.[578] The essential features of these disorders are given in Table 31-5.

In the *Crigler-Najjar syndrome,* there is unconjugated hyperbilirubinemia as a result of hepatic glucuronyl transferase deficiency. A similar disease is seen in the Gunn rat. The disease occurs in two forms, types 1 and 2. In type 1, there is absence of glucuronyl transferase; severe hyperbilirubinemia, usually greater than 20 mg per 100 ml; the bile is almost completely colorless and contains only traces of unconjugated bilirubin (UCB). In type 2, the patients have a partial deficiency of glucuronyl transferase, the hyperbilirubinemia is less severe, and the bile contains some bilirubin glucuronide. The conjugation defect in the first type is transmitted as an autosomal recessive character and in the second type as an autosomal dominant character.[22] The jaundice appears in the neonate and persists with high concentrations of unconjugated bilirubin in the blood serum. Patients in type 1 often die in infancy, whereas those in type 2 have been known to survive past age 50 without neurologic disorders.[577] Administration of phenobarbital increases the hypertrophy of the smooth endoplasmic reticulum and lowers the serum UCB in type 2 patients only. As in Gilbert's disease, dietary restriction increases the UCB and a normal diet restores the former level. Interestingly, the use of intravenous glucose after dietary restriction did not lower the UCB.[597]

In the *Gilbert syndrome,* the patient usually has intermittent attacks of jaundice, lassitude, and abdominal pain. The jaundice is attributable to an increase in the unconjugated serum bilirubin. A sharp reduction of hepatic bilirubin transferase has been shown in this group.[571] Patients with Gilbert's syndrome, when fasted or when given nicotinic acid, showed an abnormal rise in their unconjugated bilirubin.[576] Electron microscopy studies have shown a remarkable hypertrophy of the SER.[579]

In the *Dubin-Johnson-Sprinz-Nelson type, or chronic idiopathic jaundice,* there is chronic or intermittent jaundice, dark urine, and an increase in both conjugated and unconjugated bilirubin. The glucuronyl transferase is presumed to be normal, but the liver cells have difficulty in secreting conjugated bilirubin. Similarly, the secretion of sulfobromophthalein and iopanoic acid is affected so that abnormal tests result. Patients excrete an abnormal amount of coproporphyrin I.[570] The parenchymal cells, especially in the centrilobular zones, contain large granules of lipochrome pigment (Fig. 31-48), often in such amounts that the liver is black. The pigment is apparently a melanin[573] and is located within lysosomes.[575] A similar disease is seen in a Corriedale sheep mutant.[574] The disease in the human is inherited as an autosomal recessive trait.[580] The study of a large family with the Dubin-Johnson trait disclosed considerable variation in the relation of pigment in the liver to hyperbilirubinemia.[572] Improvement in the handling of bilirubin and sulfobromophthalein is noted in some patients after the use of phenobarbital, an enzyme inducer.[581]

In *Rotor's syndrome,* there is likewise an increase in both conjugated and unconjugated serum bilirubin but no pigmentation of the liver cells. There is sulfobromophthalein retention but normal visualization of the gallbladder. It has been suggested that Rotor's is a variant of the Dubin-Johnson syndrome.

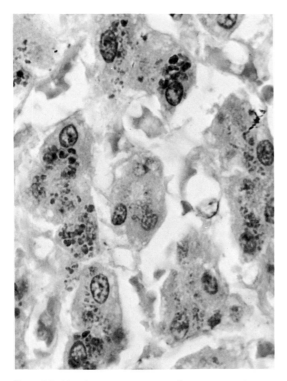

Fig. 31-48. Large masses of intracytoplasmic brown pigment in Dubin-Johnson syndrome.

CIRCULATORY DISTURBANCES
Shock

Acute hepatic changes, even centrilobular necrosis, often occur in patients who are in shock. These changes may be observed in a liver that was previously normal or be superimposed upon chronic passive congestion or cirrhosis. Trauma, hemorrhage, myocardial infarction, and endotoxin shock from septicemia are the more common causes. Shock of more than 24 hours' duration usually is associated with liver cell necrosis.[603] Jaundice is rare but does occur in endotoxin shock[386] and in cardiac conditions. The liver of the rat has been used for extensive studies on cellular metabolism during shock. According to the present hypothesis, the first step in progressive cell injury is cell membrane alteration that allows Na^+ to enter. Na^+K-ATPase is activated, ATP is used, and the mitochondria are active. Cyclic AMP decreases and a series of alterations ensues that leads to further Na^+ entering the cell, swelling of the organelles, leaking of lysosomes, and finally cell destruction with release of toxic factors.[582]

The pathologic changes in the liver that have been described are those seen at autopsy or in experimental animals. A reversible change, fatty vacuolization, has been noted[594] in patients in shock who survived more than 18 hours. *Anoxic centrilobular necrosis* is a severe lesion that occurs most often in patients with cirrhosis who die of bleeding esophageal varices. Other causes include shock attributable to myocardial infarction and exsanguinating hemorrhage from peptic ulcers. Anoxic necrosis also occurs in patients with severe heart failure who have no recognizable episode of shock. On gross examination, centrilobular necrosis may or may not be recognized, but often central zones have a characteristic dull yellow to yellow-brown appearance. The necrosis is of the coagulation type, the cells are intensely acidophilic, and the nuclei stain poorly or have disappeared. Neutrophils may be abundant, especially around the periphery of the necrotic zones. The degree of centrilobular hyperemia varies greatly; it may be so extreme that pools of blood fill the necrotic area. In many instances a distinguishing feature of anoxic necrosis is a narrow rim of intact hepatocytes that remain around the central veins. Although the necrosis is predominantly centrilobular, the midzonal area is often affected. The necrotic cells slowly disappear, and in biopsy material taken in the healing stage, only dilated sinusoids and pigmented macrophages are seen, a histologic picture difficult to distinguish from other types of healing centrilobular zonal necrosis. The cirrhotic liver is particularly prone to anoxic necrosis when there is bleeding from varices. The large pseudolobules of cirrhosis are probably poorly oxygenated as a result of an abnormal outflow pattern. Furthermore, much of the portal vein blood may be shunted around the liver, so that a fall in hepatic artery pressure during shock would lead rapidly to anoxic necrosis. The areas of necrosis are often large and pale yellow-white and may be surrounded by a thin zone of hemorrhage (Fig. 31-49). It is likely that some of the depressed scars seen in the liver of patients who have bled from varices in the past may be of anoxic origin.

Biopsy material rarely is obtained on patients in shock. In one such case, severe centrilobular necrosis was observed (Fig. 31-50). The recognition of hemorrhage within the necrotic zone is difficult, since the margins of the widened blood-filled sinusoids are difficult to distinguish.

Endotoxin shock in animals produces extensive damage to the endothelium lining the

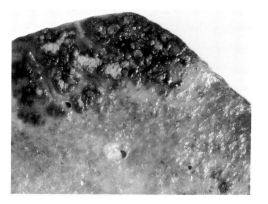

Fig. 31-49. Anoxic necrosis of liver. Alcoholic cirrhosis with fatal hemorrhage from duodenal ulcer.

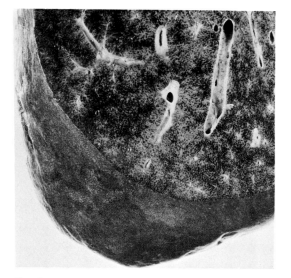

Fig. 31-51. "Nutmeg liver" in chronic passive congestion of liver.

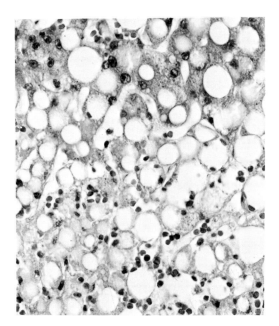

Fig. 31-50. Anoxic centrilobular necrosis in fatty liver of alcoholic who was in shock after variceal bleeding.

sinusoids, loss of microvilli in Disse's space, and the production of large intracytoplasmic vacuoles, some of which apparently contain fibrinogen and fibrin.[583] Aggregations of platelets, fibrin, erythrocytes, and leukocytes tend to accumulate in the sinusoids. Erythrocytes enter Disse's space and sometimes are seen between the hepatocytes.

Passive hyperemia and cardiac cirrhosis

Passive hyperemia of the liver is most often the result of cardiac disease with congestive failure but also may result from compression and obstruction of the inferior vena cava or obstructions of the pulmonary circulation leading to right-sided cardiac failure. Increased pressure in the venous system affects the liver severely because of the short distance between the point of entry of hepatic veins into the vena cava and the entry of the latter into the right auricle. Because the liver cells are particularly sensitive to hypoxia, the decreased oxygen content of the hepatic blood[602] and the diminished flow in congestive failure[596] are probably responsible for much of the histologic change that is observed.

In the early stages of passive congestion, only dilatation of central veins and sinusoids are seen. Later, atrophy and disappearance of liver cells lead to larger pools of blood in the dilated channels. Fragments of former sinusoidal walls remain, but the normal architectural arrangement around the central vein tends to disappear. There is often a lack of correlation between the clinical course and severity of atrophy. When the central one third to one half of the lobules has undergone atrophy, fatty change of the remaining liver cells near the margin is often present and is responsible for the gross "nutmeg" appearance (Fig. 31-51). However, in many instances, the pale peripheral lobular zones do not contain fat vacuoles. The reason for their pallor is not apparent. Coincident with the centrilobular atrophy an increase of fibrous tissue may ensue.[600] Occasionally, especially in patients with

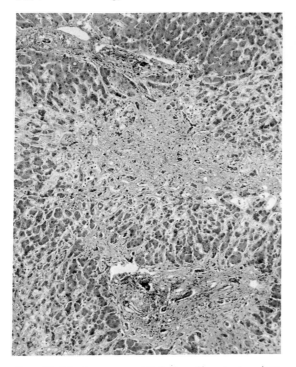

Fig. 31-52. Severe centrilobular fibrosis (cardiac cirrhosis) in patient with tricuspid stenosis and chronic heart failure.

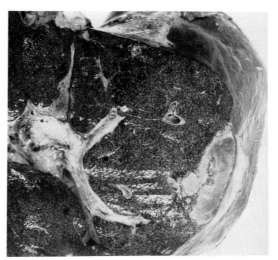

Fig. 31-53. Subcapsular infarct attributed to periarteritis nodosa.

tricuspid valvular disease, fibrosis links the centrilobular areas together and a diagnosis of cardiac cirrhosis may be made (Fig. 31-52). Portal fibrosis with communicating septa to the central fibrous areas is rare but does occur. Hyperplasia of the peripheral portions of the lobules is occasionally seen. This may or may not be in conjunction with cardiac cirrhosis.

Grossly, the liver is of normal or slightly reduced size, firm in consistency, and dark red-brown or purple-red in color. The surface is only slightly nodular, and the capsule is thickened. The cut surface shows a mottling of gray or yellow-gray areas separated by brown-red zones of variable size and shape. The hepatic veins are uniformly dilated, sometimes strikingly so, and their walls are thickened. Ill-defined nodules may be present in proximity to the portal tracts. It may be questioned whether or not true cirrhosis of congestive origin exists. A small percentage of patients with long-standing congestive failure do have esophageal varices, but these rarely bleed.[593] In our experience, the wedged hepatic vein pressure is not elevated in patients with congestive failure.

Vascular obstruction—infarction

Infarction of the liver is rare, but in most cases it is the result of *obstruction of the hepatic artery* or some of its branches by arteriosclerosis or aneurysms as well as by bland or septic emboli from the heart.[601] Obstruction of the proper hepatic artery beyond the gastroduodenal and right gastric arteries is most likely to result in infarction.[492] Ligature proximal to the latter arteries is well tolerated because of retrograde flow of blood through the right gastric artery from its anastomoses. Ligature of the hepatic artery is sometimes accidental but also may be necessary in treating severe trauma to the liver.[9] Periarteritis nodosa is a rare cause of multiple infarcts (Fig. 31-53).

Occlusion of the portal vein or of one or more of its branches is usually secondary to another disease (Fig. 31-54). These include cirrhosis of the liver, intravenous invasion by primary carcinoma of the liver that complicates cirrhosis, carcinoma of the pancreas that grows into the intrahepatic portal veins, and pylephlebitis that follows abdominal suppuration or umbilical infection of the newborn infant. Intrahepatic obstruction of the portal vein or one of the major branches usually causes only the atrophic red infarct of Zahn (Fig. 31-55), a discolored zone that does not show any necrosis on microscopic examination. Thrombosis or neoplastic invasion of the trunk of the portal vein occasionally causes areas of necrosis in the liver.

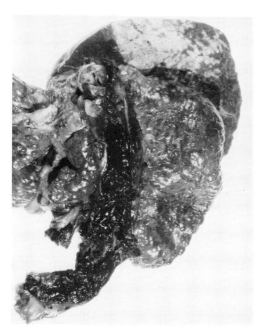

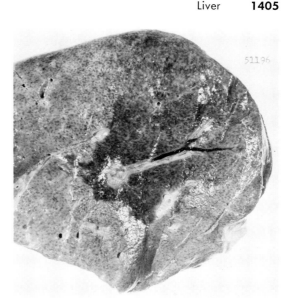

Fig. 31-54. Portal cirrhosis and thrombosis of portal vein. (Courtesy Dr. G. Lyman Duff.)

Fig. 31-55. Infarct of Zahn, area of dusky hyperemia attributed to thrombosis of branch of portal vein.

Idiopathic portal hypertension[585] is a term used for a syndrome first described by Banti.[587] In this syndrome there are esophageal varices and hypersplenism but no cirrhosis. The disease is more common in India[585] and Japan[590] than in the United States. In the United States most patients first seek medical care for bleeding esophageal varices. At this time, an enlarged spleen and mild pancytopenia are noted. Hepatic function, although initially normal, slowly deteriorates.

Grossly, the liver surface is smooth, the edges are blunted, and the parenchyma is slightly firmer than normal. Microscopically, the relationship between central veins and portal areas is inconstant. Often, two to four central veins are found in a lobule. The portal area is widened within an intact limiting plate, and there are increased numbers of dilated, thin-walled angiomatous structures (Fig. 31-56). As the disease progresses, collagen becomes more dense in portal areas and may extend beyond the confines of the limiting plate to other portal areas. The portal vein radicles may become thickened. The end stage of idiopathic portal hypertension results in a fibrotic, shrunken liver without regenerative nodules.

A number of patients with the foregoing findings will have thrombotic or sclerotic occlusion of the extrahepatic portal vein. This occlusion is considered by many investigators to be the cause of *extrahepatic portal hypertension,* whereas others[595] have suggested that

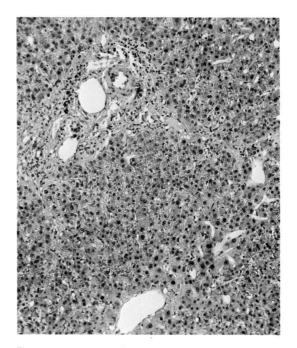

Fig. 31-56. Banti's disease with large vessels and increase of connective tissue in portal areas. Central veins enlarged and prominent.

the portal vein occlusion occurs after idiopathic portal hypertension, just as it occasionally occurs after portal hypertension associated with cirrhosis.

Banti and many subsequent investigators[586, 598,599,607] believed that primary splenic enlargement resulted in increased portal blood flow and consequent portal hypertension. However, the possibility of the development of abnormal arteriovenous communications either within the liver or in the peripheral splanchnic bed has not been excluded as the cause of the portal hypertension. It has been demonstrated that portal hypertension occurring after traumatically acquired extrahepatic arterioportal venous fistulas produces intrahepatic morphologic changes similar to those in Banti's disease. After such morphologic changes have developed, the portal hypertension is not reversible by surgical correction of the fistula.[586] It is likely that increased pressure on the intrahepatic portal bed produces irreversible change as arterial hypertension does in the arterial vascular bed.[584] A suggestion that the syndrome occurs after viral hepatitis is not supportable by data from the United States.

Budd-Chiari syndrome. Small segments of the hepatic veins may be closed by thrombi, or even tumors, and produce small areas of infarction, but these are nearly always symptomless. Primary carcinomas of the liver often grow into the hepatic veins, but rarely fill the entire system. In Budd-Chiari's syndrome, a large portion of the hepatic venous system may be more or less completely obstructed by thromboses or a combination of thrombosis and sclerosis that does produce symptoms of an acute or chronic nature. Polycythemia and paroxysmal nocturnal hemoglobinuria[589] have increased coincidence with Budd-Chiari syndrome, and the use of oral contraceptives[592,606] has been reported in association with hepatic vein thrombosis. However, the widespread use of oral contraceptives has produced no recognizable increase in incidence of this rare lesion. A fibrous membrane in the inferior vena cava is also capable of blocking the mouth of the hepatic veins.[605] Hepatic scintiscan and inferior venacavography are helpful in diagnosis.[606]

In the acute type, there is an enlarged, tender, and sometimes painful liver associated with severe ascites. Esophageal varices may develop quickly. An enlarged caudate lobe[606] may develop that presses on the inferior vena cava causing large collateral veins to develop over the abdomen as well as various degrees of edema and venous engorgement in the legs.[591] There is usually no jaundice. In the chronic type, essentially the same symptoms develop slowly. In most instances, the hepatic veins are both sclerosed and thrombosed. The remarkable fibrous tissue proliferation in the veins, plus the extreme congestion of the lobules that leads to atrophy of the central one third to one half of the lobule, is diagnostic of the Budd-Chiari syndrome. Biopsies taken in the more acute stages of the disease often disclose centrilobular zones of coagulative necrosis or even larger areas of necrosis resembling infarcts. Surgery may be successful in patients who have a membrane in the inferior vena cava.[591] Side-to-side portacaval shunt has also been used in the treatment of the Budd-Chiari syndrome.[597]

In *congenital capillary telangiectasis* (Osler-Rendu-Weber syndrome), the lesions in the liver may produce a bruit as a result of portacaval shunting. Fibrosis, cirrhosis, and even carcinoma may develop.[604]

CHRONIC INFECTIONS

Many of the granulomatous diseases, fungal infections, and parasitic infestations are capable of causing liver disease. The term *granulomatous hepatitis* often is used for this group. After the most complete laboratory and clinical study, the etiology of many of the noncaseating granulomas remains obscure.[613] The patient is often febrile, and a needle biopsy of the liver frequently is performed for diagnostic purposes. As a rule, most of the granulomas that involve the liver will cause a rise in the serum alkaline phosphate level and at least a mild retention of sulfobromophthalein. Jaundice is unusual and, when present, is of short duration. The granulomas that are observed on needle biopsy or at autopsy include lesions of tuberculosis, sarcoidosis, larval granulomatosis, Q fever, brucellosis, leprosy, histoplasmosis, secondary syphilis, and tularemia.

Tuberculous and sarcoid granulomas are the most frequently seen, and their differentiation is of practical importance. The lesion of sarcoidosis is composed of epithelioid cells with no particular arrangement. Caseation necrosis is not seen, and a few lymphocytes usually surround the granulomas (Fig. 31-57). Larger lesions are composed of multiple units, often with an occasional multinucleated giant cell. In some instances, the noncaseating lesions of sarcoidosis are observed in the walls of the central and sublobular veins. In healing, sarcoid granulomas usually become surrounded by concentric layers of connective tissue. Tubercles often have a caseous center, the epithelioid cells are arranged in a radial fashion at the periphery, and the exudate contains

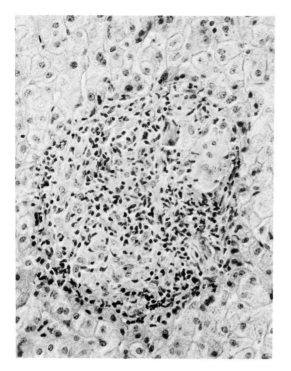

Fig. 31-57. Irregular arrangement of epithelioid cells and scanty lymphoid infiltrate in sarcoid granuloma of liver.

both lymphocytes and other mononuclear cells. Fibrin is often present, which helps to distinguish tuberculosis from sarcoidosis. In the small early lesions of tuberculosis, there may be no caseation, and the differentiation from sarcoidosis and leprosy is most difficult. An acid-fast stain should always be done on any granulomatous lesion that resembles tuberculosis. Occasionally, the tubercles are concentrated along the portal tracts, and the bile ducts may be destroyed. In a patient so affected, jaundice may occur. More rarely, solitary or multiple tuberculomas have been observed. Tubercle bacilli may reach the liver from either an active pulmonary or abdominal focus. Sarcoidlike lesions have been observed in a number of different conditions, including Hodgkin's disease and primary biliary cirrhosis.[617] Liver granulomas containing copper have also been reported.[618] Talc granulomas in narcotic addicts[616] is common. We have noted a decrease in talc crystals in biopsies on intravenous drug users in recent years.

All types of leprosy may spread to the liver, producing granulomas that closely resemble the lesions in the skin.[612] Studies with the electron microscope have shown that the lysosomes in Kupffer cells fuse with vacuoles containing lepra bacilli and apparently destroy the organisms.[614]

In *visceral larva migrans,* the presence of the larvae of *Toxocara canis, Toxocara cati,* or other parasites in the liver causes rather distinctive granulomas that may reach a diameter of several millimeters and are composed of a necrotic center surrounded by epithelioid cells having a radial arrangement, many eosinophils, and giant cells (Fig. 14-32). The larvae may be identified on serial sectioning. The disease is seen in children, usually from 1½ to 6 years of age, who eat dirt (pica) and are closely associated with dogs or cats. The syndrome is featured by fever, hepatomegaly, eosinophilia, and hyperglobulinemia.[615] A reliable intradermal test using *Toxocara* antigen has been found useful.[620]

Q fever may cause hepatic enlargement and jaundice. The ringlike necrosis of sinusoidal walls, with the formation of tiny rod-shaped fragments, is characteristic. Large necrotic granulomatous lesions with giant cells and epithelioid cells are also present.[609] Brucellosis occasionally produces caseation necrosis and even abscesses[619] (p. 401). Secondary syphilis is a rare cause of jaundice but can result in small granulomas that are of short duration, and areas of nonspecific necrosis and pericholangitis.[611] Tularemia and leprosy are discussed on pp. 402 and 415. Among the fungal infections, actinomycosis frequently produces hepatic abscesses. Blastomycosis and coccidioidomycosis occasionally may produce small hepatic lesions. Histoplasmosis often involves the liver, with the encapsulated organisms being found in large numbers in the Kupffer cells. *Toxoplasma gondii* occasionally causes a granuloma-like lesion of the liver.[610]

Several helminths commonly or characteristically produce lesions in the liver. The larval form of the dog tapeworm, *Taenia echinococcus,* often lodges in the liver, producing there a hydatid cyst (p. 1409). Schistosomal infection produces hepatic lesions because of ova that are carried to the liver in the portal blood and produce irritation (p. 543). The liver fluke, *Clonorchis sinensis,* and *Fasciola hepatica* lodge in the bile ducts, which they tend to obstruct (p. 539).

POSTMORTEM CHANGES

Postmortem autolytic changes develop rapidly in the liver, producing a soft, even mushy, organ. Microscopically, all cell detail may be lost. Portions of the liver adjacent to the transverse colon often develop a bluish black discoloration. The most striking postmortem change is the so-called "foamy" liver, which is caused by postmortem growth in the liver of anaerobic gas-producing organisms from the intestinal tract. The liver becomes soft and spongy, with the bubbles of gas produced honeycombing the hepatic tissue. Numerous bacilli may be evident, particularly in blood vessels.

CYSTS

Cysts in the liver are commonly of three types: congenital, solitary, and hydatid (*Echinococcus*).

Congenital cysts are not common,[624] but sometimes are found associated with congenital cystic disease of the kidneys or other organs. They are usually small and cause no disturbance, but cysts of large size do occur and patients present with an abdominal mass, hepatomegaly, and occasionally abdominal pain or jaundice.[625] They may be prominent just under the capsule, contain clear fluid, and are lined by flattened or cylindric epithelium (Fig.

31-58). In some instances, small gray-white areas are seen throughout the liver, and the cysts are barely visible or are of microscopic size. In this microcystic form of polycystic disease, the tubules are surrounded by dense connective tissue and may contain bile pigment. Rarely, the amount of connective tissue and number of ducts is so great that entire lobules are surrounded, a condition that has been called *congenital hepatic fibrosis*. Under these circumstances, a presinusoidal type of hypertension may develop, and variceal bleeding that necessitates shunt surgery ensues.[622]

Solitary or nonparasitic cysts occur at any age but mostly in middle-aged females, in a ratio of four or five females to one male. Abdominal enlargement and a palpable mass are the usual findings. The cysts usually have a bluish appearance as they present beneath Glisson's capsule and may reach a diameter of 15 to 20 cm. They have a low columnar to cuboid epithelial lining and are filled with serous fluid. Occasionally a cyst is lined with squamous epithelium or it is difficult to find any well-preserved epithelium. The wall is composed of compact fibrous tissue with an outside well-vascularized layer. Surgical treatment of symptomatic cysts has been successful.[621,623]

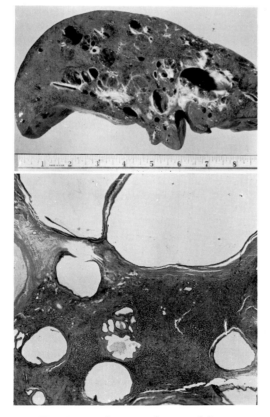

Fig. 31-58. Congenital cysts of liver.

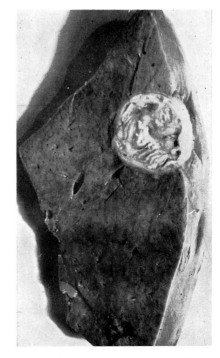

Fig. 31-59. *Echinococcus* cyst of liver. Note convoluted membranous content.

Hydatid cysts are caused by the lodgment of the larval form of the dog tapeworm, *Taenia echinococcus,* in the liver. The liver is a commonly involved organ. The cyst wall is composed of concentric hyaline laminae lined by germinal cells from which grow "daughter" cysts. Scolices and hooklets of the worm may be identified in the cyst wall or its contents by microscopic examination (Fig. 31-59).

Old cysts, in which the parasites are dead, contain a yellowish gray puttylike material.

TUMORS

The liver provides a most suitable environment for the growth of neoplastic cells, being the favorite site for metastatic cancer. In addition, the lymphomas, leukemias, and primary carcinoma all grow readily within this organ. Its size, anatomic location, and dual blood supply and the ready availability of nutritional material are factors that influence the deposition and growth of neoplasms. Between 40% and 50% of all primary cancers in the body will be noted at death to have metastases within the liver. Primary neoplasms and tumorlike lesions occur much less frequently but nevertheless are important, inasmuch as they may enter into the differential diagnosis of an enlarged liver noted clinically or observed at laparotomy. Hepatomegaly, often symptomless, is a common finding in neoplastic liver disease. Malignant tumors usually are associated with weight loss. Fever and jaundice are less common. Esophageal varices may occur as a complication of both primary and secondary tumors.[666] Laboratory findings often include an elevation of the serum alkaline phosphatase level and sulfobromophthalein retention. Angiograms made by the injection of iodine compound into the hepatic artery are most helpful in the diagnosis of neoplasms.[20] Scintiscans of the liver after the injection of colloidal gold are also useful as a diagnostic tool.

Primary growths may arise from hepatic cells, bile duct epithelium, or mesodermal structures. Benign tumors are uncommon but include cavernous hemangiomas, hemangioendotheliomas, bile duct adenomas and cystadenomas, and liver cell adenomas.

Benign tumors

Cavernous hemangiomas. Cavernous hemangiomas usually are noted incidentally at necropsy, but a few become manifest clinically,[642,677] especially in multiparous women, possibly as a result of an increase of circulating estrogenic hormones during pregnancy. Angiomatous lesions of the gingiva and skin may likewise appear. Calcified hemangiomas of the liver have been reported in older women in association with hypertension.[685] Rarely, a hemangioma may rupture into the peritoneal cavity, necessitating emergency surgery. Surgery may also be necessary for giant congenital hemangiomas.[674]

Hemangiomas appear as circumscribed, dark red-purple areas that vary from a few millimeters to several centimeters in diameter. They may bulge beneath Glisson's capsule or may be located deep within the liver (Fig. 31-60, *A*). The presence of cavernous spaces gives them a spongy appearance. Microscopically, the large, blood-filled spaces are lined by a single layer of endothelium and are separated by connective tissue that often has a myxomatous appearance (Fig. 31-60, *B*). Hemangiomas apparently grow for a limited length of time and some eventually undergo fibrosis that obliterates the cavernous spaces. Rarely, the liver may be diffusely involved by small hemangiomas. Steroid therapy has been used for cavernous hemangiomas in the newborn.[674]

Hemangioendotheliomas. The *hemangioendothelioma of infancy* is an unusual tumor that arises within the first few months of life and tends to undergo involution. However, in a large percentage of patients, an arteriovenous shunt occurs that causes hypertrophy and dilatation of the heart, with resulting congestive failure and death. In about one third of the patients there are similar growths at extrahepatic sites, especially in the skin. Radiation and steroid therapy have been used in treatment, sometimes successfully.[638,654,671] Supportive treatment alone has also been successful.[633]

Grossly, the liver contains multiple red nodules averaging 1.5 to 2 cm in diameter with uniform distribution. Microscopically, hemangioendotheliomas are characterized by anastomosing vascular channels that are lined with one or more layers of hyperchromatic endothelial cells. The tumor grows along the sinusoids of the lobules, often replacing liver tissue.

Lymphangiomatosis. Cystic lymphangiomatosis may involve the liver, spleen, and skeleton. The prognosis is poor, but some patients live to adult life. The liver contains innumerable endothelium-lined spaces filled with eosinophilic material.[629]

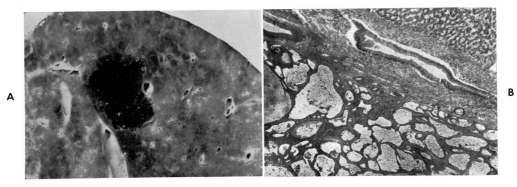

Fig. 31-60. A, Cavernous hemangioma of liver. **B,** Hepatic parenchyma seen at upper right.

Adenomas and cystadenomas. *Bile duct adenomas* are firm, gray-white areas, rarely over a centimeter in diameter, and usually located beneath Glisson's capsule. They are composed of a multitude of tiny acinar structures that are lined with bile duct type of epithelium. The connective tissue stroma is sparse.

Bile duct cystadenomas are noted almost exclusively in women, usually in the middle-aged group. They may grow 15 to 18 cm in diameter, producing abdominal enlargement and sometimes pain. Usually the tumor is composed of cysts of variable size; occasionally there is one large cyst and several smaller ones. These multilocular lesions are lined with a columnar mucin-secreting epithelium that is often arranged in folds. The connective tissue stroma, especially in the subepithelial area, is densely cellular and often contains areas of old hemorrhage. A few have undergone malignant change. The treatment is surgery.[673] Ductal cystadenomas have been reported.[694]

Adenomas derived from hepatic cells were actually rare until the use of oral contraceptives. In recent years many women with adenomas have been treated by surgery. Although adenomas occasionally occur in infants, in children, or in men, they are not complicated by hemorrhage and rupture as are those in women taking contraceptive pills. In the last, the tumors may be solitary or multiple; they are encapsulated and are usually somewhat lighter in color than the surrounding liver. About two thirds will have varying degrees of infarction and hemorrhage, particularly in their central portions (Fig. 31-61, *A*). Microscopically, the neoplastic hepatocytes have a pronounced cordlike arrangement with tiny canaliculi (Fig. 31-61, *B*). Bile formation and fatty change are sometimes observed. There are no bile ducts or other evidence of portal triads. Adenomas occur most often in women who have taken one of the contraceptives containing mestranol for 5 years or more. They appear to be hormone dependent as two of the women in our experience had remission of biopsy-proved multiple tumors after ceasing the use of oral contraceptives. A few adenomas in women not taking contraceptives have been reported. These rarely undergo infarction and hemorrhage. Malignant change in adenomas has not been proved.

• • •

Aberrant adrenal tissue is sometimes seen beneath the capsule of the right lobe, and at least one functioning adrenocortical tumor of the liver has been reported.[640]

Several tumorlike lesions are seen in the liver, many of which are of importance because they may be palpable and lead to surgery. Among these are focal nodular hyperplasia, nodular hyperplasia of cirrhosis, mesenchymal hamartoma, and peliosis hepatis.

Focal nodular hyperplasia. Focal nodular hyperplasia occurs predominantly in women between the ages of 20 and 50 years, the average age being about 32 years. In focal nodular hyperplasia, there is a firm, circumscribed, gray-brown tumor that usually measures from 1 to 8 cm in diameter. It is always lighter in color than the surrounding liver. Although sharply circumscribed, the tumors do not have a true capsule. They may be single or multiple. Most often, they are seen beneath the capsule, but they can arise deep within the liver.

Rarely are the tumors pedunculated. Ordinarily, there is a stellate-shaped mass of connective tissue in the center of the lesion with radiation of the connective tissue toward the periphery. The nodules are composed of fairly normal-appearing liver cells arranged in small

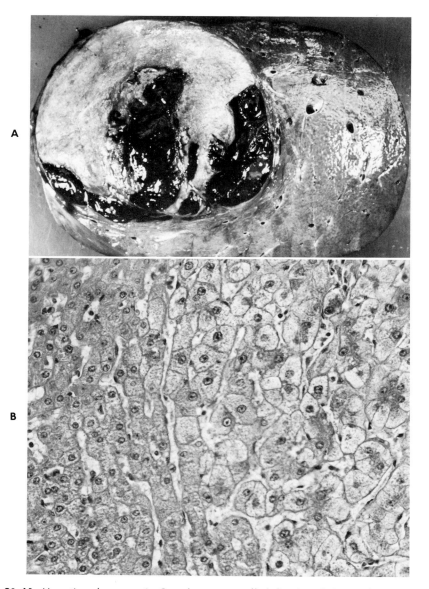

Fig. 31-61. Hepatic adenoma. **A,** Grossly, mass well defined with hemorrhage into tumor. **B,** Microscopically, transition zone between adjacent liver and adenoma cells. Note larger size of adenoma cells and more distinct cord arrangement around canaliculi.

pseudolobules. Often, the liver cells are arranged in individual units that surround small ducts and vessels. The larger lesions have an abundant arterial supply.

Adenomatous hyperplasia. In both cirrhosis and submassive necrosis large nodules of adenomatous hyperplasia may occur. These may assume tumorlike proportions and become palpable. Sometimes this has led to unnecessary surgery. The large areas of hyperplasia that occur after submassive necrosis are usually lighter in color and sometimes bile stained.

They stand out in sharp contrast to the surrounding dark brown collapsed parenchyma. Areas of adenomatous hyperplasia in cirrhosis may reach a size of several centimeters. These are outlined by surrounding septa that contain blood vessels and bile ducts and thus do not form a true capsule. Adenomatous hyperplasia differs from a true adenoma in that small bile ducts and blood vessels ramify into its interior from the periphery. The same is true of adenomatous hyperplasia in submassive necrosis. Large areas of hyperplasia in regenerating liver has a characteristic angiographic pattern.[687] Rarely, in cirrhosis the large nodules are composed entirely of hepatocytes and may be termed an *adenoma*.

Mesenchymal hamartomas. Mesenchymal hamartomas are gray-white to red-purple cyst-like lesions that most often arise at the lower margin of the right lobe of the liver in the first 2 years of life. They tend to grow rapidly because of accumulation of fluid in the cystlike areas.[682]

Microscopically, they are composed of remnants of triads with bile ducts, periportal hepatocytes, and fluid-filled spaces.[643] Electron microscopic studies disclose that the bile ducts and hepatocytes are typical of those in the normal liver, whereas the myxomatous foci consist of fibroblasts, mature collagen, and a few endothelium-lined spaces.[637] It is probable that these lesions represent an abnormal development of mesenchymal tissue in the infant.[643]

Peliosis hepatis. Peliosis hepatis is a rare, diffuse angiomatoid change of the liver.[706] Minute angiomatoid spaces of hemorrhagic appearance are distributed throughout the liver, The pathogenesis is uncertain, but it possibly stems from miliary necrosis.

A severe form of the disease, sometimes fatal, has been noted after the use of androgenic-anabolic steroid therapy.[630] Several other drugs have been implicated in its production.[639] It has also been produced experimentally with the 9H virus.[21]

Peliosis hepatis must be distinguished from hereditary hemorrhagic telangiectasis (Osler-Rendu-Weber disease). In the latter, there is ectasia of the blood vessels, both in the portal and intralobular areas. These vessels have a distinct endothelial lining and may be accompanied by fibrosis and occasionally by cirrhosis.[675]

Primary carcinoma

Primary carcinoma of the liver occupies a unique position among neoplasms because of its propensity for arising in an organ that is already severely damaged by another disease—cirrhosis. More rarely, cancer may arise in a noncirrhotic liver. Carcinomas most often are derived from the hepatic cells, but a small percentage (15% to 25%) are of bile duct origin. No unanimity of opinion exists regarding the nomenclature of malignant tumors derived from hepatocytes, since the terms "hepatocellular carcinoma (HCC)," "hepatoma," and "liver cell carcinoma" continue

to be used. Great interest in these tumors has evolved over the past few decades but especially in recent years because of the high frequency of carcinoma in certain geographic areas and the etiologic role of foodstuffs and viral hepatitis. The liver also continues to be a favored model in experimental oncology.[631]

Clinically, carcinoma of the liver complicating cirrhosis is difficult to distinguish from cirrhosis alone. An enlarging abdominal mass, pain in the right upper quadrant (often severe), weight loss, rapidly accumulating ascites, and blood-stained ascitic fluid on paracentesis point toward a diagnosis of carcinoma of the liver. Jaundice is usually not severe and occurs in a third or less of patients. The liver is enlarged in nearly every patient and is often hard and tender.

Among patients with primary liver cell carcinoma, an amazing number of abnormal laboratory findings have been noted. Some of these are helpful in diagnosis, especially the α_1-fetoprotein. This test is positive in 70% to 98% of patients.[21] This sensitive test is helpful not only in diagnosis, but also in following the course of patients who have had their tumor resected, since recurrence of growths causes the test to become positive.[681] Recently a leukocyte adherence–inhibition test has proved helpful in diagnosis.[656] Many other anomalous laboratory findings have been described, including cystathioninuria,[704] dysfibrinogenemia,[701] erythrocytosis,[668] a unique isoferritin,[693] gonadotropin,[648] elevated serum proline hydroxylase,[664] hypercalcemia,[665] hypercholesterolemia,[627] and hypoglycemia.[631] Two types of neoplasms causing hypoglycemia have been reported. In one of these there is acquired glycogenosis.[669] Acquired porphyria has been noted in patients with liver cell tumors, both benign and malignant. Porphyrins were demonstrated in the cytoplasm of the tumor cells.[698] A specific variant of alkaline phosphatase has been noted in some patients wtih hepatocellular carcinoma.[657] Angiograms and liver scans have been helpful in diagnosis of all types of liver tumors.[72]

Etiology

The etiology of liver cell carcinoma is not known, but recent research on the role of aflatoxins and hepatitis B virus strongly suggests that they may be involved. It is well known that liver cell carcinoma most often arises in a cirrhotic liver, and this is true in all parts of the globe. In geographic areas of high frequency, such as subsaharan Africa and

Southeast Asia,[641] does contaminated food or hepatitis B infection augment the frequency of carcinoma that arises in preexisting cirrhosis? Is one or both of these agents capable of taking a "shortcut" and incite the growth of liver cell carcinoma in a noncirrhotic but not necessarily a normal liver? These considerations are pertinent because of the striking geographic differences in frequency of liver cell carcinoma and the attack rate in patients with cirrhosis. The frequency of liver cell carcinoma in various parts of the world may differ by as much as a hundredfold.[641] In Europe and the United States the frequency varies from 0.1% to 0.7% of all autopsies. In portions of Southeast Asia, there is also a high frequency of carcinoma of the liver that includes both liver cell carcinoma and bile duct carcinoma.[652] Where the incidence of carcinoma of the liver is low, usually between 4% and 6% and rarely 10% of patients with cirrhosis eventually develop a carcinoma of the liver. This contrasts with some areas in Africa where the frequency is about 40% of all men with cirrhosis.[652]

A high familial incidence of HBsAg-positive liver cell carcinoma has been studied in Japan, where the family members without carcinoma have an unusually high incidence of PVH-B, CAVH-B, or inactive viral cirrhosis B.[679] Epidemiologically related cases may reflect transplacental transmission with subsequent lifelong asymptomatic chronic viral B infection.

At our liver unit in Los Angeles there has been an increase in the incidence of liver cell carcinoma over the past 30 years, both in cirrhotic and noncirrhotic livers. The percentage of cases in which HBsAg can be demonstrated in liver tissue has also risen (Fig. 31-62) and is currently found in sera of 71% of nonalcoholic but cirrhotic patients who have liver cell carcinoma and in 30% of all patients with hepatocellular carcinoma.[74]

Exactly how cirrhosis predisposes to carcinoma of the liver is not known. Carcinoma most often arises in advanced cirrhosis, especially when large regenerative nodules are present. Precancerous changes, in the form of large atypical cells that contain hyperchromatic nuclei and even binucleate forms, are common in these nodules. The term "liver cell dysplasia" has been used for such changes.[628] It seems that cirrhosis in the native African has a more progressive and intense course, occurs in younger people, and proceeds more often to carcinoma.[653] Increased gamma globulin and serum transaminase values are associated with a short survival time.[651]

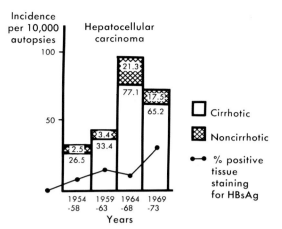

Fig. 31-62. Chart of increasing incidence of hepatocellular carcinoma per 10,000 autopsies and concomitant increase of related HBsAg positivity in involved patients. (From Okuda, K., and Peters, R. L.: Hepatocellular carcinoma, New York, 1976, John Wiley & Sons.)

In hemochromatosis, cirrhosis evolves slowly and the disease is of long duration. As might be expected, the frequency of carcinoma in this group is high.[705] At the Los Angeles County–University of Southern California Medical Center, the frequency of carcinoma in pigmentary cirrhosis is at least twice as great as carcinoma complicating alcoholic cirrhosis. It is of interest that in Wilson's disease, primary carcinoma has not been reported. Carcinoma may arise in a cirrhotic liver in patients with α_1-antitrypsin deficiency,[646] but protease inhibitor abnormalities do not form a significant basis for hepatocellular carcinoma in the United States. Liver cell carcinoma has also been associated with the carcinoid syndrome.[686]

Many research endeavors indicate that aflatoxins, the metabolic product of the fungus *Aspergillus flavus*, may be involved in the etiology of liver cell carcinoma. This fungus has widespread distribution. Its growth on peanuts, soybeans, and cereals in humid parts of the world has been studied extensively. Aflatoxin B_1 is the most toxic of the aflatoxins. It is highly carcinogenic for some species, including the rat. As little as 15 μg per kilogram daily will produce cancer. The relationship of aflatoxin intake to primary carcinoma of the liver has been studied in Kenya,[692] Thailand,[683] and Mozambique. The last country has the highest frequency of primary carcinoma of the liver in the world and also has the highest daily intake of aflatoxins. It has been estimated that one male in each 40 households will die of liver cell carcinoma. It has been suggested that there may be a short induction time after exposure to aflatoxins.[702,703] Some studies indicate that a number of liver changes in the human may be caused by aflatoxin. In studies of both biopsy and autopsy material in the Bantu of Lourenço Marques, toxic changes that differed from viral hepatitis seen in the same population were observed. It has been suggested that these changes may be the forerunner of carcinoma.[699]

Many other natural carcinogens have been considered, but so far proof is lacking that they are related to a high incidence of cancer. Among these are the alkaloids derived from plants that have a wide distribution in Africa, Asia, and South and Central America, such as *Senecio jacobaea, Crotalaria, Cynoglossum, Heliotropium,* and *Trichoderma.*

Among the parasitic infestations, only the liver fluke, *Clonorchis sinensis* or *Opisthorchis felineus* are considered to be precursors of bile duct carcinoma.[652] These lead to epithelial hyperplasia of the bile ducts and to bile duct carcinoma. Radiation injury is a known precursor of carcinoma, especially after the use of the now-abandoned diagnostic tool Thorotrast. However, it is estimated that there are 50,000 to 100,000 carriers.[691] Thorotrast is a particulate suspension of thorium dioxide in a dextrin colloid. It has a half life of almost 50 years. It emits alpha rays, which are supposed to be the most damaging. About 70%

of injected Thorotrast is taken up by the liver. In time, necrosis, fibrosis, and even cirrhosis may develop. Many tumors have been observed, especially hemangioendothelial sarcoma but also liver cell carcinoma and bile duct carcinoma.[691] Carcinoma has also been reported after the use of radioactive phosphorus.[634] A large number of agents have been used in production of experimental tumors of the liver. The steps in pathogenesis include the process of initiation followed by neoplastic development that leads to nodules in which the hepatocytes have lost some of their normal functions.[647] A new marker, preneoplastic (PN) antigen, for both the premalignant and malignant cells has been found, as it localizes to every hepatocyte.[647]

Carcinoma of the liver may occur in infancy and childhood, especially in male infants before the age of 2 years. Among adults, the disease is seen most often in men between the ages of 40 and 60 years in Europe and the United States, whereas in Africa the average is nearer 30 years of age. Carcinoma rarely arises in the absence of cirrhosis, but when it does, females are affected as often as males and they usually live less than 6 months.

Pathologic anatomy

Primary carcinomas may be massive, nodular, or diffuse. They usually arise in a liver that is the seat of advanced cirrhosis.[644] The liver usually weighs between 2 and 3 kg, but

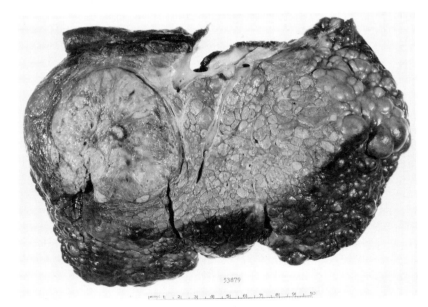

Fig. 31-63. Large nodular liver cell carcinoma of right lobe arising in liver of 38-year-old Oriental man.

some may be of normal size and weight. The right lobe is the more frequently involved in both the massive and the nodular forms. The cancer nodules often bulge beneath Glisson's capsule and are much softer to palpation than are areas of nodular regeneration. The nodules are rarely umbilicated. In the massive form of carcinoma, the right lobe particularly may be largely replaced by a well-circumscribed, soft yellow-brown tumor. This type is the more common in noncirrhotic livers. Small secondary nodules are sometimes present in other parts of the liver.

In the nodular type, there is usually one mass that is larger, appears older, and is more circumscribed than any other lesion. Such a tumor may be regarded as the primary lesion (Fig. 31-63). Ordinarily, nodules of smaller size are present throughout the remainder of the liver. Invasion of branches of the portal vein is usually demonstrable and is probably responsible for the rapid spread to all parts of the liver. Hemorrhage, necrosis, and bile-staining may produce a wide variety of color changes within the nodules. It would appear that the nodular type may arise in multicentric foci. This has been emphasized by the African investigators.[650]

The growth of carcinoma in the branches of the portal vein may lead to a tumor thrombus of the portal trunk and portal hypertension. Less often, the hepatic veins are invaded,

and a tumor thrombus extends into the inferior vena cava. By this route, the cancer may spread to the lungs and more distant structures.

Fully 75% of primary carcinomas are derived from the hepatic cell. These have variously been termed "liver cell carcinoma," "hepatocellular carcinoma," and "hepatoma." They simulate normal liver cells, being characterized by large, round, hyperchromatic nuclei, prominent nucleoli, abundant granular eosinophilic cytoplasm, and a tendency toward arrangement in trabeculae that are usually two to eight cells in width (Fig. 31-64). They retain another feature indicative of their origin; i.e., the trabeculae are covered (as are liver cords) by a thin basement membrane envelope having, external to this, endothelial cells. This arrangement is particularly well noted when the cancer grows into blood vessels. In the massive carcinomas, the trabecular pattern is not so obvious. But regardless of variations in pattern, most liver cell carcinomas are composed only of malignant cells and a capillary stroma. The excess connective tissue that characterizes most adenocarcinomas is usually absent. Some carcinomas will form acini that may or may not contain bile. Many of the functions of normal liver cells are retained in carcinomas, such as the ability to secrete bile and to store fat and glycogen. It has been suggested that the large amount of glycogen stored in a liver cell carcinoma is not available to form glucose, and this may result in hypoglycemia. Cytoplasmic hyaline inclusions, either globular or small Mallory bodies, are present in some carcinomas.[663] A few carcinomas of liver cell origin are highly undifferentiated, forming spindle and giant cell types. In some carcinomas complicating cirrhosis, there is a combination of liver cell and bile duct carcinoma, with the former predominating as a rule. Rarely, calcification of the stroma in liver cell carcinoma has been observed.[676]

Liver cell carcinomas in infants and children are large, multinodular lesions that, with rare exception, arise in noncirrhotic livers. Congenital defects have been noted in an abnormally high percentage of these patients.[650] These tumors were classified as hepatoblastoma and hepatocarcinomas.[661] The cell type is smaller than that seen in adults, and bile plugs are frequent. Some of the tumors contain mesenchymal sarcoma and osteoid tissue. The name *mixed hepatoblastoma* has been suggested for this type.[661] The electron microscopic studies

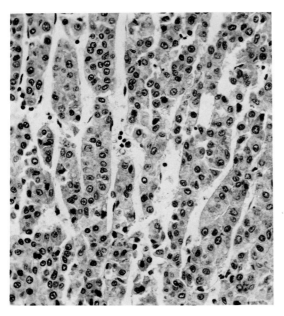

Fig. 31-64. Trabecular liver cell carcinoma with characteristic capillary pattern.

of the epithelial component of these hepatoblastomas disclose a variable degree of organelle development.[655] Biochemical studies have shown a lack of zinc in hepatoblastomas.[678] Surgical treatment of malignant tumors in infants affords the only chance for cure.[645] Rupture of hepatocellular carcinoma with abdominal bleeding may result in emergency surgery.[680] Inoperable patients may receive chemotherapy.[658]

Carcinomas may arise from bile ducts within the liver, most often from the large perihilar ducts or ducts of intermediate size. These are usually mucin-producing, well-differentiated sclerosing adenocarcinomas that, on histologic examination, are difficult to distinguish from metastatic adenocarcinomas. Some of these arise in cirrhotic livers. A cholangiolar type of carcinoma has been described.[696] Bile duct carcinoma is known to arise in patients who have had Thorotrast injection,[684,695] *Clonorchis sinensis* infestation, hemochromatosis, or polycystic disease,[659] and occasionally in patients with chronic ulcerative colitis.[688] Bile duct cancer is not so likely to grow within branches of the portal and hepatic veins, although it metastasizes just as widely to the lungs and other organs.

The surgical treatment for carcinoma of the liver has resulted in only a few 5-year survivals. Hepatic artery ligation and intensive chemotherapy have produced improvement in some patients.[649,660]

Mesodermal tumors

Malignant tumors of mesodermal origin are rare. Hemangioendothelial sarcomas form rather bulky hemorrhagic masses and may metastasize to the lungs, portal lymph nodes, and spleen. It has been possible to surgically remove some of these vascular sarcomas.[626] Microscopically, they are vasoformative tumors characterized by malignant endothelial lining cells. They may occur after ionizing radiation from Thorotrast.[691] They also have been seen after exposure to arsenic, both in vineyard workers and after the ingestion of arsenic used for therapeutic purposes.[667] In recent years much publicity has been given the occurrence of angiosarcoma in vinyl chloride workers.[632,635] Nonmalignant lesions in vinyl chloride workers consist of portal fibrosis, sinusoidal dilatation, and atypical sinusoidal lining cells. The toxicity of vinyl chloride and polyvinyl chloride has been the subject of a conference.[636] Hemochromatosis associated with hemangioendothelial sarcoma has been reported.[697]

Embryonal rhabdomyosarcoma, malignant mesenchymoma, and *hepatic mixed tumors* occasionally are seen, especially in infancy and childhood.[642] Although Kupffer cell sarcomas have been reported, this term may be restricted to vasoformative tumors in which the malignant cells are actively phagocytic. Some highly vascular sarcomas of the liver contain large stromal cells in variable quantity that appear to be myosarcomatous. A few cases of fibrosarcoma[700] and leiomyosarcoma have been reported.[690]

Metastatic tumors

In *metastatic cancer,* both lobes of the liver usually are involved, producing an enlarged nodular organ that is easily palpable in life. The cancer cells may reach the liver through the portal vein, hepatic artery, or the hilar lymphatics or, occasionally, by direct extension. Once implanted, the cells may, with growth, form small or large nodules or grow diffusely throughout the liver. Metastatic carcinoma often grows within sinusoids. The sinusoidal lining cells may be seen on biopsy around tiny metastatic growths (Fig. 31-65). In about 10% of cases, metastatic nodules are

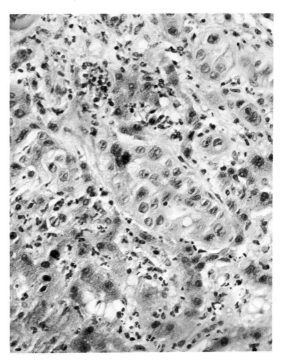

Fig. 31-65. Intrasinusoidal growth of metastatic carcinoma of liver.

solitary. Characteristically, nodules of irregular size bulge beneath Glisson's capsule and are consistently depressed in their central portions (umbilicated) because of necrosis or fibrosis with contraction. Umbilication is practically never seen in liver cell carcinoma.

The pattern of growth of metastatic cancer appears to depend somewhat on the source; e.g., carcinoma of the colon or stomach often produces large mucin-containing nodules that have a pebbled appearance (Fig. 31-66). Breast cancer often forms smaller, discrete lesions, often oval in outline, as seen beneath Glisson's capsule.

Metastatic carcinoma is usually gray to grayish white, but necrosis, hemorrhage, and mucus may add a variety of colors. Extensive hemorrhagic lesions are characteristic of choriocarcinoma, pancreatic carcinoma, and metastatic carcinoid. Malignant melanoma is black or brown but sometimes only faintly so.

Occasionally, metastatic carcinoma may grow from the hilum outward along the portal tracts, causing them to be unusually prominent. Cancer from the gallbladder may grow directly into the liver, forming a solid mass, along with smaller satellite deposits that decrease in size with increase in distance from their origin.

A needle biopsy of the liver in patients with metastatic carcinoma has proved to be positive in some 60%. If possible, a biopsy should be taken from a palpable nodule.

Metastatic carcinoma usually grows rapidly in the liver, with patients rarely living more than a year after the diagnosis is made.[662] There are two notable exceptions: metastatic malignant carcinoid is not incompatible with survival of 5 to 25 years, and metastatic neuroblastoma of the adrenal gland in infancy may apparently be cured with roentgen therapy. Satterlee[689] has given tables indicating the frequency of metastatic tumors in the liver and the probabilities regarding the original site. According to his figures, metastasis to the liver occurs in 36% of all cancers, in 50% of cancers of the portal areas, in 48% of breast cancers, and in 44% of gastric cancers.

Surgical treatment of metastatic cancer is limited to palliative procedures although, on occasion, a solitary metastasis may be resected. Hepatic dearterialization[672] has been performed in some cases, since metastatic carcinoma, like its primary form, derives its blood from the hepatic artery. These operations may prolong life somewhat and have caused amelioration of symptoms in metastatic carcinoids.[670]

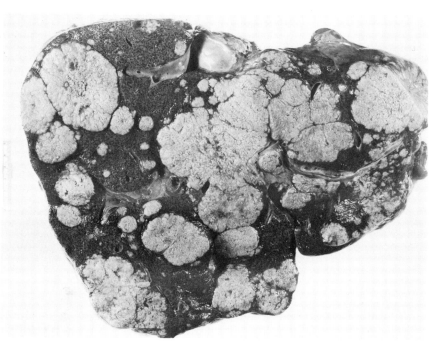

Fig. 31-66. Large metastatic nodules from primary carcinoma of stomach.

INTERPRETATION OF NEEDLE BIOPSIES

The interpretation of needle biopsies of the liver is of such practical importance in the diagnosis and treatment of liver disease that the pathologist should always follow an orderly method of microscopic examination.[43] The following comments are based upon some 19,000 needle biopsies studied by us over the past 12 years.

First, each anatomic subunit is carefully scrutinized for normality. The structures in the triads must be recognized and studied. The size of the hepatic artery approaches that of the bile duct, whereas the portal vein branch is much larger. The connective tissue within the portal triad is scanty in infants, develops with maturity, and often increases moderately in old age. The borderline between a normal and an abnormal amount of portal lymphoid tissue is difficult to establish. The triads may be considered somewhat analogous to the submucosa of the gut, where the lymphoid tissue has the capacity to become hyperplastic under conditions that cause lymphoid hyperplasia elsewhere. Such hyperplasia may widen the triads, but the limiting plate is intact. Although lymphoid and reticular elements may proliferate, follicles rarely appear. In the absence of intralobular disease, this hyperplasia should not be considered an infiltrate or exudate, and the term "triaditis" is misapplied to this nonspecific lymphoid response.

The lobules are examined for size, cord pattern, sinusoidal appearance, and the presence of central veins. Individual attention must be given to the hepatocytes, bile canaliculi, and Kupffer cells.

Normally, hepatocytes do not differ greatly from one biopsy to another. In old age, atrophy of the cells, as well as decrease in individual size, may decrease lobular diameter. Liver cells may lose glycogen and appear shrunken in starvation, in conditions causing negative nitrogen balance, and in biliary tract obstruction. The hydropic change in any one of many acute liver diseases already has been mentioned. A similar hydropic change occurs in patients with a high fever, in a liver undergoing regeneration, and in diabetic patients treated for hyperglycemia where there is a strong glycogen influx. There may be considerable variation in hepatocytic nuclear size both in specific diseases such as viral hepatitis and in nonspecific reactions. Often, centrilobular liver cells have numerous polyploid nuclei that may be related to an abortive attempt at regeneration in those who are extremely ill, elderly, or undergoing chemotherapy. Vacuolated glycogen-filled nuclei are observed in a variety of metabolic disorders, especially in diabetic patients.

Kupffer cells, as part of the reticuloendothelial system, proliferate in any chronic inflammatory reaction. Inflammatory conditions within the liver, extrahepatic infections, and fever of unknown origin may be responsible for Kupffer cell hyperplasia.

The differential diagnosis of cholestasis often arises in the various forms of acute liver disease. Rarely is viral hepatitis difficult to diagnose, but the differentiation between drug-induced jaundice, extrahepatic biliary obstruction, and simple cholestasis is often difficult or impossible. In extrahepatic bile duct obstruction, the prominence of the small interlobular bile ducts, infiltration of a few circumductal neutrophils, and centrilobular cholestasis are most often seen. In drug cholestasis, the findings are variable, but usually the inflammatory changes in and around the small bile ducts are absent. Simple centrilobular bile stasis is seen in some forms of drug jaundice, occasionally in heart failure, and in some instances of metastatic carcinoma of the liver.

A centrilobular type of zonal necrosis may occur after exposure to halothane anesthesia, ingestion of carbon tetrachloride, or drug therapy and is occasionally seen in a needle biopsy. Peripherolobular change attributable to phosphorus or to eclampsia is extremely rare. In a small percentage of biopsies, occasional foci of cellular dropout marked by a few round cells are present, usually with mild Kupffer cell hyperplasia. An increase of round cells in the triads is often present. These biopsies are taken, as a rule, in febrile patients who have minimal or no laboratory evidence of liver disease. No etiologic factors have been established.

Because of the small size of a needle biopsy, the diagnosis of cirrhosis should be made with care, unless unequivocal septa and nodules are seen. The diagnosis of specific types of cirrhosis may or may not be possible. In alcoholic liver disease, the fatty change and sclerosis of the centrilobular area are the most helpful criteria. In chronic active hepatitis, the diffuse round cell infiltrate, continuing focal necrosis, and areas of collapse are the chief indicators. Septa and nodules composed of fairly normal hepatocytes without infiltrate suggest cryptogenic cirrhosis. In primary biliary cirrhosis, the lack of bile ducts and peripherolobular cholestasis accompanied by penetration of the lobules by proliferation of connective tissue should be kept in mind. Biopsies on patients with cirrhosis often contain only fragments of pseudolobules, apparently because the needle fails to penetrate thick septa. These fragments are often larger than normal lobules and contain no bile ducts. A few islands of liver cell cancer present among cirrhotic nodules on a biopsy is easy to overlook.

Granulomas were seen in about 4% of our specimens. Occasionally, there is only a solitary lesion, best seen in only one fragment. An acid-fast stain and PAS stains should always be done.

Increased quantities of intracytoplasmic pigment may pose a diagnostic problem. Since it is not always possible to distinguish parenchymal cell iron from lipochrome, an iron stain should be performed. Iron deposition is usually greatest in the periportal zones. Lipochrome predominates in the centrilobular areas. A large quantity of fine brown pigment is usually lipochrome and of no diagnostic concern, but occasionally such pigment is seen in patients who have ingested large quantities of analgesic compounds containing phenacetin, salicylate, and caffeine. The chronic use of cascara compounds also may cause a pigmented liver. Large globules of pigment are seen in Dubin-Johnson syndrome (Fig. 31-48). Recently, lipofuscinosis of the liver was reported in patients with a specific central nervous system disease.[707]

Mild degrees of passive congestion, indicated by dilatation of the central veins and sinusoids, should always be reported. Needle biopsies rarely are performed on patients with advanced passive congestion. Massive congestion with disappearance of liver cells and conversion of large portions of the lobules to blood channels is seen in Budd-Chiari syndrome and radiation damage of the liver. An unusually intense congestion with preservation of cord pattern occasionally is observed in sickle-cell disease. The sickled cells form sludged clumps and apparently are unable to move through the sinusoids in a normal manner.

In reporting biopsies, when all structures appear normal, a diagnosis of "needle biopsy of liver, apparently normal" can be made. This does not mean, however, that a few centimeters from the location where the specimen was taken that a local lesion such as a neoplasm or abscess might not be present.

Any abnormalities noted in the specimen should be carefully described and reported to the clinician, along with the pathologist's interpretation. Some lesions are specific and involve only a single microscopic subunit, such as Gaucher's disease and periarteritis nodosa. Others, such as neoplasms and amyloidosis, have identifiable features that allow a positive diagnosis. However, in most diseases seen on biopsy, there is more than one microscopic alteration, so that a discussion of the diagnostic probabilities is in order. Such suggestions are often helpful to the clinician.

REFERENCES
General
1 Schiff, L., editor: Diseases of the liver, ed. 4, Philadelphia, 1974, J. B. Lippincott Co.
2 Sherlock, S.: Diseases of the liver and bilary system, ed. 4, Philadelphia, 1968, F. A. Davis Co.
3 Tanikawa, K.: Ultrastructural aspects of the liver and its disorders, New York, 1968, Springer-Verlag.

Structure and circulation
4 Bhathal, P. S., and Christie, G. S.: Fluorescence microscopy of terminal and subterminal portions of biliary tree, Lab. Invest. **20:**472-487, 1969.
5 Ham, A. W.: Histology, ed. 7, Philadelphia, 1974, J. B. Lippincott Co.
6 Hoyes, A. D., Riches, D. J., and Martin, B. G. H.: The fine structure of haemopoiesis in human fetal liver. I. Haemopoietic procursor cells, J. Anat. **115:**99-111, 1973.
7 Koga, A.: Morphogenesis of intrahepatic bile ducts of human fetus—light and electron microscopic study, Z. Anat. Entwicklungsgesch. **135:**156-184, 1971.
8 Ma, M. H., and Biempica, L.: Normal human liver cell—cytochemical and ultrastructural studies, Am. J. Pathol. **62:**353-390, 1971.
9 Madding, G. F., and Kennedy, P. A.: Trauma to the liver, ed. 2, Philadelphia, 1971, W. B. Saunders Co.
10 Michels, N. A.: Variant blood supply and collateral circulation of liver, Am. J. Surg. **112:** 337-347, 1966.
11 Mills, D. M., and Zucker-Franklin, D.: Electron microscopic study of isolated Kupffer cells, Am. J. Pathol. **54:**147-166, 1969.
12 Palmer, E. D.: Palpability of liver edge in healthy adults, U.S. Armed Forces Med. J. **9:** 1685-1690, 1958.
13 Rappaport, A. M.: Microcirculatory hepatic unit, Microvasc. Res. **6:**212-228, 1973.
14 Severn, C. B.: A morphologic study of development of human liver. II. Establishment of liver parenchyma, extrahepatic ducts, and associated venous channels, Am. J. Anat. **133:**85-108, 1972.
15 Steiner, J. W., and Carruthers, J. S.: Structure of terminal branches of biliary tree; morphology of normal bile canaliculi, bile preductules, and bile ductules, Am. J. Pathol. **38:** 639-661, 1961.

16 Tygstrup, N., Winkler, K., Mellemgaard, K., and Andreassen, M.: Hepatic arterial blood flow and oxygen supply during surgery, J. Clin. Invest. **41:**447-454, 1962.

17 Zamboni, L.: Ultrastructure of fetal liver, J. Ultrastruct. Res. **12:**509-524, 1965.

18 Zamboni, L.: Hemopoietic activity of fetal liver, J. Ultrastruct. Res. **12:**525-541, 1965.

Function and laboratory diagnosis

19 Afroudakis, A., Liew, C.-T., and Peters, R. L.: Immunoperoxidase technic for demonstration of hepatitis B surface antigen in human livers, Am. J. Clin. Pathol. **65:**533-539, 1976.

20 Alfidi, R. J., Ratogi, H., Buonocore, E., and Brown, C. H.: Hepatic arteriography, Radiology **90:**1136-1142, 1968.

21 Alpert, E.: In Okuda, K., and Peters, R. L., editors: Hepatocellular carcinoma, New York, 1976, John Wiley & Sons, Inc. (human α_1-fetoprotein).

22 Arias, I. M.: Bilirubin metabolism and inheritable jaundice, Isr. J. Med. Sci. **9:**1419-1426, 1973.

23 Arias, I. M.: Hepatic aspects of bilirubin metabolism, Annu. Rev. Med. **17:**257-274, 1966.

24 Barnhart, M. I.: Prothrombin synthesis, J. Histochem. Cytochem. **13:**740-751, 1965.

25 Bauer, J. P., Ackerman, P. G., and Toro, G.: Bray's Clinical laboratory methods, ed. 7, St. Louis, 1968, The C. V. Mosby Co., p. 309.

26 Bessman, S. P.: In McElroy, W. D., and Glass, B.: editors: Inorganic nitrogen metabolism, Baltimore, 1956, Johns Hopkins Press (ammonia metabolism in animals).

27 Bessman, S. P., and Bessman, A. N.: Cerebral and peripheral uptake of ammonia in liver disease with hypothesis for mechanism of hepatic coma, J. Clin. Invest. **34:**622-628, 1955.

28 Bouvier, C. A., and Maurice, P. A.: In Rouiller, C., editor: The liver, New York, 1964, Academic Press, Inc. (liver and blood coagulation).

29 Boyd, J. W.: Intracellular distribution, latency, and electrophoretic mobility of L-glutamate-oxaloacetate transaminase, Biochem. J. **81:**434-441, 1961.

30 Boyd, J. W.: Glutamate-oxaloacetate transaminase isoenzymes, Clin. Chim. Acta **7:**424-431, 1962.

31 Boyde, T. R. C., and Latner, A. L.: Starch-gel electrophoresis of transaminases, Biochem. J. **82:**51P, 1962.

32 Breen, K. J., and Schenker, S.: Liver function tests, C.R.C. Crit. Rev. Clin. Lab. Sci. **12:**573-599, 1971.

33 Brensilver, H. L., and Kaplan, M. M.: Significance of elevated liver alkaline phosphatase in serum, Gastroenterology **68:**1556-1562, 1975.

34 Bundy, H. F., and Mehl, J. W.: Trypsin inhibitors of human serum, J. Biol. Chem. **234:**1124-1128, 1959.

35 Campra, J., Ashcavai, M., Peters, R. L., and Redeker, A.: Editorial: serum antitrypsin levels in acute hepatic necrosis, Br. Med. J. **1:**616, 1972.

36 Campra, J. L., Craig, J. R., Peters, R. L., and Reynolds, T. B.: Cirrhosis associated with partial deficiency of α_1-antitrypsin in an adult, Ann. Intern. Med. **78:**233-238, 1973.

37 Colowick, S. P., and Kaplan, N. D.: Methods in enzymology, vol. 2, New York, 1955, Academic Press, Inc.

38 Craig, J. R., Dunn, A. E. G., and Peters, R. L.: Cirrhosis associated with partial deficiency of α_1-antitrypsin—a clinical and autopsy study, Hum. Pathol. **6:**113-120, 1975.

39 Diamond, L. S.: Techniques of axenic cultivation of *Entamoeba histolytica* Schaudinn, 1903, and *E. histolytica*-like amebas, J. Parasitol. **54:**1047-1056, 1968.

40 Dowling, R. H.: Enterohepatic circulation, Gastroenterology **62:**122-140, 1972.

41 Dudley, F. J., Fox, R. A., and Sherlock, S.: Cellular immunity and hepatitis-associated Australia antigen liver disease, Lancet **1:**723-726, 1972.

42 Edgington, T. S., and Ritt, D. J.: Intrahepatic expression of serum hepatitis virus–associated antigens, J. Exp. Med. **134:**871-885, 1971.

43 Edmondson, H. A.: Needle biopsy. In Schiff, L., editor: Diseases of the liver, ed. 4, Philadelphia, 1975, J. B. Lippincott Co.

44 Erlinger, S., Berthelot, P., and Dhumeaux, D.: Role in bile formation in rodents of process independent of organic anion secretion. Proceedings of the Fourth Meeting of the International Association for Study of the Liver, 1970, p. 46 (unpublished).

45 Fleisher, G. A., and Wakim, K. G.: Presence of two glutamic-oxalacetic transaminases, Proc. Soc. Exp. Biol. Med. **106:**282-286, 1961.

46 Fleisher, G. A., Potter, C. S., and Wakim, K. G.: Separation of 2 glutamic-oxalacetic transaminases, Proc. Soc. Exp. Biol. Med. **103:**229-231, 1960.

47 French, S. W., and Davies, P. L.: Ultrastructural localization of actin-like filaments in rat hepatocytes, Gastroenterology **68:**765-774, 1975.

48 Gabbiani, G., Ryan, G., Lamelin, J.-P., Vassalli, P., Majno, G., Bouvier, C. A., Cruchaud, A., and Luscher, E. F.: Human smooth muscle autoantibody—its identification as antiactin antibody and study of its binding to "non-muscular" cells, Am. J. Pathol. **72:**473-484, 1973.

49 Gartner, L. M., and Arias, I. M.: Formation, transport, metabolism, and excretion of bilirubin, New Eng. J. Med. **280:**1339-1345, 1969.

50 Gudat, F., Bianchi, L., Sonnabend, W., and Thiel, G.: Pattern of core and surface expression in liver tissue reflects state of specific immune response in hepatitis B, Lab. Invest. **32:**1-9, 1975.

51 Hadziyannis, S., Gerber, M. A., Vissoulis, C., and Popper, H.: Cytoplasmic hepatitis B antigen in "ground-glass" hepatocytes of carriers, Arch. Pathol. **96:**327-330, 1973.

52 Hadziyannis, S. T., Vissoulis, C. H., Moussouros, A., and Afroudakis, A.: Cytoplasmic localization of Australia antigen in the liver, Lancet **1:**976-979, 1972.

53 Hargreaves, T.: The liver and bile metabolism, New York, 1968, Appleton-Century-Crofts, chap. 3 (bilirubin metabolism).

54 Hoofnagle, J. H., Gerety, R. J., and Barker, L. F.: Antibody to hepatitis B virus core in man, Lancet **2**:869-872, 1973.

55 Hourani, B. T., Hamlin, E. M., and Reynolds, T. B.: Cerebrospinal fluid glutamine as a measure of hepatic encephalopathy, Arch. Intern. Med. **127**:1033-1036, 1971.

56 Huang, S.-N.: Immunohistochemical demonstration of hepatitis B core and surface antigens in paraffin sections, Lab. Invest. **33**:88-95, 1975.

57 Hurwitz, A. L., Gueller, R., and Pugay, P.: Fine-needle aspiration of malignant hepatic nodules for cytodiagnosis, J.A.M.A. **229**:814-815, 1974.

58 Itzchak, Y., Adar, R., Bogokowski, H., Mozes, M., and Deutsch, V.: Intrahepatic arterial portal communications—angiographic study, Am. J. Roentgenol. Radium Ther. Nucl. Med. **121**:384-387, 1974.

59 Kaplan, M. M.: Alkaline phosphatase, Gastroenterology **62**:452-468, 1972.

60 Karvountzis, G. G., and Redeker, A. G.: Relation of alpha-fetoprotein in acute hepatitis to severity and prognosis, Ann. Intern. Med. **80**:156-160, 1974.

61 Kessel, J. F., Lewis, W. P., Pasquel, C. M., and Turner, J. A.: Indirect hemagglutination and complement fixation tests in amebiasis, Am. J. Trop. Med. Hyg. **14**:540-550, 1965.

62 Klatskin, G., and Kantor, F. S.: Mitochondrial antibody in primary biliary cirrhosis and other diseases, Ann. Intern. Med. **77**:533-541, 1972.

63 Kueppers, F.: α_1-Antitrypsin: physiology, genetics, and pathology, Humangenetik **11**:177-189, 1971.

64 Lee, W. M., Reed, W. D., Mitchell, C. G., Galbraith, R. M., Eddleston, A. L. W. F., Zuckerman, A. J., and Williams, R.: Cellular and humoral immunity to hepatitis-B surface antigen in active chronic hepatitis, Br. Med. J. **1**:705-708, 1975.

65 Leevy, C. M.: Dye extraction by liver, Progr. Liver Dis. **1**:174-186, 1961.

66 Lester, R.: In Taylor, W., editor: The biliary system, Oxford, 1965, Blackwell Scientific Publications (why conjugation is necessary for excretion).

67 Lester, R., and Troxler, R. F.: Recent advances in bile pigment metabolism, Gastroenterology **56**:143-169, 1969.

68 Levitt, M., Schacter, B. A., Zipursky, A., and Israils, L. G.: Nonerythropoietic component of bilirubin, J. Clin. Invest. **47**:1281-1294, 1968.

69 Man, B., Kraus, L., and Pikielny, S.: Investigation of portal circulation via umbilical vein, Vasc. Surg. **8**:193-202, 1974.

70 Morrissey, K. P., and Javitt, N. B.: Extrahepatic biliary atresia: diagnosis by serum bile acid pattern and response to cholestyramine, Surgery **74**:116-121, 1973.

71 Mueller, A. F., and Leuthardt, F.: Conversion of glutamic acid to aspartic acid in liver mitochondria, Helv. Chim. Acta **33**:268-273, 1950.

72 Muroff, L. R., and Johnson, P. M.: Use of multiple radionuclide imaging to differentiate the focal intrahepatic lesion, Am. J. Roent-genol. Radium Ther. Nucl. Med. **121**:728-734, 1974.

73 Panveliwalla, D., Lewis, B., Woottoon, I. D. P., and Tabaqchali, S.: Determination of individual bile acids in biological fluids by thin-layer chromatography and fluorimetry, J. Clin. Pathol. **23**:309-314, 1970.

74 Peters, R. L.: In Okuda, K., and Peters, R. L., editors: Hepatocellular carcinoma, New York, 1976, John Wiley & Sons.

75 Pritchard, J. H., Winston, M. A., Berger, H. G., and Blahd, W. H.: Diagnosis of focal hepatic lesions—combined radioisotope and ultrasound techniques, J.A.M.A. **229**:1463-1465, 1974.

76 Read, A. E.: Clinical physiology of the liver, Br. J. Anaesth. **44**:910-917, 1972.

77 Rizzetto, M., Bianchi, F. B., and Doniach, D.: Characterization of the microsomal antigen related to a subclass of active chronic hepatitis, Immunology **26**:589-601, 1974.

78 Rizzetto, M., Swana, G., and Doniach, D.: Microsomal antibodies in active chronic hepatitis and other disorders, Clin. Exp. Immunol. **15**:331-344, 1973.

79 Roberts, H. R., and Cederbaum, A. I.: The liver and blood coagulation: physiology and pathology, Gastroenterology **63**:297-320, 1972.

80 Robinson, S. H.: Origins of bilirubin, New Eng. J. Med. **279**:143-149, 1968.

81 Rowsell, E. V.: Transaminations with L-glutamate and L-oxoglutarate, Biochem. J. **64**:235-245, 1956.

82 Rutenburg, A. M., Banks, B. M., Pineda, E. P., and Goldbarg, J. A.: Comparison of serum aminopeptidase and alkaline phosphatase in detection of hepatobiliary disease in anicteric patients, Ann. Intern. Med. **61**:50-55, 1964.

83 Scheuer, P. J.: Liver biopsy interpretation, London, 1968, Ballière, Tindall & Cassell.

84 Schmid, R.: In Taylor, W., editor: The biliary system, Oxford, 1965, Blackwell Scientific Publications (studies of congenital nonhemolytic jaundice with ^{14}C-bilirubin).

85 Schmid, R., and Hammaker, L.: Metabolism and disposition of ^{14}C bilirubin in congenital nonhemolytic jaundice, J. Clin. Invest. **42**:1720-1734, 1963.

86 Shikata, T., Uzawa, T., Yoshiwara, N., Akatsuka, T., and Yamazaki, S.: Staining methods of Australian antigen in paraffin section—detection of cytoplasmic inclusion bodies, Jap. J. Exp. Med. **44**:25-36, 1974.

87 Smith, M. G. M., Williams, R., Walker, G., Rizzetto, M., and Doniach, D.: Hepatic disorders associated with liver and kidney microsomal antibodies Br. Med. J. **2**:80-84, 1974.

88 Tong, M. J., Wallace, M. A., Peters, R. L., and Reynolds, T. B.: Lymphocyte stimulation in hepatitis B infections, New Eng. J. Med. **293**:318-322, 1975.

89 Williams, W. D., and Fajardo, L. F.: α_1-Antitrypsin deficiency, Am. J. Clin. Pathol. **61**:311-320, 1974.

90 Zeltzer, P. M., Neerhout, R. C., Fonkalsrud, E. W., and Stiehm, E. R.: Differentiation between neonatal hepatitis and biliary atresia by measuring serum alpha-fetoprotein, Lancet **1**:373-375, 1974.

Necrosis

91 Bearcroft, W. G. C.: Yellow fever, J. Pathol. Bacteriol. **80**:19-31, 421-426, 1960.

92 Ferreyra, E. C. de, Castro, J. A., Díaz Gómez, M. I., D'Costa, N., de Castro, C. R., and de Fenos, O. M.: Prevention and treatment of carbon tetrachloride hepatotoxicity by cysteine —studies about its mechanism, Toxicol. Appl. Pharmacol. **27**:558-568, 1974.

93 Fletcher, G. F., and Galambos, J. T.: Phosphorus poisoning, Arch. Intern. Med. (Chicago) **112**:846-852, 1963.

94 Francis, T. I., Moore, D. L., Edington, G. M., and Smith, J. A.: A clinicopathologic study of human yellow fever, Bull. W.H.O. **46**:659-667, 1972.

95 Goldberg, L. I.: Monoamine oxidase inhibitors, J.A.M.A. **190**:456-462, 1964. phenylhydantoin sodium hepatitis, J.A.M.A. **203**:1015-1018, 1968.

97 Kerr, J. F. R.: Shrinkage necrosis: a distinct mode of cellular death, J. Pathol. **105**:13-20, 1971.

98 Recknagel, R.: Carbon tetrachloride hepatotoxicity, Pharmacol. Rev. **19**:145-208, 1967.

99 Recknagel, R. O., and Ghoshal, A. K.: Lipoperoxidation as vector in carbon tetrachloride hepatotoxicity, Lab. Invest. **15**:132-148, 1966.

100 Salfelder, K., Seelkopf, C., and Inglessis, G.: Phosphorus poisoning, Zentrabl. Allg. Pathol. **108**:524-529, 1966.

101 Smetana, H. F.: Histopathology of drug-induced liver disease, Ann. N.Y. Acad. Sci. **104**:821-846, 1963.

102 Trump, B. F., Goldblatt, P. J., and Stowell, R. E.: Studies of necrosis in vitro of mouse hepatic parenchymal cells, Lab. Invest. **14**:1946-1968, 1965.

103 Wiggers, K. D., French, S. W., French, B. A., and Carr, B. N.: The ultrastructure of Mallory body filaments, Lab. Invest. **29**:652-658, 1973.

Viral hepatitis

104 Afroudakis, A., and Peters, R. L.: Unpublished data, 1975.

105 Allen, J. G., and Sayman, W. A.: Serum hepatitis from transfusions of blood, J.A.M.A. **180**:1079-1085, 1962.

106 Allen, J. G., Sykes, C., Enerson, D. M., Moulder, P. V., Elghammer, R. M., Grossman, B. J., McKeen, C. L., and Galluzi, N. J.: Homologous serum jaundice, J.A.M.A. **144**:1069-1074, 1950.

107 Alter, H. J., Holland, P. V., Purcell, R. H., Lander, J. J., Feinstone, S. M., Morrow, A. G., and Schmidt, P. J.: Posttransfusion hepatitis after exclusion of commercial and hepatitis B antigen–positive donors, Ann. Intern. Med. **77**:691-699, 1972.

108 Alter, H. J., Holland, P. V., and Schmidt, P. J.: Hepatitis-associated antigen, Lancet **2**:142-143, 1970.

109 Ashcavai, M., and Peters, R. L.: Hepatitis-associated antigen, improved sensitivity in detection, Am. J. Clin. Pathol. **55**:262-268, 1971.

110 Barker, L. F., Chisari, F. V., McGrath, P. P., Dalgard, D. W., Kirschstein, R. L., Almeida, J. D., Edgington, T. S. M., Sharp, D. J., and Peterson, M. R.: Transmission of type B viral hepatitis to chimpanzees, J. Infect. Dis. **127**:648-662, 1973.

111 Bearn, A. G., Kunkel, H. G., and Slater, R. L.: Chronic liver disease in young women, Am. J. Med. **21**:3-15, 1956.

112 Bergman L. A., Thomas, W., Reddy, C. R., Ellison, M. R., Smith, E. C., and Dunea, G.: Nonviral hepatitis in patients maintained by long-term dialysis, Arch. Intern. Med. **130**:96-103, 1972.

113 Bettley, F. R.: LE cell phenomenon in active chronic hepatitis, Lancet **2**:724, 1955.

114 Biava, C., and Mukhlova-Montiel, M.: Electron microscopic observations on Councilman-like acidophilic bodies, Am. J. Pathol. **46**:775-802, 1965.

115 Blumberg, B. S., Alter, H. J., and Visnich, S.: "New" antigen in leukemia sera, J.A.M.A. **191**:541-546, 1965.

116 Boeve, N. R., Winterscheid, L. C., and Merendino, K. A.: Fibrinogen-transmitted hepatitis in surgical patient, Ann. Surg. **170**:833-838, 1969.

117 Bosch, E., and Kolk-Vegter, A. J.: Control of serum hepatitis in a dialysis unit, Neth. J. Med. **16**:200-211, 1973.

118 Boyer, J. L., and Klatskin, G.: Pattern of necrosis in acute viral hepatitis—prognostic value of bridging, New Eng. J. Med. **283**:1063-1071, 1970.

119 Bradley, D. W., Hornbeck, C. L., Gravelle, C. R., Cook, E. H., and Maynard, J. E.: CsCl banding of hepatitis A–associated virus–like particles, J. Infect. Dis. **131**:304-306, 1975.

120 Briggs, W. A., Lazarus, J. M., Birtch, A. G., Hampers, C. L., Hager, E. B. Merrill J. P.: Hepatitis affecting hemodialysis and transplant patients, Arch. Intern. Med. **132**:21-28, 1973.

121 Brodersen, M., Stegmann, S., Klein, K.-H., Trulzsch, D., and Rensch, P.: Salivary HbAg detected by radioimmunoassay, Lancet **1**:675-676, 1974.

122 Bucher, N. L. R., Swaffield, M. N., and DiTroia, J. F.: Incorporation of thymidine-2-^{14}C into DNA of regenerating rat liver, Cancer Res. **24**:509-512, 1964.

123 Bulkley, B. H., Heizer, W. D., Goldfinger, S. E., Isselbacher, K. J., and Shulman, N. R.: Distinctions in chronic active hepatitis based on circulating hepatitis-associated antigen, Lancet **2**:1323-1326, 1970.

124 Carr, J. B., de Guesada, A. M., and Shires, D. L.: Decreased incidence of transfusion hepatitis after exclusive transfusion with reconstituted frozen erythrocytes, Ann. Intern. Med. **78**:693-695, 1973.

125 Chaudhary, R. K., and Perry, E.: Frequency of hepatitis B infection in artificial kidney unit and blood procurement staff, Lancet **1**:1194, 1975.

126 Child, P. L., and Ruiz, A.: Acidophilic bodies, Arch. Pathol. (Chicago) **85**:45-50, 1968.

127 Christoffersen, P., Poulsen, H., and Scheuer, P.: Abnormal bile duct epithelium in chronic aggressive hepatitis and primary biliary cirrhosis, Hum. Pathol. **3**:227-235, 1972.

128 Chung, W. K., Moon, S.-K., and Popper, H.: Anicteric hepatitis in Korea, Gastroenterology **48**:1-11, 1965.

129 Cohen, S. N., and Dougherty, W. J.: Transfusion hepatitis arising from addict blood donors, J.A.M.A. **203**:427-429, 1968.

130 Committee on Viral Hepatitis, National Academy of Science: Nomenclature of antigens associated with viral hepatitis type B, J. Infect. Dis. **130**:92, 1974.

131 Cooper, W. C., Gershon, R. K., Sun, S.-C., and Fresh, J. W.: Anicteric viral hepatitis in Taiwan, New Eng. J. Med. **274**:585-595, 1966.

132 Councilman, W. T.: In Sternberg, G. M.: Acidophilic bodies, U.S. Marine Hosp. Pub. Health Bull. **2**:151-153, 1890.

133 Dane, D. S., Cameron, C. H., and Briggs, M.: Viruslike particles in serum of patients with Australia antigen–associated hepatitis, Lancet **1**:695-698, 1970.

134 Darani, M., and Gerber, M.: Hepatitis B antigen in vaginal secretions, Lancet **2**:1108, 1974.

135 Davis, M. A., Peters, R. L., Redeker, A. G., and Reynolds, T. B.: Appraisal of mortality in acute fulminant viral hepatitis, New Eng. J. Med. **278**:1248-1253, 1968.

136 DeGroote, J., Desmet, V. J., Gedigk, P., Korb, G., Popper, H., Poulsen, H., Scheuer, P., Schmid, M., Thaler, H., Uehlinger, E., and Wepler, W.: Classification of chronic hepatitis, Lancet **2**:626-628, 1968.

137 Deinhart, F., Holmes, A. W., Capps, R. B., and Popper, H.: Studies on transmission of human viral hepatitis to marmoset monkeys. I. Transmission of disease, serial passages, and description of liver lesions, J. Exp. Med. **125**:673-688, 1967.

138 Desmyter, J., Bradburne, A. F., Vermylen, C., Daneels, R., and Boelaert, J.: Hepatitis B immunoglobulin in prevention of HBs antigenemia in hemodialysis patients, Lancet **2**:377-379, 1975.

139 Dougherty, W. J., and Altman, R.: Viral hepatitis in New Jersey 1960-1961, Am. J. Med. **32**:704-716, 1962.

140 Dunn, A. E. G., Peters, R. L., Schweitzer, I. L., and Spears, R. L.: Virus-like particles in livers of infants with vertically transmitted hepatitis, Arch. Pathol. **94**:258-264, 1972.

141 Edgington, T. S., and Chisari, F. V.: Immunological aspects of hepatitis B virus infection, Am. J. Med. Sci. **270**:213-227, 1975.

142 Feinstone, S. M., Kapikian, A. Z., and Purcell, R. H.: Detection by immune electron microscopy of viruslike antigen associated with acute illness, Science **182**:1026-1028, 1973.

143 Feinstone, S. M., Kapikian, A. Z., Purcell, R. H., Alter, H. J., and Holland, P. V.: Transfusion-associated hepatitis not due to viral hepatitis type A or B, New Eng. J. Med. **292**:767-770, 1975.

144 Feizi, T.: Immunoglobulin in chronic liver disease, Gut **9**:193-198, 1968.

145 Friedmann, C. T. H., Dinnes, M. R., Bernstein, J. F., and Heidbreder, G. A.: Chimpanzee-associated infectious hepatitis among personnel at an animal hospital, J. Am. Vet. Med. Assoc. **159**:541-545, 1971.

146 Gerber, M. A., Hadziyannis, S., Vissoulis, C., Schaffner, F., Paronetto, F., and Popper, H.: Electron microscopy and immunoelectron microscopy of cytoplasmic hepatitis B antigen in hepatocytes, Am. J. Pathol. **75**:489-502, 1974.

147 Gitnick, G. L., Gleich, G. J., Schoenfield, L. J., Baggenstoss, A. H., Sutnick, A. I., Blumberg, B. S., London, W. T., and Summerskill, W. H. J.: Australia antigen in chronic active liver disease with cirrhosis, Lancet **2**:285-288, 1969.

148 Gocke, D. J., Greenberg, H. B., and Kavey, N. B.: Correlation of Australia antigen with posttransfusion hepatitis, J.A.M.A. **212**:877-879, 1970.

149 Goldstein, L., Reynolds, T., Redeker, A., Schweitzer, I., and Peters, R. L.: Chronic liver disease from viral hepatitis, Calif. Med. **114**:26-35, 1971.

150 Grady, G.: Prevention of posttransfusion hepatitis by gamma globulin, J.A.M.A. **214**:140-142, 1970.

151 Havens, W. P.: Viral hepatitis: multiple attacks in narcotic addict, Ann. Intern. Med. **44**:199-203, 1956.

152 Held, J. R.: Scientific proceedings of 100th annual meeting of American Veterinary Medical Association, 1963, pp. 183-185 (publication data not found) (public health implication of nonhuman primates in transmission of hepatitis to man).

153 Heller, P., Zimmerman, H. J., Rozengvaig, S., and Singer, K.: L.E.-cell phenomenon in chronic hepatic disease, New Eng. J. Med. **254**:1160-1165, 1956.

154 Henigst, W.: Sexual transmission of infections associated with hepatitis B antigen, Lancet **2**:1395, 1973.

155 Hersh, T., Melnick, J. L., Goyal, R. K., and Hollinger, F. B.: Nonparenteral transmission of viral hepatitis B (Australia antigen–associated serum hepatitis, New Eng. J. Med. **285**:1363-1364, 1971.

156 Hilleman, M. R., Provost, P. J., Miller, W. J., Villarejor, V. M., Ittensohn, O. L., and McAleer, W. J.: Development and utilization of complement-fixation and immune adherence tests for human hepatitis A virus and antibody, Am. J. Med. Sci. **270**:93-98, 1975.

157 Hilleman, M. R., Provost, P. J., and Miller, W. J.: Communication from authors on material presented at the International Association of Biological Standardization at Symposium on Viral Hepatitis in Milan, Italy, 1974 (immune adherence and complement-fixation tests for human hepatitis A—diagnostic and epidemiologic investigations).

158 Holmes, A. W., Wolfe, L., Deinhardt, F., and Gurad, M. E.: Transmission of human hepatitis to marmosets—further coded studies, J. Infect. Dis. **124**:520-521, 1971.

159 Huang, S. N.: Hepatitis-associated antigen hepatitis. Electron microscopic study of viruslike particles in liver cells, Am. J. Pathol. **64**:483-494, 1971.

160 Huang, S. N., Groh, V., Beaudoin, J. G., Dauphinee, W. D., Guttmann, R. D., Morehouse, D. D., Aronoff, A., and Gault, H.: Study of relationship of virus-like particles and Australia antigen in liver, Hum. Pathol. **5**:209-222, 1974.

161 Ishak, K. G.: In Gall, E. A., and Mostofi, F. K., editors: The liver, Baltimore, 1973, The Williams & Wilkins Co. (viral hepatitis—the morphologic spectrum).

162 Iwarson, S., Lundin, P., and Holmgren, J.: Multiple attacks of hepatitis in drug addicts: biochemical, immunochemical, and morphologic characteristics, J. Infect. Dis. **127:**544-550, 1973.

163 Joske, R. A., and King, W. E.: LE cell phenomenon in active chronic viral hepatitis, Lancet **2:**477-480, 1955.

164 Karvountzis, G., Redeker, A., and Peters, R.: Long-term follow-up studies on patients surviving fulminant viral hepatitis, Gastroenterology **67:**870-877, 1974.

165 Kim, C. Y., and Tillis, J. G.: Immunologic and electrophoretic heterogeneity of hepatitis-associated antigen, J. Infect. Dis. **123:**618-628, 1971.

166 Kliman, A.: Australia antigen in volunteer and paid blood donors, New Eng. J. Med. **284:**109, 1971.

167 Klion, F. M., and Schaffner, F.: Ultrastructure of acidophilic Councilman-like bodies in the liver, Am. J. Pathol. **48:**755-767, 1966.

168 Krawczyński, K., Nazarewicz, T., Brzosko, W. J., and Nowoslawski, A.: Cellular localization of hepatitis-associated antigen in livers of patients with different forms of hepatitis, J. Infect. Dis. **126:**372-377, 1972.

169 Krugman, S., and Giles, J. P.: Viral hepatitis—new light on an old disease, J.A.M.A. **212:**1019-1029, 1970.

170 Krugman, S., and Giles, J. P.: Viral hepatitis, type B (MS-2 strain). Further observations on natural history and prevention, New Eng. J. Med. **288:**755-760, 1973.

171 Krugman, S., Giles, J. P., and Hammond, J.: Infectious hepatitis, J.A.M.A. **200:**365-373, 1967.

172 Krugman, S., Giles, J. P., and Hammond, J.: Viral hepatitis type B (MS-2 strain)—prevention with specific hepatitis B immune serum globulin, J.A.M.A. **218:**1665-1670, 1971.

173 Krugman, S., Ward, R., and Giles, J. P.: Natural history of infectious hepatitis, Am. J. Med. **32:**717-728, 1962.

174 Kunkel, H. G., Ahrens, E. H., Jr., Eisenmenger, W. J., Bongiovanni, A. M., and Slater, R. J.: Hypergammaglobulinemia in young women, J. Clin. Invest. **30:**654, 1951 (abstract).

175 Kunst, V. A. J. M., and Rosier, J. G. M. C.: Au antigen in at-risk patients, Lancet **1:**423-424, 1970.

176 LeBouvier, G. L.: Heterogeneity of Australia antigen, J. Infect. Dis. **123:**671-675, 1971.

177 LeBouvier, G. L., and Williams, A.: Serotypes of hepatitis B antigen (HBsAg)—problem of new determinants, as exemplified by *t*, Am. J. Med. Sci. **270:**165-171, 1975.

178 Levine, R. A., and Payne, M. A.: Homologous serum hepatitis in youthful heroin users, Ann. Intern. Med. **53:**164-178, 1960.

179 London, W. T., DiFiglia, M., Sutnick, A. I., and Blumberg, B. S.: Hepatitis in hemodialysis unit: Austria antigen and host response, New Eng. J. Med. **281:**571-578, 1969.

180 MacCallum, F. O., Stewart, A., and Bradley, W. H.: In Medical Research Council, Great Britain, Spec. Rep. Ser. No. 273, London, 1951, H. M. Stationery Office (transmission experiments in man).

181 Mackay, I. R., Weiden, S., and Hasker, J.: Autoimmune hepatitis, Ann. N.Y. Acad. Sci. **124:**767-780, 1955.

182 MacLachlan, M. J., Rodnan, G. P., Cooper, W. N., and Fennell, R. H.: Chronic active "lupoid" hepatitis, Ann. Intern. Med. **62:**425-462, 1965.

183 MacQuarrie, M. B., Forghani, B., and Wolochow, D. A.: Hepatitis B transmitted by a human bite, J.A.M.A. **230:**723-724, 1974.

184 Magnius, L. O., Lindholm, A., Lundin, P., and Iwarson, S.: New antigen-antibody system—clinical significance in long-term carriers of hepatitis B surface antigen, J.A.M.A. **231:**356-359, 1975.

185 Magnius, L. O., and Espmark, J. A.: New specificities in Australia antigen–positive sera distinct from LeBouvier determinants, J. Immunol. **109:**1017-1021, 1972.

186 Mosley, J. W.: Epidemiology of viral hepatitis—overview, Am. J. Med. Sci. **270:**253-269, 1975.

187 Mosley, J. W., Edwards, V. M., Wapplehorst, B., and Hajduk, P.: Hepatitis B virus subtypes *ad* and *ay* among blood donors in Greater Los Angeles, Transfusion **14:**372-377, 1974.

188 Mosley, J. W., and Galambos, J. T.: In Schiff, L., editor: Diseases of the liver, ed. 3, Philadelphia, J. B. Lippincott Co. (viral hepatitis).

189 Murray, R., and Ratner, F.: Safety of immune serum globulin, Proc. Soc. Exp. Biol. Med. **83:**554-555, 1953.

190 Nielsen, J. O., Dietrichson, O., and Juhl, E.: Incidence and meaning of the *e* determinant among hepatitis B antigen–positive patients with acute and chronic liver diseases, Lancet **2:**913-915, 1974.

191 Ohta, Y.: Viral hepatitis and hepatocellular carcinoma. In Okuda, K., and Peters, R. L., editors: Hepatocellular carcinoma, New York, 1976, John Wiley & Sons.

192 Peters, R. L.: Viral hepatitis, a pathologic spectrum, Am. J. Med. Sci. **270:**17-31, 1975.

193 Peters, R. L., and Ashcavai, M.: Immunoglobulin levels in detection of viral hepatitis, Am. J. Clin. Pathol. **54:**102-109, 1970.

194 Plainos, T. C., Chloros, G., Tripatzis, I., Luciano, L., Kourepi-Logetheti, M., and Tsilivi, N.: Dane particles in homogenates of mosquitoes fed with HBsAg-positive human blood, Lancet **1:**1334-1335, 1975.

195 Polakoff, S., Cossort, Y. E., and Tillett, H. E.: Hepatitis in dialysis units in the United Kingdom, Br. Med. J. **3:**94-99, 1972.

196 Potter, H. P., Cohen, N. N., and Norris, R. F.: Chronic hepatic dysfunction in heroin addicts, J.A.M.A. **174:**2049-2051, 1960.

197 Poulsen, H., and Christoffersen, P.: Abnormal bile duct epithelium in chronic aggressive hepatitis and cirrhosis, Hum. Pathol. **3:**217-225, 1972.

198 Prince, A. M., Brotman, B., Grady, G. F., Kuhns, W. J.: Long-incubation posttransfusion hepatitis without serological evidence of exposure to hepatitis B virus, Lancet **2:**241-246, 1974.

199 Prince, A. M., Metselaar, D., Kafuko, G. W., Mukwaya, L. G., Ling, C. M., and Overby,

L. R.: Hepatitis in wild-caught mosquitoes in Africa, Lancet 2:247-250, 1972.

200 Provost, P. J., Wolanski, B. S., Miller, W. J., Ittensohn, O. L., McAleer, W. J., and Hilleman, M. R.: Physical, chemical, and morphologic dimension of human hepatitis A virus strain CR326 (38578), Proc. Soc. Exp. Biol. Med. **148**:232-539, 1975.

201 Redeker, A. G.: Viral hepatitis: clinical aspects, Am. J. Med. Sci. **270**:9-16, 1975.

202 Redeker, A., and Carpio, N.: In Diller, J. J., editor: Present concepts internal medicine, vol. 2, San Francisco, 1969, Letterman General Hospital, pp. 107-112 (hippie hepatitis).

203 Redeker, A. G., Hopkins, C. E., Jackson, B., and Peck, P.: Controlled study of safety of pooled plasma, Transfusion **8**:60-64, 1968.

204 Redeker, A. G., and Yamahiro, H. S.: Controlled trial of exchange transfusion therapy in fulminant hepatitis, Lancet **1**:3-6, 1973.

205 Reynolds, T. B., Edmondson, H. A., Peters, R. L., and Redeker, A. G.: Lupoid hepatitis, Ann. Intern. Med. **61**:650-666, 1964.

206 Reynolds, T. B., Peters, R. L., and Yamada, S.: Chronic active and lupoid hepatitis caused by a laxative, oxyphenisatin, New Eng. J. Med. **285**:813-820, 171.

207 Ringertz, O., Nystrom, B., and Strom, J.: Clinical aspects of an outbreak of hepatitis among personnel in hemodialysis units, Scand. J. Infect. Dis. **1**:51-56, 1969.

208 Rogers, J. A.: Outbreak of jaundice in army, Milit. Surg. **91**:386-393, 1942.

209 Sapira, J. D., Jasinski, D. R., and Gorodetzky, C. W.: Liver disease in narcotic addicts. II. The role of needle, Clin. Pharmacol. Ther. **9**:725-739, 1968.

210 Schweitzer, I. L., Dunn, A. E. G., Peters, R. L., and Spears, R. L.: Viral hepatitis B in neonates and infants, Am. J. Med. **55**:762-771, 1973.

211 Schweitzer, I. L., and Spear, R. L.: Hepatitis-associated antigen in mother and infant, New Eng. J. Med. **283**:570-572, 1970.

212 Shikata, T.: Australia antigen in liver tissue, Jap. J. Exp. Med. **43**:231-245, 1973.

213 Shikata, T.: Primary liver cell carcinoma and liver cirrhosis. In Okuda, K., and Peters, R. L., editors: Hepatocellular carcinoma, New York, 1976, John Wiley & Sons.

214 Shikata, T.: In Okuda, K., and Peters, R. L., editors: Hepatocellular carcinoma, New York, 1976, John Wiley & Sons (primary liver carcinoma and liver cirrhosis).

215 Stein, O., Fainaru, M., and Stein, Y.: Visualization of viruslike particles in endoplasmic reticulum of hepatocytes of Australia antigen carriers, Lab. Invest. **26**:262-269, 1972.

216 Stevens, C. E., Beasley, R. P., and Tsui, J.: Vertical transmission of hepatitis B antigen in Taiwan, New Eng. J. Med. **292**:771-774, 1975.

217 Sun, S. C., Anderson, K. E., Hsu, C. P., Kau, S. L.: Hepatocellular ultrastructure in asymptomatic hepatitis B antigenemia, Arch. Pathol. **97**:373-379, 1974.

218 Sutnick, A. I., London, W. T., Gerstley, J. S., Cronlund, M. M., and Blumberg, B. S.: Anicteric hepatitis associated with Australia antigen—occurrence in patients with Down's syndrome, J.A.M.A. **205**:670-674, 1968.

219 Szmuness, W., Prince, A. M., Goodman, M., Ehrick, C., Pick, R., and Manzoor, A.: Hepatitis B immune serum globulin in prevention of nonparenterally transmitted hepatitis B, New Eng. J. Med. **290**:701-706, 1974.

220 Szmuness, W., Prince, A. M., Grady, G. F., Mann, M. K., Levine, R. W., Friedman, E. A., Jacobs, M. J.: Hepatitis B infection—point prevalence study in 15 U.S. hemodialysis centers, J.A.M.A. **227**:901-906, 1974.

221 Taswell, H. F., Shorter, R., Poncelet, T. K., and Maxwell, N. G.: Hepatitis-associated antigen in blood donor population, J.A.M.A. **214**: 142-144, 1970.

222 Teodori, U., Gentilini, P., and Surrenti, C.: Electron microscope observations of forms of viral hepatitis, Gastroenterologia (Basel) **108**: 105-120, 1967.

223 Tisdale, W. A.: Subacute hepatitis, New Eng. J. Med. **268**:85-89, 138-142, 1963.

224 Tong, M. J., Bischel, M. D., Scoles, B., and Berne, T. U.: T and B lymphocytes in uremic patients with type B hepatitis infection, Nephron (in press).

225 Tong, M. J., Sun, S., Schaeffer, B. T., Lo, K., Chang, N., and Peters, R.: Hepatitis-associated antigen in patients with hepatocellular carcinoma in Taiwan, Ann. Intern. Med. **75**:687-691, 1971.

226 Trey, C., Lipworth, L., Chalmers, T. C., Davidson, C. S., Gottlieb, L. S., Popper, H., and Saunders, S. J.: Fulminant hepatic failure, presumable contribution of halothane, New Eng. J. Med. **279**:798-801, 1968.

227 Villarejos, V. M., Visoná, K. A., Gutiérrez, D. A., and Rodríguez, A.: Role of saliva, urine, and feces in the transmission of type B hepatitis, New Eng. J. Med. **291**(26):1375-1378, 1974.

228 Vogel, C. L., Moody, N., Anthony, P. P., and Barker, L. F.: Hepatitis-associated antigen in Uganda patients with hepatocellular carcinoma, Lancet **2**:621-624, 1970.

229 Ware, A. J., Luby, J. P., Eigenbrodt, E. H., Long, D. L., and Hull, A. R.: Spectrum of liver disease in renal transplant recipients, Gastroenterology **68**:755-764, 1975.

230 Whittingham, S., Irwin, J., Mackey, I. R., and Smalley, M.: Smooth-muscle autoantibody in "autoimmune" hepatitis, Gastroenterology **51**: 499-505, 1966.

231 Wright, R., McCollum, R. W., and Klatskin, G.: Australia antigen in acute and chronic liver disease, Lancet **2**:117-121, 1969.

232 Zebe, H., Senwald, R., and Ritz, E.: Insect vectors in serum hepatitis, Lancet **1**:1117-1118, 1972.

Encephalopathy

233 Adams, R. D., and Foley, J. M.: Neurologic disorders associated with liver disease, Assoc. Res. Nerv. Ment. Dis. Proc. (1952) **32**:198-237, 1953.

234 Davidson, C. S., and Gabuzda, G. J.: Hepatic coma. In Schiff, L., editor: Diseases of the liver, ed. 4, Philadelphia, 1975, J. B. Lippincott Co.

235 Dubin, I. N., Sullivan, B. H., Jr., LeGolvan, P. C., and Murphy, L. C.: Cholestatic form of viral hepatitis, Am. J. Med. **29:**55-72, 1960.

236 Fischer, J. E.: Hepatic coma in cirrhosis, portal hypertension, and following portacaval shunt: its etiologies and the current status of its treatment, Arch. Surg. **108:**325-336, 1974.

237 Kardel, T., Ramsoe, K., and Rasmussen, S. N.: Preoperative liver function tests correlated with encephalopathy after portacaval anastomosis, Scand. J. Gastroenterol. **10:**29-32, 1975.

238 Rudman, D., DeFulco, T. J., Galambos, J. T., Smith, R. B., III, Salam, A. A., and Warren, W. D.: Maximal rates of excretion and synthesis of urea in normal and cirrhotic subjects, J. Clin. Invest. **52:**2241-2249, 1973.

239 Warren, W. D., Rudman, D., Millikan, W., Galambos, J. T., Salam, A. A., and Smith, R. B.: Metabolic basis of portasystemic encephalopathy and the effect of selective versus nonselective shunts, Ann. Surg. **180:**573-579, 1974.

Other acute infections

240 Brun, C., Madsen, S., and Olsen, S.: Infectious mononucleosis with hepatic and renal involvement, Scand. J. Gastroenterol. (suppl.) **7:**89-95, 1970.

241 Chang, M. Y., and Campbell, W. G., Jr.: Fatal infectious mononucleosis: association with liver necrois and herpeslike virus particles, Arch. Pathol. **99:**185-191, 1975.

242 Henson, D. E., Grimley, P. M., and Strano, A. J.: Postnatal cytomegalovirus hepatitis. An autopsy and liver biopsy study, Hum. Pathol. **5:**93-103, 1974.

243 Orenstein, J. M., Castadot, M. J., and Wilens, S. L.: Fatal herpes hepatitis associated with pemphigus vulgaris and steroids in an adult, Hum. Pathol. **5:**489-496, 1974.

244 Reller, L. B.: Granulomatous hepatitis associated with cytomegalovirus in acute mononucleosis, Lancet **1:**20-22, 1973.

Chemical and drug injury

245 Bassi, M.: Electron microscopy of rat liver after carbon tetrachloride, Exp. Cell Res. **20:**313-323, 1960.

246 Breitenbucher, R., and Crowley, L.: Hepatorenal toxicity of tetracycline, Minn. Med. **53:**949-955, 1970.

247 Brown, B. R., Jr.: Enzymatic activity and biotransformation of anesthetics, Int. Anesthesiol. Clin. **12:**25-34, 1974.

248 Conn, H. O.: Halothane-associated hepatitis—disease of medical progress, Isr. J. Med. Sci. **10**(pt. 1):404-415, 1974.

249 Dahl, M. G. C., Gregory, M. M., and Scheuer, P. J.: Methotrexate hepatotoxicity in psoriasis—comparison of different dose regimens, Br. Med. J. **1:**654-656, 1972.

250 Deo, M. G., Roy, H., and Ramalingaswami, V.: Protein deficiency in carbon tetrachloride–induced hepatic lesions, Arch. Pathol. **99:**147-151, 1975.

251 Drill, V. A.: Benign cholestatic jaundice of pregnancy and benign cholestatic jaundice from oral contraceptives, Am. J. Obstet. Gynecol. **119:**165-174, 1974.

252 Emond, M., Erlinger, S., Berthelot, P., Benhamou, J.-P., and Fauvert, R.: Effect of novobiocin on liver function, Can. Med. Assoc. J. **94:**900-904, 1966.

253 Hallén, B., and Johansson, G.: Inhalation anesthetics and cytochrome P$_{450}$–dependent reactions in rat liver microsomes, Anesthesiology **43:**34-40, 1975.

254 Hoyumpa, A. M., Jr., Schiff, L., and Helfman, E. L.: Budd-Chiari syndrome in women taking oral contraceptives, Am. J. Med. **50:**137-140, 1971.

255 Hruban, Z., Russell, R. M., Boyer, J. L., Glagov, S., and Bagheri, S. A.: Ultrastructural changes in the livers of two patients with hypervitaminosis A, Am. J. Pathol. **76:**451-468, 1974.

256 Iancu, T., and Elian, E.: Aspirin-induced abnormalities of liver function, Am. J. Dis. Child. **128:**116-117, 1974.

257 Lewis, J. E., Mello, P., and Knauer, C. M.: Isoniazid-associated hepatitis; serum enzyme determinations and histologic features, Western J. Med. **122:**371-376, 1975.

258 Maddrey, W. C., and Boitnott, J. K.: Isoniazid hepatitis, Ann. Intern. Med. **79:**1-12, 1973.

259 Maddrey, W. C., and Boitnott, J. K.: Severe hepatitis from methyldopa, Gastroenterology **68:**351-360, 1975.

260 Metreau, J.-M., Dhumeaux, D., and Berthelot, P.: Oral contraceptives and the liver, Digestion **7:**313-335, 1972.

261 Mitchell, J. R.: Drugs and the liver, Viewpoints on Dig. Dis., vol. 6, no. 5, 1974.

262 Mitchell, J. R., and Jollows, D. J.: Metabolic activation of drugs to toxic substances, Gastroenterology **68:**392-410, 1975.

263 Panner, B. J., and Hanss, R. J.: Hepatic injury in mushroom poisoning, Arch. Pathol. (Chicago) **87:**35-45, 1969.

264 Peters, R. L., Edmondson, H. A., Mikkelsen, W. P., and Tatter, D.: Tetracycline-induced fatty liver in nonpregnant patients, Am. J. Surg. **113:**622-632, 1967.

265 Popper, H., and Schaffner, F.: Pathophysiology of cholestasis, Hum. Pathol. **1:**1-24, 1970.

266 Rehder, K., and Sessler, A. D.: Biotransformation of halothane, Int. Anesthesiol. Clin. **12:**41-53, 1974.

267 Remmer, H.: Induction of drug-metabolizing enzyme system in the liver, Eur. J. Clin. Pharmacol. **5:**116-136, 1972.

268 Smith, R. L.: Biliary excretion and hepatotoxicity of contraceptive steroids, Acta Endocrinol. (Suppl.) **185:**149-161, 1973.

269 Smuckler, E. A., Iseri, O. A., and Benditt, E. P.: Intracellular defect in protein synthesis induced by CCl$_4$, J. Exp. Med. **116:**55-72, 1962.

270 Storms, W. W.: Chloroform parties, J.A.M.A. **225:**160, 1973.

271 Toghill, P. J., Smith, P. G., Benton, P., Brown, R. C., and Matthews, H. L.: Methyldopa liver damage, Br. Med. J. **3:**545-548, 1974.

272 Walker, C. O., and Combes, B.: Biliary cirrhosis induced by chlorpromazine, Gastroenterology **51:**631-640, 1966.

273 Weinstein, G., Roenigk, H., Maibach, H., Cosnides, J., and Millard, M.: Psoriasis-liver-

methotrexate interactions, Arch. Dermatol. **108:**36-42, 1973.

274 Wepler, W., and Opitz, K.: Histologic changes in the liver biopsy in *Amanita phalloides* intoxication, Hum. Pathol. **3:**249-254, 1972.

275 Winter, S. L., and Boyer, J. L.: Hepatic toxicity from large doses of vitamin B₃ (nicotinamide), New Eng. J. Med. **289:**1180-1182, 1973.

Radiation injury

276 Hendee, W. R., Alders, M. A., and Garciga, C. E.: Development of ultrastructural radiation injury, Am. J. Roentgenol. **105:**147-151, 1969.

277 Lewin, K., and Millis, R. R.: Human radiation hepatitis, Arch. Pathol. **96:**21-26, 1973.

278 Reed, G. B., Jr., and Cox, A. J., Jr.: Human liver after radiation injury, Am. J. Pathol. **48:**597-611, 1966.

Biliary obstruction and liver abscess

279 Biava, C. G.: Fine structure of normal human bile canaliculi, Lab. Invest. **13:**840-864, 1964.

280 Brown, J. R.: Human actinomycosis—study of 181 subjects, Hum. Pathol. **4:**319-330, 1973.

281 Case records of Massachusetts General Hospital: Subacute bacterial endocarditis, aortic insufficiency, renal and hepatic polycystic disease, New Eng. J. Med. **279:**932-940, 1968.

282 Charcot, J. M.: Leçons sur les maladies du foie; des voies biliaires et des reins, Recueillies et publiées par Bourneville et Sévestre, Paris, 1877, Progrès Médical, pp. 178-179.

283 Dehner, L. P., and Kissane, J. M.: Pyogenic hepatic abscesses in infancy and childhood, J. Pediatr. **74:**763-773, 1969.

284 Futch, C., Zikria, B. A., and Neu, H. C.: Bacteroides liver abscess, Surgery **73:**59-65, 1973.

285 Gall, E. A., and Dobrogorski, O.: Obstructive jaundice, Am. J. Clin. Pathol. **41:**126-139, 1964.

286 Holt, J. M., and Spry, C. J. F.: Solitary pyogenic liver abscess in patients with diabetes mellitus, Lancet **2:**198-200, 1966.

287 Lazarchick, J., deSouza e Silva, N. A., Nichols, D. R., and Washington, J. A., II: Pyogenic liver abscess, Mayo Clin. Proc. **48:**349-355, 1973.

288 Lin, C. S.: Suppurative pylephlebitis and liver abscess complicating colonic diverticulitis—report of two cases and review of literature, Mt. Sinai J. Med. N.Y. **40:**48-55, 1973.

289 McCarty, E., Pathmanand, C., Sunakorn, P., and Scherz, R. G.: Amebic liver abscess in childhood, Am. J. Dis. Child. **126:**67-70, 1973.

290 Murray-Lyon, I. M., Shilkin, K. B., Laws, J. W., Illing, R. C., and Williams, R.: Cholangitis complicating congenital hepatic fibrosis, Gut **13:**319, 1972 (abstract).

291 Rubin, R. H., Swartz, M. N., and Malt, R.: Hepatic abscess: changes in clinical, bacteriologic, and therapeutic aspects; a review, Am. J. Med. **57:**601-610, 1974.

292 Sabbaz, J., Sutter, V. L., and Finegold, S. M.: Anaerobic pyogenic liver abscess, Ann. Intern. Med. **77:**629-638, 1972.

293 Schoenfield, L. J., Sjovall, J., and Perman, E.: Bile acids on skin of patients with pruritic hepatobiliary disease, Nature (London) **212:**93-94, 1967.

294 Scott, A. J., and Khan, G. A.: Origin of bacteria in bile-duct bile, Lancet **2:**790-792, 1967.

295 Sheehy, T. W., Parmley, L. F., Jr., Johnston, G. S., and Boyce, H. W.: Resolution time of an amebic liver abscess, Gastroenterology **55:**26-34, 1968.

296 Takada, T., Hanyu, F., Mikoshiba, Y., Kobayashi, S., and Nakayama, K.: Severe choledochocholangitis causing numerous cystlike hepatic abscesses, Int. Surg. **59:**180-182, 1974.

Cirrhosis

297 Adson, M. A., and Wychulis, A. R.: Portal hypertension in secondary biliary cirrhosis, Arch. Surg. (Chicago) **96:**604-612, 1968.

298 Ahrens, E. H., Payne, M. A., Kunkel, H. G., Eisenmenger, W. J., and Blondheim, S. H.: Primary biliary cirrhosis, Medicine (Balt.) **29:**299-364, 1950.

299 Alarcón-Segovia, D., Diaz-Jouanen, E., and Fishbein, E.: Features of Sjøgren's syndrome in primary biliary cirrhosis, Ann. Intern. Med. **79:**31-36, 1973.

300 Andrade, Z. A., and Cheever, A. W.: Alterations of the intrahepatic vasculature in hepatosplenic schistosomiasis mansoni, Am. J. Trop. Med. Hyg. **20:**425-432, 1971.

301 Ashkar, F. S., Miller, R., Smoak, W. M., III, and Gilson, A. J.: Liver disease in hyperthyroidism, South. Med. J. **64:**462-465, 1971.

302 Baggenstoss, A. H., Foulk, W. T., Butt, H. R., and Bahn, R. C.: Pathology of primary biliary cirrhosis, Am. J. Clin. Pathol. **42:**259-276, 1964.

303 Baker, A., Kaplan, M., and Wolfe, H.: Congenital congestive fibrosis of liver in myxedema ascites, Ann. Intern. Med. **77:**927-929, 1972.

304 Barry, M., and Sherlock, S.: Measurement of liver-iron concentration in needle-biopsy specimens, Lancet **1:**100-103, 1971.

305 Bartholomew, L. G., Cain, J. C., Winkelmann, R. K., and Baggenstoss, A. H.: Liver disease in scleroderma, Am. J. Dig. Dis. **9:**43-55, 1964.

306 Bean, W. B.: Vascular "spiders" and palmar erythema, Am. Heart J. **25:**463-477, 1943.

307 Bennett, H. S., Baggenstoss, A. H., and Butt, H. R.: Testis, breast, and prostate of men who die of cirrhosis of liver, Am. J. Clin. Pathol. **20:**814-828, 1950.

308 Berenyi, M. R., Straus, B., and Avila, L.: T rosettes in alcoholic cirrhosis of liver, J.A.M.A. **232:**44-46, 1975.

309 Berg, P. A., Doniach, D., and Roitt, I. M.: Mitochondrial antibodies in primary biliary cirrhosis, J. Exp. Med. **126:**277-290, 1967.

310 Berthelot, P., Walker, J. G., Sherlock, S., and Reid, L.: Arterial changes in lungs in cirrhosis of liver, New Eng. J. Med. **274:**291-298, 1966.

311 Bianchi, F. B., Penfold, P. L., and Roitt, I. M.: Mitochondrial antibodies in primary biliary cirrhosis. Ultrastructural localization of antigen to inner mitochondrial membrane using direct peroxidase conjugate, Br. J. Exp. Pathol. **54:**652-665, 1973.

312 Board for classification and nomenclature of cirrhois of liver, Fifth Pan-American Congress of Gastroenterology, La Habana, Cuba, Jan.

1956, Gastroenterology **31:**213-216, 1956 (report).

313 Bothwell, T. H., and Isaacson, C.: Siderosis in Bantus, Br. Med. J. **1:**522-524, 1962.

314 Bradford, W. D., Elchlepp, J. G., Arstila, A. U., Trump, B. F., and Kinney, T. D.: Iron metabolism and cell membrane, Am. J. Pathol. **56:**201-228, 1969.

315 Butt, E. M., Nusbaum, R. E., Gilmour, T. C., and DiDio, S. L.: Hemochromatosis and refractory anemia, Am. J. Clin. Pathol. **26:**225-242, 1956.

316 Butt, E. M., Nusbaum, R. E., Gilmour, T. C., and DiDio, S. L.: Trace metal pattern in disease states, Am. J. Clin. Pathol. **30:**479-497, 1958.

317 Calabresi, P., and Abelmann, W. H.: Portopulmonary anastomoses, J. Clin. Invest. **36:**1257-1265, 1957.

318 Charley, P., Rosenstein, M., Shore, E., Saltman, P.: Role of chelation and binding equilibria in iron metabolism, Arch. Biochem. Biophys. **88:**222-226, 1960.

319 Chedid, A., Spellberg, M. A., and DeBeer, R. A.: Ultrastructural aspects of primary biliary cirrhosis and other types of cholestatic liver disease, Gastroenterology **67:**858-869, 1974.

320 Cohen, S., Kaplan, M., Gottlieb, L., and Patterson, J.: Liver disease and gallstones in regional enteritis, Gastroenterology **60:**237-245, 1971.

321 Craig, J. R., Dunn, A. E. G., and Peters, R. L.: Cirrhosis associated with partial deficiency of α_1-antitrypsin—clinical and autopsy study, Hum. Pathol. **6:**113-120, 1975.

322 Davis, A. E., and Biggs, G. C.: Pancreas and iron absorption, Gut **6:**140-142, 1965.

323 Davis, P. S., Luke, C. G., and Deller, D. J.: Reduction of gastric iron-binding protein in hemochromatosis: a previously unrecognized metabolic defect, Lancet **2:**1431-1433, 1966.

324 Dobbins, W. O., III, Rollins, E. L., Brooks, S. G., and Fallon, H. J.: A quantitative morphologic analysis of ethanol effect upon rat liver, Gastroenterology **62:**1020-1033, 1972.

325 Doberneck, R. C., Nunn, D. B., Johnson, D. G., and Chun, B. K.: Iron metabolism and portacaval shunt in dogs, Arch. Surg. (Chicago) **87:**751-756, 1963.

326 Dunn, G. D., Hayes, P., Breen, K. J., and Schenker, S.: Liver in congestive heart failure—a review, Am. J. Med. Sci. **265:**174-189, 1973.

327 Eade, M. N.: Liver disease in ulcerative colitis. I. Analysis of operative liver biopsy in 138 consecutive patients having colectomy, Ann. Intern. Med. **72:**475-487, 1970.

328 Eade, M. N., Cooke, W. T., Brook, B. N., and Thompson, H.: Liver disease in Crohn's colitis. A study of 21 consecutive patients having colectomy, Ann. Intern. Med. **74:**518-528, 1971.

329 Edmondson, H. A.: Needle biopsy of the liver. In Schiff, L., editor: Diseases of the liver, ed. 4, Philadelphia, 1975, J. B. Lippincott Co.

330 Edmondson, H. A., Peters, R. L., Frankel, H. H., and Borowsky, S.: Early stage of liver injury in alcoholics, Medicine (Balt.) **46:**119-129, 1967.

331 Edmondson, H. A., Peters, R. L., Reynolds, T. B., and Kuzma, O. T.: Sclerosing hyaline necrosis, Ann. Intern. Med. **59:**646-673, 1963.

332 Eisenmenger, W. J.: Ascites in patients with cirrhosis, Ann. Intern. Med. **37:**261-272, 1952.

333 Eriksson, S., and Larsson, C.: Purification and partial characterization of PAS-positive inclusion bodies from liver in α_1-antitrypsin deficiency, New Eng. J. Med. **292:**176-180, 1975.

334 Evans, G. W., Dubois, R. S., and Hambidge, K. M.: Wilson's disease—identification of an abnormal copper-binding protein, Science **181:**1175-1176, 1973.

335 Fleming, C. R., Dickson, E. R., Baggenstoss, A. H., and McCall, J. T.: Copper and primary biliary cirrhosis, Gastroenterology **65:**93, 1973.

336 Fox, R. A., Dudley, F. J., Samuels, M., Milligen, J., and Sherlock, S.: Lymphocyte transformation in response to phytohemagglutination in primary biliary cirrhosis—search for plasma inhibitory factor, Gut **14:**89-93, 1973.

337 Frommer, D. J.: Defective biliary excretion of copper in Wilson's disease, Gut **15:**125-129, 1974.

338 Ganrot, P. O., Laurell, C. H., Eriksson, S.: Obstructive lung disease and trypsin inhibitors in α_1-antitrypsin deficiency, Scand. J. Clin. Invest. **19:**205-208, 1967.

339 Glenn, F.: Indications for operation in biliary tract disease among elderly, Geriatrics **24:**98-103, 1969.

340 Goldfischer, S., and Sternlieb, I.: Changes in distribution of hepatic copper in relation to progression of Wilson's disease, Am. J. Pathol. **53:**883-901, 1968.

341 Grace, N. D., and Powell, L. W.: Iron-storage disorders of the liver, Gastroenterology **67:**1257-1283, 1974.

342 Grace, N. D., and Balint, J. A.: Hemochromatosis associated with end-to-end portacaval anastomosis, Am. J. Dig. Dis. **11:**351-358, 1966.

343 Grahn, E. P., Dietz, A. A., Stefani, S. S., and Donnelly, W. J.: Burr cells, hemolytic anemia, and cirrhosis, Am. J. Med. **45:**78-87, 1968.

344 Guynn, R. W., Veloso, D., Harris, R. L., Lawson, J. W. R., and Veech, R. L.: Ethanol administration and relationship of malonyl coenzyme A concentrations to the rate of fatty acid synthesis in rat liver, Biochem. J. **136:**639-647, 1973.

345 Hales, M. R., Allan, J. S., and Hall, E. M.: Injection corrosion studies of normal and cirrhotic livers, Am. J. Pathol. **35:**909-941, 1959.

346 Hamamoto, K., Tauxe, W. N., Novak, L. P., and Goldstein, N. P.: Use of whole-body counter to study body retention of radiocopper in Wilson's disease, J. Lab. Clin. Med. **72:**754-759, 1968.

347 Herbert, V.: Hematopoietic factors in liver diseases, Progr. Liver Dis. **2:**57-68, 1965.

348 Hidayat, M. A., and Wahid, H. A.: A study of vascular changes in bilharzic hepatic fibrosis and their significance, Surg. Gynecol. Obstet. **132:**997-1004, 1971.

349 Hoenig, V., Brodanova, M. R., and Kordac, V.: Effect of ethanol on iron tolerance, Scand. J. Gastroenterol. **3:**334-338, 1968.

350 Hultman, E.: Metabolism of alcohol, Acta Anaesthesiol. Scand. 55 (suppl.):58-65, 1974.

351 Ishak, K. G., Jenis, E. H., Marshall, M. L., Bolton, B. H., and Battistome, G. C.: Cirrhosis of liver associated with α_1-antitrypin deficiency, Arch. Pathol. 94:445-455, 1972.

352 Jeppsson, J.-O., Larsson, C., and Eriksson, S.: Characterization of α_1-antitrypsin in inclusion bodies from liver in α_1-antitrypsin deficiency, New Eng. J. Med. 293:576-579, 1975.

353 Jolliffe, N., and Jellinek, E. M.: Alcoholic cirrhosis, Q. J. Stud. Alcohol 2:544-583, 1941.

354 Jones, W. A., Rao, D. R. G., and Braunstein, H.: Renal glomerulus in cirrhosis of liver, Am. J. Pathol. 39:393-404, 1961.

355 Kallai, L.: Liver changes in rheumatoid arthritis, Rheumatism 20:20-26, 1964.

356 Kelty, R. H., Baggenstoss, A. H., and Butt, H. R.: Portal hypertension, Gastroenterology 15:285-295, 1950.

357 Kent, G., and Popper, H.: Secondary hemochromatosis and its association with anemia, Arch. Pathol. (Chicago) 70:623-639, 1960.

358 Kent, G., and Popper, H.: Editorial: liver biopsy in diagnosis of hemochromatosis, Am. J. Med. 44:837-841, 1968.

359 Klatskin, G.: Alcoholic cirrhosis, J.A.M.A. 170:1671-1676, 1959.

360 Klatskin, G.: Hepatitis associated with systemic infections. In Schiff, L., editor: Diseases of the liver, ed. 3, Philadelphia, 1969, J. B. Lippincott Co.

361 Klatskin, G., and Kantor, F. S.: Mitochondrial antibody in primary biliary cirrhosis and other diseases, Ann. Intern. Med. 77:533-541, 1972.

362 Krebs, H. A., and Perkins, J. R.: The physiologic role of liver alcohol dehydrogenase, Biochem. J. 118:635-644, 1970.

363 Kueppers, F.: α_1-Antitrypsin—physiology, genetics, and pathology, Humangenetik 11:177-189, 1971.

364 LaMont, J. T., and Isselbacher, K. J.: Postoperative jaundice, New Eng. J. Med. 288:305-307, 1973.

365 Laurell, C. B., and Eriksson, S.: Electrophoretic α_1-globulin pattern of serum in α_1-antitrypsin deficiency, Scand. J. Clin. Lab. Invest. 15:132-140, 1963.

366 Levi, A. J., Sherlock, S., Scheuer, P. J., and Cumings, J. N.: Presymptomatic Wilson's disease, Lancet 2:575-579, 1967.

367 Levine, R. A., Briggs, G. W., and Lowell, D. M.: Chronic chlorpromazine cholangiolitis hepatitis, Gastroenterology 50:665-670, 1966.

368 Lieber, C. S.: Hepatic and metabolic effects of alcohol (1966-1973), Gastroenterology 65:821-846, 1973.

369 Lieber, C. S., and deCarli, L. M.: Hepatic microsomal ethanol-oxidizing system—in vitro characteristics and adaptive properties in vivo, J. Biol. Chem. 245:2505-2512, 1970.

370 Lieberman, F. L., Ito, S., and Reynolds, T. B.: Effective plasma volume in sclerosis of ascites, J. Clin. Invest. 48:975-981, 1969.

371 Liebowitz, H. R.: Pathogenesis of ascites in cirrhosis of liver, N.Y. J. Med. 69:2012-2014, 1969.

372 Lisboa, P. E.: Experimental hepatic cirrhosis in dogs caused by chronic massive iron overload, Gut 12:363-368, 1971.

373 Lundquist, F., Tygstrup, N., Winkler, K., Mellemgaard, K., and Munck-Petersen, S.: Ethanol metabolism and production of free acetate in the human liver, J. Clin. Invest. 41:955-961, 1962.

374 MacDonald, R. N.: Wine as source of iron in hemochromatosis, Nature (London) 199:922, 1963.

375 MacSween, R. N. M.: Mallory's ("alcoholic") hyaline in primary biliary cirrhosis, J. Clin. Pathol. 26:340-342, 1973.

376 MacSween, R. N. M., Galbraith, I., Thomas, M. A., Watkinson, G., and Ludlam, G. B.: Phytohaemagglutinin (PHA)–induced lymphocyte transformation and Toxoplasma gondii antibody studies in PBC, Clin. Exp. Immunol. 15:35-42, 1973.

377 McDermott, W. V., Jr.: Surgery of the liver and portal circulation, Philadelphia, 1974, Lea & Febiger, pp. 117-123.

378 Madding, G. F., and Kennedy, P. A.: Trauma to the liver, ed. 2, Philadelphia, 1971, W. B. Saunders Co.

379 Maderazo, E. G., Ward, P. A., and Quintiliani, R.: Defective regulation of chemotaxis in cirrhosis, J. Lab. Clin. Med. 85:621-630, 1975.

380 Mendel, G. A.: Studies on iron absorption. III. Increased iron absorption during liver regeneration induced by partial hepatectomy, J. Lab. Clin. Med. 66:627-640, 1965.

381 Merritt, A. D., and Fetter, B. F.: Toxic hepatic necrosis (hepatitis) due to isoniazid: report of a case with cirrhosis and death due to hemorrhage from esophageal varices, Ann. Intern. Med. 50:804-810, 1959.

382 Mikkelsen, W. P., Edmondson, H. A., Peters, R. L., Redeker, A. G., and Reynolds, T. B.: Hepatoportal sclerosis, Ann. Surg. 162:602-620, 1965.

383 Mikkelsen, W. P., Turrill, F. L., and Pattison, A. C.: Portacaval shunt in cirrhosis of liver, Am. J. Surg. 104:204-215, 1962.

384 Mistilis, S. P.: Diseases of liver associated with ulcerative colitis. In Schiff, L., editor: Diseases of the liver, ed. 4, Philadelphia, 1975, J. B. Lippincott Co.

385 Monroe, S., French, S. W., and Zambone, L.: Mallory bodies in case of primary biliary cirrhosis, Am. J. Clin. Pathol. 59:254-262, 1973.

386 Mullane, J. F., and Gliedman, M. L.: Elevation of pressure in inferior vena cava, Surgery 59:1135-1146, 1966.

387 Nelson, R. S., and Sears, M. E.: Massive sarcoidosis of liver, Am. J. Dig. Dis. 13:95-106, 1968.

388 Okamura, K., Harwood, T. R., and Yokoo, H.: Isolation and electrophoretic study on Mallory bodies from the livers of alcoholic cirrhosis, Lab. Invest. 33:193-199, 1975.

389 Oliver, R. A. M.: Siderosis after transfusions of blood, J. Pathol. Bacteriol. 77:171-194, 1959.

390 Olling, S., and Olsson, R.: Congenital absence of portal venous system in a 50-year-old woman, Acta Med. Scand. 196:343-345, 1974.

391 Orloff, M. J., Ross, T. H., Baddeley, R. M., Nutting, R. O., Spitz, B. R., Sloop, R. D.,

Neesby, T., and Halasz, N. A.: Experimental ascites, Surgery **56:**83-98, 1964.

392 Palmer, E. D.: Management of esophageal varices, Progr. Liver Dis. **1:**329-337, 1961.

393 Papper, S.: Role of kidney in Laennec's cirrhosis, Medicine (Balt.) **37:**299-316, 1958.

394 Patek, A. J., Jr.: In Schiff, L., editor: Diseases of the liver, ed. 3, Philadelphia, 1969, J. B. Lippincott Co. (portal cirrhosis—Laennec's cirrhosis).

395 Peters, R. L., Gay, T., and Reynolds, T. B.: Postjejunal bypass hepatic disease—its similarity to alcoholic hepatic disease, Am. J. Clin. Pathol. **63:**318-331, 1975.

396 Peters, R. L., Redeker, A. G., Starzl, T., and Putnam, C. W.: α₁-Antitrypsin production by transplanted liver in patient, Gastroenterology **69:**A-52/852, 1975.

397 Powell, L. W.: Iron storage in relatives of patients with haemochromatosis and in relatives of patients with alcoholic cirrhosis, Q. J. Med. **34:**427-442, 1968.

398 Powell, L. W., Alpert, E., and Isselbacher, K. J.: Abnormality in tissue isoferritin distribution in idiopathic haemochromatosis, Nature **250:** 333-335, 1974.

399 Powell, L. W., Mortimer, R., and Harris, O. D.: Cirrhosis of the liver—a comparative study of four major aetiological groups, Med. J. Aust. **1:**941-950, 1971.

400 Prieto, J., Barry, M., and Sherlock, S.: Serum ferritin in patients with iron overload and with acute and chronic liver diseases, Gastroenterology **68:**525-533, 1975.

401 Rasmussen, R. W., and McGill, D. B.: Fat embolism and postoperative jaundice—case report, J.A.M.A. **233:**271-272, 1975.

402 Ratnoff, O. D.: Hemostatic mechanisms in liver disease, Med. Clin. N. Am. **47:**721-736, 1963.

403 Reppart, J. T., Peters, R. L., Edmondson, H. A., and Baker, R. F.: Electron and light microscopy of sclerosing hyaline necrosis, Lab. Invest. **12:**1138-1161, 1963.

404 Reynolds, T. B.: Editorial: Jaundice: medical or surgical? Ann. Intern. Med. **83:**114-115, 1975.

405 Reynolds, T. B.: Portal hypertension. In Schiff, L., editor: Diseases of the liver, ed. 4, Philadelphia, 1975, J. B. Lippincott Co.

406 Reynolds, T. B., Denison, E. K., Frankl, H. D., Lieberman, F. L., and Peters, R. L.: Primary biliary cirrhosis with scleroderma, Raynaud's phenomenon, and telangiectasia, Am. J. Med. **50:**302-312, 1971.

407 Reynolds, T. B., Hidemura, R., Michel, H., and Peters, R.: Portal hypertension without cirrhosis in alcoholic liver disease, Ann. Intern. Med. **70:**497-506, 1969.

408 Reynolds, T. B., Redeker, A. G., and Geller, H. M.: Wedged hepatic pressure, Am. J. Med. **22:**341-350, 1957.

409 Risdon, R. A., Barry, M., and Flynn, D. M.: Transfusional overload: the relationship between tissue iron concentration and hepatic fibrosis in thalassemia, J. Pathol. **116:**83-95, 1975.

410 Rolleston, H. D.: Diseases of the liver, gallbladder, and bile ducts, Philadelphia, 1905, W. B. Saunders Co.

411 Ross, C. E., Muir, W. A., Ng, A. B. P., Graham, R. C., Jr., and Kellermeyer, R. W.: Hemochromatosis: pathophysiologic and genetic considerations, Am. J. Clin. Pathol. **63:** 179-191, 1975.

412 Rubin, E., Kros, S., and Popper, H.: Pathogenesis of postnecrotic cirrhosis in alcoholics, Arch. Pathol. **73:**288-299, 1962.

413 Rubin, E., and Lieber, C. S.: Alcohol-induced hepatic injury in nonalcoholic volunteers, New Eng. J. Med. **278:**869-876, 1968.

414 Rubin, E., and Lieber, C. S.: Fatty liver, alcoholic hepatitis, and cirrhosis produced by alcohol in primates, New Eng. J. Med. **290:** 128-135, 1974.

415 Sedgwick, P. E., and Pultzan, A.: Portal hypertension, Boston, 1967, Little, Brown & Co.

416 Sharp, H. L., Freier, E., and Bridges, R.: α₁-Globulin deficiency in familial infantile liver disease, Pediatr. Res. **2:**298, 1968.

417 Sherlock, S.: Portal hypertension, Progr. Liver Dis. **1:**145-161, 1961.

418 Sherlock, S.: Liver in circulatory failure. In Schiff, L., editor: Diseases of the liver, ed. 4, Philadelphia, 1975, J. B. Lippincott Co.

419 Sherlock, S., and Scheuer, P. J.: Presentation and diagnosis of 100 patients with primary biliary cirrhosis, New Eng. J. Med. **289:**674-678, 1973.

420 Shorter, R. G., and Baggenstoss, A. H.: Biliary cirrhosis, Am. J. Clin. Pathol. **32:**10-17, 1959.

421 Silber, R., Amorosi, E., Lhowe, J., and Kayden, H. J.: Spur-shaped erythrocytes in Laennec's cirrhosis, New Eng. J. Med. **275:**639-643, 1966.

422 Song, Y. S.: Hepatic lesions in sickle-cell anemia, Am. J. Pathol. **33:**331-351, 1957.

423 Stanley, N. N., Fox, R. A., Whimster, W. F., Sherlock, S., and James, D. G.: Primary biliary cirrhosis or sarcoidosis, or both, New Eng. J. Med. **287:**1282-1284, 1972.

424 Sternlieb, I.: Mitochondrial and fatty changes, Gasroenterology **55:**354-367, 1968.

425 Sternlieb, I., and Scheinberg, I. H.: Chronic hepatitis as a first manifestation of Wilson's disease, Ann. Intern. Med. **76:**59-64, 1972.

426 Sternlieb, I., van den Hamer, C. J. A., Morell, A. G., Alpert, S., Gregoriadis, G., and Scheinberg, I. H.: Lysosomal defect of hepatic copper excretion in Wilson's disease (hepatolenticular degeneration), Gastroenterology **64:**99-105, 1973.

427 Strickland, G. T., Frommer, D., Leu, M.-L., Pollard, R., Sherlock, S., and Cumings, J. N.: Wilson's disease in United Kingdom and Taiwan—general characteristics of 142 cases and prognosis and genetic analysis of 88 cases, Q. J. Med. **42:**619-638, 1973.

428 Symmers, D., and Spain, D. M.: Hepar lobatum, Arch. Pathol. (Chicago) **42:**64-68, 1946.

429 Tauxe, W. N., Goldstein, N. P., Randall, R. V., and Gross, J. B.: Radiocopper studies in patients with Wilson's disease and their relatives, Am. J. Med. **41:**375-380, 1966.

430 Terris, M. L.: Epidemiology of cirrhosis of liver, Am. J. Public Health **57:**2076-2088, 1967.

431 Theron, J. J., Hawtrey, A. O., Liebenberg, N.,

and Schirren, V.: Experimental dietary siderosis, Am. J. Pathol. 43:73-91, 1963.

432 Van Thiel, D. H., Lester, R., and Sherins, R.
J.: Hypogonadism in alcoholic liver disease:
evidence for a double defect, Gastroenterology
67:1188-1199, 1974.

433 Visfeldt, J., and Poulsen, H.: Histopathology
of liver and liver tumors in thorium dioxide
patients, Acta Pathol. Scand. 80 (sect. A):97-
108, 1972.

434 Walshe, J. M.: In Schiff, L., editor: Diseases
of the liver, ed. 4, Philadelphia, 1975, J. B.
Lippincott Co. (liver in hepatolenticular degeneration).

435 Waren, K. S.: Hepatosplenic schistosomiasis
mansoni: an immunologic disease, Bull. N.Y.
Acad. Med. 51:545-550, 1975.

436 Wasastjerna, C., Reissell, P., Karjalainen, J.,
and Ekelund, P.: Fatty liver in diabetes. A
cytological study, Acta Med. Scand. 191:225-
228, 1972.

437 Webb, J., Whaley, K., MacSween, R. N. M.,
Nuki, G., Dick, W. C., and Buchanan, W. W.:
Liver disease in rheumatoid arthritis and
Sjögren's syndrome—prospective study using
biochemical and serologic markers of hepatic
dysfunction, Ann. Rheum. Dis. 34:70-81, 1975.

438 Wybran, J., Govaerts, A., and Fudenberg, H.
H.: Editorial: electrocardiographic monitoring
—bad news and good news, J.A.M.A. 232:57-
58, 1975.

Disease in infants and children

439 Aagenaes, Ø.: Hereditary recurrent cholestasis
with lymphedema—two new families, Acta
Paediatr. Scand. 63:465-471, 1974.

440 Aagenaes, Ø., Matlary, A., Elgjo, K., Munthe,
E., and Fagerhol, M. D.: Neonatal cholestasis
in α₁-antitrypsin deficient children—clinical,
genetic, histologic, and immunohistochemical,
Acta Paediatr. Scand. 61:632-642, 1972.

441 Aikat, B. K., Bhattacharya, T., and Walia, B.
N. S.: Morphological features of Indian childhood cirrhosis: the spectrum of changes and
their significance, Indian J. Med. Res. 62:953-
963, 1974.

442 Alagille, D.: Clinical aspects of neonatal hepatitis, Am. J. Dis. Child. 123:287-291, 1972.

443 Alpert, L. I., Strauss, L., and Hirschhorn, K.:
Neonatal hepatitis and biliary atresia associated
with trisomy 17-18 syndrome, New Eng. J.
Med. 280:16-20, 1969.

444 Bach, G., Friedman, R., Weissmann, B., and
Neufeld, E. F.: Defect in the Hurler and
Scheie syndromes: deficiency of α-L-iduronidase, Proc. Natl. Acad. Sci. 69:2048-2051,
1972.

445 Becker, W. B., Kipps, A., and McKenzie, D.:
Disseminated herpes simplex virus infection,
Am. J. Dis. Child. 115:1-8, 1968.

446 Beutler, E., Baluda, M. C., Sturgeon, P., and
Day, R. W.: Genetics of galactose-1-phosphate
uridyl transferase deficiency, J. Lab. Clin.
Med. 68:646-658, 1966.

447 Bourgeois, C., Olson, L., Comer, D., Evans,
H., Keschamras, N., Cotton, R., Grossman, R.,
and Smith, T.: Encephalopathy and fatty degeneration of the viscera: a clinicopathologic

analysis of 40 cases, Am. J. Clin. Pathol. 56:
558-571, 1971.

448 Bras, G., Jelliffe, D. B., and Stuart, K. L.:
Veno-occlusive disease of liver, Arch. Pathol.
(Chicago) 57:285-300, 1954.

449 Brough, A. J., and Bernstein, J.: Conjugated
hyperbilirubinemia in early infancy: reassess-
ment of liver biopsy, Hum. Pathol. 5:507-516,
1974.

450 Burke, J. A., Blair, J. D., and Kiesel, J. L.:
α₁-Antitrypsin deficiency and childhood liver
disease, Gastroenterology 66:669, 1974 (abstract).

451 Campbell, D. P., Poley, J. R., Alaupovic, P.,
and Smith, E. I.: Differential diagnosis of
neonatal hepatitis and biliary atresia, J.
Pediatr. Surg. 9:699-705, 1974.

452 Craig, J. M., Gellis, S. S., and Hsia, D. Y.-Y.:
Cirrhosis of liver in infants and children, Am.
J. Dis. Child. 90:299-322, 1955.

453 Donnell, G. N.: Pitfalls in diagnosis of galactosemia, J. Pediatr. 83:515-516, 1973.

454 Dorfman, A., and Matalon, R.: Metabolic basis
of inherited diseases. In Stanbury, J. B.,
Wyngaarden, J. B., and Fredrickson, D. S.,
editors: The mucopolysaccharidoses, ed. 3, New
York, 1972, McGraw-Hill Book Co.

455 Editorial: Phenobarbital halts rise in bilirubin,
J.A.M.A. 209:855, 1969.

456 Esterly, J. R., Slusser, R. J., and Ruebner,
B. H.: Hepatic lesions in congenital rubella
syndrome, J. Pediatr. 71:676-685, 1967.

457 Edmondson, H. A.: In Proceedings of the
Thirty-third Seminar of American Society of
Clinical Pathologists, Chicago, 1968, American
Society of Clinical Pathologists (galactosemia).

458 Feigelson, J., Pecau, Y., and Perez, J.: Liver
scanning and liver function in cystic fibrosis,
Acta Paediatr. Scand. 61:337-342, 1972.

459 Gentz, J., Jagenburg, R., and Zetterström, R.:
Tyrosinemia, J. Pediatr. 66:670-696, 1965.

460 Golden, B., Bell, W. E., and McKee, A. P.:
Disseminated herpes simplex with encephalitis
in a neonate, J.A.M.A. 209:1219-1221, 1969.

461 Grases, P. J., and Beker, S.: Veno-occlusive
disease of liver—case from Venezuela, Am. J.
Med. 53:511-516, 1972.

462 Grenier, A., and Laberge, C.: Rapid method
for screening for galactosemia and galacto-
kinase deficiency by measuring galactose in
whole blood spotted on paper, Clin. Chem. 19:
463-465, 1973.

462a Hadchovel, M., and Gautier, M.: Histopathologic study of the liver in the cholestatic phase
of alpha-1-antitrypsin deficiency, J. Pediatr.
89:211-215, 1976.

463 Halvorsen, S., Pande, H., Løken, A. C., and
Gjessing, L. R.: Tyrosinosis, Arch. Dis. Child.
41:238-249, 1966.

464 Harries, J. T., Seakins, J. W. T., Ersser, R. S.,
and Lloyd, J. K.: Recovery after dietary treatment of infant with features of tyrosinosis,
Arch. Dis. Child. 44:258-267, 1969.

465 Hashem, M.: Etiology and pathology of types
of liver cirrhosis in Egyptian children, J.
Egypt. Med. Assoc. 22:319-354, 1939.

466 Hill, H. Z., and Puck, T. T.: Detection of inborn errors of metabolism: galactosemia, Science 179:1136-1139, 1973.

467 Hochberg, F. H., Nelson, K., and Janzen, W.: Influenza type B–related encephalopathy. The 1971 outbreak of Reye syndrome in Chicago, J.A.M.A. **231**:817-821, 1975.

468 Horiguchi, T., and Bauer, C.: Ethnic differences in neonatal jaundice: comparison of Japanese and Caucasian newborn infants, Am. J. Obstet. Gynecol. **121**:71-74, 1975.

469 Hug, G., Garancis, J. C., Schubert, W. K., and Kaplan, S.: Glycogen-storage disease, Am. J. Dis. Child. **111**:457-474, 1966.

470 Hughes, J. R., Wilfert, C. M., Moore, M., Benirschke, K., and Hoyos-Guevara, E. de: Echovirus 14 infection associated with fatal neonatal hepatic necrosis, Am. J. Dis. Child. **123**:61-67, 1972.

471 Jagenburg, R. Lindblad, B., de Maré, J. M., and Rödjer, S.: Hereditary tyrosinemia: metabolic studies in a patient with partial p-hydroxyphenylpyruvate hydroxylase activity, J. Pediatr. **80**:994-1004, 1972.

472 Jevtic, M. M., Thorp, F. K., and Hruban, Z.: Hereditary tyrosinemia with hyperplasia and hypertrophy of juxtaglomerular apparatus, Am. J. Clin. Pathol. **61**:423-437, 1974.

473 Johnson, J. D.: Current concepts: neonatal nonhemolytic jaundice, New Eng. J. Med. **292**:194-197, 1975.

474 Jorgensen, M.: Stereological study of intrahepatic bile ducts. 4. Congenital hepatic fibrosis, Acta Pathol. Microbiol. Scand. **82**(sect. A):21-29, 1974.

475 Kerr, D. N. S., Harrison, C. V., Sherlock, S., and Walker, R. M.: Congenital hepatic fibrosis, Q. J. Med. **30**:91-117, 1961.

476 Kibrick, S., and Benirschke, K.: Severe generalized disease in newborn infant due to infection with coxsackievirus, group B, Pediatrics **22**:857-874, 1958.

477 Lester, R., and Troxler, R. F.: New light on neonatal jaundice, New Eng. J. Med. **280**:779-780, 1969.

478 Levi, A. J., Gatmaitan, Z., and Arias, I. M.: Deficiency of hepatic organic anion–binding protein, impaired organic anion uptake by liver, and "physiologic" jaundice in newborn monkeys, New Eng. J. Med. **283**:1136-1139, 1970.

479 Lindemann, R., Gjessing, L. R., Merton, B., Löken, A. C., and Halvorsen, S.: Amino acid metabolism in hereditary fructosemia, Acta Pediatr. Scand. **59**:141-147, 1970.

480 Linnemann, C. C., Jr., Sea, L., Partin, J. C., Schubert, W. R., and Schiff, G. M.: Reye's syndrome: epidemiologic and viral studies, 1963-1974, Am. J. Epidemiol. **101**:517-526, 1975.

481 Lynch, M. J., Glasgow, J. F., Hercz, A., Levinson, H., and Sass-Kortsak, A.: Pathology of α_1-antitrypsin deficiency in children: a study of 10 cases; occurrence of both liver and lung disease in two siblings, Am. J. Pathol. **66**:20a-21a (abstract), 1972.

482 McAdams, A. J., Hug, G., and Bove, K. E.: Glycogen-storage disease, types I to X: criteria for morphologic diagnosis, Hum. Pathol. **5**:463-487, 1974.

483 McKenzie, D., Hansen, J. D. L., and Becker, W.: Herpes simplex virus infection, Arch. Dis. Child. **34**:250-256, 1959.

484 Murray-Lyon, I. M., Ockenden, B. G., and Williams, R.: Congenital hepatic fibrosis—is it a single clinical entity? Gastroenterology **64**:653-656, 1973.

485 Okuyama, K.: Primary liver cell carcinoma associated with the biliary cirrhosis due to congenital bile duct atresia; first report of case, J. Pediatr. **67**:89-93, 1965.

486 Pagliara, A. S., Karl, I. E., Haymond, M., and Kipnis, D. M.: Hypoglycemia in infancy and childhood, J. Pediatr. **82**:365-379, 558-577, 1973. Part I.

487 Patrizi, G., Middelkamp, J. N., and Reed, C. A.: Fine structure of herpes simplex hepatoadrenal necrosis in newborn, Am. J. Clin. Pathol. **49**:325-341, 1969.

488 Petrelli, M., and Blair, J. D.: Liver in GM₁ gangliosidosis types 1 and 2—light and electron microscopical study, Arch. Pathol. **99**:111-116, 1975.

489 Phillips, M. J., Little, J. A., and Ptak, T. W.: Subcellular pathology of hereditary fructose intolerance, Am. J. Med. **44**:910-921, 1968.

490 Porter, C. A., Mowat, A. P., Cook, P. J., Haynes, D. W. G., Shilkin, K. B., and Williams, R.: α_1-Antitrypsin deficiency in neonatal hepatitis, Br. Med. J. **3**:435-439, 1972.

491 Ramboer, C., Thompson, R. P. H., and Williams, R.: Controlled trials of phenobarbitone in neonatal jaundice, Lancet **1**:966-968, 1969.

492 Ruebner, B. H., Bhagavan, B. S., Greenfield, A. J., Campbell, P., and Danks, D. M.: Neonatal necrosis, Pediatrics **43**:963-970, 1969.

493 Ruebner, B. H., and Miyai, K.: Neonatal hepatitis and biliary atresia; hemopoiesis and hemosiderin deposition, Ann. N.Y. Acad. Sci. **111**:375-391, 1963.

494 Satran, L., Sharp, H. L., Schenken, J. R., and Krivit, W.: Fatal neonatal hepatic steatosis, J. Pediatr. **75**:39-46, 1969.

495 Saxoni, F., Lapatsanis, P., and Pontelakis, S. N.: Congenital syphilis, Clin. Pediatr. (Phila.) **6**:687-691, 1967.

496 Selzer, G., and Parker, R. G. F.: *Senecio* poisoning, Am. J. Pathol. **27**:885-907, 1951.

497 Smetana, H. F., Edlow, J. B., and Glunz, P. R.: Neonatal jaundice, Arch. Pathol. (Chicago) **80**:553-574, 1965.

498 Smith, H. L., Amick, L. D., and Sidbury, J. B., Jr.: Type II glycogenosis, Am. J. Dis. Child. **111**:475-481, 1966.

499 Starzl, T. E., Porter, K. A., Brettschneider, L., Penn, I., Bell, P., Purnam, C. W., and McGuire, R. L.: Orthotopic transplantation of human liver, Surg. Gynecol. Obstet. **128**:327-339, 1969.

500 Stirling, G. A., Bras, G., and Urquhart, A. E.: Early lesion in veno-occlusive disease of liver, Arch. Dis. Child. **37**:535-538, 1962.

501 Strauss, L., and Bernstein, J.: Neonatal hepatitis in congenital rubella, Arch. Pathol. (Chicago) **86**:317-327, 1968.

502 Thaler, M. M.: Fatal neonatal cirrhosis, Pediatrics **33**:721-734, 1964.

503 Thaler, M. M., and Gellis, S. S.: Progression and regression of cirrhosis in biliary atresia, Am. J. Dis. Child. **116**:271-279, 1968.

504 Thaler, M. M., and Gellis, S. S.: Studies in neonatal hepatitis and biliary atresia, Am. J. Dis. Child. **116**:280-284, 1968.

505 Thaler, M. M., Ogata, E. S., Goodman, J. R., Piel, C. F., and Korobkin, M. T.: Congenital fibrosis and polycystic disease of liver and kidneys, Am. J. Dis. Child. **126**:374-380, 1973.

506 Tolstrup, N.: Clinical and biochemical aspects of galactosemia, Scand. J. Clin. Lab. Invest. **18**(suppl. 92):148-155, 1966.

507 Trauner, D. A., Nyhan, W. L., and Sweetman, L.: Short-chain organic acidemia and Reye's syndrome, Neurology **25**:296-298, 1975.

508 Valman, H. B., France, N. E., and Wallis, P. G.: Prolonged neonatal jaundice in cystic fibrosis, Arch. Dis. Child. **46**:805-809, 1971.

509 Wills, E. J.: Electron microscopy of the liver in infectious mononucleosis/cytomegalovirus hepatitis, Am. J. Dis. Child. **123**:301-303, 1972.

510 Wright, D. J. M., and Berry, C. L.: Liver involvement in congenital syphilis, Br. J. Vener. Dis. **50**:241, 1974.

511 Zuelzer, W. W., and Brough, A. J.: Liver disease in infancy and childhood. In Schiff, L., editor: Diseases of the liver, ed. 3, Philadelphia, 1969, J. B. Lippincott Co.

Disease in pregnancy

512 Baird, J., and Hawley, R.: Spontaneous rupture of the liver during pregnancy, J. Reproductive Med. **6**:198, 1971.

513 Block, R. A.: Pregnancy in portal cirrhosis, J. Reproductive Med. **8**:143-145, 1972.

514 Breen, K. J., Perkins, K. W., Schenker, S., Dunkerly, R. C., and Moore, H. C.: Uncomplicated subsequent pregnancy after idiopathic fatty liver of pregnancy, Obstet. Gynecol. **40**:813-815, 1972.

515 Browne, C. H., Hanson, G. C., DeJode, L. R., and Roberts, P. A.: Rupture of subcapsular haematoma of liver in a case of eclampsia, Br. J. Surg. **62**:237-238, 1975.

516 Cano, R. I., Delman, M. R., Pitchumoni, C. S., Lev, R., and Rosenthal, W. S.: Acute fatty liver of pregnancy; complication by disseminated intravascular coagulation, J.A.M.A. **231**:159-161, 1975.

517 Crawford, G., Cope, I., and Christie, A.: Liver failure in late pregnancy, Med. J. Aust. **2**:49-55, 1960.

518 Dalén, E., and Westerholm, B.: Occurrence of hepatic impairment in women jaundiced by oral contraceptives and in their mothers and sisters, Acta Med. Scand. **195**:459-463, 1974.

519 Davidson, C. S.: Hepatic disease and pregnancy, J. Reproductive Med. **10**:107-110, 1973.

520 Frederick, W. C., Howard, R. G., and Spatola, S.: Spontaneous rupture of the liver in patient using contraceptive pills, Arch. Surg. **108**:93-95, 1974.

521 Geall, M. G., and Webb, M. J.: Liver disease in pregnancy, symposium on medical gynecology, Med. Clin. North Am. **58**:817-822, 1974.

522 Kunelis, C. T., Peters, R. L., and Edmondson, H. A.: Fatty liver of pregnancy and its relationship to tetracycline therapy, Am. J. Med. **38**:359-377, 1965.

523 Mistilis, A. P.: Liver disease in pregnancy, Aust. Ann. Med. **17**:248-260, 1968.

524 Mokotoff, R., Weiss, L. S., Brandon, L. H., and Camillo, M. F.: Liver rupture complicating toxemia of pregnancy, Arch. Intern. Med. (Chicago) **119**:375-380, 1967.

525 Sheehan, H. L.: Yellow atrophy; chloroform poisoning, J. Obstet. Gynaecol. Brit. Emp. **47**:49-62, 1940.

Diseases of intrahepatic bile ducts

526 Ball, T. J., Mutchnik, M. G., Cohen, G. M., and Burrell, M.: Hemobilia following percutaneous liver biopsy, Gastroenterology **68**:1297-1299, 1975.

527 Gallagher, P. J., Millis, R. R., and Mitchinson, M. J.: Congenital dilatation of the intrahepatic bile ducts with cholangiocarcinoma, J. Clin. Pathol. **25**:804-808, 1972.

528 Hunter, F. M., Akdamar, K., Sparks, R. D., Reed, R. J., and Brown, C. L., Jr.: Congenital dilation of the intrahepatic bile ducts, Am. J. Med. **40**:188-194, 1966.

529 Katz, M. C., and Meng, C.-H.: Angiographic evaluation of traumatic intrahepatic pseudoaneurysm and hemobilia, Radiology **94**:95-99, 1970.

530 McSherry, C. K., Stubenbord, W. T., and Glenn, F.: Significance of air in biliary system and liver, Surg. Gynecol. Obstet. **128**:49-61, 1969.

531 Markoff, N.: Primary sclerosing cholangitis, Acta Hepato-Gastroenterol. **20**:77-82, 1973.

532 Mage, S., and Morel, A. S.: Surgical experience with cholangiohepatitis, Ann. Surg. **162**:187-190, 1965.

533 Mistilis, S. P.: Pericholangitis and ulcerative colitis, Ann. Intern. Med. **63**:1-16, 1965.

534 Sandblom, P.: Hemobilia: history, pathology, diagnosis, treatment, Springfield, Ill., 1972, Charles C Thomas, Publisher (biliary tract hemorrhage).

535 Thorpe, M. E. C., Scheuer, P. J., and Sherlock, S.: Primary sclerosing cholangitis, Gut **8**:435-448, 1967.

536 Thompson, B. W., and Read, R. C.: Sclerosing cholangitis and other intra-abdominal fibroses, Am. J. Surg. **128**:777-781, 1974.

Regeneration; transplantation

537 Bengmark, S., Engevik, L., and Rosengren, K.: Angiography of regenerating human liver after extensive resection, Surgery **65**:590-596, 1969.

538 Editorial: Liver transplantation, Lancet **2**:29, 1974.

539 Fennell, Robert H., Jr.: Personal communication (transplantation, liver), 1974.

540 Harkness, R. D.: Spatial distribution of dividing cells in the liver of the rat after partial hepatectomy, J. Physiol. **116**:373-379, 1952.

541 Hays, D. M.: Surgical research aspects of hepatic regeneration, Surg. Gynecol. Obstet. **139**:609-619, 1974.

542 Lane, B. P., and Becker, F. F.: Regeneration of mammalian liver, Am. J. Pathol. **50**:435-445, 1967.

543 Levi, J. U., and Zeppa, R.: The response of normal rat hepatocytes when exposed to hu-

moral (regenerating) factor, J. Surg. Res. **12:** 114-119, 1972.

544 Lilly, J. R., and Starzl, T. E.: Liver transplantation in children with biliary atresia and vascular anomalies, J. Pediatr. Surg. **9:**707-714, 1974.

545 Max, M. H., Price, J. B., Jr., Takeshige, K., and Voorhees, A. B., Jr.: Role of factors of portal origin in modifying hepatic regeneration, J. Surg. Res. **12:**120-123, 1972.

546 Porter, K. A.: Pathology of the orthotopic homograft and heterograft, In Starzl, T. E., editor: Experiments in hepatic transplantation, Philadelphia, 1969, W. B. Saunders Co.

547 Price, J. B., Jr., Takeshige, K., Max, M. H., and Voorhees, A. B., Jr.: Glucagon as the portal factor modifying hepatic regeneration, Surgery **72:**74-82, 1972.

548 Starzl, T. E., Francavilla, A., Halgrimson, C. G., Francavilla, F. R., Porter, K. A., Brown, T. H., and Putnam, C. W.: Origin, hormonal nature, and action of hepatotrophic substances in portal venous blood, Surg. Gynecol. Obstet. **137:**179-199, 1973.

549 Starzl, T. E., Porter, K. A., Brettschneider, L., Penn, I., Bell, P., Purnam, C. W., and McGuire, R. L.: Orthotopic transplantation of human liver, Surg. Gynecol. Obstet. **128:**327-339, 1969.

550 Williams, R., Smith, M. G. M., Shilkin, K. B., Herbertson, B., Joysey, V., and Calne, R. Y.: Liver transplantation in man: the frequency of rejection, biliary tract complications, and recurrence of malignancy based on an analysis of 26 cases, Gastroenterology **64:**1026-1048, 1973.

Degenerations

551 Bondar, G. F., and Pisesky, W.: Complications following small intestinal short-circuiting operations for obesity, Arch. Surg. (Chicago) **94:**707-716, 1967.

552 Bozymski, E. M., Woodruff, K., and Sessions, J. T., Jr.: Zollinger-Ellison syndrome with hypoglysemia associated with calcification of the tumor and its metastases, Gastroenterology **65:**658-661, 1973.

553 Editorial: Complications of intestinal bypass for obesity, J.A.M.A. **200:**638, 1967.

554 Farber, E., Lombardi, B., and Castillo, A. E.: Prevention by adenosine triphosphate of fatty liver induced by ethionine, Lab. Invest. **12:**873-883, 1963.

555 Graham, R. L.: Sudden death and associated fatty liver, Bull. Johns Hopkins Hosp. **74:**16-25, 1944.

556 Ham, J. M.: Segmental and lobar atrophy of liver, Surg. Gynecol. Obstet. **139:**840-844, 1974.

557 Karras, B. G., Cannon, A. H., and Zanon, B., Jr.: Hepatic calcification, Acta Radiol. (Stockholm) **57:**458-468, 1962.

558 Levy, M., Polliack, A., Lender, M., and Eliakim, M.: Liver in amyloidosis, Digestion **10:**40-51, 1974.

559 Maxwell, J. G., Richards, R. C., and Albo, D., Jr.: Fatty degeneration of liver after intestinal bypass for obesity, Am. J. Surg. **116:** 648-652, 1968.

560 Miele, A. J., and Edmonds, H. W.: Calcified liver metastases, Radiology **80:**779-785, 1963.

561 Sidransky, H., and Clark, S.: Chemical pathology of acute amino acid deficiencies, Arch. Pathol. (Chicago) **72:**468-479, 1961.

562 Theron, J. J., and Liebenberg, N.: Fine cytology of parenchymal liver cells in kwashiorkor patients, J. Pathol. Bacteriol. **86:**109-112, 1963.

563 Webber, B. L., and Freiman, I.: Liver in kwashiorkor: a clinical and electron microscopical study, Arch. Pathol. **98:**400-408, 1974.

Congenital and acquired abnormalities of form and position

564 Johnstone, G.: Accessory lobe of liver, Arch. Dis. Child. **40:**541-544, 1965.

Traumatic injury

565 Charif, P.: Subcapsular hemorrhage of liver in newborn, Clin. Pediatr. (Phila.) **3:**428-431, 1964.

566 Foley, W. J., Turcotte, J. G., Hoskins, P. A., Brant, R. L., and Ause, R. G.: Intrahepatic arteriovenous fistulas between the hepatic artery and portal vein, Ann. Surg. **174:**849-855, 1971.

567 Mays, E. T.: Editorial: Hepatic artery, Surg. Gynecol. Obstet. **139:**595-596, 1974.

568 Richardson, R. E., Gumbert, J. L., and Gale, S. A.: Traumatic intrahepatic hematoma, Arch. Surg. (Chicago) **95:**940-943, 1967.

569 Trunkey, D. D., Shires, G. T., and McClelland, R.: Management of liver trauma in 811 consecutive patients, Ann. Surg. **179:**722-728, 1974.

Hereditary hyperbilirubinemia

570 Ben-Ezzer, J., Blonder, J., Shani, M., Seligsohn, U., Post, C. A., Adam, A., and Szeinberg, A.: Dubin-Johnson syndrome: abnormal excretion of the isomers of urinary coproporphyrin by clinically unaffected family members, Isr. J. Med. Sci. **9:**1431-1436, 1973.

571 Black, M., and Billing, B. H.: Hepatic bilirubin UDP-glucuronyl transferase activity, New Eng. J. Med. **280:**1266-1271, 1969.

572 Butt, H. R., Anderson, V. E., Foulk, W. T., Baggenstoss, A. H., Schoenfield, L. J., and Dickson, E. R.: Studies of chronic idiopathic jaundice, Gastroenterology **51:**619-630, 1966.

573 Cornelius, C. E., and Arias, I. M.: Editorial: Biomedical models in veterinary medicine, Am. J. Med. **40:**165-169, 1966.

574 Cornelius, C. E., Arias, I. M., and Osburn, B.: Syndrome in Corriedale sheep resembling Dubin-Johnson, J. Am. Vet. Med. Assoc. **146:** 709-713, 1965.

575 Essner, E., and Novikoff, A. B.: Human hepatocellular pigments and lysosomes, J. Ultrastruct. Res. **3:**374-391, 1960.

576 Fromke, V. L., and Miller, D.: Constitutional hepatic dysfunction (CHD, Gilbert's disease); a review with special reference to a characteristic increase and prolongation of the hyperbilirubinemic response to nicotinic acid, Medicine **51:**451-464, 1973.

577 Gollan, J. L., Huang, S. N., Billing, B., and Sherlock, S.: Prolonged survival in three brothers with severe type 2 Crigler-Najjar syn-

drome—ultrastructural and metabolic studies, Gastroenterology 68:1543-1555, 1975.

578 Herman, J. D., Cooper, E. B., Takeuchi, A., and Sprinz, H.: Constitutional hyperbilirubinemia with unconjugated bilirubin—serum and pigment deposition in liver, Am. J. Dig. Dis. 9:160-169, 1964.

579 McGee, J. O'D., Allan, J. D., Russell, R. I., and Patrick, R. S.: Liver ultrastructure in Gilbert's syndrome, Gut 16:220-224, 1975.

580 Shani, M., Seligsohn, U., and Adam, A.: Inheritance of Dubin-Johnson syndrome, Isr. J. Med. Sci. 9:1427-1430, 1973.

581 Shani, M., Seligsohn, U., and Ben-Ezzer, J.: Effect of phenobarbital on liver functions in patients with Dubin-Johnson syndrome, Gastroenterology 67:303-308, 1974.

Circulatory disturbances

582 Baue, A. E., Chaudry, I. H., Wurth, M. A., and Sayeed, M. M.: Cellular alterations with shock and ischemia, Angiology 25:31-42, 1974.

583 Boler, R. K., and Bibighaus, A. J., III: Ultrastructural alterations of dog livers during endotoxin shock, Lab. Invest. 17:537-561, 1967.

584 Boyer, J. L., Hales, M. R., and Klatskin, G.: Idiopathic portal hypertension due to occlusion of intrahepatic portal veins by organized thrombi: study based on postmortem Vinylite injection corrosion and dissection of the intrahepatic vasculature in four cases, Medicine 53:77-91, 1974.

585 Boyer, J. L., Sen Gupta, K. P., Biswas, S. K., Pal, N. C., Basu Mallick, K. C., Iber, F. L., and Basu, A. K.: Idiopathic portal hypertension, Ann. Intern. Med. 66:41-68, 1967.

586 Donovan, A. J., Reynolds, T. B., Mikkelsen, W. P., and Peters, R. L.: Systemic portal arteriovenous fistulas, Surgery 66:474-482, 1969.

587 Editorial: Guido Banti—1852-1925, J.A.M.A. 201:693-695, 1967.

588 Grannis, F. W.: Guido Banti's hypothesis and its impact on the understanding and treatment of portal hypertension, Mayo Clin. Proc. 50: 41-48, 1975.

589 Grossman, J. A., and McDermott, W. V., Jr.: Paroxysmal nocturnal hemoglobinuria associated with hepatic and portal venous thrombosis, Am. J. Surg. 127:733-736, 1974.

590 Imanaga, H., Yamamoto, S., and Kuroyanagi, Y.: Surgical treatment of portal hypertension, Ann. Surg. 155:42-50, 1962.

591 Kimura, C., Matsuda, S., Koie, H., and Hirooka, M.: Membranous obstruction of the hepatic portion of inferior vena cava: clinical study of nine cases, Surgery 72:551-559, 1972.

592 Langer, B., Stone, R. M., Colapinto, R. F., Meindok, H., Phillips, M. J., and Fisher, M. D.: Clinical spectrum of Budd-Chiari syndrome and its surgical management, Am. J. Surg. 129:137-145, 1975.

593 Luna, A., Meister, H. P., and Szanto, P.: Esophageal varices in absence of cirrhosis, Am. J. Clin. Pathol. 49:710-717, 1968.

594 Mallory, T. B.: Systemic pathology consequent to traumatic shock, J. Mt. Sinai Hosp. N.Y. 16: 137-148, 1949.

595 Mikkelsen, W. P., Edmondson, H. A., Peters, R. L., Redeker, A. G., and Reynolds, T. B.: Extrahepatic and intrahepatic portal hypertension without cirrhosis, Ann. Surg. 162:602-620, 1965.

596 Myers, J. D., and Hickam, J. B.: Hepatic blood flow and splanchnic oxygen consumption in heart failure, J. Clin. Invest. 27:620-627, 1948.

597 Prandi, D., Rueff, B., and Benhamou, J.-P.: Side-to-side portacaval shunt in treatment of Budd-Chiari syndrome, Gastroenterology 68: 137-141, 1975.

598 Ravenna, P.: Banti syndrome, Arch. Intern. Med. (Chicago) 66:879-892, 1940.

599 Rousselot, L. M.: Role of congestion—portal hypertension—in so-called Banti's syndrome, J.A.M.A. 107:1788-1793, 1936.

600 Safran, A. P., and Schaffner, F.: Chronic passive congestion of liver in man, Am. J. Pathol. 50:447-463, 1967.

601 Seeley, T. T., Blumenfeld, C. M., Ikeda, R., Knapp, W., and Ruebner, B. H.: Hepatic infarction, Hum. Pathol. 3:265-276, 1972.

602 Seneviratne, R. D.: Physiologic and pathologic responses in blood vessels of liver, Q. J. Exp. Physiol. 35:77-110, 1949.

603 Sherlock, S.: Liver in circulatory failure. In Schiff, L., editor: Diseases of the liver, ed. 4, Philadelphia, 1975, J. B. Lippincott Co.

604 Sussman, E. B., and Sternberg, S. S.: Hereditary hemorrhagic telangiectasia: a case with hepatocellular carcinoma and acquired hepatocerebral degeneration, Arch. Pathol. 99:95-100, 1975.

605 Takeuchi, J., Takada, A., Hasumura, Y., Matsuda, Y., and Ikegami, F.: Budd-Chiari syndrome associated with obstruction of the inferior vena cava: a report of seven cases, Am. J. Med. 51:11-20, 1971.

606 Tavill, A. S., Wood, E. J., Kreel, L., Jones, E. A., Gregory, M., and Sherlock, S.: Budd-Chiari syndrome: correlation between hepatic scintigraphy and the clinical, radiological, and pathological findings in nineteen cases of hepatic venous flow obstruction, Gastroenterology 68:509-519, 1975.

607 Tisdale, W. A., Klatskin, G., and Glenn, W. W.: Portal hypertension in bleeding esophageal varices, New Eng. J. Med. 261:209-218, 1959.

608 Weil, M. H., and Spink, W. W.: Shock syndrome associated with bacteremia, Arch. Intern. Med. (Chicago) 101:184-193, 1958.

Chronic infections

609 Bernstein, M., Edmondson, H. A., and Barbour, B. H.: Liver lesion in Q fever, Arch. Intern. Med. (Chicago) 116:491-498, 1965.

610 Böhm, W., and Willnow, U.: Granulomartige Hepatitis bei konnataler Toxoplasmose, Z. Kinderheilkd. 88:215-225, 1963.

611 Editorial: Secondary syphilis and hepatitis, Br. Med. J. 1:112, 1975.

612 Gupta, M. C., Kumar, S., and Tyagi, S. P.: Reappraisal of functional and structural changes in liver in leprosy, J. Assoc. Physicians of India 22:13-18, 1974.

613 Israel, H. L., and Goldstein, R. A.: Hepatic

granulomatosis and sarcoidosis, Ann. Intern. Med. 79:669-678, 1973.

614 Kramarsky, B., Edmondson, H. A., Peters, R. L., and Reynolds, T. B.: Lepromatous leprosy in reaction, Arch. Pathol. (Chicago) 85:516-531, 1968.

615 Kuzemko, J. A.: Toxocariasis, Arch. Dis. Child. 41:221-222, 1966.

616 Min, K.-W., Gyorkey, F., and Cain, G. D.: Talc granulomata in liver disease in narcotic addicts, Arch. Pathol. 98:331-335, 1974.

617 O'Connell, M. J., Wiernik, P. H., Sklansky, B. D., Greene, W. H., Abt, A. B., Kirschner, R. H., Ramsey, H. E., and Murphy, W. L.: Staging laparotomy in Hodgkin's disease: further evidence in support of its clinical utility, Am. J. Med. 57:86-91, 1974.

618 Pimentel, J. C., and Menezes, A. P.: Liver granulomas containing copper in vineyard sprayer's lung; new etiology of hepatic granulomatosis, Am. Rev. Resp. Dis. 111:189-195, 1975.

619 Spink, W. W.: Host-parasite relationship in human brucellosis, Am. J. Med. Sci. 247:129-136, 1964.

620 Woodruff, A. W., and Thacker, C. K.: Infection with animal helminths, Br. Med. J. 1:1001-1005, 1964.

Cysts

621 Jones, W. L., Mountain, J. C., and Warren, K. W.: Symptomatic non-parasitic cysts of liver, Br. J. Surg. 61:118-123, 1974.

622 Kerr, D. N. S., Harrison, C. V., Sherlock, S., and Walker, R. M.: Congenital hepatic fibrosis, Q. J. Med. 30:91-117, 1961.

623 Longmire, W. P., Jr., Trout, H. H., II, Greenfield, J., and Tompkins, R. K.: Elective hepatic surgery, Ann. Surg. 179:712-720, 1974.

624 Melnick, P. J.: Polycystic liver, Arch. Pathol. (Chicago) 59:162-172, 1955.

625 Sanfelippo, P. M., Beahrs, O. H., and Weiland, L. H.: Cystic disease of liver, Ann. Surg. 179:922-925, 1974.

Tumors

626 Adam, Y. B., Huvos, A. G., and Hajdu, S. I.: Malignant vascular tumors of liver, Ann. Surg. 175:375-383, 1972.

627 Alpert, M. E., Hutt, M. S. R., and Davison, C. S.: Primary hepatoma in Uganda—prospective clinical and epidemiologic study of forty-six patients, Am. J. Med. 46:794-802, 1969.

628 Anthony, P. P.: Liver cell dysplasia: a premalignant condition, J. Pathol. 109:pxvii, 1973.

629 Asch, M. J., Cohen, A. H., and Moore, T. C.: Hepatic and splenic lymphangiomatosis with skeletal involvement: report of case and review of literature, Surgery 76:334-339, 1974.

630 Bagheri, S. A., and Boyer, J. L.: Peliosis hepatis associated with androgenic-anabolic steroid therapy—severe form of hepatic injury, Ann. Intern. Med. 81:610, 1974.

631 Becker, F. F.: Hepatoma—nature's model tumor—a review, Am. J. Pathol. 74:179-200, 1974.

632 Block, J. B.: Angiosarcoma of liver following vinyl chloride exposure, J.A.M.A. 229:53-54, 1974.

633 Braun, P., Ducharme, J. C., Riopelle, J. L., and Davignon, A.: Hemangiomatosis of liver in infants, J. Pediatr. Surg. 10:121-126, 1975.

634 Chudecki, B.: Primary cancer of liver following treatment of polycythaemia vera with radioactive phosphorus, Br. J. Radiol. 45:770-774, 1972.

635 Creech, J. L., Jr., and Johnson, M. N.: Angiosarcoma of liver in manufacture of polyvinyl chloride, J. Occup. Med. 16:150-151, 1974.

636 Current intelligence: Angiosarcoma of liver in vinyl chloride/polyvinyl chloride workers, J. Occup. Med. 16:809, 1974.

637 Dehner, L. P., Ewing, S. L., and Sumner, H. W.: Infantile mesenchymal hamartoma of liver—histologic and ultrastructural observations, Arch. Pathol. 99:379-382, 1975.

638 Dehner, L. P., and Ishak, K. G.: Vascular tumors of liver in infants and children, Arch. Pathol. 92:101-111, 1971.

639 Delage, C., and Lagace, R.: La péliose hépatique: rôle étiologique possible des médicaments, L'Union médicale du Canada 102:1888-1893, 1973.

640 Dolan, M. F., and Janovski, N. A.: Adrenal dystopia, Arch. Pathol. (Chicago) 86:22-24, 1968.

641 Doll, R., Muir, C., and Waterhouse, J. A. H.: Cancer incidence in five continents, UICC Publication, Berlin, 1970, Springer-Verlag.

642 Edmondson, H. A.: Tumors and tumorlike lesions in infancy and childhood, Am. J. Dis. Child. 91:168-186, 1956.

643 Edmondson, H. A.: In Atlas of tumor pathology, Sect. VII, Fasc. 25, Washington, D.C., 1958, Armed Forces Institute of Pathology (tumors of liver and intrahepatic bile ducts).

644 Edmondson, H. A., and Steiner, P. E.: Primary cancer, Cancer 7:462-503, 1954.

645 Ein, S. H.: Malignant liver tumors in children, J. Pediatr. Surg. 9:491-494, 1974.

646 Eriksson, S., and Hägerstrand, I.: Cirrhosis and malignant hepatoma in α_1-antitrypsin deficiency, Acta Med. Scand. 195:451-458, 1974.

647 Farber, E.: Pathogenesis of liver cancer, Arch. Pathol. 98:145-148, 1974.

648 Floyd, W. S., and Cohn, S. L.: Gonadotropin-producing hepatoma, Obstet. Gynecol. 41:665-668, 1974.

649 Fortner, J. G.: Treatment of primary and secondary liver cancer by hepatic artery ligation and infusion chemotherapy, Ann. Surg. 178:162-172, 1973.

650 Fraumeni, J. F., Miller, R. W., and Hill, J. A.: Primary carcinoma of liver in childhood, J. Natl. Cancer Inst. 40:1087-1099, 1968.

651 Geddes, E. W., and Falkson, G.: Malignant hepatoma in the Bantu, Cancer 25:1271-1278, 1970.

652 Gibson, J. B.: In Liver cancer, Lyon, 1971, I.A.R.C. Scientific Publication No. 1.

653 Gillman, J., and Payet, M.: Primary cancer of liver, Acta Unio. Int. Contra Cancr. 13:860-868, 1957.

654 Goldberg, S. J., and Fonkalsrud, E.: Successful treatment of hepatic hemangioma with corticosteroids, J.A.M.A. 208:2473-2474, 1969.

655 Gonzalez-Crussi, F., and Manz, H. J.: Structure of hepatoblastoma of pure epithelial type, Cancer 29:1272-1280, 1972.

656 Halliday, W. J., Halliday, J. W., Campbell, C. B., Maluish, A. E., and Powell, L. W.: Specific immunodiagnosis of hepatocellular carcinoma by leucocyte adherence inhibition, Br. Med. J. 2:349-353, 1974.

657 Higashino, K., Ohtani, R., Kudo, S., Hashinotsume, M., Hada, T., Kang, K.-Y., Ohkochi, T., Takahashi, Y., and Yamamura, Y.: Hepatocellular carcinoma and variant alkaline phosphatase, Ann. Intern. Med. 83:74-78, 1975.

658 Holton, C. P., Burrington, J. D., and Hatch, E. I.: Multiple chemotherapeutic approach to management of hepatoblastoma—preliminary report, Cancer 35:1083-1087, 1975.

659 Homer, L. W., White, H. J., and Read, R. C.: Neoplastic transformation of von Meyenberg complexes of liver, J. Pathol. Bacteriol. 96:499-502, 1968.

660 Honjo, I.: Primary carcinoma of liver, Am. J. Surg. 128:31-36, 1974.

661 Ishak, K. G., and Glunz, P. R.: Hepatoblastoma and hepatocarcinoma in infancy and childhood, Cancer 20:396-422, 1967.

662 Jaffe, B. M., Donegan, W. L., Watson, F., and Spratt, J. S., Jr.: Factors influencing survival in patients with untreated hepatic metastases, Surg. Gynecol. Obstet. 127:1-11, 1968.

663 Keeley, A. F., Iseri, O. A., and Gottlieb, L. S.: Ultrastructure of hyaline cytoplasmic inclusions in a human hepatoma; relationship to Mallory's alcoholic hyalin, Gastroenterology 62:280-293, 1972.

664 Keiser, H. R., Vogel, C. L., and Sadikali, F.: Protocollagen proline hydroxylase in sera of Ugandans with hepatocellular carcinoma, J. Natl. Cancer Inst. 49:1251-1255, 1972.

665 Kiely, J. M., Titus, J. L., and Orvis, A. L.: Thorotrast-induced hepatoma presenting as hyperparathyroidism, Cancer 31:1312-1314, 1973.

666 Kurtz, R. C., Sherlock, P., and Winawer, S. J.: Esophageal varices; development secondary to primary and metastatic liver tumors, Arch. Intern. Med. 134:50-51, 1974.

667 Lander, J. J., Stanley, R. J., Sumner, H. W., Boswell, D. C., and Aach, R. D.: Angiosarcoma of liver associated with Fowler's solution (potassium arsenite), Gastroenterology 68:1583-1586, 1975.

668 Lizzi, F. A., Tartaglia, A. P., and Adamson, J. W.: Hemochromatosis, hepatoma, erythrocytosis, and erythropoietin, N.Y. State J. Med. 73:1098-1100, 1973.

669 McFadzean, A. J. S., and Yeung, R. T. T.: Observations on hypoglycemia, Am. J. Med. 47:220-235, 1969.

670 McDermott, W. V., Jr., and Hensle, T. W.: Metastatic carcinoid to the liver treated by hepatic dearterialization, Ann. Surg. 180:305-308, 1974.

671 McLean, R. H., Moller, J. H., Warwick, W. J., Satran, L., and Lucas, R. V., Jr.: Multinodular hemangiomatosis of liver in infancy, Pediatrics 49:563-573, 1972.

672 Madding, G. F., and Kennedy, P. A.: Hepatic artery ligation, Surg. Clin. North Am. 52:719-728, 1972.

673 Marsh, J. L., Dahms, B., and Longmire, W. P., Jr.: Cystadenoma and cystadenocarcinoma of the biliary system, Arch. Surg. 109:41-43, 1974.

674 Matolo, N. M., and Johnson, D. G.: Surgical treatment of hepatic hemangioma in newborn, Arch. Surg. 106:725-727, 1973.

675 Michaeli, D., Ben-Bassat, I., Miller, H. I., and Deutsch, V.: Hepatic telangiectases and portosystemic encephalopathy in Osler-Weber-Rendu disease, Gastroenterology 54:929-932, 1968.

676 Moenandar, I. M.: Extensive calcification in stroma of a primary hepatic carcinoma, J. Pathol. 114:53-56, 1974.

677 Muehlbauer, M. A., and Farber, M. G.: Hemangioma of liver, Am. J. Gastroenterol. 45:355-365, 1966.

678 Murthy, A. S. K., Vawter, G. F., Kopito, L., and Rossen, E.: Biochemical studies on liver tumors of children, Arch. Pathol. 96:48-52, 1972.

679 Ohbayashi, A.: Genetic and familial aspects of liver cirrhosis and hepatocellular carcinoma. In Okuda, K., and Peters, R. L., editors: Hepatocellular carcinoma, New York, 1976, John Wiley & Sons.

680 Ong, G. B., and Taw, J. L.: Spontaneous rupture of hepatocellular carcinoma, Br. Med. J. 4:146-149, 1972.

681 Parks, L. C., Baer, A. N., Pollack, M., and Williams, G. M.: Alpha fetoprotein: an index of progression or regression of hepatoma, and a target for immunotherapy, Ann. Surg. 180:599-605, 1974.

682 Patil, S. D., Talib, V. H., Sultana, Z., Talib, N. S., and Bhagwat, D. S.: Mesenchymal hamartoma of liver, Indian J. Pediatr. 41:283-286, 1974.

683 Peers, F. G., and Linsell, C. A.: Dietary aflatoxins and liver cell cancer—a population based study in Kenya, Br. J. Cancer 27:473-484, 1973.

684 Person, D. A., Sargent, T., and Isaac, E.: Thorotrast-induced carcinoma of liver, Arch. Surg. (Chicago) 88:503-510, 1964.

685 Plachta, A.: Triad syndrome inherent to calcified cavernous hemangioma of liver, Angiology 16:594-599, 1965.

686 Primack, A., Wilson, J., O'Connor, G. T., Engelman, K., Hull, E., and Canellos, G. P.: Hepatocellular carcinoma with the carcinoid syndrome, Cancer 27:1182-1189, 1971.

687 Rabinowitz, J. G., Kinkabwala, M., and Ulreich, S.: Macro-regenerating nodule in cirrhotic liver: radiologic features and differential diagnosis, Am. J. Roentgenol. Rad. Ther. Nucl. Med. 121:401-411, 1974.

688 Rankin, J. G., Skyring, A. P., and Goulston, S. J. M.: Liver in ulcerative colitis—bile duct carcinoma, Gut 7:433-437, 1966.

689 Satterlee, R. C.: Primary site of carcinoma of liver, lungs and bone, U.S. Naval Med. Bull. 40:133-136, 1942.

690 Selikoff, I. J., and Hammond, E. C., editors: Toxicity of vinyl chloride–polyvinyl chloride, Ann. N.Y. Acad. Sci. 246:1-137, 1975.

691 Selinger, M., and Koff, R. S.: Thorotrast and the liver; a reminder, Gastroenterology **68**:799-803, 1975.

692 Shank, R. C., Gordon, J., Wogan, G. N., Nondasuta, A., and Subhamani, B.: Dietary aflatoxins and human liver cancer. III. Field survey of rural Thai families for ingested aflatoxins, Food Cosmet. Toxicol. **10**:71-84, 1972.

693 Alpert, E., Coston, R. L., and Drysdale, J. W.: Carcino-foetal human liver ferritin, Nature **242**:194-196, 1973.

694 Short, W. F., Nedwich, A., Levy, H. A., and Howard, J. M.: Biliary cystadenoma: report of case and review of the literature, Arch. Surg. **102**:78-80, 1971.

695 Smoron, G. L., and Battifora, H. A.: Thorotrast-induced hepatoma, Cancer **30**:1252-1259, 1972.

696 Steiner, P., and Higginson, J.: Cholangiocellular carcinoma of liver, Cancer **12**:753-759, 1959.

697 Sussman, E. B., Nydick, I., and Gray, G. F.: Hemangioendothelial sarcoma of liver and hemochromatosis, Arch. Pathol. **97**:39-42, 1974.

698 Tio (Tiong Hoo), Leijnse, B., Jarrett, A., and Rimington, C.: Acquired porphyria from a liver tumour, Clin. Sci. **16**:517-527, 1957.

699 Torres, F. O., Purchase, I. F. H., and Van der Watt, J. J.: Aetiology of primary liver cancer in the Bantu, J. Pathol. **102**:163-169, 1970.

700 Totzke, H. A., and Hutcheson, J. B.: Primary fibrosarcoma of the liver, South. Med. J. **58**:236-238, 1965.

701 von Felten, A., Straub, P. W., and Frick, P. G.: Dysfibrinogenemia in patient with primary hepatoma, New Eng. J. Med. **280**:405-409, 1969.

702 Editorial: Aflatoxin and primary liver cancer, S. Afr. Med. J. **48**:2495-2496, 1974.

703 Van Rensburg, S. J., Van der Watt, J. J., Purchase, S. F. H., Continho, L. P., and Markham, R.: Primary liver cancer rate and aflatoxin intake in a high cancer area, S. Afr. Med. J. **48**:2506a-2508d, 1974.

704 Voute, P. A., Jr., and Wadman, S. K.: Cystathioninuria in hepatoblastoma, Clin. Chim. Acta **22**:373-378, 1968.

705 Warren, S., and Drake, W. L., Jr.: Hepatic carcinoma in hemochromatosis, Am. J. Pathol. **27**:573-609, 1951.

706 Yanoff, M., and Rawson, A. J.: Peliosis hepatis, Arch. Pathol. (Chicago) **77**:159-165, 1964.

Interpretation of needle biopsies

707 Feldman, R. G., Iseri, O. A., Gottlieb, L. S., and Greenberg, J. P.: Familial intention tremor, ataxia, and lipofuscinosis, Neurology (Minneap.) **19**:503-509, 1969.

32/Gallbladder and biliary ducts

BÉLA HALPERT

STRUCTURE AND FUNCTION

The right and left hepatic ducts as they reach the porta hepatis join at an obtuse angle to form the common hepatic duct. This continues as the common bile duct after giving off the cystic duct at an acute angle. The cystic duct gradually widens into the S-shaped neck of the gallbladder, and the common bile duct terminates in the duodenum at the papilla of Vater.

The biliary ducts, as well as the gallbladder, are lined by tall columnar epithelium. Acinar glands producing a mucinous secretion open into the ducts and into the neck of the gallbladder but are absent in its body and fundus. Beneath the epithelium, a delicate lamina propria contains the capillaries. The mucosal surface of the gallbladder is immensely enlarged by deep polygonal spaces bordered by ridges of varying heights. Microscopically, the ridges are richly branching, delicate, connective tissue stalks covered by tall columnar cells (Fig. 32-1). External to the lamina propria is a fairly dense, fibrous connective tissue making up the wall of the extrahepatic biliary ducts. In the gallbladder external to the lamina propria are smooth muscle bundles arranged longitudinally and then obliquely or circularly. The muscular coat is surrounded by the perimuscular layer composed of a narrow zone of loose connective tissue, sometimes interspersed with adipose tissue cells. Serosa covers the perimuscular layer over the peritoneal surface of the gallbladder. The opposite surface is attached to the liver. Particularly on the surface toward the liver, aberrant bile ducts (Luschka ducts) frequently occur in the perimuscular layer.[39]

The closeness of the lining epithelium to the muscular layer and the absence of a submucosa suggest that the muscular coat of the gallbladder is genetically a tunica muscularis mucosae. This is further supported by the observation that the glands in the neck of the gallbladder penetrate the muscular coat just as Brunner's glands traverse the muscularis mucosae of the duodenum.[17] Furthermore, in the course of development, the muscular coat of the gallbladder appears simultaneously with that of the muscularis mucosae and later than the muscular coats of the intestine.[26] This derivation of the muscular coat would explain why direct mechanical, chemical, and electrical stimuli that cause an immediate and powerful contraction of the intestines have no demonstrable effect on the gallbladder.

The blood for the extrahepatic biliary ducts is derived from the hepatic arteries, the right supplying the cystic artery to the gallbladder. The common bile duct receives its main blood supply from the retroduodenal artery, a branch of the gastroduodenal artery.[25,30] The return from the gallbladder is through the cystic vein that empties into the portal vein.

The network of lymph channels in the wall of the gallbladder drains into the lymph node at the neck of the viscus. From here, the flow is toward the porta hepatis and to the peripancreatic lymph nodes. Enlargement of the nodes within the hepatoduodenal ligament may impede or obstruct the flow of bile through the common bile duct.

The nerve supply is parasympathetic and sympathetic. Whether the pattern of distribution in the gallbladder is that of the myenteric plexus (Auerbach's) or that of the submucous plexus (Meissner's) is at yet undetermined.

The function of the extrahepatic biliary ducts is to provide passage of bile into the duodenum. Bile is the product of the liver cells and is a complex liquid. It apparently is produced continually, with its quantity and composition subject to wide variations.[35,61] According to a conservative estimate, about 0.6 ml of bile is produced per hour per kilogram of body weight in man,[33] and about 3 ml in rabbits.[20] Bile contains an average of 3% solids. The rest is water.[11] The substances it

1439

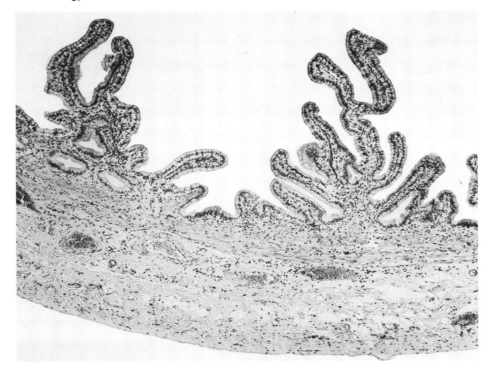

Fig. 32-1. Normal gallbladder (33-year-old woman). In cross section of midportion, delicate connective tissue stalks are covered by tall columnar epithelium. Beneath tunica propria is muscular coat with smooth muscle bundles arranged longitudinally and then obliquely or circularly. External to muscular coat is perimuscular layer. (40×.)

contains are alkali salts of the bile acids, bile pigments, cholesterol, mucoprotein, and the electrolytes common to all body fluids: sodium, calcium, potassium, and magnesium, as chlorides, bicarbonates, carbonates, and phosphates.[33] The pH of the bile is between 7.1 and 7.3.[31] In the bile from the gallbladder, the range may be between 5.79 and 7.55.[15]

A mechanism at the choledochoduodenal junction regulates the flow of bile into the duodenum. It has long been postulated that an anatomic sphincter exists here and that it has a reciprocal innervation with the gallbladder so that, when the sphincter relaxes, the gallbladder contracts and evacuates its content.[28] Clinical tests assuming the existence of this mechanism are still in use.[27] It is, however, not fully established that an *anatomic sphincter* exists at the choledochoduodenal junction.[13,19] There is also doubt whether the anatomic arrangement of the biliary ducts and the gallbladder and the distribution and strength of the muscular coat of the viscus permit complete evacuation of the gallbladder by muscle contraction. Occasionally in man and frequently in animals (rhesus monkey),

the gallbladder is completely or almost completely embedded in the liver, without obvious interference with its function.[18]

The function of the gallbladder is to receive and dispose of the overflow of bile while its passage into the duodenum is being negotiated. The bile reaches the gallbladder through the funnel-shaped cystic duct that widens toward the gallbladder. The course of the duct appears somewhat twisted because its lumen is ridged by a series of folds, the valves of Heister.[18] The last of these narrows the lumen toward the gallbladder, offering interference to the flow of bile from the gallbladder. The main force driving the bile into the gallbladder is the pressure on the liver during inspiration.[21] The muscular coat of the gallbladder adjusts the size of the viscus to the change in its content.[22] Overdistention is prevented by ability of the gallbladder to resorb half the volume of its content per hour.[24] According to one concept, mainly water is resorbed.[32] Others believe that the mucosa of the gallbladder can resorb all constituents of the bile, some constituents more rapidly than others. Accordingly, the increased concentration of bile in the gallbladder is attributable to variations in rates of resorption.[57,58]

Certain substances when injected intravenously or given by mouth appear in the bile and reach the gallbladder.[16] Some substances so administered accumulate in the gallbladder in concentrations not attained in the bile coming from the liver.[21] Cholecystography, the visualization of the gallbladder roentgenographically, is based on this selective resorbing ability of the gallbladder. Radiopaque substances (sodium tetraiodophenolphthalein, Priodax,[14] Telepaque,[10] and others) after reaching the gallbladder are resorbed more slowly than the bile, eventually attaining a concentration sufficient to cast a shadow on an x-ray film. The shadow becomes smaller after a fatty meal.[12,29] This has been interpreted as being caused by evacuation of the viscus. Diminution of the shadow may as well be accomplished by selective resorption of the content.[23,34]

LESIONS

Inflammations, concretions, neoplasms, and anomalies are the important lesions affecting the extrahepatic biliary ducts and the gallbladder. Acute cholecystitis, chronic cholecystitis, and acute cholecystitis superimposed on a chronic cholecystitis are the common inflammatory processes involving the gallbladder. Tuberculous, syphilitic, actinomycotic, and parasitic[42] lesions, when encountered, usually are associated with similar changes in the intrahepatic biliary ducts and in the liver.

Inflammations

Acute cholecystitis. Acute cholecystitis is a nonspecific inflammation caused by streptococci, staphylococci, or the enteric groups of microorganisms. These may reach the viscus in the bile, in the blood, through the lymphatics, or by direct extension from neighboring organs. In the latter instance, the process extends from the outer layers inward and may barely reach the mucosa—pericholecystitis. A temporary increase in bile salt content in the gallbladder also may cause acute cholecystitis, as has been shown experimentally.[44] Enzyme action from reflux of pancreatic secretion into the gallbladder may induce inflammation of the viscus.[37] The gallbladder may become involved in an inflammatory process as part of an allergic reaction, in polyarteritis nodosa, in endarteritis obliterans, and in terminal uremia. Chemical, enzymatic, and perhaps allergic factors probably excite or play a contributory role in exciting cholecystitis more

often than suspected. Vascular obstruction may result in hemorrhagic infarction of the gallbladder, with subsequent acute cholecystitis, and may terminate in acute diffuse peritonitis. The exact mechanism by which acute inflammation of the gallbladder is initiated is, as yet, unknown. However, in acute cholecystitis from whatever cause, the involvement usually starts within the mucosa and extends outward.

In acute cholecystitis, the viscus is enlarged, firm, and discolored reddish brown, with an increase in thickness of its wall up to tenfold. This is caused by spreading of the tissue elements and filling of the spaces with edema fluid and extravasated blood. The lumen usually contains a mixture of bile, blood, and pus. Gallstones usually are not present.

Microscopically, the epithelium may be preserved over extensive areas. Elsewhere it is either shed or missing. All the layers are spread apart and are densely infiltrated with erythrocytes and neutrophilic granulocytes in fibrin or in an amorphous pink substance. In the distended capillaries, margination of white blood cells is conspicuous. The changes are more pronounced about blood vessels and involve all the layers, including the perimuscular layer and the serosa.

Commensurate with the intensity of the inflammatory process, the clinical signs and symptoms, too, are severe. There is intense pain in the right upper abdomen radiating toward the right shoulder, associated with abdominal rigidity, malaise, nausea, and other signs of beginning peritonitis. The acute process is usually progressive and may end in perforation of the gallbladder with focal abscess or diffuse peritonitis. In rare instances, the inflammation may subside.

Chronic cholecystitis. Various conditions may induce chronic cholecystitis. It usually is assumed to be the sequel of an acute inflammation of the gallbladder (i.e., the healing state of subsiding acute cholecystitis). In other instances, the chronic cholecystitis is caused by the presence in the viscus of pure gallstones or of the mulberry-shaped mixed gallstones. Chronic cholecystitis also may be induced by intermittent or continuous abnormal composition of the bile. Attenuated or usually nonpathogenic enteric organisms also may produce chronic cholecystitis. Since so many variables operate in the production of the chronic inflammtory reaction, practically no two gallbladders with chronic cholecystitis are exactly alike, although they have certain

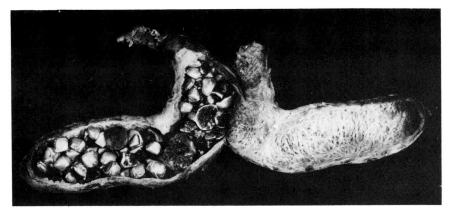

Fig. 32-2. Gallbladder with chronic cholecystitis containing mixed gallstones (40-year-old man). Noticeable trabeculations on mucosal surface. Calculi faceted and yellow with brown centers.

features in common. The most important of these is the almost invariable presence of gall-stones. In some instances the gallstones are the cause of and in others the sequel to the chronic inflammatory state of the gallbladder. Familiarity with the chemical composition and structure of gallstones aids, therefore, in interpreting their role in the inflammatory process.

The wall of the gallbladder with chronic cholecystitis is increased to several times its usual thickness. The mucosal folds are coarse and in advanced stages are obliterated or absent, with the surface trabeculated (Fig. 32-2). Occasionally, the wall may become impregnated with calcium (Fig. 32-3) so that a crackling sound (porcelain gallbladder) may be elicited on touch. The lumen of the cystic duct is invariably increased to several times its usual diameter, permitting the passage of calculi into the common bile duct.

Microscopically, the epithelium is usually intact and is mounted on coarse folds. At intervals, it dips to line outpouchings of the mucosa toward the external layers. These outpouchings, the Rokitansky-Aschoff sinuses,[39] usually form along blood vessels and penetrate the thickened muscular coat to varying depths. Their fundi frequently reach the perimuscular layer (Fig. 32-4). They are more numerous in the body and fundus than about the neck of the viscus. The muscular coat is hypertrophied, being increased to several times its usual thickness.[41] The perimuscular layer becomes dense with many coarse collagenous bundles. It may increase to a thickness greater than that of the entire wall of the normal gallbladder. There is also an increase of connective tissue in the lamina propria and between the

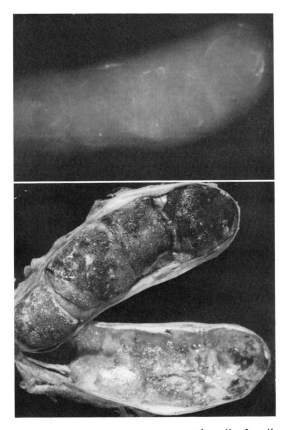

Fig. 32-3. Calcium impregnation of wall of gallbladder (73-year-old black man). Combined calculi with articulating faceted surfaces fill lumen. (Courtesy Dr. William R. Schmalhorst, Bakersfield, Cal.)

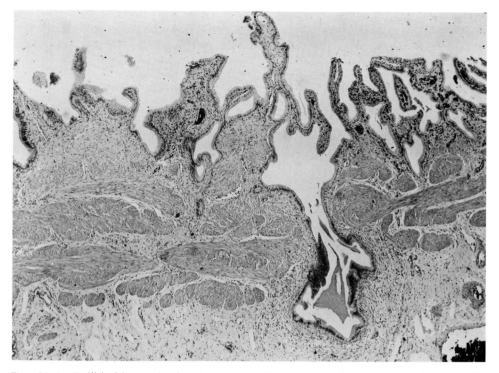

Fig. 32-4. Gallbladder with chronic cholecystitis that contained mixed gallstones (57-year-old woman). In longitudinal section from body of viscus, folds of mucosa are coarse or delicate. Rokitansky-Aschoff sinus extends through entire thickness of greatly hypertrophied muscular coat. Increase in connective tissue in tunica propria and between muscle bundles. Perimuscular layer broad. In all layers, slight infiltration with lymphocytes, plasma cells, large mononuclear cells, and some eosinophilic granulocytes. (32×.)

muscle bundles. All the connective tissue is infiltrated with lymphocytes, plasma cells, large mononuclear cells, and eosinophilic granulocytes. Rarely, there is prominence of lymphocytic infiltration in all the layers, with the formation of lymph follicles with large germinal centers—cholecystitis lymphofollicularis[36] (Fig. 32-5). Sometimes, the *Salmonella* group of organisms appears to be responsible[43]; at other times, the cause remains uncertain.

Chronic cholecystitis usually produces vague right upper abdominal distress and distaste for fatty foods. The calculous content of the viscus may occasionally be felt by bimanual palpation. Usually, the gallstones may be visualized roentgenographically. The presence of biliary calculi within the viscus lends clinical importance to chronic cholecystitis. Gallstones may pass through the dilated cystic duct and obstruct the common bile duct, producing jaundice. They also predispose to the development of acute cholecystitis that becomes grafted on the chronic process.

Chronic cholecystitis with superimposed acute cholecystitis. Acute cholecystitis more frequently occurs in a gallbladder with chronic cholecystitis containing biliary calculi than in an intact gallbladder. Occurrence of chronic and acute cholecystitis in the same gallbladder often is referred to as acute exacerbation of the chronic process, although actually the acute inflammation is superimposed on the chronic inflammatory process.

Grossly, such a gallbladder differs little from one with acute cholecystitis except for the presence of calculi within the viscus. Red, brown, or creamy pus fills the lumen. The calculi may be of any variety, although mixed gallstones of the faceted type are most common. The mucosa is angry red, velvety, and ragged, with frequent erosions. The waterlogged wall is many times the usual thickness, and the serosa is discolored red and brown, with flakes of fibrin giving the peritoneal surface a ground-glass opacity.

Microscopically, the mucosal folds are

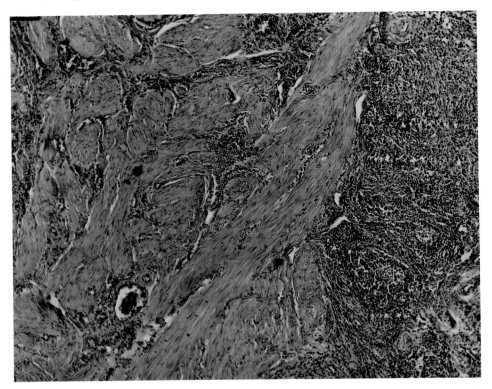

Fig. 32-5. Gallbladder with cholecystitis lymphofollicularis, cholelithiasis (calcium bilirubinate calculi), and acute cholecystitis (52-year-old man). Dense lymphocytic infiltration with formation of lymph follicles having germinal centers. Lymphocytic infiltration mostly in intermuscular connective tissue and in perimuscular layer. Superimposed are edema, extravasation of erythrocytes, and infiltrations with neutrophilic granulocytes. (60×.)

coarse, low, or absent. The epithelium varies in height. Rokitansky-Aschoff sinuses are numerous. The muscular coat is greatly hypertrophied with an increase of the intermuscular connective tissue and thickening of the perimuscular layer. In all the layers there is a scattering of lymphocytes, plasma cells, and large mononuclear cells. In addition, a hemorrhagic fibrinopurulent exudate covers denuded areas of the mucosa. All the layers are greatly spread apart by inflammatory edema and infiltrated with freshly extravasated erythrocytes and neutrophilic granulocytes. The serosal surface is covered by fibrin.

Chronic cholecystitis with superimposed acute cholecystitis is a well-known entity. This is the lesion that most commonly necessitates surgical intervention and removal of the gallbladder.[40] The clinical signs and symptoms are those of acute cholecystitis. Because of the presence of biliary calculi, obstruction of the common bile duct may occur, and jaundice may accompany the process. In acute cholecystitis without cholelithiasis, jaundice does not occur unless there is concomitant hepatitis or cholangitis. Perforation of the gallbladder, with subsequent focal or diffuse peritonitis, is a common sequel of acute cholecystitis superimposed on chronic cholecystitis with cholelithiasis.

Concretions

Gallstones usually form in the gallbladder and only occasionally in the biliary ducts. The presence of biliary calculi or gallstones in the gallbladder or in the biliary ducts is called cholelithiasis. The roles played in the formation of gallstones by faulty composition of the bile, stagnation of bile in the gallbladder, and inflammation of the gallbladder and biliary ducts are, as yet, not definitely determined.[45,61] Gallstones are best grouped according to their composition. Chemical analysis or infrared spectroscopy[50] reveals that three normal constituents of the bile—cholesterol, calcium bilirubinate, and calcium carbonate—are the principal stone-forming substances.[51] Gallstones may be composed almost entirely

Table 32-1. Classification of gallstones

Type	Composition	Appearance	Factors in origin	Changes in gallbladder
Pure gallstones (10%)	Cholesterol (crystalline)	Solitary; crystalline surface	Increased cholesterol content in bile	Cholesterolosis
	Calcium bilirubinate	Multiple; jet black; crystalline or amorphous	Increased pigment content in bile	No change
	Calcium carbonate	Grayish white; amorphous	Unknown	No change
Mixed gallstones (80%)	Cholesterol and calcium bilirubinate	Multiple, faceted or lobulated, laminated, and crystalline on cut surfaces; hue depends on content: cholesterol, yellow; calcium bilirubinate, black; calcium carbonate, white	Chronic cholecystitis plus increased content in bile of cholesterol, calcium bilirubinate, or calcium carbonate	Chronic cholecystitis
	Cholesterol and calcium carbonate			
	Calcium bilirubinate and calcium carbonate			
	Cholesterol, calcium bilirubinate, and calcium carbonate			
Combined gallstones (10%)	Pure gallstone nucleus with mixed gallstone shell	Largest of gallstones, when single; hue depends on composition of shell	As in pure gallstones, followed by chronic cholecystitis	Chronic cholecystitis
	Mixed gallstone nucleus with pure gallstone shell		As in mixed gallstones, followed by increased content in bile of cholesterol, calcium bilirubinate, or calcium carbonate	Chronic cholecystitis

of one of these substances (pure gallstones), of a mixture of them in varying proportions (mixed gallstones), or of a combination in which one kind of gallstone forms the nucleus and another the shell (combined gallstones) (Table 32-1).

Pure gallstones. About 10% of biliary calculi in surgically removed gallbladders are pure gallstones. Pure gallstones form when the bile contains intermittently or continually an excess of one of the stone-forming substances. This excess is caused by disturbances of metabolism or of liver function rather than by an inflammatory reaction of the gallbladder or of the biliary ducts. Pure gallstones are composed almost entirely of cholesterol or of calcium bilirubinate and, rarely, of calcium carbonate.

The *crystalline cholesterol stone* is the most common and is always solitary and remains so as long as its surface is crystalline (Fig. 32-6). It may vary from 0.5 to 5 cm in diam-

eter. The smaller ones are spheric, and the larger ones ovoid. Eventually, the crystalline surface becomes obscured, the crevices are filled in, and the entire calculus becomes permeated with calcium carbonate so as to cast a faint radiographic shadow. Yet, the cut surfaces remain crystalline with a glistening radiating pattern. A metabolic disturbance causing an increased cholesterol content of the bile results in the formation of the crystalline cholesterol stone.[46] The gallbladder containing such a stone may present no other change in the mucosa than a delicate network of yellowish white lines corresponding to the slightly broadened ridges of the primary and secondary folds. Microscopically (Fig. 32-7), in the connective tissue stalks of the folds are many large mononuclear cells with doubly refractile lipoid substances (cholesterol esters) in their cytoplasm (cholesterolosis, p. 1450). Electron microscopic studies reveal that the cholesterol accumulates mainly in the foam

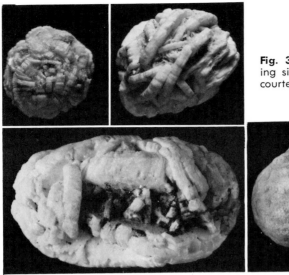

Fig. 32-6. Crystalline cholesterol stones of varying sizes, each from a different gallbladder. (2×; courtesy Dr. Malcolm A. Hyman, New York, N.Y.)

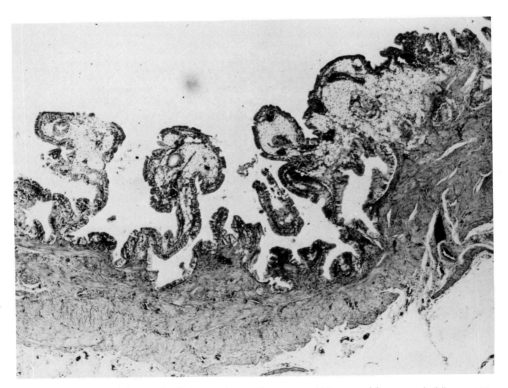

Fig. 32-7. Gallbladder with cholesterolosis of mucosa (46-year-old woman). Viscus contained crystalline cholesterol stone. In cross section from near neck, folds are enlarged and rounded. Connective tissue stalks contain many large mononuclear cells with light-stained cytoplasm and eccentric nuclei. These cells contain anisotropic lipoid substances that can be demonstrated by fat stains. (60×.)

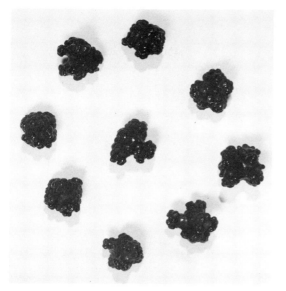

Fig. 32-8. Calcium bilirubinate calculi from gallbladder (78-year-old black man).

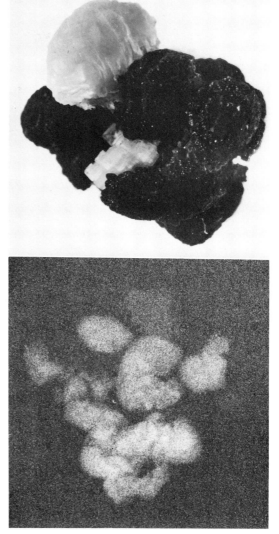

Fig. 32-9. "Paired" pure gallstone from gallbladder (41-year-old woman). Calculus 0.9 cm in diameter. Attached to black calcium bilirubinate concretion are clusters of crystalline cholesterol. Calcium bilirubinate portion radiopaque. (Courtesy Dr. Malcolm A. Hyman, New York, N.Y.)

cells and that microphages most probably participate in its transport from the epithelium into the lamina propria.[57]

The *calcium bilirubinate stones* are encountered less frequently than are the crystalline cholesterol stones. Usually, the former are multiple, jet black, with the shape of jackstones, and rarely over 1 cm in diameter (Fig. 32-8). Some are firm and preserve their shape. Others are fragile and readily crumble into small fragments. Their calcium content renders them radiopaque. The principal factor in the production of calcium bilirubinate calculi appears to be an intermittent or continuous increase in the bilirubin content of the blood serum attributable to hemolysis from whatever case.[53] Hereditary defects in the erythrocytes such as are assumed to occur in hemolytic icterus and sickle-cell anemia[64] probably play a role in some instances. In others, hemolysis may be caused by hemolysins (antibodies or chemicals) or by infections (malaria).

A "paired" pure gallstone composed of calcium bilirubinate and crystalline cholesterol has been observed (Fig. 32-9).

The *calcium carbonate stone* is the rarest of the pure gallstones (Fig. 32-10). It is usually grayish white and amorphous.[47] The source of the calcium is undetermined, and the appearance of such calculous material in the bile is not related to any known distur-

bance of calcium metabolism. Its precipitation may be caused by changes in the pH of the gallbladder content. The relation between the amorphous calcium carbonate calculus and the precipitation of a paste of lime salts, "milk of calcium bile," still remains to be investigated.[59]

Mixed gallstones. About 80% of the biliary calculi in surgically removed gallbladders are mixed gallstones; i.e., they are composed in varying proportions of all three of the stone-

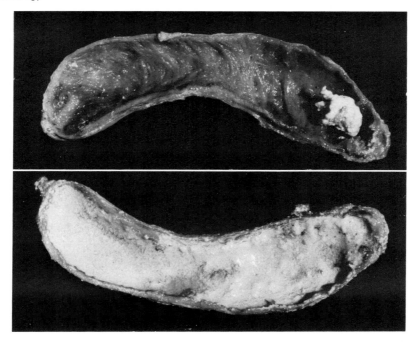

Fig. 32-10. Calcium carbonate stone and "lime paste" in gallbladder (34-year-old man).

forming constituents of the bile. They form when the function of the gallbladder is so altered that the solvents (bile acids) are resorbed faster than the stone-forming substances they hold in solution. This creates opportunities in the gallbladder for further concentration, precipitation, and crystallization of these substances. Mixed gallstones have the greatest variety in size, number, external appearance, and structure. They vary from 0.1 to 2 cm in diameter and are always multiple. When they are small, several thousands of them may be contained in a single gallbladder.[63] Their surfaces usually are faceted, with adjacent stones articulating (Fig. 32-11). Some mixed gallstones have a lobulated surface with the contour of a mulberry. These are twisted, petrified, and broken-off polypoid projections of the gallbladder mucosa that contained lipoid substances (Fig. 32-12). They usually are about 0.5 cm in diameter and rarely reach the size of 1 cm.

The appearance and structure of mixed gallstones depend largely on their chemical composition. Cholesterol lends a yellow hue, calcium bilirubinate a black hue, and calcium carbonate a white hue. Predominance of the color is a fair indication of the chemical composition. Accordingly, mixed gallstones may be grouped as having a predominant content of cholesterol and calcium bilirubinate (yellow

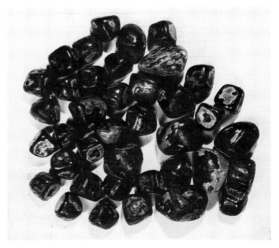

Fig. 32-11. Mixed gallstones from gallbladder (68-year-old black man). Calculi of almost equal size with articulating faceted surfaces. Black with lighter black-brown centers.

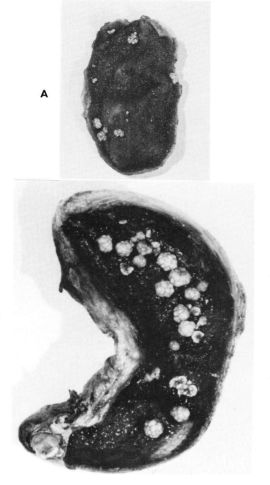

Fig. 32-12. Mixed gallstones, mulberry type. **A,** Gallbladder (46-year-old man). Petrified polypoid projections attached to mucosa (natural size). **B,** Gallbladder (42-year-old man). Calculi have same appearance and composition as polypoid projections in **A.**

and black), of cholesterol and calcium carbonate (yellow and white), of calcium bilirubinate and calcium carbonate (black and white), or of cholesterol, calcium bilirubinate, and calcium carbonate (yellow, black, and white).

Radiopacity of mixed gallstones depends on their calcium content in the form of calcium bilirubinate, calcium carbonate, or both. When the calcium content is high and the calculi are large enough or numerous enough, they cast a shadow without the aid of cholecystography.

The mode of the formation of mixed gall-stones appears to be more complicated than that of pure gallstones. It seems certain that disturbance of the resorptive activity of the gallbladder plays a leading part. Electron microscopic studies of gallbladders from patients with chronic cholecystitis and chole-lithiasis revealed a tendency for the epithelium to assume a secretory rather than the usual absorptive function.[38] Whether a disturbance that allows resorption of the solvents faster than that of the stone-forming constituents is alone responsible for the formation of mixed gallstones is uncertain. A coincidental increase in stone-forming substances in the bile would certainly accelerate the formation of mixed gallstones and would determine the relative amounts of the various components. It is also uncertain whether the process causing the mixed gallstones to form is also the cause of the chronic cholecystitis that is almost always observed in a gallbladder containing mixed gallstones. It is, however, more likely that chronic cholecystitis itself is the principal cause of the formation of mixed gallstones.

Combined gallstones. About 10% of the biliary calculi in surgically removed gallbladders are combined gallstones; i.e., they are composed of a combination of the ingredients of pure and mixed gallstones, with the one forming the nucleus and the other the shell. They form when the two principal conditions favorable to the formation of gallstones prevail in one or the other sequence. Most commonly, the combined gallstone is solitary, and its nucleus is a pure cholesterol stone; the shell, any one of the mixed gallstones. In some instances, in addition to the large combined stone, a crop of smaller mixed gallstones having the same composition as the shell of the large stone is present in the same gallbladder. Calcium bilirubinate stones may acquire a shell of mixed stone. Conversely, mixed gallstones may acquire shells composed of cholesterol or of calcium bilirubinate or of calcium carbonate. A solitary combined gallstone attains the largest size, sometimes filling the entire lumen of the viscus. The gallbladder containing a combined gallstone or combined gallstones always discloses evidences of chronic cholecystitis, not unlike gallbladders containing mixed gallstones.

Incidence. Cholelithiasis rarely is observed in the first and second decades of life.[60] Mixed gallstones occur about four times more frequently in women than in men. The child-bearing period in its second half appears to predispose to cholelithiasis. Combined gallstones occur more frequently in the older age groups.[52]

Effects. Calculi within the gallbladder need not produce clinical manifestations. This is true particularly of pure gallstones (the crystalline cholesterol stone and the calcium bilirubinate stones). Their presence, however, may induce chronic cholecystitis, or acute cholecystitis with appropriate clinical signs and symptoms.

A solitary cholesterol stone in the gallbladder may float in the bile and become imprisoned in the neck between the folds of Heister. This occurs only after the cystic duct has become permanently dilated to several times its usual diameter. The dilatation is brought about by prolonged closure of the common bile duct into the duodenum causing increased pressure in the biliary ducts. Bile produced against increased pressure contains little or no coloring matter (white bile). After the biliary ducts have reached a state of distention, valvelike action of the stone imprisoned in the neck may permit passage of bile into the viscus (hydrops of the gallbladder). A predisposition to the formation of white bile exists in a patient whose cystic duct has a low insertion and whose common bile duct therefore is short. A pure gallstone imprisoned in the neck of the gallbladder, producing intermittent distention of the viscus by its ball-valve action, may cause only transient discomfort in the right upper abdomen. Later, a chronic inflammatory reaction develops, interfering with the resorptive function of the viscus. Thereafter, three clinical courses are possible: the gallbladder becomes nonfunctioning and no signs and symptoms of cholecystic disease appear; or signs and symptoms of chronic cholecystitis develop; or, if bacterial invasion occurs, empyema of the gallbladder develops.

Calcium bilirubinate stones and calcium carbonate precipitates are usually silent; i.e., they produce no clinical manifestations whatsoever.[62]

Mixed gallstones are contained in gallbladders with chronic cholecystitis. The cystic duct of such a gallbladder is always enlarged to several times its usual diameter. This occurs because of intermittently increased intravesical pressure. As a result of this intravesical hypertension, there develops hypertrophy of the muscular coat, with outpouchings of the mucosa toward the external layers producing the Rokitansky-Aschoff sinuses.[41] The dilatation of the cystic duct with eventual incompetence

of its folds at times allows passage of mixed calculi from the gallbladder into the common bile duct, causing obstruction of the flow of bile into the duodenum. The clinical manifestations produced by the passage of gallstones are intense pain in the right upper abdomen, often radiating to the right shoulder, and sometimes associated mild fever and leukocytosis. A gradually deepening jaundice with clay-colored stools occurs after obstruction of the common bile duct.

Combined gallstone or gallstones, like mixed gallstones, are contained in gallbladders with chronic cholecystitis. A gallbladder with a large combined gallstone may become fused with the duodenum or with the transverse colon, causing a communication between the gallbladder and the duodenum or the colon. Through a cholecystoduodenal fistula, the calculus may pass from the gallbladder into the duodenum and onward through the jejunum; and, if of sufficient size, it may cause obstruction in the narrow portion of the ileum.[48,49] Communication with the colon opens a way for retrograde infection of the gallbladder and biliary ducts.

The presence of any kind of gallstones in the gallbladder predisposes to the development of acute cholecystitis. In a gallbladder containing mixed or combined stones, the acute process is superimposed on an already existing chronic cholecystitis. In such patients the possible passage of calculi into the biliary ducts or intestine may result in obstruction and is an additional hazard. Although any kind of gallstones may at times be silent, the presence of mixed or combined stones is a valid indication for surgical removal of the viscus.

Cholesterolosis. When the cholesterol content of the bile is within physiologic limits, resorption of the cholesterol apparently leaves no demonstrable trace in the mucosa of the gallbladder. When there is an increased cholesterol content, the folds of the mucosa of the gallbladder become streaked with yellow, suggesting the pattern of the surface of a ripe strawberry ("strawberry gallbladder").[54] This condition precedes and is usually concomitant with the presence of the crystalline cholesterol stone and also is observed with mixed gallstones having high cholesterol content. This cholesterolosis may be seen in otherwise normal gallbladders containing no calculi, in gallbladders containing a crystalline cholesterol stone, and in gallbladders with chronic cholecystitis containing mixed or combined gallstones. Up to 20% of all gallbladders removed surgically disclose some degree of cholesterolosis.

Cholecystography. Visualization of the gallbladder by means of radiopaque substances may reveal whether the resorptive function of the viscus is intact or impaired. Occasionally, the Rokitansky-Aschoff sinuses may be visualized.[55] Cholecystography also may disclose anomalies in the shape and position of the gallbladder and the presence of gallstones and occasionally of neoplasms.[56,73,75]

Among the biliary calculi, the crystalline cholesterol stone is nonopaque. It may occasionally visualize as a negative shadow in the opaque medium filling the viscus. Calcium bilirubinate stones are radiopaque and, if of sufficient size and number, may cast a shadow without any contrast medium. The radiopacity of mixed gallstones depends on their calcium content. Their visualization with the aid of a contrast medium may be unsuccessful because of the usually impaired resorptive function of the gallbladder. Combined gallstones usually visualize without the aid of cholecystography (scout film).

Neoplasms

In the extrahepatic biliary ducts, neoplasms are rarely encountered.[70] They are more frequent in the gallbladder.

Papilloma, adenoma, and adenomyoma

Soft projections on the mucosa of the gallbladder, papillomas,[65,77] may occur singly or in groups or may be scattered over a large part of the surface. The cauliflower-like, or seaweed-like, readily movable projection is composed microscopically of delicate or coarse connective tissue stalks covered by columnar epithelium like that of the rest of the mucosa. In the connective tissue stalks, there may be infiltrations with large mononuclear cells filled with doubly refractile lipoid substances. Sometimes these projections may become inspissated, petrified, twisted, or broken off and form the center or framework of berry-like mixed calculi. The papillomas are not precursors of, nor do they predispose to, carcinoma of the gallbladder. However, the possibility of malignant change in a preexisting neoplasm cannot be entirely dismissed.[76]

Adenoma is a low, flat elevation on the mucosal surface, usually of the body of the gallbladder, causing some thickening of the wall. Microscopically, acinar tubular structures lined by cuboid or columnar epithelium are within a scanty connective tissue stroma.

Some of the acini may open into the lumen of the viscus. They do not usually extend into the muscular coat. An adenoma is not a precursor of carcinoma.

Adenomyoma occurs on or near the fundus, causing slight thickening in that region.[65,66] Microscopically, there is a system of acinar tubular structures lined by cuboid or columnar cells in a scanty connective tissue stroma between interlacing smooth muscle bundles (Fig. 32-13). Adenomyomas are malformations rather than neoplasms. They probably represent the anlage either of a part of the fundus that did not develop or of the fundus of an undeveloped bifid or bilobed gallbladder.

Carcinoma

Carcinoma of the extrahepatic biliary ducts usually arises in either of the hepatic ducts, near their junction, or in the common hepatic or common bile ducts, where the cystic duct branches off, or at the papilla of Vater.[78] When the carcinoma involves the intraduodenal portion of the common bile duct, it is frequently difficult or impossible to determine whether the growth originated in the common bile duct, in the papilla of Vater, in the pancreas, or in the duodenum proper.[71] Although carcinoma of the head of the pancreas usually obstructs the common bile duct, possible origin of the carcinoma in the other sites is to be considered. Carcinomas of the biliary ducts produce a local stiffening, thickening, distortion of the wall, and gradual obstruction of the lumen of the duct without necessarily involving its entire circumference. The growth usually enlarges by direct extension and spreads to regional lymph nodes. After obstruction of the common bile duct occurs, jaundice appears. When the obstruction is gradual, the proximal tributaries, including the intrahepatic biliary ducts, become dilated, with the eventual production of "white bile" (hydrohepatosis).[68] While still small, these carcinomas cause obstruction, and the patient develops jaundice early and usually dies with cachexia. Practically all carcinomas of the extrahepatic biliary ducts, like those of the intrahepatic biliary ducts, are columnar cell carcinomas.[69] They exhibit considerable variation in the height of the cells lining the acinar tubular structures or covering papillary projections (Fig. 32-14). The degree of differentiation of the cells, the number of cells in a state of division, and the amount and character of the stroma also vary in the individual growths.

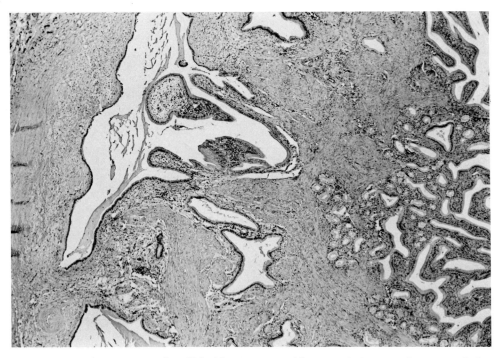

Fig. 32-13. Adenomyoma of gallbladder (56-year-old woman). System of acinar tubular structures lined by cuboid or columnar cells in scanty connective tissue stroma between interlacing smooth muscle bundles. (32×; courtesy Dr. Malcolm A. Hyman, New York, N.Y.)

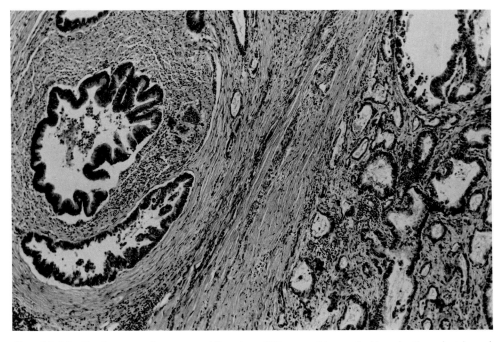

Fig. 32-14. Carcinoma of common bile duct (83-year-old man). Neoplastic cuboid and columnar cells form acinar tubular structures or are mounted on delicate connective tissue stalks. Neoplastic cells are within sheath of nerve. There was complete obstruction of common bile duct, but no involvement of regional lymph nodes and no distant metastasis. (60×.)

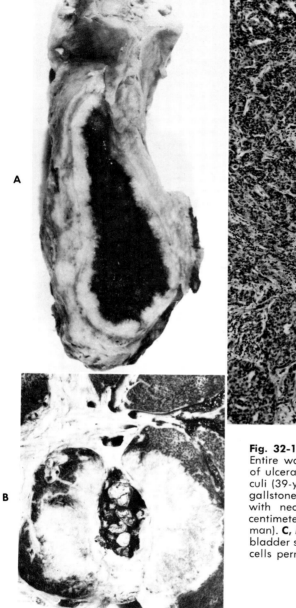

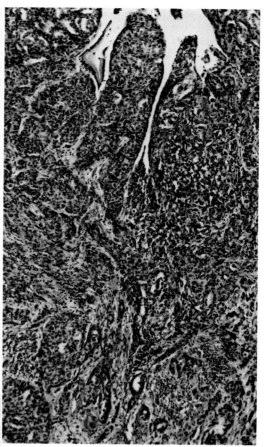

Fig. 32-15. **A** to **C**, Carcinoma of gallbladder. **A**, Entire wall diffusely involved with multiple areas of ulceration in mucosa. Viscus contained no calculi (39-year-old man). **B**, Lumen filled with mixed gallstones that are faceted. Wall of viscus blends with neoplastic tissue that forms crust several centimeters thick about gallbladder (55-year-old man). **C**, Microscopic appearance of growth in gallbladder shown in **A**. Sheets of neoplastic epithelial cells permeate entire thickness of wall. (60×.)

Carcinoma of the gallbladder[67,72,74] usually originates in the fundus or neck of the viscus and occasionally in the cystic duct. It infiltrates the viscus locally, causing thickening and stiffening of the wall at the site of involvement. It may involve the entire gallbladder (Fig. 32-15, *A*). Some growths protrude into the lumen as irregular, small or bulky, firm or soft masses. More frequently, the growth infiltrates the entire viscus and by direct extension involves the liver about the fossa of the gallbladder, forming a crust, several centimeters thick, of solid neoplastic tissue (Fig. 32-15, *B*). In rare instances in which the entire wall is diffusely involved with multiple areas of ulceration in the mucosa, the extension of the growth is toward the porta hepatis and down the course of the common bile duct, involving the pancreas and duodenum as well. It is estimated that in about 90% of carcinomas of the gallbladder there is cholelithiasis. This has led to the assertion that cholelithiasis predisposes to the development of carcinoma of the gallbladder.

Microscopically, over 90% of carcinomas of the gallbladder are columnar cell carcinomas. Their pattern and structure are similar to those of carcinomas that occur in the biliary ducts. Neoplastic columnar cells of varying heights are mounted on delicate connective tissue stalks or form acinar tubular structures in a scanty or more abundant, loose or dense, fibrous connective tissue stroma (Fig. 32-15, *C*). Occasionally, the columnar cells produce mucin in abundance. In rare instances, the mucin-producing cells have a signet-ring appearance. Occasionally, a squamous cell carcinoma is encountered in the gallbladder and, quite rarely, the growth may be a columnar cell and squamous cell carcinoma (adenoacanthoma).

Anomalies

Some of the anomalies of the extrahepatic biliary ducts[83,85] are incompatible with extrauterine existence. Anomalies of the gallbladder usually do not interfere with its function. Hypoplasia to the degree of stenosis or atresia of the lumen of the common bile duct is sometimes seen in newborn infants. A large cystlike outpouching of the common bile duct (idiopathic cyst) has been observed and in some instances, successfully removed.[84] Variations occur in the number of the hepatic ducts and in the manner of their junction with one another and with the cystic duct. Variations occur also in the manner of distribution of the arteries.[82]

There may be no anlage for the gallbladder, resulting in absence (agenesis) of the viscus, or there may be a double anlage, resulting in partial or complete duplication. Both conditions are rare. Bilobed, double, and septate fundi appear in man but are more common in animals, particularly cats.[79] A "stocking cap" reflection with a septum protruding into the lumen is observed in about 5% of gallbladders. Sometimes, the septum is near the center, giving the viscus the shape of a dumbbell. Variations in form, size, and peritoneal relations are frequent. The gallbladder may be small and end several centimeters short of the inferior margin of the liver (hypoplasia). In such instances, the cystic duct is usually short, while the common bile duct is long. The reverse is usually true of large gallbladders. The cystic duct runs parallel with the common bile duct, sometimes for a distance of several centimeters, and is fused with it, being separated only by a septum. Usually, about half of the surface of the human gallbladder is covered by peritoneum. Rarely, the entire circumference is surrounded by liver tissue. Occasionally, the viscus is covered by peritoneum with a mesentery-like peritoneal attachment. All transitions between these two extremes may be observed. In rare instances, a small accessory lobe completely detached from the liver is encountered on the surface of the gallbladder.[80] It has been inferred that there is a relation between such an accessory lobe of liver and aberrant bile ducts (Luschka ducts)[39] in the perimuscular layer of the gallbladder. Other heterotopic structures, such as pancreatic and thyroid tissue or gastric and intestinal epithelium, also have been observed.[81,86]

REFERENCES
General

1 Aschoff, L., and Bacmeister, A.: Die Cholelithiasis, Jena, 1909, Gustav Fischer.
2 Bockus, H. L.: Gastroenterology, Philadelphia, 1946, W. B. Saunders Co.
3 Graham, E. A., Cole, W. H., Copher, G. H., and Moore, S.: Diseases of the gallbladder and bile ducts, Philadelphia, 1928, Lea & Febiger.
4 Hargreaves, T.: The liver and bile metabolism, New York, 1968, Appleton-Century-Crofts.
5 Lichtman, S. S.: Diseases of the liver, gallbladder and bile ducts, ed. 3, Philadelphia, 1953, Lea & Febiger.
6 Michels, N. A.: Blood supply and anatomy of the upper abdominal organs, Philadelphia, 1955, J. B. Lippincott Co.
7 Rolleston, H. D., and McNee, J. W.: Diseases of the liver, gallbladder and bile-ducts, ed. 3, London, 1929, The Macmillan Co.
8 Sherlock, S.: Diseases of the liver and biliary system, ed. 4, Oxford, 1968, Blackwell Scientific Publications.

9 With, T. K.: Bile pigments: chemical, biological, and clinical aspects (translated by J. P. Kennedy), New York, 1968, Academic Press, Inc.

Structure and function

10 Berti, A. D., and Posse, D. R.: Am. J. Roentgenol. **75:**354-359, 1956 (visualization of biliary ducts).

11 Bollman, J. L.: In Walters, W., and Snell, A. M., editors: Diseases of the gallbladder and bile ducts, Philadelphia, 1940, W. B. Saunders Co.

12 Boyden, E. A.: Anat. Rec. **40:**147-191, 1928 (reaction of gallbladder to food).

13 Boyden, E. A.: Surgery **1:**25-37, 1937 (sphincter of Oddi).

14 Einsel, I. H., and Einsel, T. H.: Am. J. Dig. Dis. **10:**206-208, 1943 (roentgenologic examination).

15 Gilleland, J. L., Gast, J. H., and Halpert, B.: Proc. Soc. Exp. Biol. Med. **94:**118-119, 1957.

16 Graham, E. A., and Cole, W. T.: J.A.M.A. **82:**613-614, 1924 (roentgenologic examination).

17 Halpert, B.: Bull. Johns Hopkins Hosp. **40:**390-408, 1927.

18 Halpert, B.: Arch. Surg. (Chicago) **19:**1037-1060, 1929.

19 Halpert, B.: Anat. Rec. **53:**83-102, 1932 (choledochoduodenal junction).

20 Halpert, B.: Proc. Soc. Exp. Biol. Med. **39:**115-119, 1938 (rate of bile flow).

21 Halpert, B., and Hanke, M. T.: Am. J. Physiol. **88:**351-361, 1929.

22 Halpert, B., and Lewis, J. H.: Am. J. Physiol. **93:**506-520, 1930.

23 Halpert, B., Russo, P. E., and Cushing, V. D.: Proc. Soc. Exp. Biol. Med. **63:**102-104, 1946 (roentgenologic studies).

24 Halpert, B., Thompson, W. R., and Marting, F. L.: Am. J. Physiol. **111:**31-34, 1935 (resorption).

25 Henley, F. A.: Br. J. Surg. **43:**75-80, 1955 (blood supply of common bile duct).

26 Lee, H., and Halpert, B.: Anat. Rec. **54:**29-43, 1932 (development).

27 Lyon, B. B. V.: Non-surgical drainage of gall tract, Philadelphia, 1923, Lea & Febiger.

28 Meltzer, S. J.: Am. J. Med. Sci. **153:**469-477, 1917.

29 Park, C. Y., Pae, Y. S., and Hong, S. S.: Ann. Surg. **171:**294-299, 1970 (radiologic studies).

30 Parke, W. W., Michels, N. A., and Ghosh, G. M.: Surg. Gynecol. Obstet. **117:**47-55, 1963.

31 Reinhold, J. G., and Ferguson, L. K.: J. Exp. Med. **49:**681-694, 1929 (reaction of bile).

32 Rous, P., and McMaster, P. D.: J. Exp. Med. **34:**47-73, 1921 (concentrating activity).

33 Sobotka, H.: Physiological chemistry of the bile, Baltimore, 1937, The Williams & Wilkins Co.

34 Sugiyama, Y.: Jap. J. Smooth Muscle Res. **8:**55-70, 1972 (gallbladder motility, photo-optical observations).

35 Thureborn, E.: Acta Chir. Scand. suppl. 303, pp. 1-63, 1962 (composition of human bile).

Lesions
Inflammations

36 Anderson, W. A. D.: Personal communication, 1953.

37 Bisgard, J. D., and Baker, C. P.: Ann. Surg. **112:**1006-1034, 1940 (pathogenesis).

38 Fox, H.: J. Pathol. **108:**157-164, 1972 (ultrastructure of gallbladder epithelium).

39 Halpert, B.: Bull. Johns Hopkins Hosp. **41:**77-103, 1927 (morphologic studies).

40 Halpert, B.: Surgery **33:**444-445, 1953 (editorial).

41 Halpert, B.: Am. J. Gastroenterol. **35:**534-539, 1961 (significance of Rokitansky-Aschoff sinuses).

42 Hou, P. C.: J. Pathol. Bacteriol. **70:**53-64, 1955 (*Clonorchis sinersis* infestation).

43 Mallory, T. B., and Lawson, G. M., Jr.: Am. J. Pathol. **7:**71-76, 1931 (typhoid cholecystitis).

44 Womack, N. A., and Bricker, E. M.: Arch. Surg. (Chicago) **44:**658-676, 1942 (pathogenesis).

Concretions

45 Andrews, E., Schoenheimer, R., and Hrdina, L.: Arch. Surg. (Chicago) **25:**796-810, 1932 (etiology).

46 Aschoff, L.: Lectures on pathology, New York, 1924, Paul B. Hoeber, Inc.

47 Báron, J.: Radiology **35:**741-742, 1940.

48 Buetow, G. W., and Crampton, R. S.: Arch. Surg. (Chicago) **86:**504-511, 1963.

49 Coffey, R. J., and Wilcox, G. D.: Am. Surg. **18:**286-296, 1952 (gallstone obstruction of intestinal tract).

50 Edwards, J. D., Jr., Adams, W. D., and Halpert, B.: Am. J. Clin. Pathol. **29:**236-238, 1958 (infrared spectrums).

51 Halpert, B.: Arch. Pathol. (Chicago) **6:**623-631, 1928 (classification).

52 Halpert, B., and Lawrence, K. B.: Surg. Gynecol. Obstet. **62:**43-49, 1936.

53 Illingworth, C. F. W.: Edinburgh Med. J. **43:**481-497, 1936 (pathogenesis).

54 Mackey, W. A.: Br. J. Surg. **28:**462-467, 1941 (cholesterolosis).

55 March, H. C.: Am. J. Roentgenol. **59:**197-203, 1948 (visualization of Rokitansky-Aschoff sinuses).

56 Moore, R. D.: Am. J. Roentgenol. **75:**360-365, 1956.

57 Nevalainen, T., and Laitio, M.: Virchows Arch. (Zellpathol.) **10:**237-242, 1972 (cholesterolosis; ultrastructure).

58 Ostrow, I. D.: J. Lab. Clin. Med. **78:**255-264, 1971 (absorption by injured gallbladder).

59 Phemister, D. B., Day, L., and Hastings, A. B.: Ann. Surg. **96:**595-614, 1932.

60 Potter, A. H.: Surg. Gynecol. Obstet. **66:**604-610, 1938 (young subjects).

61 Redinger, R. N., and Small, D. M.: Arch. Intern. Med. (Chicago) **130:**618-630, 1972 (bile composition, bile salt metabolism, and gallstones).

62 Robertson, H. E.: Gastroenterology **5:**345-372, 1945.

63 Schenken, J. R., and Coleman, F. C.: Gastroenterology **4:**344-346, 1945.

64 Weens, H. S.: Ann. Intern. Med. **22:**182-191, 1945 (in sickle-cell anemia).

Neoplasms

65 Bricker, D. L., and Halpert, B.: Surgery **53:**615-620, 1963.

66 Christensen, A. H., and Ishak, K. G.: Arch. Pathol. (Chicago) **90**:423-432, 1970 (tumors and pseudotumors).
67 Cooper, W. A.: Arch. Surg. (Chicago) **35**:431-448, 1937 (carcinoma).
68 Counseller, V. S., and McIndoe, A. H.: Surg. Gynecol. Obstet. **43**:729-740, 1926.
69 D'Aunoy, R., Ogden, M. A., and Halpert, B.: Surgery **3**:670-678, 1938 (carcinoma).
70 Gray, G. F., and McDivitt, R. W.: Pathol. Ann. **4**:231-251, 1969.
71 Heaney, J. P., Wise, R. A., and Halpert, B.: Cancer **4**:737-744, 1951.
72 Illingworth, C. F. W.: Br. J. Surg. **23**:4-18, 1935 (carcinoma).
73 Kirklin, B. R.: Am. J. Roentgenol. **29**:8-16, 1933 (roentgenologic examination).
74 Kirschbaum, J. D., and Kozoll, D. D.: Surg. Gynecol. Obstet. **73**:740-754, 1941 (carcinoma).
75 Ochsner, S., and Carrera, G. M.: Gastroenterology **31**:266-273, 1956.
76 Sawyer, K. C.: Am. J. Surg. **120**:570-578, 1970 (significance of papillomas, polyps, and adenomas).

77 Shepard, V. D., Walters, W., and Dockerty, M. B.: Arch. Surg. (Chicago) **45**:1-18, 1942.
78 Thorbjarnarson, B.: Cancer **12**:708-713, 1959 (carcinoma of bile ducts).

Anomalies

79 Boyden, E. A.: Am. J. Anat. **38**:177-222, 1926.
80 Cullen, T. S.: Arch. Surg. (Chicago) **11**:718-764, 1925.
81 Curtis, L. E., and Sheahan, D. G.: Arch. Pathol. **88**:677-683, 1969 (heterotopic tissues in gallbladder).
82 Grant, J. C. B.: An atlas of anatomy, ed. 5, Baltimore, 1962, The Williams & Wilkins Co.
83 Ladd, W. E.: Ann. Surg. **102**:742-751, 1935.
84 McWhorter, G. L.: Arch. Surg. (Chicago) **38**:397-411, 1939.
85 Redo, S. F.: Arch. Surg. (Chicago) **69**:886-897, 1954.
86 Williams, M. J., and Humm, J. J.: Surgery **34**:133-139, 1953.

33/Pancreas and diabetes mellitus

PAUL E. LACY
JOHN M. KISSANE

NORMAL FORM AND DEVELOPMENT

The human pancreas is an elongated gland that extends from the concavity of the duodenal loop obliquely cephalad and to the left in the retroperitoneal space at the level of the junction between the first and second lumbar vertebrae, toward the hilum of the spleen. The adult gland measures 12 to 15 cm in length and weighs 60 to 100 gm. The pancreas is subdivided into three topographic parts: (1) the head dorsoventrally flattened, lies in the concavity of the duodenum; the uncinate (hooklike) process projects ventromedially from the head of the pancreas to encompass the superior mesenteric artery and vein; (2) the body, the main portion of the gland; and (3) the thin, tapered tail extending toward the hilum of the spleen.

The pancreas is subdivided into rhomboid lobules by delicate connective tissue septa in which are found blood and lymphatic vessels, nerves, and ducts. The acini within the lobules are formed by pyramid-shaped acinar cells that contain numerous zymogen granules at their apices. Enzymes such as chymotrypsin, carboxypeptidase, and elastase have been demonstrated within individual zymogen granules by the fluorescent antibody technique. The basal portions of the acinar cells are basophilic and free of zymogen granules. Acini are intimately related to minute centroacinar ducts into which secretion products are discharged. Centroacinar ducts converge to form lobular ducts, which enter the major named pancreatic ducts. Islets possess no ductal system but release their secretory products, insulin, glucagon, gastrin, and perhaps others, directly into the circulation.

Ultrastructurally, zymogen granules appear as dense spheric structures encased within smooth membranous sacs. The basal portions of acinic cells are filled with a lamellar type of ergastoplasm with numerous ribonucleopro-

tein granules attached to the membranes. The ergastoplasm is responsible for the basophilic reaction of these cells. Recent electron microscopic and biochemical studies indicate that the zymogen granules are formed within the ergastoplasmic sacs, are subsequently transmitted to the Golgi zone where they apparently undergo further maturation, and finally move to the apical portion of the cell. After stimulation, the zymogen granules with their encompassing sacs move to the apical surface of the cell; the membranous sacs fuse with the plasma membrane and rupture, and the zymogen granules are liberated into the lumens of the acini. The acinar and ductal cells are firmly attached by distinct desmosomes that prevent the enzymes within the zymogen granules from passing into the interstitial tissue. The precise intracellular metabolic changes that initiate the migration and liberation of the zymogen granules are unknown.

Development. Among several segmental diverticula of the foregut that appear in 3 to 4 mm embryos, two persist and give rise to the definitive pancreas. The larger *dorsal pancreatic diverticulum* arises from the foregut just cephalad to the hepatic diverticulum and elongates to the left in the retroperitoneal space. The smaller *ventral pancreatic diverticulum* arises in the angle between the hepatic diverticulum and foregut and, after more rapid growth of the hepatic diverticulum, comes to arise from that structure. Differential growth rotates the developing duodenum to the right and shifts the ventral pancreatic anlage into the dorsal mesentery, where it fuses with the dorsal anlage and contributes the uncinate process and most of the head to the definitive organ.

Each pancreatic anlage possesses an axial duct. The distal end of the duct of the ventral pancreas ordinarily anastomoses with the duct of the dorsal pancreas and, as the duct

1457

of Wirsung, provides the major drainage for pancreatic secretions into the duodenum at the major duodenal papilla (of Vater). Distal to the point of anastomosis with the duct of Wirsung, the duct of the dorsal pancreas persists in about half of all individuals and, as the duct of Santorini, enters the duodenum at the minor duodenal papilla cephalad to the major papilla. In about 10% of individuals, the duct of the ventral pancreas regresses, and the duct of Santorini provides the entire drainage into the duodenum. These relationships are important in the pathogenesis of acute pancreatitis (see p. 1462).

Pancreatic acini appear initially as buds from the ducts and subsequently differentiate into acinar cells containing zymogen granules. Lumens of the acini retain communication with the centroacinar ducts that converge and form a passageway for exocrine secretions of the pancreas into the duodenum. The islets of Langerhans also develop from the outer surfaces of the ultimate radicles of the pancreatic ducts. Solid masses of islet cells detach from the ducts and are vascularized by capillary sprouts. The first islets to be formed, primary islets, contain specific granules of beta cells as well as of delta cells. Insulin and several pancreatic enzymes have been identified very early in the primordial pancreas of rat embryos.[3] During the last 6 months of embryonic development, the primary islets undergo degeneration, and a second generation of islet tissue originates from the ductal cells. Both primary and secondary islets arise from ductal tissue, not from acinar cells.

ABNORMALITIES OF FORM AND DEVELOPMENT
Annular pancreas

Annular pancreas results from failure of rotation of the ventral pancreas. When the ventral pancreas fuses with the dorsal, it therefore forms a ring of pancreatic tissue that envelops the second portion of the duodenum. Usually the encirclement is complete, but occasionally a gap may be found anteriorly. In children, an annular pancreas may be associated with atresia or stenosis of the duodenum that results in intestinal obstruction.[7] In adults, an annular pancreas usually produces no symptoms, although in some instances duodenal obstruction, peptic ulceration, and pancreatitis may be present. The relationship of annular pancreas to these symptoms is not clearly understood.

Ectopic pancreas

Pancreatic tissue may be found in the gastrointestinal tract in loci other than its normal anatomic area. The most common locations of ectopic pancreas are the duodenum, stomach, jejunum, and Meckel's diverticulum. Usually, nodules of ectopic pancreatic tissue are small, less than 1 cm in diameter, located in the submucosa as circumscribed, mobile masses of firm yellow-white lobular tissue superficially suggesting a neoplasm. Microscopically, the masses consist of normal-appearing pancreatic tissue, often including islets of Langerhans. Usually, pancreatic heterotopias are asymptomatic. Rarely, such masses may produce pyloric or duodenal obstruction, lead an

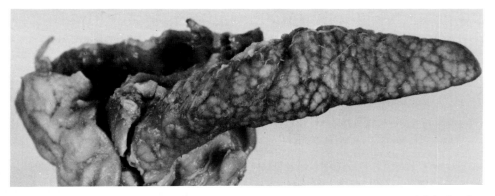

Fig. 33-1. Pancreas from child with cystic fibrosis showing accentuation of lobules but general preservation of size and contour of organ. (From Kissane, J. M., and Smith, M. G.: Pathology of infancy and childhood, ed. 2, St. Louis, 1975, The C. V. Mosby Co.)

intussusception, ulcerate and bleed, or serve as the site for an ectopic islet cell neoplasm.

Cystic fibrosis

Cystic fibrosis (fibrocystic disease) of the pancreas is a hereditary disorder characterized by increased viscosity of mucous secretions, including those of the pancreas, intestinal glands, tracheal and bronchial glands, and mucous salivary glands, and by increased concentrations of electrolytes, especially sodium and chloride, in secretions of other glands, notably eccrine sweat glands and also parotid salivary glands. The disease is transmitted as a mendelian recessive trait with clinical consequences only in homozygotes. The frequency of heterozygous carriers in most white populations must range between 2% and 5%. Factors that contribute toward maintaining this very high gene frequency despite the virtually lethal aspect of the homozygous state may include an as yet uncharacterized reproductive advantage in heterozygotes. Cystic fibrosis has been referred to as the commonest hereditary disease in white populations.[18] The disease is very rare in blacks and almost unknown in Orientals. It is responsible for approximately 5% of all deaths in infants and children who are born alive. Meticulous clinical management has conspicuously improved the prognosis of the disease so that approximately half of affected individuals reach adulthood.

The nature of the basic biologic defect in cystic fibrosis is not known.[16a,19a] The initially attractive hypothesis that the essential disorder consists of increased viscosity of mucous secretions gave rise to the early designation "mucoviscidosis" but could not be supported when more widespread disturbances, including those of eccrine sweat glands and serous glands such as parotid salivary glands, were discovered. Lines of investigation of the basic defect in cystic fibrosis are currently directed in four, not necessarily exclusive, directions.

Biochemical composition of mucous secretions

Although results are not unanimous, the consensus is that mucous secretions of many origins from patients with cystic fibrosis are higher in the ratio of fucose to sialic acid than are secretions of normal individuals. Further information regarding a defect in biosynthesis of mucoid secretions is not available.

Autonomic function

Many of the deviations from normal in the eccrine secretions of patients with cystic fibrosis resemble those that result from exhaustive parasympathetic stimulation of normal secretory mechanisms. Such nonsecretory autonomic mechanisms as the speed of pupillary mydriasis in the dark appear to be impaired in patients with cystic fibrosis.[30]

Electrolyte-concentrating mechanism

In the normal formation of sweat, a solution with composition essentially that of an ultrafiltrate of plasma accumulates in the coiled portions of eccrine sweat glands. Preferential absorption of sodium and chloride in excess of water from the duct results in the excretion of the normally hypotonic sweat. Micropuncture studies[26] suggest that primary secretion in the coil is normal in those with cystic fibrosis and that defective absorption of solute from the duct results in hypertonicity of the sweat. Recently, diminished resorption of sodium and chloride has been demonstrated in rat parotid glands perfused with sweat from patients with cystic fibrosis.[26] Sweat from normal children had no effect on the absorptive mechanism.

Effect on ciliary motility

Asynchronous and uncoordinated ciliary motility has been observed in cultured explants of rat tracheal mucosa exposed to serum from patients with cystic fibrosis. The factor responsible for this disturbance in ciliary motility is heat labile and nondialyzable. Similar effects were produced by sera from some parents of patients with cystic fibrosis.[32]

Metachromasia in cultured fibroblasts

Recent studies have demonstrated that cultured fibroblasts from patients with cystic fibrosis elaborate metachromatic material either as discrete cytoplasmic granules or as diffuse cytoplasmic metachromasia. Cultured fibroblasts from parents and other relatives of patients showed the same type of metachromasia.[18]

Clinical features

Clinical features of cystic fibrosis are highly variable, even among affected siblings. From 10% to 15% of affected individuals present in the newborn period with intestinal, usually distal ileal, obstruction by chalky masses of inspissated intestinal contents, *me-*

conium ileus. The frequency of associated ileal atresia supports an acquired mechanism for intestinal atresia. Intestinal perforation *in utero* with production of sterile meconium peritonitis may occur. Acute or episodic intestinal obstruction beyond infancy is increasingly reported as "meconium ileus equivalent."

Failure to gain weight despite adequate appetite, nonspecific feeding problems, steatorrhea, or other manifestations of intestinal malabsorption characterized one fourth to one third of all patients with cystic fibrosis. Rectal prolapse occurs in as many as one sixth of all patients. Heat prostration may be an early manifestation. In older children, ascites, bleeding from esophageal varices, or unexplained splenomegaly may be the first symptoms of cystic fibrosis.

Beyond infancy, respiratory complications are by far the commonest manifestations of cystic fibrosis and comprise its chief threat to life. Recurrent bouts of pneumonia, bronchiolitis, or bronchitis are usual but not invariable manifestations of the disease. Signs and symptoms of chronic respiratory insufficiency or of right ventricular failure occasionally may precede any indication of infection of the lower respiratory tract. The finding of inflammatory nasal polyps in the upper respiratory tract of a prepubertal child compels consideration of the diagnosis of cystic fibrosis.

Pathologic changes

Most pathologic changes in fibrocystic disease are interpretable as secondary to obstruction by abnormally viscid mucus in a variety of viscera.

Pancreas. The pancreas is almost never normal in cystic fibrosis, although the degree of pancreatic involvement varies widely from case to case and correlates only crudely with age. Grossly, especially in infancy, the pancreas may appear deceptively normal (Fig. 33-1). Close examination even then, however, may disclose an almost too tidy demarcation of lobules and an increase in consistency. Later, pancreatic lobules come to assume an ovoid rather than a rhomboid or polyhedral contour and to bulge from the cut surface. Ultimately, the pancreas, still preserving relatively normal size and contour, represents gross fatty replacement of parenchyma. Fibrosis is

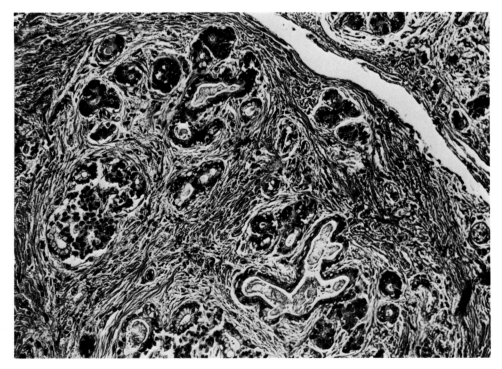

Fig. 33-2. Pancreas in cystic fibrosis showing dilated centrilobular ducts containing laminated concretions. Acini almost totally replaced by fibrous tissue that still reflects lobular pattern of organ.

rarely pronounced grossly, and macroscopic cysts are rarely discernible.

Microscopically, acinar atrophy and interlobular fibrosis are far out of proportion to the gross abnormality. Centroacinar ducts frequently contain laminated, eosinophilic concretions, and distal to these, acini are conspicuously atrophic although stromal recapitulation of lobular architecture may be well preserved (Fig. 33-2). Islets persist until late in the evolution of the disease. Inflammation, fat necrosis, and pseudocyst formation are rarely prominent.

Intestine. In 12% to 15% of patients with cystic fibrosis, intestinal obstruction occurs in the newborn period. The obstructing lesion in *meconium ileus* is a plug of chalky, inspissated meconium in the distal ileum. Ileal atresia, volvulus, or perforation with the development of meconium peritonitis may occur secondarily, and total intestinal length usually is shortened. The occurrence of meconium ileus correlates more with dilatation of intestinal glands by inspissated mucus secretions than with the extent of pancreatic lesions.

Attention has been called to the occurrence of peptic ulcers in patients with cystic fibrosis.[15] Above-normal frequency of peptic ulcer in parents of patients with cystic fibrosis has been claimed.

Respiratory tract. In a typical case, the lungs present gross compensatory overexpansion anteriorly, alternating posteriorly with areas of atelectasis and overt consolidation. Bronchi are dilated and contain inspissated mucopurulent exudate. Dilated small bronchi containing similar material usually can be appreciated in the centers of consolidated pulmonary lobules. Microscopically, the pulmonary lesion is a purulent bronchitis and bronchiolitis with resulting bronchiectasis and bronchiolectasis accompanied by a limited peribronchiolar pneumonia. Parenchymatous purulent necrosis with abscess formation is distinctly unusual. (See also p. 1084.)

Larynx, trachea, and major bronchi show chronic inflammation, often with foci of squamous metaplasia. Submucous glands are distended with inspissated secretions. In the upper respiratory tract, inflammatory nasal polyps may be found.

Liver. The liver is usually of normal size. Significant fatty metamorphosis is not common. Focal stellate areas of portal fibrosis and ductular proliferation may be seen, occasionally sufficiently extensive to justify the designation *focal biliary cirrhosis*. The lesion may produce portal hypertension with its consequences—ascites, congestive splenomegaly, and gastroesophageal varices (p. 1395).

Sweat glands. In view of the constancy and diagnostic importance of hypersecretion of sodium and chloride in the sweat, microscopic alterations in sweat glands are disappointingly scanty. Munger et al.[27] described diminished vacuolation of mucoid cells.

Reproductive system. The frequent finding of azoospermia in postpubertal males with cystic fibrosis is attributable to discontinuity of the male sex ducts. There is no anatomic correlate for the high maternal mortality among pregnant women with cystic fibrosis.

PANCREATITIS

Inflammation of the pancreas constitutes a spectrum of disorders that ranges from acute hemorrhagic pancreatitis, a prostrating, catastrophic disease with a high mortality, to chronic relapsing pancreatitis, a disorder characterized by recurring episodes of upper abdominal pain and eventual pancreatic insufficiency. Elaborate clinical systems of classification reflect the tendency of the disorder to recur.

Acute hemorrhagic pancreatitis

Acute hemorrhagic pancreatitis is almost entirely a disease of adults between 40 and 70 years of age, slightly commoner in females than in males. The onset is abrupt and calamitous, often occurring after a heavy meal or an alcoholic debauch. Severe epigastric pain, especially radiating to the back, nausea, vomiting, and shock are prominent clinical features. Peculiar ecchymotic mottling of the skin of the flanks, Grey-Turner spots, may be seen in severe cases. Early in the disease, pancreatic enzymes are liberated into the bloodstream, and increased levels of amylase and lipase in the serum are important in establishing the diagnosis. The mortality, even with vigorous supportive measures, is between 15% and 25%.

Pathologic changes. In the first few days, the pancreas is swollen and edematous. After a day or two, friable foci of necrosis appear, followed by interstitial hemorrhage that varies from reddish reticulation between pancreatic lobules to obliteration of grossly recognizable pancreatic tissue in a massive retroperitoneal hematoma. Foci of fat necrosis in the peripancreatic tissue, mesentery, and omentum appear rapidly as small ovoid yellow-white

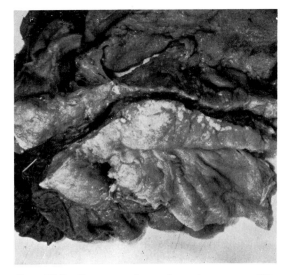

Fig. 33-3. Fat necrosis and acute pancreatitis. White opaque areas represent fat necrosis. Small white rod is in duct opening into duodenum.

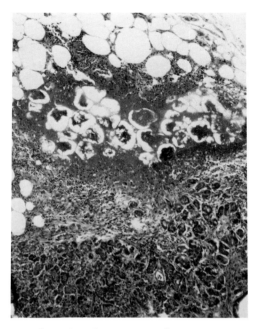

Fig. 33-4. Fat necrosis of pancreas.

nodules of pasty, gritty material (Fig. 33-3). The peritoneal cavity usually contains a moderate effusion of turbid rusty fluid with high amylase activity. Rarely, remote adipose tissues such as subcutaneous fat and fatty marrow may contain foci of necrosis attributable to lipolysis by enzymes borne in the plasma.

Very early in the disease, the pancreas microscopically shows only interstitial edema. Later, the pancreas contains patches of coagulative necrosis rimmed by infiltrates of polymorphonuclear leukocytes (Fig. 33-4). Still later, necrosis of arteries and arterioles is responsible for gross hemorrhages. Veins often are thrombosed. Eventually, as bacteria lodge in the necrotic pancreas, either via the ducts or the bloodstream, frank suppuration may occur.

A late complication of acute pancreatitis is the occasional development of a pseudocyst— an accumulation of enzyme-rich fluid, necrotic debris, and altered blood confined, not by an epithelial capsule, but by retroperitoneal connective tissue, adherent upper abdominal viscera, and the peritoneal components of the lesser omental sac. Pancreatic pseudocysts also may occur after blunt trauma to the abdomen.

Pathogenesis. The destructive changes that occur in the pancreas can be attributed to the liberation and activation of the proteolytic and lipolytic enzymes normally secreted by this organ. Active proteolytic enzymes such as trypsin and elastase produce necrosis of blood vessels, with resultant thrombosis and hemorrhage. Lipase liberated into the interstitial tissue causes necrosis of adipose tissue and the breakdown of triglycerides into fatty acids. Fatty acids combine with calcium in the interstitial tissue to form insoluble calcium soaps. This may produce a significant decrease in the level of serum calcium and lead to symptoms of hypocalcemia.

The pathogenesis of this sequence of events is not entirely clear. Experimentally, pancreatitis can be produced by injection of bile into the pancreatic duct at a pressure sufficient to rupture the ductal system. Opie's early report[45] of acute pancreatitis resulting from impaction of a gallstone in the ampulla of Vater directed perhaps undue attention toward the necessity for a "common channel" for biliary and pancreatic secretions to provide anatomically possible regurgitation of bile into the pancreatic duct. Detailed anatomic studies show that the configuration of the pancreatic ducts and common bile duct allows regurgitation of bile into the pancreatic duct in about 90% of specimens.[2]

Even in the presence of an anatomic "common channel," measurements of pressures in the pancreatic duct and in the common bile duct indicate that the higher pressure in the pancreatic duct normally prevents the reflux of bile into the pancreatic duct. Increased pancreatic secretory pressure is clearly an important factor in the pathogenesis of pancreatitis.

The frequent association of chronic alcoholism suggests that alcohol functions not only by producing edema and partial obstruction of the sphincter of Oddi but also by stimulating pancreatic secretion.

Vascular ischemia has been implicated in the production of hemorrhagic pancreatitis, since it has been demonstrated experimentally that the pancreatic edema that occurs after ligation of the pancreatic duct in the dog can be transformed into acute hemorrhagic pancreatitis by the production of temporary ischemia in the pancreas. This factor alone is apparently not sufficient to produce the sequence of events, since vascular necroses in the pancreas in malignant hypertension are accompanied by only focal areas of necrosis, not a fulminating hemorrhagic pancreatitis.

Trauma also has been implicated as an etiologic factor. Acute pancreatitis is a recognized complication of closed abdominal trauma such as may result from "steering wheel" injuries to the abdomen. Acute pancreatitis also may complicate extensive surgery in the gastroduodenal area. On historical grounds, trauma can be excluded as a pathogenic mechanism in most cases.

Circulating antibodies to pancreatic tissue have been demonstrated in the bloodstream of patients with pancreatitis. It is not clear whether these antibodies have an etiologic role in the production of pancreatitis or whether they are simply immunologic byproducts occurring after pancreatic necrosis to other factors.

The central themes that underlie most of the numerous suggested etiologic factors are partial or complete pancreatic ductal obstruction and increased pancreatic secretion. Further detailed studies of experimental models and of the human disease are needed to clarify the etiology of acute hemorrhagic pancreatitis.

Chronic pancreatitis

Chronic pancreatitis produces progressive destruction of the pancreas as the result of repeated episodes of necrosis of the parenchyma. Approximately one third of all patients who survive an episode of acute pancreatitis sustain subsequent acute episodes that ultimately progress to chronic pancreatitis. Some patients arrive at the stage of pancreatic insufficiency without sustaining a documented attack of acute pancreatitis. Chronic pancreatitis is a recognized manifestation of hyperparathyroidism and of a hereditary metabolic disorder usually, but not always, ac-

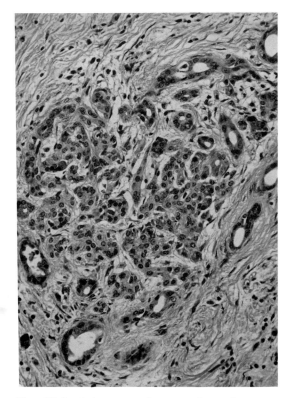

Fig. 33-5. Acinar atrophy occurring after pancreatic duct obstruction.

companied by aminoaciduria. The latter disorder account for only a small percentage of cases of chronic pancreatitis. Chronic relapsing pancreatitis occurs most frequently in the fourth or fifth decade. The disease is frequently associated with biliary tract disease or alcoholism.

Pathologic changes in the pancreas depend on the stage of the development of the disease. In acute exacerbations, diffuse edema, local areas of necrosis, and peripancreatic inflammation may be present. After the acute attacks, the pancreas will be firm and nodular, with areas of dense fibrosis, loss of acinar and islet tissue (Fig. 33-5), calcification in the interstitial tissue and pancreatic ducts, infiltration with plasma cells and lymphocytes, and formation of pseudocysts. The destruction of the pancreas eventually results in exocrine pancreatic insufficiency and, ultimately, diabetes mellitus.

Hereditary pancreatitis is a form of chronic pancreatitis that is transmitted as a mendelian dominant autosomal gene. In contrast to sporadic chronic pancreatitis, hereditary pancreatitis begins in childhood, and there is a relative infrequency of alcoholism and chronic biliary disease.[40]

PANCREATIC LESIONS IN SYSTEMIC DISEASE

Dilatation of acini and ducts of the pancreas occurs in approximately 40% to 50% of patients with uremia. The dilated structures contain eosinophilic inspissated material. In some instances, the individual lobules are separated by edematous tissue with a mild infiltrate of neutrophils.

Histologic changes in the acinar cells of the pancreatic lobules may be present in chronic congestive heart failure. Peripheral acinar cells in the pancreatic lobules appear atrophic, with diminished zymogen granules and decreased basophilia of their cytoplasm, whereas cells adjacent to islets retain their normal appearance. These histologic changes are apparently related to increased venous pressure and vascular stasis within the pancreatic venous circulation.

NEOPLASMS OF EXOCRINE PANCREAS
Cystadenoma

Cystadenomas of the pancreas are rare, slow-growing neoplasms that arise from ductal epithelium. They occur more commonly in females and usually are located in the tail of the pancreas. The tumor appears as a round,

coarsely lobulated mass comprised of multilocular cysts (Fig. 33-6). The cystic spaces are filled with fluid that may be clear, hemorrhagic, or gelatinous. The multiloculated cysts are lined by a cuboid or flattened epithelium. Papillary projections may be present.[71] A rare malignant counterpart, cystadenocarcinoma, has been described.[58]

Carcinoma

Carcinoma of the pancreas ranks fourth in frequency among fatal neoplastic diseases in the United States and is responsible for approximately 5% of all deaths caused by cancer. As a cause of death in the United States, carcinoma of the pancreas now exceeds such neoplastic diseases as carcinoma of the stomach, malignant lymphoma of all types, carcinoma of the prostate, and carcinoma of the cervix. Significantly increased risk of carcinoma of the pancreas has been attributed to and associated with disease of the gallbladder and extrahepatic biliary tree, cigarette smoking, consumption of alcoholic beverages, high levels of consumption of animal protein, and high daily average total caloric intake.[76] There is an increased risk of carcinoma of the pancreas among members of the American Chemical Society. Experimental models have been developed in animals.[59,63,71a] Carcinoma of the pancreas is extremely rare before 40 years of age. Approximately two thirds of patients are over

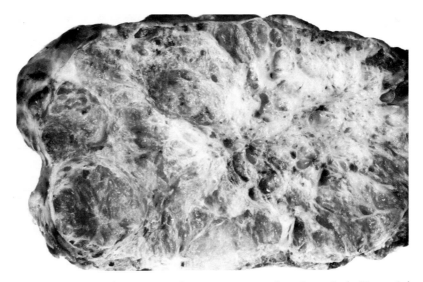

Fig. 33-6. Cystadenoma of pancreas. Coarse porous surface is typical. (From Ackerman, L. V., and Rosai, J.: Surgical pathology, ed. 5, St. Louis, 1974, The C. V. Mosby Co.)

the age of 60 years. An uncommon, sluggishly malignant, histologically characteristic carcinoma of the pancreas has been described in children.[60] Its cell of origin appears to be the acinic cell.

Clinical symptoms of carcinoma of the pancreas depend on the site of the origin of the tumor. If it arises in the head of the pancreas, obstruction of the common bile duct occurs early, producing obstructive jaundice (Fig. 33-7, *A*). Clinical recognition of carcinoma of the body and tail is difficult because of the paucity of distinctive signs and symptoms. Pain is the most common initial symptom of carcinoma of the pancreas, regardless of its location. Symptoms that appear later in the disease include anorexia, weight loss, cachexia, and weakness. The majority of patients with carcinoma of the pancreas are dead within a year after the onset of symptoms. The very high rate of failure of excisional surgery in the treatment of carcinoma of the pancreas has several possible explanations: initial symptoms are inconspicuous and nonspecific so that early diagnosis is difficult; the organ lies deep in the retroperitoneum intimately related to vital struc-

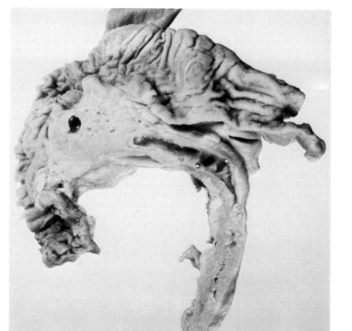

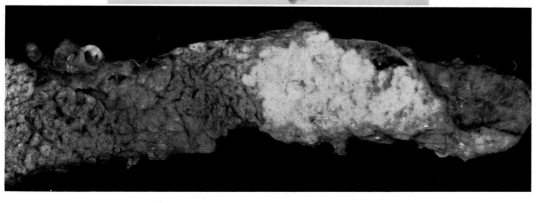

Fig. 33-7. Carcinoma of pancreas. **A,** Lesion of head of pancreas accompanied by atrophy of body and tail and dilatation of pancreatic duct. **B,** Lesion of body and tail of pancreas. (Courtesy Dr. Béla Halpert, Silver Spring, Md.)

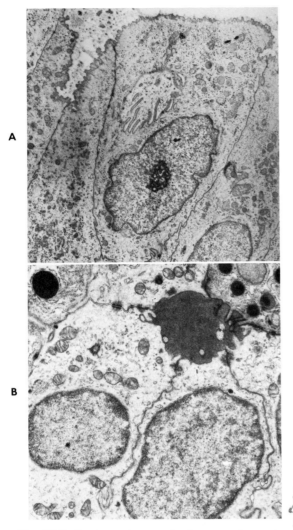

A

B

Fig. 33-8. Electron micrograph of pancreatic carcinoma compared with normal pancreatic ductule. **A,** Pancreatic adenocarcinoma. Cytoplasm of cell in center of field is traversed by canaliculus into which microvilli protrude. **B,** Normal pancreas shows a canaliculus with microvilli.

tures so that a conventional radical cancer operation is difficult; multiple sites of origin within the pancreas have been described.[57]

Approximately one half of all deaths from carcinoma of the pancreas occur within 3 months of the onset of symptoms. Among selected patients with carcinoma of the pancreas who are subjected to radical pancreaticoduodenectomy, some 12% survive longer than 5 years.[74] This figure approaches 40% in cases of (usually well-differentiated) ampullary carcinoma, a lesion that should be distinguished from pancreatic carcinoma.

Approximately 70% of carcinomas of the pancreas occur in the head of the organ. The proximity of the neoplasm to the common bile duct results in neoplastic invasion of the wall of the duct, producing obstruction and dilatation. Obstruction of the common bile duct also occurs in cases of carcinoma of the body and tail of the pancreas. However, this is usually a late complication.

Carcinomas of the body and tail of the pancreas are, on the average, larger than those of the head. Metastases occur most frequently in the regional lymph nodes, liver, lungs, peritoneum, and adrenal glands. The incidence of metastases is higher in cases of carcinoma of the body and tail than that of the head of the pancreas.

Grossly, the neoplasm is an ill-defined, firm expansion of a portion of the pancreas, with no sharp line of demarcation between the neoplasm and the surrounding parenchyma (Fig. 33-7). Most carcinomas of the pancreas are moderately well differentiated adenocarcinomas believed to arise from ductal epithelium (Fig. 33-8). These tumors recapitulate tubular and ductlike structures lined by one or several layers of neoplastic cells supported by dense fibrous stroma (Fig. 33-9, *A*). Although histochemical demonstration of mucin secretion by neoplastic cells can often be demonstrated, conspicuous extracellular production of mucin is uncommon. Occasional carcinomas of the pancreas present a peculiar histologic dimorphism between tubular and ductular structures and a sarcomatous stroma[62] (Fig. 33-9, *B*). The pancreas is one of the more common sites for the occurrence of *adenoacanthoma,* a carcinoma with both squamous and glandular elements.[56] Pure epidermoid carcinoma occurs. Undifferentiated small cell carcinoma of the pancreas may closely resemble the similar neoplasms of the lung[55] (Fig. 33-9, *C*). Acinic carcinoma is a rare neoplasm that recapitulates the pattern of acini in the normal pancreas. It may contain zymogen granules and manifest local features of lipolytic and proteolytic activity.[52,54] Peculiar giant cell tumors are rare.[73]

Adenocarcinoma of the pancreas frequently invades the perineural lymphatics (Fig. 33-9, *D*). This invasion of the nerves accounts for the frequency of abdominal pain in these patients. Multiple venous thromboses may be associated with carcinoma of the pancreas and occur more frequently when the neoplasm is in the body or tail of the pancreas. The veins most frequently involved are the iliac and femoral. The mechanism of thrombosis is not clearly defined.

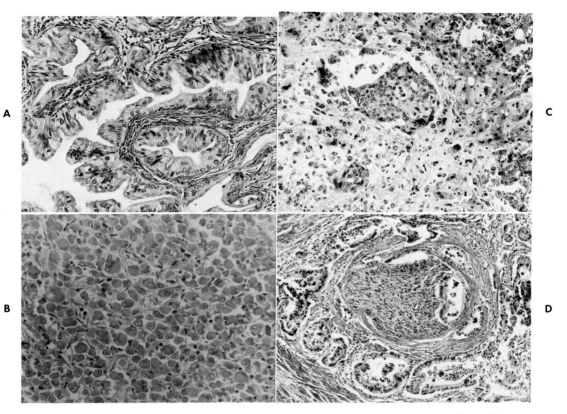

Fig. 33-9. Microscopic features of pancreatic carcinoma. **A,** Well-differentiated papillary adenocarcinoma. **B,** Adenoacanthoma in which areas of epidermoid carcinoma occur in otherwise typical adenocarcinoma. **C,** Pleomorphic carcinoma, an anaplastic carcinoma consisting of large anaplastic cells in no particular architectural pattern. **D,** Invasion of nerve by pancreatic adenocarcinoma, a common microscopic feature.

ENDOCRINE PANCREAS
Diabetes mellitus

Diabetes mellitus is a hereditary disease that affects approximately 2% to 4% of the population of the United States. The discovery of insulin and the use of this hormone in treatment has saved and prolonged the lives of diabetic patients but has not cured the disease. Today the major problems associated with diabetes are the complications that may affect the eye with resultant blindness, the kidney with resultant renal failure, the cardiovascular system with accelerated arteriosclerosis, and the peripheral nervous system with the development of neuropathy. Clinically the disease is subdivided into two categories—juvenile-onset and maturity-onset diabetes. In juvenile-onset diabetes, the disease usually begins abruptly, early in life, with a gradual loss of insulin reserve in the pancreas; thus exogenous insulin is required for therapy. Maturity-onset diabetes usually occurs in older individuals and

has an insidious onset, and the insulin reserve in the pancreas may be normal or moderately decreased.

Since diabetes mellitus affects so many different organ systems, it has been extremely difficult to determine the primary abnormality in these patients. Recent clinical studies indicate that the primary defect is in the beta cells of the pancreas. The evidence for this concept is as follows: (1) The administration of glucose to a nondiabetic patient results in a biphasic pattern of insulin secretion with an immediate release of insulin after glucose stimulation. In the early stages of diabetes, the beta cells do not respond promptly to glucose stimulation with a resultant delay in the release of insulin and development of hyperglycemia. (2) The use of sulfonylurea compounds in the treatment of diabetic patients has shown that these agents will stimulate insulin release from the islets, whereas the hyperglycemia in the diabetic subject is incapable of releasing sufficient insulin to maintain normoglycemia. (3) Transplantation of the normal human pancreas into diabetic patients has been accomplished, and in those patients in whom the transplant survived, the carbohydrate metabolism was returned to normal without the need of exogenous insulin or dietary therapy. These three findings indicate that the primary defect is in the beta cells and may involve the release mechanism of these cells. The cause of this abnormal beta cell function is probably a genetic defect or defects within the beta cells. The expression of this genetic abnormality as overt clinical diabetes is extremely variable, and the mode of genetic transmission is unknown.

Environmental factors may play a role in the expression of clinical diabetes as well as in the inception of the disease process. For example, nutrition may play a role since obesity is an important factor in the conversion of a latent diabetic state to overt diabetes. Viruses may play a role in the development of diabetes. It is possible that certain viruses may destroy beta cells in patients who have a genetic susceptibility to infection by the virus. Experimentally, infection with encephalomyocarditis virus will produce destruction of beta cells and diabetes in certain strains of mice. Epidemiologic studies in man have provided suggestive evidence of a greater incidence of coxsackie B virus infection in juvenile diabetics in comparison with controls. Autoimmunity may also play a role in the development of diabetes since antibodies to islet cells have been demonstrated in diabetic subjects.

The elucidation of the specific defect or defects in beta cell secretion in diabetics and the possible role of the environment in the development of diabetes mellitus requires an understanding of the normal mechanism of insulin secretion. This information will permit a search for defects in the insulin-secretory process of diabetic subjects. While these investigations are in progress, attempts are also being made to replace the defective beta cells with normal islet cells by transplantation.

Structure and function of beta cells

The islets of Langerhans comprise about 1% to 3% of the weight of the pancreas, and the concentration of islets is greater in the tail than in the head or body of the pancreas. By the use of special stains and electron microscopy, the islet cells of the human pancreas can be subclassified into alpha, beta, and delta cells (Fig. 33-10). The beta cells comprise 60% to 70% of the islet cell population; alpha cells, 20% to 30%; and delta cells, 2% to 8%. The alpha cells contain glucagon and the beta cells contain insulin. Gastrin has also been demonstrated in human islets; however, the specific cell type containing gastrin has not been established as yet. In other species, additional cell types and hormones have been demonstrated within the islets. An E cell has been described in the opossum pancreas and an F cell in the uncinate process of the dog pancreas. The hormones that have been localized to the islets but not to a specific cell type are somatostatin, avian pancreatic polypeptide, and human pancreatic polypeptide. Undoubtedly new endocrine disorders that involve hypersecretion or hyposecretion of these islet cell hormones will be discovered in the future.

Insulin synthesis. Insulin is stored in the beta cell as beta granules. Ultrastructurally the matrix of the mature beta granule contains a crystalline structure with lines of repeating periodicity of 50 Å, which corresponds closely to the size of the hexameric, crystalline form of zinc insulin. Zinc is also present in the beta granules. Thus it would appear that the storage form of insulin is essentially a microcrystal of zinc insulin.

Stimulation of the beta cell with glucose results in the immediate release of stored insulin and also initiates a series of events that lead to new formation of insulin. After glucose stimulation, proinsulin production is initiated in the endoplasmic reticulum. Bovine proinsulin is a single chain of 81 amino acids that consists of the A and B chains of insulin that are linked by a connecting peptide segment of 26 amino acids. This connecting segment is called the C peptide. Proinsulin is transferred by an energy-requiring mechanism to the Golgi complex where apparently the C peptide is split off by a specific proteolytic enzyme or enzymes. The newly formed insulin and C peptide are packaged into secretory granules in the Golgi complex where they are released into the cytoplasm after acquiring a membranous sac derived from the Golgi membranes. At some point in this process, zinc is transported into the beta granule resulting in the formation of zinc insulin crystals.

Since proinsulin does not produce hyperglycemia, studies have been accomplished to determine whether proinsulin is present in significant quantities in the bloodstream of diabetic individuals. These investigations have failed to reveal any elevation of proinsulin

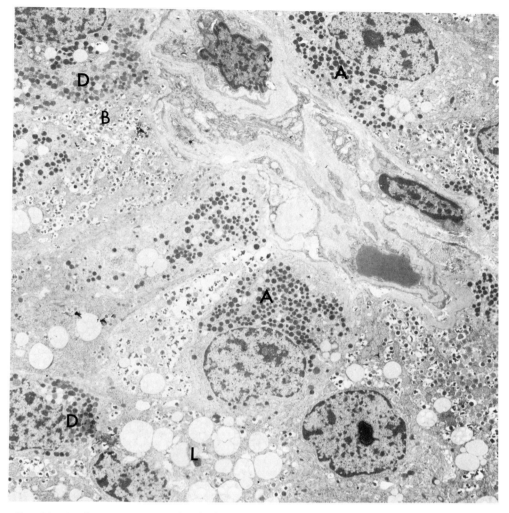

Fig. 33-10. Electron micrograph of islet cells of normal human pancreas. **A,** Alpha cell. **B,** Beta cell. **D,** Delta cell. Lipochrome pigment, **L,** present in cells. (Courtesy Dr. Marie Greider, St. Louis, Mo.)

levels in juvenile- and maturity-onset diabetics. The search for an abnormal form of insulin in the pancreas of diabetic patients has also been accomplished and no difference was found in the amino acid composition of peptide fragments of insulin extracted from the pancreases of nondiabetic and diabetic patients. These findings indicate that the primary defect in the beta cells of diabetic subjects does not involve insulin synthesis.

Insulin secretion. Understanding the biochemical and macromolecular events that link glucose stimulation with insulin release from the beta cell is of vital importance in the search for defects in this mechanism in beta cells of diabetic subjects. Glucose is the primary stimulus for insulin release in man. In the nondiabetic subject, glucose stimulates an immediate burst of insulin release followed by a second phase of secretion. Until recently, it had been assumed that the induction of insulin release from the beta cell was attributable to the metabolism of glucose. This concept was shown to be incorrect since biochemical studies indicated no significant changes in substrate and ATP levels in isolated islets after acute glucose stimulation. Indirect evidence from several sources now indicates that glucose is probably interacting with specific receptors on the plasma membrane of the beta cell, and as a result of this interaction, it initiates the chain of events leading to insulin release. Extracellular calcium is an absolute requirement for the induction of insulin release from the beta

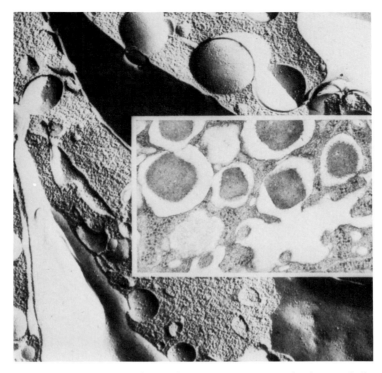

Fig. 33-11. Electron micrograph of freeze-fracture preparation of a beta cell demonstrating emiocytosis. *Inset,* Electron micrograph of section of stimulated beta cell demonstrating release of beta granule by emiocytosis. (Courtesy Dr. Lelio Orci, University of Geneva.)

cell. Studies on isolated islets using ^{45}Ca have shown that calcium accumulates in the beta cells in proportion to the degree of stimulation with glucose and the amount of insulin released. The biochemical events linking the interaction of glucose with receptors on the beta cell membrane and the accumulation of calcium in the cell are unknown.

The next step in the secretory process is to convey the packets of insulin to the beta cell surface. This is accomplished by the microtubule-microfilament system in the beta cell. In appropriate preparations examined with electron microscopy, linear bundles of microtubules separating columns of beta granules can be demonstrated. It has been suggested that calcium interacts with the microtubule-microfilament system, an interaction that results in a contraction or a change in physical conformation of the system with the resultant displacement of beta granules to the cell surface. Studies with transmission and freeze-fracture electron microscopy have demonstrated that the final step in the secretion of insulin is by emiocytosis (Fig. 33-11). This is accomplished by a fusion of the membranous

sacs surrounding the beta granules with the plasma membrane of the cell, resulting in the liberation of the beta granules and C peptide into the extracellular space where insulin and C peptide are then transported into the capillary system of the islets. The excess membrane incorporated into the plasma membrane as a result of emiocytosis is apparently recycled into the cytoplasm of the beta cell. It is unknown whether this recycling involves a specific removal of the membranous sacs inserted into the plasma membrane.

The involvement of the microtubule-microfilament system in the intracellular transport of the granules could also explain the biphasic pattern of insulin release. Those granules already associated with the system would be released immediately after glucose stimulation, whereas other stored granules and newly formed secretory granules would join the system at a later time forming the second phase of insulin release.

This simple but elegant model for insulin secretion is shown in Fig. 33-12. It would appear that this model of endocrine secretion would be applicable to other endocrine glands,

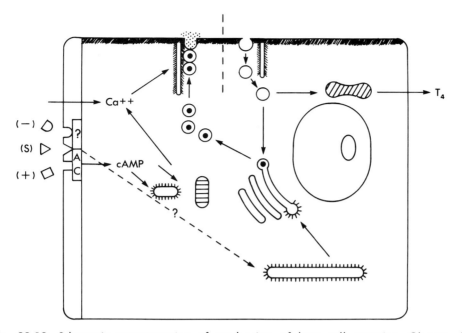

Fig. 33-12. Schematic representation of mechanism of beta cell secretion. Glucose, **S,** interacts with a presumed glucoreceptor on beta cell membrane resulting in stimulation of adenylate cyclase system, **AC,** and influx of calcium into beta cell, which results in displacement of beta granules to cell surface by microtubular-microfilament system. Granules are released by emiocytosis, and membrane is recycled into cell. Thyroid secretion, **T₄,** would involve only recycling phase of secretory process. Proinsulin forms in endoplasmic reticulum, is transferred to Golgi complex, is converted to insulin, and is stored as beta granules.

which may use either the entire system or only a portion of it. For example, in the thyroid gland only a portion of the mechanism would appear to be used. Stimulation with thyrotropic hormone results in increased pinocytosis of the apical portion of follicular cells with resultant accumulation of thyroglobulin droplets. The cytoplasm and the droplets are conveyed to lysosomes and degraded to thyroxin. Thus it would appear that only the recycling portion of the secretory process is used in the secretion of thyroxin in the thyroid gland.

An abnormality of this secretory mechanism for the release of insulin has been found in a hereditary form of diabetes in the spiny mouse. In these animals, the beta cells are deficient in microtubular protein, and it is presumed that this deficiency may play a role in the development of the diabetic state by interfering with the intracellular transport of beta granules.

Pathologic changes in islets

The specific, pathologic lesion or lesions of the islet cells that would explain the etiology and pathogenesis of diabetes mellitus have not

been elucidated. Despite this lack of specific knowledge, a number of pathologic changes have been demonstrated in the islets in association with diabetes. These changes include degranulation of beta cells, amyloidosis, glycogenosis, and leukocytic infiltration. Beta cell degranulation is not a specific pathologic change, since it occurs as a result of hyperglycemia and simply represents a depletion of insulin reserve.

Distinct differences exist in the pathologic changes observed in the pancreases of individuals with classic juvenile- and maturity-onset diabetes. In juvenile-onset diabetes, the number of islets is usually reduced, degranulation of beta cells and fibrosis may be present, and, in occasional instances, lymphocytic infiltration is observed. In maturity-onset diabetes, the number of islets may be normal, the degree of beta cell degranulation may be normal or moderately reduced, and amyloidosis may be present within the islets. In approximately 20% of patients with maturity-onset diabetes, no distinct light microscopic changes can be observed in the islets.

Amyloidosis of islets. By light microscopy,

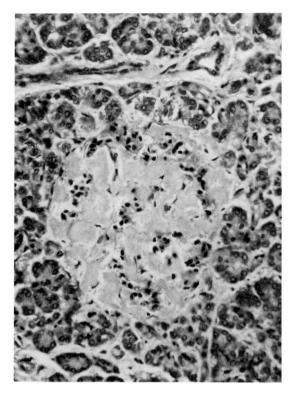

Fig. 33-13. Amyloidosis of islet of Langerhans in diabetic patient.

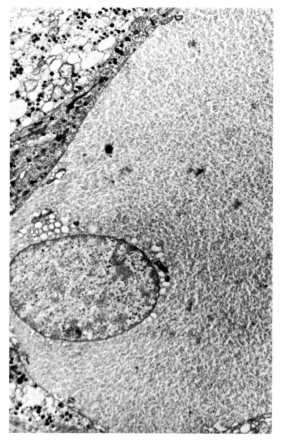

Fig. 33-14. Electron micrograph of beta cell containing massive accumulation of glycogen in diabetic hamster. Glycogen accumulation presents appearance of hydropic degeneration in ordinary microscopic preparations.

amyloid appears as an eosinophilic, amorphous material deposited around the capillaries of the islets, compressing and displacing the islet cells (Fig. 33-13). Previously, this change was called hyalinization of the islets of Langerhans and was one of the earlier morphologic findings observed in diabetic patients.

By electron microscopy, the amyloid has a fibrillar appearance and is deposited between the two basement membranes, separating the islet cells from the capillaries. Amyloidosis does not involve all the islets within a single pancreas but has a patchy distribution. Amyloidosis of the islets is not limited to diabetic patients but has been found, to a minor degree, in about 2% of nondiabetic individuals over 40 years of age. It is unlikely that this pathologic change has a primary role in the etiology of the diabetic state in man; however, it may play a role in the pathogenesis of the disease process once it is established.

Spontaneous diabetes has been described in many different species of animals. Amyloidosis of the islets has been described in spontaneous diabetes in the monkey and in cats. In the cat, occasional cases have been reported in which nearly all of the islets were replaced with amyloid, and, in some instances, calcification of the amyloid was present. Amyloidosis of the islets has not been produced experimentally and no information is available on the etiology and mechanism of development of this lesion.

Glycogenosis of beta cells. Glycogen is deposited in beta cells of the islets when there is a persistent hyperglycemia for a long period of time. Previously this lesion was called hydropic degeneration of beta cells since the cells appeared greatly vacuolated and it was assumed that the vacuoles contained water. The use of special stains demonstrated that the vacuoles actually contained glycogen. Glycogenosis of beta cells occurs in diabetes in man as well as in experimental animals with diabetes (Fig. 33-14). Prior to the insulin era, glycogenosis of beta cells was a common finding at autopsy in diabetic patients, but now it is rarely observed, since relatively few patients expire in diabetic acidosis and severe hyperglycemia. Nevertheless, this lesion undoubtedly does occur during the life of diabetic subjects when there are periods of uncontrolled hyperglycemia.

The deposition of glycogen is attributable to a change in the intracellular metabolism of glucose, which shifts the metabolism to the deposition of glycogen. Electron microscopic studies indicate that glycogen accumulates first as small focal masses within the beta cell, and as the hyperglycemic state becomes more severe, the masses increase in size and displace the normal intracellular organelles. In addition to the biochemical abnormalities that must exist in these cells, the mere presence of the mass of glycogen would interfere with the organized production of insulin by the beta cell, thus increasing the severity of the diabetic state. Glycogenosis of the beta cell is apparently a reversible change, since the glycogen disappears after treatment with insulin and maintenance of normoglycemia. The role of this reversible lesion in the pathogenesis of diabetes is difficult to understand, since it is presumed that continued hyperglycemia in the diabetic individual would result in destruction of beta cells. Experimentally, permanent diabetes has been produced in the.cat simply by maintaining hyperglycemia through repeated injections of glucose.

Electron microscopic studies have revealed a second pathologic change in beta cells of dogs with experimental diabetes induced by the administration of growth hormone and glucose. This lesion is called "ballooning degeneration," since multiple vacuoles are present in the cytoplasm, the vacuoles do not contain glycogen, and the cells appeared to be undergoing degeneration. Glycogenosis was evident in other beta cells of the islets. This degenerative change may represent the initial stages in the destruction of beta cells during prolonged hyperglycemia. The mechanism of development of this change and the relationship to glycogenosis is unknown.

Lymphocytic and eosinophilic infiltration of islets. Lymphocytic infiltration of the islets of Langerhans may be observed in juvenile diabetes. It is particularly evident in those patients who come to autopsy within days or weeks after the onset of the disease process. Experimentally, a similar type of lymphocytic infiltration occurs in virus-induced diabetes mellitus. Lymphocytic infiltration of the islets has also been observed in cattle and rabbits

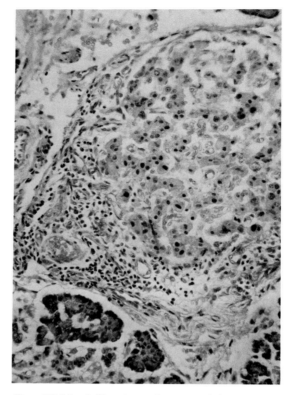

Fig. 33-15. Infiltration of eosinophils in peri-insular tissue of newborn infant of diabetic mother.

that were immunized with beef insulin. A permanent diabetic state was induced in some of the immunized rabbits. Both of these experimental findings raised the qeustion of a possible viral and autoimmune phenomenon in the pathogenesis of diabetes mellitus in man. Circulating antibodies to islet tissue have been observed in juvenile diabetes.

Infiltration of eosinophils and lymphocytes within and around the islets and in the interstitial tissue of the pancreas is observed in approximately 25% of infants who are born to diabetic mothers and who expire within 1 to 2 weeks after birth (Fig. 33-15). This infiltration is invariably associated with islet hypertrophy and hyperplasia and is diagnostic of diabetes mellitus in the mother. The appearance of eosinophilic infiltration is not related to the severity of the diabetes or the form of therapy received by the mother. In some instances, the mother has no clinical evidence of diabetes during pregnancy and may become diabetic within a period of months or years subsequently. Experimentally, a morphologic counterpart of this lesion has been produced by acute injections of anti-insulin serum into rats. In these animals, a severe diabetic state is produced and an infiltration of eosinophils and lymphocytes is present in the interstitial tissue and peri-insular areas of the pancreas. In monkeys with streptozotocin-induced diabetes, hyperpalsia of the islets has been observed in the fetuses of the diabetic mothers; however lymphocytic and eosinophilic infiltration was not present. It would appear that the hyperplasia of the beta cells is attributable to the hyperglycemia; however the lymphocytic and eosinophilic infiltration is caused by another factor involving an infectious agent or the transfer of specific antibodies to the fetus.

Hemochromatosis

Hemosiderin may be evident within acinar and beta cells of the pancreas in hemochroma-

tosis. The alpha cells are greatly reduced in number and do not contain hemosiderin. Atrophy of the acinar cells and interstitial fibrosis are usually present. The term "bronze diabetes" is sometimes used, since increased pigmentation of the skin, diabetes mellitus, and cirrhosis of the liver may be present in hemochromatosis. (See also pp. 115 and 1372.)

Diabetic microangiopathy

Pathologic changes in the small blood vessels and capillaries of the eye and kidney are responsible for the development of diabetic retinopathy and Kimmelstiel-Wilson syndrome in patients with diabetes mellitus. An important question was whether the changes in these small vessels in diabetics was limited to these two organs or whether these changes occurred in small vessels throughout the body. The

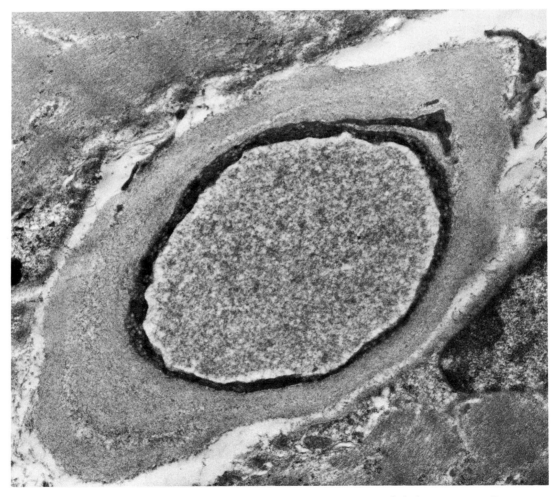

Fig. 33-16. Electron micrograph of capillary in skeletal muscle of diabetic patient. Basement membrane surrounding capillary tremendously thickened. (Courtesy Dr. Joseph R. Williamson, St. Louis, Mo.)

application of quantitative techniques to electron microscopic studies of capillaries in muscle biopsies from a large group of diabetic and nondiabetic patients has helped resolve this question as well as several others. Ultrastructural studies of the capillaries of the eye, kidney, muscle, and skin of diabetic patients have demonstrated a significant thickening of the basement membrane in each of these organs, and the basement membrane thickening is specific for diabetes mellitus (Fig. 33-16). In nondiabetic patients, thickening of muscle capillary basement membranes occurs in a linear fashion in males with increasing age, whereas in the female, the basement membrane thickness increases until about 40 to 50 years of age, then reaches a plateau, and increases again between 60 and 70 years of age. In the diabetic, the basement membrane is significantly thicker than appropriate age- and sex-matched controls, the thickening occurs segmentally, and it increases in thickness and in frequency with the duration of the disease.

A most significant question was whether the thickening of the basement membrane in diabetes was the result of a separate genetic defect or was actually a complication of diabetes mellitus. In the initial studies with insufficient control material, it appeared as though it was a separate defect. Now with adequate controls and with detailed studies on children born of diabetic mothers and fathers, it is apparent that the thickened basement membrane is a true complication of diabetes and is not a separate genetic defect.

The structural components of a capillary are the endothelial cell, the basement membrane, and a supporting cell embedded in the basement membrane. This supporting cell is called a pericyte in skeletal muscle, a mural cell in the capillaries of the eye, and a mesangial cell in the glomerulus of the kidney. It is unknown whether the supporting cell or the endothelial cell is responsible for either the formation or the removal of the basement membrane. These fundamental questions must be resolved before one can attempt to understand why excess basement membrane is produced in patients with diabetes mellitus.

Kidney in diabetes

The nodular lesions of the glomeruli described by Kimmelstiel and Wilson are characteristic pathologic changes found in the kidney in diabetes mellitus. This lesion is the result of focal thickening of the basement membrane. Quantitative ultrastructural studies of the glomeruli in diabetic patients have demonstrated that the earliest change occurs in the mesangial area of the glomerulus. Initially there is a thickening of the basement membrane in this area and an increase in the number of mesangial cells. Serial renal biopsies on these diabetic patients over a period of years have shown that the amount of basement membrane in the kidney gradually increases and results in the formation of the nodular lesions. These findings clearly indicate that the basement membrane changes are secondary to the diabetic process. In experimentally induced diabetes in rats, an increase in the number of mesangial cells, a slight increase in basement membrane thickness, and the deposition of gamma globulin in the basement membrane have been observed. Islet transplants into these diabetic animals have returned the diabetic state to normal and have completely reversed the pathologic changes in the glomeruli. (See also p. 955.)

Vacuolization of the pars recta of the proximal convoluted tubules at the corticomedullary junction may be observed in patients dying from uncontrolled diabetes and severe hyperglycemia. These vacuoles represent areas of glycogen deposition within the tubules that disappear when the diabetic state is treated. This condition is called the Armanni-Ebstein lesion of the kidney.

Necrotizing renal papillitis is a rare but serious complication of diabetes mellitus. This condition is not limited to diabetic patients but also may occur in nondiabetic individuals with obstructive lesions of the urinary tract. The condition is characterized clinically in the diabetic patient by the rapid onset of uremia and subsequent death caused by infarction and sloughing of the renal papillae.

Eye in diabetes

Diabetic retinopathy is presently the second and will soon become the first most common cause of blindness in the United States. The sequence of events in the development of this lesion are changes in the pattern of blood flow through the retina with resultant areas of ischemia, occurrence of microaneurysms in the retinal capillaries, new formation of capillaries within the retina, subsequent hemorrhage into the vitreous, and formation of granulation tissue. The development of these lesions requires many years with a varying degree of severity in individual patients and long periods of remission with no further impairment of vision.

The earliest change observed in the retina

of diabetic patients is a loss of mural cells in the capillaries. Ghostlike remnants of these cells will persist for long periods of time. It is presumed that the loss of these cells affects the capillary tone and leads in some way to the change in the pattern of blood flow through the retina and the subsequent development of microaneurysms of the retina. The mechanism of destruction of the mural cells in the diabetic is unknown. The enzyme aldose reductase is present in the retina, and it has been suggested that the utilization of this pathway for glucose metabolism in the presence of hyperglycemia may result in the accumulation of sorbitol in the mural cells with a subsequent destruction of these cells.

Experimentally, microaneurysms and intraretinal hemorrhage have been observed in dogs with alloxan-induced diabetes. Tight control of these diabetic animals with insulin results in a sharp diminution in the number of microaneurysms, which adds further support to the concept that the vascular changes in the retina are secondary to the diabetic state.

Peripheral nerves in diabetes

Peripheral neuropathy is particularly prone to occur in the older diabetic patient, with approximately 30% to 50% of the patients showing minor reflex changes and evanescent pains in the extremities. The basic pathologic change in the peripheral nerves is a segmental demyelination. The autonomic nervous system may also be involved in diabetic patients with resultant development of severe diarrhea and abdominal pain. Greatly elevated levels of sorbitol and fructose have been demonstrated in peripheral nerves of animals with experimentally induced diabetes. The accumulation of sorbitol and fructose is apparently attributable to a partial shunting of the metabolism of glucose through the aldose reductase pathway. It is unknown whether this abnormal metabolism of glucose with the formation of sorbitol is responsible for the decreased nerve conduction and segmental demyelination in diabetic subjects.

Arteriosclerosis and diabetes

Diabetes mellitus accelerates the development of arteriosclerosis with a resultant earlier onset of coronary arteriosclerosis and atherosclerosis in general. The arteriosclerotic process also involves the vessels to the lower extremity with resultant production of gangrene of the toes and feet. Elucidation of the mechanism by which diabetes mellitus accelerates arterio-

sclerosis may provide insight into the etiology and pathogenesis of arteriosclerosis in general. The recent development of techniques for the in vitro culture of human endothelial cells and smooth muscle cells provides excellent tools for the pursuit of this problem.

The precipitating causes of gangrene of the lower extremities are usually mechanical, thermal, or chemical trauma resulting in ulceration, infection, and subsequent gangrene. Comparison of the ultrastructure of dermal capillaries of the toes of amputated specimens from diabetic and nondiabetic individuals indicates that thickening of the basement membrane of the capillaries is limited to the diabetic group. The pronounced thickening in the basement membranes of the capillaries in diabetic patients may play some role in the inception and complication of the vascular insufficiency of the lower extremities, possibly by interference with nutrition and response of the tissues to injury.

Transplantation of pancreas and islets

Since the present therapeutic regime for the treatment of diabetes mellitus does not prevent the complications of the disease process, studies are in progress to attempt to replace the defective beta cells in the diabetic subject with normal-functioning beta cells. The first approach to this problem was to transplant the whole pancreas into diabetic patients receiving kidney transplants for renal failure. A few of these pancreatic transplants have continued to function, and it will be of great interest to determine whether these transplants had any effect on the progression of the vascular complications in the diabetic subjects.

The ideal approach to transplantation would be to implant only the islet cells of Langerhans. The development of the collagenase technique for the isolation of intact islets from the rest of the pancreas has made this approach feasible in the experimental animal. Using an inbred strain of rats, islets have been transplanted into the muscle, abdominal cavity, and spleen of diabetic animals with a resultant improvement in the diabetic state. Recently it has been shown that injection of isolated islets directly into the portal system of the liver results in a complete remission of the diabetic state and a return of carbohydrate metabolism to normal. The isolated islets are injected into the portal vein, and because of their size, the islets lodge in the portal tracts where they function normally.

Several problems must be resolved before

isolated islet transplantation can be attempted in diabetic patients. The major problems are the development of procedures for mass isolation of intact islets from the human pancreas and delineation of the optimal site for transplantation in man. Allografts of isolated islets are rejected; thus initial islet transplants will probably be attempted in patients who are receiving a kidney transplant and are already on immunosuppressive agents. Studies are in progress to attempt the development of artificial chambers that will permit the maintenance of the implanted islets and prevent their destruction by the immune mechanisms of the host.

A second approach to this problem is to attempt to develop an artificial beta cell. A gross version of an artificial beta cell has been developed to permit the continuous monitoring of the blood glucose and the injection of the appropriate amount of insulin into the diabetic individual during hospitalization. Studies are in progress to develop miniaturized glucose sensors and a computer system that will activate a micropump for the administration of the appropriate amount of hormone dependent on the level of blood glucose.

NEOPLASMS OF PANCREATIC ISLETS

Several different types of islet cell tumors occur in the pancreas and produce specific hormones. These tumors cannot be differentiated on the basis of their morphologic appearance using hematoxylin-and-eosin preparations. To establish the specific identity of an islet cell tumor, special stains, electron microscopy, and immunoassay of the tumor for specific hormones is required. All these procedures are readily available and should be applied to the diagnosis of islet cell tumors to permit accurate identity of the tumor and appropriate therapy of the patient.

Beta cell tumors

Funtioning beta cell neoplasms retain the capacity to form, store, and release insulin into the bloodstream. The neoplastic beta cells differ from the normal in that they are no longer responsive to the normal control mechanisms affecting insulin release and thus will release insulin at an uncontrolled rate, resulting in repeated attacks of hypoglycemia. Circulating levels of insulin are usually elevated in these patients during fasting and are increased during periods of hypoglycemia. Stimulation of insulin release from these neoplasms can usu-

ally be produced by the administration of either tolbutamide or arginine.

Beta cell tumors are most commonly found in the body and tail of the pancreas. Grossly, the tumors are usually encapsulated and well circumscribed, varying from 5 mm to 10 cm in diameter. They have a homogeneous color and increased consistency, thus one can delineate them from the surrounding normal pancreas.

Microscopically, the tumors usually have a gyroform pattern with ribbons or cords of cells passing between vascular sinusoids (Fig. 33-17). It is extremely difficult to assess the degree of malignancy of these neoplasms based upon the presence of anaplasia and hyperchromatism of the nuclei, since these changes may be present in a circumscribed adenoma or in one that has metastasized. The degree of beta granulation within the neoplasms may vary from a few scattered granules to an intense

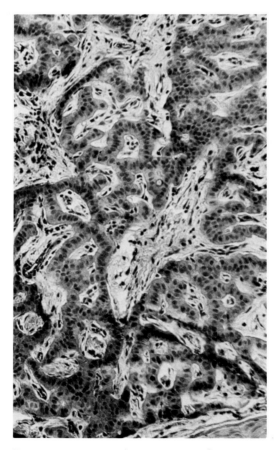

Fig. 33-17. Beta cell tumor. Gyroform pattern resulting from anastomising cords of beta cells. (Courtesy Dr. Marie Greider, St. Louis, Mo.)

degree of granulation similar to the normal beta cell. Measurements of insulin in micro-dissected neoplastic cells from freeze-dried sections confirm this striking variability in insulin content of the cells. Electron microscopically, the neoplastic cells contain the typical, crystalline, rectangular granules that are present in normal beta cells, and the number of crystalline granules varies noticeably within different neoplasms. Amyloid frequently is observed between the two basement membranes separating the neoplastic cells from the capillaries and, in some instances, calcification may be present in this area.

Alpha cell tumors

Alpha cell tumors are rare neoplasms of the islet cells. These tumors contain glucagon and usually the level of circulating glucagon in the patient is greatly elevated. By light microscopy, the neoplasms have a gyriform pattern similar to the beta cell tumors. Electron microscopically, the neoplastic cells have the ultrastructural appearance of normal alpha cells and contain numerous secretory granules. The secretory granules of the tumors are round with an extremely dense core and have a diameter of 225 to 425 nm.

Ulcerogenic tumors of pancreas

Zollinger and Ellison described a diagnostic triad that consists of a fulminating peptic ulcer diathesis persisting despite medical therapy or other radical procedures, gastric acid hypersecretion, and the presence of a non–beta cell tumor in the pancreas. Approximately one third of the ulcers observed in these patients have been found in unusual locations, such as the esophageal, postbulbar, and jejunal areas. The tumors most frequently occur in the body and tail of the pancreas and, in a few instances, the neoplasm was found in the wall of the duodenum, apparently originating in heterotopic foci of pancreatic tissue. Multiple adenomas involving the pituitary, adrenal, and parathyroid glands and islets of Langerhans have been found in approximately one third of the patients.

Histologically, the ulcerogenic tumors do not have a gyriform pattern as observed in alpha and beta cell tumors, but, in contrast, the tumors contain large, solid nests of cells containing glandular structures (Fig. 33-18). Electron microscopically, the tumor cells contain stored granules that are of two types. In type 1, the granules are round and homogeneous with a diameter ranging from 150 to 200 nm. In

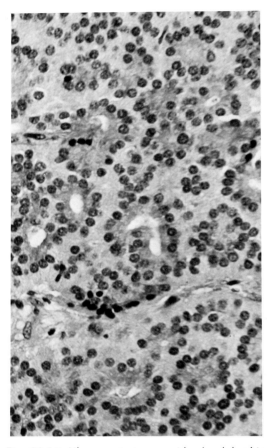

Fig. 33-18. Ulcerogenic tumor with glandular histologic pattern. (Courtesy Dr. Marie Greider, St. Louis, Mo.)

type 2, the granules have a pleomorphic shape with a diameter range up to 350 nm. Both types of granules may be present in the same neoplasm.

Ulcerogenic tumors contain gastrin, which can be demonstrated by immunoassay and by the fluorescent-antibody technique. The level of circulating gastrin is greatly elevated in these individuals. The cell of origin of ulcerogenic tumors has not been clearly established. By the fluorescent-antibody procedure, gastrin-containing cells have been demonstrated within normal human islets. Initially the cell of origin was assumed to be the delta cell; however, ultrastructurally the secretory granules within the ulcerogenic tumors are much smaller than those of delta cells. A fourth type of cell has been observed in normal human islets and contains granules resembling those present in ulcerogenic tumors and in gastrin-containing cells of the gastric mucosa. Presumably this is the cell of origin of these tumors; however, electron microscopic immunoperoxidase techniques will be required to identify this cell specifically.

Diarrheogenic tumors of pancreas

Verner and Morrison described a second type of syndrome associated with non–beta cell tumors of the pancreas. These patients had profuse diarrhea with hypokalemia and achlorhydria. The tumors usually occurred in the head and tail of the pancreas and were solitary or occasionally multiple in the pancreas. Histologically, the tumors had a pattern similar to the ulcerogenic tumors with glandular structures present in large solid nests of neoplastic cells. Electron microscopically, the tumor cells contained secretory granules that were similar to the type 1 and type 2 granules observed in ulcerogenic tumors. The hormone produced by these tumors has not been identified with certainty. It has been suggested that the tumors may contain a secretin-like substance or a gastric inhibitory polypeptide that would compete with gastrin for receptor sites on the gastric parietal cell and therefore produce achlorhydria. The specific type of islet cell responsible for the development of the tumors has not been established.

REFERENCES
Normal form and development

1 Liu, H. M., and Potter, E. L.: Development of human pancreas, Arch. Pathol. (Chicago) **74:**439-452, 1962.
2 Milbourn, E.: On the excretory ducts of the pancreas in man with special reference to their relationships to each other, to the common bile duct, and to the duodenum, Acta Anat. (Basel) **9:**1-34, 1950.
3 Rutter, W. J., Clark, W. R., Kemp, J. D., Bradshaw, W. S., Sanders, T. G., and Ball, W. D.: Epithelial-mesenchymal interactions, Baltimore, 1968, The Williams & Wilkins Co.
4 Wessells, N. K., and Cohen, J. H.: Early pancreas organogenesis: morphogenesis, tissue interactions, and mass effects, Develop. Biol. **15:**237-270, 1967.
5 Wessells, N. K., and Evans, J.: Ultrastructural studies of early morphogenesis and cytodifferentiation in the embryogenic mammalian pancreas, Develop. Biol. **17:**413-446, 1968.

Abnormalities of form and development

6 Barbosa, J. J. de C., Dockerty, M. B., and Waugh, J. M.: Pancreatic heterotopia: review of the literature and report of 41 authenticated surgical cases of which 25 were clinically significant, Surg. Gynecol. Obstet. **82:**527-542, 1946 (ectopic pancreas).
7 Elliott, G. B., Kliman, M. R., and Elliott, K. A.: Pancreatic annulus: a sign or cause of duodenal obstruction, Can. J. Surg. **11:**357-364, 1968.

8 Feldman, M., and Weinberg, T.: Aberrant pancreas; cause of duodenal syndrome, J.A.M.A. **148:**893-898, 1952 (ectopic pancreas).
9 Huebner, G. D., and Reed, P. A.: Annular pancreas, Am. J. Surg. **104:**869-873, 1962 (annular pancreas).
10 Lundquist, G.: Annular pancreas: pathogenesis, clinical features, and treatment with a report on two operation cases, Acta Chir. Scand. **117:** 451-454, 1959 (annular pancreas).
11 Pearson, S.: Aberrant pancreas; review of literature and report of three cases, one of which produced common and pancreatic duct obstruction, A.M.A. Arch. Surg. (Chicago) **63:**168-184, 1951 (ectopic pancreas).
12 Van Der Horst, L. F.: Annular pancreas, Arch. Surg. (Chicago) **83:**249-252, 1961 (annular pancreas).

Fibrocystic disease

13 Andersen, D. H.: Cystic fibrosis of pancreas and its relation to celiac disease; clinical and pathologic study, Am. J. Dis. Child. **56:**344-399, 1938.
14 Andersen, D. H.: Pancreatic enzymes in duodenal juice in celiac syndrome, Am. J. Dis. Child. **63:**643-658, 1942.
15 Aterman, K.: Duodenal ulceration and fibrocystic pancreas disease, Am. J. Dis. Child. **101:** 210-215, 1961.
16 Bodian, M.: Fibrocystic disease of the pancreas, New York, 1953, Grune & Stratton, Inc.
16a Changus, H. C., and Pitot, H. C.: Cystic fibrosis: a dilemma in metabolic pathogenesis of genetic disease, Arch. Pathol. Lab. Med. **100:**7, 1976.
17 Clarke, J. T., Elian, E., and Shwachman, H.: Components of sweat cystic fibrosis of the pancreas compared with controls, Am. J. Dis. Child. **101:**490-500, 1961.
18 Danes, B. S., and Bearn, A. G.: Cystic fibrosis of the pancreas. A study in cell culture, J. Exp. Med. **129:**775-793, 1969.
19 di Sant'Agnese, P. A., and Lepore, M. J.: Involvement of abdominal organism cystic fibrosis of the pancreas, Gastroenterology **40:** 64-74, 1961.
19a di Sant'Agnese, P. A., and Davis, P. B.: Research in cystic fibrosis, New Eng. J. Med. **295:** 481, 534, 597, 1976.
20 di Sant'Agnese, P. A., and Talamo, R. C.: Pathogenesis and physiopathology of cystic fibrosis of the pancreas. Fibrocystic disease of the pancreas (mucoviscidosis), New Eng. J. Med. **277:**1287-1294, 1344-1352, 1399-1408, 1967.
21 Dische, Z., di Sant'Agnese, P. A., Pallavicini, C., and Youlos, J.: Composition of mucoprotein fractions from duodenal fluid of patients with cystic fibrosis of pancreas and from controls, Pediatrics **24:**74-91, 1959.
22 Farber, S.: Pancreatic function and disease in early life; pathologic changes associated with pancreatic insufficiency in early life, Arch. Pathol. (Chicago) **37:**238-250, 1944.
23 Farber, S.: Relation of pancreatic achylia to meconium ileus, J. Pediatr. **24:**387-392, 1944.
24 Kaplan, E., Shwachman, H., Perlmutter, A. D., Rule, A., Khow, K.-T., and Holsclaw, D. S.:

Reproductive failure in males with cystic fibrosis, New Eng. J. Med. **279**:65-69, 1968.

25 Macdonald, J. A., and Trusler, G. A.: Meconium ileus: an eleven-year review at the Hospital for Sick Children, Toronto, Can. Med. Assoc. J. **83**:881-885, 1960.

26 Mangos, J. A., and McSherry, N. R.: Sodium transport inhibitory factor in sweat of patients with cystic fibrosis, Science **158**:135-136, 1967.

27 Munger, B. L., Brusilow, S. W., and Cooke, R. E.: An electron microscopic study of eccrine sweat glands in patients with cystic fibrosis of the pancreas, J. Pediatr. **59**:497-511, 1961.

28 Oppenheimer, E. H., and Esterly, J. R.: Pathology of cystic fibrosis. Review of the literature and comparison with 146 autopsied cases, Perspect. Pediatr. Pathol. **2**:241, 1975.

29 Roberts, G. B.: Familial incidence of fibrocystic disease of the pancreas, Ann. Hum. Genet. **24**:127-135, 1960.

30 Rubin, L. S., Barbero, G. J., Cherwick, W. S., and Sibinga, M. S.: Papillary reactivity as a measure of autonomic balance in cystic fibrosis, J. Pediatr. **63**:1120-1129, 1963.

31 Smoller, M., and Hsia, D. Y.: Studies on the genetic mechanism of cystic fibrosis of the pancreas, Am. J. Dis. Child. **98**:277-292, 1959.

32 Spock, A., Heick, H. M. C., Cress, H., and Logan, W.: In vitro study of ciliary motility to detect individuals with active cystic fibrosis and carriers of disease, Mod. Probl. Pediatr. **10**:200-206, 1967.

Acquired diseases

33 Baggenstoss, A. H.: Pancreas in uremia, histopathologic study, Am. J. Pathol. **24**:1003-1017, 1948.

34 Blumenthal, H. T., and Probstein, J. G.: Pancreatitis, Springfield, Ill., 1959, Charles C Thomas, Publisher.

35 Ciba Foundation Symposium: The exocrine pancreas, Boston, 1961, Little, Brown & Co.

36 Dreiling D. A.: Pancreatic disease: a review, J. Mt. Sinai Hosp. N.Y. **36**:388-407, 1969.

37 Edmonson, H. A., and Berne, C. J.: Calcium changes in acute pancreatic necrosis, J. Surg. Gynecol. Obstet. **79**:240-244, 1944 (calcium changes in pancreatic necrosis).

38 Elliott, D. W., Williams, R. D., and Zollinger, R. M.: Alterations in the pancreatic resistance to bile in the pathogenesis of acute pancreatitis, Ann. Surg. **146**:669-682, 1957.

39 Gambill, E. E.: Pancreatitis, St. Louis, 1973, The C. V. Mosby Co.

40 Gross, J. B., and Comfort, M. W.: Chronic pancreatitis, Am. J. Med. **33**:358-364, 1962.

41 Gross, J. B., Gambill, E. E., and Ulrich, J. A.: Hereditary pancreatitis. Description of a 5th kindred and summary of clinical features, Am. J. Med. **33**:358-364, 1962.

42 Hanna, W. A.: Rupture of pancreatic cysts. Report of a case and review of the literature, Br. J. Surg. **47**:495-498, 1960 (rupture of pseudocysts).

43 Hranilovich, G. T., and Baggenstoss, A. H.: Lesions of the pancreas in malignant hypertension; review of 100 cases at necropsy, Arch. Pathol. (Chicago) **55**:443-456, 1953.

44 Murphy, R. F., and Hinkamp, J. F.: Pancreatic

pseudocysts. Report of 35 cases, A.M.A. Arch. Surg. (Chicago) **81**:564-568, 1960 (pseudocysts).

45 Opie, E. L.: The etiology of acute hemorrhagic pancreatitis, Bull. Johns Hopkins Hosp. **12**:182-188, 1901 (common channel).

46 Ponka, J. L., Landrum, S. E., and Chaikof, L.: Acute pancreatitis in the postoperative patient, Arch. Surg. (Chicago) **83**:475-490, 1961.

47 Popper, H. L., Necheles, H., and Russell, K. C.: Transition of pancreatic edema into pancreatic necrosis, Surg. Gynecol. Obstet. **87**:79-82, 1948 (ischemia).

48 Rich, A. R., and Duff, G. L.: Experimental and pathologic studies on pathogenesis of acute hemorrhagic pancreatitis, Bull. Johns Hopkins Hosp. **58**:212-259, 1936.

49 Szymanski, F. J., and Bluefarb, S. M.: Nodular fat necrosis and pancreatic disease, Arch. Dermatol. (Chicago) **83**:224-229, 1961.

50 Thal, A. P.: The occurrence of pancreatic antibodies and the nature of the pancreatic antigen, Surg. Forum **11**:367-369, 1960.

51 Tumen, H. J.: Pathogenesis and classification of pancreatic disease, Am. J. Dig. Dis. **6**:435-440, 1961.

52 Auger, C.: Acinous cell carcinoma of pancreas with extensive fat necrosis, Arch. Pathol. (Chicago) **43**:400-405, 1947.

53 Bell, E. T.: Carcinoma of the pancreas, Am. J. Pathol. **33**:499-523, 1957.

54 Burns, W. A., Matthews, M. J., Hamosh, M., Vander Werde, G., Blum, R., and Johnson, F. D.: Lipase-secreting acinar cell carcinoma of the pancreas with polyarthropathy. A light and electron microscopic, histochemical and biochemical study, Cancer **33**:1002, 1974.

55 Carrin, B., Gilby, E. D., Jones, N. F., and Patrick, J.: Oat cell carcinoma of the pancreas with ectopic ACTH secretion, Cancer **31**:1523, 1973.

56 Cihak, R. W., Kawashima, T., and Steer, A.: Adenoacanthoma (adenosquamous carcinoma) of the pancreas, Cancer **29**:1133, 1972.

57 Collins, J. J., Jr., Craighead, J. E., and Brooks, J. R.: Rationale for total pancreatectomy for carcinoma of the pancreatic head, New Eng. J. Med. **274**:599, 1966.

58 Cornes, J. S., and Azzopardi, J. C.: Papillary cystadenocarcinoma of the pancreas with report of two cases, Br. J. Surg. **47**:139-144, 1959.

59 Druckrey, H., Ivankovic, S., Bücheler, J., Preussmann, R., and Thomas, C.: Erzeugung von Magen- und Pankreas-Krebs beim Meerschweinchen durch Methylnitroso-harnstoff und -urethan, Z. Krebsforschung **72**:167, 1968.

60 Frable, W. J., Still, W. J. S., and Kay, S.: Carcinoma of the pancreas, infantile type. A light and electron microscopic study, Cancer **27**:667, 1971.

61 Frantz, V. K.: In Atlas of tumor pathology, Sect. VII, Fasc. 27 and 28, Washington, D.C., 1959, Armed Forces Institute of Pathology (tumors of pancreas).

62 Guillan, R. A., and McMahon, J.: Pleomorphic adenocarcinoma of the pancreas, Am. J. Gastroenterol. **60**:379, 1973.

63 Hayashi, Y., and Hasegawa, T.: Experimental

pancreatic tumor in rats after intravenous injection of 4-hydroxyaminoquinoline 1-oxide, Gann 62:329, 1971.

64 Hermreck, S., Thomas, C. Y., and Friesen, R.: Importance of pathologic staging in the surgical management of adenocarcinoma of the exocrine pancreas, Am. J. Surg. 127:654, 1974.

65 Kaplan, N., and Angrist, A.: Mechanism of jaundice in cancer of the pancreas, Surg. Gynecol. Obstet. 77:199-204, 1943.

66 Kenney, W. E.: Association of carcinoma in body and tail of pancreas with multiple venous thrombi, Surgery 14:600-609, 1943.

67 Kissane, J. M.: Carcinoma of the exocrine pancreas: pathologic aspects, J. Surg. Oncology 7:167, 1975.

68 Lafler, C. J., and Hinerman, D. L.: A morphologic study of pancreatic carcinoma with reference to multiple thrombi, Cancer 14:944-952, 1961.

69 Mikal, S., and Campbell, A. J. A.: Carcinoma of the pancreas; diagnostic and operative criteria based on 100 consecutive autopsies, Surgery 28:963-969, 1950.

70 Miller, J. R., Bagenstoss, A. H., and Comfort, M. W.: Carcinoma of the pancreas; effects of histological types and grade of malignancy on its behavior, Cancer 4:233-241, 1951.

71 Piper, C. E., Jr., Remine, W. H., and Priestley, J. T.: Pancreatic cystadenomata. Report of 20 cases, J.A.M.A. 180:648-652, 1962.

71a Pour, P., Mohr, U., Cardesa, A., Althoff, J., and Krüger, F. W.: Pancreatic neoplasms in an animal model: morphological, biological, and comparative studies, Cancer 36:379, 1975.

72 Probstein, J. G., and Blumenthal, H. T.: Progressive malignant degeneration of a cystadenoma of the pancreas, Arch. Surg. (Chicago) 81:683-689, 1960.

73 Rosai, J.: Carcinoma of pancreas simulating giant cell tumor of bone. Electron microscopic evidence of its acinar cell origin, Cancer 22:333, 1968.

74 Warren, K. W., Baasch, J. W., and Thum, C. W.: Carcinoma of the pancreas, Surg. Clin. North Am. 48:601-618, 1968.

75 Weinstein, J. J.: Carcinoma of the head of the pancreas and pariampullary area, Am. J. Gastroenterol. 37:629-641, 1962.

76 Wynder, E. L., Mabuchi, K., Maruchi, N., and Fortner, J. G.: Epidemiology of cancer of the pancreas, J. Natl. Cancer Inst. 50:645, 1973.

Diabetes mellitus

77 Allen, A. C.: So-called intercapillary glomerulosclerosis—a lesion associated with diabetes mellitus, Arch. Pathol. 32:33-51, 1941.

78 Banson, B. B., and Lacy, P. E.: Diabetic microangiopathy in human toes (with emphasis on the ultrastructural change in dermal capillaries), Am. J. Pathol. 45:41-58, 1964.

79 Bloodworth, J. M., Jr.: Diabetic microangiopathy, Diabetes 12:99-114, 1963.

80 Cerasi, E., and Luft, R.: The plasma insulin response to glucose infusion in healthy subjects and in diabetes mellitus, Acta Endocrinol. (Kbh) 55:278-304, 1967.

81 Cogan, D. G., and Kuwabara, T.: Capillary

shunts in the pathogenesis of diabetic retinopathy, Diabetes 12:293-300, 1963.

82 Craighead, J. E., and Steinke, J.: Diabetes mellitus–like syndrome in mice infected with encephalomyocarditis virus, Am. J. Pathol. 63:119-134, 1971.

83 Ehrlich, J. C., and Ratner, I. M.: Amyloidosis of the islets of Langerhans, Am. J. Pathol. 38:49-59, 1961.

84 Ellenberg, M.: Current status of diabetic neuropathy, Metabolism 22:657-662, 1973.

85 Howell, S. L., Kostianovsky, M., and Lacy, P. E.: Beta granule formation in isolated islets of Langerhans: A study by electron microscopic radioautography, J. Cell Biol. 42(3):695-705, 1969.

86 Kemp, C. B., Knight, M. J., Scharp, D. W., Ballinger, W. F., and Lacy, P. E.: Transplantation of isolated pancreatic islets into the portal vein of diabetic rats, Nature 244:447, 1973.

87 Kilo, C., Vogler, N., and Williamson, J. R.: Muscle capillary basement membrane changes related to aging and to diabetes mellitus, Diabetes 21:881-905, 1972.

88 Kimmelstiel, P., and Wilson, C.: Intercapillary lesions in the glomeruli of the kidney, Am. J. Pathol. 12:83-97, 1936.

89 Lacy, P. E., and Wright, P. H.: Allergic interstitial pancreatitis in rats injected with guinea pig anti-insulin serum, Diabetes 14(10):634-642, 1965.

90 Lacy, P. E., Howell, S. L., Young, D. A., and Fink, C. J.: A new hypothesis of insulin secretion, Nature 219:1177-1180, 1968.

91 Lacy, P. E.: Beta cell secretion—from the standpoint of a pathobiologist, Diabetes 19(12):895-905, 1970.

92 Lacy, P. E.: Endocrine secretory mechanisms, Am. J. Pathol. 79(1):170-188, 1975.

93 Lazarus, S. S., and Volk, B. W.: The pancreas in human and experimental diabetes, New York, 1962, Grune & Stratton, Inc.

94 Malaisse, W. J.: Insulin secretion: multifactorial regulation for a single process of release, Diabetologia 9:167-173, 1973.

95 McGavran, M. H., and Hartroft, W. S.: The predilection of pancreatic beta cells for pigment deposition in hemochromatosis and hemosiderosis, Am. J. Pathol. 32:631, 1956.

96 Nagler, W., and Taylor, H.: Diabetic coma with acute inflammation of islets of Langerhans, J.A.M.A. 184:723-725, 1963.

97 Orci, L.: A portrait of the pancreatic B cell, Diabetologia 10:163-187, 1974.

98 Silverman, J. L.: Eosinophile infiltration in the pancreas of infants of diabetic mothers, Diabetes 12:528-537, 1963.

99 Steiner, D. F., Cunningham, D. D., Spigelman, L., and Aten, B.: Insulin biosynthesis: evidence for a precursor, Science 157:697-700, 1967.

100 Steiner, D. F., Kemmler, W., Clark, J. L., Oyer, P. E., and Rubenstein, A. H.: The biosynthesis of insulin. In Steiner, D. F., and Freinkel, N., editors: Handbook of physiology. Vol. 1. Endocrine pancreas, Baltimore, 1972, The Williams & Wilkins Co., pp. 175-198.

101 Toreson, W. E.: Glycogen infiltration (so-called hydropic degeneration) in the pancreas

in human and experimental diabetes mellitus, Am. J. Pathol. **27:**327-347, 1951.

102 Toreson, W. E., Lee, J. C., and Grodsky, G. M.: The histopathology of immune diabetes in the rabbit, Am. J. Pathol. **52:**1099-1115, 1968.

103 Volk, B. W., and Lazarus, S. S.: Ultramicroscopic evolution of B-cell ballooning degeneration in diabetic dogs, Lab. Invest. **12:**697-711, 1963.

Neoplasms of pancreatic islets
Beta cell tumors

104 Duff, G. L.: The pathology of islet cell tumors of the pancreas, Am. J. Med. Sci. **203:**437-451, 1942.

105 Frantz, V. K.: Tumors of islet cells with hyperinsulinism; benign, malignant, and questionable, Ann. Surg. **112:**161-176, 1940.

106 Greider, M. H., and Elliott, D. W.: Electron microscopy of human pancreatic tumors of islet cell origin, Am. J. Pathol. **44:**663-678, 1964.

107 Howard, J. M., Moss, N. H., and Rhoads, J. E.: Hyperinsulinism and islet cell tumors of the pancreas, Int. Abstr. Surg. **90:**417-455, 1950.

108 Laidlaw, G. F.: Nesidioblastoma, the islet tumor of the pancreas, Am. J. Pathol. **14:**125-134, 1938.

109 Markowitz, A. M., Slanetz, C. A., Jr., and Frantz, V. K.: Functioning islet cell tumors of the pancreas: 25-year follow-up, Ann. Surg. **154:**877-884, 1961.

110 Porta, E. A., Yerry, R., and Scott, R. F.: Amyloidosis of functioning islet cell adenomas of the pancreas, Am. J. Pathol. **41:**623-631, 1962.

111 Sieracki, J., Marshall, R. B., and Horn, R. C., Jr.: Tumors of the pancreatic islets, Cancer **13:**347-357, 1960.

Glucagonoma, ulcerogenic tumors,
diarrheogenic tumors

112 Greider, M. H., and McGuigan, J. E.: Cellular localization of gastrin in the human pancreas, Diabetes **20:**389-396, 1971.

113 Greider, M. H., Rosai, J., and McGuigan, J. E.: The human pancreatic islet cells and their tumors. II. Ulcerogenic and diarrheogenic tumors, Cancer **33**(5):1423-1443, 1974.

114 Greider, M. H., Steinberg, V., and McGuigan, J. E.: Electron microscopic identification of the gastrin cell of the human antral mucosa by means of immunocytochemistry, Gastroenterology **63:**572-583, 1972.

115 McGavran, M. H., Unger, R. H., Recant, L., Polk, H. C., Kilo, C., and Levin, M. E.: A glucagon-secreting alpha cell carcinoma of the pancreas, New Eng. J. Med. **274:**1408-1413, 1966.

116 McGuigan, J. E., and Trudeau, W. L.: Immunochemical measurement of elevated levels of gastrin in the serum of patients with pancreatic tumors of the Zollinger-Ellison variety, New Eng. J. Med. **278:**1308-1313, 1968.

117 Sanzenbacher, L. J., Mekhjian, H. S., King, D. R., and Zollinger, R. M.: Studies on the potential role of secretin in the islet cell tumor diarrheogenic syndrome, Ann. Surg. **176:**394-402, 1972.

118 Zollinger, R. M., and Ellison, E. H.: Primary peptic ulcerations of the jejunum associated with islet cell tumors of the pancreas, Ann. Surg. **142:**709-728, 1955.

34/Hemopoietic system: reticuloendothelium, spleen, lymph nodes, bone marrow, and blood

JOHN B. MIALE
ARKADI M. RYWLIN

The hemopoietic and reticuloendothelial system is a physiologic and pathophysiologic unit rather than an anatomic entity. Traditionally, some of its discrete anatomic subunits (spleen, lymph nodes, bone marrow) receive separate discussion. However, aside from some differences in anatomic location or in special physiologic functions, most of the functions of the system and the cellular changes accompanying benign and malignant proliferation are the same regardless of location. It is preferable, therefore, to discuss first the function and cellular changes common to the entire reticuloendothelial system. When, for convenience, the anatomic subunits are considered separately, the student will appreciate the physiologic common denominators and the interrelationship between the subunits.

Reticuloendothelial system

DEFINITION AND TERMINOLOGY

The term "reticuloendothelial system" (RES) was coined by Aschoff and Kiyono[4] to cover, by an inclusive term, a system of cells found within and outside of organs and characterized functionally by phagocytosis and staining by vital dyes. Only cells that showed avidity for the vital dyes were included in the RES (see outline below).[112] Polymorphonuclear leukocytes were excluded because they did not take up carmine in solutions, even though they did phagocytose carmine granules. The endothelial cells of most of the blood and lymph vessels and the fibroblasts were not included because they took the dye only when vital staining had been carried to an advanced degree. Aschoff named phagocytic cells in direct contact with blood or lymph "reticuloendothelia." Reticulum cells and reticuloendothelia share both the property of phagocytosis and of forming argyrophilic fibers.[3]

Cellular components of RES
1. Intravascular cells
   a. Monocytes
   b. Endothelial cells:
      (1) Liver capillaries—Kupffer cells
      (2) Lymph node sinuses
      (3) Splenic sinuses
      (4) Adrenal capillaries
      (5) Hypophyseal capillaries
2. Extravascular cells
   a. Reticulum cells—fixed macrophages, related to reticulum fibers
   b. Histiocytes—wandering macrophages of connective tissue

Although there is general agreement that it is important to individualize a system of cells possessing the ability to phagocytose particulate material and colloidal solutions, there continues to be disagreement as to what cells should belong to this system and what this system should be named. Recently the term "mononuclear phagocyte system" has been introduced to include all avidly phagocytic mononuclear cells and their precursors. The microglia of the central nervous system, alveolar macrophages, and serous membrane macrophages are all included in this system.[69]

There is also controversy about the origin and nomenclature of mononuclear phagocytic cells. Gall found the term "reticulum cell" inexact and prefers to use "histiocyte" instead. "Histiocyte" was introduced by Aschoff and Kiyono[4] to denote the tissue origin of the mobile tissue macrophage, which was believed by Metchnikoff to be derived from the peripheral blood. However, recently evidence has been developed to show that tissue macrophages are derived from blood monocytes originating in the bone marrow.[136] This consideration renders the term "histiocyte" somewhat inappropriate. For this reason many investigators prefer Metchnikoff's term "macrophage."

What seems reasonably well established is that there are fixed and mobile macrophages. The *fixed* macrophages are related to reticulum fibers and can be called "reticulum cells." The *mobile* tissue macrophages may be called "histiocytes." Since in fixed, stained sections we cannot be sure whether a cell is mobile or fixed, the terms reticulum cell and histiocyte are often interchanged. These cells can be called macrophages, though some pathologists reserve this term for cells that have actually phagocystosed a substance, rather than for cells that are capable of phagocytosis.

According to some investigators, a very important cellular component of the reticuloendothelial system is a primitive mesenchymal cell that is neither phagocytic nor stainable

with vital dyes. This, in our opinion, occupies the central position in the many functions and transformations of the system, for it is multipotential and able to differentiate into macrophages, into fibroblasts, and into precursors of lymphocytes and other blood and tissue hemopoietic cells.

Provided that this multipotentiality is appreciated, it matters little which nomenclature is used. The scheme and nomenclature used in this chapter is shown in Fig. 34-1.

PATHOPHYSIOLOGY

The functions of the reticuloendothelial system in the broad sense—the reticulum cell, is cellular derivatives, and, in the anatomic sense, the organs and specialized tissues that contain them (spleen, liver, lymph nodes, thymus, bone marrow)—can be classified as follows:

1. Hemopoiesis, the production and maintenance at physiologic levels of the cells of the blood and bone marrow
2. Phagocytosis, of senescent blood cells, cellular breakdown products and other particulate matter, bacteria, fungi, and

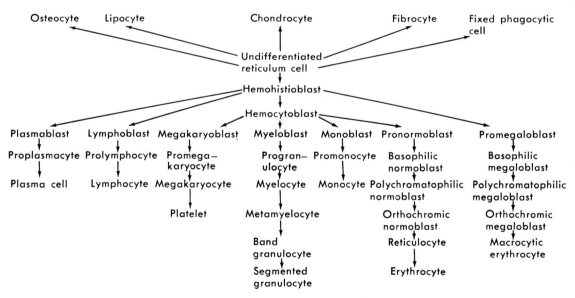

Fig. 34-1. Reticuloendothelial system from standpoint of its multipotentiality. According to this scheme, the most primitive and still undifferentiated cell is called "undifferentiated reticulum cell." This cell is neither phagocytic nor stainable with vital dyes. It is capable of differentiating into various types of connective tissue cells (osteocytes, lipocytes, chondrocytes, and fibrocytes) as well as into "classic" cell of reticuloendothelial system—fixed and mobile phagocytic cell. It is also able to differentiate in hemopoietic direction, at which time it may be considered to be hemopoietic reticulum cell in general sense, or, more specifically, hemohistioblast or hemocytoblast. Undifferentiated reticulum cell, hemocytoblast, and hemohistioblast cannot be distinguished from one another on morphologic criteria alone. (From Miale, J. B.: Laboratory medicine—hematology, St. Louis, 1972, The C. V. Mosby Co.)

parasites, and storage and clearance from the blood and interstitial tissues of certain chemical by-products of normal and abnormal métabolism (hemoglobin, hemosiderin, bilirubin, lipids, glycogen)
3. Role in immune reactions
4. Proliferative disorders of the RES

Hemopoiesis

In the embryo, the mesenchymal stem cells of the yolk sac differentiate into groups of cells characterized by a large nucleus containing spongy chromatin, one or two nucleolar chromatin condensations, and a deeply basophilic cytoplasm. This primitive cell is committed by differentiation to form blood cells, becoming a hemopoietic reticulum cell. As shown in Fig. 34-1, this is the *hemohistioblast*, normally giving rise to the plasma cell and lymphocyte series and to megaloblasts in the abnormal erythropoiesis of pernicious anemia and other megaloblastic dysplasias. In the early hemopoiesis of the yolk sac phase (Fig. 34-2), only a primitive type of nucleated erythrocyte precursor is formed, the *primitive erythroblast*. These do not survive beyond a few weeks, being replaced by the definitive type of erythroid precursor, the *normoblast*. In the yolk sac of a 9-week-old embryo, half of the cells are primitive erythroblasts while the other half are definitive normoblasts.

By the third month of fetal life, *mesoblastic* (yolk sac) hemopoiesis has gradually ceased and the liver has become the chief site of blood cell formation. This second phase is referred to as the period of *hepatic hemo-poiesis*. It reaches peak activity during the fifth to sixth month and remains active until shortly before birth. Only a few hemopoietic foci are normally present in the liver of full-term infants. However, many are present in the liver of the premature infant. Although about four fifths of the hemopoietic activity in the liver is related to the production of erythrocytes (erythropoiesis) (Fig. 34-3), there is also production of leukocytes (leukopoiesis) and platelets (thrombocytopoiesis). There is also, during the middle and last third of fetal life, hemopoiesis in the spleen, thymus, and lymph nodes. The spleen is at first active in the production of all three types of blood cells, but later it is primarily a site for erythropoiesis and lymphopoiesis. The lymph nodes are essentially sites for lymphopoiesis, although an occasional granulocyte can be seen.

From birth on, the bone marrow is the chief hemopoietic organ. It becomes increasingly active during the later months of gestation, during which time the marrow cavities (sternum, vertebrae, pelvis, ribs, skull, and proximal portions of the long bones) enlarge to accommodate more and more bone marrow cells. During the same period, the hemopoietic activity in the liver diminishes, so that at birth the bone marrow accounts for all the erythrocytes, all the granulocytes, all the platelets, most of the plasma cells, and a significant number of lymphocytes. This, then, is the situation in the normal adult: the bone marrow is the chief hemopoietic tissue, the hemopoietic activity outside of the bone marrow being limited to lymphocytopoiesis in the spleen, lymph nodes, and other lymphoid tissue.

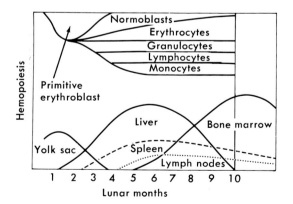

Fig. 34-2. Hemopoietic sequences in fetus. Degree and site of hemopoietic activity (lower portion) and appearance of blood cells in peripheral blood (upper portion). (From Miale, J. B.: Laboratory medicine—hematology, St. Louis, 1972, The C. V. Mosby Co.)

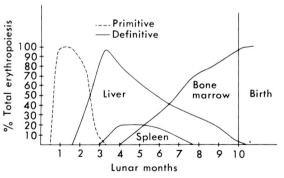

Fig. 34-3. Erythropoiesis in fetus. Comparison of primitive and definitive erythroid precursors and estimate of relative contribution of liver, spleen, and bone marrow. (From Miale, J. B.: Laboratory medicine—hematology, St. Louis, 1972, The C. V. Mosby Co.)

It is of great interest to note that the sequence of events in the development of fetal and adult hemopoiesis is recapitulated and exaggerated in some hematologic diseases in the adult. When hemopoietic activity ceases in the liver and spleen of the fetus, the primitive mesenchymal cells remain in a dormant state. At any later time, these can be stimulated again to form blood cells, at which time we see the phenomenon of *extramedullary hemopoiesis,* i.e., hemopoiesis outside of the normal adult hemopoietic organ, the bone marrow. When this occurs, the liver, spleen, and whatever other tissue involved becomes very much enlarged and, when studied under the microscope, much of the enlargement seen is attributable to proliferating blood cells. This situation is seen in both benign (the so-called myeloproliferative syndromes) and malignant (leukemic and lymphomatous) proliferation.

Phagocytosis, storage, and clearance

The second function of the reticuloendothelial system (phagocytosis, storage, and clearance) is involved in several important physiologic activities. For example, phagocytosis of senescent erythrocytes and other blood cells eliminates those cells that are no longer useful or functioning. When an erythrocyte is "worn out" at the end of its normal life span of about 120 days, it is disposed of by the phagocytic cells of the reticuloendothelial system. Since there are many phagocytes in the spleen and also in the liver, most of the phagocytic activity occurs in these organs. When disintegrating erythrocytes are removed from the blood by phagocytic cells in the spleen, the hemoglobin is broken down into the pigment moiety (bilirubin), the protein moiety (globin), and iron (Fig. 34-4).

Although this is a function common to all phagocytic reticuloendothelial cells regardless of location, it is difficult for us to ascribe such important activities to a diffuse, anatomically indistinct tissue. It is more comfortable to ascribe these functions to specific organs such as the spleen, for this has the respectability of a distinct organ, can be palpated at the bedside to the accompaniment of the medical student's admiring murmurs, and is subject to excision by the surgeon. Thus, when it seems that there is an accelerated destruction of blood cells, it is tempting to visualize this as occurring in the spleen and then to avail oneself of the term "hypersplenism." Nevertheless, there is justification for the term, for the anatomic structure of

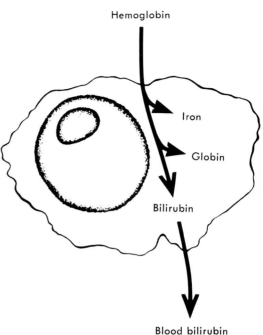

Fig. 34-4. Breakdown of hemoglobin within phagocytic reticuloendothelial cell (splenic macrophage, Kupffer cell in liver, alveolar macrophage of lung, etc.) Hemoglobin iron in form of hemosiderin is stored in phagocyte to various degrees, depending on body's need for iron, and is in equilibrium with plasma iron pool. Globin passes into plasma protein pool, whereas unconjugated bilirubin liberated into blood will be cleared and conjugated in parenchymal cells of liver.

the spleen is such that there is a sluggish flow of blood through the complex of sinuses and, because of this, erythrocytes particularly are exposed in a semistagnant situation to the lytic and other functions of this organ.

In some situations, the phagocytic and cytolytic role of the spleen is striking. In congenital spherocytic hemolytic anemia, for example, the erythrocytes are spherocytic rather than biconcave discs, and this aberration in shape is recognized by the spleen, which promptly destroys them. The slow passage through the cords of Billroth is a major factor in the apparent localization of this destructive activity in that organ and, indeed, splenectomy in such cases is dramatically beneficial. One more example will suffice. It was noted that splenectomized dogs often succumb to an overwhelming infection with *Bartonella,* an organism previously tolerated as long as the spleen destroyed the infected erythrocytes in numbers sufficient to keep the infection under control.[67]

Role in immune reactions

The RES plays a major role in immune processes. It is the interaction between macrophages and lymphocytes that constitutes the cornerstone of immune responses. Though much knowledge in this field has been acquired in recent years, many unanswered questions remain.

Immune reactions can be subdivided into two types: (1) humoral immunity related to B lymphocytes (p. 573), associated with circulating immunoglobulins responsible for the immediate type of skin reactions and the Arthus phenomenon, and (2) cell-bound immunity depending on T lymphocytes (p. 573), associated with the delayed type of skin reaction and graft rejection.

In humoral immunity, the macrophage plays a dual role: it protects the host against an overload of antigens by catabolizing them, and it presents the lymphocytes with antigenic material, which stimulates them to produce immunoglobulins. How the macrophage decides which antigen will be catabolized and which will be presented to lymphocytes is unknown.

In cell-bound immunity the macrophage becomes the effector cell. This is well illustrated by the Prausnitz-Küstner phenomenon in which a nonhypersensitive recipient is rendered hypersensitive by the injection of lymphocytes from a sensitized individual. These sensitized donor lymphocytes, when stimulated by the appropriate antigen, attract the recipient's macrophages with a resultant granulomatous inflammation characteristic of delayed hypersensitivity. The sensitized lymphocytes elaborate factors that attract monocytes (macrophages), inhibit their migration (migration inhibitory factor), and cause monocytic proliferation (blastogenic factor).[84]

Proliferative disorders of the RES

A classification of proliferative disorders of the RES is presented in the outline below. Proliferation of histiocytes (macrophages, reticulum cells, monocytes) may be localized, multicentric, or systemic. It may be reactive (inflammatory) or neoplastic.

Proliferative disorders of histiocytes (reticulum cells, macrophages, monocytes)*
1. Localized
   a. Reactive or inflammatory: granulomatous inflammation

---

*From Rywlin, A.: Histopathology of the bone marrow, Boston, 1976, Little, Brown & Co., p. 114.

   b. Neoplastic
      (1) Benign, e.g., fibrous histiocytoma, reticulohistiocytic granuloma
      (2) Malignant, e.g., malignant fibrous histiocytoma
   c. Uncertain whether reactive or neoplastic, e.g., juvenile xanthogranuloma, xanthomas
2. Multicentric or generalized
   a. Reactive or inflammatory, e.g., generalized miliary tuberculosis, sarcoidosis
   b. Neoplastic:
      (1) Eosinophilic granuloma, Hand-Schüller-Christian disease
      (2) Histiocytic lymphoma (reticulum cell sarcoma)
      (3) Multicentric reticulohistiocytosis[8]
3. Systemic (reticulosis, histiocytosis, reticuloendotheliosis)
   a. Reactive:
      (1) Storage diseases: Gaucher's disease, Niemann-Pick's disease
      (2) Ceroid histiocytosis
   b. Neoplastic:
      (1) Letterer-Siwe disease
      (2) Histiocytic medullary reticulosis
      (3) Leukemic reticuloses:
           Monocytic leukemia
           Leukemic reticuloendotheliosis
               (hairy cell leukemia)

The reactive or inflammatory proliferation of histiocytes is the familiar granulomatous inflammation. Histiocytes may proliferate diffusely or may be aggregated into fairly discrete nodules. Histiocytes are referred to as epithelioid cells when they resemble epithelial cells because they touch each other and possess abundant cytoplasm. The formation of giant cells (multinucleated cells) is frequent and is one of the characteristics of histiocytes. The aggregation of epithelioid cells into discrete nodules is referred to as tuberculoid inflammation, a variant of granulomatous inflammation. Granulomatous inflammation is seen under many different circumstances, including acute bacterial infections such as typhoid fever and listeriosis and chronic mycobacterial and fungal infections.

The localized neoplastic proliferations of the RES are discussed under soft tissues and skin.

Multicentric or generalized proliferative disorders are characterized by several or many lesions without involvement of the entire RES. Sarcoidosis is a good example of a multicentric or generalized inflammatory reaction of the RES.

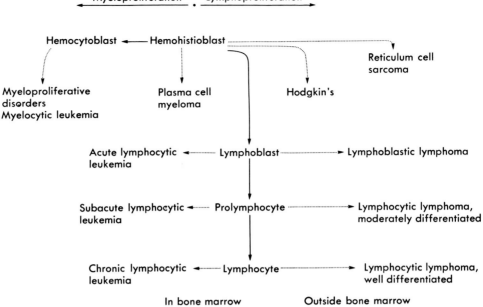

Fig. 34-5. Proliferative potential of reticuloendothelial system. Note that this scheme is concerned primarily with neoplastic proliferation. Benign proliferations (granulocytes, lymphocytes, plasma cells, etc.) differ only in that they are usually not life-threatening. Definition of myeloproliferative syndromes given on p. 1556. (From Miale, J. B.: Laboratory medicine—hematology, St. Louis, 1972, The C. V. Mosby Co.)

Neoplastic multicentric proliferative disorders are again characterized by multiple lesions without involvement of the entire RES. In a multicentric proliferative disorder such as histiocytic lymphoma, the patient presents with a dominant mass rather than with the symmetric lymphadenopathy and hepatosplenomegaly characteristic of systemic proliferation. When a histiocytic lymphoma generalizes, lesions appear away from the main mass. There is still some debate as to whether this generalization represents autochthonous multicentricity or metastatization. The secondary tumor nodules, whether autochthonous or metastatic, are usually sufficiently large to be visible with the naked eye. This contrasts with what is seen in the systemic proliferative disorders, where the proliferation of the RE cells is diffuse, causing enlargement of the liver and spleen without macroscopically visible nodules.

The hematopoietic and RES are unique in exhibiting a systemic proliferation of its cells. Systemic proliferation differs from multicentric proliferation in that all the cells of the system participate. This results in symmetric enlargement of lymph nodes, liver, and spleen. The proliferating cells are also found in the bone marrow. Systemic proliferation of the RE cells is often referred to as either reticulosis, histiocytosis, or reticuloendotheliosis depending on the terminology.

A systemic proliferation may be reactive such as seen in the storage diseases or it may be neoplastic. A reactive systemic proliferation of histiocytes is seen in response to the accumulation of a catabolic product, which accumulates because the patient is deficient in a specific enzyme necessary for the further degradation of the metabolite. Thus in Gaucher's disease the proliferated macrophages contain ceramide glucoside (glucocerebroside) because the patient is deficient in β-glucosidase.

In neoplastic systemic proliferations the proliferating cells may spill over into the peripheral blood giving rise to a leukemia.

The general scheme of the proliferative capabilities of the reticuloendothelial system is shown in Fig. 34-5.

SUMMARY

The reticuloendothelial system is a system of cells that, though present in large numbers in the spleen, liver, and lymph nodes, are in fact present in many tissues and organs in the body. The main characteristic of these cells is phagocytosis. The primitive reticuloendothelial cell, included by some in the RES, is capable of differentiating along many lines. In addition the RES participates in immune reactions and in various proliferative disorders. Neoplasms of the RES may appear to be localized in those organs richest in reticuloendothelial cells (lymph nodes, spleen, liver, bone marrow) but may be found in any organ or tissue in the body. Because of the frequently striking involvement of the spleen, lymph nodes, and bone marrow, it is traditional to describe the anatomic pathologic condition of these individual organs. It should be obvious, however, aside from special and individual characteristics of these organs, that the common denominator is their content of reticuloendothelial cells.

Spleen

STRUCTURE

The spleen comprises the largest single collection of lymphocytes and reticuloendothelial cells in the body. However, it is supplied by arterial blood by the splenic artery and is therefore in the vascular rather than the lymphatic system. It is roughly ovoid, with a convex upper surface and a concave surface below where the hilar vessels enter the organ. It lies beneath the ninth, tenth, and eleventh ribs, its long axis is parallel to them, and in the adult it weighs about 140 gm (range 100 to 170 gm). The capsule consists of a thin band of connective tissue with elastic fibers, covered by serous mesothelium. In man, there is little, if any, smooth muscle in the capsule and thus, unlike in some animal species, there is no intrinsic contractile capability.

Grossly, the surface is purple and the consistency friable. The cut surface shows tiny gray-white islands of *white pulp* scattered throughout the soft red-purple *red pulp* that makes up the bulk of splenic tissue. Scraping the normal surface with the edge of a knife yields a moderate amount of bloody cellular material.

The tiny nodules of the white pulp are collections of small lymphocytes that form a sheath around arterioles of about 0.2 mm diameter and usually extend around even smaller arterioles. The lymphoid nodules are often called malpighian corpuscles. They may or may not show germinal centers.

The red pulp as usually seen under the microscope does not seem particularly exciting,

for the sinusoids are collapsed and one sees only many erythrocytes scattered, among which are a few neutrophils and phagocytic histiocytes. If the spleen is distended by injecting fixative through the splenic vein, however, the true structure is revealed. The framework of the organ consists of a mesh of argyrophilic reticulum fibers that are continuous with the collagen fibers of the capsule and trabeculae. Supported by this framework are many sinusoids lined with long narrow endothelial cells. The spaces between the sinusoids are referred to as the "cords of Billroth," which contain red cells, reticulum cells, macrophages, some granulocytes, and plasma cells.

The vascular system of the spleen (Fig. 34-6) is not like that in any other organ. The splenic artery usually divides into several branches, which enter the organ at different points along the hilum. Each arterial branch enters the spleen within one of the large trabeculae of the capsule. When it leaves the trabecula, it becomes ensheathed with nodular collections of lymphocytes. The nodules of periarterial lymphocytes have been described previously as the "white pulp" of the spleen. The artery and arterioles within the white pulp are called "follicular arteries." These leave the white pulp and enter the red pulp as straight arterioles called "penicillary arteries."

There are several opinions as to the nature of the transition between the arterial and the venous vessels. It is agreed that between the two lie the sinusoids, but one opinion is that the penicillary arteries open directly into the sinusoids (the "closed" theory), whereas others believe that the artery opens into the pulp cords from which the blood enters the sinusoids through a discontinuous endothelial lining (the "open" theory). Knisely[66] described yet another system (in other species) made up of two portions: the arteriole empties directly into the sinusoid and a capillary shunt connects arterioles and venules.

It seems that both modes of microcirculation, the "open" and the "closed," occur in man. The open circulation, in which cells from the peripheral blood percolate slowly through the cords of Billroth prior to entering the sinusoids seems to account better for the functions of the spleen. Indeed, during the slow circulation through the cords, the cellular elements of the peripheral blood are in close association with the macrophages allowing for phagocytosis of abnormal cells, removal of abnormal inclusions, and fragmentation of abnormal erythrocytes. The veins leave the spleen at the hilum

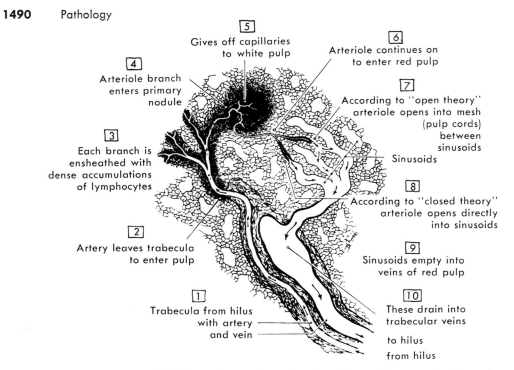

Fig. 34-6. Diagram of blood circulation through spleen. (From Blaustein, A.: The spleen, New York, 1963, copyrighted by McGraw-Hill Book Co.; used with permission.)

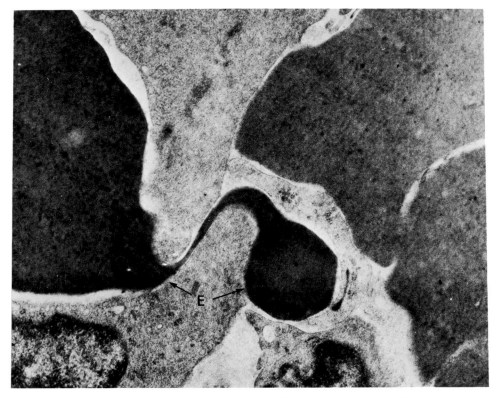

Fig. 34-7. Erythrocyte, **E,** lying partially within (smaller portion) and partially outside sinusoid. Spleen, hemoglobulin H disease, electron microphotograph. (From Wennberg, E., and Weiss, L.: Blood **31:**778-790, 1968; by permission.)

in association with the arteries that enter it.

The structure of the sinusoids deserves special mention. They do not have a basement membrane. They have been likened to a barrel, with the endothelial cells being arranged longitudinally, touching but not cemented together, with "ring fibers" running at right angles and binding them together. The ring fibers have cytochemical characteristics similar to those of the basement membrane of the renal glomerulus and have been shown by King et at.,[65] not to have the properties of reticulum in the classic sense. It has been suggested that the absence of a basement membrane makes the sinusoidal wall discontinuous, allowing blood cells to pass through the spaces between the endothelial cells (Fig. 34-7).

The extent of the lymphatics in the spleen has been debated for many years. Goldberg,[46] on the basis of the location of tumor metastases, has presented evidence that lymphatic vessels do indeed extend deeply into the splenic parenchyma and that they are present in the adventitia of arteries and arterioles and in the subintima of trabecular veins.

FUNCTION

The function of the spleen can be classified under two general headings: (1) functions of the white pulp and (2) functions of the red pulp. The white pulp contains T lymphocytes in the periarteriolar sheaths and B lymphocytes in the malpighian corpuscles proper. The functions of the B and T lymphocytes are discussed on p. 573. The functions of the red pulp are those of the RES.

Because the spleen represents the largest localization of lymphoid and reticuloendothelial tissue and also because it is surgically accessible, this organ is sometimes excised when it is suspected to be hyperactive in the production of antibodies. Splenectomy per se has no effect on antibody production. For example, if an adult who has had a splenectomy for nonhematologic reasons (i.e., traumatic rupture) is challenged with a variety of antigens, it is found that he forms antibodies in no less titer than a normal person with an intact spleen. Supposedly, the antibody-producing role is assumed by other immunologically competent tissues. However, this is not true in children. Smith et al.[124] presented 19 cases of severe and often fulminating infection in children who had been subjected to splenectomy. In two children, the splenectomy was performed for traumatic ruptures. In the others, the spleen was excised because of various

hematologic disorders. Baumgartner[9] explains the different susceptibility to infection to "serologic immaturity" in infants, whereas in the adult the entire immunologic system has matured and is capable of assuming the additional stress of splenectomy.

Phagocytosis of erythrocytes and breakdown of the hemoglobin occurs in the entire reticuloendothelial system, but roughly half of this catabolic activity is localized in the normal spleen. In splenomegaly, the major portion of hemoglobin breakdown occurs in the spleen. The iron that is liberated is stored in the splenic phagocytes. These can be seen to be engorged with hemosiderin when erythrocyte destruction is accelerated, as in the hemolytic anemias. When there is a increase in stored iron, the spleen is said to be "siderotic." Iron stored in the spleen can be used again for the synthesis of hemoglobin.

In addition to storing iron, the spleen participates in the "storage diseases" such as Gaucher's disease and Niemann-Pick disease (see discussion on reticuloendothelioses). Abnormal lipid metabolites accumulate in all phagocytic reticuloendothelial cells but may so involve the many phagocytes in the spleen as to produce huge splenomegaly.

The functions of the spleen that are characteristic of this organ relate primarily to the circulation of erythrocytes through it. In a normal person, the spleen contains only about 20 to 30 ml of erythrocytes, but in splenomegaly the reservoir function is increased greatly and the abnormally enlarged spleen contains many times this volume of red blood cells. The transit time through the cords of Billroth is lengthened, allowing for a longer exposure of red blood cells, granulocytes, and platelets to splenic macrophages. In part, stasis causes consumption of glucose, upon which the erythrocyte is dependent for the maintenance of normal metabolism, and the erythrocyte is destroyed. Selective destruction of abnormal erythrocytes is also accelerated by the splenic pooling.

As erythrocytes pass through the spleen, the organ inspects them for imperfections and destroys those that it recognizes as abnormal or senescent. This is called the "culling" function. Even more remarkable is the "pitting" function, by which the spleen removes granular inclusions (Howell-Jolly bodies, siderotic granules, etc.) without destroying the erythrocyte. This normal function of the spleen keeps the number of circulating erythrocytes with inclusions to a minimum. By the same token, after splenectomy the peripheral blood reflects the loss of the pitting effect. Thus the post-splenectomy peripheral blood film shows Howell-Jolly bodies, siderotic granules, and flat target cells. The last is a consequence of the loss of normal surface membrane maturation, for the spleen is responsible for the rearrangement of lipid molecules at the surface of the erythrocyte to form the adult surface membrane.

The spleen also pools platelets in large numbers. The entry of platelets into the splenic pool and their return to the circulation is extensive. In splenomegaly, the splenic pool may be so large as to produce thrombocytopenia. This lowering of the platelet count in splenomegaly has been erroneously interpreted as increased destruction of platelets in the spleen. The pooled platelets may be identified in the cords of Billroth as a granular eosinophilic material. Sequestration of leukocytes in the enlarged spleen in similar fashion may produce leukopenia.

The concept of *hypersplenism,* then, is that in some cases the sequestering effect on one or more of the three types of circulating blood cells (erythrocytes, granulocytes, and platelets) is so striking as to reduce the content of these cells in the peripheral blood. This sequestering effect can be demonstrated by the finding that isotope-labeled erythrocytes and platelets accumulate in the enlarge spleen, as evidenced by increased radioactivity of the organ.

ASPLENIA AND POLYSPLENIA

Asplenia refers to congenital absence of the spleen. In polysplenia, there are several, more or less equal, splenic masses instead of a single spleen. Accessory spleens differ from polysplenia in that they are present in addition to the normal spleen. Asplenia and polysplenia are associated with extensive malformations. Moller et al.[89] state that polysplenia was a complex of bilateral left-sidedness (levoisomerism) in contrast to asplenia, which showed bilateral right-sidedness (dextroisomerism). Thus, in asplenia, the liver appears symmetric, as if made up of two right lobes, with each lung having three lobes and both bronchi being eparterial. In polysplenia, each lung may have two lobes, and the bronchi are hyparterial. Patients with asplenia and polysplenia may present a complete or partial situs inversus associated with complex cardiac malformations resulting in cyanotic heart disease.

REGRESSIVE CHANGES
Hyalinization

Hyaline degeneration of the arterial wall may be found in persons of any age, even the very young, and is nonspecific in nature. In young persons, hyaline thickening often accompanies hypertension. This degenerative change is most prominent in the sheathed arterioles of the lymphoid follicles. Central hyaline deposits in malpighian follicles of the spleen were studied by Stutte and Schulter.[132] These authors found them in 34% of their autopsies and view them as being made up predominantly of fibrin.

Amyloidosis

Amyloid is deposited in the spleen under the same conditions as in other organs and is therefore found mainly when amyloid occurs in other sites. In systemic diseases leading to amyloidosis, the spleen is the organ most frequently involved.

The spleen may be normal in size, or it may be considerably enlarged, depending on the amount and distribution of amyloid. Two types of involvement are seen: nodular and diffuse.

In the nodular or sago type, amyloid is found in the walls of the sheathed arteries and within the follicles but not in the red pulp. When so distributed, the nodules of amyloid are prominent on cut surface, and their waxy translucent appearance suggests the appearance of sago grains, hence the term "sago spleen."

In the diffuse type, the follicles are not involved, the red pulp is prominently involved, the spleen is usually greatly enlarged and firm, and the cut surface is characteristically waxy and translucent.

Atrophy

Atrophy of the spleen (50 to 70 gm) is not uncommon in elderly individuals. It also may occur in wasting diseases. In chronic hemolytic anemias, particularly sickle-cell anemia, there is progressive loss of pulp, increasing fibrosis, scarring from multiple infarcts, and incrustation with iron and calcium deposits (Fig. 34-8, *A*). In the final stage of atrophy, the spleen may be so small as to be hardly recognizable (Fig. 34-8, *B*). Advanced atrophy sometimes is referred to as *autosplenectomy.*

Pigmentation

The pigments found in the spleen are (1) hemosiderin and hematoidin, derived from

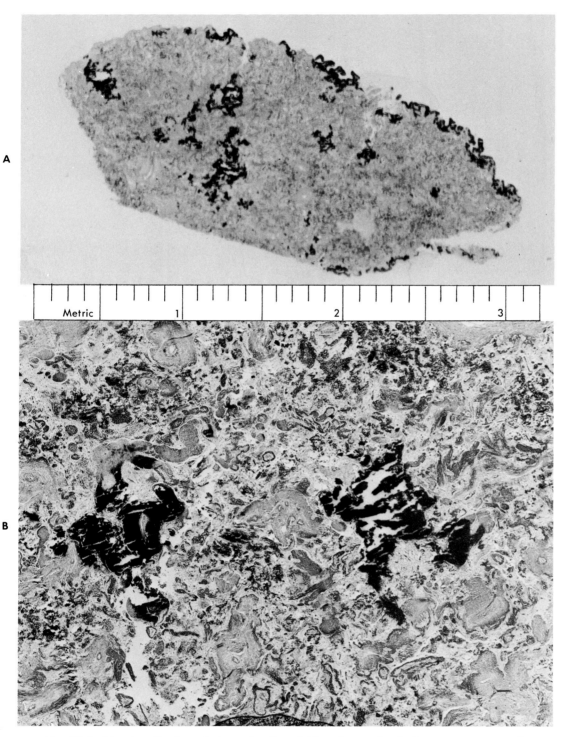

Fig. 34-8. Atrophy of spleen in long-standing sickle-cell anemia. **A,** Gross appearance of bisected organ showing actual size of spleen bisected along its greatest dimension. **B,** Paraffin section. Note complete loss of normal architecture and replacement by fibrous tissue, pigment, and calcium deposits. (**B,** Hematoxylin and eosin; 25×.)

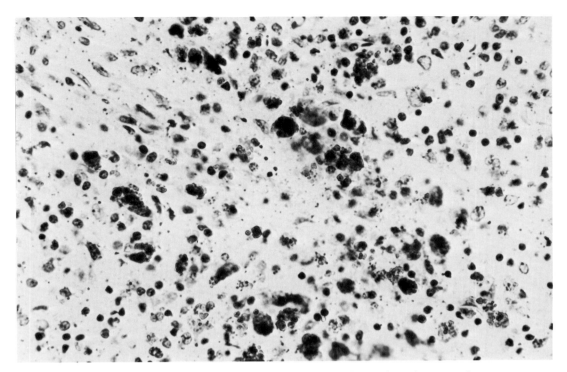

Fig. 34-9. Hemosiderosis of spleen. Most of hemosiderin lies within phagocytic histiocytes. (Hematoxylin and eosin; 125×.)

hemoglobin, (2) malarial pigment, (3) anthracotic pigment, and (4) ceroid.

Hemosiderin is the pigment form of excess iron, whether this is derived from endogenous or exogenous sources. It is seen readily in tissue sections as coarse golden brown granules within phagocytic cells. It gives a positive Prussian blue reaction and therefore contains ferric iron. Large amounts of hemosiderin are deposited in all phagocytic cells of the reticuloendothelial system when there is iron excess, as in chronic hemolytic anemia or after many blood transfusions. Deposition of hemosiderin iron in the spleen in abnormally large amounts is called *siderosis* or *hemosiderosis* of the spleen (Fig. 34-9). The same descriptive terms are used for other organs. In moderate amounts, hemosiderin produces little reaction in the tissues. In large amounts, it stimulates proliferation of fibrous tissue. Siderosis sometimes has been called secondary hemochromatosis to distinguish it from primary hemochromatosis, a primary metabolic defect in iron utilization and storage, but siderosis is the preferred term.

The nature of the pigment called hematoidin is largely unknown. It is not related to iron metabolism in the same way as hemosiderin, in that it is not deposited as a consequence of systemic iron overload. Rather, it is formed in areas of hemorrhage or infarction, possibly in a hypoxic environment. It appears as golden brown burrlike or crystalline masses and does not give the Prussian blue reaction for ferric iron but gives a positive Gmelin reaction for bile pigments. From this one must infer for the present that hematoidin is a non–iron containing breakdown product of hemoglobin. The Gmelin reaction, positive with various bile pigments, does not help better to define this pigment. Contrary to hemosiderin, hematoidin is an extracellular pigment.

In malaria, the black pigment imparts a dark brown color to the pulp of the spleen. The pigment is of the acid hematin type and is found within phagocytes.

Anthracotic pigmentation of the spleen is rare. Askanazy[5] describes finding anthracotic pigment in the bone marrow, liver, and spleen (his term *Kohlenmetastase*) in necropsy studies of anthracosis. The spread from the respiratory system is probably hematogenous.

Ceroid pigment is discussed in detail in the reticuloendothelioses.

Rupture

Rupture of a normal spleen may result from severe blunt trauma to the abdomen. An enlarged soft spleen, such as that seen in infec-

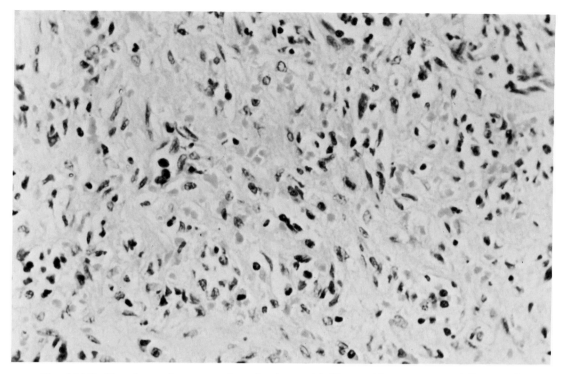

Fig. 34-10. Chronic passive congestion of spleen with fibrosis. Note pronounced fibrosis of red pulp. (Hematoxylin and eosin; 125×.)

tious mononucleosis, leukemia, malaria, or typhoid fever, ruptures easily with minimal trauma. The trauma may be so slight that the rupture is believed to be "spontaneous." It is not unusual for such a spleen to be ruptured as the result of enthusiastic palpation maneuvers by the physician, straining at the stool, or even violent retching. In some cases, rupture is delayed for some days after the trauma. The reason is that trauma causes an intrasplenic hematoma. As the hematoma enlarges, the capsule is put under tension and eventually ruptures.

One consequence of splenic rupture is auto-implantation of splenic tissue on the peritoneal surfaces, forming multiple implants (splenosis). Splenosis can be confused at the time of operative discovery with endometriosis, metastatic carcinoma or hemangioma, and, if unrecognized, may lead to unnecessary surgical procedures.[16]

CIRCULATORY DISTURBANCES
Active hyperemia

Active hyperemia accompanies the reaction in the spleen to acute systemic infections. This is called *septic splenitis, acute splenic tumor,* or *acute reactive hyperplasia of the spleen* (p. 1497). The spleen is moderately enlarged, the capsule is tense even though the organ is soft, and the cut surface is dark red and bulging, and its architecture is obscured by the bulging, cellular, bloody pulp.

Passive hyperemia and fibrocongestive splenomegaly

Passive hyperemia (chronic passive congestion) is caused by interference with the venous return through the portal circulation. This may be caused by an increase in systemic venous pressure, as in cardiac decompensation, or to increased pressure in the portal circulation alone.

In passive hyperemia caused by cardiac disease, the spleen is only moderately enlarged and rubbery. The cut surface is dry, the cut edges are sharp, and the trabecular markings are increased. In long-standing cases, there is thickening of the trabeculae, fibrosis of the red pulp (Fig. 34-10), and atrophy of lymphoid tissue.

Portal hypertension has many causes. The most frequent is cirrhosis of the liver, which is accompanied by splenomegaly in about 80%

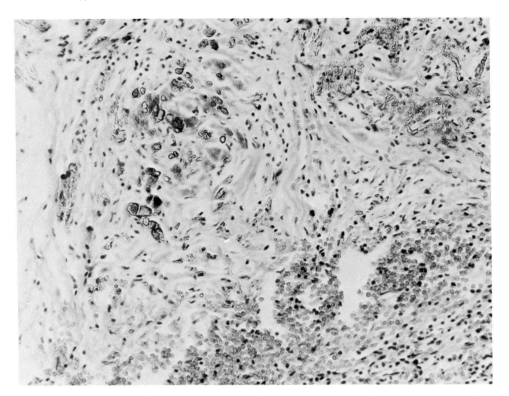

Fig. 34-11. Gamna-Gandy body consisting of fibrous tissue, hemosiderin, and hematoidin. (Hematoxylin and eosin; 125×.)

of the cases. Here, the obstruction to blood flow is intrahepatic. The obstruction may be essentially extrahepatic as in (1) the right-sided heart failure of tricuspid insufficiency, pulmonary disease, or constrictive pericarditis, (2) splenic vein sclerosis or thrombosis, (3) portal vein thrombosis, or (4) idiopathic portal hypertension where neither intrahepatic nor extrahepatic obstruction is demonstrable.

In contrast to passive hyperemia from congestive heart failure, passive hyperemia from increased portal pressure causes considerable splenomegaly, often to 500 gm or more. The spleen displays the full-blown picture of fibrocongestive splenomegaly. The malpighian follicles are atrophic and exhibit some periarterial fibrosis. Perifollicular hemorrhages may be present. As the latter get organized, "siderotic nodules" also known as "tobacco nodules," or Gamna-Gandy bodies, are formed (Fig. 34-11). They consist of areas of fibrosis containing collagen fibers encrusted with iron and calcium. The cords of Billroth contain an increased number of macrophages, fibroblasts, and irregulaly thickened reticulum fibers. The appearance of the sinuses may vary depending

on the cause of the portal hypertension. They may be dilated and empty.[102] In portal hypertension from splenic vein thrombosis, the sinuses are narrower than normal but are greatly elongated.[131] The endothelial cells are prominent.

The term "Banti's syndrome" has been used for fibrocongestive splenomegaly associated with hypersplenism. Actually Banti described a disease characterized by enlargement of the spleen and anemia followed by digestive hemorrhages, cirrhosis of the liver, and ascites. The pathologic changes in the spleen, according to Banti, were characterized by "fibroadenia." Fibroadenia included fibrosis of malpighian corpuscles (lymphadenoid tissue) and glandlike appearance of the sinusoids, because of prominent endothelial cells. The histologic appearance of the spleen is identical with that of fibrocongestive splenomegaly from splenic vein thrombosis.[131]

Whether Banti's disease exists is moot. Some observers apply the term to instances of splenomegaly with hypersplenism in which there are no demonstrable pathologic findings in the liver, portal, and splenic veins. The spleen in these instances shows varying degrees of fibro-congestive splenomegaly. Often there is only an increase in the red pulp. Some of these cases are associated with "idiopathic" portal hypertension; in others portal hypertension was not documented during the operation. We have followed a few such patients for several years. They remain cured of their hyper-splenism and have not developed any evidence of cirrhosis of the liver. Whether they would have developed Banti's sequence with ascites and cirrhosis of the liver, if the spleen had not been removed, cannot be ascertained. (See also p. 1405.)

Infarction

Infarction results from occlusion of the splenic artery or branches. Occlusion may be caused by thrombosis, by localized occlusion on the basis of sclerosis, by subendothelial infiltration with leukemic cells in chronic myelocytic leukemia, or by obstruction of the microcirculation attributable to conglutination and sludging of red blood cells such as is seen in sickle-cell anemia, sickle-cell trait, and sickle cell–hemoglobin C disease. Occlusion on the basis of emboli is most commonly seen in heart disease, either from mural thrombi in the left auricle or ventricle or vegetations on the valves on the left side of the heart. Occasionally, infarcts are found at necropsy without apparent cause for thrombosis and embolism.

Infarcts are sometimes conic, with the base at the capsular surface, and sometimes irregular in shape. Although they are classified as anemic or hemorrhagic on the basis of gross appearance (pale or red, respectively), most are hemorrhagic at first. Later, dehemoglobinization occurs and the infarcted area becomes pale, gray-white with a hyperemic border (Fig. 34-12). Later still, the necrotic tissue is replaced by fibrous tissue, which contracts and gives rise to a depressed scar.

If the embolus contains bacteria, as from vegetative endocarditis of the mitral or aortic valve, the infarct undergoes rapid softening and suppuration as the bacteria multiply. This is called a *septic infarct.*

A special type of ischemic necrosis was described by Feitis as a terminal event in uremia. The necrotic areas are white or yellowish and of varied sizes and irregular shapes, central as well as peripheral. The diffuseness of the necrosis gives the cut surface a spotted appearance—hence the term *"Fleckmilz"* (spotted spleen). Although not uncommon in uremia, this distribution of necrotic areas also is seen

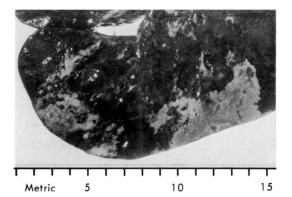

Metric   5   10   15

Fig. 34-12. Multiple infarcts of spleen. (From Rezek, P. R., and Millard, M.: Autopsy pathology, Springfield, Ill., 1963, Charles C Thomas, Publisher.)

in systemic infections, with or without vascular occlusion. The term is thus purely descriptive.

Occasionally patients with sickle-cell trait deprived of an adequate supply of oxygen, such as occurs when traveling at high altitudes, will undergo infarction of their spleen. Such a spleen may present the picture of a pseudocyst filled with a brown, mushy, semifluid material.[114] The hypoxia reduces the hemoglobin S and leads to the formation of sickled cells. As a result the viscosity of the blood is increased, producing erythrostasis and further deoxygenation. In addition, a decrease in the tissue pH favors the production of sickled cells. The capillary circulation is blocked by the conglutinated sickled erythrocytes. The result is necrosis of tissue and formation of a pseudocyst. Electrophoretic studies of hemoglobin should be performed on all patients with pseudocysts of the spleen.

SPLEEN IN SYSTEMIC INFECTIONS
General features

Enlargement of the spleen (250 to 350 gm) is common in acute systemic infections. The enlarged, soft, even diffluent, cellular organ is then said to show *acute reactive hyperplasia.* Other terms used are *acute inflammatory splenomegaly, septic splenitis,* or *acute splenic tumor.*

The splenomegaly is caused in part by a true reactive hyperplasia of the myeloid and lymphoid cells of the pulp and in part by congestion with erythrocytes. The reaction may be to pathogenic organisms, but most often it is to the products of inflammation, substances responsible for the mobilization of neutrophils, lymphocytes, and eosinophils.[47] The spleen also

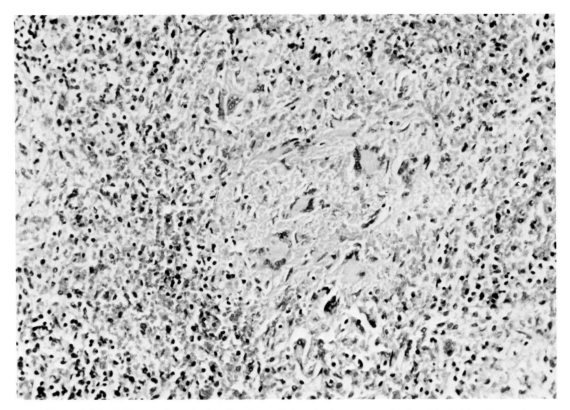

Fig. 34-13. Miliary tuberculosis of spleen. Tubercle is composed of epithelioid cells and Langhans' giant cells, and there is no caseous necrosis. (Hematoxylin and eosin; 125×.)

can react to foreign substances not the product of inflammation, such as foreign protein or a distant focus of necrotic tissue. The spleen is never enlarged in bacterial peritonitis.

Acute reactive hyperplasia is characterized by an increase in the cells of the red pulp. Grossly, the cut surface is purple-red, and the gray follicles are prominent. Microscopically, neutrophils are found without difficulty, and some may be of intermediate maturity. There is also an increase in phagocytic cells, both of the mononuclear type and of the fixed histiocyte type. These contain ingested debris from dead leukocytes and erythrocytes and sometimes bacteria and other organisms. A number of plasma cells also can be found. The lymphoid follicles are usually hyperplastic, although the lymphoid hyperplasia may be obscured by the congestion of the red pulp. Sometimes, the follicles have large reactive centers showing much phagocytic activity.

These general features are modified slightly in various infectious diseases but usually not sufficiently to enable one to make an etiologic diagnosis solely on the basis of morphologic changes.

Bacteremia and septicemia

In typhoid fever, the spleen is greatly enlarged, soft, and congested. Infiltration with granulocytes is minimal, but mononuclear cells are numerous. There is much phagocytic activity. Focal necrosis, hemorrhage, and rupture are not uncommon.

In the septicemia of *Clostridium welchii,* there is intense hyperemia and congestion of the red pulp, the sinusoids are collapsed, and there is evidence of extensive hemolysis of erythrocytes.

In streptococcal septicemia (whether acute or of the subacute type), as in subacute bacterial endocarditis, the spleen is large and extremely soft and flabby. In subacute bacterial endocarditis, infarcts (both bland and septic) are not uncommon.

Infectious mononucleosis

As mentioned earlier, the large soft spleen in infectious mononucleosis is easily subject to rupture. This complication, necessitating splenectomy, has provided most of the material studied.[125] The spleen is enlarged to three or four times the normal size. Characteristic changes are as follows:

1. Large numbers of atypical lymphocytes (virocytes) like those found in the peripheral blood, bone marrow, and lymph nodes are seen in the red pulp and in the sinusoids.
2. The follicles are usually not hyperplastic.
3. The virocytes usually infiltrate the capsule, trabeculae, adventitia of the arteries, and subintima of the veins and sinusoids.

Probably the cellular infiltration and edema of the capsule account for the high incidence of rupture.

Granulomatous inflammation

There are few features of granulomatous inflammation of the spleen that are not common to a given granulomatous inflammation in another organ or tissue. The spleen is normal in size or unusually enlarged, depending on the extent of the infection. A few special features deserve mention.

In fibrocaseous *tuberculosis* of the lungs, the spleen is usually normal, but in tuberculous pneumonitis, it may be hyperplastic as part of the generalized reaction to severe acute infection. In miliary tuberculosis, the spleen is involved almost always (Fig. 34-13). The tubercles may be few or very numerous, minute or readily visible. In either case, splenomegaly is slight. When numerous, the tubercles can be readily seen on cut surface or through the capsule. Occasionally, a large tumorlike *tuberculoma,* usually single and measuring several centimeters in diameter, is the only lesion found (see chapter on lung, pleura, and mediastinum).

The lesions in *syphilis* depend on the stage of the disease. In congenital syphilis, there is splenomegaly with hyperplastic changes in the red pulp that contains an increased number of granulocytes, plasma cells, and phagocytic histiocytes. Spirochetes are very numerous and easily demonstrated by special staining techniques. In the acquired disease, the spleen is normal during the primary stage. In the secondary stage, it is enlarged and shows follicular hyperplasia and many plasma cells in the red pulp. In the tertiary stage, it is generally normal except for the rare occurrence of the large spheroid lesions, called *gummas,* characteristic of tertiary syphilis. Occasionally, splenomegaly in tertiary syphilis is secondary to syphilitic cirrhosis of the liver with obstruction of the portal blood flow.

In *sarcoidosis,* the spleen is involved quite often as part of the generalized disease, but occasionally the splenic involvement is so severe in proportion to lesions in other organs as to appear primary. The lesions vary from microscopic to grossly nodular. In the former, they may be merely aggregates of epithelioid cells. In the latter, they show the noncaseating type of granulomatous inflammation characteristic of sarcoidosis. It must be noted that sarcoidlike lesions (i.e., noncaseating granulomas) may be found in a variety of conditions: leprosy, tularemia, histoplasmosis, brucellosis, berylliosis, splenic deposition of silica, lipid-storage diseases, Hodgkin's disease, and some reactions to parasites. To be distinguished from sarcoidosis are the rare cases of tuberculosis in which the tubercles fail to show central caseation. In granulomatous inflammation, calcification is common only in chronic brucellosis and in histoplasmosis.[120]

PARASITIC INFESTATION

Enlargement of the spleen is so common in malaria that this physical sign is used as presumptive evidence of infection when epidemiologists survey inhabitants of endemic areas. In the acute stages of malaria, the febrile episodes are accompanied by reactive hyperplasia of the spleen. In chronic malaria, the spleen is greatly enlarged, even up to 6 kg, despite fibrosis. It is firm, the capsule usually is studded with pearly white thickenings (the "ague cake spleen"), and the cut surface is slate gray because of large amounts of malarial pigment (hematin). Under the microscope, one sees malarial parasites and hematin in the sinus endothelium and the phagocytic cells of the red pulp. This pigment gives a negative reaction when stained for ferric iron. Fibrosis is prominent in infection of long duration. Rupture is not uncommon.

The spleen also enlarges in *leishmaniasis* (kala-azar). Except for the absence of pigmentation, the spleen is the same as described for malaria. Definitive diagnosis is based on identifying the many parasites (*Leishmania donovani*) in phagocytic cells.

Splenomegaly in schistosomiasis is secondary to cirrhosis of the liver and portal hypertension. Only rarely are parasites to be found in the red pulp. The parasites provoke a tuberculoid inflammation. Occasionally, there is hemorrhage in the red pulp and, in the later stages of resolution, siderotic nodules are formed.

SPLEEN IN HEMOLYTIC ANEMIA

Hemolytic anemia is the general term applied to anemia referable to decreased life span of the erythrocytes. When the rate of destruction is greater than can be compensated for by the bone marrow, anemia results. When there is accelerated destruction of erythrocytes, the spleen's normal role in disposing of damaged erythrocytes is exaggerated and so, in that sense, the spleen plays an important role in hemolytic disease.

Hemolytic anemia is a complex subject that cannot be covered here. For details, the student is referred to standard texts in hematology. Some generalizations, however, can be made.

Decreased erythrocyte survival is the result of one of two abnormal situations: the erythrocyte is itself abnormal, an *intrinsic* defect, and therefore not able to survive normally, or there is an *extrinsic* influence that damages an otherwise normal erythrocyte and shortens its life span. In either case, the spleen seems to dispose of the defective erythrocytes, but especially when the erythrocytes are intrinsically abnormal.

In *congenital spherocytic hemolytic anemia (hereditary spherocytosis)*, an intrinsic abnormality of the erythrocytes gives rise to erythrocytes that are small and spheroid rather than the normal flattened biconcave discs. Although there is evidence that intracellular glycolysis and phosphorylation are abnormal, the nature of the intrinsic defect is not known. The two components of the disease are the production by the bone marrow of spherocytic erythrocytes and increased destruction of these cells in the spleen. The spleen destroys spherocytes selectively, as shown by the following observations:

1. Normal erythrocytes transfused into a person having hereditary spherocytosis survive for a normal time.
2. Erythrocytes from hereditary spherocytosis tranfused into a normal recipient are rapidly destroyed.
3. Erythrocytes from hereditary spherocytosis transfused into a recipient previously subjected to splenectomy survive for a normal time.
4. In hereditary spherocytosis, splenectomy cures completely the hemolytic disease, even though the bone marrow continues

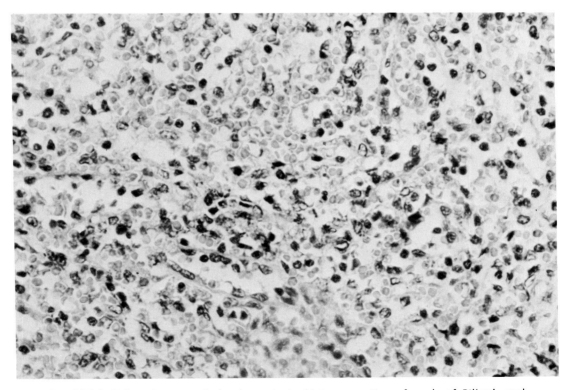

Fig. 34-14. Spleen in congenital spherocytosis. Note congestion of cords of Billroth and hyperplasia of endothelial cells lining sinusoids. (Hematoxylin and eosin; 125×.)

to make spherocytes and the appearance of the peripheral blood smear is unchanged.

The spleen is always enlarged, and weights of 500 to 1000 gm are not uncommon. The cut surface is deep red and hemorrhagic. The microscopic features (Fig. 34-14) that are characteristic are as follows:

1. Pronounced congestion of the cords of Billroth, possibly because the spheroid erythrocytes do not pass readily through the sinusoidal walls
2. Hyperplasia of the endothelial cells lining the sinusoids
3. Relatively empty sinusoids
4. Little or no hemosiderin, in contrast to many other hemolytic anemias

If accessory spleens are present, they not only show the same morphology but also, if not excised along with the principal spleen, will take over the destructive function and the original splenectomy will be ineffective.

In *sickle-cell disease,* as well as in some severe variants such as hemoglobin S, hemoglobin C, or hemoglobin S thalassemia combinations, the spleen is severely involved. The changes are progressive and are most severe in long-standing cases. As in hereditary spherocytosis, the defect in the erythrocytes is intrinsic, the content of hemoglobin S causing them to assume rigid, bizarre, sicklelike shapes under hypoxic conditions. The rigidity and peculiar shape of the erythrocytes cause them to plug up small blood vessels, and most of the clinical findings can be explained on the basis of obstruction of the microcirculation by conglutinated red cells. In the spleen, they do not pass out of the splenic cords, so that they are congested and contain many sickled erythrocytes (Fig. 34-15). Later, the spleen shows the effect of repeated hemorrhages and infarcts; the hemorrhages lead to diffuse fibrosis with scattered siderotic nodules, whereas repeated infarction produces many large depressed scars. The most severe degree of fibrosis and atrophy has already been discussed and illustrated (Fig. 34-10).

The microscopic features that distinguish the spleen in sickle-cell disease are as follows:

1. The sickled erythrocytes, always prominent in formalin-fixed tissue
2. The large amount of hemosiderin (as op-

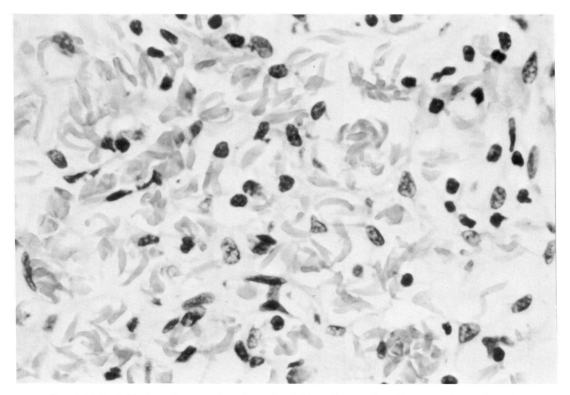

Fig. 34-15. Sickled erythocytes in spleen in sickle-cell anemia. (Hematoxylin and eosin; 450×.)

posed to the spleen in congenital sphero-cytosis)

3. Progressive fibrosis
4. Numerous infarcts

It should be noted that some sickled erythrocytes are seen in any hemoglobinopathy in which hemoglobin S is one of the hemoglobins. Thus they may be seen in sickle-cell trait (hemoglobin S plus hemoglobin A). Here, however, the spleen is relatively normal. Infarcts and pseudocysts of the spleen may occur in patients with sickle-cell trait.

Patients with sickle-cell anemia and its genetic variants are subject to periodic exacerbations or "crises" of their disease. In "hemolytic crises" there is an increase in the severity of the anemia because of a further shortening of the life span of the red cells. In "aplastic crises" the anemia becomes more severe because the bone marrow stops producing red blood cells. Nucleated red blood cells disappear from the marrow. In "visceral or pain crises" deoxygenation causes sludging of red cells in the microcirculation in different organs simulating a variety of clinical conditions. Massive sickling involving large capillary territories may be responsible for sudden death.

In contrast to sickle-cell disease, patients with hemoglobin C disorders (homozygous hemoglobin C and hemoglobin C and S disease) have large spleens exhibiting congestion of the cords of Billroth. Pregnancy is particularly dangerous for patients with hemoglobin C and S disease. Such patients may develop severe visceral crises in the third trimester of pregnancy, which may result in bone marrow necrosis with extensive fat and bone marrow emboli.[115]

The spleen also is severely involved in *thalassemia* (Cooley's anemia, Mediterranean anemia). This hemoglobinopathy differs from the others in that an abnormal molecular form of hemoglobin is not present. Rather, there is a suppression of synthesis of β-polypeptide chains (β-thalassemia) or α-polypeptide chains (α-thalassemia) resulting in deficient synthesis of normal hemoglobin. Suppression of normal hemoglobin synthesis is accompanied by increased amounts of hemoglobin A_2 or hemoglobin F. The erythrocytes are not only deficient in normal hemoglobin (hypochromic) but are also abnormal in shape, many being

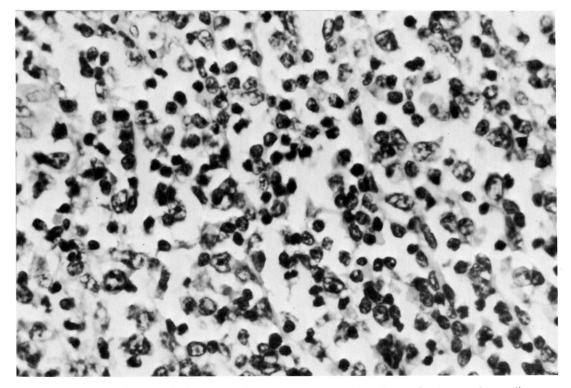

Fig. 34-16. Spleen in thalassemia. There are numerous large hyperplastic reticulum cells and some normoblasts. (Hematoxylin and eosin; 250×.)

target cells, whereas the others vary greatly in size and shape. Their life span is short because they are destroyed in large number by the spleen.

The disease ranges in severity from mild to very severe. The changes in the spleen are greatest in the severe form called thalassemia major. The spleen is very large, often seeming to fill the abdominal cavity. The organ is firm and the capsule often thickened. The cut surface is dark red. Microscopically, there is congestion, fibrosis, and hyperplasia of reticuloendothelial cells (Fig. 34-16). The one feature that is characteristic is the presence of foci of blood cell formation, extramedullary hemopoiesis. Also characteristic, but not so frequent, is the presence of foam cells in the red pulp. These are large and show a foamy cytoplasm that may contain ceroid. Siderotic nodules sometimes are found, but these are seen also in other hemolytic anemias.

SPLEEN IN OTHER DISEASES OF BLOOD AND BLOOD-FORMING ORGANS

The spleen, as one organ of the reticuloendothelial system, seldom escapes being involved in proliferative reactions that, classically, are described as having their genesis in other organs, such as lymph nodes or bone marrow. Thus, in addition to the conditions already discussed, which may be considered to involve primarily some special splenic function, splenomegaly is found in hematologic disorders involving granulocytopoiesis, lymphopoiesis, erythropoiesis, and proliferation of other cell types (see accompanying classification). For convenience, the involvement of the spleen in these diseases will be discussed in subsequent sections (granulocytic leukemia, lymphocytic leukemia, myeloproliferative syndromes, and lymphomas).

Splenomegaly primarily caused by hemopoietic activity

1. Granulocytopoiesis
   a. Reactive hyperplasia to acute and chronic infections
      (1) "Acute splenic tumor" of various acute infections
      (2) Tuberculosis
      (3) Congenital syphilis
      (4) Malaria
      (5) Trypanosomiasis
      (6) Histoplasmosis
      (7) Schistosomiasis
      (8) Leishmaniasis
      (9) Echinococcosis
   b. Myeloproliferative syndromes
   c. Granulocytic leukemia

2. Lymphopoiesis
   a. Generalized lymphocytic reactions
      (1) Infectious mononucleosis
      (2) Other viral infections
      (3) Hyperthyroidism
   b. Lymphocytic leukemia
   c. Lymphocytic lymphomas
3. Erythropoiesis
   a. Hemolytic anemias
   b. Myeloproliferative syndromes including polycythemia vera
   c. Erythroleukemia
4. Other cell types
   a. Plasmocytosis, reactive
   b. Multiple myeloma
   c. Monocytic leukemia

Splenomegaly primarily caused by destructive activity

1. Hemolytic anemias
2. Thrombocytopenic purpura (rare)
3. Splenic neutropenia

Splenomegaly caused by reticuloendothelial hyperactivity

1. Reticuloendothelial hyperplasia in acute and chronic infections
2. Disseminated lupus erythematosus
3. Rheumatoid arthritis
4. Felty's syndrome
5. Hemochromatosis and hemosiderosis
6. Gaucher's disease
7. Niemann-Pick disease
8. Amyloidosis
9. Diabetes mellitus
10. Gargoylism
11. Reticulum cell sarcoma

Splenomegaly caused by vascular factors (congestive splenomegaly)

1. Cirrhosis of liver
2. Portal vein blockage
3. Splenic vein thrombosis and other obstructions
4. Cardiac failure
5. Infarction

Splenomegaly caused by nonspecific afflictions

1. Primary neoplasms and cysts
2. Metastatic neoplasms
3. Macrosomia

PRIMARY TUMORS

The spleen is only rarely the site of primary tumor in the strict sense of the word. Thus most of the leukemias and lymphomas, being multicentric in origin, are excluded as being primary splenic tumors. Rarely, lymphoma of varying cell types seems to originate in the spleen and nowhere else. These have been called primary lymphomas of the spleen, but in the few cases we have seen that seem to fall into this category, a careful search revealed that there was also, although less obvious, involvement of the lymph nodes and bone marrow. A review of the literature on supposedly primary lymphomas of the spleen re-

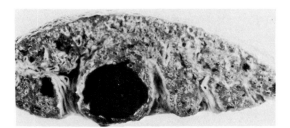

Fig. 34-17. Hemangioma of spleen with fibrosis.

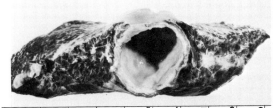

Fig. 34-19. Dermoid cyst of spleen.

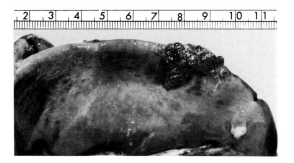

Fig. 34-18. Lymphangioma of spleen.

veals that this diagnosis is not supported by negative lymphangiographic studies.

The most common primary tumor is the cavernous hemangioma. These are sometimes only a few millimeters in diameter, more often measuring 1 to 2 cm and occasionally are so large as to cause splenomegaly (Fig. 34-17). Next in frequency are the lymphangiomas. These may also be very large and may present as multicystic lesions (Fig. 34-18). Other benign tumors (fibroma, chondroma, osteoma) are extremely rare. Also rare are malignant endotheliomas.

Occasionally well circumscribed, but not encapsulated, nodules made up of splenic tissue are seen within the splenic parenchyma. These have been called hamartomas, splenomas, splenic adenomas, and intrasplenic accessory spleens.[98-101]

METASTATIC TUMORS

The frequency of involvement of the spleen by metastatic tumor ranges from rare to 50% in the various series reported. The higher values probably reflect the true incidence of metastases, for the more care taken to examine all portions of the spleen, both grossly and microscopically, the higher the incidence of metastatic tumor.

Metastases occur late in the course of the primary cancer and are not found in the absence of metastases to other organs. The primary tumors that metastasize to the spleen are many. The most common types, in order of decreasing frequency, are lung, breast, prostate gland, colon, and stomach. Metastases may be either nodular or diffuse. Most represent hematogenous spread from the primary lesion, but some of the metastases are undoubtedly by lymphatic dissemination. Spleens showing only microscopic metastases range in weight from 60 to 400 gm. Those showing large nodules of metastatic tumor range from 70 to 1100 gm. Those showing diffuse gross involvement range from 100 to 3000 gm.

CYSTS

Cysts of the spleen are rare. They include parasitic cysts, of which those caused by *Taenia echinococcus* are the most frequent, and neoplastic (benign) cysts, which are usually cystic lymphangiomas, cavernous hemanigomas, or dermoid cysts (Fig. 34-19). The latter may contain sebum and hair and may be lined with well-preserved squamous epithelium and sebaceous glands. Pseudocysts do not show an epithelial lining. They are the result of hemorrhage or necrosis (p. 1497).

SPLEEN IN AUTOIMMUNE DISEASES

The concept of "autoimmune disease," a direct and noxious attack by specific immunologic agents against cells and tissues, is based on firm experimental evidence. For example, allergic encephalomyelitis and thyroiditis can be produced by injecting organ extracts into animals, whereas graft-versus-host reactions may involve evidence of generalized disease such as Coombs-positive hemolytic anemia, polyarthritis, myocarditis, and nephritis. Although the experimental autoimmune diseases usually are characterized by the presence of tissue-specific antibodies in the blood, it does not necessarily follow that autoimmune antibodies in the blood in human diseases are in

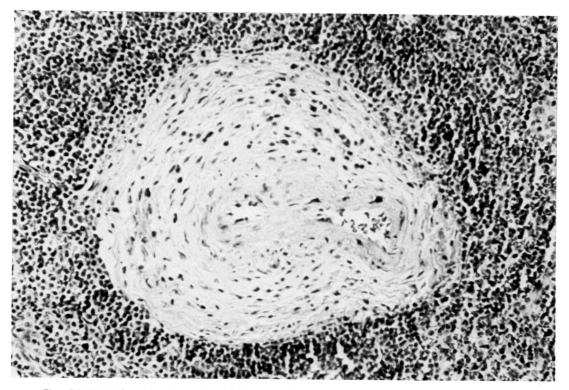

Fig. 34-20. Spleen in disseminated lupus erythematosus. Note onionskin appearance of arteriolar wall. (Hematoxylin and eosin; 125×.)

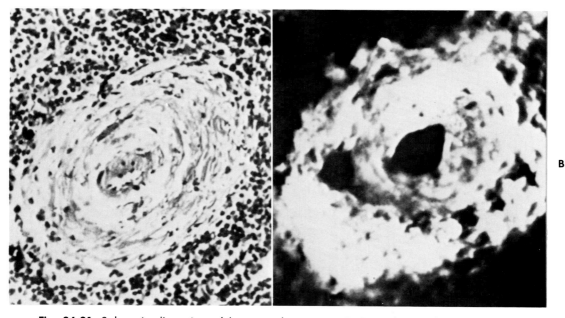

A   **B**

Fig. 34-21. Spleen in disseminated lupus erythematosus. **A,** Typical onionskin appearance of arteriole. **B,** Immunofluorescence reaction with anti–gamma globulin serum showing deposition of gamma globulin. (From Miescher, P. A., and Muller-Eberhard, H. J.: Textbook of immunopathology, New York, 1968-1969, Grune & Stratton, Inc.; by permission.)

every instance directly toxic on cells and tissues. Nevertheless, it would seem that a common denominator in these diseases is the reaction of connective tissue. Since the spleen often is involved, the pathologic changes in this organ deserve brief mention.

Splenomegaly, with or without characteristic histologic alterations, is common to the entire group. In *rheumatoid arthritis*, for example, the spleen usually is enlarged but presents no characteristic histologic changes. On the other hand, the spleen in *systemic lupus erythematosus* usually shows foci of degenerating collagen in the capsule and the characteristic periarterial "onionskin" lesion (Fig. 34-20) that affects the central and penicillary arteries. By immunofluorescence, gamma globulin (Fig. 34-21), complement, and fibrinogen can be demonstrated in the laminae of the lesion.

There are two types of thrombocytopenic purpura in which the spleen shows recognizable involvement. In *idiopathic thrombocyto-penic purpura*, an immunologic thrombocytopenia, the spleen is usually unremarkable. Occasionally, the lymphoid follicles are hyperplastic (Fig. 34-22), megakaryocytes may be found in the red pulp, and there may also be occasional foamy histiocytes, with or without ceroid pigment. *Thrombotic thrombocytopenic purpura*, on the other hand, is believed not to be caused by an immunologic reaction. There is diffuse thrombosis of small blood vessels, once believed to be caused by platelet thrombi, but we have come to appreciate that the occlusion is caused by intravascular deposition of fibrin with secondary entrapment of platelets. The lesions can be found in the spleen as well as in most other organs.

SPLEEN IN RETICULOENDOTHELIOSES

Systemic proliferations of reticuloendothelial cells (histiocytoses, reticuloses, or reticuloendothelioses) may be reactive or neoplastic (see outline on p. 1487). The reactive systemic reticuloendothelioses are associated with the

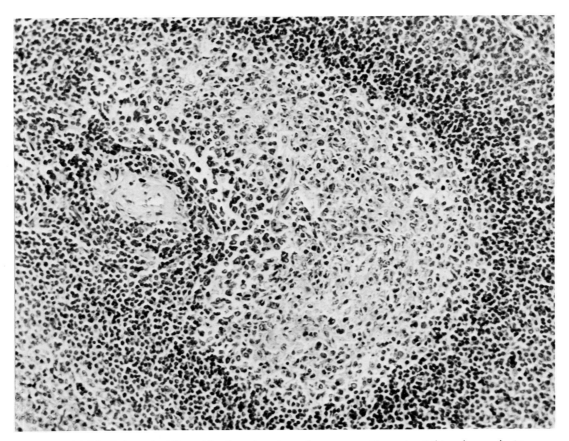

Fig. 34-22. Spleen in idiopathic thrombocytopenic purpura. There is striking hyperplasia of lymphoid follicle. (Hematoxylin and eosin; 125×.)

storage of a catabolite and are therefore also called storage diseases. Involvement of the spleen in these disorders occurs as part of a generalized reaction of the RES, so that other reticuloendothelial tissues (bone marrow and lymph nodes) are also involved. We will only discuss storage diseases involving primarily the RES: Gaucher's disease, Niemann-Pick disease, and ceroid histiocytosis. The RES is involved, to a much lesser degree, in other sphingolipidoses, mucopolysaccharidoses, and mucolipidoses.[127] Histiocytosis X, histiocytic medullary reticulosis, and leukemic reticuloendotheliosis will be discussed as examples of neoplastic proliferative disorders of the reticuloendothelial system.

Gaucher's disease

The dominant clinical features of Gaucher's disease are splenomegaly, hepatomegaly, erosion of cortices of the long bones, and generally mild anemia, leukopenia, and thrombocytopenia. Infantile, juvenile, and adult forms of

Gaucher's disease are recognized.[14] Gaucher's disease is the result of a deficiency of β-glucocerebrosidase, a catabolic enzyme required for the hydrolysis of the β-glucosidic bond of glucocerebroside. The substance that accumulates in the histiocytes is a glucocerebroside.[15] It is a derivative of sphingosine to which a long-chain fatty acid is joined through an amide bond to the nitrogen atom on C-2. This N-acylsphingosine complex is called ceramide and is common to all the sphingolipids that accumulate in sphingolipidoses. In glucocerebroside a single molecule of glucose is joined by a β-glycosidic bond to C-1 of ceramide. The major precursors of the glucocerebroside that accumulates in the histiocytes appear to be glycolipids from senescent red and white blood cells. Gaucher's disease is most prevalent in Ashkenazi Jews.

The spleen is greatly enlarged. The organ is firm and the cut surface is red-gray and greasy. Microscopically the splenic cords and sinusoids show a diffuse and nodular infiltra-

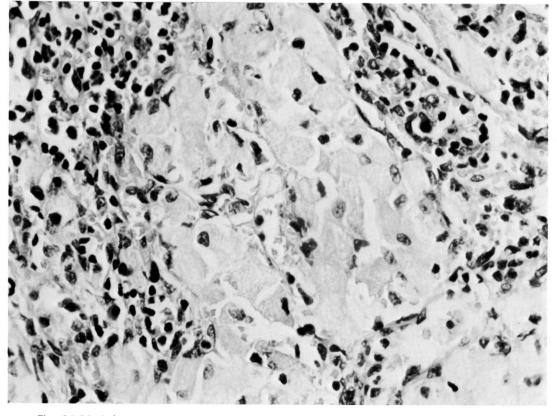

Fig. 34-23. Spleen in Gaucher's disease. Note nodule of Gaucher cells. (Hematoxylin and eosin; 250×.)

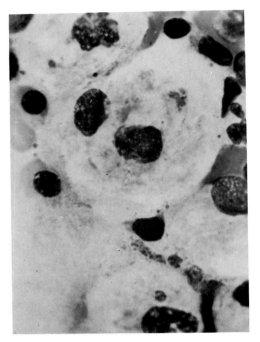

Fig. 34-24. Gaucher cell. (Spleen imprint. Wright's stain; 950×; from Miale, J. B.: Laboratory medicine—hematology, St. Louis, 1972, The C. V. Mosby Co.)

tion with Gaucher cells (Figs. 34-23). These are histiocytes whose cytoplasm is engorged with glucocerebroside (Fig. 34-24). These histiocytes are also present in the medullary portions of the lymph nodes, in sinusoids of the liver, and in the bone marrow. Gaucher cells measure 20 to 80 μm, have a relatively small nucleus, and have a cytoplasm made up of a faintly eosinophilic, striated material often containing vacuoles. The cytoplasm is PAS positive and shows autofluorescence. With the Prussian blue reaction for iron, the cytoplasm frequently exhibits a diffuse, pale blue hue. Acid phosphatase is readily demonstrated in Gaucher cells using phenylphosphate substrates.[135] Acid phosphatase is found in all histiocytes but not to the extent that it is present in Gaucher cells. Ultrastructural studies of Gaucher cells reveal spindle- or rod-shaped membrane-bound cytoplasmic inclusions measuring 0.6 to 4 μm in diameter (Fig. 34-25). Gaucher-like cells have been described in chronic granulocytic leukemia.[70]

Niemann-Pick disease

Niemann-Pick (NP) disease classically affects infants and is characterized by hepatosplenomegaly, cachexia, and impaired mental development. Five types of the disease are distinguished depending on age of onset, degree of central nervous system involvement, and rapidity of progression.[42] The disease is characterized by the accumulation of sphingomyelin in histiocytes. Sphingomyelin is a ceramide derivative containing phosphorylcholine linked to C-1 of ceramide. The accumulating sphingomyelin may be derived from cell membranes, subcellular organelles of senescent cells, and myelin sheaths. In two of the types of Niemann-Pick disease the patients lack sphingomyelinase. In the other types the cause of the sphingomyelin accumulation is unknown.[42]

Histiocytes containing sphingomyelin appear as foam cells in paraffin-embedded, hematoxylin-and-eosin–stained sections. These cells are scattered throughout the spleen, bone marrow, liver, lymph nodes, and lungs. Hepatocytes as well as Kupffer cells are involved. The foam cells seen in Niemann-Pick disease may have a pale yellow to brown yellow hue because of the presence of granules of ceroid. When stained with the Giemsa reaction, these ceroid-containing histiocytes appear sea-blue and have been called sea-blue histiocytes.[117,121] The sphingomyelin that accumulates in the histiocytes is easily removed by fixation and embedding of tissues. Luxol fast blue, which stains phospholipids, should be applied to unfixed, frozen sections. Baker's acid hematin for phospholipids, and the Schultz reaction for cholesterol are also positive. Ultrastructurally, concentrically laminated, myelin-like figures are seen in addition to granular lipid bodies.

Contrary to the Gaucher cell, the foam cell of Niemann-Pick disease is not diagnostic of this condition. A diagnosis of Niemann-Pick disease should not be based exclusively on morphologic and histochemical considerations. There is no stain that is pathognomonic for sphingomyelin. Chemical and enzymatic analyses should be performed to confirm the diagnosis.

Idiopathic ceroid histiocytosis of spleen and bone marrow (syndrome of the sea-blue histiocyte)[116,117]

In 1970 Silverstein et al. described the "syndrome of the sea-blue histiocyte" characterized by a relatively benign course, splenomegaly, thrombocytopenia, and the presence of sea-blue histiocytes in the bone marrow. Rywlin et al.[116,117] showed that the sea-blue granules observed in bone marrow smears with the Giemsa-Wright stains were made up of

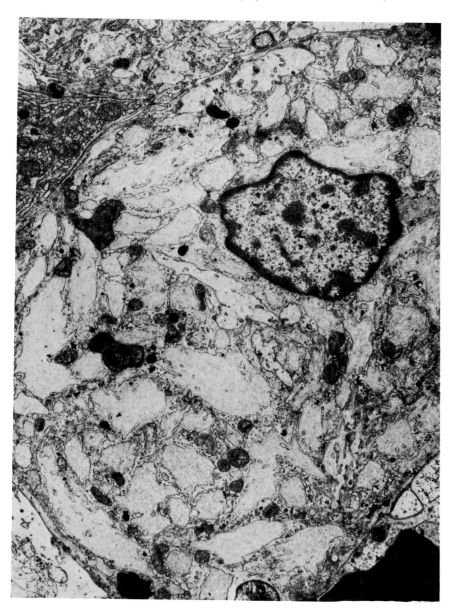

Fig. 34-25. Gaucher cell as seen by electron microscopy. Nucleus is irregular body in upper right area. Remainder is cytoplasm that contains lipid. (From Miale, J. B.: Laboratory medicine—hematology, St. Louis, 1972, The C. V. Mosby Co.)

ceroid. Ceroid is a pale yellow to dark brown pigment that results from the peroxidation and polymerization of unsaturated lipids.[53] Ceroid is defined by its insolubility in hydrocarbon lipid solvents and its reactivity with fat stains such as oil red O and Sudan black. The other histochemical reactions develop as the pigment ages: autofluorescence first, followed by diastase-resistant PAS positivity and acid-fastness.[53] Ceroid and lipofuscin share many physical and histochemical characteristics. Whether they are identical is still debated. At the present time lipofuscin seems the preferred term for naturally occurring, age-related pigment, whereas ceroid is used for a similar pigment seen in a variety of pathologic conditions. Ceroid-containing histiocytes (sea-blue histiocytes, blue-pigment macrophages) may be seen in the spleen and bone marrow in many different conditions (see list below).

The histiocytes may contain fat vacuoles only (foam cells), fat vacuoles and ceroid granules, or ceroid granules only. Before a diagnosis of idiopathic ceroid histiocytosis of the spleen and bone marrow can be made, all the known diseases that can give sea-blue histiocytes have to be eliminated by careful history and laboratory tests. Thus patients have to be tested for sphingomyelinase deficiency (to check for Niemann-Pick disease), for hyperlipoproteinemia, and for lecithin : cholesterol acyltransferase deficiency[58] before a diagnosis of idiopathic ceroid histiocytosis can be accepted.

*Conditions with ceroid-containing histiocytes in spleen or bone marrow**

Batten's disease
Niemann-Pick disease
Tay-Sachs disease
Adult lipidosis resembling Niemann-Pick disease
Wolman's disease
Ceroid-storage disease
Chronic granulomatous disease of childhood
Familial lipochrome histiocytosis
Ceroid histiocytosis of spleen with rupture in a vegetarian
Vascular pseudohemophilia associated with ceroid pigmentophagia in albinos
Hyperlipoproteinemia
Ceroid histiocytosis of spleen and bone marrow in idiopathic thrombocytopenic purpura
Syndrome of the sea-blue histiocyte (idiopathic ceroid histiocytosis of spleen and marrow)
Familial lecithin : cholesterol acyltransferase deficiency
Chronic granulocytic leukemia
Sickle-cell anemia
Cirrhosis of the liver

Histiocytosis X (eosinophilic granuloma, Hand-Schüller-Christian disease, and Letterer-Siwe disease)

Lichtenstein views eosinophilic granuloma of bone, Hand-Schüller-Christian disease, and Letterer-Siwe disease as related manifestations of a single nosologic entity, which he named "histiocytosis X."[75] Other authors consider Hand-Schüller-Christian disease to be a multifocal or systemic variant of eosinophilic granuloma, unrelated to Letterer-Siwe disease.[76,92] Eosinophilic xanthomatous granulomatosis has been proposed as a better term for these two

---

*Modified from Rywlin et al.,[116] which contains references for all the listed disorders.

entities.[92] The final word on the exact relationship of these disorders is not yet available.

The term "eosinophilic granuloma" is used for frequently solitary, bone-destroying lesions usually occurring in children. Histologically the lesion is characterized by sheets of well-differentiated histiocytes with interspersed eosinophils. The histiocytes contain an abundant eosinophilic cytoplasm.

Hand-Schüller-Christian disease consists of a multifocal or systemic proliferation of mature histiocytes with abundant cytoplasm and varying amounts of intracytoplasmic lipids consisting of cholesterol, cholesterol esters, and neutral fats (Fig. 34-26). The accumulation of intracellular lipid is not related to a primary derangement of lipid metabolism but appears to be attributable to phagocytosed lipids normally present in blood and tissues. A characteristic triad that helps to suspect a diagnosis of Hand-Schüller-Christian disease consists of punched-out bone lesions, exophthalmos, and diabetes insipidus. The spleen may be involved in a diffuse or nodular fashion. The infiltrates often have a yellow hue. Histologically there are sheets of mature histiocytes with varying numbers of foam cells, eosinophils, and fibroblasts. We emphasize again that foam cells by themselves are not diagnostic of Hand-Schüller-Christian disease and can be seen with or without ceroid-containing histiocytes in many different conditions. Transitions between eosinophilic granuloma and Hand-Schüller-Christian disease have been observed, and some authors believe that there is no justification in using the term "Hand-Schüller-Christian disease" for multifocal eosinophilic granuloma.[76]

Letterer-Siwe disease is defined by Rappaport as an acute or subacute progressive systemic proliferation of differentiated histiocytes.[98-101] The disease affects infants and rarely develops in children of more than 3 years of age. It is characterized by fever, prominent skin rash, and varying degrees of lymphadenopathy and hepatosplenomegaly. Those authors who consider Letterer-Siwe disease as distinct from Hand-Schüller-Christian disease point to the rapid course, the prominent involvement of the skin, and the lack of lipids in the diffusely proliferating histiocytes.[92] Those who view these diseases as part of a spectrum call attention to cases of Letterer-Siwe disease with a more chronic course and with partial lipidization of proliferating histiocytes.[98-101] The spleen in Letterer-Siwe disease

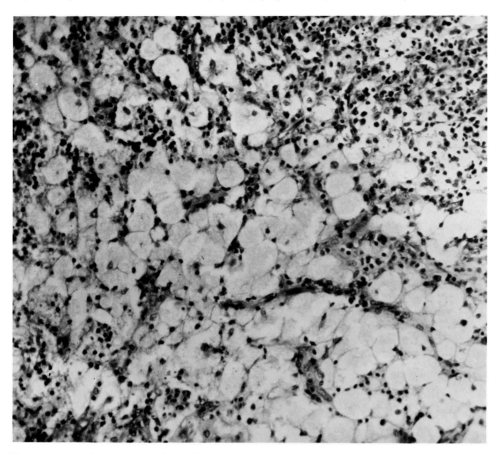

Fig. 34-26. Spleen in Hand-Schüller-Christian disease. (Hematoxylin and eosin; 250×.)

may be greatly enlarged (Fig. 34-27, *A*). Foci of necrosis may be present. Microscopically there is a diffuse proliferation of differentiated histiocytes with a well-defined eosinophilic cytoplasm (Fig. 34-27, *B*). Mitoses are rare. Multinucleated cells are frequent. Phagocytosis by the proliferating histiocytes is not a prominent feature, at least in the early stages.

An additional argument in favor of a relationship between these three diseases is the presence of a distinctive ultrastructural, rod-shaped inclusion in the cytoplasm of histiocytes in histiocytosis X. These inclusions are identical to those observed in the Langerhans cells of the epidermis.[133]

Histiocytic medullary reticulosis

Histiocytic medullary reticulosis is a rapidly fatal disease characterized by fever, weight loss, generalized lymphadenopathy, hepatic and splenic enlargement, jaundice, and pancytopenia. The disease is also known as malignant reticulosis, aleukemic reticulosis, and malignant histiocytosis.[20] The last term was introduced by Rappaport who described the disorder as a "systemic, progressive, invasive proliferation of morphologically atypical histiocytes and of their precursors."[98-101] The spleen is greatly enlarged and shows on cut section, vague, ill-defined bulging lesions. Discrete tumor nodules are not seen; so the pattern resembles leukemia rather than lymphoma.[138] Microscopically there is extensive involvement of the red pulp with atypical histiocytes showing varying degrees of phagocytosis of red blood cells. Multinucleated cells resembling Reed-Sternberg cells are also seen. The white pulp may be preserved or be partially or even completely obliterated. The lymph nodes are diffusely infiltrated or may show a sinusoidal involvement with residual intact lymphoid tissue. Leukemic forms of this disease have also been described.[23]

Leukemic reticuloendotheliosis (LRE)

This disease has been described in the literature under terms such as lymphoid myelofibrosis,[32] histiolymphocytosis of the bone

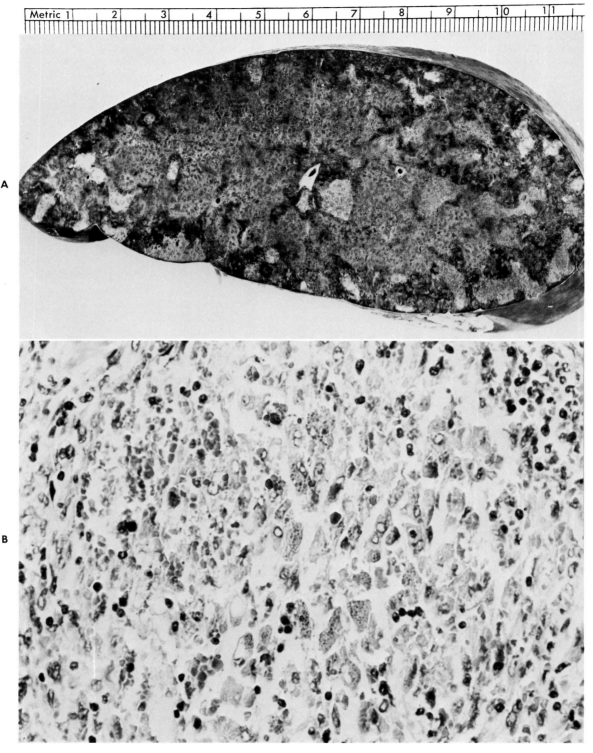

Fig. 34-27. Spleen in Letterer-Siwe disease. **A,** Gross appearance. **B,** Paraffin section. (**B,** Hematoxylin and eosin; 250×.)

marrow and spleen,[39] and hairy cell leukemia.[18,121] There is no general agreement at present whether the proliferating cell belongs to the lymphoid or monocytic series.[22,59] The onset of the disease is insidious. Splenomegaly is frequently massive. Enlargement of lymph nodes is usually absent. Pancytopenia is frequent and a "dry tap" or hypocellular specimen is obtained on bone marrow aspiration. In the peripheral blood, mononuclear cells with irregular, hairlike cytoplasmic projections are particularly well seen with phase microscopy. These cells contain a tartrate-resistant acid phosphatase isoenzyme.[143] They may also exhibit ultrastructurally a characteristic cytoplasmic inclusion referred to as ribosome-lamellar complex.[38,63] These can be recognized with the light microscope in Giemsa-stained smears as rod-shaped inclusions that are also pyroninophilic.[39,63]

The cut surface of the enlarged spleen does not reveal any tumor nodules. The trabecular and follicular pattern may be attenuated. Microscopically there is a diffuse infiltration of the splenic cords by the neoplastic cells.

The bone marrow biopsy shows a diffuse but loose infiltration with cells resembling lymphocytes. A reticulum stain reveals a sharp increase in reticulin fibers.

The prognosis of leukemic reticuloendotheliosis is relatively good. The patients benefit from splenectomy and may be harmed by chemotherapy.

Lymph nodes

STRUCTURE
Normal structure—histologic

Lymph nodes are discrete nodules of lymphoid tissue located at anatomically constant points along the course of lymphatic vessels. Lymphoid tissue is not found exclusively in lymph nodes, for lymphoid aggregates are present in the submucosa of the intestinal tract and bronchi, in normal bone marrow, in the spleen, and diffusely in the thymus. However, as in the case of the spleen, lymph nodes represent circumscribed and identifiable structures whose enlargement is easily discovered by palpation. As discrete structures, they can be excised and subjected to detailed bacteriologic, cytologic, and histologic study.

Lymph nodes have a fibrous capsule from which connective tissue trabeculae extend into the node in a roughly radial arrangement. The connective tissue framework between the trabeculae consists of a network of reticulum fibers, and this stroma supports primitive reticuloendothelial cells, scattered phagocytic histiocytes, and the predominant lymphocytes. In the central or *medullary* portion of the lymph node, the small lymphocytes are packed tightly in sheets and cords separated by medullary sinuses. In the peripheral or cortical portion, the lymphocytes are condensed into roughly spheric *lymphoid nodules* (primary follicles). These may consist entirely of small lymphocytes when the lymph node is in a completely resting or nonreactive state. When stimulated, the primary lymphoid nodules develop germinal or reactive centers (secondary follicles) that consist of small, medium, and large lymphoid cells. The germinal centers also contain dendritic, desmosome-containing reticulum cells, and macrophages with cytoplasmic inclusions known as "tingible bodies" (starry-sky macrophages).

The relationship between the small and large lymphoid cells has to be revised in the light of modern concepts (Fig. 34-28). When the small perifollicular lymphocytes are stimulated by antigens or mitogens, they enlarge and take on the appearance of "blasts," i.e., cells with round open nuclei, prominent nucleoli, large nuclear cytoplasmic ratios, and a rim of basophilic (Giemsa stain) and pyroninophilic cytoplasm. Such "blast" cells occur in normal germinal centers and have been called "large noncleaved cells" by Lukes and Collins[80] and "germinoblasts" and "centroblasts" by Lennert.[73] According to Lennert the germinoblast is characterized by a round to oval nucleus with multiple nucleoli that are situated close to the nuclear membrane. The cytoplasm is narrow and basophilic and often contains vacuoles. The germinoblast evolves into an immunoblast that is larger and contains a bigger nucleolus. The immunoblast possesses a wider rim of cytoplasm that ultrastructurally contains more rough endoplasmic reticulum and more polysomes that does the germinoblast. The B immunoblast gives rise to plasma cells. The germinoblasts and immunoblasts also seem to participate in lymphopoiesis by becoming lymphoblasts, undergoing mitosis, and then developing into small, "mature" lymphocytes. This sequence is in line with the classical concept of lymphopoiesis: lymphoblast → prolymphocyte → lymphocyte. T lymphocytes when stimulated are transformed into T immunoblasts, which probably also participate in T lymphopoiesis. T immunoblasts cannot be distinguished cytologically from B immuno-

CORTEX

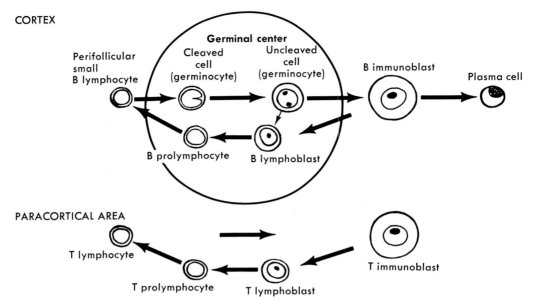

Fig. 34-28. Schematic representation of transformation of B and T lymphocytes.

blasts. They differ from B immunoblasts by their localization in the paracortical areas. Morphologically, at present, lymphoblasts cannot be distinguished with certainty from germinoblasts and immunoblasts.

The proliferating germinal *center* is usually pale-staining and sharply circumscribed by the crowded dark-staining small lymphocytes at the periphery that form a *corona* around the reactive center. When studied in serial sections, the germinal centers can be shown to be spheroid with two poles. The superficial hemisphere, adjacent to the marginal sinus in a lymph node or epithelium in the intestine, is directed toward the nearest source of antigen and stains lightly because the cells are larger and have a more abundant cytoplasm. The deep hemisphere stains dark because the cells have scantier cytoplasm, and the corona of small lymphocytes is usually less distinct than at the upper pole. The polar structure corresponds to immunologic reactions, for it has been shown[91] that bacterial antigens injected intravenously localize first in the perifollicular region and then migrate to the superficial or light area of the reactive center.

The area of the lymph node located between germinal centers and the subcapsular sinus is called the far cortical region. The deep cortex, or paracortex, is situated between the peripheral cortex with its germinal centers and the medulla of the lymph node. The deep cortex contains lymphocytes grouped around post-

capillary venules (tertiary follicles). The bursa-dependent, or B, area of the lymph node includes the far cortical and germinal center regions, whereas the thymus-dependent, or T, area lies in the deep cortex (see p. 1576).

Lymph enters the node through afferent vessels and empties into a subcapsular sinus that is continuous with sinuses running along the trabeculae. These ultimately form efferent lymphatics that leave the node at the hilum. The sinuses are lined by flat *littoral* or *lining* cells sometimes called endothelial, but littoral and endothelial cells are quite different when studied by electron microscopy.[12] The chief difference is that littoral cells are phagocytic, and, as such, they are active in performing a housecleaning function on the lymph. Under pathologic conditions, these cells hypertrophy, multiply, and become detached as free phagocytes in the lymph sinus, the *Sinuskatarrh* of German authors.

Normal structure—cytologic

Study of the morphology of individual cells, as seen in imprints from the freshly cut surface of a lymph node or from smears of aspirated material, is a useful adjunct to the histopathologic appearance. Histologic sections are essential for determining the relationship of cells to each other and to the architecture of the tissue, but cellular details are partially obscured by fixation and by the thickness of the section. On the other hand, imprints make

Table 34-1. Differential counts from normal lymph node imprints*

Cell	%
Reticulum cells	0-0.1
Mast cells	0-0.5
Lymphoblasts	0.1-0.9
Prolymphocytes	5.3-16.4
Lymphocytes	67.8-90
Monoblasts	0-0.5
Promonocytes	0-0.5
Monocytes	0.2-7.4
Plasmoblasts	0-0.1
Proplasmocytes	0-0.5
Plasma cells	0-4.7
Neutrophils	0-2.2
Eosinophils	0-03
Basophils	0-0.2

*Slightly modified from Lucas, P. F.: Blood **10**:1030-1054, 1955; by permission; from Miale, J. B.: Laboratory medicine—hematology, St. Louis, 1972, The C. V. Mosby Co.

possible a study of individual cells, as in a blood smear, and often reveal details of morphology that, in combination with the histologic appearance, are extremely useful in arriving at the correct diagnosis.

Imprints of a normal node show a predominance of small lymphocytes, as well as larger lymphoid cells, and scattered cells of other types (Table 34-1). When the node is abnormal, quantitative and qualitative abnormalities will be found. Some of these will be illustrated in later discussions.

FUNCTION

The functions of the lymph nodes are three: (1) formation of lymphocytes, (2) production of antibodies, and (3) filtration of the lymph.

The lymph nodes are responsible for a portion of the total lymphocyte-producing capacity of lymphoid tissue. There is as yet no information on how many lymphocytes enter the total lymphocyte pool from lymph nodes and how many are produced elsewhere. On the basis of weight, lymph nodes contain about 100 gm of lymphoid tissue as compared to 70 gm in the bone marrow and 1300 gm scattered throughout other tissues. Lymphocytes originating in lymph nodes enter the lymph channels on the efferent side. Some enter the bloodstream directly by passing through the walls of capillary vessels. According to modern concepts of lymphocytopoiesis and immunology, the lymphoid system is divided into a "central" portion, consisting of lymphoid tissue in Peyer's patches, appendix, and tonsils plus the lymphoid tissue in the thymus, and a "peripheral" portion consisting of spleen and lymph nodes. The spleen and lymph nodes not only generate new lymphocytes, but also are populated by lymphocytes originating in the central tissues. The functional and anatomic characteristics of lymphoid cells and monocytes (M cells) are summarized in Table 34-2.

Lymph nodes play an obvious but relatively unimportant role as filters of particulate matter (anthracotic pigment, cellular debris, bacteria). Tumor cells carried by the lymph from the primary site to regional lymph nodes may implant and grow to form metastases.

LYMPHADENITIS

Since primary tumors other than lymphomas or leukemias are never found in lymph nodes (with the exception of primary Kaposi's sarcoma), the pathologist examining a stained section of a node usually must decide whether the histologic changes represent a nonspecific or specific inflammatory reaction, a lymphoma or leukemia, or metastatic neoplasm. In most instances, an enlarged lymph node is excised for pathologic examination in order to rule out a lymphomatous process or metastatic involvement.

Nonspecific reactive hyperplasia of lymph nodes

This group includes a number of histologic reaction patterns that are nonspecific, in the sense that they can be caused by a variety of stimuli.

Nonspecific reactive hyperplasia of the *follicular type* (Fig. 34-29) is characterized by lymphoid follicles with large germinal centers exhibiting a high mitotic activity and numerous macrophages with tingible bodies. Plasma cells are numerous. The lymphoid follicles vary considerably in size but have well-defined margins surrounded by a mantle of small lymphocytes. This type of reaction pattern is caused by the stimulation of B lymphocytes. It may be seen in secondary syphilis and rheumatoid arthritis. It may simulate a malignant follicular lymphoma.

Nonspecific reactive hyperplasia of the *sinus histiocytosis type* displays distention of the sinusoids by well-differentiated histiocyte-like cells. The significance of this reaction pattern is unknown. It is often observed in axillary lymph nodes from patients with carcinoma of the breast. In these cases, the presence of a "sinus histiocytosis" pattern appears to indicate a more favorable prognosis.

Table 34-2. Functional and anatomical characteristics of lymphoid cells*

Cell type	Function	Location
T cells	Initiation of delayed hypersensitivity reactions Initiation of solid-tissue allograft rejection Initiation of graft versus host reactions Elaboration of lymphokines Defense against facultative intracellular bacterial and rickettsial pathogens, fungi, and many viruses Responsive to phytohemagglutinin or allogeneic cell stimulation in vitro ? Immunosurveillance against cancer	Blood (65% to 80% of blood lymphocytes) Lymph node: deep cortical areas (paracortex) Spleen: perivascular areas of the white pulp (perivascular lymphocyte sheath)
B cells	Synthesis and secretion of immunoglobulins and specific antibodies (IgM, IgG, IgA, IgD, IgE) Progenitor of plasma cells Primary defense against high-grade encapsulated bacterial pathogens Detoxification of certain proteins, polypeptides, and other toxins Neutralization of viruses (especially secretory IgA in respiratory tract and gut) Interference with absorption of foreign proteins from respiratory tract and gut	Blood (15% to 25% of blood lymphocytes) Lymph node: germinal centers (lymphoid follicles, pyroninophilic cells) and medullary cords (secretory lymphocytes and plasma cells) Spleen: lymphoid follicles of white pulp and red pulp cords (chief site of splenic antibody production)
M cells (monocytes)	Phagocytosis of organisms and particles Major effector mechanism in defense against most bacterial, fungal, and probably viral pathogens Processing and presentation of antigen Removal of cellular debris	Blood: monocyte Tissue: macrophages, histiocytes, Kupffer cells of sinusoids of liver Lymph node: germinal center macrophage (tingible body macrophage) and medullary cord macrophages Spleen: present in both white pulp and red pulp
Dendritic reticulum cells	Apparently play crucial role in development of antibody response through adherence and presentation of antigen	Origin unknown; appear within germinal centers; extensive dendritic processes interdigitate with lymphocytes of the germinal center

*From Hansen, J. A., and Good, R. A.: Hum. Pathol. **5:**567-593, 1974.

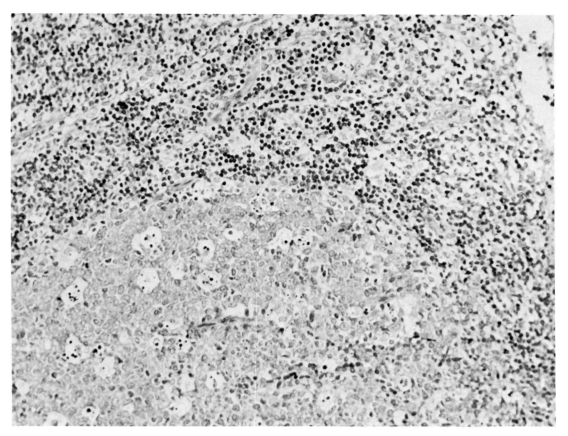

Fig. 34-29. Lymph node. Reactive hyperplasia, follicular type. (Hematoxylin and eosin; 125×.)

This nonspecific sinus histiocytosis has to be distinguished from histiocytic medullary reticulosis, histiocytosis X, and sinus histiocytosis with massive lymphadenopathy.

Paracortical lymphoid hyperplasia (T-area lymphoid hyperplasia) may be seen in antigenically stimulated lymph nodes. The paracortical areas show varying degrees of hyperplasia, which may attenuate the follicular and sinusoidal architecture of the lymph node. The paracortical areas display a considerable number of large lymphoid cells with prominent nucleoli and a basophilic cytoplasm with the Giemsa stain ("immunoblasts"). These cells impart under low-power magnification a mottled appearance to the lymph node since they are scattered among small lymphocytes.

Combination patterns between follicular, paracortical hyperplasia, and sinus histiocytosis may be seen.

Suppurative lymphadenitis

An acute suppurative inflammatory reaction in a lymph node is secondary to an inflamma-tion in the area it drains. When the primary infection is caused by a pyogenic organism such as staphylococcus or streptococcus, the regional lymph node is enlarged and tender, and the pulp between follicles is hyperemic and infiltrated with neutrophilic leukocytes. Later, there is an exudation of monocytes and phagocytes, the latter containing ingested cellular debris. When bacteria have been carried to the node, they may multiply and produce hemorrhage and abscesses.

Postvaccinial lymphadenitis and viral lymphadenitis

Hartsock[54] (see also Lukes et al.[83] and Rappaport[98-101]) has shown that the lymph nodes draining the site of smallpox vaccination undergo an intensive reaction that might, if not recognized, lead to an erroneous diagnosis of lymphoma. Similar reactions may occur after use of other vaccines such as in tetanus, typhoid fever, diphtheria, pertussis, influenza, and poliomyelitis. Although there should be no reason to excise for biopsy a node draining a vaccination site, the history of vaccination may be overlooked. Of the 20 cases reviewed by Hartsock,[54] nine had been diagnosed as lymphoma, and in 14 the history of vaccination had been overlooked.

Histologically, such a node shows (1) nodular or diffuse hyperplasia, (2) an increased number of immunoblasts (reticular lymphoblasts), (3) vascular and sinusoidal changes, and (4) a mixed cellular response. The hyperplasia involves primarily a proliferation of immunoblasts that, interspersed among other lymphocytes, produce a mottled appearance under low magnification. The immunoblasts have a single nucleus and one or more irregularly shaped acidophilic nucleoli but lack the strict characteristics of Sternberg-Reed cells. The inconstant findings of focal dilation of lymph sinuses, a mixed cellular response with scattered eosinophils, neutrophils, and plasma cells, and hypertrophy and hyperplasia of endothelial cells are not seen in non-Hodgkin's lymphoma.

Changes as described above may occur after the administration of live attenuated measles virus vaccine.[31] In such cases the lymph nodes contain Warthin-Finkeldey (mulberry cells)

giant cells, which are seen in the lymphoid tissue in the prodromal phase of measles.

Regional lymphadenopathy associated with or preceding herpes zoster skin lesions may mimic postvaccinial lymphadenitis.

Anticonvulsant-drug lymphadenopathy (Dilantin lymphadenopathy)

Ingestion of anticonvulsant drugs (used in the treatment of epilepsy) sometimes produces an illness resembling malignant lymphoma both in the hematologic picture and in the histologic changes in lymph nodes and skin. One or more of the following may occur at any time after 1 week to many months of therapy: morbilliform skin rash, lymphadenopathy, fever, hepatosplenomegaly, and painful joints. Eosinophilia in the peripheral blood is not uncommon. The commonest offending drugs are diphenylhydantoin (Dilantin) and mephenytoin (Mesantoin), but several other drugs of the same type also have been implicated.

The histologic appearance of the lymph nodes resembles postvaccinial lymphadenitis and may be mistaken for Hodgkin's disease. There is moderate to complete loss of normal

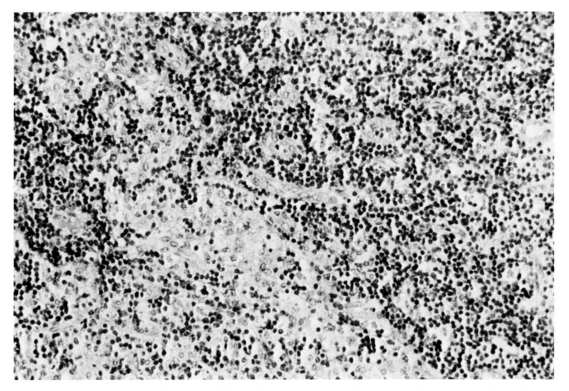

Fig. 34-30. Lymph node in pseudolymphomatous lymphadenitis secondary to ingestion of anticonvulsant drug. (Hematoxylin and eosin; 125×.)

architecture, focal or diffuse hyperplasia of immunoblasts, which may show pleomorphic nuclei, and diffuse infiltration with eosinophils, neutrophils, and plasma cells (Fig. 34-30). Mitotic figures are found, and infiltration of the capsule is common. One of the most common features is focal areas of necrosis accompanied by phagocytosis of nuclear debris.

In the differentiation of this lesion from the lymphomas, the clinical history is most important. It has been estimated that there are one million epileptic patients in the United States. Most of these are receiving anticonvulsive therapy, so that pseudolymphomatous lymphadenitis may challenge the pathologist at any time. It also must be noted that an individual with epilepsy under treatment can develop, independent of other circumstances, a true lymphoma. It has been suggested, indeed, that the incidence of lymphoma is higher in epileptic patients under treatment than in the general population, but this is not based on good statistical evidence. Hyman and Sommers[56] have described the development of lymphoma in patients on prolonged diphenylhydantoin therapy.

Tuberculous lymphadenitis

Tuberculous involvement of lymph nodes presents the entire spectrum of the histopathology of tuberculosis, from the typical small tubercle to caseous necrosis, fibrosis, and calcification (Fig. 34-31). Lymph node involvement is usually secondary to drainage from a primary site, as in involvement of hilar and peribronchial lymph nodes in the primary complex of pulmonary tuberculosis. In bronchogenic pulmonary tuberculosis or in organ tuberculosis, active lesions in satellite lymph nodes are unusual. Even when the lesion is typical, with caseous necrosis and giant cells, it is well to confirm the diagnosis by bacteriologic culture of homogenized tissue. One should note that the demonstration of acid-fast bacilli in paraffin-embedded tissue is often disappointing. Furthermore, bacteriologic studies are necessary to identify the mycobacterium as being the typical *Mycobacterium tuberculosis* or one of the atypical varieties (see chapter on lung, pleura, and mediastinum).

Sarcoidosis

The lymph nodes are involved in sarcoidosis as part of the generalized disease. Character-

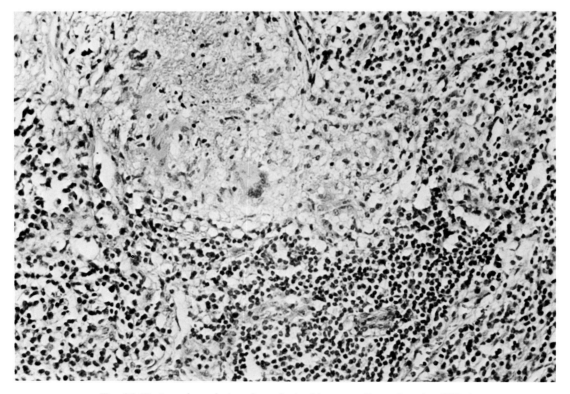

Fig. 34-31. Lymph node in tuberculosis. (Hematoxylin and eosin; 125×.)

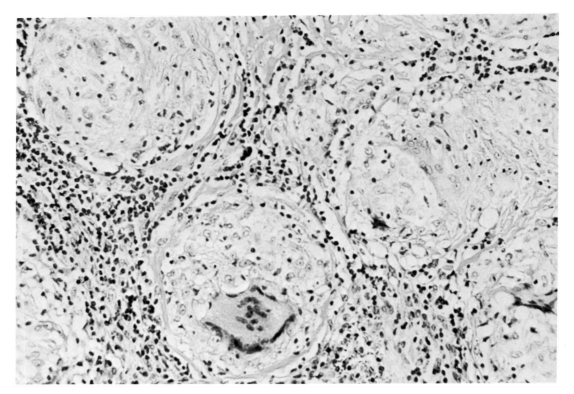

Fig 34-32. Lymph node in sarcoidosis. (Hematoxylin and eosin; 125×.)

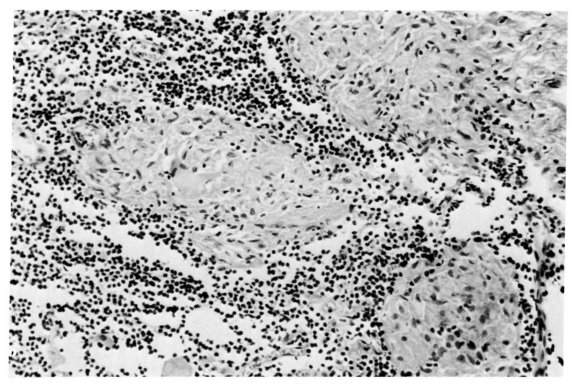

Fig. 34-33. Lymph node. Sarcoidosis-like lesions in cervical lymph node draining carcinomatous area. (Hematoxylin and eosin; 125×.)

istically, the lesions are granulomatous and noncaseous and, in the later stages, fibrotic and hyalinizing. The early granuloma is composed of epithelioid cells and may contain giant cells of the Langhans type (Fig. 34-32). At this stage, it may not be possible to determine the nature of the granuloma, for similar lesions are sometimes found in fungal infections, berylliosis, leprosy, toxoplasmosis, Hodgkin's disease, and early noncaseous tuberculosis and even in nodes draining a carcinomatous area (Fig. 34-33). Special mention should be made of the not uncommon occurrence of sarcoidosis-like lesions in scalene lymph nodes (lower deep jugular) draining a primary carcinoma of the lung.

Sarcoid lesions may contain foreign body formations (Schaumann's bodies, Fig. 34-34, and asteroids) that are not diagnostic of sarcoidosis, since they may be found in berylliosis as well. Furthermore, sarcoid lesions do, at times, undergo central necrosis. One will note that the specific diagnosis of granulomatous inflammation is, at times, difficult and requires the correlation of clinical and laboratory data with the histologic appearance of the lesion.

"Sinus histiocytosis with lymphadenopathy"

Rosai and Dorfman[109] have described a benign disease characterized clinically by massive predominantly cervical lymphadenopathy, fever, and leukocytosis. The lymph nodes show pronounced dilatation of the subcapsular and medullary sinuses. These are filled with proliferating histiocytes with prominent eosinophilic nucleoli and in some cases, foamy lipid-filled histiocytes. They believe that phagocytosis of lymphocytes by the proliferating histiocytes is one of the features that distinguishes this lesion from others that show histiocytic proliferation.

The lymphadenopathy usually persists for months or years, but the clinical course is entirely benign. Some cases with extrasinusoidal proliferation of histiocytes resulting in apparent effacement of nodal architecture may mimic malignant histiocytic proliferations.

Necrotizing lymphadenitis

An extensive hemorrhagic and necrotizing lymphadenitis is characteristic of bubonic plague. Focal necrosis of lymph nodes is also seen in lupus erythematosus where it is as-

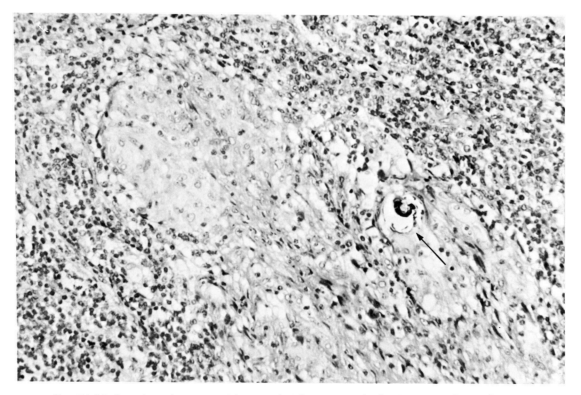

Fig. 34-34. Lymph node in sarcoidosis with Schaumann's body. (Hematoxylin and eosin; 125×.)

sociated with the deposition of hematoxylino-philic material. It has also been observed in Dilantin hypersensitivity and infectious mono-nucleosis.

Massive necrosis of lymph nodes has been attributed to thrombosis of hilar veins.[26] Varying degrees of necrosis are also seen in suppurative and granulomatous lymphadenitis.

Infectious mononucleosis

Infectious mononucleosis is an infection caused by the Epstein-Barr virus[55] and is characterized by a reaction of lymphoid tissue with the formation of "atypical" lymphocytes that have been called infectious mononucleosis cells.

More properly, these are called *virocytes*, for similar cells are produced by a variety of viral infections or even stress. The virocyte appears in the peripheral blood and is found in the lymph nodes from which it originates. Generalized or cervical lymphadenopathy is a characteristic presenting sign.

Histologically there is predominantly a paracortical lymphoid hyperplasia with the appearance of "blasts" and intermediate lymphoid cells. These cells are also seen in the sinusoids and are the source of the virocytes (Fig. 34-35). Some of the "blast" cells are binucleated and cannot always be distinguished from Reed-Sternberg cells.[85,134] Classical Reed-

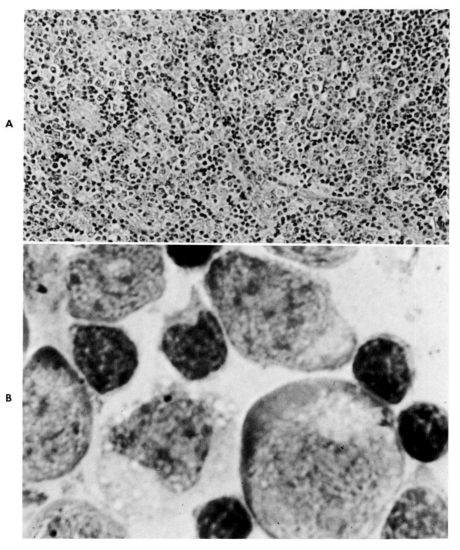

Fig. 34-35. Lymph node in infectious mononucleosis. **A,** Paraffin section. **B,** Imprint. (**A,** Hematoxylin and eosin; 100×; **B,** Wright's stain; 1080×; **A** and **B,** courtesy Dr. Joseph C. Sieracki, Pittsburgh.)

Sternberg cells of Hodgkin's disease tend to have an acidophilic cytoplasm and prominent eosinophilic inclusion–like nucleoli.[31] When the histologic picture is interpreted with the help of all available clinical and hematologic data, the diagnosis usually is obvious. It is a reckless pathologist indeed who does not take advantage of all available data when examining any tissue, particularly lymph nodes.

Enlarged lymphoid follicles with germinal centers and increased numbers of plasma cells are often present.

Immunoblastic lymphadenopathy[43,81]

Immunoblastic,[81] or angioimmunoblastic lymphadenopathy with dysproteinemia,[43] is an entity that may resemble Hodgkin's disease clinically and histologically. It is a disease of unknown etiology and pathogenesis. Clinically, it is manifested by fever, sweats, weight loss, skin rash, generalized lymphadenopathy, and often hepatosplenomegaly. There is a polyclonal hyperglobulinemia and frequently hemolytic anemia. Histologically it is characterized by the abundant proliferation of arborizing small vessels, the presence of numerous immunoblasts and plasma cells, and the deposition of varying amounts of a homogeneous, eosinophilic, PAS-positive material. Occasionally there may be abundant clusters of epithelioid cells.[31] The normal lymph node architecture is usually effaced, and lymphoid follicles and sinusoids are inconspicuous. The course of the disease is usually progressive, with a median survival of 18 months reported in 18 fatal cases.[81] In three of the reported cases the disease evolved into a malignant lymphoma.[81]

Toxoplasmic lymphadenitis

Toxoplasmic lymphadenitis involves primarily the cervical lymph nodes.[95] There is good correlation between toxoplasmic lymphadenitis and the Sabin-Feldman dye test and the IgM immunofluorescent antibody test.[30]

Histologically the involved lymph nodes show a striking degree of reactive follicular hyperplasia with large germinal centers containing many macrophages. The interfollicular zones contain small foci of epithelioid cells usually without giant cells. The epithelioid cells may be located within the germinal centers. An additional distinctive feature is the focal distention of sinuses by immature histio-

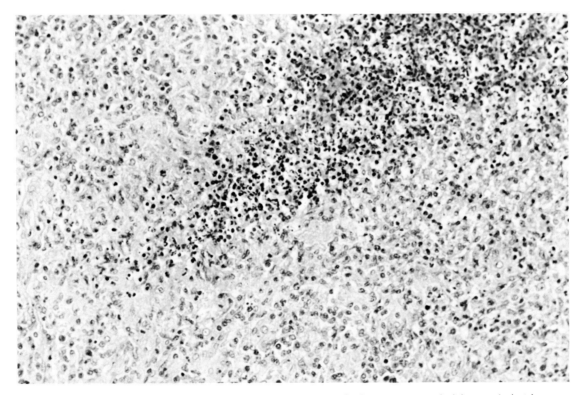

Fig. 34-36. Lymph node in cat-scratch disease; central abscess surrounded by epithelioid cells. (Hematoxylin and eosin; 125×.)

cytes. The medullary cords may contain increased numbers of plasma cells and immunoblasts. Toxoplasmic cysts are found very rarely in lymph nodes.

Cat-scratch disease

Cat-scratch disease is one of the causes of enlargement of regional lymph nodes. The causative agent is unknown, but there is a highly suggestive serologic relationship to a virus of the psittacosis-lymphogranuloma group. The infectious agent is inoculated percutaneously by a cat scratch (60% of the cases), a cat bite (10%), or various injuries such as from splinters, thorns, pins, fishhooks, rabbit claws, and porcupine quills (5%), whereas in about one fourth of the cases there is no known skin injury, although most of the patients are known to have had a cat in the household.

Since regional lymphadenopathy is the cardinal sign of cat-scratch disease, this disease must be considered in the differential diagnosis of lymphadenopathy. The histologic appearance of the lymph nodes is characterized by suppurative granulomas. These consist of a central necrotic area infiltrated with polymorphonuclear leukocytes surrounded by palisading epithelioid cells with occasional Langhans' giant cells (Fig. 34-36). This granulomatous inflammation is most noticeable in the cortical area of the lymph node. It usually extends to the perinodal tissue and to the medullary portion of the node. The remaining lymph nodal tissue shows follicular hyperplasia with prominent germinal centers, immunoblasts, plasma cells, and eosinophils. Suppurative granulomas are also characteristic of other diseases[72]: mesenteric adenitis attributable to *Yersinia enterocolitica*, tularemia, lymphopathia venereum, fungal infections, and melioidosis.

Dermatopathic lymphadenitis

Sometimes called *lipomelanotic reticulosis,* dermatopathic lymphadenitis is associated with chronic dermatoses particularly of the exfoliative type. It is characterized by the presence of numerous macrophages with vacuolated or foamy cytoplasm, which contains fat. Some macrophages also contain melanin and some hemosiderin (Fig. 34-37). The cortex of such lymph nodes appears to be widened and pale

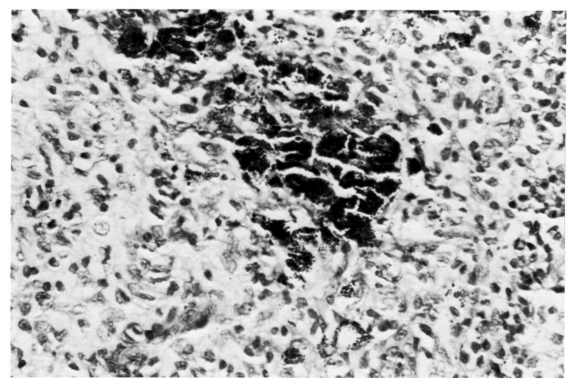

Fig. 34-37. Lymph node in dermatopathic lymphadenitis. Note macrophages containing melanin. (Hematoxylin and eosin; 250×.)

staining when viewed with low magnification. In addition to the macrophages, there are increased numbers of eosinophils, plasma cells, and immunoblasts.

The distinction between dermatopathic lymphadenitis and lymph-nodal mycosis fungoides may be difficult. For the diagnosis of mycosis fungoides of the lymph node there must be at least focal infiltration of the node by atypical cells with cerebriform nuclei with effacement of normal lymph node architecture.[137]

Postlymphangiography lymphadenitis

The angiographic contrast media used for studying the roentgenographic morphology of superficial and deep lymph nodes (lymphangiography) produce characteristic histologic changes.[106] They range from the early reaction consisting of exudation of neutrophils, eosinophils, and a few plasma cells through the chronic reaction characterized by foreign body giant cells surrounding droplets of contrast medium plus plasma cell infiltration.

GIANT LYMPH NODE HYPERPLASIA

This lesion has been described by a variety of names reflecting the different opinions concerning its histogenesis: angiomatous lymphoid hamartoma, angiofollicular lymph node hyperplasia, lymphoid hamartoma, and benign giant lymphoma.[64a] Clinically the patients present most often with a mediastinal mass discovered on routine roentgenograms of the chest or because of pressure symptoms. Occasionally a palpable mass is present outside of the thorax. Keller et al.[64a] have studied 81 cases of this entity and have divided it into two histologic types, the hyaline-vascular type and the plasma cell type. The hyaline-vascular type is characterized by small lymphoid follicles that are rich in vessels, some of which enter the follicle in a radial fashion. The centers of the follicles contain varying amounts of hyaline material and resemble superficially Hassall's corpuscles of the thymus. The follicles show a tight concentric ("onionskin") layering of small lymphocytes. The interfollicular tissue is vascular and contains varying numbers of plasma cells, eosinophils, and immunoblasts.

The plasma cell type is much less frequent. It displays prominent germinal centers devoid of the rich vascularity of the hyaline-vascular type. The interfollicular tissue is vascular and contains sheets of plasma cells and some immunoblasts.

In our experience a clear separation of the two types is not always possible and transitions between the two types exist.

It is of interest that systemic manifestations such as fever, anemia, and hyperglobulinemia were observed in association with the plasma cell type of giant lymph node hyperplasia. These clinical signs disappeared after excision of the lesion.

METASTATIC NEOPLASMS

Since lymph drains from the site of a primary neoplasm to the regional lymph nodes, the latter are frequently the site of metastases. Carcinomas and malignant melanomas metastasize to lymph nodes much more frequently than do sarcomas. The tumor tissue in the lymph node usually, but not always, reproduces the cellular and architectural features of the primary tumor. Tumor cells or small nodules are first found in the subcapsular or paratrabecular lymph sinuses (Fig. 34-38). When there is extensive involvement, the normal architecture of the lymph node is completely destroyed.

When the surgeon excises a primary neoplasm, he also is concerned with this potential involvement of the regional lymph nodes. In some circumstances, however, one may excise and examine a lymph node histologically to establish whether a primary neoplasm exists in the area or organ it drains. For example, intra-abdominal carcinoma, particularly carcinoma of the stomach, sometimes metastasizes to the left supraclavicular lymph nodes by way of the thoracic duct. An enlarged supraclavicular node containing tumor tissue sometimes is called *"Virchow's node."* Another example is involvement of the scalene lymph nodes in intrathoracic tumors.

KAPOSI'S SARCOMA

Lymphadenopathy related to Kaposi's sarcoma (KS) may be attributed to four distinct causes.[77] First, nonspecific inflammatory changes can be seen in a lymph node draining an area of ulcerated cutaneous Kaposi's sarcoma. Second, malignant lymphomas of various types occur significantly more frequently in patients with Kaposi's sarcoma.[107] Third, lymph nodes are frequently involved by Kaposi's sarcoma. This type of lymph node involvement may be seen in association with or without cutaneous Kaposi's sarcoma. It is particularly frequent in African children.[27] Grossly these lymph nodes show purple or brown nodules, which may be mistaken for

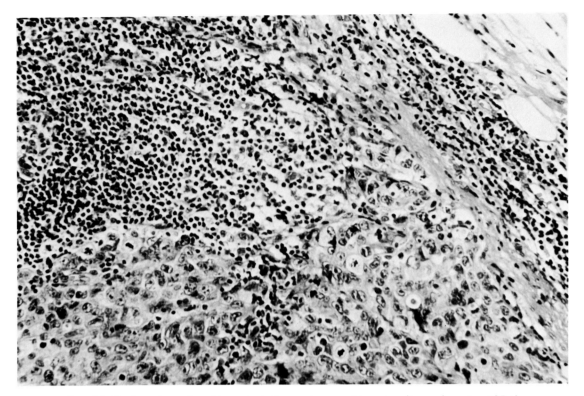

Fig. 34-38. Lymph node with metastatic carcinoma. (Hematoxylin and eosin; 125×.)

melanoma. Microscopically the typical appearance of Kaposi's sarcoma with spindle cells, vascular slits, hemosiderin, and red cells is found (see p. 1860). Fourth, lymphadenopathy may be caused by an impressive, highly vascular follicular hyperplasia, associated with hypervascularity of the interfollicular tissue and a striking increase of plasma cells. Numerous sections may have to be examined before a diagnostic focus of Kaposi's sarcoma is found. This lesion has been mistaken grossly for follicular lymphoma and histologically for plasmacytoma, giant lymph node hyperplasia, Felty's syndrome, and luetic lymphadenitis. Clinically it presents like a malignant lymphoma with lymphadenopathy, fever, weight loss, anemia, and hypergammaglobulinemia.[119]

Vascular transformation of lymph node sinuses from venous obstruction[50] and nodal angiomatosis[37] should not be mistaken for Kaposi's sarcoma though the former may be seen in association with this sarcoma. The characteristic proliferation of spindle cells with formation of vascular slits is not seen in these entities.

MALIGNANT LYMPHOMAS
General considerations

Neoplastic proliferations of lymphocytes, monocytes (reticulum cells, histiocytes), and plasma cells are listed below. By convention and somewhat arbitrarily the term "malignant lymphoma" is used collectively for some of the neoplastic proliferations listed below: Hodgkin's disease, lymphocytic lymphomas, histiocytic lymphoma (reticulum cell sarcoma), Burkitt's tumor, and mycosis fungoides. Primarily it includes malignant lymphoreticular neoplasms that are localized at the time of diagnosis and arise preferentially in lymph nodes. The systemic and leukemic proliferations are not included under the lymphomas. One should also note that Burkitt's tumor occurs usually outside of lymph nodes and that mycosis fungoides is primarily, though not exclusively, a cutaneous neoplasm.

Neoplastic proliferations of lymphocytes, monocytes (reticulum cells, histiocytes), and plasma cells

Hodgkin's disease

Lymphocytic lymphomas, follicular and diffuse

Lymphocytic leukemias
Histiocytic lymphoma (reticulum cell sarcoma)
Reticuloses (see outline, p. 1487)
Monocytic leukemias
Burkitt's tumor
Mycosis fungoides
Multiple myeloma
Waldenström's macroglobulinemia
Heavy-chain disease
    α chain—Mediterranenan lymphoma
      (Seligman's disease)
    γ chain—Franklin's disease
    μ chain—disease

The term "lymphosarcoma" was coined by Virchow to describe primary malignant neoplasms originating in lymph nodes. Kundrat[68] believed that "lymphosarcomatosis" was more appropriate for these neoplasms, since they did not metastasize like other sarcomas. For the same reason other pathologists preferred the term "malignant lymphomas" for these neoplasms. Indeed hematopoietic and lymphoreticular malignancies exhibit a unique feature among malignant neoplasms: a tendency to multicentricity and systemic involvement with or without a leukemic blood picture. Systemic involvement has to be distinguished from widespread metastases. Metastases form grossly visible nodules that may involve many different tissues, whereas systemic involvement tends to be diffuse and limited to organs normally housing lymphoreticular tissues. Transition stages between a localized tumor mass, systemic involvement, and leukemia exist for neoplasias of lymphocytes, reticulum cells, plasma cells, and granulocytes. Transition stages between lymphoma and leukemia are sometimes called "leukosarcoma." Tumors formed by immature granulocytes are known as chloromas or granulocytic sarcomas.[105]

Virchow's lymphosarcomas were composed of small or large cells. Some pathologists believed that the large cell lymphosarcomas were derived from reticulum or reticuloendothelial cells rather than from lymphocytes and that they should be called "reticulum cell sarcomas." Others referred to them as "lymphosarcoma, reticulum cell type." Rappaport[105] views the large cell lymphomas as derived from histiocytes and calls them "histiocytic lymphomas." The term "histiocyte" was introduced by Aschoff and Kiyono[4] to denote that the wandering macrophages were of tissue rather than peripheral blood origin as believed by Metchnikoff. Modern investigators consider the wandering macrophages to be derived from monocytes arriving from the bone marrow in the peripheral blood.[136] The substitution of histiocytic lymphoma for reticulum cell sarcoma has not been universally accepted, because it is impossible to determine by microscopic examination if a neoplasm has arisen from fixed macrophages (reticulum cells) or wandering macrophages (histiocyte). Also the term "histiocyte" appears to some investigators as inappropriate for wandering macrophages arriving from the peripheral blood. Furthermore some "histiocytic" lymphomas either contain or secrete increased amounts of immunoglobulins indicating that they are of lymphoid rather than histiocytic origin. Malignant lymphomas made up of smaller cells were subdivided by Rappaport et al.[105] into well differentiated and poorly differentiated lymphocytic lymphomas (Table 34-3). These terms have also been criticized, because from a functional point of view the larger cells are more differentiated than are the smaller lymphocytes. Indeed, when the small lymphocytes are stimulated by antigens or mitogens, they enlarge and take on the appearance of "blasts" (p. 1513).[73,80] Based on such considerations a number of different terms have been proposed for malignant lymphomas believed to be derived from these cells: cleaved cell

Table 34-3. Classification of lymphomas*

Nodular	Diffuse
I. Lymphocytic lymphoma	I. Lymphocytic lymphoma
1. Poorly differentiated	**1.** Poorly differentiated
2. Moderately differentiated	**2.** Moderately differentiated
3. Well differentiated	**3.** Well differentiated
II. Lymphoma, mixed cell type	II. Lymphoma, mixed cell type
III. Reticulum cell sarcoma (histiocytic lymphoma, Gall)	III. Reticulum cell sarcoma (histiocytic lymphoma, Gall)

*After Rappaport, H., Winter, W. J., and Hicks, E. B.: Cancer **9:**792-821, 1956.

lymphoma (germinocytoma, centrocytic lymphoma), germinoblastoma (centroblastic lymphoma), immunoblastic sarcoma, and others (Table 34-6).

Another lymphoma that has given rise to considerable controversy was first described by Brill, Baehr, and Rosenthal[17] as "giant lymph follicle hyperplasia." It was later renamed "giant follicle lymphoblastoma."[6] The difficulty of distinguishing this entity from reactive follicular hyperplasia, the relatively good prognosis as compared to other lymphomas, and the tendency to develop a diffuse growth pattern and lose the nodular appearance were all recognized. Rappaport et al.[105] believed that follicular lymphoma is not a distinct lesion related to germinal centers but represents a nodular growth pattern of a lymphocytic or a histiocytic lymphoma. On the basis of cytologic and ultrastructural studies a number of recent investigators have contradicted this view.[73,74,80] They present evidence that follicular (nodular) lymphomas arise from or differentiate into germinal center lymphocytes, which according to Lukes and Collins[80] are derived from small B lymphocytes at the periphery of the germinal center. This small B lymphocyte is transformed into the noncleaved cell (germinoblast of Lennert[73]) with intermediate cleaved cell (germinocyte) stages (see p. 1513). Follicular (nodular) lymphomas are composed of these cells in relatively pure forms (germinocytoma, germinoblastoma) or varying mixtures of the two.[73]

In recent years markers have been developed to characterize B lymphocytes, T lymphocytes, and monocytes.[33,52] T cells can be identified by their ability to bind sheep erythrocytes, thus forming rosettes. Phytohemagglutinin causes transformation of T cell in vitro. They can also be identified by cytotoxicity or immunofluorescence by use of specific anti-T sera. Under the scanning electron microscope T cells appear relatively smooth surfaced.[96] B cells are characterized by surface-bound immunoglobulin, a receptor for the third component of complement and a receptor for the Fc portion of IgG. On scanning electron microscopy they exhibit a villous surface.[96] Monocytes also carry membrane receptors for the third component of complement and for the Fc fragment of IgG. However, in distinction to B lymphocytes, the Fc receptor in monocytes will bind an antigen-antibody complex when presented as an IgG-coated erythrocyte. Monocytes have a ruffled surface on scanning electron microscopy.[96]

Applying these criteria to lymphoreticular neoplastic proliferative disorders, one can classify them as in the outline below. A word of caution is necessary. Neoplastic cells do not have to imitate normal cells in all their characteristics. It is likely that as more studies become available a clear-cut assignment to B lymphocytes, T lymphocytes, or monocytes will not always be possible. This is the case with leukemic reticuloendotheliosis (p. 1511).

*Classification of lymphoreticular malignancies by functional markers**

1. B Lymphocytes
   Chronic lymphocytic leukemia
   Malignant lymphoma, small cell type, nodular and diffuse
   Malignant lymphoma, large cell type, nodular and diffuse
   Burkitt's tumor
   Multiple myeloma
   Heavy-chain diseases
2. T Lymphocytes
   Mycosis fungoides
   Sézary's syndrome
   Mediastinal lymphoma of children
   Acute lymphoblastic leukemia (some cases)
3. Monocytes
   Leukemic reticuloendotheliosis (?)
   Histiocytic medullary reticulosis

Clinical presentation and staging

The most common clinical presentation of malignant lymphoma is painless lymphadenopathy. The "lump" feels rubbery firm and the diagnosis is established by biopsy and histologic examination. The lymph node or nodes involved may be in any of the lymph node–bearing areas of the body. If internal lymph nodes are involved, the presenting symptoms may be the result of pressure by the nodes on important structures, such as pressure by hilar nodes on bronchi causing cough. If the disease is widespread, the patient may present with systemic symptoms such as fever and weight loss. Mycosis fungoides is a special type of malignant lymphoma that presents with cutaneous plaques and tumors (p. 1863). Burkitt's tumor or lymphoma is predominantly a tumor of childhood that presents as a rapidly growing tumor, usually extranodal in location.

A detailed scheme for the clinical staging of Hodgkin's disease has been worked out.[21] It correlates well with prognosis and helps in deciding whether radiotherapy or chemother-

---

*Modified from Hansen, J. A., and Good, R. A.: Human Pathol. 5:567, 1974.

apy should be used. The same clinical staging is also applicable to the non-Hodgkin's lymphomas, though less experience is available with staging in these entities. It must be emphasized that clinical and pathologic staging classifications apply only to the patient at the time of disease presentation and prior to definitive therapy. The lymphatic structures are defined as the lymph nodes, spleen, thymus, Waldeyer's ring, appendix, and Peyer's patches. Stage I is involvement of a single lymph node region or of a single extralymphatic organ or site (I_E). Stage II is involvement of two or more lymph node regions on the same side of the diaphragm or localized involvement of an extralymphatic organ or site in addition to one or more lymph node regions on the same side of the diaphragm (II_E). Stage III is involvement of lymphatic structures on both sides of the diaphragm that may be associated with localized involvement of an extralymphatic organ or site (III_E), involvement of the spleen (III_S) or both (III_{SE}). Stage IV is diffuse or disseminated involvement of one or more extralymphatic organs or tissue with or without associated lymph node involvement. Each stage is further subdivided into A or B categories, B for those with defined general symptoms and A for those without. General symptoms include patients with (a) unexplained weight loss of more than 10% of the body weight in the 6 months previous to examination, (b) unexplained fever with temperatures above 38° C, and (c) night sweats.[21]

Gross appearance

Lymphomatous lymph nodes are enlarged and rubbery as contrasted with lymph nodes containing metastatic carcinoma, which may be stony hard. Not uncommonly, several enlarged nodes are matted together into a large, firm nodular mass, which, on cut surface, shows the outline of the fused nodes. The cut surface is gray-cream in color, and the tissue has been likened to fish flesh. Foci of necrosis are common when the nodes are large. The different types of lymphoma cannot be distinguished grossly.

Histopathology

The first, and most important, decision the pathologist must make when examining a section of a lymph node is whether the histologic changes represent a reactive process or a lymphoma. Some general features can be outlined that, although not always present, help in making the distinction.

The most common feature of lymphoma is the effacement of the normal architecture of the node. The sinusoids, particularly the subcapsular, are no longer seen. There is no longer a distinction between the cortex of the node, with regularly spaced and clearly defined lymphoid nodules, and the medulla. Reticulum stains may be helpful in demonstrating loss of the normal pattern. In most of the lymphomas, there is infiltration of the capsule and pericapsular fat by neoplastic cells. Infiltration of the capsule by normal lymphocytes sometimes is seen in reactive lymphadenitis, but the infiltration is seldom severe and the infiltrating cells are normal lymphocytes.

When sections are studied under high magnification, one notes that the population of cells in lymphoma varies, according to the disease, from well-differentiated small lymphocytes to highly pleomorphic and obviously malignant cells. The cell population in a reactive lymphadenitis is made up of small and large lymphocytes, histiocytes, neutrophil leukocytes, and some plasma cells. Of the lymphomas, only the mixed type of Hodgkin's disease shows eosinophils, neutrophils, and plasma cells. The final differential feature is the type of involvement of blood vessels. In lymphoma (and leukemia), the vessel wall is often infiltrated by neoplastic cells, whereas in benign hyperplasia, there is no infiltration but frequently there is hyperplasia of endothelial cells.

Lymph nodes should be sectioned at a thickness no greater than 4 μm. Poor fixation of the tissue, too thick a section, and poor staining can make what is always a difficult problem one that cannot be resolved. We also believe, strongly, that when a lymph node is excised for biopsy, it should be sent to the surgical pathology laboratory promptly and nonfixed. The pathologist, in turn, should in each case make imprints from the freshly cut surface and, whenever possible, freeze half or a portion of the node for culture should this be indicated.

HODGKIN'S DISEASE

Contrary to the lymphocytic and histiocytic lymphomas there is fairly good agreement as to the histologic classification of Hodgkin's disease. The current classification (Rye classification) is a simplification of the classification proposed by Lukes et al. (Tables 34-4 and 34-5). It was established at a conference on Hodgkin's disease held in Rye, New York, in

Table 34-4. Histologic types of Hodgkin's disease—comparison of old nomenclature, that proposed by Lukes et al. in 1966, and modified Lukes et al. classification recommended at the Conference of Hodgkin's Disease, Rye, N.Y., September 1965*

Old terminology	Lukes et al., 1966†	Conference on Hodgkin's Disease, Rye classification, 1965‡
	I. Lymphocytic and histiocytic	**I.** Hodgkin's disease, lymphocytic predominance
Hodgkin's paragranuloma Lymphoreticular medullary reticulosis Benign Hodgkin's disease Reticular lymphoma	**A.** Diffuse (lymphocytes predominant)	
Follicular lymphoma, Hodgkin's type	**B.** Nodular (lymphocytes predominant)	
Hodgkin's granuloma Lymphocytic Hodgkin's	**C.** Nodular or diffuse (histiocytes predominant)	
Hodgkin's granuloma Fibromyeloid medullary reticulosis	**II.** Mixed	**II.** Hodgkin's disease, mixed type
Hodgkin's granuloma with sclerosis	**III.** Nodular sclerosis	**III.** Hodgkin's disease, nodular sclerosis type
	IV. Diffuse fibrosis	**IV.** Hodgkin's disease, lymphocytic depletion type
Hodgkin's granuloma	**V.** Reticular **A.** With nonpleomorphic Reed-Sternberg cells	
Hodgkin's sarcoma	**B.** With pleomorphic Reed-Sternberg cells	

*From Miale, J. B.: Laboratory medicine—hematology, St. Louis, 1972, The C. V. Mosby Co.
†Slightly modified from Lukes, R. J., Butler, J. J., and Hicks, E. B.: Cancer **19**:317-344, 1966.
‡From Lukes, R. J., et al.: Cancer Res. **26**:1311, 1966.

Table 34-5. Schematic representation of variation in morphologic features in histologic types of Hodgkin's disease*

Histologic groups	Lymphocyte	Histiocytes	Eosinophils	Plasma cells	Fibrillar reticulum	Collagen	Sternberg-Reed cells
Lymphocytic and histiocytic							
Nodular	++++++++	+	0	0	0	0	+
Diffuse	++++++	+++	0	0	0	0	+
Nodular sclerosis	+ to ++++	+ to ++	+	+	+	+ to ++++	+
Mixed	+	+++	++	+	++	0	++
Diffuse fibrosis	0	+	+	+	+++++	0	++
Reticular	+	0	++	+	+	0	++++

*From Lukes, R. J., Butler, J. J., and Hicks, E. B.: Cancer **19**:317-344, 1966.

1965. The older classification of Jackson and Parker[57] divided Hodgkin's disease into paragranuloma, granuloma, and sarcoma. It was not clinically useful because the majority of the cases were included in the granuloma group. A comparison of these three classifications is presented in Table 34-4.

According to the Rye classification, which has been almost universally adopted, Hodgkin's disease is subdivided into four types:

(1) lymphocyte predominance, (2) nodular sclerosis, (3) mixed cellularity, and (4) lymphocyte depletion.[79] In general, the more mature lymphocytes there are, the better the prognosis. The various histologic types of Hodgkin's disease should not be considered as fixed and rigid categories.[79] Thus a patient who initially presents with the lymphocyte-predominance type, in time may change to the mixed and finally to the lymphocyte-

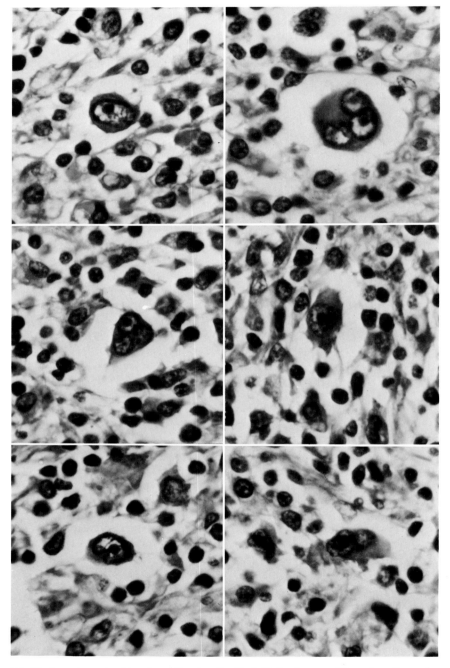

Fig. 34-39. Lymph node. Sternberg-Reed cells, Hodgkin's disease. (Hematoxylin and eosin; 450×.)

depletion type. However, nodular sclerosis type of Hodgkin's disease remains nodular sclerosis type Hodgkin's disease, even though during its cellular phase it may present, in addition to the nodular structure, the bands of collagen and the lacunar Reed-Sternberg cells, the diverse histologic appearance of the other types of Hodgkin's disease.

A histologic diagnosis of Hodgkin's disease requires the demonstration of Reed-Sternberg cells (Fig. 34-39). The classical or diagnostic type of Reed-Sternberg cell is a large cell with an abundant acidophilic to amphophilic cytoplasm, which is often pyroninophilic. It may contain two or more nuclei or a lobated nucleus with prominent, large, acidophilic, round, inclusion-like nucleoli that are surrounded with perinucleolar halos. In addition

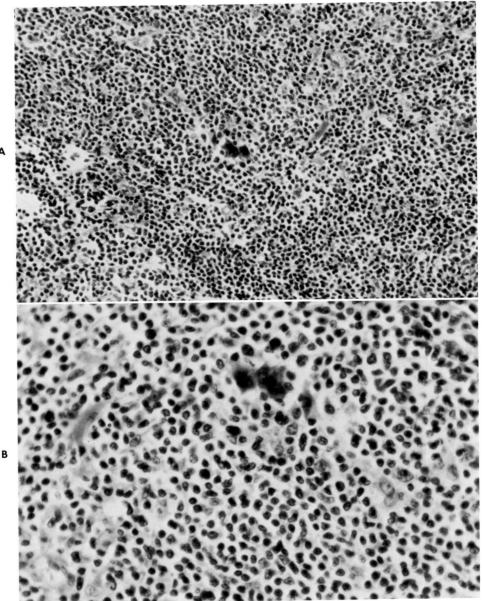

Fig. 34-40. Lymph node. **A,** Hodgkin's disease, lymphocytic predominance type. **B,** Note polyploid Reed-Steinberg cell, characteristic of Hodgkin's disease with lymphocytic predominance. (**A** and **B,** Hematoxylin and eosin; **A,** 125×; **B,** 250×.)

to this diagnostic type of Reed-Sternberg cell, there are three variants: (1) the lacunar type of Reed-Sternberg cell, characteristic of nodular sclerosis type of Hodgkin's disease; (2) a polyploid type of Reed-Sternberg cells seen in the lymphocyte predominance type, and (3) the pleomorphic, sarcomatous variant seen in the lymphocyte depletion type.[79] In general the number of Reed-Sternberg cells found is inversely proportional to the number of lymphocytes present. One should remember that Reed-Sternberg cells by themselves are not sufficient for a diagnosis of Hodgkin's disease, since they can be seen in other diseases, such as infectious mononucleosis. They have to be found in association with other characteristic histologic features before a diagnosis of Hodgkin's disease can be established.

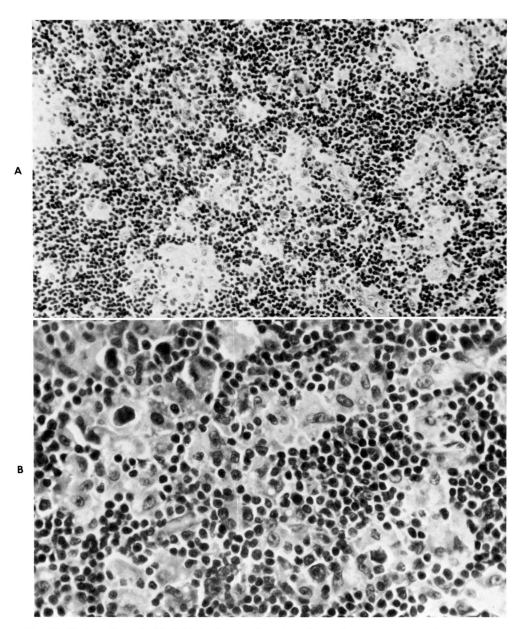

Fig. 34-41. Lymph node. Hodgkin's disease, lymphocytic predominance type. Note presence of numerous histiocytes. (**A** and **B**, Hematoxylin and eosin; **A**, 125×; **B**, 250×.)

Lymphocyte-predominance type of Hodgkin's disease

The proliferation of small lymphocytes with a varying number of mature histiocytes may involve the lymph node diffusely or focally (Figs. 34-40 and 34-41). When the node is involved diffusely, it resembles a malignant lymphoma of the small (well-differentiated) lymphocytic type or chronic lymphocytic leukemia. The diagnosis of Hodgkin's disease is made when classical Reed-Sternberg cells are found. These are rare, and many sections may have to be examined before one is found. The scarcity of diagnostic Reed-Sternberg cells is as important for the diagnosis of lymphocyte-predominance type of Hodgkin's disease as is the abundance of lymphocytes. Besides the rare diagnostic Reed-Sternberg cell, a rather characteristic variant is more frequently found in lymphocyte-predominance type of Hodg-

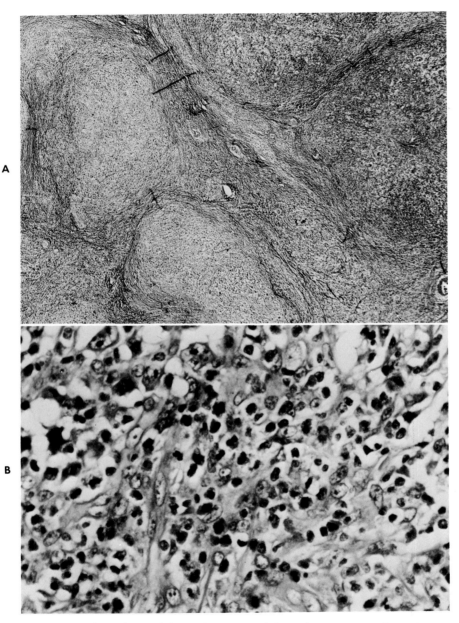

Fig. 34-42. Lymph node. Hodgkin's disease, nodular sclerosis. (**A** and **B**, Hematoxylin and eosin; **A**, 90×; **B**, 250×.)

kin's disease. It consists of a large, polyploid, twisted nucleus with fine nuclear chromatin and only small nucleoli. Varying numbers of histiocytes may also infiltrate the lymph node.

Nodular sclerosis type of Hodgkin's disease
(Figs. 34-42 and 34-43)

Two criteria are essential for the diagnosis of this type: bands of collagen and the lacunar type of Reed-Sternberg cell. The most dis-tinctive feature of the lacunar Reed-Sternberg cell is a pericellular halo that is seen in formalin-fixed tissue and is caused by the re-traction of the cytoplasm leaving only a small amount of perinuclear, acidophilic cytoplasm. The nuclei of the lacunar cells are hyper-lobated and vary in size. Prominent nucleoli are always present. With Zenker's fixation the pericellular halo is not present and these cells may be overlooked.[79]

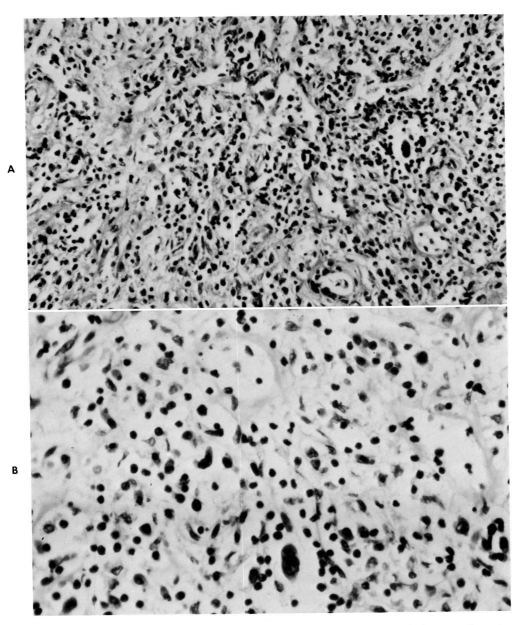

Fig. 34-43. Lymph node. Hodgkin's disease, nodular sclerosis type. Note halo around Reed-Sternberg cells. (**A** and **B,** Hematoxylin and eosin; **A,** 125×; **B,** 250×.)

In addition to these two criteria, nodular sclerosis exhibits diverse histologic appearances resembling the other histologic types of Hodgkin's disease. Occasionally the entire node may be replaced by dense, hyalinized collagen.

Nodular sclerosis is the most common histologic type of Hodgkin's disease. It is seen more frequently in women than in men and affects predominantly the mediastinal, supraclavicular, and cervical lymph nodes.

Mixed cellularity type of Hodgkin's disease

In this type the architecture of the lymph node is obliterated by proliferating lymphocytes, histiocytes, eosinophils, polymorphonuclear leukocytes, and plasma cells (Fig. 34-44). Focal necrosis may be present. There is usually some fibrosis that varies in degree in different portions of the node. Diagnostic Reed-Sternberg cells are frequent. Mixed cellularity also serves as an unclassified type and includes all

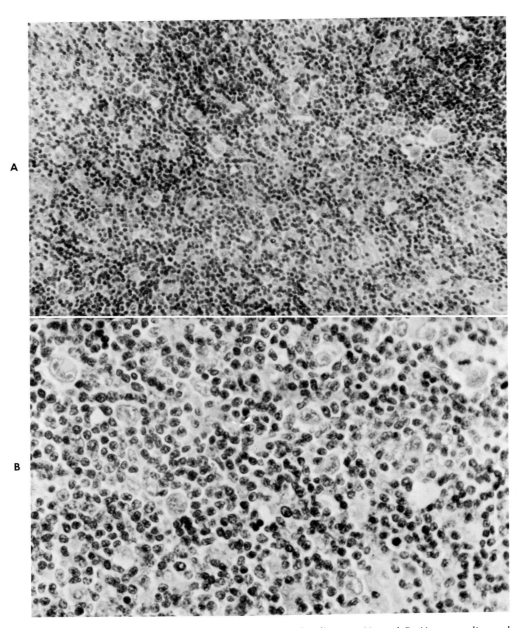

Fig. 34-44. Lymph node. Hodgkin's disease, mixed cell type. (**A** and **B**, Hematoxylin and eosin; **A,** 125×; **B,** 250×.)

cases that lack the typical features for the remaining types.[79]

Lymphocyte-depletion type of Hodgkin's disease

This group contains the diffuse fibrosis and reticular types in the classification by Lukes and his co-workers. Diffuse fibrosis is an inaccurate term for the histologic alteration observed. The lymph nodes are depleted of lymphocytes and exhibit a deposit of a homogeneous, nonfibrillary, nonbirefringent eosinophilic material, best described as hyalin. Stains for amyloid are negative. This hyalinosis is often associated with the reticular type of Hodgkin's disease, which shows proliferation, focal or diffuse, of highly atypical reticulum cells with varying numbers of diagnostic Reed-Sternberg cells (Fig. 34-45). In addition, there may be numerous pleomorphic Reed-Sternberg

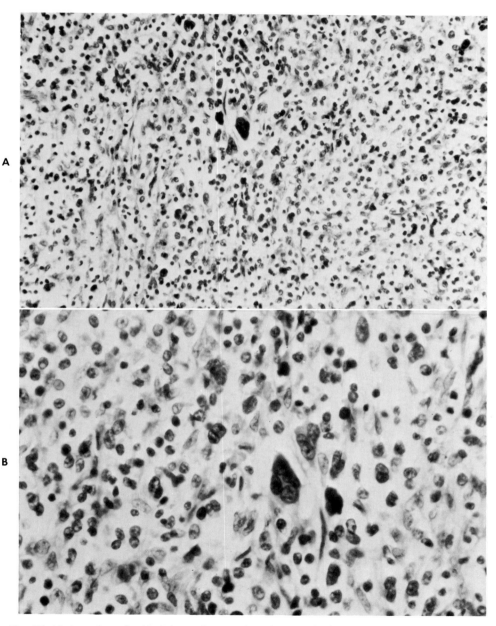

Fig. 34-45. Lymph node. Hodgkin's disease, lymphocyte depletion type, with pleomorphic Sternberg-Reed cells. (**A** and **B,** Hematoxylin and eosin; **A,** 125×; **B,** 250×.)

cells with bizarre nuclei and absent or giant eosinophilic nucleoli.

Lymphocyte-depletion Hodgkin's disease often presents clinically as a rapidly fatal disease with fever, pancytopenia, and lymphocytopenia, frequently without peripheral lymphadenopathy.[90] The distribution of the lesions is predominantly subdiaphragmatic with extensive involvement of liver, spleen, retroperitoneal lymph nodes, and bone marrow.[90]

Staging laparotomy and criteria for the diagnosis of extranodal Hodgkin's disease

Staging laparotomy with splenectomy and biopsy of liver, retroperitoneal nodes, and bone marrow is performed to determine the extent of the disease, as well as the extent of radiotherapy or chemotherapy. This procedure is performed most often to confirm the extent of the disease in patients who clinically appear to have stage I or II disease. Approximately 25% of spleens, clinically unsuspected, contain Hodgkin's disease when studied by the pathologist.[111] Also, about 50% of spleens that are clinically enlarged, will not exhibit Hodgkin's disease on detailed pathologic examination.[111] It is unusual for the liver to be involved in the absence of splenic Hodgkin's disease. The overall demonstration of liver involvement by laparotomy is about 5%.[111] The bone marrow has to be examined histologically, not cytologically, to establish a diagnosis of Hodgkin's disease. Marrow for histologic examination may be obtained by aspiration[118] or by biopsy. The latter may be performed with a needle or by an open surgical technique. The yield of abnormal bone marrow biopsies is 9% in untreated patients whose disease is beyond stage II.[110]

Staging laparotomies resulting in the submission to the pathologist of relatively small biopsies of liver and bone marrow have raised the question as to minimal criteria necessary for the diagnosis of Hodgkin's disease.[103] The criteria are not so stringent as for the initial diagnosis of Hodgkin's disease, and diagnostic Reed-Sternberg cells with eosinophilic, inclusion-like nucleoli are not required. Mononuclear cells with nuclear features of Reed-Sternberg cells (Hodgkin cells) in one of the characteristic cellular environments of Hodgkin's disease, should be regarded as indicative of liver or bone marrow involvement. The presence of atypical lymphoreticular cells that fall short of these criteria should be reported as "suggestive of Hodgkin's disease." The presence of nonspecific lymphoreticular infiltrates or sarcoidosis-like granulomas should not be considered as evidence for Hodgkin's disease.[61] Focal fibrosis of the bone marrow associated with lymphoreticular cells, in the absence of mononuclear or multinuclear cells with nuclear features of Reed-Sternberg cells, should be regarded as strongly suggestive of Hodgkin's disease in an untreated patient with histologically proved Hodgkin's disease.

Hodgkin's disease of the spleen involves primarily the white pulp and varies from microscopic foci to grossly visible nodules. In untreated patients, features of any of the histologic types of Hodgkin's disease may be identified, with the possible exception of lymphocyte predominance.[79] In the lymphocyte-depletion type the malpighian corpuscles are hyalinized and Reed-Sternberg cells are scarce. In the reticular variant of lymphocyte depletion, bizarre, pleomorphic Reed-Sternberg cells

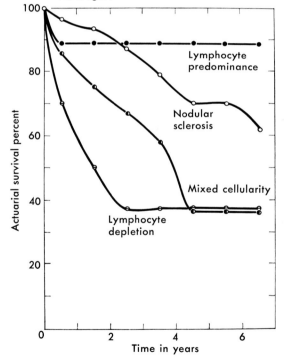

Fig. 34-46. Actuarial survival in 176 cases of Hodgkin's disease according to histologic types. Survival of nodular sclerosis and mixed cellularity groups at 5 years is significantly different (p < 0.02). (From Keller, A. R., Kaplan, H. S., Lukes, R. J., et al.: Cancer **22:**487, 1968.)

are frequent and are associated with varying numbers of diagnostic Reed-Sternberg cells.

When vascular invasion is observed in lymph node biopsies or in the spleen, there is a greater prevalence of disseminated and extranodal Hodgkin's disease.[129]

Clinical correlations

Fig. 34-46 shows the correlation between the histologic type of Hodgkin's disease and survival as obtained from a study of 176 previously untreated cases of Hodgkin's disease.[64] After 6 years the highest number of survivors were in the lymphocyte-predominance group. The largest histologic group, comprising half the cases, was in the nodular sclerosis group. The second largest group was mixed cellularity. The lymphocyte-predominance and lymphocyte-depletion groups were about equal in frequency and constituted together approximately 10% of the patients. Patients with

lymphocyte predominance were almost entirely in clinical stages I and II, whereas lymphocyte-depletion cases were largely in stages III and IV. Fig. 34-47 shows survival in relation to clinical stages.

There is a high degree of correlation between extensive disease and systemic symptoms. Thus nearly four fifths of stage IV cases had systemic symptoms, whereas three fourths of stage II cases had none.

The majority of patients with active Hodgkin's disease display a defect in cell-mediated immunity. This defect contributes to the variety of bacterial, viral, fungal, and protozoal infections to which these patients are prone.[1]

MALIGNANT LYMPHOMAS: FOLLICULAR AND DIFFUSE

At the present time there is no generally accepted classification of the so-called non-Hodgkin's lymphomas. The original classification included lymphosarcoma, reticulum cell sarcoma, and giant follicular lymphoblastoma (p. 1528). This was gradually replaced by Rappaport's classification[98] (Table 34-3). Rappaport's classification is simple and fairly well reproducible and has proved prognostically significant. There is however increasing evidence that it is histogenetically incorrect. Recent ultrastructural and immunofluorescent studies supplemented by techniques for membrane receptor sites (p. 1528) provide evidence for the origin of nodular lymphomas from follicular B lymphocytes.[45,71,73,74] The arguments against substitution of histiocytic lymphoma for reticulum cell sarcoma have been presented (p. 1527). There is also increasing evidence that many lymphomas regarded as reticulum cell sarcomas (histiocytic lymphomas) are in fact derived from transformed B or T lymphocytes.

Many different classifications of the non-Hodgkin's lymphomas have been published in recent years (Table 34-6).[10,29,45] Despite the diversity of termniology used, there is general agreement that non-Hodgkin's lymphomas may exhibit a follicular or a diffuse growth pattern and that they may be composed of small and large cells. Based on these two accepted observations and the evidence of the relationship of follicular (nodular) lymphoma to germinal center cells, we propose the classification below. Some of the large cell lymphomas exhibit round nuclei with prominent nucleoli and a rim of fairly well defined cytoplasm. The cytoplasm of these cells is

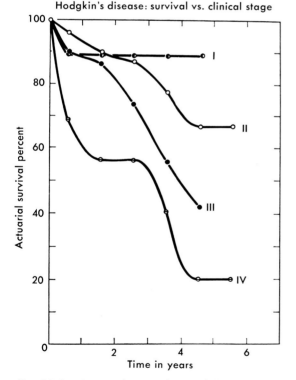

Hodgkin's disease: survival vs. clinical stage

Fig. 34-47. Actuarial survival in Hodgkin's disease according to anatomic stages; 154 patients, all with lymphangiograms. Survival at 5 years of stages I and II, II and IV, and I and IV are significantly different (p < 0.02). (From Keller, A. R., Kaplan, H. S., Lukes, R. J., et al.: Cancer **22:**487, 1968.)

Table 34-6. Various classifications of non-Hodgkin's lymphomas

Kiel classification[45]	British classification[10]	Dorfman's classification[6]

Low-grade malignancy—malignant lymphoma (ML)
ML-lymphocytic
ML-lymphoplasmacytoid (immunocytic)
ML-centrocytic
ML-centroblastic-centrocytic
  Follicular*
  Follicular* and diffuse
  Diffuse*
 	
High-grade malignancy
ML-centroblastic
ML-lymphoblastic
  Burkitt type
  Convoluted-cell type
  Others
ML-immunoblastic
	Grade 1
	Follicular lymphomas
	  Follicle cell, predominantly small
	  Follicle cell, mixed (small and large)
	  Follicle cell, predominantly large
	Diffuse lymphomas
	  Lymphocytic, well-differentiated (small round lymphocyte)
	  Lymphocytic, intermediately differentiated (small follicle cell)
	
	Grade 2
	Lymphocytic, poorly differentiated (lymphoblast)
	  Non-Burkitt's lymphoma
	  Burkitt's tumor
	  Convoluted-cell mediastinal lymphoma
	Lymphocytic cell, mixed (small and large) (mixed follicle cells)
	"Undifferentiated" large cell (large lymphoid cell)
	Histiocytic cell (mononuclear phagocytic cells)
	Plasma cell (extramedullary plasma cell)
	
	Unclassified
	Plasmacytoid differentiation in lymphocytic tumors and banded or fine sclerosis are recorded
		Follicular lymphomas (follicular or follicular and diffuse)
		
		Small lymphoid
		Mixed small and large lymphoid
		Large lymphoid
		
		Diffuse lymphomas†
		  Small lymphocytic‡
		  Atypical small lymphoid
		  Lymphoblastic
		    Convoluted
		    Nonconvoluted
		  Large lymphoid‡
		  Mixed small and large lymphoid
		  Histiocytic
		  Burkitt's lymphoma
		  Mycosis fungoides
		  Undefined

*With or without sclerosis.

†Composite lymphomas comprise the following four types: two well-defined and apparently different types of lymphoma within the same tissue; lymphomas associated with sclerosis; lymphomas showing plasmacytoid differentiation‡; those associated with epithelioid cells.

‡See this footnote symbol just above.

pyroninophilic and deeply basophilic with the Giemsa stain. These lymphomas we call "blastic" lymphomas. Other large cell lymphomas with more pleomorphic and bizarre nuclei but without a pyroninophilic or deeply basophilic cytoplasm with the Giemsa stain, we call reticulum cell sarcomas (histiocytic lymphomas).[113] This classification is to be regarded as temporary and will help the student to follow the developments in this rapidly changing field.

Non-Hodgkin's malignant lymphomas
  I. Follicular lymphomas*
     1. Intermediate cell type†
     2. Large cell type
        "Blastic"‡
        Reticulum cell type (histiocytic)
     3. Mixed cell type
 II. Diffuse lymphomas
     1. Small cell type
     2. Intermediate cell type§
     3. Large cell type
        "Blastic"‖
        Reticulum cell type (histiocytic)
     4. Mixed cell type

Follicular lymphomas

These are defined as malignant lymphomas arising from, or differentiating toward, germinal center cells. They exhibit a follicular or nodular growth pattern. This follicular pattern may be associated with a diffuse pattern. Occasionally a diffuse pattern only is seen, but a reticulin stain may still reveal remnants of a follicular pattern.

Lymphomas with a follicular pattern have to be distinguished from reactive follicular hyperplasia. The criteria for separating these two entities are well summarized by Rappaport and co-workers.[105] They are based on architectural and cytologic features. In follicular lymphomas the architecture is partially or completely effaced. This is true of all malig-

---

*Follicular lymphomas exhibit a nodular growth pattern and originate from, or differentiate into, germinal center cells.
†This is the cleaved cell of Lukes or the germinocyte of Lennert. A follicular lymphoma made up of small, round, "mature" lymphocytes has not been described.
‡Identification of "blasts" is based on the presence of narrow, blue rims of cytoplasm with the Giemsa stain in association with prominent nucleoli. The cytoplasm is also pyroninophilic.
§This is the germinal center cell described under (†); however the growth pattern is diffuse.
‖This includes the convoluted lymphocytic thymic lymphoma and Burkitt's tumor.

---

nant lymphomas and is best appreciated by a study of the subcapsular area normally occupied by the peripheral sinus. Obliteration of the subcapsular sinus is particularly well seen with reticulin stains. Neoplastic follicles vary moderately in size and shape and are evenly distributed throughout cortex and medulla. Reactive follicles are especially prominent in the cortical portion of the lymph node and vary considerably in size and shape. Reaction centers are more sharply demarcated than are neoplastic follicles. Reticulin fibers may be condensed at the periphery of neoplastic nodules, whereas they are slightly altered around reactive follicles. Cytologically, reactive follicles show debris-containing macrophages and frequent mitotic figures. In neoplastic follicles macrophages are inconspicuous and mitotic figures are scarce.

Follicular lymphoma, intermediate cell type

SYNONYMS: Nodular lymphoma, lymphocytic poorly differentiated; follicular lymphoma, small lymphoid type; prolymphocytic lymphoma, nodular; B cell lymphoma, cleaved cell type; germinocytoma; centrocytic lymphoma.

This lymphoma consists of cells that are somewhat larger than the small, "mature" perifollicular lymphocyte, hence the term "intermediate cell." The nuclear membranes are distorted, partially collapsed, and cleaved. A few "blasts" are invariably present (Fig. 34-48).

Follicular lymphoma, large cell type

SYNONYMS: Nodular lymphoma, histiocytic type; follicular lymphoma, large lymphoid type; B-cell lymphoma. large noncleaved cell type; germinoblastoma; centroblastic lymphoma.

These lymphomas exhibit a predominantly follicular or a follicular and diffuse growth pattern. When the large cells have a dark blue rim of cytoplasm with the Giemsa stain, they fall into the "blast" category. We believe that it is impossible, at the present stage of our knowledge, to clearly distinguish in neoplastic processes germinoblasts, immunoblasts, and lymphoblasts. The large cell lymphoma whose cells fail to exhibit pyroninophilia and basophilia of the cytoplasm is classified as a reticulum cell (histiocyte) type (Fig. 34-49).

Follicular lymphoma, mixed cell type

SYNONYMS: Malignant lymphoma, nodular, mixed lymphocytic-histiocytic; follicular lym-

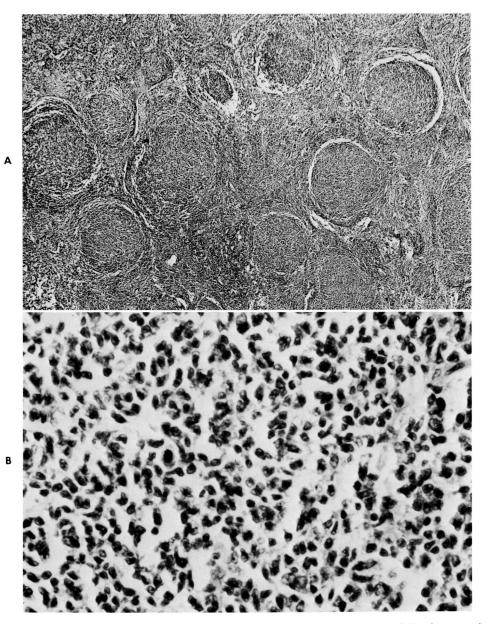

Fig. 34-48. Lymph node. Follicular lymphoma, intermediate cell type. Note follicular growth pattern, **A,** and distorted, irregular nuclear membranes, **B.** (**A** and **B,** Hematoxylin and eosin; **A,** 100×; **B,** 250×.)

phoma, mixed small and large lymphoid; centroblastic-centrocytic lymphoma.

This malignant lymphoma exhibits a follicular growth pattern and is composed cytologically of approximately equal numbers of the small and large cells described above. Varying degrees of sclerosis may be present in this lymphoma (Figs. 34-50 and 34-51).

Diffuse lymphomas
Diffuse lymphoma, small cell type

SYNONYMS: Malignant lymphoma, well-differentiated lymphocytic diffuse; diffuse lymphoma, small lymphocytic type; B-cell lymphoma, small lymphocytic type; lymphoplasmacytoid lymphoma; immunocytic lymphoma.

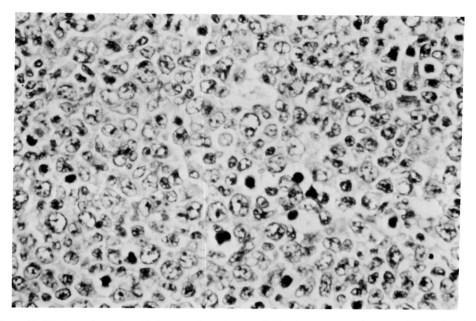

Fig. 34-49. Lymph node. Malignant lymphoma, follicular, large cell type. The follicular pattern cannot be appreciated under this magnification. (250×.)

This lymphoma exhibits a diffuse growth pattern only. The architecture of the lymph node is effaced. The lymph node is diffusely infiltrated with small, "mature" lymphocytes, exhibiting round to oval, hyperchromatic nuclei without any cleft formation (Fig. 34-52). The appearance of this lymph node is not distinguishable from chronic lymphocytic leukemia. A thorough search for Reed-Sternberg cells should be performed to exclude Hodgkin's disease, lymphocytic predominance. This type of malignant lymphoma is rare. In our experience most cases are examples of chronic lymphocytic leukemias.

This lymphoma may be associated with plasma cells, plasmacytoid lymphocytes, and cells with PAS-positive cytoplasmic and intranuclear inclusions. A high percentage of such cases will exhibit a monoclonal macroglobulinemia.

Diffuse lymphoma, intermediate cell type

SYNONYMS: Malignant lymphoma, diffuse, poorly differentiated lymphocytic; diffuse lymphoma, lymphocytic, intermediate differentiation (small follicle cell); malignant lymphoma, centrocytic, diffuse; malignant lymphoma, diffuse, cleaved cell or germinocytic type; malignant lymphoma, diffuse, prolymphocytic.

This lymphoma exhibits a diffuse growth pattern and is identical cytologically with the follicular lymphoma of the intermediate cell type. It may have started with a follicular growth pattern that became diffuse as the disease evolved. When this type of lymphoma becomes leukemic, the neoplastic cells in the peripheral blood correspond to "lymphosarcoma cells."

Diffuse lymphoma, large cell type

SYNONYMS: Malignant lymphoma, diffuse, histiocytic type; reticulum cell sarcoma; diffuse lymphoma, large lymphoid (pyroninophilic) type; B or T cell immunoblastic sarcoma; lymphoblastic sarcoma.

This type of malignant lymphoma exhibits a diffuse growth pattern. On the basis of the Giemsa stain it can be subdivided into two types: "blastic" lymphoma and reticulum cell sarcoma (histiocytic lymphoma). In the "blastic" lymphoma, the Giemsa stain reveals that the neoplastic cells possess a rim of dark blue cytoplasm (Figs. 34-53 and 34-54). The cytoplasm is also pyroninophilic. Pyroninophilia and basophilia with the Giemsa stain are indicative of high RNA content. Furthermore the cells exhibit round to oval nuclei and prominent nucleoli. In the reticulum cell sarcoma (histiocytic lymphoma), no dark blue rim of cytoplasm can be demonstrated. Also the nuclei are more pleomorphic than those in the "blastic" type, and the cytoplasm is more irregular and eosinophilic (Fig. 34-55).

The convoluted, lymphocytic thymic lym-

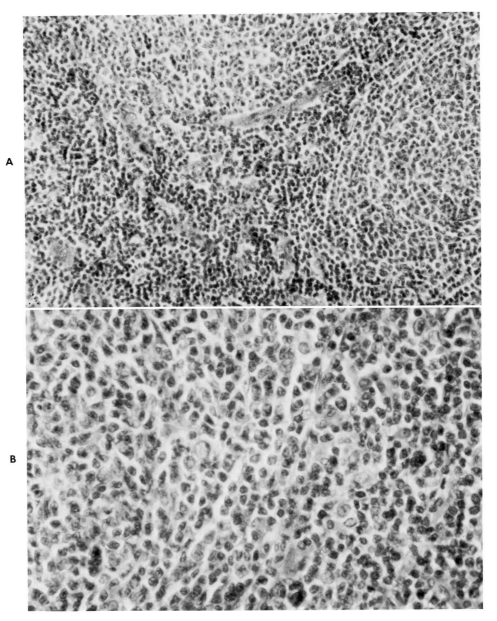

Fig. 34-50. Lymph node. Malignant lymphoma, follicular, mixed cell type. (**A** and **B,** Hematoxylin and eosin; **A,** 125×; **B,** 250×.)

phoma is essentially a diffuse "blastic" lymphoma with special clinical and histologic features.[62,126] It is a tumor of children, arising in the anterior mediastinum and associated with a "blastic" leukemia. Histologically the nuclei have a characteristic convoluted or cerebriform appearance. This tumor is supposedly derived from T lymphocytes.[62,126]

Burkitt's tumor (malignant lymphoma, undifferentiated, Burkitt type) is also a diffuse,

"blastic" lymphoma with characteristic clinical and histologic features. Burkitt's tumor was first reported as a jaw sarcoma of East African children.[19] It was identified as a malignant lymphoma by O'Connor and Davies.[93] In American patients, abdominal and pelvic involvement is far more frequent than jaw involvement. Bone marrow involvement is also more frequent in American patients. In a series of 30 American cases,[2,7] 23 presented

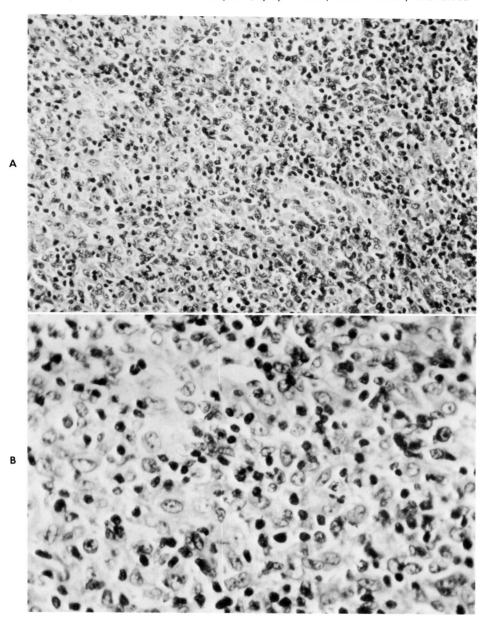

Fig. 34-51. Lymph node. Lymphoma, mixed cell type. (**A** and **B**, Hematoxylin and eosin; **A**, 100×; **B**, 250×.)

with an abdominal tumor; 4 showed ovarian involvement. In only 3 was lymphadenopathy the sole presenting physical finding. Facial bones were involved in 5 cases. Involvement of the bone marrow was documented in 5 of the 26 patients whose bone marrows were available. Good correlation between lactic dehydrogenase values and stage of Burkitt's tumor has been reported.[2] Complete remissions were obtained in 13 of the 30 patients treated with chemotherapy.[2] Metabolic complications related to therapy included azotemia, hyperkalemia, hyperuricemia, hyperphosphatemia, and hypocalcemia. Of the 13 patients who had a complete remission, 9 were free of disease for 37 to 80 months.[2]

Histologically Burkitt's tumor is composed of "blasts" with pyroninophilic and Giemsa-positive cytoplasmic rims. Nucleoli are prominent. Characteristic of this neoplasm is a

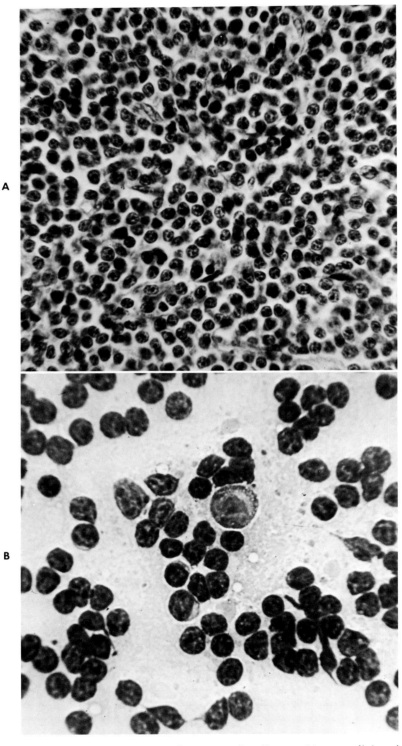

Fig. 34-52. Lymph node. Diffuse lymphoma, small cell type. Note small lymphocytes in imprint preparation, **B.** (**A,** Hematoxylin and eosin; 450×; **B,** Wright's stain; 1080×; **A** and **B,** courtesy Dr. Joseph C. Sieracki, Pittsburgh.)

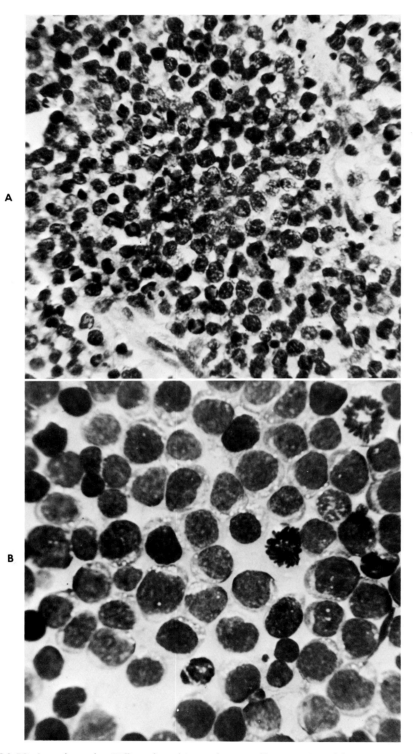

Fig. 34-53. Lymph node. Diffuse lymphoma, large cell type. Note blastic appearance of cell in imprint preparation, **B.** (**A,** Hematoxylin and eosin; 450×; **B,** Wright's stain; 950×; **A** and **B,** courtesy Dr. Joseph C. Sieracki, Pittsburgh.)

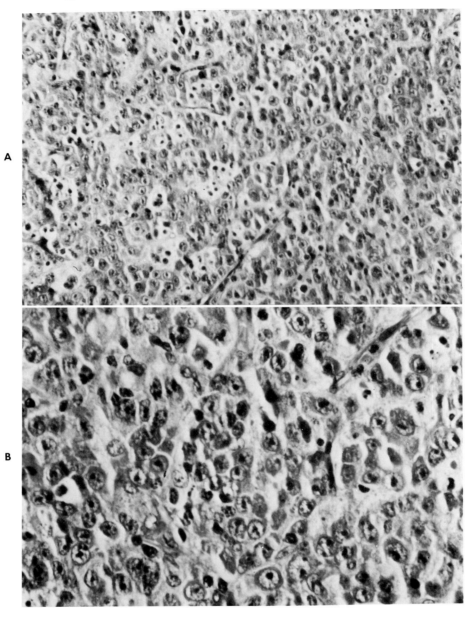

Fig. 34-54. Lymph node. Diffuse lymphoma, large cell type, "blastic." (**A** and **B**, Hematoxylin and eosin; **A**, 125×; **B**, 250×.)

"starry-sky" appearance because of benign-appearing phagocytic cells containing debris. Some PAS-positive material can be identified in these macrophages. The histologic features of Burkitt's tumor have been defined by the World Health Organization[11] and have been reviewed in detail by Wright.[142]

In 17 autopsied cases of Burkitt's tumor the most consistent feature was widespread organ involvement, predominantly in the extralymphatic sites.[7] All 17 patients had tumor in

two or more gastrointestinal organs. Twelve patients had hepatic involvement, and 16 had tumor in the kidneys. Involvement of lungs was present in 11 cases, and of the central nervous system in 9. Cardiovascular organs and the musculoskeletal system were infiltrated with tumor in 6 patients. Diffuse peripheral lymph node involvement was seen in only 1 patient. The spleen was involved in 10 and the bone marrow in 12 of the 17 autopsied cases. Chemotherapeutic agents appeared to

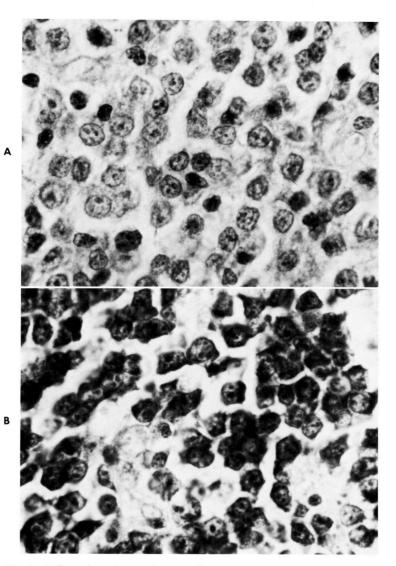

Fig. 34-55. A, Diffuse lymphoma, large cell type, reticulum cell (histiocytic). **B,** Diffuse lymphoma, diffuse blastic. Note dark blue rim of cytoplasm. (**A** and **B,** Giemsa stain, 882×.)

alter the cytologic appearance of the tumor. The cells exhibited pronounced pleomorphism resembling malignant histiocytes. Reed-Sternberg–like cells were seen occasionally.

Diffuse lymphoma, mixed cell type

SYNONYMS: Malignant lymphoma, diffuse, mixed lymphohistiocytic; malignant lymphoma, diffuse, mixed, small and large lymphoid; diffuse lymphoma, mixed, small lymphoid and undifferentiated large cell.

This variety of lymphoma exhibits a diffuse growth pattern and is composed of approximately equal numbers of intermediate cells and large cells of the blast type. In every malignant lymphoma a few large cells can be found. Some of them are reticulum cells and perhaps are the result of an inductive effect of neoplastic lymphocytes on the stroma. Other large cells exhibit the characteristics of blasts. The presence of only a few large cells does not justify the diagnosis of a malignant lymphoma, mixed cell type.

Clinical correlations

There is less information available on clinicopathologic correlations for the non-Hodgkin's lymphomas than for Hodgkin's disease. In a large series of cases studied at Stanford University Medical Center[60] follicular lymphomas were found in 44% of the group and diffuse lymphomas in 56%. Patients under the age of 35 and those over 60 tended to have diffuse lymphomas. Thirty-nine percent of the patients had stage IV disease at the time they were first diagnosed. Systemic symptoms did not adversely affect survival. They were present in 24% of patients with diffuse and 18% with follicular lymphomas. Patients with follicular lymphomas survived significantly longer than patients with diffuse lymphomas. Malignant lymphomas whether nodular or diffuse have a better prognosis if they exhibit a tendency to sclerosis.[88] A comparative study of survival of diffuse germinal center cell lymphomas and non–germinal center cell lymphomas is not available. The small cell lymphomas fare better than do the large cell lymphomas.

It is of interest that left lower cervical or supraclavicular lymphadenopathy was significantly more often correlated with para-aortic lymphadenopathy than with involvement in the right lower neck region.

All patients with malignant lymphomas should have a serum protein electrophoresis and immunoelectrophoresis. Monoclonal gammopathies of various types may be encountered in the different forms of malignant lymphomas.

HEAVY-CHAIN DISEASES

Heavy-chain diseases are lymphocellular and plasmacellular proliferative disorders associated with an overproduction of Fc fragments of gamma (γ), alpha (α), or mu (μ) heavy chains.

Franklin's disease (gamma heavy-chain disease)[41]

The most frequent clinical presentation of Franklin's disease consists of painless cervical or axillary lymphadenopathy. Occasionally there is only thoracic or abdominal lymphadenopathy. Prominent involvement of Waldeyer's ring with erythema and swelling of the uvula was described in several cases. Hepatosplenomegaly was observed clinically or at autopsy in many of the cases. Fever was present in about half the reported cases. In the fatal cases the disease lasted from 6 months to a year. Anemia, leukopenia with lymphocytosis, atypical lymphocytes, peripheral blood plasmacytosis, and thrombocytopenia have all been reported. Most patients with Franklin's disease have hypoalbuminemia with a normal total serum protein level. An abnormal band of protein is usually present on electrophoresis:

Immunoelectrophoresis of serum and urine reveals a precipitin arc with anti-IgG and anti-Fc serum. No light chains are found in the urine.

The infiltrate in the lymph nodes and other tissues consists of a varying mixture of lymphocytes, plasma cells, plasmacytoid cells, and reticulum cells (histiocytes). Occasionally Reed-Sternberg–like cells have been reported.[36] The pathologist examining a lymph node may have considerable difficulties to decide whether an inflammatory or a neoplastic process is involved. It is essential that all the clinical and laboratory data are available before committing oneself to a definite diagnosis.

Seligman's disease (Mediterranean lymphoma, alpha heavy-chain disease)[122]

Mediterranean lymphoma is a term applied to a lymphoplasmacellular proliferative disorder occurring primarily in Mediterranean populations involving the small intestine with villous atrophy and malabsorption. In some patients with Mediterranean lymphoma alphachain proteins were demonstrated in the serum on immunoelectrophoresis.[122] Whether all cases of Mediterranean lymphoma are associated with an alpha-chain peak remains unknown, since in many of the earlier cases alpha chains were not looked for. Also, the amount present in the serum may be so small that it can be overlooked on routine electrophoresis.[41]

Morphologic findings in Mediterranean lymphoma are not uniform, and it is not settled whether we are dealing with different stages of one disease or with different lymphoproliferative disorders. Ramot[97] has divided 20 cases into three groups: (1) Cases with massive plasma cell infiltration of the gut and lymph nodes without evidence of lymphoma (4 cases). In two of these patients protein studies were performed and alpha heavy chains were found in the serum. (2) Plasma cell infiltration of the intestine and malignant lymphoma in the mesenteric lymph nodes (2 cases). (3) Malignant lymphoma of small intestine with a heavy plasma cellular response (14 cases). No data on the presence of alpha chains were available on these patients. Reviewing this material, Rappaport et al.[104] concluded that the plasma cell infiltration, rather than the malignant lymphomas, were responsible for the malabsorption syndrome. There was no morphologic evidence that the malignant lymphomas were histogenetically related to the plasma cell infiltration. The possibility was suggested that the proliferation of plasma cells was a morphologic manifestation of an immune-deficiency state that predisposes patients to the development of malignant lymphoreticular neoplasms.[104] Ramot[104] believes that the massive intestinal plasma cell infiltration should be considered neoplastic and classified as an extramedullary plasmacytoma.

Recently alpha heavy-chain disease has been reported with a diffuse lymphoplasmacellular infiltrate of the respiratory tract without intestinal involvement.[128]

Mu heavy-chain disease

Mu heavy-chain disease is the rarest of the heavy-chain diseases. The cases reported presented with a long-standing chronic lymphocytic leukemia.[40,41] They had hepatosplenomegaly without peripheral lymphadenopathy. Routine electrophoresis revealed hypogammaglobulinemia; an abnormal component reacting with antisera to mu chains was discovered on immunoelectrophoresis. Mu chains have not been reported in the urine of these patients. Two of the reported patients had light chains in the urine.[41] There is evidence that the defect in mu-chain disease is a lack of normal coupling of light and heavy chains, rather than an overproduction of heavy chains, as is the case in alpha and gamma heavy-chain diseases.[70] Two of the reported cases had pathologic fractures and one had amyloidosis.[41] All the patients had vacuolated plasma cells in addition to lymphocytosis of the bone marrow.

Bone marrow and blood
FUNCTION

We have already discussed two of the three identifiable morphologic entities in the reticuloendothelial system, the spleen and the lymph nodes. The third, the bone marrow, also has some functions that are common to other tissues rich in reticuloendothelial cells. Also like the others, it has a special function, in this case to serve as the chief site of blood cell formation in the normal adult. This is medullary. hemopoiesis. It is sometimes said that medullary hemopoiesis is involved in the production of erythrocytes, granulocytes, and platelets, whereas lymphocytes and monocytes are formed outside the marrow. However, as shown in Table 34-7, the lymphocytic and monocytic population in the bone marrow is considerable. Note that there is 13 times more lymphoid tissue outside than there is within lymph nodes and spleen.

As discussed on p. 1485, the spleen and liver are active sites of normal hemopoiesis in the fetus. Hemopoietic activity in the liver stops by the end of full-term gestation; in the spleen it is greatly reduced. However, these organs retain their content of primitive mesenchymal cells capable of differentiating, when stimulated to do so, into hemopoietic cells. In the adult, therefore, certain hematologic disorders are characterized by formation of blood cells at sites outside of the bone marrow. This is *extramedullary hemopoiesis.* A consequence of hepatic and splenic involvement in extramedullary hemopoietic activity is hepatomegaly and splenomegaly.

STRUCTURE

At birth, all possible bone cavities contain active red marrow. By the age of 4 years, there is beginning replacement of red marrow by fatty marrow, and at the age of 20 years red marrow is found only in the skull, clavicles, scapulae, sternum, ribs, pelvis, and proximal

Table 34-7. Number and distribution of blood cells in normal person weighing 70 kg*

Cell type	In hemopoietic organs		Outside hemopoietic organs			Total blood cells in body (gm)
	Bone marrow (gm)	Lymphoid tissue and spleen (gm)	In peripheral blood and hemopoietic organs (gm)	Outside peripheral blood and hemopoietic organs (gm)	Ratio of cells within blood to cells outside blood	
Erythrocytic	100	0	2,500	0	—	2,600
Granulocytic	900	0	10	600	1:60	1,500
Lymphocytic	100	100	3	1,300	1:433	1,500
Monocytic, plasmocytic, thrombocytic, and disintegrated cells	200	200	1	400	1:400	800

*Slightly modified from Osgood, E. E.: Blood **9:**1141-1154, 1954; by permission; from Miale, J. B.: Laboratory medicine—hematology, St. Louis, 1972, The C. V. Mosby Co.

ends of the long bones, whereas the distal portions of the long bones contain only fatty marrow. In the normal adult, the ratio of red to fatty marrow is 1:1. Ellis[35] gives the total amount of active red marrow in a man weighing 70 kg as 1459 gm, about equal to the weight of the liver, and gives data for distribution in various bones (Table 34-8). When

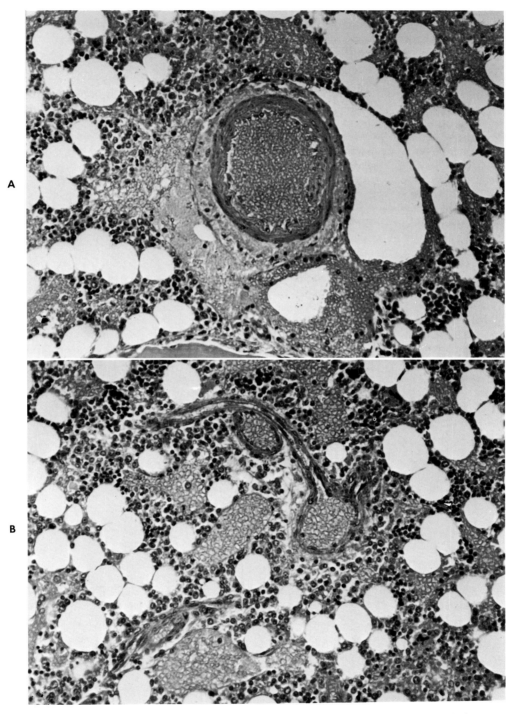

Fig. 34-56. Arterial supply of bone marrow. **A,** Thick-walled artery. **B,** Thin-walled artery. (Hematoxylin and eosin; 125×.)

marrow volume and cellularity are determined by means of radioisotopes of iron and gold, the values for the normal distribution are not changed appreciably, but these methods give interesting data in hematologic abnormalities.

The vascular bed of the bone marrow is unusual in several respects. For one thing, the rigid cortical bone that encases it makes in the marrow an unyielding hydrostatic system unlike that in any other organ. The arteries entering the marrow cavity have a normal structure (Fig. 34-56, *A*), but soon after entering the marrow, the thick-walled arteries change abruptly into thin-walled arteries (Fig. 34-56, *B*), the wall of which consists of a flattened thin tunica media and flat endothelium. The thin-walled arteries in turn open into large sinuses. The sinus walls are not easily distinguished in routine sections but by electron microscopy they can be seen to consist of lining endothelium, basement membrane, and adventitial cells. Furthermore, the sinus walls appear not to be continuous, and there are long segments in which the absence of a complete sinus wall permits open communication with the hemopoietic tissue of the marrow.

The combination of a rigidly enclosed system and discontinuous sinus walls is ideally suited to free exchange of cells and plasma between the sinuses and the hemopoietic tissue. This, plus the inherent motility of some of the blood cells, accounts for the entrance of newly formed cells into the systemic circulation. The patency of the system is illustrated by the finding that materials injected into the bone marrow (colloidal thorium dioxide, ^{22}sodium chloride, ^{131}I albumin, ^{131}I hippuran) are dispersed throughout the marrow in a few minutes, whereas the isotopically labeled materials are detectable in the systemic circulation in a matter of seconds.

Table 34-8. Distribution of red marrow by weight in bones of normal 40-year-old man*

	Weight of red marrow (gm)	% total red marrow
Cranium and mandible	136.6	13.1
Humeri, scapulae, and clavicles	86.7	8.3
Sternum	23.4	2.3
Ribs	82.6	7.9
Vertebrae	297.8	28.4
Pelvis	418.6	40.0

*Slightly modified from Ellis, R. E.: Phys. Med. Biol. **5:**255-258, 1961; from Miale, J. B.: Laboratory medicine—hematology, St. Louis, 1972, The C. V. Mosby Co.

METHODS OF STUDY
Biopsy

Biopsy of bone marrow is performed most commonly by aspiration. The sternum, anterior and posterior iliac crests, and the vertebral spinous processes all give representative specimens. After the marrow is entered, 5 to 10 ml of marrow is aspirated. Almost all the aspirated marrow is immediately ejected into 10% neutral buffered formalin. The remaining drops of marrow are used to prepare smears. The bone marrow–formalin mixture is filtered, and a button of concentrated bone marrow particles are left to be fixed and sectioned.[118] Routine sections are cut at 5 μm and stained with hematoxylin and eosin. Special stains such as the Giemsa stain can be used, but cellular morphology is best studied in the thin smears stained with Wright's stain.

If aspiration biopsy is unsuccessful, a core of bone marrow can be obtained by trephine with a modified Vim-Silverman needle. Details of biopsy techniques are given by Miale.[10] A particle of bone marrow should be teased out of the core and used for a crush smear. The remainder of the specimen is fixed and used for routine sections.

It is sometimes necessary to obtain bone marrow by open surgical biopsy. The sample obtained in this case usually consists of cortical bone and bone marrow and requires decalcification. Since decalcification often produces cytologic alterations, it is recommended that before the specimen is processed particles of marrow be teased out for smears and, if possible, sectioned without decalcification.

Necropsy

Bone marrow cells undergo degeneration soon after death. There is no relationship between rate of degeneration and age, sex, storage temperature, and mode of death, although some investigators believe that cellular damage is more rapid when death is the result of an infectious disease. Within the first 3 hours after death, the marrow cells are well preserved and can be identified easily in smears from aspirated material. After 3 hours, there is progressive degeneration of the cells, the oldest cells such as mature granulocytes and mature normoblasts degenerating earlier than immature cells, lymphocytes, and plasma cells. After 15 or more hours from the time of death, cellular damage is so far advanced that aspirated material is practically worthless.

The degenerative change usually is called autolysis of the cells, but this may not be an accurate definition of what happens. For one thing, routine sections of paraffin-embedded marrow do not show much loss of cellular detail even when the tissue is obtained many hours after death. Also, it has been shown that if marrow is suspended in 5% bovine albumin and then smeared, the cells are well preserved and easily identified many hours after death. It would seem, then, that the postmortem change is not a true autolysis, which would be irreversible, but rather an increased fragility of the cytoplasm and possibly of the nucleus as well.

RELATION TO PERIPHERAL BLOOD

The cellular population of the peripheral blood reflects the net of several effects: (1) rate of hemopoiesis in the bone marrow, (2) rate of release of cells from the bone marrow, and (3) rate of survival of cells in the peripheral blood. Hematologic diagnosis is based on making full use of all data that are pertinent to these basic mechanisms.

The hemopoietic activity of the bone marrow can be determined from the cellularity of the tissue sections and from the distribution of cells, according to type and degree of maturation, in the thin smears. One should note that the bone marrow in infants and young children is normally rich in cells and poor in fat, that in normal adults the distribution is half cells and half fat, and that in normal elderly persons the distribution is about one-third cells and two-thirds fat.

The rate of release of blood cells from the bone marrow into the peripheral blood is more difficult to establish. The presence in the blood of immature granulocytes indicates that leukocytic release is normal. Likewise, the presence of reticulocytes in normal number indicates normal release of erythrocytes. When the reticulocyte count is high, we can conclude that more young erythrocytes are being released than normal, and in this case the marrow will show hyperplasia of erythrocyte precursors. In special situations, such as the "aplastic crisis" of hemolytic anemia, the peripheral blood contains no reticulocytes, and we know that either the marrow maturation is arrested or that no new cells are being released. It is not always possible to distinguish maturation arrest from lack of release. In pernicious anemia, for example, the marrow is hyperplastic, but the peripheral blood shows anemia and a low reticulocyte count. It can be shown that in this example the failure is partially in the release mechanism, for the marrow is full of reticulocytes that are not liberated into the blood. When vitamin B_{12} is given, one of the effects is to unblock the release mechanism and induce a shower of reticulocytes into the peripheral blood.

Finally, the rate of survival of erythrocytes can be established accurately by a variety of radioisotope methods; these also detect whether a decreased life span is attributable to an intrinsic defect in the erythrocytes or to extracorpuscular hemolytic mechanisms. Thus hemolytic disease is related to shortened life span of the erythrocytes and can be classified into two major categories, one related to intrinsic abnormality of the erythrocyte (hemoglobinopathy, enzyme deficiency, etc.) and the other to extracorpuscular factors (autoantibodies, isoantibodies, etc.). Life span of platelets is determined with only fair accuracy. Life span of leukocytes has so far defied an exact and direct definition. Unlike the erythrocytes, which once in the peripheral blood do not normally leave it except when they die, leukocytes wander in and out of the blood, spending variable time in organs such as the spleen, liver, and lungs. To further complicate the problem, each type of white blood cell has a cycle and history different from the others.

HYPOPLASIA, APLASIA, AND HYPERPLASIA

The bone marrow can be hypoplastic or aplastic as the result of a variety of toxic and suppressive effects:

1. Bone marrow injury caused by physical or chemical agent
   a. Ionizing radiation
   b. Chemical agents (partial list)
      Aminopyrine
      Arsenicals, organic
      Atabrine
      Benzol
      Bismuth salts
      Chloramphenicol
      Chlorpromazine
      Colchicine
      Dinitrophenol
      Diphenylhydantoin sodium
      Folic acid antagonists
      Gold salts
      Mepazine
      Mercury salts
      Methimazole
      Methylethylphenylhydantoin
      Naphthalene
      Nitrogen mustard and derivatives
      Paraphenylenediamine (hair dyes)
      Perphenazine
      Phenindione

Phenylbutazone
Prochlorperazine
Promazine
Promethazine
Pyrimethamine
Quinacrine
Quinidine
Ristocetin
Sulfonamides
Streptomycin
Stoddard's solvent
Thiouracils
Triflupromazine
Trimethadione
Trinitrotoluene
Tripelennamine HCl
2. Congenital aplastic anemia (Diamond-Blackfan type)
3. Familial aplastic anemia
   a. Associated with developmental anomalies (Fanconi type)
   b. Without developmental anomalies (Estren and Dameshek type)
4. Chronic erythrocytic hypoplasia in adults
5. Aplastic anemia associated with thymoma
6. Metabolic inhibition of bone marrow
   a. Malignancy
   b. Infection
   c. Renal failure
   d. Endocrinopathies
   e. Chronic liver disease

f. Allergy
g. Pancreatic insufficiency
7. Erythroid hypoplasia of bone marrow in hemolytic disease
8. Idiopathic aplastic anemia
9. Aplastic anemia in myeloproliferative disorders (myelophthisic anemia)

Sectioned tissue shows a greatly hypocellular marrow (Fig. 34-57) with a preponderance of fat. The remaining cells are lymphocytes and reticulum cells. When the tissue section shows such a severe degree of hemopoietic failure, one is justified in calling the marrow aplastic. One should note, however, that representative sections from many sites may still fail to reveal some remaining foci of hemopoietic activity, and it is probable that complete aplasia of the entire bone marrow is a very rare occurrence.

Hypoplasia can affect only one or two cell types, particularly when the offending agent is a myelotoxic drug. Such selective hypoplasia is reflected in the peripheral blood by a reduction of the corresponding circulating cells. Thus the peripheral blood may show leukopenia with neutropenia, or thrombocytopenia,

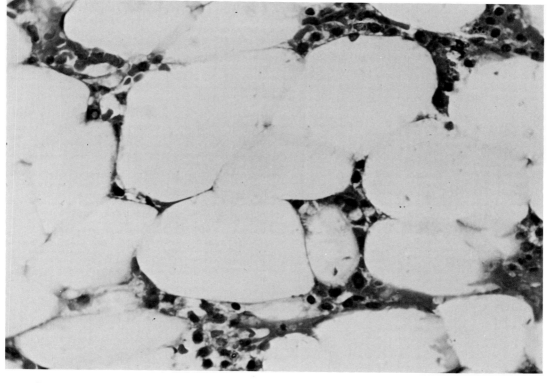

Fig. 34-57. Aplastic bone marrow caused by chloramphenicol. (Hematoxylin and eosin; 125×.)

or anemia, or combinations of these. The term "aplastic anemia" refers specifically to the anemia secondary to bone marrow depression but is sometimes used loosely to refer to aplasia of the marrow and suppression of all cell types in the peripheral blood (pancytopenia). We know, however, that the pancytopenia in some cases is accompanied by hyperplasia of the bone marrow. This anomalous finding is one

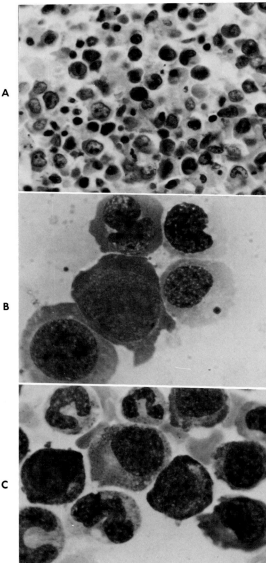

Fig. 34-58. Megaloblastic dyspoiesis in bone marrow. **A,** Paraffin section. **B,** Smear. All cells are megaloblasts. **C,** Smear. Note giant neutrophil metamyelocytes and stab cells. (**A,** Hematoxylin and eosin; 400×; **B** and **C,** Wright's stain; 950×.)

of the situations that brought about a reconsideration of the pathophysiology of the "myeloproliferative syndromes."

Hyperplasia of the bone marrow may be selective or generalized. In most instances, the hyperplasia is the result of a specific stimulation of one type of cell and is therefore selective. In anemia of whatever etiology, there is hyperplasia of erythroid cells to compensate for the anemia.

A special type of erythroid hyperplasia is seen in those anemias caused by a deficiency of folic acid or vitamin B_{12}. Instead of the usual normoblastic maturation, there is a profound abnormality of maturation that affects all cell types, a *dyspoiesis*. The erythroid cells are large and atypical, resembling reticulum cells, and are called megaloblasts (Fig. 34-58, *A* and *B*). There is also abnormal maturation of granulocytes, and the metamyelocytes and bands are two or three times normal size (Fig. 34-58, *C*). Megakaryocytes are even more bizarre than usual. In infectious diseases characterized by leukocytosis, there is granulocytic hyperplasia. Hyperplasia of all cell types usually is seen in the myeloproliferative syndromes, although even in these, one series may be more hyperplastic than the others.

MYELOPROLIFERATIVE SYNDROMES

The concept of the "myeloproliferative syndromes" was expressed by Dameshek,[25] who speculated on the possibility of a common etiologic agent for myelocytic leukemia, polycythemia vera, agnogenic myeloid metaplasia, thrombocythemia, megakaryocytic leukemia, and erythroleukemia. His suggestion that these diseases have a common myeloproliferative stimulus, hormonal or steroid, remains only a speculation and, in fact, an unlikely possibility. However, the concept that apparently dissimilar diseases are related insofar as each is a manifestation of abnormal hemopoietic proliferation has deepened our understanding of the clinical and hematologic findings.

Previously, pathologists and hematologists had focused attention on criteria to distinguish among and identify diseases showing in various combinations features such as (1) leukocytosis or leukopenia with immature cells (myeloid or erythroid) in the peripheral blood, (2) bone marrow that might be aplastic, sclerotic, hyperplastic, infiltrated with tumor cells, or normal, (3) various degrees of splenomegaly and hepatomegaly, (4) anemia, and (5) polycythemia. The question of leukemia versus a benign process was always a serious concern.

The terms to be found in the literature for the various "diseases" showing one or several of these abnormalities reflect the most striking presenting finding and the principal concern of the investigator with the "atypical" nature of these diseases. These may be grouped as follows:

Differentiation from leukemia
    Pseudoleukemia
    Aleukemic myelosis
    Chronic nonleukemic myelosis
    Atypical myelosis
    Megakaryocytic myelosis
    Aleukemic megakaryocytic myelosis
    Myeloid megakaryocytic myelosis
Splenomegaly and hepatomegaly
    Agnogenic myeloid metaplasia of spleen
    Splenomegaly with myeloid transformation
    Splenomegaly with sclerosis of bone marrow
    Splenomegaly with anemia
    Myelophthisic splenomegaly
    Splenomegaly with anemia and myelemia
    Myeloid splenomegaly without myelocythemia
    Aleukemic hepatosplenic myelosis
    Myeloid megakaryocytic hepatosplenomegaly
Abnormalities in peripheral blood
    Leukanemia
    Myeloid splenic anemia
    Leukoerythroblastic anemia
    Leukoerythroblastosis
    Osteosclerotic anemia
    Polycythemia vera
    Thrombocythemia
    Leukemoid reaction
    Pancytopenia
    Erythroleukemia
    Erythremic myelosis
    Di Guglielmo's disease
Abnormalities in bone marrow
    Myelosclerosis
    Myelofibrosis
    Osteosclerosis
    Atypical aplastic anemia
    Myelophthisic anemia
    Myelopathic anemia
    Panmyelophthisis

This impressive list could be extended into a meaningless triumph of descriptive pathology by combining several of the features of a given disease. In any case, there is implicit in any list of "diseases" or "syndromes" the supposition that each disease can be characterized by a set of features that distinguish it from the others. Experience has shown that this usually is impossible. The final blow to the concept of individual and characteristic diseases is dealt by the realization that, when one has the opportunity to follow the course of these patients over a period of time, the disease often progresses through a series of clinical and morphologic variants. At any given time, the diagnostic term that is applicable may well be different from that used a year previously or a year hence (Figs. 34-59 to 34-62).

What, then, is the common denominator and how does one face the problem of diagnosis?

We have postulated that a proliferation-inducing stimulus (or stimuli with selective effects) acts on undifferentiated mesenchymal cells and their immediate derivatives to produce medullary and extramedullary hemopoietic and connective tissue proliferation (Fig. 34-63). Proliferation and differentiation along one or several lines would account for the many variants observed, the changing patterns as the disease progresses, and the concomitant occurrence of fibrosis and hemopoietic proliferation. This last is, in my opinion, a strong point in favor of the hypothesis. Otherwise, how can we explain the simultaneous proliferation of connective tissue and blood cells in the bone marrow in acute leukemia. Support for the hypothesis also can be derived from noncontroversial reactions that are accepted by all. For example, when the stimulus is of known infectious origin, stimulation of the marrow may result in such a striking increase in the number of circulating leukocytes, and a shift toward immature forms as well, as to mimic leukemia (hence, *leukemoid* reaction). In chronic myelocytic leukemia we have an example of involvement of more than one cell type at the same time: granulocytes (leukocytosis) and platelets (thrombocytosis). We know also that hypoxia, as from a prolonged sojourn at high altitudes, cyanotic heart disease, etc., is a specific stimulus for proliferation of erythroid cells with resultant secondary polycythemia.

The splenomegaly and hepatomegaly seen so frequently in the myeloproliferative disorders are not "compensatory," as is sometimes said. If this were the case, then massive splenomegaly and hepatomegaly should be seen in cases of complete marrow aplasia, as in chloramphenicol toxicity. In fact, extramedullary hemopoiesis does not occur in such cases. Rather, hepatosplenomegaly (extramedullary hemopoiesis also may occur in other tissues) reflects the stimulation of primitive mesenchymal cells dormant in the adult organ (p. 1486). One should note that in rare cases, the spleen is not enlarged, even though all the histologic features of extramedullary hemopoiesis are present (Fig. 34-59).

We might speculate a little on the nature of the proliferation-inducing stimulus or stimuli. Many of the myeloproliferative syndromes

Text continued on p. 1562.

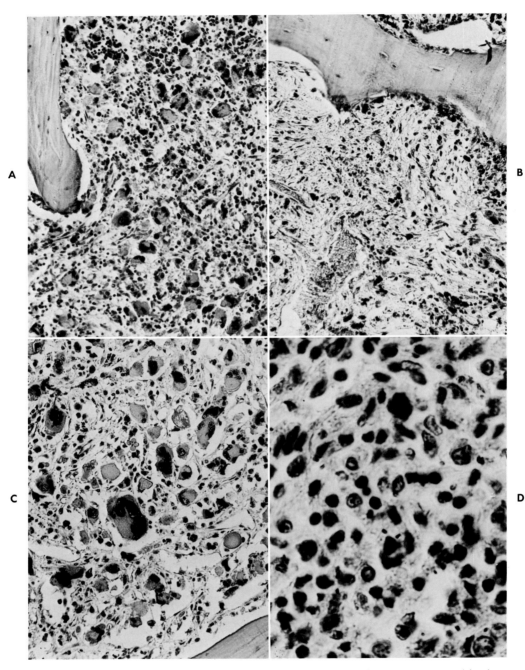

Fig. 34-59. Myelosclerosis with megakaryocytic myelosis of spleen in 61-year-old white man. Onset occurred 6 months before death, with pancytopenia, fatigue, and weight loss. There was progressive pancytopenia, and death was attributed to thrombocytopenia and hemorrhage. Bone marrow was fibrotic, with striking megakaryocytic proliferation. Spleen was small, weighing 60 gm, but showed striking megakaryocytic myelosis. **A** to **C,** Bone marrow. **D,** Spleen. (**A** to **D,** Hematoxylin and eosin; **A** and **B,** 130×; **C,** 350×; **D,** 585×.)

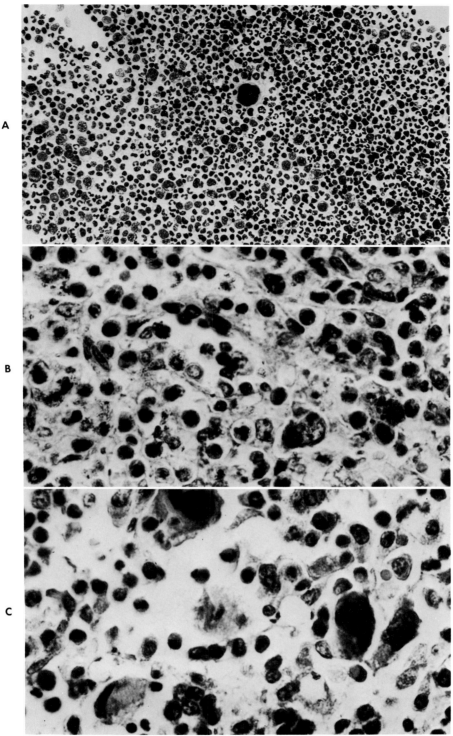

Fig. 34-60. Leukemoid reaction with hepatosplenomegaly and megakaryocytic myelosis of spleen in 71-year-old white man. Patient admitted to hospital because of mental confusion and leukocytosis 1 year before death. Leukocyte count at admission was 74,000 per cubic millimeter, and there was shift to left with immature granulocytes. Bone marrow during life was hyperplastic. There was striking splenomegaly. Necropsy revealed glioblastoma multiforme of right frontal lobe, splenomegaly (960 gm), and cardiac failure. **A,** Antemortem bone marrow aspiration. **B** and **C,** Paraffin sections of spleen. (**A,** Wright's stain; 130×; **B** and **C,** hematoxylin and eosin; **B,** 450×; **C,** 585×.)

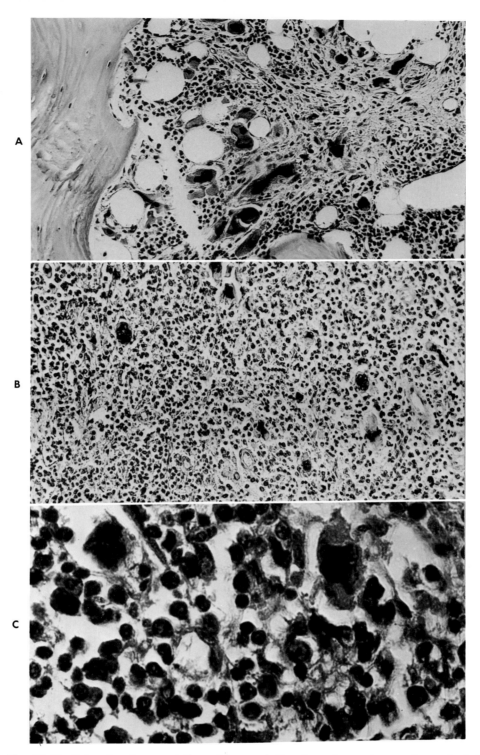

Fig. 34-61. Polycythemia vera followed by myelofibrosis and megakaryocytic myelosis in 77-year-old white man. Diagnosis of polycythemia vera was established 7 years before death and patient treated with ^{32}P. Five years later, white blood cell count rose to 45,000 per cubic millimeter and peripheral blood picture was leukemoid. One year later, peripheral blood picture changed again to leukoerythroblastic form with many immature leukocytes and 17% normoblasts. During last year of life, patient developed progressive anemia characterized by sharply decreased ^{51}Cr-erythrocyte survival. Splenectomy was performed. Death occurred postoperatively. **A,** Postmortem bone marrow. **B** and **C,** Antemortem spleen. (**A** to **C,** Hematoxylin and eosin; **A** and **B,** 130×; **C,** 585×.)

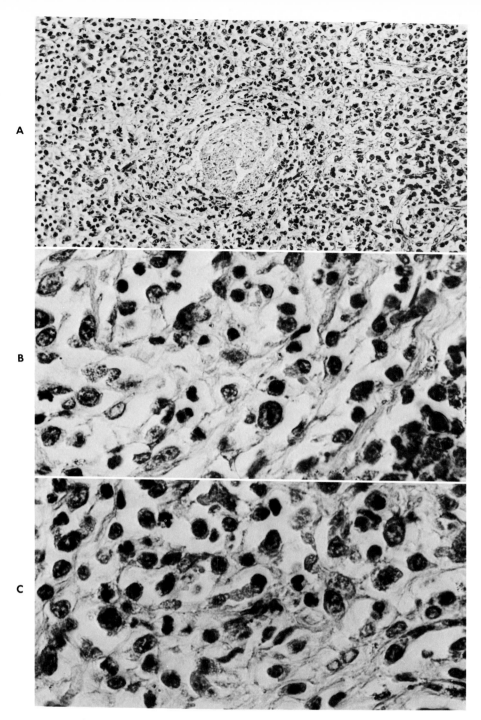

Fig. 34-62. Chronic myelocytic leukemia (?) with hypersplenism in 38-year-old white man. There was 11-year history of leukocytosis before gastrectomy for peptic ulcer. At operation, spleen found to be moderately enlarged but was not removed. White cell count at that time was 49,700. Differential count showed 2% blasts, 24.5% myelocytes, 13% meta-myelocytes, 40% segmented neutrophils, and 2% normoblasts. One year before death (4 years after gastrectomy), patient treated with cobalt irradiation, following which he developed pancytopenia. Simultaneously, there was sudden enlargement of spleen. Al-though leukopenic, differential count on peripheral blood showed 20% blasts. ^{51}Cr-erythrocyte survival was very short (half-life of 7 days). Splenectomy was performed. Death occurred from staphylococcus septicemia. Spleen weighed 3300 gm (normal spleen weight is 150 gm). Necropsy did not reveal typical histopathologic lesions of leukemia. **A** to **C**, Spleen. Note siderosis in **B** and **C**. (**A** to **C**, Hematoxylin and eosin; **A**, 130×; **B** and **C**, 585×.)

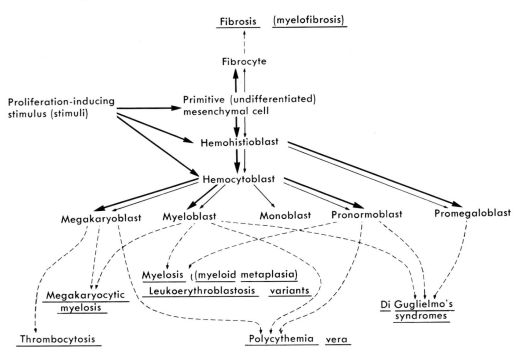

Fig. 34-63. Hypothesis that fundamental proliferation-inducing stimulus acts first on undifferentiated mesenchymal cells and, through these, to other cell lines to produce various myeloproliferative syndromes. (From Miale, J. B.: Laboratory medicine—hematology, St. Louis, 1972, The C. V. Mosby Co.)

mimic leukemia, and, in fact, many have a terminal leukemic phase. In experimental animals, variants of leukemogenic viruses produce nonleukemic myeloproliferative disease. If human leukemia is caused by viruses as many believe, then it is tempting to postulate that, at least in some of the myeloproliferative syndromes, we see either an attenuated viral stimulus or an altered host response to a leukemogenic virus.

LEUKEMIA

Leukemia is a neoplastic disease characterized by the proliferation of hemopoietic cells in the bone marrow and other organs. By definition, the term leukemia refers to the appearance of these cells in the peripheral blood. The disease is uniformly fatal. There are some very few cases on record of suppressed spontaneous cure. Most of these can be attributed to the original diagnosis being in error. Since spontaneous cures of other malignant tumors have been seen, we can accept that one or two cases of leukemia (usually chronic lymphocytic) may fall into this category.

Incidence

The incidence of leukemia has shown a steady increase during the past 40 years (Fig. 34-64). In the United States, the mortality from leukemia has risen from 3.9 per 100,000 in 1940 to 6.5 per 100,000 in 1954 and to 8 per 100,000 in 1964. An upward trend is seen in other countries as well. Perhaps a portion of the increase can be ascribed to better diagnosis but, even when allowance is made for this and other factors, there remains what appears to be a true increase in incidence. There has been a proportionately greater increase in incidence in the older age groups. Only a small fraction of this can be ascribed to greater longevity. The remarkable figures for improved longevity given by the biostatisticians reflect almost entirely improved neonatal and childhood survival, and the life expectancy for the middle-aged has improved only a little. In any case, if the incidence of all leukemias is plotted according to age (Fig. 34-65), two peaks are noted: one between the third and fourth year and one between the ages of 70 and 80 years. In the older age group, the incidence in men is significantly

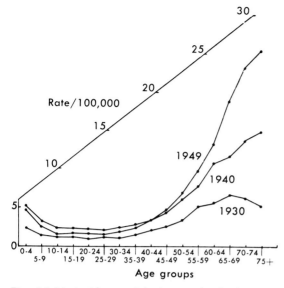

Fig. 34-64. Incidence of leukemia deaths by age in 1930, 1940, and 1949. (From Cooke, J. V.: Blood **9:**340-347, 1954; by permission.)

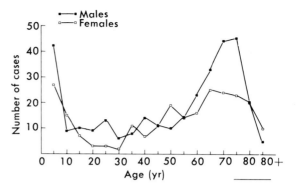

Fig. 34-65. Age and distribution of 553 cases of leukemia. Data from Gunz, F. W., and Hough, R. F.: Blood **11:**882-901, 1956; from Miale, J. B.: Laboratory medicine—hematology, St. Louis, 1972, The C. V. Mosby Co.)

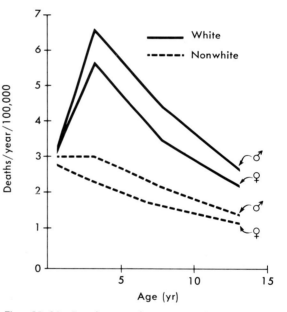

Fig. 31-66. Death rate from acute leukemia in white and black children, 1950-1959. (Data from Ederer, F., Miller, R. W., and Scotto, J.: J.A.M.A. **192:**593-596, 1965; from Miale, J. B.: Laboratory medicine—hematology, St. Louis, 1972, The C. V. Mosby Co.)

higher than in women. In the younger age group, the incidence in white children is significantly greater than in black children (Fig. 34-66).

Although any type of leukemia can occur at any age, a consistent pattern is found in most large series. Acute leukemia is more common than chronic leukemia at all ages and is most frequent in children and in elderly persons. Chronic myelocytic leukemia is rare in childhood, becoming increasingly more frequent in older age groups. Chronic lymphocytic leukemia is rare before the age of 35 years but is the most common type in elderly individuals. The overall distribution by type in the United States is as follows: chronic lymphocytic, 25%; chronic myelocytic, 22%; chronic myelomonocytic, 3%; acute lymphocytic, 20%; acute myelocytic, 20%; and acute myelomonocytic leukemia, 10%. Chronic lymphocytic leukemia is rare in China, Japan, and India. In children, almost all leukemias are acute lymphocytic (225 of 258 cases, with 13 acute myelocytic, 13 acute monocytic, 4 blast cell, and 3 chronic myelocytic leukemia).

Etiology and epidemiology

The etiology of leukemia is not known. There are four partially overlapping approaches to the investigation of etiology: epidemiologic, the leukemogenic effect of ionizing radiation, the role of viruses, and the genetic (chromosomal) determinants.

Epidemiology. The epidemiology of leukemia shows some interesting but unexplained features. We know that there are some true differences in incidence among special groups:

1. The incidence in black children is lower than in whites and does not peak at 3 to 4 years of age.
2. The incidence of leukemia in Japan is about half of that in the United States, partly because of a lower incidence in

middle-aged persons and partly because of the rarity of chronic lymphocytic leukemia in older Japanese.

3. African children have the lowest incidence of leukemia, even though the incidence of Burkitt's lymphoma is high.

4. There are occasional families with a high incidence of leukemia; it is noteworthy however that in these families the leukemia is sometimes of the same type (chronic lymphocytic) and sometimes of different types (the next most frequent association is chronic lymphocytic and chronic myelocytic leukemia).

5. The incidence of leukemia in both identical and nonidentical twins may be higher than in only one of the twins.

Leukemogenic effect of ionizing radiation. There is no longer doubt that ionizing radiation is leukemogenic. Among survivors of the atomic explosion over Hiroshima, the first cases of leukemia appeared 18 months later and the peak incidence ocurred 5 years later. The highest incidence was in those receiving the greatest dose of radiation. Of great interest is the finding that, in line with the low incidence of chronic lymphocytic leukemia in the Japanese, no case of chronic lymphocytic leukemia developed in the survivors. Therapeutic and diagnostic x radiation also can be leukemogenic. The mechanism by which irradiation induces leukemia is not known.

Role of viruses. The induction by viruses of leukemia in fowls has been studied for over a half century. Gross[48] showed that mouse leukemia can be transmitted to newborn mice by cell-free filtrates. A viral etiology for human leukemia remains a likely possibility, but as yet no proof has been forthcoming. Direct transfusion of leukemic blood into normal recipients does not transmit leukemia. If a viral etiology is operative in human leukemia, one must suppose that there are other interacting factors such as genetic predisposition, ionizing radiation, and the latency of the virus until activated by intrinsic or extrinsic factors.

Chromosomal abnormalities. The association of chromosomal abnormalities with leukemia is well established. The most constant and characteristic change involves chromosome 21. In chronic myelocytic leukemia, a characteristic small chromosome, called the Philadelphia or Ph[1] chromosome (Fig. 34-67) is formed by deletion or translocation of portions of the normal 21 chromosome. This abnormal chromosome is not found in normal persons or in those with nonleukemic myeloproliferative syndromes. Some cases of chronic myelocytic leukemia without the Ph[1] chromosome also have been found. The high incidence of leukemia in mongoloids (17 times greater than in normal children) also suggests that abnormalities of chromosome 21 (mongoloids have trisomy 21) is related to the development of leukemia.

Classification

Leukemia is classified according to (1) clinical duration of the disease, (2) cell type in the blood and bone marrow, and (3) leukocyte count in the peripheral blood.

On the basis of duration, *acute* leukemia has a short life expectancy (12 months or more). The term *subacute* is used by some for cases of intermediate duration and by others for cases in transition between chronic and acute. The use of chemotherapy and improved supportive therapy makes this clinical classification a retrospective one.

Classification of leukemia on the basis of cell type is as follows:

1. Blast cell leukemia (acute)*
2. Lymphocytic leukemia
3. Myelocytic leukemia†
4. Monocytic leukemia
   a. Myelomonocytic (Naegeli type)‡
   b. Histiocytic (Schilling type)
5. Plasmacytic leukemia and multiple myeloma
6. Erythroleukemia
7. Mast cell leukemia

Generally the more immature the cells, the more acute the clinical course.

On the basis of the leukocyte count in the peripheral blood, leukemia is classified as *leukemic* (high leukocyte count), *subleukemic* (low leukocyte count but abnormal cells present), and *aleukemic* (low leukocyte count with no abnormal cells). It is improbable that truly aleukemic cases exist. Abnormal cells usually can be found if smears of the buffy coat of centrifuged blood are examined.

Acute leukemia

Morphologically, acute leukemia is characterized by the preponderance of immature cells classified as blasts (Fig. 34-68). These may belong to one or another of the cell types and

---

*Predominant cell is a blast that cannot be otherwise identified at the time; "stem cell leukemia."
†Includes neutrophilic, eosinophilic, and basophilic types that are variants and need not be classified separately.
‡Some classify this under myelocytic leukemia.

therefore can be subclassified as acute lymphocytic leukemia, acute myelocytic leukemia, etc. Sometimes the cells are so immature that they cannot be classified, and then the term "stem cell" leukemia is applied. In most cases, however, cell identification is possible on morphologic grounds or from the presence of other more mature cells.

Clinically, the onset is characterized by one or several of the following: pallor, fever, purpura, malaise, bone pain, splenomegaly, lymphadenopathy, and central nervous system involvement. Lymphadenopathy is common in acute lymphocytic leukemia and uncommon in acute myelocytic leukemia. Splenomegaly may be present in any type but is most common in acute lymphocytic leukemia.

The leukocyte count is moderately or strikingly elevated, and thrombocytopenia is common. Anemia is sometimes severe. When the leukocyte count is not elevated, the onset may mimic idiopathic thrombocytopenia purpura or aplastic anemia.

Chronic myelocytic leukemia

Most cases of chronic myelocytic leukemia occur in adults. Splenomegaly, sometimes with the spleen so large as to seemingly fill the abdomen, is the most striking clinical finding. Lymphadenopathy is rare.

The leukocyte count usually is very high, and the differential count shows many immature granulocytes (metamyelocytes, myelocytes, and progranulocytes) and only a slight increase in myeloblasts. Characteristically

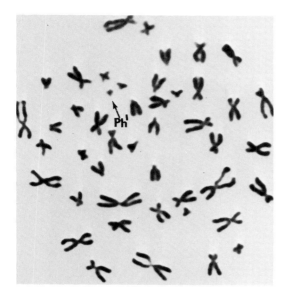

Fig. 34-67. Philadelphia chromosome (Ph¹). Metaphase of diploid marrow cell in chronic myelocytic leukemia. (Courtesy Dr. Jacqueline Whang and Dr. J. H. Tjio, Bethesda, Md.)

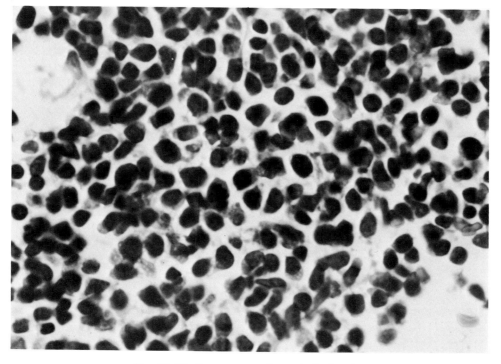

Fig. 34-68. Bone marrow in acute leukemia.

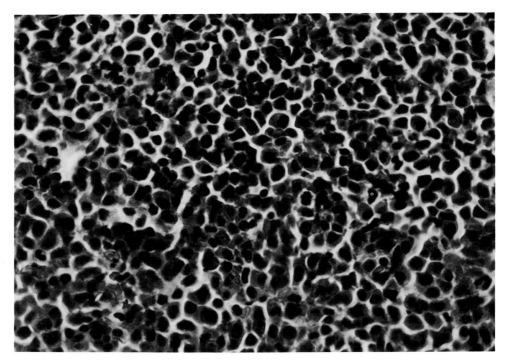

Fig. 34-69. Bone marrow in chronic myelocytic leukemia.

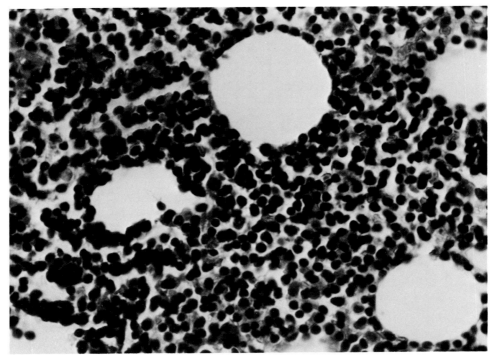

Fig. 34-70. Bone marrow in chronic lymphocytic leukemia.

many basophils are present, but this also may be seen in myeloproliferative syndromes. The leukocytes show reduced alkaline phosphatase activity. In myeloproliferative syndromes, alkaline phosphatase is high except when in transition to the leukemic phase. Thrombocytosis is common. The bone marrow is hypercellular and contains a preponderance of myeloid cells (Fig. 34-69).

Chronic lymphocytic leukemia

Chronic lymphocytic leukemia is usually so benign as to raise the question of whether it is a true leukemia. It is often discovered when a routine blood count is done in a person who is asymptomatic. Sometimes, usually late in the disease, there is lymphadenopathy and splenomegaly. Death is quite often the result of some other disease.

The leukocyte count in the peripheral blood is moderately to strikingly elevated—from 40,000 to several hundred thousand per cubic millimeter. The differential count shows a preponderance of small lymphocytes. Characteristically, there are many "smudge" or degenerated cells. Anemia is not common and, when present, is of the acquired autoimmune type. The bone marrow shows solid sheets of small lymphocytes as the predominant cell (Fig. 34-70). The histopathology of the lymph nodes is that of a diffuse well-differentiated lymphocytic lymphoma.

Monocytic leukemias

Monocytic leukemia occurs in two basically unrelated forms. The more common, myelomonocytic leukemia (Naegeli type) is believed by some to be a variant of myelocytic leukemia, but we believe it to be a morphologic and clinical entity. Morphologically, the myelocytes and progranulocytes show a delicate, folded nucleus unlike that of a typical myeloid cell. The granules in the cytoplasm are not unusual. True *monocytic* leukemia or *histiocytic* leukemia (Schilling type) is very rare. The cells have a true monocytic nucleus, and the granules in the cytoplasm are of the pink monocytic type.

Mast cell leukemia

Mast cell leukemia is the rarest of the leukemias and was described relatively recently. The leukemic cell is the tissue mast cell, and the release of histamine from these cells gives symptoms of flushing, palpitation, nausea, vomiting, and diarrhea. The clinical course is acute.

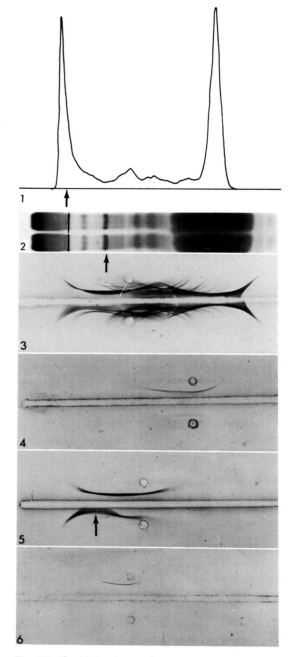

Fig. 34-71. Multiple myeloma. **1,** Electrophoretic pattern showing abnormal gamma peak (*arrow*). **2,** Starch gel electrophoresis showing abnormal gamma band (*arrow*). **3** to **6,** Immunoelectrophoresis: control subject, *top;* patient, *bottom.* **3,** Polyvalent antiserum showing abnormal gamma components. **4,** Anti-IgA serum showing reduction of IgA. **5,** Anti-IgG serum showing abnormal and increased IgG component (*arrow*). **6,** Anti-IgM serum showing decreased IgM. (From Miale, J. B.: Laboratory medicine—hematology, St. Louis, 1972, The C. V. Mosby Co.)

MULTIPLE MYELOMA

Myelomas are neoplasms of proliferating plasma cells. They may present as solitary tumors involving bone or other tissues, the *solitary myeloma,* or as neoplasms involving the bone marrow and other organs, *multiple myeloma.* Solitary myeloma may remain localized or may change into multiple myeloma. Multiple myeloma may show a terminal leukemic phase, *plasma cell leukemia.* Multiple myeloma can be classified either as a leukemia or a lymphoma (see also p. 1526).

Proliferation of plasma cells at extramedullary sites accounts for splenomegaly (present in about 10% of the patients) and hepatomegaly (present in about 30% of the patients). Hyperproteinemia accounts for the characteristic renal lesion, the *myeloma kidney,* consisting of tubular degeneration with proteinaceous casts. Atypical amyloid deposits (paramyloidosis) are formed by a combination of protein and polysaccharide. Proliferation of plasma cells in the bone marrow produces destruction of cortical bone. This results in pain, swelling, deformity, or pathologic fracture. Roentgenographic evidence of bone destruction can be found in about 80% of the patients, with the ribs, sternum, and vertebral bodies being involved most commonly.

Abnormal protein metabolism is characteristic of multiple myeloma. The laboratory evidence for protein abnormalities is one or more of the following:

1. Hyperproteinemia
2. Hyperglobulinemia
3. Electrophoretic evidence of an abnormal protein component in the serum
4. Bence Jones protein in the urine
5. Electrophoretic evidence of an abnormal globulin component in the urine with or without Bence Jones protein
6. Cryoglobulinemia
7. Pyroglobulinemia
8. Macroglobulinemia
9. Identification and quantitation of the excess globulin by immunoelectrophoresis (Fig. 34-71)

Multiple myeloma is one of the diseases having an abnormal globulin component that, because of its relation to antibody globulin, now falls into the group called *immunoglobulins.* In addition to myeloma, there are other diseases (Waldenström's macroglobulinemia is one) in which there is an immunoglobulin

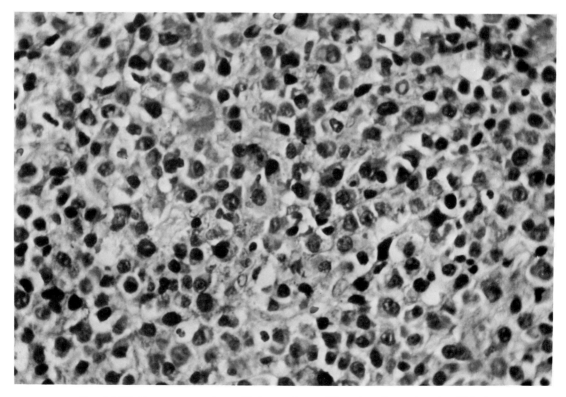

Fig. 34-72. Bone marrow in multiple myeloma. (Hematoxylin and eosin; 250×.)

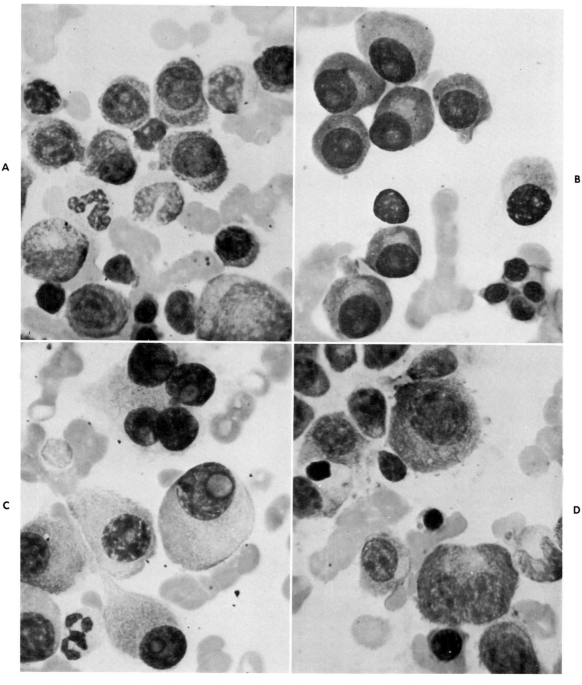

Fig. 34-73. Different degrees of maturity of plasma cells in multiple myeloma. Bone marrow smears. **A,** Most mature. **D,** Least mature. (**A** to **D,** Wright's stain; 950×; from Miale, J. B.: Laboratory medicine—hematology, St. Louis, 1972, The C. V. Mosby Co.)

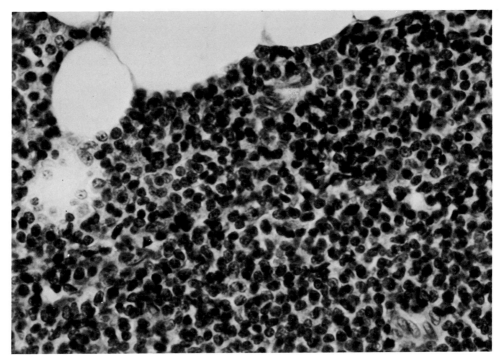

Fig. 34-74. Bone marrow infiltrated by malignant lymphoma, intermediate cell type. (Hematoxlin and eosin; 250×.)

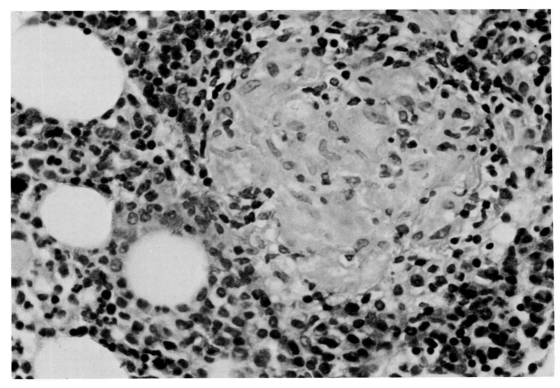

Fig. 34-75. Bone marrow in sarcoid granuloma. (Hematoxylin and eosin; 250×.)

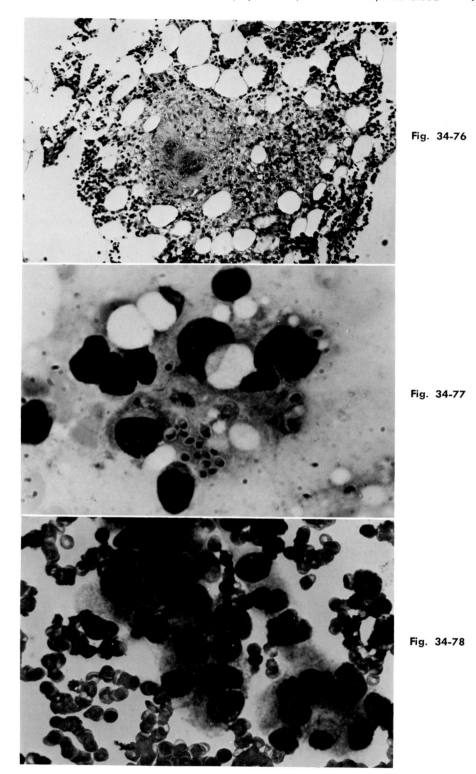

Fig. 34-76

Fig. 34-77

Fig. 34-78

Fig. 34-76. Bone marrow in miliary tuberculosis. (Hematoxylin and eosin; 120×.)
Fig. 34-77. Bone marrow in histoplasmosis. Smear. (Wright's stain; 950×.)
Fig. 34-78. Bone marrow in metastatic carcinoma of prostate. Smear. (Wright's stain; 950×.)

abnormality. There are now five known classes of immunoglobulins: IgG, IgA, IgM, IgD, and IgE. Most commonly, multiple myeloma shows an increase in IgA or IgG, but other types have been described. Rarely, in about 1% of all patients with myelomas, there is no demonstrable immunoglobulin increase in either the serum or the urine.

Morphologically, from aspiration biopsy of the bone marrow, spleen, or a lesion identified by roentgenography, the diagnosis is made on the basis of the tissue being infiltrated by plasma cells (Fig. 34-72). These are sometimes essentially normal in appearance. Sometimes they are immature (plasmablasts) and, characteristically, have a very large pale-staining nucleolus (Fig. 34-73).

MISCELLANEOUS ABNORMALITIES

Tissue from the bone marrow may show a number of other abnormalities. These include involvement by lymphomas (Fig. 34-74), sarcoidosis (Fig. 34-75), tuberculosis (Fig. 34-76), histoplasmosis (Fig. 34-77), and metastatic tumor (Fig. 34-78). Since the morphology of these lesions is not different from that in other tissues, they are not discussed further.

REFERENCES

1 Aisenberg, A. C.: J.A.M.A. **222**:1301-1302, 1972.
2 Arseneau, J. E., Canellos, G. P., Banks, P. M., et al.: Am. J. Med. **58**:314-321, 1975.
3 Aschoff, L.: Ergeb. Inn. Med. Kinderheilkd. **26**:1, 1924.
4 Aschoff, L., and Kiyono: Folia Haematol. **15**:385-390, 1913.
5 Askanazy, M.: In Henke, F., and Lubarsch, O., editors: Handbuch der speziellen pathologischen Anatomie und Histologie, Berlin, 1927, Julius Springer Verlag, vol. 1.
6 Baehr, G., and Klemperer, P.: N.Y. State J. Med. **40**:7-11, 1940.
7 Banks, P. M., Arseneau, J. E., Gralnick, H. R., et al.: Am. J. Med. **58**:322-329, 1975.
8 Barrow, M. V., and Holubar, K.: Medicine **48**:287, 1969.
9 Baumgartner, L.: Yale J. Biol. Med. **6**:403-434, 1934.
10 Bennett, M. H., Farrer-Brown, G., Henry, K., and Jelliffe, A. M.: Lancet **2**:405-406, 1974.
11 Berard, C., O'Connor, G. T., Thomas, L. B., and Torloni, H.: Bull. WHO **40**:601-607, 1969.
12 Bernhard, W., and Leplus, R.: Fine structure of the normal and malignant human lymph node, New York, 1964, The Macmillan Co.
13 Blaustein, A.: The spleen, New York, 1963, The McGraw-Hill Book Co.
14 Brady, R. O., and King, F. M.: Gaucher's disease. In Hers, H. G., and Van Hoof, F., editors: Lysosomes and storage diseases, New York, 1973, Academic Press, Inc., pp. 381-394.
15 Brady, R. O., Kanfer, J. N., Bradley, R. M.,

and Shapiro, D.: J. Clin. Invest. **45**:1112-1115, 1966.
16 Brewster, D. C.: Am. J. Surg. **126**:14-19, 1973.
17 Brill, N. E., Baehr, G., and Rosenthal, N.: J.A.M.A. **84**:668-671, 1925.
18 Burke, J. S., Byrne, G. E., Jr., and Rappaport, H.: Cancer **33**:1399-1410, 1974.
19 Burkitt, D.: Br. J. Surg. **46**:218-223, 1958.
20 Byrne, G. E., Jr., and Rappaport, H.: Malignant histiocytosis. In Akazaki, K., Rappaport, H., Berard, C. W., Bennett, J. M., and Ishikawa, E., editors: Malignant disease of the hematopoietic system, Gann Monogr. Cancer Res., no. 15, pp. 145-162, 1973, University of Tokyo Press.
21 Carbone, P. P., Kaplan, H. S., Musshoff, K., Smithers, D. W., and Tubiana, T.: Cancer Res. **31**:1860-1861, 1971.
22 Catovsky, D., Petit, J. E., Galetto, J., Okos, A., and Galton, D. A. G.: Br. J. Haematol. **26**:29-37, 1974.
23 Clark, B. S., and Dawson, P. J.: Am. J. Med. **47**:314-317, 1969.
24 Cook, J. V.: Blood **9**:340-347, 1954.
25 Dameshek, W.: Blood **6**:372-375, 1951.
26 Davies, D. J., and Stansfeld, A. G.: J. Clin. Pathol. **25**:689-696, 1972.
27 Davies, J. N. P., and Lothe, F.: Kaposi's sarcoma in African children. In Ackerman, L. V., and Murray, J. F., editors: Symposium on Kaposi's sarcoma, Basel, 1963, S. Karger AG, pp. 81-86.
28 Donaldson, V. H.: J. Exp. Med. **127**:411-429, 1968.
29 Dorfman, R. F.: Lancet **6**:1295-1296, 1974.
30 Dorfman, R. F., and Remington, J. S.: New Eng. J. Med. **289**:878-881, 1973.
31 Dorfman, R. F., and Warnke, R.: Hum. Pathol. **5**:519-550, 1974.
32 Duhamel, G.: Acta Haematol. **45**:89-98, 1971.
33 Edelson, R. L., Smith, R. W., Frank, M. M., and Green, I.: J. Invest. Dermatol. **61**:82-89, 1973.
34 Ederer, F., Miller, R. W., and Scotto, J.: J.A.M.A. **192**:593-596, 1965.
35 Ellis, R. E.: Phys. Med. Biol. **5**:255-258, 1961.
36 Ellman, L. L., and Block, K. J.: New Eng. J. Med. **278**:1195-1201, 1968.
37 Fayemi, A. O., and Toker, C.: Arch. Pathol. **99**:170-172, 1975.
38 Flandrin, G., Daniel, M. T., Foucarde, M., and Chelloul, N.: Nouv. Rev. Fr. Hematol. **13**:609-640, 1973.
39 Flandrin, G., and Ripault, J.: Actualités hématologiques, ser. 3, pp. 18-29, Paris, 1969, Masson & Cie.
40 Forte, F. A., Prelli, F., Yount, W. J., et al.: Blood **36**:137-144, 1970.
41 Frangione, B., and Franklin, E. C.: Semin. Hematol. **10**:53-64, 1973.
42 Fredrickson, D. S., and Sloan, H. R.: Sphingomyelin lipidoses: Niemann-Pick disease. In Stanbury, J. B., Wyngaarden, J. B., and Fredrickson, D. S., editors: The metabolic basis of inherited disease, ed. 3, New York, 1972, McGraw-Hill Book Co., pp. 783-807.
43 Frizzera, G., Moran, E. M., and Rappaport, H.: Lancet **1**:1070-1073, 1974.

44 Gall, E. A.: Ann. N.Y. Acad. Sci. **73**:120-130, 1958.

45 Gerard-Marchant, R., Hamlin, I., Lennert, K., et al.: Lancet **2**:406-408, 1974.

46 Goldberg, G. M.: Lab. Invest. **6**:383-388, 1957.

47 Gordon, A. S., Handler, E. S., Siegel, C. D., Dornfest, B. S., and LoBue, J.: Ann. N.Y. Acad. Sci. **113**:766-789, 1964.

48 Gross, L.: Proc. Soc. Exp. Biol. Med. **76**:27-32, 1951.

49 Gunz, F. W., and Hough, R. F.: Blood **11**:882-901, 1972.

50 Haferkamp, O., Rosenau, W., and Lennert, K.: Arch. Pathol. **92**:81-83, 1971.

51 Halpert, B., and Györkey, F.: Am. J. Clin. Pathol. **32**:165-168, 1959.

52 Hansen, J. A., and Good, R. A.: Hum. Pathol. **5**:567-593, 1974.

53 Hartroft, W. S., and Porta, E. A.: Am. J. Med. Sci. **250**:324-345, 1965.

54 Hartsock, R. J.: Cancer **21**:632-649, 1968.

55 Henle, W., Henle, G. E., and Horowitz, C. A.: Hum. Pathol. **5**:551-565, 1974.

56 Hyman, G. A., and Sommers, C.: Blood **28**:416-427, 1966.

57 Jackson, H., and Parker, F.: Hodgkin's disease and allied disorders, New York, 1947, Oxford University Press, pp. 3-11.

58 Jacoben, C. D., Gjone, E., and Hovig, T.: Scand. J. Haematol. **9**:106-113, 1972.

59 Jaffe, E. S., Shevach, E. M., Frank, M. M., and Green, I.: Am. J. Med. **57**:108-114, 1974.

60 Jones, S. E., Fuks, Z., Bull, M., et al.: Cancer **31**:806-823, 1973.

61 Kadin, M. D., Donaldson, S. S., and Dorfman, R. F.: New Eng. J. Med. **283**:859-861, 1970.

62 Kaplan, J., Mastrangel, R., and Peterson, W. D.: Cancer Res. **34**:521-525, 1974.

63 Katayama, I., Nagy, G. K., and Balogh, K., Jr.: Cancer **32**:843-846, 1973.

64 Keller, A. R., Kaplan, H. S., Lukes, R. J., and Rappaport, H.: Cancer **22**:487-499, 1968.

64a Keller, A. R., Hochholzen, L., and Castleman, B.: Cancer **29**:670-683, 1972.

65 King, J. T., Puchtler, H., and Sweat, F.: Arch. Pathol. **85**:237-245, 1968.

66 Knisely, M. H.: Anat. Rec. **65**:23-50, 1936.

67 Knutti, R. E., and Hawkins, W. B.: J. Exp. Med. **61**:115-125, 1935.

68 Kundrat, H.: Wien. Klin. Wochenschr. **6**:211-216, 1893.

69 Langevoort, H. L., Cohn, Z. A., Hirsch, J. G., Humphrey, J. H., Spector, W. G., and van Furth, R.: The nomenclature of phagocytic cells. In van Furth, R., editor: Mononuclear phagocytes, Oxford, 1970, Blackwell Scientific Publications.

70 Lee, R. E., and Ellis, L. D.: Lab. Invest. **24**:261-264, 1971.

71 Lee, S. L., Rosner, F., Ruberman, W., and Glasberg, S.: Ann. Intern. Med. **75**:407-414, 1971.

72 Lennert, K.: In Uehlinger, E., editor: Handbuch der speziellen pathologischen Anatomie und Histologie, 1961, Heidelberg, Springer Verlag, pp. 206-248.

73 Lennert, K.: Follicular lymphoma—a tumor of the germinal centers. In Akazaki, K., Rappaport, H., Berard, C. W., Bennett, J. M., and

Ishikawa, E., editors: Malignant diseases of the hematopoietic system, Gann Monogr. Cancer Res., no. 15, pp. 217-225, 1973, University of Tokyo Press.

74 Levine, G. D., and Dorfman, R. F.: Cancer **35**:148-164, 1975.

75 Lichtenstein, L.: Arch. Pathol. **56**:84-102, 1953.

76 Lieberman, P. H., Jones, C. R., Dargeon, H. W. K., and Begg, C. F.: Medicine **48**:375-400, 1969.

77 Lubin, J., and Rywlin, A. M.: Arch. Pathol. **92**:338-341, 1971.

78 Lucas, P. F.: Blood **10**:1030-1054, 1955.

79 Lukes, R. J.: Cancer Res. **31**:1755-1767, 1971.

80 Lukes, R. J., and Collins, R. D.: New observations on malignant lymphoma. In Akazaki, K., Rappaport, H., Berard, C. W., Bennett, J. M., and Ishikawa, E., editors: Malignant diseases of the hematopoietic system, Gann Monogr. Cancer Res., no. 15, pp. 209-215, 1973, University of Tokyo Press.

81 Lukes, R. J., and Tindle, B. H.: New Eng. J. Med. **292**:1-8, 1975.

82 Lukes, R. J., Butler, J. J., and Hicks, E. B.: Cancer **19**:317-344, 1966a.

83 Lukes, R. J., Craver, L. F., Hall, T. C., Rappaport, H., and Ruben, P.: Cancer Res. **26**:1311, 1966b.

84 Mackaness, G. B.: Semin. Hematol. **7**:172-184, 1970.

85 McMahon, N. J., Gordon, H. W., and Rosen, R. B.: Dis. Child. **120**:148-150, 1970.

86 Miale, J. B.: Laboratory Medicine—hematology, St. Louis, 1972, The C. V. Mosby Co.

87 Miescher, P. A., and Muller-Eberhard, H. J.: Textbook of immunopathology, New York, 1968, Grune & Stratton, Inc., vol. 2.

88 Millett, Y. L., Bennett, M. H., Jelliffe, A. M., and Farrer-Brown, G.: Br. J. Cancer **23**:683-692, 1969.

89 Moller, J. H., Nakib, A., Anderson, R. C., and Edwards, J. E.: Circulation **36**:789-799, 1967.

90 Neiman, R. S., Rosen, P. T., and Lukes, R. J.: New Eng. J. Med. **288**:751-754, 1973.

91 Nossal, G. J. V., Austin, C. M., Pye, J., and Mitchell, J.: Int. Arch. Allergy Appl. Immunol. **29**:368-383, 1966.

92 Nyholm, K.: Acta Pathol. Microbiol. Scand. (A) Suppl. No. 216, 1971.

93 O'Connor, G. T., and Davies, J. N. P.: J. Pediatr. **56**:526-535, 1960.

94 Osgood, E. E.: Blood **9**:1141-1154, 1954.

95 Piringer-Kuchinka, A., Martin, I., and Thalhammer, O.: Virchows Arch. (Pathol. Anat.) **331**:522-535, 1958.

96 Polliack, A., Lampen, N., Clarkson, B. D., et al.: J. Exp. Med. **138**:607-624, 1973.

97 Ramot, B.: Isr. J. Med. Sci. **7**:1488-1490, 1971.

98 Rappaport, H.: Tumors of the hematopoietic system. In Atlas of tumor pathology, Sect. III, Fasc. 8, Washington, D.C., 1966a, Armed Forces Institute of Pathology, pp. 49 and 64.

99 Rappaport, H.: Tumors of the hematopoietic system. In Atlas of tumor pathology, Sect. III, Fasc. 8, Washington, D.C., 1966b, Armed Forces Institute of Pathology.

100 Rappaport, H.: See reference 98, 1966c, pp. 99 and 241.

101 Rappaport, H.: See reference 98, 1966d, Washington, D.C., p. 380.

102 Rappaport, H.: In Lennert, K., and Harms, D., editors: The spleen, Berlin, 1970, Springer Verlag, p. 425.

103 Rappaport, H., Berard, C. W., Butler, J. J., et al.: Cancer Res. 31:1864-1865, 1971.

104 Rappaport, H., Ramot, B., Hulu, N., and Park, J. K.: Cancer 29:1502-1511, 1972.

105 Rappaport, H., Winter, W. J., and Hicks, E. B.: Cancer 9:792-821, 1956.

106 Ravel, R.: Am. J. Clin. Pathol. 46:335-340, 1966.

107 Reynolds, W. A., Winkelman, R. K., and Soule, E. H.: Medicine 44:419-443, 1965.

108 Rezek, P. R., and Millard, M. M.: Autopsy pathology, Springfield, Ill., 1963, Charles C Thomas, Publisher.

109 Rosai, J., and Dorfman, R. F.: Arch. Pathol. 87:63-70, 1969.

110 Rosenberg, S. A.: Cancer Res. 31:1733-1736, 1971.

111 Rosenberg, S. A., Boiron, R., DeVita, V. T., et al.: Cancer Res. 31:1862-1863, 1971.

112 Rywlin, A. M.: The reticuloendothelial system—distribution and function. In Gilson, A. J., Smoak, W. M., and Weinstein, M. B., editors: Hematopoietic and gastrointestinal investigations with radionuclides, Springfield, Ill., 1972, Charles C Thomas, Publisher.

113 Rywlin, A. M.: Lancet 2:106, 1973.

114 Rywlin, A. M., and Benson, J.: Am. J. Clin. Pathol. 36:142-150, 1961.

115 Rywlin, A. M., Block, A. L., and Werner, C. S.: Am. J. Obstet. Gynecol. 86:1055-1059, 1963.

116 Rywlin, A. M., Hernandez, J. A., Chastain, D. E., and Pardo, V.: Blood 37:587-593, 1971a.

117 Rywlin, A. M., Lopez-Gomez, A., Tachmes, P., and Pardo, V.: Am. J. Clin. Pathol. 56:572-579, 1971b.

118 Rywlin, A. M., Marvan, P., and Robinson, M. J.: Am. J. Clin. Pathol. 53:389-393, 1970.

119 Rywlin, A. M., Recher, L., and Hoffman, E.: Arch. Dermatol. 93:554-561, 1966.

120 Salfelder, K., and Schwarz, J.: Dtsch. Med. Wochenschr. 92:1468-1471, 1967.

121 Schrek, R., and Donnelly, W. J.: Blood 27:199-211, 1966.

122 Seligmann, M., Mihaesco, E., and Frangione, B.: Ann. N.Y. Acad. Sci. 190:487-500, 1971.

123 Silverstein, M. N., Ellefson, R. D., and Ahern, E. J.: New Eng. J. Med. 282:1-4, 1970.

124 Smith, C. H., Erlandson, M., Schulman, I., and Stern, G.: Am. J. Med. 22:390-404, 1957.

125 Smith, E. B., and Custer, R. P.: Blood 1:317-333, 1946.

126 Smith, J. L., Clein, G. P., Barker, C. P., and Collins, R. O.: Lancet 1:74-77, 1973.

127 Spranger, J. W., and Wiedemann, H. R.: Humangenetik 9:113-139, 1970.

128 Stoop, J. W., Ballieux, R. E., Hijmans, W., and Zegers, B. J. M.: Clin. Exp. Immunol. 9:625-635, 1971.

129 Strum, S. B., Hutchinson, G. B., Park, J. K., and Rappaport, H.: Cancer 25:1-6, 1971.

130 Stuart, A. E.: The reticuloendothelial system, Edinburgh, 1970, E & S Livingstone.

131 Stutte, H. J.: In Lennert, K., and Harms, D., editors: The spleen, Berlin, 1970, Springer Verlag, p. 425.

132 Stutte, J. H., and Schülter, E.: Virchows Arch. (Pathol. Anat.) 356:32-41, 1972.

133 Tarnowski, W. M., and Hashimoto, K.: Arch. Dermatol. 96:298-304, 1967.

134 Tindle, B. H., Parker, J. W., and Lukes, R. J.: Am. J. Clin. Pathol. 58:607-617, 1972.

135 Tuchman, L. R., Goldstein, G., and Clyman, M.: Am. J. Med. 27:959-975, 1959.

136 van Furth, R.: Semin. Hematol. 7:125-141, 1970.

137 Variakojis, D., Rosas-Uribe, A., and Rappaport, H.: Cancer 33:1589-1600, 1974.

138 Warnke, R. A., Kim, H., and Dorfman, R. F.: Cancer 35:215-230, 1975.

139 Wennberg, E., and Weiss, L.: Blood 31:778-790, 1968.

140 Williams, W. J., Beutler, E., Erslev, A. J., and Rundles, R. W.: Hematology, New York, 1972, McGraw-Hill Book Co.

141 Wintrobe, M. W., Lee, G. R., Boggs, D. R., Bithel, T. C., Athens, J. W., and Foerster, J.: Clinical hematology, Philadelphia, 1974, Lea & Febiger.

142 Wright, D. H.: Pathol. Annu. 6:337-363, 1971.

143 Yam, L. T., Li, C. Y., and Finkel, H. E.: Arch. Intern. Med. 130:248-256, 1972.

35 / Thymus

STANLEY B. SMITH

STRUCTURE AND FUNCTION[9]

The thymus is a lymphoepithelial organ located in the anterior mediastinum. In the past few years it has been suggested that it is the master gland of the immune system. Morphologic differences between thymus and lymph nodes are outlined in Table 35-1. The thymus is divided into two lobes covered by a capsule of loose connective tissue. Septa from the capsule divide the lobes into lobules, which measure approximately 1 to 2 mm in diameter. Each lobule is composed of a cortex and medulla, which Clark[14] further divides, on the basis of cell population and structure, into the following four geographic areas: (1) the outermost subcapsular cortex populated by large lymphocytes, (2) the inner cortex composed of a dense population of small non-proliferating lymphocytes and occasional large mitotic cells, (3) the medulla—an area in which emigrating lymphocytes are observed in the thymic veins on their way to colonize the peripheral lymphoid tissue, and (4) the perivascular connective tissue—the final exit for emigrating thymocytes. Small numbers of scattered larger mononuclear cells, termed "reticular cells," are seen in the medulla and in the inner cortex. These cells have pale-staining nuclei and abundant pale-staining cytoplasm. They are particularly prominent during acute episodes of thymic involution, when they are seen to contain ingested lymphocytes. Recently electron micrographic studies have demonstrated a second type of reticular cell.[34] It has an irregularly shaped nucleus, narrow cisterns of rough endoplasmic reticulum, and

Table 35-1. Morphologic differences between thymus and lymph nodes*

Characteristics	Normal thymus	Normal lymph node
Histogenesis	Foregut endoderm	Mesoderm
Histologic maturity attained	First trimester	Childhood
Growth rate at maximum	During gestation	After birth
Age involution	Depletion of all cell types	Depletion of cortical lymphocytes only
	Fatty and fibrous replacement	
	Increase in PAS-positive cells	
	Increase in spindled cells	
Lymphatic channels	Efferent only, of uncertain significance	Afferent and efferent united by sinusoids
Connective tissue	Scanty	Abundant
	Enters from septa and capsule	Radiates from a hilum
	Isolated from parenchyma	In continuity with parenchyma
Hassall's corpuscles	Unique to thymus	None
Stem cell	Reticular epithelial	Reticulum cells of mesenchyme
	Possibly secretory as well as phagocytic	Phagocytic
Lymphocytes	Form mast cells readily	Form mast cells less readily
	High glycogen content	High protein content
Morphologic behavior	Suppressed maximally by steroids	Suppressed maximally by radiation
	No specific change on antigenic stimulation	Germinal center formation on antigenic stimulation
	Exceptionally high mitotic rate and DNA incorporation	Less mitotic activity

*From Chatten, J.: Am. J. Med. Sci. **248**:715-727, 1964.

widespread interdigitation and invagination of the cell membrane. The surfaces of these interdigitating reticulum cells were observed in contact with the cell surfaces of small lymphocytes, polysomal lymphatic cells, and epithelial cells and sometimes with lymphatic cells containing ergastoplasm. Similar cells have been seen in the thymus-dependent areas[30,35] of the lymph nodes and spleen, a finding that suggests that they may contribute to the microenvironment needed for the differentiation of T cells.

The development of T cells within the thymus is stepwise rather than continuous, with each step occupying a different region of the thymus.[14] In the outermost or subcapsular cortex, stem cells proliferate and differentiate to produce the thymocytes of the inner cortex. These thymocytes are coated with thymus-specific antigens of their own making and are small, inactive lymphocytes lacking most of the characteristics of T cells. Moving slowly through the cortex, thymocytes reach the medulla where they lose some of their thymus-specific surface antigenicity, grow larger and more active looking, and show the characteristics of T cells. These new T cells move into the connective tissue surrounding medullary blood vessels, enter venules and lymphatics, and leave the thymus. From the incomplete evidence available it seems possible that thymocytes develop all the potentialities of T cells while still in the subcapsular cortex but that these potentialities are masked or suppressed by some surface coating such as thymus-specific antigens, as long as thymocytes remain in the cortex. Upon reaching the medulla, this coat is lost and uncovers the nascent T cell beneath.

The role of the intrathymic environment in these events is not yet clear, but the two most obvious characteristics of that environment are its secludedness and its (presumptive) secretion by thymic epithelial cells.

Hassall's corpuscles, found in the medulla, are spheric structures 30 to 100 μm in diameter composed of concentric layers of epithelial cells that may be seen to form keratin. Hassall's corpuscles frequently undergo cystic degeneration and calcification. Eosinophils, neutrophils, and lymphocytes are found within Hassall's corpuscles from time to time. On electron micrographs,[36] as well as in fluorescent-antibody studies,[7,46] it appears that Hassall's corpuscles are derived from thymic epithelial cells. The first appear in the human embryo at 12 weeks. During the first few weeks after birth a rapid increase in their number takes place. They increase in number until about 11 years of age. Between 15 and 25 years of age there is a rapid decline in the number of Hassall's corpuscles. After 60 years of age the number of Hassall's corpuscles is about the same as that of a 24-week-old fetus.

The thymus is derived embryologically from the third and sometimes the fourth branchial pouches in association with the parathyroid glands. The parathyroid glands normally remain in the neck, as the thymus migrates downward into the anterior part of the mediastinum. Sometimes, residual thymic tissue remains in the neck in close association with parathyroid tissue, or parathyroid tissue may be found in the mediastinum.

The thymus is prominent in infancy and childhood but begins to atrophy after puberty, a fact that has long suggested that the thymus plays a role in developmental biology. Largely by extirpation of the thymus in the neonatal period and then restoration of the function with thymic grafts, it has been shown that the thymus plays an essential role in the development of cellular immunity (delayed hypersensitivity).[6,31,44]

According to current concepts, there are two general types of lymphoid tissue: central and peripheral. The central lymphoid tissue is composed of the thymus and the mucosal gastrointestinal lymphoid tissue. The peripheral lymphoid tissue is composed of lymph nodes and spleen. The two types are functionally related in that precursor lymphoid cells are believed to originate in the bone marrow and migrate to either the thymus or to the mucosa-related gastrointestinal lymphoid tissue, where they are induced to develop their genetic potential into particular cell lines. Lymphocytes that have transited the thymus are known as "T cells." They migrate to the peripheral lymphoid tissues and express thymus-dependent functions. Among these functions are delayed hypersensitivity, graft-versus-host reactivity, homograft rejection, resistance to certain viral and fungal diseases and to tuberculosis, and possibly a role in the rejection of tumors.

The gastrointestinal mucosa-related central lymphoid tissue has been termed "bursa-derived system." This term came into use after the discovery of Glick et al.[21] that the bursa of Fabricius in birds, a mucosa-related lymphoid organ, was necessary for the development of lymphoid cells capable of producing antibodies. They found that removal

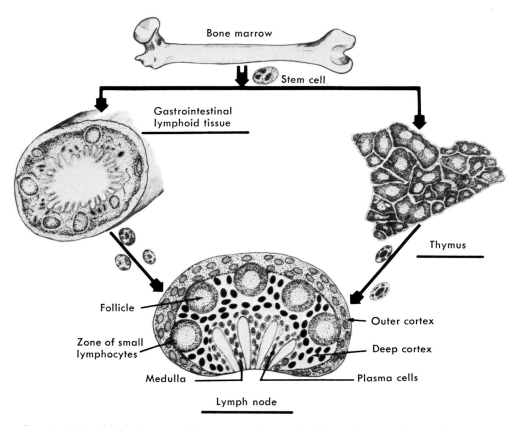

Fig. 35-1. Simplified schematic diagram showing traffic of lymphocytes. Stem cells originate in bone marrow and migrate to thymus or gastrointestinal lymphoid tissue. Thymus derived cells migrate chiefly to deep cortical areas of lymph nodes. Outer cortex, mantle zone around germinal centers, and medulla of lymph node are dependent on functioning gastrointestinal lymphoid system. Some cells may migrate directly from bone marrow to lymph nodes.

of the bursa from a newborn chicken resulted in its failure to develop circulating immunoglobulins in a normal manner. Peyer's patches, vermiform appendix, pharyngeal tonsils, and bone marrow itself have all been considered as possible bursal equivalents in man. Lymphocytes that have been influenced by this system are known as "B cells." T lymphocytes form the major fraction of the recirculating lymphocyte pool and are the main cellular component of the periarteriolar sheaths of the splenic white pulp and of the deep cortex (paracortical areas) of the lymph nodes. B lymphocytes are the main cellular constituent of outer follicular regions and medullary cords of lymph nodes and of the splenic white pulp.

Fig. 35-1 shows that absence or abnormality of bone marrow–derived stem cells can result in a defect of both immunoglobulin production and cellular sensitivity. Absence or abnormality of the thymus results in a defect in cellular sensitivity, but, in general, production of immunoglobulins remains normal. On the other hand, an individual with a normal thymus and a defective or absent bursa-derived system has a defect involving only production of immunoglobulins. One should also note that any congenital or acquired defect involving recognition of antigen, engulfment of antigen, or processing of antigen, or a defect in one of the steps involved in subsequent production of the immune response, would lead to a deficiency of one or more classes of the immune response.

The concept of B lymphocytes and T lymphocytes has been extended in recent years.[3,4,][25,28,51] Human B lymphocytes[13,17,18,26,33] can be identified in the clinical laboratory by the presence of surface immunoglobulins, surface receptors for complement, their retention by nylon columns, and a blastogenic response to pokeweed mitogen. T cells[13] give negative responses to the descriptors of B cells, but they can be identified by the formation of rosettes with sheep cell erythrocytes, by thymus-dependent antigens on the cell surface, and by a mitogenic response when exposed to phytohemagglutinin. Several investigators[38,48,49] have suggested that human B and T lymphocytes can be distinguished on the basis of an analysis of surface architecture with the scanning electron microscope. According to these authors the T lymphocyte is relatively smooth whereas the B lymphocyte has numerous microvilli on the surface. More recent observations with the scanning electron microscope in which lymphocytes have been carefully fixed in suspension with minimal cell loss reveal that both types are villous and hence indistinguishable by this method.[5]

T cells are believed to have the following four major functions:

1. Mediators of cellular immunity–activated[42] or "killer" T cells[29] directly attack and kill foreign antigens. This mechanism also presumably plays a role in tumor surveillance, graft-versus-host reaction, and transplantation immunity. In the course of mediating cellular immunity, T lymphocytes produce and secrete lymphokines (B lymphocytes may also produce several types of lymphokines), which are soluble nonantibody products produced by lymphocytes when activated by a specific antigen. In general lymphokines have a molecular weight varying from 20,000 to 60,000 Daltons; they are heat stable and can be degraded by proteolytic enzymes. The activities of lymphokines can be classified into three major groups—those that cause cell proliferation (usually of other lymphocytes), those that destroy target cells (lymphotoxins), and those that affect inflammatory cells. A partial list of known lymphokines[45] is as follows:
   a. Lymphocyte mitogenic factor
   b. Inflammatory factors
   c. Cytotoxic factors
   d. Migration-inhibition factor
   e. Macrophage-agglutinating factor
   f. Macrophage-spreading factor
   g. Chemotactic factor
   h. Lymph node–activating factor
   i. Macrophage-activating factor
   j. Interferon-like factor
2. Helper function. B cells need the cooperation of helper T cells in order to respond with antibody production to many antigens.

3. Suppressor function.[41] Suppressor T cells are believed to play an important role as regulators of the immune response. There is evidence that either an excess or deficiency of suppressor T cells can result in serious disease. It has been hypothesized that malfunction of suppressor T cells could result in excess of antibodies as an allergic reaction or production of aberrant antibodies such as autoantibodies found in autoimmune conditions, or a lack of antibodies and consequent immune deficiency. (For example, too many suppressor cells could result in an immune deficiency that is characterized by inability to make adequate antibodies.)
4. Amplifier function. Amplifier cells are not required for antibody production but are believed to enhance it under certain conditions.

The advances in characterization of lymphocyte subpopulations have been applied to further defining of immune deficiencies, malignant lymphomas, and autoimmune diseases. The subject of immune deficiencies are dealt with later in this chapter. The following lymphomas and leukemias are T cell diseases:

1. Sézary syndrome[11,19,59]
2. Mycosis fungoides[2]
3. Childhood acute lymphocytic leukemia[10,53] (T cells demonstrated in 2 of 14 patients. Both were boys, ages 7 years and 11 years, with high initial blast counts. One had an anterior mediastinal mass, probably the thymus.
4. T cell lymphoma[40]

Chronic lymphocytic leukemia is an example of a B cell disease.[1,50,57,58] Multiple myeloma, Waldenström's macroglobulinemia, Burkitt's lymphoma,[8] and some cases of lymphosarcoma are also examples of B cell malignancies.

Gell and Coombs[20] have divided immune damage into four general categories: type I (anaphylaxis), type II (damage caused by cytotoxic antibody, e.g., autoimmune hemolytic anemia and Goodpasture's syndrome), type III (damage caused by antigen antibody complexes, e.g., some types of glomerulonephritis), type IV (damage to cellular immune reactions). From this discussion it is obvious that damage from reactions of types I, II, and III can be considered as damage caused by B cell activity, whereas damage from type IV reactions is a result of T cell activity. Two or more mechanisms of tissue damage are operational in some diseases. For example, hypersensitivity pneumonitis is a result of both type I and probably type III damage.

Lesions of the thymus have been reported in many so-called autoimmune diseases. An autoimmune disease[52] may be viewed as one in which there is a loss of immunologic tolerance to antigens present in one's own body constituents (i.e., to one's own "self" antigens). In the normal individual there is neither a humoral nor a cellular immune response to self-antigens. This failure of an immune response to self-antigens is known as self-tolerance. The variation in pathologic findings and symptomatology in autoimmune diseases is dependent on the type and location of antigen to which there is a loss of tolerance, as well as to the type of immune response mounted against the individual's own tissue. Experimental findings indicate that the thymus has a role in some forms of immune tolerance.

THYMIC HORMONES

Thymic hormones are the subject of several excellent recent reviews.[15,39,55] Numerous thymic hormones and inhibitors have been characterized with varying degrees of completeness. These include (1) lymphocyte-stimulating hormone (LSH), (2) thymosin, (3) homeostatic thymic hormone (HTH), (4) thymic humoral factor (THF), (5) thymic protein (TP), (6) hypocalcemic component (CaC), (7) thymus-specific antigen (TSA), (8) thymin, (9) thymotoxin, and (10) thymosterin. These are all proteins or peptides except for thymosterin, which is a steroid. Of these thymin, which depresses neuromuscular transmission, and thymosin have received the most attention.

Thymosin, a protein with a molecular weight of 12,600, was first described in 1972.[22,27] When thymosin is incubated with precursor cells derived from mouse bone marrow and spleen, there is a resultant differentiation of lymphocytes with T-cell characteristics. Touraine et al.[54] subsequently showed that a fraction of human bone marrow cells, incubated with thymosin, differentiated into lymphocytes with T-cell markers. Wara et al.[56] partially restored thymic function and achieved clinical improvement in a child with thymic hypoplasia by giving her injections of thymosin. Other studies[23] in patients with a number of clinical disorders including thymic hypoplasia, ataxia, telangiectasia, Wiscott-Aldrich syndrome and lupus erythematosus, cancer, and virus infections show that incubation of peripheral blood lymphocytes with thymosin increases the number of T cells (by the sheep erythrocyte rosette technique). Thymosin, however, does not appear to increase the number of erythrocyte rosette–forming cells in patients with combined immunodeficiency, a disease in which the defect is apparently at the level of the stem cell. Goldstein's[24] working hypothesis on the basic mechanism of action of thymosin is that it can act on bone marrow–derived or bone marrow–dwelling primitive stem cell populations as well as on more mature T cells that may transiently reside within the thymus gland. The short time period required for thymosin to convert a primitive lymphoid cell into a more mature T cell indicates that thymosin probably derepresses or activates a cell that is already genetically programmed for T-cell differentiation. Phase I clinical trials with thymosin in patients with primary and secondary immunodeficiency disease are under way and early results are promising.[24]

INVOLUTION[60-63]

There is a considerable variation in weight of the thymus according to age, and a relatively large variation occurs within each age group. For this reason, there is difficulty in defining thymic hyperplasia or hypertrophy solely in terms of weight (Table 35-2).

The thymus increases in weight until puberty, at which time it begins to decrease in size (physiologic involution). Decrease in size secondary to stress, such as occurs in infection, is termed "accidental thymic involution" (Figs.

Table 35-2. Weight of thymus*

Age (yr)	Weight (gm)		
	Minimum	Average	Maximum
Newborn	7.3	15.2	25.5
1-5	8.0	25.7	48.0
5-10	13.0	29.4	48.0
10-15	19.0	29.4	43.3
15-20	15.9	26.2	49.7
21-25	9.5	21.0	51.0
26-30	8.3	19.5	51.5
31-35	9.0	20.2	37.0
36-43	5.9	19.0	36.0
47-55	6.0	17.3	45.0
56-65	2.1	14.3	27.0
66-90	3.0	14.0	31.0

*According to Hammar, J. A.: Die Menschenthymus in Gesundheit und Krankheit, Leipzig, 1926, Akademische Verlagsgesellschaft; from Fisher, E. R.: Pathology of the thymus and its relation to human disease. In Good, R. A., and Gabrielsen, A. E., editors: The thymus in immunobiology, New York, 1964, Paul B. Hoeber Medical Division, Harper & Row, Publishers.

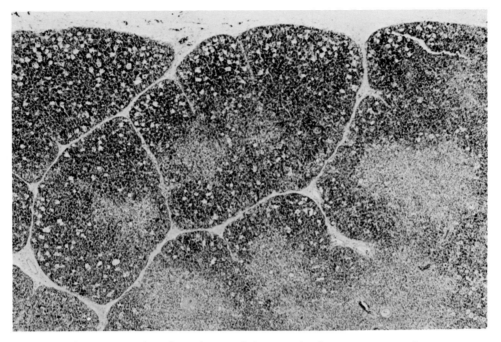

Fig. 35-2. Acute or accidental involution of thymus of infant. Note starry-sky appearance in cortex and lack of chronic involution. Except for this acute stress reaction, gland is normal (55×.)

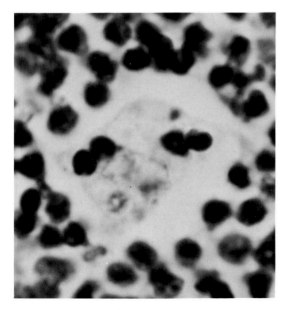

Fig. 35-3. View of cortex shown in Fig. 35-2. Lymphocytes within large cortical mononuclear cell. It is not known whether this results from phagocytosis or lymphocytic migration into mononuclear cell. (1890×.)

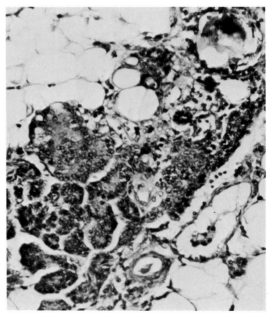

Fig. 35-4. Chronic involution of thymus with rosettes and microcysts. (207×.)

35-2 and 35-3), and a striking decrease in thymic size as observed by roentgenogram of the chest may occur within 12 hours of onset of severe stress. Caution should be used in interpreting a roentgenogram showing a small thymus in an acutely ill child suspected of having an immunologic deficiency disorder.

In physiologic involution, the thymic parenchyma gradually decreases in size, cortical lymphocytes are scanty, and the lobules are separated by adipose tissue. Epithelial elements of the medulla may have a fusiform or spindle shape. In occasional glands, epithelial rosettes are seen. Hassall's corpuscles vary in number, sometimes are closely packed, and occasionally appear partially calcified or cystic. The thymus in adults, particularly those of advanced age, often contains cysts ranging in size up to about 1 cm and is lined by flat cells. It is presumed that some of these are the end stage of cystic Hassall's corpuscles (Figs. 35-4 and 35-5).

In accidental involution, the early changes include clumping and fragmentation of lymphocytes and phagocytosis of lymphocytes by large cortical cells, sometimes giving the so-called starry-sky appearance (Fig. 32-2). These cortical phagocytes accumulate nuclear debris, PAS-positive material, phospholipid, and neutral lipid, all probably the result of cellular breakdown. The lympholysis is accompanied by depletion of lymphocytes from the cortex of the gland. There is an early increase in plasma cells and mast cells, followed by a later decrease in these elements. Accidental involution also is characterized by progressive collapse of the reticulin lobular network and fibrosis (Fig. 35-6). In the final stage, the lobule is completely collapsed and surrounded by fibrous septa. The extent of the capacity for regeneration may decrease with the degree of collapse and fibrosis (Fig. 35-7).

HYPERPLASIA[64,65]

Hyperplasia of the thymus cannot be defined with weight as the only criterion. The presence of germinal centers in the medulla has been considered to be histologic evidence of thymic hyperplasia (Fig. 35-8). The presence of lymph follicles in the medulla frequently has been reported in association with

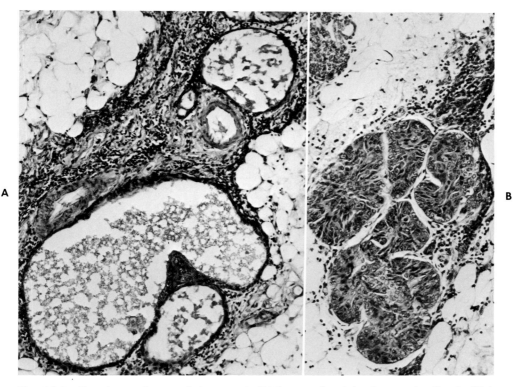

Fig. 35-5. Chronic involution of thymus. **A,** With cysts lined by flattened cells. **B,** With prominent rosettes similar to those seen in some thymomas. Patient had no known immunologic abnormalities, and there was no evidence of primary carcinoma. (**A** and **B,** 165×.)

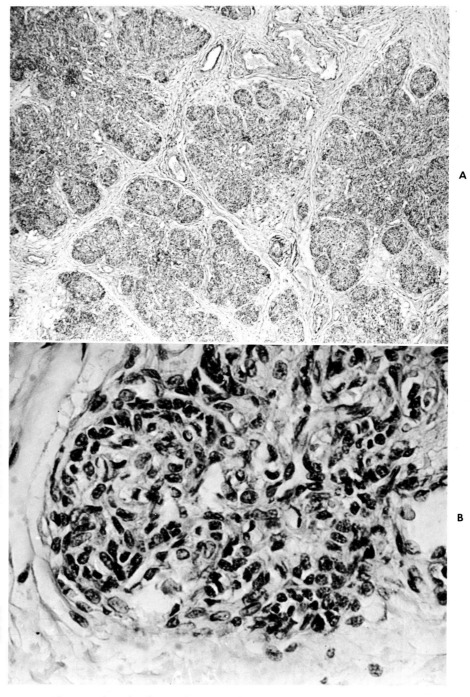

Fig. 35-6. Thymic alymphoplasia showing fibrous septa separating poorly developed lobules and absence of small lymphocytes and Hassall's bodies. (**A,** 52×; **B,** 486×· courtesy Dr. David Gitlin and Dr. John M. Craig, Boston, Mass.)

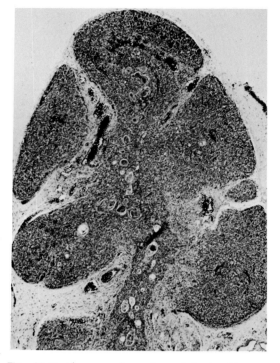

Fig. 35-7. Thymus of newborn infant with considerable depletion of cortical lymphocytes in acute involution probably secondary to infection in utero. Presence of Hassall's corpuscles distinguishes this from thymic alymphoplasia. (60×.)

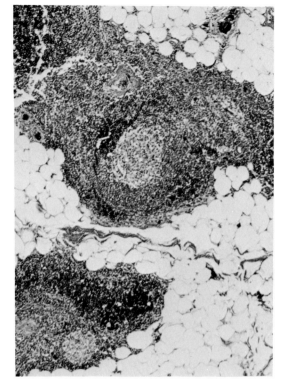

Fig. 35-8. Germinal centers in involuted gland. This can be viewed as hyperplasia in atrophic gland. Patient had myasthenia gravis.

various diseases in which there is an immunologic abnormality such as myasthenia gravis, systemic lupus erythematosus, Hashimoto's disease, thyrotoxicosis, and chronic glomerulonephritis. Although thymic germinal centers have been considered suggestive of an autoimmune disorder, their occurrence in cases of accidental death indicates that their presence is not diagnostic.

IMMUNOLOGIC DEFICIENCY DISEASES

As has been previously mentioned, there are two major subpopulations of lymphocytes known as B lymphocytes and T lymphocytes. These can be recognized on the basis of both surface markers and blastogenic response to various mitogens. About 70% to 80% of peripheral blood lymphocytes are T cells and about 20% are B cells.

The primary immune deficiencies can thus be approached as defects in B cells or T cells or both. The disorders are discussed here as classified by a committee of the World Health Organization.[88]

Infantile sex-linked agammaglobulinemia (Bruton's disease)

Infantile sex-linked agammaglobulinemia is a B-cell disorder occurring in males and is characterized by recurring infections, usually with pyogenic organisms. Onset is usually in the second year of life. Common offending organisms are pneumococci, staphylococci, streptococci, and *Haemophilus influenzae*. The most common types of infections are sinusitis, pneumonia, meningitis, furunculosis and sepsis. Infections recur frequently unless proper prophylactic therapy is given. The thymus is morphologically normal. A normal number of lymphocytes are found in the blood, bone marrow, and thymus-dependent areas of lymph nodes. In most cases circulating B lymphocytes are decreased. In some cases circulating B lymphocytes without detectable surface Ig have been found. Functionally, the patients have normal cell-mediated responses. Plasma cells are absent in the tissues even after stimulation by potent antigens. The lymphoid tissue shows an absence of plasma cells and germinal centers. Tonsils are small, with absence of germinal centers and poorly developed crypts. Peyer's patches are poorly developed and lack follicles. Plasma cells are not seen in the lamina propria of the intestinal tract. There is a pronounced deficiency in all classes of immunoglobulins, as well as a deficiency of production of antibodies to all antigens.

Many of the boys with the disorder develop arthritis, particularly of the large joints. Replacement therapy with gamma globulin usually relieves this complication. Sometimes a fatal syndrome resembling dermatomyositis is seen. It is characterized by weakness and a rash generally over the extensor surfaces of the joints with edema and ligneous induration of muscles. Lymphocytes are seen around small blood vessels. Sometimes the central nervous system is involved similarly.

In some cases hemolytic anemia, atopic eczema, asthma, allergic rhinitis, poison ivy, and drug eruptions have been seen.

Transient hypogammaglobulinemia of infancy[104,148]

Newborn infants begin to synthesize IgM at birth. Synthesis of IgA is generally observed by the third week of life. IgG levels at birth are the result of transplacental passage of maternal IgG. The IgG level at birth therefore approximates the level of the maternal IgG. IgG is catabolized in the infant and reaches a low point of about 300 mg per 100 ml by the end of the second month of life. At that time the normal infant begins to synthesize IgG and achieves adult levels by the end of 1 year of age. In transient hypogammaglobulinemia of infancy there is a prolonged delay in onset of IgG synthesis. This condition is evenly distributed between males and females who usually recover between 18 and 30 months of age. Before recovery occurs, they have an increased susceptibility to infections of the skin, meninges, or respiratory tract. Grampositive organisms are particular offenders. This then is a disorder limited to B cells capable of producing IgG.

Selective immunoglobulin deficiency[72,81,89,140,150,154]

An isolated lack of IgA is seen in a small number of apparently normal individuals (4 to 7 per 1000). Some individuals with selective IgA deficiency are subject to recurrent sinusitis, bronchitis, and exudative enteropathy. Those with exudative enteropathy present with steatorrhea or nontropical sprue and lack IgA-producing cells in the lamina propria of the intestinal tract. Some patients have familial lack of IgA. Cases have been documented in which there are anti-IgA antibodies associated with the lack of IgA, which may result in rapid catabolism of IgA. These patients may develop transfusion reactions on receiving plasma.

A few cases of septicemia associated with selective IgM deficiency have been reported. Chronic progressive bronchiectasis has been seen in patients with IgG subclass deficiencies. Decreases in IgG_4 subclass results in more severe disease than in other IgG subclass deficiencies. An increased incidence of collagen disease is seen in patients with selective immunoglobulin deficiencies, especially in IgA deficiency.

Sex-linked immunodeficiency with hyper-IgM[142,152]

In this condition there is a deficiency of IgA and IgG with increased levels of IgM. The IgM is composed of normally distributed molecules with antibody activity and a normal distribution of lambda (λ) and kappa (κ) chains. A few of the patients have had increased levels of IgD. They have an increased susceptibility to infection. Some of the patients develop hemolytic anemia, aplastic anemia, renal lesions, neutropenia, and thrombocytopenia. Many of the patients develop a malignant proliferation of IgM-producing B cells, usually starting in the gastrointestinal tract. Some cases of increased levels of IgM associated with immune deficiency have been seen in children with congenital rubella. This then is a B-cell disorder.

Thymic aplasia (DiGeorge's syndrome, congenital absence of thymus and parathyroid glands)[70,83,91,108,139]

Thymic aplasia is characterized by a failure of development of both the third and fourth pharyngeal pouches, with resulting absence of both thymus and parathyroid glands. Anomalies of the aortic arch, which originate in the fourth branchial arch, also have been seen in this syndrome. A right-sided aortic arch and tetralogy of Fallot are seen. These infants have often been noted to have low-set ears with notched pinnae, nasal clefts, a shortened lip philtrum and hypertelorism. There is depletion of lymphocytes in the thymus-dependent areas (Fig. 35-9). Germinal centers are present. The lymphoid sheaths in the spleen are depleted of lymphocytes. No T cells are seen in the peripheral blood. Plasma cells are present, and immunoglobulins are normal.

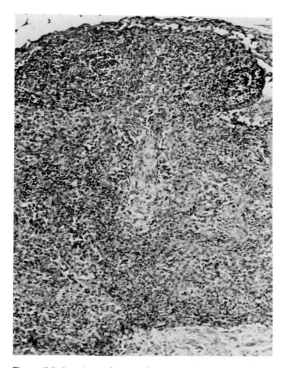

Fig. 35-9. Lymph node in thymic aplasia (DiGeorge's syndrome). Note absence of lymphocytes in deep cortical areas and small germinal centers with thin mantle zone of lymphocytes. (165×.)

Serum levels of immunoglobulins are normal and the primary antibody response is normal. Cell-mediated immune responses such as skin tests to *Candida* and to streptokinase, ability to respond to sensitization to dinitrofluorobenzene, skin allograft rejection, and blastogenic responses to phytohemagglutinin are all abnormal. Infants with this syndrome usually present with signs of tetany in the newborn period. No genetic abnormality has been described.

Restoration of T-cell function has been shown to be possible by transplantation of a fetal thymus. Robinson[139] postulates that premature involution of the thyroidea ima artery, the principal embryonic blood source of the third and fourth pharyngeal pouches, may be the critical event in the embryogenesis of this syndrome.

Immune deficiency with thrombocytopenia and eczema (Wiskott-Aldrich syndrome)[76,85,86,112]

Immune deficiency with thrombocytopenia and eczema is a sex-linked genetic disease in which male children develop thrombocytopenia, eczema, and frequent infections from gram-positive and gram-negative organisms,

viruses, and fungi. The cause of death usually is attributable to either infection or hemorrhage or malignant reticuloendotheliosis. IgG and IgA levels are normal or elevated, but IgM levels are usually low. Commonly, there is a deficiency in the ability to produce isohemagglutinins or to produce antibodies to carbohydrate antigens. Plasma cells are present. In some individuals, the thymus has been normal, but in others, there is a decrease in thymic lymphocytes, an indistinct corticomedullary relationship, and numerous Hassall's corpuscles. This constellation of histologic findings is characteristic of involutional atrophy of the thymus. The number of circulating lymphocytes is usually low, and cellular immunity usually is impaired. Normal percentages of lymphocytes forming T-cell rosettes have been reported by one laboratory. Monocyte function as measured by chemotactic assay in the Boyden chamber and by cytophilic antibody receptor is normal. It has been speculated that there is a defect in the initiation of specific immune responses.

Ataxia-telangiectasia (Louis-Bar syndrome)[79,93,110,126,129-132,136,144]

Ataxia telangiectasia is transmitted as an autosomal recessive trait. The infant appears normal at birth, but at about 2 years of age the child is noted to have ataxia and prominent oculocutaneous blood vessels. By the age of 16 years, the patient is generally confined to a wheelchair. By that time, telangiectases, which at first involved only bulbar conjunctivas, extend to the butterfly area of face, ears, antecubital fossae, and neck. The chief finding in the brain is degeneration of Purkinje cells in the cerebellum. Gonadal dysgenesis is a commonly associated defect. There is an increased incidence of malignancy in these patients (tumors of the lymphoid system, ovarian dysgerminomas, cerebellar medulloblastoma, and frontal lobe gliomas). Many of the children develop sinopulmonary infections, progressive bronchiectasis, respiratory insufficiency, and pneumonia.

The condition is accompanied by an embryonic type of thymus that is small and lacks cortical and medullary organization. Hassall's corpuscles have been lacking in all but one reported case. Lymphocytes are deficient in the thymus-dependent areas of the lymph node in most cases. In a few cases, the lymph nodes appear relatively normal, but in others they consist almost entirely of stromal cells with an absence of follicles and lymphocytes. The number of circulating lymphocytes tends to be slightly decreased. As would be expected from these pathologic findings, the cell-mediated responses are constantly deficient with decreased numbers of T cells and decreased in vitro blast transformation of lymphocytes exposed to phytohemagglutinin. There is also usually a lack of response to attempts to sensitize patients with dinitrochlorobenzene and a decreased ability to reject skin grafts. Levels of IgA are low or absent, as are levels of IgE. There is a deficient antibody response to viral and bacterial antigens.

Immune deficiency with normal or hyperimmunoglobulinemia[97,98]

An infant with recurrent bacterial infections who lacked IgM and IgA but had normal levels of IgG was described by Giedion and Scheidegger in 1957. The child was unresponsive to a variety of antigenic stimuli. They designated this entity "immunoparesis." It is considered to be a disorder of B cells and possibly also of T cells.

Thymoma with agammaglobulinemia (Good's syndrome)[105]

In thymoma with agammaglobulinemia, there is epithelial or spindle cell type of thymoma and an associated decrease or absence of plasma cells. The number of circulating lymphocytes is low. Immunoglobulins are reduced, and there is a deficiency of humoral antibody production to all antigens, as well as a deficient response of cell-mediated immunity to all antigens. Eosinophils are absent or decreased in the blood and bone marrow. Some cases also have an associated pure red cell aplasia. This then is both a T cell and B cell disorder.

Immunodeficiency with short-limbed dwarfism[113]

T cell defects with lymphopenia and decreased blastogenic responses to specific antigens and to phytohemagglutinin have been associated with short-limbed dwarfism and cartilage-hair hypoplasia. Some of these children have developed fatal vaccinia or varicella.

Severe combined immune deficiency[70,75,79,90, 95,96,99,100,106,111,114,125,134,143,145,152]

This is a severe immune deficiency in which both sex-linked recessive and autosomal recessive patterns of inheritance have been described. The onset of symptoms is usually between 3 and 6 months of age. These children present with thrush, severe diarrhea, and a morbilliform rash. Enteropathic *Escherichia coli* and *Salmonella* are frequent isolates. Pulmonary infection is common with *Pseudomonas aeruginosa* frequently isolated. *Pneumocystis carinii* pneumonia is seen with some frequency. Fatalities have resulted from infections with adenovirus, cytomegal virus, Hecht's giant cell pneumonia, chickenpox, and measles.

Usually agammaglobulinemia is seen. Leukopenia with a low lymphocyte count is seen. Decreased numbers of plasma cells and lymphocytes are present in the bone marrow. Lymph nodes show a lack of germinal centers, plasma cells, and lymphocytes. The spleen and gastrointestinal lymphoid tissue are depleted of lymphocytes. Cell-mediated immune responses to all antigens are deficient. The thymus is very small and is composed chiefly of epithelial or spindle cells and lacks lymphocytes and Hassall's corpuscles. Some of these infants have a variant of severe combined immunodeficiency with normal plasma cells and immunoglobulins (Nezelof's syndrome). These infants with Nezelof's syndrome also have hypoplastic thymuses lacking both lymphocytes and Hassall's corpuscles. Some of these children develop a Coombs-positive hemolytic anemia and other autoimmune phenomena.

In another variant known as reticular dysgenesis there is a stem-cell defect with a total myelopoietic failure. Recently an intrathymic defect has been demonstrated.

The discovery of several of the preceding defects led to the investigation of other areas of host resistance to microbial disorders.

A number of defects of phagocytosis have been brought to light.[155] In considering these defects, one should realize that for the neutrophils to play an effective role in host resistance they must be present in adequate numbers and have adequate random movement and adequate directional movement (chemotaxis) to reach the invading microorganism where they must then be able to ingest and kill the organism. Defects in each of these activities have been described. Some patients[146,149] with recurrent episodes of pyoderma, recurrent otitis media, and pneumonia have been found to have a circulating inhibitor affecting leukocyte mobility but not associated with any abnormality of ingestion or killing phases of phagocytosis. These patients were successfully treated with plasma infusions. Some[123] but apparently not all persons with congenital ichthyosis have a defect in neutrophil chemotaxis associated with cutaneous infections with *Trichophyton rubrum*. Other facets of neutrophil function such as random mobility, opsonizing activity of the serum, and the ability to ingest and kill organisms were all normal. In the "lazy leukocyte syndrome" described by Miller et al.,[121] children with recurrent gingivitis, otitis media, and stomatitis were found to have similar abnormalities of the release of neutrophils from storage from both the marrow and the intravascular pools, accompanied by both impaired chemotaxis and random mobility, but their serum was capable of generating chemotactic factors. Furthermore, neutrophil bactericidal activity was normal.

Myeloperoxidase deficiency[109] is a rare hereditary disorder in which an increased susceptibility to candidosis is seen. Chronic granulomatous disease is the prototype of neutrophil function disorders. Children suffering from it develop severe recurrent infections of the lungs, subcutaneous tissue, liver, skin, lymph nodes, and bones. *Staphylococcus aureus,* gram-negative enteric bacteria, and some fungi are common offending agents. Histologic examination[106] of these lesions reveals abscess formation and granulomas containing giant cells. In a classic paper, Quie, White, and Holmes[135] demonstrated a defect in the capacity of neutrophils to kill selected bacterial species, including those previously mentioned. Neutrophils from these patients[74,101] have an impairment of the hexose monophosphate shunt, of oxygen consumption, and in the production of hydrogen peroxide. Decreased level of glutathione peroxidase or decreased activity of NADH or NADPH oxidase may be the cause of decreased production of hydrogen peroxide with the resultant failure of iodination of bacteria by the neutrophils.[73,101,107] As might be expected, those organisms, such as pneumococci, streptococci and *Haemophilus influenzae* that generate hydrogen peroxide within the confines of the phagocytic vacuole commit suicide and are therefore not a clinical problem in these children.

Of the complement components C3 and C5 are particularly important in resistance to infection. In patients deficient in C3 there is an increased susceptibility to pyogenic organisms. Such a deficiency can result from hypercatabolism of C3.[66,67,69,70] The clinical problem is a result of impaired chemotactic and opsonic activity. Children with a defect in C5[119,120] present with generalized seborrheic dermatitis, intractable severe diarrhea, severe wasting, and recurrent infections usually caused by gram-negative organisms and *Staphylococcus aureus.* Opsonic activity is deficient and chemotactic activity is normal in some patients and abnormal in others.

Chediak-Higashi syndrome[77,78,82,141,153]

The Chediak-Higashi syndrome is characterized by photophobia, oculocutaneous albinism, and frequent episodes of skin and respiratory infections usually caused by gram-positive organisms. It is an autosomal recessive disorder. Leukocytes have giant lysosomes that degranulate slowly and show a decrease in the release of lysosomal enzymes into the phagocytic vacuole with a reduction of intracellular killing. Chemotaxis is also decreased.

Since 1973 at Variety Children's Hospital (Miami, Florida) we have seen six patients with defects of the ingestion phase of neutrophil phagocytosis. Three of the patients presented with recurrent staphylococcal infections. Other clinical pictures encountered were asthma with recurrent respiratory infections and frequent mild respiratory infections. Two children had an imbalance of IgG subclasses, one had low levels of IgG, another appears to have sex-linked agammaglobulinemia. In two others the reasons for the abnormality are not clear.

The previously described deficiencies of host resistance can be likened to the top of an iceberg. The bottom of the iceberg is represented by numerous conditions of moderately depressed host resistance. Some of these conditions are transient and potentially treatable. Newborn infants[115,137] have a defect in chemotaxis probably caused by low levels of C3 and C5 and by an abnormality in their leukocytes. Infants with low birth weight[94,116] have decreased serum opsonins attributable in part to low levels of C3. Even full-term infants have been shown to have deficient serum opsonic activity.[92] Another study has demonstrated an intracellular defect in the killing of *Staphylococcus aureus.*[84] An increased susceptibility to salmonella, osteomyelitis, pneumococcal sepsis, and meningitis[102] is seen in children with sickle-cell anemia. Heat-labile opsonic activity to pneumococci is decreased, but opsonic activity for *Salmonella* is normal. A functional defect of the spleen has been demonstrated.[127] Neutrophils obtained from diabetic patients show decreased chemotactic responsiveness.[124]

Migration of their cells into a Rebuck skin window is abnormal,[128] and their serum has a decreased ability to generate chemotactic factors.[122] Neutrophils obtained from diabetics in ketoacidosis have a decreased ability to ingest staphylococci.[80] Children suffering from protein and calorie malnutrition are prone to infections because of impaired immunity, granulocytic dysfunction, and defective epithelial barriers.[117,147] These children develop a nutritional thymectomy and usually die of infections including tuberculosis, varicella, herpes simplex, measles, malaria, and diseases caused by *Pneumocystis carinii, Staphylococcus, Salmonella, Shigella, Strongyloides,* and hookworm.[153] The epidemic of gram-negative sepsis and bronchopneumonia seen as terminal events in cancer patients, as well as in other diseases of later life, reflects a huge population of persons with acquired deficiencies of host resistance.

It should be pointed out that a lymph node removed for evaluation of immune deficiency should be handled by cutting the node transversely through its short axis in order to permit penetration of fixative. To assess immunologic function, transverse sections cut along the short axis from the middle portion of the nodes should be examined. This will permit evaluation of representative areas of the cortex and medulla as shown in Fig. 35-9. The description and nomenclature used to describe the histology should follow a standardized system.[88]

RELATIONSHIP OF THYMUS TO MYASTHENIA GRAVIS

Myasthenia gravis is characterized clinically by weakness and easy fatigability of voluntary muscle. The symptoms are aggravated by exercise and are ameliorated by rest. Since the first description of a thymic tumor in association with myasthenia gravis in 1901 by Laquer and Weigert, numerous examples have been recorded. Later, the presence of germinal centers in the thymus in myasthenia gravis was noted.[161,220] Early descriptions of a lymphocytic infiltrate in skeletal muscle (lymphorrhages), together with other degenerative muscle changes, are recorded.[166]

There is recent evidence suggesting altered cell populations in the thymus in myasthenia gravis.[156,221] In mixed leukocyte reactions, thymic cells from myasthenic patients with hyperplastic thymuses stimulated blastogenesis in autologous peripheral blood lymphocytes. This type of reactivity was not seen in thymocyte–peripheral blood lymphocyte cultures from patients with myasthenia gravis and thymoma or in control patients undergoing cardiac surgery. No difference was found in the percentage of T lymphocytes, as estimated by the E-rosette technique, in patients with either thymocytes or peripheral blood lymphocytes obtained from controls versus patients with myasthenia gravis. Increased numbers of B lymphocytes were found in the thymus of myasthenics compared to controls. This increase in B cells predominantly carried IgM receptors. The thymic cells from myasthenic patients also responded more vigorously to pokeweed mitogen. Abdou expressed the opinion that the demonstration of increased numbers of B cells in the thymus and the demonstration of new antigens on the surface of thymocytes strongly suggest an occult virus infection. A later study showed a modest decrease in peripheral-blood T lymphocytes in myasthenics. The antigenic disparity between the thymic lymphocytes and the peripheral blood lymphocytes was not enhanced by autologous plasma and was not the result of HL-A differences between the two cell populations.[199] This increase in the thymus may be associated with a break in immunologic tolerance within the gland and could account for immunologic and clinical aberrations seen in myasthenia gravis.[176,183] In another study[160] thymic lymphocytes from patients with myasthenia gravis, when stimulated with phytohemagglutinin, induced cytotoxicity for fetal muscle. Inhibition of migration of lymphocytes and monocytes from a capillary tube (an in vitro correlate of delayed hypersensitivity) in the presence of muscle antigen occurred more frequently in the myasthenics than in controls. No difference in response to nonspecific mitogens was noted. A study by Kott et al.[192,193] suggests that "delayed hypersensitivity to muscle appears to be the most significant immune response in myasthenia gravis." By use of the leukocyte-migration technique, abnormalities of delayed hypersensitivity to muscle antigen were noted in 40 of 46 myasthenics, and by use of monkey thymus as an antigen, 21 of 42 myasthenics showed an abnormal response. Namba et al.[295] found that serum from patients with myasthenia gravis reacted with skeletal muscle membranes greater than sera obtained from controls. They also observed that lymphocytes of myasthenia gravis patients did not show greater blast transformation after addition of isolated human skeletal muscle membranes. Their studies also indicated that the proportion of T cells in myasthenia gravis patients were lower than normal. Both T and B cells increased after thymectomy. Lymphocytes from patients with myasthenia gravis were stimulated when cultured in vitro with an electric-eel extract enriched in acetylcholine receptor. No stimulation was noted with use of other antigens obtained from nerve or muscle. These findings suggest that an in vivo sensitization of lymphocytes to self–acetylcholine receptor may occur.[157]

Rose et al.[213] found a depressed lymphocyte blastogenic response to concanavalin A (Con A) in 8 of 20 patients, to phytohemagglutinin in 4 of 22 patients, to pokeweed mitogen (PWM) in 4 of 20 patients with myasthenia gravis. In the same group of patients they also found antibodies to double-stranded DNA in 3 of 22 patients and to single-stranded DNA in 9 of 20 patients. Antinuclear antibody was found in 3 of 22 patients. Antibody against normal thymocytes was seen in 20 of 22 patients, which demonstrated T-cell defects, as well as autoantibodies, which was interpreted as supporting the concept of a defect in immunoregulation. Another study[217] found that the population of T cells in the peripheral blood of myasthenics is normal and uninfluenced by thymectomy.

Strauss demonstrated antibodies to striations of skeletal muscle. The antimuscle antibodies may be directed against the sarcoplasmic reticulum of I bands.[222]

Several studies have suggested that in myasthenia gravis antibody may also exist against thymic myoid cells, thyroid, aggregated gamma globulin, parietal cells, and various cell nuclei.[223,227]

McFarlin et al.[200] found no antibody binding to the neuromuscular junction.

Using the direct labeling approach (patients' globulins were fluorescein labeled and made to react with the tissue), Kornguth[191] found antineuronal nuclear antibodies in myasthenia gravis. These studies were not confirmed by Whitaker[228] using the indirect labeling method. (The patients serum was unlabeled. After reaction between the myasthenic serum and the tissue section, fluorescein-labeled anti–human globulin was reacted with the preincubated tissue section.)

Most recently, however, Martin et al.,[198] using indirect immunofluorescence analysis, detected selective antineuronal nuclear antibodies present in the serum of some patients with myasthenia gravis. They believed that the results of Whitaker and Engel might be attributable to a nonspecific reaction of anti–human globulin with nuclei similar to that detected with commercial antiglobulin preparation or possibly that the sera of patients of Whitaker may have had a low antibody titer.

Oosterhuis[203] and later Rowland[214] found

that the presence of antibody to skeletal muscle correlates with the presence of a thymoma and with inflammatory lesions in muscle.

Patients with antimuscle antibodies have all mediated myotoxicity similar to that found in polymyositis, and the fiber of the antibody is related to the degree of lymphocyte cytotoxicity.[168]

Dawkins[169,170] has recently reviewed autoallergic myositis, myasthenia gravis, and autoimmune disease of muscle associated with immune deficiency and neoplasia.

RELATIONSHIP OF MYASTHENIA GRAVIS WITH HL-A ANTIGENS

Recently there have been numerous studies attempting to define associations between antigens of the major human transplantation or histocompatibility antigen system (the HL-A system, or the human leukocyte antigen) and specific diseases. HL-A antigens are glycoproteins with a molecular weight of about 50,000 and are found in the plasma membranes of leukocytes, as well as other types of cells. HL-A8 has been associated with myasthenia gravis[182,209,215] as well as with coeliac disease, Graves' disease, dermatitis herpetiformis, active chronic hepatitis, hayfever, and idiopathic Addison's disease.[199] HL-A8 is increased in females with early age of onset of myasthenia gravis and in addition is significantly correlated with the presence of thymic follicular hyperplasia.[182] In a recent analysis of 159 myasthenics, Pirskanen[210] also found an increase of HL-A8 in females with onset of myasthenia gravis before age 35. He also found that in myasthenics with thymic hyperplasia HL-A8 was present in 28/35 or in 73.7%. The myasthenics with HL-A8 rarely have a thymoma or autoantibodies to skeletal muscle. In contrast to patients with early-onset myasthenia gravis, those with late-onset disease show no prevalance of HL-A8 but have an increased incidence of HL-A2, HL-A3, thymoma, and antibodies to skeletal muscle,[178,210] leading Feltkamp to suggest two genetically different forms of myasthenia gravis.

Oosterhuis et al.[204] recently examined the sera of 67 patients with thymomas: 43 patients also had myasthenia gravis and 24 did not have myasthenia gravis. These sera were examined by the indirect immunofluorescence test for the presence of antibodies reacting with skeletal muscle, thyroid tissue, gastric parietal cells, adrenocortex, and antinuclear antibodies. The data were compared with 83 patients with myasthenia gravis in whom a thymoma was excluded. HL-A antigens were tested in 24 patients with thymoma plus myasthenia, in 23 of those with thymoma but without myasthenia, and in 43 of those with myasthenia but without thymoma, and in 533 controls. Antimuscle antibody was found in all patients with thymoma plus myasthenia gravis, in 42% of those with thymoma but without myasthenia, in 11% of myasthenics without thymoma, and in less than 1% of controls. Antinuclear antibodies were found in 54%, 18%, and 4%, respectively, of these groups. The frequencies of antithyroid antibodies were low and showed no differences between groups. The frequencies of HL-A8 were significantly decreased in both thymoma groups. Patients with myasthenia gravis without antimuscle antibodies did not have thymomas, a fact that should be of practical value in management of these patients.

Germinal center hyperplasia in the thymuses of some myasthenic patients was first noted by Sloan.[220] It has been reported that after thymectomy patients with proliferation of thymic germinal centers improved but those who had an atrophic thymus did not improve.[196] Alpert[159] reported that patients with many germinal centers in the thymus have a higher morbidity than thymectomized myasthenic patients whose thymuses show few germinal centers. The fact that four other studies[164,167,189,212] fail to show any definite correlation between the relative proportion of germinal centers and the degree or rapidity of improvement after thymectomy casts doubt upon the validity of basing prognosis on the determination of the number of germinal centers in the thymus.

After the observation of Blaylock,[164] in 1939, that thymectomy relieved symptoms in a patient with myasthenia gravis, numerous other reports[190,202,208,218,224-226] advocated thymectomy in selected patients.

In the Mount Sinai Hospital of New York series of patients without tumor, the indications for thymectomy are an increasing need for anticholinesterase drugs or a poor response to medications.[205]

The indications for surgery of the Liverpool group[172] are noticeable weakness and incapacity despite anticholinesterase therapy, frequent respiratory infections associated with one or more myasthenic or cholinergic crises, and recently married women who hope to have children. At the Royal Free Hospital in London[188] the operation is offered to most patients early in the course of the disease, with the exception of patients with the purely ocular form of the disease.[181] It is of note that patients with the ocular form may respond to alternate-day prednisone therapy.

It is generally accepted that the anatomic site of the abnormality in myasthenia gravis involves the neuromuscular junction, but the exact site is not settled. Considerable debate as to whether the nerve terminal[171,173] or the postsynaptic region of the muscle[186] or both[219] are the site of the lesion. An abnormality of acetylcholine receptors[175] has been found by use of alpha bungarotoxin (obtained from the snake *Bungarus multicinctus*), a specific molecular probe for the nicotinic acetylcholine receptor molecule. The alpha toxin of the Taiwanese cobra *(Naja naja atra)*, a substance believed to block acetylcholine receptors, given intravenously to rats produced electrophysiologic and pharmacologic changes typical of myasthenia gravis, a result supporting the concept that a reduction of acetylcholine receptors may play an important role in myasthenia gravis. Recent evidence indicates that the acetylcholine receptor is located postsynaptically[179,186] and therefore Satymurto et al.[216] have postulated the myasthenic abnormality as being postsynaptic.

Three possibilities about the receptor abnormality have been suggested: (1) the receptor protein is defective, (2) the receptor packing in the postsynaptic membrane is abnormal, and (3) the receptor is damaged or blocked, perhaps by an autoimmune mechanism. In regard to the last possibility, it has been observed that the globulin fraction of the sera of some myasthenic patients will show an inhibitory effect to the binding of ^{125}I-labeled bungarotoxin to the acetylcholine receptors.[158] Bender[163] has shown that sera from myasthenia gravis patients will block the alpha bungarotoxin binding to acetylcholine receptors of normal human neuromuscular junctions and to the diffuse acetylcholine receptors of denervated human fibers. Guinea pigs and rats immunized with purified eel electroplax acetylcholine receptor protein and adjuvant develop a syndrome resembling myasthenia gravis based upon physiologic and pharmacologic criteria[174,194] again suggesting a postsynaptic autoimmune disorder. Electron micrographic studies,[211] using tritiated alpha bungarotoxin to label the acetylcholine receptors of mammalian end plates, show that these receptors are distributed asymmetrically along the postsynaptic membrane, being concentrated at the fold crests—that portion nearest to the presynaptic membrane.

In regard to etiology of myasthenia gravis, it has been suggested that there is a genetically determined breakdown of immunologic tolerance[219] with immunologic damage to the motor end plates. An alternative suggestion is that it is an autoimmune disease with production of neuromuscular disease by release of a blocking substance from the thymus.

The constellation of immunologic abnormalities described have led to the use of steroid therapy in myasthenics with some success.[197]

STATUS THYMICOLYMPHATICUS[230-234]

According to the concept of status thymicolymphaticus, there is a constitutional abnormality in certain persons (usually infants and children) characterized by generalized lymphoid hyperplasia, hypoplasia of the aorta, atrophy of the adrenal glands, and underdevelopment of the gonads. Such children were supposedly subject to sudden death as a result of some trivial stimulus. It is now recognized that sudden infant deaths are attributable to other causes and not to status thymicolymphaticus.[235] The concept is now discredited, but it has left an unhappy memory. Following the original description of status thymicolymphaticus, it was found that the thymus shrunk after x-ray treatments. Large numbers of children were given x-ray therapy to the chest in order to shrink the thymus. This resulted in a high incidence of carcinoma, particularly of the thyroid and of the breast, in the treated individuals. This should serve as a warning against premature therapeutic adventures.

TUMORS
Thymoma

Tumors of the thymus are uncommon lesions. In one third of the patients, the tumors are asymptomatic and are discovered on a routine chest roentgenogram.[281] Roentgenographic features[263,303] suggesting a thymoma are an anterior mediastinal mass with an oval or lobulated shape sometimes showing calcification. Sometimes the tumor is plaque-like and closely attached to pericardium and large blood vessels. In these cases the plain chest roentgenogram may show a widening of the upper part of the mediastinal shadow on the right and left margin. In frontal and oblique views the tumor may be seen to be a peculiar shape with a slightly curved oblique upper border, ending in a more noticeable hooked lower contour. It may show a decrease in size on deep inspiration. In another third of cases the symptoms present as an anterior mediastinal mass, such as cough, dysphasia, dyspnea, retrosternal pain, or signs of compression of the superior vena cava. In one third the tumors are found in association with myasthenia gravis.

Gross features

Most thymic tumors are lobulated or multinodular and appear well encapsulated, although some are nonencapsulated and appear to extend by local invasion. There is considerable variation in size, ranging from 1 to 20 cm in diameter. The cut surfaces show varying colors of pink, gray, or yellow and show fibrous septa. Cystic degeneration is seen occasionally in larger tumors.

Histologic classification

Lattes and Jones[282] proposed a classification of thymomas into four major groups according to the predominant cell: lymphoid, spindle cell, epithelial, and rosette-forming types (Fig. 35-10).

The most common is the lymphoid type, which shows thymic lymphocytes separated into lobules by fibrous septa. Follicles and germinal centers are not seen within the tumor. Epithelial cells are singly scattered or are present in small islands of spindle-shaped or squamoid cells.

The spindle cell type is the second most common variety. It is generally believed that these cells are of epithelial origin,[251,278] although there may be two types of spindle cell tumor, with one type arising from pericytes. The cells are plump with oval vesicular nuclei. Cytoplasmic boundaries frequently are indistinct. The cells may be arranged in whorls or elongated bundles and show areas of pseudorosette formation. In some areas, there may be a cribriform or microcystic appearance. These areas also have been described as lymphangiomatous. Spindle cell thymomas are more likely to show calcification, cyst formation, and fibrosis than are other histologic types. Reticulin stains usually fail to show reticulin fibers between individual cells. Spindle cell tumors are infrequently associated with myasthenia gravis.[243,251,281,309]

In the epithelial type of thymoma, the cells are arranged in sheets. Occasional areas of palisading are seen. Individual cells are squamoid or cuboid and frequently have clear cytoplasm. There is an inconstant mixture of

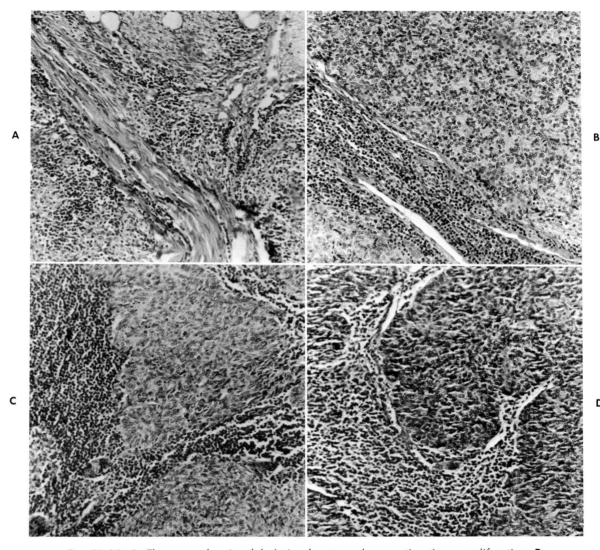

Fig. 35-10. A, Thymoma showing lobulation by stromal connective tissue proliferation. **B,** Thymoma showing rosette-forming area. **C,** Thymoma with lymphoid and epithelium-appearing areas. **D,** Thymoma with lymphoid areas and spindle cell masses.

epithelial cells and lymphocytes (Fig. 35-11). Sometimes there is a suggestion of Hassall's corpuscles. Occasionally, the cells, in part, may be arranged in an organoid pattern.

The pseudorosette is the least common pattern. In this variety, the epithelial cells appear to be arranged in clusters surrounding a central area without a true lumen.

The term "granulomatous thymoma"[256, 273,296] is now obsolete, as it is now recognized to represent Hodgkin's disease, usually of the nodular sclerosis type, of the thymus.

Prognosis

In Batata's series[242] of 54 cases at The Memorial Hospital features indicating a poor

prognosis were nonencapsulated tumor of predominantly epithelial type, a superior vena cava syndrome, malignant pleural effusion, involvement of the supraclavicular lymph nodes, dysphagia, hoarseness, myasthenia gravis, erythroid hypoplasia, and hypogammaglobulinemia. All 18 patients with completely encapsulated noninvasive lesions were considered to be benign and were treated by surgery alone. None had recurrences. This is in agreement with the experience of others indicating that benign thymomas can be treated by surgery alone.[247,252,305,309,310,322,323]

In some series[323] invasion and the presence of myasthenia gravis are considered the most important factors in evaluating prognosis with

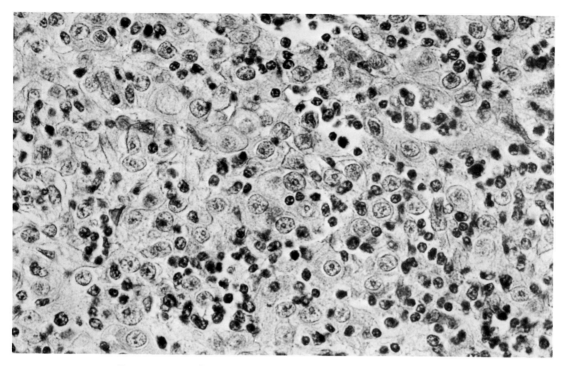

Fig. 35-11. Predominantly epithelial type of thymoma. (585×.)

invasion[271] being the most important factor. Local invasion and lymphatic spread are the two main forms of spread in malignant thymomas.[239,255,264,309]

In the series of 181 Mayo Clinic patients[243] invasion occurred in 15% of spindle cell thymomas, in 27% of lymphocytic thymomas, in 55% of predominantly epithelial thymomas, and in 60% of the mixed cell type. In this series of patients myasthenia gravis, if present, did not affect survival if the tumor was invasive but did shorten survival if there was no invasion. Others have also noted that spindle cell tumors tend to be localized and slow growing[309] but that epithelial tumors tend to be invasive.[305,309]

In addition to myasthenia gravis, thymic tumors have been associated with a number of other diseases, as follows:

1. Pure red cell aplasia (more than 50% of adults with red blood cell aplasia had thymoma and 70% of these were of spindle cell type)[236,237,257,261,267,272,291,294,307,308,317]
2. Hypogammaglobulinemia[248,262,288,292,316] and an inhibitor to antigen-induced lymphocyte transformation[261]
3. Multiple neoplasms and IgA deficiency[265]
4. Giant cell polymyositis[295]
5. Megakaryocytopenia[314]
6. Erythrocytosis[313]
7. Multiple myeloma[237,258]
8. Cushing's syndrome[268,284,289,290,301,308,321,324]
9. Pancytopenia[250,302]
10. Thyroiditis[253]
11. Lichen planus and alopecia areata[316]
12. Pemphigus erythematosus[286]
13. Autoimmune hemolytic anemia[266]
14. Monoclonal gammopathy[318]
15. Pemphigus vulgaris and internal malignancy[245,247,270,276,299,311]
16. Myositis and granulomatous myocarditis[259,280,320]
17. Meningoencephalitis[279]
18. Generalized cutaneous candidosis[240,260,287,293,312]
19. Dermatomyositis[275] with Sjögren's syndrome and scleroderma

Seminoma

A few seminomas of the thymus have been reported.[319] These resemble seminomas of the testis or dysgerminomas of the ovary. These are not always pure and may be mixed with malignant teratomatous elements.[297,298] Primary choriocarcinoma[298] and endodermal sinus tumors[300] of the anterior mediastinum have also been described. Two theories of origin of mediastinal seminomas have been proposed. According to one theory, there is faulty thymic embryogenesis (somatic aberration).[306] The other theory proposes histogenesis from germ cells.[258]

On gross examination the tumors are lobulated, with the lobules being separated by thin fibrous septa. Histologically they are composed of large numbers of round or polygonal cells with either clear or eosinophilic cytoplasm. The nuclei tend to be large, round, and hyperchromatic. Sometimes nucleoli are prominent. In some tumors, nonspecific granulomatous foci are seen. Areas of thymic tissue surrounded by tumor may be seen. Cystic degeneration may occur.

The distinction of mediastinal seminoma from epithelial thymoma is important because the former is radiosensitive[241] whereas surgery[281] is the primary form of treatment of the latter. In most cases histologic analysis is sufficient to make the correct diagnosis[269] with the presence of perivascular spaces, frequently containing lymphocytes, broad collagen trabeculae subdividing the lesions into lobules, occasional formation of rosettes, and vesicular tumor nuclei favoring the diagnosis of epithelial thymoma. The seminoma is subdivided into numerous islands by fine reticulin fibers, granulomatous inflammation may be seen, the nuclei show coarse chromatin stippling, and there is much cytoplasmic glycogen. In addition, islands of seminoma may be separated by lymphoid cells. It is advisable to fix a portion of the tumor for electron microscopy because if difficulty is encountered in the histologic diagnosis the two can be distinguished ultrastructurally,[283] with the seminoma showing regular round to partially flattened nuclei, bizarre complex nucleoli, short cytoplasmic processes, absent tonofibrils, only rare desmosomes and an absent basal lamina, relatively scanty organelles, and abundant glycogen. In contrast, the epithelial thymoma has irregular oval nuclei, relatively simple nucleoli, elongated cytoplasmic processes, and prominent tonofibrils, desmosomes, and basal lamina, in addition to well-developed organelles and absent glycogen.

Thymolipoma (lipothymoma)[244,246]

The thymolipoma is a rare benign tumor that is generally curable by local excision. The majority of reported cases have been in men. Only a few cases have been described in black people. Brown and Smith have recently reviewed the literature on thymolipomas. The tumors are composed mostly of mature fatty tissue separated into distinct lobules by bands of fibrous tissue. Some tumors are composed chiefly of lobules of thymic tissue with preservation of corticomedullary architecture and numerous Hassall's corpuscles. Although most cases are unassociated with other diseases, single case associations have been described with Graves' disease, aplastic anemia, and a pharyngeal lipoma.

Cysts

Cysts of the thymus large enough to produce symptoms are rare (Fig. 35-12). Cystic degeneration of Hassall's corpuscles is common, particularly in infections. A recent review of anterior mediastinal fat pads in several hundred autopsies revealed that small cysts measuring up to 5 mm in diameter are common (an incidence of approximately 3% in adults over 50 years of age). Since these have atrophic thymic tissue in their wall, they probably should be classified as thymic cysts. As of 1974, 34 cases of cervical thymic cyst have been described. Therefore, thymic derivatives should be included in the differential diagnosis of cystic masses in the neck.[289]

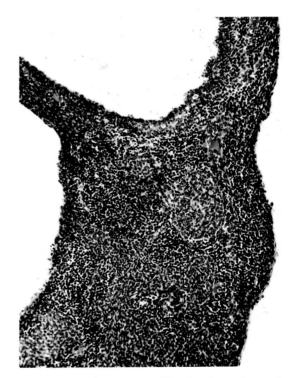

Fig. 35-12. Thymic cyst. Thymic tissue in wall shows lymphoid tissue and Hassall's bodies. (125×.)

REFERENCES
Structure and function

1 Aisenberg, A. C., Kurt, J. B., Long, J. C., and Colvin, R. B.: Blood **41**:417-423, 1973.
2 Aisenberg, A. C., Bloch, K. J., and Long, J. C.: Am. J. Med. **55**:184-191, 1973.
3 Aiuti, F., Cerottini, J. C., Coombs, R. R. A., et al.: Scand. J. Immunol. **3**:521-532, 1974.
4 Aiuti, F., Cerottini, J. C., Coombs, R. R. A., Cooper, M., Dickler, H. B., et al.: Report of a WHO committee on identification, enumeration, and isolation of band T lymphocytes from human peripheral blood, Clin. Immunol. Immunopathol. **3**:584-597, 1975.
5 Alexander, E. L., and Wetzel, B.: Science **188**:732-734, 1975.
6 Arnason, B. G., Jankovic, B. D., Waksman, B. H., and Wennersten, C.: J. Exp. Med. **116**:177-186, 1962.
7 Beletskaya, L. V., and Gnezditskaya, E. V.: Bull. Exp. Biol. Med. (of U.S.S.R.) **77**:678-681, 1974.
8 Binder, R. A., Jencks, J. A., Chun, B., and Rath, C. E.: "B" cell origin of malignant cells in a case of American Burkitt's lymphoma, Cancer **36**:161-168, 1975.
9 Bloodworth, Jr., J. M. B., Hiratsuka, H., Hickey, R. C., and Wu, J.: Pathol. Annu. **10**:329-391, 1975.
10 Borella, L., and Sen, L.: Cancer **34**:646-654, 1974.
11 Broome, J. D., Zucker-Franklin, D., Weiner, M. S., Bianco, C., and Nussenzweig, V.: Clin. Immunol. Immunopathol. **1**:319-329, 1973.
12 Brown, G., and Greaves, M. F.: Eur. J. Immunol. **4**:302-310, 1974.
13 Brown, G., and Greaves, M. F.: Scand. J. Immunol. **3**:161-172, 1974.
14 Clark, S. L.: The intrathymic environment. In Davies, A. J. S., and Carter, R. L., editors: Contemporary topics in immunobiology. Vol. 2. Thymus dependency, pp. 77-99, New York, 1973, Plenum Press.
15 Comsa, J.: The thymic hormones, Hormones **2**:226-255, 1971.
16 Cooper, M. D., Perey, D. Y., Peterson, R. D. A., Gabrielsen, A. E., and Good, R. A.: Birth defects, Original Article Ser. **IV**(1):7-16, 1968, The National Foundation, New York.
17 Cooper, M. D., Keightley, R. G., Wu, L. F., and Lawton, A. R.: Transplant Rev. **16**:51-84, 1973.
18 Dickler, H. B., and Kunkel, H. G.: J. Exp. Med. **136**:191-196, 1972.
19 Ding, J. C., Adams, P. B., Patison, M., and Cooper, I. A.: Cancer **35**:1325-1332, 1975.
20 Gell, P. G. H., and Coombs, R. R. A.: Clinical aspects of immunology, ed. 2, Philadelphia, 1968, F. A. Davis Co., pp. 575-596.
21 Glick, B., Chang, T. S., and Jaap, R. G.: Poult. Sci. **35**:224-225, 1956.
22 Goldstein, A. L., Guha, A., and Zatz, M. M., et al.: Proc. Natl. Acad. Sci. USA **69**:1800-1803, 1972.
23 Goldstein, A. L., Thurman, G. B., Cohen, G. H., and Hooper, J. A.: The role of thymosin and the endocrine thymus on the ontogenesis and function of T-cells. In Smith, E. E., and Ribbons, D. W., editors: Molecular approaches to immunology, New York, 1975, Academic Press, Inc., pp. 1-20.
24 Goldstein, A. L.: Personal communication, 1975.
25 Greaves, M. F., Owen, J. J. T., and Roff, M. D.: T and B lymphocytes, New York, 1973, American Elsevier Publishing Co., Inc.
26 Greaves, M. F., Brown, G., and Rickinson, A. B.: Clin. Immunol. Immunopathol. **4**:67-84, 1975.
27 Guha, A., Goldstein, A. L., and White, A.: Fed. Proc. **31**:418, 1972.
28 Hallberg, T.: Acta Pathol. Microbiol. Scand., Sect. C, Suppl. **250**:1-54, 1975 (extensive review).
29 Henney, C. S.: New Eng. J. Med. **291**:1357-1358, 1974.
30 Heusermann, U., Stutte, H. J., and Müller-Hermelink, H. K.: Cell Tissue Res. **153**:415-417, 1974.
31 Jankovic, B. D., Waksman, B. H., and Arnason, B. G.: J. Exp. Med. **116**:159-176, 1962.
32 Janower, M. L., and Miettinen, O. S.: J.A.M.A. **215**:753-756, 1971.
33 Jondal, M., Wigzell, H., and Aiuti, F.: Transplant Rev. **16**:163-195, 1973.
34 Kaiserling, E., Stein, H., and Müller-Hermelink, H. K.: Cell Tissue Res. **155**:47-55, 1974.
35 Kaiserling, E., and Lennert, K.: Virchows Arch. (Zellpathol.) **16**:51-61, 1974.
36 Kameya, T., and Watanabe, Y.: Acta Pathol. Jap. **15**:223-246, 1965.
37 Komuro, K., and Boyse, E. A.: Lancet **1**:740-743, 1973.
38 Lin, P. S., Cooper, A. G., and Wortis, H. H.: New Eng. J. Med. **289**:548-551, 1973.
39 Luckey, T. D., editor: Thymic hormones, Baltimore, Md., 1973, University Park Press.
40 Mann, R. B., Jaffee, E. S., Braylan, R. C., Eggleston, J. C., Ransom, L., Kaizer, H., and Berard, C. W.: Am. J. Med. **58**:307-313, 1975.
41 Marx, J. L.: Science **188**:245-247, 1975 (role of suppressor T cells in immune regulation).
42 McCluskey, R. T., and Cohen, S.: Mechanisms of cell mediated immunity, New York, 1974, John Wiley & Sons, Inc.
43 Meuwissen, H. J., Stutman, O., and Good, R. A.: Semin. Hematol. **6**:28-66, 1969 (functions of lymphocyte).
44 Miller, J. F. A. P.: Lancet **2**:748-749, 1961.
45 Morley, J., Wolstencroft, R. A., and Dumonde, D. C.: In Weir, D. M., editor: Handbook of experimental immunology, ed. 2, Oxford, 1973, Blackwell Scientific Publications, pp. 28.1-28.26.
46 Pertschuk, L. P.: Tissue Antigens **4**:446-451, 1974.
47 Pfizer, J. W., Hempelmann, L. H., Dodge, H. J., and Hodges, F. J.: Am. J. Roentgenol. Radium Ther. Nucl. Med. **103**:13-18, 1968.
48 Polliack, A., Lampen, N., Clarkson, B. D., DeHarven, E., Bentwich, Z., Siegel, F. P., and Kunkel, H. G.: J. Exp. Med. **138**:607-624, 1973.
49 Polliack, A., Fu, S. M., Douglas, S. D., Bentwick, Z., Lampen, N., and DeHarven, E.: J. Exp. Med. **140**:146-158, 1974.
50 Preud'homme, J. L., and Seligmann, M.: Blood **40**:777-794, 1972.

51 Raff, M. D.: Nature **242**:19-23, 1973.

52 Rose, N. R.: Semin. Thrombosis Hemostasis **1**:319-335, 1975.

53 Sen, L., and Borella, L.: New Eng. J. Med. **292**:828-832, 1975.

54 Touraine, J. L., Incefy, G. S., Touraine, F., et al.: Clin. Exp. Immunol. **17**:151-158, 1974.

55 Trainin, N.: Thymic hormones and the immune response, Physiol. Rev. **54**:272-315, 1974.

55a Valdes-Dapena, M.: Bull. Int. Acad. Pathol. **16**:15-25, 1975.

56 Wara, D. W., Goldstein, A. L., Doyle, .N. E., and Amman, A. J.: New Eng. J. Med. **292**:70-74, 1975.

57 Wilson, J. D., and Nossal, G.: Lancet **2**:788-791, 1971.

58 Wilson, D., and Nossal, G.: **2**:1153-1154, 1971.

59 Zucker-Franklin, D., Melton, J. W., Jr., and Quagliata, F.: Proc. Natl. Acad. Sci. U.S.A. **71**:1877-1881, 1974.

Involution

60 Davis, J. H., Reiss, E., Artz, C. P., and Amspacher, W. H.: Armed Forces Med. J. **5**:545-548, 1954 (involution after burns).

61 Fisher, E. R.: Pathology of the thymus and its relation to human disease. In Good, R. A., and Gabrielson, A. E., editors: The thymus in immunobiology, New York, 1969, Paul B. Hoeber Medical Division, Harper & Row, Publishers.

62 Henry, L.: J. Pathol. Bacteriol. **93**:661-671, 1967 (involution).

63 Henry, L.: J. Pathol. Bacteriol. **96**:337-343, 1968 (accidental involution).

Hyperplasia

64 Middleton, G.: Aust. J. Exp. Biol. Med. Sci. **45**:189-199, 1967.

65 Okabe, H.: Acta Pathol. Jap. **16**:109-130, 1966.

Immunologic deficiency diseases

66 Alper, C. A., Abramson, N., Johnston, R. B., Jr., et al.: New Eng. J. Med. **282**:349-354, 1970.

67 Alper, C. A., Abramson, N., Johnston, R. B., Jr., et al.: J. Clin. Invest. **49**:1975-1985, 1970.

68 Alper, C. A., Black, K. J., and Rosen, F. S., New Eng. J. Med. **288**:601-606, 1973.

69 Alper, C. A., Rosen, F. S., and Lachman, P. J.: Proc. Natl. Acad. Sci. U.S.A. **69**:2910-2913, 1972.

70 August, C. S., Rosen, F. S., Filler, R. M., et al.: Lancet **2**:1210-1211, 1968.

71 Ammann, A. J., Meuwissen, H. J., Good, R. A., and Hong, R.: Clin. Exp. Immunol. **7**:343-353, 1970.

72 Bachmann, R.: Scand. J. Clin. Invest. **17**:316-320, 1965.

73 Baehner, R. L., and Karnovsky, M. L.: Science **162**:1277-1279, 1968.

74 Baehner, R. L., Nathan, D. G., and Karnofsky, M. L.: J. Clin. Invest. **49**:865-870, 1970.

75 Berry, C. L., and Thompson, E. N.: Arch. Dis. Child. **43**:579-584, 1968.

76 Blaese, R. M., Strober, W., Brown, R. S., et al.: Lancet **1**:1056-1060, 1968.

77 Blume, R. S., Bennett, J. M., and Yankee, R. A.: New Eng. J. Med. **279**:1009-1015, 1968.

78 Blume, R. S., and Wolff, S. M.: Medicine **51**:247-280, 1972.

79 Boder, E., and Sedgwick, R. P.: Pediatrics **21**:526-554, 1958.

80 Bybee, J. D., and Rogers, D. E.: J. Lab. Clin. Med. **64**:1-13, 1964.

81 Cassidy, J. T., Burt, A., Petty, R., et al.: New Eng. J. Med. **280**:275, 1968.

82 Clark, R. A., and Kimball, H. R.: J. Clin. Invest. **50**:2645-2652, 1971.

83 Cleveland, W. W., Fogel, B. J., and Kay, H. E.: J. Clin. Invest. **47**:20a-21a, 1968.

84 Coen, R., Grush, O., and Kauder, E.: J. Pediatr. **75**:400-406, 1969.

85 Cooper, M. D., Chase, H. P., Lowman, J. T., et al.: Am. J. Med. **44**:499-513, 1968.

86 Cooper, M. D., Chase, H. P., Lowman, J. T., Krivit, W., and Good, R. A.: Birth Defects, Original Article Ser. **IV**(1):378-387, 1968, The National Foundation, New York.

87 Cooper, M. D., Faulk, W. P., Fudenberg, H. H., Good, R. A., Hitzig, W., Kunkel, H. G., Roitt, I. M., Rosen, F. S., Seligmann, M., and Soothill, J. F.: New Eng. J. Med. **288**:966-967, 1973.

88 Cottier, H., Turk, J., and Sobin, L.: Bull. WHO **47**:375-408, 1972.

89 Crabbe, P. A., and Heremans, J. F.: Am. J. Med. **42**:319-326, 1967.

90 deVaal, O. M., and Seynhaeve, V.: Lancet **2**:1123-1125, 1959.

91 DiGeorge, A. M.: Discussion of Cooper, M. D., Peterson, R. D. A., and Good, R. A.: J. Pediatr. **67**:907-908, 1965.

92 Dossett, J. H., Williams, R. C., and Quie, P.: Pediatrics **44**:49-57, 1969.

93 Eisen, A. H., Karpati, G., Laszlo, T., Andermann, F., Robb, J. P., and Bacal, H. L.: New Eng. J. Med. **272**:18-22, 1965.

94 Forman, M. L., and Stiehm, E. R.: New Eng. J. Med. **281**:926-931, 1969.

95 Fulginiti, V. A., Hathaway, W. E., Pearlman, D. S., Blackburn, W. R., Reiquam, C. W., Githens, J. H., Chamand, H. N., and Kempe, C. H.: Lancet **2**:5-8, 1966.

96 Gatti, R. A., Meuwissen, H. J., Allen, H. D., et al.: Lancet **2**:1366-1369, 1968.

97 Giedion, A., and Scheidegger, J. J.: Helvet. Paediatr. Acta **12**:241-259, 1957.

98 Gilbert, C., and Hong, R.: Am. J. Med. **37**:602-609, 1964.

99 Gitlin, D., Vanter, G., and Craig, J. M.: Pediatrics **32**:517-530, 1963.

100 Hitzig, W. H., and Willi, K.: Schweiz. Med. Wochenschr. **91**:1625-1633, 1961.

101 Holmes, B., Park, B. H., Malawista, S. E., et al.: New Eng. J. Med. **283**:217-221, 1970.

102 Hook, E. W., Campbell, C. G., Weens, H. S., et al.: New Eng. J. Med. **257**:403-407, 1957.

103 Jacobs, J. C., and Miller, M. E.: Pediatrics **49**:225-232, 1972.

104 Janeway, C. A., and Gitlin, D.: Adv. Pediatr. **9**:65-136, 1957.

105 Jeunet, F. S., and Good, R. A.: Birth Defects, Original Article Ser. **IV**(1):192-206, 1968, The National Foundation, New York.

106 Johnston, R. B., Jr., and Baehner, R. L.: Pediatrics **48**:730-739, 1971.

107 Klebanoff, S. J., and White, L. R.: New Eng. J. Med. **280**:460-466, 1969.

108 Kretschmer, R., Burhan, S., Brown, D., and Rosen, F. S.: New Eng. J. Med. **279**:1295-1301, 1968.

109 Lehrer, R. I., and Cline, M. J.: J. Clin. Invest. **48**:1478-1488, 1969.

110 Leikin, S. L., Bazelon, M., and Parks, K. H.: J. Pediatr. **68**:477-479, 1966.

111 Levey, R. H., Gelfand, E. W., Batchelor, J. R., et al.: Lancet **2**:571-575, 1971.

112 Levin, A. S., Spitzler, L. E., Stiles, D. P., et al.: Proc. Natl. Acad. Sci. U.S.A. **67**:821-828, 1970.

113 Lux, S. E., Johnston, R. B., Jr., August, C. S., et al.: New Eng. J. Med. **282**:231-236, 1970.

114 Matsaniotis, N., and Economou-Mavrou, C.: Pediatrics **34**:138-139, 1964.

115 McCracken, G. H., Jr., and Shinefeld, H. R.: Am. J. Dis. Child **112**:33-39, 1966.

116 McCracken, G. H., Jr., and Eichenwald, H. F.: Am. J. Dis. Child. **121**:120-126, 1971.

117 McFarlane, H.: Lancet **2**:1146-1147, 1971.

118 Middleton, G.: Aust. J. Exp. Biol. Med. Sci. **45**:189-199, 1967.

119 Miller, M. E., Seals, J., Kaye, R., et al.: Lancet **2**:60-63, 1968.

120 Miller, M. E., and Nilsson, U. R.: New Eng. J. Med. **282**:354-358, 1970.

121 Miller, M. E., Oski, F. A., and Harris, M. B.: Lancet **1**:665-669, 1971.

122 Miller, M. E., and Baker, L.: J. Pediatr. **81**:979-982, 1972.

123 Miller, M. E., Norman, M. E., Koblenzer, P. J., et al.: J. Lab. Clin. Med. **82**:1-8, 1973.

124 Mowat, A. G., and Baum, J.: New Eng. J. Med. **284**:621-627, 1971.

125 Nezelof, C., Jammet, M. L., Lortholary, P., et al.: Arch. Franc. Pediatr. **21**:897-920, 1964.

126 Oppenheim, J. J., Barlow, M., Waldman, T. A., and Block, J. B.: Br. Med. J. **2**:330-333, 1966.

127 Pearson, H. A., Spencer, R. P., and Cornelius, E. A.: New Eng. J. Med. **281**:923-926, 1969.

128 Perillie, P. E., Nolan, J. P., and Finch, S. C.: J. Lab. Clin. Med. **59**:1008-1015, 1962.

129 Peterson, R. D. A., Kelley, W. D., and Good, R. A.: Lancet **1**:1189-1193, 1964.

130 Peterson, R. D. A., Cooper, M. D., and Good, R. A.: Am. J. Med. **41**:343-359, 1966.

131 Peterson, R. D. A., and Good, R. A.: Birth Defects, Original Article Ser. **IV**(1):370-377, 1968, The National Foundation, New York.

132 Pump, K. K., Dunn, H. G., and Meuwissen, H.: Dis. Chest **47**:473-486, 1965.

133 Purtilo, D. T., and Connor, D. H.: Arch. Dis. Childhood **50**:149-152, 1975.

134 Pyke, K. W., Dosch, H.-M., Ipp, M. M., and Gelfand, E. W.: New Eng. J. Med. **293**:424-428, 1973.

135 Quie, P. G., White, J. G., and Holmes, B.: J. Clin. Invest. **46**:668-679, 1967.

136 Reed, W. B., Epstein, W. L., Boder, E., and Sedgwick, R.: J.A.M.A. **195**:746-753, 1966.

137 Robbins, J. B., and Pearson, H. A.: J. Pediatr. **66**:877-882, 1965.

138 Robinson, M. G., and Watson, R. J.: New Eng. J. Med. **274**:1006-1008, 1966.

139 Robinson, H. B., Jr.: Review of pathology and pathogenesis of DiGeorge's syndrome, Perspect. Pediatr. Pathol. **2**:173-206, 1975.

140 Rockey, J. H., Hanson, L. A., Heremans, J. F., et al.: J. Lab. Clin. Med. **63**:205-212, 1964.

141 Root, R. K., Rosenthal, A. S., and Balestra, D. J.: J. Clin. Invest. **51**:649-665, 1972.

142 Rosen, F. S., Kevy, S. V., Merler, E., et al.: Pediatrics **28**:182-195, 1961.

143 Rosen, F. S., and Janeway, C. A.: New Eng. J. Med. **275**:709-715, 1966.

144 Rosenthal, I. M., Markowitz, A. S., and Medinis, R.: Am. J. Dis. Child. **110**:69-75, 1965.

145 Rubenstein, A., Speck, B., and Jeannet, M.: New Eng. J. Med. **285**:1399-1402, 1967.

146 Smith, C. W., Hollers, J. C., and Dupree, E.: J. Lab. Clin. Med. **79**:878-885, 1972.

147 Smythe, P. M., Schomland, M., Brereton-Stiles, G. G., Cooradia, H. M., et al.: Lancet **2**:939-943, 1971.

148 Soothill, J. F., Hayes, K., and Dudgeon, J. O.: Lancet **1**:1385-1388, 1966.

149 Soriano, R. B., South, M. A., Goldman, A. S., et al.: J. Pediatr. **83**:951-958, 1973.

150 Steiner, M. L., and Pearson, H. A.: J. Pediatr. **68**:562-568, 1966.

151 Schur, P. H., Borel, H., Gelfand, E. W., Alper, C. A., and Rosen, F. S.: New Eng. J. Med. **283**:631-636, 1970.

152 Stiehm, E. R., Lawlor, G. J., Kaplan, M. S., et al.: New Eng. J. Med. **286**:797-803, 1972.

153 Stossel, T. P., Root, R. K., and Vaughan, M.: New Eng. J. Med. **286**:120-123, 1972.

154 Vyas, G. N., Perkins, H. A., and Fudenberg, H. H.: Lancet **2**:312-315, 1968.

155 Winkelstein, J. A., and Drachman, R. H.: Pediatr. Clin. North Am. **21**:551-569, 1974 (review article).

Relationship of thymus to myasthenia gravis

156 Abdou, N. I., Lisak, R. P., Zweiman, B., Abrahamsohn, I., and Penn, A. S.: New Eng. J. Med. **291**:1271-1275, 1975.

157 Abramsky, O., Aharonov, A., Webb, C., and Fuchs, S.: Clin. Exp. Immunol. **19**:11-16, 1975.

158 Almon, R. R., Andrew, C. G., and Appel, S. H.: Science **186**:55-57, 1974.

159 Alpert, L. I., Papatestas, A. E., Kark, A. E., et al.: Arch. Pathol. **91**:55-61, 1971.

160 Armstrong, R. M., Nowak, R. M., and Falk, R. E.: Neurology **23**:1078-1083, 1973.

161 Barton, F. E., and Branch, C. F.: J.A.M.A. **109**:2044-2048, 1937.

162 Behan, P. O., Simpson, J. A., and Dick, H.: Lancet **2**:1033, 1973.

163 Bender, A. N., Ringel, S. P., Engel, W. K., Daniels, M. P., and Vogel, Z.: Lancet **1**:607-609, 1975.

164 Blaylock, A., Mason, M. F., and Morgan, H. J., et al.: Ann. Surg. **110**:544-561, 1939.

165 Buckberg, G. D., Herrmann, C., Dillon, J. B., and Mulder, D. G.: J. Thorac. Cardiovasc. Surg. **53**:401-411, 1967.

166 Buzzard, E. F.: Brain **28**:438-483, 1905.

167 Castleman, B., and Norris, E. H.: Medicine (Balt.) **28**:27-58, 1949.

168 Dawkins, R. L., Robinson, J., and Wetherall, J. D.: In Bradley, G., Gardener, D., and Walton, J. N., editors: Recent advances in myology, Third International Congress on Muscle Diseases, Amsterdam, 1975, Excerpta Medica Foundation (ICS no. 360).

169 Dawkins, R. L., and Zelko, P. J.: Lancet **1**:200-202, 1975.

170 Dawkins, R. L.: Clin. Exp. Immunol. 21:185-201, 1975.

171 Desmedt, J. E.: In Desmedt, J. E., editor: New developments in EMG and clinical neurophysiology, Basel, 1973, S. Karger AG.

172 Edwards, F. R., and Wilson, A.: Thorax 27:513-516, 1972.

173 Elmqvist, D., Hofman, W. W., Kugelberg, J., and Quastel, D. M. J.: J. Physiol. 174:417-434, 1964.

174 Engel, A. G., Tsujihata, M., Lambert, E. H., Lindstrom, J. M., and Lennon, V. A.: Ann. N.Y. Acad. Sci. 274:60-79, 1976.

175 Fambrough, D. M., Drachman, D. B., and Satyamurti, S.: Science 182:293-294, 1973.

176 Feltkamp, T. E. W., van den Berg-Loonen, P. M., Nijenhuis, L. E., et al.: Relations between HL-A antigens, myasthenia gravis and autoantibodies. In Kunze, K., and Desmedt, J. E., editors: Studies on neuromuscular diseases, Proceedings of an International Symposium, Giessen, 1973; Basel, 1973, S. Karger AG.

177 Feltkamp, T. E. W., van den Berg-Loonen, P. M., Nijenhuis, L. E., Engelfriet, C. P., van Rossum, A. L., van Loghem, J. J., and Oosterhuis, H. J. G. H.: Br. Med. J. 1:131-133, 1974.

178 Feltkamp, T. E. W., van den Berg-Loonen, P. M., Oosterhuis, H. J. G. H., et al.: In Bradley, G., Gardener, D., and Walton, J. N., editors: Recent advances in myology, Third International Congress on Muscle Diseases, Amsterdam, 1975, Excerpta Medica Foundation (ICS no. 360).

179 Fertuck, H. C., and Salpeter, M. M.: Proc. Natl. Acad. Sci. U.S.A. 71:1376-1378, 1974.

180 Fields, W. S.: Ann. N.Y. Acad. Sci. 183:3-4, 1971.

181 Fischer, K. C., and Schwartzman, R. J.: Neurology 24(2):795-798, 1974.

182 Fritze, D., Naeim, F., Herrmann, C., Jr., Smith, G. S., and Walford, R. L.: Lancet 1:240-243, 1974.

183 Goldstein, G., and Whittingham, S.: Lancet 2:315-318, 1966.

184 Goldstein, G., and Manganaro, A.: Ann. N.Y. Acad. Sci. 183:230-240, 1971.

185 Goust, J. M., Castaigne, A., and Moulias, R.: Clin. Exp. Immunol. 18:39-47, 1974.

186 Grob, D., and Johns, R. J.: In Viets, H. R., editor: Myasthenia gravis, Springfield, Ill., 1961, Charles C Thomas, Publisher, p. 127.

187 Grob, D., and Namba, T.: Ann. N.Y. Acad. Sci. 274:143-173, 1976.

188 Havard, W. H.: Br. Med. J. 3:437-440, 1973.

189 Henson, R. A., Stern, M., and Thompson, V. C.: Brain 88:11-28, 1965.

190 Keynes, G.: Lancet 266:1197-1202, 1954.

191 Kornguth, S. E., Hanson, J. C., and Chun, R. W. M.: Neurology (Minneap.) 20:749-755, 1970.

192 Kott, E., and Rule, A. H.: Neurology (Minneap.) 23:745-748, 1973.

193 Kott, E., Genkins, G., and Rule, A. H.: Neurology (Minneap.) 23:374-380, 1974.

194 Lennon, V. A., Lindstrom, J. M., and Seybold, M. E.: J. Exp. Med. 141:1365-1375, 1975.

195 Lisak, R. P., Abdou, N. I., Zweiman, B., Zmijewski, C. M., and Penn, A. S.: Ann. N.Y. Acad. Sci. 274:402-410, 1976.

196 Mackay, I. R., Whittingham, S., and Goldstein, G., et al.: Aust. Ann. Med. 17:1-11, 1968.

197 Mann, J. D., Johns, T. R., Campa, J. F., and Muller, W. H.: Ann. N.Y. Acad. Sci. 274:608-622, 1976.

198 Martin, L., Herr, J. C., Wanamaker, W., and Kornguth, S.: Neurology (Minneap.) 24:680-683, 1974.

199 McDevitt, H. O., and Bodmer, W. F.: Lancet 1:1269-1275, 1974 (review of HL-A antigens in association with various disease states).

200 McFarlin, D. E., Engel, W. K., and Strauss, A. J. L.: Ann. N.Y. Acad. Sci. 135:656-663, 1966

201 Mendell, J. R., Whitaker, J. N., and Engel, W. K.: J. Immunol. 111:847-856, 1973.

202 Mulder, D. G., Braitman, H., and Li Wei-I: J. Thorac. Cardiovasc. Surg. 63:109-113, 1972.

203 Oosterhuis, H. J., Bethlem, J., and Feltkamp, T. E. W.: J. Neurosurg. Psychiatry 31:460-463, 1968.

204 Oosterhuis, H. J., Feltkamp, T. E. W., van Rossum, A. L., van den Berg-Loonen, P. M., and Nijenhuis, L. E.: Ann. N.Y. Acad. Sci. 274:468-474, 1976.

205 Papatestas, A. E., Alpert, L. I., Osserman, K. E., Osserman, R. S., and Kark, A. E.: Am. J. Med. 50:465-474, 1971.

206 Patrick, J., and Lindstrom, J.: Science 180:871-872, 1973.

207 Penn, A. S., Schotland, D. L., and Rowland, L. P.: Res. Publ. Assoc. Res. Nerv. Ment. Dis. 49:215-240, 1971.

208 Perlo, V. P., Poskanzer, D. C., Schwab, R. S., Viets, H. R., Osserman, K. E., and Genkins, G.: Neurology (Minneap.) 16:431-439, 1966.

209 Pirskanen, R., Tiilikainen, A., and Hokkanen, E.: Ann. Clin. Res. 4:304-306, 1972.

210 Pirskanen, R.: Ann. N.Y. Acad. Sci. 274:451-460, 1976.

211 Porter, C. W., and Barnard, E. A.: Ann. N.Y. Acad. Sci. 274:85-107, 1976.

212 Reinglass, J. S., and Brickel, A. C. J.: Neurology (Minneap.) 23:69-72, 1973.

213 Rose, J. W., Huang, S. W., and Mayer, R. F.: Abstract presented at American Neurologic Association, 1975.

214 Rowland, L. P., Lisak, R. P., Schotland, D. L., De Jesus, P. V., and Berg, P.: Neurology (Minneap.) 23:282-288, 1973.

215 Safwenberg, J., Lindblom, J. B., and Osterman, P. O.: Tissue Antigens 3:465-469, 1973.

216 Satyamurti, L., Drachman, D. B., and Sloan, F.: Science 187:955-957, 1975.

217 Sandilands, G. P., Gray, K., Cooney, A., Anderson, J. R., Simpson, J. A., and Behan, P. O.: Lancet 1:171-172, 1975.

218 Schwab, R. S., Wilkins, E. W., Head, J. M., Pontoppidan, H., and Viets, H. R.: J.A.M.A. 187:850-851, 1964.

219 Simpson, J. A.: Scott. Med. J. 5:419-436, 1960.

220 Sloan, H. E., Jr.: Surgery 13:154-174, 1943.

221 Strauss, A. J. L., Seegal, B. C., and Hsu, K. C., et al.: Proc. Soc. Exp. Biol. Med. 105:185-191, 1960.

222 Strauss, A. J. L.: Adv. Intern. Med. 14:241-280, 1968.

223 Starber, F. G., Fink, U., and Sack, W.: New Eng. J. Med. **292**:1032-1033, 1975.
224 Viets, H.: J.A.M.A. **153**:1273-1280, 1953.
225 Viets, H.: Am. J. Med. **19**:658-660, 1955.
226 Viets, H. R., and Schwab, R. S.: Thymectomy for myasthenia gravis, Springfield, Ill., 1960, Charles C Thomas, Publisher.
227 White, R. G., and Marshal, A. H. E.: Lancet **2**:120-123, 1962.
228 Whitaker, J. N., and Engel, W. K.: Neurology (Minneap.) **24**:61-63, 1974.
229 Zeldowicz, L. R., and Saxton, G. D.: Can. Med. Assoc. J. **101**:609-613, 1969.

Status thymicolymphaticus

230 Conti, E. A., Patton, G. D., Conti, J. E., and Hempelmann, L. H.: Radiology **74**:386-391, 1960.
231 Friedlander, A.: Arch. Pediatr. **24**:490-501, 1907.
232 Saenger, E. L., Silverman, F. N., Sterling, T. D., and Turner, M. E.: Radiology **74**:889-904, 1960.
233 Simpson, C. L., and Hempelmann, L. H.: Cancer **10**:42-56, 1957.
234 Simpson, C. L., Hempelmann, L. H., and Fuller, L. M.: Radiology **64**:840-845, 1955.
235 Valdes-Dapena, M.: Bull. Int. Acad. Pathol. **16**:15-25, 1975.

Tumors

236 Al-Mondhiry, H., Zanjani, E. D., Spisak, M., Zalusky, R., and Gordon, A. S.: Blood **38**:576-582, 1971.
237 Andersen, E. T., and Vye, M. V.: Ann. Intern. Med. **66**:141-149, 1967.
238 Andersen, S. B., and Ladefoged, J.: Acta Haematol. (Basel) **30**:319-325, 1963.
239 Andritsakis, G. D., and Sommers, S. C.: J. Thorac. Surg. **37**:273-290, 1959.
240 Baer, R. L., Bart, R. S., Stritzler, R. L., et al.: Hautarzt **15**:413-418, 1964.
241 Bagshaw, M. A., McLaughlin, W. T., and Earle, J. D.: Am. J. Roentgenol. **105**:86-94, 1969.
242 Batata, M. A., Martini, N., Huvos, A. G., Aguilar, R. I., and Beattie, E. J., Jr.: Cancer **34**:389-396, 1974.
243 Bernatz, P. E., Khonsari, S., Harrison, E. G., Jr., and Taylor, W. F.: Surg. Clin. North Am. **53**:885-892, 1973.
244 Bernstein, A., Klosk, E., Simon, F., and Brodkin, H. A.: Circulation **3**:508-513, 1951.
245 Beutner, E. H., Chorzelski, T. P., and Jordan, R.: Autosensitization in pemphigus and bullous pemphigoid, Springfield, Ill., 1970, Charles C Thomas, Publisher, pp. 85-86.
246 Boetsch, C. H., Swoyer, G. B., Adams, A., and Walker, J. H.: Dis. Chest **50**:539-543, 1966.
247 Braitman, H., Herrmann, C., Jr., and Mulder, D. G.: Arch. Surg. **103**:14-16, 1971.
248 Brasher, G. W., Howard, P. H., Jr., and Brindley, G. V., Jr.: Surg. Clin. North Am. **52**:429-438, 1972.
249 Brown, W., and Smith, S. B.: (Submitted for publication.)
250 Burrows, S., and Caroll, R.: Arch. Pathol. **92**:465-468, 1971.
251 Castleman, B.: In Atlas of tumor pathology, Sec. V, Fasc. 19, Washington, D.C., 1955, Armed Forces Institute of Pathology.
252 Cohn, L. H., and Grimes, D. F.: Surg. Gynecol. Obstet. **131**:206-216, 1970.
253 Dawson, M. A.: Am. J. Med. **52**:406-410, 1972.
254 Edland, R. W., Levine, S., Serfas, L. S., and Flair, R. C.: Am. J. Roentgenol. **103**:25-31, 1968.
255 Effler, D. B., and McCoronack, L. J.: J. Thorac. Surg. **31**:60-82, 1956.
256 Fechner, R. E.: Cancer **23**:16-23, 1969.
257 Fernandez, B. B., and Hartman, C.: Ill. Med. J. **145**:121-124, 1974.
258 Friedman, N. B.: Cancer **4**:265-276, 1951.
259 Funkhouser, J. W.: New Eng. J. Med. **264**:34-36, 1961.
260 Gafni, J., Michaeli, D., and Heller, H.: New Eng. J. Med. **263**:536-541, 1960.
261 Geary, C. B., Byron, P. R., Taylor, G., MacIver, J. E., and Zervas, J.: Br. J. Haematol. **29**:479-486, 1975.
262 Good, R. A.: Bull. Univ. Minn. Hosp. **26**:1-19, 1954.
263 Good, C. A.: Am. J. Roentgenol. Radium Ther. Nucl. Med. **57**:305-312, 1947.
264 Guillan, R. A., Zelman, S., and Iglesias, P. A.: Cancer **27**:823-830, 1971.
265 Hamoudi, A. B., Ertel, I., Newton, W. A., Jr., Reiner, C. B., and Clatsworthy, H. W., Jr.: Cancer **33**:1134-1144, 1974.
266 Hennemann, H. H., and Beck, T.: Dtsch. Med. Wochenschr. **99**:1869-1871, 1974.
267 Hirst, E., and Robertson, T. I.: Medicine (Balt.) **46**:225-264, 1947.
268 Hubble, D.: Q. J. Med. **18**:133-147, 1949.
269 Iverson, L.: Am. J. Pathol. **32**:695-719, 1956.
270 Jablonska, S., Chorzelski, T., and Blaszyk, M.: Br. J. Dermatol. **83**:315-323, 1970.
271 Jain, U., and Frable, W. J.: J. Thorac. Cardiovasc. Surg. **67**:310-321, 1974.
272 Jepson, J. H., and Vas, M.: Cancer Res. **34**:1325-1334, 1974.
273 Katz, A., and Lattes, R.: Cancer **23**:1-15, 1969.
274 Kough, R., and Barnes, W. T.: Ann. Intern. Med. **61**:308-315, 1964.
275 Klein, J. J., Gottlieb, A. J., Mones, R. J., Oppel, S. H., and Osserman, K. E.: Arch. Intern. Med. **113**:142-152, 1964.
276 Krain, L. S.: Br. J. Dermatol. **90**:397-405, 1974.
277 Krain, L. S., and Bierman, S. M.: Cancer **33**:1091-1099, 1974.
278 Kuhn, C., and Rosai, J.: Arch. Pathol. **88**:653-663, 1969.
279 Lambie, J. A., and Pilot, R.: J. Lancet **88**:315-318, 1968.
280 Langeton, J. D., Wagman, G. F., and Dickeman, R. C.: Arch. Pathol. **68**:367-373, 1959.
281 Lattes, R.: Cancer **15**:1224-1260, 1962.
282 Lattes, R., and Jonas, S.: Bull. N.Y. Acad. Med. **33**:145-147, 1957.
283 Levine, G. D., and Bensch, K. G.: Cancer **31**:729-741, 1973.
284 Leyton, O., Turnbull, M., and Bratton, A. B.: J. Pathol. Bacteriol. **34**:635-660, 1931.
285 Lindstrom, F. D., Williams, R. C., and Brunning, R. D.: Arch. Intern. Med. **122**:526-531, 1968.
286 Lynfield, Y. L., Pertschuk, L. P., and Zimmerman, A.: Arch. Dermatol. **108**:690-693, 1973.

287 Maize, J. C., and Lynch, P. J.: Arch. Dermatol. **105**:96-98, 1972.

288 Mallinson, W. J., and Beck, E. R.: Proc. Roy. Soc. Med. **64**:1305-1306, 1971.

289 Mikal, S.: Arch. Surg. **109**:558-562, 1974.

290 Miura, K., Sasaki, C., Katsushima, I., Ohtoma, T., Sato, S., et al.: J. Clin. Endocrinol. **27**:631-637, 1967.

291 Miyata, M., Matsuyama, R., Ito, T., and Yoshiki, T.: Acta Haematol. Jap. **34**:438-451, 1971.

292 Monagen, E. S., Kern, W. A., and Terry, R.: Ann. Intern. Med. **65**:548-554, 1966.

293 Montes, L. F., Carter, E., Moreland, N., and Aballos, R.: J.A.M.A. **204**:351-354, 1968.

294 Murray, W. D., and Webb, J. N.: Am. J. Med. **41**:974-980, 1966.

295 Namba, T., and Brunner, N. G.: Arch. Neurol. **31**:27-30, 1974.

296 Nickels, J., Franssila, K., and Hjelt, L.: Acta Pathol. Microbiol. Scand., Sect. A. **81**:1-5, 1973.

297 Oberman, H. A., and Libcke, J. H.: Cancer **17**:498-507, 1964.

298 Pachter, M. R., and Lattes, R.: Dis. Chest **45**:301-310, 1964.

299 Peck, S. M., Osserman, K. E., Weiner, L. B., et al.: New Eng. J. Med. **279**:951-958, 1968.

300 Pederson, H.: Acta Pathol. Microbiol. Scand., Suppl. **212**:128-142, 1970.

301 Pimstone, B. L., Uys, C. J., and Vogelpoel, L.: Am. J. Med. **53**:521-528, 1972.

302 Rogers, B. H. G., Manaligod, J. R., and Blazer, W. V.: Am. J. Med. **44**:154-164, 1968.

303 Rosenthal, T., Hertz, M., Samra, Y., and Shakin, N.: Chest **65**:428-430, 1974.

304 Rundle, L. D., and Sparks, F. P.: Arch. Pathol. **75**:276-283, 1963.

305 Sawyers, J. L., and Foster, J. H.: Arch. Surg. **96**:814-817, 1968.

306 Schlumberger, H. G.: Arch. Pathol. **41**:398-444, 1946.

307 Schmid, J. R., Kiely, J. M., Harrison, E. G., Jr., Bayrd, G. L., and Peas, G. L.: Cancer **18**:216-230, 1965.

308 Scholz, D. A., and Bahn, R. C.: Mayo Clin. Proc. **34**:433-441, 1959.

309 Sellors, T. H., Thackery, A. C., and Thomson, A. D.: Thorax **22**:193-220, 1967.

310 Shields, T. W., Fox, R. T., and Lees, M. W.: Arch. Surg. **92**:617-622, 1966.

311 Stillman, M. A., and Baer, R. I.: Acta Dermatol. Venereol. (Stockh.) **52**:393-397, 1972.

312 Stillman, M. A., and Baer, R. L.: J.A.M.A. **224**:628-629, 1973.

313 Sundstrom, C., Lundberg, D., and Werner, I.: Acta Pathol. Microbiol. Scand. **80**:487-490, 1972.

314 Sundstrom, C.: Acta Pathol. Microbiol. Scand. **80**:235-240, 1972.

315 Takigawa, M., and Hayakawa, M.: Arch. Dermatol. **110**:99-102, 1974.

316 Tan, R. S.: Proc. Roy. Soc. Med. **67**:196-198, 1974.

317 Teoh, P. C., Tan, D. K., DaCosta, J. L., and Chew, B. K.: Med. J. Aust. **2**:373-376, 1973.

318 Tsunematsu, K., Nagese, K., Maekawa, I., Shiraishi, T., and Nakamura, K.: Acta Haematol. Jap. **34**:468-474, 1971.

319 Viets, H.: Med. Hist. **9**:184-186, 1965.

320 Waller, J. V., Shapiro, M., and Paultauf, R.: Am. Heart J. **53**:479-484, 1957.

321 Warter, J., Batzenschlager, A., Asch, L., and Wiederkehr, J. L.: Presse Med. **73**:1831-1834, 1965.

322 Watson, R. R., Weisel, W., and O'Connor, T. M.: Arch. Surg. **97**:230-238, 1968.

323 Wilkins, E. W., Edmunds, L. H., and Castleman, B.: J. Thorac. Cardiovasc. Surg. **52**:322-330, 1966.

324 Yalow, R. S., and Berson, S. A.: Biochem. Biophys. Res. Comm. **44**:439-445, 1971.

36/Pituitary gland

NANCY E. WARNER

EMBRYOLOGY

The pituitary gland arises from two quite separate primordia that meet and join early in embryonic life to form the definitive organ. The adenohypophysis, or anterior lobe, is an ectodermal derivative that arises from Rathke's pouch, a midline diverticulum of the roof of the stomodeum, or primitive buccal cavity. The pouch grows upward through the transient craniopharyngeal canal to fuse with the infundibulum, the downgrowth from the floor of the diencephalon that forms the neurohypophysis. By rupture of its attachment, Rathke's pouch loses its connection with the roof of the pharynx and comes to lie within the developing sphenoid bone. Cells of Rathke's pouch proliferate to form the adenohypophysis; thus the lumen of the pouch is reduced to a narrow cleft, which eventually is obliterated, though remnants may persist as small cysts. The anterior part of the pouch becomes the definitive pars distalis. An upward extension of the developing adenohypophysis forms a cuff that surrounds the pituitary stalk, known as the pars tuberalis. The portion of the pouch that lies in contact with the neurohypophysis becomes the pars intermedia, which thus is delimited by the cleft from the developing pars distalis. In the human, the pars intermedia remains rudimentary. The developing neurohypophysis differentiates into the infundibulum, the infundibular stem (or stalk), and the infundibular process, or neural lobe. Whereas the adenohypophysis loses its connection with the pharynx as the craniopharyngeal canal closes, the neurohypophysis permanently retains direct connections with the brain by the infundibular stalk (Fig. 36-1).

The adenohypophysis of the human fetus begins to produce growth hormone sometime between the twelfth and seventeenth week of pregnancy, as demonstrated by immunofluorescent staining (Fig. 36-2). Hormones produced by the fetal hypophysis appear to have a crucial role in normal development of the thyroid and adrenal glands, since (1) congenital absence or hypoplasia of the human anterior lobe invariably leads to hypoplasia of thyroid and adrenals, and (2) experimental destruction of the fetal pituitary in the rat, mouse, and rabbit leads to reduction in size of the thyroid and adrenals, which can be avoided by injection of TSH or ACTH into the fetus.[5,13]

Remnants of Rathke's pouch regularly persist into postnatal life. The pharyngeal (caudal) end of the ruptured stalk of Rathke's pouch forms the pharyngeal pituitary.[3,6] The pharyngeal pituitary, which is present consistently in all age groups, is a small cylindric

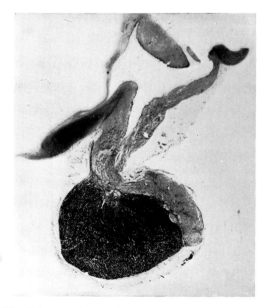

Fig. 36-1. Midsagittal section of pituitary gland to show neural attachments. (Hematoxylin and eosin; 4×; courtesy Dr. Dorothy S. Russell and Dr. A. R. Currie.)

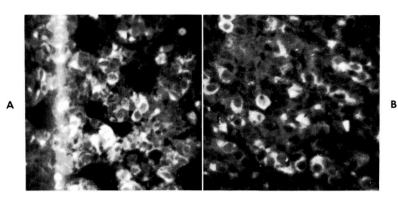

Fig. 36-2. Growth hormone–containing cells in fetal human adenohypophysis. **A,** 15-week-old fetus. **B,** 20-week-old fetus. Note increase in amount of cytoplasm with increasing age and compare with Fig. 36-5. (**A** and **B,** Indirect immunofluorescence technique; 400×; from Ellis, S. T., Beck, J. S., and Currie, A. R.: J. Pathol. Bacteriol. **92:**179-183, 1966.)

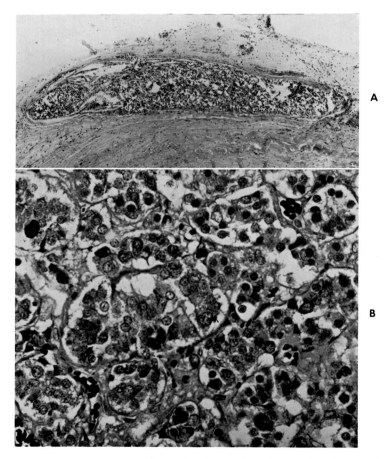

Fig. 36-3. A, Pharyngeal pituitary gland. **B,** Showing mainly chromophobe cells. (**A,** Hematoxylin and eosin, 44×; **B,** acid fuchsin and aniline blue; 350×; **A** and **B,** courtesy Dr. Dorothy S. Russell and Dr. A. R. Currie.)

body 5 to 6 mm in length, located in the midline in the midline in the roof of the nasopharynx, beneath the mucoperiosteum inferior to the vomerosphenoid junction[14] (Fig. 36-3). The extent of its function is uncertain. Other epithelial remnants include parapituitary epithelial residues, persistent Rathke's cleft within the gland, and remains of the craniopharyngeal stalk within the sphenoid bone[14]; these elements may be the source of cysts or tumors (see p. 1621).

ANATOMY

The pituitary gland in the adult is a small, bean-shaped, bilaterally symmetric organ that weighs 500 to 900 mg.[9] The gland usually is heavier in women, and its weight may reach 1100 mg or more in pregnancy[4] when hyperplasia normally occurs. The gland has two major anatomic divisions, the reddish brown adenohypophysis and the pale gray neurohypophysis. The adenohypophysis consists of the pars distalis (or pars anterior), the pars intermedia, and the pars tuberalis, which is an upward extension forming a cuff around the infundibular stem. The neurohypophysis consists of the pars nervosa (also known as the neural lobe, or infundibular process), the infundibular stem, and the infundibulum proper. The gland is attached to the brain by the stalk, which contains the nerve tracts and blood vessels, vital links to the hypothalamus. The stalk in turn merges with the infundibulum, a cone-shaped projection of the tuber cinereum of the hypothalamus; this region is referred to as the median eminence.

The pituitary gland is located in the hypophyseal fossa of the sella turcica, a midline cavity in the sphenoid bone. In this position deep inside the head, the gland is unusually well protected, but at the same time surgical approach is difficult. An extension of the dura mater lines the hypophyseal fossa and spreads out to form an incomplete covering for the sella, known as the diaphragma sellae. An extension of the leptomeninges blends with the surface of the pituitary, and a subarachnoid space of variable size may be present.

Knowledge of the anatomic relationships of the pituitary to its environs is essential in understanding the symptoms caused by pituitary tumors, which often compress the vital structures adjacent. The optic chiasm, hypothalamus, and third ventricle lie directly above the gland. Just lateral to the pituitary on each side are the cavernous sinuses, each containing the internal carotid artery and cranial nerves 3, 4, 5, and 6. Minor anatomic variations of these relationships are common, a matter of great concern to the neurosurgeon who is operating for tumor or palliative ablation of the hypophysis.[2,8]

The arterial supply of the pituitary gland is derived from the internal carotids by way of paired superior and inferior hypophyseal arteries. The neurohypophysis is supplied by direct branches of these arteries, which supply the superior and inferior regions of the neurohyphophysis, respectively.[15] In contrast, the arterial supply of the adenohypophysis is small[12] and probably insignificant.[1] Instead, the major blood supply of the adenohypophysis is derived from the hypophyseal portal system. The primary capillary bed of this portal system consists of capillaries in the infundibulum and infundibular stem; the secondary bed is the network of capillaries in the adenohypophysis.[16] The capillaries in the infundibulum and upper region of the stem are drained by the long portal veins, which course to the adenohypophysis through the stalk. The capillaries of the lower part of the stem are drained by the short portal veins, which are contained within the body of the gland. Therefore transsection of the stalk will destroy the long portal veins, but the short veins may remain intact, unless the stalk is divided at its junction with the gland.[10] The portal veins deliver blood to the secondary capillary bed of the adenohypophysis, each group of vessels supplying a specific territory in the pars distalis.[1] The capillaries of both the pars distalis and the pars nervosa drain into the dural venous sinuses surrounding the pituitary.

The neural and vascular pathways that link the hypothalamus to the pituitary warrant special consideration, since they are crucial in the regulation of the secretion of hormones by both neurohypophysis and adenohypophysis. The pathway between the hypothalamus and the neurohypophysis is a direct neural connection, the hypothalamo-hypophyseal tract, which originates from neurons in the supraoptic and paraventricular nuclei, traverses the pituitary stalk, and terminates in the pars nervosa. The supraoptic and paraventricular nuclei secrete vasopressin and oxytocin, octapeptide hormones with antidiuretic and oxytocic effects. These hormones become attached to carrier substances, the neurophysins, and are transported down the axons of the hypothalamo-hypophyseal tract to the pars nervosa,

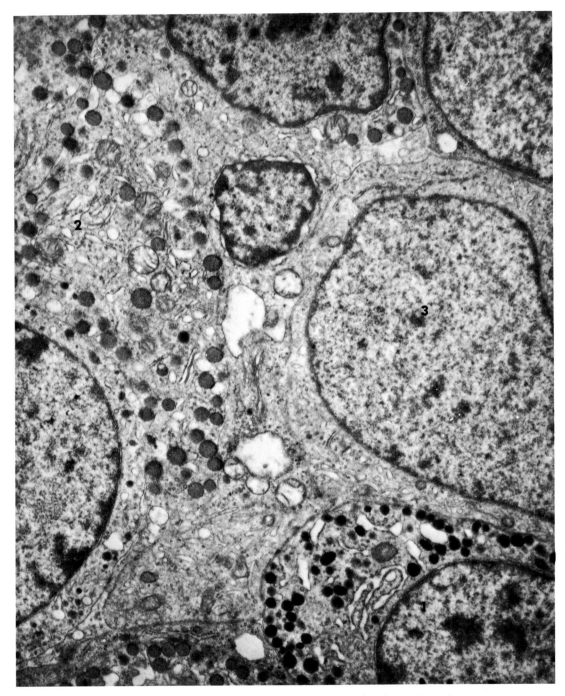

Fig. 36-4. Electron micrograph of 18-week-old fetal human adenohypophysis showing granular cells and one agranular cell. **1,** Granule size approximately 280 nm—consistent with basophil. **2,** Granule size approximately 500 nm—consistent with acidophil. **3,** Agranular—chromophobe. (Glutaraldehyde and Palade-Karnovsky; 12,600×; from Ellis, S. T.: Ph.D. thesis, University of Aberdeen; courtesy Dr. A. R. Currie.)

where they are stored prior to release into the capillaries of the neural lobe. Whereas the neurohypophysis is connected directly to the hypothalamus by a single link, the hypothalamo-hypophyseal nerve tract, the adenohypophysis is connected to the hypothalamus by a path consisting of two components, the tuberohypophyseal neural tract and the hypophyseal portal system. The tuberohypophyseal tract originates from neurons in the tuberal and other nuclei of the hypothalamus and terminates in the infundibulum, adjacent to the primary capillary beds of the hypophyseal portal system. Releasing and inhibiting factors synthesized in the cell bodies of tuberal nuclei pass down its axons and are deposited at the capillaries of the infundibulum, to be transported through the portal veins to the sinusoids of the adenohypophysis, where they control the release of hormones in the pars distalis.

The recognition of the hypothalamus as a higher center for integration of the pituitary has clarified the regulation of hypophyseal function.[7,11] That part of the hypothalamus concerned with the hormonal regulation of pituitary function has been aptly termed the "endocrine hypothalamus." The releasing and inhibiting substances produced by the endocrine hypothalamus are peptides. Those releasing substances that have been recognized to date include corticotrophin-releasing factor (CRF), thyrotrophin-releasing hormone (TRH), and luteotrophin-releasing hormone (LRH, also referred to as luteotrophic hormone–releasing factor, LH-RF). Whether LRH is the sole hypothalamic hormone regulating gonadotrophins and releasing both LH and FSH is uncertain. The inhibiting substances established at present are somatotrophin release–inhibiting factor (SRIF, or somatostatin) and prolactin-inhibiting factor (PIF). Proof of a series of hypothalamic regulating factors can be anticipated.

HISTOLOGY AND FUNCTION
Adenohypophysis

The pars distalis is composed of cords and clumps of epithelial cells separated by a network of capillaries, the secondary plexus of the hypophyseal portal bed. The capillaries are surrounded by perivascular spaces (best shown by electron microscopy) into which the secretory granules are released from the epithelial cells by exocytosis. Some of these cells are arranged in follicles, with a small central lumen containing colloid.

By light microscopy, the epithelial cells can be separated into chromophils, which have cytoplasmic secretory granules with a strong affinity for dyes, and chromophobes, smaller cells with cytoplasm having no visible granules by light microscopy, and a lesser affinity for dyes. In hematoxylin-eosin sections, three types of epithelial cells can be distinguished: chromophil cells with acidophilic granules (about 40%), chromophil cells with basophilic granules (about 10%), and chromophobe cells with no visible granules (about 50%). Efforts to subclassify the acidophils and basophils on the basis of special stains led to a succession of classifications[22,40] and resulted in chaos, principally for the reason that full understanding of functional cytology of the hypophysis was not possible without access to a broad range of techniques, some only recently available. These techniques include histochemistry, enzyme histochemistry, electron microscopy of normal (Fig. 36-4) and abnormal hypophysis, ultrastructural analysis of cytoplasmic granules obtained by ultracentrifugation, autoradiography, and the histologic

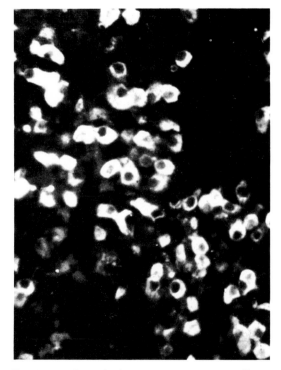

Fig. 36-5. Growth hormone–containing cells in adult human adenohypophysis. (Indirect immunofluorescence technique; 400×; from Porteous, I. B., Beck, J. S., and Currie, A. R.: J. Pathol. Bacteriol. **91:**539-543, 1966.)

Table 36-1. Cells of adenohypophysis and corresponding hormones

Hormone	Hematoxylin and eosin	Periodic acid Schiff—orange G	Herlant's Tetrachrome[28]
Simple proteins 1. STH (somatotrophic hormone, growth hormone)	*Acidophils* (α cells)	*Acidophils* Orange G+	*Somatotrophs* Orange G+
2. LTH (lactogenic hormone, mammotrophic hormone, prolactin)			*Lactotrophs* Erythrosin+ (η cell)
Mucoproteins 3. FSH (follicle-stimulating hormone) 4. ICSH (interstitial cell–stimulating hormone, luteinizing hormone, LH) 5. TSH (thyroid-stimulating hormone)	*Basophils* (β cells)	*Mucoid cells* PAS+	*Basophils*
Polypeptides 6. ACTH (adrenocorticotrophic hormone) 7. MSH (melanocyte-stimulating hormone)			
(None)	*Chromophobes*	*Chromophobes* (No visible granules)	*Chromophobes* (No visible granules)

*PM-AT-PAS-orange G = permanganate–aldehyde thionin–periodic acid Schiff–orange G.

†PFA-AB-PAS-orange G = performic acid–alcian blue–periodic acid Schiff–orange G.

analysis of antigen-antibody reactions by immunofluorescence (Fig. 36-5). In recognition of the problems in terminology, an international committee for nomenclature proposed a functional classification, in which each cell was named according to its secretory activity.[41] This functional classification has been widely accepted. Although a corresponding standard system of morphologic nomenclature has not been formally proposed yet, a tentative system gradually has emerged.[25] Previous classifications and recent developments are summarized in Table 36-1.

The designation alpha and beta granules instead of acidophil and basophil followed recognition that the staining reactions of chromophils were capricious and varied with fixation and pH of the medium. McManus[30] first reported PAS-positive granules in hypophyseal cells, and Pearse identified the adenohypophyseal cells as basophils[35] (Fig. 36-6). These discoveries marked the beginning of the histo-

chemical studies that led ultimately to the demonstration of distinct classes of basophils.

The acidophils include somatotrophs and lactotrophs, which produce STH (somatotrophic hormone) and LTH (lactogenic hormone, or prolactin), respectively. Both hormones are simple proteins. In a horizontal section of the adenohypophysis, the acidophils are localized in the lateral wings.[25, 33] Acidophils are identified readily by their affinity for eosin and other acid dyes, such as orange G, erythrosin, and carmoisine.[19] Differentiation between the somatotrophs and the lactotrophs is based upon simultaneous use of orange G and erythrosin or carmoisine.[24,34] By electron microscopy, the somatotrophs have abundant granules averaging 350 nm in diameter.[25] The lactotrophs have large, sparse granules measuring up to 750 nm and the most abundant rough endoplasmic reticulum of all the adenohypophyseal cells.[25] Concentric whorls of rough endoplasmic reticulum known as neben-

PM-AT-PAS-orange G*[22, 32]	PFA-AB-PAS-orange G†[17,36]	Immunocytologic stains	Electron microscopy
cidophils Orange G+	Acidophils Orange G+	STH cell	Granules 350 nm and abundant; well-developed rough endoplasmic reticulum[26]
		LTH cell	Granules up to 750 nm[25] and sparse; abundant and distinctive rough endoplasmic reticulum
Gonadotrophs PAS+ (magenta granules); cell contour round[25] (δ cells)	S$_1$ cells[36] Blue; granules PFA-susceptible	FSH/LH cell	Granules 200 to 250 nm[26]; density variable
hyrotroph[21] Thionin+ (blue purple granules); cell contour angular[25] (β$_2$ cell)	S$_2$ cells[36] Purple; granules PFA-susceptible	TSH cell	Granules 150 to 200 nm[26]; may be located peripherally
orticomelanotrophs PAS+ (red granules); cell contour oval[25] (β$_1$ cell)	R cells[36] Red; granules PFA-resistant	ACTH/MSH cell	Granules 300 to 400 nm[60]; density variable[42]; cytoplasmic filaments[20]
hromophobes (No visible granules)	Chromophobes (No visible granules)		Sparse, fine granules[27] 150 nm or less
		Chromophobes (No reaction)	No granules

kern are a prominent feature. In pregnancy, the distinction between the somatotrophs and lactotrophs can be made with hematoxylin-and-eosin stain alone, since the lactotrophs are considerably enlarged (pregnancy cells of Erdheim).[4]

The basophils include three kinds of cells: (1) gonadotrophs, which are the source of FSH (follicle-stimulating hormone) and LH (luteinizing hormone; synonymous with ICSH, interstitial cell–stimulating hormone), (2) thyrotrophs, which produce TSH (thyrotrophic hormone), and (3) the corticomelanotrophs, which produce ACTH (adrenocorticotrophic hormone) and MSH (melanotrophic hormone). Separation of the basophils has evolved from application of histochemistry, immunohistology, and electron microscopy, together with indirect evidence based upon pathologic states, including deficiency, hyperactivity, and neoplasia. FSH, LH, and TSH are mucoproteins, and the basophils that produce them

are known collectively as mucoid cells, after Pearse.[35] These cells contain glycoprotein, a combination of protein and polysaccharide, and they can be demonstrated by the periodic acid–Schiff (PAS) reaction. Oxidation with periodic acid results in formation of free aldehyde groups in the polysaccharide, and the aldehyde groups then can be demonstrated by Schiff's reagent, which forms visible purple complexes with the aldehydes. Further separation of the mucoid cells was accomplished by Adams and Swettenham.[17] They described two types of granules, S (susceptible) and R (resistant), based upon preliminary oxidation by performic acid, followed by alcian blue, PAS, and orange G. The R granules are resistant to extraction by performic acid and stain red with Schiff's reagent. S granules have a high content of cystine, are susceptible to extraction with performic acid, and stain with alcian blue but not with PAS. Pearse and van Noorden[36] divided the S cells into two types—blue S$_1$

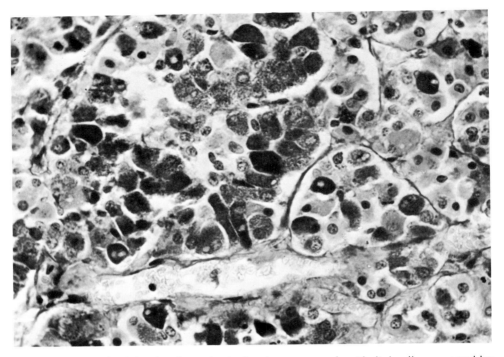

Fig. 36-6. Normal adult adenohypophysis showing groups of epithelial cells supported by connective tissue and sinusoids. "Dark" cells are basophils. (PAS-trichrome; 500×; courtesy Dr. A. R. Currie.)

cells, associated with gonadotrophins, and purple S_2 cells, associated with thyrotrophic hormone.

The important characteristics of the three types of basophils may be summarized as follows. The gonadotrophs are cells with round or oval contour and an eccentric nucleus; in horizontal section they are most numerous in the posterior portion of the median wedge. Phifer et al.[37] showed that antisera to FSH and LH reacted with the same cell types, suggesting that both FSH and LH are secreted by the same cell, hence the designation FSH-LH cell. With electron microscopy, the granules of gonadotrophs are 200 to 250 nm in diameter[26]; some workers have described two types of gonadotrophs.[42] The thyrotrophs are angular cells with granules that can be demonstrated selectively by Ezrin and Murray's permanganate–aldehyde thionin–PAS–orange G stain.[22] In horizontal section, the thyrotrophs are found in the median wedge, mainly in an anterior and subcapsular location. With immunohistologic techniques, the thyrotrophs stain with antibodies against TSH.[39] By electron microscopy, the cells are elongated and contain dense granules 150 to 200 nm in

diameter,[26] which may have a peripheral distribution. The corticomelanotrophs, or ACTH-MSH cells, are large oval cells that in horizontal section are concentrated in the anterior median wedge and adjacent lateral wings. A second group of ACTH-MSH cells may be found infiltrating the pars nervosa, just next to the pars distalis. MSH occurs in two forms, α-MSH and β-MSH; in the human, β-MSH is the principal hormone. α-MSH and β-MSH share amino acid sequences with ACTH, resulting in immunologic cross reactivity. Nevertheless, Phifer et al.[38] succeeded in demonstrating that the corticomelanotroph contains both α-MSH and β-MSH, in addition to ACTH, by using a combination of histochemical techniques and the immunostaining of serial sections. With the electron microscope, the ACTH-MSH cell contains granules 100 to 200 nm in diameter[26] and typical filaments are found in the cytoplasm.[20] Variations in size and density of granules have been reported.[42]

The classic chromophobes are small cells with scanty cytoplasm and no visible granules by light microscopy. Originally, chromophobes were believed to be cells having no secretory function, though it was postulated that some might be primordial or resting cells. The finding of nongranulated cells with strongly basophilic cytoplasm suggested to earlier workers that some chromophobes might be actively secreting cells that failed to store granules. This hypothesis was supported by the subsequent finding that basophilia depends on RNA content, and the observation that an increase in granules is associated with a decrease in RNA.[29] With the advent of electron microscopy, a large subpopulation of chromophobes was shown to consist of poorly granulated chromophils that had fine granules 150 nm or less and thus were invisible by light microscopy. These cells are associated with secretion of ACTH.[27] A second subclass of chromophobes contains a few fine granules but is not associated with secretion of any known hormone. A third subgroup are the follicular, or stellate cells; these are best seen with the electron microscope. These elongated stellate elements are associated with follicles. Distinctive features include microvilli, cilia, junctional complexes at the apical (follicular) pole, stacking of organelles, and elongated mitochondria.[18,31] Recent evidence suggests that follicular cells may have a phagocytic function[23] or may act as a transport system from the blood to the adenohypophyseal secretory cells.[29]

Neurohypophysis

The pars nervosa consists of interlacing nerve fibers and specialized glial elements known as pituicytes, together with interspersed blood vessels. Granules of neurosecretory material, made up of the octapeptides vasopressin and oxytocin in association with carrier proteins termed "neurophysins," are present throughout the neurohypophysis. The neurophysins are a useful marker of neurosecretion, since they can be stained by the chrome alum–hematoxylin, the aldehyde fuchsin, or the performic acid–alcian blue technique.[10] Vasopressin, or antidiuretic hormone (ADH), causes reabsorption of water from the renal tubules, and it is essential for maintaining osmolality of the plasma. Deficiency of ADH results in the condition known as diabetes insipidus, which is characterized by uncontrolled diuresis and polydipsia. Oxytocin is responsible for the ejection of milk from the lactating breast, by causing contraction of the mammary myoepithelium. It also stimulates contraction in the uterus at term.

The function of the pituicytes is unknown.

Electron microscopy has revealed that pituicytes are closely apposed to neurosecretory fibers, and in lower animals, a phagocytic function for disposal of neurophysins and membranes of granules has been suggested.[29]

PITUITARY IN PREGNANCY

The hypophysis undergoes a striking enlargement duuring pregnancy and lactation, when it may reach 1100 mg or more. Although involution occurs subsequently, the weight of the gland remains heavier in multiparas.[4] The basis for the enlargement is the pronounced hypertrophy and hyperplasia of the lactotrophs (LTH, or prolactin cells). In the pituitary of nonpregnant, nonlactating adults, the lactotrophs are sparsely granulated and are inconspicuous except by immunostaining.[24,34] However, during pregnancy and lactation, the hypertrophic, hyperplastic lactotrophs can be recognized in hematoxylin-eosin section as enlarged acidophils, termed "pregnancy cells" by Erdheim and Stumme.[4] The lactotrophs also may be stained selectively with erythrosin by Herlant's tetrachrome method[28] or Brookes' carmoisine technique.[19]

PITUITARY IN DISORDERS OF OTHER ENDOCRINE GLANDS
Hypothyroidism

In untreated or inadequately treated myxedema caused by primary disease of the thyroid, the pituitary gland is enlarged because of hypertrophy and hyperplasia of the thyrotrophs; weights up to 1.21 gm have been recorded.[44] Historically, such abnormal thyrotrophs also have been designated thyreopriva cells,[67] large chromophobes,[67] or hypertrophic amphophils.[45] With the light microscope, the thyrotrophs can be recognized as large cells containing coarse vesicles, or droplets, in the cytoplasm; the typical basophil granules are lacking (Fig. 36-7). These droplets are PAS- and aldehyde thionin–positive.[21] In rats, high resolution radioautography has demonstrated that the thyroidectomy cells originate from division of preexisting TSH cells.[66] In hypothyroid mice after administration of ^{131}I, the thyroidectomy cells by electron microscopy show ballooning of the ergastoplasmic cisternae, and the secretory granules are decreased or absent, resulting in a chromophobic appearance.[31] In hypothyroid mice, hyperplasia of thyrotrophs is followed by appearance of microadenomas and then gross tumors.[21,31] In humans with untreated primary hypothyroid-

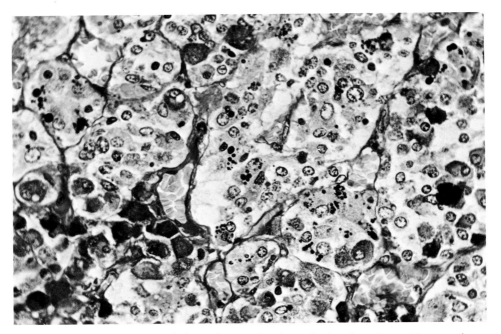

Fig. 36-7. Vesiculate chromophobe cells in adenohypophysis of patient with myxedema. Note variation in size of PAS-positive granules. (PAS-trichrome; 500×; courtesy Dr. A. R. Currie.)

ism, microadenomas composed of thyrotrophs also have been described.[21,57,58]

Hyperthyroidism

Ezrin has described regression of thyrotrophs in patients who died of hyperthyroidism.[21,59] The regressed TSH cells have small nuclei, a thin rim of cytoplasm, and a few aldehyde thionin–positive droplets. These alterations in the TSH cells are reversible. In contrast to the characteristic findings in the adenohypophysis in myxedema, the abnormalities in hyperthyroidism are not considered diagnostic.[25]

Addison's disease

In Addison's disease, gross enlargement of the hypophysis has been recorded, with a weight of 1.2 gm.[61] The granulated basophils are reduced in number, the chromophobes are increased, and transitional forms of basophils are present.[48] Mitotic figures may be found.[61] Using special stains, Ezrin demonstrated that the apparent reduction in basophils is attributable to degranulation of those basophils associated with production of ACTH; these are transformed into actively secreting cells that resemble chromophobes by light microscopy.[22] A similar sequence of events occurs in rats subjected to adrenalectomy; the ACTH cells

enlarge and secretory granules are strikingly reduced.[65]

In patients with Addison's disease, the number of thyrotrophs may be greatly increased.[22] This increase in thyrotrophs may be a reflection of the frequent association of idiopathic atrophy of the adrenals with atrophy of the thyroid, a condition known as Schmidt's syndrome, which apparently has an autoimmune basis[43,46,53] (see also p. 1665).

Hyperadrenocorticism

A typical cytoplasmic alteration known as Crooke's hyaline change was observed first in the basophils in cases of Cushing's syndrome.[47] Subsequently, the abnormality was found in other conditions characterized by excess circulating adrenocortical hormones, including therapy with exogenous glucocorticoids[55] and hypercorticism resulting from ectopic production of ACTH in lung cancer.[54] The basophils that are affected are the ACTH-MSH cells, or corticomelanotrophs.[52] In Crooke's change, the granules disappear and the cytoplasm gradually becomes PAS-negative.[52,64] In hematoxylin-eosin section, the cytoplasm assumes a ground-glass, pale gray appearance. The nucleus and the cell body enlarge, and a few cytoplasmic vacuoles may be present (Fig. 36-8). By electron microscopy, the hyaline

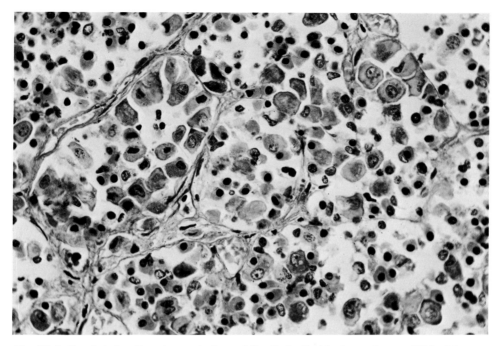

Fig. 36-8. Crooke's hyaline change in basophil cells in Cushing's syndrome. (PAS-trichrome; 500×; courtesy Dr. A. R. Currie.)

substance is made up of a dense feltwork of fine filaments[60] of the same type that is found in the normal corticomelanotroph.

Hyperadrenocorticism also affects the population of thyrotrophs, or TSH cells. Halmi and McCormick found that the thyrotrophs were scanty or undetectable at autopsy in patients with elevated levels of glucocorticoids, whether exogenous or endogenous.[51] They postulated that the paucity of thyrotrophs was the morphologic basis for the tonic depression of TSH secretion that is observed clinically in sustained hyperadrenocorticism (see also p. 1667).

Deficiency of gonadal hormones

In rodents, ovariectomy removes the negative feedback exerted by ovarian steroids upon the pituitary gonadotrophs. In such animals, the degranulated, hyperactive gonadotrophs acquire large vacuoles, assume a signet-ring appearance, and are known as castration cells. By electron microscopy, the signet-ring morphology results from fusion of distended elements of the endoplasmic reticulum and enlargement of individual cisternae.[23,50]

Although the same feedback action exists in humans, distinctive signet-ring castration cells such as those found in rodents do not occur. Nonetheless, changes are found in the gonadotrophs of patients with deficiency of gonadal hormones. Russfield[62] observed cellular hypertrophy and enlargement of the Golgi complex in the gonadotrophs of patients with gonadal deficiency; the changes were reversible by hormone therapy. In a man who underwent castration for carcinoma of the prostate, Russfield and Byrnes[63] found hyperplasia of sparsely granulated, PAS+ cells, but the staining method did not differentiate between the types of basophils. Phifer et al.[37] observed an increase in the size and number of gonadotrophs in a woman castrated 5 years previously. Ezrin[49] noted enlarged, vacuolated gonadotrophic basophils resembling chromophobes by light microscopy in patients with hypogonadism and in postmenopausal women. With the electron microscope, extreme dilatation of cisternae of the endoplasmic reticulum of these hypertrophied cells has been observed.[56]

HYPOPHYSECTOMY

Hypophysectomy has been shown to produce temporary remission of symptoms in about one third of women with disseminated mammary cancer.[76,77] Relief from bone pain is especially gratifying. In treatment of metastatic carcinoma, total ablation of adenohypophyseal function is the goal. Thus hypophysectomy for palliation of breast cancer is an important cause of hypofunction of the pituitary.

The ability to predict the patient who will have a favorable response to endocrine ablation more accurately has been enhanced recently by the recognition of estrogen receptors in some mammary tumors. Evidence is incomplete, but it appears that women whose tumors contain such receptors are more likely to have a remission.[68,70,71]

Several lines of evidence suggest that the pharyngeal hypophysis is capable of active secretion of adenohypophyseal hormones. Müller[75] has reported "activation" of the cells of the pharyngeal pituitary in patients whose sellar hypophysis was destroyed by tumor or hypophysectomy. In such patients, Müller found typical acidophils and chromophobes in the pharyngeal pituitary, in contrast to the undifferentiated cells in the "inactive" state. McGrath[73] noted that acidophils were predominant in the pharyngeal hypophysis after hypophysectomy; basophils and chromophobes were present as well. Also, in extracts of pharyngeal hypophyses, she demonstrated prolactin and growth hormone.[74] Using an immunofluorescence technique, McPhie and Beck[72] demonstrated human growth hormone in the acidophils of the pharyngeal pituitary of patients without endocrine disease. These findings strongly suggest that the pharyngeal hypophysis is an actively secreting, extrasellar adenohypophyseal tissue. However, the extent to which this organ is capable of compensating for the absence of the sellar hypophysis is uncertain.[69]

HYPOPITUITARISM

Hypopituitarism, or pituitary insufficiency, may involve the neurohypophysis, the adenohypophysis or both. The pathology of the major causes of insufficiency is discussed in detail in the later sections; some of the clinical features are described briefly here.

Deficiency of the neurohypophysis results in the syndrome known as diabetes insipidus because of the loss of vasopressin. The condition is characterized by diuresis, polyuria, and uncontrollable thirst.

Deficiency of the adenohypophysis may involve one, several, or all of the trophic hormones. Deficiency of all hormones (panhypopituitarism) follows destruction of 70% or more of the adenohypophysis. Infarction and tumor are the most common causes. Isolated hormonal deficiency may be associated with incomplete adenohypophyseal destruction, but it also may occur in the absence of a recognizable pathologic lesion. In such cases, a functional disorder of the hypothalamus has been postulated.

The classic clinical syndrome of panhypopituitarism in the adult is known as Simmonds' disease. The advanced cachexia that characterized the cases observed by Simmonds now is rarely observed, probably because of the advances in medical care since then.[78] From this heterogeneous group of cases described by Simmonds, Sheehan separated the clinicopathologic entity of postpartum necrosis of the adenohypophysis, and this syndrome now bears his name.[80]

The effects of isolated hormone deficiency depend on the hormone involved and to some extent on the age of the patient. Deficiency of gonadotrophic hormones leads to hypogonadotrophic eunuchoidism in men and amenorrhea in women; before the age of puberty there are no clinical signs, but secondary sexual development fails to occur at adolescence.[79] Deficiency of corticotrophin secretion leads to anorexia, weakness, weight loss, and hypoglycemia; in women axillary and pubic hair may be lost, and in girls it fails to appear. Isolated deficiency of thyrotrophic hormone causes hypothyroidism in adults but has not been described in children. Isolated deficiency of growth hormone results in ateliotic dwarfism in children and microsplanchnia in adults.[49]

ANOMALIES
Agenesis

Agenesis of the pituitary is a rare anomaly that is almost always associated with cyclopia, a gross malformation involving the neural tube and axial skeleton. Even in this condition, agenesis is not universal, occurring in only about half the cases reported.[83] Agenesis of the anterior lobe has been described in a few normocephalic infants; in males, the penis is unusually small, a finding that has been suggested as an external marker of this condition.[85] In such normocephalic infants, the sella turcica may appear normally formed but empty, or it may be smaller than normal with a persistent craniopharyngeal canal.[88] In all cases in which the anterior lobe of the pituitary is absent, the adrenal glands are hypoplastic and the thyroid gland often is similarly affected. The adrenals lack a fetal or "X" zone, and the layers of the cortex are irregular and disordered. That the function of these abnormal adrenal glands is defective is supported by the observation of stable, low maternal urinary estriol levels in the last weeks of pregnancy.[85] The hypoplastic thyroid is small and it may lack an isthmus. The testes also may be hypoplastic, and absence of interstitial cells of Leydig has been reported.[82] Several of these infants have survived a decade or more, exhibiting mental deficiency, dwarfism, failure of development, myxedema, hypoglycemic convulsions, and undeveloped genitalia.[87]

Agenesis of the anterior pituitary may occur without any anomaly of the posterior pituitary.

Hypoplasia

Hypoplasia of the pituitary is a constant finding in anencephaly. In this condition, the sella turcica is flattened and the exposed base of the skull is covered by a mat of spongy, vascular tissue. The hypophysis usually cannot be recognized grossly, but it can be found by en bloc removal of the entire sella, decalcification, and vertical sectioning of the central portion.[81] The size and shape of the gland are quite variable. Whereas the pars anterior nearly always is present, the pars nervosa often is absent.

The adrenals in anencephaly invariably are hypoplastic and the "X" zone, or fetal cortex, is absent, so that the glands resemble miniature replicas of those of older infants,[86] with orderly cortical layers. The thyroid gland, gonads, and genitalia are unaffected.

Malposition

Malposition, or dystopia of the hypophysis is a rare occurrence. Lennox and Russell[84] reviewed the literature and added two cases in which the pars nervosa lay between the infundibulum and the sella, being connected to the pars anterior by a stalk composed of pars tuberalis. No disorder of pituitary function was recognized. Another rare malposition occurs as a result of failure of contact between Rathke's pouch and the developing diencephalon, leading to displacement of the pituitary tissue into a persistent craniopharyngeal duct.[75] In such cases, polypoid protrusion of the pituitary anlage into the pharynx may occur.

HEMORRHAGE

Severe trauma to the skull frequently injures the hypophysis, causing hemorrhage, laceration, and necrosis.[90] The patients who survive such injury may have diabetes insipidus as a result of damage to the neurohypophysis.[89,90] Hemorrhage in the posterior pituitary also occurs in patients who have cerebral hemorrhage, tumors of the brain, or "respirator brain" (the deterioration of the brain that occurs as a complication of mechanical respirator therapy).[91]

Acute hemorrhage into a pituitary tumor is responsible for the condition known as pituitary apoplexy. This condition is characterized by sudden headache, ophthalmoplegia, meningismus, and signs of compression of the optic nerves or chiasm.[92] Sudden pituitary failure may result.[49] In some patients, pituitary apoplexy may be the first manifestation of a pituitary tumor. Impaction of the pituitary by the expanding neoplasm has been cited as the mechanism.[92]

INFARCTION AND NECROSIS

Foci of ischemic necrosis occasionally are observed post mortem, with an incidence of 1% to 3% in unselected autopsies.[96] These almost always involve the adenohypophysis. The associated conditions are varied[97] and include such diverse entities as obstetric shock,[100] elevated intracranial pressure, diabetes mellitus,[95,98] craniocerebral trauma, cerebrovascular accident, shock, mechanical respirator therapy ("respirator brain"),[91,94,101] transection of the hypophyseal stalk,[10,93] overwhelming sepsis, and carcinomatous permeation of local blood vessels.[9] The common denominator in most of these conditions appears to be inadequate perfusion of the adenohypophysis, resulting in ischemia and coagulative necrosis. The "life support" of the adenohypophysis is the hypophyseal portal system, and the direct arterial supply to the anterior pituitary is not sufficient to sustain the cells.[1,10] This arrangement renders the adenohypophysis more vulnerable to episodes of stasis and ischemia. The pathogenesis of the ischemia has been ascribed to such mechanisms as embolism, thrombosis, Shwartzman phenomenon, vascular spasm, and vascular compression.[97] In many patients with infarcts, the lesions occur as a terminal complication of a severe systemic illness; hence they are of little importance clinically whether large or small. Survivors with microinfarcts do not have symptoms of hypopituitarism because insufficiency is not apparent until 70% of the adenohypophysis is destroyed.[62] However, survivors of large infarcts do suffer from hypopituitarism.

The most important cause of pituitary in-

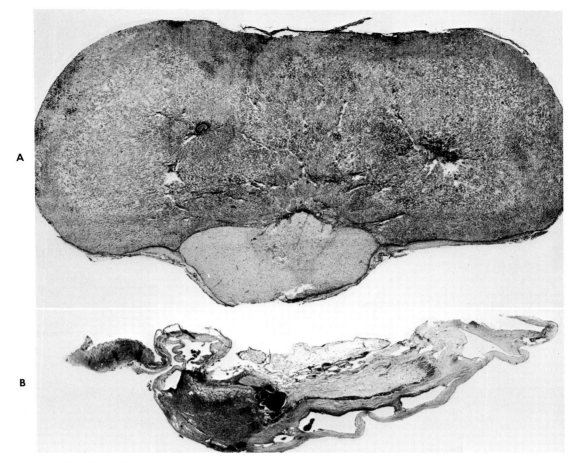

Fig. 36-9. Postpartum necrosis of pituitary gland. **A,** Most of anterior lobe affected. **B,** Gland shriveled and deformed. Patient survived for many years. (**A** and **B,** Hematoxylin and eosin; 10x; courtesy Prof. H. L. Sheehan and Dr. A. R. Currie.)

sufficiency from massive infarction is obstetric shock, usually related to hemorrhage at the time of delivery. Postpartum necrosis of the pituitary is known as Sheehan's syndrome. In severe cases, the extent of necrosis of the adenohypophysis approaches 99%[11] (Fig. 36-9). A narrow zone of tissue at the periphery may survive. The necrotic anterior lobe gradually shrivels and becomes replaced by a thin, semilunar collagenous scar (Fig. 36-9). The posterior lobe is unaffected. The degree of hypopituitarism depends on the extent of destruction. Failure of lactation may be the first sign, followed by amenorrhea and eventually by adrenocortical insufficiency and hypothyroidism.[99]

ACUTE INFLAMMATION

Acute purulent inflammation of the hypophysis may occur by direct extension of inflammation in an adjacent structure, or by hematogenous dissemination during the course of overwhelming sepsis. Purulent meningitis causes acute hypophysitis as a consequence of direct spread into the subarachnoid space surrounding the pituitary; inflammation in such a case may be limited to the surface of the gland. Rarely, the hypophysis is converted into a pus-filled sac.[102,103] Other causes include sphenoid sinusitis, osteomyelitis of the sphenoid bone, thrombophlebitis of the cavernous sinus, and suppurative otitis media. In the case of hematogenous dissemination, microabscesses may form within the substance of either adenohypophysis or neurohypophysis.[111]

CHRONIC INFLAMMATION
Granuloma

Granulomatous diseases may involve the pituitary and cause destruction of both adenohypophysis and neurohypophysis. Symptoms of hypopituitarism are proportional to the extent of destruction and localization of the involvement. Tuberculosis occurs by hematogenous dissemination, or by direct extension from tuberculous meningitis; miliary tubercles or areas of caseous necrosis are found at autopsy. Syphilis of the pituitary may be congenital or acquired; in the acquired cases, the lesion may be a diffuse fibrosis or gummatous necrosis.[109] Boeck's sarcoid can affect the central nervous system, with involvement of the base of the brain, hypothalamus, and pituitary including both neurohypophysis and adenohypophysis.[110] Noncaseating tubercles composed of epithelioid cells, lymphocytes, and giant cells of Langhans' type, which may contain asteroid bodies and Schaumann bodies, characterize the lesions. No etiologic agent can be demonstrated, and special stains for acid-fast organisms and fungi are negative.

The entity known as giant cell granuloma of the pituitary presents a histologic picture similar to Boeck's sarcoid, but unlike sarcoidosis, giant cell granuloma is not a disease of multiple systems. This rare disorder affects the anterior pituitary, and the involvement may progress to destruction of the adenohypophysis with consequent hypopituitarism and secondary atrophy of thyroid and adrenals. The hypophyseal lesions consist of noncaseating tubercles with Langhans' giant cells and associated chronic inflammatory cells. The condition occurs chiefly in middle-aged and elderly women.[104] The pathogenesis is obscure. In a few reported cases, similar granulomas were observed in the adrenals, and it has been suggested that giant cell granuloma may be an autoimmune or an infectious disorder.[104]

Lymphocytic hypophysitis

More recently, another variant of chronic inflammatory disease of the pituitary known as lymphocytic hypophysitis has been described.[106-108] The adenohypophysis is the seat of extensive diffuse or nodular infiltration by lymphocytes, sometimes with fibrosis. Concomitant hypothyroidism and adrenal insufficiency have been observed, with lymphoid infiltration in these organs. An autoimmune basis for anterior hypophysitis has been postulated.[105,108]

INFILTRATIONS AND METABOLIC DISORDERS
Amyloid

Generalized secondary amyloidosis may involve the pituitary.[114] In this condition, amyloid is deposited in the walls of the blood vessels of the adenohypophysis (Fig. 36-10). Amyloid also may be deposited in the pituitary

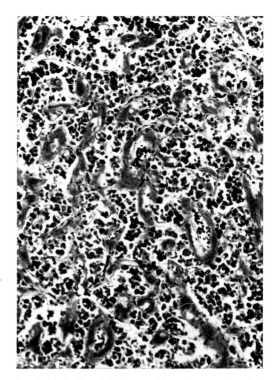

Fig. 36-10. Amyloid deposition in anterior lobe of pituitary gland. (Hematoxylin and eosin; 140×; courtesy Dr. Dorothy S. Russell and Dr. A. R. Currie.)

in multiple myeloma.[112] Amyloid in the form of laminated concretions has been described in pituitary adenomas.[112,113,115,116]

Hand-Schüller-Christian disease

The posterior lobe, infundibular stem, and the infundibulum often are involved by the xanthomatous deposits that characterize this disorder.[11] Usually, the skull and dura mater adjacent to the hypophysis also are involved, with bony destruction. The infundibular lesions interfere with neurosecretion and Hand-Schüller-Christian disease is an important cause of diabetes insipidus in children (see also p. 1510).

Hurler's syndrome (gargoylism)

The adenohypophyseal cells in Hurler's syndrome display a characteristic vacuolation with a foamy appearance, corresponding to the abnormal storage of mucopolysaccharides characteristic of this disorder. By electron microscopy, the majority of the affected cells contain numerous membrane-bound vesicles. Lipid cytosomes with parallel-stacked or concentric osmiophilic lamellae known as "zebra bodies" also are present.[117]

TUMORS

Tumors of the pituitary are not common, constituting about 6% of intracranial neoplasms,[142,166] but these lesions are of great interest because of their clinical manifestations. Tumors of the pituitary give rise to symptoms in two ways: (1) local effects, which result from expansion of the lesion, and (2) distant effects, caused by hypersecretion or hyposecretion of trophic hormones or hypothalamic principles. The local growth and expansion of hypophyseal tumors enlarge the sella turcica, with loss of the clinoid processes, resulting in its typical x-ray appearance. Extension of the tumor upward into the suprasellar region compresses the optic chiasm, optic nerves, neurohypophysis, hypothalamus, and adjacent cranial nerves (Fig. 36-11). At the same time, the uninvolved pituitary may become compressed and attenuated, with insufficiency of trophic hormones or diabetes insipidus as a result of pressure on the adenohypophysis or

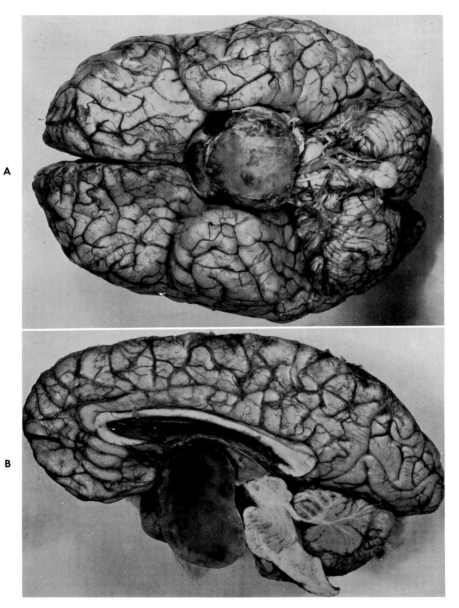

Fig. 36-11. A, Basal view of intrasellar part of large chromophobe adenoma. Note distortion of optic chiasm. **B,** Midsagittal view of same specimen shown in **A.** (Courtesy Dr. Dorothy S. Russell and Dr. A. R. Currie.)

neurohypophysis, respectively. Displacement of the hypothalamus may impair production and transport of releasing substances and inhibitory factors, with further endocrine imbalance and abnormality. In fact, analysis of the effects of tumors has given considerable insight into the function of the hypophysis and hypothalamus.

Adenomas

Adenomas are the most common of the pituitary tumors and their incidence is cited as 4.4% in a recent series of 5000 cases of intracranial tumors.[166] A simple classification of adenomas as acidophil, basophil, or chromophobe was proposed by earlier workers.[125] For many years it has been apparent that such a classification was inadequate, since chromophobe tumors sometimes were accompanied by hyperpituitarism. No solution for this paradox was apparent until the remarkable advances of the past two decades clarified the correlation of morphology of the pituitary cells in relation to their function (specific hormone production) and resulted in the tentative functional classification summarized in Table 36-1. Using the functional classification, one can recognize a parallel series of neoplastic cells and construct a similar table of tumors (Table 36-2). In light of this information, many of the tumors that formerly were designated "chromophobe adenomas" in reality are tumors with granules too small to be seen with the light microscope. This finding has explained the paradoxical occurrence of "chromophobe" tumors in patients who had clear-cut syndromes of hyperpituitarism such as acromegaly, Cushing's syndrome, or hyperthyroidism.

Some observers have suggested total rejection of the older classification in which adenomas were designated acidophil, basophil, or chromophobe. Instead, it seems more reasonable to retain this terminology when one uses light microscopy and the hematoxylin-eosin section as a screening procedure in the analysis of a pituitary adenoma, recognizing that this technique alone is not sufficient for final diagnosis. With this approach, the old terminology then is the point of departure for the application of the more advanced techniques necessary for the functional classification of the cell type.

Adenomas originate in the adenohypophysis, and therefore they arise in the hypophyseal fossa in the majority of cases. A few instances in which an adenoma originated outside the sella turcica, in an anomalous remnant of the adenohypophysis, have been reported.[14]

Grossly, adenoma varies in size from a small nodule just barely visible (Fig. 36-12) to a massive tumor with a smooth or bosselated surface. The larger tumors bulge upward from the sella turcica to encroach upon the hypothalamus and third ventricle (Fig. 36-11). In such cases, the tumor does not invade the brain, and it can be easily shelled from its bed in the compressed, invaginated cerebral tissue. Whereas small tumors are solid, the larger tumors may be cystic, containing turbid or clear fluid. The larger neoplasms may undergo infarction and hemorrhage, resulting in the syndrome of pituitary apoplexy.

Microscopically, three patterns are observed: diffuse, sinusoidal, and papillary. The diffuse form is composed of polygonal cells arranged in sheets and masses, with an inconspicuous stroma (Fig. 36-13). The sinusoidal form more or less resembles the structure of the normal adenohypophysis. The cells tend to be columnar or fusiform, and the stroma has fibrovascular septa with sinusoidal blood vessels to which the cells are oriented, creating a perisinusoidal arrangement (Fig. 36-13). In the

Table 36-2. Classification of tumors of adenohypophysis

Hormone	Cell type		Syndrome
	Hematoxylin and eosin	Functional classification	
STH	Acidophil or chromophobe*	Somatotroph	Acromegaly
LTH		Lactotroph	Amenorrhea-galactorrhea
FSH-LH	Basophil or chromophobe*	Gonadotroph	— *not seen*
TSH		Thyrotroph	Hyperthyroidism
ACTH-MSH		Corticomelanotroph	Cushing's syndrome
			Nelson's syndrome
None	Chromophobe	(No secretory function)	Local compression: Impaired vision, Hypopituitarism

*Granules too small to be seen with light microscope.

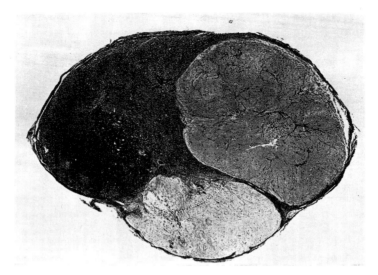

Fig. 36-12. Small chromophobe adenoma of anterior lobe of pituitary gland. Clinically silent. (Acid fuchsin and aniline blue; 6×; courtesy Dr. Dorothy S. Russell and Dr. A. R. Currie, London.)

papillary form, which is a variant of the sinusoidal pattern, cuboid or columnar neoplastic cells are arranged radially about papillae with a vascular core. In all three types, the cells are quite orderly and mitoses are rare.

Acidophil adenoma

The acidophil tumors make up approximately one third of adenomas of the pituitary.[121,154] These neoplasms usually do not reach massive proportions and are confined to the sella, though compression of the uninvolved hypophysis with hypophyseal insufficiency, and suprasellar extension with compression of the optic chiasm and blindness, may occur.

Two major forms of acidophil adenomas are recognized, the STH cell, or somatotroph type, and the less common LTH cell, or lactotroph type. Special stains and electron microscopy are required to differentiate the two on morphologic grounds. In some cases, granules are quite sparse, and by light microscopy alone, the neoplasm may appear to be a chromophobe adenoma. By electron microscopy, the cells closely resemble their normal counterparts.[31,158] Thus the STH cell has abundant, well-developed rough endoplasmic reticulum, a prominent Golgi apparatus, and spheric secretory granules measuring 350 to 450 nm. The LTH cells, which are erythrosin-positive by light microscopy, possess well-developed rough endoplasmic reticulum, nebenkern, a prominent Golgi apparatus, and spheric or pleomorphic

secretory granules 500 nm or larger.[31,140,148,154]

The acidophil adenomas often are functional, although production of hormones is not invariable. Two distinctive syndromes are associated with functioning acidophil tumors: (1) gigantism or acromegaly, produced by excess growth hormone, and (2) amenorrhea-galactorrhea, produced by excess prolactin. The STH-cell adenoma producing excess growth hormone in a prepubertal patient whose epiphyses have not closed results in proportionate growth of the body and gigantism. In the adult, epiphyses are closed, and abnormal growth is confied to the skull, jaw, hands, feet, and soft tissues, with enlargement of supraorbital ridges, mandible, and phalanges, together with a characteristic coarsening of the features, thickening of the heel pads, and enlargement of the viscera.

The functioning LTH tumor produces prolactin, and the excess prolactin causes lactation. In women, the increased prolactin somehow blocks the cycling center in the hypothalamus, so that ovulation fails to occur and amenorrhea results. The clinical picture of amenorrhea and galactorrhea produced by a functioning LTH-cell tumor is known as the Forbes-Albright syndrome.[31,128,148] In men, galactorrhea, gynecomastia, and impotence have been reported with functioning LTH-cell tumors.[150]

Acidophil tumors containing both STH and LTH cells can be produced experimentally in the rat,[130] and at least one such tumor in a

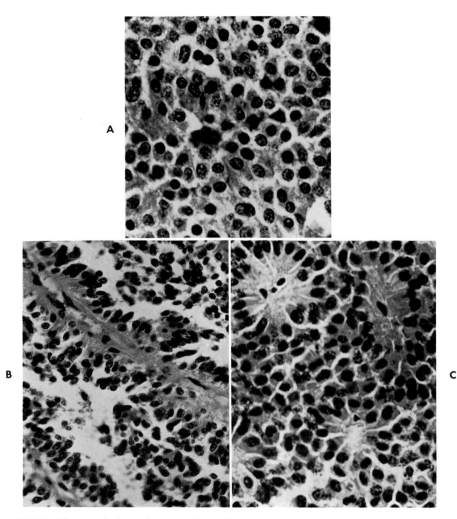

Fig. 36-13. Chromophobe adenoma. **A,** Diffuse type. **B** and **C,** Perisinusoid type, with cells arranged about sinusoids. (**A** to **C,** Hematoxylin and eosin; **A,** 490×; **B,** 350×; **C,** 540×; courtesy Dr. Dorothy S. Russell and Dr. A. R. Currie, London.)

human has been reported.[134] Other reports of human cases can be anticipated.

Basophil adenoma

Basophil tumors are the rarest of the functioning adenomas, constituting less than 5% in most series. These neoplasms also are the smallest of the functional tumors, and adenomas only a few millimeters in diameter that produced hyperpituitarism have been reported.

On theoretic grounds, three functional types of basophil tumors would be expected, corresponding to the functional categories of basophils, namely gonadotrophs, thyrotrophs, and corticomelanotrophs. In fact, only the tumor of ACTH-MSH–producing cells is well known in

humans. A few cases of presumptive human TSH-cell adenomas and one case of adenoma associated with elevated serum TSH levels and hyperthyroidism have been reported,[57,120,135,147,165] but none has been studied by electron microscopy. However, TSH adenomas and the sequence of events in their pathogenesis are well known in animals.[31,124] Experimental tumors of gonadotrophs also have been described in animals,[133] but this tumor remains to be established as an entity in the human.

The histologic patterns of the basophil adenomas present no unusual features. The morphology of the neoplastic ACTH-MSH cell closely resembles that of its normal counterpart. The granules have the staining reactions of R cells with the performic acid–alcian blue–PAS–orange G technique. In many cases, granules appear quite sparse, and the cells may appear to be chromophobes by light microscopy. With the electron microscope, the granules are small and of variable density.[31] The cytoplasm may contain microfilaments.

Two distinctive clinical disorders are associated with functioning basophil tumor composed of corticomelanotrophs—Cushing's disease[122] and Nelson's syndrome.[146] In Cushing's disease, the tumor of basophils produces excess ACTH, which in turn causes hyperplasia of the adrenal cortex.[152] The overproduction of adrenocortical hormones leads to the distinctive clinical findings, which include truncal obesity, moon face, purple striae, muscular wasting, hypertension, and abnormal glucose tolerance. Although Cushing believed pituitary adenoma to be the principal cause of this condition, experience has shown that a pituitary tumor is found only in a small percentage of cases, and the majority are attributable to idiopathic adrenal hyperplasia (see also p. 1667).

The second disorder associated with a tumor of corticomelanotrophs is Nelson's syndrome. In this condition, the patient initially has the classic clinical picture associated with adrenocortical hyperplasia and overproduction of adrenocortical hormones; the sella turcica is normal by x ray. However, some time after bilateral adrenalectomy has been done, signs and symptoms of a pituitary tumor appear, together with brown pigmentation of the skin and elevated levels of plasma ACTH. Whether the tumor was present at the outset, and was the original cause of the adrenal hyperplasia, is not known at present.

Chromophobe adenoma

Chromophobe tumors formerly were regarded as the most common of the adenomas of the pituitary, constituting well over half according to most authors.[126,137] However, their incidence has been revised downward since the application of electron microscopy to their morphology. One recent study of a series of 85 cases investigated with light and electron microscopy lists the incidence of chromophobe tumors as 37%.[155]

Chromophobe tumors arise in adults, with a peak incidence of 30 to 50 years and a preponderance in men.[121] These neoplasms tend to reach the largest size of all the adenomas and are more prone to become cystic.[126] As they slowly enlarge, they erode the sella turcica and extend both laterally and upward, impinging upon the chiasm and other suprasellar structures. With the larger tumors, the uninvolved hypophysis is almost invariably compressed, causing hypopituitarism.

With light microscopy, the cells are small with scanty cytoplasm; they are arranged in the usual diffuse, sinusoidal or papillary patterns. Typically, the cytoplasm fails to stain with hematoxylin, eosin, PAS, or orange G. With electron microscopy, the cells have a variable number of mitochondria and other cytoplasmic organelles and may contain a few small secretory granules.[31,140,157] In some chromophobe tumors, Kovacs et al.[140] have found nebenkern formation and other features suggesting that certain sparsely granulated chromophobe tumors are capable of prolactin secretion.

Since some of the chromophobe tumors have fine granules but no known secretory activity, the question that naturally arises is, Why do such neoplasms have no endocrine function? Olivier et al.[31] suggest several hypotheses: (1) the secretory product may be a substance that is hormonally inactive; (2) the secretory product may be too weak to have biologic significance; and (3) the granules may be lysed in situ rather than be released.

Rarely, a true chromophobe tumor associated with galactorrhea has been observed. In such cases, the mechanism is ascribed to damage to the hypothalamus, interfering with formation or transport of prolactin-inhibiting factor. Thus the production of prolactin by the adenohypophysis no longer is inhibited, and the level of prolactin rises, causing galactorrhea.

Multiple endocrine adenomatosis

Adenomas of the pituitary occur as an integral part of Wermer's syndrome, or multiple endocrine adenomatosis type I.[118] This condition is a genetic disorder that is inherited as an autosomal dominant, and familial involvement is the rule.[164] The disease is characterized by multiple adenomas involving pancreatic islets, parathyroids, and pituitary. Clinically, the patient usually presents with some combination of Zollinger-Ellison syndrome, hyperparathyroidism, and acromegaly. Hypopituitarism sometimes is observed instead of acromegaly. It is important to note that the endocrine involvement may be sequential rather than simultaneous.

The associated pituitary lesion is an adenoma of acidophil or chromophobe type by light microscopy.[162] At least one case of a malignant pituitary tumor has been recorded in association with multiple endocrine adenomatosis.[145]

Oncocytic adenoma

Recently, adenomas composed of oncocytes have been described.[139,141,155] The cells of these tumors are eosinophilic and finely granular by light microscopy, resembling acidophils except for their fine granulation. With electron microscopy, the cytoplasm is found to be densely packed with abnormal mitochondria, which is the basis for the acidophilia observed with the light microscope. Thus positive identification of this tumor depends on electron microscopy. Secretory granules are exceedingly sparse, and symptoms of hypersecretion are absent.

Carcinoma

Primary carcinoma. To identify a primary tumor of the adenohypophysis with distant metastases as a carcinoma presents no problem.[123,149] However, the characteristic tendency of tumors of the adenohypophysis to erode bone and displace or compress soft tissues as the tumors expand, which already has been emphasized, has led to considerable debate on the criteria for malignancy of tumors without distant spread. Evans[126] takes the sensible approach that all tumors that burst their capsules and directly invade the adjacent structures, especially the cavernous sinuses, the base of the cranium, and the sphenoidal sinuses, should be labeled malignant. It is clear that cytologic criteria are not absolute, since pleomorphism, hyperchromatism, and mitotic activity have been observed in tumors that are not infiltrative and tumors with none of these qualities have exhibited invasiveness.[126]

Carcinomas may originate from chromophobe or chromophil cells; chromophobe neoplasms are the rule. However, functioning tumors usually producing adrenocortical hyperplasia and Cushing's syndrome have been reported.[149]

Metastatic carcinoma. Metastases to the pituitary gland occur in patients having widespread metastatic carcinoma. The usual primary site is the breast, and carcinoma of the lung is the second most common.[138,151] Most observers have found the pars nervosa to be involved more frequently than the pars distalis. Destruction of the posterior pituitary by metastatic carcinoma is a significant cause of diabetes insipidus in patients with carcinomatosis.[136]

Craniopharyngioma

This benign tumor is believed to originate in remnants of Rathke's pouch that persist into postnatal life. An alternate explanation that the neoplasm arises by metaplasia of adenohypophyseal cells has been proposed. The onset of these tumors in childhood favors the origin from embryologic rests.[126] Whichever theory is correct, it is a fact that most craniopharyngiomas originate outside the sella turcica and usually are suprasellar in location. Occurrence within the sphenoid bone also has been reported.

Craniopharyngiomas make up 1% to 3% of intracranial tumors.[142,166,167] They are most common in children and young adults but may occur in older persons as well.

Grossly, the tumor is encapsulated and firmly adherent to surrounding tissues, which suffer compression as the neoplasm slowly enlarges. Thus the structures comprised are the brain above, the pituitary below, the optic chiasm anteriorly, and the circle of Willis at the periphery. The typical tumor is cystic, with intervening solid areas (Fig. 36-14). The content is fluid or semisolid dark brown, greasy material containing cholesterol crystals, altered blood, and calcified debris.

Microscopically, the patterns are distinctive. The solid areas contain anastomosing cords of well-differentiated stratified squamous epithelium with a palisaded peripheral layer, set in a stroma of connective tissue (Fig. 36-15). Within the epithelium, areas composed of loosely arranged stellate cells may be found. Mitoses and cellular pleomorphism are uncommon. The cystic regions may be lined by similar epithelial cords, with lipid histiocytes in the stroma, and desquamated keratin in the cysts. The ultrastructure of craniopharyngioma has been described by Ghatak et al.[132]

The histologic patterns may strikingly resemble those of adamantinoma, an epithelial odontogenic tumor of the jaw.[159] Consequently, craniopharyngioma also is known as adamantinoma. That a craniopharyngioma should resemble an adamantinoma is not surprising, since the adenohypophysis itself arises in primitive buccal epithelium. It follows that neoplasms of its developmental remnants might be expected to reflect kinship with other buccal derivatives.

Although craniopharyngioma is histologically benign and grows slowly, ablation is very difficult because of its location, and progressive enlargement is the rule.

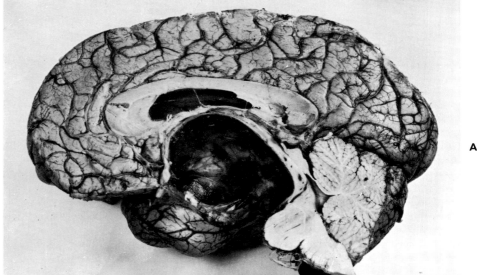

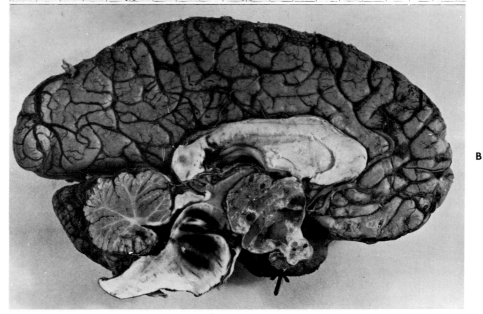

Fig. 36-14. A, Cystic suprasellar craniopharyngioma. **B,** Solid and cystic suprasellar cranio-pharyngioma. *Arrow,* Pituitary gland. (Courtesy Dr. Dorothy S. Russell and Dr. A. R. Currie.)

Intrasellar cyst

Colloid-filled, epithelium-lined, asymptomatic benign cysts of microscopic size are commonly found at the junction of the pars distalis and the pars nervosa.[160] Such cysts are interpreted as remnants of Rathke's pouch. Rarely, benign larger cysts producing symptoms occur. They may be located entirely within the sella, or they may protrude above it, producing a dumbbell shape.

The intrasellar cysts usually are lined by simple cuboid epithelium, which may be ciliated.[115,160] The suprasellar portion of a dumbbell cyst may be lined by stratified squamous epithelium.[9]

Granular cell tumor (choristoma)

The granular cell tumor arises in the neurohypophysis, and it is the most common primary tumor of the posterior lobe. Nearly always

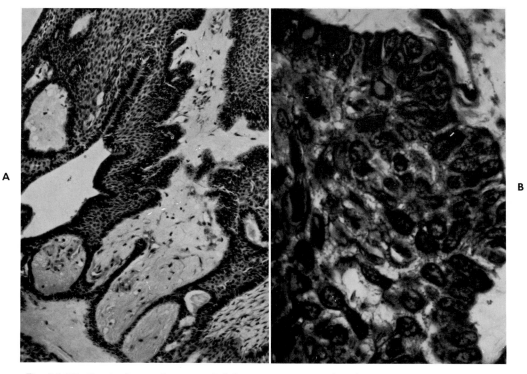

Fig. 36-15. Craniopharyngioma. **A,** Solid anastomosing trabeculae of cells. **B,** Surface cells of basal type and squamous cells. (**A,** Hematoxylin and eosin, 140×; **B,** phosphotungstic acid and hematoxylin, 850×; courtesy Dr. Dorothy S. Russell and Dr. A. R. Currie.)

asymptomatic, granular cell tumor usually is identified as an incidental finding at autopsy in individuals past the age of 30 years.[143] The incidence in Luse and Kernohan's series of autopsies was 6.4%. Originally, the name "choristoma" was proposed in the belief that the condition was a developmental anomaly. More recently, origin from Schwann cells[127] or pituicytes[119] has been suggested.

Grossly, the lesion generally is too small to be seen. Microscopically, it is composed of orderly, large polygonal cells with abundant granular pale pink cytoplasm and small, oval, eccentrically placed nuclei. The resemblance to the tumor known as granular myoblastoma found in extracranial locations is striking.

Rarely, granular cell tumor of the neurohypophysis may be large enough to produce symptoms. Such patients present with signs and symptoms of a space-occupying intracranial lesion[161] or with loss of vision as a result of compression of the optic chiasm.[156,163]

Germinal tumors

Tumors histologically identical to germinoma (seminoma) and teratoma of the gonads may occur within and adjacent to the sella turcica.[131,153] Because these tumors are more common in the pineal region, formerly they were designated ectopic pinealoma when they occurred in the hypothalamic region or the sella. However, the identity of the pinealoma with the germinoma (seminoma) of the testis was recognized by Friedman,[129] who emphasized their unmistakable morphologic congruity, and the term "germinoma" has become accepted.[153]

Grossly, the germinoma is a fleshy, soft gray, diffusely infiltrating mass, frequently associated with hemorrhage. Microscopically, the tumor is composed of large polygonal cells with abundant cytoplasm, a large vesicular nucleus, and one or more prominent nucleoli (Fig. 36-16). Mitoses are numerous. The cells are arranged in sheets or clusters separated by fibrovascular septa. Numerous small lymphocytes usually are present in the stroma. The resemblance to germinoma (seminoma) of the testis and dysgerminoma of the ovary is remarkable.

Teratomas also may occur in a suprasellar location. These neoplasms typically are cystic and are lined by ectodermal derivatives; bone and cartilage may be found in the wall.[153]

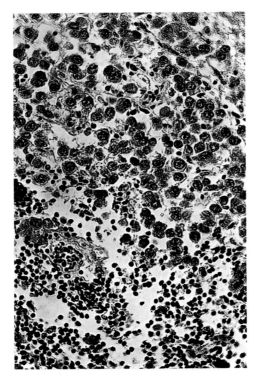

Fig. 36-16. Germinoma of pituitary stalk and posterior lobe of pituitary gland. (Hematoxylin and eosin; 260×; courtesy Dr. Dorothy S. Russell and Dr. A. R. Currie.)

REFERENCES
Structure

1 Adams, J. H., Daniel, P. M., and Prichard, M. M. L.: Observations on the portal circulation of pituitary gland, Neuroendocrinology 1:193-213, 1965-1966.
2 Bergland, R. M., Ray, B. S., and Torack, R. M.: Anatomical variations in the pituitary gland and adjacent structures in 225 human autopsy cases, J. Neurosurg. 28:93-99, 1968.
3 Boyd, J. D.: Observations on the human pharyngeal hypophysis, J. Endocrinol. 14:66-77, 1956.
4 Erdheim, J., and Stumme, F.: Über die Schwangerschaftsveränderungen bie der Hypophyse, Beitr. Pathol. Anat. 46:1-32, 1909.
5 Jost, A.: Anterior pituitary function in foetal life. In Harris, G. W., and Donovan, B. T., editors: The pituitary gland, Berkeley, Cal., 1966, University of California Press.
6 Melchionna, R. H., and Moore, R. A.: The pharyngeal pituitary gland, Am. J. Pathol. 14:763-771, 1938.
7 Pantić, V. R.: The specificity of pituitary cells and regulation of their activities, Int. Rev. Cytol. 40:153-195, 1975.
8 Renn, W. H., and Rhoton, A. L., Jr.: Microsurgical anatomy of the sellar region, Neurosurgery 43:288-298, 1975.
9 Russell, D. S.: Pituitary gland (hypophysis). In Anderson, W. A. D., editor: Pathology, ed. 4, St. Louis, 1961, The C. V. Mosby Co.
10 Russell, D. S.: Effects of dividing the pituitary stalk in man, Lancet 1:466-468, 1956.
11 Sheehan, H. L.: Neurohypophysis and hypothalamus. In Bloodworth, J. M. B., Jr., editor: Endocrine pathology, Baltimore, 1968, The Williams & Wilkins Co., Chap. 3.
12 Stanfield, J. P.: The blood supply of the human pituitary gland, J. Anat. 94:257-273, 1960.
13 Wells, L. J., and Highby, D. N.: Experimental evidence of production of adrenotrophin by the fetal hypophysis, Proc. Soc. Exp. Biol. Med. 68:487-488, 1948.
14 Willis, R. A.: The borderland of embryology and pathology, London, 1958, Butterworth & Co., Chap. 7 (developmental vestiges and their pathology).
15 Xuereb, G. P., Prichard, M. M. L., and Daniel, P. M.: Arterial supply and venous drainage of human hypophysis cerebri, Q. J. Exp. Physiol. 39:199-217, 1954.
16 Xuereb, G. P., Prichard, M. M. L., and Daniel, P. M.: The hypophysial portal system of vessels in man, Q. J. Exp. Physiol. 39:219-230, 1954.

Histology and function

17 Adams, C. W. M., and Swettenham, K. V.: Histochemical identification of two types of basophil cell in the normal human adenohypophysis, J. Pathol. Bacteriol. 75:95-103, 1958.
18 Bergland, R. M., and Torack, R. M.: An ultrastructural study of follicular cells in the human anterior pituitary, Am. J. Pathol. 57:273-297, 1969.
19 Brookes, L. D.: A stain for differentiating two types of acidophil cells in the rat pituitary, Stain Technol. 43:41-42, 1968.
20 deCicco, F. A., Dekker, A., and Yunis, E. J.: Fine structure of Crooke's hyaline change in the human pituitary gland, Arch. Pathol. 94:65-70, 1972.
21 Ezrin, C.: Embryology and anatomy of thyrotrophin-secreting cell, the thyrotroph. In Werner, S. C., and Ingbar, S. H., editors: The thyroid, ed. 3, Hagerstown, Md., 1971, Harper & Row, Chap. 12.
22 Ezrin, C., and Murray, S.: The cells of the human adenohypophysis in pregnancy, thyroid disease and adrenal cortical disorders. In Benoit, J., and DaLage, C., editors: Cytologie de l'adénohypophyse, Paris, 1963, Centre National de la Recherche Scientifique, pp. 183-199.
23 Farquhar, M. G., Skutelsky, E. H., and Hopkins, C. R.: Structure and function of dispersed anterior pituitary cells: in vitro studies. In Tixier-Vidal, A., and Farquhar, M. G., editors: The anterior pituitary, New York, 1975, Academic Press, Inc., pp. 123-126.
24 Goluboff, L. G., and Ezrin, C.: Effect of pregnancy on the somatotroph and the prolactin cell of the human adenohypophysis, J. Clin. Endocrinol. 29:1533-1538, 1969.
25 Halmi, N. S.: Curent status of human pituitary cytophysiology, N.Z. Med. J. 80:551-556, 1974.
26 Ham, A. W.: Histology, ed. 7, Philadelphia, 1974, J. B. Lippincott Co.

27 Herlant, M.: In Tixier-Vidal, A., and Farquhar, M. G., editors: The anterior pituitary, New York, 1975, Academic Press, Inc. (introduction).

28 Herlant, M., and Pasteels, J. L.: Histophysiology of human anterior pituitary, Methods Achiev. Exp. Pathol. 3:250-305, 1967.

29 Holmes, R. L., and Ball, J. N.: The pituitary gland, Cambridge, 1974, Cambridge University Press (comparative account of structure and function).

30 McManus, J. F. A.: Histological demonstration of mucin after periodic acid, Nature 158:202, 1946.

31 Olivier, L., Vila-Porcile, E., Racadot, O., Peillon, F., and Racadot, J.: Ultrastructure of pituitary tumor cells: a critical study. In Tixier-Vidal, A., and Farquhar, M. G., editors: The anterior pituitary, New York, 1975, Academic Press, Inc., pp. 231-276.

32 Paget, G. E., and Eccleston, E.: Simultaneous specific demonstration of thyrotroph, gonadotroph, and acidophil cells in anterior hypophysis, Stain Technol. 35:119-122, 1960.

33 Paiz, C., and Hennigar, G. R.: Electron microscopy and histochemical correlation of human anterior pituitary cells, Am. J. Pathol. 59:43-73, 1970.

34 Pasteels, J. L., Gausset, P., Danguy, A., Ectors, F., Nicoll, C. S., and Varavudhi, P.: Morphology of lactotropes and somatotropes of man and Rhesus monkeys, J. Clin. Endocrinol. 34:959-967, 1972.

35 Pearse, A. G. E.: Cytochemistry and cytology of the normal anterior hypophysis investigated by the trichrome–periodic acid–Schiff method, J. Pathol. Bacteriol. 64:811-826, 1952.

36 Pearse, A. G. E., and van Noorden, S.: The functional cytology of human adenohypophysis, Can. Med. Assoc. J. 88:462-471, 1963.

37 Phifer, R. F., Midgley, A. R., and Spicer, S. S.: Immunohistologic and histologic evidence that follicle-stimulating hormone and luteinizing hormone are present in the same cell type in the human pars distalis, J. Clin. Endocrinol. 36:125-141, 1973.

38 Phifer, R. F., Orth, D. N., and Spicer, S. S.: Specific demonstration of human hypophyseal adrenocortico-melanotropic (ACTH/MSH) cell, J. Clin. Endocrinol. 39:684-692, 1974.

39 Phifer, R. F., and Spicer, S. S.: Immunohistochemical and histologic demonstration of thyrotrophic cells of the human adenohypophysis, J. Clin. Endocrinol. 36:1210-1221, 1973.

40 Romeis, B.: In von Möllendorff, W., editor: Handbuch der mikroskopischen Anatomie des Menschen, vol. 6, part 3, Berlin, 1940, Julius Springer Verlag (hypophysis).

41 van Oordt, P. G. W. J.: Nomenclature of the hormone-producing cells in the adenohypophysis. A report of the International Committee for Nomenclature of the Adenohypophysis, Gen. Comp. Endocrinol. 5:131-134, 1965.

42 von Lawzewitsch, I., Dickmann, G. H., Amezua, L., and Pardal, C.: Cytological and ultrastructural characterization of the human pituitary, Acta Anat. 81:286-316, 1972.

Pituitary in endocrine disorders

43 Bloodworth, J. M. B., Jr., Kirkendall, W. M., and Carr, T. L.: Addison's disease associated with thyroid insufficiency and atrophy (Schmidt syndrome), J. Clin. Endocrinol. 14:540-553, 1954.

44 Boyce, R., and Beadles, C. F.: Enlargement of the hypophysis cerebri in myxoedema; with remarks upon hypertrophy of the hypophysis, associated with changes in the thyroid body, J. Pathol. Bacteriol. 1:224-239, 1893.

45 Burt, A. S., Landing, B. H., and Sommers, S. C.: Amphophil tumors of hypophysis induced in mice by I¹³¹, Cancer Res. 14:497-502, 1954.

46 Carpenter, C. C. J., Solomon, N., Silverberg, S. G., Bledsoe, R., Northcutt, R. C., Klinenberg, J. R., Bennett, I. L., Jr., and Harvey, A. M.: Schmidt's syndrome (thyroid and adrenal insufficiency): a review of the literature and a report of fifteen new cases including ten instances of coexistent diabetes mellitus, Medicine 43:153-180, 1964.

47 Crooke, A. C.: A change in the basophil cells of the pituitary gland common to conditions that exhibit the syndrome attributed to basophil adenoma, J. Pathol. Bacteriol. 41:339-349, 1935.

48 Crooke, A. C., and Russell, D. S.: The pituitary gland in Addison's disease, J. Pathol. Bacteriol. 40:255-283, 1935.

49 Ezrin, C.: The adenohypophysis. In Ezrin, C., Godden, J. O., Volpe, R., and Wilson, R., editors: Systematic endocrinology, Hagerstown, Md., 1973, Harper & Row, Chap. 4 (basophils in hypogonadism).

50 Farquhar, M. G., and Rinehart, J. F.: Electron microscopic studies of the anterior pituitary gland of castrate rats, Endocrinology 54:516-541, 1954.

51 Halmi, N. S., and McCormick, W. F.: Effects of hyperadrenocorticism on pituitary thyrotrophic cells in man, Arch. Pathol. 94:471-474, 1972.

52 Halmi, N. S., McCormick, W. F., and Decker, D. A., Jr.: The natural history of hyalinization of ACTH/MSH cells in man, Arch. Pathol. 91:318-326, 1971.

53 Irvine, W. J.: Autoimmunity in endocrine disease, Proc. Roy. Soc. Med. 67:548-555, 1974.

54 Ketelbant-Balasse, P., Herlant, M., and Pasteels, J. L.: Modifications hypophysaires dans un cas d'hypercorticisme para-néoplastique, Ann. Endocrinol. (Paris) 34:743-752, 1973 (Crooke's change due to hyperadrenocorticism caused by lung cancer: report of a case).

55 Kilby, R. A., Bennett, W. A., and Sprague, R. G.: Anterior pituitary gland in patients treated with cortisone and corticotropin, Am. J. Pathol. 33:155-173, 1955.

56 Kovacs, K., and Horvath, E.: Gonadotrophs following removal of ovaries: a fine structural study of human pituitary glands, Endokrinologie 66:1-8, 1975.

57 Melnyk, C. S., and Greer, M. A.: Functional pituitary tumor in an adult possibly secondary to long-standing myxedema, J. Clin. Endocrinol. 25:761-766, 1965.

58 Mösli, P., and Hedinger, C.: Noduläre Hyperplasie und Adenome des Hypophysenvorderlappens bei Hypothyreose, Acta Endocrinol. **58:**507-520, 1968.

59 Murray, S., and Ezrin, C.: Effect of Graves' disease on the "thyrotroph" of the adenohypophysis, J. Clin. Endocrinol. **26:**287-293, 1966.

60 Porcile, E., and Racodot, J.: Ultrastructure des cellules de Crooke observées dans l'hypophyse humaine au cours de la maladie de Cushing, C. R. Acad. Sci. (Paris) Series D, **263:**948-951, 1966.

61 Russfield, A. B.: The endocrine glands after bilateral adrenalectomy compared with those in spontaneous adrenal insufficiency, Cancer **8:** 523-537, 1955.

62 Russfield, A. B.: Adenohypophysis. In Bloodworth, J. M. B., Jr., editor: Endocrine pathology, Baltimore, 1968, The Williams & Wilkins Co., Chap. 4, pp. 92-93 (basophils in hypogonadism).

63 Russfield, A. B., and Byrnes, R. L.: Some effects of hormone therapy and castration on the hypophysis in men with carcinoma of the prostate, Cancer **11:**817-828, 1958.

64 Schochet, S. S., Jr., Halmi, N. S., and McCormick, W. F.: PAS-positive hyalin change in ACTH/MSH cells of man, Arch. Pathol. **93:**457-463, 1972.

65 Siperstein, E. R., and Miller, K. J.: Hypertrophy of ACTH-producing cell following adrenalectomy: a quantitative electron microscopic study, Endocrinology **93:**1257-1268, 1973.

66 Stratmann, I. E., Ezrin, C., Sellers, E. A., and Simon, G. T.: The origin of thyroidectomy cells as revealed by high resolution radioautography, Endocrinology **90:**728-734, 1972.

67 Thornton, K. R.: The cytology of the pituitary gland in myxoedema, J. Pathol. Bacteriol. **77:** 249-255, 1959.

Hypophysectomy

68 Block, G. E., Jensen, E. V., and Polley, T. Z., Jr.: The prediction of hormonal dependency of mammary cancer, Ann. Surg. **182:**342-352, 1975.

69 Crome, L.: Underdevelopment of the pituitary, Dev. Med. Child Neurol. **16:**222-224, 1974.

70 Horwitz, K. B., McGuire, W. L., Pearson, O. H., and Segaloff, A.: Predicting response to endocrine therapy in human breast cancer: a hypothesis, Science **189:**726-727, 1975.

71 Lipsett, M. B.: Endocrine responsive cancers of man. In Williams, R. H., editor: Textbook of endocrinology, ed. 5, Philadelphia, 1974, W. B. Saunders Co., Chap. 28.

72 McPhie, J. L., and Beck, J. S.: Growth hormone in the normal human pharyngeal pituitary gland, Nature (London) **219:**625-626, 1968.

73 McGrath, P.: Extra-sellar post-hypophysectomy remnant, Br. J. Surg. **56:**64-67, 1969.

74 McGrath, P.: Prolactin activity and human growth hormone in pharyngeal hypophyses from embalmed cadavers, J. Endocrinol. **42:** 205-212, 1968.

75 Müller, W.: On the pharyngeal hypophysis. In Currie, A. R., and Illingworth, C. F. W., editors: Endocrine aspects of breast cancer, Edinburgh, 1958, E. & S. Livingstone, Ltd.

76 Pearson, O. H., and Ray, B. S.: Hypophysectomy in the treatment of metastatic mammary cancer, Am. J. Surg. **99:**544-552, 1960.

77 Ratzkowski, E., Adler, B., and Hochman, A.: Survival time and treatment results of patients with disseminated breast cancer especially after adrenalectomy and hypophysectomy, Oncology **28:**385-397, 1973.

Hypopituitarism

78 Daughaday, W. H.: The adenohypophysis. In Williams, R. H., editor: Textbook of endocrinology, ed. 5, Philadelphia, 1975, W. B. Saunders Co., Chap. 2.

79 Laron, Z.: The hypothalamus and the pituitary gland (hypophysis). In Hubble, D., editor: Paediatric endocrinology, Philadelphia, 1969, F. A. Davis Co., Chap. 2.

80 Sheehan, H. L.: Post-partum necrosis of the anterior pituitary, J. Pathol. Bacteriol. **45:**189-214, 1937.

Anomalies

81 Angevine, D. M.: Pathologic anatomy of hypophysis and adrenals in anencephaly, Arch. Pathol. **26:**507-518, 1938.

82 Blizzard, R. M., and Alberts, M.: Hypopituitarism, hypoadrenalism, and hypogonadism in newborn infant, J. Pediatr. **48:**782-792, 1956.

83 Edmonds, H. W.: Pituitary, adrenal and thyroid in cyclopia, Arch. Pathol. **50:**727-735, 1950.

84 Lennox, B., and Russell, D. S.: Dystopia of the neurohypophysis: two cases, J. Pathol. Bacteriol. **63:**485-490, 1951.

85 Moncrieff, M. W., Hill, D. S., Archer, J., and Arthur, L. J. H.: Congenital absence of pituitary gland and adrenal hypoplasia, Arch. Dis. Child. **47:**136-137, 1972.

86 Potter, E. L., and Craig, J. M.: Pathology of the fetus and the infant, ed. 3, Chicago, 1975, Year Book Medical Publishers, Inc., Chap. 16, p. 331.

87 Steiner, M. W., and Boggs, J. D.: Absence of pituitary gland, hypothyroidism, hypoadrenalism and hypogonadism in a 17-year-old dwarf, J. Clin. Endocrinol. **25:**1591-1598, 1965.

88 Willard, D., Sacrez, R., Messer, J., Korn, R., Krug, J.-P., and Vors, J.: La dysgénésie antéhypophysaire primitive, Nouv. Presse Med. **1:**2237-2242, 1972 (agenesis of pituitary).

Hemorrhage

89 Goldman, K. P., and Jacobs, A.: Anterior and posterior pituitary failure after head injury, Br. Med. J. **5217:**1924-1926, 1960.

90 Kornblum, R. N., and Fisher, R. S.: Pituitary lesions in craniocerebral injuries, Arch. Pathol. **88:**242-248, 1969.

91 McCormick, W. F., and Halmi, N. S.: Hypophysis in patients with coma dépassé ("respirator brain"), Am. J. Clin. Pathol. **54:**374-383, 1970.

92 Rovit, R. L., and Fein, J. M.: Pituitary apoplexy: review and reappraisal, J. Neurosurg. **37:**280-288, 1972.

Infarction and necrosis

93 Adams, J. H., Daniel, P. M., Prichard, M. M. L., and Schurr, P. H.: The volume of the infarct in pars distalis of a human pituitary gland, 30 hr after transection of the pituitary stalk, J. Physiol. **166:**39P, 1963.

94 Daniel, P. M., Spicer, E. J. F., and Treip, C. S.: Pituitary necrosis in patients maintained on mechanical respirators, J. Pathol. **111:**135-138, 1973.

95 Frey, H. M.: Spontaneous pituitary destruction in diabetes mellitus, J. Clin. Endocrinol. **19:**1642-1650, 1959.

96 Kovacs, K.: Adenohypophysial necrosis in routine autopsies, Endokrinologie **60:**309-316, 1972.

97 Kovacs, K.: Necrosis of anterior pituitary in humans, Neuroendocrinology **4:**170-241, 1969.

98 Kovacs, K.: Pituitary necrosis in diabetes mellitus, Acta Diabetol. Lat. **9:**958-970, 1972.

99 Purnell, D. C., Randall, R. V., and Rynearson, E. H.: Postpartum pituitary insufficiency (Sheehan's syndrome: review of 18 cases, Mayo Clin. Proc. **39:**321-331, 1964.

100 Sheehan, H. L., and Davis, J. C.: Pituitary necrosis, Br. Med. Bull. **24:**59-70, 1968.

101 Towbin, A.: The respirator brain death syndrome, Hum. Pathol. **4:**583-594, 1973.

Inflammation

102 Askenasy, H. M., Israeli, J., Karny, H., and Dujovny, M.: Intrasellar abscess simulating pituitary adenoma, Neurochirurgia **14:**34-37, 1971.

103 Brenner, J. H.: Abscess of the pituitary gland in a diabetic patient, Diabetes **4:**223-225, 1955 (Houssay phenomenon in man).

104 Doniach, I.: Diseases of endocrine glands. In Harrison, C. V., editor: Recent advances in pathology, Boston, 1960, Little, Brown & Co., Chap. 7.

105 Goudie, R. B.: Anterior hypophysitis associated with autoimmune disease, Proc. Roy. Soc. Med. **61:**275, 1968.

106 Goudie, R. B., and Pinkerton, P. H.: Anterior hypophysitis and Hashimoto's disease in a young woman, J. Pathol. Bacteriol. **83:**584-585, 1962.

107 Hume, R., and Roberts, G. H.: Hypophysitis and hypopituitarism: report of a case, Br. Med. J. **2:**548-550, 1967.

108 Lack, E. E.: Lymphoid "hypophysitis" with end organ insufficiency, Arch. Pathol. **99:**215-219, 1975.

109 Oelbaum, M. H.: Hypopituitarism in male subjects due to syphilis, Q. J. Med. **21:**249-264, 1952.

110 Plair, C. M., and Perry, S.: Hypothalamic-pituitary sarcoidosis, Arch. Pathol. **74:**527-535, 1962.

111 Simmonds, M.: Über embolische Prozesse in der Hypophyse, Virchows Arch. Pathol. Anat. Physiol. **217:**226-239, 1914.

Infiltrations and metabolic disorders

112 Barr, R., and Lampert, P.: Intrasellar amyloid tumor, Acta Neuropathol. **21:**83-86, 1972.

113 Bilbao, J. M., Horvath, E., Hudson, A., and

114 Kraus, E. J.: In Henke, F., and Lubarsch, O., editors: Handbuch der speziellen Anatomie und Histologie, vol. 8, Berlin, 1926, Julius Springer Verlag (diseases of the hypophysis).

Kovacs, K.: Pituitary adenoma producing amyloid-like substance, Arch. Pathol. **99:**411-415, 1975.

115 Russell, D. S., and Rubinstein, L. J.: Pathology of tumours of the nervous system, London, 1963, E. Arnold & Co.

116 Schober, R., and Nelson, D.: Fine structure and origin of amyloid deposits in pituitary adenoma, Arch. Pathol. **99:**403-410, 1975.

117 Schochet, S. S., Jr., McCormick, W. F., and Halmi, N. S.: Pituitary gland in patients with Hurler syndrome, Arch. Pathol. **97:**96-99, 1974.

Tumors

118 Ballard, H. S., Frame, B., and Hartsock, R. J.: Familial multiple endocrine adenoma–peptic complex, Medicine **43:**481-516, 1964.

119 Burston, J., John, R., and Spencer, H.: "Myoblastoma" of neurohypophysis, J. Pathol. Bacteriol. **83:**455-461, 1962.

120 Caughey, J. E., and Lester, M. J.: Hypothyroidism and pituitary tumors, N.Z. Med. J. **60:**486-489, 1961.

121 Currie, A. R.: Pituitary gland. In Anderson, W. A. D., editor, Pathology, ed. 6, St. Louis, 1971, The C. V. Mosby Co., Chap. 33.

122 Cushing, H.: The basophil adenomas of the pituitary body and their clinical manifestations (pituitary basophilism), Bull. Johns Hopkins Hosp. **50:**137-195, 1932.

123 D'Abrera, V. S. E., Burke, W. J., Bleasel, K. F., and Bader, L.: Carcinoma of pituitary gland, J. Pathol. **109:**335-343, 1973.

124 Dingemans, K. P.: Development of TSH-producing pituitary tumours in mouse, Virchows Arch. (Zellpathol.) **12:**338-359, 1973.

125 Dott, N. M., Bailey, P., and Cushing, H.: Hypophysial adenomata, Br. J. Surg. **13:**314-366, 1925.

126 Evans, R. W.: Histological appearances of tumours, ed. 2, Edinburgh, 1966, E. & S. Livingstone, Ltd., Chap. 21 (tumors of pituitary gland).

127 Fisher, E. R., and Wechsler, J.: Granular cell myoblastoma—a misnomer, Cancer **15:**936-954, 1962.

128 Forbes, A. P., Henneman, P. H., Griswold, G. C., and Albright, F.: Syndrome characterized by galactorrhea, amenorrhea and low urinary FSH: comparison with acromegaly and normal lactation, J. Clin. Endocrinol. **14:**265-271, 1954.

129 Friedman, N. B.: Germinoma of pineal—its identity with germinoma ("seminoma") of the testis, Cancer Res. **7:**363-368, 1947.

130 Furth, J., Clifton, K. H., Gadsden, E. L., and Buffett, R. F.: Dependent and autonomous mammotropic pituitary tumors in rats; their somatotropic features, Cancer Res. **16:**608-616, 1956.

131 Ghatak, N. R., Hirano, A., and Zimmerman, H. M.: Intrasellar germinomas: a form of ectopic pinealoma, J. Neurosurg. **31:**670-675, 1969.

132 Ghatak, N. R., Hirano, A., and Zimmerman,

H. M.: Ultrastructure of a craniopharyngioma, Cancer **27**:1465-1475, 1971.

133 Griesbach, W. E., and Purves, H. D.: Basophil adenomata in the rat hypophysis after gonadectomy, Br. J. Cancer **14**:49-59, 1960.

134 Guyda, H., Robert, F., Colle, E., and Hardy, J.: Histologic, ultrastructural, and hormonal characterization of pituitary tumor secreting HGH and prolactin, J. Clin. Endocrinol. **36**: 531-547, 1973.

135 Hamilton, C. R., Jr., Adams, L. C., and Maloof, F.: Hyperthyroidism due to thyrotrophin-producing pituitary chromophobe adenoma, New Eng. J. Med. **283**:1077-1080, 1970.

136 Houck, W. A., Olson, K. B., and Horton, J.: Clinical features of tumor metastasis to pituitary, Cancer **26**:656-659, 1970.

137 Kernohan, J. W., and Sayre, G. P.: In Atlas of tumor pathology, Sect. X, Fasc. 36, Washington, D.C., 1956, Armed Forces Institute of Pathology.

138 Kovacs, K.: Metastatic cancer of pituitary gland, Oncology **27**:533-542, 1973.

139 Kovacs, K., and Horvath, E.: Pituitary chromophobe adenoma composed of oncocytes. A light and electron microscopic study, Arch. Pathol. **95**:235-239, 1973.

140 Kovacs, K., Horvath, E., Corenblum, B., Sirek, A. M. T., Penz, G., and Ezrin, C.: Pituitary chromophobe adenomas consisting of prolactin cells, Virchows Arch. (Pathol. Anat.) **366**:113-123, 1975.

141 Landolt, A. M., and Oswald, U. W.: Histology and ultrastructure of an oncocytic adenoma of human pituitary, Cancer **31**:1099-1105, 1973.

142 Leibowitz, U., Yablonski, M., and Alter, M.: Tumors of nervous system—incidence and population selectivity, J. Chron. Dis. **23**:707-721, 1971.

143 Luse, S. A., and Kernohan, J. W.: Granular-cell tumors of the stalk and posterior lobe of the pituitary gland, Cancer **8**:616-622, 1955.

144 Markesberry, W. R., Duffy, P. E., and Cowen, D.: Granular cell tumors of the central nervous system, J. Neuropathol. Exp. Neurol. **32**:92-109, 1973.

145 Marshall, A. H. E., and Sloper, J. C.: Pluriglandular adenomatosis of pituitary, parathyroid and pancreatic islet cells associated with lipomatosis, J. Pathol. Bacteriol. **68**:225-229, 1954.

146 Nelson, D. H., Meakin, J., and Thorn, G. W.: ACTH-producing pituitary tumors following adrenalectomy for Cushing's syndrome, Ann. Intern. Med. **52**:560-569, 1960.

147 Nyhan, W. L., and Green, M.: Hyperthyroidism in patient with a pituitary adenoma, J. Pediatr. **65**:583-589, 1964.

148 Peake, G. T., McKeel, D. W., Jarett, L., and Daughaday, W. H.: Ultrastructural, histologic, and hormonal characterization of a prolactin-rich human pituitary tumor, J. Clin. Endocrinol. **29**:1383-1393, 1969.

149 Queiroz, L. de S., Facure, N. B., Facure, J. J., Modesto, N. P., and Lopes de Faria, J.: Pituitary carcinoma with liver metastases and Cushing syndrome, Arch. Pathol. **99**:32-35, 1975.

150 Racadot, J., Vila-Porcile, E., Peillon, F., and Olivier, L.: Adénomes hypophysaires à cellules à prolactine: étude structural et ultrastructurale, corrélations anatomocliniques, Ann. Endocrinol. **32**:298-305, 1971.

151 Roessmann, U., Kaufman, B., and Friede, R. L.: Metastatic lesions in the sella turcica and pituitary gland, Cancer **25**:478-480, 1970.

152 Rovit, R. L., and Duane, T. D.: Cushing's syndrome and pituitary tumors, Am. J. Med. **46**:416-427, 1969.

153 Rubenstein, L. J.: Tumors of the central nervous system, Ser. 2, Fasc. 6, Atlas of tumor pathology, Washington, D.C., 1972, Armed Forces Institute of Pathology.

154 Saeger, W.: Hypophysenadenome bei Galactorrhoe, Virchows Arch. (Pathol. Anat.) **368**: 123-139, 1975.

155 Saeger, W.: Licht- und elektronenmikroskopische Untersuchungen zur Klassifikation von Hypophysenadenomen, Z. Krebsforsch. **84**:105-128, 1975.

156 Satyamurti, S., and Huntington, H. W.: Granular cell myoblastoma of the pituitary: case report, J. Neurosurg. **37**:483-486, 1972.

157 Schecter, J.: Electron microscopic studies of human pituitary tumors. I. Chromophobe adenomas, Am. J. Anat. **138**:371-385, 1973.

158 Schechter, J.: Electron microscopic studies of human pituitary tumors. II. Acidophilic adenomas, Am. J. Anat. **138**:387-399, 1973.

159 Seemayer, T. A., Blundell, J. S., and Wiglesworth, F. W.: Pituitary craniopharyngioma with tooth formation, Cancer **29**:423-430, 1972.

160 Shuangshoti, S., Netsky, M. G., and Nashold, B. S., Jr.: Epithelial cysts related to sella turcica—proposed origin from neuroepithelium, Arch. Pathol. **90**:444-450, 1970.

161 Symon, L., Ganz, J. C., and Burston, J.: Granular cell myoblastoma of neurohypophysis. Report of 2 cases, J. Neurosurg. **35**:82-89, 1971.

162 Underdahl, L. O., Woolner, L. B., and Black, B. M.: Multiple endocrine adenomas: report of 8 cases in which the parathyroids, pituitary and pancreatic islets were involved, J. Clin. Endocrinol. **13**:20-47, 1953.

163 Waller, R. R., Riley, F. C., and Sundt, T. M., Jr.: A rare cause of the chiasmal syndrome, Arch. Ophthalmol. **88**:269-272, 1972 (granular cell myoblastoma of neurohypophysis).

164 Wermer, P.: Endocrine adenomatosis and peptic ulcer in a large kindred, Am. J. Med. **35**: 205-212, 1963.

165 Werner, S. C., and Stewart, W. B.: Hyperthyroidism in a patient with pituitary chromophobe adenoma and a fragment of normal pituitary, J. Clin. Endocrinol. **18**:266-270, 1958.

166 Zimmerman, H. M.: Ten most common types of brain tumor, Semin. Roentgenol. **6**:48-58, 1971.

167 Zülch, K. J.: Brain tumors, their biology and pathology, ed. 2, New York, 1965, Springer Verlag.

37/Thyroid gland

SHELDON C. SOMMERS

STRUCTURE AND FUNCTION

The normal weight of the adult thyroid gland is 15 to 35 gm, or not more than 0.35 gm per kilogram of body weight. In the newborn infant, the normal weight is 1.4 to 3.5 gm. The functional unit comprises a main thyroid follicle and satellite follicles, which together form lobules. On gross examination, the bilobed thyroid gland, isthmus, and variable pyramidal lobe have a translucent capsule. Sectioning shows homogeneous, moist, tan, slightly gelatinous tissue. Histologically, the normal thyroid gland is composed of uniform, regularly arranged follicles filled with colloid and lined by low cuboid follicular epithelium with a thin basement membrane. The interfollicular vascular stroma is delicate. Increased colloid storage of the two major thyroid hormones, thyroxine (T_4) and triiodothyronine (T_3), is reflected by a flattening and secretion by a columnar hypertrophy of the epithelial cells. Their microvilli, secretory or resorptive vacuoles, lysosomes, and other organelles alter with thyroid function.

The thyroid gland preferentially absorbs iodide from the blood and concentrates it 40 times or more. By five important enzymatic reactions, the iodide is trapped and organified, iodotyrosines are coupled and deiodinated, and thyroglobulin is formed, to be resorbed subsequently and secreted as T_3 and T_4. Enzymatic defects are the cause of most familial goiters. In the circulation, some 80% of T_4 is attached to the plasma thyroid-binding globulin and thyroid-binding prealbumin. When this globulin is increased, as by estrogens, thyroid gland hypertrophy ensues to maintain the normal plasma concentration of free T_4. The parafollicular or C cells in the human thyroid gland are not identifiable by ordinary light or electron microscopy. Calcitonin secreted by these cells is a polypeptide hormone of low molecular weight with a hypocalcemic effect that counterbalances parathyroid hormone.

CONGENITAL ABNORMALITIES

Lingual thyroid gland is a persistent undescended embryonic anlage forming a mass at the base of the tongue. Its removal usually renders the patient athyrotic. Normally, the anlage descends in the anterior cervical midline, and incomplete descent results in aberrant subhyoid or intratracheal thyroid tissue. Heterotopic thyroid tissue also has been found in the larynx, pericardium, heart, porta hepatis, vagina, scrotum, and inguinal canal.

Thyroglossal duct cysts are commonly thin walled, 1 to 2 cm in diameter, and contain sticky yellow fluid. The cyst wall is formed either by mature thyroid epithelium or by ciliated columnar or metaplastic stratified squamous epithelium. Because of its propinquity, the hyoid bone also is often removed surgically to prevent recurrent cyst formation.

Substernal thyroid tissue is the result of embryologic descent into the anterior mediastinum. Substernal goiters may rise with respiration into the suprasternal notch or become incarcerated there. Lingual and subhyoid thyroid tissue sometimes also forms goiters. Papillary adenomas and carcinomas occur in thyroglossal duct cysts, but few of these cancers have metastasized. "Lateral aberrant thyroid" ordinarily refers to microscopic groups of mature follicles in lymph nodes, cervical strap muscles, or fat located a few millimeters from the thyroid capsule. When larger lateral thyroid masses are removed, practically all prove to be prominent metastases of an unrecognized intrathyroid carcinoma.

Failure of thyroid organogenesis may result in a mixture of ducts, lymphatic nodules, connective tissue, and a few folllicles. Abundant fat mingled with mature thyroid tissue is termed "adenolipomatosis" or "hamartomatous thyroid adiposity." Minor malformations of branchial pouch differentiation include intrathyroidal parathyroid glands or portions of thymus. Ducts or squamous cell cysts in otherwise well-formed thyroid glands may represent remnants of the embryonic ultimobranchial body.

Cretinism centers around congenital thyroid deficiency. Cretins typically have a large head, broad nose, wide-set eyes, low forehead, large, thick tongue, and dry skin. The most serious clinical aspect is failure of central nervous system development. If infantile hypothyroidism is not discovered and treated within 6 months, irreversible mental retardation may result. Cretins show stunted growth, enamel dysplasia, umbilical hernia, and sexual infantilism, and they may have other defects of the central nervous system, such as deaf-mutism.

Thyroid aplasia, so-called athyrotic cretinism, is the usual type in the United States. Hypoplasia of either a normally located or ectopic thyroid gland also occurs. Together, these conditions comprise sporadic, nongoitrous cretinism.

GOITER AND ALTERED HORMONAL BIOSYNTHESIS

Goiter means persistent thyroid enlargement. Different terms for thyroid disease are sometimes used by clinicians and pathologists, but interpretation is not difficult (Table 37-1). Most goiters weigh over 40 gm, but some are as small as 25 gm.

Simple goiter also is called diffuse or colloid-storage goiter. Adolescent girls and pregnant women and other women exposed to increased estrogens may develop the symmetric thyroid enlargement and swanlike neck depicted in Renaissance paintings. Colloid-storage goiters ordinarily involute. Grossly, the tissue is homogeneous and notably gelatinous. Microscopically, the follicles generally are enlarged with excessive colloid content, and the lining epithelium is flattened.

Nodular goiter is the most familiar thyroid disease. It also is called, among various names, adenomatous, endemic, nodular colloid, and nontoxic multinodular goiter. Iodine deficiency is the ordinary cause of nodular goiter. Before the widespread use of iodized salt, iodine-poor diets predisposed to goiter, particularly in mountainous areas or around inland fresh waters. In southern Austria (Styria) and some areas of the Andes mountains, nodular goiter is still commonplace. Women are affected more than men in a ratio of about 6:1. With iodine deficiency, at first the entire thyroid gland becomes enlarged and more vascular. Follicles shrink, and their epithelium proliferates. An opportunity to see this early diffuse hyperplastic reaction is uncommon except experimentally.

Typical nodular goiters are large, weighing from 60 to over 1000 gm. Grossly and microscopically, they have four characteristics: nodules, hemorrhage, fibrosis, and calcification (Fig. 37-1). The nodules vary in size and colloid content, and some are colored red or brown by recent or old hemorrhage. Histologically, the appearance also is varied, with undemarcated rounded masses of abnormally large colloid-filled follicles compressing the intervening normal-sized or small so-called fetal follicles that contain very little colloid. Practically no unaltered follicles remain. In questionable cases, individual follicles larger than 2 mm in diameter, or four times the upper limit of normal, indicate a nodular goiter. The follicular epithelium is predominantly flat cuboid. Locally thickened areas, either small polsters or large reticulated epithelial papillary structures protruding into the follicles are common (Fig. 37-2). These have no known functional importance. The capillary network is reduced. Among the follicles are focal hemorrhages attributable to pressure and ischemic necrosis. Consequences of the necrosis and hemorrhage are interfollicular infiltrates of macrophages, organized hematomas, cholesterol crystals, atheromas, foreign body giant cells, and irregular fibrosis with focal calcification.

In established nodular goiters, the major processes are irregular degeneration and regeneration, hypertrophy, and colloid storage. The characteristic nodules are nonneoplastic and have no known precancerous significance.

Table 37-1. Classification of some diseases of the thyroid gland with different clinical and pathologic designations

Clinical diagnosis	Pathologic diagnosis
Euthyroidism with:	
Nontoxic diffuse goiter	Simple or colloid-storage goiter
Nontoxic uninodular goiter	Thyroid nodule
Nontoxic multinodular goiter	Nodular goiter
Hyperthyroidism with:	
Toxic diffuse goiter (Graves' disease)	Primary thyroid hyperplasia
Toxic uninodular goiter	Nodular thyroid or adenoma with hyperplasia
Toxic multinodular goiter	Nodular goiter with secondary hyperplasia
Hypothyroidism with:	
Idiopathic myxerema	Thyroid atrophy

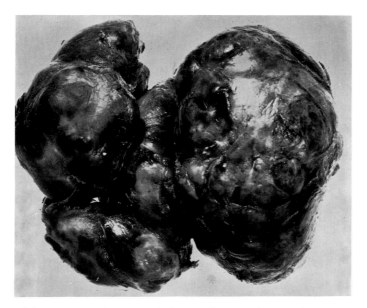

Fig. 37-1. Nodular goiter with areas of degeneration and hemorrhage. (From Anderson, W. A. D., and Scotti, T. M.: Synopsis of pathology, ed. 9, St. Louis, 1976, The C. V. Mosby Co.)

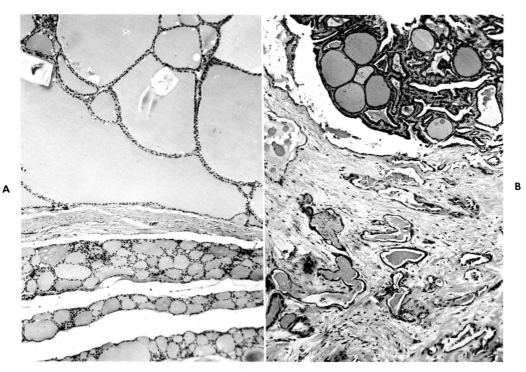

Fig. 37-2. Nodular goiter. **A,** Abundant colloid, flat epithelium, and fibrosis around upper nodule. **B,** Fibrosis and nodule with hyperplasia. (**A** and **B,** 85×.)

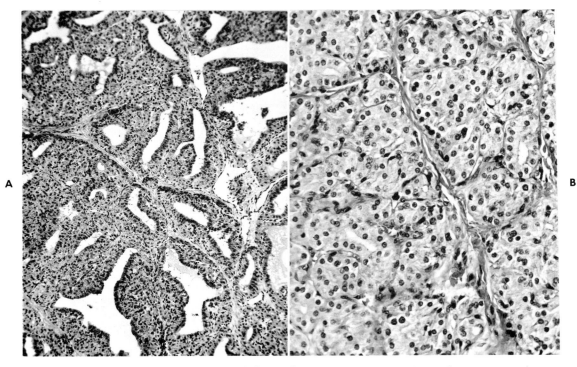

Fig. 37-3. A, Congenital goiter with hyperplastic appearance. **B,** Goiter from cretin with pale and notably hyperplastic epithelium. (**A,** 85×; **B,** 240×.)

Two important complications are local hemorrhage with sudden enlargement of the goiter and secondary hyperthyroidism, which is considered later.

Goitrous cretinism classically reflects severe maternal and critical fetal iodine deficiency with a functionally inadequate compensatory embryonic thyroid enlargement. The endemic type has become rarer with the availability of iodized salt. Iodine lack is not the sole cause however. Genetic factors contribute to both sporadic and endemic goitrous cretinism. Some cretins represent instances of familial goiter, with the histologic peculiarities described below (Fig. 37-3). Older cretins may be euthyroid.

Genetically mutant human beings or animals may lack an enzyme involved in one of the major biosynthetic reactions necessary for the secretion of thyroxine (T_4). The metabolic blocks generally are believed to be caused by autosomal recessive genes. Familial goiter may result, either with euthyroidism or with hypothyroidism. Following are six identified metabolic defects:

1. Iodide trapping
2. Iodide conversion to organically bound iodine (peroxidase deficiency)
3. Iodide organification, partially like the defect noted in (2), with eighth nerve deafness (Pendred's syndrome)
4. Monoiodotyrosine and diiodotyrosine conversions to T_3 and T_4
5. Iodotyrosine deiodination (dehalogenase deficiency)
6. T_4 release in a nonbutanol extractable form

Additional metabolic defects are still unidentified. Peripheral tissue resistance to thyroid hormones has also been reported.

Familial goiters are grossly indistinguishable from other nodular goiters. Microscopically, their recognizable peculiarities occasionally include nodules of bizarre embryonal or fetal appearance and striking cytologic atypia with irregular nuclei or large hydropic cells (Fig. 37-3, *B*). Hyperplastic epithelium occurs unaccompanied by hyperthyroidism. Genuine anaplasia and some features of carcinoma such as calcospherites and local invasion may be present, but the clinical course is ordinarily benign.

Dietary nodular goiters may develop after excessive ingestion of cabbage, which contains cyanates, or turnips, soybeans, and other foods containing goitrogens.

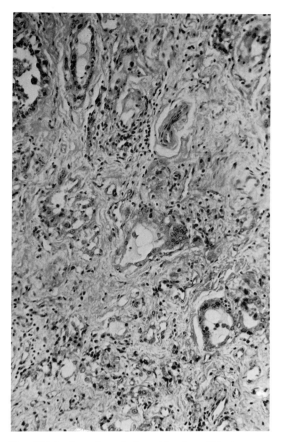

Fig. 37-4. Atrophy of thyroid after ^{131}I therapy. Abnormal epithelial cells at upper left. (85×.)

IATROGENIC ABNORMALITIES

Medications such as cyanates, thiocyanates, salicylates, and sulfonylureas may induce nodular goiter formation. Unrelated substances, some of which inhibit oxidative enzymes, including resorcinol, potassium perchlorate, lithium chloride, and cobalt chloride, are also sometimes goitrogenic. Treatment with such drugs or with thiouracil compounds during pregnancy may result in the birth of a goitrous cretin infant.

Iodide goiter may be congenital if the mother received considerable potassium iodide or iodopyrine. The fetus is evidently more sensitive than its mother to the goitrogenic effects of excess iodide. A few adults treated with iodides or iodine-containing compounds also have developed iodide goiter because of an unusual susceptibility to thyroid peroxidase inhibition. After birth, or in adults after discontinuance of therapy, iodide goiters usually regress, with colloid resorption and a transient epithelial hyperplasia accompanied by hyperfunction. Thyroid hormones administered dur-

ing pregnancy occasionally may cause an infantile goiter with epithelial hyperplasia. At least 25 other drugs affect thyroid function tests.

Ionizing radiation has notable effects on the thyroid gland from the fetal stage until adulthood. Thereafter, the thyroid is less radiosensitive, probably because its cell turnover becomes slower. After x irradiation, atomic irradiation, or exposure to isotopic ^{131}I, histologic evidence of irradiation includes an irregular hyaline fibrosis of interstitial thyroid tissue and vessel walls. Cytologically, the size, arrangement, and staining of its epithelial cells vary, with nuclei of irregular sizes and chromatin content (Fig. 37-4). Thyroid regeneration after irradiation may be nodular. Adenomas or carcinomas may develop. Neonatal or childhood x irradiation of the thyroid area is a major carcinogenic stimulus identified in more than half the children and adolescents who develop thyroid carcinomas.

HYPERPLASIA
Primary hyperplasia

An "exophthalmic goiter" removed surgically usually weighs 35 to 60 gm. The thyroid gland is diffusely enlarged, firm, red brown, opaque, and nongelatinous. Microscopically, the colloid is depleted. The follicular epithelium is columnar and folded in places to form papillae projecting inward. Typically, the colloid margins are scalloped, an artifact of aqueous fixation that reflects increased proteolysis of the peripheral colloid prior to its accelerated resorption (Fig. 37-5).

Hyperthyroidism typically goes through cycles of exacerbation with depletion or disappearance of the stored colloid and increased epithelial height, followed by remission accompanied by decreased epithelial hyperplasia and enhanced colloid storage. The epithelial papillae persist permanently even in involuted or hyperinvoluted glands. In young persons, intrathyroid lymph follicles are common, possibly related to lymphoid cell production of LATS (long-acting thyroid stimulator). This antithyroid immunoglobulin G is increased in about half the individuals with Graves' disease. LATS titers correlate with the presence of exophthalmos and pretibial myxedema.

Recurrent primary thyroid hyperplasia, either untreated or occurring after surgical or medical therapy, manifests an irregular interfollicular fibrosis and nodularity. Postoperatively, follicles may become mingled with the cervical strap muscles. Long-neglected cases merge in appearance with nodular goiter, but the intrafollicular papillae remain to indicate antecedent primary hyperplasia. Thiouracil type of medication produces no distinctive human thyroid alterations. However, since it has been in use, irregularly involuted primary thyroid hyperplasia has become more frequent.

Thyroid storm or crisis is a life-threatening exacerbated thyrotoxicosis. Psychosis, shock, and death from cardiopulmonary complications may occur. Severe primary thyroid hyperplasia is usually responsible, but rarely it is thyroiditis with hyperplasia. After trauma or infection, the normal thyroid gland responds subclinically by increased hormone secretion, with localized thickenings of the follicular epithelium (Sanderson polsters) and vacuolization of the overlying colloid.

Secondary hyperplasia

Nodular goiter complicated by hyperthyroidism chiefly affects older people. Grossly, red-tan granular thyroid tissue is found either in or between the nodules. Microscopically, nodular goiter with secondary hyperplasia is characterized by some follicles containing peripherally scalloped colloid and columnar epithelial cells. Papillae formed in secondary hyperplasia are distinguished by small follicles enclosed in their stroma (Fig. 37-6). In difficult cases, individual abnormally large follicles and papillae with follicles in their stalks indicate secondary hyperplasia rather than recurrent primary thyroid hyperplasia with irregular involution.

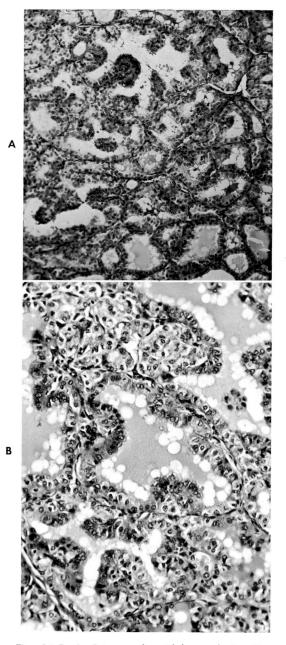

Fig. 37-5. A, Primary thyroid hyperplasia. Note scanty colloid and epithelial papillae. **B,** In primary hyperplasia with Graves' disease, follicular epithelium is tall with papillary infoldings and peripheral vacuolation of colloid. (**A,** 85×; **B,** 200×.)

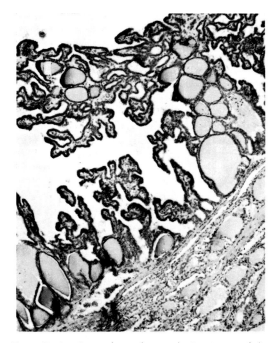

Fig. 37-6. Secondary hyperplasia in nodular goiter, with characteristic follicles in stalks of papillae. (85×; AFIP 59-6958.)

Table 37-2. Clinicopathologic features of noninfective chronic thyroiditis

Type	Sex	Age (year)	Weight of gland (gm)	Salient histopathology	Eventual hypothyroidism
Lymphocytic	F (90%)	6-35 (av. 31)	Av. 19	Lymphocytes	0-2%
Nonspecific	F (85%)	Av. 40	35-60	Plasma cells	50%
Hashimoto's struma	F (98%)	8-71 (av. 50)	60-225	Lymph follicles, epithelial damage	80%
Granulomatous	F (84%)	20-40	45-60	Foreign body granulomas	6%-20%
Riedel's struma	M = F	20-70	Bulky	Dense local fibrosis	Uncommon

Iodine treatment of a person with nodular goiter may be followed by secondary hyperthyroidism, called *jodbasedow*.

The clinical term "hot nodule" usually refers to a focus of secondary hyperplasia in a nodular goiter that concentrates ^{131}I with or without demonstrable hyperthyroidism. Over 90% of these prove pathologically to be merely the dominant nodule of a diffusely nodular thyroid gland. Until surgical removal, it may not be evident that the entire gland is nodular and either enlarged or of normal weight. A genuine follicular adenoma with secondary hyperplasia is uncommon. Secondary hyperthyroidism sometimes also complicates a follicular thyroid adenocarcinoma.

THYROIDITIS
Acute thyroiditis

Acute thyroiditis appears often to be a complication of bacterial or viral infection of the oropharynx or salivary glands. The thyroid gland becomes temporarily enlarged and tender but rarely requires operation except for drainage of suppuration. Biopsy specimens show interstitial neutrophils and some follicle degeneration.

Chronic thyroiditis

Chronic thyroiditis represents a more difficult problem, since there is no agreement on its classification or pathogenesis. The distinctive clinicopathologic features of five recognized noninfective types are listed in Table 37-2.

Hashimoto's struma. Hashimoto's struma, or struma lymphomatosa, is characterized by a firm, rubbery, enlarged gland that weighs 60 to 225 gm and is covered by an unaltered, thin capsule. On section, the thyroid tissue has a uniform, faintly lobulated, opaque yellow-tan surface unlike the grayish pink granularity of cancer (Fig. 37-7). It is often difficult microscopically to recognize thyroid follicles because of a notable lymphocytic infiltrate in sheets and follicles with germinal centers. Remnants of thyroid follicles and epithelial nests persist, often with metaplastic granular acidophilic cytoplasm, termed "Hürthle cells" (Fig. 37-8). They are more precisely named Askanazy or oxyphil cells, which are apparently nonfunctional but packed with mitochondria. Hürthle cells are common in Hashimoto's struma but also accompany other thyroid diseases and types of thyroiditis. In the fibrous variant of Hashimoto's thyroiditis one third or more of the thyroid parenchyma is replaced by dense hyaline connective tissue, which clinically may be confused with thyroid cancer.

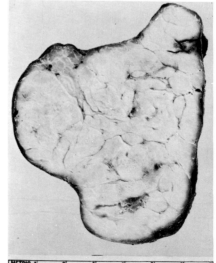

Fig. 37-7. Thyroid gland in Hashimoto's struma. (From Anderson, W. A. D., and Scotti, T. M.: Synopsis of pathology, ed. 8, St. Louis, 1972, The C. V. Mosby Co.)

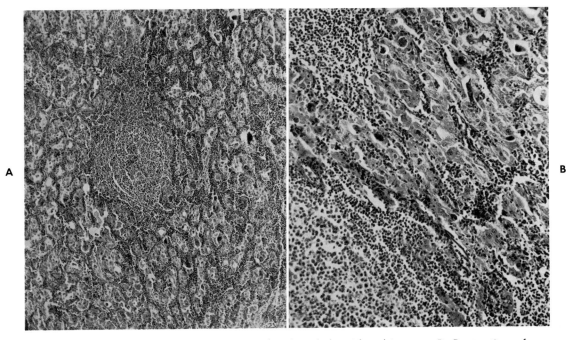

Fig. 37-8. Hashimoto's struma. **A,** Greatly altered thyroid architecture. **B,** Destruction of follicles, lymphocytic infiltrate, and oxphilic cells characteristic of Hashimoto's struma. (**A,** 50×; **B,** 150×.)

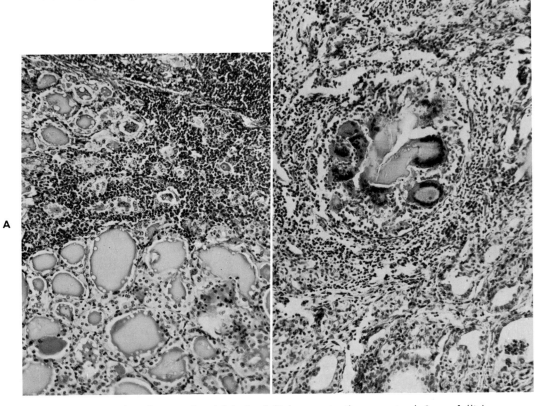

Fig. 37-9. A, In lymphocytic thyroiditis the follicles are easily recognized. Some follicles are intact and others are degenerated, with infiltration of lymphocytes. **B,** Granulomatous thyroiditis has a foreign body giant cell reaction around colloid, granuloma formation, and fibrosis. (**A** and **B,** 150×.)

Lymphocytic thyroiditis. In lymphocytic thyroiditis, also called juvenile or adolescent thyroiditis, the gland is less enlarged than in Hashimoto's struma or is of normal weight. Microscopically, the lymphocytic infiltration is less extensive than in Hashimoto's struma, with little or no thyroid epithelial destruction or fibrosis (Fig. 37-9, *A*). The follicles may appear unaltered or hyperplastic. Perhaps this condition represents an earlier or milder manifestation of Hashimoto's struma affecting a young population.

Nonspecific chronic thyroiditis. Nonspecific chronic thyroiditis, also called chronic sclerosing thyroiditis, is the most common type of thyroiditis and often is confused with Hashimoto's struma. However, it differs from the latter in three ways. The gland is smaller, weighing 35 to 60 gm. Microscopically, the thyroid parenchyma is easily recognized despite some follicular disruption, mild fibrosis, and infrequent lymph follicles. The most distinctive feature is an abundance of interstitial plasma cells. There also may be focal squamous metaplasia. In brief, an ordinary chronic inflammatory reaction is present, possibly subsequent to an infectious, chemical, immunologic, or vascular injury.

Granulomatous thyroiditis. Granulomatous thyroiditis is synonymous with giant cell, pseudotuberculous, de Quervain's, or so-called subacute thyroiditis. Neither clinically nor pathologically is it subacute. Grossly, the thyroid gland is moderately enlarged, but the tissue is pale and hard like a raw turnip. Histologically, a striking multifocal foreign body giant cell reaction surrounds colloid escaped from disorganized follicles, mingled with granulomas composed of epithelioid macrophages (Fig. 37-9, *B*). An intervening chronic inflammatory infiltrate is present, sometimes containing microabscesses and calcium oxalate crystals. One third of the cases involve the gland asymmetrically. Palpation may induce granulomas.

Riedel's struma. Riedel's struma (struma fibrosa or invasive fibrous thyroiditis) is the rarest type of thyroiditis. It produces a localized hard cervical mass that on resection proves to be a dense fibrous scar involving the thyroid gland and contiguous tissues. Histologically, this appears like an exaggerated fibrous connective tissue response to unilateral injury.

• • •

Specific types of chronic thyroiditis include sarcoidosis, tuberculosis, syphilis, and echinococcosis, all of which are uncommon.

The clinical diagnosis of chronic thyroiditis is assisted by serum antithyroid antibody tests. T lymphocytes in the blood are increased. Basement membrane deposits like antigen-antibody complexes may be seen ultrastructurally. Lymphocytes may also infiltrate the pituitary and adrenal glands. Whether Hashimoto's struma and the other types are true autoimmune diseases is uncertain. They appear equally likely to be nonimmunologically initiated diseases, which may be perpetuated and exaggerated by immune reactions. Further investigations are necessary to understand these lesions.

AGE CHANGES, DEGENERATION, AND ATROPHY

Beyond 50 years of age, about half of normal-sized thyroid glands contain single or multiple nodules with increased colloid storage, mostly clinically impalpable. Irregular colloid repletion and depletion appear responsible. The nodular thyroid gland has no known clinical significance. Mild interstitial fibrosis, calcium oxalate crystals, and medial calcification of the thyroid arteries also are common in elderly persons.

Hyaline interstitial fibrosis and follicle shrinkage represent the most familiar thyroid degeneration. When the hyalin is abundant and partly involves vessel walls, special staining may demonstrate amyloid. Amyloid goiter is a massive deposit predominantly restricted to the thyroid gland (Fig. 37-10).

Cytoplasmic iron-positive pigment is usual in hemochromatosis and occasionally in hemosiderosis. Lipofuscin is increased in mucoviscidosis. Ochronosis also pigments the thyroid gland.

Mild thyroid atrophy with small follicles may accompany aging or chronic systemic diseases. Moderate atrophy reduces the gland weights to 10 or 12 gm. In severe atrophy, the thyroid gland weighs only 3.5 to 6 gm, representing mostly capsule, vessels, and infiltrative fibroadipose connective tissue. A few miniature follicles or nests of Hürthle cells remain (Fig. 37-11, *A*).

Myxedema results from subtotal or total thyroid inactivity. The characteristic facies of myxedema comprise a puffy, pasty complexion, sparse eyebrows, coarse hair, and large tongue. Menorrhagia and increased sensitivity to cold are common. Mental activity is sluggish, frequently with irritability. Deep tendon reflexes are slow. Coma may complicate myxedema, associated with hypothermia, carbon dioxide retention, and hyponatremia. Skin biopsy dem-

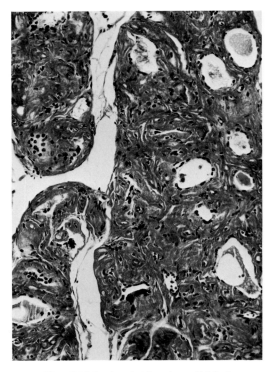

Fig. 37-10. Amyloid goiter. (120×.)

onstrates increases in hyaluronic acid and neutral mucoprotein ground substance in the upper dermis (Fig. 37-11, *B*).

Usually, myxedema appears because of idiopathic thyroid failure. Fewer cases are secondary to TSH insufficiency or panhypopituitarism, whereas hypothalamic myxedema is rare. In all three situations, the thyroid gland is moderately or severely atrophied. Hypothyroidism or myxedema after thyroid operations or ^{131}I therapy for thyrotoxicosis is not unusual. Chronic thyroiditis also causes hypothyroidism.

Pretibial myxedema is a localized bilateral swelling of the shins caused by excessive myxoid dermal connective tissue. Paradoxically, it usually accompanies hyperthyroidism and increased LATS titer.

NEOPLASMS
Benign neoplasms

Thyroid adenomas are true neoplasms, usually solitary and predominating in women, with a sex ratio of 5:1 or 6:1. Thyroid nodules outnumber adenomas at least 10:1, but adenomas require special scrutiny because they are sometimes precancerous. About 10% show invasive characteristics. Five diagnostic criteria of thyroid adenoma are complete fibrous en-

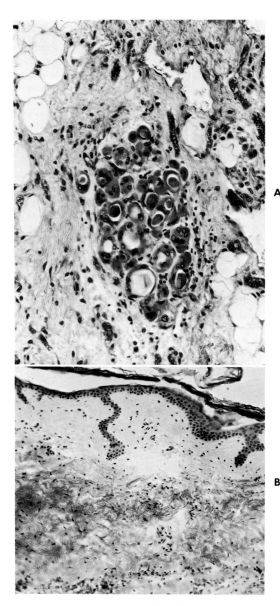

Fig. 37-11. A, Atrophic thyroid gland in myxedema. Few small follicles remain, surrounded by fibroadipose tissue. **B,** Skin in myxedema, with edematous thickening of upper dermis. (**A** and **B,** 120×.)

capsulation, a different architecture inside and outside the capsule, a uniform internal growth pattern, compression of follicles outside the capsule into crescentic shapes, and singleness (Fig. 37-12). Genuine multiple adenomas occur postirradiation and in inbred individuals.

Adenomas

Adenomas are divided most simply into follicular, papillary, and atypical types.

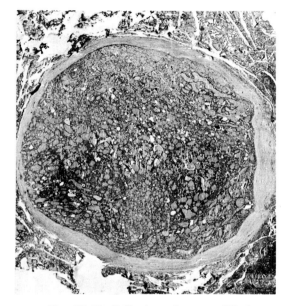

Fig. 37-12. Follicular adenoma. (50×.)

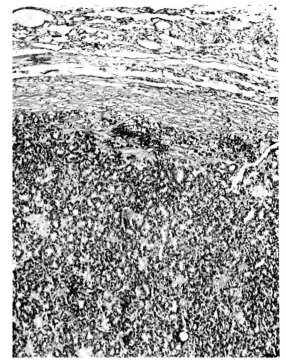

Fig. 37-13. Fetal adenoma composed of miniature follicles and fibrous capsule. (85×.)

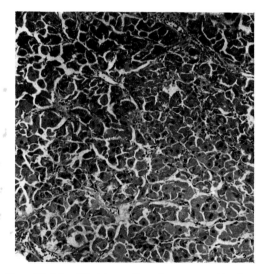

Fig. 37-14. Hürthle cell adenoma with large acidophilic cells. (100×.)

Follicular adenomas. Follicular adenomas have five variants. In order of decreasing frequency, there are fetal, colloid, simple, embryonal, and Hürthle cell types. Grossly, an adenoma usually measures 1.5 to 5 cm in diameter, and on section the tan, smooth tissue everts, a sign that indicates compression by the fibrous capsule. In the center of larger adenomas may be a dense white fibrous scar. Fetal adenoma is by far the most common. The miniature "fetal" follicles contain small colloid masses and lie closely packed or loosely arranged in an edematous fibrovascular stroma (Fig. 37-13). In embryonal adenoma the epithelium grows in branching cords with little or no follicle formation. Simple adenomas have follicles of normal adult size. This is the type that, on rare occasions, develops hyperplasia and constitutes the genuine "toxic adenoma." In colloid adenoma, the follicles are unusually large. Hürthle cell adenoma is characterized by large granular oxyphil cells that form cords and follicles containing scanty colloid (Fig. 37-14). The cytoplasm is rich in mitochondria. Because Hürthle cells are metaplastic, it may be preferable to designate these as follicular adenomas with oxyphilic (Hürthle cell) metaplasia.

Follicular adenomas require careful study of the capsule and the vessels within and outside of it to determine the presence of invasion. Some specialists believe eight to 12 blocks should be examined microscopically for evidence of capsular and blood vessel invasion.

Elastic tissue stains simplify the identification of veins. Tumor that penetrates a vessel wall and also occupies its lumen is most clearly acceptable as invasive.

Follicular adenoma with capsular or vascular invasion is an older designation now re-

Table 37-3. Adenomas of thyroid gland—invasion, metastasis, and death

Adenoma	Cases	% invasion	% metastasis (5 years)	% death (10 years)
Follicular types	1,105	5.1	15*	10*
Fetal	459	4.8	—	—
Embryonal	134	25	—	—
Simple	204	0	0	0
Colloid	288	0	0	0
Hürthle cell	20	5	0	0
Atypical	70	4.3	0	0
Papillary	138	46	11	15
Total adenomas	1,313	9.5	14*	11*

*Percentage of metastasis or death from cancer in adenomas with invasion.

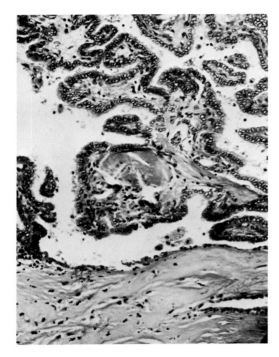

Fig. 37-15. Papillary adenoma with fibrous capsule below. (120×.)

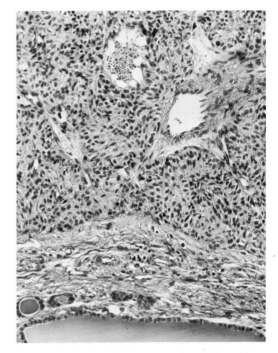

Fig. 37-16. Atypical adenoma of spindle cell pattern. (120×; AFIP 68-9551.)

garded as undesirable by many. Angioinvasive adenoma and encapsulated follicular carcinoma are two related terms. In effect, it is usually an early stage of follicular adenocarcinoma. As such, there is an excellent chance of cure by a simple excision that includes some extracapsular thyroid tissue. The recurrence rate thereafter is 15% or less after 5 years. The comparative frequency of invasion and malignant behavior for adenomas of different growth patterns is given in Table 37-3.

Papillary adenoma. Papillary adenoma is grossly distinctive, since on sectioning it typically contains wine-red fluid and a capsule lined by granular gray tissue nodules. Micro-

scopically, few papillary adenomas are completely encapsulated. If this diagnostic criterion is satisfied, only 0.5% of adenomas are papillary. Expert opinion differs on what designation should be applied to papillary adenomas with capsular invasion. Similar disagreements exist on classifying papillary neoplasms of the urinary bladder, ovary, and breast. In the absence of any significant cytologic dysplasia and other evidence of invasive activity, it is not clear that incomplete encapsulation of a papillary adenoma indicates cancer (Fig. 37-15). Statistically, extensive surgery appears unnecessary for well-differentiated papillary adenomas.

Atypical adenoma. Atypical adenoma is a rarity, making up 2% to 5% of the adenomas. Grossly, the tissue is more opaque and grayish pink than in other adenomas. Microscopically, closely packed spindle cells form bundles separated by stromal bands, unlike the usual thyroid patterns (Fig. 37-16). A few atypical adenomas are composed of clear cells or pale follicles resembling parathyroid tissue ("parastruma") or possess bizarre giant nuclei without other indications of carcinoma. Despite the peculiar and somewhat ominous cytology, their course is benign.

Teratoma

Teratoma of the thyroid gland is a curiosity usually affecting newborn infants. Grossly, teratomas are partly cystic with mesodermal components, including muscle, glia, and glandular or other epithelial elements of ectodermal and endodermal origin. The benign thyroid teratoma is dangerous chiefly because of its strategic cervical location.

Malignant neoplasms
Carcinoma

Papillary carcinoma. The most common thyroid cancer, papillary carcinoma comprises over 60% of thyroid carcinomas in a large series. The incidence is high in Hawaii and in atomic bomb survivors. Generally, it has a long, sluggish natural history, corresponding to grade I carcinomas elsewhere. Most affected children and adolescents have been exposed to ionizing radiation. Grossly, papillary carcinomas may not be discernible. Larger carcinomas are either partly encapsulated or unencapsulated, or the tumor may massively involve the thyroid and adjacent tissues.

Papillary carcinomas of microscopic size usually are discovered by recognition of the more prominent metastases in lateral cervical lymph nodes. After resection of the homolateral thyroid lobe, careful study by multiple or subserial sections reveals the primary carcinoma, which is sometimes less than 1 mm in diameter. At autopsy, the smallest papillary carcinomas may be circumscribed and noninvasive.

Partly encapsulated papillary carcinomas may originate from papillary adenomas. In carcinomas, anaplastic epithelium is piled up on papillae or growing in solid masses, with clear-cut invasion of the adjacent gland (Fig. 37-17). The nuclei often have a clear or ground-glass appearance with relatively scanty chromatin. Use of this criterion as a marker for

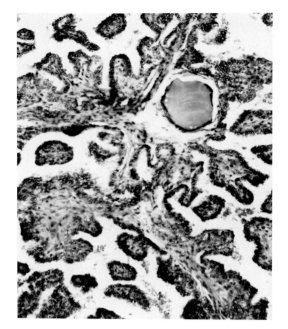

Fig. 37-17. Papillary carcinoma of thyroid gland with atypical layered epithelium. (85×.)

papillary carcinoma notably increases its frequency at the expense of follicular carcinoma. Unencapsulated papillary carcinomas are histologically identical but show no indication of an original adenoma. Over one third are multicentric and bilateral. Patients with localized varieties of papillary carcinoma survive after treatment as well as the normal population, based on 20-year to 40-year postoperative follow-up of 700 cases. Seventeen deaths from thyroid carcinoma (2.3%) were reported by Woolner et al.[99] Metastases are relatively radiosensitive.

Nonencapsulated sclerosing carcinoma (Hazard-Crile tumor) is discovered in a thyroid gland removed for another reason, when sectioning shows a minute stellate scar. Histologically, this is a very localized papillary carcinoma, incidentally discovered and ordinarily nonrecurrent.

Massive papillary carcinoma spreading into the extrathyroid tissues and lymph nodes is lethal in about one third of patients within 20 years and compares to stage III, grade I carcinomas elsewhere. Peculiar to papillary carcinoma are its notable tendency to lymphatic invasion with metastasis to regional cervical lymph nodes and the calcospherites ("psammoma bodies") found in the stroma. Calcospherites may remain in areas of local tumor regression, and their presence suggests

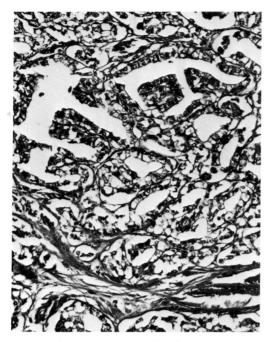

Fig. 37-18. Papillary and follicular carcinoma, including some clear cells. (120×.)

nearby papillary carcinoma. However, such calcospherites occasionally occur in thyroid hyperplasia and other conditions.

Papillary carcinoma may grow purely in this pattern, or papillary and follicular carcinoma may be found together in the original site, in metastases, or in both (Fig. 37-18). Sometimes, an apparently pure papillary carcinoma has lymph node metastases with predominant follicular carcinoma. Squamous foci also sometimes are present. No difference in prognosis

has been found between these papillary carcinoma variants; this is better than for follicular carcinoma. The stages and grades of papillary and other thyroid carcinomas are summarized in Table 37-4. The overall death rate within 5 years of diagnosis is about 10%.

Follicular carcinoma. Follicular carcinoma of the thyroid gland is generally comparable to stage II, grade II adenocarcinomas in other tissues. Pure follicular carcinoma is rare. Two varieties of follicular carcinoma are the most favorable:

1. Encapsulated follicular carcinoma. This merges with follicular adenoma manifesting capsular or vascular invasion. Acceptable cases have cytologic anaplasia. Only about 15% of the patients develop metastases and die of cancer.
2. Langhans' struma. This is a sluggish tumor that grows in continuity to fill the anterior part of the neck and finally compromises respiration. Microscopically, its monotonous appearance resembles fetal adenoma but is unconfined. It is too rare to give prognostic figures.

Grossly, a follicular thyroid carcinoma is ordinarily a hard, gritty, grayish pink unencapsulated mass 2 cm or more in diameter, not unlike a breast carcinoma in appearance. Microscopically, it may vary from an obviously anaplastic solid epithelial growth that forms a few follicles to a well-differentiated follicle-forming tumor recognizable as carcinoma by glands with disproportionately large nuclei growing back to back (Fig. 37-19). Sometimes, the best differentiated follicular carcinomas metastasize to lymph nodes, bones, or else-

Table 37-4. Carcinomas of thyroid gland—pathologic grades and clinical stages*

Type	Pathologic grade	Clinical stage†	Survival	
			10 years	15 years
Follicular adenoma with invasion	0-I	IB		
Papillary adenoma with invasion	0-I	IA or B	For total 694 stage I cases	
Papillary carcinoma	I	IA or B, II or III	89%	83%
Papillary and follicular carcinoma	I or II	IB, II, or III		
Nonencapsulated sclerosing carcinoma	I or II	IA		
Langhans' struma	I or II	III		
Follicular carcinoma	II	IB or II	For total 151 stage II cases	
Medullary carcinoma	II	I, II, or III	54%	42%
Small cell compact carcinoma	III	III or IV	For total 101 stage III cases	
Small cell diffuse carcinoma	III	II, III, or IV	29%	16%
Giant cell carcinoma	III	III or IV	For total 60 stage IV cases	
			10%	10%

*Modified from Pub. 8, American Joint Committee for Cancer Staging and End Results Reporting, 1967.
†Stage I tumors are less than 5 cm in diameter, with or without cervical lymph node metastases; A, impalpable; B, palpable. Stage II tumors are 5 cm in diameter or larger, with or without cervical lymph node metastases. Stage III tumors extend directly into adjacent structures. Stage IV tumors have distant metastases.

where and, focally, are of practically normal thyroid appearance. However, a careful study usually reveals some neoplastic qualities. "Benign metastasizing thyroid" is largely a myth.

Blood vessel invasion, which is common in follicular carcinoma, contributes to the likelihood of osseous and pulmonary metastases. A few cases concentrate sufficient iodine to make ^{131}I therapy worthwhile. Survival rates are 34% at 10 years and 16% at 20 years, according to the data of Woolner et al.[99] One fifth of follicular carcinomas are of Hürthle cell type, and these have shown no distinctive clinical behavior.

Medullary carcinoma. Medullary carcinoma of the thyroid gland with amyloid stroma, also called solid carcinoma, was first distinguished in 1959 by Hazard et al.[76] Grossly, medullary carcinoma varies from less than 1.5 cm to massive size. It has a rounded, demarcated outline without encapsulation, and the tumor tissue is gray or white with focal hemorrhages. Microscopically, the structure is solid and cellular. Most typically, medullary carcinoma is composed of spindle cells, unlike any pattern expected in a thyroid neoplasm but sometimes

resembling a carcinoid. The stroma is irregularly hyalinized. Special staining regularly demonstrates amyloid, but this often is not diffuse or obvious (Fig. 37-20). Amyloid occurs also in the metastases. Despite the rather undifferentiated appearance of medullary thyroid carcinomas and a tendency to bilaterality, these tumors behave like moderately malignant (grade II) neoplasms. If there are no lymph node metastases, the 10-year and 20-year survival rates are as good as for the age-matched population without cancer. With metastases, the 10-year survival is reduced to 42%.

Electron microscopy shows that the medullary carcinoma cells contain specialized granules of calcitonin, indicating the tumor to be a parafollicular or C cell carcinoma. Blood calcitonin excess and increased histaminase have been found, and some cases are accompanied by parathyroid hyperplasia. Intestinal and bronchial carcinoid tumors also are capable of calcitonin secretion.

Several unusual syndromes are related to medullary thyroid carcinoma. These include pheochromocytoma, especially familial or bilateral, and parathyroid hyperplasia or adenoma (Sipple's syndrome). Further, neurofibromatosis, neurofibromas, or multiple mucosal neuromas, and sometimes Marfan's syndrome are correlated. Occasionally diarrhea,

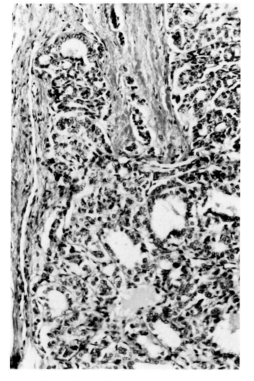

Fig. 37-19. Well-differentiated follicular carcinoma invading thyroid capsule. (150×.)

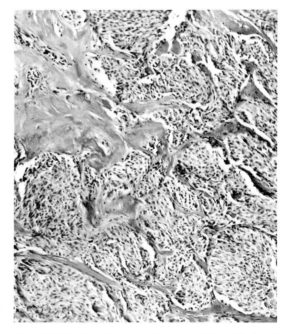

Fig. 37-20. Medullary carcinoma of thyroid gland with amyloid-positive stroma. (85×.)

the carcinoid syndrome, and Cushing's syndrome attributable to medullary thyroid carcinoma have been recognized. In its aberrant endocrine peptide hormonal activities, medullary carcinoma rivals oat cell lung carcinomas and certain pancreatic islet tumors, all of which are believed derived from cells of Pearse's APUD* neuroectodermal endocrine system.

C cell hyperplasia in the upper two thirds of both lobes of the thyroid gland occurs in some families with type II multiple endocrine adenomatosis before medullary carcinoma develops. The C cells possess cresyl violet, Giemsa-stained, and argyrophil granules and may have adjacent stromal amyloid. Plasma and urine immunoreactive calcitonin is increased, and plasma gastrin is decreased.

Undifferentiated carcinoma. Undifferentiated carcinomas also are termed anaplastic. Ordinarily, they are obviously malignant clinically, grossly, and microscopically because of their hard consistency and rapid growth. Older people are affected. Regardless of the histologic type, in the series reported by Woolner et al.,[99] half of the patients were dead of cancer in 5 months and nearly all by 3 years. Four of 160 patients lived over 5 years. Occasionally, a long history begins with an invasive adenoma, progresses to follicular carcinoma, and ends with death from undifferentiated carcinoma 25 years or more thereafter.

Small-cell compact undifferentiated carcinoma in some series is the most common grade III variety. Grossly and microscopically, it resembles a scirrhous breast carcinoma except for a few neoplastic follicles. Giant cell carcinoma, also called spindle and giant cell carcinoma or carcinosarcoma, is the other relatively well-known undifferentiated carcinoma. Some arise from adenomas. The bizarre and disorderly neoplastic cells are unrecognizable as thyroid, and tumor giant cells of striking variability are present (Fig. 37-21, *A*). Ultrastructural details of epithelial cells are found.

Small-cell diffuse carcinoma is uncommon and not easily distinguished from malignant lymphoma, even in well-prepared sections. Both in the thyroid and nodal metastases, the small cells retain some epithelial characteristics, such as cordlike growth and compression of the preexisting reticulin (Fig. 37-21, *B*).

Rarer and ordinarily lethal carcinomas include adenoacanthoma, squamous cell carci-

---

APUD is amine precursor uptake and decarboxylation.

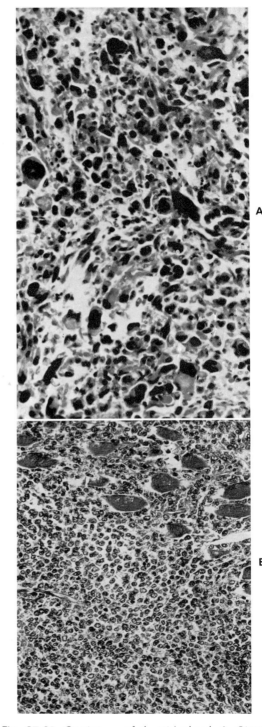

Fig. 37-21. Carcinoma of thyroid gland. **A,** Giant cell carcinoma. **B,** Small cell diffuse carcinoma invading striated muscle at upper right. (**A** and **B,** 150×; **A,** AFIP 59-6950; **B,** AFIP 59-6943.)

noma, and mixed carcinoma that includes intermingled components of a moderately differentiated grade II and an undifferentiated grade III carcinoma.

Stromal tumors

Sarcoma of the thyroid gland most often is malignant lymphoma of histiocytic type, lymphosarcoma, or Hodgkin's disease. Elderly women usually are the victims of either primary or secondary thyroid lymphomas. The histopathologic features used to distinguish thyroid lymphoma from carcinoma or thyroiditis are essentially the same as those employed in lymph nodes. Plasmacytoma restricted to the thyroid gland is said to have the same benign course observed in certain other extramedullary sites.

Fibrosarcoma, rhabdomyosarcoma, osteosarcoma, and angiosarcoma, or hemangioendothelioma, have been described in thyroid glands. Benign mesenchymal thyroid tumors include lipoma, hemangioma, neurilemoma, and leiomyoma.

Metastatic cancer

Metastatic cancer of the thyroid gland is fairly common at autopsy with widely disseminated tumors. Breast or lung carcinomas and malignant melanoma are the most common sources of thyroid metastases.

REFERENCES
General

1 Committee on Nomenclature, American Thyroid Association: J. Clin. Endocrinol. 29:860-862, 1969.
2 Klinck, G. H., Oertel, J. E., and Winship, T.: Lab. Invest. 22:2-22, 1970.
3 McGowan, G. K., editor: J. Clin. Pathol. 28:205-254, 1975.

Structure and function

4 Berg, G.: J. Ultrastruct. Res. 42:324-336, 1973 (thyroglobulin ultrastructure).
5 Braunstein, H., and Stephens, C. L.: Arch. Pathol. (Chicago) 86:659-666, 1968 (parafollicular cells).
6 Copp, D. H., Cockcroft, D. W., Kueh, Y., and Melville, M.: In Calcitonin: Proceedings of the symposium on thyrocalcitonin and C cells, New York, 1968, Springer Verlag, p. 306.
7 Goldberg, H. M., and Harvey, P.: Br. J. Surg. 43:565-569, 1956 (squamous cysts).
8 Heimann, P.: Acta Endocrinol. (Kbh) 53 (suppl. 110):1-102, 1966 (ultrastructure).
9 Joseph, T. J., and Komorowski, R. A.: Hum. Pathol. 6:717-729, 1975 (thyroglossal duct carcinoma).
10 Kurman, R. J., and Prabha, A. C.: Am. J. Clin. Pathol. 59:503-507, 1973 (vaginal thyroid).

11 Larkander, O., Larsson, L. G., and Ottosson, J.: Acta Psychiatr. Scand. (suppl.) 221:103-110, 1971 (hereditary goitrous cretinism).
12 Little, G., Meador, C. K., Cunningham, R., and Pitman, J. A.: J. Clin. Endocrinol. 25:1529-1536, 1965 (sporadic cretinism).
13 Meyer, J. S., and Steinberg, L. S.: Cancer 24:302-311, 1969 (aberrant thyroid in lymph nodes).
14 Meyers, E. N., and Pantangco, I. P., Jr.: Laryngoscope 85:1833-1838, 1975 (laryngeal thyroid).
15 Sherman, P. H., and Shabbahrami, F.: Am. Surg. 32:137-142, 1966 (substernal goiter).
16 Tremblay, G.: Lab. Invest. 11:514-517, 1962 (Askanazy cells).

Goiter and altered hormonal biosynthesis

17 Bartuska, D.: Am. J. Med. Sci. 266:249-252, 1973 (thyroid disease genetics).
18 Fierro-Benitez, R., Penafiel, W., De Groot, L. J., and Ramirez, I.: New Eng. J. Med. 280:296-302, 1969 (Andean goiter and cretinism).
19 Lupulescu, A., Negoescu, I., Petrovici, A., Nicolae, M., Stoian, M., Balan, M., and Stancu, H.: Acta Anat. (Basel) 66:321-338, 1967 (ultrastructure in cretin).
20 Marine, D., and Kimball, O. P.: J.A.M.A. 77:1068, 1921 (simple goiter).
21 Miller, J. M., Horn, R. C., and Block, M. A.: J. Clin. Endocrinol. 27:1264-1274, 1967 (nodules and activity).
22 Stanbury, J. B., Wyngaarden, J. B., and Fredrickson, D. S., editors: The metabolic basis of inherited disease, ed. 2, New York, 1966, Blakiston Division, McGraw-Hill Book Co. (familial goiter).
23 Thould, A. K., and Scowen, E. F.: J. Endocrinol. 30:69-77, 1964 (Pendred's syndrome).
24 Weaver, D. K., Nishiyama, R. H., Burton, W. D., and Batsakis, J. G.: Arch. Surg. (Chicago) 92:796-801, 1966 (nodular goiter).

Iatrogenic abnormalities

25 Domphin, G. W.: Health Phys. 15:219-228, 1968 (radiation carcinogenesis).
26 Doniach, I., Eadie, D. G. A., and Hope-Stone, H. F.: Br. J. Surg. 53:681-685, 1966 (post-irradiation adenomas).
27 Galina, M. P., Avnet, N. L., and Einhorm, A.: New Eng. J. Med. 267:1124-1127, 1962 (fatal newborn iodide goiter).
28 Greig, W. R., Crooks, J., and Macgregor, A. G.: Proc. Roy. Soc. Med. 59:599-602, 1966 (radiation effects).
29 Guinet, P., Tourniaire, J., and Peyrin, J. O.: Ann. Endocrinol. (Paris) 28:199-206, 1967 (resorcinol goiter).
30 Roy, P. E., Bonenfant, J. L., and Turcot, L.: Am. J. Clin. Pathol. 50:234-239, 1968 (cobalt).
31 Schottstaedt, E. S., and Smollers, M.: Ann. Intern. Med. 64:847-849, 1966 (thyroid tablet poisoning).
32 Singer, I., and Rotenberg, D.: New Eng. J. Med. 289:254-257, 1973 (lithium goiter).
33 Wolff, J.: Am. J. Med. 47:101-124, 1969 (iodide goiter).
34 Wood, J. W., Tamagaki, H., Neriishi, S., Sato, T., Sheldon, W. F., Archer, P. G., Hamilton,

H. B., and Johnson, K. G.: Am. J. Epidemiol. 89:4-14, 1969 (atomic radiation carcinoma).

Hyperplasia
Primary hyperplasia

35 Buckle, R. M., Mason, A. M. S., and Middleton, J. E.: Lancet 1:1128-1130, 1969 (hypercalcemia).
36 Gluck, F. B., Nusynowitz, M. L., and Plymate, S.: New Eng. J. Med. 293:624-628, 1975 (thyroiditis and thyrotoxicosis).
37 Hamilton, C. R., and Maloof, F.: Medicine 52:195-215, 1973 (jodbasedow).
38 Hershman, J. M., Givens, J. R., Cassidy, C. E., and Astwood, E. B.: J. Clin. Endocrinol. 26:803-807, 1966 (recurrent hyperthyroidism).
39 McKenzie, J. M.: Metabolism 21:883-894, 1972 (LATS and Graves' disease).
40 Menendez, C. E., and Rivlin, R. S.: Med. Clin. North Am. 57:1463-1470, 1973 (thyrotoxic crisis).

Secondary hyperplasia

41 Charkes, N. D.: J. Nucl. Med. 13:885-892, 1972 (functioning nodules).
42 McKenzie, J. M.: J. Clin. Endocrinol. 26:779-781, 1966.
43 Molnar, G. D., Wilbur, R. D., Lee, R. E., Woolner, L. B., and Keating, F. R., Jr.: Mayo Clin. Proc. 40:665-684, 1965.
44 Vagenakis, A. G., Wang, C.-A., Burger, A., Maloof, F., Braverman, L. E., and Ingbar, S. H.: New Eng. J. Med. 287:523-527, 1972 (jodbasedow).

Thyroiditis

45 Carney, J. A., Moore, S. B., Northcutt, R. C., Woolner, L. B., and Stillwell, G. K.: Am. J. Clin. Pathol. 64:639-647, 1975 (palpation granulomas).
46 Farid, N. R., Munro, R. E., Row, V. V., and Volpe, R.: New Eng. J. Med. 288:1313-1317, 1973 (T lymphocytes).
47 Hall, R., and Stanbury, J. B.: Clin. Exp. Immunol. 2:719-725, 1967 (familial autoimmune thyroiditis).
48 Kalderson, A. E., Bogaars, H. A., and Diamond, I.: Am. J. Med. 55:485-491, 1973 (Hashimoto's struma ultrastructure).
49 Katz, S. M., and Vickery, A. L., Jr.: Hum. Pathol. 5:161-170, 1974 (fibrous Hashimoto's variant).
50 Kiaer, W., and Norgaard, J. O.: Acta Pathol. Microbiol. Scand. 76:229-238, 1969 (thyroiditis, hypophysitis, and adrenalitis).
51 Ling, S. M., Kaplan, S. A., Weitzwan, J. J., et al.: Pediatrics 44:695-708, 1969 (lymphocytic thyroiditis).
52 Meyer, S., and Hausman, R.: Am. J. Clin. Pathol. 65:274-283, 1976 (Riedel's struma).
53 Reidbord, H. E., and Fisher, E. R.: Am. J. Clin. Pathol. 59:327-337, 1973 (thyroiditis ultrastructure).
54 Tung, K. S. K., Ramos, C. V., and Deodhar, S. D.: Am. J. Clin. Pathol. 61:549-555, 1974 (antithyroid antibodies).

Degeneration and atrophy

55 Blum, M.: Am. J. Med. Sci. 264:432-443, 1972 (myxedema coma).
56 Borel, D. M., and Reddy, J. K.: Arch. Pathol. 96:269-271, 1973 (lipofuscin).
57 Dube, V. E., and Joyce, G. T.: Cancer 27:434-437, 1971 (squamous metaplasia).
58 Dubin, I. N.: Am. J. Clin. Pathol. 25:514-542, 1955 (hemochromatosis and siderosis).
59 James, P. D.: J. Clin. Pathol. 25:683-688, 1972 (amyloid goiter).
60 Johnson, W. C., and Helwig, E. B.: Arch. Dermatol. (Chicago) 93:13-20, 1966 (pretibial myxedema).
61 Lynch, P. J., Maize, J. C., and Sisson, J. C.: Arch. Dermatol. 107:107-111, 1973 (pretibial myxedema).
62 Patchefsky, A. S., and Hoch, W. S.: Am. J. Clin. Pathol. 57:551-552, 1972 (psammoma bodies).
63 Richter, M. N., and McCarty, K. S.: Am. J. Pathol. 30:545-553, 1974 (oxalate crystals).
64 Roth, S. I., Olen, E., and Hansen, L. S.: Lab. Invest. 11:933-941, 1962 (Hürthle cells).
65 Hazard, J. B.: In Young, S., and Inman, D. R., editors: Thyroid neoplasia; proceedings of the second Imperial Cancer Research Fund symposium, London, April 1967, New York, 1968, Academic Press, Inc., pp. 3-37.
66 Horn, R. C., Jr.: Arch. Pathol. (Chicago) 69:481-492, 1960.
67 Knowlson, G. T. G.: Br. J. Surg. 58:253-254, 1971 (cancer in solitary nodule).
68 Meissner, W. A., and Warren, S.: Atlas of tumor pathology, Ser. 2, Fasc. 4, Washington, D.C., 1969, Armed Forces Institute of Pathology.
69 Spigelman, M.: Med. J. Aust. 1:53-54, 1969 (thyroid teratoma).

Neoplasms
Carcinoma

70 Beaugié, J. M., Brown, C. L., Doniach, I., and Richardson, J. E.: Br. J. Surg. 63:173-181, 1976.
71 Baylin, S. B., Beaven, M. A., Engelman, K., and Sjoerdma, A.: New Eng. J. Med. 283:1239-1244, 1970 (medullary carcinoma histaminase).
72 Feldman, P. S., Horvath, E., and Kovacs, K.: Cancer 30:1279-1285, 1972 (Hürthle cell tumors).
73 Franssila, K. O.: Cancer 32:853-864, 1973 (papillary versus follicular carcinoma).
74 Goltzman, D., Potts, J. T., Jr., Ridgway, E. C., and Maloof, F.: New Eng. J. Med. 290:1035-1039, 1974 (medullary carcinoma calcitonin).
75 Gould, V. E., and Jao, W.: Cancer 35:1280-1292, 1975 (giant cell carcinoma ultrastructure).
76 Hazard, J. B., Hawk, W. A., and Crile, G., Jr.: J. Clin. Endocrinol. 19:152-161, 1959 (medullary carcinoma).
77 Heitz, P., Moser, H., and Staub, J. J.: Cancer 37:2329-2337, 1976.
78 Jaques, D. A., Chambers, R. G., and Oertel, J. E.: Am. J. Surg. 120:439-446, 1970 (in thyroglossal duct).

79 Key, C. R.: Hum. Pathol. **2**:521-523, 1971 (radiation carcinogenesis).
80 Lindahl, F.: Cancer **36**:540-552, 1975 (papillary carcinoma).
81 Ljungberg, O.: Acta Pathol. Microbiol. Scand. A. (suppl. 231):1-57, 1972 (medullary carcinoma).
82 Melvin, K. E. W.: Ann. N.Y. Acad. Sci. **230**:378-390, 1974 (paraneoplastic syndromes).
83 Mortensen, J. D., Woolner, L. B., and Bennett, W. A.: Cancer **9**:306-309, 1956 (metastases to thyroid).
84 Nishiyama, R. H., Dunn, E. L., and Thompson, N. W.: Cancer **30**:113-127, 1972 (giant cell carcinoma).
85 Noguchi, S., Noguchi, A., and Murakami, N.: Cancer **26**:1053-1064, 1970 (papillary carcinoma).
86 Pearse, A. G. E.: Pathol. Annu. **9**:27-42, 1974 (APUD cells).
87 Rayfield, E. J., Nishiyama, R. H., and Sisson, J. C.: Cancer **28**:1023-1030, 1971 (small cell tumors).
88 Russell, W. O., and Ibanez, M. L.: In Endocrine and nonendocrine hormone-producing tumors, Chicago, 1973, Year Book Publishing Co., pp. 363-397.
89 Saito, R., and Shanma, K.: Am. J. Clin. Pathol. **65**:623-630, 1976 (small cell carcinoma).
90 Sampson, R. J., Woolner, L. B., Bahn, R. C., and Kurland, L. T.: Cancer **34**:2072-2076, 1974 (smallest papillary carcinoma).
91 Silverberg, S. G., Hutter, R. V. P., and Foote, F. W., Jr.: Cancer **25**:792-802, 1970.
92 Sizemore, G. W., Go, V. L. W., Kaplan, E. L., et al.: New Eng. J. Med. **288**:641-644, 1973 medullary carcinoma calcitonin and gastrin).

93 Steinfeld, C. M., Moertel, C. G., and Woolner, L. B.: Cancer **31**:1237-1239, 1973 (diarrhea and medullary carcinoma).
94 Tashjian, A. H., Jr., Wolfe, H. J., and Voelkel, E. F.: Am. J. Med. **56**:840-849, 1974 (C cell calcitonin).
95 Task Force on Carcinoma of Thyroid Gland: Clinical staging system, Chicago, 1967, American Joint Committee for Cancer Staging and End-Results Reporting.
96 Thomas, C. G., Jr., and Buckwalter, J. A.: Ann. Surg. **177**:632-642, 1973.
97 Wilson, S. M., Platz, C., and Block, G. M.: Arch. Surg. **100**:330-335, 1970.
98 Wolfe, H. J., Melvin, K. E. W., Cervi-Skinner, S. J., et al.: New Eng. J. Med. **289**:437-441, 1973 (C cell hyperplasia).
99 Woolner, L. B.: Semin. Nucl. Med. **1**:481-502, 1971.
100 Zehbe, M.: Virchows Arch. (Pathol. Anat.) **197**:240-291, 1909 (Langhans' struma).

Stromal tumors

101 Bisbee, A. C., and Thoemy, R. H.: Cancer **35**:1296-1299, 1975 (lymphoma).
102 Haegert, D. G., Wang, N. S., Farrer, P. A., et al.: Am. J. Clin. Pathol. **61**:561-570, 1974.
103 More, J. R. S., Dawson, D. W., Ralston, A. J., and Craig, I.: J. Clin. Pathol. **21**:661-667, 1968 (plasmacytoma).
104 Roberts, C.: J. Pathol. Bacteriol. **95**:537-540, 1968 (sarcoma).
105 Shimkin, P. M., and Sagerman, R. H.: Radiology **92**:812-816, 1969 (lymphoma).
106 Woolner, L. B., McConahey, W. M., Beahrs, O. H., and Black, B. M.: Am. J. Surg. **111**:502-523, 1966.

38/Parathyroid glands

JAMES E. OERTEL

The parathyroid glands are important regulators of the metabolism of calcium and phosphorus and act to maintain normal levels of these elements in the blood.

DEVELOPMENT AND STRUCTURE

The parathyroid glands, usually four in number, are developed from endoderm of the third and fourth branchial pouches, in intimate relationship to portions of the thymus, but quite independent of the thyroid gland.[3-5] The superior pair of glands is derived from the fourth pharyngeal pouches, whereas the inferior pair, derived from the third pouches, outdistances the superior pair and the thyroid gland in caudal migration and hence takes the lower position. Their close connection with the development of the thymus explains the occasional occurrence of one or more parathyroid glands near or even embedded in thymic tissue. This possibility should be borne in mind during search for parathyroid tissue or a parathyroid adenoma by surgical procedures or at autopsy.

Although four parathyroid glands are usually present, variations in number from two to ten have been reported. The superior pair are situated rather constantly on the medial part of the dorsal surface of each lobe of the thyroid gland, about the junction of the middle and upper thirds, and lie close to ascending branches of the inferior thyroid artery. They often are embedded in thyroid substance but separated from it by a connective tissue capsule. The inferior parathyroid glands, more inconstant in position, are found usually on the dorsal surface of the lateral lobes of the thyroid gland, near the lower pole.

The parathyroid glands are brownish yellow, oval, somewhat flattened bodies, each measuring, in the adult, about 1.5 by 3.5 by 6.5 mm and having a combined weight of about 120 to 130 mg (four glands). The amount of interstitial tissue is quite variable, but the mean weight of parenchymal tissue has been estimated to be about 80 to 90 mg (four glands).[6]

Each parathyroid gland possesses a capsule of connective tissue, from which bands pass through the gland. The parenchymal cells may be arranged in solid masses but frequently appear in cords or columns. Acinar or follicular structures may be found, tending to increase in frequency with age. These may contain colloid. Interstitial adipose tissue is present after puberty and tends to increase in proportionate amount with age until the middle of the fifth decade. This interstitial fat is replaced and decreases or disappears when there is hyperplasia or adenomatous growth of the parenchyma.

The parenchymal cells appear in three main forms: chief cells, water-clear cells, and oxyphil cells. Transitional forms occur.

The chief cell (6 to 8 μm in diameter) is the most numerous. Its cytoplasm is weakly acidophilic and may appear vacuolated by light microscopy. Electron microscopy indicates that the chief cell has cycles in which it changes from an inactive form to an actively synthesizing phase and again to an inactive form.[7] In the inactive phase the cell contains abundant glycogen, dispersed sacs of rough endoplasmic reticulum, a small Golgi apparatus, and rare secretory granules. The actively synthesizing cell has the expected increase of granular endoplasmic reticulum. This form is followed by a phase in which the cellular structures suggest transfer and packaging of the hormone into secretory granules. After releasing the hormone, the cell returns to the inactive phase. Individual cells do not appear to synchronize their cycles with their neighbors,

The opinions or assertions contained herein are the private views of the author and are not to be construed as official or as reflecting the views of the Department of the Army or the Department of Defense.

which may account for the subtle differences in the appearance of adjacent cells that are visible with the light microscope.

The water-clear cell is larger (10 to 15 μm), has abundant clear cytoplasm and a relatively small pyknotic nucleus, and has well-defined cell borders, a feature often evident in all varieties of parathyroid cells. This cell is rare in normal glands. Large membrane-limited cytoplasmic vacuoles are the most conspicuous aspect of its fine structure. Dense secretory granules are sparse.

The oxyphil cell is 8 to 14 μm in diameter. Its eosinophilic granular cytoplasm is packed with mitochondria, secretory granules are rare, and glycogen is present in moderate amounts. Before puberty, oxyphil cells are uncommon. They increase in number with age and in certain diseases, such as chronic renal failure.[2]

PARATHYROID HORMONE

Parathyroid hormone is a polypeptide that acts to elevate serum calcium and reduce serum phosphate. Reduction of serum ionized calcium promptly causes increased secretion of the hormone, whereas elevation of serum calcium results in decreased secretion. Elevation of magnesium ions in serum also causes decreased secretion of the hormone, but the effects of magnesium deficiency are uncertain.

Parathyroid hormone acts on the tubular cells of the nephrons to inhibit reabsorption of phosphate and to promote absorption of calcium and magnesium, causes resorption of bone matrix and bone mineral, and with vitamin D enhances the absorption of calcium and magnesium from the small intestine.

REGULATION OF CALCIUM METABOLISM

The regulation of the metabolism of calcium is a complex mechanism involving the effects of hormones and ions on bone, the absorption of calcium and phosphate from the small intestine, and the loss of calcium and phosphate in the urine and feces. Parathyroid hormone maintains the level of calcium in the blood and other extracellular fluids by the actions mentioned in the previous section. Calcitonin partly opposes parathyroid hormone by preventing resorption of bone and by enhancing renal excretion of sodium, calcium, and phosphate. It is released in response to elevations of serum calcium and probably also by certain hormones of the alimentary tract. Calcitonin may play a more important role in children than in adults.

Vitamin D_3 plays an important but poorly understood role in calcium metabolism. Its active metabolite, 1,25-dihydroxycholecalciferol, undergoes its final step in synthesis in the kidney. Vitamin D_3 appears to be essential for the fully effective action of parathyroid hormone on the skeleton and the intestine but apparently not for its action on the kidney.

Calcium metabolism is also affected by the corticosteroids, by some of the hormones of the alimentary tract, and by thyroid hormone. Estrogens, androgens, and growth hormone also have long-term effects on the skeleton, but their short-term influence on divalent cation metabolism is unknown.

PATHOLOGIC CALCIFICATION

Pathologic calcification is the deposition of calcium salts in tissues not normally calcified as well as in excretory or secretory ducts. Calcium salts occur in some soft tissues quite regularly, however (e.g., the pineal gland after puberty). Calcium phosphate and calcium carbonate are the salts usually found. They are present most often as hydroxyapatite. Calcium oxalate deposits also may be present.

Pathologic calcification usually has been described under four categories: dystrophic calcification, metastatic calcification, calcinosis, and calciphylaxis.

Dystrophic calcification is the deposition of calcium salts in injured or dead tissue. The systemic chemical balance is normal, but the local environment is altered to encourage precipitation of the salts. Metastatic calcification is the deposition of calcium salts in soft tissue as a result of a systemic disturbance of calcium and phosphate metabolism. Calcinosis is local or generalized calcification in or under the skin, sometimes including muscles, fasciae, nerves, and tendons, and occasionally is associated with scleroderma. Tumoral calcinosis refers to a localized, often cystic, calcific mass in the soft tissue next to a large joint, usually solitary. Calciphylaxis is an experimental process whereby hypercalcemia is produced by a "sensitizing" agent (vitamin D, parathyroid hormone) followed by a "challenging" agent that produces calcification either in the soft tissues at the site of injection or application or in a distant tissue if injected intravenously.

It is likely that these categories of calcification are somewhat artificial. Metastatic calcification associated with vitamin D intoxication, uremia, or hyperparathyroidism, for example, is probably occurring in tissues already damaged by the systemic disease and is therefore related to dystrophic calcification. The possible relationships to Selye's calciphylaxis are also apparent.

Calcification of soft tissues is a complex process that is poorly understood and depends on the local balance of inhibitor substances and of compounds promoting calcification as well as the systemic chemical environment. Major factors promoting calcification include elevation of the calcium-phosphate product (Ca × P in mg per 100 ml) resulting from higher levels of calcium or phosphate or both, elevation of pH locally or systemically, and the presence of circulating substances that may cause tissue damage.[50] The local elevation of pH in the eye and kidney (because the cells establish a hydrogen-ion gradient across their membranes) may enhance calcification. Whether a similar mechanism occurs in the stomach, lungs, and bursae is controversial.[19] Other possible factors leading to deposition of calcium salts are local increases in calcium or phosphate concentrations as a result of intracellular transport mechanisms, concentration of calcium ions in mucopolysaccharides, removal of inhibiting pyrophosphate by pyrophosphatases, decrease in inhibitor peptides (especially in urine), and the action of collagen and elastin as nucleating substances for crystal formation.

HYPOPARATHYROIDISM

Diminution or absence of circulating parathyroid hormone causes a reduction of serum calcium (to as little as half the normal level) and an elevation of serum phosphate (to as much as three or four times normal levels). Little or no calcium appears in the urine. Tetany and other evidence of neuromuscular irritability are the most important clinical manifestations of hypoparathyroidism. If the disease is of long duration, the persons affected may have (in addition to tetany) skin disorders, abnormal nail growth, loss of hair, cataracts, a variety of disorders of the central nervous system, and roentgenographic evidence of increased bone density and calcification in the vessels of the basal ganglia of the brain. Convulsions, papilledema, and gastrointestinal disturbances may be present.

The most common cause of hypoparathyroidism is the removal of all or part of the parathyroid tissue during surgery of the neck, especially during thyroidectomy. If only part of the gland tissue is removed, or if the glands are partially injured by impairment of their blood supply or by postoperative edema, then the hormonal deficiency will be temporary.

Complete removal or more severe damage results in permanent impairment of function.

Temporary neonatal hypocalcemia may be a manifestation of the hypoparathyroidism that occurs normally in many infants for a brief period after birth. This state may persist in sick or injured infants and may become manifest as symptomatic hypocalcemia.[22]

So-called idiopathic hypoparathyroidism is a rare disease that is sporadic or familial and, in some instances, may be an autoimmune disorder. The glands are either replaced by fat or cannot be found.[23,24] Permanent idiopathic hypoparathyroidism developing during the first year of life may be associated with congenital hypoplasia or absence of the parathyroid glands and thymus, and the children usually die.[26] Another type of hypoparathyroidism that also occurs in childhood may be familial or sporadic and is associated with a variety of disorders, some of which are accompanied by autoimmune phenomena. These include idiopathic adrenocortical atrophy, lymphocytic thyroiditis, oophoritis, diabetes mellitus, gastric mucosal atrophy, hepatitis, alopecia totalis, and severe *Candida* infections.

PSEUDOHYPOPARATHYROIDISM

Pseudohypoparathyroidism and pseudopseudohypoparathyroidism are related disorders and may be called Albright's hereditary osteodystrophy. Pseudohypoparathyroidism is familial, with a female predominance, and is characterized by clinical and chemical features suggestive of idiopathic hypoparathyroidism. Brachydactyly, short stature, and multiple foci of soft-tissue calcification and ossification are additional distinctive features. Renal glomerular function is normal. Pseudo-pseudohypoparathyroidism is similar, but the serum calcium and phosphate levels are normal.

In these disorders, the parathyroid glands are normal or hyperplastic. Parathyroid function is intact. Levels of circulating parathyroid hormone are increased. The disease results from the inability of the renal tubules and the skeleton to respond to parathyroid hormone.

HYPERPARATHYROIDISM

Excessive production of parathyroid hormone results from several different disorders: from a disturbance of calcium and phosphorus metabolism originating elsewhere in the body (renal failure, vitamin D deficiency) and leading to secondary hyperplasia of parathyroid tissue, from primary hyperplasia of the parathyroid tissue, from benign and malignant tumors of the parathyroid glands, and from neoplasms not of parathyroid origin, such as carcinoma of the lung or of the kidney.

Hyperparathyroidism may occur at any age but is more likely after the age of 30 years. It is more common in women, and there is evidence that primary hyperparathyroidism is especially likely to occur in women about the time of the menopause.

In some patients, there is no clinical evidence of disease. Laboratory tests reveal the presence of the disorder. The most common signs and symptoms in hyperparathyroidism are those related to urinary calculi. Renal manifestations also include nephrocalcinosis and uremia. Less common are signs and symptoms of skeletal disease, such as pathologic fractures, bone pain, and generalized demineralization of the skeleton. Gastrointestinal disorders occur, including epigastric discomfort, constipation, and vague abdominal complaints. More important, peptic ulcers occur in 10% to 15% of hyperparathyroid patients, especially men, and acute pancreatitis is also fairly common. Central nervous system disturbances may constitute an important part of the clinical picture. These include depressive reactions, confusion, stupor, and personality changes. Additional manifestations of hypercalcemia include weakness, polydipsia, and polyuria. The ophthalmologist may find band keratopathy, a corneal opacity extending across the cornea from within the limbus, and also may note crystals in the conjunctivas. Some patients have hypertension, often the result of renal damage, but in some instances the relationship to kidney disease is unclear because impairment of renal function cannot be demonstrated.[34]

Elevated levels of circulating parathyroid hormone cause increased urinary excretion of inorganic phosphate, decreased serum phosphate, and increased serum calcium. Intestinal absorption of calcium rises. If skeletal lesions are present, serum alkaline phosphatase is elevated, and the urinary excretion of hydroxyproline rises (see also p. 1922).

Hyperparathyroidism must be differentiated from other causes of hypercalcemia, such as hypervitaminosis D and A, hyperthyroidism, adrenocortical insufficiency, the milk-alkali syndrome (excessive ingestion of milk and absorbable alkalis, leading to hypercalcemia, alkalosis, and azotemia without hypophosphatemia or hypercalciuria), sarcoidosis, tuberculosis, multiple myeloma, leukemia, lympho-

ma, and some other malignant neoplasms with and without metastatic foci in bone. Idiopathic hypercalciuria with normal serum calcium and repeated formation of renal stones and the hypercalciuria present in renal tubular acidosis are conditions that also must be distinguished from hyperparathyroidism.

Hyperplasia

Disturbances in calcium and phosphorus metabolism not primarily involving the parathyroid glands may, in time, cause changes in the glands as they respond to the metabolic abnormalities. Chronic renal glomerular insufficiency resulting in retention of phosphate and depression of intestinal absorption of calcium is the most common cause of compensatory parathyroid hyperfunction and hyperplasia. Very high levels of circulating parathyroid hormone may be present, but the glands are still responsive to changes in serum calcium. Hyperplasia may occur in rickets and osteomalacia caused by vitamin D deficiency, with intestinal malabsorption syndromes causing deficiencies of calcium and vitamin D, and in pseudohypoparathyroidism. The hyperplasia present with some medullary thyroid carcinomas producing calcitonin may be secondary to the calcitonin excess or may be primary hyperplasia as a part of multiple endocrine adenopathy.

Parathyroid hyperplasia may occur in the absence of an obvious underlying metabolic disease. This type of parathyroid hyperplasia is called "primary hyperplasia," which implies that the cause is not known. Primary hyperplasia probably accounts for less than one half the total cases of hyperparathyroidism that are not known to be secondary to metabolic disorders such as renal disease and vitamin D deficiency. Sometimes the disorder is familial, and it may be part of a syndrome of multiple abnormalities of the endocrine glands.

Hyperplastic glands range from normal size to striking enlargement. Variations in the size of the individual glands in any one person may be evident. The lower pair are often larger. The glands are not adherent to the surrounding tissues, as a rule, even though they may have quite irregular contours. The cut surfaces may be smooth or nodular. There is a sharp decrease or even absence of stromal fat, and the glands are cellular, composed usually of pale and vacuolated chief cells (Fig. 38-1). Transitional oxyphil cells or transitional water-clear cells may predominate occasionally. The cells often are arranged in solid masses,

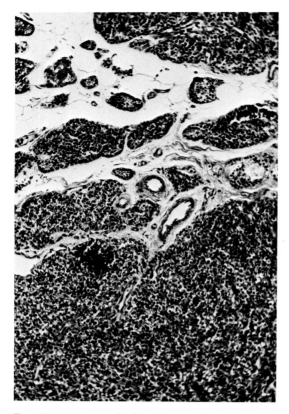

Fig. 38-1. Primary chief-cell hyperplasia. Irregular involvement of gland can occur. Several small groups of cells appear to be normal.

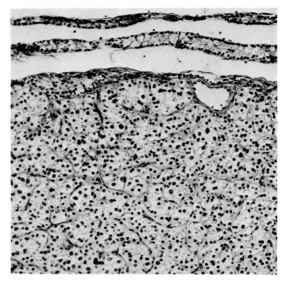

Fig. 38-2. Adenoma. Two delicate strands of remaining glandular tissue above tumor.

but nests, cords, or acinar patterns may occur. Nuclei are about normal size or somewhat enlarged; giant nuclei and multinucleated cells are rare. It is not possible to distinguish between primary and secondary hyperplasia on histologic grounds alone. Nevertheless, the presence of irregular involvement of an individual gland or the presence of nodules of hyperplastic tissue separated from one another by more nearly normal parathyroid tissue are characteristics much more likely to occur in primary hyperplasia than in secondary hyperplasia. On the other hand, oxyphil cells are more likely to be numerous in cases of secondary hyperplasia caused by chronic renal disease.

Primary water–clear cell hyperplasia is rare and may be related to the chief-cell type.[29] All of the glands are irregularly enlarged, but the upper pair is usually the larger. The glands are chocolate brown and not adherent to the surrounding tissue, and their surfaces are irregular. Cut surfaces are soft, smooth, and uniform. All of the glands are composed entirely of large water-clear cells 10 to 40 μm in diameter. They have nearly uniform, small, dark-staining nuclei about 4 to 8 μm in diameter. Cellular patterns include diffuse solid masses, acini with basal orientation of the nuclei, and irregular trabeculae. Giant nuclei may be present in small numbers.

Neoplasms
Parathyroid adenoma

Parathyroid adenoma (Fig. 38-2) is the cause of primary hyperparathyroidism in one half or more of patients with the disorder. Two or more adenomas are rare. They are more common in the lower pair of glands. Adenomas range in weight from less than 100 mg to several hundred grams (rarely), but most weigh only a few grams. A few are palpable on physical examination. There is a rough correlation between the size of the tumor and the degree of hyperfunction. The tumors are spheric to ovoid, soft, tan to reddish brown, or occasionally gray, have a smooth capsule, and are usually not adherent to the surrounding tissues. The cut surface may be focally hemorrhagic or cystic, and zones of fibrosis and calcification may be present. Deposits of brown pigment mark the sites of old hemorrhage.

The majority of adenomas are composed of chief cells, either normal or abnormal in appearance, but any cell type can predominate and any single tumor can contain a variety of cell types. Oxyphil cell tumors are often nonfunctional (not always), but with this exception, there is no correlation between the degree of hyperfunction and the cell type. Giant nuclei, bizarre nuclei, and multinucleated cells are fairly common. Mitoses are rare.

The cells may be arranged as simply a solid mass or they may form cords, nests, acini, or follicles resembling thyroid follicles. Nodules of single or mixed patterns may be evident. Commonly one histologic pattern predominates, but in some tumors a variety of patterns is visible.

The remaining tissue of a gland containing an adenoma often forms a "rim" of normal or somewhat atrophic-appearing parathyroid cells outside the capsule of the adenoma. Such tissue usually contains fat and is composed of small chief cells and perhaps some oxyphil cells. It may be difficult or impossible to decide whether adenoma or irregular hyperplasia is present, especially if only limited tissue is available to the pathologist. In distinguishing these two entities it is of paramount importance to have information regarding the gross appearance of the other glands. The problem is aggravated by the possibility that diffuse hyperplasia and adenoma may represent only polar ends of a spectrum of parathyroid proliferative disorders.[33,41]

Carcinoma

Nonfunctional parathyroid carcinomas are difficult to separate from thyroid carcinomas, so that most pathologists require the presence of hyperparathyroidism to make the diagnosis. These rare neoplasms are frequently palpable on physical examination. Parathyroid hyperfunction may be pronounced. At surgery, carcinoma is nearly always tightly adherent to surrounding tissue and is irregular in shape, but some have resembled typical adenomas. The cut surface is gray, light tan, or brown and is firm, largely as a result of fibrous septa running through the tumor.

Microscopically, the carcinoma consists of solid masses of cells separated by irregular fibrous septa and surrounded by a thick, fibrous capsule. The cells may be large chief cells, clear cells, or elongated cells with eosinophilic to amphophilic cytoplasm and large nuclei. Perivascular palisading and trabecular patterns are common. Mitotic figures are usually present.

The only certain criteria of malignancy are the presence of local invasion of adjacent tissues and distant metastatic lesions. Recurrence is common, and death may occur. Management of the patient is difficult because of the persistent or recurring hyperparathyroidism.

Hyperparathyroidism with tumors of other organs

A variety of malignant neoplasms, including carcinoma of the lung, liver, and kidney, have produced parathyroid hormone and are thus responsible for ectopic hyperparathyroidism.

Lesions associated with hyperparathyroidism

The hypercalcemia of hyperparathyroidism may result in the deposition of calcium salts (known as metastatic calcification) in a variety of soft tissues. Renal calculi occur in at least half the patients with symptomatic hyperparathyroidism and often are the reason the patient seeks medical aid. A considerably smaller number of patients have osteoporotic lesions of the skeletal system, the fully developed condition being known as generalized osteitis fibrosa cystica.

Metastatic calcification

The kidneys and blood vessels are the most frequent sites of metastatic calcification, but some deposits, especially in acute hyperparathyroidism, may be found in the lungs, stomach, heart, eyes, and other tissues. Calcific deposits are particularly abundant when there is renal failure with phosphate retention.

In blood vessels, the calcification is mainly in the media and particularly involves elastic tissue, so that the internal elastic lamella is often prominently calcified. The adjacent intima may be thickened by hyperplasia but is usually without calcification. Vascular calcification may be particularly severe in secondary renal hyperparathyroidism in which there is an increased level of blood phosphate. In some patients, ischemic muscle pains in the extremities and even gangrene have resulted.

Generalized osteitis fibrosa cystica

Osteitis fibrosa cystica (Recklinghausen's disease) (Fig. 38-3) is essentially an osteoclastic resorption of bone and its replacement by connective tissue in which there are abortive attempts at new bone formation. When mild, the gross change in the bones is merely a slight porosity and, microscopically, mild generalized osteoporosis and marrow fibrosis. As the condition progresses, there is more loss of osseous tissue, with replacement by connective tissue. Immature and poorly calcified bone develops in the connective tissue. The newly

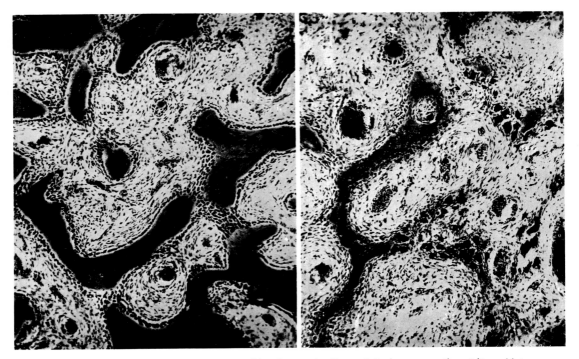

Fig. 38-3. Osteitis fibrosa cystica (Recklinghausen's disease) in hyperparathyroidism. Note irregular arrangement of newly formed bone trabeculae, which exhibit narrow osteoid zones and osteoclastic resorption. Marrow is fibrous and hyperemic. (Courtesy Dr. Walter H. Bauer, Boston.)

formed bone soon may again undergo resorption. Osteoclasts are abundant. Large fibrous scars develop in the place of the original spongy bone. Brown tumors, usually in the jaws or long bones, are colored by blood pigment and consist of multinucleated giant cells in a cellular fibrous stroma. Cysts lined by connective tissue may result from degeneration or hemorrhage but are not always present. Characteristic early roentgenographic changes include subperiosteal resorption of bone, most frequently seen along the margins of the middle phalanges of the fingers. Plasma alkaline phosphatase is increased. Because skeletal collagen is resorbed, urinary hydroxyproline excretion is increased.

Renal lesions

The kidneys may be severely damaged in hyperparathyroidism as a result of the deposition of calcium salts (nephrocalcinosis) and the formation of renal stones. Excess parathyroid hormone apparently interferes with the ability of the tubules to concentrate urine. In acute hyperparathyroidism, some of the nephrons show calcification of tubular epithelial cells and tubular basement membranes. Calcific casts are formed.

In the milder chronic cases, patchy calcification usually involves cells of the ascending limb of the loop of Henle, the distal convoluted tubule, and the collecting tubule.[32] Casts, usually calcific, are formed partly from desquamated cells and cellular debris and may cause obstruction of the nephron. Some interstitial calcification may occur. Foci of fibrosis with tubular and glomerular atrophy and infiltration by chronic inflammatory cells are common.

In advanced cases fibrosis, inflammation, and nephron destruction are extensive, and calcification of interstitial tissue may be striking. Both atrophy and cystic dilatation of the tubules proximal to obstructing calcific masses may be evident. (See Fig. 38-4.)

Although hyperparathyroidism is an uncommon cause of renal calculi, investigation for its presence should be made in every patient with renal stones. In some clinics, 4% of individuals with renal stones have hyperparathyroidism. The calculi are predominantly calcium oxalate or calcium phosphate. Kidneys

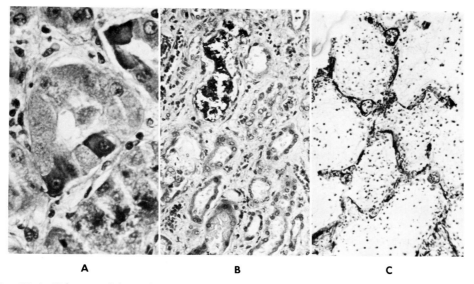

Fig. 38-4. Kidney and lung from 35-year-old man with large parathyroid adenoma. **A,** Several renal tubular cells have undergone calcification. **B,** Calcific material fills a renal tubule. **C,** Walls of alveoli and of blood vessels are calcified.

containing stones may have only minor tubular damage, or they may be extensively involved by calcific deposits and the associated parenchymal damage. Hydronephrosis may occur. Pyelonephritis is common in kidneys damaged by stones and by calcinosis.

Renal osteodystrophy and secondary hyperparathyroidism

The osteodystrophy occurring in chronic renal failure is characterized by varying degrees of osteitis fibrosa, osteomalacia, osteoporosis, and osteosclerosis.[50] The clinical and pathologic features in a single patient depend on the pathologic process that predominates during a particular time period. The pathologic processes, in turn, depend on which of the complex metabolic disturbances of uremia are most important in the person affected and how these disturbances are altered by therapeutic measures. Renal lesions of a type in which large amounts of renal parenchyma are lacking or destroyed and those that are stationary or very slowly progressive (renal insufficiency over a prolonged period) may result in these skeletal changes. Hemodialysis and renal transplantation prolong life and thereby have substantially increased the possibility that skeletal disease may develop.

One of the most important complications of the secondary hyperparathyroidism usually present in chronic renal disease is soft-tissue calcification. Sites commonly involved are the arteries, heart, kidneys, lungs, stomach, soft tissues around joints, eyes, and skin and subcutaneous tissues. Arterial, myocardial, and renal calcification may have grave clinical effects.

In children, remarkable skeletal deformities and growth disturbances (dwarfism) may result because bone growth is incomplete and the epiphyses are not united. The underlying renal lesion is most commonly a developmental malformation in the kidneys or urinary tract, such as congenital hypoplasia, congenital polycystic disease, strictures of the ureters, or congenital valves of the urethra. Infection (pyelonephritis) may be added to hydronephrotic atrophy in cases of obstruction in the lower urinary tract and still further decrease the functioning renal parenchyma.

The characteristic changes occurring in the epiphyseal cartilages are probably the result of abnormal metabolism of vitamin D as well as of hyperparathyroidism. The epiphyseal cartilages are greatly increased in bulk but show degenerative changes, defects of calcium deposition, and distortion. The cartilage may be bent and twisted and displaced from its normal position at the end of the shaft. Extreme deformity often results. The skull may be greatly thickened, and the appearance of the calvaria closely resembles that in Paget's disease of bone.

The kidneys show less calcium deposition

than in primary hyperparathyroidism, and renal calculi are less frequent.

OTHER ABNORMALITIES

Parathyroid cysts large enough to be clinically apparent are rare. They may occur within the thyroid gland and the mediastinum as well as in the lower neck near the thyroid gland (p. 1271).

Inflammatory processes in parathyroid tissue are unusual. Sometimes, inflammation in the thyroid gland extends into one or several glands. Rarely, part of the gland tissue is replaced by amyloidosis or by secondary carcinoma, such as carcinomas of the lung and the thyroid gland.

REFERENCES
General; development and structure

1 Castleman, B.: Tumors of parathyroid glands. In Atlas of tumor pathology, Sect. IV, Fasc. 15, Washington, D.C., 1952, Armed Forces Institute of Pathology.
2 Christie, A. C.: J. Clin. Pathol. **20**:591-602, 1967.
3 Gilmour, J. R.: J. Pathol. Bacteriol. **45**:507-522, 1937.
4 Gilmour, J. R.: J. Pathol. Bacteriol. **46**:133-149, 1938.
5 Gilmour, J. R.: J. Pathol. Bacteriol. **48**:187-222, 1939.
6 Gilmour, J. R., and Martin, W. J.: J. Pathol. Bacteriol. **44**:431-462, 1937.
7 Roth, S. I., and Capen, C. C.: Int. Rev. Exp. Pathol. **13**:161-221, 1974.

Hormones, regulation of calcium metabolism

8 Chase, L. R., and Aurbach, G. D.: Science **159**:545-547, 1968.
9 Copp, D. H.: J. Endocrinology **43**:137-161, 1969.
10 Epstein, F. H.: Am. J. Med. **45**:700-714, 1968.
11 Kyle, L. H.: New Eng. J. Med. **251**:1035-1040, 1954 (milk-alkali syndrome).
12 MacIntyre, I.: Curr. Top. Exp. Endocrinol. **2**:179-193, 1974.

Pathologic calcification

13 Anderson, W. A. D.: J. Pediatr. **14**:375-381, 1939.
14 Anderson, W. A. D.: J. Urol. **44**:29-34, 1940.
15 Barr, D. P.: Physiol. Rev. **12**:593-624, 1932.
16 Lutz, J. F.: Ann. Intern. Med. **14**:1270-1282, 1941 (calcinosis).
17 Mortensen, J. D., and Baggenstoss, A. H.: Am. J. Clin. Pathol. **24**:45-63, 1954 (nephrocalcinosis).
18 Mulligan, R. M.: Arch. Pathol. (Chicago) **43**:177-230, 1947 (metastatic calcification).
19 Parfitt, A. M.: Arch. Intern. Med. (Chicago) **124**:544-556, 1969.
20 Selye, H.: Calciphylaxis, Chicago, 1962, University of Chicago Press.

Hypoparathyroidism, pseudohypoparathyroidism

21 Chase, L. R., Melson, G. L., and Aurbach, G. D.: J. Clin. Invest. **48**:1832-1844, 1969.
22 David, L., and Anast, C. S.: J. Clin. Invest. **54**:287-296, 1974.
23 Drake, T. G., Albright, F., Bauer, W., and Castleman, B.: Ann. Intern. Med. **12**:1751-1765, 1939.
24 Mann, J. B., Alterman, S., and Hills, A. G.: Ann. Intern. Med. **56**:315-342, 1962.
25 Spinner, M. W., Blizzard, R. M., and Childs, B.: J. Clin. Endocrinol. **28**:795-804, 1968.
26 Taitz, L. S., Zarate-Salvador, C., and Schwartz, E.: Pediatrics **38**:412-418, 1966.

Hyperparathyroidism

27 Castleman, B., and Mallory, T. B.: Am. J. Pathol. **11**:1-72, 1935.
28 Cope, O.: Ann. Surg. **114**:706-733, 1941.
29 Hellström, J., and Ivemark, B. I.: Acta Chir. Scand. suppl. 294, pp. 1-113, 1962.
30 Lloyd, H. M.: Medicine (Balt.) **47**:53-71, 1968.
31 Pugh, D. G.: Am. J. Roentgenol. **66**:577-586, 1951.
32 Pyrah, L. N., Hodgkinson, A., and Anderson, C. K.: Br. J. Surg. **53**:245-316, 1966.
33 Reiss, E., and Canterbury, J. M.: Am. J. Med. **56**:794-799, 1974.
34 Rienhoff, W. F., Jr., Rienhoff, W. F., III, Brawley, R. K., and Shelley, W. M.: Ann. Surg. **168**:1061-1074, 1968.
35 Rogers, H. M., Keating, F. R., Jr., Morlock, C. G., and Barker, N. W.: Arch. Intern. Med. (Chicago) **79**:307-321, 1947 (peptic ulcer).
36 Turchi, J. J., Flandreau, R. H., Forte, A. L., French, G. N., and Ludwig, G. D.: J.A.M.A. **180**:799-804, 1962 (hyperparathyroidism and pancreatitis).

Hyperplasia
Secondary hyperplasia

37 Castleman, B., and Mallory, T. B.: Am. J. Pathol. **13**:553-574, 1937 (renal disease).

Primary hyperplasia

38 Albright, F., Bloomberg, E., Castleman, B., and Churchill, E. D.: Arch. Intern. Med. (Chicago) **54**:315-329, 1934.
39 Black, W. C., III, and Utley, J. R.: Am. J. Clin. Pathol. **49**:761-775, 1968.
40 Cope, O., Keynes, W. M., Roth, S. I., and Castleman, B.: Ann. Surg. **148**:375-388, 1958.
41 Golden, A., Canary, J. J., and Kerwin, D. M.: Am. J. Med. **38**:562-578, 1965.

Neoplasms

42 Arnold, B. M., Kovacs, K., Horvath, E., Murray, T. M., and Higgins, H. P.: J. Clin. Endocrinol. **38**:458-462, 1974.
43 Schantz, A., and Castleman, B.: Cancer **31**:600-605, 1973.
44 Sherwood, L. M., O'Riordan, J. L. H., Aurbach, G. D., and Potts, J. T., Jr.: J. Clin. Endocrinol. **27**:140-146, 1967 (nonparathyroid tumors).
45 Woolner, L. B., Keating, F. R., Jr., and Black, B. M.: Cancer **5**:1069-1088, 1952.

Lesions associated with hyperparathyroidism

46 Andersen, D. H., and Schlesinger, E. R.: Am. J. Dis. Child. **63:**102-125, 1942.

47 Anderson, W. A. D.: Arch. Pathol. (Chicago) **27:**753-778, 1939.

48 Follis, R. H., Jr., and Jackson, D. A.: Bull. Johns Hopkins Hosp. **72:**232-241, 1943 (skeletal changes).

49 Herbert, F. K., Miller, H. G., and Richardson, G. O.: J. Pathol. Bacteriol. **53:**161-182, 1941.

50 Kleeman, C. R., Massry, S. G., Coburn, J. W., and Popovtzer, M. M.: Arch. Intern. Med. (Chicago) **124:**261-268, 1969.

51 Pappenheimer, A. M., and Wilens, S. L.: Am. J. Pathol. **11:**73-91, 1935.

52 Williams, H. E.: New Eng. J. Med. **290:**33-38, 1974.

Other abnormalities
Cysts

53 Wood, J. W., Johnson, K. G., and Hinds, M. J. A.: Arch. Surg. (Chicago) **92:**785-790, 1966.

39/Adrenal glands

SHELDON C. SOMMERS

STRUCTURE AND FUNCTION

The adrenal glands are glands of mystery and adventure. Biochemical and functional investigations recently have outdistanced adrenal morphology.

Embryologically, the adrenal medulla is of neural crest ectodermal origin. The cortex originates from urogenital ridge mesoderm. Accessory cortical nodules are commonly present in the adrenal capsule. They also are scattered throughout the retroperitoneal space, in the testicular region in 7.5% and beneath the renal capsule in 1.2% of autopsies, and less often in the ovaries or broad ligaments. Celiac accessory adrenal glands were found in 32% of autopsies. Tissue foci resembling the adrenal medulla and termed "paraganglia" are peppered throughout the retroperitoneum, forming the prominent infant organ of Zuckerkandl, which is more difficult to find after puberty.

The human adrenal gland passes through three major developmental phases—fetal, childhood, and adult. The prenatal cortex has an inner fetal zone, similar in location to the X zone in mice, which disappears within months after birth. Relative to body weight, the adrenal glands are large at birth, weighing 2 to 4 gm each, or 8.2 ± 3.4 gm together. In anencephalics, the fetal cortical zone atrophies prematurely after the twentieth week of pregnancy, and at birth each adrenal gland weighs only about 8% of normal, with closely packed cortical cells that lack ultrastructural indications of steroidogenesis.

In late childhood, the adrenarche occurs, with increased prepubertal secretion of androgens and related compounds. By then, the adult cortical zonation of glomerulosa, fasciculata, and reticularis has become established. At 11 to 15 years of age, the normal aggregate weight is 8.5 gm in boys and 7.5 gm in girls. Apparently normal adult adrenal glands removed surgically weigh 4.8 ± 0.8 gm in men

and 4.1 ± 0.8 gm in women. After sudden death, the aggregate adrenal weight is 9.2 ± 1.8 gm in the United States. In other autopsies, the normal range is 12 to 16 mg, or 0.21 to 0.26 gm per kilogram of body weight. The increase is ascribed to cortical hypertrophy in response to the stress of illness. Crowding of experimental animals leads to adrenocortical hypertrophy and gonadal shrinkage. Comparable effects may occur in human beings. Most autopsies do not include careful stripping of the periadrenal fat or accurate weighing of the glands and, except for a few series, satisfactory baseline weights are difficult to find.

The flattened right and pyramidal left human adrenal glands each have a head, body, and tail region, with the medulla in the more medial aspect of the head and body. The zona fasciculata accounts for 69.3% of the total cortical volume. Medulla, capsule, connective tissue, and vessels make up about 21.5% of the whole gland volume. The normal cortex measures 1 to 2 mm in width. The total cortical width and zona fasciculata width are statistically significantly correlated with their volumes. The human zona glomerulosa is normally discontinuous.

On section, the adrenal cortex is golden yellow with a brown pigmented inner zona reticularis and a gray medulla. In women of menopausal age, the zona reticularis is often prominent. Abundant sudanophilic lipid and cholesterol are present in all three adrenocortical zones. The cells normally appear finely vacuolated in paraffin sections. Zonation may not be obvious histologically, but with experience aided by reticulin stains, the outer glomerulosa pattern, the linearly arranged fasciculata, and the diagonal network of slightly pigmented reticularis cells can be recognized. The irregularly arranged medullary cells have prominent nuclei and abundant amphophilic cytoplasm. Chromaffinity is a mahogany brown medullary tissue color produced by the oxidant effect of chromate salts or Helly's solution on epinephrine in unfixed tissues.

Electron microscopy demonstrates characteristic platelike mitochondrial cristae in the zona glomerulosa cells, in contrast to tubular mitochondria of zona fasciculata cells. Cortical cells have abundant smooth endoplasmic reticulum like other steroid-secreting cells and a less prominent rough endoplasmic reticulum. Although it contains isolated adrenocortical cells, the adrenal medulla is separated completely from the cortex by a basement membrane. Osmiophilic cytoplasmic catecholamine-storage granules in medullary cells comprise pure epinephrine and norepinephrine types, each surrounded by limiting membranes. The latter have a clear peripheral halo.

Adrenocortical function involves the synthesis and secretion of steroids formed from cho-

lesterol (Fig. 39-1). In the human adult, these include aldosterone, chiefly from the zona glomerulosa, hydrocortisone (cortisol) from the zona fasciculata, and androgens and estrogens predominantly from the zona reticularis. The human fetal cortex responds to both ACTH and chorionic gonadotropin but has relatively little 3β-hydroxysteroid dehydrogenase activity, which prevents the formation of progesterone and hence of aldosterone and cortisol. Instead, dehydroepiandrosterone and its derivatives are the major steroids secreted, contributing to the placental synthesis of estrogens, particularly estriol.

At birth, the fetal cortical zone degenerates, shrinks, and completely involutes within 3 to 12 months. Failure of the fetal cortex to involute or to develop 17-hydroxylase, 21-hydroxylase, and 11β-hydroxylase, which normally

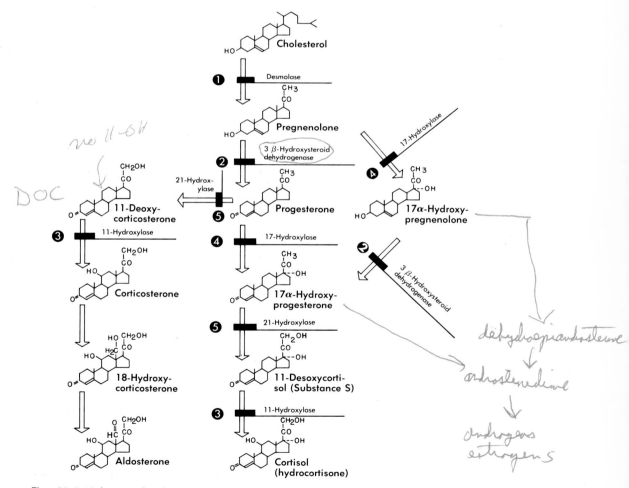

Fig. 39-1. Scheme of adrenocorticosteroid synthetic pathways. Enzymes underlined and numbered correspond to congenital enzymatic deficiencies that block reactions, as discussed in text.

occur after the first 10 weeks of pregnancy, may result in some instances of congenital adrenal hyperplasia.

CONGENITAL ANOMALIES

Absence of both adrenal glands is compatible with life if accessory cortical tissue is present in the retroperitoneum or testes or if sufficient corticosteroids are produced by the brown fat. Aberrant adrenal tissue also may occur in the pancreas or liver. Only one adrenal gland may develop, the two glands may be fused, or there may be bilaterally double adrenal glands. Minor anomalies include adrenohepatic or adrenorenal fusion, usually unilateral and without functional importance.

Hypoplasia

Hypoplasia of the fetal cortical zone associated with anencephaly has been mentioned, and similar effects occur in pregnancies with subnormal maternal urinary estriol, preeclampsia, or both, as well as with prenatal pituitary or nervous system degeneration. Neonates with the respiratory distress syndrome had adrenal weights 19% less than normal, and their plasma cortisol was one third the expected levels. Cystic degeneration of the outer cortex is common in premature infants of less than 35 weeks of gestation.

Congenital hypoplasia

Three types of adrenal hypoplasia are recognized in liveborn infants:
1. Precocious involution of the fetal cortex, which is found in postmaturity or various newborn illnesses. Destructive necrosis and hemorrhage of the fetal cortex are extensive, with infiltrates of neutrophils, and may destroy parts of the definitive cortex.
2. Idiopathic hypoplasia, in which the glands weigh only 0.3 to 1.8 gm each, with miniature adult type of cortices some eight cells thick. Fetal cortex is decreased or absent. An ACTH-resistant familial variety develops regularly in females. The affected infants typically suffer weight loss, dehydration, hyponatremia, hypoglycemia, and convulsions and die of adrenocortical insufficiency within 10 days.
3. Cytomegalic adrenocortical hypoplasia, which is rare, usually in males, and evidently involves failure of the fetal cortical zone to involute and a related hypoplasia of the permanent outer cortex. Some instances are familial.

Anaplastic fetal adrenocortical cells are found in about 5% of infants at autopsy. Ordinarily, this focal cytomegaly and irregular nuclear polyploidy may only represent an atypical involutional change. Fetal adrenocortical cytomegaly is a characteristic of Beckwith's syndrome, which also includes macroglossia, abnormal umbilicus, somatic gigantism, and severe hypoglycemia. Three children with this syndrome developed adrenocortical carcinoma. If bilateral adrenocortical cytomegaly is extensive, death from adrenal insufficiency may follow in about 1 month. The cytomegalic cells may be functional; ultrastructural features of steroidogenesis also are found.

Congenital hyperplasia

Congenital adrenal hyperplasia with the adrenogenital syndrome is an uncommon condition believed attributable to autosomal recessive genes. Its importance lies in the associated anomalies of the external genitalia, the enzyme blocks responsible for the syndrome, and the interrelations of embryonic adrenal and genital tract differentiation thus revealed. The following classification of Bongiovanni et al.[13] is useful, since it permits correlation of the individual enzyme deficiencies indicated in Fig. 36-1 with clinicopathologic alterations.
1. Desmolase deficiency is a rarity associated with lipid adrenal hyperplasia. The cortical cells contain excessive cholesterol and neutral lipid. Since practically all types of corticosteroid synthesis are blocked, there is no virilization, the blood pressure is low, salt and water loss are common, and death in infancy is frequent. Males usually are hypospadiac and may be regarded as pseudohermaphrodites. Urinary ketosteroids are low.
2. 3β-Hydroxysteroid dehydrogenase deficiency is also rare and usually fatal. The affected males are hypospadiac or may possess a vagina. Normal development of the male external genitalia is inhibited since the testis also lacks the enzyme, so that testosterone and related steroids are not produced. Females may be moderately virilized at birth by the weakly androgenic effects of dehydroepiandrosterone and related Δ^5-3β-hydroxysteroid compounds, which comprise almost all the urinary steroids. Ordinarily, low blood pressure, salt loss, hypoadrenal crises, failure to respond to treatment, and death ensue.
3. 11-Hydroxylase deficiency is the chief virilizing and hypertensive type of con-

genital adrenal hyperplasia. The dominant steroid is compound S, urinary 17-ketosteroids are increased, and salt wastage is uncommon. Urinary pregnanetriol is slightly elevated. Similar clinical and laboratory findings occur in some children with hypertension, adrenal adenoma, malnutrition, or diarrhea. A few postpubertal girls with polycystic ovaries and some with hypertension may have incomplete 11-hydroxylase deficiency. Adrenal hyperplasia is not always demonstrated.

4. 17-Hydroxylase deficiency is rare. No androgens or estrogens are produced. The urinary 17-ketosteroids are low. Aldosterone and cortisol are deficient. Hypertension is present without salt wastage, since the major steroids produced are deoxycorticosterone and corticosterone. Amenorrhea, incompletely developed secondary sex characteristics, and polycystic ovaries have been found. It is uncertain whether the enzyme deficiency is congenital or is associated with adrenal hyperplasia.

5. 21-Hydroxylase deficiency accounts for about 90% of all congenital adrenal hyperplasias. It produces the most familiar type of adrenogenital syndrome in infants and children. Virilization in both sexes is moderate or notable. Af-

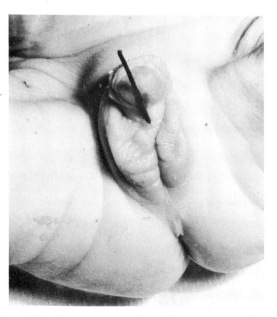

Fig. 39-2. External genitalia of female infant with 21-hydroxylase deficiency and adrenocortical hyperplasia. Appearance typical of female pseudohermaphroditism with adrenogenital syndrome.

fected females have clitoral hypertrophy, and labial fusion may simulate a scrotum (Fig. 39-2). In males, there may be precocious penile enlargement (macrogenitosomia). Both sexes have accelerated somatic growth. The dominant steroid is 17-hydroxyprogesterone, and over 20 urinary steroids that lack C-21 hydroxyl groups are present, with androsterone and etiocholanolone predominant among the increased 17-ketosteroids. Pregnanetriol is one urinary 17-hydroxyprogesterone metabolite. The virilizing androgen is testosterone.

6. The last type of enzyme deficiency involves 18-oxidase without cortical hyperplasia.

In embryos, androgens inhibit differentiation of the genital tract along female lines, except in testicular feminization. One consequence is external genitalia of female pseudohermaphroditic appearance. The internal genitalia of embryos and children are less affected by androgens, whereas after puberty luteinized ovarian cysts or testicular Leydig cell hyperplasia may occur. In some cases there is testicular proliferation of accessory adrenocortical cells, but usually the testicular masses are hyperplastic Leydig cells. Female pseudohermaphroditism occasionally follows maternal therapy with progesterone, androgens, or estrogens. Since masculinization is progressive, early diagnosis and continuous cortisone type of steroid therapy are desirable.

In about 30% of patients with 21-hydroxylase deficiency, there is salt loss, a tendency to low blood pressure, sudden collapse with water restriction, and low serum sodium and high potassium levels, as well as hypoglycemia, susceptibility to infections, and brown skin pigmentation. Episodic fever may be attributable to etiocholanolone secretion. Supported by cortisone therapy, the individuals may survive to middle age or beyond.

Except for desmolase deficiency, the adrenal glands appear similar in all the congenital hyperplasias. The glands are up to five times normal size and may weigh 40 to 50 gm each. The cortex is thickened and convoluted, with cells resembling the zona reticularis comprising two thirds of its total volume (Fig. 39-3). Apparently, the hyperplasia does not represent persistent fetal adrenocortical tissue. In children, the cells generally are not pigmented or stained by fuchsin. The zona fasciculata usually is identifiable microscopically. In adult female pseudohermaphrodites, the hyperplastic zona reticularis is both pigmented and fuch-

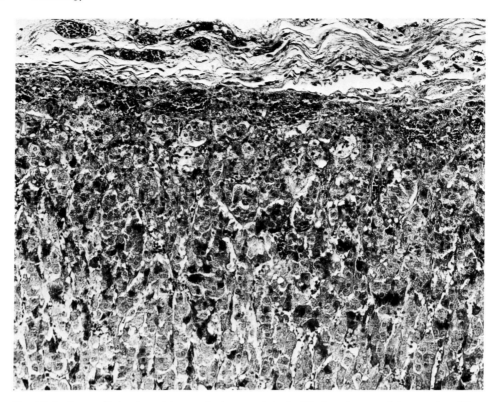

Fig. 39-3. Congenital adrenal hyperplasia associated with female pseudohermaphroditism. Cortical cells irregularly enlarged, with acidophilic granular cytoplasm. (120×.)

sinophilic. The characteristically increased ACTH that accompanies congenital adrenal hyperplasia has been ascribed to insufficient feedback control by cortisol.

At least three other conditions with adrenal hyperplasia in the newborn infant have been reported. Infants of diabetic mothers may have increased urinary corticoids as part of an edematous, pseudoerythroblastosis syndrome, sometimes with an apparent increase of fetal cortical width. In infants dying of erythroblastosis fetalis or α-thalassemia, the fetal cortex is both thick and excessively vacuolated; the accompanying thymic atrophy suggests adrenal hyperfunction, possibly because of chronic intrauterine hypoxia. Antenatal infection also is reported associated with adrenocortical hyperplasia in the newborn.

CHILDHOOD ABNORMALITIES

Hemorrhage. Certain adrenal lesions are more common before puberty, without necessarily being limited to children. Adrenal hemorrhage that destroys both the cortex and medulla may reflect birth trauma, particularly after breech delivery. Waterhouse-Friderichsen syndrome involves bilateral, ordinarily fatal, destructive adrenal hemorrhages, classically associated with meningococcemia. Other gram-negative organisms such as colon bacilli may be responsible, and, less often, diphtheria, varicella, or measles. Gram-negative endotoxin shock, endothelial necrosis, sinusoidal thrombi, and intravascular consumption coagulopathy are implicated in the pathogenesis.

Necrosis. Hepatoadrenal necrosis is another usually fatal lesion, especially in premature infants with systemic herpes simplex infection acquired at birth, probably from maternal vaginitis. Both the adrenocortical and hepatic cells are extensively destroyed. Some contain intranuclear Cowdry type A inclusion bodies. Cytomegalic inclusion disease is accompanied by typical, large, acidophil intranuclear viral inclusions and cortical necrosis in about one third of generalized cytomegalovirus infections. A comparable adrenal involvement may occur in adults as a complication of lymphoma, leukemia, or peptic ulcer. Systemic pneumocystis or cryptococcus infections may localize in the adrenals. Varicella and herpes zoster of the adrenal glands produce medullary intranuclear inclusions.

Granulomas. In about half of the autopsied cases of infantile toxoplasmosis, adrenal granulomas with or without recognizable organisms are found. In generalized histoplasmosis, coccidioidomycosis, and brucellosis, there occur epithelioid, caseous, or partly calcified adrenal granulomas, sometimes extensive enough to cause death from adrenocortical insufficiency. Congenital syphilis may show subcapsular adrenal fibrosis and abundant treponemes. Tuberculous Addison's disease of children is like the adult condition described below.

Hypoplasia. Adrenocortical cytotoxic hypoplasia, occasionally with persistent cytomegalic cortical cells, characterizes idiopathic Addison's disease of infancy. Histologically, the adrenocortical cells are degenerated, with intermingled lymphocytes and macrophages. Several familial syndromes include childhood Addison's disease, most frequently combined with hypoparathyroidism and candidosis or pernicious anemia. Adrenoleukodystrophy comprises ballooning degeneration and cytoplasmic striations affecting the cells of the zona fasciculata and zona reticularis accompanying cerebral demyelinization. Another rare, sex-linked recessive condition is adrenocortical atrophy and cerebral sclerosis in males. Adrenocortical insufficiency and death from malnutrition at the age of 4 months or less occur in primary familial xanthomatosis (Wolman's disease). Among various xanthomatous lesions ascribed to inborn lysosomal acid lipase deficiency, the adrenal glands are notably enlarged by cortical foam cells. Adrenal cholesterol, over 90% esterified, is increased twentyfold. There is also adrenocortical necrosis, foreign body reaction to crystallized lipid, and diffuse punctate calcifications that may be radiologically diagnostic. In children, adrenal calcification also follows hemorrhage from birth trauma.

Cortical insufficiency. Partial adrenocortical insufficiency with selective familial cortisol deficiency in a child was correlated with absence of the zonae fasciculata and reticularis. Adrenal cortisol unresponsiveness to ACTH, mental retardation, typical facies, dwarfism, and obesity comprise the Prader-Willi syndrome. Familial hypoaldosteronism in infants with 18-oxidase deficiency is accompanied by hyponatremia and hyperkalemia. Urinary corticosterone and related dehydro and tetrahydro compounds are increased. At autopsy, the adrenal glands are not enlarged. Small cells form tubular cords in the peripheral cortex.

Functional, sometimes transient, hypoaldosteronism is reported in a few children and young adults but lacks a distinctive lesion.

Cortical hyperfunction. Adrenocortical hyperfunction in children is more often attributable to adrenal neoplasms than to hyperplasia. Boys may show the "infant Hercules" syndrome of pronounced muscular and somatic development with precocious pseudopuberty, comprised of macrogenitosomia and hirsutism but without testicular tubular or Leydig cell maturation. Girls with either neoplasms or adrenal hyperplasia are more often virilized, with some attributes comparable to Cushing's syndrome in adults. Adrenal medullary hyperplasia has been correlated with hypertension in two children and reported in pancreatic cystic fibrosis and in the sudden infant death syndrome.

Neuroblastoma. Neuroblastoma of the medulla is the chief infantile adrenal neoplasm, varying from incidentally found seedlings to massive retroperitoneal tumors. Next to retinoblastoma, this is the most common congenital cancer. The age at diagnosis is less than 1 year in 30% and below 5 years in 80%. Less than 5% of the patients are over 15 years old. Extra-adrenal neuroblastomas arise elsewhere, particularly in the retroperitoneum and posterior mediastinum. When the primary tumor is small, metastases may first attract attention. Typical profuse osseous metastases, which include the skull and orbit, with resulting exophthalmos, are called the Hutchison type of neuroblastoma. Large hepatic neuroblastomatous metastases constitute the Pepper syndrome.

Adrenal neuroblastomas are grossly or finely nodular, soft, gray-red, and vascular with a peripheral rim of persistent yellow adrenal cortex. Necrosis, hemorrhage, cystic degeneration, and calcification are seen. Microscopically, the viable tumor is composed of small, dark-stained, rounded or unipolar cells, practically without cytoplasm or architecture, arranged among thin-walled sinusoidal vessels (Fig. 39-4). Rosettes with distinctive neuroblastic palisading around spaces resembling primitive neural canals or pseudorosettes similar to those in embryonic sympathetic ganglia distinguish about half of neuroblastomas. Neurites and rosettes are formed in neuroblastoma tissue cultures. Ultrastructurally, most neuroblastomas contain cytoplasmic catecholamine granules, and they occasionally secrete excessive epinephrine (Fig. 39-4, *inset*).

In related better differentiated and less lethal

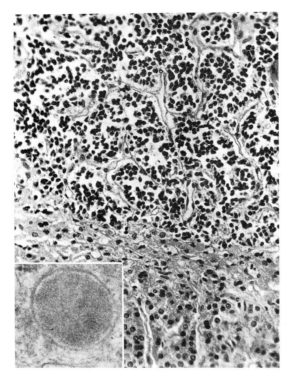

Fig. 39-4. Adrenal medullary neuroblastoma in newborn infant. (200×.) *Inset,* Membrane-enclosed catecholamine granule. (50,000×.)

neoplasms classified as ganglioneuroblastomas, foci of immature or mature neurons and nerve fibers are present. Fully differentiated ganglioneuromas are benign. In 11 cases, maturation has been observed from malignant neuroblastoma to benign ganglioneuroma. Sometimes, neuroblastoma and the histologically indistinguishable retinoblastoma regress spontaneously.

HEMORRHAGE AND NECROSIS

Adult adrenal apoplexy involves massive, usually bilateral adrenal hemorrhage, complicating trauma, infections, malignant hypertension, myocardial infarction, toxemia of pregnancy, septic abortion, or anticoagulant therapy. Vascular injury, parenchymal degeneration, venous thrombi, and generalized hemorrhagic or intravascular coagulative states are considered responsible.

Adrenocortical shrinkage or coagulative necrosis occurs focally in malaria, tetanus, typhus, Rocky Mountain spotted fever, epidemic hemorrhagic fever, and gram-negative bacterial infections, may accompany acute peptic ulcers, and occurs after abdominal operations. Diffuse bilateral adrenal necrosis and cortical insufficiency are more common in

children than in adults but may complicate infected abortion, obstetric shock, and fatal pemphigus vulgaris. Focal necrosis more often occurs after thromboses of afferent capsular vessels and outer zonal sinusoids, whereas diffuse bilateral adrenocortical necrosis results from long-lasting sinusoidal obstruction and medullary venous thromboses. Combined arterial and venous damage exaggerates both parenchymal necrosis and the subsequent hemorrhage.

INFLAMMATION, ATROPHY, AND ADDISON'S DISEASE

Exudative inflammation is uncommon in the adrenal cortex because of the antiphlogistic effects of corticosteroids. Necrosis exceeds leukocytic infiltration in various viral, mycotic, and bacterial infections that involve the adrenal glands. Granuloma formation is retarded in adrenal tuberculosis, leprosy, coccidioidomycosis, and histoplasmosis, with relatively more organisms and parenchymal destruction and less epithelioid or giant cell reaction and fibrosis than in other tissues. In lesions of extra-adrenal infections, corticoid therapy also reduces granulomas and promotes increased organisms and necrosis.

Foci of lymphocytes and plasma cells localized around adrenal medullary veins usually are associated with comparable infiltrations in the splenic red pulp and surrounding the renal and retroperitoneal veins. These commonly indicate chronic pyelonephritis with retroperitoneal chronic phlebitis rather than intrinsic adrenal disease.

Bilateral destructive adrenocortical tuberculosis is the classic cause of Addison's disease. Weakness, pigmentation of the skin and mucous membranes, hypotension, hypoglycemia, hyponatremia and hyperkalemia, a tendency to dehydration, and adrenal crises with shock after trauma or infections are its salient characteristics. Both adrenal glands are enlarged and largely replaced by caseous granulomas (Fig. 39-5). Forty years ago, 70% of Addison's disease was tuberculous, but idiopathic adrenocortical atrophy now predominates. Amyloidosis accounts for 1% and adrenal replacement by metastatic carcinoma for less than 0.5% of Addison's disease. Lymphoid tissues and pancreatic islets tend toward hyperplasia because of their release from adrenocortical control.

In idiopathic adrenal atrophy, the gland weights are reduced to a range of 1.2 to 2.5 gm each and the cortices are narrowed and largely

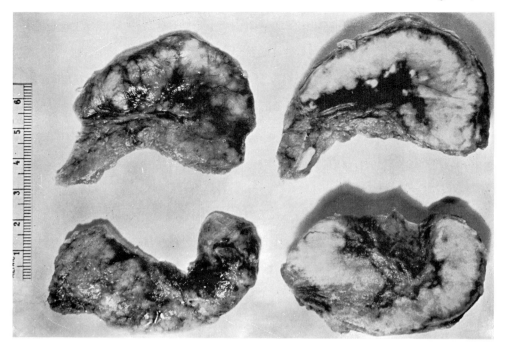

Fig. 39-5. Tuberculosis of adrenal glands in Addison's disease.

replaced by fibrous tissue (Fig. 39-6). Sometimes, nonspecific granulomas, giant cells, or
infiltrates of lymphocytes are present in the
cortices and medullae. These lesions comprise
so-called cytotoxic atrophy. Lymphocytic adrenalitis is associated with familial immune disorders, antibodies to adrenal, thyroid, and
gonadal cells, and sometimes with other endocrine deficiencies. Periadrenal brown fat may
be conspicuous.

Combined nontuberculous Addison's disease, hypothyroidism from chronic thyroiditis,
and occasionally hypopituitarism associated
with pituitary lymphoid infiltrates constitute
Schmidt's syndrome. Circulating antiadrenal
mitochondrial and microsomal antibodies are
found in the sera of half of the patients with
nontuberculous Addison's disease. Diabetes
mellitus, chronic hepatitis, gonadal failure, or
pernicious anemia may accompany Addison's
disease, a relationship that also suggests autoimmune reactions. Experimental allergic adrenalitis can be transferred passively by lymphoid cells.

Adenocortical atrophy secondary to hypophysectomy or pituitary destruction by disease
may be extreme. In one adult with panhypopituitarism, the combined weight of the adrenal
glands was only 0.8 gm, with cortices 10 to 12
cells thick. Giant mitochondria occur after

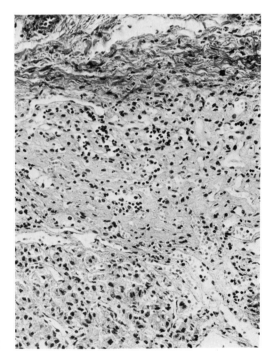

Fig. 39-6. Idiopathic adrenocortical atrophy with
Addison's disease. Cortical cells have practically
disappeared and stroma is collapsed. Adrenal
medulla and central veins can be seen below.
(120×.)

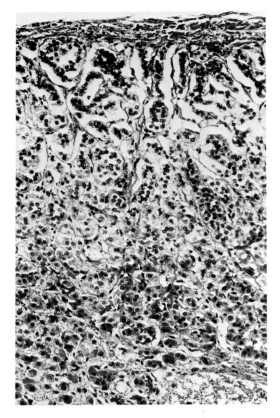

Fig. 39-7. After prolonged cortisone therapy, zona fasciculata cells become shrunken and cortical thickness reduced to 0.5 mm, half the normal width. Zona glomerulosa and zona reticularis unaffected and appear prominent. (120×.)

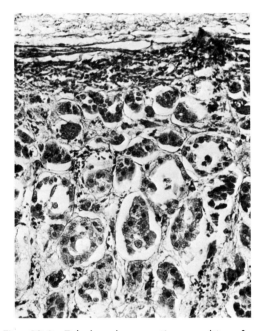

Fig. 39-8. Tubular degeneration resulting from cytolytic degeneration of zona fasciculata with regeneration to form hollow cylinders of cortical cells. (120×.)

hypophysectomy in the zona fasciculata, reflecting a high progesterone : corticosterone ratio. Long-term cortisone type of therapy for connective tissue diseases, arthritis, or asthma reduces the gland weights by about half, with notable shrinkage of the zona fasciculata and sometimes the zona glomerulosa (Fig. 39-7). In iatrogenic adrenocortical atrophy, the collapsed, condensed cortical stroma may simulate fibrosis. Patients treated with both ACTH and cortisone demonstrate zona fasciculata cytolysis.

DEGENERATIONS AND INFILTRATIONS

As corticosteroids are secreted in acute diseases, the adrenal cortex becomes rapidly depleted of both birefringent and sudanophilic lipid. After 6 days, the cortical lipid is restored, but in the interval lipid depletion reflects recent hypersecretion. In chronically ill individuals, adrenal lipid also is frequently depleted. The outer zona fasciculata cells may be reduced in size, producing a lipid-depletion reversion

pattern. In severe acute trauma, burns, toxemias, and infections like diphtheria, besides the loss of lipid, hyaline protein droplets are found in cortical cells with necrobiosis. The outer zona fasciculata regenerates around the cytolysis, resulting in a hollow cylindric appearance of the fasciculata cell cords termed "Rich's tubular degeneration" (Fig. 39-8). Excessive ACTH stimulation is considered responsible for tubular degeneration, but hyaline droplet change has been produced experimentally by methyl androstenediol. Similar hyaline droplets in adrenal medullary cells occur in various chronic diseases. Spironolactone, an aldosterone antagonist, produces laminated sudanophilic whorled membranous myelin-like bodies in the zona glomerulosa cells and aldosterone-secreting adenomas.

Less specific degenerative changes include adrenal lymphocytic infiltrates near the corticomedullary junction associated with fragmented basement membranes. Hyaline fibrotic areas beneath the capsule or in the medulla are commonly secondary to arteriolosclerosis. Heavy roentgenotherapy results in fibrosis of the juxtamedullary zona reticularis. In old age relatively little identifiable adrenal medulla may remain. Rarely, there is also medullary calcification and functional insufficiency.

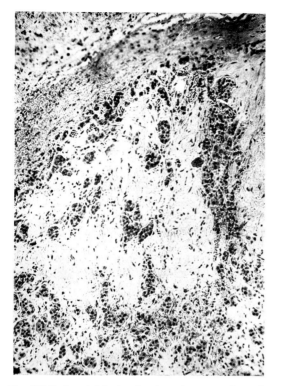

Fig. 39-9. Amyloidosis of adrenal cortex. Capsule at top and adrenocortical cells largely replaced by deposits. (100×.)

Amyloid is deposited in the zona fasciculata in about 80% of patients with generalized amyloidosis, with such deposition augmenting the adrenal weights. The zona glomerulosa is infiltrated last, and adrenocortical insufficiency is uncommon (Fig. 39-9). Purely localized adrenal deposits of amyloid have been found in 6% of autopsies. In primary amyloidosis, only the adrenal arteries may be involved.

The zona glomerulosa becomes pigmented in hemosiderosis, and additional hemosiderin is deposited here in hemochromatosis.

Fat replaces parts of the adrenal zonae fasciculata and reticularis occasionally without affecting adrenal weight. A few lymphocytes or hematopoietic foci may be associated with fatty infiltration. The adrenal cortex also is a site of myeloid metaplasia; hematopoiesis is evident in sinusoids of the deep zona fasciculata, compressing the cell cords without significant gland enlargement.

CORTICAL NODULARITY

Approximately half of persons over 50 years of age have nonuniform adrenal cortices with multiple small rounded nodules of zona fas-

ciculata. Regeneration after segmental ischemic adrenocortical atrophy attributable to local vascular disease accounts for many cortical nodules in older people. The nodular foci may possess more or less lipid than the uninvolved cortex and also differ in histochemical succinic dehydrogenase, esterase, and acid phosphatase reactions. Nodularity is more common with cirrhosis, hypertension, and cancer than with other chronic conditions. Its functional importance is unknown.

HYPERPLASIA, CUSHING'S SYNDROME, AND ADRENAL VIRILISM

Adrenocortical hyperplasia may be either diffuse or nodular (finely or grossly), and it is usually bilateral. Criteria for the diagnosis include gland weights exceeding the top 5% or above twice the standard deviation from the mean of normal weights and cortices thicker than 2 mm. Usually, hyperplasia involves the zona fasciculata. Exceptions in aldosteronism and adrenal virilism are noted below. Additional less conclusive indications of hyperplasia are irregular extracapsular proliferations of cortical cells, nodules that bulge into the medulla, and prominent cortical cell cuffs around the central veins.

Nonspecific adrenocortical hyperplasia is most common with acromegaly, thyrotoxicosis, hypertension associated with arteriolosclerosis and arteriosclerosis, cancer, and diabetes mellitus. Some cases are unexplained. The adrenal glands of acromegalic patients usually are enlarged and nodular, with exaggerated androgen secretion after ACTH stimulation. Hyperplasia accompanies hyperthyroidism in about 40% of the patients, essential hypertension and arteriosclerosis in 16%, and diabetes mellitus in 3.4%. In both hyperthyroidism and hypertension, increased adrenal weights may be ascribed partly to the frequent terminal complication of congestive heart failure.

The best understood specific adrenocortical hyperplasia accompanies Cushing's syndrome. As originally described, Cushing's disease is caused by an ACTH-secreting basophil pituitary adenoma, but in the much more common *syndrome,* no pituitary tumor is found. The typical patient has a rounded, moon-shaped face, obesity with a "buffalo hump" around the shoulders or a girdle distribution, a plethoric complexion associated with polycythemia, thin skin with easy bruising and abdominal striae, muscle weakness, hypertension, osteoporosis, and a diabetic type of glucose tolerance test. Hirsutism in women, amenor-

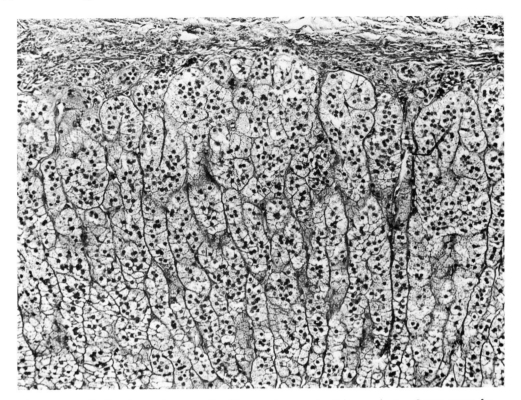

Fig. 39-10. Cushing's syndrome with diffuse adrenocortical hyperplasia. Outer zona fasciculata cells typically enlarged to form club-shaped cords. (120×.)

rhea, and mental disturbances are frequent, and acne may be present. Since practically all these changes occur after sufficient cortisone or cortisol administration, Cushing's syndrome is attributable to hypercortisolism. Women are affected more frequently than men in a ratio of about 3:1 (see also p. 1620).

In children, Cushing's syndrome is about equally commonly associated with adrenocortical hyperplasia and tumors, but after the age of 10 years, zona fasciculata hyperplasia accounts for approximately 70% of cases. The zona reticularis also may be increased. Cortical adenoma is responsible for about 20% of the cases of adult Cushing's syndrome and adrenocortical carcinoma for 10%. The uninvolved and contralateral cortices are atrophic. Surgically removed glands with diffuse hyperplasia together weigh 14 to 26 gm or more in three fourths of the patients with Cushing's syndrome and 10 to 12 gm in one fourth. The cortices are usually thicker than 2 mm. In equivocal cases, volumetric studies demonstrate zona fasciculata hyperplasia. A distinctive cytologic enlargement and increased cytoplasmic lipid are observed, producing clublike

thickenings of the outer zona fasciculata cell cords, with occasional very large cells (Fig. 39-10). Ultrastructurally the mitochondria are increased in size and complexity, smooth endoplasmic reticulum is increased and dilated, and pericellular basal laminae are reduplicated. The hyperplastic zona fasciculata may compress, infiltrate, or replace the zona glomerulosa and zona reticularis and penetrate into the medulla. Hyperplasia also includes the zona reticularis in women with virilization, so that in clinical Cushing's syndrome the endocrine hyperfunction is not necessarily restricted to the zona fasciculata and hypercortisolism.

Nodular hyperplasia involves increased adrenal weights and cortices thickened by rounded zona fasciculata nodules, usually 1 to 6 mm and occasionally up to 2 cm in diameter. Some individuals are apparently normal endocrinologically. Others have hypertension, edema, and hyperaldosteronism. Grossly, nodular hyperplasia with Cushing's syndrome involves bilateral adrenal hypertrophy up to triple the normal weight and multiple adenomatous nodules that are 1 to 5 cm in diameter and yellow, brown, black, or red according to their lipid

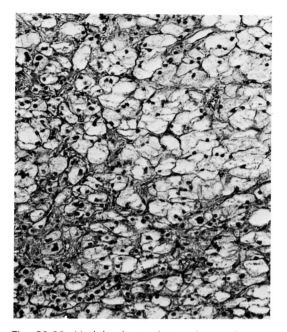

Fig. 39-11. Nodular hyperplasia of zona fasciculata with Cushing's syndrome associated with irregular cellular enlargement and locally increased lipid in adrenocortical cells. (120×.)

content and lipochrome or heme pigmentation from hemorrhages. The nodules have variable lipid content and decreased glucose-6-phosphate dehydrogenase activity (Fig. 39-11). On electron microscopy, the hyperplastic adrenocortical cells possess an abundant smooth endoplasmic reticulum and tubulovesicular mitochondria characteristic of the zona fasciculata.

Nodular adrenocortical dysplasia is an unusual lesion in infants or children with Cushing's syndrome. The glands are not enlarged, and the cortex contains multiple minute nodules up to 2 mm in diameter, notably pigmented by lipochrome and apparently arising from the zona reticularis. The intervening cortical tissue is atrophic. The cortical hyperfunction is unresponsive to ACTH or dexamethasone, unlike the more common ACTH-dependent hyperplasia with Cushing's syndrome.

Ectopic ACTH production by non–endocrine tissue tumors is considered responsible for approximately 20% of the cases of Cushing's syndrome. Often, the clinical findings are incomplete or absent, perhaps because the condition has developed rapidly, but hypokalemic alkalosis is a usual finding. Edema, skin pigmentation, and severe diabetes mellitus are more common than in idiopathic Cushing's syndrome. Oat cell carcinoma of the lung is the most frequently associated tumor. Pituitary hyaline basophils are increased, indicating increased circulating cortisone. Other recognized ACTH-secreting tumors include thymic oat cell carcinomas, pancreatic islet cell tumors, thyroid medullary carcinomas, and carcinoids of the lung or stomach, among diverse foregut endodermal neoplasms. Neuroblastomas and ovarian, testicular, and other neoplasms also have been implicated.

The adrenal glands in the ectopic ACTH syndrome usually are notably enlarged, two to five times the normal weight. Microscopically, the zona fasciculata cells, particularly near the capsule, are distinctively enlarged, depleted of lipid, and acidophilic (Fig. 39-12). These are effects of maximal ACTH stimulation. Besides ACTH, some neoplasms also produce excessive melanocyte-stimulating hormone, parathyroid hormone, gastrin, glucagon, antidiuretic hormone, norepinephrine, calcitonin, or serotonin. Pancreatic tumors appear the most versatile. Patients with lung carcinomas that do not produce ACTH may secrete excessive 17-hydroxycorticosteroids and cortisone after ACTH administration, as occurs nonspecifically in other severe illnesses.

Iatrogenic adrenocortical hyperplasia has followed prolonged ACTH therapy in leukemic children and in adults with various chronic diseases. Gland weights are nearly doubled. Both the zonae fasciculata and reticularis are thicker, the individual cells are enlarged, and cholesterol and lipid are reduced. The clinical and laboratory findings resemble Cushing's syndrome.

Cushingoid states have some attributes of Cushing's syndrome such as obesity, diabetes mellitus, hirsutism, or hypertension, without a clear-cut correlated hypercortisolism, pituitary and adrenocortical hyperplasia, or neoplasia.

Hyperplasia of the inner zona fasciculata and zona reticularis together characterize adrenal virilism, sometimes called the acquired or adult adrenogenital syndrome. In women, hirsutism, acne, temporal alopecia, squared body contours, deep voice, and clitoral enlargement to some degree frequently accompany Cushing's syndrome. Androgen secretion, particularly dehydroepiandrosterone and 11β-hydroxyandrostenedione, is responsible. Cortisol and corticosterone also are increased. Pure adrenal zona reticularis hyperplasia is unusual. When mild, it may produce only hirsutism. Adrenal hirsutism is estimated to explain about 1% of excessive hair growth in women. Two

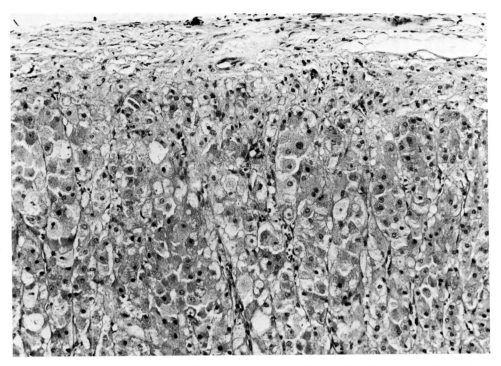

Fig. 39-12. Enlargement and lipid depletion of maximally stimulated outer zona fasciculata cells produced by ectopic ACTH. (120×.)

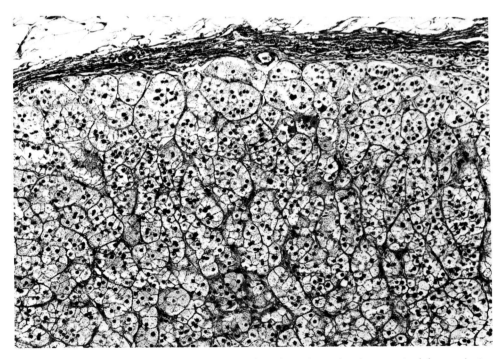

Fig. 39-13. Primary aldosteronism associated with unilateral adrenocortical hyperplasia. Zona glomerulosa cells enlarged and finely granular. (120×.)

distinctive characteristics of hyperplastic zona reticularis cells are lipochrome pigment and fuchsinophilia.

Zona glomerulosa hyperplasia, with enlarged lipid-containing cells forming a continuous subcapsular layer at least 100 μm wide, is associated with secondary aldosteronism fully developed as a complication of malignant or renovascular hypertension, nephrotic syndrome, cirrhosis with ascites, and other conditions. Nodular hyperplasia of both zonae glomerulosa and fasciculata accompanies cases variously classified as secondary, nontumorous, idiopathic, or pseudoprimary aldosteronism. Unilateral nodular hyperplasia is a rare acceptable cause of primary aldosteronism (Fig. 39-13). In sodium restriction the zona glomerulosa ordinarily is increased in thickness with depletion of the cytoplasmic lipid and cholesterol.

NEOPLASMS
Adenoma, primary aldosteronism, and carcinoma

Adrenocortical adenoma is usually a relatively large, single, rounded mass of yellow-orange adrenocortical tissue, measuring 1 to 5 cm in diameter (Fig. 39-14). Larger adenomas up to 12 cm in diameter may show hemorrhages, cystic degeneration, and calcification. The tissue bulges from the cut surface, an indication of compression. Most adenomas

are surrounded by a rim of stretched, uninvolved adrenal cortex and have an incomplete fibrous capsule or none. Histologically, adenomas are composed of relatively regular large cells with uniformly abundant lipid, arranged in nodules and cords with a vaguely fasciculate pattern. The margins of contact with uninvolved adrenal cortex are evident, since cells of the latter are zonated and smaller and contain less lipid. Giant cells with prominent nuclei and cellular polymorphism often present in adrenocortical adenomas are not considered evidence of cancer.

Nodules smaller than 9 mm in diameter sometimes are considered adenomas, but if they are multiple, bilateral, or zonated and lie in the capsule or outside, it is doubtful that they are true adenomas. A genuine adrenocortical adenoma usually is associated with either a normal or atrophic homolateral and contralateral uninvolved gland. When the adrenal cortices are multinodular or hyperplastic, the largest masses represent dominant nodules rather than adenomas.

Adenomas located centrally in the adrenal gland may be difficult to distinguish from pheochromocytomas, and in extra-adrenal sites such as the retroperitoneum or ovary they may be confused with nonchromaffin paragangliomas, Leydig cell tumors, and hypernephroid or other neoplasms. Some differential diagnostic features are given in Table 39-1.

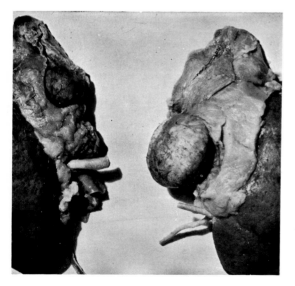

Fig. 39-14. Bilateral cortical adenomas of adrenal glands showing their location in relation to kidneys.

Table 39-1. Differential diagnostic features

Features	Adrenocortical tumor	Pheochromocytoma
Gross appearance	Yellow or orange	Grey, red, or brown
Histology	Cordlike arrangement	Sheets, nests, mosaic or twisted cord pattern
Cytology	Uniform size, squared shapes	Variable size, polyhedral shapes
	Cytoplasmic lipid vacuoles, Sudan- and cholesterol-positive	No lipid vacuoles
	Occasional mitoses	No mitoses
Chromaffinity	Negative	Positive
Ultrastructure	No catecholamine granules	Catecholamine granules

An adrenal adenoma is found in 2% to 8% of autopsies on adults. In the absence of overt endocrine effects and hormonal analyses, these are called "nonfunctional adenomas." Adenomas have been found most commonly in autopsies of elderly, obese, diabetic patients, 30%; women averaging 81 years of age, 29%; hypertensive individuals, 20%; and patients with the familial multiple endocrine adenomatosis syndrome that also involves the pancreatic islets and the parathyroid, pituitary, and thyroid glands besides peptic ulcerations, gastric mucosal hyperplasia, and colonic villous adenomas.

About three fourths of functioning adrenal tumors in children are benign adenomas, 10% of which are bilateral. The remaining quarter are carcinomas. Practically all the carcinomas metastasize and prove fatal. Dehydroepiandrosterone is the chief steroid secreted by virilizing adenomas, and the urinary 17-ketosteroids are increased. Androgens also promote somatic growth and maturation. The testicular tubules and Leydig cells remain undeveloped, or there is no menstrual activity, unlike the situation in precocious puberty. Cortisol hypersecretion typifies Cushing's syndrome. Combined virilization and estrogenization are associated with adrenocortical conversion of dehydroepiandrosterone partly to estradiol.

In adults with Cushing's syndrome, functioning adrenal adenomas characteristically reduce the plasma ACTH, unlike adrenocortical hyperplasia. Hirsutism and acne accompany adenoma less commonly than they do adrenal carcinoma. Virilizing and feminizing adrenal tumors more often are carcinomas than adenomas. Adenomas may produce testosterone and respond functionally to ACTH, dexamethasone, or chorionic gonadotropin.

Primary aldosteronism is associated with an adrenocortical adenoma in about 90% of cases and with carcinoma, multiple adenomas, and unilateral cortical hyperplasia in the remainder. Few authentic cases with adenomas have been reported in children. Before the age of 20 years, most instances of aldosterone hypersecretion have been associated with either bilateral diffuse or nodular cortical hyperplasia. Conn's syndrome (Conn et al.[91]) describes the combination of hypokalemic alkalosis, renal potassium loss, and hypertension, which may be cured by removing an aldosterone-secreting adrenal adenoma. Renin is characteristically suppressed, and the renal juxtaglomerular cells are atrophic. Aldosteronomas often are flattened tumors 0.9 cm to 1.5 cm in diameter. They may be impalpable and unidentified until multiple sections of the gland are made. A few are larger, and some have

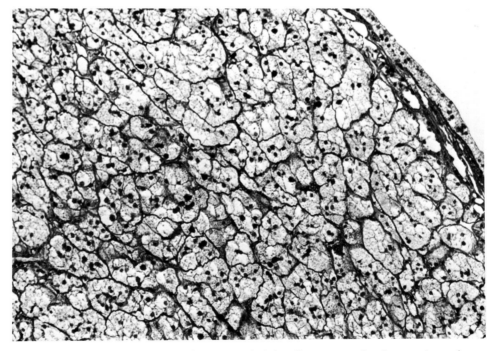

Fig. 39-15. Enlarged lipid-rich cells surrounded by fibrous capsule characterize adrenocortical adenomas, in this instance aldosteronoma. (120×.)

weighed more than 30 gm. Characteristically, they are more orange than yellow, rich in lipid, and histologically resemble other adrenal adenomas, with either a fasciculate or glomerulosal architecture (Fig. 39-15). Biosynthesis of cortisol, corticosterone, and aldosterone is demonstrable. Electron microscopy has shown the tumor mitochondria to possess the platelike cristae of zona glomerulosa cells, or tubulovesicular cristae like the zona fasciculata, or a combined "hybrid cell" type. Histochemically 3β-hydroxysteroid dehydrogenase activity is reportedly intense.

Hypertension also occurs associated with adenomas that produce corticosterone, deoxycorticosterone, or, more rarely, tetrahydrodeoxycorticosterone. Unlike adenomas, adrenal carcinomas with aldosteronism usually show increased 17-ketosteroids and 17-hydroxycorticosteroids, and biosynthesis in vitro of hydrocortisone, cortisone, and corticosterone also is found.

Primary aldosteronism without hypokalemia or an aldosteronoma exists but is uncommon enough to question the diagnosis. The nature of cases with hyperaldosteronism and one or multiple cortical nodules 0.3 to 0.8 cm in diameter or bilateral hyperplasia is disputed. Conceivably, they represent transitions from adrenocortical hyperplasia to genuine adenomas. In contrast to other functioning adrenocortical neoplasms, the uninvolved homo-lateral and the contralateral zonae glomerulosa and fasciculata in primary aldosteronism have been reported as atrophic, normal, or hyperplastic.

Hypoaldosteronism as an isolated adult abnormality is also a puzzling condition. Instances have been observed with an adenoma containing compound S, or with postoperatively recurrent hypercortisolism, prolonged heparin therapy, or excessive licorice ingestion, or as a functional deficiency with orthostatic hypotension. Some cases have accompanied hypopituitarism. Deficient renin secretion, a failure of angiotensin to stimulate aldosterone secretion, or renal tubular unresponsiveness to this hormone have been reported.

Pigmented adrenocortical adenoma, or so-called black adenoma, is usually without functional significance. Grossly and microscopically, the cells contain so much brown pigment that they resemble a melanoma, but special stains demonstrate a PAS-positive lipochrome like that of the zona reticularis. Rarely, Cushing's syndrome or hyperaldosteronism is associated with a black adenoma.

Adrenal carcinomas are distinguished from

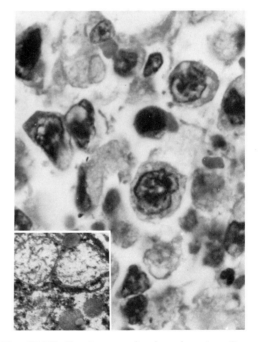

Fig. 39-17. Carcinoma of adrenal cortex. Tumor cells show considerable variation in size, shape, and intensity of staining (900×). *Inset,* Cytoplasmic lipid droplets and mitochondria of adrenocortical type. (5080×.)

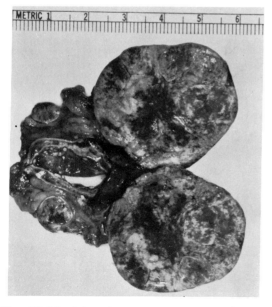

Fig. 39-16. Adrenal carcinoma associated with Cushing's syndrome.

adenomas by capsular or blood vessel invasion and metastasis. Carcinomas are usually large when first discovered, 7 to 20 cm in diameter, and weigh 100 to 2400 gm. Hemorrhage, necrosis, and calcification are more common in adrenal carcinomas than in adenomas (Fig. 39-16). Nuclear atypia, large nucleoli, multinucleated cells, mitoses, and compact acidophilic cells are typical of adrenocortical carcinomas, but demonstrable invasion, metastasis, or both, are necessary for definite diagnosis (Fig. 39-17). Most adrenal carcinomas metastasize widely and cause death. Large anaplastic adrenocortical carcinomas may be difficult to recognize histologically, and the ultrastructural features may aid in their diagnosis (Fig. 39-17, *inset*). Judged from reported cases, about half of adrenal carcinomas are functional. Of these, 50% are associated with combined Cushing's syndrome and virilization, 30% with virilization, 12% with feminization, and 4% with aldosteronism and related conditions. Fever may attract attention to the nonfunctioning type. Some 12 large carcinomas have been observed in association with severe hypoglycemia.

About three fourths of feminizing adrenal neoplasms are carcinomas, and one fourth are adenomas. Most develop in men between 20 and 60 years of age, with bilateral gynecomastia, loss of libido, and atrophy of the testes and penis. Obesity, attributes of Cushing's syndrome, and feminine distribution of body hair may be present. The tumors are not distinguishable histopathologically from other adrenal neoplasms. Estrogen biosynthesis is demonstrable from pregnenolone, progesterone, androstenedione, and testosterone. In women, estrogen-producing adrenal tumors are associated with amenorrhea, hirsutism, and clitoral enlargement. No feminizing adrenocortical hyperplasia is known in adults.

Feminizing and virilizing adrenal neoplasms that arise in extra-adrenal rests are difficult or impossible to distinguish morphologically from Leydig cell tumors, ovarian lipid cell tumors, Sertoli cell type of androblastomas, or luteomas of pregnancy. These primary gonadal tumors are ordinarily virilizing and benign, whereas adrenocortical neoplasms that produce sex hormones are predominantly malignant.

One adrenal theca-granulosa cell tumor has been described, possibly arising from ectopic ovarian stroma in the gland.

Metastatic cancer in the adrenal glands is often bilateral, with tumors commonly less than 2.5 cm in diameter. Initially, the medulla usually is involved. Carcinomas of the lung, particularly of the squamous cell type, form adrenal metastases in one third of cases. Carcinomas of the breast show metastases in 25% of adrenalectomy specimens and 30% at autopsy. Carcinomas of the stomach, large intestine, and pancreas frequently metastasize to the adrenal glands. Also melanomas, renal cell carcinomas, and thyroid carcinomas often spread to the adrenal glands.

Cysts

Aside from rare echinococcal cysts, found in less than 0.5% of patients with echinococcosis, most adrenal cysts are noninflammatory. Pseudocysts lined by fibrous tissue represent residues of remote hematomas or degenerated adenomas. Genuine cysts may be lined by glandular epithelium or by endothelium indicating a cavernous lymphangioma or hemangioma. Angiomas may exceed 20 cm in diameter and constitute the largest adrenal cysts. They may have partly calcified walls.

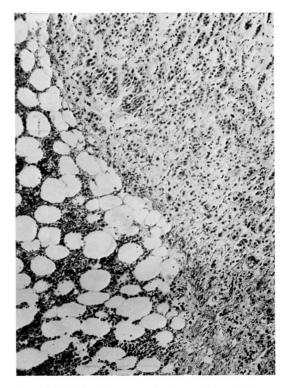

Fig. 39-18. Myelolipoma of adrenal gland. Tissue resembling bone marrow surrounded by adrenal cortex. (100×.)

Myelolipoma

Myelolipoma of the adrenal gland is a fatty, gray or red spheroid mass apparently originating in the inner zona fasciculata, usually measuring 0.5 to 6 cm in diameter. One such tumor measuring 25 cm in diameter produced pressure symptoms. Histologically, the structure simulates adult hematopoietic bone marrow, with comparable amounts of adipose and myeloid cells (Fig. 39-18). Myelolipomas are not clearly neoplasms and may represent enlarged mesenchymal rests. Sometimes they accompany obesity or bone marrow failure and may occur also in the intercostal spaces and retroperitoneal or pelvic connective tissue. One woman has been reported with bilateral adrenal tumors composed of brown fat or hibernomas.

Pheochromocytoma and chromaffin paraganglioma

A pheochromocytoma is a medullary adrenal neoplasm that typically secretes epinephrine, norepinephrine, or both. Similar extra-adrenal tumors, conventionally termed "chromaffin paragangliomas," may be retroperitoneal, above the aortic bifurcation or celiac in location, or attached to the urinary bladder, in the ovary, or within mediastinal, intrathoracic, or intracranial areas. Sporadic pheochromocytomas may be unsuspected and often are found after an elective operation in an individual who develops acute hypertension and subsequent lethal shock under anesthesia. Patients with preoperatively recognized pheochromocytomas have paroxysmal or persistent hypertension, with increased urinary vanilmandelic acid and other catecholamine metabolites. About two thirds have hyperglycemia ascribable to decreased insulin release, and three fourths are hypermetabolic. Occasionally, diabetes mellitus is cured by removal of a pheochromocytoma.

The tumors vary from incidental microscopic findings to masses over 2 kg in weight, but the average weight is 90 gm and the size 5 to 6 cm in diameter. Grossly, pheochromocytomas are rounded, gray or red, and circumscribed and are surrounded by stretched adrenal cortex. Hemorrhages, cystic areas, calcification, or a central dense fibrous scar are common (Fig. 39-19). Chromaffin tests on fresh tissue characteristically color pheochromocytomas dark brown. Occasional tumors containing pure norepinephrine are chromaffin-negative; these pheochromocytomas are more common in childhood. Tissue fixed in Helly's or Zenker's fluid demonstrates chromaffinity both grossly and microscopically.

Histologically, pheochromocytomas show notable variability of cell and nuclear size and arrangement. Basic twisted cell cord patterns, basophilic or acidophilic staining, and the presence of fine or coarse intracytoplasmic pigment granules and PAS-stained secretory droplets aid in making the diagnosis (Fig. 39-20). Ultrastructurally identified epinephrine-containing cytoplasmic granules in pheochromocytomas are larger than in the normal medulla. Similar organelles in neuroblastomas and ganglioneuroblastomas explain their occasionally

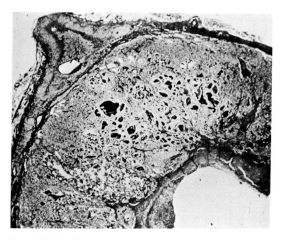

Fig. 39-19. Pheochromocytoma enclosed by adrenal cortex at upper left. Central cystic degeneration and rich sinusoidal vascularity demonstrated. (×8.)

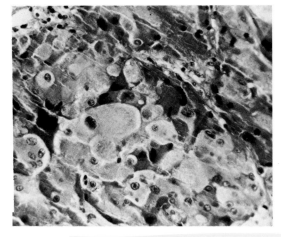

Fig. 39-20. Irregular size and shape of pheochromocytoma cells and nuclei, as well as variable staining of their cytoplasm, are characteristic. Darker colored cells are brown because of the chromaffin reaction. (350×.)

excessive secretion of catecholamines. Catecholamines are stored and secreted from osmiophilic cytoplasmic granules. Differentiation from adrenocortical neoplasms may be difficult microscopically (Table 39-1). Adrenocortical adenoma and pheochromocytoma may occur in the same gland. The periadrenal adipose tissue in cases of pheochromocytoma typically has an excess of brown or hibernating fat.

Whether pheochromocytomas originate from adrenal medullary hyperplasia is uncertain. Homolateral and contralateral hyperplasia of the predominant pheochromocytoma cell type has been reported. In the absence of reliable criteria for identifying hyperplasia of the adrenal medulla, these reports are difficult to evaluate.

Malignant pheochromocytomas constitute about 6% of all cases. Some are microscopically atypical, more closely resembling neuroblastomas. Others are typical except for gross or microscopic invasion of the periadrenal fat or blood vessels. However, neither gross invasion nor microscopic pleomorphism is a reliable indication of likely recurrence of pheochromocytomas or metastasis, and the metastatic tumor histologically may still appear benign. Multiple benign chromaffin paragangliomas are to be distinguished from malignant pheochromocytoma.

Several syndromes associated with pheochromocytoma include Recklinghausen's neurofibromatosis, von Hippel–Lindau disease and cerebellar hemangioblastoma, Albright's syndrome, multiple mucocutaneous neuromas, and familial multiple endocrine neoplasms that include medullary thyroid carcinoma and hyperparathyroidism caused by parathyroid hyperplasia or adenomas. This last combination is also called Sipple's syndrome, or multiple endocrine neoplasia type 2, to distinguish it from multiple adenomas of the pituitary gland, parathyroid glands, and pancreatic islets (type 1) and combined papillary thyroid carcinoma and parathyroid adenoma (type 3). Pheochromocytomas are bilateral in about half the cases of familial pheochromocytoma, compared to 5% of sporadic cases. Autosomal dominant inheritance appears responsible for familial multiple endocrine neoplasia.

Cushing's syndrome caused by a cortisol-secreting pheochromocytoma has been recognized in about 12 cases, including one intrapancreatic chromaffin paraganglioma. Both catecholamines and cortisol were produced by a single tumor.

Malignant melanoma and other adrenal neoplasms

Primary malignant melanoma in the adrenal gland has been recognized in 12 cases. Usually, multiple metastases are present elsewhere. The pigment is identified as melanin, and other possible primary sites are excluded. Neural crest melanoblasts are probably the cells of origin.

Other adrenal neoplasms are usually small benign connective tissue tumors, including neurilemoma, neurofibroma, lipoma, leiomyoma, osteoma, and angioma, as well as mixed mesenchymoma.

REFERENCES
Structure and function

1 Bech, K., Tygstrup, I., and Nerup, J.: Acta Pathol. Microbiol. Scand. 76:391-400, 1969 (involution of fetal cortex).
2 Beisel, W. R., and Rapport, M. L.: New Eng. J. Med. 280:541-546, 596-604, 1969 (response to infections).
3 Falls, J. L.: Cancer 8:143-150, 1955 (accessory adrenal in broad ligament).
4 Johannisson, E.: Acta Endocrinol. (Kbh) 58 (suppl. 130):7-107, 1968 (adrenal development).
5 Kadair, R. G., Block, M. B., Katz, F. H., and Hofeldt, F. D.: Am. J. Med. 62:278-282, 1977 (steroidogenesis defects).
6 Naeye, R. L., and Blanc, W. A.: Arch. Pathol. 91:140-147, 1971 (adrenal in anencephaly).
7 Neville, A. M., and MacKay, A. M.: Clin. Endocrinol. Metab. 1:361-395, 1972 (functional correlations).
8 Schulz, D. M., Giordano, D. A., and Schulz, D. H.: Arch. Pathol. (Chicago) 74:244-250, 1962 (weights in infants).
9 Stirling, G. A., and Keating, V. J.: Br. Med. J. 2:1016-1018, 1958 (weights in Jamaicans).
10 Symington, T.: Functional pathology of the adrenal gland, Baltimore, 1969, The Williams & Wilkins Co.
11 Villee, D. B.: New Eng. J. Med. 281:473-484, 1969 (fetal adrenal function).

Congenital anomalies

12 Biglieri, E. G., Herron, M. A., and Brust, N.: J. Clin. Invest. 45:1946-1954, 1966 (17-hydroxylase deficiency).
13 Bongiovanni, A. M., Eberlein, W. R., Goldman, A. S., and New, M.: Recent Progr. Hormone Res. 23:375-449, 1967 (congenital adrenocortical hyperplasia).
14 Borit, A., and Kosek, J.: Arch. Pathol. (Chicago) 88:58-64, 1969.
15 Clayton, B. E., Edwards, R. W., and Makin, H. L.: J. Endocrinol. 43:xlvi-xlvii, 1969 (other 11-hydroxylase deficiencies).
16 Dolan, M. F., and Janovski, N. A.: Arch. Pathol. (Chicago) 86:22-24, 1968 (adrenohepatic fusion).
17 Ehrlich, E. N., Straus, F. H., II, Hunter, R. L., and Wiest, W. G.: J. Clin. Endocrinol.

29:523-538, 1969 (cytomegalic hypoplasia in adult).

18 Favara, B. E., Franciosi, R. A., and Miles, V.: Am. J. Clin. Pathol. 57:287-296, 1972 (congenital hypoplasia).

19 Filippi, G., and McKusick, V. A.: Medicine 49:279-298, 1970 (Beckwith-Wiedemann syndrome).

20 Laqueur, G. L., and Harrison, M. B.: Am. J. Pathol. 27:231-245, 1951 (brown fat).

21 Mallin, S. R.: Ann. Intern. Med. 70:69-75, 1969.

22 O'Donohoe, N. V., and Holland, P. D. J.: Arch. Dis. Child. 43:717-723, 1968 (familial congenital hypoplasia).

23 Oppenheimer, E. H.: Arch. Pathol. (Chicago) 87:653-659, 1969 (adrenal in prematurity).

24 Sherman, F. E., Bass, L. W., and Fetterman, G. H.: Am. J. Clin. Pathol. 30:439-446, 1958 (cytomegaly and carcinoma).

25 Silverman, W. A., editor: Dunham's Premature infants, ed. 3, New York, 1961, Paul B. Hoeber Medical Division, Harper & Row, Publishers (edema in infants of diabetics).

26 Wiener, M. F., and Dallgaard, S. A.: Arch. Pathol. (Chicago) 67:228-233, 1959 (intracranial adrenal).

27 Zondek, L. H., and Zondek, T.: Acta Paediatr. Scand. 57:250-254, 1968 (cytomegalic adrenal hypoplasia).

Childhood abnormalities

28 deBaecque, C. M., Pollack, M. A., and Suzuki, K.: Arch. Pathol. Lab. Med. 100:139-145, 1976 (lipofuscinosis).

29 Cheatham, W. J., Weller, T. H., Dolan, T. F., Jr., and Dower, J. C.: Am. J. Pathol. 32:1015-1035, 1956 (varicella).

30 Crocker, A. C., Vawter, G. F., Neuhauser, E. B. D., and Rosowsky, A.: Pediatrics 35:627-640, 1965 (familial xanthomatosis).

31 Forsyth, C. C., Forber, M., and Cumings, J. N.: Arch. Dis. Child. 46:273-284, 1971 (adrenal atrophy and cerebral sclerosis).

32 Hawkins, E., and Singer, D. B.: Am. J. Clin. Pathol. 66:710-714, 1976 (cystic fibrosis).

33 Hortnagl, H., Hortnagl, H., Winkler, H., et al.: Lab. Invest. 27:613-619, 1972 (neuroblastoma catecholamines).

34 Kidder, L. A.: Am. J. Clin. Pathol. 22:870-878, 1952 (cytomegalovirus disease).

35 Margaretten, W., Nakai, H., and Landing, B. H.: Am. J. Dis. Child. 105:346-351, 1963 (septicemic adrenal hemorrhage).

36 Misugi, K., Misugi, N., and Newton, W. A., Jr.: Arch. Pathol. (Chicago) 86:160-170, 1968 (neuroblastoma ultrastructure).

37 Naeye, R. L.: Am. J. Clin. Pathol. 66:526-530, 1976 (sudden infant death).

38 Powers, J. M., and Schaumber, H. H.: Arch. Pathol. 96:305-310, 1973 (adrenoleukodystrophy).

39 Rudd, B. T., Chance, G. W., and Theodoridis, C. G.: Arch. Dis. Child. 44:244-247, 1969 (Prader-Willi syndrome).

40 Templeton, A. C.: J. Clin. Pathol. 23:24-30, 1970 (generalized herpes simplex).

41 Turkel, S. B., and Itabashi, H. H.: Am. J.

Pathol. 76:225-244, 1974 (fetal neuroblastic cells).

42 Wilkerson, J. A., Van De Water, J. M., and Goepfert, H.: Cancer 20:1335-1342, 1967 (benign transformation of neuroblastoma).

43 Young, E. P., and Patrick, A. D.: Arch. Dis. Child. 45:664-668, 1970 (Wolman's disease).

Hemorrhage and necrosis

44 Fox, B.: J. Pathol. 119:65-89, 1976.

45 Kaufman, G.: Arch. Pathol. 97:395-398, 1974 (adrenocortical necrosis).

46 Kerr, J. F. R.: J. Pathol. 107:217-219, 1972 (adrenal shrinkage necrosis).

47 Lever, W. F.: Medicine (Baltimore) 32:1-123, 1953 (pemphigus).

48 Redman, J. F., and Faas, F. H.: Am. J. Med. 61:533-536, 1976 (hemorrhage).

49 Robboy, S. J., Colman, R. W., and Minna, J. D.: Hum. Pathol. 3:327-343, 1973 (disseminated intravascular coagulation).

Inflammation, atrophy, and Addison's disease

50 Carpenter, C. C. J., Solomon, N., and Silverberg, S. G.: Medicine (Baltimore) 43:153-180, 1964 (Schmidt's syndrome).

51 Das, G., and Becker, M.: J.A.M.A. 207:2438, 1969 (oral contraceptives and adrenal insufficiency).

52 DeLellis, R. A., Wolfe, H. J., Gagel, R. F., Feldman, Z. T., Miller, H. H., Gaug, D. L., and Reichlin, S.: Am. J. Pathol. 83:177-196, 1976 (medullary morphometry).

53 Goudie, R. B., Anderson, J. R., Grav, K. K., and Whyte, W. G.: Lancet 1:1173-1176, 1966 (adrenal autoantibodies).

54 Jantet, G., Crocker, D. W., Shiraki, M., and Moore, F. D.: New Eng. J. Med. 269:1-7, 1963 (posthypophysectomy atrophy).

55 Kiaer, W., and Norgaard, J. O. R.: Acta Pathol. Microbiol. Scand. 76:229-238, 1969 (cytotoxic adrenalitis).

56 Nichols, J., and Delp, M.: J.A.M.A. 185:643-646, 1963 (atrophy with hypopituitarism).

57 Petri, M., and Nerup, J.: Acta Pathol. Microbiol. Scand. 79:381-388, 1971 (lymphocytic adrenalitis).

58 Pousset, G., Monier, J. C., and Thivolet, J.: Ann. Endocrinol. 31:995-1002, 1970 (adrenal autoantibodies).

59 Sunder, J. H., Bonessi, J. V., Balash, W. R., and Danowski, T. S.: New Eng. J. Med. 272:818-824, 1965 (familial Addison's disease).

60 Wuepper, K. D., Wegienka, L. C., and Fudenberg, H. H.: Am. J. Med. 46:206-216, 1969.

Degenerations and infiltrations, cortical nodularity

61 Braunstein, H., and Yamaguchi, B. T., Jr.: Am. J. Pathol. 44:113-126, 1964 (nodularity in chronic illness).

62 Dekker, A., and Oehrle, J. S.: Arch. Pathol. 91:353-364, 1971 (medullary hyaline globules).

63 Dobbie, J. W.: J. Pathol. 99:1-18, 1969 (cortical nodules and hyperplasia).

64 Hart, M. N., and Cyrus, A., Jr.: Am. J. Clin. Pathol. 49:387-391, 1968.

65 Kovacs, K., Korvath, E., and Singer, W.: J. Clin. Pathol. 26:949-957, 1973 (spironolactone bodies).

66 Rodin, A. L., Hsu, F. L., and Whorton, E. B.: Arch. Pathol. Lab. Med. **100**:499-502, 1976 (cystic degeneration).

67 Sommers, S. C., and Carter, M.: Arch. Pathol. **100**:421-423, 1975 (radiation reaction).

68 Sugihara, H., Kawai, K., and Tsuchiyama, H.: Acta Pathol. Jpn. **23**:253-260, 1973 (cortical nodules).

69 Wilbur, O. M., Jr., and Rich, A. R.: Bull. Johns Hopkins Hosp. **93**:321-347, 1953 (tubular degeneration).

Hyperplasia, Cushing's syndrome, and adrenal virilism

70 Azzopardi, J. G., and Williams, E. D.: Cancer **22**:274-286, 1968 (ectopic ACTH syndrome).

71 Baer, L., Sommers, S. C., and Krakoff, L. R.: Circ. Res. **27**(suppl. I):203-216, 1970 (pseudoprimary aldosteronism).

72 Choi, Y., Werk, E. E., and Sholiton, L. J.: Arch. Intern. Med. **125**:1045-1049, 1970 (autonomy of adrenal nodules in Cushing's syndrome).

73 Cohen, R. B.: Cancer **19**:552-556, 1966 (histochemistry of Cushing's syndrome—adrenals).

74 Cushing, H.: Bull. Johns Hopkins Hosp. **50**:137-195, 1932.

75 Dobbie, J. W.: J. Pathol. **99**:1-18, 1969 (nodular adrenal hyperplasia).

76 Granger, P., and Genest, J.: Can. Med. Assoc. J. **103**:34-36, 1970 (adrenals in hypertension).

77 Hashida, Y., Kenny, F. M., and Yunis, E. J.: Hum. Pathol. **1**:595-614, 1970 (adrenal ultrastructure in Cushing's syndrome).

78 Lim, N. Y., and Dingman, J. F.: New Eng. J. Med. **271**:1189-1194, 1964 (acromegaly).

79 Meador, C. K., Bowdoin, B., Owen, W. C., Jr., and Farmer, T. A., Jr.: J. Clin. Endocrinol. **27**:1255-1263, 1967 (nodular dysplasia and Cushing's syndrome).

80 Neville, A. M., and Symington, T.: J. Pathol. Bacteriol. **93**:19-35, 1967.

81 O'Neal, L. W., Kipnis, D. M., Luse, S. A., Lacy, P. E., and Jarett, L.: Cancer **21**:1219-1232, 1968 (ectopic ACTH and other hormones).

82 O'Riordan, J. L. H., Blanshard, G. P., Moxham, A., and Nabarro, J. D. N.: Q. J. Med. **35**:137-147, 1966.

83 Parker, T. G., and Sommers, S. C.: Arch. Surg. (Chicago) **72**:495-499, 1956 (hyperplasia and cancer).

84 Reidbord, H., and Fisher, E. R.: Arch. Pathol. (Chicago) **86**:419-426, 1968 (ultrastructure of adrenal in Cushing's syndrome).

85 Ross, E. J., Marshall-Jones, P., and Friedman, M.: Q. J. Med. **35**:149-192, 1966 (Cushing's syndrome).

86 Russell, R. P., and Masi, A. T.: Ann. Intern. Med. **73**:195-205, 1970 (hyperplasia and hypertension).

87 Visser, J. W., and Axt, R.: J. Clin. Pathol. **28**:298-304, 1975 (medullary hyperplasia).

Neoplasms
Adenomas, primary aldosteronism, and carcinoma

88 Alterman, S. L., Dominguez, C., Lopez-Gomez, A., and Lieber, A. L.: Cancer **24**:602-609, 1969 (adrenal carcinoma and aldosteronism).

89 Besser, G. M., and Landon, J.: Br. Med. J. **4**:552-554, 1968 (tumors with Cushing's syndrome).

90 Caplan, R. H., and Virata, R. L.: Am. J. Clin. Pathol. **62**:97-103, 1974 (black adenoma and Cushing's syndrome).

91 Conn, J. W., Knopf, R. F., and Nesbit, R. M.: Am. J. Surg. **107**:159-172, 1964 (primary aldosteronism).

92 Cussen, L. J.: Med. J. Aust. **47**(1):39-41, 1960 (metastases to adrenal).

93 Davis, W. W., Newsome, H. H., Jr., Wright, L. D., Jr., Hammond, W. G., Easton, J., and Bartter, F. C.: Am. J. Med. **42**:642-647, 1967 (pseudoprimary aldosteronism).

94 De Lima, C. R., Capuano, Y., Ciscato, J. G., Carvalhal, S., and Chiorboli, E.: Obstet. Gynecol. **28**:209-212, 1966 (ovarian adrenal rest tumor).

95 Dhom, G., and Stadtler, F.: Virchows Arch. (Pathol. Anat.) **345**:176-199, 1968 (aldosteronism).

96 Gabrilove, J. L., Nicolis, G. L., Hausknecht, R. U., and Wotiz, H. H.: Cancer **25**:153-160, 1970.

97 Hajjar, R. A., Hickey, R. C., and Samaan, N. A.: Cancer **35**:549-554, 1975.

98 Harrison, J. H., Mahoney, E. M., and Bennett, A. H.: Cancer **32**:1227-1235, 1973 (tumors of the adrenal cortex).

99 Huvos, A. G., Hajdu, S. I., Brasfield, R. D., and Foote, F. W.: Cancer **25**:354-361, 1970.

100 Kaplan, N. M.: J. Clin. Invest. **46**:728-734, 1967 (aldosteronoma steroids).

101 Kenny, F. M., Hashida, Y., Askari, H. A., Sieber, W. H., and Fetterman, G. H.: Am. J. Dis. Child. **115**:445-458, 1968 (virilizing adrenal tumors).

102 Le Compte, P. M.: Am. J. Pathol. **20**:689-707, 1944 (adenoma versus pheochromocytoma).

103 Lewinsky, B. S., Grigor, K. M., Symington, T., and Neville, A. M.: Cancer **33**:778-790, 1974 (nonfunctioning adrenal carcinoma).

104 Lufkin, E. G., Katz, F. H., and Herman, R. H.: Am. J. Med. Sci. **264**:367-374, 1972 (primary adrenal hyperplasia and aldosteronism).

105 Reidbord, H., and Fisher, E. R.: Arch. Pathol. (Chicago) **88**:155-161, 1969 (aldosteronoma ultrastructure).

106 Robinson, M. J., Pardo, V., and Rywlin, A. M.: Hum. Pathol. **3**:317-325, 1972 (black adenoma).

107 Schteingart, D. E., Oberman, H. A., Friedman, B. A., and Conn, J. W.: Cancer **22**:1005-1013, 1968 (adenoma versus carcinoma).

108 Silverstein, M. N.: Cancer **23**:142-144, 1969 (hypoglycemia with adrenal tumors).

109 Sommers, S. C., and Terzakis, J. A.: Am. J. Clin. Pathol. **54**:303-310, 1970.

110 Spain, D. M., and Weinsaft, P.: Arch. Pathol. (Chicago) **78**:231-233, 1964 (adenoma in aged women).

111 Tannenbaum, M.: Pathol. Annu. **5**:145-171, 1970.

112 Werk, E. E., Jr., Sholiton, L. J., and Kalejs, L.: New Eng. J. Med. **289**:767-770, 1973 (adenoma secreting testosterone).

Cysts, myelolipoma

113 Hodges, F. V., and Ellis, F. R.: Arch. Pathol. (Chicago) **66:**53-58, 1958.

114 McGregor, A. L.: Acta Med. Scand., suppl. 306, pp. 107-110, 1955 (hibernoma).

115 Mikail, M., and Kirshbaum, A.: J. Urol. **99:** 361-365, 1968.

116 Tulcinsky, D. B., Deutsch, V., and Bubis, J. J.: Br. J. Surg. 57:465-467, 1970 (myelolipoma).

Pheochromocytoma, other neoplasms

117 Carney, J. A., Sizemore, G. W., and Sheps, S. G.: Am. J. Clin. Pathol. **66:**279-290, 1976 (type 2 adrenal lesions).

118 Edmunds, L. H., Jr.: Ann. Thorac. Surg. **2:** 742-751, 1966 (mediastinal pheochromocytoma).

119 Onuigbo, W. I. B.: Arch. Pathol. **99:**342-346, 1975 (lung cancer metastases).

120 Orselli, R. C., and Bassler, T. J.: Cancer **31:** 474-477, 1973 (adrenal theca granulosa cell tumor).

121 Ransom, C. L., Landes, R. R., and Gaddy, C. G.: J. Urol. **79:**368-376, 1958 (malignant pheochromocytoma).

122 Sharp, W. V., and Platt, R. L.: Angiology **22:** 141-146, 1971 (pheochromocytoma and von Hippel–Lindau disease).

123 Sherwin, R. P.: Am. J. Surg. **107:**136-143, 1964.

124 Steiner, A. L., Goodman, A. D., and Powers, S. R.: Medicine (Baltimore) **47:**371-409, 1968 (familial endocrine neoplasms).

125 Tang, C.-K., and Hajdu, J. I.: N.Y. State J. Med. **75:**1434-1438, 1975 (adult neuroblastoma).

126 Tannenbaum, M.: Pathol. Annu. **5:**145-171, 1970.

40/Female genitalia

FREDERICK T. KRAUS

Abnormalities and diseases of the female genitalia have been the object of fascination for centuries and the basis for one of the oldest of medical specialties. An abnormal external physical appearance may provide the clues to significant underlying malformations some of which are life threatening. The genital tract is the portal of entry of infectious diseases of remarkable variety and far-reaching effects on the patient and sometimes on her progeny. Neoplasms of the female genitalia are unsurpassed for bizarre appearance, variety of systemic effects and size; they also represent the second most common source of fatal cancer in women. Many important insights into the biology of infections and neoplasms are afforded by a study of these conditions as they occur in the female genitalia; the correct application of principles of prevention and treatment of these diseases may offer a greater prospect for relief of suffering and extension of life than is possible in any other area of the body.

EMBRYOLOGY OF FEMALE GENITAL TRACT

Knowledge of the anatomic changes in the early development of the female genitalia is helpful in understanding various pathologic conditions. Some malformations become recognizable as a failure in the completion of a developmental sequence. There is a close relationship between primitive urinary and genital structures, so that malformations often affect both systems, sometimes in predictable ways. For instance, recognition of ambiguous sexual differentiation of the vulva may be the first evidence of the potentially fatal, but curable, adrenogenital syndrome. Finally, the histologic similarities in neoplasms are understandable in terms of the embryologic relationships that form the basis of their classification. A brief summary of female genital tract embryology is supplied as a basis for such an understanding;

for more detailed descriptions see standard texts.[7]

Genital ridges and müllerian ducts

With the exception of the germ cells, the internal genitalia arise from the mesoderm (celomic epithelium and adjacent mesenchyme) of the posterior body wall. Bilateral *urogenital ridges* are formed, parallel to the body axis. In a 6 mm embryo (about 5 weeks old) each of these has become segregated longitudinally into a lateral *mesonephric ridge* and a medial *genital ridge* (Fig. 40-1).

By the end of the sixth week the primitive gonad is represented by proliferating surface epithelial cells and an inner blastema of loose mesenchymal cells. A lateral groove forms in the surface epithelium of each urogenital ridge, rolls inward, and closes to form the müllerian (paramesonephric) duct on each side. The cranial ends remain open and eventually become the fimbriated open ends of the uterine tubes. The caudal ends burrow medially in front of the mesonephric ducts, and farther caudad toward the urogenital sinus. The point at which they end in the dorsomedial aspect of the urogenital sinus is transiently marked by a swelling, *Müller's tubercle.* The distal ends of the müllerian ducts fuse to become the uterus, cervix, and upper vagina. The myometrium and endometrial stroma differentiate from the surrounding mesenchyme (Fig. 40-2).

In a 60 mm embryo the ovary is suspended by its mesovarium from the ventral surface of the *mesonephros,* which is still prominent (Fig. 40-3). The mesonephric ducts are functional at this time and pass into the urogenital sinus through the lateral walls of the developing myometrium.

Differentiation of ovary

Each ovarian blastema is covered by a surface layer of celomic epithelium, closely related but not identical to the cells that form the

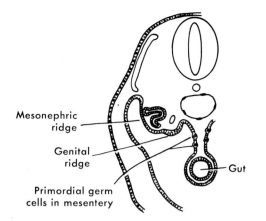

Fig. 40-1. Diagrammatic cross section of a 6 mm embryo showing migrating germ cells, genital ridge, and mesonephros. (From Kraus, F. T.: Gynecologic pathology, St. Louis, 1967, The C. V. Mosby Co.)

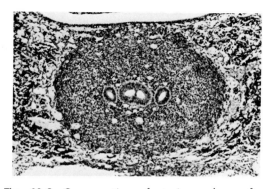

Fig. 40-2. Cross section of uterine anlage of a 60 mm embryo. Müllerian ducts have nearly fused at center. Mesonephric ducts are situated on each side. Peritoneum of cul-de-sac is at top. (150×; from Kraus, F. T.: Gynecologic pathology, St. Louis, 1967, The C. V. Mosby Co.)

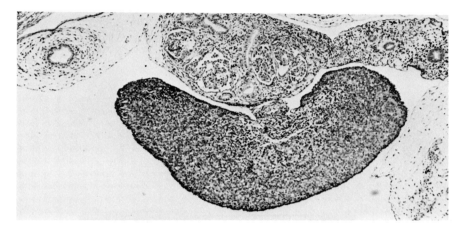

Fig. 40-3. Transverse section of ovary and adjacent mesonephros. Mesonephric glomeruli persist at this 60 mm stage. (90×; from Kraus, F. T.: Gynecologic pathology, St. Louis, 1967, The C. V. Mosby Co.)

müllerian ducts. Perhaps because of this close relationship in early development, the adenocarcinomas that arise from ovarian surface epithelium closely resemble typical adenocarcinomas of the tube, endometrium, cervix, and vagina. As a result of this similarity of patterns, it has become customy to regard the common ovarian epithelial neoplasms as "müllerian," even though the ovary does not actually form from the müllerian duct. The advantage of conceptual understanding overshadows the sacrifice of conformity to rigid embryologic fact.

The germ cells originate in the yolk sac endoderm near the hind gut, move through the primitive hind gut mesentery, and finally settle in the blastemas of the primitive ovaries.[17] The segregation of an occasional straggler along the way may explain some retroperitoneal germ cell tumors and the development of heterotopic ovarian tissue along the trail of this migration. This migration is completed by the tenth week. The germ cells begin to proliferate by mitosis upon arrival, notably after the eighth week; by the twelfth week some begin the first meiotic division. At birth, germ cell mitosis has ceased and most ova, at this time called "oogonia," are in the dictyotene stage of meiosis. The adjacent stromal cells differentiate into a single layer of flattened granulosa cells, forming a *primary follicle*. The granulosa cells proliferate; a cavity, the *antrum* appears, forming a *graafian follicle;* follicles may be numerous and some are large at birth. The ovaries descend into the pelvis attached to connective tissue strands, the *gubernacula,* which will become the medial *ovarian ligaments* and the *round ligaments,* extending from the uterine horns to the labia majora.

Differentiation of müllerian ducts

The separate proximal portions of the müllerian ducts develop into the uterine (fallopian) tubes. The fused mid and distal portions complete their merger by the twelfth week, forming the uterus and upper vagina, respectively. The myometrium differentiates from the surrounding mesenchyme, enveloping the adjacent segments of the withering mesonephric ducts.

Between the eighth and eleventh weeks the primitive vagina is a solid cord of epithelial cells ending distally in the urogenital sinus at Müller's tubercle. Evaginations of the urogenital sinus on either side of Müller's tubercle enlarge, fuse, and merge to form the hymen and very distal vaginal wall. The lining of the vagina is formed by proliferation of epithelial cells from the dorsum of the urogenital sinus, extending craniad toward the cervix, which is lined by simple columnar epithelium. This process occurs between the twelfth and eighteenth weeks, which proves to be a crucial period for female infants exposed in utero to the drug diethylstilbestrol and its derivatives.

Differentiation of vulva

The primitive hind gut, urinary ducts, and genital ducts all empty into a common chamber, the cloaca. By the sixth week the urorectal septum has formed as a transverse ridge separating the urogenital sinus and rectum. Müller's tubercle moves progressively caudad. The urinary bladder forms from the allantois, so that the müllerian and urinary orifices empty as separate orifices into the shallow remains of the urogenital sinus, now represented as the vestibule of the vulva (Figs. 40-4 and 40-5).

The development of the vulva begins at a sexually indeterminate stage.[24] At about 36 days (9 mm) the external structures are represented by a *genital tubercle,* a conic anterior midline protuberance, and the *labioscrotal swellings,* two broad lateral elevations located just caudad to the genital tubercle on either side of the *cloacal groove* (Fig. 40-6). The cloacal groove at first is closed by the *cloacal membrane.* After the urorectal septum grows down to

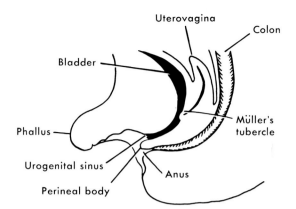

Fig. 40-4. Diagrammatic sagittal section showing relationship between urinary bladder, urogenital sinus, and Müller's tubercle. Age approximately 10 weeks. (Redrawn from Arey, L. B.: Developmental anatomy, ed. 6, Philadelphia, 1954, W. B. Saunders Co.)

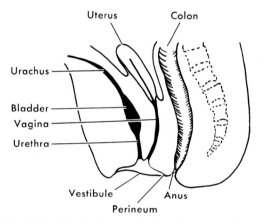

Fig. 40-5. Caudad growth of perineum and urovaginal septum separates bladder and vagina and enlarges separation between vulvar vestibule and anus. (Redrawn from Arey, L. B.: Developmental anatomy, ed. 6, Philadelphia, 1954, W. B. Saunders Co.)

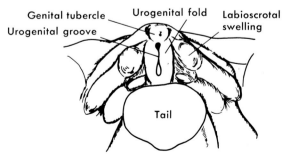

Fig. 40-6. External genitalia at about 7 weeks are sexually indeterminate. (Redrawn from Arey, L. B.: Developmental anatomy, ed. 6, Philadelphia, 1954, W. B. Saunders Co.)

Table 40-1. Correlation of age, size, and sequence of development of female urogenital organs

Age (approximately*)	Crown-rump length (mm)	Developmental levels in female urogenital tract
25 days	25	Pronephros formed; pronephric ducts grow caudad as blind tubes; cloaca and cloacal membrane present; embryo has 14 somites
32 days	5	Pronephros degenerated; mesonephric tubules forming; pronephric (now mesonephric) ducts reach cloaca; metanephric bud forms at distal end of mesonephric duct
35 days	8	Genital ridge bulges; ureteric and renal pelvic primordia formed
40 days	13	Urorectal septum begins to subdivide cloaca; genital tubercle and labioscrotal swellings evident; müllerian duct begins to form
7 weeks	22	Urogenital membrane dissolves; cloaca separated into urogenital sinus and rectum; glans of phallus is evident
8 weeks	30	Testis and ovary become recognizable as such; müllerian ducts approach urogenital sinus and begin to fuse (distal portion) to become uterovaginal primordium
10 weeks	46	Mesonephric ducts atrophy; glands of urogenital sinus (vulvo-urethral and vestibular glands) appear
12 weeks	56	Uterine horns absorbed; muscular walls appear in uterus, vagina, and fallopian tubes; distinction of sex from external genitalia becomes possible
16 weeks	112	Uterus and vagina become distinctive structures
5 months	150	Primary ovarian follicles are found; vagina develops lumen; urogenital sinus becomes shallow vestibule
7 months	230	Uterine glands appear

*There is no accurate way of determining embryonic age from the length; the figures given represent a composite or average and are based upon the stages described by Hamilton, W. J., Boyd, J. D., and Mossman, H. W.: Human embryology, Baltimore, 1962, The Williams & Wilkins Co., and by Van Wagenen, G., and Simpson, M. E.: Embryology of the ovary and testis, New Haven, 1965, Yale University Press.

meet it, the cloacal membrane becomes divided into an anterior urogenital groove, closed by the urogenital membrane, and a posterior anal membrane. The urogenital membrane disintegrates at about 42 days; a glans becomes evident on the genital tubercle in the 46-day-old (19 mm) embryo. The urogenital groove extends anteriorly on the caudal aspect of the phallus thus formed. A sexual distinction is made evident by the *urethral groove,* which extends onto the phallus from the urogenital groove; the urethral groove extends distally onto the glans in the male but not in the female. This distinction is probably not a reliable indicator of sex until after the eleventh week (50 mm) is attained. The *urethral folds* lateral to the urethral groove fuse to form the male penile urethra; they persist as separate structures, the *labia minora,* in the female. The labioscrotal swellings enlarge to form the labia majora; they fuse posteriorly at the posterior commissure at about 50 mm. In the 4-month-old (100 mm) embryo the prepuce forms around the glans of the clitoris.

The most significant events in the embryology of the female genital tract are summarized in Table 40-1. This timetable of development is useful in relating malformations to possible teratogenic events such as maternal infection with a virus or exposure to a teratogenic drug.

Sexual differentiation: male and female

Although this section is concerned with the development of female genitalia, some knowledge of the parallel development in the male genitalia is crucial to any understanding of the complex intersex anomalies discussed below.

The gonadal blastemas begin similarly in both sexes and at first are morphologically indistinguishable from one another. The definitive ovary and testis have been identified by Van Wagenen and Simpson in 23 mm embryos, after the age of 42 days. In the female the müllerian ducts and vulva develop appropriately, but this progression is *not* dependent on the presence of one or both ovaries. In males, however, the persistence and development of the mesonephric (wolffian) duct system, together with atrophy of the müllerian ducts and the structures that form from them, are dependent on two factors: a local-acting *müllerian regression factor* and circulating *testosterone,* both produced by the testis.[9] Development of an epididymis, a vas deferens, and a seminal vesicle does not occur in the absence of a testis *on the same side;* this development may be deficient if the gonad is an ovotestis or a dysgenetic testis. Development of male external genitalia and prostate gland depends on *circulating testosterone,* secreted by the testes. Testosterone is required to produce the glans and shaft of the penis, cause the urethral folds to fuse forming the penile urethra with its orifice in the glans, and produce fusion of the labioscrotal folds to **form** a scrotum into which the testes descend. Male structures also fail to develop when the somatic cells of a fetus are insensitive to androgen stimulation as in the *testicular feminization syndrome.*

Because the action of the müllerian regression factor is local, it must be produced in adequate amounts by both testes to prevent the development of both tubes, uterus, and upper vagina completely. Therefore an individual with a testis on one side and a streak (no gonad), an ovary, or ovotestis, on the other will usually have a uterus and upper vagina, and possibly a tube on the side opposite that occupied by the testis.

In the strongly estrogenic maternal environment, genital development is female independently of the presence of a fetal ovary. Therefore a fetus with no gonadal tissue on either side (bilateral streaks or bilateral agenesis) will have at birth a uterus, vagina, tubes, and the female pattern of external genitalia. Individuals with abnormal (dysgenetic) testes, which may not produce either müllerian regression factor or testosterone in adequate amounts will have some degree of müllerian tract development and either female external genitalia or incompletely formed male external genitalia. A single testis might be expected to inhibit müllerian development on the same side, but not on the opposite side, or the uterus; however, it could produce enough circulating testosterone to masculinize the external genitalia.

Congenital anomalies

Congenital anomalies of the genitalia are extremely varied. Because of the importance of sex in social development, they may have as devastating an impact as many anomalies carrying a more serious threat to survival.

Any classification of female genital tract anomalies must reflect the current incomplete knowledge of genetics and of other teratogenic factors such as viruses and toxic chemicals or drugs. At the present time it is convenient to divide genital malformations into two broad groups: (1) those related to intersex states, in which a genetic abnormality of a sex chromosome is demonstrable or suspected, and (2) those more simply structural and localized developmental abnormalities in which one of the processes of the growth, fusion, canalization, or separation of developing tubular structures is incomplete. A detailed classification in relation to biochemical and cytogenetic anomalies has been prepared by Park et al.[16]

Intersex states and cytogenetic abnormalities

Normal sexual development is determined first of all by the presence in the zygote of a normal set of sex chromosomes, XX for a female and XY for a male. The initial factor in many genital anomalies is the contribution of abnormal or deficient genetic material by one of the gametes. Alternatively, during the first division of the zygote some genetic material may be lost or unevenly distributed in the daughter cells *(nondisjunction)* resulting in a mixture *(mosaic)* of two or more types of cells as the organism develops further. Although the loss or severe alteration or duplication of an autosome is usually lethal, most sex chromosomal abnormalities exert their most notable effects in the form of altered genital structure and function.

A significant chromosomal abnormality can be detected in about 50% of spontaneous abortions when the fetus is either absent or morphologically abnormal,[22] and 5% of perinatal deaths or stillbirths have a chromosomal anomaly.[12] In adults, among 50 women who failed to begin to menstruate (primary amenorrhea), Sarto[19] found chromosomal anomalies in 19.

A bewildering array of intersex states has been described, together with associated cytogenetic analyses and deranged endocrine physiology. Extensive clinical descriptions and genetic studies are available in monographs such as those by Federman,[5] and Mittwoch.[14] This discussion is limited to a summary of the usual findings in a few of the more common intersex syndromes, with Table 40-2 for comparison. This table is a generalization. There is no perfect correspondence between phenotype, karyotype, and other features of these syndromes at the present state of the art: many patients will not fit the chart.

Certain commonly used terms require definition, as follows.

hermaphrodite An inexact term that indicates that an individual has some kind of mixture

Table 40-2. Intersex syndromes affecting females, apparent females, or female genitalia*

Syndrome	Gonads	Karyotype (genotype)	Inheritance	Internal genitalia	External genitalia	Habitus (phenotype)	Comment
Pure gonadal dysgenesis	Bilateral streaks	XX, mosaics	Autosomal recessive	Vagina, uterus, and tubes	Female	Female	Nerve deafness
Turner's syndrome	Bilateral streaks	XO, mosaics	No	Vagina, uterus, and tubes	Female	Female	Multiple malformations
Gonadal agenesis	Absent	XY	Uncertain	Rudimentary tubular structures No uterus or vagina	Ambiguous or female	Female	Minor malformations in some cases
Mixed gonadal dysgenesis	Streak and dysgenetic testis	XO/XY	No	May be uterus and tubes	Variable male-female	Female	Gonadal neoplasms Virilization
True hermaphrodite	Ovary and testis Ovotestis Ovotestis with ovary or testis	Majority XX Some XY Many mosaics	No	Usually or may be vagina, uterus, and tubes	Ambiguous, variable	Variable male-female	
Female pseudohermaphrodite (chiefly adrenogenital syndrome)	Ovaries	XX	Autosomal recessive	Vagina, uterus, and tubes	Ambiguous	Female	Some infants virilized by iatrogenic androgens
Male pseudohermaphrodite (chiefly androgen insensitivity syndrome, partial or complete)	Testes	XY	X-linked recessive or sex-limited autosomal dominant	Vagina partial; no uterus or tubes	Female	Female	Testes in inguinal hernias Less pubic and axillary hair
47 XXX syndromes	Ovaries	XXX, XXXX, and a variety of mosaics	No	Uterus, vagina, and tubes	Female	Female	Some have been mentally retarded

*Courtesy Dr. Robert H. Shikes, Denver, Colorado.

of both male and female gonads, external genitalia, and sex characteristics. A *"true" hermaphrodite* has both ovarian and testicular tissue, either or both of which may be functional.

pseudohermaphrodite An inexact, confusing, and often unnecessary *general* term for an individual with gonads and genotype of one sex and external genitalia more consistent with the opposite sex. A *male pseudohermaphrodite* has testes but otherwise appears to be female (typically represented by the androgen-insensitivity syndrome). A *female pseudohermaphrodite* has ovaries, but the external genitalia are masculinized (typically represented by congenital adrenal hyperplasia). It is nearly always possible, desirable, and sufficient to name the specific condition or syndrome.

genotype An expression of the genetic characteristics of an individual cell as determined by analysis of the number and morphologic characteristics of the chromosomes examined at metaphase; e.g., 46 XX indicates that the individual has 44 normal autosomes and two normal X chromosomes, the genotype of a normal female; 46 XY is the normal male genotype; and 45 XO indicates 44 autosomes, one X, and deletion of the second sex chromosome, as seen in Turner's syndrome.

phenotype Refers to the external habitus and general appearance of the individual; in intersex states, it refers more specifically to the appearance of the external genitalia (male or female). In the postpubertal individual it generally includes also secondary sex characteristics such as hair distribution, wide or narrow hips, laryngeal enlargement, and hirsutism.

dysgenetic gonad An ovary or testis that has been abnormal from the beginning, usually as the result of the absence or other abnormality of a sex chromosome complement of the cells. The streak gonad (Turner's syndrome) can be regarded as a dysgenetic ovary. Neoplasms, especially gonadoblastoma, are likely to occur in dysgenetic gonads.[21]

gonadal dysgenesis The gonads are "streaks" composed of fibrous ovarian stroma with no follicles and no ova (Fig. 40-7). The phenotype is female, and fallopian tubes, uterus, and vagina are present. Patients with associated short stature, webbing of the neck, widely spaced nipples, and, less frequently, coarctation of the aorta and red-green color blindness are said to have *Turner's syndrome.* Those with the gonadal lesion only are classified as having "pure gonadal dysgenesis." The cytogenetic lesion is some kind of abnormality—usually absence—of the second sex chromosome in at least some of the cells; typically 45 XO.

Hilus cells, mesonephric duct remnants, and a fibrous stroma reminiscent of ovarian stroma are usually identifiable. The presence of a few ova suggests that the patient is a mosaic: the XO karyotype has been leavened with a few XX (or other karyotype with a second X) cells. Cordlike structures reminiscent of immature testis argue the existence of at least a few Y chromosomes.[13]

mixed gonadal dysgenesis One gonad is a fibrous streak as in Turner's syndrome, and the other is a testis, usually an immature or rudimentary testis, but occasionally the dysgenetic gonad opposite the streak is replaced by a tumor. The internal genitalia include a uterus, upper vagina, and, despite the influence of the testis, usually two fallopian tubes. The phenotype varies considerably, from normal male to normal female with variable degrees of ambiguity in many instances; a few have the appearance of Turner's syndrome. The chromosomal lesion varies but commonly includes mosaicism with both XO and XY stem lines.

Gonadal agenesis

Gonads and internal genitalia are completely absent. Phenotype is female; genotype is XY. This is an extremely rare condition; the absence of müllerian duct derivatives is unexplained.[5]

True hermaphroditism

Recognizable ovarian and testicular tissues are both present, either together in the same gonad (an ovotestis) or on opposite sides, or in such combinations as ovotestis on one side with ovary or testis on the other. There is nearly always a uterus. The side with a testis has a vas deferens; the side with an ovary has a tube. A wide variety of internal genitalia combinations occur, and the phenotypes and external genitalia are also extremely variable. Most patients have a 46 XX karyotype, but 46 XY and a variety of mosaics have been reported.

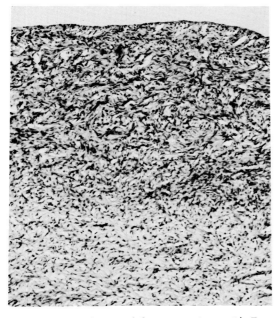

Fig. 40-7. Streak gonad from a patient with Turner's syndrome. (85×; from Kraus, F. T.: Gynecologic pathology, St. Louis, 1967, The C. V. Mosby Co.)

Testicular feminization, androgen insensitivity syndrome, and other male pseudohermaphrodites

The gonads are testes and the genotype is indistinguishable from that of a normal male. The general appearance is that of a normally developed woman, except for absence of pubic hair and axillary hair as well as body hair generally. Breasts develop normally at puberty; they usually have small nipples with normal-sized but pale areolae. The vagina is less deep and ends blindly, sometimes with a mass of smooth muscle at the apex.[15]

Androgen production is apparently normal; the defect seems to be the result of androgen insensitivity of somatic cells. The exact nature of the defect is still unknown but is probably the result of an intracellular abnormality of protein receptors for androgen.[2,28] The existence of a comparable syndrome in rats and mice has facilitated the study of the molecular biology of this lesion.[2]

Various incomplete forms of the defect occur; inheritance is probably based upon a sex-linked recessive trait, although an autosomal defect has not been excluded.

Congenital adrenal hyperplasia and other hormonally induced causes of female pseudohermaphroditism

This is fundamentally an adrenal abnormality in which defective hydrocortisone synthesis leads to androgen excess (see p. 1660). The gonads are normal ovaries; the uterus and tubes are likewise normal. The morphologic genital defect involves the external genitalia only and is the result of excessive androgen production by hyperplastic adrenal glands. This is the commonest cause of ambiguous genitalia; it is also the most effectively treatable so that fertility and all other aspects of a normal sex role can usually be achieved. Because of the hydrocortisone deficiency, it is also likely to be fatal if unrecognized and is therefore the most important abnormality of sexual development to recognize at birth.

Rarely a similar masculinization of the external genitalia has been caused by the androgenic effect of progestogens administered to pregnant women in the hope of preventing abortion.

Other chromosomal syndromes

Other cytogenetic abnormalities affecting the sex chromosomes are less likely to present as malformations of female genitalia. The female with one or more extra X chromosomes (47 XXX, etc.) is phenotypically normal; some have mental retardation. Klinefelter's syndrome (usually 47 XXY) involves a malformation of the male genitalia.

Localized developmental anomalies

Ovary. An ovary may be absent. The tube and uterine horn on the same side are usually also absent, and, of great clinical significance, the kidney and ureter on the affected side may also be absent. Supernumerary ovaries and accessory ovarian tissue are most commonly found adjacent to a normally situated ovary and should be distinguished from lobulation of a single ovary. In rare instances ovarian tissue has been identified in the retroperitoneum, in the posterior bladder wall, and in the omentum and sigmoid mesentery.[18,27] Occasionally a cystic teratoma has arisen at such a site; the rare finding of other neoplasms of ovarian type that seem to have arisen in the pelvic retroperitoneum may in some instances be explained on a similar basis.

Fallopian tube. Duplication and atresia occur rarely. Occasionally tiny accessory ostia, like miniature representatives of the fimbriated end, sprout from the side of the fallopian tube, especially the distal half.[29] Small patches of mucinous and endometrial epithelium may occur, especially when there is inflammation or endometriosis, so that it may not be clear whether this change in the tubal lining is congenital or acquired by metaplasia.

Unilateral absence is uncommon and is associated with ureteral and renal abnormalities, including absence.

Uterus, vagina, and vulva. The commonest anomaly of the uterus, vagina, and vulva is the result of failure of fusion of some or all of the lower müllerian ducts. All gradations may occur, from complete separation causing the development of two complete genital tracts, to minimal failure with an incomplete sagittal septum at the uterine fundus. In the presence of a complete double vagina, a double cervix and uterus is usual, but duplication of a distal structure such as the cervix does not invariably indicate that the uterine corpus is duplicated.[25] Pregnancy may occur in either side, or both. Both elements of a duplicated structure may not be of equal size. Development of one side may be discontinuous; a semidetached uterine horn may form a muscular walled cyst connected to the cervix by a fibrous cord.

Anomalies involving failure of fusion or establishment of patency in the lower müllerian system are often associated with urinary tract anomalies, including unilateral renal agenesis and misplaced ureters that discharge into the bladder at an abnormal site such as the uterus or vagina.

Transverse septa and atresias in the vagina probably result from the failure of canalization of the distal end of the müllerian duct. Retention of fluid (hydrocolpos or hematocolpos) is usually caused by a transverse septum situated proximal to a patent hymen.

Nearly all patients with congenital absence of the vagina have no uterus; however, when the vagina is apparently absent and accumulated menstrual blood forms a bulging cystic mass, the obstruction is almost always below the cervical level.

An extreme degree of hypoplasia of the cervix—or apparent absence or atresia of the cervix—will occasionally also cause a cystic accumulation of menstrual blood in the normally formed uterine corpus; successful term pregnancy is possible after surgical reconstruction.[4]

Associated with internal duplications, there may be even more rarely a duplication of the external genitalia, including both labia, clitoris, and urethra. Congenital fistulas between the anus or rectum and vestibule, anterior displacement of the anus, and vestibular location of the anus have been described in detail by Stephens.[23] These anomalies are dependent chiefly on the extent of the contribution by the uroanal septum to the formation of the perineum.

VULVA
Anatomy

The vulva is composed of the labia majora, labia minora, mons veneris, clitoris, vestibule, hymen, Bartholin's glands, and the minor vestibular glands. The mons veneris and labia majora externally are covered by skin with hair follicles, sebaceous glands, and sweat glands, including apocrine sweat glands. The inner surfaces of the labia majora, the labia minora, and vestibule have sebaceous glands but no hair and are covered by a less keratinized epidermis. The vulva is profusely permeated by lymphatics that cross the midline extensively so that a lesion on one side is very likely to affect the lymph nodes on the opposite side. Lymph from the labia flows to the superficial inguinal nodes; lymph from the vestibule and clitoris may flow directly to the deep femoral nodes. An inconspicuous layer of specific stroma similar to that beneath the epithelium of the vagina and cervix extends also beneath the vulvar epithelium.

The vulvar epithelium is subject to all of the dermatoses that affect the body skin generally, as well as specific dystrophic conditions that may also affect the perineum and perianal skin. Reactive changes expressed as atrophy and inflammation with pruritus that occur in women with diabetes mellitus and pernicious anemia, are relieved by control of the primary disease.

Inflammation

The vulva represents the portal of entry and the site of destructive results of most venereal infections. The inflammatory patterns vary considerably; though none are entirely specific, the pathologic changes are often sufficiently distinctive to suggest the agent responsible. Confirmation by culture or serologic techniques will usually be possible.

The specific pathologic features of venereal diseases and other specific infectious diseases of the vulva are described in the chapters devoted to venereal diseases (p. 428), bacterial diseases (p. 391), viral diseases (p. 452), and fungal diseases (p. 497). Crohn's disease of the intestinal tract (p. 1286) may produce destructive vulvar granulomas and abscesses.[38]

Bartholin's gland cyst and abscess

Bartholin's glands may be invaded by any bacterial agent; the ducts may become dilated behind an obstruction, so that an abscess, which may be acutely swollen and painful, may be produced. A less severe chronic bacterial infection may evolve more slowly into a fluid-filled cyst. The commonest cause of Bartholin's gland abscesses and cysts is gonorrhea, but other pathogenic bacteria can cause the same reactions. The mass must be distinguished from a neoplasm, and therefore a biopsy at the time of drainage is desirable, especially in the absence of any antecedent symptoms of acute inflammation.

Herpes simplex

Herpes simplex infection of the vulva deserves special attention in the context of the female genital tract. There has been a remarkable increase in the incidence of genital herpes. A distinctly specific strain of virus (herpesvirus, type II) that is indigenous to the genital tract has emerged; this virus has become implicated in the etiology of cervical and vulvar cancer.

Vulvar herpetic lesions begin as painful vesicles, ulcerate, and heal in about 2 weeks (Fig. 40-8). The lesions are more numerous and slightly larger in primary infections. The

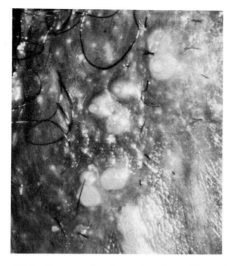

Fig. 40-8. Herpes simplex of vulva. Ulcers have yellow shaggy necrotic base and surrounding erythema. (Courtesy Dr. Ernst R. Friedrich, St. Louis, Mo.)

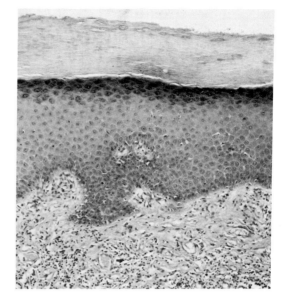

Fig. 40-9. Hyperkeratosis and chronic inflammation. Note dense keratin layer at surface, and fibrosis and chronic inflammation in the underlying dermis. Cytologic pattern is benign. (85×.)

symptoms frequently respond to topical application of light-sensitive dyes such as neutral red or proflavine. The dye is incorporated into the viral DNA; exposure to light inactivates the virus. Whether its putative carcinogenic properties are also inactivated remains to be seen.

Cells with viral inclusions are easily identifiable in vaginocervical smears (see vagina, p. 1697).

Dystrophies, keratoses, and atrophy
Terminology

The vulvar epithelium is subject to a group of chronic conditions of unknown origin, affecting chiefly older women. The skin appears white, mottled red and white, or less commonly, red. There are variable degrees of atrophy of the subcutaneous tissue so that at an advanced stage the labia are obliterated and the introitus is stenotic. Pruritus is common and may be severe and unremitting. The perineum and perianal skin may also be affected.

The term *leukoplakia* is often used by the clinician to describe the patchy areas of whitened skin. In a similar way, the term *kraurosis* indicates that the atrophy and shrinkage are advanced. As the result of extremely varied usage in the past, both terms have no specific pathologic diagnostic meaning at this time. Their use by a pathologist now is undesirable, as the reader of his report may interpret the terms as signifying benign disease, malignant disease, or (correctly) total ambiguity and confusion.

The following lesions of the vulvar skin have the appearance and symptoms noted above:
Hyperkeratosis and chronic inflammation.
Lichen sclerosus et atrophicus.
Specific intraepithelial neoplasms: carcinoma in situ, Bowen's disease, Paget's disease.
Specific dermatoses, especially psoriasis, neurodermititis, allergic or contact dermatitis, and lichen planus, as described in Chapter 39.
Systemic diseases such as pernicious anemia and diabetes with or without candidosis.
The spectrum of clinical significance varies from benign to malignant; the treatment varies from excision to insulin injections. The lesions must be biopsied to be identified correctly and treated appropriately.

Hyperkeratosis and chronic inflammation

The combination of a thick layer of surface keratin, hyperplastic but cytologically benign squamous epithelium, and a mixture of chronic inflammatory cells distributed through the underlying dermis (Fig. 40-9) causes the vulva to appear thickened and white and usually to itch unremittingly. Scratching adds trauma and chronic inflammation and thereby probably reinforces the pruritus. In areas where the keratin layer is lacking, the physical appearance is red. The epidermis is usually hyperplastic; elongation of rete ridges in obliquely oriented microscopic sections may falsely suggest an invasive lesion. Either hyperkeratosis or parakeratosis may occur at the surface.

The cause is unknown. Symptomatic relief has resulted from use of topical creams containing hydrocortisone or other corticoid hormone preparations.[56]

Lichen sclerosus et atrophicus

This specific dermatosis is not confined to the vulva and may affect both sexes at any age. However the majority of patients who consult a gynecologist are postmenopausal women whose lesion and symptoms are either confined to the vulva or associated with perianal and perineal involvement.

The lesions appear first as small coalescent macules, which may have central pits resulting from follicular plugging. There is progressive shrinkage of the vulvar connective tissues so that the skin becomes smooth, shiny, and thin. Eventually the atrophic connective tissue changes obliterate the labia and produce stenosis of the introitus. Although usually white and opaque, the skin may appear mottled red and white.

The microscopic appearance is specific and characteristic: the epidermis in cross section is a thin atrophic band without rete ridges. The surface layer is hyperkeratotic. The most distinctive feature is the amorphous homogeneous degenerative change in the dermal collagen, usually in a wide band beneath the epidermis. Elastic fibers are absent; the collagen that remains may stain densely or faintly and is relatively acellular, except for scattered lymphocytes. A band of lymphocytes with a few plasma cells lies beneath, in the middermis. There is often separation at the epidermal-dermal junction, at least in focal areas (Fig. 40-10). Kaufman et al.[56] have reported considerable success with topical application of ointments containing testosterone or other androgenic steroids; response to vulvectomy is poor, as the lesions recur consistently.[52]

Clinicopathologic correlation

Lichen sclerosus and hyperkeratosis with chronic inflammation may occur together, and other more threatening lesions may also be present in the same patient. Multiple biopsies are necessary to evaluate an extensive lesion, especially if its appearance varies from place to place. The use of a colposcope in selecting areas for biopsy may prove to be useful.[58]

The frequency of subsequent malignant change has been much debated. In the few large series of patients whose original lesion

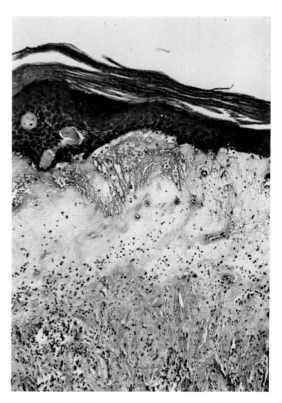

Fig. 40-10. Lichen sclerosus et atrophicus. Epidermis is thin and atrophic; underlying dermal collagen is hyalinized and edematous. Beneath this area of degenerative change there is moderate chronic inflammation. There is surface hyperkeratosis. (85×.)

was a benign dystrophy, subsequent malignant change has been uncommon, in the range of 1% to 3%,[53,56,60] even after follow-up periods of many years. Detailed pathologic studies have failed to show any evidence that lichen sclerosus et atrophicus predisposes vulvar epithelium to the development of cancer.[48] Much of the controversy has probably been fired by misunderstandings based upon semantics. Authors whose experience suggests that vulvar cancer commonly occurs after vulvar dystrophies have apparently included patients with dysplastic epithelial lesions or carcinoma in situ in their study of "leukoplakic vulvitis." Unquestionably many patients with vulvar carcinoma have a dystrophic lesion in the skin next to it (but not necessarily antecedent to it). Both sides of this polemic have been reviewed by Gardner and Kaufman.[44]

It is important to emphasize that vulvectomy for a chronic vulvar dystrophy is not likely to relieve the symptoms, remedy the disease, or exclude the possibility of subsequent can-

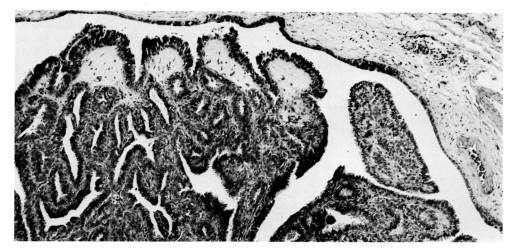

Fig. 40-11. Hidradenoma papilliferum. All the papillary processes have a delicate fibrovascular support, and there is a double layer of epithelial cells covering each of the papillary processes. (90×.)

cer.[53] The best results to date have occurred after topical treatment with corticosteroids for hyperkeratosis and androgens for lichen sclerosus et atrophicus; none of the treated patients has developed a carcinoma.[55]

Neoplasms
Benign tumors and tumorlike conditions

Hidradenoma (Hidradenoma papilliferum). This small papillary neoplasm forms a nodule in the subcutaneous tissue of the vulva. The papillary fronds are covered by a double layer of epithelial cells, supported by a delicate fibrovascular stalk, an arrangement that resembles papilloma of the breast (Fig. 40-11). As in the breast, clusters of pink "apocrine" cells may form a part of the pattern. The labia are the usual location; about one fifth of the cases reported[64] occurred in the perianal region.

Granular cell tumor (granular cell myeloblastoma). More commonly found in other sites such as tongue, breast, and respiratory tract, granular cell tumor occasionally produces a poorly circumscribed indurated gray or yellow solid mass in the subcutaneous tissue of the vulva. The tumor cells are large, with abundant pink granular cytoplasm and benign uniform round nuclei. Ultrastructural studies show a varied appearance that suggests a cell full of secondary lysosomes. Some of the cells contain larger granular structures, called angulate bodies, that are packed with fibrillar material and sometimes lipid.[74]

Because the general pattern suggests organelles and membrane arrangements found in Schwann cells, especially the degenerative changes found in Schwann cells during wallerian degeneration, it is likely that most granular cell tumors are of Schwann cell origin. However similar cytoplasmic changes have been described in smooth muscle cells of the appendix,[74] in the irradiated myometrium, and in one tumor of the urinary bladder.[35] The characteristic histologic and cytologic features probably represent one type of cellular response to injury that may occur in a variety of neoplastic or nonneoplastic cells.

All vulvar lesions, and virtually all those located elsewhere as well, have been benign.

Breast tissue and fibroadenoma

The vulva is at the caudal end of the embryonic milk line, and nodular masses of breast tissue measuring as much as 10 cm in diameter have been reported. Sometimes the lesion first becomes evident during lactation as the result of rapid and alarming enlargement. The various patterns associated with chronic cystic disease of the breast also occur in vulvar breast tissue. Fibroadenomas in the vulva resemble breast fibroadenomas. A primary adenocarcinoma of the vulva with the patterns of breast adenocarcinoma would be most unusual; the finding of such a lesion in the vulva strongly suggests metastatic and disseminated breast adenocarcinoma.[37]

Stromal polyps

Cutaneous polyps are invested externally by an orderly epidermis that covers a loose fibrous connective tissue stroma with a variable com-

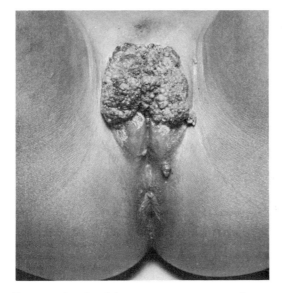

Fig. 40-12. Condyloma acuminatum. Exuberant keratotic papillary processes may cover and obliterate large areas of vulva.

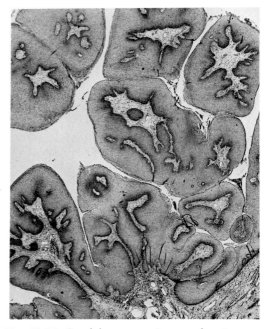

Fig. 40-13. Condyloma acuminatum showing papillary processes covered by orderly squamous epithelium, each supported by a fibrovascular connective tissue stalk. (20×.)

ponent of adipose tissue and vessels, and most polyps of the vulva have this pattern.

Rarely a stromal polyp may include scattered large giant cells of the type encountered more commonly in the vagina (see p. 1699). The specific subepithelial stroma of the cervix and vagina also extends beneath the epithelium of the vulva.[85]

Condyloma acuminatum

This papillary lesion of squamous epithelium occurs chiefly as multiple soft warty masses. They may be large or small and can be distributed about the anus, perineum, vaginal wall, and cervix, as well as the vulva (Fig. 40-12).

The squamous epithelium that covers the papillary fronds is histologically benign and is supported by a uniformly distributed fibrovascular stroma that ramifies into all of the papillary projections (Fig. 40-13). Perinuclear vacuolation is common and characteristic. The presence of occasional pyknotic or hyperchromatic nuclei should not be interpreted as evidence of malignant change, especially if there has been prior treatment with podophyllin.

The etiologic agent is a papovavirus closely related to the virus of the ordinary cutaneous wart. Malignant change is the subject of an occasional anecdotal reference; such lesions have probably in fact been instances of papillary carcinoma in situ, verrucous carcinoma, or well-differentiated epidermoid carcinoma from the outset. Participation of the condyloma, or wart, virus in the pathogenesis of carcinoma is a highly speculative possibility.

Most lesions respond to podophyllin, cautery, excision, or freezing. The surprising effectiveness of an autogenous vaccine in eradicating large or resistant condylomas is at present unexplained.[70]

Miscellaneous

Benign mucinous cysts lined by a single layer of endocervical type of columnar cells are more common than generally appreciated. Most have appeared in the vicinity of the vestibule. Tissue of origin has been considered to be paramesonephric duct[47] or urogenital sinus vestiges.[43]

A collection of 34 benign vulvar neoplasms studied by Lovelady[62] included 16 fibromas, 7 lipomas, 5 hemangiomas, 2 neurofibromas, 2 leiomyomas, 1 ganglioneuroma, and 1 lymphangioma. Such cutaneous lesions as pyogenic granuloma, seborrheic keratosis, nevi of various types, and single squamous papillomas have no distinctive features when encountered in the vulva and are discussed in Chapter 42.

Endometriosis occurs in the vulva usually as the result of implantation of endometrial tissue in minor operative wounds, notably episiotomy scars.

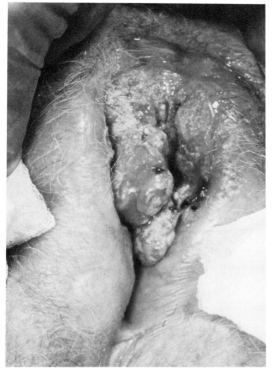

Fig. 40-14. Carcinoma of vulva. Tumor forms nodular erythematous mass with ulceration and erythema. Adjacent labia are edematous.

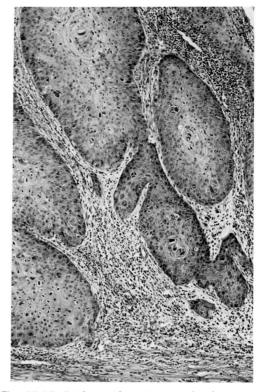

Fig. 40-15. Epidermoid carcinoma of vulva. Irregular rounded masses of well-differentiated keratinizing epidermoid carcinoma with well-circumscribed margin and associated inflammatory changes. (80×.)

Malignant tumors

The predominant malignant tumor of the vulva is epidermoid carcinoma (at least 96%). Malignant melanomas make up another 2%, and the rest are a mixture of rare adenocarcinomas, soft-tissue sarcomas, and an occasional basal cell carcinoma. Vulvar carcinomas comprise less than 1% of all cancers; they accounted for 657 (5%) of 12,688 women with genital cancer admitted to Radiumhemmet, the well-known cancer hospital in Stockholm.[39]

Epidermoid carcinoma

Invasive epidermoid carcinoma is chiefly a disease of postmenopausal women. Smaller lesions are usually elevated and superficial with an irregular granular, nodular, or ulcerated surface. Larger lesions tend to protrude as an outward growing warty mass with a weeping ulcerated surface and a mottled red-gray or yellow surface (Fig. 40-14). More aggressive poorly differentiated infiltrating tumors have ulcerated surfaces with elevated, undermined margins.

Associated carcinoma in situ or dystrophic changes in the adjacent skin are commonly present. The usual location is the labia majora, especially the inner aspect, and most carcinomas begin on the anterior two thirds of the vulva.

Most vulvar epidermoid carcinomas are well differentiated, produce keratin, and have well-circumscribed margins (Fig. 40-15). Lesions with this pattern are more likely to remain localized and have a better prognosis. Poorly differentiated carcinomas have a more diffusely infiltrating pattern, invade nerve sheaths and lymphatics, grow in narrow strands, and have a more aggressive natural history. The loose fibroblastic stroma in such cases is usually relatively abundant, and the tumor margin is indistinct.

It is important to emphasize that physical examination is an unreliable indicator of metastatic spread; even a very experienced examiner is likely to miss metastases or overdiagnose their presence in about 40% of patients.[76] The presence of a hyperkeratotic dysplastic lesion in the adjacent skin is associated with a significantly better prognosis.[46]

Size of the primary tumor is not a reliable indicator of metastasis; in the experience of Green and associates[45] one third of the lesions 1 cm in maximum diameter or smaller and half of the well-differentiated grade I epidermoid carcinomas were associated with lymph node metastases. Even the earliest "microinvasive" changes may occasionally be the source of lymph node metastasis.[66] On the other hand it appears that the risk of lymph node metastases is limited if the primary cancer invades no further than a depth of 5 mm.[77] Lymph node metastases commonly appear in the opposite side of the vulva so that bilateral inguinal lymph node dissections are necessary. Lesions located anteriorly or on the clitoris are more likely to spread to deeper (pelvic, iliac) lymph nodes. Frozen-section evaluation of Cloquet's node may be a logical way to select the patients who will require bilateral iliac and pelvic lymph node dissection, in addition to bilateral inguinal node dissection.

There is a distinct association with other areas of carcinoma of the lower genital tract, notably the cervix[31,36] and upper vagina, as well as the anus and perineum.

Verrucous carcinoma

This extremely well differentiated form of epidermoid carcinoma was first described by Ackerman as a lesion occurring chiefly in the oral cavity. It may become quite large and will expand inexorably into adjacent tissues.

Although the histologic and cytologic pattern appears benign, it is possible to distinguish verrucous carcinoma from condyloma acuminatum by the uneven distribution of the fibrovascular stromal support in comparison with that of condyloma acuminatum.

Lymph node metastases occur only rarely if at all, but any tissue including lymph nodes and nerve sheaths may be involved by direct extension. A satisfactory response to radiation therapy is unusual.[59]

Epidermoid carcinoma in situ and Bowen's disease

The lesions are white patches, or mottled red and white, and often form plaque-like elevations. Some lesions have a warty papillomatous appearance ("papillary carcinoma in situ"). Pruritus is common. Distinction between benign dystrophy and carcinoma in situ is impossible without biopsy.

The affected epithelium is composed almost entirely of dysplastic or anaplastic squamous epithelial cells that lie typically beneath a keratotic surface of variable thickness (Fig. 40-16). It is important to identify invasion if it is present; the magnification possible with a colposcope should improve diagnostic accuracy because invasion in the vulva, as in the cervix, is associated with an abnormal vascular pattern of vessels oriented parallel to the epithelial surface.[58]

Dysplastic lesions resembling carcinoma in situ have occurred in association with herpetic infection in pregnant women; the lesions have regressed spontaneously after delivery.[41,73] It will be important to learn the ultimate fate of these women.

Most studies have emphasized a high frequency of multifocal carcinoma in situ, with other areas located especially in the cervix and upper vagina, and less frequently in the perineal and perianal skin.

Gosling and Abell[46] distinguish Bowen's disease as a variant of epidermoid carcinoma in situ of the vulva that is detectable by the presence of scattered large bizarre cells, bizarre mitoses, keratin "pearls," and pyknotic nuclei (corps ronds). The terms are used inter-

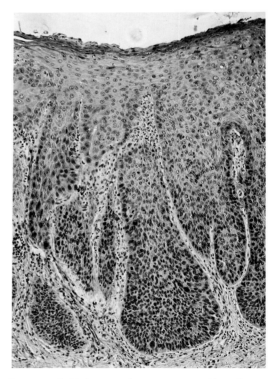

Fig. 40-16. Vulvar carcinoma in situ. Note hyperchromatic dysplastic nuclei, mitoses, and disorderly pattern in comparison with hyperkeratosis. (140×.)

changeably by most pathologists, and an accurate histologic distinction is often difficult.

Extramammary Paget's disease

Vulvar Paget's disease begins as an intraepidermal, noninvasive adenocarcinoma. The affected skin is mottled red and white, scaling, elevated, and slightly indurated. Characteristically there are small white keratotic patches separated by red fissures or irregular bands from which the superficial epidermis has exfoliated. The neoplastic cells infiltrate into adjacent epidermis. Extensive lesions may eventually spread onto the pubic area, thighs, or sacral region.

The epidermis is infiltrated by large pale adenocarcinoma cells, scattered between compressed but normal-appearing squamous epithelial cells (Fig. 40-17). The epithelium of hair follicles and apocrine sweat glands is characteristically involved. Many, but not all of the Paget cells contain stainable epithelial mucin. In ultrastructural studies various patterns of cytologic differentiation, resembling

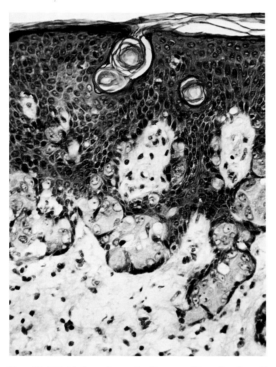

Fig. 40-17. Vulvar Paget's disease. Neoplastic cells infiltrate epidermis individually and in small clumps. Squamous cells of epidermis itself are histologically benign and compressed by tumor. There is no infiltration of underlying dermis. (260×.)

eccrine, apocrine, and squamous cell patterns have been described. It is probable that the cell of origin is very primitive and capable of differentiation into any cell type specific to the epidermis and its appendages.

If there is no invasion, the prognosis is good. Margins are difficult to see, and local recurrence is therefore common. The colposcope may refine the planning of surgical margins.

Approximately one patient in three may have an underlying tumor mass composed of infiltrating adenocarcinoma, usually poorly differentiated; foci of squamous differentiation are commonly present. In the presence of invasion, metastases are likely and the prognosis is very poor.

Adenocarcinoma and Bartholin's gland carcinoma

Adenocarcinomas of the vulva are uncommon; they may arise in Bartholin's gland or in the minor vestibular glands. The initial appearance is a subcutaneous lump. The microscopic pattern may be adenoid cystic adenocarcinoma, papillary adenocarcinoma, mucoepidermoid carcinoma, or mucinous adenocarcinoma. About one third of Bartholin's gland carcinomas are epidermoid carcinomas.

The principles of treatment are the same as for other vulvar carcinomas. Many patients are premenopausal: half of the lesions studied by Chamlian and Taylor[34] were originally underestimated as Bartholin's gland cysts. Adenoid cystic adenocarcinomas characteristically do not metastasize to lymph nodes but invade widely along nerve sheaths.

Malignant melanoma

Most are located anteriorly near the midline. The prognosis in recent years (30% 5-year survival) is less bleak than formerly. Local recurrence is usually at vaginal and urethral margins where the impulse to temporize is greatest. The bilateral distribution of lymph node metastases and surgical approach are the same as for epidermoid carcinoma.

Metastatic carcinoma

Metastatic carcinoma was the third most common malignant tumor encountered in a study by Dehner,[37] comprising 22 of 262 primary malignant neoplasms (8%). The most common primary sources are cervix and endometrium. Metastatic cancers from the colon, breast, and ovary also are found in the vulva and should not be mistaken for primary vulvar cancer.

Rare neoplasms

Instances of *fibrosarcoma, liposarcoma, leiomyosarcoma, rhabdomyosarcoma,* and *malignant lymphoma* may occur in the soft tissues of the vulva.[51] *Basal cell carcinomas* of the vulvar skin resemble those occurring in more common cutaneous locations (see Chapter 42).

VAGINA
Anatomy and physiology

The vagina is a collapsed cylinder, situated between the vestibule externally and the cervix internally. It has an inner lining of nonkeratinized squamous epithelium surrounded by a layer of connective tissue stroma, all supported by a double layer of smooth muscle.

There are no named glands, but small glandular remnants of the mesonephric ducts occasionally persist and may form cysts.

The histology and cytology of the squamous epithelium are affected by hormonal stimuli. During the reproductive years estrogens increase the thickness of the epithelium and the amount of cytoplasmic glycogen. The epithelium is thin in childhood and atrophic after menopause, when estrogen stimulation is minimal.

Cytologic patterns, as seen in the vaginal smear vary with age and undergo cyclic changes with the menstrual cycle. During the first 14 days of the menstrual cycle, a period of estrogen predominance, the exfoliated cells, called "superficial cells," are large, flattened, and have pyknotic nuclei. After ovulation, under the superimposed influence of progesterone, the nuclei are larger and vesicular, and the cell margins are folded; these are called "intermediate cells" (Fig. 40-18). The amount of cytoplasmic glycogen is greatly increased and cytoplasmic margins are dense and accentuated in pregnancy. In childhood, after menopause, and after childbirth, the mucosa is atrophic and the predominant exfoliated cells are small, round or oval parabasal cells that have very little glycogen. Small amounts of estrogen administered at these times will induce maturation to the estrogenic pattern of superficial cell predominance.

Knowledge of the normal cytologic variations is important in the identification of neoplastic cells and other pathologic states.

Cytologic manifestations of pathologic states
Endocrine disturbances

The vaginal cell population in precocious puberty shows pronounced maturation with superficial cell predominance as the result of estrogen stimulation. Exposure to any *estrogenic drug,* including estrogen-containing face creams, will have a similar effect. Digitalis is said to have an estrogenic effect upon the vaginal smear of some postmenopausal women. Death of a fetus with *inevitable abortion* results in a reversion of the pregnancy pattern to superficial cell smear of estrogen predominance.

Women taking *artificial progestogens* cyclically (the contraceptive pill) may have increased numbers of large parabasal cells or intermediate cells with very large but cytologically benign nuclei. Syndromes of ovarian dysfunction such as the Stein-Leventhal syndrome are associated with continuous exfoliation of

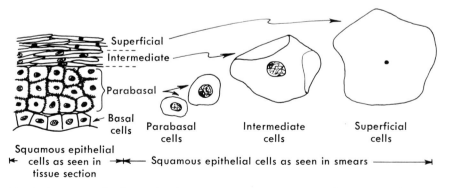

Fig. 40-18. Diagram of relationship between squamous mucosa of vagina and ectocervix, and parabasal, intermediate, and superficial cells exfoliated and seen in smears. Superficial cells predominate in estrogenic smears of first 2 weeks of menstrual cycle, and intermediate cells predominate in second 2 weeks after ovulation under influence of progesterone. (Redrawn from Frost, J. K.: Concepts basic to general cytopathology, Baltimore, Md., 1972, The Johns Hopkins Press.)

intermediate cells, without any sort of cyclic change.

Cytology of vaginal inflammation

The vaginal smears of women with active *gonorrhea* contain the typical intracellular diplococci of *Neisseria gonorrhoeae* located in the cytoplasm of polymorphonuclear leukocytes. Streptococci, staphylococci, and *Escherichia coli*, as well as a number of other bacteria, may cause vulvovaginitis. Vaginitis caused by *Haemophilus vaginalis*, is associated with malodorous leukorrhea.

The most common causes of symptomatic vaginitis are a fungus, *Candida albicans*, and a protozoan, *Trichomonas vaginalis*. Hyphae of *Candida* species, and trichomonads are easily identified in smears (Fig. 40-19). In *Trichomonas* infections the vagina has a red punctate appearance with abundant frothy discharge. Candidosis is associated in typical cases with white patches of mycelia attached to an inflamed mucosa and is more common in pregnancy and in women with diabetes.[91] The vulva and cervix are usually involved simultaneously.

The most important viral disease identifiable by vaginal cytology is herpes simplex. The infected epithelial cells form a mutinucleated syncytium, like a cluster of bubbles. Ng et al.[102] have described two types of intranuclear inclusions and found that one type with a homogeneous ground-glass appearance was more common in primary infections, whereas the typical eosinophilic inclusions surrounded by a clear zone were seen more frequently in secondary or recurrent infections (Fig. 40-20).

Cysts and nonneoplastic growths
Subepithelial cysts

Vaginitis emphysematosa is a remarkable process characterized by the presence of numerous subepithelial gas-filled cysts, which may pop audibly when traumatized (Fig. 40-21). They are essentially stromal bubbles with no epithelial lining, associated with a slight inflammatory response, including scattered giant cells. Many patients have been pregnant and a significant association with *Trichomonas* infection has been suggested.[90]

Epithelial cysts

Gartner's duct cysts of the lateral vaginal wall are lined by cuboid glandular epithelium without cytoplasmic mucin; they are considered to arise from dilated vestiges of the mesonephric ducts. *Mucinous cysts*, considered to be of paramesonephric duct origin seem to be more commonly situated near the vestibule[88] and are actually more common.[84] An occasional paramesonephric cyst contains ciliated tubal epithelium with ciliated cells.

Squamous epithelial inclusion cysts, lined by squamous epithelium and filled with keratin,

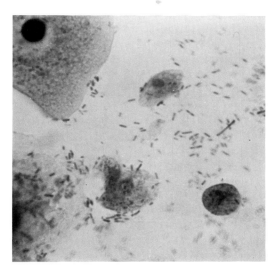

Fig. 40-19. *Trichomonas* organisms as seen in cervicovaginal smear. Organisms are above and below the center. Portion of superficial squamous cell is present at top left, indicating relative size. (1000×.)

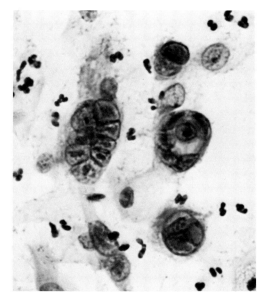

Fig. 40-20. Vaginal smears showing epithelial cells containing typical herpes simplex viral inclusions. Note syncytial clustering of nuclei. (600×.)

occur in the vaginal muosa as they do in the skin. *Endometriosis* of the vagina forms multiple blue mucosal cysts, which may even rupture and bleed during menses. The usual cause is implantation of endometrium in an incision, especially an episiotomy.

Adenosis, clear-cell carcinoma, and in utero diethylstilbestrol exposure

Adenosis in the context of vaginal pathologic conditions refers to the presence of histologi-

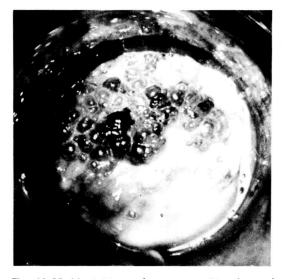

Fig. 40-21. Vaginitis emphysematosa. Vesicles and vaginal discharge as photographed through a cylindrical speculum. (From Close, J. M., and Jesurun, H. M.: Obstet. Gynecol. **19**:513-516, 1962.)

cally benign mucinous epithelium of typical endocervical pattern in an area that is normally covered by stratified squamous vaginal mucosa. The extent ranges from tiny foci 1 or 2 mm in greatest diameter to a virtual conversion of the entire vaginal lining to a surface of columnar mucous epithelium.

The affected mucosa has a reddened, velvety appearance, in contrast to the more opaque pale pink of the normal squamous mucosa (Fig. 40-22, *A*). Focal lesions require a colposcope for identification; larger patches are visible in ordinary physical examination.

The epithelium in areas of adenosis is composed of a single layer of mucinous columnar epithelial cells, but glandular crypts and slight papillary projections produce a more complicated pattern in some areas (Fig. 40-22, *B*). Occasional patches of epithelium are composed of ciliated columnar cells without mucin vacuoles, resembling tubal mucosa.[110] Some degree of squamous metaplasia is often present, beginning as a proliferation of reserve cells beneath the gland cell layer, as in the cervix; a complete conversion to a squamous epithelial lining probably occurs eventually in most cases.

Adenosis in adolescent girls received considerable notoriety after the demonstration of a causal relationship with exposure in utero to diethylstilbestrol ingested by the mother. It has been shown that the crucial period of exposure to the fetus is prior to the eighteenth week of gestation.[108]

After this time formation of the vagina is completed and susceptability to the effects of

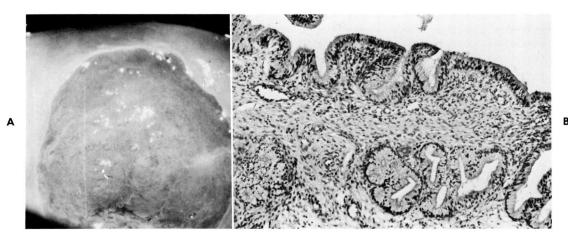

Fig. 40-22. Vaginal adenosis. **A,** Glandular mucosa covers ectocervix and adjacent vaginal mucosa in place of normal squamous epithelium. **B,** Photomicrograph of abnormal epithelium shown in **A.** Epithelial surface is covered by columnar mucinous epithelium, thrown into tiny clefts and folds. (**B,** 150×; **A** and **B,** courtesy Dr. James G. Blythe, St. Louis, Mo.)

diethylstilbestrol is apparently lost. Adenosis may also occur in the mucosa of the portio vaginalis of the cervix. About one third of the patients have an anomalous ridge or "hood" of muscular connective tissue surrounding the cervix. Forsberg[87] has produced identical lesions experimentally in neonatal mice with diethylstilbestrol.

The incidence of adenosis in diethylstilbestrol-exposed infants is probably very high, if minute areas are searched for carefully with a colposcope. A much more significant but fortunately less common association is clear-cell adenocarcinoma of the vagina and cervix.[94,95] Both the mucinous epithelium of adenosis and the clear-cell adenocarcinomas are probably of müllerian duct origin.

Neoplasms
Benign tumors

Fibroepithelial polyp (stromal polyp). The subepithelial connective tissue of the vagina may form single or multiple polypoid masses, covered by orderly vaginal squamous mucosa. This stroma characteristically has a loose myxoid appearance, interspersed with giant cells (Fig. 40-23). Benign polyps lack the subepithelial crowded zone of proliferating immature cells found in sarcoma botryoides, and they are found in young adults, especially during pregnancy.[85,104] Rarely there is a component of mucinous epithelial glands intermixed with the stroma.

Leiomyoma. The most common benign connective tumor of the vagina is leiomyoma, and even these are rare. Bennet and Ehrlich[81] found 12 in a series of 50,000 gynecologic le-

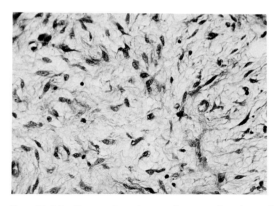

Fig. 40-23. Connective tissue of stromal polyp of vagina has loose myxoid appearance. Cells are spindle shaped or stellate and may be multinucleated. (260×.)

sions. The morphologic features are like those of more common uterine leiomyomas.

Other benign tumors. Other benign tumors include neurofibroma and neurilemoma. A benign *cystic teratoma* has also been reported.[98]

Occasionally after hysterectomy, the *tubal fimbria* may herniate into the vaginal apex, simulating a neoplasm.[111] *Granulation tissue,* which may contain rapidly proliferating blood vessel sprouts can produce sizable lumps at the vaginal apex after surgery.

Malignant tumors

Most cancers encountered in the vaginal wall are metastatic. According to the definition adopted by the International Federation of Gynecology and Obstetrics, a lesion that extends to the cervical os is classified as a cancer of the cervix and a lesion that extends to the vulva is designated a vulvar carcinoma. The remaining true primary vaginal carcinomas comprise slightly less than 1% of female genital cancers.

Over 95% of vaginal cancers are epidermoid carcinomas; of these, 10% have not invaded and are called in situ carcinomas. The remaining 5% is composed of adenocarcinomas, malignant melanomas, and sarcomas.

Epidermoid carcinoma in situ. It is uncommon to find carcinoma in situ first in the vagina. In most instances there has been a prior or concurrent carcinoma, either in situ or invasive located in the cervix or vulva.

The histologic and colposcopic features are identical to epidermoid carcinoma of the cervix. If there is no invasion, local excision of involved areas is adequate treatment; the use of a colposcope is a useful and important way to identify all areas of involvement and their margins. An associated carcinoma of the vulva or cervix, or both, is highly probable and must be excluded before therapy is planned.

Vaginal carcinoma in situ may appear ten or more years after treatment of carcinoma in situ of the cervix or vulva. The prognosis for in situ lesions is good even if superficial invasion is present,[107] a fact that emphasizes the importance of continued cytologic follow-up of women treated for carcinoma of the cervix or vulva.

Invasive epidermoid carcinoma. Most invasive vaginal epidermoid carcinomas are indurated, ulcerated nodules; a few are elevated, soft, and papillary. The histologic pattern is commonly (about 50%) moderately differentiated, without keratinization.[106] Well and moderately differentiated carcinomas with keratinization account for about 15% each, and the rest are poorly differentiated, without keratinization. Moderately differentiated keratinizing lesions with large anaplastic nuclei seemed to be more aggressive, in the series studied by Perez et al.[106] Most patients are elderly postmenopausal women; the usual location is the upper posterior vaginal wall. Significant etiologic factors have not been identified. Lesions of the distal vagina may metastasize to inguinal lymph nodes.

For purposes of evaluating the prognosis and comparing the results of treatment the extent of spread is classified by stages, according to criteria agreed upon by the International Federation of Gynecology and Obstetrics as follows:

Stage 0 Carcinoma in situ
Stage I Limited to vaginal wall
Stage II Involving subvaginal tissue without extension to pelvic wall
Stage III Extension to pelvic wall
Stage IV Extension beyond true pelvis or to mucosa of bladder or rectum

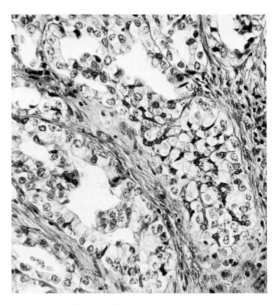

Fig. 40-24. Clear-cell carcinoma arising in adenosis of vagina of young woman exposed to diethylstilbestrol in utero. Tumor cells contain glycogen but not mucin. (300×; courtesy Dr. Robert E. Scully, Boston, Mass.)

Radiation therapy has been selected for most patients; about 75% of those with stage I disease survive for 5 years. Unfortunately less than one third of the patients have stage I lesions; less than half of the patients of all stages survive for 5 years.

Metastatic cancer. The most frequent primary source of metastatic carcinoma in the vagina is the uterine cervix, often by direct extension. Carcinomas of the urinary bladder, rectum, vulva, urethra, or anus may infiltrate directly into the vagina. Embolic metastases from the endometrium, ovary, kidney, breast, or intestinal tract occur less frequently. The first evidence for choriocarcinoma may be a vaginal metastasis.

Adenocarcinoma. Adenocarcinomas of the vagina are rare.

Clear-cell adenocarcinoma associated with adenosis in adolescent girls exposed in utero to diethylstilbestrol or its derivatives (see above) is at this time the most frequently encountered pattern. Similar tumors also occur rarely in older women not exposed to diethylstilbestrol. The tumors are usually superficial and either papillary or nodular. Most have been located in the upper or middle third, primarily on the anterior wall.

The histologic pattern, like that of clear-cell carcinomas found elsewhere in the female genitalia, is composed of tubules or small cysts, with inconspicuous stroma (Fig. 40-24). The tumor cells are large, with variable degrees of nuclear anaplasia. There is abundant clear cytoplasm, containing much glycogen and no mucin; there may be some intraluminal mucin. The nuclei of cells lining cystic spaces may protrude into the lumens; the cells are separated and produce a pattern that is said to resemble hobnails in a boot.

Vaginal adenosis has been found in almost all cases. Factors associated with recurrence and poor prognosis are large size, proximity to resection margins, and penetration more than 3 mm into the wall of the vagina.[108] A total of 300 cases have been accumulated.

Mucinous adenocarcinomas also occur in the vagina. Although usually very well differentiated, they are characteristically aggressive and may metastasize widely. Some tumors of this type have been associated with adenosis[109]; these lesions occurred in older women whose birth dates preceded any possibility of diethylstilbestrol exposure in utero.

Embryonal rhabdomyosarcoma (sarcoma botryoides). This malignant tumor of very undifferentiated muscle cells tends to produce ovoid masses that protrude into the vagina, covered by normal epithelium (Fig. 40-25). There is a "cambium" zone of very immature round or spindle cells crowded beneath the

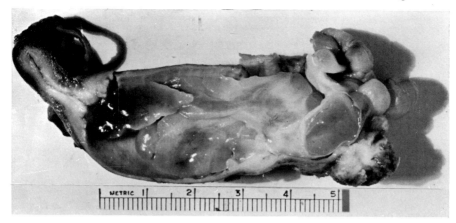

Fig. 40-25. Embryonal rhabdomyosarcoma of vagina (sarcoma botryoides), seen in sagittal section. Tumor arose in and filled vagina of a 16-month-old infant and invaded adjacent pelvic tissues including base urinary bladder. (Courtesy Dr. Sidney Farber, Boston, Mass.)

epithelium, and it contrasts with the looser, more myxoid pattern of the central core. The cambium layer is seen best in smaller polyps.

Most of the patients are infants; 90% are under age 5. After puberty there is an overwhelming probability that a polypoid lesion with myxoid-appearing stroma is a benign stromal polyp (p. 1691). Embryonal rhabdomyosarcoma has a predilection for the anterior vaginal wall and tends to invade extensively in the pelvis and metastasize to regional lymph nodes and distant sites such as lung and liver.[96] Most instances of successful treatment have resulted from early diagnosis and radical surgery. Similar tumors may arise also in the orbit, urinary bladder, external auditory canal, and biliary tract. There is probably no relationship to malignant mixed müllerian tumor; heterologous elements, such as bone or cartilage, and glandular components have been absent in nearly all cases reported.[96]

Distinctive adenocarcinoma of infant vagina (endodermal sinus tumor). This tumor arises as multiple polypoid masses, resembling the botryoid gross appearance of embryonal rhabdomyosarcoma. The histologic pattern is identical to that of a type of germ cell carcinoma that has been called the endodermal sinus tumor, arising in the ovary (see Fig. 40-75) or infant testis.[103] The prognosis has been poor, although promising results have been reported with chemotherapy.[80]

Other neoplasms. Rare instances of leiomyosarcoma[100] and malignant melanoma[105] have been reported. The pathologic features do not differ significantly from those of similar lesions in more common locations.

CERVIX
Anatomy and physiology

The distal third of the adult uterus is channeled by a central endocervical canal that communicates superiorly, at an ill-defined *internal os* with the endometrial cavity and inferiorly through an equally ill-defined *external os* with the vagina. The endocervical canal is lined by a single layer of tall columnar mucin-producing cells. The endocervical mucosa is thrown into redundant longitudinally oriented folds, separated by clefts. Opposing walls of clefts tend to fuse in an irregular manner, forming irregular tunnels that may reenter the endocervical canal or end blindly. These grooves and tunnels may produce an intricate pattern on cross section and are commonly referred to as "glands"; in fact, they represent extensions of the endocervical mucosa.

The physical properties of the cervical mucus vary during the menstrual cycle. After menses the mucus is at first viscous and sticky; under the influence of estrogen it becomes thin, glossy, and permeable to spermatozoa; when it dries on a glass slide the sodium chloride crystallizes in delicate arborizing patterns (fern test). After ovulation and in pregnancy, as progesterone predominates, this crystallization is inhibited.

The portio vaginalis is part of the cervical mucosa exposed to the vagina; these surfaces are covered by stratified squamous epithelium, which is resistant to infection. Variable areas of exposed cervical mucosa may be covered by glandular endocervical mucosa at birth ("congenital erosion"). Of greater significance

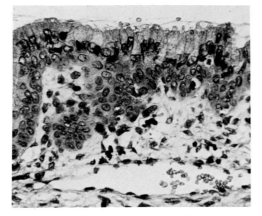

Fig. 40-26. Squamous metaplasia of cervix begins by proliferation of reserve cells beneath columnar epithelium. This new layer thickens, keratinizes, and will become a squamous mucosal surface when surface gland cells ultimately are sloughed away. (300×.)

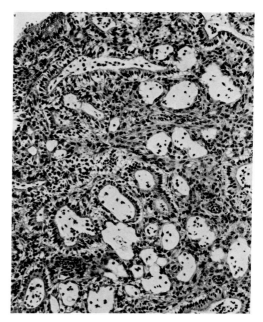

Fig. 40-27. Microglandular hyperplasia of cervix has complicated pattern produced by many small glandular spaces surrounded by immature proliferating reserve cells and squamous epithelial cells intermixed with inflammatory cells and strands of fibrous stroma. This pattern should not be confused with a neoplasm. (150×.)

is the fact that cervical reconstitution and healing after parturition leaves variable areas of endocervical glandular surfaces everted into the vagina and exposed to its contents. Such areas of *eversion* appear red and have been called "erosions." This expression is misleading because the mucosal layer is actually intact; glandular mucosa is transparent and the visible underlying vessels give a red color.

The exposed glandular surfaces are less resistant to infections of all kinds; a discharge is common, and the subepithelial layers are infiltrated by chronic inflammatory cells. The resulting *chronic cervicitis* is the invariable experience of women with a normal reproductive life.

Squamous metaplasia (squamous prosoplasia). The normal response to eversion is the gradual conversion of exposed glandular epithelium to squamous epithelium. Local factors such as pH and estrogen[143] stimulate the proliferation of an underlying layer of *reserve cells* that eventually forms a multilayered covering several cells thick (Fig. 40-26). The surface gland cells slough away to leave mature stratified squamous epithelium. The area involved in these changes is called the *transition zone*.

Hyperkeratosis. The squamous epithelium of the portio vaginalis may develop a thick surface layer of keratin, especially in patients with uterine prolapse. Biopsy is important especially if the process is patchy, for some well-differentiated carcinomas may have a similar appearance. The keratotic process is itself benign, as in the vulva.

Microglandular hyperplasia. A very characteristic pattern of gland cell hyperplasia occurs in young women taking oral contraceptives.[157,185] The larger lesions are polypoid. They are formed of masses of small endocervical gland cells intermixed with reserve cells in an early stage of squamous metaplasia producing an intricate but recognizable pattern (Fig. 40-27) that should never be confused with carcinoma. Similar changes occur in pregnancy. Less commonly, gland cells with large, dark, but cytologically benign polyploid nuclei may be found. This change is analogous to the secretory gestational hyperplasia described in the endometrium by Arias-Stella[195] (see p. 1710). At this time there is no evidence that birth control pills have any direct carcinogenic effect on the cervix.[190]

Vestigial and heterotopic structures

Vestiges of the mesonephric ducts commonly persist in the lateral walls of the cervix and occasionally produce sizable collections. These are distinguished from well-differentiated cervical adenocarcinoma by the absence of cytoplasmic mucin and benign cytologic pattern. A few sizable mesonephric cysts have been reported.[179]

Roth and Taylor[173] described heterotopic hyaline cartilage in the cervix. Benign stromal polyps containing well-differentiated skeletal muscle, like those described in the vagina,[129] also occur on the cervix. In most instances it is possible to show that apparent heterotopic tissues are the result of implantation of aborted fetal tissues.[122,162] Endometriosis of the cervix may appear as one or more blue hemorrhagic nodules or blisters on the portio vaginalis.

The startling occurrence of sebaceous glands, hair, and sweat glands[189] is harder to explain in this mesodermal organ. Similar "Fordyce spots" occurred in the mouth of the patient described by Watson and Cochran.[187]

Inflammation

Acute cervicitis may be associated with an acute gonococcal infection, or in puerperal sepsis. Caustic substances used as abortifacients, such as potassium permanganate, produce extensive ulceration and hemorrhage. Occasionally a primary chancre will be biopsied to exclude carcinoma. Acute cervicitis occurs also with herpes simplex infection; the characteristic multinucleated cells and intranuclear viral inclusions are only infrequently demonstrated. Ulcerated lesions may resemble cancer on visual inspection. The clinical and pathologic features have been beautifully illustrated by Kaufman[149] and by Naib.[160] The relationship between herpes simplex infections and cervical cancer is discussed on p. 1705.

Chronic cervicitis is so common in sexually active women that the term is essentially useless as an informative pathologic diagnosis. Characteristically the everted endocervical mucosa may have a slightly papillary appearance, and the stroma is infiltrated by lymphocytes and plasma cells. The epithelium is intact and usually some degree of squamous metaplasia is in progress, at least focally.

Exotic inflammatory lesions. Amebiasis may cause painful ulcerative lesions in the cervix and vagina.[133] Schistosomiasis is common in some parts of Africa[125]; the finding of calcified ova in the stroma is characteristic. The tiny vessels in which they are lodged may be difficult to identify in most histologic preparations.

Polyps and papillomas

Endocervical polyps represent the growth of redundant folds of endocervical mucosa, including both stroma and epithelium. There is often squamous metaplasia of the epithelium, especially at the tip. Much of the substance of the polyp may be the result of cystic dilatation of endocervical glands.

Stromal polyps of the cervix resemble those already described in the vagina (p. 1691).

Condyloma acuminatum may occur on the cervix, nearly always in association with multiple similar lesions of the vulva, vagina, and perianal area.

Coxcomb polyps occur but rarely in the transitional zone of the cervix in pregnancy. They are often papillary, covered by moderately or even severely dysplastic-looking squamous epithelium, and regress spontaneously after delivery.

True papilloma is described by Hertig and Gore[51] as an extremely rare lesion that may be potentially malignant. The histologic appearance is essentially indistinguishable from coxcomb polyp.

Neoplasms
Benign tumors

Leiomyomas of the cervix resemble those described below in the myometrium. They may cause cervical stenosis with secondary pyometra or hematometra. The occasional polypoid smooth muscle mass with an admixture of endocervical or endometrial glands and stroma is called an *adenomyoma*.

Rarely a glandular papilloma, said to be of mesonephric duct origin, has been described in children.[148] The stroma is inconspicuous and the epithelial component is cytologically benign. *Hemangiomas* include the cervix in their ubiquitous distribution; the cervix itself is very vascular and many reported "hemangiomas" are nothing more than a conspicuous demonstration of local vascularity.

Dysplasia, carcinoma in situ, microinvasion, and pathogenesis of epidermoid carcinoma of cervix

In some women the sequence of repair by squamous metaplasia in the transition zone does not proceed in an orderly manner to form mature stratified squamous epithelium. Instead the proliferating epithelial surface contains many cells that resemble carcinoma cells. These abnormal cells are confined to the surface epithelium and do not invade the stroma. There is at this time a consensus that an intraepithelial lesion, carcinoma in situ, is an important stage in the development of invasive epidermoid carcinoma of the cervix. An estimated 40,000 new cases are diagnosed and treated annually in the United States.[181]

Definitions

The term *dysplasia* indicates that many but not all of the cells resemble cancer cells; it is possible to recognize a sequence of maturation from basal layer to surface, although it may be very disorderly (Fig. 40-28).

The term *carcinoma in situ* indicates that all of the cells in the affected area from basement membrane to surface resemble cancer cells (Fig. 40-29), and they tend to resemble one another. Both dysplasia and carcinoma in situ occur within endocervical glandular crypts; such a locus may represent a separate focus of involvement but is not evidence for invasion or that the process is more aggressive.

Although there is general agreement about the definitions of dysplasia and carcinoma in situ,[145] the histologic distinction between the two is necessarily subjective. Complete agreement among a group of pathologists will occur in about 65% of the cases they examine.[151]

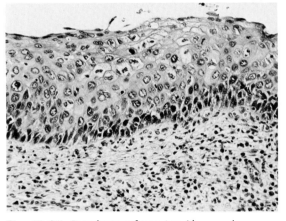

Fig. 40-28. Dysplasia of cervix. Abnormal squamous epithelial cells appear anaplastic, but they vary considerably in size and shape and have a relatively abundant amount of cytoplasm. Sequence of maturation is evident as the surface is approached. (150×.)

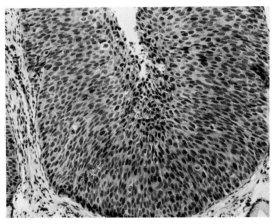

Fig. 40-29. Carcinoma in situ of cervix. Abnormal cells have a more uniform size and shape, relatively scant cytoplasm, and sequence of maturation is lost. (130×.)

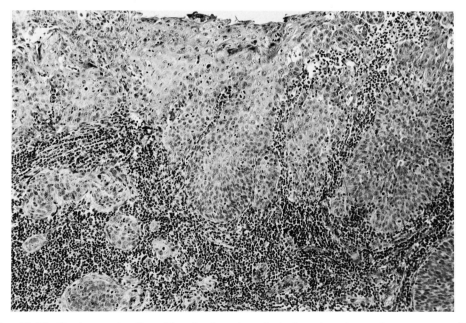

Fig. 40-30. Carcinoma in situ with microinvasion. Early invasive clumps have a more differentiated appearance with more abundant cytoplasm. Prominent inflammatory infiltrate in adjacent stroma is characteristic. (130×.)

A *microinvasive carcinoma* is a small carcinoma that has invaded the cervical stroma to a limited extent. The maximum allowable depth of penetration and how to measure it are debated; a majority of reports favor a limit of 5 mm.[126,132,159,164] Measurement from the surface of the lesion to the point of maximum penetration gives the most reproducible figure in most cases.[159]

The earliest invasive changes have the appearance of tiny irregular sprouts of neoplastic epithelial cells projecting into the cervical stroma, usually beneath an area of carcinoma in situ (Fig. 40-30). The cells at the interface between infiltrating epithelium and stroma appear more differentiated, have more cytoplasm, and are often degenerated. The adjacent stroma is infiltrated by lymphocytes and plasma cells. No metastases or deaths from such lesions have been reliably documented.

Small confluent growths composed of nests of invasive epidermoid carcinoma cells in the cervical stroma deserve to be classified separately as *occult invasive carcinoma,* even if they are only 1 to 2 mm in diameter, because intravascular emboli occur and metastases to lymph nodes have been demonstrated, rarely with a fatal outcome.[126] The presence of histologically apparent involvement of lymphatic spaces did not correlate with demonstrable lymph node metastases in 30 cases studied by Roche and Norris.[172] It is rare to find lymph node metastases in radical hysterectomy specimens that include nodes,[159] and long-term follow-up after simple hysterectomy has shown favorable results in nearly every case.[132]

Pathogenesis

Studies of epidemiology, viral culture, cytogenetics, marker enzymes, and tumor-specific immune response have added many dimensions to our understanding of the biology of carcinoma in situ and its relationship to invasive carcinoma of the cervix.

Cytogenetic studies have shown that dysplastic cells not only look different but have profoundly altered chromosomes. A relatively small proportion of cells from dysplasia of the cervix show this change.[150] Both the number of chromosomes and their appearance vary widely among the abnormal cells; there is no consistent pattern in the genetic derangement.

In contrast, many or most of the cells from an area of carcinoma in situ are cytogenetically abnormal, and furthermore the abnormal genetic patterns, though not identical, tend to be similar in a sizable proportion of the cells. Apparently, an aggressive strain of cells (modal group) has emerged and managed to proliferate more rapidly than do other cell types.

One or more modal groups are characteristically present in carcinoma in situ; in microinvasive carcinoma there is usually a single modal group. Marker chromosomes having a distinctive and recognizable shape are also often present in early invasive lesions.[184b] This suggests that all the affected cells are closely related, possibly members of a clone originating from a single cell.

Radioautographic studies of epithelium incubated with tritiated thymidine confirm increased DNA replication in large numbers of cells scattered throughout the epithelium.[177] Replication normally occurs only in the parabasal cells in the nonneoplastic cervical epithelium. The most striking increases in DNA replication occur in areas of early "budding" areas of microinvasion.[175]

The ultrastructure of the cells of dysplasia and carcinoma in situ is similar. Nuclei are enlarged, with more irregular profiles than those of normal squamous cell nuclei. At the cell surface, microvilli are more numerous, whereas desmosomes and tonofibrils are decreased in size and numbers. Mitochondria remain numerous even in surface layers, there are many free ribosomes, and the glycogen accumulation normally found in surface cells does not occur. These changes together reflect increased metabolic activities in the individual cells and decreased organization and surface maturation of the epithelium as a whole.[180]

Epidemiologic analyses of large populations of women with carcinoma of the cervix indicate that a considerable increase in risk is associated with early and promiscuous sexual activity, especially involving multiple partners.[124,174] This observation prompted a search for a venereally transmissible etiologic factor. A variety of possible pathogenic agents have been investigated, including spermatozoa, mycoplasma, and various other organisms.[118]

Virologic and immunologic studies of women with in situ and invasive cervical cancer implicate *herpesvirus 2* as the most promising etiologic agent. Antibodies to herpesvirus 2 are present in the sera of women with cervical carcinoma more often than in controls; furthermore the titers are higher and the high titers appear at an earlier age.[170] Membrane antigens extracted from cervical carcinoma cells seem to be specific markers for the presence of the virus genome in the tumor cells.[147] Aurelian[120] has shown that latent virus can be unmasked from cultured cervical cancer cells and that 90% of patients with cervical cancer have antibody to a virus-specific antigen (AG-4) that is not found in controls or in successfully treated patients. Even inactivated herpes virus seems to have the capacity to transform cells in vitro.[169] Ultimately, viral hydridization methods should provide the most conclusive evidence implicating herpes virus as the most important cause of carcinoma of the cervix.[142]

Immunopathology. Epidermoid carcinoma of the cervix, like other cancers, produces circulating tumor-specific antigens, and pa-

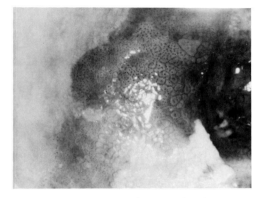

Fig. 40-31. Colposcopic photograph of carcinoma in situ of cervix. This mosaic pattern and accentuated punctate vessels emphasized against a background of opaque whitened epithelium are characteristic. (Courtesy Dr. James G. Blythe, St. Louis, Mo.)

tients form antibodies to them.[158] Circulating antigens appear before invasion occurs. Cell-mediated immune response is unimpaired,[131] and lymphocytes of patients with cervical carcinoma are sensitized to epidermoid carcinoma cells and can destroy them in vitro.[137] Using a specific erythrocyte absorption test, Davidsohn et al.[135] have shown that A, B, and H blood-group surface antigens normally also found in squamous epithelium are lost or masked in invasive and metastatic epidermoid carcinomas.

Colposcopy. The use of a magnifying instrument, the colposcope, has remarkably improved the accuracy of physical diagnosis of lesions of the cervix.[58,134] Based chiefly upon differences in vascular pattern, distinctions can be made between squamous metaplasia, dysplasia, carcinoma in situ, and early invasive carcinoma (Figs. 40-31 and 40-32). Used in conjunction with cytology, biopsy, and conization, the colposcope has significantly improved the accuracy of diagnosis and the effectiveness of local treatment.[130,134,186]

Clinical significance of dysplasia and carcinoma in situ of cervix

Opinions about the significance of carcinoma in situ of the cervix vary widely. The name implies a threat of death, poised, yet momentarily held in check. The usual management, hysterectomy, is usually swiftly applied.

Dysplasia, left undisturbed, may progress to carcinoma in situ.[171] If there is no intervention of any sort, the observed conversion of dys-

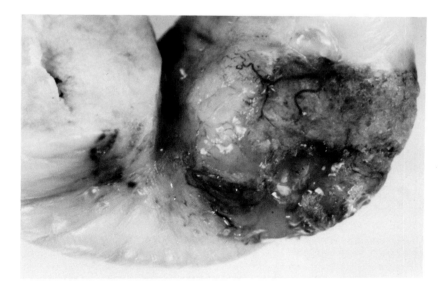

Fig. 40-32. Invasive carcinoma of cervix. Dark granular appearance and abnormal blood vessels running over surface of lesion are features of an invasive process.

plasia and carcinoma in situ to invasive carcinoma is nearly constant: 21% in 5 years, 28% in 10 years, 33% in 15 years, and 38% in 20 years.[184a] However, local treatment in the form of conization or cautery effectively interrupts the process in a high percentage of patients.[130,144,156,186] Residual in situ carcinoma has been identified in as many as one third of the patients in hysterectomy specimens obtained after cervical conization.[178] Those who require more extensive treatment can be identified by colposcopy and cytology, if one assumes that meticulous follow-up examinations will be carried out. Prospective studies designed to show the best form of treatment have not been carried out.[151] In a carefully conducted long-term study of 1121 women with carcinoma in situ, subsequent invasive carcinoma was found in 2.1% of those treated by hysterectomy and in 0.9% of those treated only by conization.[152] The popularity of hysterectomy may be related to the fact that it solves other problems.

The screening of large populations of women has identified hundreds of women with carcinoma in situ, as well as early invasive carcinomas. Treatment of the lesion at this stage has considerably reduced the number of women with advanced cervical cancer, for which treatment is much less effective, and improved survival.[132]

On the other hand, there is a definite but apparently small group of invasive cervical carcinomas that originate from the basal layer of histologically normal squamous epithelium. There may be no detectable surface abnormality at any point in the cervix, until (presumably) the lesion ulcerates, sloughing the surface and exposing the cancer lurking beneath.[161] Approximately 10% to 15% of cervical carcinomas may arise in this manner.[115]

Adenocarcinoma in situ. This rare lesion is characterized by replacement of the gland cells of endocervical mucosa and its crypts by cytologically malignant gland cells. The columnar pattern is usually retained, but the basal polarity of the nuclei is lost, the cytoplasmic mucin is replaced by amphophilic cytoplasm, and the nuclei have malignant cytologic features. If involved gland-space outlines resemble those lined by normal epithelium in the same cervix, and if only part of the gland-space lining is affected, it is reasonable to conclude that stromal invasion has not occurred. Associated epidermoid carcinoma in situ is often present. The histologic pattern has been extensively illustrated by Burghardt.[128] In nearly every case, the lesion is discovered when malignant gland cells are found in the cervical cytologic smear.[168] Mixed adenosquamous carcinoma in situ is rare.[184d]

Invasive carcinoma of cervix

In contrast to the remarkable increase in the numbers of women treated for in situ carcinoma of the cervix, it was estimated that the number of patients with invasive cervical carcinoma had decreased to 19,000 in 1975, from more than 20,000 in 1970. After several decades as the most common gynecologic cancer, cervical carcinoma is now encountered less often than endometrial carcinoma, which has increased to first place in many institutions in the United States.[181]

Gross appearance

Cervical carcinomas large enough to be visible and palpable have one of three growth patterns, sometimes in combination. The *ulcerating* type has an infiltrative pattern of growth that eventually becomes necrotic in the center and sloughs, leaving a cavity surrounded by invasive cancer. The *exophytic type* is often papillary and may form a bulky mass of considerable size while still confined to the superficial portions of the cervix. The *nodular type* originates typically in the endocervix forming multiple firm masses that expand the cervix and isthmus. The mass may be large, and when it is distributed circumferentially, it has been called the barrel-shaped cervix. The gross relationships are important clinically because they affect the placement of radioactive sources used in treatment.

Clinical stage

The extent of involvement of the cervix and pelvic tissues is determined by physical examination. The clinical staging of extent of disease must be determined prior to beginning treatment. It is in part the basis of selection of the best treatment for the patient and forms the standard for comparison of results of treatment of large groups of patients.

Definitions of the different clinical stages in carcinoma of the cervix uteri, as established by the Cancer Committee of the International Federation of Gynecology and Obstetrics[153]:

Stage 0 Carcinoma in situ, intraepithelial carcinoma.

Stage I Carcinoma strictly confined to the cervix (extension to the corpus should be disregarded).
  a. Microinvasive carcinoma (early stromal invasion).
  b. All other cases of stage I. Occult cancer should be marked *Occ*.

Stage II The carcinoma extends beyond the cer-

vix but has not extended on to the pelvic wall. The carcinoma involves the vagina, but not the lower third.
  a. No obvious parametrial involvement.
  b. Obvious parametrial involvement.

Stage III The carcinoma has extended to the pelvic wall. On rectal examination there is no cancer-free space between the tumor and the pelvic wall. The tumor involves the lower third of the vagina. There is presence of hydronephrosis or nonfunctioning kidney.
  a. No extension to the pelvic wall.
  b. Extension to the pelvic wall and/or hydronephrosis or nonfunctioning kidney.

Stage IV The carcinoma has extended beyond the true pelvis or has involved the mucosa of the bladder or rectum. A bullous edema as such does not permit a case to be alloted to stage IV.
  a. Spread to adjacent organs.
  b. Spread to distant organs.

Microscopic appearance

The majority of cervical carcinomas, about 80%, are epidermoid carcinoma; adenocarcinomas comprise about 10%, and the remainder is a variety of unusual adenocarcinoma patterns or mixtures.[115]

Epidermoid carcinoma. A moderately differentiated nonkeratinizing large cell *epidermoid carcinoma* is the most common pattern (70%) and in some series, at least, has the best prognosis (Fig. 40-33). Well-differentiated *keratinizing epidermoid carcinoma* occurs less frequently (25%); *small-cell undifferentiated carcinoma* is uncommon (about 5%) and has a distinctly poor prognosis.[163]

Adenocarcinoma. Although they are much less common than epidermoid carcinoma, the proportion of cervical carcinomas arising from gland cells doubled in the decade from 1960 to 1970.[115,116] The patterns vary from a well-differentiated mucinous adenocarcinoma (Fig. 40-34), sometimes papillary, to a clear-cell pattern containing glycogen but no mucin. A mixed *adenosquamous* carcinoma apparently arises from subcolumnar reserve cells capable of both squamous and gland cell differentiation.

Spread of carcinoma of cervix

It is important to recognize simultaneous involvement of cervix and endometrium because this distribution affects principles of treatment; the prognosis is not so good as that for carcinoma limited to the cervix. Hysterectomy, with radiation therapy, improves results, probably because the more extensive distribution of some lesions interferes with the spatial arrangement of intrauterine radiation sources.

Carcinoma of the cervix spreads by direct extension into contiguous tissues, through lymphatics to regional lymph nodes, and less often by blood vessel invasion to embolize throughout the body. Because of their close anatomic relationship to the cervix, the ureters may be obstructed; secondary hydronephrosis, pyelonephritis, and renal failure remain the most common cause of death.[123] Distant metastases to lungs and liver are found in about 25% of fatal cases at autopsy. In patients dying of cancer of the cervix, central pelvic recurrences are more common after surgery and distant metastases are more common after radiation therapy.[123] Less than 2% of patients with stage I or IIa carcinoma of the cervix treated by megavoltage radiation therapy with adequate dosage and distribution of the radiation will develop central pelvic recurrence.[166]

Local recurrence occurs in 5% of patients with stage IIb disease, 7.5% in stage IIIa, and 17% in stage IIIb. Over half of the distant metastases become evident within the first year after treatment, and 95% have appeared by the end of the fifth year after treatment. Because most of the patients without evidence of cancer 5 years after treatment die of unrelated causes, this follow-up period is customarily used in evaluating effectiveness of therapy.

Rare tumors

Verrucous carcinoma, an extremely well differentiated form of epidermoid carcinoma, resembles and behaves like the same lesion in the vulva. *Clear-cell* adenocarcinomas identical to those described in the vagina (p. 1700) also occur occasionally in the cervix after in utero exposure to diethylstilbestrol. This pattern of adenocarcinoma has also been called "mesonephroma"; in fact, origin from mesonephric remnants is rarely if ever demonstrable. Very rarely a cervical adenocarcinoma may have a histologic pattern identical to *adenoid cystic carcinoma,* a highly specific lesion more common in the salivary gland. The prognosis is poor.[141] An extremely *well differentiated mucinous adenocarcinoma* may be very difficult to recognize because the epithelial pattern closely resembles benign endocervical epithelium even in metastases. If one assumes that there is adequate treatment, the prognosis is probably the same as that of any adenocarcinoma at the same stage.[182]

Malignant mixed müllerian tumors, carcinosarcomas, and *leiomyosarcomas* of the cervix resemble those occurring in the endometrium

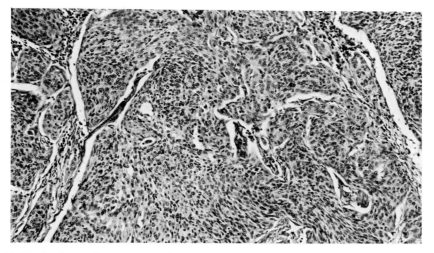

Fig. 40-33. Epidermoid carcinoma of cervix. This poorly differentiated nonkeratinizing pattern is most common histologic type. (150×.)

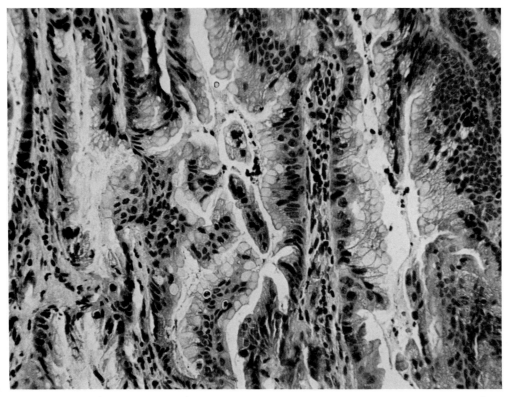

Fig. 40-34. Well-differentiated adenocarcinoma of cervix. Cytologic pattern appears deceptively benign, but bridges formed by epithelial cells without stromal support identify lesion as a carcinoma. (275×.)

(p. 1718) and share the same unfavorable prognosis.[117]

Metastatic adenocarcinoma in the cervix is not common, but one should not mistake it for a primary lesion, thereby exposing the patient to a lengthy, painful, and expensive treatment that would be inappropriate. A cervical metastasis is usually the harbinger of rapid dissemination and death. The most common primary sites have been ovary, colon, and breast.[116,136]

ENDOMETRIUM

The function of the normal endometrium is to produce a satisfactory substrate in which a healthy blastocyst may implant and flourish. Many of the pathologic changes that occur in the endometrium reflect its responsiveness either to hormonal stimulation or the lack of it.

Normal cyclic changes

The endometrial cycle starts with a phase of proliferation for about 14 days under the influence of estrogen. If ovulation occurs, it then undergoes prominent secretory changes for the next 7 days in time for implantation if the ovum has been fertilized. If not, the secretion wanes slowly during the following 7 days, after which the endometrium sloughs away and the whole cycle begins anew.

The histologic, ultrastructural, and histochemical changes of the endometrial cycle have been reviewed in detail by Noyes,[240] Ferenczy and Richart,[213] and Boutselis,[202] respectively. By convention, the first day of a cycle begins with the onset of menstrual flow, which results from ischemic necrosis of the inner layer of the endometrial stroma. The denuded surface heals after about 4 days. Under the influence of estrogen the stromal cells and endometrial gland cells proliferate rapidly (Fig. 40-35, *A*). The associated histochemical events are related chiefly to protein synthesis; RNA, glucose-6-phosphatase, alkaline phosphatase, β-glucuronidase, and nonspecific esterase are especially abundant.

After ovulation, under the influence of progesterone, there is a rise in enzymes related to carbohydrate synthesis. Lactic dehydrogenase, glucose-6-phosphate dehydrogenase, and isocitric, succinic, and malic dehydrogenases are active as increasing amounts of glycogen become evident in the gland cells.

The morphologic changes related to secretion follow a distinctive sequence. Thirty-six hours after ovulation prominent basal vacuolation appears in the glandular epithelial cells,

representing an accumulation of glycogen (Fig. 40-35, *B*). Ultrastructural studies have related the appearance of a unique and specific nucleolar channel system to ovulation. It is seen in endometrium on the sixteenth day and for several days thereafter.[213,253] Giant mitochondria with tubular cristae also appear and increase in numbers in step with the secretory process.[198] During the next 3 days secretion increases, occupying the entire cytoplasmic mass. Coincident with the time of implantation (day 20 or 21), abundant edema is present in the stroma (Fig. 40-35, *C*). If implantation does not occur, there follows a progressive decrease in secretion and stromal edema, as the activity of the corpus luteum wanes. During the 2 or 3 days before menses, cytoplasmic secretion is exhausted and stromal cells undergo a predecidual reaction, i.e., become progressively plump and prominent, especially around the spiral arterioles and beneath the surface epithelium (Fig. 40-35, *D*). On the twenty-eighth day of a typical cycle the spiral arterioles contract, the stroma crumbles, and menstrual bleeding and expulsion of the functional endometrial lining occurs.

If implantation occurs, the presence of a gestation is reflected in the endometrial pattern by the twenty-fifth day, 3 days before the next period of bleeding is expected to begin. Hertig[219] has shown that this early gestational hyperplastic pattern is a highly characteristic combination of recrudescence of glandular secretion and accentuation of stromal edema, together with normal predecidual reaction and increased vascular prominence. A distinctive pattern of gestational glandular hyperplasia, emphasized by Arias-Stella,[195] especially in ectopic pregnancy and in abortions, is formed by masses of enlarged gland cells with abundant clear cytoplasm and large bizarre nuclei; there is no decidual reaction in the intervening stroma.

The importance of relative proportions of estrogen to progesterone in producing the normal sequence of menstrual patterns has been shown by Good and Moyer[216] in a study of endometrial biopsies in *Macaca mulatta* monkeys.

Pathologists vary in their willingness to ascribe a specific day in the cycle to an endometrial biopsy; physicians vary in their request for and acceptance of a specific date supplied by a pathologist.[247] In the course of infertility investigations, endometrial biopsy may be used to confirm that ovulation has occurred and that the morphologic development of the endometrium is sufficiently normal to support implantation. In general, the finding of a pathologic process such as atrophy or hyperplasia indicates that the prospects for pregnancy are very poor.[252] Some patients who are unable to develop an adequate secretory response may be helped by hormonal therapy.[234]

Effects of hormone therapy

Physicians treat women with estrogens or progestogens or both, most frequently to alleviate the symptoms of estrogen deficiency (especially after menopause) and for control of conception. The morphologic changes that result

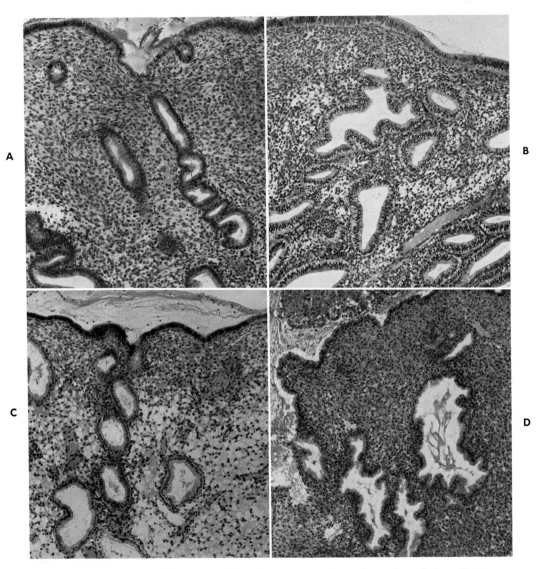

Fig. 40-35. A, Late proliferative endometrium at or about time of ovulation. Tortuous, pseudostratified glands with many mitoses are characteristic. Stroma, without predecidual reaction, may have variable degree of edema. **B,** Sixteen-day secretory endometrium. This early postovulatory endometrium is characterized by tortuous growing glands with irregular vacuolization caused by accumulation of glycogen in cytoplasm beneath nuclei. **C,** Twenty-two-day secretory endometrium. Significant features of this stage are massive stromal edema, tortuosity of glands nearing secretory exhaustion, thin-walled blood vessels, and absence of predecidua. This coincides with peak of corpus luteum activity during which time ovum is in process of implanting. **D,** Premenstrual endometrium. This phase is characterized by nearly complete predecidual transformation of stroma, secretory exhaustion of glands (which have serrated pattern), and inspissation of secretion. There is also leukocytic infiltration—both polymorphonuclear and monocytic. (150×; from Noyes, R. W., Hertig, A. T., and Rock, J.: Fertil. Steril. **1:**3-25, 1950.)

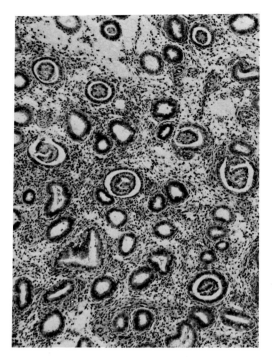

Fig. 40-36. Anovulatory endometrium. Irregular gland outlines and intraglandular epithelial protrusions are frequently found after anovulatory cycles, especially at time of menopause. (85×.)

in the endometrium vary with dosage and according to the sequence with which different combined preparations are used.

Estrogens. The characteristic changes of the proliferative phase are produced by estrogen. The estradiol produced by the ovarian follicle and synthetic estrogens have similar effects. Unremitting estrogen stimulation may occur with approximately physiologic estrogen concentrations at the time of menopause, in the postmenopausal woman treated with estrogen, or in younger women after multiple anovulatory cycles, as in the Stein-Leventhal syndrome. In such cases proliferative activity continues, producing a characteristic anovulatory pattern with intraglandular protrusions of redundant epithelium and a compact stroma (Fig. 40-36). After longer periods, or with higher degrees of estrogen stimulation, the endometrium may become hyperplastic. The pattern in some cases may resemble atypical hyperplasia. Very high doses of estrogen, in animal experiments, actually cause endometrial atrophy.

Progestogens. The therapeutic addition of progesterone or artificial progestogens causes *estrogen-primed* endometrial gland cells to differentiate into a secretory pattern and further growth is inhibited. This effect is produced if the endometrium has become hyperplastic, even in the case of atypical hyperplasia

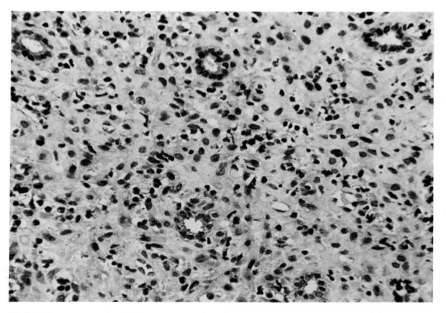

Fig. 40-37. Secretory atrophic pattern after long-term exposure to combination type of contraceptive hormonal preparation. Stromal cells are large, decidua-like; glands are small, atrophic, with faint traces of secretion. (350×.)

or carcinoma in situ.[226] The secretory changes induced are followed by regression, gland cell atrophy, and a decidua-like reaction in the stroma.

Estrogens and progestogens. If dosages and sequences are regulated carefully, it is possible to reproduce physiologically normal cycles with a normal morphologic sequence in the endometrium. This fact has had some application in treatment of functional bleeding, dysmenorrhea, endometriosis, menopausal symptoms, infertility, and some intersex states.

Unquestionably the most common application of hormonal therapy in gynecology is in conception control. Estrogen-progestogen *combination* regimens produce secretion at an early point in the cycle, arresting the proliferative stimulus of estrogen at an incompletely developed stage. Continuation of the same stimulus leads to further gland atrophy, with a relatively pronounced decidua-like stromal reaction at the end of the cycle. Estrogen-progestogen *sequential* regimens operate in a different manner. The estrogen stimulus is carried past the time of ovulation and implantation so that secretion is delayed until about the twenty-fifth day and does not exceed the early secretory pattern of endometrium of the eighteenth day. Predecidual stromal changes do not appear.

After several months of cyclic therapy with combination type of agents, the endometrial lining becomes thin and atrophic. Stromal cells are plump, with abundant cytoplasm. Vessels are small. The glands are generally small, lined by small, low columnar cells with traces of cytoplasmic secretion (Fig. 40-37).

The atrophy is less pronounced after long-term exposure to sequential agents. Perhaps because of the stimulative effects of estrogen, occasional patients have developed hyperplasia and even carcinoma at a relatively young age, after long-term exposure to sequential agents.[233,251]

Metaplasia. Squamous metaplasia occasionally appears in the endometrium much as it does in the endocervix. Small clusters of cells proliferate beneath the glandular epithelium and eventually replace it. Actual keratinization is unusual. Chronic inflammation of various causes has been the most common associated factor; squamous metaplasia may occur after long continued estrogen therapy and in hyperplasia. More exotic tissues such as cartilage,[244] bone,[215a] and glial tissue[258] probably also arise as metaplastic foci sometimes, but implanted aborted fetal tissue may be the commonest

cause. It is also possible that the endometrial stroma may react to organizing substances produced by an aborted embryo.

Hysterectomy and normal uterus

The uterus is one of the most commonly resected organs in any institution in which major surgical procedures are performed on women. There is surprisingly little objective data or discussion on the measurements, appearance, and significance of the "normal" uterus, a fact that accounts for some pointless disagreement in hospital tissue committees.

Langlois[229] has reviewed sizes and weights of a series of 461 uteri considered to have a "normal" gross appearance in the sense that there was no dectectable lesion known to have an effect on uterine size. The principal factor determining uterine weight in this population was parity. In general, it was found that the weight above which a uterus is *probably* abnormal was 130 gm for the nulliparous uterus, 210 gm for parity 1 to 3, and 250 gm for parity of 4 and above.

As a practical matter, objective pathologic data about the uterus frequently have little relevance to the reason for hysterectomy. Nearly half the "normal" uteri in the series reported by Langlois[229] were resected for relief of symptoms related to prolapse or abnormal bleeding. Assuming that the associated symptoms and abnormal physical findings are truthfully reported, one can state that hysterectomy is an extremely valuable means of providing relief for these patients. The uterus itself, however, usually shows no morphologic changes commensurate with the degree of preoperative symptoms. Review of the pathologists reports alone in these circumstances does not provide the data required to audit the desirability of the surgical procedure. The endometrium examined by prior curettage is either normal, especially in the case of prolapse, or has one of the types of benign anovulatory or mixed patterns discussed below.

A more controversial basis for hysterectomy is that it is undeniably an effective form of contraception. In certain ethnic and religious backgrounds it may actually be the only available approach to contraception although other diagnoses and symptoms are necessarily and even sincerely offered and believed by both patient and doctor.

Dysfunctional uterine bleeding

Uterine bleeding that occurs at irregular intervals in excessive or scant amounts, espe-

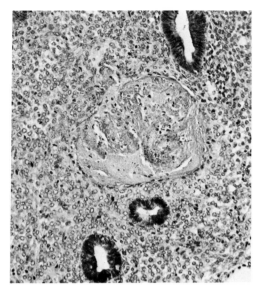

Fig. 40-38. This large fibrin thrombus distending a thin-walled vessel, with intact surrounding stroma and irregular gland outlines, indicates abnormal endometrial bleeding. (150×.)

cially when prolonged, is said to be "dysfunctional" when there is no easily assignable cause such as hyperplasia, neoplasm, polyps, trauma, blood dyscrasia, pregnancy, or hormone administration.

The morphologic findings are variable. The presence of a mixed proliferative and secretory pattern ("irregular shedding") is believed to be the result of continued progesterone secretion from a corpus luteum that fails to involute. Another common pattern is that of irregular nonsecretory glands with intraluminal protrusions of epithelial folds, a somewhat disorganized proliferative pattern that is common after a series of anovulatory cycles. Pathologic findings that confirm the history of bleeding include fragmentation of the stroma into compact ball-like masses, stromal fibrin accumulations, hemosiderin, and scattered tiny fragments of nuclear material sometimes called "nuclear dust" (Fig. 40-38).

A majority of the patients are in the perimenopausal period, have elevated follicle-stimulating hormone levels, and tend to have anovulatory cycles. A second group is young perimenarcheal women with the Stein-Leventhal syndrome, obesity, stress, or ovarian anomalies; most have abnormal luteinizing hormone levels, either elevated or prolonged.[193] A detailed classification has been presented by Arronet and Arrata.[199]

Inflammation

Chronic endometritis. The finding of an infiltrate of plasma cells in the endometrial stroma is the pathologic basis for this diagnosis. Most patients have menstrual disturbances and about half may have pelvic pain or tenderness. The most common etiologic factors are recent abortion or recent delivery, coexisting pelvic inflammatory disease, and the presence of an intrauterine contraceptive device (IUD).[203]

The finding of hyalinized thick-walled stromal vessels and stellate glands with moderate secretory changes are sufficiently characteristic to identify a recent abortion as the most likely cause even in the absence of villi.[241] Although the endometrium seems to be sterile in the presence of most IUDs, serious infections do occur, some of which have been fatal.[221]

Tuberculous endometritis is rare in the United States in comparison with other countries; the disparity is so far unexplained by such factors as variations in sophistication of treatment or public health control.[220] Granulomas are usually small, sparse, and without caseation. Patients are usually sterile; tubal infection usually occurs first.

Organisms implicated as possible causes of endometritis that deserve more study include *Mycoplasma*[232] and *Listeria*[194] species, especially with respect to chronic endometrial infection and infertility or repeated abortion. Rare causes of endometritis have been reviewed by Dallenbach-Hellweg.[209]

Acute endometritis. The most significant form of acute endometritis is postpartum bacterial sepsis originating in the endometrium. The pathologic lesion is an acute invasive suppurative infection with progressive infiltration of the endometrium, myometrium, and parametrium by polymorphonuclear leukocytes. The portal of entry is the vagina. The classical agent is the streptococcus, but anaerobic bacteria, notably *Bacteroides* species, have more recently been implicated.[201] The precise role of anaerobes is controversial. Because of the prevalence of these organisms in the lower genital tract, the significance of a positive culture may be difficult to interpret.[215]

Hyperplasia

Abnormally prolonged profuse, and irregular uterine bleeding in the menopausal or postmenopausal woman is commonly associated with proliferative glandular and stromal patterns called *hyperplasia*. Hyperplastic endometrial patterns vary, and the terms used are

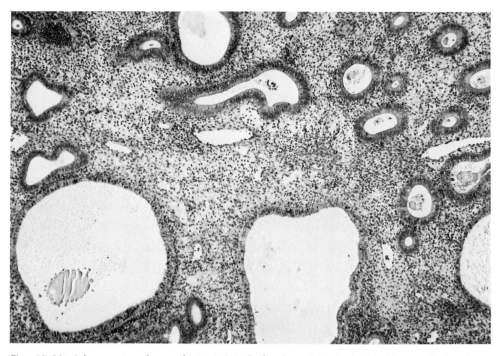

Fig. 40-39. Adenomatous hyperplasia. Dilated glands with irregular outlines and abundant stroma. (150×; from Kraus, F. T.: Gynecologic pathology, St. Louis, 1967, The C. V. Mosby Co.)

confusing. Unfortunately different terms are used by various authors. It is believed that the following terms and definitions are those most widely used and accepted.

Cystic hyperplasia is characterized by large dilated gland spaces with rounded profiles lined by relatively atrophic epithelium, separated by edematous, sparsely cellular stroma. Cystic atrophy would be a more apt designation.

Adenomatous hyperplasia is represented by a more distinctly proliferative pattern; the glands are lined by tall columnar epithelial cells with large nuclei often distributed at different levels but basal polarity of nuclei is generally maintained. The gland outlines are made irregular by outpouchings and papillary infoldings of glandular epithelium. The stroma is dense, cellular, and compact. There are numerous mitoses in both glands and stroma (Fig. 40-39).

Atypical hyperplasia refers to a similar histologic pattern in addition to dysplastic cytologic changes and further loss of nuclear polarity. The nuclei are generally larger, vary in size, and have irregular outlines and prominent nucleoli. The terms "pronounced hyperplasia," "anaplasia," and "carcinoma in situ" have also been used synonymously for this process (Fig. 40-40).

Carcinoma in situ is a term reserved by Hertig to describe irregular glands composed of large cells with abundant eosinophilic cytoplasm, with complete loss of nuclear polarity and frequent papillary intraglandular tufts of cells. The nuclear chromatin is sparse and clumped near the nuclear membrane; nucleoli are often present and may be very large. This pattern is considered to be a variant of atypical hyperplasia by some authorities[191] because the abnormal cells will still respond to the differentiating effects of progesterone[226] and because endometrial carcinomas do not have this pattern.

The etiology and significance of these lesions is debated, and the varied use of terms has not clarified understanding of the subject. Unquestionably, estrogen administration will produce hyperplasia.[227] Prolonged periods of anovulation with steady estrogen secretion that omit the periodic differentiating stimulus of progesterone have a similar effect, even in young women.[205,217,254] Atypical hyperplastic patterns may occur after prolonged anovulation in the Stein-Leventhal syndrome, and will regress after therapeutic induction of ovulation.[222]

Actual progression to carcinoma has been observed, as reviewed by Gore and Hertig[218]

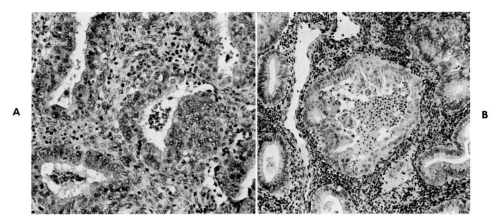

Fig. 40-40. Atypical hyperplasia. **A,** Epithelium two or three cells thick, loss of polarity, and atypical cytologic pattern (not evident at this magnification, 175×). **B,** Piled-up masses of large cells with abundant dense pink cytoplasm, small round nuclei, loss of polarity and inflammatory cells, characteristic of Hertig's carcinoma in situ. (75×.)

and by Vellios,[254] but not frequently; most patients have been treated with progestogens or by hysterectomy, usually to control bleeding, within a few months or years of the diagnosis of hyperplasia. The lesions classified here as atypical hyperplasia and carcinoma in situ apparently respond completely to the differentiating effect of progestogens.[226] For this reason the term "carcinoma in situ" as applied to the endometrium may be semantically unfortunate. Despite reversal of the morphologic lesion, abnormal bleeding often resumes and eventually is the basis for hysterectomy in most patients treated for endometrial hyperplasia.

Benign polypoid lesions

Endometrial polyps are composed of a mixture of endometrial glands and stroma organized into a circumscribed mass that protrudes into the endometrial cavity. The histologic pattern usually resembles that of so-called cystic hyperplasia, as described above. There may be variable degrees of stromal fibrosis, and traces of smooth muscle are commonly present. When smooth muscle is abundant, the lesion is classified as a *pedunculated adenomyoma*.

Endometrial polyps may be a source of abnormal uterine bleeding. An isolated carcinoma arising in an endometrial polyp is rare; the patients who had focal carcinoma in a polyp, described by Salm,[246] also had focal carcinoma elsewhere in the endometrium. Armenia[196] found that 17 of 482 women with endometrial polyps subsequently were shown to have carcinoma of the endometrium. This is a greater incidence than expected in all women of the same age, but such an association is not commonly demonstrable.

Neoplasms

Adenocarcinoma

Carcinoma of the endometrium is primarily a disease of menopausal and postmenopausal women. The patients are more commonly nulliparous and as a group are more likely to be obese, diabetic, and hypertensive than a comparable group of women with normal endometrium. Although endometrial carcinoma occurred with one tenth the frequency of cervical carcinoma 40 years ago, it has become increasingly common and has finally surpassed the incidence of cervical carcinoma.[236]

The etiology is unknown, but long-continued noncyclic endometrial stimulation by estrogen even at normally occurring concentrations seems to be an important factor, especially when unopposed by the periodic differentiating stimulus provided by progestogen.

Estrone appears to be the most significant estrogenic hormone in this postulated relationship to cancer.[233a] Estrone is produced by conversion from adrenal (or ovarian) androstenedione in the menopausal woman, the polycystic ovary syndrome, and in obesity. Conversion apparently occurs in peripheral adipose tissue. Statistical studies indicate that the postmenopausal woman who takes estrogens is from four to eight times more likely to develop endometrial carcinoma than is a group of matched controls,[251a] especially with estrogens composed principally of estrone.[258a] It has been suggested that the lower incidence of carcinoma of the

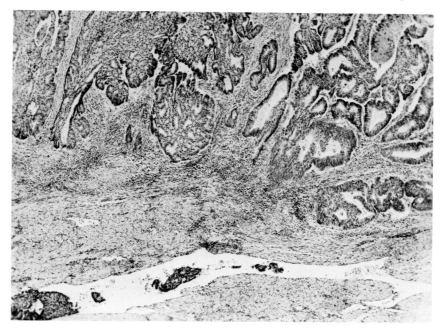

Fig. 40-41. Endometrial adenocarcinoma, moderately differentiated, invading myometrium and dilated lymphatic. (46×; AFIP 264087-2.)

endometrium (and breast) in some populations of women may be the result of the "protective" effect of a relatively greater production of estriol, which apparently does not have the prolonged stimulative effect of estrone.[248a]

Hyperstimulation by high levels of estrogen may produce an extremely hyperplastic pattern that may be difficult to distinguish from well-differentiated carcinoma. Such a pattern has also been produced by exogenous estrogens and by endogenous estrogen from ovarian neoplasms, especially granulosa-theca cell tumors. Lesions of this type seem to be estrogen dependent, for they may regress when the stimulus is removed, and there are few if any documented reports of death or metastases. More recently, a relationship between the use of the sequential type of contraceptive hormone preparations and endometrial cancer has been suggested. The relatively extended exposure to estrogen may be responsible. Some kind of constitutional predisposition may also be a necessary factor; very few cases have thus far been identified.[233,251]

Gross appearance. Endometrial adenocarcinoma forms large irregular masses of friable, granular, gray-tan tissue that protrude into the endometrial cavity. Extension into the muscular wall of the uterus is identified in cut sections by the presence of softer, bulging masses of lighter gray granular tissue that replaces the myometrium.

Microscopic appearance. Most endometrial adenocarcinomas are well differentiated and composed of festoons and ribbons of columnar epithelium, forming multiglandular masses. The gland spaces are typically bridged by strands of epithelium that lack stromal support (Fig. 40-41). Nuclei are large and have irregular outlines, clumped chromatin, and prominent nucleoli. Focal histologically benign squamous metaplasia is common especially in well-differentiated tumors, a pattern that is designated "adenoacanthoma" (Fig. 40-42). Ng et al.[236] recommended that the term "adenosquamous carcinoma" be used to identify mixed carcinomas in which the squamous and glandular elements both are malignant. Rarely an endometrial carcinoma is composed of large clear cells that produce abundant glycogen; these *clear-cell adenocarcinomas* resemble the endometrial hypersecretory pattern seen during pregnancy. Ultrastructural studies indicate a müllerian histogenesis; there is no evidence for a relationship to mesonephric structures.[250]

Many endometrial carcinomas include a few cells that produce vacuoles of mucin, and occasionally adenocarcinomas limited to the fundus may be composed chiefly of typical mucinous epithelium of the cervical type. For this reason, histochemical stains for mucin are of little use in identification of the origin of an adenocarcinoma; one must examine tissue

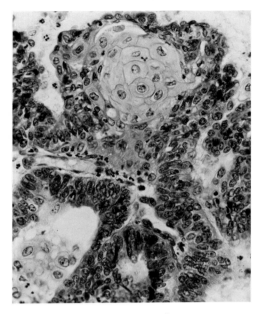

Fig. 40-42. Adenocarcinoma with squamous metaplasia (adenoacanthoma). Benign squamous epithelial pattern distinguishes this from adenosquamous carcinoma in which squamous component is malignant. (235×; AFIP 264048-1.)

from the endocervix and endometrium specifically and separately in order to localize the extent of an adenocarcinoma of the uterus. There are occasional reports of endometrial epidermoid carcinoma.[223]

Factors affecting prognosis. Nearly 90% of women with endometrial cancer limited to the endometrium survive 5 years. As invasion extends to the inner half of the myometrium, survival falls to 70%, and with cancer spread outside the uterus, survival is less than 15%. Endometrial carcinomas that involve the cervix are more likely to metastasize to pelvic lymph nodes with a similar distribution to that of cervical carcinoma. For this reason the factor of cervical involvement must be determined before treatment can be planned on a rational basis. Survival is good (85%) when the cancer is well differentiated, and bad (30%) when it is poorly differentiated.[235] Carcinomas with a mixed adenosquamous pattern are usually poorly differentiated and have a poor prognosis.[236,249]

Endometrial stromal neoplasms

Benign *endometrial stromal nodules* form single, well-circumscribed masses that can often be distinguished grossly from leiomyomas by their yellow color and softer consistency. Most

are situated in the myometrium, but some protrude into the endometrial cavity. The histologic appearance closely resembles normal endometrial stroma, with numerous evenly distributed small vessels forming a distinctive part of the pattern. Stromal lesions of similar origin that have a distinct trabecular pattern have also been called *plexiform tumorlets.*[230] The endometrial stroma can form a variety of glandlike structures, some of which mimic ovarian stromal tumor patterns, including sex cords and Call-Exner bodies.[206]

Endolymphatic stromal myosis forms multiple bulging masses of variable size, though there is often a single dominant endometrial mass. The most dramatic and characteristic feature is the presence of numerous wormlike masses of stromal tissue that extrude from vascular channels when the uterine wall is cut (Fig. 40-43). The margins of the stromal growths are well circumscribed; mitoses are infrequent. The clinical course is usually benign, but incompletely resected lesions may recur slowly in the pelvis and an occasional patient has developed a pulmonary metastasis. One of the 19 patients reported by Norris and Taylor[238] died of the tumor 12 years after the initial resection.

Endometrial stromal sarcoma is a highly malignant tumor that characteristically forms one or more polypoid endometrial masses. Margins are indistinct as the result of diffuse infiltration of the myometrium by poorly differentiated small cells (Fig. 40-44). Mitoses are numerous; more than 10 per 10 highpowered microscopic fields indicate a poor prognosis.[238]

Carcinoma and malignant mixed müllerian tumor (mixed mesodermal tumor)

An uncommon and highly malignant group of endometrial cancers is composed of a mixture of carcinoma and sarcoma patterns. The patients are usually elderly and postmenopausal. A surprisingly large proportion have experienced prior radiation therapy.[239]

Abnormal bleeding is the most common symptom; the tumor may appear as a polyp protruding through the cervical canal.

The carcinoma component includes the full range of patterns seen in endometrial carcinoma. Poorly differentiated endometrial adenocarcinoma is usually predominant. Focal components of clear-cell adenocarcinoma, epidermoid carcinoma, and even papillary serous adenocarcinoma like that in the ovary are also

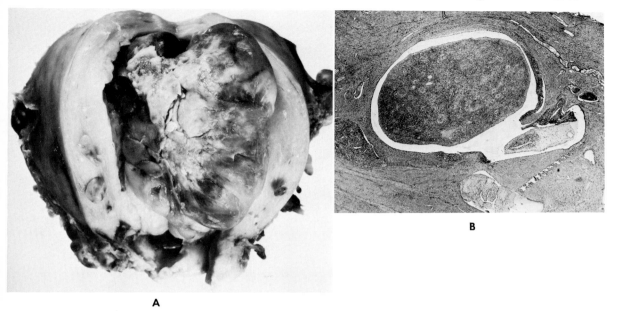

B

A

Fig. 40-43. Endolymphatic stromal myosis. **A,** Large soft polypoid mass distends endometrial cavity; extensions of mass protrude wormlike from dilated vascular spaces in sectioned uterine wall. **B,** Photomicrograph of neoplastic stroma extending through vascular space in uterine wall. Myometrium is not infiltrated.

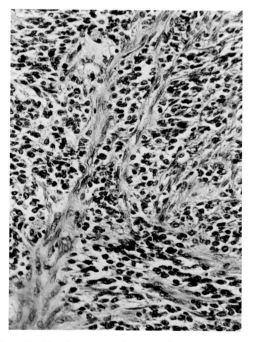

Fig. 40-44. Endometrial stromal sarcoma. Myometrial fibers are separated by infiltrating anaplastic endometrial stromal cells. (150×.)

common, and occasional embryonic-appearing gland structures are characteristic. If the stromal component is an undifferentiated sarcoma, the tumor is said to be a *homologous mixed müllerian tumor* or *carcinosarcoma* (Fig. 40-45). *Heterologous mixed müllerian tumors* are those that contain also chondrosarcoma, osteosarcoma, or rhabdomyosarcoma.

The prognosis is extremely poor. Metastases occur early. The few survivors have had small lesions confined to the uterus, but even with such limited involvement, the tumor often may disseminate widely, rapidly, and fatally. The presence or absence of heterologous elements has not affected prognosis significantly in most series.

An uncommon variant with a benign epithelial component mixed with a sarcomatous stroma has been called *adenosarcoma* by Clement and Scully.[207] Most of their patients survived.

Metastatic carcinoma

Carcinoma metastatic from distant primary sites is rare in the endometrium. The most common site noted is usually breast cancer identified at autopsy.[228] Gastrointestinal cancer has also been reported[251b] and may be identified in endometrial curettings. The simultaneous finding of areas of neoplastic change in the endometrium together with cancer of the

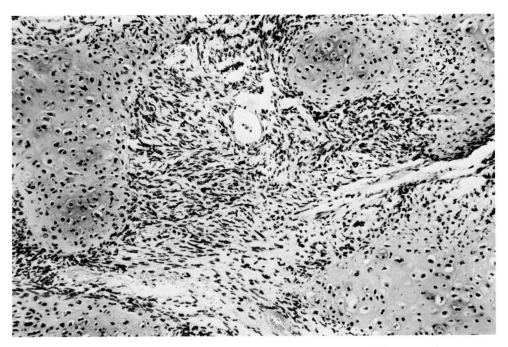

Fig. 40-45. Malignant mixed müllerian tumor. Sarcoma pattern, undifferentiated at center, with chondrosarcoma at margins. (150×; from Kraus, F. T.: Gynecologic pathology, St. Louis, 1967, The C. V. Mosby Co.)

tube, cervix, or ovary may occasionally represent a metastasis, but in most instances probably represents multifocal origin.[257]

MYOMETRIUM

The myometrium exists to provide a tough envelope for the developing fetus and to propel it into independent life at parturition. It is painful when ischemic as in the case of prolonged contraction and perhaps with infarction of a smooth muscle neoplasm.

Adenomyosis

The abnormal distribution of nests of histologically benign endometrial tissue within the myometrium is called "adenomyosis." It may be focal or diffuse. The involved portions of myometrial smooth muscle are hypertrophied.

The typical uterus is enlarged and globular, often with lateral humps at the cornua. The posterior wall is most commonly affected and is more extensively involved when the process is diffuse. The cut surface of areas of adenomyosis bulges, has ill-defined margins, and a coarse trabecular appearance. The scattered foci of endometrial tissue appear depressed, soft, and occasionally hemorrhagic (Fig. 40-46).

The islands of ectopic endometrium appear

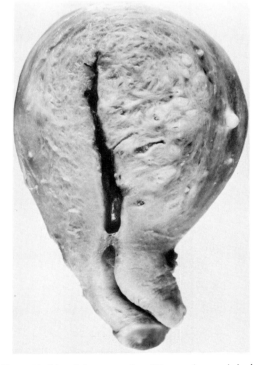

Fig. 40-46. Adenomyosis. Uterus has globular shape. In sagittal section, myometrial mass is poorly circumscribed. Soft depressions are composed of heterotopic endometrium; some are hemorrhagic.

normal on histologic examination, except that orientation of glands is lacking. Both glands and stroma are present. Recent hemorrhage and hemosiderin in macrophages, indicating the residue of past hemorrhage, are usually found only in occasional areas. Both glands and stroma may respond to hermonal stimulation, but not in all cases or in all parts of the same lesion.

The minimal criteria for diagnosis are vague. Most texts refer to the depth of more than "one low-powered microscopic field" as the borderline beyond which endometrium qualifies for the diagnosis of adenomyosis. Microscopes vary. It is probable that the occasional superficial foci of endometrial growth that retain cystic accumulation of old blood are symptomatic and significant even if they do not qualify as adenomyosis by the above criterion. The presence of associated muscle hypertrophy, as detected by bulges on the fresh cut surface, also probably indicates a pathologic process. The common extensions of endometrium that retain continuity with the surface but reach a depth of 1 to 2 mm are probably not significant. Some judgment is required in evaluation of the possibility that a superficial process may have been the cause of symptoms; rigid criteria of measurement alone will probably never classify all cases reliably.

The symptoms ascribed to adenomyosis are pain, especially with menstrual periods, cramps, and abnormally prolonged and profuse menstrual bleeding. Correlation of degree of symptoms with extent of the pathologic process is frequently poor. Occasionally a uterus is found to be extensively involved, with no history of menstrual difficulty. Just as often, an enlarged uterus is removed for all of the appropriate reasons, but no adenomyosis can be demonstrated by the pathologist to justify the symptoms or the hysterectomy.[263]

The pathogenesis is unexplained. Adenomyosis is not seen in children and is much less common in young women, a finding that makes it unlikely to be a congenital malformation. The most popular concept is that the endometrium extends into the myometrium; a metaplasia of myometrium is equally tenable. It is possible that estrogen stimulation may be an important etiologic factor. Adenomyosis is not usually associated with endometriosis, even when the endometriosis is extensive. It does seem to occur more frequently in women with endometrial hyperplasia or endometrial carcinoma.[271] In such cases the foci of adenomyosis may occasionally also appear hyperplastic or neoplastic, in step with the endometrial lesion.

Neoplasms of smooth muscle

Leiomyoma. The commonest lesion of the myometrium is a benign neoplasm composed of smooth muscle with a variable fibrous tissue component. Leiomyomas are well-circumscribed, rounded, firm or hard rubbery masses of gray-white tissue with a characteristic whorled appearance on cut surface. They are often multiple and vary considerably in size (Fig. 40-47). Most occur during the years of active reproductive life; growth may be stimulated by pregnancy or hormone therapy.

Symptoms vary with location. Subserosal leiomyomas may impinge upon the bladder or the sacral plexus, for instance, causing urinary frequency or pain. Submucous leiomyomas that protrude into the endometrial cavity cause abnormal bleeding. Rarely, very large leiomyomas have been associated with

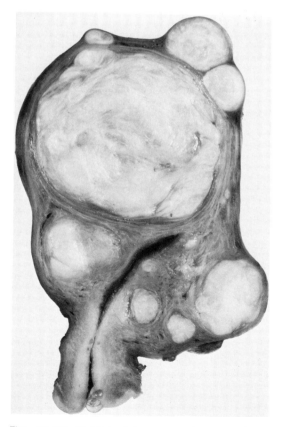

Fig. 40-47. Multiple leiomyomas in sagittal section. Typical well-circumscribed solid light gray nodules distort uterus.

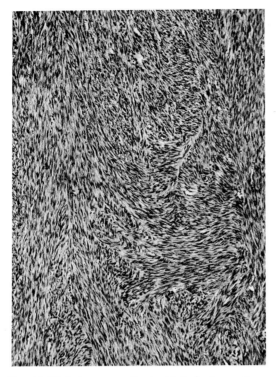

Fig. 40-48. Leiomyoma. Typical interlacing pattern. (140×; from Kraus, F. T.: Gynecologic pathology, St. Louis, 1967, The C. V. Mosby Co.)

polycythemia[275,278]; whether the leiomyoma secretes an erythropoietic factor itself or stimulates the kidney to do it remains to be shown. Leiomyomas undergoing infarction or hemorrhage may be painful. Hysterography may amplify physical findings in establishing diagnosis and sites of involvement with considerable accuracy.[277]

The histologic pattern is a familiar one, with streaming masses of smooth muscle separated by strands or masses of collagen (Fig. 40-48). Some remarkable variations occur, with pronounced edema or massive calcification or hyalinization. Leiomyomas that have a sizable adipose tissue component have been called *lipoleiomyomas*.[269]

Cellular leiomyomas have a threatening histologic appearance because of the absence of fibrotic areas and the large size of the individual cells and their nuclei. They are distinguished from leiomyosarcoma by the absence of mitoses.[262]

Bizarre leiomyomas have an even more frightening microscopic appearance because of the many large giant cells with very large cytologically malignant-looking nuclei, which may be multiple. These lesions also lack the mitoses that characterize leiomyosarcoma and have proved to be benign after many years of follow-up.[262] Fechner[264] has described bizarre leiomyomas in a few younger women using oral contraceptives. A direct relationship has not been established; the prognosis has been good.

Clear-cell leiomyomas (leiomyoblastomas) are rare uterine counterparts of a similar tumor found in the stomach,[285] characterized histologically by abundant clear cytoplasm. Nearly all are benign; the few aggressive lesions have had more numerous mitoses.

Borderline smooth muscle lesions. Rarely proliferating masses of smooth muscle may behave in an aggressive manner that belies their benign microscopic appearance.

Peritoneal leiomyomatosis refers to the extensive spread of histologically benign masses of smooth muscle about the peritoneal surfaces, but limited to the peritoneal cavity. There seems to be a close relationship to pregnancy; it is possible that the origin is metaplastic rather than metastatic from the uterus.[276,286]

Metastasizing leiomyoma. Rarely a histologically benign leiomyoma may seem to be the source of lymph nodal or pulmonary metastases.[268] Mitoses are not seen. In some cases progression seems related to hormonal factors, including pregnancy.[261] Intravenous extensions of the uterine tumor are absent.

Intravenous leiomyomatosis is a benign smooth muscle neoplasm that produces fleshy outgrowths of histologically benign smooth muscle into pelvic veins. Mitoses are absent. The prognosis is good even if all of the intravenous extensions cannot be resected.[274,282] The changes are dramatic when extensive; less obvious cases are probably often overlooked.

Leiomyosarcoma. This most common of uterine sarcomas arises from the muscular wall of the uterus; although origin from a leiomyoma is possible and associated leiomyomas are present in a minority of cases, it is unusual to be able to prove such an occurrence.[224,262,274,283] The incidence is approximately 0.6 per 100,000 women over 20.[262,280] The mean age of patients at the time of diagnosis in most series is over 50, with an age range of 40 to 80 years. Nonspecific symptoms related to uterine enlargement and abnormal uterine bleeding form the usual basis for exploration; only occasionally will tissue obtained by curettage establish a preoperative diagnosis.

Most leiomyosarcomas are large and soft; the yellow or tan color, lack of a trabeculated pattern, at least in some areas, and poorly

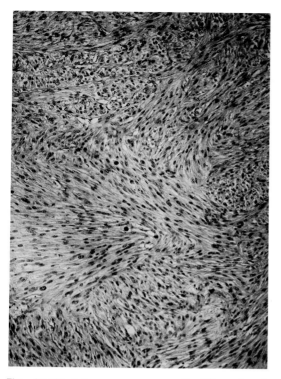

Fig. 40-49. Leiomyosarcoma, well differentiated. Tumor cells are only moderately pleomorphic, but mitoses are numerous. (150×; from Kraus, F. T.: Gynecologic pathology, St. Louis, 1967, The C. V. Mosby Co.)

circumscribed margins may suggest the diagnosis on gross inspection.

The histologic pattern nearly always includes areas with typical swirling masses of spindle-shaped smooth muscle cells containing identifiable myofibrils (Fig. 40-49). Nuclei are large and hyperchromatic with irregularly clumped chromatin. Most leiomyosarcomas include a few areas with large pleomorphic or anaplastic tumor cells. The most significant indicator of malignant behavior is the number of mitoses found in microscopic sections. Lesions that contain areas with more than 10 mitoses per 10 high-powered fields (hpf) are classified as sarcomas.[262,288] Lesions with less than 5 mitoses per 10 hpf have been associated with a good prognosis.[224,262,280,283] Those lesions in which the numbers of mitoses lie between 5 and 10 per hpf constitute a borderline group of whom most will survive, at least for 5 years, but several reports have recorded a few deaths in this category.

Extension beyond the uterus is associated uniformly with a fatal prognosis. About 20% of patients will survive 5 years; the lesions in

these cases are usually small, confined to the uterus, and have relatively fewer mitoses. Chemotherapy with doxorubicin (Adriamycin) has seemed to produce a transient antitumor effect in a few patients.[259]

Other neoplasms. *Lipomas,* composed entirely of adipose tissue are rare, and probably result from metaplasia in smooth muscle or stromal cells.[281] *Adenomatoid tumor* is an uncommon benign nodular mass that resembles a leiomyoma grossly but microscopically has a microcystic honeycomb appearance caused by numerous small spaces lined by vacuolated cells.[289] Similar lesions occur in the fallopian tube. Ultrastructural and histochemical studies support a mesothelial origin.[265,287]

Uterine *hemangiopericytoma* is another rare benign nodular tumor. It resembles endometrial stromal nodule grossly and microscopically; the photomicrographs of many reported cases appear more consistent with stromal nodule. Reticulin stains accentuate the pericapillary growth of plump, spindle-shaped pericytes that comprise the tumor. This histogenetic concept is supported by ultrastructural study.[284]

FALLOPIAN TUBE
Anatomy and physiology

The paired fallopian tubes are divided into specific regions each of which has somewhat different functions. The *interstitial portion* is a narrow channel through the cornual wall of the uterine fundus. The *isthmic portion,* about 2 to 3 cm long is immediately distal to the tubouterine junction. The muscular wall, both longitudinal and circular, is especially prominent in this portion and probably functions as a sphincter. The *ampullary portion,* about 5 to 8 cm long, has a much wider lumen and an extensive mucosa as the result of the complex folds or plicae, which greatly increase its surface and secretory capacity. The *infundibulum* is the trumpetlike distal portion that terminates in the tubal fimbria. The infundibular muscle also has the capacity to act as a sphincter.

The tubal mucosa is composed of three types of cells. The *ciliated cells* have an obvious function in transport through the tube. The *secretory cells* are columnar; they become especially tall and actively secreting during the secretory half of the menstrual cycle. Also present are narrow, dark *intercalated* cells, which apparently represent secretory cells at an inactive or exhausted stage. Both scanning and transmission electron microscopy have contributed considerably to current concepts of tubal mucosal morphology.[213]

The outer serosal covering is a mesothelial structure; tiny nodular masses of mesothelial proliferation may glisten like dewdrops on the outer surface of the tube; these so-called Walthard rests should not be confused with tumor implants. The ultrastructural pattern is similar to urinary transitional epithelium, apparently a metaplastic change in mesothelial cells.

The fallopian tubes clearly are complex structures that represent considerably more than conduits from ovary to endometrial cavity. The fringe-like fimbriae are actively approximated to the ovary at ovulation by a fold of smooth muscle.

Coordination of muscular activity, epithelial proliferation, ciliary activity, and mucosal secretion is under endocrine control and varies with the phases of the menstrual cycle. Muscular activity is also probably affected by coitus. Mitochondria are greatly increased in both ciliated and secretory cells during the secretory half of the menstrual cycle; granular endoplasmic reticulum and secretion granules appear in the secretory cells at this time.

The circular smooth-muscle layer can have a peristaltic effect under appropriate stimulation; spermatozoa are conveyed to the ampullary portion of the tube where fertilization takes place faster than their unaided locomotive powers can achieve. The secretions of the tubal epithelium are indispensible for capacitation of both spermatozoa and ova, without which fertilization cannot take place. The speed of transport of the zygote cannot be unduly accelerated or retarded if the blastocyst is to develop properly and implant.

Inflammation

Acute salpingitis and pelvic inflammatory disease. Acute inflammation of the fallopian tube originates chiefly as a complication of venereally transmitted infections of the lower genital tract. Puerperal or postabortal salpingitis occurs especially after intrauterine instrumentation. Intra-abdominal infections such as appendicitis with peritonitis may secondarily affect the tube. Hematogenous spread is important in the pathogenesis of tuberculosis of the tube and some cases of pneumococcal salpingitis occurring in children.

The most common agent, at least initially, is *Neisseria gonorrhoeae;* about 10% of women with gonorrhea of the lower genital tract develop gonococcal salpingitis.[299] Subse-quently, with the formation of more extensive pelvic tubo-ovarian abscess, numerous other organisms, notably anaerobes have been cultured. Intrauterine contraceptive devices may increase the potential for salpingitis and more extended pelvic infection after lower genital tract infections, including gonorrhea.[309]

Meticulous culture techniques are important because the most common anaerobes identified have been *Bacteroides* species, which are not sensitive to penicillin,[304] and pose a considerable threat to the patient if inadequately controlled. Mycoplasms also represent important organisms that will not be cultured by "routine" bacteriologic cultural techniques in most laboratories unless the possibility is specifically stressed by the physician performing the culture.[296] Laparoscopic examinations are especially effective in establishing an accurate diagnosis.[295]

The fallopian tubes are nearly always affected bilaterally. The fimbriated ends are sealed by organizing inflammatory exudate and the lumens are dilated, especially the ampullary portion, producing a retort-shaped deformation (Fig. 40-50). The serosa is red and covered with purulent exudate, which extends to the ovaries and pelvic wall. Loculated pockets of pus may accumulate, producing a *tubo-ovarian abscess,* for which the tube, uterus, broad ligament, and ovary form parts of the surrounding abscess wall.

Microscopically, the lumen of the tube is filled with polymorphonuclear leukocytes, which also extensively infiltrate the tubal mucosa and wall. The mucosal epithelium may be focally ulcerated but generally remains intact.

Chronic salpingitis. After approximately 10 days plasma cells, macrophages, and lymphocytes begin to dominate the inflammatory cell pattern. Fibrosis becomes progressively more apparent as the exudate organizes. The tubal

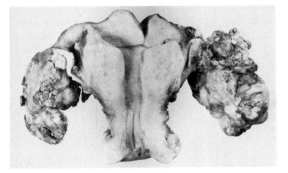

Fig. 40-50. Note bilateral retort-shaped, swollen, sealed tubes and adhesions of ovaries.

plicae form adhesions in many areas, sometimes producing a complicated multiglandular pattern. As the inflammatory process finally resolves, this arrangement persists. The epithelium lining spaces thus formed by inflammatory entrapment produces secretions, eventually forming small cysts, which in aggregate form a multicystic structure sometimes termed *follicular salpingitis*.

It must be emphasized that active inflammation is not a self-perpetuating process, and the expression "sterile pus" is a fallacy. The causative organisms, often anaerobes, may be difficult to culture, but they are there and can be identified and treated effectively.[305] Anaerobes are especially likely to be present in the most serious and life-threatening pelvic infections.

Granulomatous salpingitis. Granulomatous salpingitis is most commonly caused by *Mycobacterium tuberculosis*. The tube is dilated, with a thickened wall. The exudate within the lumen usually appears purulent rather than caseous. Typical caseating granulomas are identified in microscopic sections, however. The glandlike pattern produced by the combination of adhesions of plicae and epithelial hyperplasia may be remarkably proliferative and has been mistaken for adenocarcinoma (Fig. 40-51).

Foreign body granulomas in the tube may occur after instillation of oily contrast media used in hysterosalpingography, and talc granulomas have occurred after laparotomy. Rare

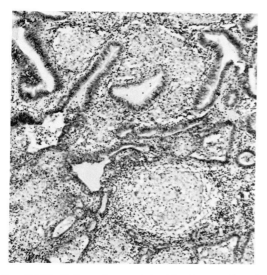

Fig. 40-51. Tuberculous salpingitis. Severe chronic inflammation, inconspicuous granulomas, and exuberant glandular epithelial proliferation. (90×.)

instances of sarcoidosis, actinomycosis, and schistosomiasis have been reported.[308]

Endometriosis

Ectopic growth of endometrial glands and stroma can occur in all parts of the tube. Serosal implants appear as small red or red-brown patches or nodules with hemorrhage and fibrous adhesions. They are most common as a part of more generalized pelvic endometriosis. Involvement of the muscular wall stimulates muscle proliferaton, and a nodular enlargement results. In about 10% of cases the tubal mucosa is replaced by endometrial glandular epithelium and stroma.[300]

In pregnancy, focal *decidual reaction* may involve the serosa or mucosal stroma, especially in the plicae of the ampullary portion of the tube. The cells are large with refractile borders and closely resemble endometrial decidual cells; they must not be confused with granulomas or metastatic carcinoma.

Salpingitis isthmica nodosa

The characteristically bilateral nodular enlargements of salpingitis isthmica nodosa are located in the tubal isthmus and may be multiple. They vary from a few millimeters to a few centimeters in diameter, are firm, and appear gray, yellow, or brown on cut surface.

Microscopically, the nodules are composed of channels or spaces, lined by benign tubal epithelium separated by bundles of smooth muscle, which forms the major component of the mass. Inflammatory changes are inconspicuous or absent. The glandular channels communicate with the tubal lumen and therefore can be demonstrated by hysterosalpingography.[306]

The lesions are apparently acquired, but the pathogenesis is unknown. Benjamin and Beaver[291] considered inflammation to be an unlikely cause and suggested that the process is analogous to adenomyosis. Most patients are sterile.

Ectopic pregnancy

Implantation of a fertilized ovum may occur in the tube especially when tubal structure or function has been altered or impaired by inflammation. The muscular wall is weakened by trophoblastic infiltration and attenuated because the lumen is distended by hemorrhage (Fig. 40-52). Vascular invasion by trophoblast is invariably present.

The diagnosis is not always easy because only a minority of the patients report the "typical"

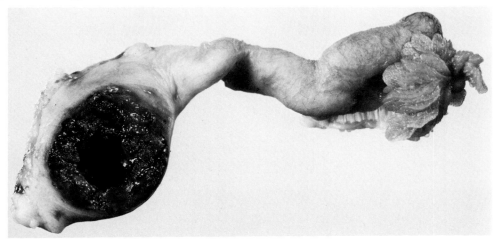

Fig. 40-52. Tubal ectopic pregnancy. Placental villi and trophoblast have infiltrated muscular wall, forming a hemorrhagic mass.

clinical picture of amenorrhea, pain, and vaginal bleeding, and at least half will have a negative pregnancy test.[308] Salpingectomy is done to control the massive hemorrhage that often results from rupture of the tube. Repeat tubal pregnancy occurs in about 10% of patients.

Attempts to enhance fertility in the future by a more conservative procedure than salpingectomy have been disappointing; although the prospects for future pregnancy are somewhat greater, the higher incidence of abortion and repeat tubal pregnancy tends to cancel any gains.[307]

Benign tumors and cysts

Hydatids of Morgagni are unilocular thin-walled cysts that hang from the tubal fimbria. Ferenczy and Richart[213] have shown that the epithelium is like that of the tube and undergoes cyclic changes in step with tubal epithelium; these are true "tubal cysts."

Mesonephric (paratubal or parovarian) cysts are also unilocular thin-walled cysts filled with clear straw-colored fluid. The epithelium of these cysts resembles that of the mesonephric duct remnants of the mesovarium and does not undergo cyclic changes as does tubal epithelium.[213] The larger cysts spread the mesovarium and mesosalpinx so that the tube is often compressed and attenuated into a longer structure.

Adenomatoid tumors of the tube are histologically identical to those already described in the uterine wall (p. 1723). In the tube they form a small nodular mass that compresses the tubal lumen to one side. It is important to recognize the pseudoglandular pattern in order

to avoid a mistaken diagnosis of adenocarcinoma.[310]

Leiomyomas of the tube are surprisingly rare in view of their common occurrence in the adjacent uterus and the shared origin of the smooth muscle of both organs. Of the 60 or 80 cases reported, a few have been remarkably large.[308]

Teratomas, in rare instances, have originated from within the tube.[297] Most have been intraluminal and cystic and have resembled ovarian cystic teratomas (dermoid cysts). A few have been solid. A single instance of malignant teratoma is recorded.[303]

The histogenesis of these lesions is much debated. I have seen one instance of ovarian tissue including ova and typical ovarian stroma located within tubal mucosa. The patient had been subjected to prior pelvic surgery, but the wall of the tube appeared to be intact. Such a finding may also explain the unique report of a Sertoli-Leydig cell tumor of the tube,[292] but a satisfactory explanation for the ovarian tissue itself at this location is still lacking.

Malignant tumors

Adenocarcinoma. This least common of female genital tract carcinomas is also one of the most aggressive.

The symptoms of pain and vaginal discharge are more characteristic of tubal inflammation, which is commonly also present. The inflammatory changes usually affect only the tube containing the neoplasm, a finding that suggests that the neoplasm appears first; primary inflammation of the tube usually affects both sides at the same time. The often mentioned

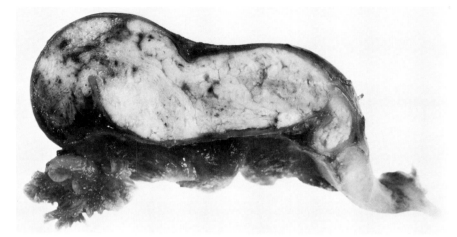

Fig. 40-53. Adenocarcinoma of fallopian tube, distending tubal lumen with soft gray tissue.

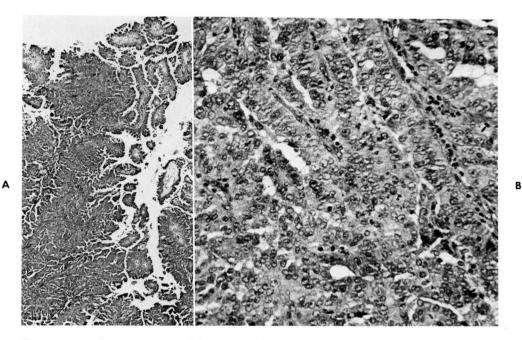

Fig. 40-54. Adenocarcinoma of fallopian tube. **A,** Typical papillary pattern. **B,** Higher magnification showing poorly differentiated adenocarcinoma. (**A,** 40×; **B,** 350×; from Kraus, F. T.: Gynecologic pathology, St. Louis, 1967, The C. V. Mosby Co.)

symptom of sudden copious watery discharge accompanied by relief of pain, dignified by the Latin term *hydrops tubae profluens,* is not commonly encountered. In about one patient in five, both tubes are affected.

Because of the nonspecific nature of the symptoms, the diagnosis is rarely made prior to laparotomy. Cancer cells were found in the vaginal smears of 24 of the 40 patients collected by Sedlis[302]; but a lower incidence is reported in most series.

The affected tube resembles a distorted sausage and tends to feel firm instead of fluctuant (Fig. 40-53). The appearance of the tumor in the opened tube is usually papillary but may be soft or solid. Simultaneous involvement of tube and ovary may occur, in which case the lesion is considered by convention to be of ovarian origin.

The histologic appearance closely resembles the various patterns of papillary serous adenocarcinoma of the ovary (Fig. 40-54). Better differentiated lesions may contain psammoma bodies. It is common to see invasion of the tubal stroma and muscle.

The prognosis is poor; about one patient in five lives for 5 years after the diagnosis is established. The few survivors have tended to have well-differentiated lesions confined to the tubal mucosa, situated within a sealed tube.

Malignant mixed müllerian tumor of the tube is extremely rare. It has no gross distinguishing features. The histologic patterns and clinical correlations are similar to those described under carcinosarcoma and malignant mixed müllerian tumors of the endometrium.[290] The prognosis is very poor.

Metastatic carcinoma involving the tube is more common than primary carcinoma. The most common primary site is from one of the more common female genital tract carcinomas, but breast and gastric adenocarcinoma are also encountered. The conspicuous lymphatic involvement and lack of neoplastic change in the tubal epithelium distinguish metastatic from primary carcinomas easily in most instances.

OVARY

The ovary has a complex structure and operates on a multiphasic schedule. Its function is to produce eggs to implant, after fertilization, in an endometrium whose preparation is coordinated afresh each time by the ovarian hormones. To do this, the ovary must react appropriately to a set of trophic substances (hormones, prostaglandins) whose stimulation schedules these activities.

The disarray of body structure and function that can occur when the ovarian hormonal stimuli appear inappropriately is often devastating and in many cases still incompletely explained. The bizarre collection of neoplasms and their fascinating effects on the patient rival the repertory of any other organ.

Both the disorders of physiology and the tumors are more easily understood when the morphology and activities of the cellular components of the ovary have been explained.

Anatomy and physiology

The two bean-shaped ovaries hang from either tube posterior to the broad ligament, attached to the tube by a mesentery, the mesovarium. The blood vessels and lymphatics enter and leave through the lateral suspensory ligaments and thence through long channels to terminate at the level of the kidneys. The first order of lymph nodes that drain the ovaries is therefore in the aortic chain at the level of

the kidneys, a fact that must be remembered when the possible extent of an ovarian neoplasm is being investigated.

Cells of ovary

Germ cells. At birth the germ cells are represented by oocytes, in a resting stage of the first meiotic division, a process that will not be completed until ovulation occurs and fertilization is in process. Ultrastructural features of these events have been beautifully compiled by Ferenczy and Richart.[213] Germ cells have the potential for reproducing tissues of all germ layers and are considered to be the cell of origin of *teratomas*. They do not themselves produce ovarian hormones, but organize the cells that do; adjacent ovarian stromal cells are induced to specialize and form the granulosa and theca cells that produce estrogens and progestogens.

Specialized gonadal stroma

Granulosa cells. In the primary follicle of an infant the granulosa cells lie in a single layer around the oocyte. Under the influence of follicle-stimulating hormone (FSH) they proliferate, forming a fluid that contains the precursor of the *zona pellucida,* a dense capsule that surrounds the maturing oocyte. Cytoplasmic projections of granulosa cells extend through the zona pellucida and abut upon the

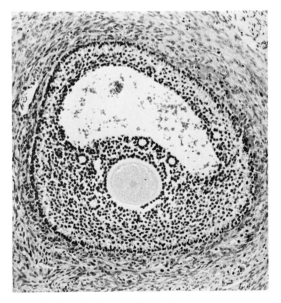

Fig. 40-55. Ovarian follicle. Large ovum is surrounded by mass of granulosa cells in which four Call-Exner bodies can be seen. Concentrically surrounding plump spindle cells compose theca externa. (150×.)

oocyte cell membrane. As the graafian follicle enlarges, a fluid-filled space, the antrum, forms. The oocyte, surrounded by a hillock of granulosa cells, lies eccentrically near the wall of the follicle (Fig. 40-55). Small round masses of dense pink material surrounded by a rosette of granulosa cells are usually evident in sections; these *Call-Exner bodies* are a specific product of granulosa cells, normal and neoplastic. The granulosa layer is avascular until ovulation.

Granulosa cells can synthesize estrogen (estrone) and various intermediates, including dehydroepiandrosterone.[390] At the time of ovulation, they enlarge and form the corpus luteum, described below.

Theca cells. As the maturing graafian follicle enlarges, the immediately surrounding stromal cells also enlarge and become rounded and plump. This change in an ovarian stromal cell is called *luteinization.* The luteinized theca layer becomes noticably more vascular than does adjacent stroma. Follicle-associated theca cells thus activated produce estrogen (both estrone and estradiol) and are considered to be the primary source of estrogen in the preovulatory stage of the menstrual cycle.

Corpus luteum. In response to the midcyclic peak of pituitary *luteinizing hormone* (and with local help from prostaglandins[322]), the graafian follicle ruptures, expels the oocyte, and rapidly becomes a corpus luteum. The granulosa layer becomes vascularized, the granulosa cells enlarge to accommodate a massive accumulation of cytoplasm, and are then said to be luteinized (Fig. 40-56). This transformation probably results from luteinizing hormone stimulation alone.[353] Electron micrographs show abundant cytoplasmic agranular reticulum and mitochondria with tubular cristae typical of steroid hormone–producing cells. The corpus luteum is the principal source of progesterone (which stimulates the secretory endometrial pattern) and estrone and estradiol as well. If a pregnancy does not occur, the corpus luteum rapidly regresses. The morphologic changes attending the growth and decline of the corpus luteum have been extensively illustrated by Adams and Hertig.[313] The roles of gonadotropins in the rise, and prostaglandins in the fall, of the corpus luteum have been reviewed by Hammerstein.[344]

Unspecialized ovarian stroma. The unspecialized ovarian stroma is a deceptively innocent-appearing mass of spindle-shaped cells. They produce collagen and are also capable of responding to gonadotropic stimuli to become luteinized producers of steroid hormones. They are considered to be the cells of origin from which hyperplastic and stromal tumors (granulosa-theca cell, Sertoli-Leydig cell, etc.) arise. The ovarian stroma also contains smooth muscle fibers, which respond to prostaglandins, cholinergic agents, and oxytocin; contractile

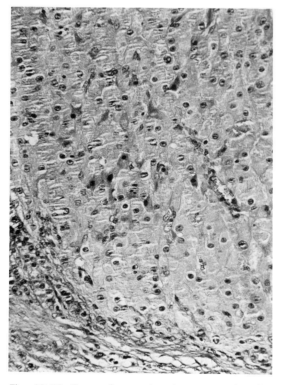

Fig. 40-56. Corpus luteum late in menstrual cycle. Luteinized granulosa cells are large and pale. Luteinized theca cells are smaller, intermixed with stromal cells at peripheral margin (lower left). (275×.)

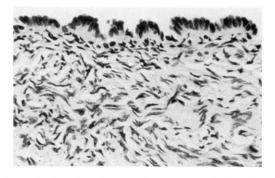

Fig. 40-57. Ovarian surface, covered by low columnar or cuboid celomic epithelium; cortical stroma immediately below has fibrotic appearance. (300×.)

responses to drugs vary with the stage of the menstrual cycle.[331]

Surface mesothelium. The ovary is invested with a mesothelial covering, like other organs of the abdominal cavity (Fig. 40-57). It is the mesothelium of the urogenital ridge from which the müllerian ducts arise; the surface covering of the ovary seems to share or retain some specialized potential for differentiation with the related müllerian cells that form the lining of tube, endometrium, cervix, and upper vagina. This relationship seems to be the basis for the close similarity between the epithelial cell types found in hyperplastic, metaplastic, and neoplastic growths that occur in or on the ovary.

Focal decidual reaction is regularly present on the surface of the ovaries in pregnancy and may be extensive on peritoneal surfaces generally. These areas look like tiny pink patches of serosal thickening. Rarely a similar change

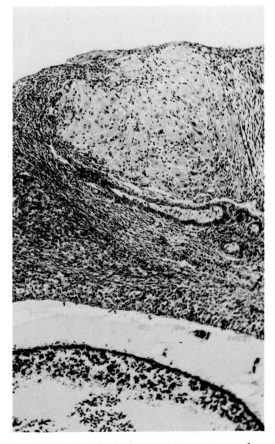

Fig. 40-58. Decidual change at ovarian surface. Multiple foci are found in ovaries of all pregnant patients and rarely in postmenopausal women. (100×; AFIP 294919-17074.)

is seen in postmenopausal women[374] (Fig. 40-58).

Hilum cells (hilar Leydig cells). Clusters of large cells with abundant pink cytoplasm are commonly found associated with nonmyelinated nerve fibers in the hilum of the ovary at the insertion of the mesovarium. Hilum cells regularly contain proteinaceous *crystalloids of Reinke,* a feature shared with testicular Leydig (interstitial) cells but not with luteinized stromal cells in the ovary. The physiologic significance of hilum cells in the ovary has not been demonstrated; they are increased in the newborn in association with such pregnancy complications as toxemia, diabetes, and multiple pregnancy, perhaps as a response to increased amounts of placental chorionic gonadotropin.[418]

Vestigial structures. Traces of the mesonephros persist as isolated small ducts in the mesovarium; a more plexiform glandular structure, the rete ovarii, is situated at the margin of the ovarian-hilar junction. It is homologous with the rete testis; confusion with focal neoplastic change is to be avoided.

Tiny nodules of heterotopic adenocortical tissue occur in the ovarian suspensory ligament, broad ligament, and mesovarium. They are common if carefully sought, especially in children.[334] Although there is some potential for neoplastic change in any cell, no important type of neoplasm has been consistently related to either mesonephric or adrenal rests.

Ovarian senescence, failure, atrophy

The ovary at birth contains about one-half million oocytes.[323] Between 300 and 400 oocytes may mature as potential gametes. Some of the rest will form small follicles, which undergo atresia, but the majority lyse and disappear without a trace.

As the age of menopause approaches, the number of oocytes diminishes and the number of anovulatory cycles increases. The follicles undergoing atresia leave behind a thin convoluted skein of hyalinized tissue. A few residual oocytes can be identified during the sixth decade in about 25% of ovaries studied; functional corpora lutea with secretory endometrial changes are present in about 10%.[372]

The postmenopausal ovary is composed chiefly of stroma, which remains biochemically active, and may be slightly or moderately hyperplastic. It produces chiefly the androgenic steroids dehydroepiandrosterone, androstenedione, and testosterone; it does not aromatize androgens to estrogen.[364]

Menopausal changes may occur prematurely

in young women in the group 15 to 25 years of age. The ovaries are small, atrophic, and usually contain no follicles. A few or no oocytes are present.[402] Gonadotropin titers are characteristically elevated, and the ovaries do not respond to gonadotropin therapy.

The basis of premature ovarian atrophy has not been explained by morphologic study, except in some instances of autoimmune ovarian failure. Thus far, the patients with autoimmune ovarian destruction have had other well-recognized forms of autoimmune disease, notably Addison's disease and Hashimoto's thyroiditis.[365] At an active stage of the antiovarian immune response, the follicles are infiltrated by lymphocytes and plasma cells.

A form of ovarian atrophy that is usually reversible is that caused by prolonged use of contraceptive progestogen-estrogen drugs. The ovaries are small and contain essentially no graafian follicles, but numerous oocytes persist.[363,390]

Nonneoplastic cysts and hyperplasia
Surface inclusion cysts

The ovary gradually develops a convoluted surface, perhaps as the result of contraction after ovulation, when the stigma of rupture heals, leaving a crevice with buried epithelium and delicate surface adhesions.[413] The buried epithelium may proliferate and often undergoes metaplastic changes, typically to a tubal epithelial pattern.[266] With accumulation of fluid, small cysts result. The resulting surface-inclusion cysts usually remain tiny; an occasional large unilocular cyst may also originate in this fashion.

Follicle cyst, corpus luteum cyst

Follicles and corpora lutea generally do not exceed 2 cm in diameter; when either exceeds a diameter of 3 cm, it may be regarded as "cystic," i.e., larger than usual. Symptoms that can be related to such a cyst are unusual, though menstrual irregularities have been attributed to corpus luteum cysts in some reports.[379] Rarely a large follicle cyst may be a source of excessive estrogen secretion; such a lesion in a child has been reported as a cause of sexual precocity.[404] Severe hemorrhage may originate from the site of rupture in an early corpus luteum.[311]

Luteoma of pregnancy and other luteinized cysts and nodules

Theca lutein cysts. Hyperplasia of luteinized theca cells regularly occurs in pregnancy, usually without significant disturbance in the gross morphology of the ovary. Occasionally the process is greatly accentuated, producing multiple large cysts, with prominent luteinization of theca cells but not granulosa cells. This change, sometimes called *hyperreactio luteinalis*, is seen in association with hydatidiform mole, multiple pregnancy, erythroblastosis fetalis, and conditions in which chorionic gonadotropin titers are increased.[340] Occasional cases have been associated with otherwise uncomplicated pregnancy.[330] A remarkable degree of theca-lutein cystic hyperplasia can be produced when clomiphene or gonadotropin administration is used to stimulate ovulation.[393]

Luteoma of pregnancy. Nodular masses of theca-lutein hyperplasia have been discovered chiefly as incidental findings during cesarean section.[405] They are solid, have an orange-brown color, and may be bilateral or multiple within the same ovary.

The cells are large and uniform, about half the diameter of a luteinized granulosa cell, and form solid masses or, less commonly, microcystic follicle-like structures. Mitoses may be numerous (Fig. 40-59).

A minority of women and a few female infants have been virilized; testosterone levels may be elevated.[380] Luteomas of pregnancy regress when the pregnancy terminates.

Stromal luteoma. Scully[394] has described nodular theca-lutein proliferation of the ovarian stroma, chiefly in postmenopausal women. Associated endometrial changes suggested estrogen or progesterone production. In view of the somewhat elevated gonadotropin secretion at this age, the pathogenesis may be analogous to that of pregnancy luteoma; the original lesions were considered to be neoplastic. The lesions reported have been small and benign.

Polycystic ovary (Stein-Leventhal) syndrome

The syndrome described by Stein and Leventhal in 1935[403] included infertility, secondary amenorrhea, hirsutism, and obesity in a group of young women whose only notable endocrine lesion was enlarged pale cystic ovaries. Actual masculinization with clitoral hypertrophy, frontal balding, and deep voice, and changes of body habitus does *not* occur. Since that time a great many facts have been accumulated, but a fully satisfactory explanation remains to be found. In any series there is a general similarity in the endocrine problems, but only a minority of patients present with all the criteria listed above. The condition is sometimes hereditary.[326]

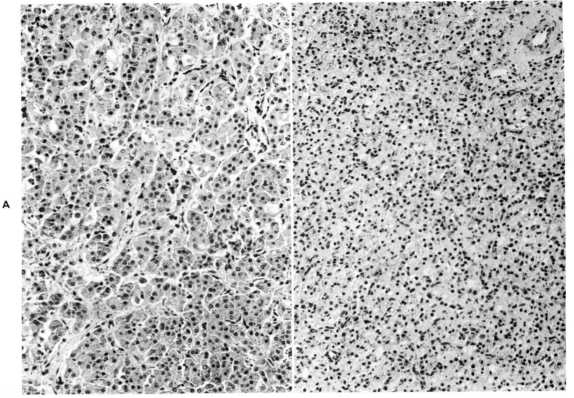

Fig. 40-59. A, Pregnancy luteoma composed of large luteinized stromal cells, occurred as multiple red-brown nodules, identified at cesarean section. Female infant was temporarily masculinized. **B,** Section from ill-defined yellow area in opposite ovary 2 months later. (Courtesy Dr. L. R. Malmak and Dr. George V. Miller.)

The ovarian lesion is not specific; it is almost certainly just a reactive change like the other features of the syndrome. The appearance is essentially that of an *anovulatory ovary*. Numerous follicles are present; typically they form a layer beneath the thickened white cortex. The medullary stroma that forms the central core is solid, gray, and somewhat edematous (Fig. 40-60). Microscopically the follicles and atretic follicles are all surrounded by a relatively prominent luteinized theca-cell layer. The stromal cells themselves may be focally luteinized. Except in rare cases there is no corpus luteum. The ovaries are usually enlarged, sometimes more than 6 cm in diameter, but may be of normal size.

Unquestionably more than one basic physiologic defect will trigger the entire symptom complex and physical changes, including those in the ovary. For instance, androgens from adrenal hyperplasia or neoplasm can do it; a similar syndrome has resulted from use of contraceptive steroids.[316,412] A common thread

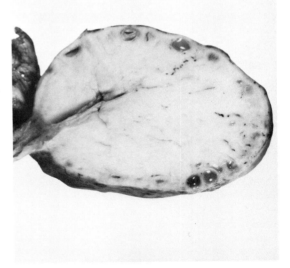

Fig. 40-60. Enlarged ovary from young woman with Stein-Leventhal (polycystic ovary) syndrome. Note abundant central stroma and peripheral subcapsular follicles.

seems to be consistently elevated androgen secretion, especially testosterone. It is necessary to identify the concentration of the protein-bound testosterone component as well as the total because only the unbound component reacts biologically; women with the polycystic ovary syndrome have low levels of testosterone-binding protein, which will rise as they respond to treatment.[332]

Greenblatt and Mahesh[342] note that the pituitary follicle-stimulating hormone (FSH) is inhibited to low levels by testosterone but luteinizing hormone (LH) is not always so affected. The levels of LH are sufficient to stimulate the ovarian theca and stromal cells to luteinize[337]; they may then secrete androgens inappropriately because of the abnormal pattern of initial gonadotropin stimulation, perpetuating the abnormal anovulatory state.

Any intervention that will elicit a surge of FSH sufficient to stimulate maturation of a follicle and ovulation will correct this abnormal state of affairs, at least temporarily. This has been done by direct injection of gonadotropins, by stimulation of their production with hypothalamic FSH/LH–releasing factors,[328,408,417] and by reduction of ovarian steroid feedback effect through ovarian injury (chiefly wedge resection), clomiphene,[389] or suppression with corticoids.

Hyperthecosis and stromal hyperplasia

The amount of ovarian stroma varies and may be abundant even at menopause and thereafter. When stromal proliferation is excessive, it is said to be hyperplastic.

In some young women stromal hyperplasia is sufficiently pronounced to cause enlargement or displacement of follicles and other structures. Variable degrees of stromal luteinization may occur. The abnormal stromal cells produce androgens, especially testosterone; in some patients masculinization may be severe. The ovaries may be solid or partly cystic. Both the clinical and pathologic features tend to overlap with the polycystic ovary syndrome, except that hyperthecosis produces masculinization, which may be severe. This condition is harder to treat than the polycystic ovary syndrome. Some patients have responded to oophorectomy.[321]

Massive edema

This rare form of ovarian enlargement usually occurs in young women who present either with severe abdominal pain or with severe masculinization. The ovarian enlargement may be unilateral or bilateral. There often seems to be some degree of torsion, especially in the patients who have pain. The masculinizing lesions have histologic evidence of stromal luteinization that resembles hyperthecosis. Both types of ovaries are massively edematous so that water leaks copiously from the cut surface. The pathogenesis is unknown; it has been suggested that torsion is responsible.[351] Total ovariectomy is probably unnecessary for this benign condition; resection to a normal-sized remnant has been recommended.[325]

Endometriosis

Ectopic endometrium in the ovary is troublesome because it forms fibrous adhesions and hemorrhagic cysts, which are painful and a cause of infertility. Accumulated hemorrhage results from stromal breakdown at the time of menstrual bleeding. Cysts may become large and typically are filled with semisolid dark brown altered blood. Endometrial tissue can usually be found somewhere in the fibrous wall, but a search may be necessary. Smaller foci of hemorrhage organize and contract, leaving a characteristic puckered scar tinged yellow-brown with hemosiderin (Fig. 40-61).

The pathogenesis has been debated. Implants from a reflux of menstrual blood have been shown to occur and implants have been observed to grow from such material. Serosal metaplasia is another possibility and almost

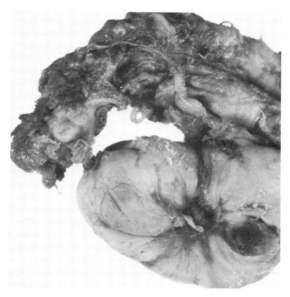

Fig. 40-61. Ovarian endometriosis forming characteristic puckered hemorrhagic scar and extensive tubal adhesions.

certainly has been the cause in some cases. In a given case it is usually impossible to demonstrate the origin of the lesion.

Heterotopic ovarian tissue

Misplaced ovarian tissue is rare. The usual sites lie near the migratory route of the germ cells, in the pelvic retroperitoneum and mesosigmoid[414]; unquestionable nodules of ovarian stroma with oocytes have been encountered beneath the uterine serosa.[314] Heterotopic ovarian tissue has been the site of neoplasm[356] (see fallopian tube) and a source of unexpected ovarian function after bilateral ovariectomy.[356]

Neoplasms
Classification

Because of their remarkable diversity, ovarian tumors seem to present a bewildering array. Natural history annd response to treatment vary considerably from one group of tumors to another. Especially in the area of chemotherapy and radiation therapy, the best therapeutic approach may be highly specific for a single type of neoplasm; accordingly, accurate histologic diagnosis is often a critical factor in achieving an optimal treatment response. It is extremely important therefore that the pathologist responsible for diagnosis and physician responsible for therapy communicate clearly. Similarly, the classification used in any discussion of new therapeutic techniques must be understandable or the report is useless.

Neoplasms arise from and tend to resemble any of the normally occurring cellular components of the ovary described at the beginning of this section. This classification is based upon histogenesis; the cell or tissue of origin. It is essentially the classification presented by the World Health Organization[399] with minor abridgments in the interest of clarity for this introduction to the subject.

I. Tumors of surface epithelium
   A. Serous tumors
     1. Benign cystadenoma, cystadenofibroma, and papillary cystadenoma
     2. Borderline serous tumors
     3. Malignant serous cystadenocarcinomas, papillary carcinomas
   B. Mucinous tumors
     1. Benign mucinous cystadenoma
     2. Borderline mucinous tumors
     3. Malignant mucinous carcinomas
   C. Endometrioid tumors
     1. Benign (cystic endometriosis?)
     2. Borderline; rare lesions resembling atypical endometrial hyperplasia(?)
     3. Malignant
       a. Adenocarcinomas, well differentiated, poorly differentiated, and adenosquamous carcinoma
       b. Endometrioid stromal sarcoma (?)
       c. Malignant mixed müllerian tumor
   D. Clear-cell tumors
     1. Benign clear-cell tumor (chiefly cystadenofibroma)
     2. Borderline clear-cell tumors
     3. Malignant clear-cell adenocarcinoma
   E. Brenner tumor
     1. Benign
     2. Borderline (proliferating Brenner tumor)
     3. Malignant
   F. Mixed (serous and mucinous, etc.)
   G. Undifferentiated carcinoma (always malignant)
II. Sex cord stromal tumors
   A. Granulosa-theca cell tumors
     1. Granulosa cell tumor
     2. Thecoma
     3. Fibroma
     4. Mixed and indeterminate types
   B. Sertoli-Leydig cell tumors (androblastomas, "arrhenoblastomas")
     1. Well differentiated; tubular and Leydig cell types
     2. Intermediate differentiation
     3. Poorly differentiated (sarcomatoid)
   C. Gynandroblastoma
III. Lipid cell tumors (hilum cell tumor, "adrenal rest" tumor, etc.)
IV. Germ cell tumors
   A. Dysgerminoma
   B. Endodermal sinus tumor
   C. Embryonal carcinoma, polyembryoma
   D. Choriocarcinoma
   E. Teratomas
     1. Mature: chiefly benign cystic teratoma (dermoid cyst)
     2. Immature (malignant teratoma)
     3. Specialized (struma, carcinoid, etc.)
   F. Mixed forms
V. Gonadoblastoma

It has been estimated that about 17,000 women in the United States would be found to have ovarian cancer in 1975, and in the same year about 10,800 would die of ovarian cancer. The yearly death rate from ovarian cancer has remained about 8.5 per 100,000 women from 1950 to 1975.[181]

The relative frequency with which different types of ovarian neoplasms occur is summarized in Table 40-3. The proportions indicated are approximate, and represent a synthesis of numerous reports. This is necessary because older studies use uncertain criteria for malignancy and do not distinguish important tumor categories, especially endometrioid carcinoma. More recent reports from cancer treatment centers do not reflect the true incidence of common benign neoplasms, which are usually treated in less specialized institutions.

Tumors of surface epithelium

This is the most common group of ovarian neoplasms and includes the majority of ovarian carcinomas (Table 40-3). The tissue of origin is considered to be the surface celomic mesothelium that covers the ovary (Fig. 40-62); it seems to retain, in neoplasms, the capacity to recapitulate tumor patterns that resemble the epithelial components of the müllerian ducts. For example, the epithelium of serous tumors resembles that which lines the tube; the cells that line mucinous cystadenomas resemble endocervical mucosa. These neoplasms usually have a prominent cystic component with single or multiple loculations, often a variable amount of fibrous stroma, and an epithelial lining that often is thrown into papillary tufts.

It is necessary to recognize a spectrum of aggressiveness that is divided into benign, malignant, and borderline categories. Clearly *benign* cystic tumors are lined by a single layer of well-oriented columnar epithelial cells; papillary projections, if present, are supported by fibrovascular stromal stalks and covered by the same type of epithelium. Obviously *malignant* tumors of this group have an anaplastic

Table 40-3. General classification of primary ovarian neoplasms

Cell of origin (representative tumor types)	Relative incidence, all ovarian neoplasms*	Relative incidence, malignant neoplasms only
Surface epithelium (serous, mucinous, endometrioid, clear cell, etc.)	65%	95%
Germ cells (immature ova) (cystic teratoma, solid teratoma, dysgerminoma, etc.)	20%	1%
Stromal cells (sex cords) (granulosa-theca cells, Sertoli-Leydig cells, lipid cells, fibroma, etc.)	12%	2%
Tumors in dysgenetic gonads (gonadoblastoma)	1%	—
Unclassified (chiefly undifferentiated carcinoma)	2%	4%

*The relative incidence figures noted here represent an approximation (see text).

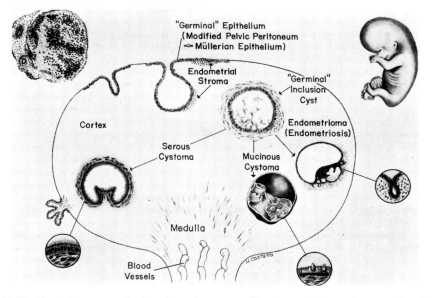

Fig. 40-62. Semidiagrammatic drawing of ovary to illustrate origin and types of cystomas derived from "germinal" epithelium. Note papillary growth on surface and various types of cystic tumors derived from infolding of this type of epithelium. Embryonic ovary and müllerian duct *(top left)* is drawn from 35 mm embryo *(top right)* and illustrates embryonic similarity of müllerian duct to germinal epithelium. The three types of cystomas (and their malignant counterparts) derived from "germinal" inclusion cysts are serous, endometrial, and mucinous—all recapitulating müllerian system, to which germinal epithelium is embryologically very closely related. Low-power and high-power drawings are from actual specimens. (From Hertig, A. T., and Gore, H. M.: Rocky Mountain Med. J. **55:**47-50, 1958.)

epithelial component that *invades* the stroma of the tumor or other structures, in addition to forming the epithelial lining. The epithelial cells are often several layers thick and have anaplastic nuclei, with a loss of polarity. The prognosis is very poor; about 15% of patients survive for 5 years, regardless of treatment.

The important intermediate, or *borderline* group is identified chiefly by the *absence of invasion* in an otherwise highly proliferative neoplasm. A complex papillary pattern is often present, and the epithelium may be two or

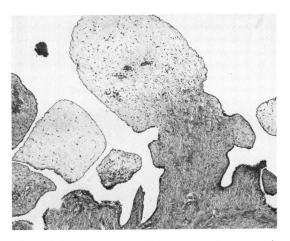

Fig. 40-63. Benign papillary serous tumor, with abundant fibrous stroma covered by single layer of small flattened epithelial cells. (85×.)

three cells thick. The epithelial cells generally appear only moderately dysplastic and maintain some degree of columnar orientation in some degree of columnar orientation in most areas.

Although the behavior of borderline tumors is unpredictable in individual cases, as a group they have a much better prognosis than do malignant tumors of the ovary. More than 80% of patients survive 5 years and almost as many survive 10 years, even in the presence of implants on peritoneal surfaces.[391] Recurrences, if they occur, typically appear after several years; the minority of tumors that have a malignant course tend to progress slowly. Radical therapy has not improved survival. It is important, therefore, to avoid radical or extensive therapeutic methods with significant morbidity and mortality for patients in this group unless it can be shown that the prospective benefits overweigh the risks.

Serous tumors. Benign serous cysts and cystadenomas may form single or multiple loculations, lined by low columnar epithelium, which is sometimes ciliated, often distinctly resembling tubal epithelium (Fig 40-63). The cyst fluid is watery or viscous and clear and contains a variety of mucins; however the epithelial cells that secrete the fluid do not have the characteristic vacuolated pattern of mucinous epithelium. Papillary processes are common and may be numerous and complicated.

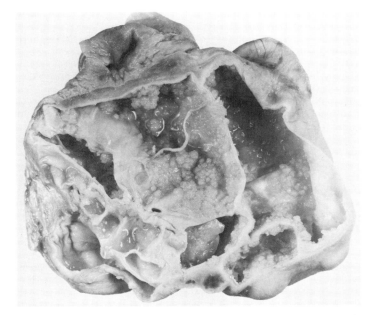

Fig. 40-64. Borderline serous tumor of ovary, a multilocular cystic mass with spaces lined by papillary epithelial masses.

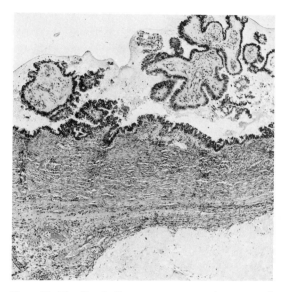

Fig. 40-65. Borderline serous cystodenoma of ovary without invasion. Epithelium is pleomorphic and forms small papillary processes. (46×; AFIP 264082-1.)

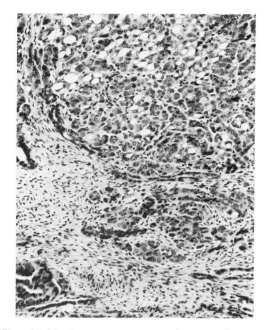

Fig. 40-66. Serous carcinoma of ovary showing invasion of stroma by strands and small clusters of adenocarcinoma cells. (100×.)

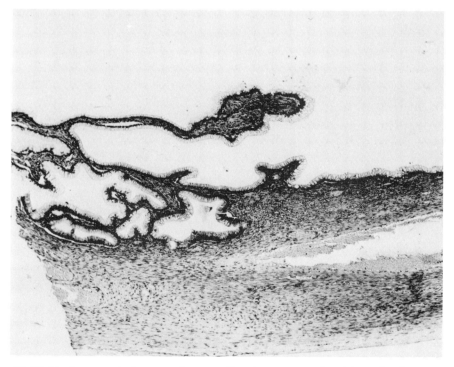

Fig. 40-67. Mucinous cystadenoma of ovary. Gland spaces are lined by tall columnar cells with basal nuclei and large apical mucin vacuoles. Note resemblance to cervical mucosa. (70×; AFIP 316189-23112.)

The epithelial component of serous tumors, unlike other neoplasms of surface epithelium, may appear on the external surfaces; occasional lesions are composed entirely of a surface papillary growth with no cystic component. It is common to find tiny round laminated calcific concretions called *psammoma bodies* in the stroma of the papillary processes.

The presence of a relatively prominent or abundant fibrous tissue stroma produces plump papillae and large solid fibrous masses as well as cysts. The resulting growths are called papillary adenofibromas and cystadenofibromas.

Borderline serous tumors are often multilocular (Fig. 40-64) and have a more complex papillary pattern; fine papillae, closely packed, may resemble solid epithelial proliferation. Variable degrees of dysplastic nuclear change and mitotic activity are present (Fig. 40-65).

The presence of stromal invasion is the basis for identifying a serous tumor as a serous *carcinoma* (Fig. 40-66). Bilateral ovarian involvement occurs in about two thirds of both borderline and malignant serous tumors, and in one third of tumors that have not spread beyond the uterus, tubes, and ovaries.[355] Because microscopic foci of cancer may lurk in an apparently normal ovary when serous carcinoma is present on the opposite side, Kottmeier favors bilateral oophorectomy in every case.[355]

Mucinous tumors. Mucinous tumors are also typically unilocular or multilocular cystic masses. The epithelium that lines the cysts is composed of tall columnar "goblet" cells with basal nuclei and prominent mucin vacuoles; it resembles endocervical mucosa (Fig. 40-67). In some instances the pattern appears even more like intestinal epithelium, including argentaffin cells and even Paneth cells.[396] Rarely, a mucinous tumor has produced enough gastrin to cause the Zollinger-Ellison syndrome.[327] Since about 5% of mucinous tumors are associated with cystic teratomas, it has been suggested that some, at least, originate from germ cells; an intestinal metaplasia of these exotic cell types seems more likely, despite the apparent production of endodermal derivatives by mesodermal cells.[336] A larger number, however, may have endometrioid or serous elements, which supports their classification with surface epithelial tumors. Since the biologic activity of mucinous tumors is more like that of other surface epithelial tumors, their inclusion in this section has a solid practical basis, which outweighs the latent quibble over histogenesis.

In carcinomas, the mucin vacuoles are less prominent and nuclear polarity is lost, but the typical pattern is usually evident in better differentiated parts of the tumor. Stromal invasion is sometimes considerably more difficult to evaluate in mucinous tumors, when small glandular spaces are distributed through fibrous stroma. Hart and Norris[345] have noted that a multilayered epithelial proliferation more than three cells thick also correlates well with malignant behavior. *Borderline mucinous tumors,* then, are defined as mucinous tumors in which there is no stromal invasion, and the epithelial proliferation, although sometimes cytologically atypical, remains no more than two or three cells thick.[345] In cases selected by these criteria, more than 90% of women with borderline tumors survive for 10 years; in the same report[345] 59% of patients with mucinous carcinoma (all stage I) survived for 10 years. Survival at 10 years in mucinous carcinoma (all stages) is 34%.[396]

Bilateral ovarian involvement occurs in about one fifth of both borderline and malignant mucinous tumors, but only in 10% of cases in which there is no spread beyond the uterus, tubes, and ovaries.[355] Kottmeier found no instance of microscopic involvement of an apparently normal ovary on the side opposite a mucinous carcinoma.

Mucinous ascites (pseudomyxoma peritonei) occasionally occurs in association with a well-differentiated borderline mucinous tumor. The ovarian tumor characteristically contains mucin-filled cystic spaces that dissect the ovarian stroma. The neoplastic epithelium in the ovary and in the peritoneal lesion as well is sparse and well differentiated.[345] Chemotherapy with alkylating agents has provided symptomatic improvement and prolonged survival in some patients.[359]

Endometrioid tumors. Endometrioid carcinomas are so named because the histologic pattern closely resembles that of uterine endometrial adenocarcinoma. The distinction is most easily recognized in well-differentiated carcinomas (Fig. 40-68). Less-differentiated lesions may have a typical endometrioid pattern only in focal areas or a few patches of squamous metaplasia as the only clues to their identity, which accounts for some of the variation in the frequency with which they are reported. They probably comprise between 15% and 20% of ovarian cancers.

The *benign* counterpart is probably repre-

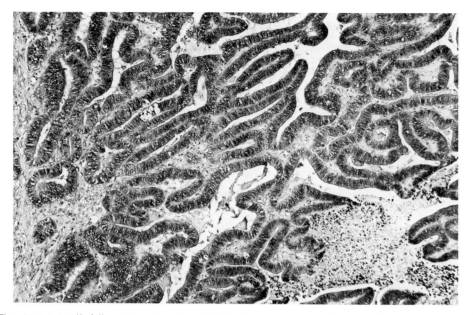

Fig. 40-68. Well-differentiated endometrioid adenocarcinoma of ovary. Pattern is identical to that of uterine endometrial adenocarcinoma. (150×.)

sented by some cases of cystic endometriosis of the ovary. A clearly defined concept of the *borderline* endometrioid tumor is lacking; certainly such lesions are quite rare.

Endometrioid carcinomas are often partly cystic frequently with prominent solid areas; The cyst fluid is often brown or bloody. The cyst lining has a velvety or papillary appearance. Association with endometriosis is demonstrable in about one third of cases,[392] but the presence of endometriosis is not the basis for inclusion of a tumor within this group. Endometriosis is a common lesion of the ovary and occurs together with other ovarian neoplasms, especially clear-cell tumors.

The prognosis for well-differentiated carcinomas is good; about 60% of patients survive for 5 years as compared to 23% survival for poorly differentiated carcinomas.[392]

In about one third of the patients there is a coexistent adenocarcinoma of the endometrium. It is generally accepted that both lesions are separate primary cancers because the survival rate in the presence of endometrial involvement is not appreciably lower.[355] Furthermore the two lesions commonly occur together without evidence of any other metastatic lesion; the common presence of multiple foci of dysplastic endometrial change is further evidence for a multifocal process.

Other endometrioid neoplasms such as *stromal sarcoma, malignant mixed müllerian tumor,* and *adenosarcoma* have rarely been reported as primary tumors of the ovary. The histologic features and prognosis (poor) do not differ significantly from similar lesions occurring in the endometrium.

Clear-cell tumors. The gross appearance is often a combination of solid and cystic components that is very much like that of endometrioid carcinoma. The cyst is usually unilocular; the fluid is commonly brown and the solid areas form nodular masses that protrude into the lumen.

The histologic pattern is characterized by masses of large epithelial cells with abundant clear cytoplasm, supported by delicate fibrous trabeculae (Fig. 40-69). The cytoplasm contains abundant glycogen. A variation in pattern is the presence of small cystic spaces lined by a single layer of large cuboid cells that are somewhat separated from one another; the nuclei may be oriented toward the cyst lumen rather than the basal area, producing what is called a "hobnail" pattern.

Less than 10% are bilateral. Benign, borderline, and malignant varieties occur, but the malignant variety is much more common. Association with endometriosis is six times as great as with ovarian carcinoma in general.[396]

Because the clear-cell histologic pattern resembles that of renal adenocarcinoma and the proximity of adjacent mesonephric structures, the term *mesonephroma* has also been used to

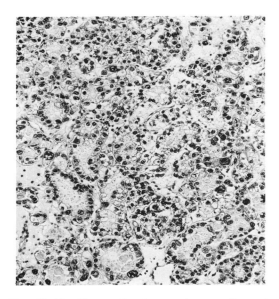

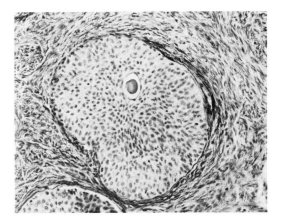

Fig. 40-70. Brenner tumor. Typical sharply circumscribed nest of uniform cytologically benign cells surrounded by dense fibrous stroma. (140×; AFIP 305334-1-4-2.)

Fig. 40-69. Clear-cell adenocarcinoma. There is abundant cytoplasmic glycogen; mucin is found only in extracellular secretions. (100×.)

designate this type of neoplasm. There is no convincing evidence to support the concept of mesonephric origin.[397] On the other hand, ovarian clear-cell carcinomas and identical neoplasms of the endometrium, cervix, and vagina seem to be related to tumors of müllerian epithelial type, especially endometrioid tumors. Endometrioid and clear-cell patterns occur together in ovarian and endometrial carcinomas, and clear-cell tumors have been shown to arise in endometriosis.[397] Clear-cell carcinoma patterns also occur in many malignant mixed müllerian tumors. Survival rates are in an intermediate range; 37% survive 5 years.[391]

Brenner tumor. Brenner tumors are solid gray or yellow-gray masses of fibrous tissue; occasionally it is possible to find scattered tiny cysts on cut section. The external serosal surface is smooth and shiny.

The microscopic appearance of scattered epithelial masses on a field of fibrous stroma is distinctive (Fig. 40-70). The epithelial component is composed of ovoid cells with clear cytoplasm, vesicular nuclei, and a characteristic nuclear groove. Mucinous epithelial cells form tiny cysts in the epithelial masses in about one third of the tumors, and one fifth have a conspicuous cystic mucinous component.

In the borderline variety of Brenner tumor (called proliferating Brenner tumor) the epithelial masses form larger cysts with a redundant, sometimes papillary lining of cells that look identical to transitional cell papilloma of the urinary bladder. Malignant Brenner tumors have an anaplastic epithelial component that resembles poorly differentiated transitional cell carcinoma or epidermoid carcinoma and invades the stroma of the tumor. Borderline and malignant Brenner tumors are both extremely rare; one needs to identify a well-differentiated Brenner tumor pattern in some part of the lesion in order to establish the diagnosis.

Arey's wax model reconstruction preparations have shown that the epithelial islands are actually anastomosing cords of epithelial cells, in continuity with the covering serosal epithelium of the ovary. The ultrastructural appearance of Brenner epithelial cells resembles that of urinary bladder transitional epithelium and the Walthard cell nests of the tubal serosa. On the basis of these studies it is generally accepted that Brenner tumors probably represent a neoplastic proliferation of ovarian surface epithelial cells that further differentiate into urinary type of transitional epithelium.[329,387,400]

Fewer than 10% are bilateral. The stromal component is not always inert. In occasional cases the stromal cells appear luteinized and contain birefringent lipid; associated endometrial hyperplasia has suggested secretion of estrogen by the tumor.[333]

Mixed forms. Surface epithelial tumors often include a combination of the foregoing types. Unless two or more patterns form a distinct and prominent component, the neoplasm is usually and most reasonably classified after the predominant cell type represented.

Undifferentiated carcinoma. Nearly all adenocarcinomas too undifferentiated for subclassification probably belong to the group of tumors originating from surface epithelium. About 54% are bilateral; they comprise about 4% of ovarian carcinomas.[355] The prognosis is extremely poor. Many are composed of small cells of nearly uniform size. Mitoses are extremely numerous; nuclei are anaplastic. It is a mistake to classify such lesions as "granulosa cell carcinomas." Confusion of this highly malignant group of neoplasms with granulosa cell tumors serves only to blur the distinctive clinical correlations associated with these two very different neoplastic diseases.

Sex cord stromal tumors (sex cord–mesenchyme tumors)

This group of neoplasms arises from specialized ovarian stromal cells. The general designation of *sex cord–mesenchyme tumors* is favored by Scully[396] because the assumption that the embryonic sex cords and their derivatives are mesenchymal or stromal derivatives (as opposed to celomic epithelium) remains unproved. It is the specialized stromal cells that produce ovarian steroid hormones. The tumors that arise from them produce the full range of the ovarian and testicular steroid hormonal repertory, including intermediates, and occasionally adrenal steroids as well.

Granulosa-theca cell tumors. About half of the tumors in this group are thecomas, one fourth are composed only of granulosa cells, and the remaining one fourth are a mixture of both.

Granulosa cell tumors are often partly cystic, and multiple areas of hemorrhage are common. Solid areas have a yellow-brown color. Thecomas are solid, firm, and have a yellow or yellow-white color with dense streaks and patches of hyalinized white tissue. *Mixed granulosa-theca tumors* are made firm and solid by the fibrotic thecal component.

Granulosa cells have uniform, small, oval or rounded nuclei, with a fold or cleft in the nuclear membrane. The cells are distributed in masses with little intervening stroma. Ultrastructural studies support and extend the resemblance to normal granulosa cells.[377] Characteristic rosette-like structures called Call-Exner bodies are nearly always present; they are rounded masses of pink inspissated material surrounded by a circular row of typical granulosa cells and resemble similar structures found in the normal graafian follicle (Fig. 40-71). Unlike acini, with which they are often

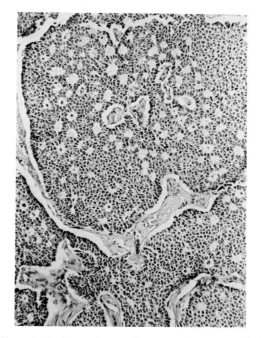

Fig. 40-71. Granulosa cell tumor. Many rounded spaces (Call-Exner bodies) containing amorphous eosinophilic material are scattered among uniform small cells with compressed-appearing nuclei. Compare with Fig. 40-55. Strands of hyalinized stroma are characteristic feature. (70×.)

confused, the central cytoplasmic margins are indistinct, there is no stainable mucin, and the nuclei tend to lie adjacent to the inner rim of the space.

A variety of microscopic patterns occur; microfollicular and macrofollicular tumors resemble clusters of small or large graafian follicles. The descriptive terms trabecular, insular, gyriform, solid-tubular, and diffuse are often applied, without significant clinical correlations. Paradoxically, the cystic macrofollicular tumors produce androgenic effects.[371] The so-called sarcomatoid variety, in which large masses of granulosa cells tend to form swirling patterns of somewhat spindle-shaped cells, may have a more aggressive natural history.[358] Norris and Taylor[370] could not correlate aggressive lesions with pattern, cellular atypism, or mitoses but noted that lesions that ultimately recurred tended to invade the tumor capsule and lymphatics when originally excised.

Thecomas are solid fibrotic masses in which some of the spindle-shaped cells that form the tumor are plump and rounded and contain abundant cytoplasm that reacts with lipid stains. Another characteristic feature is the presence of hyaline plaques.

Granulosa-theca cell tumors characteristically produce estrogenic hormones, but they are occasionally androgenic. Since the type of hormonal effect is not a reliable criterion for establishing the nature of an ovarian neoplasm, it is a poor basis for classification. Even metastatic carcinomas may be associated with hormone production.

The most common symptom is uterine bleeding. Women with estrogen-secreting granulosa-theca cell tumors often have endometrial hyperplasia. Well-differentiated endometrial adenocarcinoma occurs in from 9%[370] to 24%[362] of cases in postmenopausal women. Although the morphologic features of these adenocarcinomas meet the criteria of well-differentiated adenocarcinoma, they have a remarkably good prognosis; reports of death or metastasis related to these cancers are very difficult to find. It is possible that some of these endometrial carcinomas are highly estrogen-dependent and therefore fail to progress when the source of estrogen is withdrawn.

Granulosa-theca cell tumors are bilateral in less than 5% of cases. About two thirds occur after menopause. The prognosis is very good; over 90% will survive for 10 years.[370] Even malignant granulosa cell tumors act out their aggressive natural history over a period of many years; recurrences or metastases may appear more than 20 years after the original treatment, and the recurrences themselves respond well to treatment. For these reasons most authorities recommend that the opposite ovary in a young woman be preserved.[355,370,396] If malignant thecomas exist, they are extremely rare; Norris and Taylor found one acceptable case, but Scully[396] has seen none.

Fibroma. Large fibrous tumors of the ovary without clinical or morphologic evidence of endocrine activity are relatively common, forming about 5% of all ovarian tumors in most large series. Densely collagenized fibrous tissue forms a monotonous histologic pattern, broken by areas of calcification in some cases. Occasionally there may be an associated benign ascites and pleural effusion, which disappear when the tumor is resected (Meigs' syndrome).

Fibrosarcoma is extremely rare.

Sertoli-Leydig cell tumors (arrhenoblastoma, androblastoma). Although many tumors in this group produce androgens and masculinize the patient, many are hormonally inert and some even have estrogenic effects.[366] Testosterone and a variety of androgenic precursors may be produced in variable proportions.

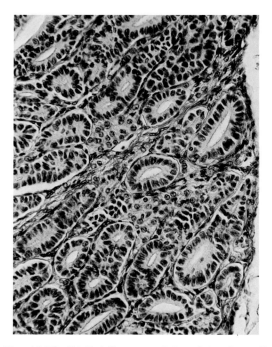

Fig. 40-72. Well-differentiated Sertoli-Leydig cell tumor, forming small tubules composed of Sertoli cells. Leydig cells are scattered through stroma (center). (250×.)

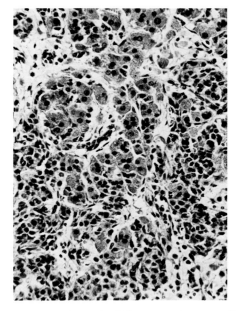

Fig. 40-73. Moderately differentiated intermediate type of Sertoli-Leydig cell tumor. Large, dense, eosinophilic Leydig cells are intermixed with cord-like strands of smaller Sertoli cells in a loose, sparsely cellular stroma. (275×.)

Although their histologic patterns resemble developing male gonadal structures, Sertoli-Leydig cell tumors arise from the same female sex cord stromal cells as granulosa-theca cell tumors and consistently contain female sex chromatin.[375] Some ultrastructural studies confirm a closer relationship to ovarian stroma than to the testis,[348,352] however the finding of cilia and other structures[350] leaves the subject unsettled.

Three histologic types are distinguished. Well-differentiated tumors form tubular structures composed of Sertoli cells, separated by a fibrous stroma, intermixed with large round Leydig cells in poorly circumscribed clumps (Fig. 40-72). Tumors of intermediate differentiation have a biphasic pattern in which large pink Leydig cells are prominent, separated by a spindly stroma in which the abortive tubule formation resembles early sex cords of the embryonic testis (Fig. 40-73).

Least differentiated is the sarcomatoid variety, composed of spindle cells that condense focally into a vague trabecular arrangement, separated by a looser myxoid component composed of the same type of cell. Leydig cells may or may not be present.

About half of the well-differentiated tumors, three fourths of intermediate tumors, and all sarcomatoid tumors are androgenic. Sertoli cell tumors in children, however, are estrogenic and cause precocious puberty.[312] Nearly all Sertoli-Leydig cell tumors are benign, despite reports indicating malignant behavior in more than 20%; it has been suggested that the higher figures resulted from inclusion of other kinds of adenocarcinoma, primary and metastatic, with functioning stroma.[375] Malignant behavior takes the form of intra-abdominal implantation, ordinarily without distant metastases.

Gynandroblastoma. Rarely, a sex cord stromal tumor may include both granulosa-theca cell and Sertoli-Leydig cell patterns.[373] Most have been benign. Those with hormonal function have produced androgens. Authentic examples are extremely rare.

Lipid cell tumors (hilum cell tumors, "adrenal rest" tumors, luteomas, etc.)

This distinctive group of neoplasms occurs in the form of soft yellow or yellow-brown nodules. The cells that comprise them may be relatively small and rounded with dense pink cytoplasm, or larger with foamy or clear cytoplasm. Occasionally the smaller cells may con-

tain crystalloids of Reinke, like testicular Leydig cells and ovarian hilum cells. Both types of cell may occur in the same tumor. The ultrastructure is consistent with ovarian stromal origin; the cytoplasmic organelles resemble those of steroid-secreting cells,[352] like the cells of the adrenal cortex.

Most are benign. The few that behave aggressively are likely to be larger and invade contiguous structures and may have atypical cytologic features.[407] The most common endocrine abnormality is virilization; a few have caused Cushing's syndrome.

Germ cell tumors

Ovarian germ cells are those that produce the female gametes—ova. They retain the capacity to produce in tumors an extremely diverse group of tissues. Most are benign cystic teratomas and occur chiefly in the young; malignant teratomas nearly always occur in children and young women. Optimal therapy depends on accurate identification and knowledge of the natural history of each type of neoplasm; various combinations of the different types are likely to occur together.

Dysgerminoma. Dysgerminomas are large solid encapsulated masses of soft gray-white

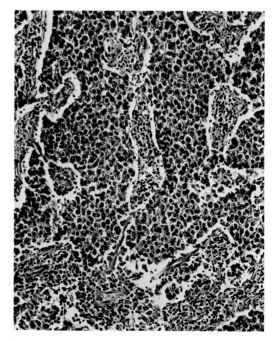

Fig. 40-74. Dysgerminoma. Masses of large uniform germ cells are separated by fibrous trabeculae that are infiltrated by lymphocytes. (130×.)

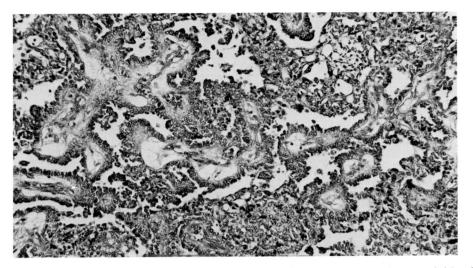

Fig. 40-75. Endodermal sinus tumor. Tangle of papillary processes with central blood vessel, usually covered by single layer of anaplastic germ cells; stroma is inconspicuous. (150×.)

tissue, often with foci of hemorrhage and necrosis. They are composed of large vesicular cells indistinguishable from the primordial germ cells of the embryonic gonad, distributed in large clumps and masses separated by fibrous trabeculae (Fig. 40-74). The fibrous stroma is almost always infiltrated by lymphocytes and may contain sarcoidosis-like granulomas. This pattern is indistinguishable from testicular seminoma. About 10% are bilateral.[317] The opposite ovary may contain microscopic foci of dysgerminoma even when it appears grossly normal (Table 40-4); if it is to be preserved, biopsy with frozen-section examination is desirable.

Dysgerminoma is extremely radiosensitive and radiocurable even in the presence of metastases. For this reason, since most patients are young, unilateral oophorectomy is desirable and sufficient when the opposite ovary is normal. The 5-year survival rate is between 70% and 90%. Some dysgerminomas produce chorionic gonadotropin (HCG), which should be detected, if present, by radioimmunoassay. HCG may indicate a more aggressive lesion and in any case serves as a tumor marker for early detection of recurrence.

Endodermal sinus tumor. Teilum[409] has established endodermal sinus tumor as a morphologically distinct entity. The most specific feature of this rare neoplasm is the presence of isolated papillary projections with a central blood vessel and peripheral sleeve of malignant embryonic epithelial cells (Fig. 40-75). Cross sections of this structure were once erroneously compared to immature glomeruli. In fact, they closely resemble invaginations of yolk sac endoderm, as seen best in the rat placenta, forming the endodermal sinuses of Duval.[409] Another distinctive feature is the presence of PAS-positive, diastase-resistant hyaline globules partly composed of alpha-fetoprotein.[410] Some tumors contain multiple gland spaces with an hourglass constriction resembling yolk sac vesicles, a pattern that Teilum has designated *polyvesicular vitelline tumor*.

The gross appearance is much like dysgerminoma except for the presence of more extensive yellow and red areas of hemorrhage and necrosis, and often there are cystic areas. Endodermal sinus tumors consistently produce alpha-fetoprotein, which can be demonstrated in tissue sections by immunohistochemical techniques[410] and in the patient's serum.[320] This substance is produced in the yolk sac of the developing embryo and may serve as a tumor marker in evaluating the course of the patient after treatment. All of the patients have been children or young adults. The prognosis is very poor; remissions have occurred in some patients treated postoperatively with multiple chemotherapeutic agents. Bilateral involvement in stage I is unlikely (Table 40-4).

Choriocarcinoma. Nongestational primary choriocarcinoma of the ovary is rare and malignant. The histologic pattern and clinical correlations are similar to gestational choriocarcinoma (p. 1764), except that the remark-

Table 40-4. Status of contralateral ovary in patients with stage I germ cell tumors of ovary*

Tumor	Number of patients		Number of stage Ia patients with microscopic involvement of opposite ovary	
	Stage Ia	Stage Ib	Number examined microscopically	Number positive
Dysgerminoma	71	7	21	4
Endodermal sinus tumor	51	0	24	0
Immature teratoma	40	0	6	0
Embryonal carcinoma	9	0	0	0
Mixed germ cell tumor	20	0	5	1

*Courtesy Dr. Robert J. Kurman and Dr. Henry J. Norris, Washington, D.C.

able response to chemotherapy usually does not occur. There have been occasional survivors.[346]

Teratomas. Teratomas are composed of recognizable tissues of ectodermal, mesodermal, and endodermal origin, in any combination. They are common and usually benign and inert but rarely produce remarkably bizarre and varied syndromes, reflecting the diverse potentials of the germ cell.

Benign cystic teratoma (dermoid cyst). Cystic teratomas are composed of mature somatic tissues of almost every description. Most cysts are unilocular and the tissue that forms the lining is usually skin (Fig. 40-76). The desquamated keratin and secretions, notably from sebaceous glands, accumulate with masses of hair to fill the lumen of the cyst. This disagreeable mixture is liquid at body temperature but solidifies when chilled. Other common components are salivary gland; bronchus; fat; smooth muscle; cartilage; bone; neural tissue including ganglia, glia, and choroid plexus; retina; pancreas; thyroid; and teeth. Characteristically a protuberance from the inner surface is the locus of growth of most of the hair and the richest depository of odd tissues. Uncommon tissues are skeletal and cardiac muscle, kidney, and liver.

In collected series bilateral teratomas occur in 8% to 15% of cases. Cystic teratomas comprise 20% of all ovarian tumors in adults and 50% of all ovarian tumors in children. Most patients are between 20 and 40 years, but they occur at all ages. Roentgenograms often are diagnostic, especially when teeth or bone are present. Most patients are operated on because a mass has been discovered during a physical examination.

The pathogenesis of teratomas has always excited speculation because of their exotic composition; Blackwell et al.[324] have made an

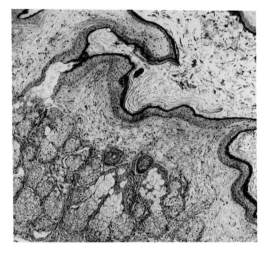

Fig. 40-76. Lining of typical benign cystic teratoma (dermoid cyst) is composed chiefly of skin with sebaceous glands, hair follicles, and sweat glands. (75×; AFIP 510588-07023.)

interesting historical review of this subject. Analysis of more recent cytogenetic studies using chromosome-banding techniques indicates that ovarian teratomas are parthenogenetic tumors that must originate from a single germ cell after its first meiotic division.[357]

Malignant change in a cystic teratoma is certainly less frequent than the 1.8% of cases reported,[378] because most benign teratomas are not reported. Almost any component may become malignant; epidermoid carcinoma is most common, but sweat gland carcinoma, thyroid carcinoma, malignant melanoma, and various sarcomas including osteosarcoma occur rarely.

Solid teratomas (teratomas with abundant solid tissue and relatively small cysts) are nearly all malignant (see below), but a few benign solid teratomas have been reported.[411]

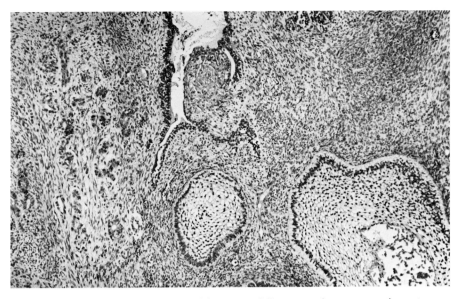

Fig. 40-77. Malignant teratoma. In addition to differentiated structures there is an embryonic stroma resembling sarcoma *(upper right)*. (80×.)

All the tissue components of a benign solid teratoma are as mature as are the other tissues of the patient in whom they occur.

Malignant teratoma (embryonal teratoma). Malignant teratoma is a unilateral solid mass with a heterogeneous appearance on cut surface. The histologic pattern is also extremely variable; many tissues have an embryonic appearance, with numerous mitoses. Islands of immature cartilage, bone, and glandular structures are distributed through a poorly differentiated stroma of actively growing spindle-shaped myxoid or undifferentiated sarcoma cells (Fig. 40-77). Bilateral involvement in patients with stage I malignant teratoma is very unlikely (Table 40-4).

A rare and malignant interesting variant called *polyembryoma* is composed of many embryo-like structures distributed through a loose sarcoma-like stroma of embryonic connective tissue.

Relatively mature (stage I) malignant teratomas have a good prognosis, whereas immature teratomas (stage III) have an extremely poor prognosis.[356a,382] Areas of endodermal sinus tumor, embryonal carcinoma, and choriocarcinoma are extremely unfavorable. Tumors without these structures that have an abundant neural component—resembling ganglioneuroblastoma—are more unpredictable; nearly half of these patients survive for 2 years. The neural component, even in peritoneal implants may mature, leaving well-differentiated glial vestiges on the peritoneal surfaces. Although they may persist for many years, mature glial implants are innocuous and not a basis for radical treatment.[382]

Specialized teratomas. Rare teratomas composed solely of thyroid tissue are usually benign but may function and even cause thyrotoxicosis.[368] Carcinoid tumors with the insular pattern typical of midgut derivatives[381] and trabecular carcinoids of the foregut and hindgut type[383] also occur as primary ovarian tumors. The latter type may be mixed with thyroid tissue. Both are nearly always unilateral and benign; insular carcinoids especially, if large, may cause the carcinoid syndrome. On the other hand intestinal carcinoids metastatic to the ovary are usually bilateral and have a poor prognosis. It is especially important to distinguish them from granulosa cell tumors and Sertoli-Leydig cell tumors as well as from primary ovarian carcinoids.[381]

Mixed forms. Germ cell tumors occur in various combinations. Solid areas in the wall of a cystic teratoma deserve careful study as they may represent a locus of endodermal sinus tumor or other malignant category with a greatly different prognosis and implications for further treatment.

Malignant mixed germ cell tumors (stage I) have a poor prognosis if more than one third of the tumor consists of endodermal sinus tumor, choriocarcinoma, or stage III teratoma. Tumors that contain less than one third of

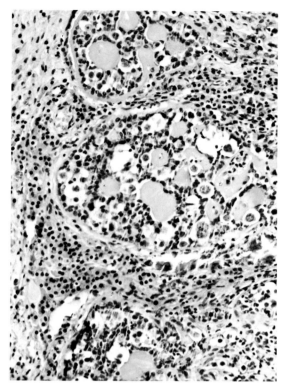

Fig. 40-78. Gonadoblastoma. Large germ cells and hyaline globules intermixed with smaller granulosa cells, forming islands or nests. Clumps of Leydig cells are scattered through intervening stroma. (160×; courtesy Dr. Jerzy Teter, Warsaw, Poland; from Scully, R. E.: In Grady, H. G., and Smith, D. E., editors: The ovary, Baltimore, 1963, The Williams & Wilkins Co.)

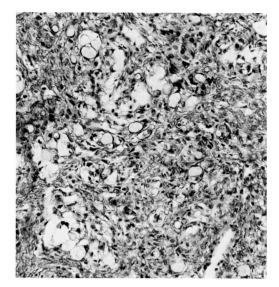

Fig. 40-79. Metastatic adenocarcinoma to ovary from stomach. Signet-ring cells and small acini are present. Stromal cells are hyperplastic. (150×.)

these components, or contain combinations of dysgerminoma, embryonal carcinoma, or stage I or II teratoma have a good prognosis.[356a] Patients with tumors less than 10 cm in diameter are more likely to survive regardless of tumor composition.[356a]

Gonadoblastoma. Gonadoblastoma is a rare tumor that may arise in a dysgenetic gonad. The patients are usually phenotypic females but nearly all are genotypic males (i.e., have a Y chromosome). The tumor contains both immature germ cells and sex cord–stromal cells, which resemble granulosa or Sertoli cells, growing in small islands, intermixed with rounded pink hyaline bodies. Leydig cells or lutein cells are distributed through the intervening stroma in about two thirds of the cases (Fig. 40-78). Small calcifications may be extensive and have a distinctive radiographic pattern. Most are benign, but dysgerminomas and other malignant germ cell tumors develop occasionally.[395]

Metastatic carcinoma, lymphoma

Metastatic carcinomas represent 6% of ovarian cancers encountered in the course of surgical exploration of the abdomen.[391] The primary site in most instances is colon, stomach, or breast; it may be small and difficult to locate, even when the ovarian metastases are large.

The characteristic pattern of growth is diffuse infiltration of the ovarian stroma by strands and small nests of poorly differentiated carcinoma cells, forming a solid mass. The external surface is knobby and smooth. The eponymic designation of *Krukenberg's tumor* is usually reserved for this typical presentation; when the tumor cells have large eccentric mucin vacuoles (signet-ring cells) and the primary site is the stomach (Fig. 40-79). The same pattern rarely occurs in a lesion that seems to be primary in the ovary, after a thorough search for extraovarian primary carcinoma.[349] Because of wide variation in the use of this name, it is essentially useless; since Krukenberg's original paper erroneously concluded that the tumors were primary in the ovary there is little point to clamoring for a "rigorous" use of this term for metastatic carcinoma. Colon cancers metastatic to the ovary may secrete enough mucin to produce cystic cavities; distinction in these cases from primary mucinous carcinoma of the ovary may be difficult.

The most important clinical correlation is the surprising fact that the ovarian metastases are often the only metastases apparent, and if they and the primary lesion are resected, the patient may live without symptoms for several years. For this reason, ovarian metastases should generally be resected.

The basis for the selective enhancement of growth of certain adenocarcinoma cells in the ovary is unexplained. It is of interest that most of the patients are in the premenopausal age group, about a decade younger than those with primary ovarian adenocarcinoma; the phenomenon may be hormone dependent.

The ovarian stroma may be stimulated to secrete both androgenic and estrogenic hormones in the presence of metastatic carcinoma, especially colon carcinoma.

Pathologic factors affecting prognosis

The foregoing discussion has emphasized that each different type of ovarian neoplasm is in fact a separate disease. There are other general characteristics that also affect the outcome of treatment.

Clinical stage. The extent of disease at the time of diagnosis is an important determinant of the outcome of therapy and must be stated in any comparison of effectiveness of different therapeutic techniques. The following internationally recognized criteria for staging primary ovarian carcinoma have been established by the International Federation of Gynecology and Obstetrics[153]:

Stage I	Growth limited to the ovaries
Stage Ia	Growth limited to one ovary; no ascites (i) capsule not ruptured (ii) capsule ruptured
Stage Ib	Growth limited to both ovaries; no ascites (i) capsule not ruptured (ii) capsule ruptured
Stage Ic	Growth limited to one or both ovaries; ascites present with malignant cells in the fluid (i) capsule not ruptured (ii) capsule ruptured
Stage II	Growth involving one or both ovaries with pelvic extension
Stage IIa	Extension or metastases to the uterus, tubes, or other ovary, or any combination
Stage IIb	Extension to other pelvic tissues
Stage III	Growth involving one or both ovaries with widespread intraperitoneal metastases
Stage IV	Growth involving one or both ovaries with distant metastases
Special category	Unexplored cases that are believed to be ovarian carcinoma

Implants. The significance of implants depends on the nature of the primary lesion. The prognosis is good, even in the presence of omental or other peritoneal implants, if the primary tumor is in the borderline category.[396] It is extremely important to examine the undersurface of the diaphragm for distant metastases in establishing the stage of an ovarian cancer because this may be the only area with grossly evident metastases.[335]

Ascites. The significance of effusions depends on the nature of the primary lesion. Effusions associated with fibromas or Brenner tumors (Meigs' syndrome) are benign and do not recur after the tumor has been resected. Effusions that contain cancer cells, originating from an invasive ovarian cancer, indicate an average survival of 7.2 months.[354]

Rupture. The significance of rupture depends on the nature of the neoplasm. It has no demonstrable effect in the case of benign or intermediate tumors. The prognosis of an invasive carcinoma, very poor in any case, may be adversely affected, but it is difficult to demonstrate such a change convincingly.[343]

Metastases. The lymphatic drainage of the ovaries is directly to the aortic lymph nodes at the level of the renal veins. Biopsies inferior to this site are generally useless. From a study of aortic lymph node biopsies it is clear that many ovarian cancers believed to be confined to the ovaries have actually produced lymph node metastases at the time of diagnosis.[360]

Role of pathologic study in management of apparently normal opposite ovary in young women. Preservation of an apparently normal ovary is extremely important in young women. A comparison of the results of ovarian conservation in the presence of apparently unilateral invasive carcinoma with a similar group of patients treated by bilateral ovariectomy shows no significant difference in survival.[367,385] On the other hand Kottmeier[355] found that invasive serous carcinomas produced microscopic metastases that were grossly undetectable in a third of the patients in his series of 71 cases and recommended bilateral oophorectomy for this specific neoplasm in all cases.

PLACENTA
Examination of placenta

The placenta is best examined fresh. The decisions to prepare for electron microscopy and to culture viruses, bacteria, or tissues for cytogenetic study must be made immediately after delivery, based upon historical data,

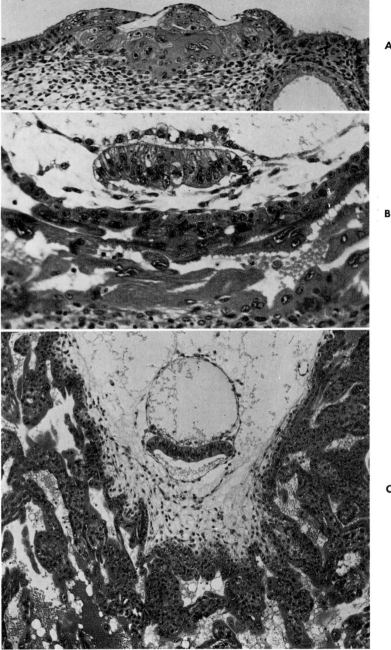

Fig. 40-80. A, Human 7½-day ovum superficially implanted for 36 hours on edematous 22-day secretory endometrium. Note solid trophoblast, derived from blastocyst wall at its contact with endometrium and composed of pale cytotrophoblast and darker syncytiotrophoblast. **B,** Human 12½-day ovum showing embryonic disc (above) and adjacent trophoblast in contact (below) with predecidual stroma of 26-day secretory endometrium. Note inner cytotrophoblast beginning to form primordial chorionic villi and outer syncytiotrophoblast whose lacunar spaces contain maternal blood, beginning of uteroplacental circulation. **C,** Human 14-day ovum showing embryo (upper center) surrounded by early chorion frondosum. Note simple unbranched primordial villi composed largely of central cytotrophoblastic core, beginning to form mesenchymal core and surrounded by syncytium, which lines intervillous space. (**A,** 150×; **B,** 250×; **C,** 100×; **A** to **C,** courtesy Department of Embryology, Carnegie Institution of Washington; **A** and **C,** Carnegie No. 7801; from Heuser, C. H., Rock, J., and Hertig, A. T.: Contrib. Embryol. **31:**85-100, 1945; **B,** Carnegie No. 7700; from Hertig, A. T., and Rock, J.: Contrib. Embryol. **29:**127-156, 1941.)

physical examination of mother and infant, and gross inspection of the placenta itself. Subsequent examination by a pathologist is not impeded seriously by refrigeration for a few hours.

The first step is to reconstruct the relationships of the membranous sac, noting the width of the narrowest margin between the site of rupture and the placental margin. Any margin at all excludes placenta previa.

After an inspection, the membranes are cut away from the placental margin, rolled into a sausage-shaped structure and held thus by transfixion with a pin; after fixation a cross section of this roll is submitted for microscopic study.

The cord is next examined and measured; the number of vessels is recorded. It is separated by a cut near the placenta, and the placenta is weighed. The surfaces are inspected for disruption or exudate. A whole mount of amnion may be examined immediately for the presence of bacteria or sex chromatin. The placenta is then sliced in cross section like a loaf of bread; representative blocks are cut for microscopic study. A detailed protocol prepared for the National Institutes of Health collaboration study has been described with further comments about more specialized techniques.[466]

Development: anatomy and physiology

Although the entire section on pathology of the female genitalia derives heavily from the towering work of Arthur T. Hertig, our debt is nowhere so immense, and obvious, as in this section on the placenta. These illustrations and the words to describe them will be recognized by anyone who has so much as glanced at the subject, for they are unique and have been published necessarily by every writer who sets out to review the morphology of the early conceptus. The best and only completely original review of the subject is the monograph in which Hertig summarizes earlier work done either by himself or in collaboration with others.[466]

Significant stages in the formation of the placenta are as follows:

1. Implantation of the 6- to 7-day blastocyst, with formation of solid trophoblast from its wall at the point of contact with the endometrium (Fig. 40-80, *A*).
2. Gradual peripheral orientation of the syncytiotrophoblast in which vacuoles appear and then coalesce to form the intervillous space; central orientation of the cytotrophoblast, which proliferates as isolated masses, forerunners of the primordial villi; these changes occur from the ninth to thirteenth day of development (Fig. 40-80, *B*).
3. Conversion of the cytotrophoblastic masses covered by syncytiotrophoblast to primordial villi from the fourteenth to seventeenth day (Figs. 40-80, *C,* and and 40-81, *D*).
4. Branching of primordial villi from the eighteenth day on through the first trimester; each primordial villus with its derivatives constitutes a cotyledon of the mature placenta (Fig. 40-81).
5. Gradual enlargement of the entire ovum from the twentieth day to the twentieth week, resulting in the following:
   a. Obliteration of the entire uterine cavity by fusion of decidua capsularis and decidua vera

---

Fig. 40-81. Gross and microscopic aspects of chorionic, embryonic, and body stalk development at developmental age of 19 days (menstrual age of 33 days). **A,** Ovisac and implantation site bisected to show embryo, chorionic cavity, and chorionic villi around entire circumference. Thin *decidua capsularis* above, *decidua vera* laterally, and *decidua basalis* below, but above myometrium. For gross details of embryo viewed at right angles, see **B. B,** Embryo showing yolk sac with blood islands (right), curved germ disc (left), and crescent-shaped amniotic cavity between chorionic membrane (extreme left) and body stalk (below). For microscopic details (in mirror image), see **C. C,** Midsagittal section of embryo, body stalk, and adjacent chorion, the last representing one-half of chorion and including both *chorion laeve* (top) and *chorion frondosum* (bottom). **D,** Detail of chorionic villus from pregnancy comparable to that shown in **A** to **C.** Note immature stroma containing developing blood vessels. Trophoblast consists of outer syncytium and inner Langhans' epithelium. Between streamers of solid trophoblast (upper right) are maternal blood cells within intervillous space. (**A,** 4×; **B** and **C,** 12×; **D,** 300×. **A** to **D,** Courtesy Department of Embryology, Carnegie Institution of Washington; Carnegie Numbers: **A,** 8671, seq. 2; **B,** 8671, seq. 6; **C,** 8671, sect. 10-4-2; **D,** 5960, sect. 5-2-1; **D,** from Hertig, A. T.: Contrib. Embryol. **25:** 37-82, 1935.)

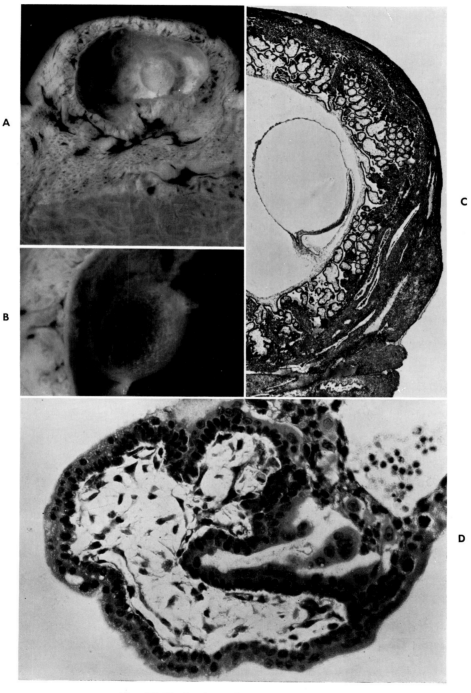

Fig. 40-81. For legend see opposite page.

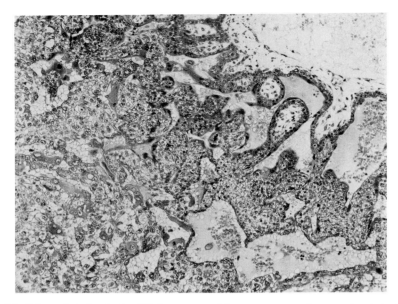

Fig. 40-82. Primordial chorionic villi from normal human ovary of approximately 15 days' gestation. These villi (upper right) are comparable to that shown in Fig. 40-31, *D*, and are continuous with cytotrophoblast of cell column and placental floor. The latter is contiguous with decidua basalis (left margin). Remnants of peripheral syncytiotrophoblast appear as giant cells (center) from which the placental site giant cells will be derived. (150×.)

b. Progressive thinning of the abembryonic chorion to become the chorion laeve

c. Progressive growth of the amnion with gradual obliteration of the chorion cavity by fusion of chorionic and amniotic fibrous tissue

d. Progressive growth of the chorion frondosum, forming 8 to 15 cotyledons, constituting the placenta (Fig. 40-82).

Amnion. Significant phases in the formation of the amnion are as follows:

1. Its in situ delamination from the adjacent cytotrophoblast of the implanting ovum during the seventh to ninth day of development.

2. Resulting formation of a veil-like membrane over and attached to the periphery of the circular concave germ disc during the ninth to thirteenth day of development (Fig. 42-80, *B*).

3. Gradual transformation of this membrane to amniotic epithelium during the fourteenth to twenty-fifth day of development (Fig. 42-80, *C*).

4. Simultaneous accumulation of a second mesoblastic layer.

5. Progressive distention of the amniotic cavity, growth of the embryo, and its "prolapse" into the amniotic cavity.

6. Gradual obliteration of the chorionic cavity by fusion of connective tissue of amnion and chorion.

Umbilical cord. Significant stages in the formation of the umbilical cord are as follows:

1. Its origin as a mass of chorionically derived mesoblast at the caudal end of the embryonic disc when the latter develops its longitudinal axis during the fourteenth to sixteenth day (Fig. 42-81, *C*).

2. Gradual shifting of the caudally located body stalk to a more ventrally situated umbilical cord as the embryo grows caudally.

3. Gradual "prolapse" of the embryo accompanied by its cord into the amniotic cavity and simultaneous covering of the cord by amniotic epithelium.

Chorionic villi. The immature villi are covered by an outer layer of syncytiotrophoblast and an inner layer of cytotrophoblast cells (Fig. 42-81, *D*). The latter divide, mature, and become incorporated into the growing syncytiotrophoblast layer, a process that is virtually completed by the sixteenth week. Only syncytiotrophoblast is evident thereafter. The capillary vessels are very small. The stromal core contains fibroblasts, collagen, and Hofbauer cells, which are macrophages with very large vacuoles that apparently result from the imbibition of large amounts of water.[452] In mature placental villi the cytotrophoblast cells have disappeared, the stroma is scant, capillaries are multiple with thin walls, and the immensely active syncytiotrophoblast layer is thin, except where nuclei accumulate into clusters or "knots." The morphology of placental anatomy and development has been described in detail in the beautifully illustrated monographs by Hertig[466] and Boyd and Hamilton.[432]

The syncytiotrophoblast cells of the villi are responsible for sorting and distributing nutrients to the fetus, fetal metabolic by-products back to the mother, and synthesis of a remarkable variety of hormones. Placental functions are so numerous and placental products so varied that a completely satisfactory clinical test of placental function remains to be elaborated. The steroid hormones include estrogens, progesterone, androgens, adrenocorticosteroids, and aldosterone. The placental peptide hormones are chorionic gonadotropin (HCG), chorionic somatomammotropin (HCS), chorionic thyrotropin, and adrenocorticotropic hormone. These placental activities have been summarized in monographs by Villee[518] and Gruenwald.[461] When the exact cell origin of substances produced in the mother during gestation involves fetal and placental tissues together, the metabolic products are considered to define the functional status of the *fetoplacental unit;* e.g., the amount of estriol in maternal urine is dependent on fetal adrenals and liver as well as the placenta, and a decline indicates a threat to survival of the fetus, although the site of the lesion responsible may not have been determined.

Chorionic gonadotropin alters maternal immune response and is probably an important factor in the survival of the placental allograft. Trophoblast is antigenic.[429,471] Circulating HCG levels throughout pregnancy are not as high as required for complete in vitro inhibition of lymphocyte transformation[420] or mixed lymphocyte culture reaction. However, local concentrations in the syncytiotrophoblast layer are very high in comparison to other tissues.[447,472] There seems to be an especially important electronegative barrier of sialic acid (an HCG moiety) at the syncytiotrophoblast surface.[489] This surface represents the interface between maternal and fetal tissues and is ultimately the locus at which accommodation between the two must be settled. Of great interest is the apparent paradox that the maternal sensitization to trophoblast, which must be blocked for the placenta to survive, actually enhances implantation and subsequent fetal growth.[427] One important line of cancer research is based upon the similarity between cancer cells and trophoblast: cancers produce HCG,[517] which can be detected in the patient's serum, and HCG has been identified in nontrophoblastic cancer cells by immunohistochemical techniques.[488]

The dynamics of placental circulation are unique. *Maternal blood* from the uterine arteries works its way through the uterine wall into the spiral arterioles of the maternal endometrium (now decidua vera) and empties in spurts into the intervillous space of the placenta. The openings of the spiral arterioles are distributed about the placental floor; between them are the openings of the decidual veins, through which blood from the intervillous space returns into the maternal venous system.

In the early weeks of pregnancy an extremely important sequence of changes enlarges the flow capacity of the decidual spiral arteries. The cytotrophoblast cells of the outer margin of the conceptus invade opened ends of these small arteries, replace the endothelium, and infiltrate the muscular walls; the muscular layer and elastic tissue are destroyed (Fig. 40-83). By the middle of the second trimester this change has extended to involve the myometrial segments of the spiral arteries. The result is a group of 100 to 150 tortuous, greatly widened funnel-shaped arterial channels, the true uteroplacental arteries, with walls composed of fibrinoid material and a lining of trophoblast. Thus the placenta must structure its vascular supply line.

The *fetal* circulation begins with the umbilical arteries, which come to the placenta through the umbilical cord. The umbilical arteries divide and redivide in the placenta, ultimately into small capillaries of the villi and return through tributaries of the umbilical vein into the umbilical cord.

The intervillous space is a single vast pool of maternal blood, in which the placental villi dangle, rootlike, with margins sealed by tight contact between decidua and placental membranes. There is no "marginal sinus" in the sense of an anatomic walled structure to collect maternal blood before its return to the uterus. A premature separation at this margin may allow maternal blood to leak out rapidly, an

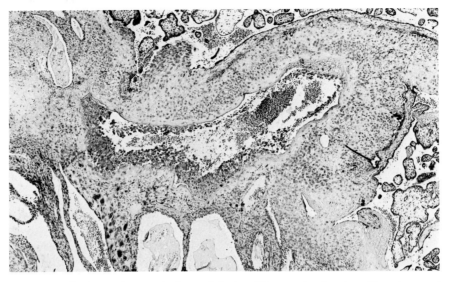

Fig. 40-83. Decidual spiral arteriole *(center)* during fifth month, showing dilatation, replacement of endothelium by cytotrophoblast, and hyalinization of vessel wall. Decidua is infiltrated by syncytiotrophoblast cells at *lower left*. Placental villi at *top*, dilated decidual glands at *bottom center*. (40×.)

alarming event that is still called *"marginal sinus tear."*

Anomalies

Abnormal shapes. The umbilical cord usually inserts near the center, but in about 10% of cases it may insert at the placental margin (battledore placenta). Less frequent (1%), but of greater potential importance, is *velamentous insertion,* in which the cord runs for variable distances through the membranes before reaching the placenta. This fixes the location of the cord and may result in compression or even rupture if the area involved passes over the cervical outlet.

A placenta divided into two parts is bipartite; a small accessory *succenturiate lobe* is important as a cause of bleeding if left behind, an event that can be detected because the vessels that extend to it will end abruptly at a tear in the membranes.

Single umbilical artery. In a series of 39,773 white and black single births 0.9% of umbilical cords contained a single umbilical artery.[456] Fourteen percent of the infants so affected were stillborn or died in the neonatal period; of those autopsied, half were found to have significant congenital anomalies, chiefly affecting the cardiovascular or genitourinary systems. Although the presence of a single umbilical artery implies a 10- to 20-fold increase in serious congenital malformations, affected in-

fants who survive the perinatal period have normal prospects, except for a 1 in 20 chance of developing an inguinal hernia.

Placenta membranacea. Persistence of villi surrounding the entire conceptus is called placenta membranacea; the situation is comparable to placenta previa, including the threat of severe hemorrhage.[455] Arteriographic studies may be misleading.[442]

Amnion nodosum. Amnion nodosum occurs with any condition resulting in extreme oligohydramnios, such as renal agenesis. Clusters of squamous cells, fibrin, and other amorphous debris become inspissated and form loosely attached plaques on the amnionic surfaces.[430] It should be distinguished from focal squamous metaplasia of the amnion, which is common around the insertion of the cord and has no known significance.

Multiple gestation

The question of genetic relationship in multiple pregnancy has increased importance because of the potential need for organ transplantation and because of the threatening implications of circulatory connections in monochorionic placentas. The relationships of the membranes are diagrammed in Fig. 40-84.

Dichorionic diamnionic twin placentas. If two separate zygotes implant concurrently, the placentas may fuse; the twins in this case are fraternal (not identical). Separate placentas

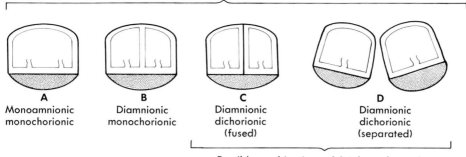

Possible combinations of fetal membranes in monozygous twin placenta (identical twins)

A	**B**	**C**	**D**
Monoamnionic monochorionic	Diamnionic monochorionic	Diamnionic dichorionic (fused)	Diamnionic dichorionic (separated)

Possible combinations of fetal membrane in dizygous twin placenta (fraternal twins)

Fig. 40-84. Diagram of common morphologic variations in twin placentation. Types **A** and **B** occur only in identical twins; types **C** and **D** are common to both. (From Kraus, F. T.: Gynecologic pathology, St. Louis, 1967, The C. V. Mosby Co.)

(chorions) also result if a single zygote divides and the two daughter cells separate completely and implant—each will mature, producing identical twins. The fused placentas will be recognizable by a persistent ridge of chorion at the base of the septum between the two amnions after the amniotic membranes are stripped away. Histologic section of the septum shows two amnions and an intervening layer of chorion. It appears that about 20% of twins with this type of placenta are monozygotic (identical), and 80% are dizygotic (fraternal).[428]

Monochorionic diamnionic twin placentas. If two germ discs form after implantation of a single zygote, the twins (always identical) will share a single placenta. Vascular connections are large and easily demonstrated and no chorionic ridge is present when the amnions are stripped away.[431] There is no layer of chorion (trophoblast) between the two amnions that fuse to form the septum between the amnionic cavities.

Monochorionic monoamnionic twin placentas. When there is no intervening septum, the twins (always identical) share the same amnionic cavity. The prospects for entanglement are great and mortality is high.

Clinicopathologic correlation. In a series of 250 twin placentas carefully correlated by all possible factors to confirm zygosity (fraternal versus identical) 56% of placentas were dizygotic and 44% were monozygotic. Thirty percent of the monozygotic twins had dichorionic placentas, and 70% had monochorionic placentas, of which 3% had monochorionic monoamnionic placentas. Eighty percent of twins with dichorionic placentas are dizygotic (fra-

ternal). Thus, by examination of a twin placenta, one can conclude that the twins are definitely *identical* in the case of a monochorionic placenta and *probably fraternal* (4 chances in 5) in the case of a dichorionic placenta.[428]

Higher orders of multiple pregnancy. The same criteria of zygosity may be applied by examination of the septal membranes between adjacent amnionic cavities.

Abnormal implantation

Extrachorial implantation. In about 18% of deliveries the margins of the placenta lie submerged beneath the decidua. If the amnionic membrane extends to the placental rim and is reflected back toward the center, it is called a *circumvallate placenta* (Fig. 40-85). The amnion of a *marginate placenta* does not follow the placental rim beneath the decidua but continues out over the decidual surface. Scott[505] found no significant risk to mother or infant attributable to this relationship; there may be a slight increase in vaginal bleeding.

Placenta accreta. Placental separation at parturition occurs by cleavage through the decidua. If there is no intervening decidua, the villi become attached to the myometrium and will not separate. The condition may be complete over the entire base of the placenta or, more commonly, only partial; the villi may extend into the myometrium (placenta increta) or entirely through it, resulting in rupture (placenta percreta).[513] In all cases the placenta cannot be delivered, the uterus cannot contract, and hemorrhage is usually brisk. In most cases hysterectomy is necessary to control bleeding.[473,480]

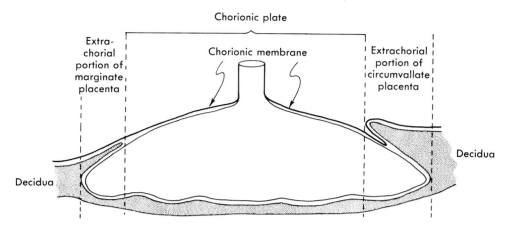

Fig. 40-85. Diagrams of placenta-uterus relationships in extrachorial placenta. (Modified after Scott, J. S.: Placenta extrachorialis. J. Obstet. Gynaecol. Br. Commonw. **67**:904-918, 1960.)

Ectopic pregnancy. Implantation may occur outside the uterine cavity. The commonest site is the uterine tube. Less frequent sites include the interstitial part of the tube, the cervix, the ovary, and the intra-abdominal peritoneal surface.

Tubal ectopic pregnancy usually occurs in a tube altered by prior inflammation, which apparently interferes with transport of the ovum. In all sites there is a threat of rupture attended by severe hemorrhage. The endometrium may or may not show gestational histologic changes, depending on the extent to which the gestation has progressed and the length of time elapsed between fetal death and onset of bleeding. An occasional abdominal pregnancy is successfully terminated by cesarean section, but the fetal mortality exceeds 90%[426]; attempts at placental removal at delivery (laparotomy) may lead to serious hemorrhage.[470]

Placenta previa. After low implantation of a normal ovum, the enlarging placenta may come to lie over the internal os of the cervix. Even before onset of labor, the exposed maternal surface may be a source of bleeding, and with the onset of labor the certainty of massive hemorrhage requires cesarean section. Variable degrees of placenta accreta often accompany placenta previa probably because of the generally deficient endometrium in the lower uterine segment.[466]

Spontaneous abortion (miscarriage)

The termination of pregnancy, regardless of the mechanism, before the fetus can survive (if it is present) is called an *abortion*. Spontaneous abortion is usually the result of a pathologic ovum, infection, or maternal disease. *Missed abortion* refers to retention of a dead fetus longer than 2 months.

By far the commonest abnormality leading to spontaneous abortion is a genetic defect of the conceptus. In about half of all spontaneous abortions the fetus is either absent or grossly malformed. Hertig[466] has written a detailed description and classification of various gross abnormalities. Cytogenetic studies have shown a chromosomal abnormality in about a third of the cases,[437] but the incidence was nearly 60% in a small series utilizing more refined chromosomal banding techniques.[481] The most common chromosomal anomalies demonstrated have been triploidy, 45 XO karyotype, and single autosomal trisomy.

The decidua associated with spontaneous abortion shows hemorrhage, necrosis, and leukocytic infiltration. The endometrium away from the implantation site often shows the pattern of secretory gestational hyperplasia described by Arias-Stella.[195]

The chorionic villi may appear nearly normal or be surrounded by dense deposits of intervillous fibrin clot. In a majority of the cases in which the embryo is absent, the villous stroma is swollen and hydropic, as the result of fluid accumulation. This is the hallmark of a "blighted" ovum and probably a result of continued trophoblast function in the absence of a vascular transport to carry the accumulated fluid, for there is no fetus. Hydropic villi have no direct significance for the mother and

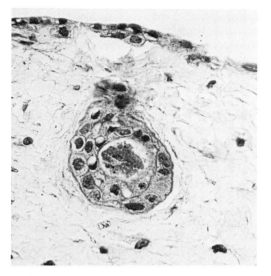

Fig. 40-86. Trophoblastic invagination in villus, shown in cross section. Chromosomal analysis of cultured cells showed a 69 XXX triploid karyotype, which correlates consistently with this morphologic abnormality. (Courtesy D. Emile Philippe, Strasbourg, France.)

especially should not be confused with hydatidiform mole.

Philippe[495] has correlated cytogenetic studies of spontaneous abortions with histologic patterns. In these studies, invagination of the surface trophoblast into the core of the villus was found chiefly in instances of triploidy (Fig. 40-86). Cases with autosomal trisomy showed migration of occasional large cytotrophoblast cells into the villous stroma. Occasional abortuses with large edematous winglike projections from the posterior neck suggesting hygromas have been shown to have a 45 XO karyotype.[496]

Maternal factors in abortion include induced abortion and its complications, often related to infection. Infectious diseases have been generally considered to be an uncommon primary cause of spontaneous abortion. With the increased utilization of sophisticated microbiologic techniques infections have been detected in increasing numbers; their role in abortion and fetal loss will have to be reevaluated. The organisms that have been implicated include herpes virus,[458,487] cytomegalic inclusion virus,[443,485] virus of rubella,[490] *Listeria monocytogenes,*[496] *Toxoplasma gondii,*[424,445] and mycoplasmas.[464,469] Anaerobic bacteria are especially important in the pathogenesis of septic abortion and its maternal complications.[504]

Toxemia of pregnancy (eclampsia and preeclampsia)

Toward the end of pregnancy about 6% of women develop salt retention, edema, albuminuria, and become hypertensive. This syndrome is called toxemia of pregnancy or preeclampsia. The most severe manifestation, eclampsia, is accompanied by convulsions; there is extensive intravascular coagulation with fibrin thrombi and focal necrosis in the liver, kidneys, and brain.

The pathogenesis of toxemia of pregnancy has been extensively studied but remains unexplained; theories are numerous.[491] The most significant pathologic lesion seems to be in the uterine spiral arteries. As described originally by Hertig,[467] there is fibrinoid necrosis of the walls of the terminal ends of the spinal arteries in the decidua. The myometrial segments of the uteroplacental arteries of the placental bed and the basal arteries that supply the decidua are also affected. In addition there is an accumulation of foamy lipophages in the necrotic vessel walls and an infiltrate of small mononuclear cells in and around the vessels. These changes, called *acute atherosis,* begin with lipid accumulation in smooth muscle cells, necrosis of smooth muscle, exudation of fibrin into the vessel wall, and infiltration of the vessel wall by phagocytic macrophages that become swollen with accumulated lipid. They are often accompanied by thrombosis.[502]

Brosens et al.[434] have found that the physiologic trophoblastic invasion of placental bed spiral arteries (see p. 1753) does not extend into the myometrial segments of these vessels. These segments cannot expand and therefore represent a constriction between the proximal radial arteries and the distended distal segments in the decidua. It is in these areas that acute atherosis occurs. The similarity between acute atherosis and vascular changes in rejected renal allografts suggests that this placental vascular lesion may be the result of a local immunologic attack, which ordinarily is blocked by the physiologic invasion of trophoblast. Immunofluorescent studies provide some support for this.[478]

Regardless of how they are produced, the lesions of acute atherosis impair blood flow to the placenta and to the decidua itself. It is in this ischemic background that placental infarction, retroplacental hematoma, premature placental separation, fetal distress, and the small fetus appear.

In experimental models of eclampsia, Mc-

Kay[483] has emphasized the similar features of the generalized Shwartzman reaction and the degenerative changes in the placental trophoblast. The placental lesions are not specific, but the ischemia and accentuation of degenerative changes produce a very abnormal pattern. Syncytiotrophoblast nuclei form tight clusters or "knots." Some are necrotic. The cytoplasm of the syncytiotrophoblast becomes vacuolated. The amount of intervillous fibrin material—always present at term—is increased. Infarcts are common and may be extensive.

Circulatory lesions

In addition to the changes more clearly related to toxemia, there are other disturbances in the vascular supply of the placenta and its decidual support. These include infarcts, hematomas, and vascular lesions resulting from systemic maternal disease unrelated to pregnancy.

Infarcts. The blood supply that supports the placenta comes from the maternal circulation. Impaired maternal circulation in local areas will produce placental infarcts; impaired fetal circulation does not.

The lesion responsible may be thrombosis of a group of decidual spiral arteries or atherosclerotic changes in branches of the uterine artery. A recent infarct appears red and granular. As the blood pigment is broken down and carried away, the infarct becomes progressively lighter, achieving eventually a pale yellow color (Fig. 40-87).

Intraplacental hematoma. Clots that develop in the intervillous space have a characteristic laminated pattern. They are red if recent and pale yellow if old. Since the villi are pushed aside as the hematoma forms, there are no villi in it, and the granularity of an infarct is not seen. The blood is of maternal origin.

A specific type of placental hematoma forms in the subchorionic area, producing a large tuberous mass. It is consistently but not always

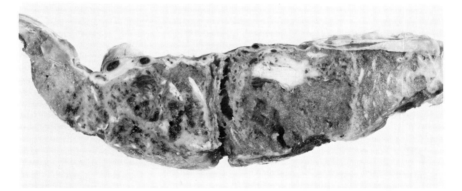

Fig. 40-87. Placental infarcts. Note granular cut surface, mottled white and red of old and recent lesions, and irregular margins. The mother had severe toxemia.

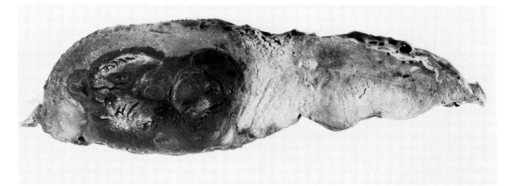

Fig. 40-88. Premature separation (abruptio placentae) with large hematoma that compresses overlying placenta.

associated with missed abortion and is called a *Breus mole;* there is no relationship to hydatidiform mole.[507]

Premature separation. The normally implanted placenta may become detached before the onset of labor. The bland decidual necrosis that disrupts the normal attachment may be the result of vascular disease such as toxemia, or possibly to poor nutrition, especially folic acid deficiency.[468]

The placenta is compressed by the clot that forms behind it (Fig. 40-88). As the result of consumption of clotting factors in this large hematoma, the circulating blood is depleted; thus there is a severe bleeding diathesis in at least one fifth of the patients. The uterine bleeding often leads to shock. The subsequent disseminated intravascular coagulation may be associated with bilateral renocortical necrosis and pituitary infarction. Any delay in delivery of the fetus results in prolonged anoxia and death; the perinatal mortality is high.

Premature separation carries an increased risk of *amniotic fluid* embolism, a grave complication with a high mortality found also in women of high parity, with intrauterine fetal death, or hypertonic labor, or such symptoms as sudden onset of dyspnea, shock, or disseminated intravascular coagulation.[494] The presence of amniotic fluid is not always easily identified at autopsy with standard histologic sections but is readily demonstrated with the colloidal iron stain for acid mucopolysaccharide.[503]

Atherosclerosis: essential hypertension and diabetes mellitus. Young women with essential hypertension who happen also to become preg-nant have hyperplastic intimal atherosclerotic lesions affecting the myometrial segments of the spiral arteries of the placental bed. The lesions here are often disproportionately severe in comparison to similar vessels elsewhere in the body. If the arterial physiologic changes of pregnancy (p. 1753) progress normally, the prognosis for the fetus is good.[502] Decidual arterioles in diabetes mellitus may be thick walled with hyalinized media.[428] Either situation may be further complicated by lesions of atherosis if the patient develops toxemia; the consequences are usually severe.

Infectious diseases

Intrauterine infection may be transplacental or ascending from the vagina. Unquestionably infection is an underestimated cause of "spontaneous" abortion. Many birth defects originally considered to be "acts of God" are now reliably ascribed to a specific infectious organism, notably viruses. The extent to which the cytogenetic alterations described in the section on abortions might be virus induced is essentially unexplored. Midtrimester abortion is especially likely to be the result of chorioamnionitis.[421] About one fourth of placentas of small-for-gestational age infants show nonspecific villitis; the mortality for this group is 16%.[422]

Bacterial infections. Rupture of the fetal membranes before onset of labor provides a path for ascending bacterial infection. If the infection is well developed by the time of delivery, purulent exudate may be obvious on gross inspection of the fetal surfaces of the placenta and membranes and similar ad-

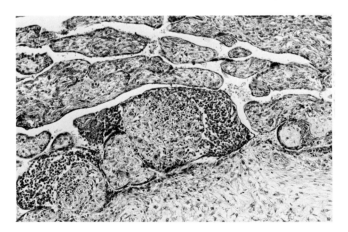

Fig. 40-89. Placental villitis associated with *Listeria monocytogenes* infection. Inflammatory cells expand villus, but a thin envelope of attenuated trophoblast persists. (130×.)

vanced infection may be presumed to exist in the infant's lungs. Microscopically a dense infiltrate of neutrophils obliterates the amniotic epithelium; bacterial colonies may or may not be present. In many instances an infiltrate of leukocytes and fibrin in the subchorionic plate of the placenta is the only histologic evidence of infection. The most common species of organisms are those that inhabit the vagina in pregnancy, including *Staphylococcus, Escherichia coli, Proteus, Pseudomonas,* and such highly virulent anaerobes as *Bacteroides* and *Peptostreptococcus.*

Placental *tuberculosis* occurs rarely as a complication of miliary spread in the mother. *Syphilis* may cause villitis and fetal endovasculitis, but none of the gross or microscopic changes is specific for *Trepenoma pallidum* infection.[482]

Listeria monocytogenes produces a severe placentitis characterized by miliary abscesses and is one of the less recognized causes of septic abortion, especially repeated abortion.[499] The histologic appearance of the abscesses is a characteristic collection of polymorphonuclear leukocytes and mononuclear cells at the tip of a villus, enveloped by an attenuated layer of trophoblast (Fig. 40-89). The organism is better known as a cause of fetal wastage in animals, especially cattle; the basis for its selective pathogenicity in pregnancy is unknown.[428] The newborn is also susceptible, developing a distinctive disseminated infection called *granulomatosis infantiseptica,* in which the liver, lungs, spleen, and adrenal glands are riddled with miliary abscesses; the cause of death in the few born alive is acute meningitis.[486] The organism is a small gram-positive rod, which must not be hastily discarded as a "diphtheroid." Maternal endometrial infection may be chronic and should be treated even though asymptomatic.

Viral infections. Transmission of viruses to the fetus may be hematogenous and transplacental or by contact at the time of delivery. Smallpox, varicella, herpes simplex, and cytomegalic inclusion virus[485] cause necrotizing villitis with typical intranuclear inclusions. Placental lesions in congenital rubella infection include acute necrotizing villitis, older fibrotic areas, and cytoplasmic viral inclusions. Ornoy et al.[490] found a close correlation between severe fetal anomalies and placental inflammation (including cytoplasmic inclusions) in pregnancies complicated by rubella infection. They have suggested that evaluation of placental biopsies would aid in the decision to continue a pregnancy in the face of maternal rubella exposure or infection.

Perinatal infection with cytomegalovirus in term infants born alive is apparently transmitted by contact with recently contracted active cervical infection in the mother.[501] First and second trimester abortion caused by necrotizing villitis and deciduitis has also been reported, but its numerical significance is uncertain.

Protozoal infections. *Toxoplasmosis* is transmitted to the infant through the placenta. Mothers who have antibodies prior to pregnancy do not have infected infants. The most serious fetal lesions are produced when maternal exposure occurs during the first two trimesters of pregnancy. The encysted organisms can be demonstrated histologically, but often with difficulty; more consistent identification is obtained by intraperitoneal injection in mice.[445] The placental lesion is focal necrosis and villitis, with a mononuclear infiltrate. When infection is severe, fetal hydrops occurs and the placental appearance mimics erythroblastosis grossly and microscopically.[424]

Malaria parasites have been identified in maternal erythrocytes in the intervillous space.

Fungus infections. The most common fungus infection of the placenta is that caused by *Candida* organisms that invade transvaginally after premature rupture of the membranes. Associated bacterial infection is common. Fungal hyphae may infiltrate the umbilical cord. Instances of *Coccidioides* infection have been reported.[428]

Mycoplasma infection. *Mycoplasma* organisms have been implicated in infertility[469] and abortion,[486] and organisms have been cultured in cases of chorioamnionitis. The lesions resemble those produced by bacteria, with a polymorphonuclear leukocytic infiltrate. Correlation between placental lesions caused by T mycoplasmas and any sort of fetal disease seems to be poor.[509]

Erythroblastosis fetalis

The placenta in erythroblastosis fetalis is greatly enlarged, from two to four times the normal size and weight. The fetal membranes are pale gray when associated with fetal hydrops. The cut surface is pale, spongy, and granular. The microscopic appearance represents a recapitulation of the immature state, with prominent cytotrophoblast cells, abundant villous stroma, and many Hofbauer cells.[465] Nucleated red blood cells in clusters may fill and distend capillary spaces.

Trophoblastic hyperplasia and neoplasia

The aggressive overgrowth of trophoblast, benign or malignant, is an unusual but always dramatic complication of pregnancy. All the lesions described below are frequently lumped together as forms of *"trophoblastic disease."*

Hydatidiform mole. This form of pathologic pregnancy is uncommon in the United States (about 1 per 2000 pregnancies) but for reasons still unknown occurs with about 10 times that frequency in various parts of Asia and Central America.[493]

The patient experiences a rapid increase in uterine size, often with symptoms of toxemia and vaginal bleeding. Ultrasound techniques can be used to confirm the absence of the fetus. By the middle of the second trimester the uterus may approach the size of a term pregnancy; bleeding begins at this time if not before.

A hydatidiform mole itself is actually a placenta, composed entirely or almost entirely of immensely swollen villi. The volume varies from about 1 to 3 liters (Fig. 40-90). There is usually an abundance of hyperplastic trophoblast covering some or all of the villi and infiltrating the decidua at the implantation site. It is possible but rare to find a fetus (Fig. 40-91). In the presence of a fetus, or in smaller abortions composed of a mixture of normal and hydropic villi, subsequent choriocarcinoma is extremely unlikely. The term "hydatidiform mole" should be avoided in such cases.

The pathogenesis is unknown. The considerably higher incidence in the lowest socioeconomic populations suggests a nutritional factor that remains undefined. Cytogenetic studies have shown a striking preponderance of female sex chromatin–positive cells, and a large percentage have triploid or other polyploid chromosomal karyotypes. Aneuploid cells are also common. Although cytogenetic anomalies have also been noted in abortions, the

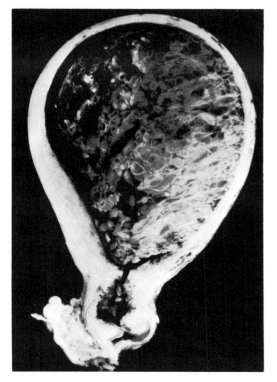

Fig. 40-90. Midsagittal section of typical molar uterus approaching term size, although of gestational age of only about 20 weeks. Uterine cavity is greatly distended but small oval, centrally located chorionic sac may still be identified. (Courtesy Dr. H. Sheehan and AFIP.)

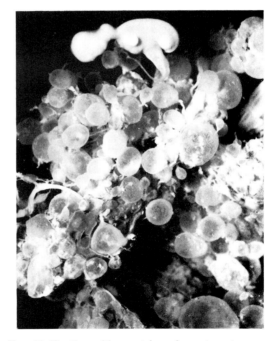

Fig. 40-91. Grapelike vesicles of varying size constituting hydatidiform mole. Stunted, macerated fetus at menstrual age of approximately 6 weeks was within intact chorionic sac (not shown here) when mole was delivered at hysterectomy. This is unusual, since chorionic sac usually is empty. (2×; Carnegie No. 8723, seq. 1; from Hertig, A. T.: In Meigs, J. V., and Sturgis, S. H., editors: Progress in gynecology, vol. II, New York, 1963, Grune & Stratton, Inc.; by permission.)

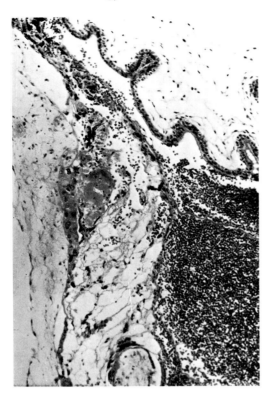

Fig. 40-92. Group II mole (probably benign). Despite benign appearance, patient developed clinically invasive mole (chorioadenoma destruens) 5 weeks after evacuation of mole. These portions of two villi show normal double-layered trophoblast on upper right and pleomorphism of Langhans' epithelium and vacuolization of syncytiotrophoblast on other villus. (110×; from Hertig, A. T., and Sheldon, W. H.: Am. J. Obstet. Gynecol. **53:** 1-36, 1947.)

presence of significant numbers of aneuploid cells suggests that hydatidiform moles are neoplastic. This is a popular concept, despite strongly argued objections.[466]

The histologic pattern of the villous core varies little; the jelly-like edematous stroma is nearly clear, traversed by thin strands of connective tissue, most of which are ruptured (Fig. 40-92). Capillary structures are not apparent in ordinary microscopic examination but can be demonstrated by electron microscopy. The most significant component is the trophoblast that covers the villi and infiltrates the implantation site. Here there is considerable variation, from thin layers of atrophic degenerated attenuated syncytiotrophoblast cells with pyknotic nuclei to piled-up hyperplastic masses of syncytiotrophoblast or cytotrophoblast, or both. The presence of large anaplastic-looking nuclei certainly often has

at least the appearance of a neoplasm and a malignant-looking one as well (Fig. 40-93, *A*). In fact, the manner in which cytotrophoblast and syncytiotrophoblast remain segregated is characteristic and resembles the trophoblast pattern in the area of the cytotrophoblast shell of a 10- to 12-day implantation.

Extreme degree of dysplastic and anaplastic nuclear change undeniably have an ominous appearance when present. As a practical matter the presence of the villi, even hydropic villi serve to classify the lesion in question as benign. Grading of moles on the basis of degrees of anaplastic change in the trophoblast has little prognostic significance in an individual case.[428,466,493]

The most important factor in the decision to treat the patient is the demonstration of a rise in chorionic gonadotropin (HCG) titers after the fall attending the removal of the mole. It is extremely important to detect this rise early. For this reason a suitably sensitive assay is absolutely necessary. The radioimmunoassay of serum samples for the presence of the beta subunit of HCG is specific and sufficiently sensitive to detect minute amounts and capable of showing changes in ranges at which the ordinary immunoassay of standard pregnancy tests will not react.[517]

Invasive mole (destructive mole). In addition to the threat that attends severe bleeding and the possibility of infection, hydatidiform mole may invade the wall of the uterus (Fig. 40-94) and molar tissue may be deported to other sites. Invasion of the uterine wall is a source of hemorrhage after the mole has been passed or removed. Molar trophoblast cells, like normal trophoblast,[423] are constantly embolizing the general circulation. Molar tissue may be deported to the lungs[474] or vaginal wall and produce local nodular lesions, which are usually hemorrhagic because of the vascular destructiveness of trophoblast. Such a lesion is regarded as benign in the sense that it is not a malignant neoplasm, but the potential for hemorrhage is a strong inducement for treatment. Before the availability of chemotherapy it was generally recognized that such lesions regressed and could usually be managed conservatively.

The most devastating complication of hydatidiform mole is the subsequent occurrence of *choriocarcinoma* (see below) in about 1.5% of patients. The morphologic findings are not so important a factor in the decision to treat the patient as continued HCG production. Demonstration of a rising HCG titer after

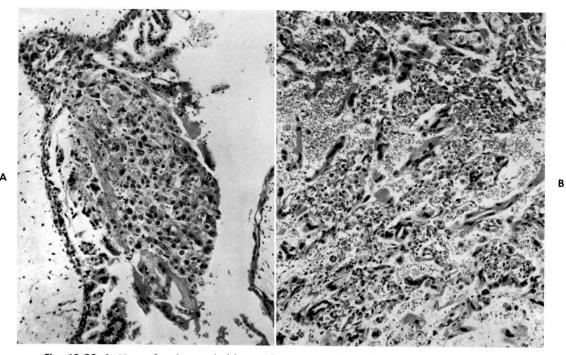

Fig. 40-93. A, Mass of molar trophoblast with pronounced anaplasia attached to villus while remainder of trophoblast is not unusually active. Although mole gave rise to choriocarcinoma, this trophoblast does not resemble that of tumor shown in **B. B,** Renal metastasis of typical choriocarcinoma occurring in patient whose original mole is shown in **A.** Patient died 16 months after delivery of hydatidiform mole. (110×; courtesy Rhode Island Hospital, Providence; AFIP 218754-562 and 218754-563.)

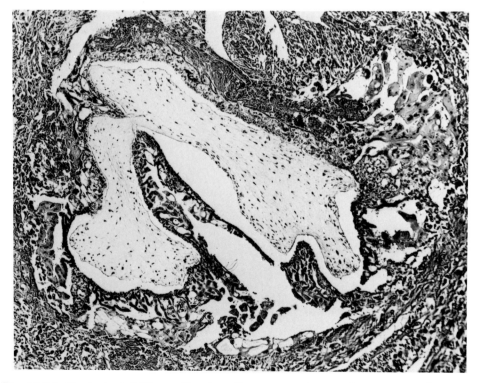

Fig. 40-94. Single hydatidiform villus invading myometrium, pathognomonic of invasive mole. (48×; AFIP No. 298593-2.)

delivery of the mole is the basis for starting chemotherapy, regardless of the presence of a demonstrable lesion. The production of HCG is a constant and consistent property of trophoblast and is generally proportional to the amount of trophoblast present in a given patient. Rising titers mean growing trophoblast. If the location of proliferating trophoblast is uncertain or inaccessible, it is not necessary or desirable for one to identify it morphologically before instituting chemotherapy. A detailed plan for the follow-up of patients after passage of a mole is obviously important; the protocols at the regional centers for treatment of trophoblastic disease are similar.[460,463] The drugs used successfully have been methotrexate and actinomycin D.

Having bowed to the overriding significance of HCG in management of clinical problems, we should give attention to some interesting morphologic correlations. Hydatidiform mole in the presence of a fetus is often associated with unusually severe toxemia and hypertension; subsequent choriocarcinoma is most unlikely.[493] *Transitional moles* (abortions of small size with a high proportion of vesicular villi) are followed only very rarely by choriocarcinoma. Women who have had one mole are somewhat more likely to have another than women who have not. The trophoblast cells of the molar implantation site occasionally persist for several months, with slowly *declining* HCG titers, and may be a source of bleeding. The histologic pattern is not that of choriocarcinoma, and demonstration of trophoblast cells at the implantation site of a mole does not mean that the patient has or ever will have a choriocarcinoma, but it is a reasonable basis for extension of the period of follow-up.

Choriocarcinoma. Gestational choriocarcinoma is a malignant neoplasm of trophoblast; it may occur after hydatidiform mole (50%), spontaneous abortion (25%), normal pregnancy (22.5%), and even rarely an ectopic pregnancy (Fig. 40-95).

Intravascular metastases occur early and disseminate widely. They are found chiefly in the lung (60%), vagina (40%), brain (12%),

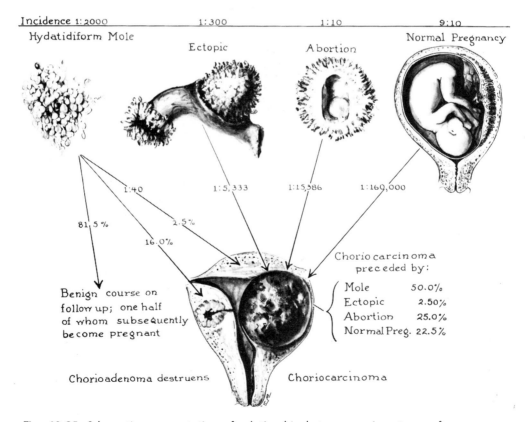

Fig. 40-95. Schematic representation of relationship between various types of pregnancy and chorioadenoma destruens and choriocarcinoma. (Adapted from Hertig, A. T.: In Meigs, J. V., and Sturgis, S. H., editors: Progress in gynecology, vol. II, New York, 1963, Grune & Stratton, Inc.; by permission.)

liver (16%), and kidney (13%), but virtually any site perfused by blood vessels is possible. The uterine lesion may be small and often no uterine lesion can be identified. Except in the unusual case of uncontrolled bleeding from a uterine mass, hysterectomy has little to offer the patient with choriocarcinoma.

The tumor masses are soft, necrotic, and hemorrhagic wherever they are found. The bulk of a nodular lesion often is a blood clot, and the trophoblastic tissue is occasionally difficult to find.

The histologic pattern varies only slightly. Plexiform masses of syncytiotrophoblast and cytotrophoblast are intimately intermixed, forming a distinctive biphasic pattern (Fig. 40-93, *B*). Nuclei of both cell types may be bizarre and anaplastic; mitoses occur in the cytotrophoblast cells.

Choriocarcinoma is the best example of a malignant tumor that responds to chemotherapy. Nearly always fatal in the past, it has now become nearly always curable; many of the patients go on to have additional children. The drugs used most successfully have been actinomycin D and methotrexate. It is important to monitor therapy with serial HCG determinations. The drugs themselves can be dangerous, and the protocol for treatment can be extremely complicated. The results in the regional centers for treatment of trophoblastic disease have been excellent.[460,463] Their consultation and support are generally available upon request and should be sought, for the results without highly specialized clinical and laboratory facilities can be disastrous.

The prognosis for the patient with cerebral or liver metastases is poor. Very high HCG titers are also a very unfavorable finding; the inhibition of the immune response by large amounts of HCG could be the responsible factor. It would be interesting to know if its removal, e.g., by plasmapheresis, would help in these grave circumstances.

Chorioangioma represents a small and insignificant hemangioma that has been reported in 0.5% to 7% of placentas. Large lesions may be associated with hydramnios, toxemia, prematurity, and even a hydrops fetalis syndrome unrelated to Rh sensitization.[510] Metastatic malignant tumors of maternal origin, notably breast and malignant melanoma occur occasionally but usually do not cross the placental barrier to the fetus.[500] Very rarely, malignant lesions of the fetus affect the placenta (leukemia, neuroblastoma), and instances of congenital giant nevus with placental metastasis have occurred.[444]

ACKNOWLEDGMENT: The continued use of Figs. 21, 25, 35, 41, 42, 58, 59, 62, 65, 67, 70, 76, 78, 80, 81, 90, 91, 92, 93, 94, and 95 in this chapter, originally prepared by Dr. Arthur T. Hertig, is gratefully acknowledged.

REFERENCES
Embryology and congenital malformations
1 Boczkowski, K.: Obstet. Gynecol. **41:**310-314, 1973 (sex anomalies).
2 Bullock, L. P., and Bardin, C. W.: J. Steroid Biochem. **4:**139, 1973 (androgen insensitivity).
3 Dewhurst, C. J.: J. Obstet. Gynaecol. Br. Commonw. **75:**377-391, 1968 (genital anomalies).
4 Farber, M., and Marchant, D. J.: Am. J. Obstet. Gynecol. **121:**414-417, 1975 (cervix absence).
5 Federman, D.: Abnormal sexual development, Philadelphia, 1967, W. B. Saunders Co.
6 Forsberg, J. G.: Obstet. Gynecol. **25:**687-691, 1965 (vaginal embryology).
7 Hamilton, W. J., Boyd, J. D., and Mossman, H. W.: Human embryology, ed. 4, Baltimore, 1972, The Williams & Wilkins Co.
8 Jacobs, P. A., Melville, M., and Ratcliffe, S.: Ann. Hum. Genet. **37:**359-376, 1974 (newborn cytogenetics).
9 Jost, A.: Cold Spring Harbor Symp. Quant. Biol. **19:**167-181, 1954 (müllerian regression).
10 Jost, A.: Recent Progr. Horm. Res. **8:**379-418, 1953.
11 Jost, A., Vigier, B., Prepin, J., and Perchellet, J. P.: Recent Prog. Horm. Res. **29:**1-41, 1973 (experimental embryology).
12 Machin, G. A.: Lancet **1:**549-551, 1974.
13 Marquez-Monter, H., Armendares, S., Buentello, L., and Villegas, J.: Am. J. Clin. Pathol. **57:**449-456, 1972 (gonadal dysgenesis).
14 Mittwoch, U.: The genetics of sexual differentiation, New York, 1973, Academic Press, Inc.
15 Naftolin, F., and Judd, H. L.: Testicular feminization, Obstet. Gynecol. Annu. **2:**25-53, 1973.
16 Park, I. J., Aimakhu, V. E., and Jones, H. W.: Am. J. Obstet. Gynecol. **123:**505-518, 1975 (hermaphroditism).
17 Pinkerton, J. H. M., McKay, D. G., Adams, E. C., and Hertig, A. T.: Obstet. Gynecol. **18:**152-181, 1961 (ovarian embryology).
18 Prinz, J. L., Choate, J. W., Townes, P. L., and Harper, R. C.: Obstet. Gynecol. **41:**246-252, 1973 (ectopic ovaries).
19 Sarto, G. E.: Am. J. Obstet. Gynecol. **119:**14-23, 1974 (amenorrhea cytogenetics).
20 Sarto, G. E., and Opitz, J. M.: J. Med. Genet. **10:**288-293, 1973 (gonadal agenesis).
21 Scully, R. E.: Cancer **25:**1340-1356, 1970 (gonadoblastoma).
22 Singh, R. P., and Carr, D. H.: Obstet. Gynecol. **29:**806-818, 1967 (abortion cytogenetics).
23 Stephens, F. D.: Aust. N.Z. J. Obstet. Gynaecol. **8:**55-73, 1968 (vulvar anomalies).
24 Spaulding, M. H.: Contrib. Embryol. **13:**67-88, 1921 (vulvar embryology).
25 Tavassoli, F.: Obstet. Gynecol. **49:**366-369, 1977.
26 van Wagenen, G., and Simpson, M. E.: New Haven, 1965, Yale University Press (ovarian embryology).

27 Wharton, L. R.: Am. J. Obstet. Gynecol. **78:** 1101-1118, 1959 (ectopic ovary).

28 Wilson, J. D., Harod, M. J., Goldstein, J. L., et al.: New Eng. J. Med. **290:**1097-1103, 1974 (androgen insensitivity).

29 Woodruff, J. D., and Pauerstein, C. J.: The fallopian tube, Baltimore, 1969, The Williams & Wilkins Co.

30 Woolf, R. M., and Allen, W. M.: Obstet. Gynecol. 2:236-265, 1953 (genital anomalies).

Vulva

31 Abell, M. R.: Am. J. Obstet. Gynecol. **86:** 470-482, 1963 (adenocarcinoma).

32 Abell, M. R., and Gosling, J. R. G.: Cancer **14:**318-329, 1961 (carcinoma in situ).

33 Burger, R. A., and Marcuse, P. M.: Am. J. Clin. Pathol. 24:965-968, 1954 (fibroadenoma).

34 Chamlian, D. L., and Taylor, H. B.: Obstet. Gynecol. 39:489-494, 1972 (adenocarcinoma).

35 Christ, M. L., and Ozzello, L.: Am. J. Clin. Pathol. 56:736-749, 1971 (myoblastoma).

36 Dean, R. E., Taylor, E. S., Weisbrod, D. M., and Martin, J. W.: Am. J. Obstet. Gynecol. 119:59-68, 1974 (carcinoma).

37 Dehner, L. C.: Obstet. Gynecol. 42:47-57, 1973 (metastatic carcinoma).

38 Devroede, G., Schlaeder, G., Sanchez, G., et al.: Am. J. Clin. Pathol. 63:348-358, 1975 (Crohn's disease).

39 Edsmyr, F.: Acta Radiol. 217(suppl.):1-135, 1963 (carcinoma).

40 Franklin, E. W., and Rutledge, F. D.: Obstet. Gynecol. 39:165-172, 1972 (carcinoma).

41 Friedrich, E. G.: Obstet. Gynecol. 39:173-181, 1972 (carcinoma in situ).

42 Friedrich, E. R., Cole, W., and Middlekamp, J. N.: Herpes simplex, Am. J. Obstet. Gynecol. 104:758-779, 1969.

43 Friedrich, E. G., and Wilkinson, E. J.: Obstet. Gynecol. 42:407-414, 1973 (cysts).

44 Gardner, H. L., and Kaufman, R. H.: Benign diseases of the vulva and vagina, St. Louis, 1969, The C. V. Mosby Co.

45 Green, T. H., Ulfelder, H., and Meigs, J. V.: Am. J. Obstet. Gynecol. 75:834-864, 1958 (carcinoma).

46 Gosling, J. R. G., Abell, M. R., Drolette, B. M., and Loughrin, T. D.: Cancer 14:330-343, 1961 (carcinoma).

47 Hart, W. R.: Am. J. Obstet. Gynecol. **107:** 1079-1084, 1970 (cysts).

48 Hart, W. R., Norris, H. J., and Helwig, E. B.: Obstet. Gynecol. 45:369-377, 1975 (lichen sclerosus).

49 Hassim, A. M.: J. Obstet. Gynecol. Br. Commonw. 76:275-277, 1969 (fibroadenoma).

50 Helwig, E. B., and Graham, J. H.: Cancer 16:387-403, 1963 (Paget's disease).

51 Hertig, A. T., and Gore, H.: In Atlas of tumor pathology, Sect. IX, Fasc. 33, Washington, D.C., 1960, Armed Forces Institute of Pathology (tumors).

52 Janovski, N. A., and Ames, S.: Obstet. Gynecol. 22:697-708, 1963 (lichen sclerosus).

53 Jeffcoate, T. N. A.: Am. J. Obstet. Gynecol. 95:61-74, 1966 (dystrophies).

54 Jimerson, G. K., and Merrill, J. A.: Cancer 26:150-153, 1970 (carcinoma).

55 Kaufman, R. H., et al.: Am. J. Obstet. Gynecol. **117:**1144-1146, 1973 (herpes simplex).

56 Kaufman, R. H., et al.: Am. J. Obstet. Gynecol. **120:**363-367, 1974 (dystrophies).

57 Kelly, J.: J. Obstet. Gynaecol. Br. Commonw. **79:**265-272, 1972 (carcinoma).

58 Kolstad, P., and Stafl, A.: Atlas of colposcopy, Baltimore, 1972, University Park Press.

59 Kraus, F. T., and Perez-Mesa, C.: Cancer **19:** 26-38, 1966 (carcinoma).

60 Langley, I. I., Hertig, A. T., and Smith, G. van S.: Am. J. Obstet. Gynecol. 62:167-169, 1951 (dystrophies).

61 Lukas, W. F., Benirschke, K., and Lebherz, T. B.: Am. J. Obstet. Gynecol. 19:435-440, 1974 (carcinoma).

62 Lovelady, S. B., McDonald, J. R., and Waugh, J. M.: Am. J. Obstet. Gynecol. 42:309-313, 1941 (benign tumors).

63 Medenica, M., and Sahihi, T.: Arch. Dermatol. 105:236-243, 1972 (Paget's disease).

64 Meeker, J. H., Neubecker, R. D., and Helwig, E. B.: Hidradenoma papilliferum, Am. J. Clin. Pathol. 37:182-195, 1962.

65 Morrow, C. P., and Rutledge, F. N.: Obstet. Gynecol. 39:745-752, 1972 (melanoma).

66 Nakao, C. Y., Nolan, J. F., DiSaia, P. J., and Futoran, R.: Am. J. Obstet. Gynecol. **120:**1122-1123, 1974 (carcinoma).

67 Neilson, D., and Woodruff, J. D.: Am. J. Obstet. Gynecol. 113:719-732, 1972 (Paget's disease).

68 Ng, A. B. P., Reagan, J. W., and Lindner, E.: Acta Cytol. 14:124-129, 1970 (herpes cytology).

69 Palladino, V. S., Duffy, J. L., and Bures, G. J.: Cancer 24:460-470, 1969 (basal cell carcinoma).

70 Powell, L. C., Jr.: Condyloma acuminatum, Clin. Obstet. Gynecol. 15:948-965, 1972.

71 Ragni, M. V., and Tobon, H.: Obstet. Gynecol. 43:658-664, 1974 (melanoma).

72 Rutledge, F., Smith, J. P., and Franklin, E. W.: Am. J. Obstet. Gynecol. 106:1117-1130, 1970 (carcinoma).

73 Skinner, M. S., Sternberg, W. H., Ichinose, H., and Collins, J.: Obstet. Gynecol. 42:40-46, 1973 (carcinoma in situ).

74 Sobel, H. J., Schwarz, R., and Marquet, E.: J. Pathol. 109:101-111, 1973 (myoblastoma).

75 Tsukada, Y., Lopez, R. G., Pickren, J. W., Piver, M. S., and Barlow, J. J.: Obstet. Gynecol. 45:73-78, 1975 (Paget's disease).

76 Way, S., and Benedet, J. L.: Gynecol. Oncol. 1:119-122, 1973 (carcinoma).

77 Wharton, J. T., Gallager, S., and Rutledge, F. N.: Am. J. Obstet. Gynecol. **118:**159-162, 1974 (carcinoma).

78 Woodworth, H. J., Dockerty, M. B., Wilson, R. B., and Pratt, J. H.: Am. J. Obstet. Gynecol. 110:501-508, 1971 (hidradenoma).

79 Yackel, D. B., Symmonds, R. E., and Kempers, R. D.: Obstet. Gynecol. 35:625-631, 1970 (melanoma).

Vagina

80 Allyn, D. L., Silverberg, S. G., and Salzberg, A. M.: Cancer 17:1231-1238, 1971 (adenocarcinoma).

81 Bennet, H. G., and Ehrlich, M. M.: Am. J. Obstet. Gynecol. **42**:314-320, 1941 (myoma).

82 Berry, A.: J. Pathol. Bacteriol. **91**:325-338, 1966 (bilharziasis).

83 Davis, B. A.: Obstet. Gynecol. **34**:40-45, 1969 (candidosis).

84 Deppisch, L. M.: Obstet. Gynecol. **45**:632-637, 1975 (cysts).

85 Elliot, G. B., and Elliot, J. D. A.: Arch Pathol. **95**:100-101, 1973 (stroma).

86 Fentanes de Torres, E., and Benitez-Bribiesca, L.: Acta Cytol. **17**:252-257, 1973 (parasites).

87 Forsberg, J. G.: Am. J. Obstet. Gynecol. **121**:101-104, 1975 (experimental adenosis).

88 Friedrich, E. G., and Wilkinson, E. J.: Obstet. Gynecol. **42**:407-414, 1973 (cysts).

89 Frost, J. K.: Concepts basic to general cytopathology, Baltimore, 1972, The Johns Hopkins Press.

90 Gardner, H. L., and Fernet, P.: Am. J. Obstet. Gynecol. **88**:680, 1964 (vaginitis emphysematosa).

91 Gardner, H. L., and Kaufman, R. H.: Benign diseases of the vulva and vagina, St. Louis, 1969, The C. V. Mosby Co.

92 Gray, L. A., and Christopherson, W. W.: Obstet. Gynecol. **34**:226-230, 1969 (carcinoma in situ).

93 Hart, W. R.: Am. J. Obstet. Gynecol. **107**:1079-1084, 1970 (cysts).

94 Herbst, A. L., Green, T. H., Jr., and Ulfelder, H.: Am. J. Obstet. Gynecol. **106**:210-218, 1970 (carcinoma).

95 Herbst, A. L., Robboy, S. J., Scully, R. E., and Poskanzer, D. C.: Am. J. Obstet. Gynecol. **119**:713-724, 1974 (adenocarcinoma).

96 Hilgers, R. D., Malkasian, G. D., Jr., and Soule, E. H.: Am. J. Obstet. Gynecol. **107**:484-502, 1970 (sarcoma).

97 Hummer, W. K., Mussey, E., Decker, D. G., and Dockerty, M. B.: Am. J. Obstet. Gynecol. **108**:1109-1116, 1970 (carcinoma in situ).

98 Johnson, H. W.: Can. Med. Assoc. J. **41**:386, 1939.

99 Koss, L. G.: Diagnostic cytology and its histopathologic bases, ed. 2, Philadelphia, 1968, J. B. Lippincott Co.

100 Malkasian, G. D., Welch, J. S., and Soule, E. H.: Am. J. Obstet. Gynecol. **86**:730-736, 1963 (leiomyosarcoma).

101 McIndoe, W. A., and Green, G. H.: Acta Cytol. **13**:158-162, 1969 (carcinoma).

102 Ng, A. B. P., Reagan, J. W., and Lindner, E.: Acta Cytol. **14**:124-129, 1970 (herpes simplex).

103 Norris, H. J., Bagley, G. P., and Taylor, H. B.: Arch. Pathol. **90**:473-479, 1970 (adenocarcinoma).

104 Norris, H. J., and Taylor, H. B.: Cancer **19**:227-232, 1966 (polyps).

105 Norris, H. J., and Taylor, H. B.: Am. J. Clin. Pathol. **46**:420-426, 1966 (melanoma).

106 Perez, C. A., Arneson, A. N., Dehner, L. P., et al.: Obstet. Gynecol. **44**:862-872, 1974 (carcinoma).

107 Perez, C. A., Arneson, A. N., Galakatos, A., and Samanth, H. K.: Cancer **31**:36-44, 1973 (cancer).

108 Robboy, S. J., Scully, R. E., Welch, W. R., and

109 Herbst, A. L.: Arch. Pathol. Lab. Med. **101**:1-5, 1977 (adenocarcinoma).

109 Sandberg, E. C., Danielson, R. W., Cauwet, R. W., and Bonar, B. E.: Am. J. Obstet. Gynecol. **93**:209-222, 1965 (adenosis).

110 Scully, R. E., Robboy, S. J., and Herbst, A. L.: Am. Clin. Lab. Sci. **4**:222-233, 1974 (adenocarcinoma).

111 Silverberg, S. G., and Frable, W. J.: Arch. Pathol. **97**:100-103, 1974 (tubal prolapse).

112 Stabler, F.: J. Obstet. Gynaecol. Br. Commonw. **74**:493-498, 1967 (adenosis).

113 Underwood, P. B., Jr., and Smith, R.: J.A.M.A. **217**:46-52, 1971 (carcinoma).

114 Vooijs, P. G., Ng, A. B. P., and Wentz, W. B.: Acta Cytol. **17**:59-63, 1973 (adenosis).

Cervix

115 Abel, M. R.: In Norris, H. J., Hertig, A. T., and Abell, M. R., editors: The Uterus, Baltimore, 1973, The Williams & Wilkins Co., pp. 413-456 (carcinoma).

116 Abell, M. R., and Gosling, J. R. G.: Am. J. Obstet. Gynecol. **83**:729-755, 1962 (adenocarcinoma).

117 Abell, M. R., and Ramirez, J. A.: Cancer **31**:1176-1192, 1973 (sarcoma).

118 Alexander, E. R.: Cancer Res. **33**:1485-1496, 1973 (carcinoma).

119 Ashley, D. J. B.: J. Obstet. Gynaecol. Br. Commonw. **73**:372-381, 1966 (carcinoma in situ).

120 Aurelian, L.: Cancer Res. **33**:1539-1547, 1973 (carcinoma).

121 Aurelian, L., Schumann, B., Marcus, R. L., et al.: Science **181**:161-164, 1973 (carcinoma).

122 Ayers, L. R., Drosman, S., and Saltzstein, S. L.: Obstet. Gynecol. **37**:755-760, 1971.

123 Badib, A. O., Kurohara, S. S., Webster, J. H., et al.: Cancer **21**:434-439, 1968 (carcinoma).

124 Beral, V.: Lancet **1**:1037-1043, 1974 (carcinoma).

125 Berry, A.: J. Pathol. Bacteriol. **91**:325-338, 1966.

126 Boyes, D. A., Worth, A. J., and Fidler, H. K.: J. Obstet. Gynaecol. Br. Commonw. **77**:769-780, 1970 (carcinoma in situ).

127 Brudnell, J. M., Cox, B., and Taylor, C.: J. Obstet. Gynaecol. Br. Commonw. **80**:673, 1973 (carcinoma in situ).

128 Burghardt, E.: Early histological diagnosis of cervical cancer (translated by E. Judith and E. A. Friedman). Major problems in obstetrics and gynecology, Philadelphia, 1973, W. B. Saunders, vol. 6, pp. 335-362 (adenocarcinoma in situ).

129 Ceremsak, R. J.: Am. J. Clin. Pathol. **52**:604-606, 1969 (rhabdomyoma).

130 Chanen, W., and Hollyock, V. E.: Obstet. Gynecol. **43**:527-534, 1974 (colposcopy).

131 Chen, S. S., Koffler, D., and Cohen, C. J.: Am. J. Obstet. Gynecol. **121**:91-95, 1975 (carcinoma).

132 Christopherson, W. M., Gray, L. A., and Parker, J. E.: Cancer **38**:629-632, 1976 (carcinoma).

133 Cohen, C.: Obstet. Gynaecol. Br. Commonw. **80**:476-479, 1973 (amebiasis).

134 Coppleson, M., Pixley, E., and Reid, B.: Col-

poscopy, Springfield, Ill., 1971, Charles C Thomas, Publisher.

135 Davidsohn, I., Norris, H. J., Stejskal, R., et al.: Arch. Pathol. 95:132-134, 1973 (carcinoma).

136 Daw, E.: Am. J. Obstet. Gynecol. 114:1104-1105, 1974 (metastatic carcinoma).

137 DiSaia, P. J., et al.: Am. J. Obstet. Gynecol. 114:979-989, 1972 (carcinoma).

138 Ehrmann, R. L.: Am. J. Obstet. Gynecol. 105:1284, 1969 (sebaceous metaplasia).

139 Fluhmann, C. F.: The cervix and its diseases, Philadelphia, 1961, W. B. Saunders Co.

140 Friedrich, E. R.: In Blandau, R. J., editor: The biology of the cervix, Chicago, 1973, University of Chicago Press (ultrastructure).

141 Gallagher, H. S., Simpson, C. B., and Ayala, A. G.: Cancer 27:1398-1402, 1971 (adenocarcinoma).

142 Goodheart, C. R.: Cancer Res. 33:1548-1551, 1973 (carcinoma).

143 Graham, C. E.: Am. J. Obstet. Gynecol. 97:1033-1040, 1967 (anatomy).

144 Green, G. H., and Donovan, J. W.: J. Obstet. Gynaecol. Br. Commonw. 77:1-9, 1970 (carcinoma in situ).

145 Govan, A. D. T., et al.: J. Clin. Pathol. 22:383-395, 1969 (carcinoma in situ).

146 Gunderson, L. L., Weems, W. S., Hebertson, R. M., et al.: Am. J. Roentgenol. 120:74-87, 1974 (carcinoma).

147 Hollinshead, A. C., and Tarro, G.: Science 179:698-700, 1973 (carcinoma).

148 Janovski, N. A., and Kasdon, E. J.: J. Pediatr. 63:211-216, 1963 (papilloma).

149 Kaufman, R. H., et al.: Cancer Res. 33:1446-1451, 1973 (herpes simplex).

150 Kirkland, J. A., Stanley, M. A., and Cellier, K. M.: Cancer 20:1934-1952, 1967 (carcinoma in situ).

151 Knapp, R. C., and Feldman, G. B.: Clin. Obstet. Gynecol. 13:889-897, 1970 (carcinoma in situ).

152 Kolstad, P., and Klem, V.: Obstet. Gynecol. 48:125-129, 1976.

153 Kottmeier, H. L., editor: Annual report, vol. 16, Stockholm, 1976, International Federation of Gynecology and Obstetric (staging).

154 Kraus, F. T.: In Norris, H. J., Hertig, A. T., and Abell, M. R., editors: The uterus, Baltimore, 1973, The Williams & Wilkins Co., pp. 348-381 (microinvasion).

155 Kraus, F. T.: In Norris, H. J., Hertig, A. T., and Abell, M. R., editors: The uterus, Baltimore, 1973, The Williams & Wilkins Co., pp. 457-488 (radiation effect).

156 Krieger, J. S., and McCormack, L. J.: Am. J. Obstet. Gynecol. 101:171-182, 1968 (carcinoma in situ).

157 Kyriakos, M., Kempson, R. L., and Konikov, N. F.: Cancer 22:99-110, 1968 (microglandular hyperplasia).

158 Levi, M.: Am. J. Obstet. Gynecol. 109:686-698, 1971 (carcinoma).

159 Leman, M. H., Benson, W. L., Kurman, R. J., and Park, R. C.: Obstet. Gynecol. 48:571-578, 1976 (microinvasion).

160 Naib, Z. M., Nahmias, A. J., Josey, W. E., and Zaki, S. A.: Cancer Res. 33:1452-1463, 1973 (herpes simplex).

161 Nangle, R., Berger, M., and Levin, M.: Cancer 16:1151-1159, 1963 (carcinoma).

162 Newton, C. W., and Abell, M. R.: Obstet. Gynecol. 40:686-691, 1972.

163 Ng, A. B. P., and Atkin, N. B.: Br. J. Cancer 28:322-331, 1973 (carcinoma).

164 Ng, A. B. P., and Reagan, J. W.: Am. J. Clin. Pathol. 52:511-529, 1969 (microinvasion).

165 Niven, P. A. R., and Stansfield, A. G.: Am. J. Obstet. Gynecol. 115:534-538, 1973 (glia).

166 Paunier, J. P., Delclos, L., and Fletcher, G. H.: Radiology 88:555-562, 1967 (carcinoma).

167 Perez, C. A., et al.: Cancer 35:1493-1504, 1975 (carcinoma).

168 Qizelbash, A. H.: Am. J. Clin. Pathol. 64:155-170, 1975 (adenocarcinoma).

169 Rapp, F., and Duff, R.: Cancer Res. 33:1527-1534, 1973 (carcinoma).

170 Rawls, W. E., Adam, E., and Melnick, J. L.: Cancer Res. 33:1477-1482, 1973 (carcinoma).

171 Richart, R. M., and Barron, B. A.: Am. J. Obstet. Gynecol. 105:386-393, 1969 (dysplasia).

172 Roche, W. D., and Norris, H. J.: Cancer 36:180-186, 1975 (microinvasive carcinoma).

173 Roth, E., and Taylor, H. B.: Obstet. Gynecol. 27:838-844, 1966 (cartilage).

174 Rotkin, E. D., and Cameron, J. R.: Cancer 21:663-671, 1968 (carcinoma).

175 Rubio, C. A., and Lagerlof, B.: Acta Pathol. Microbiol. Scand. (A) 82:411-418, 1974 (carcinoma in situ).

176 Rutledge, F. N., et al.: Am. J. Obstet. Gynecol. 122:236-245, 1975 (adenocarcinoma).

177 Schellhas, H. F., and Heath, G.: Am. J. Obstet. Gynecol. 104:617-632, 1969 (carcinoma in situ).

178 Selim, M. A., So-Bosita, J., and Neuman, M. R.: Surg. Gynecol. Obstet. 139:697-700, 1974 (carcinoma in situ).

179 Sherrick, J. C., and Vega, J. G.: Congenital intramural cysts of uterus, Obstet. Gynecol. 19:486-493, 1962 (cysts).

180 Shingleton, H. M., Richart, R. M., Wiener, J., et al.: Cancer Res. 18:695-706, 1968 (carcinoma).

181 Silverberg, E., and Holleb, A. I.: CA 25:2-7, 1975 (carcinoma).

182 Silverberg, S. G.: Am. J. Clin. Pathol. 64:192-199, 1975 (adenomyomatosis).

183 Silverberg, S. G., et al.: Am. J. Obstet. Gynecol. (adenocarcinoma). (To be published.)

184 Singer, A.: Br. J. Obstet. Gynaecol. 82:81-99, 1975 (anatomy).

184a Sorensen, H. M., Peterson, O., Nielson, J., Bang, F., and Koch, F.: Acta Obstet. Gynecol. Scand. 43 (suppl. 7):103-104, 1964 (carcinoma in situ).

184b Spriggs, A. E., Bowey, E., and Cowdell, R. H.: Cancer 27:1239-1254, 1971 (carcinoma in situ).

184c Stamler, T., Fields, C., and Andelman, S. L.: Am. J. Pub. Health 57:791-803, 1967 (carcinoma).

184d Steiner, G., and Friedell, G. H.: Cancer 18:807-810, 1965 (adenosquamous carcinoma in situ).

185 Tayor, H. B., Irey, N. S., and Norris, H. J.:

J.A.M.A. **202:**637-639, 1967 (microglandular hyperplasia).

186 Thompson, B. H., et al.: Am. J. Obstet. Gynecol. **114:**329-338, 1972 (colposcopy).

187 Watson, A. A., and Cochran, A. J.: J. Pathol. Bacteriol. **98:**87-89, 1969 (sebaceous glands).

188 Wentz, W. B., and Reagan, J. W.: Cancer **12:** 384-388, 1959 (carcinoma).

189 Willis, R. A.: The borderland of embryology and pathology, ed. 2, London, 1962, Butterworth & Co. (Publishers) Ltd., p. 534.

190 Worth, A. J., and Boyes, D. A.: J. Obstet. Gynaecol. Br. Commonw. **79:**673-679, 1972.

Endometrium

191 Ackerman, L. V., and Rosai, J.: Surgical pathology, St. Louis, 1974, The C. V. Mosby Co., page 797 (carcinoma in situ).

192 Aikawa, M., and Ng, A. B. P.: Cancer **31:**385-397, 1974 (carcinoma).

193 Aksel, S., and Jones, G. S.: Obstet. Gynecol. **44:**1-13, 1974 (abnormal bleeding).

194 Anderson, G. D.: Obstet. Gynecol. **46:**102-103, 1975 (endometritis).

195 Arias-Stella, J.: In Norris, H. J., Hertig, A. T., and Abell, M. R., editors: The uterus, Baltimore, 1973, The Williams & Wilkins Co., Chap. 10 (gestational changes).

196 Armenia, C. A.: Obstet. Gynecol. **30:**524-529, 1967 (polyps).

197 Armstrong, E. M., More, I. A. R., McSeveny, D., and Carty, M.: J. Anat. **116:**375, 1973 (ultrastructure).

198 Armstrong, E. M., More, I. A. R., McSeveney, D., and Chatfield, W. R.: J. Obstet. Gynaecol. Br. Commonw. **80:**446-460, 1973 (ultrastructure).

199 Arronet, G. H., and Arrata, W. S. M.: Obstet. Gynecol. **29:**97-107, 1967 (abnormal bleeding).

200 Baggish, M. D., and Woodruff, J. D.: Obstet. Gynecol. Survey **22:**69-116, 1967 (metaplasia).

201 Bosio, B. B., and Taylor, E. S.: Obstet. Gynecol. **42:**271-275, 1973 (endometritis).

202 Boutselis, J. G.: In Norris, H. J., Hertig, A. T., and Abell, M. R., editors: The uterus, Baltimore, 1973, The Williams & Wilkins Co., Chap. 9 (histochemistry).

203 Cadena, D., Cavanzo, F. J., Leone, C., and Taylor, H. B.: Obstet. Gynecol. **41:**733-738, 1973 (endometritis).

204 Cavazos, F., and Lucas, F. V.: In Norris, H. J., Hertig, A. T., and Abell, M. R., editors: The uterus, Baltimore, 1973, The Williams & Wilkins Co., Chap. 8 (ultrastructure).

205 Chamlian, D. L., and Taylor, H. B.: Obstet. Gynecol. **36:**659-666, 1970 (hyperplasia).

206 Clement, P. B., and Scully, R. E.: Am. J. Clin. Pathol. **66:**512-525, 1976 (sarcoma).

207 Clement, P. B., and Scully, R. E.: Cancer **34:** 1138-1149, 1975 (adenosarcoma).

208 Craig, J. M.: Arch. Pathol. **99:**233-236, 1975.

209 Dallenbach-Hellweg, G.: Histopathology of the endometrium, New York, 1975, Springer-Verlag.

210 Dutra, F. R.: Am. J. Clin. Pathol. **31:**60-65, 1959 (metaplasia).

211 Fechner, R. E., and Kaufman, R. H.: Cancer **34:**444-452, 1974 (carcinoma).

212 Fechner, R. E.: Obstet. Gynecol. **31:**485-490, 1960.

213 Ferenczy, A., and Richart, R. M.: Female reproductive system: dynamics of scan and transmission electron microscopy, New York, 1974, John Wiley & Sons, Inc.

214 Friedrich, E. G.: Obstet. Gynecol. **30:**201-219, 1967 (hormonal effects).

215 Gibbs, R. S., et al.: Am. J. Obstet. Gynecol. **121:**919-925, 1975 (endometritis).

215a Ganem, K. J., Parsons, L., and Friedell, G. H.: Am. J. Obstet. Gynecol. **83:**1592-1594, 1962 (bone).

216 Good, R. G., and Moyer, D. L.: Fertil. Steril. **19:**37-49, 1968 (hormonal effects).

217 Gore, H.: In Norris, H. J., Hertig, A. T., and Abell, M. R., editors: The uterus, Baltimore, 1973, The Williams & Wilkins Co., Chap. 13 (hyperplasia).

218 Gore, H., and Hertig, A. T.: Am. J. Obstet. Gynecol. **94:**134-155, 1966 (carcinoma in situ).

219 Hertig, A. T.: Lab. Invest. **13:**1153-1191, 1964 (gestational changes).

220 Israel, S. L., Roitman, H. B., and Clancy, E.: J.A.M.A. **183:**63-65, 1963 (tuberculosis).

221 Kahn, H. S., and Tyler, C. W.: J.A.M.A. **234:** 57-59, 1975 (intrauterine device).

222 Kaufman, R. H., Abbot, J. P., and Wall, J. A.: Am. J. Obstet. Gynecol. **77:**1271-1285, 1959 (carcinoma).

223 Kay, S.: Am. J. Clin. Pathol. **61:**264-269, 1974 (epidermoid carcinoma).

224 Kempson, R. L., and Bari, W.: Hum. Pathol. **1:**331-349, 1970 (sarcoma).

225 Kempson, R. L., and Pokorny, G. E.: Cancer **21:**650-662, 1968 (carcinoma).

226 Kistner, R. W.: In Norris, H. J., Hertig, A. T., and Abell, M. R., editors: The uterus, Baltimore, 1973, The Williams & Wilkins Co., Chap. 12 (hormonal effects).

227 Kistner, R. W., Duncan, C. J., and Mansell, H.: Obstet. Gynecol. **8:**399-407, 1956 (hormonal effects).

228 Klaer, W., and Holm-Jensen, S.: Acta Pathol. Microbiol. Scand. **80:**835, 1972 (metastatic carcinoma).

229 Langlois, P. L.: J. Reprod. Med. **4:**220-228, 1970 (normal weight).

230 Larbig, G. G., Clemmer, J. J., Koss, L. G., and Foote, F. W.: Am. J. Clin. Pathol. **44:** 32-35, 1965 (stromal tumors).

231 Laros, R. K., and Work, B. A.: Obstet. Gynecol. **46:**215-220, 1975.

232 deLouvois, J., et al.: Lancet **1:**1073-1075, 1974 (endometritis).

233 Lyon, F. A.: Am. J. Obstet. Gynecol. **123:** 299-301, 1975 (estrogens and cancer).

233a MacDonald, P. C., and Siiteri, P.: Gynecol. Oncol. **2:**259-263, 1974 (estrone and cancer).

234 deMoraes-Ruehsen, M. D., Jones, G. S., Burnett, L. S., et al.: Am. J. Obstet. Gynecol. **103:**1059-1077, 1969 (infertility).

235 Ng, A. B. P., and Reagan, J. W.: Obstet. Gynecol. **35:**437-443, 1970 (carcinoma).

236 Ng, A. B. P., Reagan, J. W., Storaasli, V. P., et al.: Am. J. Clin. Pathol. **59:**765-781, 1973 (carcinoma)

237 Nogales, F., Beato, M., and Martinez, H.: Arch. Gynaekol. **203:**45, 1966 (tuberculosis).

238 Norris, H. J., and Taylor, H. B.: Cancer **19:** 755-766, 1966 (stromal tumors).

239 Norris, H. J., Roth, E., and Taylor, H. B.: Obstet. Gynecol. **28:**57-63, 1966 (mixed müllerian tumor).

240 Noyes, R. W.: In Norris, H. J., Hertig, A. T., and Abell, M. R., editors: The uterus, Baltimore, 1973, The Williams & Wilkins Co., Chap. 7 (anatomy).

241 Philippe, E.: Rev. Franc. Gynec. **65:**413-421, 1970 (endometritis).

242 Picoff, R. C., and Luginbuhl, W. H.: Am. J. Obstet. Gynecol. **88:**642-646, 1964 (abnormal bleeding).

243 Rorat, E., Ferenczy, A., and Richart, R. M.: Cancer **33:**880-887, 1974 (clear-cell carcinoma).

244 Roth, E., and Taylor, H. B.: Obstet. Gynecol. **27:**838-844, 1966 (cartilage).

245 Ryan, G. M., Jr., Craig, J., and Reid, D. E.: Am. J. Obstet. Gynecol. **90:**715-725, 1964 (progestogens).

246 Salm, R.: J. Pathol. **108:**47-53, 1972 (polyps).

247 Shanklin, D. R.: J. Reprod. Med. **3:**179-207, 1969 (dating).

248 Sheffield, W. H., Soule, S. D., and Herzog, G. M.: Am. J. Obstet. Gynecol. **103:**828-835, 1969 (progestogens).

248a Siiteri, P., et al.: Gynecol. Oncol. **2:**228-238, 1974.

249 Silverberg, S. G., Bolin, M. G., and DeGeorgi, L. S.: Cancer **30:**1307-1314, 1972 (carcinoma).

250 Silverberg, S. G., and DeGeorgi, L. S.: Cancer **31:**1127-1140, 1973 (clear-cell carcinoma).

251 Silverberg, S. G., and Makowski, E. L.: Obstet. Gynecol. **46:**503-506, 1975 (carcinoma and hormones).

251a Smith, D. C., et al.: New Eng. J. Med. **293:** 1164-1167, 1975 (estrogens and cancer).

251b Stemmerman, G. N.: Am. J. Obstet. Gynecol. **82:**1261-1266, 1961.

252 Stevenson, C. S.: Fertil. Steril. **16:**208-222, 1965 (infertility).

253 Terzakis, J. A.: J. Cell Biol. **27:**293-304, 1965 (ultrastructure).

254 Vellios, F.: In Sommers, S. C., editor: Pathology annual, New York, 1972, Appleton-Century-Crofts, vol. 7, pp. 201-229 (hyperplasia).

255 Wienke, E. C., Cavazos, F., Hall, D. G., and Lucas, F. V.: Am. J. Obstet. Gynecol. **103:** 102-111, 1969 (hormonal effects).

256 Williamson, E. O., and Chistopherson, W. M.: Cancer **29:**585-592, 1972 (mixed müllerian tumor).

257 Woodruff, J. D., and Julian, C. G.: Am. J. Obstet. Gynecol. **103:**810-819, 1969.

258 Zettergren, L.: Glial tissue in the uterus, Am. J. Pathol. **71:**419-426, 1973.

258a Ziel, H. K., and Finkle, W. D.: New Eng. J. Med. **293:**1167-1170, 1975.

Myometrium

259 Barlow, J. J., et al.: Cancer **32:**735-743, 1973 (leiomyosarcoma chemotherapy)

260 Bartsich, E. G., Bowe, E. T., and Moore, J. G.: Obstet. Gynecol. **32:**101-106, 1968 (leiomyosarcoma).

261 Boyce, C. R., and Buddhdev, H. N.: Obstet. Gynecol. **42:**252-258, 1973 (leiomyoma).

262 Christopherson, W. M., Williamson, E. O., and Gray, L. A.: Cancer **29:**1512-1517, 1972 (leiomyosarcoma).

263 Emge, L. A.: Am. J. Obstet. Gynecol. **83:** 1541-1563, 1962 (adenomyosis).

264 Fechner, R. E.: Am. J. Clin. Pathol. **49:**697-703, 1968 (leiomyoma).

265 Ferenczy, A., Fenoglio, J., and Richart, R. M.: Cancer **30:**244-260, 1972 (adenomatoid tumor).

266 Ferenczy, A., Richart, R. M., and Okagaki, T.: Cancer **28:**1004-1018, 1971 (leiomyoma).

267 Goodhue, W. W., Susin, M., and Kramer, E. E.: Arch. Pathol. **71:**263-268, 1974 (plexiform tumor).

268 Idelson, M. G., and Dairds, A. W.: Obstet. Gynecol. **21:**78-85, 1963 (leiomyoma).

269 Jacobs, D. S., Cohen, H., and Johnson, J. S.: Am. J. Clin. Pathol. **44:**45-51, 1965 (lipoleiomyoma).

270 Konis, E. E., and Belsky, R. D.: Obstet. Gynecol. **27:**442-446, 1966 (metastasizing leiomyoma).

271 Marcus, C. C.: Am. J. Obstet. Gynecol. **82:** 408-416, 1961 (adenomyosis).

272 Mathur, B. B. L., Shah, B. S., and Bhende, Y. M.: Am. J. Obstet. Gynecol. **84:**1820-1829, 1962 (adenomyosis).

273 Murphy, E.: Am. J. Obstet. Gynecol. **103:** 403-408, 1969 (sclerosis).

274 Norris, H. J., and Parmley, T.: Cancer **36:** 2164-2178, 1975 (intravenous leiomyomatosis).

275 Paranjothy, D., and Vaish, S. K.: J. Obstet. Gynaecol. Br. Commonw. **74:**603-605, 1967 (leiomyoma).

276 Parmley, T. H., et al.: Obstet. Gynecol. **46:** 511-516, 1975 (leiomyomatosis).

277 Pietila, K.: Acta Obstet. Gynaecol. Scand. **48**(suppl. 5), 1969 (leiomyoma).

278 Rothman, D., and Rennard, M.: Obstet. Gynecol. **21:**102-105, 1963 (leiomyoma).

279 Rywlin, A. M., Recher, L., and Benson, J.: Cancer **17:**100-104, 1964 (clear-cell leiomyoma).

280 Saksela, E., Lampinen, V., and Procope, B. J.: Am. J. Obstet. Gynecol. **120:**452-460, 1974 (sarcoma).

281 Salm, R.: Beitr. Pathol. **149:**284, 1973 (lipoma).

282 Scharfenberg, J. C., and Geary, W. L.: Obstet. Gynecol. **43:**909-914, 1974 (intravenous leiomyomatosis).

283 Silverberg, S. G.: Obstet. Gynecol. **38:**613-628, 1971 (leiomyosarcoma).

284 Silverberg, S. G., Willson, M. A., and Board, J. A.: J. Obstet. Gynecol. **110:**397-404, 1971 (hemangiopericytoma).

285 Stout, A. P.: Cancer **15:**400-409, 1962 (leiomyoma).

286 Taubert, H. D., Wissner, S. E., and Haskins, A. L.: Obstet. Gynecol. **25:**561-564, 1965 (leiomyomatosis).

287 Taxy, J. B., Battifora, H., and Oyasu, R.: Cancer **34:**306-316, 1974 (adenomatoid tumor).

288 Taylor, H. B., and Norris, H. J.: Arch. Pathol. **82:**40-44, 1966 (leiomyosarcoma).

289 Youngs, L. A., and Taylor, H. B.: Am. J.

Clin. Pathol. 48:537-545, 1967 (adenomatoid tumor).

Fallopian tube

290 Acosta, A. A., Kaplan, A. L., and Kaufman, R. H.: Obstet. Gynecol. 44:84-90, 1974 (mixed müllerian tumor).

291 Benjamin, C. L., and Beaver, D. C.: Am. J. Clin. Pathol. 21:212-222, 1951.

292 Dokumov, S., and Dekov, D.: J. Clin. Endocrinol. Metab. 23:1262-1265, 1963.

293 Flege, J. B.: Arch. Surg. 92:397-398, 1966 (ectopic pregnancy).

294 Fogh, I.: Primary carcinoma of the fallopian tube, Cancer 23:1332-1335, 1969 (carcinoma).

295 Jacobson, L., and Westrom, L.: Am. J. Obstet. Gynecol. 105:1088-1098, 1969 (infection).

296 Mardh, P.-A., and Westrom, L.: Br. J. Vener. Dis. 46:179-186, 1970 (infection, mycoplasma).

297 Mazzarella, P., Okagaki, T., and Richart, R. M.: Obstet. Gynecol. 39:381-388, 1972 (teratoma).

298 Palladino, V. S., and Trousdell, M.: Cancer 23:1413-1422, 1969 (mixed müllerian tumor).

299 Rees, E., and Annels, E. H.: Br. J. Vener. Dis. 45:205-215, 1969 (gonorrhea).

300 Rubin, I. C., Lisa, J. R., and Trinidad, S.: Surg. Gynecol. Obstet. 103:469-474, 1956 (metaplasia).

301 Schiller, H. M., and Silverberg, S. G.: Cancer 28:389-395, 1971 (carcinoma).

302 Sedlis, A.: Obstet. Gynecol. Survey 16:209-226, 1961 (carcinoma).

303 Sweet, R. I., Selinger, H. E., and McKay, D. G.: Obstet. Gynecol. 45:553-556, 1975 (teratoma).

304 Swenson, R. M., et al.: Obstet. Gynecol. 42:538-541, 1973 (anaerobic infection).

305 Thadepalli, H., Gorbach, S. L., and Keith, L.: Am. J. Obstet. Gynecol. 117:1034-1040, 1973 (anaerobic infections).

306 Thomas, M. L., and Rose, D. H.: Acta Radiol. (Diagn.) 14:295-304, 1973.

307 Timonen, S., and Nieminen, U.: Acta Obstet. Gynecol. Scand. 46:337-339, 1967 (ectopic pregnancy).

308 Woodruff, J. D., and Pauerstein, C. J.: The fallopian tube, Baltimore, 1969, The Williams & Wilkins Co.

309 Wright, N. H., and Laemmle, P.: Am. J. Obstet. Gynecol. 101:979-990, 1968 (infection).

310 Youngs, L. A., and Taylor, H. B.: Am. J. Clin. Pathol. 48:537-545, 1967 (adenomatoid tumor).

Ovary

311 Abel, K. P.: Lancet 1:136-137, 1964 (infarction).

312 Abell, M. R., and Holtz, F.: Am. J. Obstet. Gynecol. 93:850-866, 1965 (carcinoma).

313 Adams, E. C., and Hertig, A. T.: J. Cell Biol. 41:716-1969 (ultrastructure).

314 Angervall, L., and Knutson, H.: Acta Obstet. Gynecol. Scand. 38:275-285, 1959 (anatomy).

315 Arey, L. B.: Am. J. Obstet. Gynecol. 81:743-751, 1961 (Brenner tumor).

316 Arrata, W. S. M., and de Alvarez, R. R.:

317 Asadourian, L. A., and Taylor, H. B.: Obstet. Gynecol. 33:370-379, 1969 (dysgerminoma).

318 Aure, J. C., Hoeg, K., and Kolstad, D.: Am. J. Obstet. Gynecol. 109:113-118, 1971 (carcinoma).

319 Aure, J. C., Hoeg, K., and Kolstad, P.: Obstet. Gynecol. 37:1-9, 1971 (carcinoma).

320 Ballas, M.: Ann. Clin. Lab. Sci. 4:267-275, 1974 (alpha-fetoprotein).

321 Bardin, C. W., Lipsett, M. B., Edgecomb, J. H., and Marshall, J. R.: New Eng. J. Med. 277:399-402, 1967 (hyperthecosis).

322 Behrman, H. R., and Caldwell, B. V.: In Greep, R. O., editor: Reproductive physiology, M.T.P. Int. Rev. Science 8:63-94, 1974, Baltimore, University Park Press (physiology).

323 Block, E.: Acta Anat. 17:201-206, 1953 (anatomy).

324 Blackwell, W. J., Dockerty, M. B., Masson, J. C., and Mussey, R. O.: Am. J. Obstet. Gynecol. 51:151-172, 1946 (teratoma).

325 Case Records of the Massachusetts General Hospital: Case 24-1971, New Eng. J. Med. 284:1369-1375, 1971 (massive edema).

326 Cooper, H. E., Spellacy, W. N., Prem, K. A., et al.: Am. J. Obstet. Gynecol. 100:371-387, 1968 (polycystic ovary).

327 Cocco, A. E., and Conway, S. J.: New Eng. J. Med. 293:485-486, 1975 (mucinous tumor).

328 Crosignani, P. G., et al.: Obstet. Gynecol. 46:15-22, 1975 (anovulation syndrome).

329 Cummins, P., Fox, H., and Langley, F. A.: J. Pathol. 110:167-176, 1973 (Brenner tumor).

330 Daane, T. A., Lurie, A. D., and Barton, R. K.: Obstet. Gynecol. 34:655-663, 1969 (lutein cysts).

331 Diaz-Infante, A., Virutamasen, P., Connaughton, J. F., et al.: Obstet. Gynecol. 44:830-838, 1974 (physiology).

332 Easterling, W. E., Talbert, L. M., and Potter, H. D.: Am. J. Obstet. Gynecol. 120:385-389, 1974 (polycystic ovary).

333 Ehrlich, C. E., and Roth, C. E.: Cancer 27:332-342, 1971 (Brenner tumor).

334 Falls, J. L.: Cancer 8:143-150, 1955 (anatomy).

335 Feldman, G. B., and Knapp, R. C.: Am. J. Obstet. Gynecol. 119:991-994, 1974.

336 Fenoglio, C. M., Ferenczy, A., and Richart, R. M.: Cancer 36:1709-1722, 1975 (mucinous tumors).

337 Gambrell, R. D., Greenblatt, R. B., and Mahesh, V. B.: Obstet. Gynecol. 42:429-440, 1973 (polycystic ovary).

338 Garcia-Bunuel, R., and Morris, B.: Cancer 17:1108-1118, 1964 (carcinoma).

339 Gillim, S. W., Christensen, A. K., and McLennan, C. E.: Am. J. Anat. 126:409-428, 1969 (ultrastructure).

340 Girouard, D. P., Barclay, D. L., and Collins, C. G.: Obstet. Gynecol. 23:513-525, 1964 (hyperreactio luteinalis).

341 Givens, J. R., Wiser, W. L., and Coleman, S. A.: Am. J. Obstet. Gynecol. 110:955-972, 1971 (hyperthecosis).

342 Greenblatt, R. B., and Mahesh, V. B.: J.

Reprod. Med. **13**:85-88, 1974 (polycystic ovary).

343 Grogan, R. H.: Obstet. Gynecol. **30**:716-720, 1967 (cysts, rupture).

344 Hammerstein, J.: In Greep, R. O., editor: Reproductive physiology, M.T.P. Int. Rev. Science **8**:279-311, 1974, Baltimore, University Park Press (physiology).

345 Hart, W. R., and Norris, H. J.: Cancer **31**: 1031-1045, 1973 (mucinous tumors).

346 Hay, D. M., and Stewart, D. B.: J. Obstet. Gynaecol. Br. Commonw. **76**:941-943, 1969 (carcinoma).

347 Hertig, A. T., and Gore, H.: Tumors of the female sex organs. Part 3. Tumors of the ovary and fallopian tube. Sect. IX, Fasc. 33, Atlas of tumor pathology, Washington, D.C., 1961, Armed Forces Institute of Pathology.

348 Jensen, A. B., and Fechener, R. E.: Lab. Invest. **21**:527-535, 1969 (Sertoli-Leydig tumor).

349 Joshi, V. V.: Cancer **22**:1199-1207, 1968 (Krukenberg's tumor).

350 Kalderon, A. E., and Tucci, J. R.: Lab. Invest. **29**:81-89, 1973 (Sertoli-Leydig tumor).

351 Kalstone, C. E., Jaffe, R. B., and Abell, M. R.: Obstet. Gynecol. **34**:564-571, 1969 (massive edema).

352 Kempson, R. L.: Arch. Pathol. **86**:492-507, 1968 (Sertoli-Leydig tumor).

353 Keyes, P. L.: Science **164**:846-847, 1969 (physiology).

354 Konikov, N., Bleisch, V., and Piskie, V.: Acta Cytol. **10**:335-339, 1966 (ascites).

355 Kottmeier, H. L.: Surgical management—conservative surgery. In Gentil, F., and Junqueira, A. C. Ovarian cancer, Unio. Int. Contra Cancr. Monogr. Ser. **11**:157-164, 1968, New York, Springer-Verlag.

356 Kriss, B. R.: J. Mt. Sinai Hosp. **14**:798-801, 1947.

356a Kurman, R. J., and Norris, H. J.: Obstet. Gynecol. **48**:579-589, 1976.

357 Linder, D., McCaw, B. K., and Hecht, F.: New Eng. J. Med. **292**:63-66, 1975 (teratoma, origin).

358 Long, M. F., and Taylor, H. C.: Am. J. Obstet. Gynecol. **90**:936-950, 1964 (endometrioid carcinoma).

359 Long, R. T. L., Spratt, J. S., and Dowling, E.: Am. J. Surg. **117**:162-169, 1969 (carcinoma).

360 Knapp, R. C., and Friedman, E. A.: Am. J. Obstet. Gynecol. **119**:1013-1017, 1974.

361 Malkasian, G. D., Dockerty, M. D., and Symmonds, R. E.: Obstet. Gynecol. **29**:719-725, 1967 (teratoma).

362 Mansell, H., and Hertig, A. T.: Obstet. Gynecol. **6**:385-394, 1955 (granulosa cell tumor).

363 Maques, M., et al.: Contraception **5**:177-185, 1972 (progestogen effect).

364 Mattingly, R. F., and Huang, W. Y.: Am. J. Obstet. Gynecol. **103**:679-693, 1969 (physiology).

365 deMoraes-Ruehsen, M., Blizzard, R. M., Garcia-Bunuel, R., and Jones, G. S.: Am. J. Obstet. Gynecol. **112**:693-703, 1972 (autoimmune disease).

366 Morris, J. M., and Scully, R. E.: Endocrine pathology of the ovary, St. Louis, 1958, The C. V. Mosby Co.

367 Munnell, E. W.: Am. J. Obstet. Gynecol. **103**: 641-650, 1969 (carcinoma).

368 Nieminen, I., von Numers, C., and Widholm, O.: Struma ovarii, Acta Obstet. Gynecol. Scand. **42**:399-424, 1964.

369 Norris, H. J., and Taylor, H. B.: Am. J. Clin. Pathol. **45**:557-566, 1967 (luteoma pregnancy).

370 Norris, H. J., and Taylor, H. B.: Cancer **21**: 255-263, 1968 (granulosa-theca cell tumors).

371 Norris, H. J., and Taylor, H. B.: Obstet. Gynecol. **34**:624-635, 1969 (granulosa cell tumor).

372 Novak, E. R.: Obstet. Gynecol. **36**:903-910, 1970.

373 Novak, E. R.: Obstet. Gynecol. **30**:709-715, 1967 (gynandroblastoma).

374 Ober, W. B., Grady, H. G., and Schoenbucher, A. K.: Am. J. Pathol. **33**:199-217, 1957 (decidua).

375 O'Hern, T. M., and Neubecker, R. D.: Arrhenoblastoma, Obstet. Gynecol. **19**:758-770, 1962.

376 Pearl, M., and Plotz, E. J.: Obstet. Gynecol. **21**:253-256, 1963 (ectopia).

377 Pedersen, P. H., and Larsen, J. F.: Acta Obstet. Gynecol. Scand. **49**:105-110, 1970 (granulosa cell tumor).

378 Peterson, W. F.: Obstet. Gynecol. Survey **12**: 793-830, 1957 (teratoma).

379 Piver, M. S., Williams, L. J., and Marcuse, P. M.: Obstet. Gynecol. **35**:740-751, 1970 (follicle cyst).

380 Polansky, S., dePapp, E. W., and Ogden, E. B.: Obstet. Gynecol. **45**:516-522, 1975 (luteoma pregnancy).

381 Robboy, S. J., Norris, H. J., and Scully, R. E.: Cancer **36**:404-418, 1975 (carcinoid).

382 Robboy, S. J., and Scully, R. E.: Hum. Pathol. **1**:643-653, 1970 (teratoma).

383 Robboy, S. J., and Scully, R. E.: Lab. Invest. **26**:488, 1972 (abstr.) (strumal carcinoid).

384 Robboy, S. J., Scully, R. E., and Norris, H. J.: Cancer **33**:798-811, 1974 (metastatic carcinoid).

385 Roberts, D. W. T., and Haines, M.: Br. Med. J. **2**:917-919, 1965 (cancer).

386 Roth, C. M.: Lab. Invest. **31**:15-23, 1974 (Brenner tumor).

387 Roth, L. M.: Cancer **27**:1482-1488, 1971 (Brenner tumor).

388 Roth, L. M., and Sternberg, W. H.: Cancer **27**:687-693, 1971 (Brenner tumor).

389 Rust, L. A., Israel, R., and Mishell, D. R., Jr.: Am. J. Obstet. Gynecol. **120**:785-790, 1974.

390 Ryan, K. J., Petro, Z., and Kaiser, J.: J. Clin. Endocrinol. **28**:355-358, 1968 (physiology).

391 Santesson, L.: Cited by Kraus, F. T.: Gynecologic pathology, St. Louis, 1967, The C. V. Mosby Co. (carcinoma).

392 Santesson, L., and Kottmeier, H. L.: In Gentil, F., and Junqueira, A. C.: Ovarian cancer, Union Int. Contre Cancer Monogr. Ser. **11**: 1-8, 1968, New York, Springer-Verlag (carcinoma).

393 Schenker, J. G., and Polishuk, W. Z.: Obstet. Gynecol. **46**:23-28, 1975 (hyperstimulation).

394 Scully, R. E.: Cancer **17**:769-778, 1964 (stromal luteoma).

395 Scully, R. E.: Gonadoblastoma, Cancer **25:** 1340-1356, 1970.

396 Scully, R. E.: Hum. Pathol. **1:**73-98, 1970 (carcinoma).

397 Scully, R. E., and Barlow, J. F.: Cancer **20:** 1405-1417, 1967 (clear-cell carcinoma).

398 Scully, R. E., and Richardson, G. S.: Cancer **14:**827-840, 1961 (metastatic carcinoma).

399 Serov, S. F., Scully, R. E., and Sobin, L. H.: Histological typing of ovarian tumours, Geneva, 1973, World Health Organization.

400 Silverberg, S. G.: Cancer **28:**588, 1971 (Brenner tumor).

401 Sjostedt, S., and Wahlen, T.: Acta Obstet. Gynecol. Scand. **40**(suppl. 6):1-26, 1961 (granulosa cell tumor).

402 Starup, J., and Sele, V.: Acta Obstet. Gynecol. Scand. **52:**259-268, 1973 (atrophy).

403 Stein, I. F., Sr., and Leventhal, M. L.: Am. J. Obstet. Gynecol. **21:**181-191, 1935 (polycystic ovary).

404 Steiner, M. M., and Hadawi, S. A.: Am. J. Dis. Child. **108:**28-36, 1964 (follicle cyst).

405 Sternberg, W. H., and Barclay, D. L.: Am. J. Obstet. Gynecol. **95:**165-181, 1966 (luteoma pregnancy).

406 Stevens, V. C.: J. Clin. Endocrinol. **29:**904-910, 1969 (physiology).

407 Taylor, H. B., and Norris, H. J.: Cancer **20:** 1953-1962, 1967 (lipid cell tumor).

408 Taymor, M. L., Berger, M. J., Thompson, I. E., et al.: Am. J. Obstet. Gynecol. **114:** 445-453, 1972 (physiology).

409 Teilum, G.: Acta Pathol. Microbiol. Scand. **64:**407-429, 1965.

410 Teilum, G., Albrechtsen, R., and Norgaard Pedersen, J.: Acta Path. Microbiol. Scand. **82:**586-588, 1974 (alpha-fetoprotein).

411 Thurlbeck, W. M., and Scully, R. E.: Cancer **13:**804-811, 1960 (teratoma).

412 Tyson, J. E., et al.: Obstet. Gynecol. **46:**1-11, 1975 (progestogen effect).

413 van Wagenen, G., and Simpson, M. E.: Postnatal development of the ovary, New Haven, 1973, Yale University Press.

414 Wharton, L. R.: Am. J. Obstet. Gynecol. **78:** 1101-1119, 1959.

415 Woodruff, J. D., et al.: Am. J. Obstet. Gynecol. **107:**202-208, 1970 (metastatic carcinoma).

416 Woodruff, J. D., Protos, P., and Peterson, W. F.: Am. J. Obstet. Gynecol. **102:**702-714, 1968 (teratoma).

417 Zanartu, J., Dabancens, A., Rodriquez-Bravo, R., et al.: Br. Med. J. **1:**605-608, 1974.

418 Zondek, L. H., and Zondek, T.: Acta Obstet. Gynaecol. Scand. **46:**392-413, 1967.

Placenta

419 Acosta-Sison, H.: Am. J. Obstet. Gynecol. **88:** 634-636, 1964 (hydatidiform mole).

420 Adcock, E. W., III, et al.: Science **181:**845-847, 1973 (HCG).

421 Altshuler, G., and McAdams, A. J.: Am. J. Obstet. Gynecol. **113:**616-626, 1972 (infections).

422 Altshuler, G., Russell, P., and Ermocilla, R.: Am. J. Obstet. Gynecol. **121:**351-359, 1975 (insufficiency).

423 Attwood, H. D., and Park, W. W.: J. Obstet. Gynaecol. Br. Commonw. **68:**611-617, 1963 (anatomy).

424 Bain, A. D., et al.: J. Obstet. Gynaecol. Br. Emp. **63:**826-832, 1956 (toxoplasmosis).

425 Banti, D., et al.: J. Clin. Pathol. **21:**322-331, 1968 (hemorrhage).

426 Beacham, W. D., Hernquist, W. C., Beacham, D. W., et al.: Am. J. Obstet. Gynecol. **84:** 1257-1270, 1962 (abdominal pregnancy).

427 Beer, A. E.: In Brosens, I. A., Dixon, G., and Robertson, W. B.: Human placentation, Amsterdam, 1975, Excerpta Medica Foundation, pp. 135-146 (immunology).

428 Benirschke, K., and Driscoll, S. G.: The pathology of the human placenta, New York, 1967, Springer-Verlag.

429 Billington, W. D.: In Brosens, I. A., Dixon, G., and Robertson, W. B.: Human placentation, Amsterdam, 1975, Excerpta Medica Foundation, pp. 147-158 (immunology).

430 Blanc, W. A.: N.Y. J. Med. **61:**1492-1496, 1961 (amnion nodosum).

431 Bleisch, V. R.: Am. J. Clin. Pathol. **42:**277-284, 1964 (twins).

432 Boyd, J. D., and Hamilton, W. J.: The human placenta, Cambridge, 1970, W. Heffer & Sons (remarkable, handsomely illustrated description of the anatomy and development of the normal human placenta).

433 Brauenstein, G. D., Grodin, J. M., Vaitukaitis, J., et al.: Am. J. Obstet. Gynecol. **115:**447-450, 1973 (HCG).

434 Brosens, I. A., Dixon, G., and Robertson, W. B.: Human placentation, Amsterdam, 1975, Excerpta Medica Foundation.

435 Brosens, I., Robertson, W. B., and Dixon, H. G.: In Wynn, R. M., editor: Obstetrics and gynecology annual, New York, 1972, Appleton-Century-Crofts, p. 177 (toxemia).

436 Burrows, S., et al.: Am. J. Obstet. Gynecol. **115:**579-580, 1973 (chorioangioma).

437 Carr, D. H.: Obstet. Gynecol. **37:**750-754, 1971 (cytogenetics).

438 Carter, B.: Obstet. Gynecol. **29:**30-33, 1967 (abruption).

439 Carter, J. E., Vellios, F., and Huber, C. P.: Am. J. Clin. Pathol. **40:**374-378, 1963 (infarcts).

440 Clark, P. B., Gusdon, J. P., and Burt, R. L.: Obstet. Gynecol. **35:**597-600, 1970.

441 Craig, J. M.: Arch. Pathol. **99:**233-236, 1975 (abortion).

442 Culp, W. C., et al.: Radiology **108:**309-310, 1973 (placenta membranacea).

443 Dehner, L. P., and Askin, F. B.: Obstet. Gynecol. **45:**211-214, 1975 (cytomegalovirus).

444 Demian, S. D. E., Donnelly, W. H., Frias, J. L., et al.: Am. J. Clin. Pathol. **61:**438-442, 1974 (giant nevus).

445 Desmonts, G., and Courreur, J.: New Eng. J. Med. **290:**1110-1116, 1974 (toxoplasmosis).

446 Douthwaite, R. M., and Urbach, G. I.: Am. J. Obstet. Gynecol. **109:**1023-1028, 1971 (immunology).

447 Dreskin, R. B., Spicer, S. S., and Greene, W. B.: J. Histochem. Cytochem. **18:**862-874, 1970 (HCG histochemistry).

448 Driscoll, S. G.: Am. J. Dis. Child. **118:**49-53, 1969 (rubella).

449 Dyke, P. C., and Fink, L. M.: Cancer 20: 150-154, 1967 (choriocarcinoma).

450 Elston, C. W.: J. Pathol. 97:261-268, 1969 (choriocarcinoma).

451 Elston, C. W., and Bagshawe, K. D.: J. Obst. Gynaecol. Br. Commonw. 79:717-724, 1972 (hydatidiform mole).

452 Enders, A. C., and King, B. F.: Anat. Rec. 167:231-252, 1970 (Hofbauer cells).

453 Faulk, W. P., Jeannet, M., Creighton, W. D., et al.: J. Clin. Invest. 54:1011-1019, 1974.

454 Ferenczy, A., and Richart, R. M.: Gynecol. Oncol. 1:95-110, 1972 (anatomy).

455 Finn, J. L.: Placenta membranacea, Obstet. Gynecol. 3:438-440, 1954.

456 Froehlich, L. A., and Fujikura, T.: Pediatrics 52:6, 1973 (single umbilical artery).

457 Gärtner, A., Larsson, L. I., and Sjöberg, N. O.: Acta Obstet. Gynecol. Scand. 54:161-163, 1975 (HCG).

458 Gagnon, R. A.: Report of 2 cases, Obstet. Gynecol. 31:682-684, 1968 (herpes simplex).

459 Goldstein, D. P.: Obstet. Gynecol. 38:817-822, 1971 (chemotherapy).

460 Goldstein, D. P., et al.: Obstet. Gynecol. 45: 527-530, 1975 (HCG).

461 Gruenwald, P.: The placenta and its maternal supply line, Baltimore, 1975, University Park Press.

462 Gruenwald, P.: Fetal deprivation and placental insufficiency, Obstet. Gynecol. 37:906, 1971.

463 Hammond, C. B., Borchert, L. G., Tyrey, L., et al.: Am. J. Obstet. Gynecol. 115:451-457, 1973 (choriocarcinoma).

464 Hawick, H. J., et al.: Am. J. Obstet. Gynecol. 99:715-727, 1967 (septic abortion).

465 Hellman, L. M., and Hertig, A. T.: Am. J. Pathol. 14:111-120, 1938 (erythroblastosis).

466 Hertig, A. T.: Human trophoblast, Springfield, Ill., 1968, Charles C Thomas, Publisher.

467 Hertig, A. T.: Clinics 4:602, 1945 (toxemia). Quoted by Robertson, W. B., et al.: see reference 502.

468 Hibbard, B. M., and Jeffcoate, T. N. A.: Obstet. Gynecol. 27:155-167, 1966 (abruption).

469 Horne, H. W., Hertig, A. T., Kundsin, R. B., and Kosasa, T. S.: Int. J. Fertil. 18:226-231, 1973 (mycoplasma).

470 Hreshchyshyn, M. M., Bozen, B., and Loughran, C. H.: Am. J. Obstet. Gynecol. 81:302-307, 1961 (abdominal pregnancy).

471 Hulka, J., and Mohr, K.: Science 161:696-698, 1968 (immunology).

472 de Ikonicoff, L., and Cedard, L.: Am. J. Obstet. Gynecol. 116:1124-1132, 1973 (HCG).

473 Irving, F. C., and Hertig, A. T.: Surg. Gynecol. Obstet. 64:178-200, 1937 (placenta accreta).

474 Jacobson, F. J., and Enzen, N.: Am. J. Obstet. Gynecol. 78:868-875, 1959 (hydatidiform mole, metastasis).

475 Jaffe, R. B., Lee, P. A., and Midgley, A. R.: J. Clin. Endocrinol. 29:1281-1283, 1969 (HCG).

476 Kaye, M. D., and Jones, W. R.: Am. J. Obstet. Gynecol. 109:1029-1031, 1971 (HCG).

477 Khudr, G., et al.: Am. J. Obstet. Gynecol. 115:530-533, 1973 (X cell and placental site giant cell).

478 Kitzmiller, J. L., and Benirschke, K.: Am. J. Obstet. Gynecol. 115:248, 1973 (toxemia).

479 Kurman, R. J., Scully, R. E., and Norris, H. J.: Cancer 38:1214-1226, 1976 (trophoblastic pseudotumor).

480 Luke, R. K., Sharpe, J. W., and Greene, R. R.: Am. J. Obstet. Gynecol. 95:660-668, 1966 (placenta accreta).

481 McConnell, H. D., and Carr, D. H.: Obstet. Gynecol. 45:547-552, 1975 (abortion, cytogenetics).

482 McCord, J. R.: Am. J. Obstet. Gynecol. 28: 743-750, 1934 (syphilis).

483 McKay, D. G., Goldenberg, V., Kaunitz, H., et al.: Arch. Pathol. 84:557-597, 1967 (toxemia).

484 Marshall, J. R., Hammond, C. B., Ross, G. T., et al.: Obstet. Gynecol. 32:760-764, 1968 (HCG).

485 Monif, G. R. G., and Dische, R. M.: Am. J. Clin. Pathol. 58:445-449, 1972 (cytomegalic inclusion virus).

486 Monif, G.: Infectious diseases in obstetrics and gynecology, New York, 1974, Harper & Row, Publishers.

487 Naib, Z. M., Nahmias, A. J., Josey, W. E., and Wheeler, J. H.: Obstet. Gynecol. 35:260-263, 1970 (herpes simplex).

488 Naughton, M. A., Merrill, D. A., McManus, L. M., et al.: Cancer Res. 35:1887-1890, 1975 (HCG).

489 Nelson, D. M., Smith, C. H., Enders, A. C., and Donohue, T. M.: Anat. Rec. 184:15-181, 1976 (ultrastructure).

490 Ornoy, A., et al.: Am. J. Obstet. Gynecol. 116: 949-956, 1973 (rubella).

491 Page, E. W.: J. Obstet. Gynaecol. Br. Commonw. 9:883-894, 1972 (toxemia).

492 Park, W. W.: In Brosens, I. A., Dixon, G., and Robertson, W. B.: Human placentation, Amsterdam, 1975, Excerpta Medica Foundation, pp. 35-46 (anatomy).

493 Park, W. W.: Choriocarcinoma, Philadelphia, 1971, F. A. Davis Co.

494 Peterson, E. P., and Taylor, H. B.: Obstet. Gynecol. 35:787-793, 1970 (amniotic fluid embolism).

495 Philippe, E.: Rev. Franc. Gynec. 68:645-653, 1973 (abortion, cytogenetics).

496 Philippe, E.: Histopathologie placentaire, Paris, 1974, Masson et Cie.

497 Philippe, E., Lefakis, P., Laedlein-Greilsammer, D., et al.: Rev. Franc. Gynec. 65:413-421, 1970 (endometritis).

498 Ramsey, E. M., Corner, G. W., and Donner, M. W.: Am. J. Obstet. Gynecol. 86:213-225, 1963 (circulation).

499 Rappaport, F., Rabinowitz, M., Toaff, R., and Krochik, N.: Lancet 1:1273-1275, 1960 (listeriosis).

500 Rewell, R. E., and Whitehouse, W. L.: J. Pathol. 91:255-256, 1966 (metastatic carcinoma).

501 Reynolds, D. W., Stagno, S., Hasty, T. S., Tiller, M., and Alford, C. A., Jr.: New Eng. J. Med. 289:1-5, 1973 (cytomegalovirus).

502 Robertson, W. B., Brosens, I., and Dixon, G.: In Brosens, I. A., Dixon, G., and Robertson,

W. B.: Human placentation, Amsterdam, 1975, Excerpta Medica Foundation, pp. 47-65 (anatomy, toxemia).

503 Roche, W. D., Jr., and Norris, H. J.: Obstet. Gynecol. **43**:729-731, 1974 (amniotic fluid embolism).

504 Rotheram, E. B., and Schick, S. F.: Am. J. Med. **46**:80-89, 1969 (septic abortion).

505 Scott, J. S.: J. Obstet. Gynaecol. Br. Commonw. **67**:904-918, 1960 (placenta extrachorialis).

506 Seeliger, H. P. R.: Some new aspects of human listeriosis. In Human listeriosis—its nature and diagnosis, U.S. Department of Health, Education and Welfare, Communicable Disease Center, Atlanta, 1957.

507 Shanklin, D. R., and Scott, J. S.: Br. J. Obstet. Gynecol. **82**:476-487, 1975 (hematoma).

508 Shanklin, D. R., and Sotelo-Avila, C.: Lab. Invest. **15**:111, 1966 (placenta extrachorialis).

509 Shurin, P. A., et al.: New Eng. J. Med. **293**: 5-8, 1975 (mycoplasma).

510 Sieracki, J. C., Panke, T. W., Horvat, B. L., et al.: Obstet. Gynecol. **46**:155-159, 1975 (chorioangioma).

511 Steigrad, S. J., James, R. W., and Osborn, R. A.: Aust. N.Z. J. Obstet. Gynaecol. **8**:79-86, 1968.

512 Taylor, H. B., and Peterson, E. P.: Obstet. Gynecol. **35**:787-793, 1970 (amniotic fluid embolism).

513 Teteris, N. J., Lina, A. A., and Holaday, W. J.: Obstet. Gynecol. **47**(suppl.):15s-18s, 1976 (placenta percreta).

514 Thomson, A. M., et al.: J. Obstet. Gynaecol. Br. Commonw. **76**:865-872, 1969 (anatomy).

515 Tominaga, T., and Page, E. W.: Am. J. Obstet. Gynecol. **96**:305-309, 1966 (hydatidiform mole).

516 Vaitukaitis, J. L.: Ann. Clin. Lab. Sci. **4**:276-280, 1974 (HCG).

517 Vaitukaitis, J. L., Brunstein, G. D., and Ross, G. T.: Am. J. Obstet. Gynecol. **113**:751-758, 1972 (HCG).

518 Villee, D. B.: New Eng. J. Med. **281**:473-484, 533-541, 1969 (endocrinology).

519 Wallenburg, H. C. S.: Obstet. Gynecol. Survey **26**:411-425, 1971 (chorioangioma).

520 Wynn, R. M.: Am. J. Obstet. Gynecol. **103**: 723-739, 1969 (anatomy).

521 Wynn, R. M.: Am. J. Obstet. Gynecol. **114**: 339-355, 1972 (anatomy).

522 Wynn, R. M., and Harris, J. A.: Am. J. Obstet. Gynecol. **99**:1125-1137, 1967 (hydatidiform mole).

41/Breast

JOSEPH F. KUZMA

Breast disease is *different*—different from all other organ-system disorders wherein many aberrations of mechanical, degenerative, inflammatory, and biochemical nature (including benign tumors) are disabling or lethal. The *absence* of conventional symptoms, which customarily direct the patient to seek medical advice and care, is the beginning of the difference. The one and only significant disease of the breast (cancer) has insignificant signs and symptoms—nothing more than the accidental discovery of a lump in the breast! At least this is the prototype case—no pain, no anemia from blood loss, no constitutional symptoms, and no perversion of function or biochemical profiles. What, then, is it all about? It is about the probability that a breast mass is cancer. Our study of breast disorders has but one purpose—to understand what is breast cancer and how to identify it. Collectively, all other breast diseases have little clinical significance. In the United States, breast cancer leads all other cancers in both incidence and mortality in the female.[4]

DEVELOPMENT, GROWTH, AND STRUCTURE

General anatomy. The adult female breast is a modified compound alveolar secretory gland derived from the skin. It is composed of approximately one dozen irregular lobes radiating from the central nipple area. Each lobe has an excretory duct with a local dilatation of the duct beneath the nipple known as the lactiferous sinus. The ducts do not anastomose, although two or more may have a common opening at the nipple. Multiple duct branchings (lobes) ending in custers of epithelial cells (lobules) constitute the parenchyma. Large ducts at the nipple are lined by stratified squamous epithelium that gradually merges with the columnar cells of the smaller ducts. The peripheral portions have low columnar cells, frequently of two layers, that blend into the cuboid cells of the lobules.

Just within the basement membrane, fibrillar elongated cells derived from epithelium (myoepithelial cells) may be seen.

The stroma immediately supporting the lobules of the breast is known as the intralobular connective tissue, which is continuous with the periductal tissue. The periductal and intralobular tissue varies with the functional state and may be considered as a part of the "parenchyma." It is loose reticular or myxomatous in appearance and is sharply defined from the more dense interlobar substance. Except during pregnancy and lactation, the bulk of the breast is made up of connective tissue and fat.

Embryology. As in all mammals, the human breast develops in a primitive epidermal thickening known as the milk line, which extends bilaterally on the ventral surface between the upper and lower limb attachments. In the human embryo, the milk line appears at about the sixth week. This primitive line then gradually atrophies, but at the ninth week the site of the permanent mammae can be recognized by the persistence of the epithelial thickening (primitive nipple buds). By the sixth month of development, about 15 to 20 solid epithelial cords extend into the corium from the basal layer of the primitive nipple. By the ninth month, these branching cords have developed a lumen and may have two or three layers of cells.

Neonatal mammary gland. In gestation the hormones that pass the placenta have an effect on the fetal breast tissue. Engorgement of the breast of the neonate, with secretory activity in the terminal portions of the ducts, is sufficiently active to produce enlargement of the breast area and active secretion. The process is self-limited, although the clinical manifestations may be misinterpreted as an inflammatory condition.

Mammary gland of adolescence. Prior to adolescence, the breast structure is similar in male and female. However, during adolescence

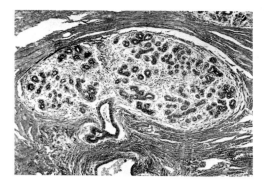

Fig. 41-1. Normal lobule. Mature, well-developed lobule with sharp distinction between lobular parenchymal connective tissue and that of general stroma. (40×.)

the breasts of the female gradually enlarge over a period of several years. The enlargement is primarily attributable to connective tissue and fat, in which elongation and active division of ducts and ductules terminate in units called lobules, with their special intralobular connective tissue.

Mammary gland of sexual maturity. The breast epithelium and stroma participate in cyclic patterns of growth and recession somewhat parallel to the events taking place in the endometrium. At the time of menstruation, the breast epithelium is chiefly that of involution and desquamation. After menstruation, the epithelial cells proliferate and increase in size. The intralobular connective tissue appears edematous, pale staining, and acellular at the time that the epithelial cells are the largest. Abortive secretory activity may be noted in the period of premenstrual epithelial hyperplasia. The breast's connective tissue also has the capacity to bind water, and patients attest to volume changes and sensations of fullness and heaviness in the premenstrual period. In the condition of amenorrhea, the cyclic breast changes are not observed (Fig. 41-1).

Mammary gland in pregnancy and lactation. In pregnancy, the earliest external change detected in the mammary gland is the moderate increase in firmness of the breast, associated with enlargement of the superficial veins, and the gradually developing pigmentation of the areola and nipple. The first 3 months of pregnancy are characterized by cellular proliferation. This is particularly noticeable at the blind ends of the branched ducts and in the sites of lobular development. As the epithelial tissue becomes more and more prominent, the periductal tissue softens and has a less intense staining character. Eventually, the

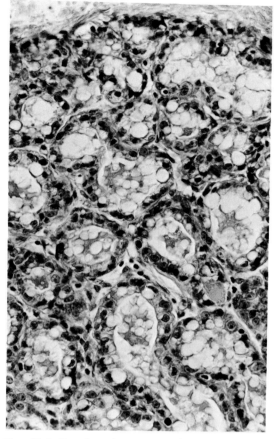

Fig. 41-2. Developed acini actively secreting (lactation) in lobule of breast at term pregnancy. (320×.)

lobular proliferation is characterized by forms of acini with their acinar ducts accompanied by a delicate vascular connective tissue bed. It has been pointed out that the centralmost parts of breast beneath the nipple develop blind duct pouches that may act as reservoirs.[9]

At term, superficial epithelial cells of the breast have differentiated into fat-containing (colostrum) cells. Such cells are shed in variable amounts and constitute what is known as the initial secretion of the breast (colostrum). Shortly after delivery, the basal cells lining the dilated acini become the secretory epithelium, with pale cytoplasm and various globules (Fig. 41-2). Quite remarkable mammotropic and lactational effects have been observed in young patients of both sexes treated with high doses of certain tranquilizing drugs.[8,10,11]

In the phase of involution after lactation, the collapse of the dilated secretory lobules and ducts may be followed by failure of adequate connective tissue growth, producing

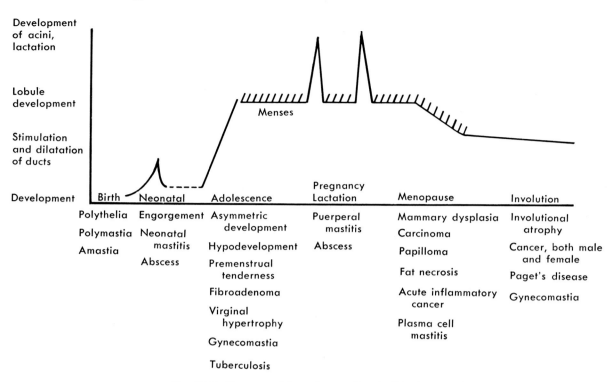

Fig. 41-3. Diseases of breast according to life stage.

thereby a breast of a flattened contour and flabby consistency. The irregularity of involution, the persistence of dilated ducts, and the periductal and perilobular lymphocytic infiltration may constitute chronic cystic mastitis. However, it is generally accepted that mastodynia disappears and cystic disease of the breast improves after lactation. This may be attributed to luteal hormone influence.

Tumor formations are adversely influenced by pregnancy and lactation (Fig. 41-3). Fibroadenomas grow rapidly and may increase remarkably. *Mammary infarcts* during pregnancy may be indistinguishable, by clinical criteria, from malignancy,[7] whereas histologically it may not be clear whether such ischemic accidents occur in focal gravid hypertrophy or other lesions such as fibroadenoma.

Control of growth and function.[6] A complex system of hormone interrelationships guides the development and physiologic activity of the mammary glands. Ovarian estrogen initiates the anatomic and histologic growth of the breast, with cooperative assistance from the pituitary's somatotropin, and adrenal glucocorticoids. Progesterone augments ductular growth and lobular organization and intermittently primes secretory function, which abates in the absence of pregnancy. However,

when pregnancy ensues, the placenta contributes chorionic gonadotropin, estrogen, progesterone, and a lactogenic stimulus. Prolactin of pituitary origin adds to the placental prolactin and continues its secretory stimulation of the breast after delivery and loss of the placenta. Participation of thyroid hormone and insulin in the process of lactation has been suggested.

Lactation in the human is limited and periodic, although frequently spaced pregnancies may be associated with prolonged uninterrupted lactation. A prolactin-inhibiting hormone from the hypothalamus eventually suppresses lactational activity, but neurogenic stimuli (nursing) tend to postpone its effects. The neurogenic stimuli of nursing and the pituitary mammotrophs also inhibit menstruation and ovulation.

Milk is an actively secreted product of breast acinar cells, which synthesize milk proteins by the abundant cisternae of rough-surfaced endoplasmic reticulum. The Golgi apparatus participates in the delivery of the protein by a system of secretory vesicles. Fat synthesized by breast cells moves to the free surfaces of the cells and leaves the cells enclosed in membranes, i.e., reverse pinocytosis.

In recapitulation, then, it may be simply stated that ovarian *estrogens* act anatomically, i.e., initiate growth, differentiation, and duct branching of the breast; ovarian *progesterone,* with estrogen, acts biochemically and physiologically, promoting a refined ductular and lobular differentiation and modulating specialized cellular activity; and *prolactin,* upon release of hypothalamic inhibition, continues and augments the highly specialized secretory influence initiated by placental prolactin.

Senile breast. After menopause, the striking change in the breast is the atrophy of the acini and lobules, with gradual epithelial involution progressing toward the nipple from the periphery. The involution is frequently irregular and quite commonly accompanied by dilated ducts lined by small, deeply stained epithelial cells. Eventually, the stroma also decreases in bulk, by nature of sclerosis and loss of cellularity. Dilatation of atrophic ducts along with retention of acellular debris, *duct ectasia,* is a common finding in this age group.

CONGENITAL ANOMALIES

Supernumerary breast parts along the milk line are the most common anomalies—polythelia (nipples), polymastia (axillary breast tissue). Ectopic breast tissue responds in pregnancy lactation and, like the conventional breast, is subject to cancer development. Amastia is absence of nipple or breast.

HYPERTROPHY

Hypertrophy of one or both breasts may take place at any time and is brought about by abnormal hormonal relationships. Before puberty, hypertrophy is usually bilateral and is frequently the physical evidence of estrogen-producing tumors. These include granulosa cell tumors of the ovary, chorioepithelioma of the ovary, adrenal gland (cortical cell) tumors, and pituitary tumors. Such changes are reversible, as evidenced by regression of the breast size after extirpation of the hormone-producing tumors.

At the time of adolescence or shortly thereafter, irreversible hypertrophy of one or both breasts may take place (juvenile hypertrophy). The breast may become extremely pendulous, the veins enlarged, and the nipple drawn into the pendulous mass. Prominent histologic change is the increase of the fibrous tissue and the attempted lobular formation.

In both the precocious hypertrophy and the true hypertrophy, the estrogenic activity is evidenced by duct epithelial hyperplasia and hypertrophy accompanied by irregular, meager secretory activity. The development of acini

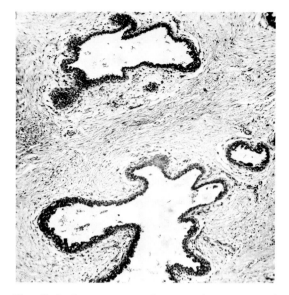

Fig. 41-4. Gynecomastia showing elongation and abortive budding of ducts, which are surrounded by loose periductal stroma in which lymphocytes are evident.

depends on luteal hormones and pituitary influence rather than on estrogens. The finding of follicular cysts of the ovary or a fibroadenoma in such a breast has been noted.

Gynecomastia (hypertrophy of the male breast).[12] A buttonlike swelling beneath the areola of one or both breasts most often occurs in the adolescent and in old men. It is characterized histologically by elongation and blunt branching of ducts, with variable infiltration by lymphocytes, mononuclear cells, and the polymorphonuclears in the pale intralobular type of connective tissue surrounding the ducts (Fig. 41-4).

Male breast hypertrophy is caused by a hormone imbalance, with actual or relative increase of estrogenic hormones or nonuniform abnormal sensitivity of the tissues to estrogen. Unilateral gynecomastia suggests a variation in end-organ responsiveness to hormones, also observed in the nonuniform lactational activity occurring with pregnancy. Pubertal male breast hypertrophy is accompanied by an elevation of serum estradiol, without significant increase in testosterone levels,[13] i.e., decrease of the testosterone : estradiol ratio. A similar hormonal relationship may explain gynecomastia occurring at other times and in other disorders such as old age, cirrhosis of the liver, starvation, or testicular atrophy, or in the hypogonadal syndrome (i.e., Klinefelter and Reifenstein). Gynecomastia may sometimes result from therapy with spironolactone (aldactone and aldactazide). A number of hormone-producing tumors have a causative association with gynecomastia. These include choriocarcinoma of the testis and other sites, Leydig or Sertoli cell tumors of the testis, pituitary adenomas, and adrenocortical cell tumors. Injury may promote the rate of growth but probably does not initiate it.

INFLAMMATIONS

Puerperal mastitis. Acute bacterial mastitis is almost always a complication of the puerperal period. It occurs after a few weeks of nursing, particularly in primiparas in whom *Staphylococcus aureus* or the *Streptococcus* becomes invasive through fissures in the nipples. All the cardinal signs of classic inflammation may be evident.

Acute puerperal mastitis must be differentiated from acute inflammatory carcinoma and vice versa. Rarely, puerperal mastitis is late-appearing, subacute, or relapsing type.

Galactocele. Galactocele is a grossly identifiable cyst occurring during lactation, containing milk products. Its wall may show necrosis, inflammation, and loss of epithelial lining.

Plasma cell mastitis. This is an uncommon chronic mastitis occurring in multiparas who had had nursing problems at one time or another. Stasis and inspissation of secretion rather than bacteria initiate the inflammatory process. At times, it is multicentric in origin and accompanied by thickened palpable ducts and enlarged axillary nodes. Although the lesion of plasma cell mastitis is firm, it is characterized by moist, reddish gray cut surfaces, with cloudy fluid or minute foci of necrosis.

The microscopy of the lesion resembles tuberculosis, and the condition has been referred to as pseudotuberculosis. However, the organized pattern of epithelioid and giant cells shows no caseation, and the cell population is a mixture of polymorphonuclear cells, histiocytes, some of lipid character, lymphocytes, and great numbers of plasma cells (Fig. 41-5).

Reparative cicatrization may so increase the hardness of the lesion and cause retraction and distortion of the nipple that it may be virtually impossible to distinguish the lesion on a clinical basis from cancer of the breast.

Ductular ectasia. Ductular ectasia, with or without mastitis, is usually a postmenopausal condition characterized by dilated ducts containing cellular and secretory debris. Inflammation, expressed by histiocytes, round cells, and plasma cells, mimics plasma cell mastitis. Ductular ectasia may, in fact, be a form of plasma cell mastitis. Periductal mastitis is another designation of the same process.

Chronic specific mastitis. Chronic mastitis, with the exception of the chronic puerperal mastitis, is a granulomatous inflammation. In most instances, it is secondary to a systemic disease, such as tuberculosis, blastomycosis, actinomycosis, or syphilis.

Fat necrosis.[14] A peculiar and unusual breast "tumor" is occasionally encountered in fat, pendulous breasts after "injury." A history of physical violence to the breast, however, is elicited in less than one half of the women with this condition. Indeed, fat necrosis may be associated with a suppurative disease of the breast, with carcinoma, with ischemia produced by pressure, and with "biopsy" breast surgery. Symptoms may be present for months or years.

Clinical characteristics of a hard, somewhat fixed lump in the absence of discoloration of the skin easily may be misinterpreted as that of a malignant tumor.[2] In the early stages, the lesion appears as a well-defined, firm, solid, homogeneous, lardaceous substance. As necrosis progresses, it may change to a light yellow, orange, brown, or brownish red color, depending on presence or absence of hemorrhage. Cyst formation, hemorrhage, calcification, stel-

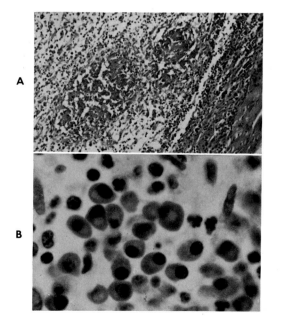

Fig. 41-5. Plasma cell mastitis. **A,** Epithelioid cell tubercles at periphery of lesion. **B,** Cellular complement. (**A,** 100×; **B,** 750×.)

late scarring, and fixation are almost constant in the old lesion.

Histologic architecture of acute inflammation in the adipose tissue may be more striking than "fat necrosis." Polymorphonuclear cells, plasma cells, lymphocytes, and monocytes are constant. The monocytes may be of epithelioid or foam type but generally form foreign body giant cells. Early stages of the disease present opaque fat cells (fat saponification), and later there is found true necrosis with the presence of cholesterol crystals (sharp, angular clefts) and calcification (Fig. 41-6).

BENIGN BREAST DISEASES

Multifocal, poorly formed lobules produce variations in the histoanatomy of the breast resulting from an abnormal interplay between epithelium, myoepithelium, intralobular connective tissue, supporting stromal connective tissue, and inflammatory cells (failure of uniform reciprocal relationships between proliferation and involution). The basic disorder is maldevelopment and maturation of the breast lobules and ductules. Certain patterns are sufficiently distinctive to be separated from others and are so labeled, i.e., adenosis, lobular sclerosis, and fibrocystic disease with or without epithelial hyperplasia. The histoanatomic aberrations probably reflect ovarian hormonal imbalance and low pregnanediol levels.[22] Administration of progesterone tends to ameliorate the condition.

Lobular fibrosis is the minimal clinical and pathologic disorder in the mammary dysplasia category. Periodic swelling, discomfort, and granularity of the breast tissue are clinical manifestations. Microscopically the process is one of intralobular sclerosis and fusion with the stromal connective tissues. Lobules vary in size, outline, and circumscription. Lobular ducts are often dilated (Fig. 41-7).

Processes that are characterized by a proliferation of ductular structures, forming gland-like patterns resulting in a mass or nodular area of the breast, are termed *adenosis*.

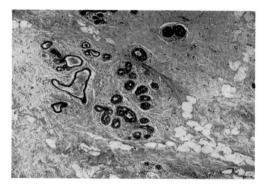

Fig. 41-7. Lobular fibrosis. Loss of distinction between lobular and stromal connective tissue and cystic dilatation of ductule. (45×.)

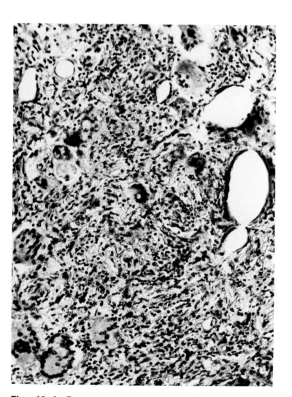

Fig. 41-6. Fat necrosis. Lesion is rather old, showing numerous multinucleated giant cells, spaces occupied by lipids, moderate fibrosis, and numerous small round cells.

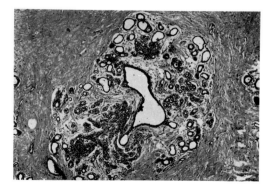

Fig. 41-8. Adenosis. Lobule with early cyst formation and "spilling out" of epithelial cells into lobular stroma. (40×.)

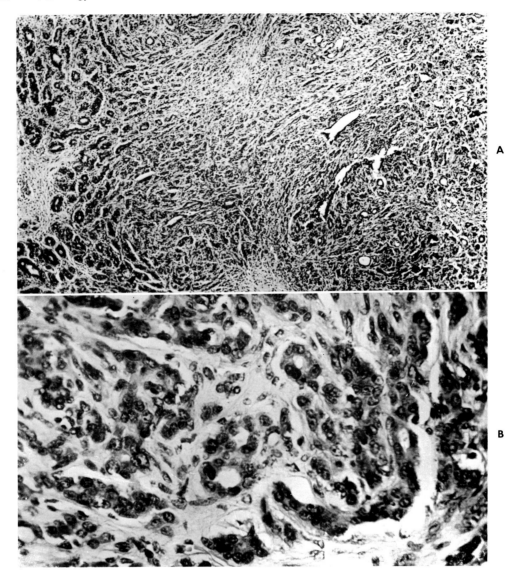

Fig. 41-9. Sclerosing adenomatosis. **A,** Four lobules of breast represented in pattern of delicate filigree architecture. **B,** High-power magnification of central portion of one lobule. Admixture of fibrous stroma with disorganized glands closely mimics pattern of infiltrating adenocarcinoma.

Glandular and nonglandular epithelial masses of ductular epithelium and myoepithelial cells have a tendency to spill outwardly from the ductules and to share an intimate relationship with growing intralobular connective tissue.[21]

Advanced intralobular fibrosis, with epithelio-myoepithelial proliferation of microglandular nature, mimics the histologic appearance of an invasive malignancy but in fact is a benign process termed *sclerosing adenosis*. Cytologic uniformity and a repetitive consistent realtionship of epithelial and myoepithelial cells to fibroblasts and circumscription

of the process are helpful criteria in the differential diagnosis (Figs. 41-8 and 41-9).

Fibrocystic disease. This condition most often develops in the later reproductive years. Variations from irregular lumps, ill-defined masses, thickening of breast substance to tense translucent cysts may characterize the clinical findings in the same patient at different times. Cysts are likely to be multiple (Fig. 41-10). Macroscopic cysts have a smooth glistening internal surface unless cyst wall inflammation is acute. Other areas of the lesion have a unique firmness and granularity because of

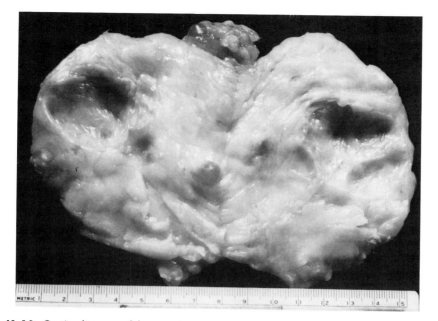

Fig. 41-10. Cystic disease of breast. Larger cyst is bisected and shows glistening smooth lining. In center is smaller bulging cyst.

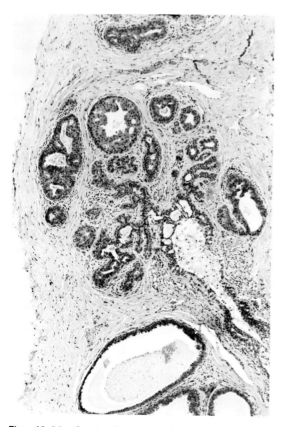

Fig. 41-11. Cystic disease with epithelial hyperplasia.

microcysts, large lobules nonuniformly distributed, sclerosis of the stroma, and inflammation. Microscopically, large cysts are noted to have an atrophic flattened epithelium or none at all. However, intracystic and intraductal epithelial hyperplasias, solid or papillary, are commonly present. Adenosis, miniature fibroadenomas and lobular hyperplasias are frequently intermixed. Reddish-staining apocrine type of glands tend to be numerous and hyperplastic.[25] These are characterized by the tall red cells with knobby luminal free edges and lipid vacuoles immediately beneath the luminal cell membrane. Inflammatory reactions of acute or chronic nature are frequently present but quantitatively tend to be insignificant (Fig. 41-11).

Epithelial hyperplasia is the single important process of fibrocystic disease of the breast that requires precise analysis. Proliferations may be solid, papillary, in ducts, or in cysts. This pattern of change must be separated from fibrocystic disease without epithelial hyperplasia because it bears a positive relationship to risk of cancer in the breast (see below).[18]

NEOPLASMS
Benign tumors
Fibroadenoma

Fibroadenoma is a breast lump formed by a local overgrowth of intralobular connective tissue and haphazardly branching ducts. Often it is associated with other forms of mammary dysplasia. Predominance of either connective tissue or epithelial ducts, or their morphologic interrelationships, form histologic patterns that vary even within a single mass. An intracanalicular fibroadenoma is characterized by a mosaic of polypoid masses of intralobular connective tissue budding into the branching duct system so that each connective tissue unit is covered by closely applied ductal epithelium (Fig. 41-12). Great variations in the epithelium may be noted. It is flat at points of physical pressure and multilayered in dilated segments of the tortuous arborizing ducts. Very large formations of this type, 10 cm or greater, are known as giant intracanalicular fibroadenomas or myxomas. Those with increased cellularity and atypicalities are designated cystosarcoma phyllodes (see the discussion on sarcoma, p. 1799).

Fibroadenoma not otherwise designated is a lesion predominantly composed of ductal branchings forming closely spaced, rather uniform, glands ((Fig. 41-13). Growth of intra-

lobular connective tissue is rather limited, and the appearance is that chiefly of glandular architecture. In certain fibroadenomas, the intralobular connective tissue forms encircling and sweeping bands about the variable duct structures. When this is prominent, the term "pericanilicular fibroadenoma" may be used.

Fibroadenomas are usually well defined or encapsulated. They are rubbery, white, and moist or mucoid and present a fine granularity or delicately fissured cut surface. Old lesions tend to undergo atrophy, hyalinization, and calcification.

This condition occurs early in reproductive life. A more rapid growth is noted during pregnancy, and rarely in pregnancy a fibroadenoma may suffer ischemic infarction. Cessation of growth occurs in menopause, but, because of atrophy of the breast tissue, the fibroadenoma may first become evident in the menopausal patient.

Papillomatosis

A papilloma is a discrete nodule of fibroepithelial character that develops within a duct

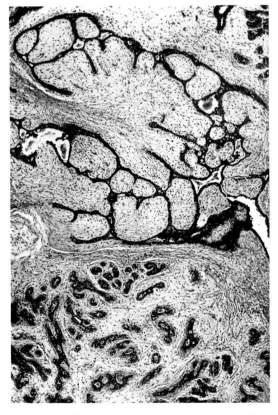

Fig. 41-12. Fibroadenoma showing intracanalicular formation at top, and pericanalicular arrangement in lobule at bottom.

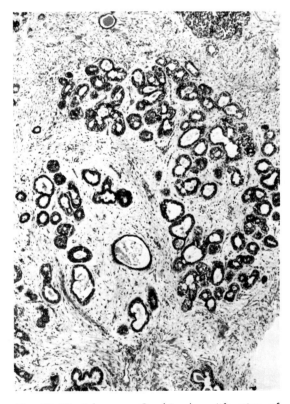

Fig. 41-13. Adenoma. Combined proliferation of young lobular connective tissue and epithelium. (40×.)

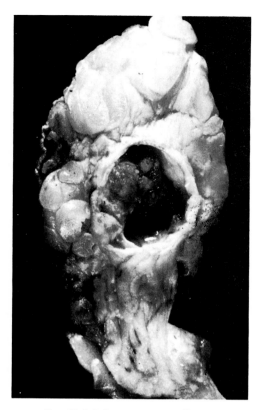

Fig. 41-14. Intracystic papilloma.

or cystic cavity. Such nodules are firm, granular, raspberry-like, projecting from the wall. The lesions are delicately fissured on the surface or villous in character (Fig. 41-14). A cloudy sanguinous fluid may fill the duct or cyst and accounts for the spontaneous or induced discharge from the nipple that occurs in more than one half the cases. In young women, the discharge is more often sanguinous, and in older women it is cloudy or milky.

Microscopically, papillomas show a complex arrangement of fibrovascular stalks bearing epithelial surfaces. The epithelial cells form a layer or two of uniform size and polarity (Fig. 41-15). The presence of broad fibrovascular stalks is indicative of a benign papilloma. On the other hand, papillomas have a great tendency to form irregular aggregates of epithelial or myoepithelial cells between the stalks. Such areas require critical histologic analysis. The occurrence of a malignant transformation within a papilloma must be recognized. Crowding of the epithelial cells, loss of cellular polarity, and cytologic features of nuclear enlargement, nucleoli, and mitotic activity, when properly quantitated, may help in the recognition of a malignant focus. Particularly important are highly cellular lesions characterized by epithelial bridging or perforated sheets of

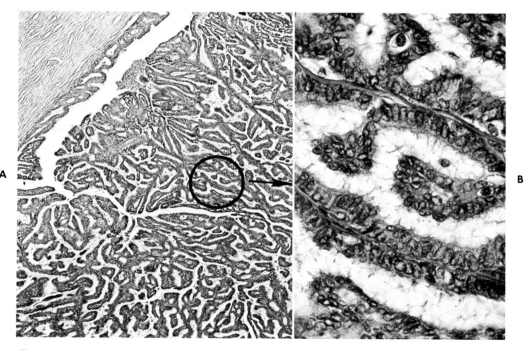

Fig. 41-15. Papilloma. **A,** Arborescent pattern of delicate papillary formations in a large papilloma. **B,** Enlargement of encircled area.

epithelial cells, referred to as the cribriform pattern. Abnormal mitotic activity and demonstrable aggressiveness by infiltration are ultimate criteria of malignancy (Fig. 41-16).

Adenoma of nipple (subareolar papillomatosis)

Papillomatosis in the major ducts at the nipple is a distinct lesion. It is benign in nature but complex in morphology. The lesion is a papillary intraductal epithelial hyperplasia with uniform cytologic appearance and with a fibromyxoid stroma tending to entrap epithelial cells. Such spurious "infiltration" should not be mistaken for a malignant process[23] (Fig. 41-17).

Grossly, the adenoma of the nipple usually appears to be sharply defined, and its papillary nature is usually clearly evident. It differs from an intraductal papilloma, being intimately "attached" in all areas.

Caution against overdiagnosis of this lesion should not be questioned. On the other hand, in rare instances a malignant process developing in nipple adenoma has been observed. This fact demands that each case be evaluated on the basis of the most precise cytologic criteria.[16,19]

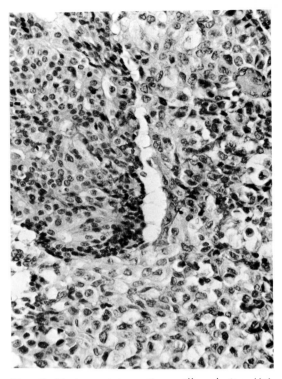

Fig. 41-16. Large intracystic papillary lesion. Uniform cellular pattern of benign lesion depicted at upper left, while remainder is cytologically malignant and histologically infiltrating. Presumed that all of lesion was benign in character at one time. (320×.)

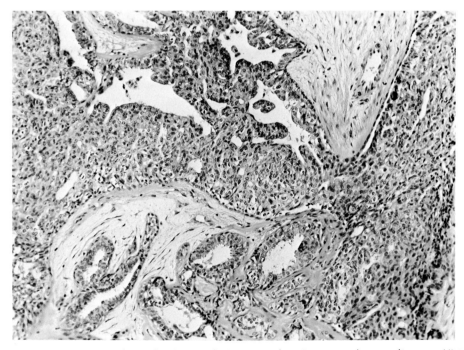

Fig. 41-17. Adenoma of nipple. Benign lesion too often interpreted as malignant. Histologically, it is mixture of papillomatosis and adenosis, but cells with benign cytologic features should be most helpful in making correct diagnosis. (125×.)

Premalignant proliferations

When a nonmalignant process is discovered in the breast, the patient and surgeon may ask, "What relationship, if any, has this condition to the risk of breast cancer in the future?" The answer is not always clear.[23]

From retrospective studies, one must be impressed by the statistical probability that a breast with "benign" disease is at greater than normal risk for breast cancer.[26] I am not suggesting that all benign epithelial proliferations terminate as a malignant process but that epithelial hyperplasia-proliferation represents a step in that direction; i.e., cancerous breasts have a much higher incidence of epithelial hyperplasia than do normal breasts, and more cancer is found in breasts previously biopsied for benign disease than in the normal population.

Common to many benign and all malignant breast disease is epithelial hyperplasia or cellular proliferation, but in neither do we recognize a sudden single event of proliferation. In fact, it takes years to develop the morphologic cellular atypicalities of a malignancy in normal boundaries, additional variable time to invade, and more time to metastasize.

Quantitation of the greater than normal risk for breast cancer in women with benign proliferation is not precise. Nonetheless, application of the principles learned in the studies of uterine cervical cancer can furnish a sound foundation. True, the breast is different from the cervix—the volume of tissue potentially affected is greater in the breast, and sampling of tissue for study is not so precise—but cytologic and histologic criteria need not be!

Proliferation in mammary ducts and lobules has been histologically and biologically classified analogous to what has been done in cervical carcinoma by Toker.[32]

Correlation between degree of "dysplasia" or cellulary atypicality and incidence of subsequent ipsilateral invasive carcinoma was made.

Type I: 4% at 10 years, 12% at 15 years
Type II: 14% at 10 years, 25% at 15 years
Type III (in situ carcinoma): 21% at 10 years, 45% at 15 years.

Studies of this kind applied to epithelial proliferations of cystic disease and duct papillomatosis and to other cellular hyperplasias are needed.

Malignant tumors

Predisposition and clinical orientation. Breasts that have not achieved full anatomic and physiologic potential early in life, or have certain benign lesions, are more prone to develop cancer. Relative levels of estrogen fractions, estrone, estradiol, and estriol in the decade after puberty may be the significant factor (estrone being most carcinogenic and estriol possibly protective). The protective effects of early pregnancy may relate to either progesterone or estriol, both of which are elevated during pregnancy.[44,57] Pregnancy early in reproductive life, frequent pregnancies, and early menopause, whether natural or artificial, decrease the lifetime risk of breast cancer. Prepubertal castration is totally protective. It is of interest to note that mammary cancer in dairy cows is almost nonexistent.[49] Prolonged lactation is not so protective against breast cancer in women as previously believed.[5]

Whether relative levels are unfavorably influenced by administration of certain estrogens is not clear, but it is known that cancer of the breast has been induced in transsexual individuals, and in males with prostatic cancer by the use of synthetic estrogens over a long period of time.[45,52] However, at this date it appears that steroidal contraceptive pills produce no distinctive morphologic breast changes and have no bearing on risk of breast cancer in the women who use them.[41,54]

Familial predisposition to breast cancer has been reported for sisters and daughters of patients with breast cancer. It has also been demonstrated that sisters of patients with breast cancer had abnormal 17-hydroxycorticosteroid and 11-deoxy-17-ketosteroid excretions as did the patients.[36] Another possible factor in high-risk patients is elevated plasma levels of prolactin.[43]

Trauma plays a negligible role in the causation of breast cancer. However, injury may induce hemorrhage and degeneration that increase the tumor size.

The risk of breast cancer for the American female is presently about 1 out of 15, or about 6%. About 70,000 new cases are diagnosed each year, and nearly 30,000 patients die of the disease in the same period. The incidence of contralateral breast cancer is much greater than that of primary breast cancer in the general female population. It is stated as 1% per year, especially in women less than 50 years old. Identification of the high-risk women and early discovery (small lesion) of breast cancer have been meritorious recent goals.[56]

Curability of breast cancer, although dependent on many factors, resides largely in the premise that dissemination (incurability) of

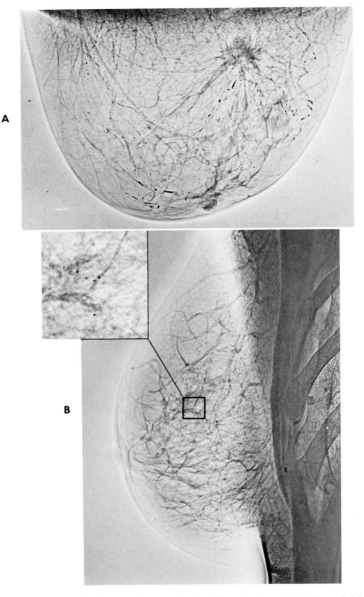

Fig. 41-18. A, Craniocaudad xeroradiograph of stellate lesion, clinically palable and malignant. **B,** Lateral xeroradiograph of a breast lesion proved by biopsy to be malignant. *Inset,* High magnification of lesion site showing pattern of stippled calcification. (Courtesy Dr. John Milbrath, Medical College of Wisconsin, Milwaukee, Wis.)

the disease is a function of duration and size of the lesion when first discovered—the most curable breast cancer is not a gross or clinical lesion, i.e., lobular carcinoma in situ. The smallest clinically detectable lesion has existed for nearly 2 years in a preclinical phase. Most breast cancers are discovered by the patient when the disease is local in less than one half the cases. Annual physical examination by physicians interested in breast cancer and xero-

mammography (Fig. 41-18) complementing patient self-examination will detect breast lesions at an early stage when the disease is local in 80% of the cases. Undoubtedly early discovery and early treatment offer the best care for survival of the patient with breast cancer.[37] However, it must be made clear that factors beyond the physician's control also play a significant role. Breast-cancer survival rates at one Japanese Institute are better than those

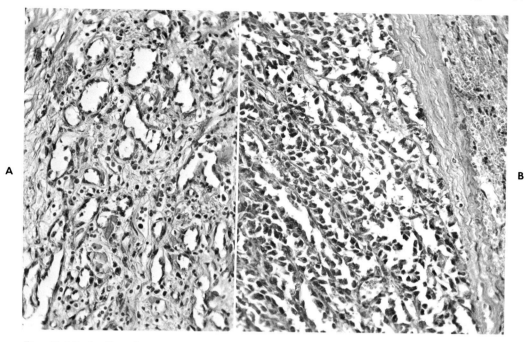

Fig. 41-19. A, Chronic postmastectomy lymph stasis or lymphangiectasis. **B,** Lymphangiosarcoma (same case).

in one New York Center.[39] Tumor-host relationships are not readily assayed, but lymph node sinus histiocytosis is reportedly greater in Japanese women![38] Among American women, nodal sinus histiocytosis and plasma cell node reactions are favorable to better prognosis.[34]

Radical mastectomy has been the standard treatment of breast cancer for many decades. At times it is followed by severe and persistent edema of the upper extremity. In rare instances a lymphangiosarcoma arises in the skin and soft tissue of such an arm (Fig. 41-19).[50]

In recent years this treatment has been challenged as "stereotyped," "excessive," "ineffectual," etc. Chemotherapy and irradiation are presently being evaluated in context with lesser surgery.[48] The ultimate answer has not yet evolved.

A clinical stage classification of cancer of the breast has been developed by the American Joint Committee on Cancer Staging and End Results Reporting[33] and by the International Union Against Cancer.

Etiology. The highly specialized biologically and biochemically active mammary tissue, under the influence of various *hormones,* undergoes periodic hyperplasia and involution. The primary hormone governing growth of the breasts is *estrogen.* It appears reasonable, then, to suggest that this hormone also plays a role

in the development of breast cancer. Precise information of target tissue response in relation to formation-excretion of estrogen and ratios of its principal fractions, estriol, estradiol and estrone, is needed.

Knowledge that many breast cancers are hormone dependent has been utilized in the clinical care of patients. More recently, however, the demonstrtaion and quantitation of estrogen-binding sites in the breast has been applied to the study of breast-cancer cells in the hope that better understanding of the "cause" of breast cancer will result. The very extensive work done in this field has been reviewed by Jensen.[57]

Probable *virus* etiology of human breast cancer also has received much attention in research laboratories. Bittner's classic contributions from the study of mammary carcinoma in mice has not been matched by studies in the human.[63] Evidence for virus etiology of human breast cancer has remained unconvincing, although data derived from epidemiologic, biochemical, immunologic, morphologic, and biologic studies are sufficiently suggestive of a positive association of virus and human breast cancer to supply the impetus for continuing study.[64]

Another area of intense interest is immunologic defense mechanisms of the host against cancer cells. Deficiencies in this system may not initiate cancers, but permit the process to be clinically evident.

Biopsy. Biopsy should be "excisional," total skillful removal of the tumor, whenever possible. "Incisional" biopsy is permissible for very large lesions. Needle-aspiration biopsy provides satisfactory documentation for infiltrating lesions, clearly benign conditions, and cysts. Spontaneous breast secretions are subject to the "Pap smear" technique of diagnosis. Specific duct canalizing and flushing, and gentle "milking," may provide a satisfactory specimen for Pap smear. Use of tranquilizers to produce secretions is presently not advisable. Radiographic studies of ducts injected with contrast material help locate lesions.[67]

In biopsy of minimal subclinical or mammographic lesions that cannot be confidently palpated by the surgeon, it is imperative to make a "mammogram" of the biopsy specimen to ensure that the lesion is present in the biopsy and that the pathologist selects the correct area for microscopy.

Pathologic anatomy. Malignant tumors arise most frequently in the upper outer quadrant of the breast. The central area is next in frequency and then the upper inner quadrant, followed by the lower quadrant. In the elderly

individual, cancer is likely to be of a hard fibrous character. In the small atrophic breast, duct carcinoma of comedo variety is seen. In the atrophic but fatty breast, early metastasis may arise from a very small focus of carcinoma.

The classic example of carcinoma of the breast is a single, hard, poorly movable, non-elastic, easily cut nodule. Sections have a dry, gritty, opaque surface marked by radiating, translucent lines of connective tissue accompanied by small yellowish or opaque grayish dots and streaks. The central portion of the tumor is slightly concave, and the margins extend into the stroma, between which the fat lobules may protrude above the level of the tumor (Fig. 41-20). Therefore, the border may be scalloped.

The lesion may be firm enough to grate on cutting, and if one cuts thin slices of the tumor, these maintain an extremely sharp edge and a flat surface. The tissue appears extremely turgid and is not elastic or flexible. The infiltration of the connective tissue produces a contraction of the dermal papillae and of Cooper's ligaments, thereby developing the orange-peel appearance of the skin. Periductal invasion causes retraction of the nipple (Fig. 41-21). Intimate fixation to breast stroma and sometimes to the underlying fascia makes the tumor limited in movement. Such cancers are "scirrhous," or carcinomas with "productive fibrosis." Other gross types include the medullary

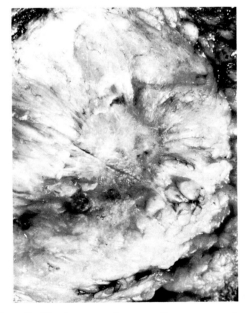

Fig. 41-20. Adenocarcinoma. Classic example of so-called scirrhous adenocarcinoma with a depressed infiltrating flat mass showing chalk streaks.

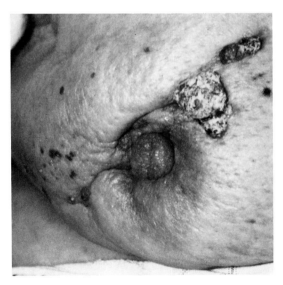

Fig. 41-21. Infiltrating adenocarcinoma producing retraction of nipple, dimpling of skin, and invasion of skin surface.

(opaque white or pink soft tumors, frequently with hemorrhage and necrosis), the mucoid or gelatinous, papillary, circumscribed, and intracystic, and the comedo.

More than 90% of the malignant mammary gland tumors arise from the epithelium of the duct system, either the large or the small channels. Lobular carcinomas and sarcomas comprise the remainder. Basic features of adenocarcinoma may be found in virtually any mammary carcinoma, although one or another modification of histologic architecture may predominate, and several varieties may occur in one tumor.

Metastasis. Not all malignant tumors are equally metastasizing. Nonmetastasizing cancers are lobular carcinoma, intraductal carcinoma (comedo), and papillary carcinoma when they are locally noninfiltrating. Some locally infiltrating carcinomas are infrequently metastasizing: medullary, papillary, intracystic, tubular, adenocystic, mucinous, juvenile, and Paget's. Lesions customarily metastasizing are lobular carcinoma (when locally invasive), adenocarcinoma (scirrhous, undifferentiated, or with mesenchymal metaplasia), inflammatory carcinoma, and carcinoma during pregnancy.

The principal route of metastasis is lymphatic, notably to the axilla, since the majority of lesions are found in the upper outer quadrant of the breast. Of the general group of carcinomas at the time of operation, 47% have axillary metastasis.[71] In instances of bilateral simultaneous mammary cancers, 71% have axillary involvement. The lesions that are diagnosed as grade IV are associated with 84% axillary metastasis.[68] Other lymphatic routes involve the lower cervical chain, the supraclavicular and infraclavicular lymph nodes, and the intercosal, retrosternal, and mediastinal routes, particularly from the medial and lower quadrants of the breast. There is also an epigastric pathway that may lead directly to the mediastinal or abdominal nodes.

Intramammary secondary foci are not uncommon, and extension across the midline to the opposite breast occurs occasionally. The skin may be involved by way of the periductal lymphatics or of the lymphatics of Cooper's ligament, or by direct continuity. Multiple nodular cutaneous metastasis of the chest wall is known as cancer *en cuirasse*. Visceral metastases are most prominent in the lungs and pleura, occurring in over one half of the patients. The liver, bone, brain, adrenal gland, and spleen follow in order of frequency. Dis-semination of tumor cells to the spine and brain may be explained by vertebral vascular communications that favor retrograde spread.[70] It is peculiar that both cutaneous and osseous metastases are very unusual distal to the elbows and knees. Symptomatic (bleeding) gastrointestinal metastases of breast cancers appear to be related to adrenal steroid therapy.[69]

Classification of mammary cancer

Mammary tumors may be classified according to gross characteristics (scirrhous, colloid, medullary), histologic characteristic (adenocarcinoma, papillary, sarcoma), histogenesis (duct, lobule, acini), or activity (infiltrating, noninfiltrating). It is obvious, therefore, that a classification can readily become both confusing and unwieldy. Terms denoting histologic appearance are based on the predominant architecture and not on purity of the lesion. One should note, therefore, that many patterns may be seen in any one carcinoma (Fig. 41-22). A working classification may well combine the various features that make a tumor histologically, clinically, or otherwise distinct. The following orientation scheme, to which benign tumors have been added, is modified from Foote and Stewart*:

Benign
1. Epithelial
   a. Papillomas
2. Mixed epithelial and mesodermal
   a. Fibroadenoma
      (1) Intracanalicular
      (2) Pericanalicular
      (3) Adenoma
3. Mesodermal—breast tumors only by location in mammary gland and in no way distinctive (lipoma, angioma, fibroma, myoma)

Malignant
1. Mammary ducts
   a. Noninfiltrating tumors
      (1) Papillary carcinoma
      (2) Comedocarcinoma or duct carcinoma
   b. Infiltrating tumors (adenocarcinoma)
      (1) Paget's disease
      (2) Papillary carcinoma
      (3) Comedocarcinoma
      (4) Adenocarcinoma with productive fibrosis (scirrhous, simplex)
      (5) Medulla carcinoma
      (6) Mucinous carcinoma
2. Mammary lobules
   a. Noninfiltrating—"in situ"
   b. Infiltrating—lobular adenocarcinoma
3. Rare carcinomas—adenoid cystic, apocrine,

---

*Modified from Foote, F. W., Jr., and Stewart, F. W.: Surgery **19:**74-99, 1946.

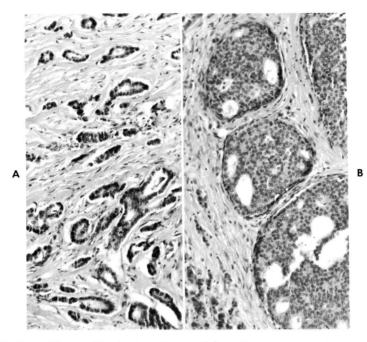

Fig. 41-22. Two different histologic patterns of breast cancer present in single primary lesion, 2.5 cm in width. Adenocarcinoma with fibrosis, **A**, and carcinoma simplex, **B**.

juvenile, and tubular carcinomas; carcinoma with mesenchymal metaplasia; carcinosarcoma

4. Epithelial or mesodermal origins such as tumors of skin, skin appendages, and supporting tissues of breast; same as found elsewhere in body— dermoid cyst, sweat gland tumors, basal or squamous cell carcinoma of skin, liposarcoma, etc.

Adenocarcinoma

Basically, malignant epithelial tumors of the breast are adenocarcinomas, but because gland patterns are not consistently evident, the site of origin designation "duct carcinoma" has gained favor (Fig. 41-22). These tumors tend to be hard, stellate in form, chalk streaked (scirrhous carcinoma), and metastasizing. Three fourths of all breast cancers are of this type. They are self-discovered lesions, 2 to 3 cm in diameter, and have about 75% incidence of axillary metastases.

Histologically, these tumors have a dense hyalinized stroma diffusely infiltrated by small glands, small clusters, and ribbons or single rows of cancer cells (Fig. 41-23). Larger cell aggregates tend to be necrotic. Inflammatory cells are sparse.

Desmoplastic stromal response furnishes the hardness so characteristic of this lesion. At times, however, epithelial or mesenchymal

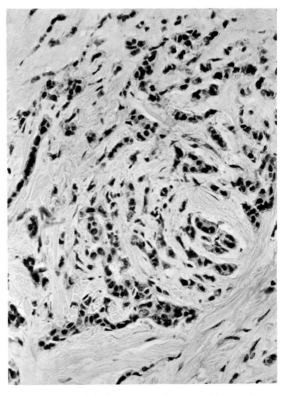

Fig. 41-23. Scirrhous carcinoma. Note dense stroma with narrow columns of tumor cells.

metaplasia compounds the histologic spectrum. Squamous epithelial metaplasia and chondroid, osseous, and spindle-cell mesenchymal metaplasias are the most common.

Medullary carcinoma

Approximately 5% of the malignant tumors belong to the group called medullary carcinoma. This tumor is characterized by a deeply situated, midzonal, circumscribed, movable mass. The skin may be stretched over the bulging mass, but it does not show dimpling and is generally free of ulceration. The gross lesion appears as a soft, partially cystic or hemorrhagic, bulky, somewhat opaque white tumor. It frequently resembles lymphoid tissue or has encephaloid characteristics. It is generally spheric and in two thirds of the patients is larger than 5 cm in diameter. Such a tumor generally grows slowly but may rapidly enlarge because of hemorrhage or necrosis. Prognosis is better than in adenocarcinoma.

The microscopic picture is that of a highly cellular tumor composed of large, oval or

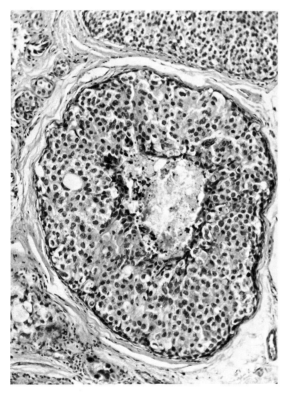

Fig. 41-24. Comedocarcinoma. Large ductlike structure has central debris and uniform small cells.

polygonal cells with slightly basophilic cytoplasm and vesicular nuclei with prominent nucleoli. The pattern may be large broad sheets or wide roughly parallel bands of tumor cells. At times, only the periphery of the tumor is viable, the remainder having been converted to a cyst by autolysis and hemorrhage. Usually, a generous lymphocyte infiltration accompanies the epithelial cells and forms an important histologic characteristic.

Circumscribed (but infiltrating) cancer is a name given to medullary carcinomas that are grossly sharply demarcated and histologically rich in plasma cells.

Noninfiltrating duct carcinoma

Intraductal carcinoma tends to be multicentric, but confined within the medium-sized duct system, and to be noninfiltrating. Ducts are enlarged by sheets of polyhedral cells (Fig. 41-24), with lightly stained or clear cytoplasm. Nuclei are chiefly round and moderately anaplastic. Perforations of the epithelial sheets (cribriform) support the interpretation of a malignant process. In the centers of the distended ducts, the tumor cells undergo necrosis. Accumulated yellowish gray cellular debris in such ducts may be expressed upon compression (*comedocarcinoma*). This gross physical characteristic separates this tumor from others. Local invasion and metastases occur infrequently, perhaps in 10% of the cases.

Duct carcinoma

Duct carcinoma is quite similar to comedocarcinoma, but it ordinarily lacks the central necrosis of the tumor cell discs. It is more rapid in its progress, with a brief period of symptoms, and is more commonly associated with pain or discharge from the nipple and involvement of axillary nodes. It arises from the central ducts.

The microscopic picture is that of a profuse growth of the duct epithelium, forming large clear cells with large nuclei, prominent nucleoli, and frequent mitoses. Minute papilla-like projections and accessory acinar formation are more prominent than in comedocarcinoma. Pleomorphism is noteworthy. In some instances, clear areas within the tumor-filled ducts are evident, but eosinophilic necrosis is not striking in the typical case. Both comedocarcinoma and duct carcinoma are of ductal origin, and both are noninfiltrating intraductal proliferations for an indefinite period of time (very good prognosis) prior to demonstrable infiltration and aggression.

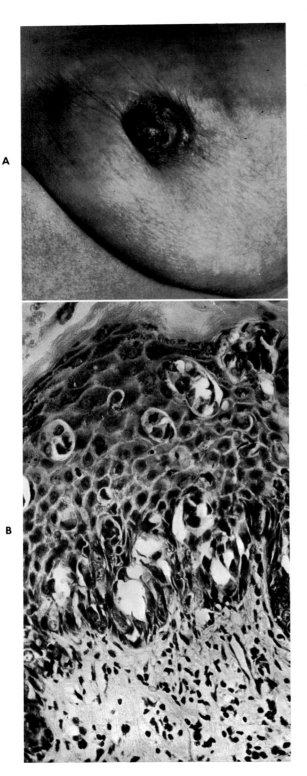

A

B

Paget's disease

Paget's disease is a chronic eczematoid thelitis associated with a central duct carcinoma. It has a course of long duration that begins with subjective symptoms of burning, itching, or soreness of the nipple, followed by physical findings of hyperemia and enlargement. This change extends to the areola and is accompanied by fissuring, weeping or oozing, crust formation, and eventually ulceration and destruction of the nipple. Paget's disease comprises less than 5% of mammary carcinomas and occurs in an older age group of women than those with the usual carcinoma. Gross examination of the tissue beneath the nipple area shows dilated thick ducts containing grumous pasty material. Some ducts also may be identified as being filled with cell masses, fixed and indurated. The periductal infiltration produces a fairly well-defined tumor not different from that previously described, although it may be very small.

The nipple and cutaneous manifestations of the disease are characterized by the presence of very large, pale, vacuolated cells (Paget cells) in the rete pegs of the epithelium. These may show large hyperchromatic nuclei and mitoses. The epidermis, therefore, has a "motheaten" histologic appearance (Figs. 41-25 and 41-26). Question still exists whether Paget cells represent an epidermoid carcinoma of the nipple arising in situ, whether they represent an intraepithelial metastasis from the constantly present underlying duct carcinoma, or whether they are just "peculiar cells" found in some cases of duct carcinoma.[1,47] It is probably correct that Paget's disease is not a primary tumor of the squamous epithelium of the nipple, since in its metastasis it does not have epidermoid characteristics. There is some evidence of intraepithelial spread of the duct cancer cells. However, not infrequent confusion with superficial melanoma, chiefly in extramammary sites, and confusion vice versa, suggests needed rethinking regarding the possible role of melanocytes in Paget's disease.[46] Electron microscopy and histochemistry have

Fig. 41-25. Paget's disease of nipple. **A,** Nipple is retracted, and surrounding its base there is scaling dermatitis associated with thickening and induration of periphery of areola. **B,** Epithelium shows surface hyperkeratosis and striking disorganization of its basal portions, numerous vacuoles, and many large extremely pale cells. Note mitotic figure.

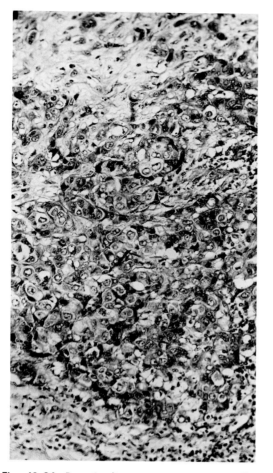

Fig. 41-26. Paget's disease metastasis to axillary lymph node. Cells are large and clear, maintaining histologic features of nipple-skin changes.

not answered the basic questions in Paget's disease.

Papillary adenocarcinoma

A centrally located tumor, papillary adenocarcinoma grows slowly and frequently is 5 cm or more in diameter. It represents about 1% of all cases. It is commonly associated with discharge from the nipple and the presence of a large, soft, bulky nodule. With central hemorrhage or cyst formation, it may be fluctuant (intracystic carcinoma). In the late stages, it loses its movable characteristics and ulcerates through the skin. Axillary node involvement is quite late and not prominent. The microscopic architecture is papillary in type, showing a communicating dendritic pattern. The cells are variable, in some instances forming large sheets and in other instances forming single cell layers. Lymphoid cells about the borders are not unusual. Histologic invasion is evident at the attachment of the papillary mass and is characterized by cells of moderate hyperchromatism, lack of polarity, and frequent mitoses. Invasion is the best evidence of malignancy. Other histologic and cytologic criteria many times fail to accurately differentiate papilloma from papillary carcinoma.

Mucinous carcinoma

Mucinous carcinoma is an adenocarcinoma also known by the name of colloid or gelatinous carcinoma. It is not a common lesion. It grows rather slowly and is associated with late metastasis and lack of nipple retraction.

Grossly, the tumor is fairly well demarcated but not encapsulated. It produces a spheric mass of moderately firm character, with a translucent, moist, gelatinous or slimy surface marked by a delicately interlacing pattern of more solid, opaque tissue. Its gross characteristics frequently closely resemble those of mixed tumor of the parotid gland. On cutting, strings of mucoid material may adhere to the knife. It is very slippery, and small particles of mucoid material can easily be removed from the tumor by scraping. The bulging droplets of slimy material are most pronounced after formalin fixation.

The typical microscopic picture is that of a multilocular cystlike formation. The spaces contain a light grayish blue–staining amorphous material. At some point around the periphery of these spaces, small clusters of deeply stained epithelial cells may be evident (Fig. 41-27). They generally are poor in detail, apparently because of mechanical pressure. Between such cystic spaces, the breast stroma and parenchyma may be infiltrated by columns and nests of deeply stained epithelial cells. These have round solid nuclei, eccentrically placed. The cytoplasm contains a single small or large vacuole. "Signet-ring" forms are produced by large amounts of intracellular mucoid substance. When the predominant picture consists of large mucoid spaces with few cells, the tumor is usually slow in its growth and metastasizes very late. However, the presence of cellular areas in which the cells are of "signet-ring" type (intracellular mucus) always makes such tumors unpredictable. Two percent of all carcinomas are mucinous.

Infrequently, mucinous carcinoma presents as an ill-defined tumor with nondestructive extensive infiltrations by large granular cells with small round nuclei. Resemblance to granular cell myoblastoma (a benign tumor of the

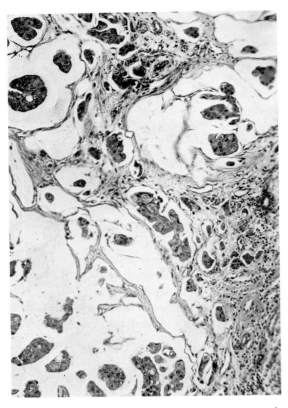

Fig. 41-27. Adenocarcinoma showing compressed clusters of tumor cells with abundant extracellular mucinous material.

breast) may be striking (Fig. 41-28). Multiple blocks should be examined to identify malignant nuclear features, cytoplasmic vacuoles, single rows of hyperplastic cells, and proliferative epithelial abnormalities.

Acute inflammatory carcinoma

Acute inflammatory carcinoma is a condition occurring in the obese pendulous breasts of young women, especially during lactation (50%). It comprises 1% of mammary carcinomas and is a special tumor only by virtue of clinical findings. It very closely resembles an acute inflammation of the breast and has been called "erysipeloid carcinoma" or "carcinomatous mastitis." It generally is associated with outstanding signs and symptoms of inflammation—both local and generalized. It is sudden in onset, showing a rapidly developing discoloration and induration of the breast. It develops an intense reddish purple hue that may extend onto the chest wall or to the opposite breast. The skin is hot and dry and frequently shows a diffuse scaling. It has a particularly indurated feel. The crusted nipple generally is retracted so as to be barely visible. Frequently, the breast substance presents no definable tumor but a diffuse brawny induration. On gross examination of such a breast, a very thick edematous skin and breast stroma are readily identified. In many instances, the

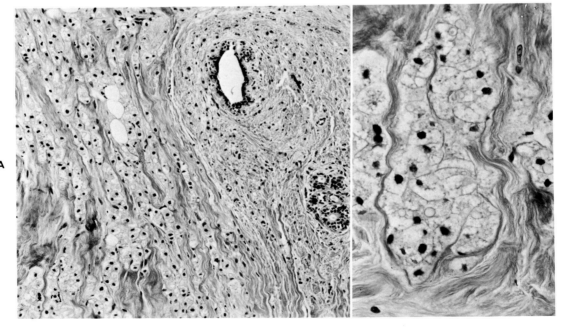

Fig. 41-28. Unusual histologic pattern of infiltrating and metastasizing mucinous carcinoma masquerading as "granular cell myoblastoma." (**A,** 160×; **B,** 390×.)

fat and stroma are poorly demarcated and there is diffuse induration of all structures. In rare instances, a large, centrally situated, poorly defined mass can be identified, and this generally has the characteristics of an infiltrating adenocarcinoma. Histologic characteristics are not specific, but infiltration of the subepidermal lymphatics and vessels is the identifying feature. This apparently represents retrograde lymphatic metastasis from blockage of the deeply situated lymph channels. Similar minute clusters of neoplastic cells infiltrate throughout the breast substance. One half of the patients develop widespread skin metastasis, and more than three fourths of the patients have axillary metastasis when seen.

Lobular carcinoma

Carcinoma originating in ductules of the histoanatomic units called lobules and distending its ductules without invasion is known as *in situ lobular carcinoma*. Multicentric independent foci of disease and bilaterality are additional characteristics. In situ lobular carcinoma frequently is demonstrable in breasts removed for clinical cancer, in the contralateral breast on biopsy, and in biopsied benign lesions. It is a presymptomatic, preclinical microscopic cancer not suspected or identified by gross examination of breast tissue. Diagnosis is histologic—epithelial filling and distention of ductules by a single type of cell population, uniform in size, shape, and round dark nuclei

in a constant repetitive pattern. Simple excision of the lesion is inadequate (Fig. 41-29). One third of such patients will develop a clinical breast cancer in the decades ahead. Clinical experience of this kind is truly impressive, but it has not established that the lobular carcinoma in situ eventually becomes the clinical breast cancer. It is known that some women with lobular carcinoma in situ subsequently develop *other* kinds of breast cancer.[2] Presence of lobular carcinoma in situ in breasts synchronously with other forms of clinical breast cancer is also known. We recognize, then, that lobular carcinoma in situ identifies the breasts that have an inordinate risk for any breast carcinoma and not infiltrating lobular carcinoma alone.[75]

Infiltrating and metastasizing lobular carcinomas comprise approximately 10% of all breast cancers and derive from in situ lobular forms.[75] Transitions between the two patterns are clear. Infiltration of fibrous and fatty stroma is by relatively small uniform cells, chiefly single or in rows, as beads on a string, reminiscent of scirrhous adenocarcinoma. Gross specimen characteristics of increased density and turgor may be ill-defined.

Rare tumors[23]

Adenoid cystic carcinoma. Microscopic morphology of this rare tumor is shared by certain sweat, salivary and respiratory mucous gland carcinomas (see Fig. 29-36). Stainable "mu-

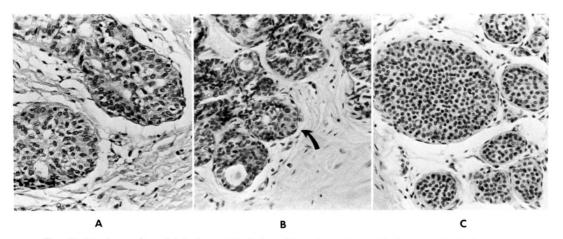

| A | B | C |

Fig. 41-29. Examples of lobular epithelial proliferations. **A** and **B,** Benign. **C,** Malignant—in situ lobular carcinoma. **A,** Terminal ductular atypical proliferation. **B,** Atypical lobular hyperplasia. Compare cytology at end of *arrow* with **C. C,** In situ lobular carcinoma. Single type of cell population with uniform dispersion in distended ductules. The specimen in **B** suggests positive relationship between atypical lobular hyperplasia and lobular carcinoma in situ by cluster of carcinoma-in-situ kind of cells. What does specimen shown in **A** mean in high-risk women? In postmenopausal women? (**A** to **C,** 320×.)

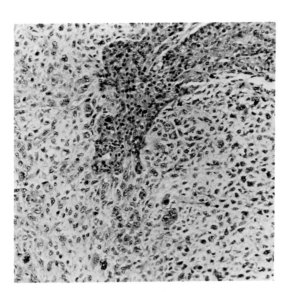

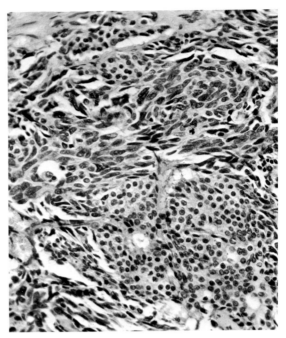

Fig. 41-30. Chondromucoid sarcomatous metaplasia in carcinoma of breast. Darker epithelial component blends with sarcomatous features just below midfield.

Fig. 41-31. So-called carcinosarcoma of breast—infiltrating carcinoma of breast having histologic features of sarcoma.

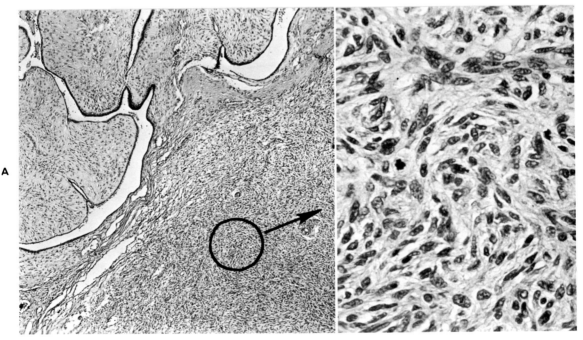

Fig. 41-32. A, Cystosarcoma phyllodes, malignant form showing cellullar atypical stroma. **B,** Enlargement of area in circle.

cinous" product in the cribriform spaces and lack of true gland cellular polarity are the histologic characteristics.

Apocrine carcinoma (sweat gland carcinoma). This lesion is glandular and micropapillary. It is formed by large or tall epithelial cells like those of apocrine metaplasia.

Juvenile carcinoma. A clear-cell infiltrating duct carcinoma has been encountered in children. PAS-positive droplets are present in the cells and homogeneous secretory material is in the spaces. Survival is good.

Tubular carcinoma. Lesions in this classification are well differentiated. Metastases are rare. Microscopy reveals single-layered tubules in moderately cellular fibrous stroma. Epithelial sheets, papillary formations, and necrosis are absent. The tubules are uniform, without the variations in size, cellularity, and dispersion that characterize sclerosing adenosis.

Carcinoma with mesenchymal metaplasia. Chondroid, osseous, and spindle-cell mesenchymal metaplasias constitute the most common patterns (Fig. 41-30).

Carcinosarcoma. Carcinosarcoma identifies the malignant tumor in which epithelial and mesenchymal components are distinct and separate, and each is malignant (Fig. 41-31).

Sarcoma

The specialized mesenchyma of the breast, along with epithelium, has the capacity to form tumors, i.e., fibroadenoma or giant myxo-fibroadenoma. Lobulations and cystic formations in very large tumors of this type are emphasized by the designation *"cystosarcoma phyllodes,"* although a very small number actually are malignant. The lesion may be very large, yet not infiltrative. Few are frankly malignant, metastasizing (to lungs rather than axillary nodes) as fibrosarcomas, liposarcomas, or mixtures including muscle tissue. To avoid errors, one should add "benign" or "malignant" to the diagnosis of cystosarcoma phyllodes (Fig. 41-32).

Other sarcomas not in context with fibroadenoma or epithelial participation are by and large much more malignant: liposarcoma, fibrosarcoma, leiomyosarcoma, soft-tissue osteogenic sarcoma, and angiosarcoma. The latter may appear deceptively innocent. Hodgkin's disease, reticulum cell sarcoma, lymphosarcoma, and malignant fibrohistiocytic proliferations in the breast are seldom local disease only. Granulocytic leukemia in the breast closely mimics an infiltrating lobular carcinoma. Great care is necessary to avoid errors in diagnosis in the instances when an enlarged breast is the first and only clinical manifestation of a leukemia. Granular cell myoblastoma may be a "tumor of the breast."

Cancer of male breast

Cancer of the male breast (Fig. 41-33), although infrequent, presents clinical and pathologic findings quite similar to those of cancer

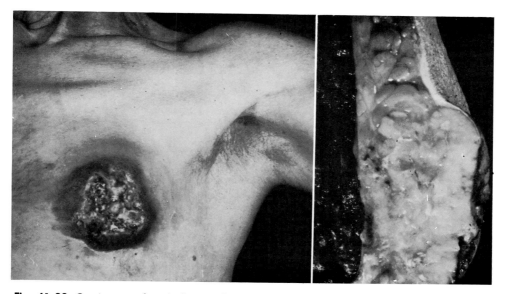

Fig. 41-33. Carcinoma of male breast showing ulceration and induration. Gross specimen reveals attachment to pectoral muscle and invasion of skin.

of the female breast. The report of Treves and Holleb presents an unusually rich experience with this disease.[72-74]

REFERENCES
General

1 Cutler, M.: Tumors of the breast, Philadelphia, 1962, J. B. Lippincott Co.
2 Haagensen, C. B.: Diseases of the breast, ed. 2, Philadelphia, 1971, W. B. Saunders Co.
3 Ham, A. W.: Histology, ed. 7, Philadelphia, 1974, J. B. Lippincott Co.
4 Seidman, H.: Statistical and epidemiological data in cancer of the breast, a professional education publication, 1972, American Cancer Society, Inc.
5 Second National Conference on Breast Cancer, Cancer 28:1368-1703, 1971.
6 Turner, C. D., and Bagnara, J. R.: General endocrinology, ed. 5, Philadelphia, 1971, W. B. Saunders Co.

Development, growth, and structure

7 Hassan, J., and Pope, C. H.: Surgery 49:313-316, 1962.
8 Khazan, N., Primo, C., Danon, A., et al.: Arch. Int. Pharmacodyn. Ther. 136:291-305, 1962.
9 Koeneke, I. A.: Am. J. Obstet. Gynecol. 27:584-592, 1934.
10 Ozzello, L.: Pathol. Annual 6:1-61, 1971.
11 Pier, W. J., Jr., Garancis, J. C., and Kuzma, J. F.: Obstet. Gynecol. 60:119-123, 1970.

Hypertrophy—gynecomastia

12 Greenblatt, R. B., and Perez-Ballester, B.: Med. Aspects Hum. Sex. 3:52-63, 1969.
13 Lee, P. A.: J. Pediatr. 86:212-215, 1975.

Inflammations

14 Adair, F. E., and Munzer, J. T.: Am. J. Surg. 74:117-128, 1947.
15 Cromar, C. D. L., and Dockerty, M. B.: Proc. Staff Meet. Mayo Clin. 16:775-783, 1941.

Benign breast diseases

16 Bhagavan, B. S., Patchefsky, A., and Koss, L. G.: Hum. Pathol. 4:289-295, 1973.
17 Brennan, M. J., et al.: Lancet 1:1076-1079, 1973.
18 Davis, J. B.: Cystic disease of breast: relationship to mammary cancer, Progr. Clin. Cancer 3:221-224, 1967.
19 Gould, E. V., and Snyder, R. W.: Pathol. Annual 9:441-469, 1974.
20 Kraus, F. T., and Neubecker, R. D.: Cancer 15:444-455, 1962.
21 Kuzma, J. F.: Am. J. Pathol. 19:473-489, 1943.
22 Lewis, D., and Geschickter, C. F.: Am. J. Surg. 24:280-304, 1934.
23 McDivitt, R. W., Stewart, F. W., and Berg, J. W.: Tumors of the breast. In Atlas of tumor pathology, Ser. 2, Fasc. 2, Washington, D.C., 1968, Armed Forces Institute of Pathology.
24 McLaughlin, C. W., Jr., Schenken, J. R., and Tamisiea, J. X.: Ann. Surg. 153:735-744, 1961.
25 Pier, W. J., Jr., Garancis, J. D., and Kuzma, J. F.: Arch. Pathol. 89:446-452, 1970.
26 Potter, J. F., Slimbaugh, W. P., and Woodward, S. C.: Ann. Surg. 167:829-838, 1968.
27 Sandison, A. T.: An autopsy study of the adult human breast, Natl. Cancer Inst. Monogr. no. 8, 1961, U.S. Public Health Service.

Neoplasms
Benign tumors—premalignant proliferations

28 Ashikari, R., Huvos, A. G., Snyder, R. E., Lucas, J. C., Hutter, R. V. P., McDivitt, R. W., and Schottenfeld, D.: Cancer 33:310-317, 1974.
29 Black, M. M., Barclay, T. H. C., Cutler, S. J., et al.: Cancer 29:338-343, 1972.
30 Gallagher, H. S.: Pathol. Annual 7:231-250, 1972.
31 Gallagher, H. S., and Martin, J. E.: In Sommers, S. C., editor: Breast cancer early and late, Chicago, 1970, Year Book Medical Publishers, Inc., pp. 37-50.
32 Toker, C.: Mt. Sinai J. Med. 40:799-805, 1973.

Malignant tumors
Predisposition and clinical orientation

33 American Joint Committee on Cancer Staging and End Results Reporting: Clinical staging system for cancer of the breast, Chicago, 1962, American College of Surgeons.
34 Berg, J.: Active host resistance cancer, Acta Unio. Int. Contra Cancrum 18:854-861, 1962.
35 Berg, J. W., Huvos, A. G., Axtell, L. M., and Robbins, G. F.: Ann. Surg. 177:8-12, 1973.
36 Bullbrook, R. D., Hayward, J. L., and Allen, D. S.: In De Bussy, J. H., editor: Hormonal aspects in the epidemiology of human breast cancer, Amsterdam, 1969, Excerpta Medica Foundation, p. 163-170.
37 Cady, B.: Lahey Clin. Found. Bull. 22:125-131, 1973.
38 Chabon, A. B., Takeuchi, S., and Sommers, S.: Cancer 33:1577-1579, 1974.
39 Devitt, J. E.: Cancer 27:12-17, 1970.
40 Dunn, J. E., Jr.: Cancer 23:775-780, 1969.
41 Fechner, R. E.: Cancer 26:1204-1211, 1970.
42 Friedell, G. H., et al.: Lancet 2:1228-1229, 1974.
43 Kwa, H. G., De Jong-Bakker, M., Engelsman, E., et al.: Lancet 1:433-435, 1974.
44 MacMahon, B., Cole, P., Lin, T. M.: et al.: Bull. WHO 43:209-221, 1970.
45 O'Grady, W. P., and McDivitt, R. W.: Arch. Pathol. (Chicago) 88:162-165, 1969.
46 Orr, J. W., and Parish, D. J.: J. Pathol. Bacteriol. 84:201-208, 1962.
47 Paget, J.: St. Bartholemew Hosp. Rep. 10:87-89, 1874.
48 Rubin, P., editor: Carcinoma of the breast, current cancer concepts, multidisciplinary review, Chicago, 1974, American Medical Association.
49 Stewart, F. W.: In Atlas of tumor pathology, Sect. IX, Fasc. 34, Washington, D.C., 1950, Armed Forces Institute of Pathology (tumors of breast).
50 Stewart, F. W., and Treves, N.: Cancer 1:64-81, 1948.
51 Strax, P., Venet, L., Shapiro, S., and Gross, S.: Cancer 20:2184-2188, 1967.
52 Symmers, W. S.: Br. Med. J. 2:83-85, 1968.
53 Vessey, M. P., Doll, R., and Sutton, P. M.: Cancer 28:1395-1399, 1971.
54 Vorherr, H.: Am. J. Obstet. Gynecol. 117:1002-1025, 1973.
55 Wynder, E. L., Bross, I. J., and Hirayama, T.: Cancer 13:559-601, 1960.

56 Zippin, C., and Petrakis, N. L.: Cancer **28**:1381-1387, 1971.

Etiology
Hormones

57 Jensen, E. V.: New Eng. J. Med. **291**:1252-1254, 1974.
58 MacMahon, B., and Austin, J. H.: Cancer **23**:275-280, 1969.
59 MacMahon, B., Cole, P., and Brown, J.: J. Natl. Cancer Inst. **50**:21-42, 1973.
60 Papaioannou, A. N.: Surg. Gynecol. Obstet. **138**:257-287, 1974.
61 Smithline, F., Sherman, L., and Kolodney, H. D.: New Eng. J. Med. **292**:784-792, 1975.
62 Wetchler, B. B., et al.: Mt. Sinai J. Med. **41**:682-686, 1974.

Virus

63 Bittner, J. J.: Cancer Res. **12**:510-515, 1952.
64 Borden, E. C.: Johns Hopkins Med. J. **134**:66-76, 1974.
65 Moore, D. H., and Charney, J.: Am. Sci. **63**:160-168, 1975.
66 Schlom, J., and Spiegelman, S.: Pathobiol. Annual **3**:269-291, 1973.

Biopsy

67 Ouimet-Oliva, D., et al.: Am. J. Roentgenol. **120**:56-61, 1974.

Metastasis

68 Adair, F. E.: N.Y. J. Med. **59**:2149-2153, 1959.
69 Asch, M. J., Wiedel, P. D., and Habif, D. V.: Arch. Surg. (Chicago) **96**:840-843, 1968.
70 Batson, O. V.: Ann. Surg. **112**:138-149, 1940.
71 Berkson, J., Harrington, S. W., Clagett, O. T., Kirklin, J. W., Dockerty, M. B., and McDonald, J. R.: Proc. Staff Meet. Mayo Clin. **32**:645-670, 1957.

Cancer of male breast

72 Norris, H. J., and Taylor, H. B.: Cancer **23**:1428-1435, 1969.
73 Treves, N., and Holleb, A. I.: Cancer **8**:1239-1250, 1955.
74 Visfeldt, J., and Scheike, O.: Cancer **32**:985-990, 1973.

Lobular carcinoma

75 Hutter, R. V. P., and Foote, F. W.: Cancer **24**:1081-1085, 1969.
76 Newman, W.: Ann. Surg. **164**:305-314, 1966.

42/Skin

ARTHUR C. ALLEN

This text was the first to devote a comprehensive chapter to the pathology of the skin, an allocation soon followed by other editors. However, we must admit that our initial objective—to help develop among colleagues a renewed interest and a practical expertise in dermatopathology—has not been realized. Because of the increasing awareness of the dermatologic manifestations of systemic disease, this failure to enlist affection for this fascinating, highly informative aspect of pathology is regrettable. The reduction rather than expansion of this chapter is, in part, an acknowledgment of this costly fragmentation of pathology.

In the interval between this and the previous edition, promising sophisticated methodology has been improved or initiated. This includes transmission and scanning electron microscopy, electron histochemistry, tissue cultures, fracture-freeze replication, diagnostic and pathogenetic fluorescent immunology, the determination of B- and T-cell markers, the observation of defective DNA repair after ultraviolet irradiation, and others. The inferences from these newer approaches do not always match the sophistication of the methodology. Nonetheless, hard data are useful, of course, but often must await maturation of interpretations.

There is a sizable group of dermatoses that have significant morphologic individuality. In many instances, the distinguishing features are so clear cut that a diagnosis may be offered on examination merely of the histologic slide. In other cases, a small range of diagnoses may be suggested by the section. In the remainder, the microscopic changes give no diagnostic help in the absence of a clinical history. Although the size of the last group will obviously be determined by the experience of the examiner, the percentage of cases that falls into it can be made sufficiently low as to merit the lagging interest of the general pathologist. One of the major difficulties in the learning of dermatopathology is that the changes usually are not of the "all-or-none" or *qualitatively* distinct variety but are often a matter of weighted *quantitative* differences. The proper judgment of these differences depends on a knowledge of the normal histologic range of the structures of the skin, as well as on an ability to add up and interpret a whole series of aberrations in these structures.

Obviously, only a small segment of cutaneous pathology can be included in this chapter. Accordingly, it would seem to underscore the applicability of dermatopathology best if some of the many lesions diagnosable by histologic characteristics alone were given preference over those less easily recognizable. For the latter, the reader may refer to the general references.[1-7]

STRUCTURE OF NORMAL SKIN

The skin normally varies in color, elasticity, thickness, blood supply, and texture depending on anatomic location, age, state of nutrition, endocrinologic status, and race of the individual. With the unaided eye, fine (Blaschko's) ridges are noted over the skin generally, and coarse folds, allowing for movement, are present, particularly over the joints. Between the ridges are *sulci of Heidenhain*. The ridges are further marked by delicate, crisscross, triangular or polygonal lines. In recent years, there has been considerable interest in the science of *dermatoglyphics*, which deals with the interpretation of detailed patterns of sulci, furrows, and ridges of the palms. Dermatoglyphic abnormalities have been observed in patients with rubella, psoriasis, neurofibromatosis, anonychia, a variety of chromosomal abnormalities, and in some disorders otherwise unassociated with cutaneous manifestations.

The ostia of sweat glands, the pores, open onto the ridges. The hair, of course, varies, too, in texture, length, density, contour, and color depending on age, race, sex, etc. The

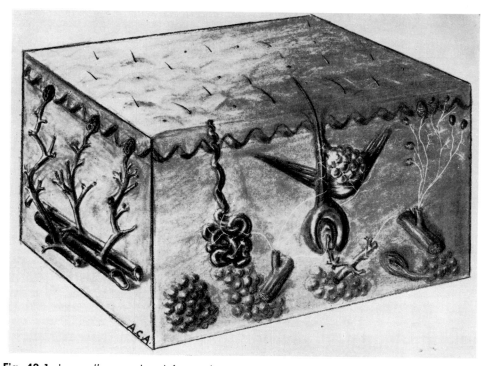

Fig. 42-1. In *smaller panel at left* are shown arteries, veins, and lymphatic vessels, along with their plexuses within papillae. In reality, plexuses of all three types of vessels overlap in same regions. In *larger front panel* are included appendages, nerves, and subcutaneous fat. Tubular sweat gland on *left* reaches surface through duct that, in its course through epidermis, maintains its own epithelial lining. Ductal ostium or sweat pore is independent of hair follicle. In *center* is pilosebaceous apparatus comprising hair follicle, sebaceous glands, and arrectores pilorum. Nerves and vessels supplying critical papillae are shown at *deep portion* of follicle. Sebaceous gland is intimately linked to hair follicle, into which its duct empties directly. Arrectores pilorum not only stiffen hair shaft but, as may be surmised from position illustrated, also help, by contraction, to expel contents of sebaceous gland and to constrict superficial vessels. On *right* are shown nerves and nerve endings—corpuscles of Merkel-Ranvier, Meissner, Ruffini, Krause, and Pacini. Nerve fibers entwined about appendages are also illustrated. (From Allen, A. C.: The skin, New York, 1967, Grune & Stratton, Inc.; by permission.)

smooth, hairless skin, or the skin with fine vellus hairs, is known as *glabrous* skin. The epidermis varies over most of the body from 0.07 to 0.12 mm and from 0.8 to 1.4 mm or more on the palms and soles. The cutis has a corresponding range of thickness. The junction of the cutis and the subcutis or subcuticular fat is usually indistinct, except in certain regions such as the forehead, ear, perineum, and scrotum.

Fig. 42-1 represents a diagram of normal skin. It is of diagnostic use to bear in mind how the skin varies in different parts of the body. For example, sebaceous glands are particularly prominent about the face, especially in the region of the nose, so that diagnoses of hyperplasia or adenoma of sebaceous glands should take this feature into account. The epidermis is normally thin and the rete ridges are relatively inconspicuous over the tibia, the breasts, and the flexor surfaces of forearms. This variant should not, therefore, be mistaken for atrophy. Similarly, the dermis over the lower legs, for example, is normally much thinner than it is in many other portions of the body, so that, again, the possibility of confusion with atrophy exists. The elastic tissue of the dermis shows such a large range in its quantity, as well as in the degree of fraying and splintering of the fibers, even in normal tissues, that considerable caution should be used in concluding that abnormalities of elastic tissue are present. Finally, the normally thick stratum corneum of the sole of the foot may prompt the diagnosis of keratoderma. These are a few of the examples of the variation in cutaneous histology, an accurate evaluation of which is clearly essential for an appraisal of some of the qualitatively similar pathologic changes.

The objective of the pathologist is to match the dermatologist's clinical observation of erythema, scales, pigmentation, blisters, and patterns of lesions with his observation of parakeratosis, acanthosis, edema, epidermal spongiosis or cleavages, vascular alterations, and type and location of inflammatory cells, along with several other ancillary histologic changes. One would hope that these factors, properly weighted and fed into the "clinical-histologic computer," will lead to the appropriate diagnosis. Undoubtedly, when the precise pattern and location of fluorescently revealed immunologic deposits, enzymatic abnormalities, and qualitative, quantitative, and topographic distribution of B and T lymphocytes are, one day soon, added to the input, the composite diagnoses will be refined.

Finally, the assessment of the intradermal cells depends on their patterns, their nature, their source, their correlation with similar cells in the peripheral blood and the regional lymph nodes, their content of immunoglobulins and complement, and their identification with categories, fulminance, and deflorescence of clinical lesions, in addition to the common antigenicity of these cells and other specific anatomic sites such as the various parts of the epidermis. These are the urgent problems that need to be resolved for a more stable insight into currently vaguely understood cutaneous disorders.[24]

Epidermis

The epidermis is composed of the following layers:
1. Basal cell layer (stratum germinativum)
2. Prickle cell layers (stratum spinosum, rete mucosum, rete Malpighii)
3. Granular layers (stratum granulosum)
4. Stratum lucidum
5. Cornified layer (stratum corneum)

Basal cell layer. The basal cell layer is one cell thick and forms the junction between epidermis and dermis. The nuclei are relatively hyperchromatic, arranged perpendicular to the epidermal "basement membrane," and normally contain a few mitoses as evidence of the activity of a layer that serves in part as the progenitor of the remainder of the epidermis. Interspersed in the basal layer are cells with a clear zone separating and often compressing most of the cytoplasm and nucleus away from the cell wall (the so-called *cellule claire*). The

cytoplasm may or may not contain melanin, but these cells are likely to be dopa-positive and, accordingly, are melanocytes. Not all melanocytes of the basal layer are "clear cells." Ultrastructurally, the melanocytes contain melanosomes but most observers believe they contain few or no desmosomes or tonofilaments. As a matter of fact, such structures may be noted, albeit often reduced in number, not only in many melanocytes but, more vividly and meaningfully, also in the marginal cells of melanocarcinomas in situ (Fig. 42-40). The fairly universal insistence that keratinocytes lack lysosomes has contributed to the circular reasoning that melanocytes are *ipso facto* nonkeratinocytes inasmuch as they contain these organelles. A directly contrary observation has recently clearly indicated that keratinocytes are characterized by *Odland bodies,* which are membrane-coated granules, keratinosomes, or lysosomes.[55]

For a long time it has been accepted, on debatable evidence, that melanocytes are really nerve endings that originated in the neural crest, became incorporated in the epidermis, and later constituted the source of normal pigment in skin as well as of pigmented nevi and melanocarcinomas. It is generally maintained that melanocytes are the same in number in both white and black skin and the pigment is transferred to neighboring keratinocytes, which "nip off" pieces of melanized dendrites attached to scattered, basally located melanocytes. Nor is it explained how epidermis, regenerated after ulceration, develops basal melanocytes spaced every tenth cell or so. In our opinion, the process of conversion of basal cells and keratinocytes into melanocytes normally takes place continuously and may be retarded (as in vitiligo) or accelerated (as in sunburn). Actually, as would be anticipated, the numbers of dopa-reactive epidermal melanocytes have been found to be increased after irradiation with ultraviolet light, although contrary results previously had been reported. In other words, the activation of basal cells and keratinocytes into melanocytes is an in situ conversion and varies in speed and extent with different age groups, races, and stimuli. However, it would be misleading to fail to acknowledge that the concept of neurogenesis of melanocytes, nevi, and melanocarcinomas is the popular one at the moment.

There has been a revival of interest in the nature of the controverted intraepidermal, aurophilic *Langerhans' cell.* To some, it is a worn-out ("effete") melanocyte with a debatable capacity to manufacture or even to phagocytose melanin. To others, it is a form of intraepidermal neural element with a spectrum of "neural enzymes," including ATPase and leucine aminopeptidase. To still others, it is a histiocyte that has wandered into the epidermis and is identical with the histiocytes of "histiocytosis X." Ultrastructurally, it was forcefully emphasized that this cell possessed a specific racquet-shaped organelle but, as was to be expected, similar organelles have been observed in other organs such as the thymus gland. More recently, it has been admitted, in a refreshing reversal of opinion, that Langerhans' cells are not related to melanocytes, that they are not derived from the neural crest, and that the whole question of their nature, derivation, and function must be regarded as wide open again.[19] It will come as no surprise that, to me, this cell as well as the melanocyte has always appeared to be a modulated keratinocyte that, like other keratinocytes, has a variable content of enzymes, pigment, and organelles depending on its functional stage. Obviously, these features are conditioned by genetics and the response to stimuli at a given time.

Prickle cell layer. The prickle cells are several layers thick, the number varying in different parts of the body. The cells are joined by cytoplasmic bridges (spines, prickles, desmosomes), which serve as the most easily recognizable identification of such cells, both in squamous cell neoplasms and in metaplastic processes. The intracellular cytoplasmic *tonofilaments* generally are regarded as the precursors of keratin. Glycogen is usually present. The generally accepted absence of lysosomes (keratinosomes) in keratinocytes has been disputed; thus the supposed differences between keratinocytes and melanocytes are narrowed.

Stratum granulosum. The *stratum granulosum* averages about two layers thick and is composed of cells with blue, round cytoplasmic granules of keratohyalin. The chemical nature of the keratohyaline granules remains essentially obscure. Although superficially resembling nuclear material, they are Feulgennegative and PAS-negative and contain no protein-bound sulfhydryl groups. They appear as electron-dense bodies and apparently contain tonofilaments. The granules are also osmophilic, are digested with elastase, and are presumed to be closely related histogenetically to keratin. The *stratum lucidum,* which is practically confined to the palms and soles, is a clear, homogeneous, acidophilic, anuclear, thin layer of "eleidin."

Stratum corneum. The *stratum corneum,* also normally without nuclei, is made up of various thicknesses of keratin. The stratum corneum, particularly its lower half, is important as the barrier in regulating the transfer of water through the skin. Fat globules may be present in the two uppermost layers.

PAS-positive, diastase-resistant mucopolysaccharides are present in the epidermis and are presumed to play a role in binding or cementing the epidermal cells together. Since keratinization normally takes place in the upper layers of epidermis, the acid mucopolysaccharides are presumably degraded, allowing the keratin to be discarded as invisible flakes. With incomplete degradation of the mucopolysaccharides, visible coherent, parakeratotic scales occur, as in psoriasis.

Basement membrane. There is convincing histologic evidence to indicate that a true epidermal basement membrane, equivalent, for example, to the one surrounding glands, does not exist. Basement membranes in other locations, such as those about sweat glands, renal tubules, etc., are argyrophilic. No such continuous epidermal basement membrane is demonstrable with silver stains, although an illusion of one occasionally is created by argyrophilic granules of melanin aligned in the basal layer. On the other hand, stains with the periodic acid–Schiff reagent do reveal what appear to be interrupted segments of a basement membrane. This simulation is caused by the presence of polysaccharides that have been irregularly concentrated by the varying densities of the subepidermal collagen, especially with edema of the upper cutis. In this connection, one other fact should be mentioned again. Basal cells do have "intercellular" bridges (desmosomes) that bind them to the overlying cells of the stratum spinosum and, in their upper portions, to each other. To the corium they are attached by semidesmosomes to an ultrastructurally visible membrane called an *"adepidermal lamina,"* visible only electron microscopically and not equivalent to the argyrophilic structures readily detectable even in routine stains, as mentioned.

Dermis

The dermis or corium is divided into the superficial pars papillaris and the deeper pars reticularis. The papillae of the dermis alternate with projections of epidermis called *rete ridges.* The length of the papillae, the thickness of the overlying epidermal plate, the vascularity, the edema, and the direction and consistency of the collagenous fibers of the papillae are all of diagnostic value. In the papillary portion, the fibers of collagen tend to run vertically. In the deeper part, the fibers are rather loosely dispersed in a horizontal direction. Accuracy in evaluating changes in the consistency, tinctorial qualities, and cellularity of the collagen and elastic tissue of the dermis furnishes the basis for many diagnoses. With electron microscopy, elastic fibers show a fibrillar structure within an otherwise almost homogeneous matrix in which dense elements are embedded but in which the characteristic periodicity of collagen is lacking.

The cutaneous *appendages* include the sweat glands, sebaceous glands, hair follicles, arrectores pilorum, and nails. The sweat glands are coiled glands of two varieties: eccrine and apocrine.

The *eccrine glands* are universally distributed in the skin and are made up of several coils of tubular glands lying deep in the dermis. These glands empty their secretion into tubules traversing the dermis and epidermis, opening into the fine ridges of the skin as pores. The coils are lined by two principal layers of cells: (1) the more superficial, basophilic, *dark,* granular mucopolysaccharide-containing cells and (2) the more basilar, acidophilic *clear* or chief cells. There may be some interdigitation between these cells. A flattened third type of cell, the myoepithelial or "basket" cell, is interposed between these secretory cells and the basement membrane. A large battery of enzymes is detectable in the eccrine glands, including oxidases, dehydrogenases, phosphorylases, alkaline phosphatase, and glucuronidases. Their presence has been utilized in defining certain of the neoplasms of sweat glands. The ducts are lined also by two layers of epithelial cells, but the myoepithelium is absent. The inner lining of the ducts of sweat glands is keratinized in their course through the epidermis, and, indeed, some of the neoplasms of sweat glands show evidence of squamous cell metaplasia. In any case, the inner hyaline membrane of the ducts often serves as a clue to the genesis of these neoplasms.

The *apocrine glands* occur in the axilla, groin, nipple, umbilicus, anus, and genital region. The apocrine glands are easily recognized by their large lumens, prominence of secretory cytoplasmic granules, and rows of myoepithelial cells longitudinally oriented below the cuboid or columnar secretory cells.

The periglandular basement membrane is especially conspicuous. Light yellow, sudanophilic granules, as well as granules of hemosiderin and a minimum of glycogen, are commonly present. Mucin normally is present within the lumen and cells of apocrine glands and is PAS-positive and diastase-resistant. Desmosomes, similar to those of keratinocytes, have been noted. The ultrastructural observation of canaliculi, particularly, suggests that an eccrine type as well as an apocrine (i.e., apically erosive) type of secretion occurs. Secretory activity varies with the menstrual cycle. The ducts of the apocrine glands usually open in close relationship to the hair follicles but may reach the surface independently, as do the eccrine glands.

The *sebaceous* or *holocrine glands* are racemose structures that serve mainly as appendages to the hair follicles to which they are attached. Each alveolus is rimmed by a basement membrane surrounding one or two layers of squamous cells, internal to which are the characteristic sebaceous cells with small round nuclei and abundant, finely latticed, fatty cytoplasm. The sebaceous cells are pushed toward the duct, wherein they finally rupture and release their fatty contents in the hair follicle. Modifications of sebaceous glands occur in the eyelids and ears, in the areolae of the nipples, and in the male and female genitalia (odoriferous glands). In these regions, they are unconnected with hairs or hair follicles. The amount of sebum secreted is about the same in the adolescent boy and girl, shows no appreciable change in the aging female, and decreases in the aging male. Ectopic sebaceous glands may be found in the salivary glands and in the glans penis. Such ectopic glands of the corona penis are often referred to as Tyson's glands. Actually, Tyson appears to have described a beaded rim of fibroepithelial pearly nodules about the corona.

The *hair* consists of a shaft that, at its lower end, enlarges into a bulb. The bulb embraces an invaginating dermal papilla, through which the hair receives its blood supply. The intracutaneous portion of the hair shaft and the bulb are enclosed in a hair follicle. The hair shaft is made up of a cuticle, a sheath, and a more or less pigmented cortex and medulla, the latter being absent in lanugo hairs.

The *arrectores pilorum* are bands of smooth muscle originating in or near the papillary layer of the dermis and inserting at several points into the outer layer of adjacent hair follicles just above their papillae. The direction of the muscle is at an angle to the hairs so that their contraction (gooseflesh) causes the hairs to be erected. At the same time, the superficial vessels are constricted to avoid cooling, and sebaceous secretion is expelled by the pressure of the contracting arrectores pilorum. However, there is some disagreement as to this last function.

The *blood* and *lymphatic vessels* of the skin are arranged in plexuses. The arterial vessels are derived from the subcutaneous arteries, which give off plexuses to the papillary layer, as well as to the reticular layer and the various appendages. It has been suggested that the selective localization of infiltrate to various components of the dermis is related to the pattern of these plexuses. In the skin of certain regions of the body, particularly the fingers, there are, normally, arteriovenous shunts or *glomera* that serve to regulate blood flow and surface temperature. The glomus is composed of an afferent arteriole, a shunt called the Sucquet-Hoyer canal, and an efferent vein. The canal is lined by layers of rounded glomus cells that have a contractile function. The veins also form plexuses in the papillary, subpapillary, and deep reticular layers, as well as about the appendages.

The lymphatic plexuses are localized principally in the papillae and at the junction of dermis and subcutaneous tissue. The deeper lymphatic vessels have valves.

The *nerves* of the skin are preponderantly medullated. A few are nonmedullated and lead to the blood vessels, smooth muscles, epidermis, hair follicles, and glands. The specialized nerve endings include the corpuscles of *Vater-Pacini,* which are found in the deep layers of the skin and subcutaneous tissue, in the mucous membranes, and in the conjunctiva and cornea. These structures are particularly numerous in the skin of the nipple and external genital organs. Other nerve endings are the *Meissner corpuscles* of the papillae of the skin of palms, soles, and tips of fingers and toes, the end bulbs of *Krause,* which are smaller than but structurally similar to the Meissner corpuscles and are found in the external genitalia, the elongated, dermal corpuscles of *Ruffini,* and the intraepidermal disclike, tactile *Merkel-Ranvier* corpuscles, which are identified with silver stains and are present in the epidermis and external root sheath of hairs. The endings are presumably receptors for touch (Merkel-Ranvier and Meissner corpuscles), pressure (pacinian corpuscles), heat (corpuscles of Ruffini), and cold (end bulbs of Krause).

DEFINITIONS
Clinical terms

macule Circumscribed flat area of altered coloration of skin; evanescent or permanent; varies in size from pinhead to several centimeters, in color from red (erythema), brown (ephelis), and the various colors of blood pigment (petechiae and ecchymoses) to white (vitiligo), and in shape from circular, polygonal, linear to the polymorphous varieties of erythema multiforme.

papule Circumscribed elevated area; varies in size from pinhead to about 5 mm, in surface contour from flat, conical, pointed circular to umbilicated, in color from red, yellow, white to violaceous, and in shape of base from round to more or less polygonal (e.g., papules of lichen planus and psoriasis); the papule, as well as the macule, may provoke pruritus, burning sensation, anesthesia, and pain or may cause no symptoms; both macules and papules may be overlain by scales.

nodule An enlarged papule varying in size from about 0.5 to 2 cm, usually deep-seated, involving the lower dermis and subcutaneous fat (e.g., the nodules of rheumatoid arthritis and leprosy).

vesicle Circumscribed, single or grouped elevations of the epidermis, beneath which are collections containing serum, plasma, or blood; surface may be flat, globoid, or umbilicated (e.g., smallpox and eczema).

pustule Vesicle containing pus predominantly (e.g., impetigo).

bulla (bleb) Similar to vesicle, except that the bullae are larger, varying from 0.5 to more than 8 cm (e.g., pemphigus).

scale Loosened, imperfectly cornified, parakeratotic superficial layer of skin that is shed as fine, branny, dirty white, yellowish keratinous dust or large pearly white flakes; distribution may be focal or universal and usually is associated with inflammation of the skin (e.g., psoriasis and exfoliative dermatitis) but need not be (as in ichthyosis).

crust Residue of dried serum, blood, pus, and epithelial, keratinous, and bacterial debris; crusts vary in color from yellow to green to dark brown, depending on the admixture of the different ingredients, and in consistency from a thin superficial and watery (as in impetigo) to a thick, bulky and loosely or firmly attached covering of a rupioid syphiloderm; crusts occur after the oozing of serum, blood, or pus in a disrupted, eroded, or ulcerated epidermis (as in eczema, impetigo, smallpox, abrasions, and other conditions).

excoriation (erosion) Superficial erosion and ulceration produced mechanically, usually by the fingernails in scratching pruritic skin or in picking at various lesions (as in "neurotic excoriations").

fissure (rhagade) Linear, often crusted, tender, painful defect in continuity of the skin, occurring usually at mucocutaneous junctions at sites where there is normally considerable elasticity of the skin (e.g., about the anus, mouth, fingers, palms, and soles) and also in certain diseases (e.g., syphilis, nonspecific anal fissures, keratoderma, intertrigo, and eczema).

ulcer Defect of the skin, deeper than an erosion or excoriation, extending at least into the dermis; the edges may be ragged, punched out in appearance, undermined or everted; the floor may be glazed or granular, puriform or hemorrhagic, and shallow or deep; the outline of an ulcer may be circular, serpiginous, crescentic, ovoid, or irregular; ulcers may be painless or exquisitely sensitive; they heal generally by concentric scarring and epithelization (e.g., tropical, diphtheritic, and varicose ulcers).

lichenification Thickening of the skin with exaggeration of its normal markings so that the striae form a crisscross pattern; occur after chronic irritation of pruritic skin.

comedo Keratinous plug, sometimes admixed with bacteria and inflammatory cells, within ducts of sebaceous glands; characteristic of acne.

Histologic terms

acanthosis Thickening through hyperplasia of the rete Malpighii; may exist without hyperkeratosis (Fig. 42-13).

hyperkeratosis Thickening of the keratinized layer, the stratum corneum; generally is associated with a prominent stratum granulosum.

parakeratosis Persistence of nuclei in the stratum corneum, signifying the presence clinically of a loosely adherent scale (e.g., dandruff); characterized by the absence or striking diminution of the stratum granulosum, except in the stage of healing (Fig. 42-13); with fluorescence microscopy (with acridine orange, rhodamine B, and thioflavine S), hyperkeratosis is reflected by orthochromasia and brilliance, and parakeratosis is reflected by dullness and metachromatic color changes.

spongiosis Intercellular edema of the epidermis which, when pronounced, progresses to vesiculation (e.g., eczema).

acantholysis Separation of individual cells from the stratum spinosum, with loss of prickle cells and consequent isolation within the fluid of a vesicle (e.g., pemphigus).

ballooning degeneration One of the diagnostic morphologic phenomena leading to vesiculation in viral diseases; characterized by the isolation of a cell from its neighbors, especially in the lower layers of the epidermis, the withdrawing of its prickles after intracytoplasmic edema and vacuolization, and the amitotic division of its nucleus so as to form a multinucleated giant cell (e.g., variola, but, particularly, herpes and varicella).

reticular colliquation A characteristic of the cutaneous vesicles because of viruses, as in ballooning degeneration; the cytoplasm of several cells becomes edematous, granular, coalescent, and partially disintegrated; the residual cytoplasm forms reticulated septa that separate multiloculated intraepidermal collections of fluid or vesicles; the nuclei become small, pyknotic, or completely karyorrhectic.

dyskeratosis Abnormality of development or distinctive alteration of epidermal cells; two types are distinguished: (1) benign dyskeratosis—e.g., the molluscum bodies of molluscum contagiosum, represented by swollen brightly eosinophilic cells, mostly of the stratum granulosum, containing virus elementary bodies, or the *corps ronds* and *grains* of the stratum granulosum and stratum corneum, respectively, as noted in Darier's disease; in molluscum contagiosum, the dyskeratosis is caused by a virus; (2) malignant dyskeratosis—anaplastic changes such as hyperchromatism, changes in polarity, increase in mitotic figures, and enlargement of nuclei and nucleoli so as to signify potential or actual development of carcinoma.

pseudoepitheliomatous hyperplasia Pronounced acanthosis with extensive downgrowth of rete ridges such as may occur at the periphery of an ulcer, in bromodermas, and after insect bites; occasionally, the exuberant epidermal hyperplasia is mistaken for carcinoma as in so-called molluscum sebaceum or keratoacanthoma (Fig. 42-45).

liquefaction degeneration Obliteration of the line of demarcation of epidermis and dermis by edema of the basal cells and subepidermal dermis, as well as by the presence of inflammatory cells at this junction (e.g., lichen planus and lupus erythematosus) (Fig. 42-10).

CUTANEOUS-VISCERAL DISEASE

The cutaneous reflection of visceral disease is finally coming to be accorded the significance it has long merited. It is relevant to note that because of the increasing awareness of the importance of the association of visceral with cutaneous diseases, graduate students of dermatology are requesting more sophisticated training in internal medicine, as recent surveys emphasize. A simple listing of some of the cutaneous manifestations of visceral lesions, many of which have become apparent within the past decade, will underscore this vital relationship:

1. Pigmentations
   a. Acanthosis nigricans of adults ("malignant" type)—commonly associated with visceral adenocarcinoma
   b. Acanthosis nigricans (juvenile)—occasionally associated with congenital lipodystrophy and insulin-resistant diabetes or with Rud's syndrome (tetany, epilepsy, anemia, and mental retardation; also with ichthyosis hystrix)
   c. Peutz-Jeghers syndrome—focal mucosal and cutaneous pigmentation with gastrointestinal polyps and, rarely, with carcinomas
   d. Hemochromatosis—with pigmentary cirrhosis of liver and diabetes mellitus
   e. Addison's disease
   f. Incontinentia pigmenti—with neurologic and cardiac abnormalities
   g. Ochronosis—with cardiac disease
   h. Phenylketonuria—with neurologic manifestations
   i. Pellagra
   j. Café-au-lait spots—with Recklinghausen's disease and fibrous dysplasia
   k. Chediak-Higashi syndrome—with specific leukocytic inclusions, semialbinism, etc.
2. Miscellaneous nonbullous dermatoses
   a. Lupus erythematosus—with nephritis, carditis, arthritis, and hypersplenism

  b. Dermatomyositis in adults—with visceral cancer
  c. Ichthyosis in adults—with lymphomas
  d. Alopecia mucinosa—with mycosis fungoides
  e. Erythema annulare (gyratum)—with rheumatic fever and cancer
  f. Pyoderma gangrenosum—with ulcerative colitis
  g. Sarcoidosis and other granulomatous diseases—with visceral involvement
3. Vesiculobullous lesions
  a. Zoster—with malignant lymphomas (occasionally, dermatitis herpetiformis, pemphigoid, and erythema multiforme bullosum are associated with visceral cancers)
  b. Acrodermatitis enteropathica
  c. Bullous lesions—with porphyrias
  d. Dermatitis herpetiformis—with intestinal disease (spruelike)
  e. Toxic epidermal necrolysis—several instances associated with malignant lymphomas
4. Urticaria
  a. Urticaria pigmentosum—with involvement of bones, liver, spleen, and lymph nodes
  b. Urticaria—with amyloidosis, nerve deafness, and renal disease
5. Diseases of collagen and elastic tissue
  a. Scleroderma—with renal, cardiac, and gastrointestinal lesions
  b. Pseudoxanthoma elasticum—with ocular and cardiac lesions
  c. Ehlers-Danlos syndrome—increased serum hexosamine; involvement of vessels, heart, and gastrointestinal tract
  d. Cutis laxa
  e. Necrobiosis lipoidica diabeticorum—with diabetes mellitus
  f. Circumscribed myxedema—with exophthalmic goiter
  g. Amyloidosis (primary and secondary)—with myeloma (primary amyloidosis), chronic infections (secondary amyloidosis), etc.
6. Vascular diseases
  a. Angiokeratoma of Fabry—with renal and vascular lesions
  b. Allergic granulomatosis—with visceral angiitis
  c. Degos' syndrome—thromboangiitis of skin and intestines
  d. Blue, rubber-bleb nevus—with intestinal angiomas
  e. Neurocutaneous-vascular syndromes
    (1) Sturge-Weber syndrome—cutaneous angiomatosis, epilepsy, etc.
    (2) Ataxia-telangiectasia
    (3) Rendu-Osler-Weber syndrome—with arteriovenous fistulas of lung, brain, etc.
7. Metabolic disorders
  a. Xanthomatoses—with diabetes mellitus, von Gierke's disease, biliary cirrhosis, lipid nephrosis, and essential familial hypercholesterolemia
  b. Lipidoses with cutaneous infiltration—reticulohistiocytic granulomas (lipid dermatoarthritis); lipid proteinosis; gangliosidoses

and other sphingolipidoses (Fabry's, Tay-Sachs, Gaucher's etc.)
  c. Mucopolysaccharidoses—e.g., Hurler's syndrome
  d. Dysproteinemias—including Waldenström's macroglobulinemia (with malignant lymphomas), cryoglobulinemias (with cutaneous infarcts), and multiple myeloma (with cutaneous infiltration)
8. Cutaneous tumors
  a. Arsenical lesions (keratoses, Bowen's disease, etc.)—with visceral cancers in limited percentage
  b. Kaposi's sarcoma—with malignant lymphomas
  c. Sebaceous adenomas—with tuberous sclerosis
  d. Basal cell nevus syndrome and other neurocutaneous syndromes

DERMATOSES

In order to be set up as what may possibly be a more workable and more orderly classification of the varieties of dermatoses than seems currently to exist for pathologists, the diseases of the skin have been divided primarily into histologic categories. Although some overlapping of criteria is present, it is hoped that the basis for the classification is, in general, sufficiently defined to be of practical value. The diseases discussed are not only those that the pathologist is most likely to encounter but also those that, with minor exceptions, are diagnosable on histologic changes alone.

Shave biopsy. Succinctly mentioned here is the "shave" or horizontal biopsy, which is used commonly by dermatologists. This method is opposed to the *vertical* biopsy performed with a punch instrument or scalpel. A case for its use was recently formally, but unconvincingly made.[40] The advantages listed include the saving of time, supplies, and equipment, the preservation of a dermal "hammock" for subsequent curettage, minimal hemorrhage, and good cosmetic results. However, the disadvantages are more serious than generally conceded. The precise histologic diagnosis of many lesions is jeopardized by a limited, superficial shaving, which, of course, also fails to disclose the involvement or clearance of the margins.

DISEASES PRINCIPALLY OF EPIDERMIS
Hyperplasias

Darier's disease. Clinically, Darier's disease (keratosis follicularis, psorospermosis) is recognized by the development early of small, uniform, firm, reddish brown, greasy keratinous papules that subsequently become coalescent, papillomatous, and crusted and acquire an offensive odor. The lesions tend to be lo-

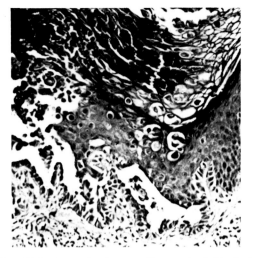

Fig. 42-2. Darier's disease (keratosis follicularis) showing suprabasilar cleavage, corps ronds, grains, and pronounced parakeratosis. (Hematoxylin and eosin.)

cated about the face and neck and spread to the chest, limbs, and loins. The palms and nails may be involved, as may the oral mucosa. The disease occurs predominantly in the second and third decades.

The histologic picture is so distinctive as to be pathognomonic and consists of the following (Fig. 42-2):

1. Focal, truncated masses of keratin, usually partially parakeratinized, especially near the surface, may be located over the ostia of hair follicles or over the interfollicular epidermis. For this reason, the term *keratosis follicularis* is inaccurate.
2. *Corps ronds,* or dyskeratotic cells, practically limited to the stratum granulosum, contain nuclei that are rounded and encircled by a clear cytoplasmic halo.
3. *The* "grains" are cells basically similar to the *corps ronds* but occur in the lower portion of the overlying keratinous masses.
4. The suprabasilar cleavage of the epidermis at the junction of the basal layer and the lowermost layer of the stratum spinosum forms a lacuna or small vesicle with a papillary base (Fig. 42-2).

The lesions that may offer some difficulty in differentiation are the isolated keratosis follicularis and benign chronic familial pemphigus (bullous Darier's disease). Verrucal or isolated keratosis follicularis, originally recorded in 1948 in the first edition of this text and elsewhere in the same year, is histologically similar to Darier's disease, although the

lesions of the latter appear more regular, smaller, and often multiple even in the same section.[10] This verrucal lesion is likely to be single and has a predilection for the scalp. Others and I have seen an identical histologic picture in the wall of the epidermal inclusion or pilosebaceous cysts.

Acanthosis nigricans. Acanthosis nigricans appears as patches of gray-black warty masses with a predilection for the axilla, groin, submammary region, elbows, knees, and, occasionally, oral mucous membranes. Two types are recognized: juvenile and adult. The distinction is based on age rather than any difference in appearance of the lesions.

The juvenile type, unlike the adult form, is rarely associated with cancer, and, in some instances, it may accompany lipodystrophies and mental retardation.[25] The adult type is prone to be associated with visceral cancer—in about 50% of the patients, particularly in those beyond the fourth decade.[25] In about 65% of the patients, the associated cancer is a gastric adenocarcinoma. Adenocarcinomas of other viscera, such as lung and infrequently uterus, may be found. Occasionally, the acanthosis nigricans may appear to antedate the visceral cancer. The association of acanthosis nigricans and abdominal cancer in elderly people is a very real (if poorly understood) phenomenon. Acanthosis nigricans may also occur after the use of oral contraceptive drugs in the absence of visceral cancer.

The histologic picture of acanthosis nigricans is that of a papillary hyperkeratosis, in most areas disproportionately greater than the underlying acanthosis. The epidermis is thrown into folds by its excessive lateral growth and in sections often appears recticulated where rete ridges have joined. The basal layer is densely pigmented with fine argyrophilic melanin granules (Fig. 42-3), and a few chromatophores lie in the upper corium. This folding of a hyperkeratotic epidermis in which the basal layer is diffusely darkened as an almost solid line of melanin is characteristic of acanthosis nigricans. There is no anaplasia of the epidermis even in those cases accompanied by abdominal neoplasms. Oral florid papillomatosis may be associated with acanthosis nigricans.

Molluscum contagiosum. Molluscum contagiosum is a mildly contagious autoinoculable disease of the skin, caused by a virus and characterized by pinhead-sized to pea-sized waxy, firm, buttonlike, often pruritic papules occurring on the face, trunk, and genital re-

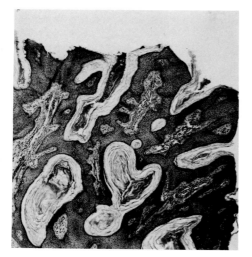

Fig. 42-3. Acanthosis nigricans with melanin pigmentation of basal layer. (Hematoxylin and eosin.)

gions particularly and on the feet rarely. The lesions develop slowly over a period of weeks and may remain indefinitely without therapy. The disease appears especially in children and may occur in epidemic proportions in institutions. Molluscum contagiosum may occur in deceptively giant forms and apparently may be transmitted venereally.

The histologic picture should be immediately recognizable. The connective tissue papillae between the lobules are compressed or altogether obliterated, so that the inwardly projecting lobules appear as a bulbous downgrowth. This lobulation of the epidermis is almost as suggestive of the diagnosis as is the pathognomonic feature, the molluscum bodies, and may serve to help differentiate this lesion from verrucae, particularly when the molluscum bodies happen to be inconspicuous. The molluscum bodies are clustered cells, principally of the stratum granulosum but also of the stratum spinosum, which are enlarged, as are virus-infected cells generally, and contain homogeneously smooth, brightly eosinophilic cytoplasm. The nucleus is inconspicuously flattened to one side of the cell, and keratohyalin granules tend to disappear. The cytoplasm, when studied with vital stains, appears actually to contain many elementary bodies (Lipschütz) embedded in a mucoid matrix. These dyskeratotic cells are enclosed in an eosinophilic, keratin-like membrane that resembles the dense cell membranes of plants. The molluscum bodies have been confused with the brightly eosinophilic cells of the stratum granu-

losum that are often prominent in verrucae vulgares. The virus seen electron microscopically measures about $300 \times 200 \times 100$ nm, is characteristically brick shaped, and contains a dumbbell-shaped nucleoid. The virus replicates in the cytoplasm rather than nucleus.[42] Specific fluorescence staining of the inclusion bodies with tagged antibodies of serum from infected human beings and rabbits has been demonstrated.

Vesicles

The vesicles of various diseases may closely simulate each other clinically. Inasmuch as the prognostication, even as to fatality, may depend on the exact diagnosis, it is clearly important that the diagnostic histologic features be definitely evaluated. In general, three types of vesicles occur: (1) eczematous, (2) cleavage (e.g., dermatitis herpetiformis, pemphigus, epidermolysis bullosa, impetigo, and burns), and (3) viral (e.g., smallpox, chickenpox, and herpes).

Eczema. Eczema may begin as an erythema and evolve through the papular, vesicular, pustular, and exfoliative stages. Some cases of eczema remain in one of the phases (e.g., eczema rubrum, eczema squamosum, eczema papulosum), but in most instances, the disease passes through the stage of vesiculation. From the histologic point of view, the vesicle of eczema, whatever the etiology, is basically the same whether caused by an external irritant, ingested food, or the product of superficial fungi, as in the epidermophytid. Moreover, the histologic picture of the eczematous vesicle differs sharply from that of pemphigus, dermatitis herpetiformis, and the viral lesions of smallpox, chickenpox, and herpes.

The vesicle of eczema begins as foci of spongiosis in the rete Malpighii. The intercellular edema progresses so as to form microvesicles that coalesce with adjacent vesicles similarly formed. The walls of such vesicles are the compressed epidermal cells that usually are arranged as septa in the large blisters. Histologic changes of this sort occur also in the vesicles of pompholyx, dyshidrosis, acrodermatitis perstans, and other eruptions of unknown etiology that are localized chiefly to the hands, as well as in the vesicles of pustular bacterids. These bacterids are usually sterile pustules of the palms and soles and are assumed to be provoked by allergic reactions to bacterial products.

Cleavage vesicles. Some years ago, we applied the term "cleavage" to those vesicles formed by the separation or "cleavage" of the epidermis or dermis through a single horizontal plane.[10] The cleavage may occur at any level of the epidermis and, occasionally, may split the upper dermis. The precise level of cleavage usually embodies a key diagnostic clue. The following discussion is of representative types of cleavage vesicles.

The lesions of *dermatitis herpetiformis (Duhring's disease)* are symmetrically distributed in groups in the scapular regions, on the buttocks, or on the extremities. The lesions may be erythematous macules or papules, but in most cases they are characterized by vesicles that may vary from those detectable only microscopically to large bullae. Oral lesions in dermatitis herpetiformis are more common than is generally indicated.[30] The disease may be accompanied by mild constitutional symptoms and signs. Itching, burning, and pricking sensations almost always are present. The disease is characterized by spontaneous remissions and relapses. The etiology is unknown. The lesions respond remarkably in most instances to penicillin and sulfapyridine but usually do not react satisfactorily to other sulfonamides.

The microscopic features of the vesicle of dermatitis herpetiformis consist of a collection of serum, fibrin, and a few neutrophilic and eosinophilic leukocytes that have cleaved and lifted the entire epidermis from the corium. The epidermis itself shows no other constant change. Of diagnostic importance is the change in the dermal base of the vesicle— i.e., particularly, the flattened papillae that are edematous and infiltrated with cells of the same type that are found in the vesicle itself (Fig. 42-4). The absence of eosinophilic leukocytes by no means precludes the diagnosis of dermatitis herpetiformis, although those cells often are noted in considerable numbers.

It has been suggested that dermatitis herpetiformis is attributable to an immunologic disorder linked with gluten sensitivity. Both the cutaneous and intestinal lesions respond to the withdrawal of gluten. Immunofluorescent studies reveal IgG in granular or fibrillary form, rarely linear, at the dermo-epidermal junction. By contrast, in pemphigoid, the immunoglobulin is mostly IgG, but it appears in linear form. So-called benign *chronic bullous dermatosis* of childhood appears to have the characteristics of dermatitis herpetiformis, except for the absence of circulating epithelial antibodies.

Pemphigus refers to a group of diseases, commonly fatal and characterized by bullous

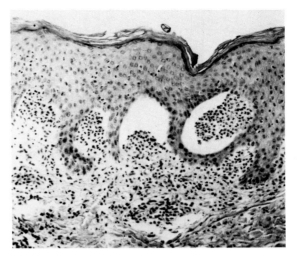

Fig. 42-4. Dermatitis herpetiformis in its early stage showing cleavage of epidermis from dermis by collections of leukocytes. (Hematoxylin and eosin.)

lesions. The cause is unknown. The disease involves both sexes equally, mainly between 40 and 70 years of age, and most frequently begins in the mucous membranes of the mouth or in the skin of the trunk. Rarely, pemphigus vulgaris is observed in children. The several varieties include pemphigus vulgaris, pemphigus foliaceus, and pemphigus vegetans. These forms are entities primarily on the basis of the acuteness of the disease or the type of lesions accompanying the vesicles, e.g., the foul-smelling scales of pemphigus foliaceus and the fungoid papillomatous masses of pemphigus vegetans. Pemphigus erythematodes (Senear-Usher syndrome) previously was regarded as a separate entity with a good prognosis. It is now believed that this condition is actually a variant of pemphigus in which the erythematous stage may be prolonged. The incidence of pemphigus vulgaris is about four times that of all the other varieties combined. Bullae are observed at some time in the course of pemphigus foliaceus and vegetans. The group name is applied also to benign chronic familial pemphigus (Hailey-Hailey disease), but there is reason to believe that this disease is quite distinct from the usually fatal varieties of pemphigus. The actual cause of death in uncomplicated pemphigus is not clear, although the loss of proteins and electrolytes in the bullous fluid is probably a significant factor. The prognosis for patients with pemphigus is better if the disease develops before the age of 40 years and is treated with steroids early in its course.

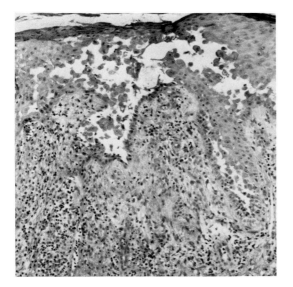

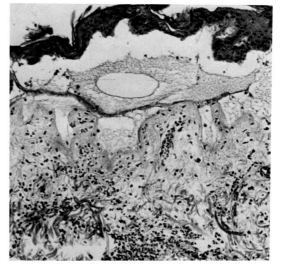

Fig. 42-5. Pemphigus vulgaris with suprabasilar cleavage and isolated clusters of epidermal cells within vesicle. These are acantholytic cells of Tzank. (Hematoxylin and eosin.)

Fig. 42-6. Pemphigoid. Cleavage vesicle between epidermis and dermis with relatively sparse dermal reaction. Tzank cells are absent. (Hematoxylin and eosin.)

The histologic picture of the cutaneous lesion of pemphigus is as follows:

1. The typical vesicle or bulla consists of a collection of serous fluid, most often at the suprabasilar layer of the epidermis. As a rule, there is little or no reaction in the dermis, although there are many exceptions in which the upper dermis or submucosa is crowded with polymorphonuclear leukocytes admixed with the various mononuclear cells (i.e., lymphocytes, plasma cells, and histiocytes). Such a vesicle or bulla characterizes *pemphigus vulgaris* but may be a part of the picture of other varieties of pemphigus (Fig. 42-5). In addition, rounded epidermal cells, loosened by "acantholysis" (Tzank cells) frequently are found in the vesicles of pemphigus, but, as stated, they are not pathognomonic of this disease. These acantholytic cells may be recognized in smears of vesicles stained with hematoxylin and eosin and may be distinguished from cells of viral vesicles, for example. They are characterized by the distintegration of desmosomes and the separation, disorganization, and loss of tonofilaments, a sequence of events accompanying acantholysis not only in other dermatoses such as Darier's disease but also in some epidermal neoplasms, particularly melanocarcinomas. The vulnerability of the desmosomes is regarded as the principal pathogenetic basis of pemphigus, a concept reinforced by immunofluorescent demonstration of the fixation of autoantibodies at these inter-cellular sites. As indicated, autoimmune antibodies may be demonstrated by fluorescence in the intercellular spaces of the epidermis of patients with pemphigus vulgaris. In bullous pemphigoid, the antibodies are localized to the position of the "basement membrane" zone. Some investigators have noted that the immunoglobulins of bullous pemphigoid are localized between the epidermis and basal lamina as contrasted with the localization deep to the basal lamina in lupus erythematosus.[59]

The histologic differentiation of pemphigus vulgaris from "bullous pemphigoid" is often not so clear cut as was implied when the latter term was coined. The early mucosal involvement, the relative lack of inflammation, the abundance of acantholysis, and the suprabasilar (versus epidermal-dermal) cleavage are features indicative of pemphigus. *Benign mucosal* pemphigoid may involve the conjunctivas, oronasal cavity, larynx, esophagus, and genitalia. The histology is like that of bullous pemphigoid except for the occurrence of cicatrization as a consequence of the submucosal inflammatory reaction. It is probable that pemphigoid is a variant of *erythema multiforme bullosum,* as is the *Stevens-Johnson syndrome.* Pemphigoid may, on occasion, be associated with visceral cancer (Fig. 42-6).

Bullae also may result after the use of anticoagulants. These bullae are subepidermal and histologically simulate erythema multiforme.

2. In *pemphigus vegetans,* in addition to

the bulla just described, there is an associated diagnostic lesion consisting of pronounced acanthosis with prominent prolongation of the rete ridges, between which are brilliantly dense collections of eosinophilic leukocytes. The eosinophils may migrate into the epidermis, which may become ulcerated and be the seat of intraepidermal microabscesses. The ulcerations, the intraepidermal abscesses, and the extensive acanthosis with winding reticulated ridges may simulate a bromoderma or the reaction to deep fungal infections such as coccidioidomycosis.

3. In *pemphigus foliaceus,* the typical bulla often is immediately adjacent to a unique acanthosis. Often, the fluid accumulates between layers of the upper rete Malpighii. If the accumulation of fluid is minimal, the cleavage may be sufficient to separate the uppermost portion of the epidermis by crude pressure of the thumb on the skin of the patient (Nikolsky's sign). The ridges are rounded and formed in congeries so that in a single section they may appear isolated in the deep dermis, as in an early squamous cell carcinoma. This type of acanthosis resembles most the epidermal proliferation often seen overlying myoblastomas. The epidermal proliferation usually is accompanied by a polymorphous cellular infiltrate of neutrophilic leukocytes and mononuclear cells. Tzank cells are present in both pemphigus foliaceus and pemphigus vegetans, and, in lesser numbers, in Hailey-Hailey disease and other vesicular dermatoses.

Circulating "intercellular" antibodies are demonstrable in the serum of patients with pemphigus and their titers tend to parallel the severity of the disease.[57] Indeed, reappearance of the antibodies may herald the recrudescence of the disease. Immunofluorescent studies of cutaneous biopsies reveal a striking, diagnostic, diffuse, intercellular localization of immunoglobulins in a characteristic polygonal pattern about the keratinocytes. Pemphigus-like antibodies occur in patients with burns, toxic epidermal necrolysis, and several other drug-induced eruptions. In sharp contrast, the immunofluorescent studies are negative in Hailey-Hailey (bullous Darier's) disease in which the acantholysis may present a differential diagnostic problem in routinely stained sections. In bullous and cicatricial pemphigoid, dematitis herpertiformis, and lupus erythematosus, immunoglobulins may be demonstrated by fluoresceinated sera in the immediate subepidermal region.

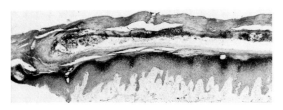

Fig. 42-7. Epidermolysis bullosa. Cleavage vesicle in stratum corneum, unlike deeper, dystrophic form. (Hematoxylin and eosin.)

Epidermolysis bullosa occurs soon after birth (congenital) or may first appear in the second or third decade (so-called acquired type). There are two varieties of epidermolysis bullosa: simple and dystrophic. In the simple type, the lesions occur, after slight trauma, on any portion of the body and regress, leaving merely temporary pigmentation but no permanent changes. The dystrophic type is characterized by lesions of the extremities, provoked by minimal trauma and associated with pigmentation, milia (epidermal cysts), atrophy, destruction of nails, cicatrizations, and syndactylism. It may be complicated by the development of epidermoid carcinomas both in the skin and in the mucosa of the mouth and esophagus. The pathogenesis may well be related to the associated desmoplasia or scarring as in other situations, e.g., burns and chronic osteomyelitis.

Both the simple and dystrophic types may be congenital or acquired. The histology is that of a pressure vesicle with cleavage often at the junction of the stratum corneum and stratum granulosum or between the epidermis and dermis, especially in the dystrophic type (Fig. 42-7). The inflammatory reaction within both the vesicle and the underlying dermis is mild except in regions, such as the feet, that are easily traumatized and infected. Small epidermal inclusions lie in the dermis beneath or at the margins of the vesicles. A congenital disturbance of the dermal elastic tissue is said to occur in the dystrophic type. The evidence for this is not satisfactory. However, necrosis of upper dermal collagen and elastic tissue may occur in the dystrophic form and may result in severe contractures of the extremities with bony absorption. Involvement of the conjunctiva, oral mucosa, and esophagus may develop, heralding a poor prognosis. The epidermal inclusion cysts are particularly prone to appear in the dystrophic form and reflect, in part, the dermal isolation of portions of sweat ducts and rete ridges that subsequently

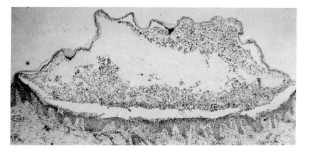

Fig. 42-8. Impetigo contagiosum. Superficial cleavage vesicle with purulent exudate. (Hematoxylin and eosin; AFIP 99848.)

form the cysts. The relative lack of inflammatory cellular response within and beneath the vesicles is of diagnostic usefulness in differentiating them from other vesicles with cleavages at corresponding sites. The bullae of dystrophic epidermolysis bullosa have been attributed to the specifically higher local production of collagenase in contrast with pemphigus vulgaris and bullous pemphigoid. A picture simulating epidermolysis bullosa may occur after the administration of penicillamine. Subepidermal cleavage vesicles (along with necrosis of the epithelium of sweat glands and ducts) may occur also, especially over traumatized pressure points, after carbon monoxide or barbiturate poisoning.[18]

Subcorneal pustular dermatosis is considered to be a special vesicular entity. The lesions, which tend to affect particularly middle-aged women, appear as minute gyrate or annular groups of erythematous, superficial vesiculopustules localized chiefly to the intertriginous areas about the breasts, axillae, and groins.

Histologically, the changes consist of cleavage vesicles and pustules located immediately beneath the stratum corneum, as the name indicates. Eosinophils are not a part of the picture, although occasionally acantholytic cells may be present. The exudate is usually sterile—unlike that of impetigo contagiosa, which the lesion otherwise resembles histologically (Fig. 42-8). *Staphylococcus aureus* is the most common offender in impetigo contagiosa; it is often mixed with β-hemolytic streptococcus. Streptococci also may occur alone or in association with a variety of organisms. Diphtheroids *(Corynebacterium pyogenes)* are responsible for about 5% of cases.

Toxic epidermal necrolysis (Lyell's disease). Toxic epidermal necrolysis (Lyell's disease) presents as a tender, painful rash resembling "scalded skin," with rapid onset and recovery

or rapid death.[44] The exotoxin of *Staphylococcus* is imputed in most diseases but drugs, viruses, and vaccinations (e.g., those against poliomyelitis, diphtheria, and measles) have also been involved. The drugs linked to this fairly new entity include allopurinol, barbiturates, sulfonamides, penicillin, phenylbutazone, hydantoins, salicylates, and antihistamines.[29] Histologically, the epidermal cleavage may develop at one of several levels: dermal-epidermal as in erythema multiforme bullosum, suprabasilar as in pemphigus, or the upper rete Malpighii. Scattered foci of necrotic keratinocytes are characteristically present and some of these may occupy the vesicles as acantholytic cells. Few or no dermal inflammatory cells appear unless secondary infection takes place, so that the simulation of erythema multiforme may be striking. Indeed some observers regard the disease as a variant of erythema multiforme bullosum. In both there has been occasional association with membranoproliferative glomerulonephritis. In sharp contrast with the good prognosis in small children, the mortality in adults is over 40% and recovery is often protracted for many months.

Pyoderma gangrenosum. Pyoderma gangrenosum refers to the ugly, large, purple-rimmed, undermined suppurative ulcerations occurring especially with ulcerative colitis but associated with other diseases, e.g., rheumatoid arthritis. Its etiology and pathogenesis are still problematic although leukocytoclastic arteriolitis, perhaps as part of a Shwartzman phenomenon, has been suspected.

Viral vesicles. Smallpox (variola), chickenpox (varicella), alastrim, vaccinia (cowpox), herpangina, herpes simplex, and herpes zoster (shingles) are described in Chapter 12. In contrast to the ease with which most of the exanthemas are differentiable clinically is the difficulty or impossibility of differentiating the vesicles histologically. Nevertheless, there are certain features common to each of these vesicles that at least permit the recognition of each, histologically, as a vesicle produced by a virus. These features include (1) *reticular colliquation* by which the epidermis becomes transformed into multiple locules bounded by a reticulum of drawn-out, stringy, cytoplasmic septa, (2) *ballooning degeneration,* the formation of multinucleated giant cells in the lower layers of the rete Malpighii, and (3) *intranuclear inclusions.*

It is stated that in the vesicle of smallpox, reticular colliquation proceeds at a faster pace, particularly at the periphery of the lesion, than does ballooning degeneration and thereby accounts for the umbilication of this vesicle. In smallpox, Guarnieri bodies are found as eosinophilic, varying-sized, round, cytoplasmic inclusions—especially in those cells that are at the base of the vesicle, including those undergoing ballooning degeneration. In addition, eosinophilic intranuclear inclusions with margination of the nuclear chromatin are common in these cells. In the vesicles of herpes, these intranuclear inclusions are referred to as "zoster bodies of Lipschütz," although they are morphologically similar to the intranuclear inclusions of the other viral vesicles.

The scarring that follows some of these vesicles (e.g., those of zoster and occasionally of smallpox) is an index of the prior inflammatory destruction of the upper corium. As a rule, edema and infiltrate of inflammatory cells are present in the upper dermis of most vesicles of the various viral diseases. The residual scaring, however, appears to reflect the greater intensity and destructiveness of the process. The virus of zoster appears capable of producing the clinical picture of varicella in susceptible individuals. It is suggested that steroids increase this susceptibility.

Relatively recently, a new entity referred to as *"herpangina"* has been described. It is a benign, febrile, self-limited disease of viral etiology, affecting children chiefly and characterized by a sudden onset of grayish white, papulovesicular, oral or pharyngeal lesions with a surrounding red areola. Histologic studies of the vesicles are not available, but one anticipates that they would resemble the vesicles of herpes.

Another controverted disease that now appears clearly virogenic is *Kaposi's varicelliform eruption*. This disease is really either disseminated herpes simplex or generalized vaccinia, often inoculated in skin made receptive by a preceding dermatosis such as eczema or atopic dermatitis. The rapid diagnosis of viral vesicles is expedited by the use of smears of the vesicular contents. This cytodiagnostic method is particularly useful with the viral vesicles as opposed to other types in which excessive dependence may be placed on acantholytic cells. It is hypothesized that the virus of varicella-zoster remains latent in sensory ganglia after a preceding varicella and hematogenous dissemination of the virus occurs with subsequent activation.

Herpes virus type 2, as opposed to type 1, tends to disseminate. They may be differentiated by cultural or immunofluorescent studies and, it is said, morphologically by the greater tendency toward ballooning degeneration by type 2 virus.

Superficial mycoses

Superficial mycoses are included in this section because of their involvement of epidermis principally. The mycoses are separated into the superficial type (ringworm, tinea corporis, and favus) and the deep type (blastomycosis, coccidioidomycosis, actinomycosis, etc.). Superficial mycoses are divided, according to the region affected, into tinea capitis, barbae, corporis, cruris, and pedis (or epidermophytosis). Several kinds of fungi may be responsible for the same clinical type of lesion. On the other hand, the form and chronicity of the ringworm may vary considerably with the causative fungus. For example, *Trichophyton* infection of the feet presents as a dry, scaly dermatosis, whereas that of *Epidermophyton* appears vesicular and moist. It has therefore been suggested that the etiology, as well as the anatomic region, be indicated in the name, e.g., tinea corporis trichophytica. However, usage sanctions the retention of additional names for varieties of ringworm infection that have distinguishing features of pattern, color, severity, or chronicity of lesions, e.g., favus, kerion (ringworm of scalp complicated by abscesses), tinea imbricata, and tinea versicolor.

Botryomycosis is merely a bacterial infection histologically confused with actinomycosis because of the eosinophilic radiate or asteroid formation about the colonies of bacteria. The etiologic agent is usually a staphylococcus, but streptococci and proteus organisms also may produce this pattern. Gram stains on histologic sections facilitate the diagnosis.

The fungus may be observed in wet smears of scrapings soaked in sodium or potassium hydroxide, or they may be cultured on special media, such as Sabouraud's agar. However, with the exceptions of tinea versicolor and favus, it is rare to observe the fungus in a routine paraffin section of a lesion of ringworm. Generally, the histologic picture comprises merely the presence of scales or vesicles along with subepidermal hyperemia and slight perivascular cuffing by mononuclear cells. In tinea versicolor, the spores and hyphae of *Pityrosporon furfur* are usually abundant and confined to the stratum corneum. In favus, the large scutula, or matted scales, contain masses of the fungus.

The vesicle of ringworm, no matter where the lesion is located, is an eczematous vesicle, usually multiloculated, and the morphologic result of excessive spongiosis. This type of vesicle is the picture of the dermatophytid or allergic manifestation of the fungal infection. The dermatophytids are sterile of fungi and are caused by the cutaneous reaction to the products of fungi transported probably through the blood or lymph. For example, the dermatophytids after ringworm of the feet often occur on the hands. It has been suggested that sensitizing antibiotic therapy with preparations from fungi such as penicillin may be responsible in some measure for the dermatophytids after superficial mycoses. The deep mycoses are described in Chapter 13.

Scabies. Another lesion of the epidermis that is often recognizable in a fortunate histologic section is caused by *Acarus scabiei.* The disease is characterized by the occurrence of intensely pruritic papules, vesicles, pustules, and excoriations usually located in relation to the burrow, cuniculus, or gallery dug by the mite of the *Acarus* into the epidermis. These lesions tend to occur in the webs of the fingers, on the wrists, in the genital regions, and beneath the breast. The disease is contagious and, in most instances, is transmitted by direct bodily contact with an infected individual. The diagnosis may be made clinically by picking the female mite out of the burrow and identifying it with the low-power lens of the microscope.

Histologically, none of the lesions of scabies is diagnostic except the burrow with the tenant mite. However, the mite often may not be included in the section, but the presence of ova or fecal material of the *Acarus* within the burrow or merely the presence of the gallery itself is strongly presumptive evidence of scabies. The burrow is a superficial epidermal defect extending obliquely through the thickened stratum corneum, which serves as a roof to shelter the *Acarus.*

A form of scabies may be transmitted to man by mites that infest dogs, cats, birds, and monkeys. So-called *Norwegian scabies* appears to be merely a more fulminant form of ordinary scabies.

The *Demodex folliculorum,* the acarid commonly found within the keratinous follicular plugs of comedones, has generally been regarded as an innocuous infestation. More recently, the innocuous nature of infestation with *Demodex folliculorum* has been questioned. Blepharitis, for example, has been attributed to this arthropod.

Diseases affecting both epidermis and dermis

In this discussion are included those histologic entities in which changes in both the epidermis and the dermis jointly contribute to the morphologic diagnosis.

Lupus erythematosus

Lupus erythematosus occurs in two principal forms: acute and chronic or discoid.

Discoid lupus erythematosus. The discoid variety is fortunately the more common and manifests itself by stationary or slowly progressive coalescent macules or plaques covered irregularly with fine, whitish or yellowish, greasy scales and associated with focal gray patches of atrophy and keratotic plugging of follicles. The lesions usually are well defined (hence, discoid) and show a predilection for the malar areas and bridge of the nose distributed in the shape of a butterfly. The process is not limited to this area but may occur also on other parts of the face, the scalp, the neck, extremities, and elsewhere. In any location, the lesions are aggravated by exposure to sunlight or other forms of irradiation. The lesions may regress completely, but usually there is residual, rather typical superficial scarring with pigmentation or leukoderma and alopecia. Acute changes also may be superimposed on the discoid lesions. Carcinomatous transformations (squamous cell) may occur in the chronic process, probably for nonspecific reasons similar to those that obtain in some other forms of chronic cicatrizing ulcerations. The lesions respond remarkably well to antimalarial drugs.

The histologic features of the discoid variety of lupus erythematosus are easily recognizable in most cases. They include the following:

1. Alternating acanthosis and atrophy of the epidermis, with the process infrequently progressing to squamous cell carcinoma
2. Liquefaction degeneration of the basal layer
3. Hyperemia or telangiectasis and edema of the papillary and subpapillary layers of the dermis
4. Dense collections of mononuclear cells, principally lymphocytes, in the upper and midportions of the dermis, most concentrated about the appendages, often with atrophy and consequent alopecia (Fig. 42-9)
5. Focal depigmentation of the basal layer along with clusters of melanophages secondary to the subepidermal inflammation

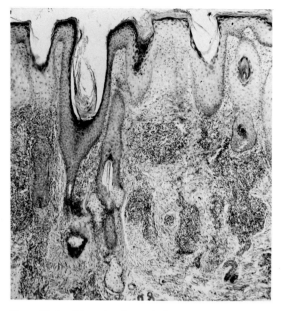

Fig. 42-9. Chronic discoid lupus erythematosus with alternating acanthosis and atrophy, liquefaction degeneration, keratinous plugs in follicles, superficial telangiectases, and dense collections of dermal lymphocytes. (Hematoxylin and eosin; from Allen, A. C.: Arch. Dermatol. Syph. [Chicago] **57:**19-56, 1948.)

Basophilic "degeneration" of collagen in the upper dermis is a completely unreliable criterion of chronic lupus erythematosus, inasmuch as it is found normally in the skin of the malar regions, especially in the older age groups of patients. Changes in vessels, other than telangiectasis, are not part of the picture of discoid lupus erythematosus. The lesions of *rosacea* may occasionally offer differential diagnostic difficulty because of the presence of keratotic plugs and erythema. The epidermal changes and mid-dermal masses of lymphocytes favor lupus erythematosus. Occasionally, the collections of lymphocytes extend into the underlying panniculus *(lupus erythematosus profundus)* and may be mistaken for Weber-Christian disease. Lupus erythematosus profundus (lupus erythematosus panniculitis) presents as a nodular involvement of the subcutis with or without overlying dermal and epidermal involvement. This lesion, too, has been attributed to injury caused by immune complexes.[63] Similar dense masses of lymphocytes in the dermis may be confused with a malignant lymphoma, the benign dermal lymphocytosis of Jessner, or the potpourri of lesions labeled Spiegler-Fendt sarcoid.

Acute lupus erythematosus. The acute (or

"subacute") lupus erythematosus may occur as a focal, transient reaction to sunlight or may be part of the frequently fatal systemization of the disease. These acute lesions may be superimposed on the chronic process or may affect previously uninvolved skin. The chronic lesion is assumed to be complicated by the disseminated form in the rarest instances. However, although this may be the impression clinically, the histologic and recent clinical data belie this impression. Moreover, antinuclear antibodies are stated to be present in over 90% of patients with systemic lupus erythematosus and in from 15 to 40% of those with discoid lupus erythematosus. Immunofluorescent studies reveal characteristic bands of immunoglobulins (IgG) and complement at the dermo-epidermal junction in both systemic and discoid lupus erythematosus. The immunofluorescence is said to be positive occasionally in rosacea and in a few other diseases in which, however, the differential histologic diagnosis may be achieved in sections stained routinely.

In the acute cases, the skin becomes reddened, edematous, and sometimes purpuric, with patchy macules that may coalesce into an erysipeloid, somewhat mottled malar flush. On the hands, the lesions may be erythematous or purpuric and macular or papular. Elsewhere, they may take other forms such as vesicles, bullae, scaling macules, and telangiectases. When the acute process complicates the discoid lesion, fresh superficial or even moderately deep ulcerations may occur, in addition to the other changes mentioned, particularly at the advancing periphery of the old lesion. As stated, the acute cutaneous alterations may be a localized reaction to sunlight without systemic complications. In the disseminated variety, which occurs particularly but by no means exclusively in young women, the constitutional signs and symptoms include fever, thrombopenia, leukopenia, excessive gammaglobulinemia, splenomegaly, arthralgias, valvular disease (Libman-Sacks disease), anorexia, vomiting, diarrhea, dysphagia, abdominal pain, and lymphadenitis. The principal causes of death are renal insufficiency, bacterial endocarditis, cardiac failure, sepsis, or pneumonia (see also pp. 797 and 1101).

The acute histologic changes in the skin are recognized in an exaggeration of the liquefaction degeneration of the basal layer of the epidermis (Fig. 42-10) with eosinophilic swelling of the cytoplasm of the basal cells, edema of the papillary and subpapillary layers, necro-

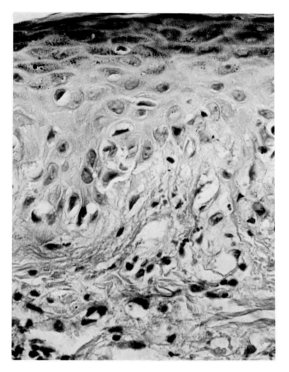

Fig. 42-10. Acute disseminated lupus erythematosus with pronounced liquefaction degeneration at epidermal-dermal junction. (Hematoxylin and eosin.)

biosis with karyorrhexis and nuclear distortion of inflammatory cells in the upper dermis, telangiectasis, and, occasionally, fibrinoid degeneration of foci of collagen in this region, as well as the walls of some of the arterioles. The last change, arteriolar involvement, is inconstant and is surely not responsible for the other cutaneous alterations.

By far, the most diagnostically revealing histologic changes occur at the dermo-epidermal junction. They are the vacuolization of the basal cells (liquefaction degeneration) and the subepidermal edema with a linear condensation of PAS-positive material simulating a basement membrane but differing by its discontinuity and nonargyrophilia in the absence of melanin. Direct immunofluorescent studies reveal in this zone an immunofluorescent band reflecting immunoglobulins (IgG, IgM), components of complement (C1q, C3), and fibrin and properdin in both clinically involved and clinically intact skin.[26,39] The presence of the immunofluorescent band in clinically uninvolved skin worsens the prognosis and has been found associated with renal disease.[33] Although such skin may appear clinically "uninvolved," careful histologic evaluation of even routinely

hematoxylin and eosin–stained sections is likely to reveal some evidence of edema in this zone. In patients who have an inherited deficiency of complement, there is likely to be an absence of C3 at the dermo-epidermal junction and low titers of antinuclear antibodies. Interestingly, systemic lupus erythematosus has been associated with porphyria in more than a fortuitous manner.

Characteristic histologic changes occur in other organs in the disseminated disease. These include the following:

1. Atypical verrucous endocarditis (Libman-Sacks disease)
2. Striking fibrinoid alteration of the interstitial collagen of the myocardium that may, but need not, be mistaken for Aschoff bodies
3. Concentric dense rings of collagen, apparently thickened reticulum, about the central splenic arterioles (Figs. 34-20 and 34-21)
4. Focal fibrinoid swelling of the walls of glomerular capillaries ("wire loops")

Viruslike, microtubular cytoplasmic inclusions have been noted in the skin, glomeruli, and other sites. These have provoked much interest but their presence in patients without systemic lupus erythematosus and even in the vascular endothelium of patients with bullous pemphigoid has dampened the initial enthusiasm for the likelihood that they represent the etiologic virus.[31]

Undoubtedly, one of the most provocative discoveries in the field of cutaneovisceral integration of the last few decades has been the phenomenon of the lupus erythematosus cell. Cytologically the phenomenon is manifested typically by a rosette of neutrophilic leukocytes about a mononuclear cell (apparently a lymphocyte) or, less typically, by a neutrophilic leukocyte with a cytoplasmic vacuole or a cytoplasmic inclusion of a nuclear fragment. Often, there is excessive clumping of platelets. The essence of this phenomenon resides in the gamma globulin of the serum of patients with disseminated lupus erythematosus and may be observed not only with cells of the patient's marrow but with cells of the peripheral blood. It also may be observed with normal cells (human or animal) after mixture with the patient's serum. Similar cells are noted in a cantharides-induced blister in the skin of individuals with disseminated lupus erythematosus. It is of interest, but by now not surprising, to record the dramatic remissions initiated by cortisone and ACTH in profoundly ill patients. With this improvement, the number of lupus erythematosus cells diminishes and may completely disappear. Some instances of a positive lupus erythematosus phenomenon have been recorded in multiple myeloma, leukemia, Hodgkin's disease, rheumatoid arthritis, viral hepatitis, acquired hemolytic anemia, and reactions to drugs (phenylbutazone and hydralazine) and in association with infection or contamination of serum with *Aspergillus niger* or *Trichophyton gypseum*. It is of interest that the lupus erythematosus cell is generally absent in scleroderma and dermatomyositis, which, together with disseminated lupus erythematosus, have been gratuitously linked as diffuse vascular or diffuse collagen disease—notwithstanding this and other discrepancies. Moreover, there is adequate reason to conclude that no one of these diseases is either a diffuse vascular disease or a generalized disease of collagen. Review of the histology of even a small number of autopsies in such cases quickly reveals that the involvement of vessels or collagen is, as a rule, neither diffuse nor itself responsible for the clinical picture, with the exception of scleroderma.

Mixed connective tissue disease

"Mixed connective tissue disease" is a designation applied to a mild form of systemic lupus erythematosus without renal involvement and with high titer levels of antinuclear antibodies exhibiting a speckled rather than membranous rim of homogeneous nuclear staining with indirect immunofluorescence tests.

Dermatomyositis

The purplish red, finely scaly edematous rash located principally about the upper face is fairly diagnostic, the histologic picture of the skin is not. It consists chiefly of spotty parakeratosis, some liquefaction degeneration at the epidermal-dermal junction, and edema of the upper dermis. However, the vacuolar sarcolysis, coagulation necrosis, and acute inflammatory changes in the swollen muscle fibers may be strongly suggestive. As stated, the search for vascular alterations is generally fruitless (Fig. 42-11).

The pathogenetic and etiologic spectra of myositides are expanding rapidly and form an intriguing chapter dealing with viruses, unresolved relationship to visceral cancer, lesions of the thymus, etc. It appears evident that some of the confusion related to dermatomyositis is that a variety of myositic disorders as well as systemic lupus erythematosus and

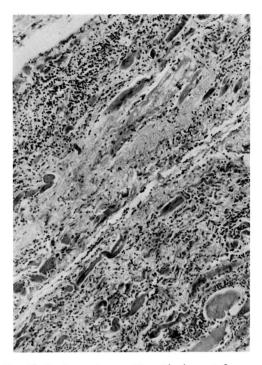

Fig. 42-11. Dermatomyositis with dense inflammatory cells interspersed among atrophic muscle fibers. (Hematoxylin and eosin.)

scleroderma are mistakenly considered to be dermatomyositis. The presence of dermal mucin in a specimen with no specific pattern is stated to be suggestive of dermatomyositis. The cutaneous eruption of dermatomyositis may occur before involvement of muscle is evident clinically or histologically. Direct immunofluorescent studies are usually negative, except for globular deposits of IgG, IgM, and IgA, in the upper dermis, which are of unknown significance.

Psoriasis

Psoriasis is characterized by reddish brown papules, covered with silvery white micaceous scales with a predilection for symmetric distribution on the extremities, especially on the knees and elbows. Lesions may occur also on the scalp, upper back, face, and genitalia and over the sacrum. The nails often are involved and become thickened, dirty white, irregularly laminated, rigid, and brittle. The disease is notoriously chronic although remissions may occur spontaneously and after certain therapy, such as x-ray or ultraviolet ray therapy.

Occasionally, a widespread erythroderma or exofoliative dermatitis may complicate psoriasis, either spontaneously or, more particularly,

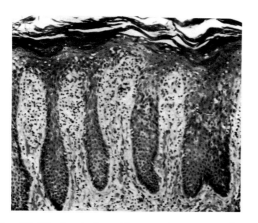

Fig. 42-12. Psoriasis with conspicuous parakeratosis, elongated, clubbed rete ridges, thinned suprapapillary epidermis, and rigid vessels in papillae. (Hematoxylin and eosin.)

after vigorous therapy. Another complication of psoriasis is arthritis, occurring usually in association with the generalized erythroderma. Occasionally, the arthritis is deforming and persistently ankylotic, as in rheumatoid arthritis.

The use of various qualifying terms such as psoriasis punctata, psoriasis guttata, psoriasis rupioides, psoriasis follicularis, psoriasis nummularis, and others reflects simply the predominant clinical pattern of the lesions.

The histologic features of psoriasis (Fig. 42-12) are as follows:

1. Acanthosis with regular downgrowth of the rete ridges to about the same dermal level
2. Rounded tips of the rete ridges
3. Prolongation of the papillae, frequently with single vessels (venules) extending the length of the papillae as if rigid rather than tortuous
4. Thin epidermal plates over the elongated papillae, which offers so little covering for the dilated vessels of the papillae that bleeding occurs when a scale is lifted (Auspitz's sign)
5. Prominent parakeratosis, usually extending the length of the lesion rather than focally
6. Absence or sparsity of stratum granulosum
7. Microabscesses (of Munro) in the upper rete Malpighii

In addition, there is an absence of spongiosis, as a rule, except in the immediate vicinity of the epidermal microabscesses. Intracellular edema in the rete Malpighii is common. The papillae are infiltrated chiefly with lymphocytes and histiocytes. In lesions that are in the early stage of development, some of these features, such as the rounding of the ridges and the elongation of the papillae with thin epidermal plates, may be absent. Furthermore, as in other dermatoses, recent therapy, trauma, or secondary infection obviously will modify the pattern. However, in patients in whom there has been a superimposed exfoliative dermatitis, the basic histologic picture of the psoriatic lesion tends to persist and thereby may help differentiation from the exfoliative stage of *mycosis fungoides,* a problem that occasionally arises. Neurodermatitis may simulate psoriasis so closely as to be histologically indistinguishable. As a rule, however, the psoriasiform features listed previously are irregular or less developed in neurodermatitis or individual changes are altogether lacking.

Parapsoriasis. Parapsoriasis, notwithstanding the name, is not otherwise related to psoriasis. The disease is characterized by erythematous macules covered with fine scales and distributed on the trunk and extremities. The lesions are extremely resistant to therapy.

The histologic changes of parapsoriasis are said to be quite nonspecific and to simulate psoriasis, seborrheic dermatitis, lichen planus, a macular syphiloderm, or the early stage of mycosis fungoides. Although the changes may simulate these other diseases, the specific diagnosis of parapsoriasis may be made with considerable assurance in many cases on the basis of the histologic changes alone. These changes include the spotty, thin areas of parakeratosis, slight to moderate acanthosis, vertical arrangement with some hyperchromatism of the basal layer along with slight liquefaction degeneration and, perhaps most revealing, the localization of inflammatory cells, mostly mononuclear, in the immediately subepidermal zone. The infiltrate hugs the epidermis tightly, and characteristically some of the inflammatory cells are located in the epidermis in their transepidermal migration. The presence of parakeratosis and a minimal stratum granulosum, as well as the shape of the ridges, easily distinguish parapsoriasis from lichen planus. One of the serious errors of histologic diagnosis is mislabeling as parapsoriasis (en plaque) the early stage of mycosis fungoides. This error is made both clinically and histologically.

Lichen planus

Lichen planus is generally easily recognized clinically by the irregular, violaceous, glistening, flat-topped, pruritic papules, covered with a thin, horny, adherent film and distributed symmetrically, particularly along the flexor aspects of the wrists, forearms, and legs. The usual form of lichen planus tends to resolve spontaneously after a year or so.

On careful examination, minute whitish points and lines (Wickham's striae) are seen on the surface of the papules. The disease is chronic, may last from months to years, and is rarely associated with constitutional reaction except in some of the hyperacute cases. The varieties include lichen planus, lichen planus hypertrophicus, and lichen planus atrophicus.

The histology of lichen planus is strikingly characteristic and comprises the following:

1. Hyperkeratosis
2. Prominence of the stratum granulosum
3. Acanthosis, with elongated, saw-toothed rete ridges
4. Liquefaction degeneration of the basal layer
5. A mononuclear infiltrate consisting mostly of lymphocytes and histiocytes, sharply limited to the papillary and subpapillary layers of the dermis (Fig. 42-13)

Many of the subepidermal macrophages are laden with melanin from the basal cells not because these cells are unable to unload their pigment into "damaged" unreceptive neighboring keratinocytes and so spill over into the dermis,[51] but because the subepidermal infil-

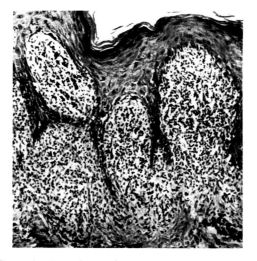

Fig. 42-13. Lichen planus with hyperkeratosis, acanthosis, pointed rete ridges, liquefaction degeneration, and dense subepidermal inflammatory zone. (Hematoxylin and eosin.)

trate provokes not only the development of the epidermal pigmentation but also its release from the epidermis into dermal histiocytes. This same phenomenon is observed in other dermatoses, such as mycosis fungoides, Atabrine dermatitis, dermal postinflammatory pigmentation, and lupus erythematosus, in each of which a subepidermal inflammatory or cellular reaction occurs.

In the atrophic form the ridges are flattened and the dermal infiltrate is sparse and replaced by an increased density of collagen containing somewhat thickened arterioles.

Immunofluorescence reflecting the presence of immunoglobulins and complement is noted in the eosinophilic, clustered, subepidermal globular bodies (Civatte's bodies). Somewhat similar foci are seen also in a variety of other dermatoses, but their diagnostic significance in these is inconsequential. Actually, the meaning of these deposits even in lichen planus is not understood. To suggest that they represent an autoimmune process is not warranted at this time. Instances of ulcerated lichen planus of the feet may exhibit positive antinuclear-antibody tests and elevated gamma globulins with resulting confusion with systemic lupus erythematosus.

Keratoderma blennorrhagicum

Infrequently, perhaps in about 1 in 5000 cases, there develops an ugly eruption after the contraction of gonnorrheal urethritis. This eruption is called "keratoderma blenorrhagicum" or "gonorrheal keratosis" and is associated with a nonsuppurative migrating arthritis and gonorrheal urethritis that persist despite chemotherapy. The cutaneous lesions appear several weeks after the urethritis, do not contain gonococci, according to most observers, and clear only after disappearance of the urethritis. The lesions of the skin are identical with those of *Reiter's syndrome,* which is associated with a presumed "nonspecific" urethritis, conjunctivitis, and nonsuppurative arthritis. In both the keratoderma and Reiter's syndrome, evolution of the disease is essentially similar. In both, the arthritis clears, as a rule, without residual damage to the joints. In the few cases tested, the complement fixation test for gonorrhea was negative in Reiter's syndrome. More recently *chlamydia trachomatis* and the pleuropneumonia or "L" organisms have been considered responsible for Reiter's syndrome.

The histologic features of keratoderma blennorrhagicum are as follows:

1. Prominent parakeratosis with excessive loosening of the scales so that they may be difficult to include in the histologic sections
2. Acanthosis with elongation and rounding of the ends of the rete ridges, very much as in psoriasis, so that pustular psoriasis may be a difficult differential diagnostic problem
3. Elongation of the papillae but generally not so strikingly as in psoriasis because the overlying epidermal plate usually is not so thinned as in the latter disease
4. Numerous polymorphonuclear leukocytes, particularly in the upper rete Malpighii and in the scales

Diseases principally of dermis
Urticaria pigmentosa

Urticaria pigmentosa is a chronic disease of the skin that begins usually in the first year of life but may start shortly after puberty or in later adult life, selecting particularly males of light complexion. In a significant number of patients with urticaria pigmentosa there is a history of asthma or hay fever. The eruption, characteristically, is made up of oval, 0.5 to 2.5 cm, pigmented, yellowish-to-reddish brown, macular, papular, and even nodular lesions occurring on the back especially but also on the face, scalp, palms, and soles. Infrequently, a patient will have merely a solitary nodule of urticaria pigmentosa. Solitary mastocytomas generally are detected by the first month of life and comprise about 10% to 15% of all instances of cutaneous mastocytosis. The disseminated cutaneous form usually develops by the next few months. About 25% of cases appear late in teenage or adult life, between the ages of 15 and 40 years, occurring equally in males and females.

Occasionally, the eruptions may be sufficiently yellow to simulate xanthomatosis. The lesions are often intensely pruritic and, when irritated, become reddened, swollen, and urticarial; i.e., they show evidence of dermographism. They may persist for years and, in many instances, disappear spontaneously. In those patients in whom the lesions of urticaria pigmentosa appear in childhood and are confined to the skin, the likelihood of spontaneous resolution during adolescence is great. In those in whom the lesions first appear in adolescence or later, the possibility of their persistence and systemization is considerable. Bullae are common in neonatal mastocytosis.

Systemic involvement (bones, liver, lymph nodes, spleen etc.) occurs in about 10% of patients, mostly in adults, and about one-third of them develop the equivalent of a mast cell leukemia. Uncommonly, a solitary nodule or mastocytoma is followed by dissemination to the viscera or to the remainder of the skin. Such dissemination is said not to occur if the nodule remains solitary for approximately two months.

The histologic picture of urticaria pigmentosa is distinctive. In the more striking examples, the upper one half of two thirds of the dermis is replaced by a compact zone of mast cells that obscure the dermal landmarks (Fig. 42-14). The mast cells should be recognized in sections stained with the routine hematoxylin and eosin, notwithstanding their simulation of ordinary histiocytes and of plasma cells. Frequently, under high magnification, even with this routine stain, the cytoplasmic granules of mast cells may be discerned. These granules are, of course, more clearly demonstrable in metachromatic stains, such as Giemsa's or toluidine blue. The granules are presumed to contain histamine, heparin, and possibly serotonin. In some cases, mast cells are present in smaller numbers and are dispersed as clumps of 10 to 20 cells about the mid-dermal vessels. In these instances, fine judgment may be required to differentiate the presence of mast cells in normal and abnormal numbers. In addition to the mast cells, there often are subepidermal edema (urticaria), chromatophores containing melanin in the

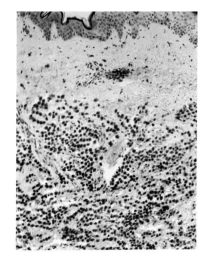

Fig. 42-14. Urticaria pigmentosa with superficial edema of cutis and extensive numbers of mast cells in remainder of dermis. (Hematoxylin and eosin.)

upper dermis, and eosinophilic leukocytes scattered among the mast cells. Melanosis of the basal layer of the epidermis also may be present. The full-blown picture of urticaria pigmentosa closely resembles the so-called mastocytoma of dogs. Systemic foci of infiltrations of mast cells are found also in the viscera, e.g., in the spleen, liver, and lymph nodes. Routine histologic sections of urticaria pigmentosa are commonly mistaken for leukemia, nevi, malignant melanomas, and Letterer-Siwe disease. Resignation to the teaching that mast cells cannot be detected or strongly suspected with stains of hematoxylin and eosin is, in large part, responsible for these serious errors.

Simple urticaria may be caused in a variety of ways: by drugs, allergenic foods, infections (melioidosis), ultraviolet irradiation (*urticaria solaris*), and, fairly commonly, emotional disturbances. Urticaria solaris occurs immediately after exposure to light of sufficient intensity and of proper wavelength, usually in the violet or blue part of the spectrum. The essential histologic picture is that of bland subepidermal edema. In the inherited angioneurotic lesion the edema may extend into the subcutis. The evidence for a deficiency in plasma protease inhibitors (α_1-antitrypsin) in patients with chronic urticaria has been stressed recently.[27]

Erysipelas

Erysipelas is described in the chapter on bacterial diseases (p. 385).

Diseases of collagen

Keloid. A keloid is a hypertrophic cutaneous scar that develops as a reaction to burns of various sorts, incisions, insect bites, vaccinations, and other stimuli. Ulcerated keloids are prone to undergo carcinomatous transformation of the epidermis after a long interval, particularly those attributable to burns or associated with chronic sinuses, as in osteomyelitis. The dermal portion of a keloid is not more likely to become sarcomatous than the dermis elsewhere. Rarely, a keloid resolves spontaneously.

The histologic features of a keloid include thick, homogeneously eosinophilic bands of collagen admixed with thin collagenous fibers and large active fibroblasts. The sweat glands, sebaceous glands, follicles, and arrectores pliorum are atrophic, destroyed, or displaced by the scar. The epidermis may be atrophic or only slightly altered by fusion and irregular pattern of the ridges. The ordinary scar of the skin is more cellular than a keloid and is composed of uniformly thinner collagenous fibers. In both instances, elastic tissue is diminished or absent. The keloidal reaction of hypertrophic collagenous bundles and large fibroblasts is characteristic of dermatitis papillaris capillitii (keloidal acne), which occurs particularly in the nuchal region and, with the associated extensive plasmacytic reaction, represents a type of response to folliculitis.

Balanitis xerotica obliterans. Balanitis xerotica obliterans constitutes another disease of collagen that appears clinically as whitish, firm, coalescent papules or a sclerotic plaque of the glans penis and foreskin and occurs, often, after circumcision. The disease is of some importance because the process tends to extend to the urethral meatus, causing stenosis of the orifice. The lesion is to be differentiated clinically from erythroplasia of Queyrat and circumscribed scleroderma. There is likelihood that balanitis xerotica obliterans is a form of lichen sclerosus et atrophicus, which tends to occur on the vulva.

The histologic picture consists of:

1. Atrophic epidermis or epithelium with loss of rete ridges
2. Striking homogenization of the collagen affecting about one third of the upper dermis
3. A more or less dense zone of lymphocytes and histiocytes beneath the homogenized collagen (Fig. 42-15)

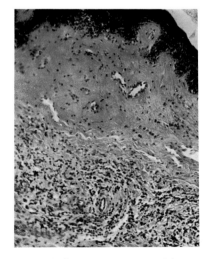

Fig. 42-15. Balanitis xerotica obliterans with homogenization of subepidermal collagen over zone of inflammatory cells. (Hematoxylin and eosin.)

The small arteries and arterioles of the upper and middle dermis may show evidence of endarteritis obliterans, but this process is sufficiently inconstant as not to warrant the use of the qualification "obliterans" in the name of the disease. Furthermore, on the basis of other cutaneous atrophy, there is considerable reason to believe that the vascular change does not initiate the collagenous change but perhaps is an incidental secondary reaction as in other kinds of chronic inflammations (e.g., chronic gastric ulcer).

In lichen sclerosus et atrophicus, the initial change is a subepidermal edema that subsequently progresses to the characteristically homogenized densely sclerotic collagen in which the elastic fibers are diminished because of their displacement downward. The edema may be so great as to cause actual vesiculation at the dermo-epidermal junction. Uncommonly lichen sclerosis et atrophicus will develop an epidermoid carcinoma. Even though the association is infrequent, the histologic appearance of transition of the two processes suggests that the carcinoma develops from the sclerosis on more than a chance basis.

Acrodermatitis chronica atrophicans. Acrodermatitis chronica atrophicans presents as atrophy of the epidermis and a subepidermal homogenized zone of collagen beneath which is a dense zone of mononuclear cells (Fig. 42-16). There is also loss of dermal elastic tissue and atrophy of appendages.

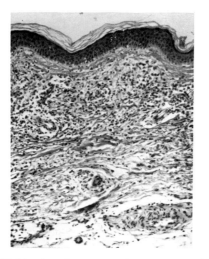

Fig. 42-16. Acrodermatitis chronica atrophicans with thin zone of hyalinized subepidermal collagen and deeper layer of inflammatory cells. (Hematoxylin and eosin.)

Acrodermatitis chronica atrophicans begins as erythematous, slightly edematous macules that later become wrinkled, atrophic, and sclerodermatoid. As the prefix *acro-* indicates, the disease tends to select the extremities, particularly the hands and feet and the extensor surfaces of the elbows and knees. The condition occurs predominantly in middle-aged women.

Granuloma annulare. Granuloma annulare is a chronic eruption made up of papules or nodules grouped in a ringed or circinate arrangement, with a tendency to occur on the dorsa of the fingers and hands and on the elbows, neck, feet, ankles, and buttocks, particularly of children and young adults. The lesions can be palpated intracutaneously rather than subcutaneously, in contrast to rheumatic nodules.

The etiology of the disease is unknown. Because of the histology, a rheumatic or rheumatoid basis for the disease comes to mind, but here, too, clinical evidence is sparse. We have seen cases associated with disseminated allergic granulomatous arteritis. The histologic picture of granuloma annulare has been observed also as a reaction to the *Culicoides furans,* a biting gnat.

Histologically, granuloma annulare is characterized by an intradermal oval or circular focus of fibrinoid degeneration of collagen. They may occasionally ulcerate and are then categorized as "perforating" granuloma annulare. These necrotic foci of dermal collagen really suggest infarcts, although corresponding occlusion of adjacent vessels is not regularly noted. About such a focus there are palisaded rows of epithelioid cells or histiocytes, some of which may be vacuolated by fat (Fig. 42-17). It is the combination of fibrinoid alteration of collagen and palisaded histiocytes that suggests a possible rheumatic etiology. In fact, the histologic features of granuloma annulare are identical with those of the *rheumatic or rheumatoid nodule*—the only difference, as indicated, being the location of the latter in the subcutaneous tissue, adjacent to or within synovial membranes. Certainly, the histologic picture is not that of tuberculosis, although the characteristic fibrinoid degeneration of the collagen of granuloma annulare and the rheumatic nodule has been mistaken for the caseation of tuberculosis, a simulation that usually can be detected easily. There may be considerable difficulty, however, in recognizing early or small lesions of granuloma annulare in which the only clue may be a minimal

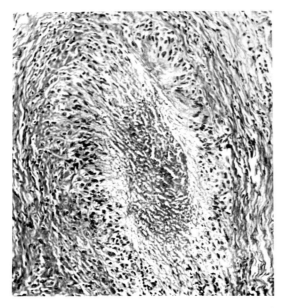

Fig. 42-17. Granuloma annulare with central fibrinoid necrosis of dermal collagen surrounded by palisaded epithelioid histiocytes. (Hematoxylin and eosin; from Allen, A. C.: Arch. Dermatol. Syph. [Chicago] **57**:19-56, 1948.)

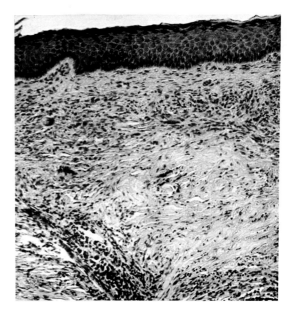

Fig. 42-18. Necrobiosis lipoidica diabeticorum with irregularly homogenized, degenerated dermal collagen and tuberculoid granulomas at periphery. (Hematoxylin and eosin.)

smudgy fibrinoid swelling of collagen with clumps of a few histiocytes, some vacuolated and others partially palisaded. These minute lesions may be confused with xanthoses, necrobiosis lipoidica diabeticorum, or leprosy. Of course, Aschoff bodies are absent in granuloma annulare, as they are in the subcutaneous rheumatic nodule; they are confined to the heart. A protease and a collagenase similar to those of rheumatoid synovial enzymes have been isolated from rheumatoid nodules. The necrosis has been attributed to these, but the greater likelihood is the primacy of vascular compromise as a cause of the infarctlike necrosis both in these nodules and in granuloma annulare.

Necrobiosis lipoidica diabeticorum. Necrobiosis lipoidica diabeticorum is a disease characterized by oval, circular, firm, sharply defined plaques with yellowish centers and violaceous peripheries, occurring predominantly on the legs but found also on the forearms, palms, soles, neck, and face. The centers of the lesions are prone to ulcerate. Trauma, often inconspicuous, may initiate the lesions. In about 50% to 80% of the patients, the disease is associated with diabetes. In about 10%, the lesions precede the onset of diabetes. In the remainder, diabetes does not develop. Obviously, the recognition of necrobiosis lipoi-

dica diabeticorum can be of prophetic importance.

Clinically, the disease must be differentiated from other such focal diseases of collagen as granuloma annulare, amyloidosis, morphea, and lipid proteinosis, as well as the granulomas of sarcoid and erythema induratum, which tend, also, to occur on the extremities. The diabetic state in some instances of necrobiosis lipiodica diabeticorum may be missed with the standard glucose tolerance test and discovered with the cortisone glucose tolerance test.

The basic histologic change of necrobiosis diabeticorum consists of ischemia-like degeneration of collagen, occurring in irregular patches, especially in the upper dermis. In well-developed foci, the altered collagen is swollen and somewhat granular, with loss of fibrils and with a diminution in nuclei of fibrocytes. At the periphery of the collagenous alteration are small collections of histiocytes often arranged about Langhans' giant cells and simulating sarcoid or tuberculosis (Fig. 42-18). This giant cell reaction occasionally may involve the walls of veins to produce a giant cell phlebitis reminiscent of the reaction in temporal arteritis. Vacuoles may be present in the cytoplasm of the giant cells and histiocytes, but fat is found infrequently within the cells of these lesions, although extracellular fat is detectable about the altered collagen.

Scleroderma. There are two basic varieties of scleroderma, the differentiation of which is of great importance prognostically: (1) morphea or circumscribed scleroderma and (2) diffuse scleroderma.

Circumscribed scleroderma occurs as well-delimited, round or oval plaques with whitish, yellowish, or ivory-colored centers and violaceous peripheries. Occasionally, the plaques correspond in distribution to the innervation of a cutaneous nerve, so that a trophic origin has been suggested. Degeneration and regeneration of dermal nerves are said to occur with characteristic patterns in scleroderma and acrosclerosis. *Morphea guttata* or *white-spot disease* is a modification of circumscribed scleroderma characterized by varying-sized chalky white patches on the chest and neck. Rarely does circumscribed scleroderma progress into the often fatal diffuse scleroderma. Usually, the lesions clear, with a barely noticeable thin atrophic area as a residuum. *Linear scleroderma* of an extremity may be associated with melorheostosis or linear hyperostosis of the underlying bone.

Diffuse scleroderma, which affects women twice as often as men, begins insidiously—usually as edema of the hands, other parts of the extremities, or neck—and extends inexorably on to sclerosis that stiffens, binds, and limits the mobility of the affected part. Ulcerations may occur over bony prominence. Calcareous cutaneous deposits and pigmentation, the latter of such a degree as to simulate Addison's disease, are frequent. The normal cutaneous lines become obliterated. Diminution in sweating, hyperesthesias, and pruritus may occur. Sclerosis limited to the hands in association with the vasospastic symptoms of Raynaud's disease is called acrosclerosis or sclerodactylia. In actuality, this symptom complex presents a phase of diffuse scleroderma, although the progress to the fatal disease is not invariable.

Systemic sclerosis refers to diffuse scleroderma with visceral involvement. Dense fibrosis may affect the myocardium and the esophagus and other portions of the gastrointestinal tract. The lungs may be affected with cystic fibrosis, particularly at the bases. Renal vessels may present the histologic picture of accelerated nephrosclerosis, and, if widespread, will indeed be associated with malignant hypertension. The glomeruli may show conspicuous diffuse membranous glomerulonephritis.

The cardiac fibrosis or the cystic pulmonary changes may lead to myocardial failure. Antibodies bound to nucleoli may be present in systemic lupus erythematosus but are more diagnostic of systemic sclerosis.

The histologic sections of morphea cannot be differentiated from those of diffuse scleroderma. The principal changes involve the collagenous fibers, which become hypertrophied through edema and then atrophy. The atrophic fibers are no longer loosely disposed as in the normal dermis but are compressed into dense, compact, collagenous masses, with diminution of fibrocytic nuclei and obliteration of spaces between collagenous bundles so that the thickness of the dermis is visibly decreased (Fig. 42-19). Inflammatory reaction tends to be absent, except in the early stages, when focal collections of mononuclear cells may be disposed about appendages. The appendages (hair, sweat glands, and sebaceous glands) are atrophic. Elastic fibers may be diminished or distorted, but they represent the least informative alteration and are unduly emphasized in the literature. The epidermis may be normal, but usually it is atrophic, with flattened rete ridges and a hyperpigmented basal layer. Subepidermal melanin-containing chromatophores may be increased. In conjunction with the collagenous change, small arteries and arterioles may become secondarily sclerotic. Calcific or even ossified foci (osteoma cutis) may replace the altered collagen of the dermis and subcutaneous septa. The deposits of calcium may be so extensive as to camouflage the primary diagnosis and be dismissed as "calcinosis." Superficial dermal telangiectasia is common, possibly as a consequence of sclerosis of deeper vessels.

Atrophic myositis may accompany the cutaneous lesions, although uncommonly to the degree found in *dermatomyositis* or *poikilodermatomyositis,* in which the inflammatory reaction in the skeletal muscles may be extreme, despite the usual nondescript subepidermal edema and focal liquefaction degeneration in the latter diseases. Here, again, it is emphasized that neither *diffuse* vascular nor *diffuse* visceral collagenous changes occur in dermatomyositis or poikilodermatomyositis any more than they do in the majority of cases of diffuse lupus erythematosus.

In view of the association between sclerosis of skin and lung (systemic sclerosis, burns, healed infarcts, etc.) on the one hand and carcinoma on the other, it may be anticipated that carcinoma of the skin would be a

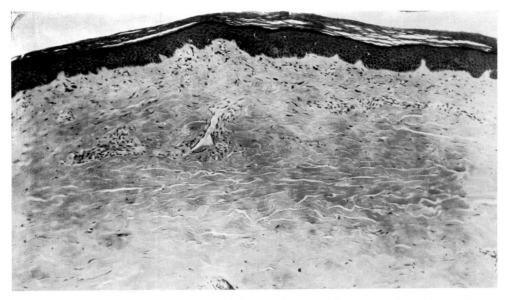

Fig. 42-19. Scleroderma with dense and thickened dermal fibers, atrophy of appendages and epidermis, and melanin pigmentation of basal layer. (Hematoxylin and eosin.)

complication of diffuse scleroderma. This latter association is rare and may, perhaps, be a reflection of the duration of the sclerosis.

Scleredema. Scleredema (Buschke's disease) is to be distinguished from scleroderma. Although the entity is commonly known as *scleredema adultorum,* it does involve children in an appreciable percentage of cases.

Scleredema is usually a self-limited disease characterized by a tough, nonpitting, uniform edema of the head and neck, producing a masklike expression and restricted motion that simulates scleroderma. The periphery of the process is readily palpable. The disease generally runs its course in from several months to a year and a half, leaving no residuum. Recurrences have been recorded.

The lesion differs from scleroderma in the absence of pigmentation, the rarity of involvement of the hands and feet, and complete resolution with rarest exceptions. The usually self-limited scleredema of Buschke is distinguished from the long-lasting, often extensive scleredema associated with diabetes mellitus.

The histologic picture of scleredema is that of striking edema and hypertrophy of tight collagenous bundles so that, despite the compactness of the bundles, the thickness of the dermis is distinctly increased over normal. The epidermis, vessels, elastic tissue, and muscle show no changes. The changes of *sclerema neonatorum* are altogether different from scleredema or scleroderma and consist of the

precipitation of fatty acid crystals and foreign body reaction in the subcutaneous fat, possibly because of a deficiency of olein in the fat, with consequent raising of its melting point. The localized, nodular sclerema, which some believe may result from birth trauma, is also self-limited. The diffuse form, which may involve also visceral (e.g., periadrenal and perirenal) fat, is a fatal disease. Scleredema and scleroderma are to be differentiated also from *myxedema* of either the circumscribed or the diffuse type.

Lipid proteinosis. Lipid proteinosis *(hyalinosis cutis et mucosae)* is another remarkable disease affecting dermal collagen and its vessels. The disorder generally manifests itself in infancy and is characterized by verrucous yellowish plaques, especially on the hands, feet, elbows, and face. The lesions may involve also the mouth and larynx. In the latter location, the woody consistency of the lesions may cause a stenosis severe enough to require tracheotomy. Persistant hoarseness is a common symptom. Disturbances in phospholipids are inconstant. A familial tendency toward diabetes mellitus is occasionally present. It does not now appear that the entity is a primary lipidosis but rather that the lipid is normal in composition incidental to other tissue changes, especially those of collagen. One form of lipid proteinosis is light sensitive and occurs with erythropoietic porphyria.

The histologic features of lipid proteinosis

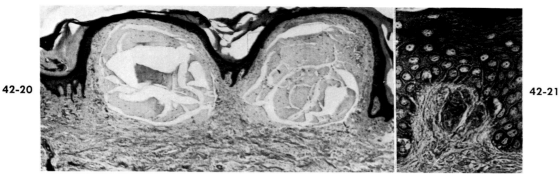

42-20

42-21

Fig. 42-20. Colloid milium with characteristic nodules of altered collagen. (Hematoxylin and eosin.)
Fig. 42-21. Amyloidosis showing metachromatic focus in papilla. (Toluidine blue stain.)

are a hyperkeratotic and acanthotic epidermis overlying eosinophilic homogenized collagen in the upper dermis. The walls of arterioles and small arteries of this region are thickened. A fat stain reveals dense sudanophilic deposits in and about their walls, as well as in the stroma. No foam cells are present such as are found in *Fabry's disease (angiokeratoma corporis diffusum)*. The serum lipids are normal, as a rule. It is stated that the fat is combined with the protein of the collagen and therefore resists ordinary fat solvents. This property was not borne out in two cases personally observed. As might be expected, the hyalinized collagen is PAS-positive and diastase-resistant. Accordingly, the entity has been designated a "lipoglycoproteinosis."

Amyloidosis. Amyloidosis may be confined to the skin, or the cutaneous lesions may represent part of a systemic process. The eruption is characterized by pruritus and brownish papules, nodules, or plaques, occurring particularly on the legs. Histologically, there are focal areas of bland homogenization of dense collagen, occasionally scattered in the dermis but often located as subepidermal round masses (lichen amyloidosis) that stain metachromatically with the ordinary stains for amyloid.

The subepidermal nodules of amyloidosis *(lichen amyloidosis)* tend to be restricted to the skin. The nodular, para-articular masses of amyloid, along with amyloidotic macroglossia, are likely to be a manifestation of primary amyloidosis (para-amyloidosis) and to be associated with myeloma or related plasmocytosis and globulinemias. The cutaneous manifestations of amyloidosis secondary to leprosy, tuberculosis, rheumatoid arthritis, Hodgkin's disease, chronic suppuration, etc. may be detectable only microscopically. The amyloid of primary amyloidosis tends to resist metachromatic stains in contrast with amyloid of secondary amyloidosis. Rarely, epidermolysis bullosa may overlay secondary amyloidosis of the skin.

The histologic picture of lichen amyloidosis may closely simulate *colloid milium,* in which, too, there is a homogeneous alteration, with swelling into nodular masses of the subepidermal collagen (Fig. 42-20). However, the collagen of colloid milium does not stain metachromatically, and, in addition, the fibers in this disease appear looser, more edematous, and more friable than do those of amyloidosis (Fig. 42-21).

Clinically, colloid milium appears as small translucent papules from 1 to 5 mm in diameter, occurring commonly on the exposed areas, particularly the face, of fair-skinned individuals, more commonly men.

Circumscribed myxedema. Circumscribed or localized myxedema occurs in association with exophthalmic Graves' disease. It appears as a fairly demarcated nonpitting, solidly edematous, usually bilateral plaque of the pretibial region, at times extending to the dorsa of the feet.

Persistently elevated serum levels of "long-acting" thyroid stimulator (LATS) are the rule in patients with pretibial myxedema. In some instances, LATS has been detected in homogenates of tissue from the affected areas in concentrations significantly higher than in unaffected tissue. It is hypothesized that LATS acts as a specific antibody that, when fixed in tissue, elicits the characteristic local edematous reaction (see also p. 1638).

Histologically, abundant basophilic mucin is found separating and fragmenting dermal collagenous bundles, without inflammatory reaction other than an occasional increase of mast cells. The diffuse myxedema of hypothyroidism is characterized by swelling of the collagenous bundles by interfibrillary mucin, which, in some instances, is demonstrable with alcian or toluidine blue. There is less disruption of the collagenous bundles in diffuse myxedema than in circumscribed myxedema of hyperthyroidism. These lesions are to be distinguished from the nonendocrinogenic subepidermal mucinous papules of *lichen myxedematosis* or *papular mucinosis*.

Mucinous cysts

Mucinous dermal cysts, often loosely referred to as "synovial cysts" or "myxoid cysts," are seen as single, smooth, and firm 5 to 6 mm nodules at the bases of distal phalanges. The overlying epidermis is likely to be slightly thinned but not otherwise significantly altered. The cyst contains a mucinous, clear material quite like that of synovial cysts, and the similarity extends to the histologic structure. The mucin is PAS-negative but contains large amounts of hyaluronic acid as reflected in the positive alcian blue stain. There is no communication of these cysts with bursae or joint cavities.

Microscopically, the cyst is found to be unilocular or multilocular and to be derived from a simple liquefaction of the dermal collagen so that no mesothelial or endothelial lining is present. Such a lining may be simulated by compressed fibrocytes of the dermal collagenous fibers. Essentially, this picture is analogous to that found in what are also loosely called synovial cysts of tendons or ganglions. These, too, do not represent cysts of expanded synovial walls with mesothelial lining but, rather, foci of mucinous degeneration of collagen of tendon or synovia. The mucinous dermal cyst may become obliterated by fibrosis and calcification.

Diseases of elastic tissue

Although alterations in elastic tissue, especially diminution and fraying, occur in many dermatoses, there are several principal, primary disorders of elastic tissue: (1) cutis hyperelastica (Ehlers-Danlos syndrome), (2) pseudoxanthoma elasticum, (3) senile elastosis, (4) elastoma dorsi, (5) elastosis perforans serpiginosa, and (6) dermatolysis (cutis laxa).

Cutis hyperelastica. Cutis hyperelastica (Ehlers-Danlos syndrome) is a familial disease characterized by hyperelastic velvety skin ("rubber skin") associated with hyperlaxity and hyperextensibility of the joints and the

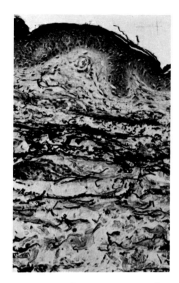

Fig. 42-22. Hyperelastosis cutis. (Weigert–van Gieson.)

tendency of the skin to bleed, tear, and scar after slight trauma. The disorder may be associated with skeletal deformities, including arachnodactyly, blue scleras (as in *Löbstein's syndrome*), dilatation of viscera (trachea, esophagus, and colon), pulmonary blebs, dissecting aneurysms, etc.

Histologically, abundant compact masses of elastic fibers throughout the dermis are demonstrable by Weigert's stain for elastic tissue (Fig. 42-22). The suggestion that the increase in elastic fibers is illusionary rather than real is not borne out by personal observations. There appears to be no qualitative alteration in these or in the collagenous fibers. The tendency for calcification, as observed in elastic fibers in pseudoxanthoma elasticum and in degenerative arterial diseases, is not apparent in the elastic fibers of Ehlers-Danlos syndrome. Edema of the superficial dermis, with disruption of the normal wavy pattern of the dermal collagenous fibers, may be observed. On the other hand, calcification within the panniculus may be present.

Pseudoxanthoma elasticum. Pseudoxanthoma elasticum is another hereditary disease in which yellowish papules and plaques symmetrically distributed are found in abnormally lax skin of the neck, axilla, groin, and cubital and popliteal spaces. Other parts of the body are less frequently involved.

In histologic sections, the elastic fibers are easily detectable, even in routine preparations stained with hematoxylin and eosin, as masses of basophilic, curved, small, partially calcified, fragmented curlicues, with a tendency toward concentration near the mid-dermis. Occasionally, there are associated disheveled, foreign body type of granulomas. In about 50% of the patients with pseudoxanthoma elasticum there occur ophthalmoscopically visible "angioid streaks" in the retina that are said to be similar to the dermal changes histologically and are attributed to cracking of Bruch's elastic membrane of the choroid. The histologic evidence, however, is limited.

Ultrastructurally, an elastic fiber appears as a central amorphous core of elastin surrounded by microfibrils. Abnormal fibers show changes in size, shape, and granularity. The presence of calcium and polyanions such as sulfates or pyrophosphates is reported.

Pseudoxanthoma elasticum may be associated with changes in the cardiovascular system, including arterial aneurysms and calcification and degeneration of elastic tissue of arteries. Other congenital cardiovascular, gastrointestinal, and genitourinary defects may occur with the syndrome. Rarely, it is associated with cutis hyperelastica and with osteitis deformans.

Senile elastosis. Senile elastosis is the term used to describe the loss of elasticity of the skin of elderly people, as noted particularly on the face and the dorsum of the hands (i.e., the exposed portions of the body). This condition is found associated also with epidermal neoplasms, discoid lupus erythematosus, radiodermatitis, and other diseases. In microscopic sections, the change is represented by a subpapillary zone of basophilic alteration of swollen elastic fibers.

This form of elastosis may or may not be associated with atrophy of the epidermis and appendages (Fig. 42-23). It is of interest that, notwithstanding the increase in elastic tissue, such skin is characterized by a loss of elasticity as if the physical properties of these fibers had been altered or as if collagenous fibers had acquired the staining properties of elastic tissue.

Elastofibroma dorsi. Elastofibroma dorsi refers to an apparently reactive fibrous tumefaction that is localized preponderantly to the scapula but occurring also near the ischial tuberosity and greater trochanter, is firm, varies in size from about 2 to 10 cm, and develops over a period of years. The surprising histologic finding is the presence of numerous clusters of thick and fragmented elastic fibers, readily recognizable by their eosinophilia even

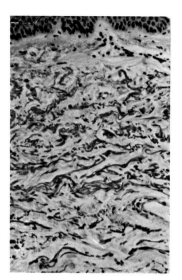

Fig. 42-23. Senile elastosis. (Hematoxylin and eosin.)

in sections stained with hematoxylin and eosin. Although these fibers lack the periodicity of collagen and are digested with elastase, there are reasons to suggest origin from denatured collagen. These fibers, which do not contain fat or calcium, exhibit differences from those of the elastic laminae of arteries, elastotic degeneration of the skin, and pseudoxanthoma elasticum.

Elastofibroma dorsi is to be distinguished from the familial fibromas or "collagenomas" recently described, in which no change in the elastic tissue was noted.

Elastosis perforans serpiginosa. There is a group of disorders that have in common the gross and histologic feature of transepidermal extrusion of plugs of keratin, collagen, and elastic tissue. These entities, which are commonly mistaken for each other, are known as reactive perforating collagenosis (RPC), perforating folliculitis, elastosis perforans serpiginosa, and Kyrle's disease. Elastosis perforans serpiginosa is characterized by groups of arciform or circinate, erythematous, acuminate keratotic papules, usually on the face and neck and has been noted to develop after long courses of penicillamine therapy.

The histology is made diagnostic by the compact packets of curled, frayed, thickened basophilic elastic fibers over which the epidermis is acanthotic and hyperkeratotic. The papule or plug is attributable chiefly to the penetration and extrusion of masses of elastic fibers through the epidermis. Lymphocytes and foreign body type of giant cells surround the lesion. The pattern simulates that of Kyrle's disease (hyperkeratosis follicularis in cutem penetrans), in which the extruded plugs are keratinous rather than elastic tissue. Further, in Kyrle's disease, the parakeratotic plug penetrates the dermis through invaginated epidermis. The lesion is not confined to follicles, is not accompanied by pseudoepitheliomatous hyperplasia, and may show a giant cell granulomatous reaction.

Specific granulomas

Of the specific granulomas of the skin, the following should be mentioned: those caused by tuberculosis, sarcoidosis, berylliosis, leprosy, brucellosis, leishmaniasis, syphilis, and granuloma inguinale, granulomas caused by atypical acid-fast bacilli, and those from deep fungi, such as sporotrichosis, blastomycosis, coccidioidomycosis, and histoplasmosis.

Tuberculosis cutis. Tuberculosis cutis may assume a large variety of clinical forms of which lupus vulgaris, scrofuloderma, tuberculosis cutis verrucosa, miliary cutaneous tuberculosis, and many kinds of tuberculids are a few examples. Although differing prognostic implications usually make the precise diagnosis of tuberculosis of significance, the important service the pathologist is expected to render is to name the overall tuberculous process. In this, the problem is complicated by the difficulty with which the sparse tubercle bacilli are demonstrable in paraffin sections of the skin, so that the tubercle is usually the chief basis for the diagnosis. Unfortunately, many agents other than tubercle bacilli are capable of producing tubercles. Moreover, the tubercle often is incompletely formed, and reliance is then placed on such suggestions as epithelioid cells clustered or palisaded in the vicinity or in a matrix of caseated tissue, with or without giant cells. The cutaneous reaction of leishmaniasis, as well as of histoplasmosis and other fungi, is often tuberculoid, but the detection of the respective organisms in histiocytes and giant cells establishes the diagnosis.

Of increasing interest are the cutaneous granulomas produced by "atypical" acid-fast bacilli or, more accurately, bacilli that, although acid-fast, are basically different in drug sensitivity as well as in cultural and pathogenetic respects from *Mycobacterium tuberculosis.* Runyon's classification of these strains into four groups—photochromogens (e.g., *Mycobacterium balnei*), scotochromogens, Battey strain, and "rapid growers"—is a workable

one. Not all of the granulomas produced by these organisms have a tuberculoid structure histologically. Some appear quite nonspecific.

Sarcoidosis. The histologic diagnosis of *Boeck's sarcoid* is made on the finding of dermal hyperplastic tubercles, with or without giant cells and Schaumann's or asteroid bodies but in the absence of caseation. Usually, the tubercules are surrounded by dense bands of collagenous stroma. No tubercle bacilli are detectable. The term *Darier-Roussy sarcoid* is reserved for an essentially similar histologic process occurring in the deep dermis and subcutaneous fat, thereby resembling erythema induratum. Confusion arises from the simulation of the tuberculous process by the tissue reaction in the tuberculoid form of leprosy, in the syphilitic gumma, and by the tissue response in blastomycosis, coccidioidomycosis, leishmaniasis, and sporotrichosis. Moreover, in some instances of sarcoid, a form of fibrinoid degeneration simulating caseation may occur (p. 1101).

Sarcoidosis responds well to cortisone. A diagnostic test for sarcoidosis, called the *Kveim test,* consists of injecting intradermally a brei of tissue known to be involved with Boeck's sarcoid and observing the delayed clinical and histologic reaction to the injection several weeks later.

Berylliosis and brucellosis. The granulomas of berylliosis (usually acquired by inoculation of the beryllium phosphors from broken fluorescent lamps) and those of *brucellosis* may be histologically indistinguishable from those of sarcoidosis or tuberculosis. Silica granulomas are distinguished by the presence of birefringent silica crystals within giant cells. Zirconium in stick deodorants may also cause giant cell granulomas.

Other granulomas. The remainder of the granulomatous lesions, including those of leprosy, syphilis and other venereal diseases, the deep mycoses and parasitic infestation, etc., are discussed in other chapters.

PIGMENTATIONS

The abnormalities of cutaneous pigmentation may be considered under two principal categories: metallic and nonmetallic.

Metallic abnormalities of cutaneous pigmentation

The exogenous pigmentations are chiefly those from metals introduced into the body in a variety of ways, including ingestion, parenteral administration, inunction, and intradermal injection. In general, the metallic pigmentations provoke at least an increased deposition of melanin in the basal layer and in dermal chromatophores. The brown **arsenic pigmentation** caused by the ingestion of, particularly, trivalent arsenicals (in Fowler's solution, sodium cacodylate, or arsenic trioxide) often is associated with keratosis of the palms and soles. Histologically, there is relative hyperkeratosis with atrophy of the remainder of the epidermis, hyperchromatism, and a tendency toward palisading of the basal cells and increased melanin deposits in these cells as well as in the chromatophores of the upper dermis, which usually is edematous. Late complications include Bowen's disease and squamous and basal cell carcinomas.

Argyria, in which the skin is discolored bluish gray, may occur after the ingestion of silver nitrate, formerly used in the treatment of peptic ulcers, or the application of this drug as well as colloidal silver compounds (Argyrol and Neo-Silvol) to mucous membranes. The pigmentation is particularly noticeable in those areas of the skin exposed to light. The black granules of silver are noted especially in the argyrophilic basement membrane of the sweat glands but also in the connective tissue about sebaceous glands and hair follicles and just beneath the epidermis.

Chrysiasis, from the parenteral use of gold preparations, as in the treatment of chronic lupus erythematosus, causes an ash-gray or mauve pigmentation characterized histologically by irregular, large granules located chiefly in chromatophores and in the walls of blood vessels. A somewhat similar histologic picture is caused by pigmentation from **bismuth** and **mercury.**

In **tattoos,** the pigmentation is the result of the deposition of various metallic and vegetable pigments (e.g., cinnabar or red mercuric sulfide) both within chromatophores and extracellularly in irregularly large clumps sometimes surrounded by foreign body reaction (Fig. 42-24). Discoid lupus erythematosus may selectively involve the red areas of tattoos (mercuric sulfide) and spare the blue. Similarly, individuals sensitive to mercury may show allergic reactions in the red portions. Conversely, syphilitic lesions may spare these mercury-impregnated red components of tattoos.

Nonmetallic abnormalities of cutaneous pigmentation

The nonmetallic abnormalities of cutaneous pigmentation include those attributable to hemochromatosis, Addison's disease, pellagra, Peutz-Jeghers syndrome, acanthosis nigricans, chloasma, melanosis of Riehl, ephelides (freckles), sunburn, purpuras, tinea versicolor, and pinta. Several of these entities illustrate once again the cutaneous reflection of visceral disease.

In **hemochromatosis** (bronze diabetes), hemosiderin and, less noticeably, hemofuscin are deposited as brownish granules in melanophores principally and diagnostically about sweat glands. In addition, there is increased melanin in the epidermis and adjacent chromatophores. This cutaneous lesion is commonly associated with deposits of the pigments in the pancreas, liver, and lymph nodes and the development of diabetes mellitus and cirrhosis of the liver. The mostly deeply pigmented areas are the exposed surfaces but may include also the genital regions and mucous membranes in 10% to 15% of cases.

In **Wilson's disease** (hepatolenticular degeneration) the pigmentation takes the form of epidermal melanosis favoring the anterior portions of the legs.

In **Addison's disease,** there is an excessive deposit of melanin in the basal layer of the epidermis and in underlying melanophores. A similar histologic picture is found in the ordinary freckle (ephelis), sunburn, and chloasma (the latter especially during pregnancy).

Melanosis of Riehl, often associated with

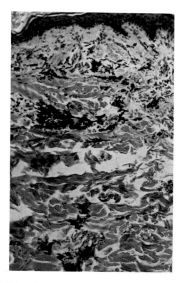

Fig. 42-24. Tattoo with irregular deposits of black-appearing pigment. (Hematoxylin and eosin.)

malnutrition, is characterized by brown macular discolorations of the face, neck, and, occasionally, hands. Histologically, there is irregular pigmentation by melanin of the basal layer and chromatophores, in addition to telangiectasis, varying degrees of hyperkeratosis, liquefaction degeneration of the basal layer, and partial obliteration of the rete ridges. A similar picture is seen in tar melanosis, the occupational dermatosis probably concerned with photosensitization.

The **Peutz-Jeghers syndrome** consists of melanosis of the lips, oral mucosa, and digits in patients with gastrointestinal polyposis and occasional carcinomas.

The association of dermatoses with intestinal disorders comprises a facet of dermatology that is as intriguing as it is puzzling. A partial list of such dermatoses includes, in addition to the Peutz-Jeghers syndrome, acrodermatitis enteropathica, dermatitis herpetiformis, Fabry's disease, and pyoderma gangrenosum (with idiopathic ulcerative colitis, systemic lupus erythematosus, and systemic sclerosis). In some of the diseases, the nature of the relationship is clear but variable for obvious reasons; in others, the connection is enigmatic.

Increased pigmentation of the skin follows a variety of cutaneous purpuras: **purpura annularis telangiectodes** (Majocchi's disease), **Schamberg's disease,** and **pigmented purpuric lichenoid dermatitis** of Gougerot and Blum. Each of these disorders occurs selectively on the lower extremities. The pigment in these cases is hemosiderin, which is deposited in chromatophores in the upper dermis. **Angioma serpiginosum,** which is also rather loosely included in the category of cutaneous purpuras, is really an inflammatory telangiectasia and usually shows little or no hemosiderin. In all of these "purpuras," which are unassociated with systemic disorders, there are inflammatory cells (principally lymphocytes and histiocytes) localized in the upper dermis, especially about arterioles and capillaries, which may have swollen and prominent endothelium. This latter finding is particularly true of Majocchi's disease. There is some question as to whether these conditions are actually different phases of the same basic vascular disease. Occasionally, these purpuric lesions, particularly those of *Majocchi's disease,* may be confused histologically with the vascular changes of **periarteritis nodosa** or bacterial and rickettsial arteritis. The changes of **thrombophlebitis migrans** and of **thromboangiitis obliterans** are discussed elsewhere (p. 1870).

Achromia should be mentioned among the abnormalities of cutaneous pigmentation. The congenital absence of pigment is referred to as partial or complete albinism or leukoderma. **Vitiligo** or acquired leukoderma is usually of unknown etiology. The depigmented patches may be rimmed by hyperpigmented borders, and the histologic sections reveal the depigmented and hyperpigmented basal layers in the respective portions. Vitiliginous areas may occur also in any lesion in which there are considerable liquefaction degeneration of the basal layer and encroachment onto this layer by inflammatory cells. *Pinta* and *lichen planus* are cases in point. In both, the melanin is extracted from the basal layer, phagocytized by chromatophores, and carried away to regional lymph nodes. Vitiliginous patches occur in patients with tinea versicolor, partly because the areas affected by the fungus prevent absorption of ultraviolet irradiation and partly because the fungus itself actively causes a degree of depigmentation. In skin that has been planed for scars of acne, there is a tendency for the unabraded skin to become hyperpigmented and for the abraded epidermis to regenerate with less pigmentation than the original.

DISEASES OF APPENDAGES

Limitations of space permit no more than the briefest mention of the nonneoplastic diseases of the cutaneous appendages.

Sweat glands

The disorders of the sweat glands include hyperhidrosis, congenital or acquired hypohidrosis, miliaria (prickly heat and tropical or thermogenic hypohidrosis with plugging of the sweat ducts by hydropic edematous epithelium), bromhidrosis (fetid sweat), chromhidrosis (colored sweat), hidradenitis suppurativa of the apocrine glands, and Fox-Fordyce disease (pruritic papular chronic adenitis of the sweat glands of the axillae, nipples, and pubic and perineal regions).

Sebaceous glands

The diseases of the sebaceous glands include varieties of seborrhea, hyposteatosis or diminished secretion, comedones, acne in its several forms, and rhinophyma.

Hair

The *abnormal conditions of the hair* are many. Hypertrichosis, the alopecias of the cicatricial types (pseudopelade, folliculitis de-

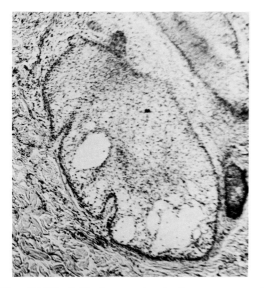

Fig. 42-25. Follicular mucinosis from a case of mycosis fungoides. (Hematoxylin and eosin.)

calvans, and chronic lupus erythematosus of the scalp) and the noncicatricial types (alopecia areata, ordinary male baldness, fungal infections, etc.), fragile hairs (fragilitas crinium), trichorrhexis nodosa, pili torti (twisted hairs), fungal infections such as piedra and trichomycosis nodosa, and trichostasis spinulosa (multiple lanugo hairs in a single follicle) constitute a few of the problems.

One of the more interesting disorders of hair follicles is called *alopecia mucinosa* or follicular mucinosis (Fig. 42-25).[50] It is characterized histologically initially by intracellular and subsequently extracellular mucin within the hair sheaths, perifollicular inflammatory cells, and loss of hair shafts. The mucin stains with alcian blue and is PAS-negative. The significant fact concerning this lesion is that in individuals over 40 years of age it represents strongly presumptive evidence of the early stage of mycosis fungoides.

Nails

The diseases of the nails are of particular interest not only for the involvement of the nails themselves but for the accessory information they reflect on systemic disorders. *Beau's lines* are transverse furrows in the nail that date periods of severe acute illnesses or of inflammations near the nail folds, leading to the arrest of function of the matrix.

The discoloration and the thickening of the nail from psoriasis, eczema, or fungi, the spoon nails *(koilonychia)* associated with trauma,

eczema, and the Plummer-Vinson syndrome, the brittleness (onychorrhexis) after the use of certain chemicals or in vitamin A deficiency, the loss of nails (onycholysis) after trauma or systemic diseases such as hypothyroidism, and the whitening of nails (leukonychia) represent some of the changes that affect the nails.

The *"yellow nail" syndrome* is associated with lymphedema and pleural effusions and, at times, with ascites. The nails not only are discolored yellow but show transverse ridging, oncholysis, curving, and defective cuticles.

PANNICULITIS

Several diseases of the subcutaneous fat simulate each other closely histologically but have different prognostic and etiologic implications: (1) erythema induratum (Bazin's disease), (2) nodular, nonsuppurative, febrile, relapsing panniculitis (Weber-Christian disease), (3) erythema nodosum, (4) nodular vasculitis, (5) erythema pernio (chilblain), and factitious panniculitis.

Erythema induratum. Erythema induratum appears as chronic, recurring, often ulcerated, bluish red nodosities (of the calves of the legs, particularly). The lesions generally are found in patients with frank tuberculosis elsewhere. Histologically, tubercles, as a rule of an incomplete or atypical variety, are found in the subcutaneous fat. Caseation may or may not be present. Fat necrosis and fat atrophy associated with nonspecific inflammation of the fibrous septa, fat, and lower dermis are present. Endarterial and endophlebitic inflammation and proliferation are seen commonly. Tubercle bacilli are rarely found in these lesions, although positive results have been reported from guinea pig inoculation of the tissue.

Subacute nodular migratory panniculitis. Subacute nodular migratory panniculitis, which may follow acute infections such as tonsillitis, appears similar to erythema induratum histologically.

Nodular, nonsuppurative, febrile, relapsing panniculitis (Weber-Christian disease). Nodular, nonsuppurative, febrile, relapsing, panniculitis is observed preponderantly in women and is characterized by bluish discoloration of the skin over firm subcutaneous nodules on the extremities and trunk, usually associated with otherwise unexplained fever. Isolated cases have responded to chemotherapy (sulfapyridine and penicillin). Fatalities have occurred in several cases, but autopsy findings were not especially enlightening except for the steatitis in the pretracheal, mediastinal, and retroperitoneal regions. The recently recorded instances of "mesenteric panniculitis" appear unrelated.

In sections of what are regarded as typical cases, the fat itself is infiltrated chiefly with lymphocytes and histiocytes, but the septa are relatively spared. Wucher atrophy of fat (replacement of atrophied fat by fat-laden histiocytes), foreign body giant cell reaction, and endophlebitis and endarteritis are also present. However, the septa, although relatively spared, often are infiltrated and edematous. Therefore, the involvement of the septa cannot be used as a criterion for excluding the possibility of Weber-Christian disease. If they are free, the evidence is considerable that the panniculitis belongs to this category.

Although "nonsuppurative" is included in the name of the entity, the fact is that sterile abscesses occasionally are noted along with cystic liquefaction necrosis and focal calcification. It has been suggested that Weber-Christian disease is of diverse etiology and in some instances is attributable to pancreatitis.

Erythema nodosum. Erythema nodosum occurs clinically as tender, pale red to livid blue nodules, principally on the anterior aspect of the lower extremities. These lesions, unlike those of erythema induratum, do not ulcerate, are transient, lasting only for several weeks on an average, and are not necessarily associated with a tuberculous process elsewhere. The disease may be one manifestation of a variety of unrelated infections, including coccidioidomycosis, leprosy, syphilis, viral diseases (e.g., measles, cat-scratch fever), and ringworm, or it may follow lymphomas, the ingestion of drugs, or the administration of a vaccine.

The histologic picture of erythema nodosum is much like that of erythema induratum with the addition that there is a greater tendency in erythema nodosum for nonspecific inflammation of the middle and lower dermis, which is practically spared in erythema induratum.

Nodular vasculitis. Nodular vasculitis occurs chiefly in older women and refers to the often recurrent nodosities that are more painful, are of shorter duration, and have less tendency to ulcerate than the lesions of erythema induratum.

The histologic picture of nodular vasculitis is the same as that of Bazin's disease.

Erythema pernio. Erythema pernio occurs usually on the hands and feet as tender, red, pruritic macules provoked by cold.

The histologic picture may closely simulate that of erythema induratum, as may the lesions produced in response to cold allergy.

Miscellaneous forms. Miscellaneous forms of panniculitis include those secondary to trauma, insulin injections, pancreatitis, allergic reactions (including those occurring after insect bites), angiitis, cold agglutinins, and sclerosing lipogranulomas.

Actually the sharp artificial segregation of the panniculitides characteristic of the bulk of the dermatologic literature appears unwarranted by the histologic evidence of transitional merging of supposedly definitive criteria. This statement of confluence of diagnosis applies particularly to acute and chronic erythema nodosum, erythema nodosum migrans, nodular vasculitis and, often, erythema induratum. This is so because tuberculoid or foreign body type of granulomas, phlebitis and arteritis, involvement or lack of involvement of septa or lobules, and the presence of microabscesses may characterize any of these entities. Otherwise, it is the weight given to one or other features, integrated with the clinical details, that leads to more informative diagnosis.

VASCULAR DISORDERS

There is a broad spectrum of vascular disorders in which the skin plays a prominent clinical and, at times, diagnostic, role. A few of these are mentioned in Chapter 21. Additional ones, with probable or clear-cut vascular involvement, include the cutaneous lesions of rheumatic fever, subacute bacterial endocarditis, typhus fevers, and other infections, Degos' syndrome, allergenic vasculitides, necrobiosis lipoidica diabeticorum, the vascular changes of diabetes mellitus and hypertension, granuloma annulare, rheumatoid granuloma, Mucha-Habermann disease, and the purpuric dermatoses.

Acute, often necrotizing arteriolitis with karyorrhexis of polymorphonuclear neutrophil leukocytes (leukocytoclasis), deposition of immune complexes, hypocomplementemia, cryoglobulinemia, and arthralgia have been linked as a syndrome. Immunoglobulins and complement were demonstrable in the vessels of the skin prior to the infiltration of leukocytes and the development of clinical lesions.[58] Moreover, IgA has been demonstrated in the acutely inflamed dermal arterioles in purpuric hyperglobulinemia of Waldenström. This local finding was associated with elevated circulating levels of IgA and suggests the immunologic pathogenesis.

Immunofluorescent studies of dermal vasculitis promise diagnostic and pathogenetic clues. At present, IgG, IgM, IgA, and several

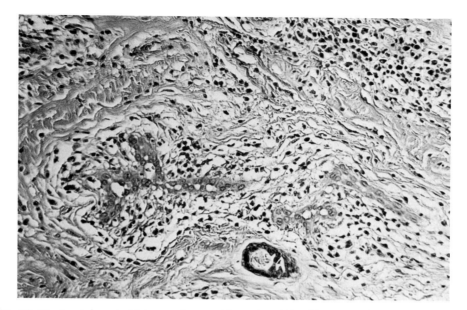

Fig. 42-26. Angiolymphoid hyperplasia with eosinophilia (Kimura's disease). Prominence of endothelium is evident. (Hematoxylin and eosin.)

components of complement have been demonstrated in and about vessels (e.g., in Henoch-Schönlein purpura), but their full significance remains to be determined.

Angiolymphoid hyperplasia with eosinophilia (Kimura's disease)

The lesion termed "angiolymphoid hyperplasia with eosinophilia" starts usually as a papule or a cluster of papules in the skin of the head and neck of adults. This lesion is as extraordinary in its behavior as it is in its histology. On occasion, the lesions may recur after excision or may spread uncontrollably to cover much of the face after the manner of a fulminant angiosarcoma. Histologically, the characteristic features include dilated dermal thin-walled vascular sprouts with conspicuously hypertrophic practically diagnostic endothelial cells with vesicular nuclei and abundant eosinophilic cytoplasm (Fig. 42-26). Often the endothelial cells appear clustered beside or at one end of a vessel that has been cut obliquely and in this pattern simulate masses of histiocytes. The stroma also is characteristically structured with loosely disposed eosinophilic leukocytes, histiocytes, lymphocytes, and mast cells. These cells are strongly positive for ATPase, indoxyl esterase, and nicotinamide adenine dinucleotide and negative for alkaline phosphatase, a pattern characteristic of endothelial cells.[20]

A form of superficial, subcutaneous thrombophlebitis known as **Mondor's disease** is characterized clinically by a linear, cordlike induration with an overlying cutaneous groove extending usually from the axilla toward the nipple. The lesion may be mistaken for a neoplasm clinically.

Thrombocytopenic verrucal angionecrosis (thrombotic thrombocytopenic purpura, TTP)

Of great interest is another truly diffuse vascular disease characterized by thrombocytopenia, purpura, a usually fulminant, fatal course (although rare protracted cases have occurred), and a specific histologic picture of fibrinoid necrosis and platelet-like *verrucal* thickening of the walls of dilated arterioles and capillaries. In the past, the disease has been called generalized platelet thrombosis or some variant of this term. However, the histogenesis of the entire lesion from the vascular walls would seem to make the designation "thrombocytopenic verrucal angionecrosis" more appropriate as was long ago suggested.[1] These cases are rarely diagnosed clinically. Inasmuch as the vascular necrosis occurs in the skin as well as the viscera, a skin or muscle biopsy is called for in obscure instances of thrombocytopenic purpura. There is strongly suggestive clinical and histologic evidence of a factor of hypersensitivity in this primarily diffuse vascular disease. Accordingly, we should attribute the thrombocytopenia to an allergic response rather than to depletion by so-called generalized thrombosis, which, as already indicated, and despite certain immunofluorescence studies, does not occur, as previously indicated.[1]

In our judgment, a somewhat obverse phenomenon exists in the syndrome called "disseminated intravascular coagulation" (DIC). Here, the coagulating factors normally residing in the blood are assumed to be depleted therefrom by universally distributed clots in small vessels. The *widespread* presence of such clots has simply not been documented.

XANTHOSES

The xanthoses may be classified as follows:

1. Normolipemic
   a. Juvenile xanthoma (or xanthogranuloma)
   b. Xanthoma disseminatum
2. Hyperlipemic
   a. Xanthoma diabeticorum
   b. Xanthoma tuberosum multiplex (Fig. 42-27)
   c. Xanthoma eruptiva (in association with lipid nephrosis, von Gierke's disease, diabetes mellitus, biliary cirrhosis, hypothyroidism, idiopathic hyperlipemia)
   d. Xanthelasma (± 50% with hyperlipemia) (Fig. 42-28)
   e. Xanthoma planum (± 50% with hyperlipemia) (in association with biliary cirrhosis, diabetes mellitus, myeloma and other dysproteinemias)

Other dermatoses characterized by the presence of lipid include lipid proteinosis, angiokeratoma of Fabry, necrobiosis lipoidica diabeticorum, lipid dermatoarthritis (reticulohistiocytoma), Hand-Schüller-Christian disease, Niemann-Pick disease, and Gaucher's disease. These are described elsewhere in this book.

Many of the lesions included in this classification are often classified with neoplasms. Actually, none is really a neoplasm in the usual sense of neoplasia. Most are obviously a reflection of disordered metabolism of lipids or lipoproteins, but it would constitute no major contribution to hasten to discard the term "xanthoma." The differentiation of these various xanthoses is often important from the prognostic and therapeutic viewpoints, although in many instances the distinction cannot be made on the basis of histology alone. Moreover, several of these types of lesions often are combined in the same patient.

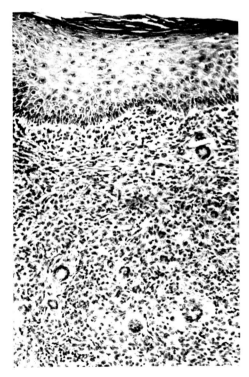

Fig. 42-27. Xanthoma tuberosum with numerous lipid histiocytes, some of which are congregated as Touton giant cells. (Hematoxylin and eosin.)

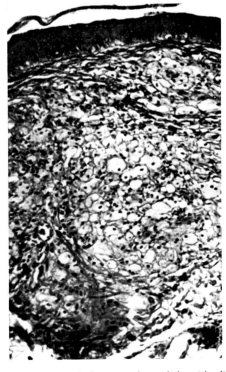

Fig. 42-28. Xanthelasma of eyelid with lipid-filled histiocytes. (Hematoxylin and eosin.)

RETICULOHISTIOCYTOMA
(RETICULOHISTIOCYTIC GRANULOMA)

The entity "reticulohistiocytoma," which was so named in 1948, produces remarkable lesions, the extent and nature of which are still being investigated.[8,10] Because of the association with arthritis, it has more recently been designated *lipid dermatoarthritis*.[8] Originally, this condition was believed to be limited to the skin and was regarded as a form of ganglioneuroma because of the superficial simulation of ganglion cells by the histiocytes.

Clinically, the disease is characterized by cutaneous papules and nodules (rarely solitary) and, often, by an associated disabling polyarthritis. The nodules may resemble xanthomas, and, indeed, xanthelasma is present in about one fourth of the patients.

Histologically, the cutaneous lesions are characterized by histiocytes with abundant basophilic cytoplasm intermingled with lymphocytes and occasionally scattered eosinophilic leukocytes (Fig. 42-29). The infiltrate tends to be confined to the upper dermis, with resulting moderate atrophy of the overlying epidermis. The cytoplasm of the histiocytes reacts positively with Sudan black B and PAS stains and is presumed to contain a glycolipid.

ANGIOLIPOMA

There are two types of angiolipomas: (1) noninfiltrating or encapsulated and (2) infiltrating. In both, there is likely to be associated pain or tenderness. The infiltrating angiolipomas tend to occur on the extremities and to ramify into the skeletal muscle. They may occur also in the spinal region and cause erosion of portions of vertebrae with resulting neurologic problems. Unlike liposarcomas, the infiltrating angiolipomas lack atypia of the fat cells. Fibrolipomas of infancy commonly show atypia.

"ATYPICAL FIBROXANTHOMA"

There has been considerable interest in the past few years in an ulceronodular lesion of the exposed skin (chiefly the ears and cheeks) of elderly people. The lesion has been called "atypical fibroxanthoma" and resembles an anaplastic sarcoma with spindle cells and multinucleated giant cells, as well as bizarre cells with single, large hyperchromatic nuclei, mitoses (often abnormal tripolar), and some intracellular lipid (Fig. 42-30). The striking feature is the disparity between the histologic anaplasia and the benign course in most instances. Some of these are undoubtedly nonpigmented spindle cell melanocarcinomas.

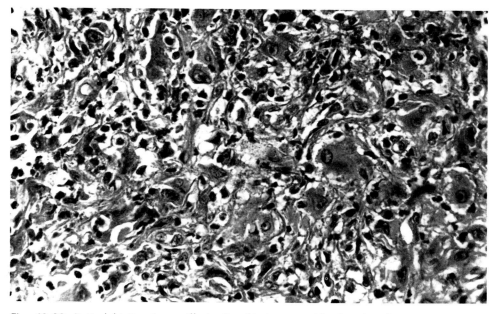

Fig. 42-29. Reticulohistiocytoma, illustrating histiocytes with abundant homogeneous cytoplasm loosely admixed with few lymphocytes and eosinophilic leukocytes. (Hematoxylin and eosin; from Allen, A. C.: The skin, ed. 2, New York, 1967, Grune & Stratton, Inc.; by permission.)

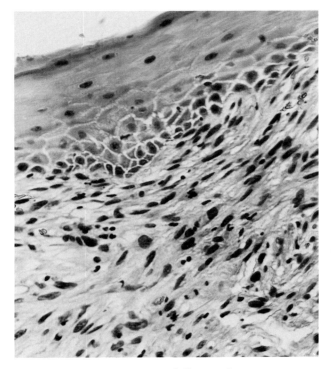

Fig. 42-30. Atypical fibroxanthoma.

One should note that fat may be present in melanocarcinomas.[1]

Although originally considered benign, instances of metastasis are accumulating. Undoubtedly more such instances will follow and, in my judgment, for the reason that they represent either spindle cell epidermoid carcinomas or malignant melanomas. The origin from the overlying epidermis may be easily missed, inasmuch as evidence is often obscure or minimal, yet pivotal, in spindle cell epidermoid carcinomas and melanocarcinomas.

NEOPLASMS OF SKIN

The following classification of neoplasms of the skin is based on the segregation of cutaneous neoplasms with respect to their location and histogenesis from epidermis, dermis proper, and appendages. In the ensuing discussion, several of the lesions are taken out of the order of the outline for purposes of clarity of presentation.

Epidermis

A. Benign
  1. Verruca (including vulgaris, digitata, filiformis, plantaris, and juvenilis)
  2. Seborrheic keratosis
  3. Condyloma acuminatum
  4. Keratoacanthoma
  5. Junctional nevus
B. Precancerous
  1. Senile keratosis
  2. Leukoplakia (with atypia)
  3. Xeroderma pigmentosum
  4. Bowen's disease
  5. Erythroplasia of Queyrat
C. Malignant
  1. Basal cell carcinoma
  2. Squamous cell carcinoma
  3. Melanocarcinoma (malignant melanoma)

Dermis

A. Nevus
  1. Intradermal nevus (common mole)
  2. Compound nevus (dermis and epidermis)
  3. Juvenile melanoma (dermis and epidermis)
  4. Blue nevus (Jadassohn-Tièche)
B. Tumors of vessels
  1. Lymphangioma
  2. Hemangioma
  3. Angiokeratoma (dermis and epidermis)
  4. Glomus tumor
  5. Hemangiopericytoma
  6. Kaposi's idiopathic hemorrhagic sarcoma
  7. Postmastectomy lymphangiosarcoma
  8. Sclerosing hemangioma (dermatofibroma lenticulare)
  9. Dermatofibrosarcoma protuberans
  10. Angiosarcoma
C. Fibroma and fibrosarcoma
D. Neurofibroma and neurofibrosarcoma
E. Tumors of muscle
  1. Leiomyoma (arrectores pilorum)

2. Angiomyoma
3. Myoblastoma (genesis?)
F. Osteoma
G. Xanthomas (discussed in previous section)
H. Lymphomas and allied diseases
I. Metastatic neoplasms

Appendages
A. Sweat glands
  1. Adenoma or epithelioma
    a. Ductal
    b. Glandular
  2. Carcinoma
B. Sebaceous glands
  1. Adenoma
  2. Carcinoma
C. Hair follicles
  1. Brooke's tumor—trichoepithelioma or epithelioma adenoides cysticum
D. Miscellaneous cysts
  1. Dermoid
  2. Epidermoid
  3. Pilosebaceous
  4. Calcifying epithelioma ("pilomatrixoma")

Benign lesions of epidermis
Verruca (wart)

The verrucae, or warts, represent thickenings or projections of epidermis to which are traditionally, if inconsistently, applied one of several adjectives in accordance with the shape, location, or other clinical feature of the lesion: verruca vulgaris, verruca plantaris, verruca digitata, verruca filiformis, verruca plana juvenilis, and verruca senilis.

The **verruca vulgaris** is the papillary wart common in children and found especially on the fingers, palms, and forearms. They occur singly or in groups. There is some question as to whether these tumors merit inclusion under "neoplasms," inasmuch as they may disappear spontaneously or, as in some reported cases, under psychotherapy, or with placebos. The possibility that these lesions are caused by viruses is still strongly considered and fortified by evidence from electron microscopy of viral particles. Wart-virus antibodies, measured by immunodiffusion and complement-fixation techniques are detectable in a high percentage of instances. The warts associated with complement-fixing antibodies seem to disappear more quickly than those with antibodies determined by immunodiffusion techniques. The titers of such antibodies as well as the effects of cell-mediated immunity may be factors in the "spontaneous" regression of warts.[52] The prevention and resolution of warts has been attributed also to cell-mediated immunity.[48]

Histologically, the verruca vulgaris is characterized by a papillary acanthosis surmounted by friable keratotic material. The cells of the stratum granulosum are often acidophilic and vacuolated. The basophilic intranuclear inclusions of the verrucae are related to the viral particles rather than the osmophilic intranuclear eosinophilic material, which is related to keratin. A loose infiltration of various mononuclear cells may be present in the papillae. Carcinomatous transformation of these lesions must occur rarely, if ever, although occasionally a verrucal form of senile keratosis or a squamous cell carcinoma with a prominent papillary hyperkeratotic surface is erroneously regarded as having arisen from a verruca vulgaris.

Oral florid papillomatosis comprises benign condylomatoid verrucal masses covering large portions of the buccal mucosa. These presumably are of viral origin.

An oral and genital lesion histologically similar to condyloma occurs with the entity called *dyskeratosis congenita*, which may be associated with a variety of ectodermal and mesodermal changes, including hyperpigmentation of the skin, reticulated poikilodermatous changes, dystrophic nails, deforming atrophic arthritic changes, dental dystrophies, cardiovascular changes, testicular atrophy, and hypersplenism.

Seborrheic keratosis

The *seborrheic keratosis* is labeled also *verruca senilis* or *pigmented papilloma*. The term "verruca senilis" is not well chosen, for the reason that the lesions often appear in young people and acanthosis is the feature of note. Seborrheic keratosis is used by the dermatologists and emphasizes the greasy feeling to the touch imparted by the abundant fatty keratinous nests within the lesion. These lesions occur particularly on the trunk and forehead and are usually dark brown, elevated, and sharply delimited. The sudden appearance of seborrheic keratoses, along with rapid increase in their size and number, may herald the presence of a visceral carcinoma, usually an adenocarcinoma. This phenomenon is known as the sign of Leser-Trélat.

The histologic picture is that of abruptly thickened epidermis that encloses nests of laminated keratin resulting from focal, irregular maturation of epidermis partially inverted within the core of the lesion. In places, the central pearls are incompletely developed and present large mature squamous cells without the keratinous nests. The surrounding cells are usually focally pigmented with fine brown granules of melanin and superficially resemble basal cells. However, close examination often reveals residual intercellular bridges that help identify them as squamous cells, notwithstanding statements to the contrary. Many of these *epithelial cells are dopa-positive.* In our judgment, the pigment is produced by the tumor cells (i.e., the keratoinocytes). Others assume, on evidence not easily acceptable, that the pigment is inoculated into the tumor cells by nonneoplastic melanocytes carried along with the tumor. This same judgment applies to the condylomatous, so-called melanoacanthoma. Rare cases of malignant transformation of the seborrheic keratosis have been recorded.[15] These have included basal cell carcinomas and malignant melanomas.[1,15] Of interest is the high concentrations of zinc in seborrheic keratoses and pigmented moles.[47]

A lesion that has many of the cellular characteristics of the verruca pigmentosum is the so-called inverted papilloma, which grows downward rather than outward from the epidermal surface. The "inverted papilloma" often is associated with an inflammatory reaction of mononuclear cells at its base, very much as are the senile keratoses (Fig. 42-31). The lesion referred to as "eccrine porotheli-oma" or "acrosyringoma" closely resembles the earliest stage of seborrheic keratosis. The *Degos* or *clear-cell acanthoma* also is reminiscent of an initial stage in the development of seborrheic keratosis. Glycogen is present in the clear cells.

Keratoacanthoma

The problem of pseudoepitheliomatous hyperplasia is directly related to the histologically difficult subject of so-called *self-healing squamous cell carcinomas,* also more or less equivalently labeled *molluscum sebaceum* and *molluscum pseudocarcinomatosum.* Most commonly, these occur in elderly males, although even adolescents may be affected, especially if there has been contact with oils. The lesions appear as single or multiple nodules that are smooth except for the characteristic umbilication of the central keratin. The nodules often regress spontaneously in about 2 months, leaving little or no scar. Recurrences have been recorded.

Histologically, as already implied, the nodules are not really carcinomas but, rather, coalescent comedones or keratinous masses with prominent pseudoepitheliomatous hyperplasia at their bases (see Fig. 42-33). Giant keratoacanthomas may become incredibly large, particularly on the face, and may recur after incomplete excision. The well-differenti-

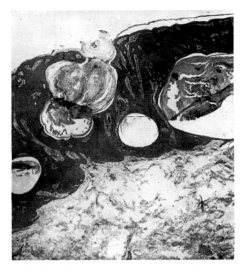

Fig. 42-31. Seborrheic keratosis. (Hematoxylin and eosin.)

ated, keratoacanthomatous pattern in the rapid recurrence supports the original diagnosis, although considerable self-confidence may be required to maintain it. An important clue is the absence of significant atypia in the epidermis at the margins of the keratoacanthomas.

Notwithstanding the occasional recurrences after incomplete removal, these lesions are benign. On the other hand, the attention that has been focused on keratoacanthomas has perforce led to misdiagnosis of squamous cell carcinomas as keratoacanthomas. An analogous problem exists in the erroneous diagnosis of melanocarcinomas as juvenile melanomas.

A variety of the lesion has been designated "generalized eruptive keratoacanthoma." These may be so numerous as to cover most of the body and involve even the oral mucosa.

It is becoming obvious from reports in the literature that prior confidence is being replaced by considerable uncertainty regarding the differential diagnosis between keratoacanthoma and verrucal, keratinizing squamous cell carcinoma. The reality of this diagnostic difficulty is expressed in both directions, i.e., unnecessarily radical surgical operations for giant keratoacanthomas, including leg amputation; and injudiciously delayed therapy for squamous cell carcinomas mistaken for keratoacanthomas.

Precancerous lesions

The precancerous lesions of the skin include senile keratosis, Bowen's disease, erythroplasia of Queyrat, and the *active* junctional nevus. Each of these entities is characterized by atypia or "dyskeratosis" of cells that, importantly, is confined to the limits of the epidermis. To such lesions the term "carcinoma in situ" is often applied. "Precancerous" as applied to these lesions connotes, in a crude measure, the relatively high degree of probability with which they are likely to undergo malignant degeneration rather than the inevitability of such a complication. *Kraurosis vulvae,* a term which has become unpopular in recent years, had been used diversely either in place of vulval lichen sclerosis et atrophicus, on the one hand, or as equivalent to epidermoid carcinoma in situ, on the other.

Senile keratosis

The senile keratoses are irregular brownish patches of epidermis roughened by horny scales, occurring characteristically on the dorsa of the hands of aged people. Histologically similar lesions may occur after irradiation and exposure to arsenic or to the elements of the weather. They may be single or several, or they may occur in great numbers over many parts of the body.

Microscopically, they are characterized chiefly by dyskeratosis of the cells of the basal layer and adjacent layers of the rete Malpighii. These cells show hyperchromatism, loss of polarity, increased numbers of mitotic figures, and irregularity of size and shape of nuclei. Hyperkeratosis and parakeratosis of varying degrees are responsible for the roughened surface. Inflammatory cells, principally mononuclear, are present in the subepidermal tissue. These cells often encroach onto the epidermis so as to obscure the integrity of the "basement membrane" and occasionally prompt the premature and erroneous impression of infiltrating carcinoma. The cutaneous horn in many instances represents a senile keratosis with an accumulation of keratinous material in the form of a projecting spur. The same type of horny projection may be superimposed also on verrucae.

Leukoplakia

Leukoplakia is a term that merits some discussion of its usage. As applied clinically, or grossly, it refers to whitish patches of mucosa that encompass not only cancerous or "precancerous" foci, but also those benign patches of mucosa thickened and whitened by mycoses, lichen planus, reaction to dentures, smoking, etc. Nevertheless, to many surgeons and pathologists (probably to most of them),

leukoplakia connotes a carcinoma in situ or a lesion morphologically approaching an intraepithelial carcinoma. The difficulty is that the diagnosis often is rendered as merely "leukoplakia" when the pathologist is not certain in his or her own mind that there is or is not sufficient atypia to warrant a designation of leukokeratosis or of carcinoma in situ. This is very much the situation with lesions of the cervix, when the diagnosis is hedged with such terms as "basal cell hyperplasia" or "dyskaryosis"—to the bewilderment of the clinician. Surely, there are instances in which the pathologist may not be certain of the malignant potential of such a "whitish patch," but it would appear more informative if this uncertainty were indicated rather than concealed euphemistically.

Xeroderma pigmentosum

Xeroderma pigmentosum is a potentially cancerous familial disease of the skin, usually first manifested early in childhood. It is characterized clinically by areas of atrophy, as well as isolated and coalescent scaly patches of keratosis showing varying amounts of pigmentation. A hyper-alpha-2-globulinemia has been found consistently in patients with xeroderma pigmentosum, and it has been hypothesized that this abnormality is related to ceruloplasmin.

Histologically, the changes in xeroderma pigmentosum are those of irregular atrophy, acanthosis, and hyperkeratosis, with excessive deposits of melanin in the basal layer and lowermost layers of the stratum spinosum, as well as in chromatophores in the upper dermis. Xeroderma pigmentosum may be complicated by junctional nevi, basal cell or squamous cell carcinomas, and melanocarcinomas.

The diagnosis of xeroderma pigmentosum may be established even before the characteristic cutaneous lesions appear, by estimation of the deoxyribonucleic acid excision repair level in cutaneous fibroblasts (after irradiation by ultraviolet light).[53] This defect in repair of DNA damaged by ultraviolet light has been detected prenatally by the use of amniotic cells cultured in vitro.[53]

Bowen's disease

Bowen's disease occurs as irregular, scaly, slowly progressive, usually brownish patches on the trunk, buttocks, and extremities. It was estimated that approximately one third of patients develop evidence of visceral cancer within 6 to 10 years after the initial diagnosis of Bowen's disease. Here again, what was regarded as a proved relationship a few years ago must now be considered moot on the basis of more recent analyses.[17]

Microscopically, the principal feature of the lesions is the presence of isolated dyskeratotic cells scattered haphazardly in all layers of the epidermis. These cells often have large, hyperchromatic single or double nuclei surrounded by cytoplasmic halos. Mitotic figures are numerous in these altered cells. Hyperkeratosis or parakeratosis may be pronounced. The acanthosis is usually uniform, but irregular thickening may be present.

Electron microscopic study of the dyskeratotic cells discloses displaced cytoplasmic fascicular aggregations of tonofilaments and separation of the desmosomal-tonofilament attachments. This desmosomal-tonofilament dissociation would be anticipated not only from the acantholytic appearance of Bowen's cells as seen under light microscopy, but also from the ultrastructural studies of acantholytic cells in other lesions such as Darier's disease, pemphigus vulgaris, etc.[21] In my judgment, as previously stated, a basically similar retraction of tonofilaments and loss of desmosomes occur in the conversion of keratinocytes to neval and melanocarcinomatous cells.

Erythroplasia of Queyrat

Erythroplasia of Queyrat is the precancerous lesion occurring principally on the glans penis but also on the vulva and on mucous membranes of the mouth.[34] In addition, the acanthotic thickening associated with erythroplasia is often characterized by long rete ridges that are psoriasiform or attached to each other in a reticulated pattern. A cytologic pattern somewhat similar to that of Bowen's disease occurs in the nipple and adjacent areas of the female breast in *Paget's disease*. However, unlike the lesions just described, Paget's disease is associated with carcinoma of the underlying mammary ducts. As indicated elsewhere, we find the evidence for the conclusion that so-called extramammary Paget's disease is associated with underlying adenocarcinoma of apocrine or eccrine glands somewhat less than convincing.[1] In my judgment, the majority of such lesions are pagetoid melanocarcinomas. The small group of remaining lesions includes epidermoid carcinomas and metastatic mucin-producing carcinomas, principally from the bowel and occasionally from other organs such as the ovaries.

The much emphasized presence of mucopolysaccharides within epidermal cells hardly precludes the possibility that they are keratinocytes. Among several kinds of evidence is the clear fact that under the influence of an excess of vitamin A, keratinocytes are modulated into mucus-secreting cells.[38]

Malignant lesions of epidermis

The malignant lesions of the epidermis include basal cell carcinoma, squamous cell carcinoma, Paget's disease, and melanocarcinoma.

Basal cell carcinoma

The term "carcinoma" is preferred to "epithelioma" in connection with the basal cell tumors that belong to the general group of rodent ulcers. If left untreated, these neoplasms will progress, erode, and infiltrate neighboring bone and cartilage in a manner that would seem to merit the designation "cancer" despite the infrequency of metastasis. Actually, over 50 instances of metastasizing basal cell carcinoma have been recorded.[23] The term "epithelioma" might best be reserved for the form of basal cell proliferation that does not show these invasive characteristics, i.e., the trichoepithelioma, otherwise known as epithelioma adenoides cysticum or Brooke's tumor (p. 1870).

Basal cell carcinomas occur predominantly in blond, fair-skinned people in the region of the face bounded by the hairline, ears, and upper lip. A tumor of the skin of the tip of the nose, however, is more likely to be a squamous carcinoma provided that it is not a keratoacanthoma. Basal cell tumors are not confined to the face, but may, in small numbers, occur in the skin of any part of the body, although there is a tendency to desmoplasia in those located away from the face. Squamous cell carcinomas of the anal canal, which are aggressive, particularly if they are located above the anal verge, may appear deceptively similar to basal cell carcinomas. Indeed, some of them are labeled "basaloid"—to the surgeon's confusion.

The basal cell carcinoma begins as a smooth, slightly elevated papule that may be scaly at first but tends soon to ulcerate centrally as the lesion spreads peripherally beneath the epidermis. Characteristically, the ulcer is rimmed by a waxy, smooth, firm, rolled border representing the intact epidermis, which is wrapped over but not yet invaded by the underlying and undermining neoplastic nests. If neglected, the tumor may advance to a grotesque erosion of large portions of the soft tissue, as well as the cartilage and bone of the face (Fig. 12-20). Early treatment by irradiation, excision, or the various other means of local destruction is usually adequate. The advantage of treatment of neoplasms by excision is that it then becomes possible to know by histologic examination not only the precise type of tumor present, but also whether the excised tumor is bounded by normal tissue.

Histologically, although there is considerable variability to the pattern of the basal cell carcinomas, there are sufficient characteristics in common so as to make them recognizable with relative ease. They are made up of nests of closely packed cells of uniform size and oval shape, with dark nuclei separated by a small amount of spineless cytoplasm. The nests often are rimmed by a single layer of similar cells arranged, however, in a neat radial pattern and strongly reminiscent of the more or less vertically arranged basal cells forming the lowermost layer of the normal epidermis or of the hair shafts. Mitotic figures are usually fairly common. Such nests may be observed arising not only from the basal portion of the epidermis, but also from the corresponding layer of the hair shaft or from both sources in the same tumor. The presence in these tumors of cells of the same type as those that line both the epidermis and the hair follicle would appear to account for the origin of these neoplasms from either of these structures. This is by no means equivalent to maintaining that embryonic rests of hair matrix, in one or another phase of its development, are the source of basal cell carcinomas. The basal cells of *adult* epidermis do have a limited range of reaction to *carcinogenic* stimulation. One major form such a reaction takes is the production of hair matrixes in the disheveled manner of a basal cell carcinoma, just as the basal cells in response to *normal* growth stimuli produce the orderly components of hair. In other words, when carcinogenic agents such as arsenic or x irradiation produce basal cell carcinomas, they do so not by activating embryonic rests of hair follicles but by provoking neoplastic change in previously normally situated *adult* basal cells. The origin of basal cell carcinomas from any part of the mature pilary complex is demonstrable also in the skin of rats to which anthramine and methylcholanthrene have been applied.

The histology of basal cell carcinomas may vary in the following ways:

1. By the presence of edematous stroma rimmed by neoplastic cells to form the *alveolar* or *cystic* type

2. By excessive, dense, hyalinized stroma between nests of basal cells to give the *morphea* type

3. By the presence of foci of squamous cells or pearls, occasionally calcified, in the centers of nests of basal cells

This last modification has been called *basosquamous cell* (transitional or metatypical cell) *carcinoma*. It is stated that the keratin produced by basal cell carcinomas differs from that produced by squamous cell carcinomas in the histochemically demonstrable presence of cystine ("hair follicle keratin") in the basal cell cancers. There is, in addition, the *comedo* type of basal cell carcinoma in which the cores of the masses of basal cells are necrotic.

In terms of prognosis, it has yet to be shown with any degree of credibility that there is any significant difference in these types. This matter is emphasized because of the general belief to the contrary. In particular, it is commonly stated that a basal cell carcinoma with areas of squamous cells represents a tumor with a more precarious prognosis than the ordinary basal cell carcinoma. This concept is based on the assumption that the squamous element of the neoplasm is prone to metastasize. This impression has no basis in fact.

Superficial epitheliomatosis, or multicentric basal cell carcinoma, is a special variety of the basal cell tumors. These lesions occur predominantly on the trunk either as dry and scaly or moist and eczematous, slowly enlarging plaques. Histologically, the lesions are small basal cell carcinomas arising from multiple foci in the basal layers of epidermis. The lesion is differentiated from the Jadassohn type of intraepidermal basal cell carcinoma, in which the neoplastic cells appear to be growing upward toward the surface from the basal cell layer instead of into the dermis. In the superficial lesions, as well as in other cutaneous "carcinomas in situ," arsenic should be suspected as a possible etiologic factor (Fig. 42-32).

The so-called premalignant fibroepithelial tumor is really part of the spectrum of variants of basal cell carcinomas and hardly merits such segregation.

In situ and, infrequently, superficially invasive basal cell carcinomas may complicate sclerosing angiomas.[35] The existence of these fairly innocuous lesions has been disputed, but in my judgment they are indistinguishable from "superficial epitheliomatosis" and we be-

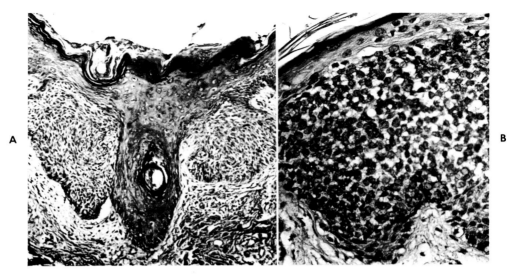

Fig. 42-32. A, Basal cell carcinoma (superficial epitheliomatosis, multicentric basal cell carcinoma). **B,** Intraepidermal basal cell carcinoma (Jadassohn type). (**A** and **B,** Hematoxylin and eosin.)

lieve would be so diagnosed if seen without the underlying angioma.

Basal cell nevus syndrome

Basal cell carcinomas, along with a variety of adnexal hamartomas, may occur as a congenital hereditary phenomenon known as the *basal cell nevus syndrome*. These lesions may vary from several on the face to hundreds on the trunk and extremities. The associated lesions or symptom complexes may include pseudohypoparathyroidism, ovarian fibromas, mesenteric cysts, dental cysts, bifid ribs, spina bifida, hypertelorism, broad nasal root, bridging of the sella turcica, calcification of the falx cerebri, and agenesis of the corpus callosum. Occasionally, granulomatous or ulcerative colitis may be present.

Isolated basal cell carcinomas in children occur more often than is generally suspected. As with the tumors of adults they are present chiefly on the face.[46]

Squamous cell carcinoma

The squamous cell carcinoma may occur in the skin of any part of the body, but there is a predilection for the exposed areas, particularly the face and hands. Certain sources of chronic irritation definitely predispose to squamous cell carcinoma. These include pipe smoking, particularly clay pipes, irritation to the scrotum as incurred by chimney sweeps, the exposure to arsenic, tar, and carcinogenic oils that soak the clothes and abdomen of the mule spinner (in textile industry), the constant contact of the abdomen with the small charcoal heaters causing the so-called kangri cancers observed in the Kashmir regions, the exposure of susceptible blond skins to actinic rays and other elements of the weather, the unexplained cancerous irritant that is present in old scars as from burns or osteomyelitis, the vague irritant of syphilitic leukoplakia, and a variety of others.

The sources of the arsenic include that used therapeutically (Fowler's solution, arsphenamine, etc.), orchard sprays, and contaminated water from artesian wells (e.g., of Taiwan). In the latter instance, the cutaneous manifestations may be endemic and include a broad spectrum comprising benign-appearing keratoses, keratoses with fronds or ridges of early basal cell carcinoma, multicentric in situ and invasive basal cell carcinomas, Bowen's disease in its many variations, epidermoid carcinomas, and combinations of any of these lesions. Scars after vaccination may be complicated infrequently by basal cell carcinomas, squamous cell carcinomas, and melanocarcinomas. The basal and squamous cell carcinomas tend to occur in individuals with the type of skin vulnerable to damage from exposure to ultraviolet light. However, in most instances of squamous cell carcinoma, the source of irritation or stimulation is not apparent.

Clinically, the lesion begins as a superficially scaly, slightly indurated area that bleeds, crusts, and resists casual therapy. With growth, the surface becomes ulcerated or hornified and the base indurated. The ulceration may extend to a deforming depth. The sectioned surface is granular and is grayish white flecked with yellow. Usually, the limits of the neoplasm may be determined even by gross inspection of the cut surface.

Microscopically, these carcinomas are characterized by irregular nests of epidermal cells that have infiltrated the dermis for varying depths. The nests of a squamous cell carcinoma may include cells representing any layer of the epidermis from the basal layer to the stratum corneum. In well-differentiated lesions, the intercellular spines and the central keratinous nests, or the "epithelial pearls," easily identify the origin of the tumor from squamous epithelium. In highly anaplastic lesions, these elements may be altogether lacking. Indeed, the anaplasia may be so extreme in occasional squamous cell carcinomas that they may be almost indistinguishable from spindle cell sarcomas. These spindle cell *carcinomas* almost always follow irradiation and are controlled with difficulty. They are not to be confused with the unimportant, focal areas of spindle cells occurring in many basal cell carcinomas or with the spindle cell melanocarcinomas. Another variety characterized by intercellular edema, particularly affecting the central cells of the neoplastic nests that are rimmed by basilar cells is occasionally mistaken for sebaceous or sweat gland carcinomas or even adamantinomas.

Often of greater practical importance than determining the precise type of carcinoma is the decision as to whether an isolated nest of cells represents actual carcinomatous invasion or is merely an obliquely cut rete ridge in an area of *pseudoepitheliomatous hyperplasia*. In some instances, the decision may be most difficult to make. However, the cells of a ridge in hyperplastic epidermis are quite differentiated and tend to resemble very closely the cells of the neighboring, obviously benign ridges and epidermis. The neighboring ridges—elongated, curved, and yet attached to the epidermis and cut perpendicularly—help to indicate that the isolated nest of cells actually represents an obliquely cut ridge rather than cancer. Another problem arises when abundant subepidermal inflammatory cells are present, some of which may have migrated across the "basement membrane" and lower epidermis, thereby obscuring the integrity of or even actually interrupting the "basement mem-

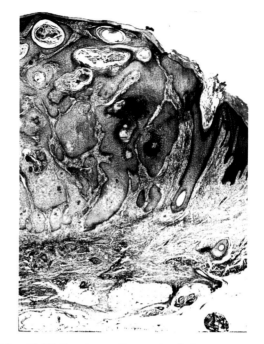

Fig. 42-33. Keratoacanthoma simulating squamous cell carcinoma. (Hematoxylin and eosin.)

brane." Since disruption of the basement membrane is one of the standard (if unreliable) criteria for provoking at least the suspicion of carcinoma, it becomes of some limited importance to judge, particularly by the anaplasia of the epidermal cells involved, whether or not the disruption is attributable merely to inflammation or to early cancer (Fig. 42-33).

The squamous cell carcinomas of the skin are, as a rule, not so anaplastic as the corresponding lesions of mucous membranes such as the lip or uterine cervix. Accordingly, metastases are considerably more common after squamous cell carcioma of the mucous membranes than of the skin. Although this difference is the rule, there are conspicuous exceptions. One of the most anaplastic squamous cell carcinomas of our experience occurred in a scar after a burn of the skin of the leg. The tumor metastasized widely to the viscera.

Effects of ionizing radiation on skin

Ionizing radiation is used therapeutically for a great variety of inflammatory diseases, including acne, psoriasis, eczema, and plantar warts. Such treatment is usually at least temporarily effective for the dermatosis, but sequelae in the form of acute and chronic radiodermatitis occur often enough to warrant serious concern. It is estimated that carcinomas complicate approximately 20% of instances of chronic radiodermatitis. This complication may occur over a wide span of years, from 3 to more than 50, with a median of 12 to 18 years. Because of the great time interval between the induction of therapy and the onset of complications, the frequency of such complications may be underestimated by therapists.

The usual type of cutaneous cancer occurring after radiotherapy is the squamous cell carcinoma, but basal cell carcinomas also may occur, particularly in areas about the face where such tumors are prone to arise "spontaneously." As previously mentioned, spindle cell carcinomas are an especially anaplastic variety of squamous cell cancers produced by irradiation (see Fig. 17-34).

Pigmented nevi

The term "nevus" is often used by dermatologists to refer to any congenital blemish. Therefore they refer not only to pigmented nevi but also to vascular nevi, sebaceous gland nevi, sweat gland nevi, and others. However, to others, "nevus" denotes a neoplasm derived from pigmented or, at least, dopa-positive cells. We have classified these nevi and their malignant counterparts as follows*:

A. Benign
   1. Junctional nevus (Fig. 42-34)
   2. Intradermal nevus
   3. Compound nevus (including halo nevus) (Fig. 42-35)
   4. Juvenile melanoma (Fig. 42-36)
   5. Blue nevus—cellular blue nevus (Fig. 42-37)
B. Malignant
   1. Melanocarcinoma (Figs. 42-39 and 42-40)
      a. In situ
      b. Superficial (including melanotic freckle of Hutchinson)
      c. Deep
   2. Malignant blue nevus

Junctional nevus

The junctional nevus, also known as dermoepidermal or marginal nevus, is of concern because in its active form it is a direct forerunner of the melanocarcinoma. Happily, this malignant transformation of junctional nevi occurs relatively infrequently.

The uncomplicated (quiescent verus active) junctional nevus appears as a flat, smooth,

*Slightly modified from Allen, A. C.: Cancer 2:28-56, 1949, and Allen, A. C., and Spitz, S.: Cancer 6:1-45, 1953.

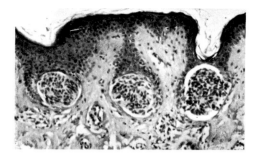

Fig. 42-34. Junctional nevus. (Hematoxylin and eosin; from Allen, A. C.: Cancer **2:**28-56, 1949.)

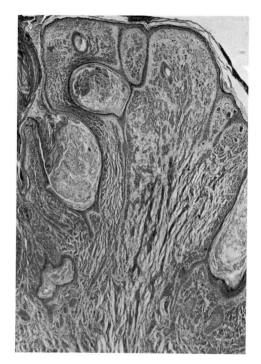

Fig. 42-35. Intradermal nevus. (Hematoxylin and eosin; from Allen, A. C.: Cancer **2:**28-56, 1949.)

generally hairless, light-brown to dark-brown mole. The lesions may be single or multiple. Their smooth appearance may be altered by their combination with an underlying intradermal nevus (compound). *Unfortunately, it is not always possible to diagnose them accurately clinically.* However, one may assume that pigmented moles on the ventral surface of the hands and the feet and on the genitalia are usually junctional nevi or, at least, have a junctional component in the form of a compound nevus.

Histologically, the junctional nevus is easily

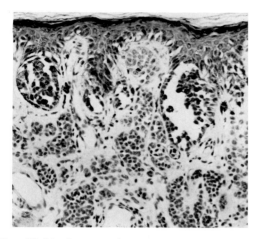

Fig. 42-36. Compound nevus showing junctional and intradermal components. (Hematoxylin and eosin.)

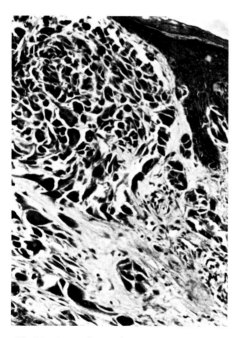

Fig. 42-37. Juvenile melanoma, special form of compound nevus simulating melanocarcinoma. (Hematoxylin and eosin; from Spitz, S.: Am. J. Pathol. **24:**591-609, 1948.)

recognized by the clusters of enlarged, rounded, loosened cells of the basal and adjacent prickle cells of the epidermis. In addition, these cells lose their prickles and cohesion with neighboring cells, and many become powdered with fine granules of melanin. This acantholysis is reflected ultrastructurally in the partial to complete loss of desmosomes and tonofilaments, although residua of these

structures are readily noted at the periphery of the "junctional" or acantholytic focus. If mitotic figures are present and the nuclei show any noteworthy anaplasia, the lesion may be assumed to have been on the verge of melanocarcinomatous transformation. Accordingly, depending on the extent of the atypia, these lesions are designated *"active junctional nevi"* or "melanocarcinomas in situ."[15] The process may be diffuse along a strip of epidermis or it may be focal, with normal or skipped areas of epidermis intervening between involved portions. In the latter case, judgment as to the adequacy of normal margin bordering the lesion must be made with caution, inasmuch as the section may be removed through one of the intervening, unaltered areas (Fig. 42-34).

It is generally believed that the cells of the junctional nevus are derived from specialized nerve endings intercalated in the basal layer as clear cells. However, it seems that such a restricted view disregards the occurrence of cells of the junctional nevus (many dopapositive) not only in a continuous row in the basal layer, but also as isolated cells high in the prickle cell layers, in the stratum granulosum, and even well into the stratum corneum. This phenomenon I believe to occur not by proliferation of neurogenic cells within the epidermis, as many believe, but, rather, by the alteration *in situ* of the preexisting basal and spinous keratinocytes, as a few formerly believed (Fig. 42-40).

It has long ago been clearly shown that the dendrites, which to many seem automatically to connote neurogenesis, may be entirely absent in many of these cells. Actually, when the dendrites of melanocytes are seen with silver stains, they are made evident *not because of an intrinsic argyrophilia* such as is possessed by cells of true neurons *but because of the argyrophilia of the contained granules of melanin.* The supranuclear localization of pigment within the prickle cells is, in itself, indicative of an *in situ* origin rather than by "a nippedoff" dendrite belonging to a neighboring cell or by the diffusion of tyrosinase from a clear cell. In the latter instances, one would expect that the granules of pigment would be diffusely or haphazardly deposited as in melanophores or histiocytes.

It is, of course, a brilliantly established fact that the pigment of skin, hair, and feathers may be controlled by the transposition of the embryonic cells of the neural crest. That neural *control* of many varieties of pigmentation exists is obvious. However, to conclude from this that the cells of the neural crest are incorporated in the epidermis as melanocytes is to fail, in effect, to distinguish the artist from his pigments.

The addition of these facts, supplemented by evidence from the direct examination of many junctional nevi and melanocarcinomas, indicates that basal cells principally, but also prickle cells or keratinocytes, may become converted to melanocytes and that the junctional nevi are derived from these cells.

Intradermal nevus

The intradermal nevus, or common mole, is the ordinary pigmented spot that few people are altogether spared. The mole may be flat or raised, with or without hairs, papillary and keratotic. Intradermal nevi may be present at birth or may develop in later years. They tend to become more prominent at the time of puberty.

Histologically, the tumor is composed of nests and cords of cells with round, moderately chromatic nuclei surrounded by an even, easily seen rim of cytoplasm. Melanin pigment, when present, usually is limited to the superficial cells in the upper dermis. Similarly, the cells in the upper part of the lesion are more likely to be dopa-positive than are the deeper ones.* Mitotic figures are seen rarely in these nevi in adults. Occasionally, hyperchromatism and enlargement of nuclei are simulated by mere agglutination of neval cells. The neval cells characteristically trail off into the depths of the dermis, and rarely into the subcutis, without sharp limitation. The overlying epidermis usually is thinned and may be flat or papillary, with or without hyperkeratosis (Fig. 42-35).

There is impressive histologic basis for the conclusion that the ordinary intradermal mole that is *not* overlain by a junctional nevus rarely becomes malignant.

The origin of the cells of the common mole is still unsettled. The possibilities include the following: (1) epidermal cells, (2) specialized

"nerve endings" similar to Merkel-Ranvier corpuscles, and (3) dermal nerves. Those who subscribe to the epidermal origin of the intradermal nevus assume, as Unna did, that the altered epidermal cells drop off *(Abtropfung)* and migrate into the dermis.[64] Those who believe in the neurogenesis of pigmented nevi suggest that the neval cells arise from dermal nerves or their sheaths, as well as from the intraepidermal nerve endings or cells that migrated from the neural crest. The frequency with which intradermal nevi are associated with loosened nests of epidermal cells that appear about to drop off (junctional changes) makes the epidermal origin of the common mole (as well as the junctional nevus) the likeliest possibility. This frequent association of the junctional change with the intradermal nevus can hardly be fortuitous, inasmuch as the change is rarely seen with blue nevi and yet is infrequently absent in the moles of children, normally diminishing in frequency and prominence after puberty.

Balloon cell nevus

Occasional intradermal nevi, called "balloon cell nevi," are characterized by large, coalescent vacuoles within the cytoplasm of nevus cells. These have been shown ultrastructurally to represent altered melanosomes rather than lipid.[36]

Compound nevus

In about 98% of the intradermal nevi occurring prior to puberty and in about 12% of nevi of adults, there is an associated junctional change[12] (Fig. 42-36). For lesions with this combination of features, the term "compound nevus" was applied by me many years ago.[12] It recently has been stated that silver stains are of appreciable help in distinguishing compound nevi from malignant melanomas. This, unfortunately, is not correct.

Clinically, as stated, there is no way to be certain as to whether or not an intradermal nevus is compounded with a junctional nevus. This fact emphasizes the importance of histologic examination of all excised nevi. As is indicated in the discussion of melanocarcinomas, the compound nevus has the capacity for undergoing malignant transformation by virtue of its junctional component. This conversion takes place relatively infrequently. The possibility exists that an intradermal nevus may, on occasion, develop overlying junctional change.

---

*Melanophores are merely phagocytes that engulf and transport melanin. Melanophores are dopa-negative. A pigmented neval cell or melanoblast may be dopa-negative because its enzyme has been completely utilized at a given time or has never been developed. The cells of a nonpigmented (amelanotic) melanoma may be dopa-positive. However, not all cells of a pigmented or nonpigmented melanocarcinoma are necessarily dopa-positive.

Juvenile melanoma

Juvenile melanoma is the name applied to a special form of compound nevus occurring predominantly in children. In the past, these lesions were considered to be histologically malignant but clinically benign. In other words, if the patient was prepubertal, these moles were arbitrarily labeled benign.

It was not until the basic histologic definition of these was first published in 1948 by the late Dr. Sophie Spitz that the morphologic distinction between the juvenile melanomas and true melanocarcinomas began to become evident[60,61] (Fig. 42-37). It is now reasonably apparent that this much-needed definition has served in a most practical way to clarify portions of a gravely confused problem.

Briefly, the distinguishing features of the juvenile melanomas are those of the compound nevi, with the addition of myogenous-appearing, occasionally spindled, single and multinucleated giant cells with abundant basophilic cytoplasm, often loosely dispersed in an edematous upper cutis. We have found no basis for believing that the juvenile melanoma, which, as indicated, is really a special form of compound nevus, is any more likely to become malignant than is the ordinary compound nevus. The juvenile melanomas undergo involutional fibrosis, as do other types of nevi.[13,14]

With increasing experience, it has become possible to recognize the juvenile melanomas for what they are on the interpretation of the histologic picture alone. On this basis, the scope of the significance of the juvenile melanoma has been extended by our confirmed discovery that this lesion may be found in adults, preponderantly in the second, third, and fourth decades but occasionally in older patients.[15] The practical importance of this observation is obvious when it is realized that, previously, benign juvenile melanomas of adults were treated as cancers.

Currently, there is unfortunately an increasing tendency to submit for histologic examination the shaved top of a pigmented lesion. Such a superficial biopsy not only complicates the problems of histologic diagnosis and the determination of cleared margins, but also leads to local recurrences of incompletely removed lesions. These local recurrences may be treacherously difficult to diagnose correctly.

There has been a good deal of objection to our use of "juvenile melanoma" (rather than "spindle cell nevus," for example) for a lesion that is benign and occurs occasionally in adults. Actually, we have always used the term in a *descriptive, histologic sense,* much as the terms embryonal rhabdomyosarcoma, fetal adenoma of the thyroid gland, juvenile cirrhosis, juvenile nasopharyngeal angiofibroma, and juvenile carcinoma of the breast are used. These terms are applied to tumors of adults by the very ones who rather inconsistently object to the corresponding designation "juvenile" in this instance. Accordingly, the use of "juvenile melanoma" serves the important practical purpose of viewing with added caution the acceptance of a given evaluation of a lesion so diagnosed. Sometimes, it seems to have been forgotten that, after all, it was not many years ago that no one claimed to be able to distinguish the juvenile melanoma from the malignant melanoma, and, in a great many laboratories, this problem has obviously been far from resolved.

Blue nevus

The blue or Jadassohn-Tièche nevus appears as a flat or slightly elevated blue or bluish black lesion, occurring particularly on the trunk and extremities and often mistaken clinically for a malignant melanoma. It is structurally essentially the same as the *mongolian spot* or the nevus of Ota. The former is found in the sacral region. The nevus of Ota occurs in the eye and on the skin of the face.

Histologically, these nevi are composed of interlacing fasciculi of spindle cells with long cytoplasmic processes and oval fibrocytoid nuclei. The cells are usually much more loosely disposed than those of the blue nevus. If the pigment were not present, the histologic picture of the blue nevus would resemble that of a dermal neurofibroma, and, indeed, it is possible that the basic morphogenesis of the two is similar. However, many of the cells of the blue nevus and the mongolian spot are dopa-positive. Abundant melanin pigment may obliterate the details of most of the cells of the blue nevus. In addition, the neoplastic cells are interspersed with numerous pigment-laden chromatophores. Usually, the neval cells lie deep in the dermis, or occasionally they are directly apposed to the epidermis. The color of the nevus is, of course, dependent not only on the amount of pigment present, but also on the distance of the lesion from the epidermis. Infrequently, the blue nevus is combined with the ordinary intradermal nevus (common mole) and with the junctional nevus.

Cellular blue nevus. There is a striking variant of the blue nevus that is frequently

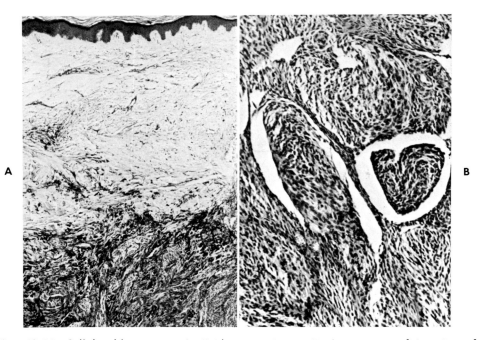

A   B

Fig. 42-38. Cellular blue nevus. **A,** Epidermis is intact. **B,** Appearance of invasion of lymphatics is an illusion characteristic of this lesion and is secondary to artifactual shrinkage. (**A** and **B,** Hematoxylin and eosin; from Allen, A. C.: Cancer **2:**28-56, 1949.)

incorrectly diagnosed as melanosarcoma. Some years ago, I termed this lesion *cellular blue nevus.*[1,12] It occurs in about 50% of cases in the skin of the buttocks and the dorsum of the hands or feet. The epidermis is unchanged. The cells of this tumor show no significant anaplasia, and mitotic figures almost always are absent. Fused nuclei often simulate the hyperchromasia of activity. One of the features that characterize the lesion is the cross sections of fasciculi surrounded by clear zones, giving the illusion that the whorls are metastases in lymphatics when they actually represent artifactitious shrinkage and cleavage of the fasciculi (Fig. 42-38). The melanosomes of the cellular blue nevus are stated to have a distinctive ultrastructure.

Blue nevi undergo malignant change with consoling rarity. We have seen somewhat over 45 examples of malignant blue nevi arising generally from cellular blue nevi. Although it appears obvious that the diagnosis of sarcomatous transformation of a blue nevus is often made unjustifiably, it is incorrect to assume, as some do, that such cancers do not occur.

• • •

Several eponyms continue to be applied to pigmented lesions that, unfortunately, are still poorly defined histologically. Among these are Hutchinson's lentigo or freckle and melanoma of Dubreuilh.

Senile lentigo

The senile lentigo is a common lesion occurring on exposed surfaces in approximately one third of individuals past middle age. It is characterized histologically by hyperkeratosis and parakeratosis and fringelike elongation of the hyperpigmented rete ridges, often showing an increase in basilar "clear cells" or minimal junctional change (Fig. 42-39).

Melanotic freckle of Hutchinson

Much attention has been given recently to essentially restatements of information concerning the melanotic freckle of Hutchinson, also known as *la mélanose circonscrite précancéreuse de Dubreuilh, senile* or *malignant freckle, precancerous* or *acquired melanosis, premalignant lentigo,* and *lentigo maligna.* Actually, this lesion is characteristically a relatively slow-growing lesion of the face, generally of elderly patients, which evolves from epidermal melanosis to a junctional nevus with varying degrees of activity and, finally, if the patient lives long enough, to a superficial and then deep (or nodular) melanocarcinoma. As we long ago documented, the mela-

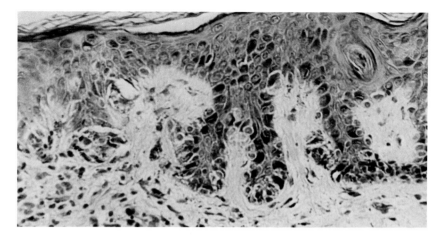

Fig. 42-39. Lentigo with pigmented rete ridges associated with junctional change. (Hematoxylin and eosin.)

nocarcinomas of the face, especially those of women, tend to be associated with a better prognosis than those of most other regions of the body.[15] Their histogenesis, however, is no different from any other junctional nevus or from the melanocarcinoma derived therefrom.

Halo nevi

Halo nevi (leukoderma acquisitum centrifugum, Sutton's nevus) refers to the progressive centripetal extension of a zone of depigmentation about a nevus. This perilesional depigmentation may encircle not only benign nevi (intradermal, compound, and blue) but also malignant melanomas, as well as cutaneous metastases. Accordingly, this leukodermatous reaction gives no hint as to whether a given lesion is benign or malignant.

It has been hypothesized that the destruction of the nevus cells may represent an immune response to the antigens of the nevus cells or, on occasion, melanocarcinomatous cells. The cellular disintegration (of nevus cells) that we have noted in juvenile melanomas may reflect a similar immunologic self-destruction. In the instance of juvenile melanomas this reaction may occur in the absence of nearby lymphocytes. The distortion generated by this reaction in both instances—halo nevi and juvenile melanomas—may lead to the mistaken diagnosis of malignant melanomas.

As stated, a spectrum of hypotheses ranging from antigen-antibody reaction to neurotropic disturbance has been suggested to explain the local vitiligo or leukoderma. The most reasonable is that the depigmentation is secondary to the underlying inflammatory reaction simi-

lar to the depigmentation that may occur with lichen planus, for example.

Malignant melanomas

In 1953, we classified malignant melanomas as indicated below.[15] Almost two decades later, others modified this classification by the addition, in effect, of more subdivisions indicated by the levels in parentheses[22]:

1. Melanocarcinoma from active junctional nevus (or junctional component of compound nevus)
   a. Melanocarcinoma in situ (level I)
   b. Superficial (level II, some in level III)
   c. Deep (those deeper in level III; IV, reticular; and V, subcuticular)
2. Malignant blue nevus

The essential modification of the parallel classifications involves the subdivision of our "deep" level into levels III, IV, and V. Actually, melanocarcinomas so advanced and neglected as to have directly invaded the panniculus (level V) are rarely seen these days, mostly on the soles where the dermis is especially thin. The debatable contribution therefore centers about deeper levels III and IV. In one large series this subdivision has not proved informative[37] although others disagree somewhat.[65] However, there are several overlooked sources of error inherent in the classification by dermal levels, as follows:

1. Because of the pseudoepitheliomatous hyperplasia frequently associated with malignant melanomas, the rete ridges may extend illusorily deep into the reticular layer (level IV) and still function as a superficial melanocarcinoma.

2. The malignant melanomas have a remarkable propensity for growing outward, or exophytically. Accordingly, the nodular melanocarcinomas may behave the worst and yet not extend below the papillary layer of the dermis. This same nodular lesion eventually complicates many "superficially spreading" or "lentiginous" melanocarcinomas.

3. The dermal papillary layer varies considerably in different parts of the body, being particularly thin and superficial in the skin of many areas of the extremities. Hence the arbitrary use of the level of the interface between papillary and reticular layers as a measure of depth of invasion of lesion in various areas is grossly inaccurate. To imply further that the reticular layer is somewhat a barrier to spread of the tumor is baseless. Finally, to state that "the subdivision of melanoma into five anatomic levels of invasion permits the accurate assignment of prognosis to each case" is patently hyperbolic. The behavior of these capriciously aggressive tumors cannot be measured predictably by boundaries of highly variable thicknesses, even if they are speciously drawn to the second decimal place. Therefore, we believe that divisions of dermal invasion other than superficial and deep lend little substance to the analysis of these cancers. The hard fact is that the least invasive superficial melanocarcinoma may be as devastatingly lethal as one that has reached the panniculus.

There is no perceptible advantage to labeling a melanocarcinoma in situ either "superficial spreading melanoma" or "lentigo maligna melanoma." The pivotal point is the presence or absence of dermal invasion, and, if present, whether it is superficial or deep. One of the disquieting consequences we are witnessing of the popularization of "superficial spreading melanoma" is its increasingly facile use as an unwarranted substitute for junctional nevus.

Clinically, the malignant melanoma is preceded usually by a flat, hairless mole, pigmented light to dark brown. When such a mole, which may have appeared the same for years, begins to darken, it probably has already undergone at least local malignant transformation. The changes of ulceration, increase in size, and bleeding lend obviously a serious increment to the prognosis. The recently promoted notion that, with few exceptions, mainly congenital, malignant melanomas arise anew, fails to reckon with the duration of the lesions and their histologic composition. These establish the frequent superimposition of malignant melanomas onto long-standing junctional or compound nevi.

A mole that is hairy, elevated, and papillary is uncommonly the site of cancer, although the insurance is by no means absolute—for the histologic reasons to be explained. In some instances, the neoplasm appears to arise anew, especially on the scrotum, palms, and soles. In these regions, the common (intradermal) mole rarely occurs, but the small, flat, often unnoticed, freckle-like junctional or compound nevus frequently is present. Because the lesions of the soles and genitalia are likely to have a junctional component, tend to escape inspection, and are located in areas that appear to have a proportionately higher incidence of malignant melanomas than other anatomic sites, it would seem reasonable to have such nevi removed electively from these sites when feasible.

In many instances, the benign deeply pigmented blue nevus is mistaken for a developing malignant melanoma. As stated, metastasizing melanomas are uncommon prior to the age of puberty, although we have recorded a number of such cases. In each of these instances, the histologic picture could be distinguished from that of the juvenile melanomas but not from the melanocarcinomas of adults.[15]

Histology and histogenesis. There is considerable variation in the cellular pattern of the melanocarcinomas. The primary lesion may simulate a squamous cell carcinoma, a spindle or basal cell carcinoma, an adenocarcinoma, a neurofibrosarcoma, or other neoplasms. The usual melanocarcinoma is composed of cells arranged as compact masses with some cords and alveoli. The cells are likely to be more or less uniform in size and shape. The nuclei of the primary lesion commonly do not exhibit the classic evidence of anaplasia. Mitotic figures may not be numerous, despite the aggressiveness of the neoplasm. Often, the nuclei are vacuolated and contain large acidophilic nucleoli resembling inclusion bodies, sometimes containing melanin. Melanin pigment may be present or absent without prognostic influence. In the neoplastic cells, the pigment tends to be of a uniform, fine granularity, whereas in the chromatophores, the pigment granules are likely to be more irregular in size and shape.

One of the most helpful histologic aids in

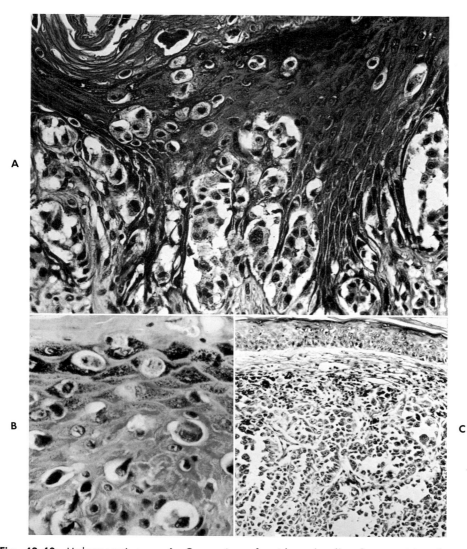

Fig. 42-40. Melanocarcinoma. **A,** Conversion of epidermal cells of pagetoid melanoma into melanocarcinomatous cells. **B,** In situ transformation of epidermal cells into melanocarcinomatous cells. **C,** Metastatic melanocarcinoma to skin showing overlying intact epidermis—criterion for primary versus metastatic melanocarcinoma. (**A** to **C,** Hematoxylin and eosin; from Allen, A. C.: Cancer **2:**28-56, 1949.)

diagnosis is the active junctional change overlying and continuous with the dermal portion of the cancer. The cells of the rete ridges may be so loosened as to be incorporated in the dermal neoplasm, with consequent partial dissolution of the ridges. Isolated, spheric, haloed cells, often powdered with fine melanin granules, may be found as far up as the stratum corneum (Fig. 42-40, *A*). Such intraepithelial cells are, in my opinion, the source of practically all melanocarcinomas of the skin and mucous membranes (blue nevi excepted) (Fig. 42-41). These cancerous cells are not related

to Langhans' cells or Merkel-Ranvier corpuscles but actually seem to have been, originally, cells derived from various layers of the epidermis. Nor is it true, as some believe, that these cells within the epidermis are metastatic from the underlying tumor within the dermis. Evidence for the autochthonous epidermal origin is found not only in the occurrence of such cells within the epidermis alone in early junctional nevi or superficial malignant melanomas but also in their absence in the epidermis overlying a snugly apposed dermal metastasis of a melanoma (Fig. 42-40),

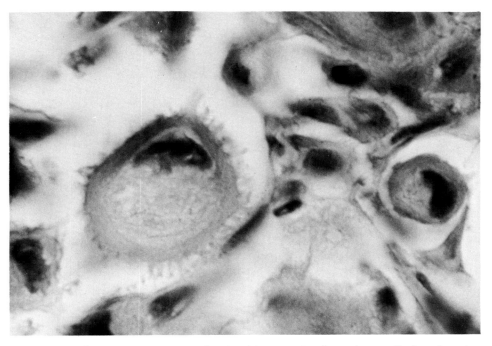

Fig. 42-41. Melanocarcinoma in situ showing histogenesis of neoplasm cells from keratino-cytes. Residue of identifying "prickles" and atypical neoplastic nuclei are evident. (Hema-toxylin and eosin; 1000×.)

a criterion that distinguishes the primary from the metastatic melanocarcinoma (Fig. 42-41).

Active junctional nevus (melanocarcinoma in situ). It is now apparent that when a malignant melanoma appears to be superimposed onto a benign intradermal nevus, there was originally present a clinically obvious or latent junctional nevus that itself was the source of the malignant melanoma. Routine studies of the epidermis of the primary melanocarcinomas of skin (and mucous membranes, including conjunctivas) demonstrate this junctional change. In other words, the melanocarcinoma arising in the skin would actually seem to be a peculiarly virulent variant of an epidermogenic carcinoma, a view originally expressed by Unna in 1893.[64] Why the malignant melanoma behaves usually more aggressively than other epidermal carcinomas is not yet known. Occasionally, it becomes a problem to decide if a given lesion is still in the stage of junctional nevus or whether it has become a melanocarcinoma in situ. The histologic diagnosis of a *superficial melanocarcinoma* must, in the last analysis, depend on finding evidence of invasion of the upper dermis by the cells of the *active junctional nevus*[15] (Fig. 42-40, *A*).

Actually, all junctional nevi, by definition, exhibit a kind of activity or dynamics in the form of varying stages of acantholysis of the intraepidermal cells. However, with this reservation, we have in the past applied the term "active junctional nevus" to the one with nuclear atypia, mitotic figures, and often with large, pagetoid cells scattered singly or in clumps to various levels of the epidermis.[1,15,16] Such a lesion is equivalent to "melanocarcinoma in situ." The presence of such an active junctional nevus should lead to a painstaking search for dermal invasion with the help of multiple sections. The histologic criteria for the distinction of a superficial melanocarcinoma—from an active junctional nevus on the one hand and a deep melanocarcinoma on the other—are essentially similar to those used for distinguishing a superficial squamous cell carcinoma from leukoplakia and from a deeply infiltrating carcinoma. Incidentally, the high degree of pseudoepitheliomatous hyperplasia so commonly associated with melanocarcinomas is largely responsible for mistaking these neoplasms for squamous cell carcinomas.[15] Patients with a melanocarcinoma appear to have a *systemic diathesis for activation* of junctional nevi, which in a considerable percentage of cases (3.5%) leads to multiple primary melanocarcinomas. Such histologic features as the content of melanin and the absence of appreciable polymorphism or mitotic figures are not significantly contributory in the evaluation of the prognosis.

Melanocarcinomas of mucous membranes. Melanocarcinomas of the mucous membranes of the oronasopharynx, larynx, bronchus, esophagus, gallbladder, and genitalia, including cervix, and anorectal region are almost uniformly fatal. Undoubtedly, some of the contributory reasons for their grave prognosis is the delay in detection and in accurate histologic diagnosis, the frequent injudicious therapy, the difficulties in adequate operative removal, and possibly such extraneous factors as chronic infection and repeated trauma. In approximately 15% of 337 patients, the tumors arose in these various mucous membranes (exclusive of the conjunctiva). The ulceration of the junctional change and the absence of appreciable amounts of pigment in about 50% of the melanomas of mucous membranes increase the difficulties of histologic diagnosis. Melanocarcinomas of mucous membranes may arise in any mucosa lined by either normally present or metaplastic stratified squamous epithelium.[1,15]

Tumors of vessels
Lymphangioma

The number of histologic and clinical variants, as well as the difficulty in distinguishing neoplasia of lymphatic vessels from ectasias, anomalies, and proliferations attributable to stasis, has led to the application of needlessly confusing names. The same situation exists with respect to the angiomas, but in both instances it has existed so long that scrapping of terminology at this point would add to the confusion.

The **lymphangioma simplex** is a soft, compressible, grayish pink nodule. The nodules are often multiple and grouped irregularly. Although the skin of the genitalia is the common site for these tumors, they are found also on the lips and tongue and may be associated with a macroglossia or macrocheilia. They are composed of varying-sized, endothelium-lined, thin-walled vessels, either empty or containing lymph with occasional leukocytes. Some of the channels may contain a few red blood cells. There is an abundant proliferation of endothelial cells in a proportion of the tumors, to which the designation **lymphangioma tuberosum multiplex** or **lymphangioendothelioma** has been applied.

Lymphangioma cutis circumscriptum occurs in the skin of the face, chest, or extremities in the form of a single tumor or of multiple, projecting, somewhat papillary, verrucose nodules. They may resemble opalescent vesicles, and there may be an associated telangiectasis. Histologically, they are composed of dilated lymphatic vessels in the upper dermis and are so closely linked to the epidermis as to appear incorporated in it. The overlying epidermis may be irregularly atrophied and acanthotic as well as hyperkeratotic in a papillary manner so as to simulate the angiokeratomas (see also p. 1859).

The **lymphangioma cavernosum** may be small and circumscribed, or it may extend diffusely over an extensive area, causing macrodactylia, for example. Histologically, the lymphatic channels are greatly dilated and may extend into fat and muscle, as do the so-called infiltrating angiomas. The unencapsulated extensions are in neither instance evidence of malignant transformation, but they do complicate local removal.

The **lymphangioma cysticum coli** or **hygroma** is a congenital lesion that arises usually in the neck and submaxillary regions and is histologically similar to the lymphangioma cavernosum in both structure and extension. The hygroma may ramify widely upward to the parotid area, downward as far as the mediastinum, and inward to lie precariously close to the trachea and adjacent structures. The lymphangioma cysticum may occur also in the region of the sacrum (p. 919).

Hemangioma

The problems of the pathogenesis and terminology of tumors of blood vessels are even more complicated than those of lymphangiomas. Theoretically, a true hemangioma is to be differentiated from a simple dilatation of blood vessels by its independence from the adjacent normal circulatory channels. A hemangioma enlarges, therefore, by growth of its own elements rather than by incorporation of nearby vessels. In practice, however, these criteria are seldom applied, and accordingly many ectasias, hyperemias, and hyperplasias are included as neoplasias. The hemangiomas may be classified simply as capillary, cavernous, or mixed (p. 919).

The **capillary angioma** corresponds clinically to the familiar port-wine stain common on the face and neck, but it exists also as simple small "vascular nevi" or birthmarks. In infants, such angiomas may be composed of compact masses of endothelial cells in which the capillary lumens are obscured in many areas. These proliferations often extend from the dermis into the subcutaneous tissue. The extension of the lesion beyond the dermis and its rich cellularity may provoke the erroneous diagnosis of angiosarcoma.[60] However, such angiomatous formations are usually sufficiently characteristic as to make possible the diagnosis of benign *infantile angioma* on the basis of histologic appearance alone. The capillary angioma may be confused histologically also with granuloma pyogenicum, particularly if the former is ulcerated and inflamed, as the latter usually is. The granuloma pyogenicum, however, is characteristically polypoid, generally has been present for no longer than a period of 1 to 3 months, and bleeds easily and repeatedly. The histology of the granuloma pyogenicum is identical with the so-called pregnancy tumor that occurs in the oral mucosa during the period of gestation. Thrombocytopenia may be associated with giant vascular tumors. The remission of the thrombocytopenia after removal of the hemangioma suggests that the tumor may occasionally serve as a reservoir for the platelets.

The *sclerosing hemangioma* appears to be a special variety of capillary angioma, although few dermatologists subscribe to this interpretation. They prefer to regard the lesion as a dermatofibroma lenticulare, histiocytoma, or merely subepidermal fibrosis. The lesions occur chiefly on the extremities and present clinically as single, firm, and slightly elevated intracutaneous nodules, averaging several millimeters to a centimeter in diameter. Their sectioned surface is smooth and yellow.

Histologically, more or less of the dermis is replaced by spindle cells, arranged generally in tight curlicues, although in some areas these cells appear to enclose tiny spaces suggestive of the lumens of capillaries. In a few cases, the lumens are so large and numerous as to make the vascular nature of this lesion obvious. Usually, the cells are vacuolated by lipid, and in some cases the fat content is the most striking feature. Dark brown granules of hemosiderin are often present in many of the cells. At times, the iron pigment may be so abundant that some observers, confusing the pigment with melanin, have succumbed to the serious error of labeling the lesion a malignant melanoma. The overlying epidermis may be normal, atrophied, moderately acanthotic, or the site of a superimposed basal cell carcinoma[35] (Fig. 42-42). In some instances, a sharply delimited subepidermal zone of the dermis is spared. A similar free zone is seen

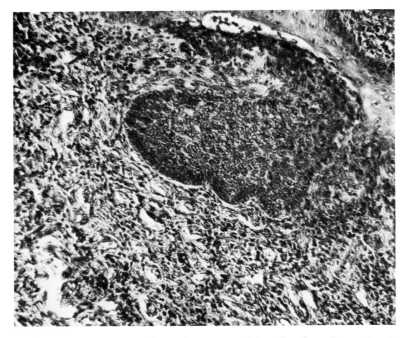

Fig. 42-42. Sclerosing angioma with overlying nest of basal cell carcinoma in situ. (Hematoxylin and eosin.)

in the dermal neurofibroma, although perhaps not so frequently. The sclerosing hemangioma may sometimes be justifiably confused with the neurofibroma when, as not infrequently occurs, the deeper portion of the lesion is composed of fasciculi of spindle cells such as characterize the neurofibroma. The impression gained by light microscopy of the hemangiomatous origin of these lesions is confirmed by the observation of Weber-Palade bodies with the electron microscope. These are intracytoplasmic tubular structures, presumably derived from the Golgi appartus and apparently specific for endothelial cells.

Occasionally, a fibrotic tumor resembling the sclerosing hemangioma, particularly of the trunk, recurs locally with formation of satellite nodules. Usually, such tumors originally extended into the subcutaneous fat and were removed incompletely. These tumors, called *dermatofibrosarcoma protuberans,* give rise to distant metastases in the rarest instances.

The **cavernous hemangiomas** are histologically similar to the cavernous lymphangiomas except for the presence of blood in the congeries of vessels. The vessels may ramify progressively in the subcutaneous fat, fascia, and intermuscular septa. The extensions may be so wide and inaccessible as to make surgical removal an exceedingly difficult procedure. The term "infiltrating angioma" is more aptly applied to such tumors than is "angiosarcoma."

Clinically, the covernous hemangiomas present on the skin surface as purple, single, globular or multilobular tumors or as the flat or slightly elevated "strawberry" nevus of infants. The angiomas may be multiple and may cause, or at least be associated with, enlargement and distortion of an area of the body in the vicinity of the tumors. The distortion from edema and hypertrophy of an arm *(Weber syndrome)* may be so great as to require amputation because of the sheer weight of the extremity.

Other syndromes associated with anomalies of blood vessels include the Sturge-Weber syndrome (nevus flammeus of the face, cerebral angiomatosis, hemiplegia, and mental retardation), Maffucci's syndrome (angiomas with dyschondroplasia), and heredofamilial angiomatosis *(Rendu-Osler-Weber disease).* Cutaneous angiomas also may be part of the complex of *multiple congenital angiomas* found in the viscera, particularly in the cerebellum and retina, and known as *Hippel's disease.* The *"blue rubber-bleb nevus"* appears to be a form of venous hamartoma involving both skin and gastrointestinal tract. It is characterized by pain, sweating, and a sensation of dermal "herniation."[56]

The *angiokeratoma* or telangiectatic wart represents a variety of cavernous hemangioma that is structurally similar to the lymphangioma cutis circumscriptum. The dilated blood channels are located high in the papillae and are so intimately associated with the epidermis as to appear actually within it in many places. The overlying epidermis is usually papillary, acanthotic, and hyperkeratotic. Clinically, the lesions are dark purplish red, firm, the size of a pinhead or split pea, and located in the scrotum, ears, fingers, and toes. The lesions often are associated with some circulatory disturbance such as might follow chilblains and varicosities. This type that tends to occur on the extensor surface of the extremities is known as the *Mibelli* type of angiokeratoma as opposed to *Fordyce's* type without associated pernio. The *angiokeratoma of Fabry* may be associated with lesions of viscera, particularly the kidneys and vessels, with characteristic foam cells. Patients with angiokeratoma of Fabry may excrete increased amounts of the glycoproteins ceramide trihexoside and dihexoside. Examination of the urine for these glycoproteins may aid in the detection of the disorder in members of the families of patients.

Spider "angiomas," which are really small telangiectases, possibly with arteriovenous shunts, occur with chronic hepatic damage as in Laennec's cirrhosis, as well as in pregnancy. They are believed to be an effect of excess of estrogenic hormones.

The term "hemangioendothelioma," as previously indicated, hedgingly applied to hemangiomas in which there is a relative prominence of endothelial cells with or without atypia. The implication in its use is that the neoplasm shows greater activity and therefore presents more likelihood of local recurrence than the ordinary hemangioma. The evidence for this presumption is questionable. A similar situation exists with respect to the use of "lymphangioendothelioma." Unfortunately, the name "hemangioendothelioma," rather than "angiosarcoma," is sometimes applied to the frankly malignant tumor.

Cutaneous meningioma

The *cutaneous meningioma* occurs as an isolated dysembryogenetic subcutaneous nodule with occasional dermal involvement, or as an ectopic extension into soft tissue corresponding in distribution to cranial and spinal nerves. The latter may cause signs and symptoms reflective of the associated nerves or those of a tumor mass such as proptosis, nasal polyp, or soft tissue mass. The histologic picture is that of a meningothelial cell tumor or sclerosing angioma with characteristic psammoma bodies.[41]

Angiosarcoma

Primary solitary angiosarcoma of the skin, exclusive of Kaposi's hemorrhagic sarcoma, is rare. However, several cases have been recorded in which visceral metastases have occurred. The metastases tend to be more cellular and anaplastic than the original growth. Others have been reported as malignant vascular tumors of skin under the title "hemangioendothelioma," but in most instances evidence of origin from dermis, as well as of the cancerous characteristics, is not convincingly presented. Knowledge of the rarity of such tumors is of practical importance because of its tempering effect on the tendency to call sarcomatous those nonmetastasizing angiomas with abundant endothelial cells or those that have infiltrated into the subcutaneous fat and beyond into the muscles. The Kaposi sarcoma, on the other hand, represents a process of vastly different significance.

Kaposi's idiopathic hemorrhagic sarcoma

Kaposi's sarcoma begins as reddish to purplish brown, discrete or grouped, painful, tender nodules varying from 1 to 2 mm in size to about 1 cm. They occur particularly on the hands and feet, although they may start in the skin of any part of the body. The incidence is about 10 times greater in men than in women, and the disease is seen especially in elderly patients, although it has been described in children. The surface of the nodules may be telangiectatic, but often it is verrucose. Local purpura and bullae may be associated with the lesions. Lymphatic blockage with elephantiasis of the extremities is common and is reminiscent of the edema associated with postmastectomy lymphangiosarcoma. The course of the disease is slow, the nodules often involuting, with resultant atrophic scarring and pigmentation. The condition may last from 1 to fully 25 years, although the average duration is from 5 to 10 years. The disease is found chiefly in Italian and Jewish people.

The lesions may involve extensive areas of the skin and nearly every organ of the body. The gastrointestinal tract, mesenteric nodes, liver, and lungs are the most common sites, although even the osseous and central nervous systems may be affected. The question is unsettled as to whether these lesions are truly metastases or actually multicentric foci of a neoplasm. The intestinal lesions of Kaposi's sarcoma, unlike most other metastatic lesions, have a predilection for the inner coats rather than the serosa. In this location, the tumors give rise to profuse hemorrhage. This difference in location in the intestinal tract between the Kaposi's sarcoma and other metastatic tumors is a bit of evidence in favor of the multicentric origin of the former. Visceral tumors histologically identical with Kaposi's sarcoma have been found infrequently without cutaneous involvement. Patients with Kaposi's sarcoma die of hemorrhage from an intestinal lesion, intercurrent infection, extensive visceral involvement, or complicating malignant lymphomas.

Kaposi's sarcoma is a form of angiosarcoma that is so varied histologically as frequently to cause difficulty in the interpretation of a given slide. In one phase, perhaps the earliest, the picture is that of a simple hemangioma or of foci of hyperemic, nonspecific granulation tissue characterized by clusters of capillaries placed closely together, with or without a sprinkling of mononuclear cells and histiocytes containing hemosiderin in the intervening and often edematous stroma. At this stage, the endothelial cells may be quite regular, without mitotic figures or other evidence of anaplasia. The important histologic clue is the disposition of these vascular foci not only near the epidermis, *but also isolated about appendages in the deeper layers of the dermis.* The presence of such vascular foci at a distance from the surface of the skin is suspiciously unlike the ordinary pattern of the response of skin to inflammation. In more advanced lesions, there occurs proliferation of spindle cells and fibroblasts in association with scattered lymphocytes and histiocytes. The cells appear to form abortive capillaries, and in the actively growing lesions these cells are large and hyperchromatic and contain mitotic figures. In the later stages, there is a tendency toward focal necrosis of the neoplastic tissue and subsequent fibrosis. These variegated pictures may be observed not only at different stages of the disease but often within a single lesion.

Relation of Kaposi's sarcoma to malignant lymphomas. There is an increasing number of reports in the literature of the simultaneous occurrence of Kaposi's sarcoma with one or another of the malignant lymphomas, including Hodgkin's disease, lymphatic leukemia, lymphosarcoma, and mycosis fungoides. For both statistical and histologic reasons (the latter reasons comprising evidence of transition of the two processes within the same lesion), the association is not considered coincidental.[1]

Postmastectomy lymphangiosarcoma

In 1948, an entity described as lymphangiosarcoma was recorded[62] as a complication of postmastectomy lymphedema of the upper extremity. The lymphangiosarcoma in the skin of the edematous arm developed 6 to 24 years after the mastectomy, with the lymphedema having existed during the entire latent period. In one instance, the tumor of the breast was benign. There was no relationship between the use of radiation and the development of the lymphangiosarcoma. As originally suspected, lymphangiosarcoma may complicate chronic edema including congenital lymphedema of extremities unassociated with mammary carcinoma or its treatment.[28]

Histologically, the sarcoma has a range of variation quite equal to that of Kaposi's sarcoma, and indeed in many sections one cannot be certain that the neoplastic elements are lymphatic vessels rather than blood sinuses. The tumor is capable of metastasizing. Rare instances of lymphangiosarcoma as a complication of the lymphedema of filariasis have been recorded. The mechanism of cancerogenesis in the cases of lymphedema is obscure (see Fig. 41-19).

Glomus tumor

In the corium of the skin of the fingertips, particularly in the nail beds, around the joints of the extremities, and over the scapulae and coccyx, there are normally arteriovenous shunts or glomera. These are composed of an afferent artery, the Sucquet-Hoyer canal or shunt, and an efferent vein. The artery is surrounded by several layers of small, spheric, uniform glomus cells that superficially resemble the cells of the intradermal nevus and that are presumed to control the flow of blood by their contractility. Nonmedullated nerves and bundles of smooth muscle are intimately associated with the shunt. Tumors of this structure are called glomangiomas, angiomyoneuromas, glomus tumors, or neuromyoarterial aneurysms. They are most common in the nail bed but occur elsewhere on the extremities and trunk and even deep to the skin in muscles and joints, as well as in viscera. No instance of tumor occurring in the coccygeal glomus has been observed.

Glomus tumors appear as purplish red spots several millimeters in diameter, which are often clinically diagnosable by a characteristically lancinating pain, remarkably severe in view of the small size of the tumors. Not all glomangiomas, however, are associated with this characteristic symptom, which occasionally is simulated by dermal angiomyomas.

Histologically, the glomus tumors range from compact masses of uniform glomus cells with few vascular channels to cavernous skeins of vessels cuffed by these cells. The vessels of the tumors tend to be small, especially in the nail bed. The identifying features are the several rows of peritheliomatously arranged glomus cells in which mitotic figures are rare or absent. These cells may be so numerous as to obliterate vascular lumens and to resemble a basal cell tumor or a variety of sweat gland adenoma. Nonmedullated nerves usually are discerned, but there appears to be no apparent relationship between the pain and the number or location of these nerves. Occasionally, glomus tumors are called simply hemangiomas or glomangioid tumors because of the presence of only two or three perivascular rows of glomus cells. However, such tumors have been observed with the typical symptomatology of glomangiomas. Ultrastructural studies reveal masses of cytoplasmic fibers suggestive of a transition from smooth muscle cells.

Tumors of muscle

Two varieties of tumors of dermal muscle are described: leiomyoma (arising from arrectores pilorum) and angiomyoma. What are called "granular cell myoblastomas" are lesions that were believed to have been myogenic.

Leiomyoma cutis

The leiomyoma cutis occurs singly or in groups of as many as dozens of firm and usually pea-sized nodules, which are often tender and painful. Histologically, they are composed of interlacing sheets of smooth muscle that may resemble a haphazard compact collection of arrectores pilorum. Infrequently, the nuclei are large, irregular in size and shape, and hyperchromatic so as to merit the term *leiomyosarcoma cutis* or *dermatomyosarcoma*. However, these lesions rarely metastasize.

Angiomyoma

The angiomyoma presents as a small nondescript nodule that, microscopically, is made up of circular masses of smooth muscle strongly reminiscent of the media of arteries. The residual arterial lumen is discernible in the core of many of the masses of muscle. These lesions remain benign. Occasionally, they may be found in the subcutaneous fat or even more deeply in the fascia or intermuscular septa of the extremities. As stated, they may cause the sharp pain generally associated with glomangiomas.

Myoblastoma

The "granular cell myoblastoma" is found as a nodule in the skin of various parts of the body, as well as on the mucous membranes, particularly of the tongue and isolated sites such as the larynx, thyroid gland, breast, gallbladder, esophagus, stomach, appendix, pituitary gland, and uvea.

Histologically, the tumors are composed of nests and alveoli of large cells with small, centrally placed nuclei in cytoplasm loosely stippled with eosinophilic granules, occasionally replaced by polyhedral crystalloids. These PAS-positive granules appear to contain lipoprotein or glycolipid and ultrastructurally may be amorphous, vesicular, vacuolar, or particulate. The cells closely resemble those of a xanthoma, but fat stains are negative. On close examination, it is observed that the cytoplasm is not actually vacuolated, as are lipid histiocytes. The loose dispersion of granules that simulate vacuoles has been believed to represent embryonic fibrils of striated muscle cells. Such a hypothesis is open to question, inasmuch as these tumors are present in the corium and other sites where striated muscle does not occur. The same objection may be leveled at the hypothesis that these cells represent degenerated adult striated fibers, although in sites where striated muscle is normally present, such as the tongue, this kind of transition occasionally is suggested. In our opinion, the evidence for the neurogenesis is not considered adequate. The concept of a fibroplastic origin has been advanced and appears far more convincing. In any event, whether or not these tumors are proved eventually to be fibroblastic, it is clear that they are easily recognizable histologic entities that rarely, if ever, metastasize. Some of the so-called malignant granular cell myoblastomas are, in reality, unrelated rhabdomyosarcomas in which a few of the cells happen to be granular.

One of the remarkable and distinctive features of many of the myoblastomas is the characteristic epithelial or epidermal acanthosis that overlies the lesion. This feature is not present in association with frank cutaneous leiomyomas. As a rule, dermal neoplasms leave the epidermis essentially unaltered or cause its atrophy through compression. The myoblastomas, on the other hand, appear to provoke

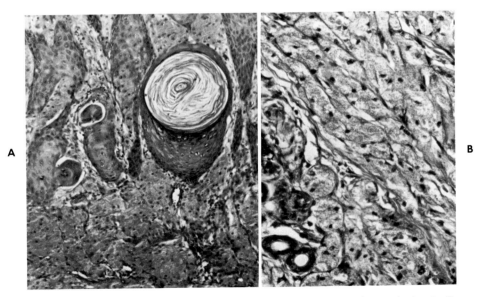

Fig. 42-43. Myoblastoma. **A,** Characteristic pseudoepitheliomatous hyperplasia. **B,** Granular cytoplasm and uniform small nuclei. (**A** and **B,** Hematoxylin and eosin.)

a degree of acanthosis that may simulate squamous cell carcinoma. It is as if some epidermal irritant were present in the cells of the myoblastoma (Fig. 42-43). An analogous epidermal proliferation overlies many of the sclerosing angiomas, as previously mentioned.

Fibroma

Cutaneous fibroma. The diagnosis of cutaneous fibroma is usually found on careful review to include dermatofibroma lenticulare or sclerosing hemangioma, neurofibroma, leiomyoma, keloids, and other scars. This confusion does not apply to the pedunculated soft lipofibromas (fibroma molle) in which the fibrous component closely simulates the normal dermal collagen. Undoubtedly, some of the spindle-shaped squamous cell carcinomas and melanocarcinomas have been mistaken for fibrosarcomas and "atypical fibroxanthomas" of the skin.

Digital fibrous tumors of childhood

Fibrous tumors involve the fingers and toes, are present at birth, and tend to recur locally. Histologically they appear to be cellular fascial or dermal fibromas.

Neurofibroma

Neurofibroma may occur in the skin as a single tumor or as multiple nodules. In the latter condition, the entity is classified as neurofibromatosis or von Recklinghausen's disease and may be associated with café-au-lait pigmented spots and neurofibromas of the sympathetic system, as well as motor and sensory nerve trunks. The tumors of the skin may be so numerous as to cover almost the entire body from scalp to feet.

The histogenesis of the tumors is complex. The axons, as well as the nerve sheaths (neurilemma) and endoneurium, participate to a varying extent, so that the histologic picture may be altered accordingly. The tumor derived predominantly from nerve sheaths (neurilemoma) tends to manifest more obvious palisading of cells (Antoni A structure), degenerating, edematous microcystic foci (Antoni B), and hyaline Verocay bodies. Occasionally, the neurilemoma presents pronounced central necrosis and such excessive telangiectasis that it can be mistaken for an angioma. An examination of the periphery of these degenerated tumors usually reveals the telltale palisading of the neurilemoma. A small percentage of the cutaneous neurofibromas show sufficient hyperchromatism and irregularity in size and

shape of nuclei as to suggest sarcomatous degeneration. However, here, too, metastases from these neoplasms of the skin are rare, although local recurrence is fairly frequent. On the other hand, malignant changes in the visceral neurofibromas are common and may take the form of extensive, fatal, local infiltrations or metastases (p. 2133). The benign neurilemoma (schwannoma) undergoes malignant change with extreme rarity. However, malignant neurilemomas do occur. These are presumed not to have developed from a benign neurilemoma but to have been malignant from the start. These, too, are uncommon.

Osteoma

Osteoma cutis, an example merely of heterotopic bone, represents a metaplastic change of dermal collagen rather than true neoplasia. The lesion occurs as small nodules, as a rule, in scleroderma or syphilis, in association with acne or intradermal nevi, with hyperparathyroidism, and after trauma or cystotomies—the latter because of the osteogenic potentialities of urinary tract epithelium or without apparent reason.

The histologic picture may include fat and even marrow cells in addition to the bony trabeculae.

Lymphomas and allied diseases

The lymphomas and allied diseases of the skin include mycosis fungoides, Hodgkin's disease, lymphosarcoma, and leukemia.

Mycosis fungoides

There has been renewed interest in the histogenesis, histology, and natural history of the entity long ago and still unhappily labeled mycosis fungoides. It is a lymphomatous disease in which the cutaneous component is characterized clinically by three stages: (1) premycotic, (2) infiltrative, and (3) fungoid tumefaction.

The premycotic stage is characterized by eczematoid, severely pruritic, erythrodermic, scaly, well-defined patches or by a generalized erythroderma. The eruption in this phase may simulate eczema, psoriasis, parapsoriasis, seborrheic dermatitis, or a nonspecific exfoliative dermatitis. This stage may persist for months or years and may be impossible to diagnose with assurance either clinically or microscopically. In the second or infiltrative stage, firm, slightly elevated, bluish-red plaques arise—both in the previously involved and the uninvolved areas. Partial or incomplete loss of hair from the scalp and other regions may occur. The last or fungoid stage follows the infiltrative period by several months.

The tumors vary in diameter up to 10 cm or larger and are prone to ulcerate. In each of the stages, spontaneous remissions may be noted, but these are temporary. Of interest in this respect is the regression—albeit temporary—of cutaneous lesions of mycosis fungoides occurring after reactions of delayed hypersensitivity provoked directly in the lesions. The diagnosis in the few reported instances of cure must be questioned. In some cases, the preliminary two stages do not develop. This form is called "mycosis fungoides d'emblée." True instances of mycosis fungoides d'emblée must be exceedingly rare. Undoubtedly, most of the recorded cases are, in reality, examples of Hodgkin's disease, reticulum cell sarcoma, or leukemia.

Sézary's syndrome disease or reticulosis is a variant of mycosis fungoides consisting of erythroderma and Sézary cells in the peripheral blood, marrow, and lymphocytes. The likelihood is that the Sézary cells and the atypical cells of mycosis fungoides, with indented, convoluted, or cerebriform nuclei, are identical and represent T lymphocytes.[43] Similar cells have been noted in normal individuals, in patients with benign dermatoses and after stimulation of lymphocytes with mitogens.[66] Actually, mycosis fungoides is being regarded as a response to antigenic persistence with malignant lymphoma developing as a consequence of immunologic imbalance. Perhaps related in principle is the occurrence of reticulum cell sarcoma in recipients of renal transplants with immunosuppressive therapy, as others have suggested.

The histologic picture of the first or premycotic stage of mycosis fungoides is usually not diagnostic and may resemble one of the many conditions simulated clinically. However, even in this phase of the disease, there is a tendency for the infiltrate to be confined as a zone in the upper dermis and for the epidermis to appear psoriasiform. Occasionally, large, single or binucleated hyperchromatic cells are observed, as well as a rare infiltrative cell in mitosis, affording a clue. In the subsequent stages, the infiltrate, still selecting the upper dermis principally, becomes dense and polymorphous. In this variegated infiltrate, the presence of eosinophilic leukocytes and cells that simulate the Sternberg-Reed cell of Hodgkin's disease and often an abundance of small and large (Marschalko) plasma cells constitute the evi-

dence for mycosis fungoides. In addition, there is a tendency toward scattered clumping of cells of the infiltrate. The epidermis tends to be moderately acanthotic and hyperkeratotic with focal spongiosis and small intraepidermal "microabscesses of Darier-Pautrier." These "microabscesses" are actually foci of tumor cells that have extended into the epidermis. Their absence does not preclude the diagnosis (Fig. 42-44). The quality of the infiltrate may be indistinguishable from that of Hodgkin's disease. The cutaneous infiltrate of Hodgkin's disease tends to be irregularly distributed in parts of the dermis. The critical point is that the histologic changes even in the "premycotic" erythrodermatous stage are usually of the pattern and quality that, if properly evaluated, permit the diagnosis to be made.

Potentially, the most revealing and yet most disputed morphologic clues to the nature of mycosis fungoides are the findings at autopsy. Recent reports indicate visceral involvement in about 70% of cases in contrast with our finding some years ago of approximately 20%.[54] It has been suggested that the lower incidence in our material may reflect the longer survival in later series because of supportive measures not previously available. The peripheral lymph nodes often are enlarged because of their drainage of pigment, etc. from the infiltrated skin. Such nodes—now called "dermatopathic lymphadenopathy"—show partial obliteration of their architecture by reticulum cell hyperplasia, deposits of melanin and fat, and—what is an especially common and presumptive clue in mycosis fungoides—numerous plasma cells. Similar plasma cells are generally in the bone marrow and spleen, and occasionally even contain Russell bodies. These nonspecifically altered lymph nodes of Pautrier and Woringer may be mistaken for those of Hodgkin's disease.

Hodgkin's disease, lymphosarcoma, leukemia

The criteria for the histologic recognition in the skin of Hodgkin's disease, lymphosarcoma, and the various leukemias are the same as those used for the visceral lesions. Additional clues are offered by the almost constant denseness of the infiltrate, immediately noted with low-power magnification, and the selectivity of the infiltrate for the upper dermis in some instances of leukemia (Fig. 42-44). An important deceptive feature of the lymphomas is the occurrence also of quite *nonspecific cutaneous reactions* in which neoplastic cells are ab-

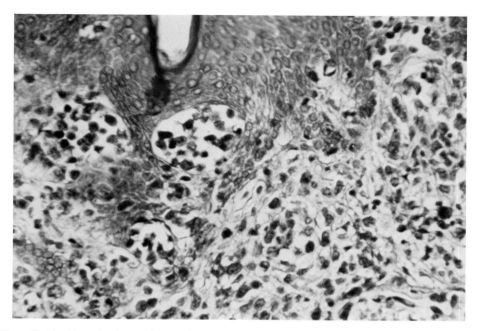

Fig. 42-44. Mycosis fungoides with "Pantrier-Darier abscesses" and characteristic sub-epidermal infiltrate. (Hematoxylin and eosin.)

sent. These reactions may take the clinical form of toxic erythema, excoriated pruritic exfoliative erythroderma, generalized pigmentation, urticaria, and herpes zoster. Severe nonspecific cutaneous reactions lead to the changes in the regional lymph nodes, dermatopathic lymphadenopathy, which may become so enlarged as to be clinically indistinguishable from lymphomas. Undoubtedly one of the most difficult neoplasms to evaluate from a biopsy specimen of skin is Letterer-Siwe disease of infancy or the related malignant histiocytoses of childhood, i.e., the so-called reticuloendothelioses, histiocytosis X, or lipid and nonlipid histiocytoses. The crux of the problem is the decision as to whether the cutaneous lesion indicates visceral involvement and a fatal prognosis or merely a local histiocytosis or variant of xanthomatosis. In the briefest terms, one may state that, in general, the degree of anaplasia and the compactness of the infiltrate of the monocytoid cells in the upper dermis are of great importance in suggesting the grave nature of the disease. However, remarkable disparities have been noted by Spitz.[61]

Another source of clinical and histologic confusion is the entity known as *Spiegler-Fendt sarcoid*, which is characterized by grouped, local or disseminated, bright red nodules. The histologic diagnosis is based principally on the finding of mature lympho-cytes, as well as reticulum cells either scattered or as germinal centers of follicles. Anaplasia of the infiltrate or histologic evidence of appreciable activity is lacking. It is obvious that differentiation of this lesion from lymphosarcoma must, at times, require a great nicety of judgment. Indeed, some of the cases originally but erroneously considered to be Spiegler-Fendt sarcoid have been recorded as having terminated in lymphosarcoma. Further confusion results from the use of the term *"benign lymphocytoma,"* which is popular in dermatologic literature. This lesion, which may be single or multiple, resembles Boeck's sarcoid, leukemic infiltration, or discoid lupus erythematosus clinically. Histologically, it consists essentially of dense masses of mature lymphocytes that may be arranged in follicles with germinal centers. As would be anticipated, the lesions are highly radiosensitive.

Reactions to arthropods

In 1948, I called attention to the remarkable diagnostically troublesome biphasic cutaneous reactions to the arthropods or "insect bites."[11] These reactions involve the epidermis and the dermis. The dermal lesion is commonly mistaken for one of the lymphomas. The reaction usually consists of eosinophilic leukocytes, histiocytes, plasma cells, and reticulum cells, with the last occasionally binucleated and even

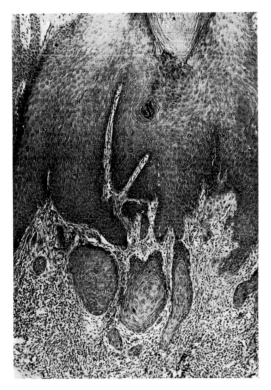

Fig. 42-45. Tick bite with pseudoepitheliomatous hyperplasia simulating squamous cell carcinoma. (Hematoxylin and eosin; from Allen, A. C.: Am. J. Pathol. **24:**367-387, 1948; AFIP 95767.)

in mitosis. In some lesions, there are also prominent lymphoid follicles with germinal centers. Many patients with such an innocuous reaction have been given the grave diagnosis of Hodgkin's disease, mycosis fungoides, or lymphosarcoma. Part of the reason for the error is that it is not generally appreciated that the reaction to arthopods may persist for many months. The presence of only a single lesion is suggestive evidence, in doubtful cases, of an insect bite. On the other hand, an isolated lesion may occur also in the neoplastic conditions.

A similar pseudolymphomatous cutaneous reaction may occur after injection of antigens for hyposensitization. The other deceptive reaction to the venom of insects and ticks is the pseudoepitheliomatous hyperplasias that may be mistaken for squamous cell carcinoma[11] (Fig. 42-45).

Eosinophilic granulomas and *Jessner's lymphocytosis* of the skin of the face also may be erroneously misinterpreted as forms of malignant lymphomas. *"Lethal midline granuloma"* refers to a fulminant, destructive ulcera-

tion of the nose and paranasal tissues often because of either *Wegener's granulomatosis* or one of the malignant lymphomas. The abundant necrosis, along with secondary vascular involvement, commonly obscures the precise histologic diagnosis.

Metastatic neoplasms

Cancerous metastases reach the skin by direct invasion or through the lymphatics or blood vessels. The most common metastases include those from carcinomas of the breast, uterus, lung, gastrointestinal tract, pancreas, thyroid gland, and prostate gland, in addition to those from melanocarcinomas, epidermoid carcinomas and lymphomas, and sarcomas of bone, muscle and fascia.

There is generally little difficulty in recognizing the metastatic character of a tumor in the skin except, of course, in the case of the lymphomas and in Kaposi's sarcoma. In both of these instances, the possibility of autochthonous multicentric origin is to be considered. Plasma cell myeloma occasionally involves skin. A nodule of malignant melanoma usually may be recognized as metastatic by the presence of an overlying intact epidermis showing no evidence of junctional change. Occasionally, a metastatic focus of adenocarcinoma is mistaken for a primary cutaneous carcinoma of sweat gland origin, or "extramammary" Paget's disease.

Tumors of dermal appendages

Following is a classification of benign tumors of the sweat apparatus:

Ductal (syringal)
  A. Eccrine
    1. Inverted, papillary syringoma ("eccrine poroma," intraepidermal or dermal or both)
    2. Lobular syringoma ("eccrine spiradenoma")
    3. Lobular hyalinized syringoma ("cylindroma")
    4. Diffuse syringoma
  B. Apocrine
    1. Syringocystadenoma papilliferum

Glandular
    1. Eccrine cystadenoma with chondral metaplasia
    2. Apocrine cystoma or cystadenoma
    3. Hamartoma

Sweat glands

There is obviously an abundance of histologic variants of tumors of sweat gland or duct origin. As a result, a great number of terms

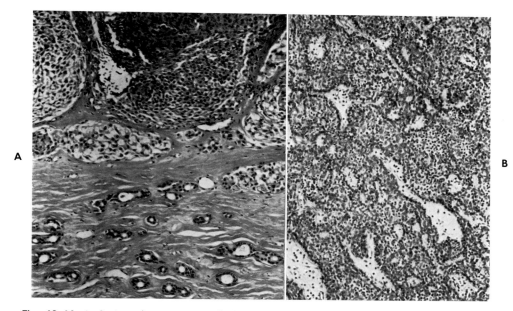

Fig. 42-46. A, Syringadenoma—usually labeled myoepithelioma on questionable evidence. **B,** Lobular syringadenoma (so-called eccrine spiradenoma). (**A** and **B,** Hematoxylin and eosin.)

have arisen that often are used ambiguously and applied inconsistently. It would seem that no practical purpose would be denied if all the neoplasms of sweat glands were labeled simply as solid or cystic syringadenoma or syringocarcinoma. However, the range of histologic variation is so great as to lead not infrequently to serious diagnostic errors—such as the mistaking of a sweat gland adenoma for a basal or a squamous cell carcinoma, malignant melanoma, or even synovioma. It may be worthwhile, therefore, at least to mention and illustrate the various sweat gland tumors. Despite their histologic variations, in almost all instances there are foci of cells that indicate their source by their resemblance to sweat glands or ducts. In many instances of the solid syringadenoma, the hard, smooth, hyalinized, collagenous stroma is a clue to the nature of the tumor. In others, large cells with abundant acidophilic cytoplasm—cells that some observers (on insecure evidence) believe to be myoepithelial—suggest origin from sweat ducts (Fig. 42-46). In a considerable number of the cystic syringadenomas, the stratified epithelium frequently is papillated, and the individual cells are vacuolated with glycogen (Fig. 42-47, *D*).

The inverted papillary syringoma (eccrine poroma) occurs as a single, slightly raised or pedunculated tumor predominantly on the soles, insteps, and palms.[49] The lesion extends

downward into the dermis from the stratum corneum as papillary, reticulated bands of compact, uniform, rarely pigmented, nonkeratinizing, phosphorylase-positive cells suggestive of origin from the sweat duct. Often, there is a fairly sharp demarcation from the adjacent epidermis. A similar lesion, comprised apparently of thickened, winding masses of ductal origin, may be confined to the dermis. The so-called clear cell hidroadenoma—the lesion that was once labeled "myoepithelioma"—is probably a partially cystic variant of the papillary syringoma in which abundant glycogen is present in the proliferating ductal cells. One might anticipate that the underlying sweat glands would be dilated as a consequence of these presumably obstructive lesions. We have, in fact, seen a single instance of grossly visible cyst formation in the sweat glands subtending this type of syringoma. We have not observed or read of other instances of such microscopic glandular dilatation.

The terms **eccrine poroepithelioma** and **acrospiroma** also have been applied to what are believed to be intraepidermal proliferations of sweat duct origin (acrosyringium) of patterns somewhat different from the syringoma. It is apparent that seborrheic keratoses and even melanocarcinomas in situ are being included in this category.

The **lobular syringoma** (eccrine spiradenoma) presents usually as a solitary firm

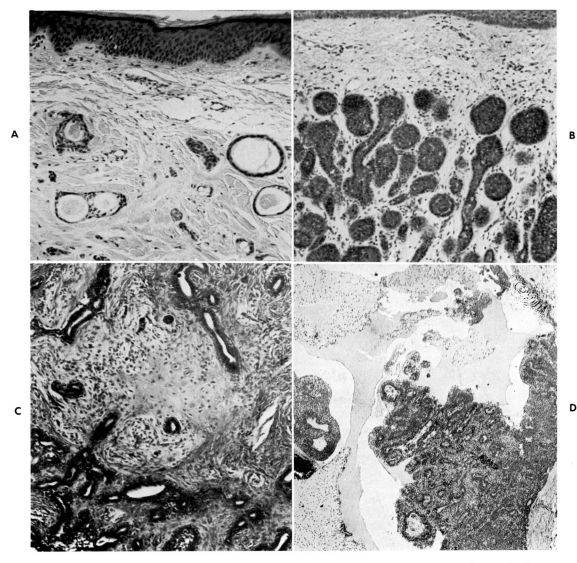

Fig. 42-47. A, Syringadenoma (hidrocystoma). **B,** Diffuse syringoma (spiradenoma). **C,** Syringadenoma with chondral metaplasia ("mixed" tumor) such as occurs in salivary and lacrimal glands. **D,** Syringocystadenoma. (**A** to **D,** Hematoxylin and eosin.)

nodule that is occasionally painful. The tumor is characteristically lobulated and composed of compact acini with predominant proliferation of the outer darker, lymphocytoid-appearing epithelial cells as distinct from the lighter, larger inner cells that often lie beneath a residual cuticle-like structure. The origin of these tumors from the sweat duct is vividly demonstrable in the early or incompletely developed lesion.

A variant of the lobular syringoma is characterized by conspicuous, *hyalinized* bands of collagen surrounding and intertwining among the lobules and its cells (Fig. 42-48). This lesion (**turban tumor, cylindroma**) tends to be multiple and may be so extensive as to cover the scalp. Both types of lobular syringoma remain benign.

The **diffuse syringoma** usually occurs as multiple, small, soft yellowish papules on the chest, back, and face. The overlying epidermis is intact or may appear glistening. Histologically, the lesion is composed of minute cysts scattered through the upper dermis (hence "diffuse" versus "lobular" syringoma). The cysts are noted to be dilated sweat ducts con-

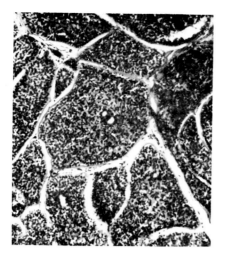

Fig. 42-48. Lobular hyalinized syringoma (turban tumor). (Hematoxylin and eosin.)

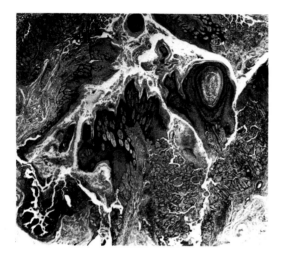

Fig. 42-49. Syringocystadenoma papilliferum. (Hematoxylin and eosin.)

taining inspissated secretion and, occasionally, keratin and characterized by epithelial spurs coming off the outer walls.

The **syringocystadenoma papilliferum** tends to occur as a solitary lesion of the scalp or forehead in patients of all ages. The overlying epidermis may be smooth or ulcerated. The histologic picture is easily recognizable by the cystic, papillary lesion projecting onto the surface from the upper dermis (Fig. 42-49). The papillary components are lined by two layers of cells, a deeper layer of small cuboid cells and an outer layer of tall columnar cells. The luminal secretion of the latter at times is mistaken for cilia, and such tumors in the cervical region have been mistaken for odd branchiogenic fistulas. Frequently, the lining is altered focally by squamous cell metaplasia that extends into underlying sweat ducts and glands. There is often considerable surrounding inflammatory reaction and a common association with hamartomas of sebaceous glands, pilary structures, and small basal cell carcinomas.

The term **hidradenoma papilliferum** is applied to the corresponding tumor of the labia majora or adjacent region that also simulates the papilloma of the subareolar mammary ducts.

The eccrine and apocrine **cystadenomas** occur on the face as solitary small translucent nodules and are easily identified by their lining epithelium. Some of these are regarded as retention cysts and are called **hidrocystomas.** Chondral metaplasia may occur in eccrine or apocrine cystadenomas. As I indicated many years ago, the genesis of such cartilage is epithelial, as it is in corresponding tumors of the salivary, lacrimal, and mammary glands.[9] These chondroid syringomas may also contain pilary components.

Cystic syringadenoma. The clear-cell, solid, or partially cystic syringadenoma or hidradenoma (unsupportably labeled "myoepithelioma") tends to be single, with a predilection for middle-aged and older women, and to occur in any region of the body. The tumors are likely to be sharply delimited and usually occur in the dermis but occasionally extend to the subcutis. In some instances, the lesions are in direct contact with the epidermis often thickened by pseudoepitheliomatous hyperplasia. The tumor cells are arranged in solid or cystic masses, the latter lined by stratified or papillary epithelium of characteristically clear, grossly vacuolated large polyhedral cells. These cells contain abundant glycogen.

In some instances, there are tubular lumens lined by cuboid cells and scattered through the lesion. Portions of the walls of the cysts may be lined by double layers of cuboid cells which, too, suggest their origin from sweat glands. These tumors contain abundant phosphorylase, esterases, and respiratory enzymes characteristic of tissue derived from sweat glands. The stroma commonly is focally homogenized and, as long emphasized, is in itself suggestive of the syringadenomatous nature of these tumors.

Syringocarcinoma. There is a tendency to diagnose sweat gland adenomas as malignant not because of anaplasia of the cells but because of the irregular ramification of nests of cells into adjacent dermis. On the other hand, some of the basal and squamous cell carcinomas characterized by small, discrete nests of cells are mistaken for sweat gland tumors—as are adenocarcinomas metastatic to skin, as well as melanocarcinomas. As a rule, the uncommon sweat gland carcinomas are of a low grade of virulence, as are carcinomas of appendages generally. There have been notable exceptions.

• • •

The diagnosis of tumors of the sweat ducts or glands is usually made without difficulty with the light microscope. Electron microscopic and histochemical studies offer supplementary information. However, electron microscopic and histochemical criteria that appear of decisive differential use in the recognition of normal structures of the sweat apparatus are apparently not always applicable to neoplasms. The widely prevalent notion that the validity of conclusions parallels the magnification needs reexamination. In general, amylophorylase, branching enzyme, succinic dehydrogenase, and leucine aminopeptidase are regarded as indicative of eccrine ducts and glands, whereas acid phosphatase and β-glucuronidase are stated to be characteristic of apocrine glands. And yet, the lobular hyalinized syringoma ("cylindroma"), for example, which is clearly of eccrine origin, has been found by some investigators histochemically to suggest apocrine as opposed to eccrine origin.

Sebaceous glands

Adenomas of sebaceous glands occur as small yellowish papules principally on and beside the nose, cheeks, and forehead. In many cases of multiple adenomas, there are associated verrucae, neurofibromas, subungual fibrosis, and "shagreen" patches. These patches of tuberous sclerosis are nodules or elevated masses of skin produced by the proliferation and sclerosis of dermal collagen. This sclerosis may easily be mistaken histologically for scleroderma. The overlying epidermis may be normal or acanthotically reticulated. In some cases, the patients develop tuberous sclerosis of the cerebral cortex and present the triad of sebaceous adenoma, mental deficiency, and epilepsy (p. 2080). These patients also may have visceral tumors, such as renal angiolipomas. Poliosis, café-au-lait spots, fibroepithelial tags, and hemangiomas also may be associated with this entity. The sebaceous adenomas are likely to

have developed during the first few years of life.

The histologic picture is that of an overgrowth of sebaceous glands without apparent linkage to the hair apparatus. Often, it is difficult to be sure that the process is not simple hyperplasia rather than neoplasia. There is another histologic form of sebaceous adenoma, characterized by a proliferation of the basal cells lining the sebaceous glands interspersed with isolated sebaceous cells. Rarely, a metastasizing sebaceous gland carcinoma develops in which at least a few scattered sebaceous cells help to identify the source.

Nevus sebaceus of Jadassohn. The term "nevus sebaceus of Jadassohn" is applied to hamartomatous or dysembryogenetic papular or nodular tumefactions of sebaceous glands or the pilosebaceous apparatus. Such malformations may be associated with other ectodermal or mesodermal malformations. Overlying or adjacent verrucal epidermal hyperplasia, a variety of sweat or lacrimal gland adenomas, focal alopecia, dermoids, dermal lipomas, angiomas, or basal cell carcinomas may accompany the lesion. Occasionally, it may be combined with ocular and cerebral lesions, with mental retardation and convulsions, as a form of *neurocutaneous* syndrome. Sebaceous gland hyperplasia, adenomas, and carcinomas have been reported in association with multiple visceral carcinomas.

Hair follicles

There is a divergence of opinion as to the types of neoplasms that may arise from hair follicles. Many observers believe that basal cell carcinomas are derived from *embryonic* hair follicles. However, as previously stated, the histologic evidence favors the view that basal cell carcinomas arise from the mature basal cells wherever they lie—at the base of the epidermis, at the periphery of sebaceous glands, or in the outermost layer of the hair follicles. However, the tumor that probably does arise from hair follicles is known synonymously as *trichoepithelioma, Brooke's tumor,* or *epithelioma adenoides cysticum* (Fig. 42-50). Some observers believe that the origin of this tumor from sweat or sebaceous glands is a possibility. The lesion tends to be familial and appears as multiple smooth nodules on the face and chest.

Histologically, unlike most basal cell carcinomas, the tumor is overlain by intact epidermis. The lesion is made up of varying-sized units of cysts filled with keratin and lined with stratified squamous epithelium, from which

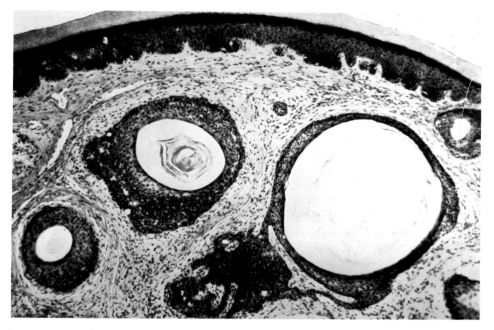

Fig. 42-50. Trichoepithelioma (Brooke's tumor; epithelioma adenoides cysticum). (Hematoxylin and eosin.)

nests of basal cells proliferate. The trichoepithelioma is benign, unlike the basal cell "epithelioma."

Cysts

The **dermoid cyst** is a congenital cutaneous inclusion occurring usually in the skin of the forehead, especially in the supraorbital region or midline. **Epidermoid cysts** also may be congenital and familial, particularly *steatocystoma multiplex,* but commonly they are the result of trauma (including insect bites) or inflammatory downgrowth, with separation and eventual isolation and encystment of a fragment of epidermis. A number originate from obstructed sweat ducts or hair follicles rather than from implantation by trauma. As previously indicated, "sebaceous cyst" is the term loosely applied to cysts that are, in actuality, derived from the entire pilary or pilosebaceous apparatus rather than from the sebaceous gland alone.[1] These keratinous cysts are lined by ordinary stratified squamous epithelium with, rarely, some residual sebaceous cells in one segment of the lining. Usually, the sebaceous cells have been obliterated in the mature cyst. Accordingly, they are labeled *pilosebaceous cysts,* although pilary cysts might be even more appropriate.

Grossly, the dermoid cannot be differentiated from pilosebaceous and epidermoid cysts.

Histologically, the wall of the cyst is actually skin with all of its appendages, often with a prominence of sebaceous glands. The epidermoid and sebaceous cysts differ from the dermoid cysts in that the former lack the appendages and their walls are made up of stratified squamous epidermis surrounded by fibrous tissue. As a rule, it is impossible to distinguish the epidermoid from the pilosebaceous cyst. Infrequently, evidence of the relation of the cyst to a contiguous sebaceous gland may persist. The criteria that have been set up for the differentiation are unreliable. The epithelium of both tends to be nonpigmented.

The contents of each of the cysts are predominantly a beige-colored, greasy keratin, representing in reality the stratum corneum, which in these instances cannot be shed but accumulates in the epidermal enclosures. There is also much fat within the laminated keratin, which either may not be demonstrable in routine sections or may be seen as cholesterin slits. In the dermoid cysts, hairs may be included. Occasionally, the lining epithelium may proliferate as papillary buds, either externally or inward toward the lumen of the cyst. Because of the irregularity of these proliferations and perhaps because of their superficial resemblance to the carcinomas of epidermis, there is a tendency to classify these hyperplasias or benign proliferations as cancer

—a tendency not warranted by their behavior.

The *calcifying epithelioma* is an exaggeration of this process of proliferation, which frequently is misinterpreted as cancer. Histologically, this lesion is usually a sharply circumscribed mass of disheveled fragments of epithelium, many of which are necrotic and often partially calcified. The epithelial cells have a basaloid character, although it is likely that they are predominantly of prickle cell origin. This pattern has suggested to some observers an attempt of cells with the ever-invoked "pluripotentiality" to form abortive hair and so has been labeled the etymologically unfortunate term "pilomatrixoma."

Actual cancerous transformation of the lining of cysts is an infrequent occurrence. The incidence of 1% to 6% quoted in the literature is probably high. A figure of about 0.5% would appear to be more representative.

REFERENCES
General

1 Allen, A. C.: The skin; a clinicopathologic treatise, St. Louis, 1954, The C. V. Mosby Co.
2 Braverman, I. M.: Skin signs of systemic disease, Philadelphia, 1970, W. B. Saunders Co.
3 Lever, W. F.: Histopathology of the skin, ed. 5, Philadelphia, 1975, J. B. Lippincott Co.
4 Montgomery, H.: Dermatopathology, Philadelphia, 1967, Paul B. Hoeber Medical Division, Harper & Row, Publishers.
5 Pinkus, H., and Mehregan, A. H.: Guide to dermatohistology, New York, 1969, Appleton-Century-Crofts.
6 Rook, A., Wilkinson, D. S., and Ebling, F. J. G.: Textbook of dermatology, Oxford, 1968, Blackwell Scientific Publications.
7 Zelickson, A. S.: Ultrastructure of normal and abnormal skin, Philadelphia, 1967, Lea & Febiger.

Specific

8 Albert, J., Bruce, W., Allen, A. C., and Blank, H.: Am. J. Med. **28:**661-667, 1960 (reticulohistiocytomas).
9 Allen, A. C.: Arch. Pathol. (Chicago) **29:**589-624, 1940 (origin of cartilage in mixed tumors).
10 Allen, A. C.: Arch. Dermatol. Syph. (Chicago) **57:**19-56, 1948 (survey of cutaneous diseases, World War II).
11 Allen, A. C.: Am. J. Pathol. **24:**367-387, 1948 (insect bites).
12 Allen, A. C.: Cancer **2:**28-56, 1949 (nevi and malignant melanomas).
13 Allen, A. C.: Surg. Gynecol. Obstet. **104:**753-754, 1957 (juvenile melanomas).
14 Allen, A. C.: Ann. N.Y. Acad. Sci. **100:**29-48, 1963 (juvenile melanomas).
15 Allen, A. C., and Spitz, S.: Cancer **6:**1-45, 1953 (nevi and malignant melanomas).
16 Allen, A. C., and Spitz, S.: Arch. Dermatol. Syph. (Chicago) **69:**150-171, 1954 (histogenesis of pigmented nevi).
17 Anderson, S., et al.: Arch. Dermatol. **108:**367-370, 1973 (Bowen's disease and visceral cancer).
18 Bandy, S., and Ackerman, G. B.: J.A.M.A. **213:**253-256, 1970 (lesions in drug-induced coma).
19 Breathnach, A. S.: J. Invest. Dermatol. **65:**2-15, 1975 (Langerhans' cells).
20 Castro, C., and Winkelmann, R. K.: Cancer **34:**1696-1705, 1974 (angiolymphoid hyperplasia).
21 Caulfield, J. B., and Wilgram, G. F.: J. Invest. Dermatol. **41:**57-65, 1963 (ultrastructure of acantholysis).
22 Clark, W. H., Jr., et al.: Cancer Res. **29:**705-726, 1969 (melanomas).
23 Coleta, D. F., et al.: Cancer **22:**879-884, 1968 (metastasizing basal cell carcinoma).
24 Cormane, R. H., et al.: Ann. N.Y. Acad. Sci. **254:**592-598, 1975 (B and T lymphocytes).
25 Curth, H. O., et al.: Cancer **15:**364-382, 1962 (acanthosis nigricans).
26 Davis, P., Atkins, B., and Hughes, G. R. V.: Br. J. Dermatol. **91:**175-181, 1974 (antibodies to DNA in discoid lupus erythematosus).
27 Douglas, H. M. G., and Bleumink, E.: Arch. Dermatol. **111:**979-985, 1975 (urticaria).
28 Dubin, H. V.: Arch. Dermatol. **110:**608-614, 1974 (lymphosarcoma and congenital lymphedema).
29 Ellman, M. A., et al.: Arch. Dermatol. **111:**986-990, 1975 (toxic dermal necrosis and allopurinol).
30 Fraser, N. G., Kerry, N. W., and Donald, D.: Br. J. Dermatol. **89:**439-444, 1973 (oral lesions in dermatitis herpetiformis).
31 Garancis, J. C., et al.: Am. J. Pathol. **64:**1-12, 1971 (microtubules).
32 Gazzolo, L., and Prunieras, M.: J. Invest. Dermatol. **51:**186-189, 1968 (lysosomes and keratinocytes).
33 Gilliam, J. N., et al.: J. Clin. Invest. **53:**1434-1440, 1974 (immunofluorescent band and renal disease in systemic lupus erythematosus).
34 Graham, J. H., and Helwig, E. B.: Cancer **32:**1396-1414, 1973 (review of erythroplasia of Queyrat).
35 Halpryn, H. J., and Allen, A. C.: Arch. Dermatol. **80:**160-166, 1959 (epidermal changes overlying sclerosing angiomas).
36 Hashimoto, K., and Bale, G. F.: Cancer **30:**530-540, 1973 (balloon cell nevi).
37 Huvos, A., et al.: Am. J. Pathol. **71:**33-45, 1973 (melanomas).
38 Jackson, S. F., and Fell, H. B.: Dev. Biol. **7:**394-419, 1963 (mucus-producing keratinocytes).
39 Jordon, R. E., et al.: Br. J. Dermatol. **92:**263-271, 1975 (dermo-epidermal deposition of complement components and properdin in systemic lupus erythematosus).
40 Kopf, A. W., and Popkin, G. L.: Arch. Dermatol. **110:**637, 1974 (shave biopsies).
41 Lopez, D. A., et al.: Cancer **34:**728-744, 1974 (cutaneous meningiomas).
42 Lutzner, M. R.: Arch. Dermatol. **87:**436-444, 1963 (molluscum bodies).
43 Lutzner, M. A., et al.: J. Natl. Cancer Inst. **50:**1145-1162, 1973 (Sézary cells).
44 Lyell, A.: Br. J. Dermatol. **68:**355-361, 1956 (toxic dermal necrolysis).
45 Mehregan, A. H.: Arch. Dermatol. **97:**381-393, 1968 (perforating elastosis).

46 Milston, E. B., and Helwig, E. B.: Arch. Dermatol. **108**:523-527, 1973 (basal cell carcinomas in children).

47 Molokhia, M. M., and Portnoy, B.: Br. J. Dermatol. **88**:347-353, 1973.

48 Morrison, W. L.: Viral warts and immunity, Br. J. Dermatol. **92**:625-630, 1975.

49 Pinkus, H., et al.: Arch. Dermatol. **74**:511-541, 1956 (eccrine poroma).

50 Pinkus, H.: Arch. Dermatol. **76**:419-426, 1957 (alopecia mucinosa).

51 Pinkus, H.: Arch. Dermatol. **107**:840-846, 1973 (lichenoid tissue reaction).

52 Pyrhönen, S., and Johannson, E.: Lancet, March 15, 1975 (regression of warts: an immunological study).

53 Ramsay, C. A., and Gianelli, F.: Br. J. Dermatol. **92**:49-56, 1975 (erythemal action spectrum and deoxyribonucleic acid repair synthesis in xeroderma pigmentosum).

54 Rappaport, H., and Thomas, L. B.: Cancer **34**:1198, 1974 (mycosis fungoides).

55 Reams, W. M., Jr., and Tompkins, S. P.: Dev. Biol. **31**:114-123, 1973 (keratinocytic nature of Langerhans' cells).

56 Rice, J. S., and Fischer, D. S.: Arch. Dermatol. **86**:503-511, 1962 (blue rubber-bleb nevus).

57 Sams, W. B., Jr.: Yearbook of dermatology, Chicago, 1973, Year Book Medical Publishers, Inc., pp. 5-27 (immunofluorescence in dermatology).

58 Sams, W. M., Jr., et al.: J. Invest. Dermatol. **64**:441-445, 1975 (vasculitis).

59 Schaumburg-Lever, G., et al.: J. Invest. Dermatol. **64**:47-49, 1975 (immunoglobulins in pemphigoid and lupus erythematosus).

60 Spitz, S.: Am. J. Pathol. **24**:591-609, 1948 (juvenile melanomas).

61 Spitz, S.: J. Am. Med. Wom. Assoc. **6**:209-219, 1951 (clinicohistologic disparities of tumors).

62 Stewart, F. W., and Treves, N.: Cancer **1**:64-81, 1948 (postmastectomy lymphangiosarcoma).

63 Tufanelli, D. L.: Arch. Dermatol. **103**:231-242, 1971 (lupus erythematosus panniculitis).

64 Unna, P.: Berl. Klin. Wochenschr. **30**:14-16, 1893 (epithelial origin of melanocarcinomas).

65 Wanebo, H. J., et al.: Cancer **35**:666-676, 1975 (clinicopathologic analysis of malignant melanoma).

66 Yeckley, J. A., et al.: Arch. Dermatol. **11**:29, 1975 (production of Sézary cells from normal human lymphocytes).

43/Mesenchymal tumors of soft tissues

RICHARD SHUMAN
W. A. D. ANDERSON

The term "soft tissues" is applied for convenience to the extraskeletal connective tissues of the body, including the organs of locomotion and their various component structures such as nerves, blood vessels, and lymphatics, but not including the glia, the reticuloendothelial system, and the supporting tissue of certain specific organs and tissues. These soft tissues comprise a variety of specific and nonspecific types, the latter retaining to some extent their embryonic potentialities, which, with a few neuroectodermal exceptions, are of mesodermal origin. Although these largely mesenchymal tissues, which are the most widespread in the body, are susceptible to a great number of pathologic and metabolic disturbances, they give rise to neoplasms (particularly malignant ones) with relative infrequency. Nevertheless, tumors of the soft parts comprise a sizable group with a wide morphologic and behavioral range. Logically, they include a number of comparable, supposedly nonneoplastic, tumorlike proliferations and hamartomatous anomalies sometimes virtually inseparable from true neoplasms on the basis of their histologic structure and clinical behavior.

In general, the cell types of the various neoplasms tend to perpetuate to a variable degree their prototype tissues. However, because they may undergo aberrant or incomplete differentiation or because their common mesenchymal derivation endows them with intimate histogenetic relationships, the various histogenetic types overlap and may present similar growth characteristics lacking in morphologic individuality. This has given rise to an impression that their diagnosis and treatment are fraught with considerable uncertainty and contradiction. Further hindering comprehensive understanding of these tumors are a lack of uniform diagnostic criteria, a divergent nomenclature, and limited clinicopathologic correlative studies in certain areas of investigation. A variety of older and newer techniques such as histochemistry, immunochemistry, tissue culture studies, and phase contrast and electron microscopy have contributed materially to the knowledge and understanding of many of the soft-tissue tumors. However, they have not reached the point of practical application for routine diagnostic purposes.

Although the majority of soft-tissue tumors are recognizable and can be classified on a histogenetic basis, so that their behavior is predictable, the interpretation of these tumors can be hazardous unless the pathologist follows a definite regional plan in order to arrive at an accurate diagnosis as a basis for appropriate treatment. For this, he must be familiar not only with the gross and microscopic features of the different tumor types but also with their relative frequency and distinctive characteristics by age groups and pattern of distribution. Naming soft-tissue tumors according to the appearance of the cell (e.g., round cell, spindle cell, or giant cell) and grading unrecognizable neoplasms on this basis—as though from these names their behavior might be inferred—is to be deprecated. Among soft-tissue sarcomas, histologic grade, in which frequency of mitoses is a major factor, correlates well with recurrence rates and is a valuable prognostic guide.

Benign and malignant mesenchymal tumors of the soft tissue are listed in Table 43-1. Those of predominantly regional or of systemic distribution are described elsewhere in this volume.

Table 43-1. Tumors and tumorlike growths of soft tissues

Type of tissue	Benign tumors	Malignant tumors

Fibrous tissue	Fibroma
	  Juvenile aponeurotic fibroma
	  Juvenile angiofibroma
	  Fibroma molle (fibrolipoma)
	  Fibroma durum
	  Elastofibroma
	Congenital generalized fibromatosis
	  (fibromatous hamartomatosis)
	Fibrous hamartoma of infancy
	Nodular fasciitis
	Fibromatosis
	  Keloid
	  Cicatricial
	  Irradiation
	  Palmar and plantar (Dupuytren's
	    contracture)
	  Fibromatosis colli
	  Penile (Peyronie's disease)
	Musculoaponeurotic fibromatosis
	  (desmoid fibromatosis)
	  Abdominal desmoid
	  Extraabdominal desmoid
		Fibrosarcoma
		  Differentiated
		    Nonmetastasizing fibrosarcoma
		    (aggressive fibromatosis)
		  Poorly differentiated

Undifferentiated and pluripotential mesenchyme	Myxoma
	Mesenchymoma (hamartoma-mixed
	  mesodermal tumor)
		Mesenchymoma (mixed mesodermal
		  tumor)

Adipose tissue	Lipoma
	Diffuse lipomatosis
	Hibernoma
	Lipoblastomatosis (embryonic lipoma,
	  fetal lipoma)
		Liposarcoma
		  Differentiated
		  Myxoid
		  Undifferentiated

Smooth muscle	Leiomyoma
	  Superficial (cutaneous, subcutane-
	    ous)
	  Deep
	  Bizarre (epithelioid) leiomyoma
		Leiomyosarcoma
		Bizarre (epithelioid) leiomyosarcoma

Striated muscle	Rhabdomyoma	Rhabdomyosarcoma
		  Embryonal
		    Mixed or botryoid type
		    Spindle cell type
		    Pseudopapillary, alveolar, or un-
		      differentiated round cell type
		  Undifferentiated adult
		    Pleomorphic type
		    Spindle cell type

Synovial tissue	Giant cell tumor of tendon sheath
	  (fibroxanthoma)
	Villonodular synovitis and bursitis
		Malignant giant cell tumor
		Synovial sarcoma
		  Monophasic type
		  Biphasic type

Mesothelial tissue	Benign mesothelioma (localized)
	  Epithelial (tubular) type
	  Fibrous (spindle cell) type
		Malignant mesothelioma (diffuse)
		  Epithelial (tubular) type
		  Spindle cell (fibrosarcoma) type
		  Mixed tubular and spindle cell
		    types
		  Pleomorphic type

Blood vessels and lymph vessels	Hemangioma
	  Capillary
	  Cavernous
	  Venous
	  Arterial
	  Arteriovenous
		Angiosarcoma

Continued.

Table 43-1. Tumors and tumorlike growths of soft tissues—cont'd

Type of tissue	Benign tumors	Malignant tumors
Blood vessels and lymph vessels—cont'd	Systemic hemangiomatosis (Osler, Surge-Weber, von Hippel, Lindau) Benign hemangioendothelioma ?Benign hemangiopericytoma Glomus tumor (glomangioma, glomangiomyoma) Lymphangioma Capillary Cystic Cavernous Lymphangiomatosis	Malignant hemangioendothelioma ?Malignant hemangiopericytoma Lymphangiosarcoma (malignant lymphangioendothelioma) Kaposi's sarcoma
Heterotopic bone and cartilage	Chondroma Osteoma Osteochondroma Myositis ossificans	Chondrosarcoma (extraosseous) Osteosarcoma (extraosseous)
Undetermined type	Granular cell myoblastoma Benign xanthogranuloma (histiocytoma)	Alveolar soft-part sarcoma (malignant organoid granular cell myoblastoma; malignant tumor of nonchromaffin paraganglia) Malignant xanthogranuloma (histiocytoma)
Peripheral nerves (nerve sheath type)	Neurofibroma Neurofibromatosis (Recklinghausen's disease) Neurilemoma (neurimoma; schwannoma)	Malignant neurofibroma (neurogenic sarcoma, neurofibrosarcoma) Malignant schwannoma Malignant mesenchymoma of nerve sheath

TUMORS OF FIBROUS TISSUE
Fibroma

Whether or not benign tumors of fibroblasts occur anywhere in the body in pure form as specific histologic entities is a matter of controversy. It is often difficult to make structurally precise distinctions between true tumors and tumorlike fibromatoid masses representing inflammatory and reparative hyperplasias, regressive metaplasias, and nonneoplastic overgrowths. Thus, because of the problems of histogenesis and terminology, usage of the term "fibroma" is not uniform.

From a descriptive standpoint, the designation fibroma is loosely applicable to the majority of localized, predominantly fibrous lesions that are without sharply separable patterns but among which recognizable variants exist. In the traditional histogenetic sense, however, the term is usually restricted to the more typical examples, which appear to have neoplastic qualities. Such tumors are characteristically described as encapsulated fibrous nodules that arise spontaneously, have limited growth potential, seldom attain a size more than a few centimeters in diameter, and do not recur after removal. Since problems of histogenesis are unsettled at present, it appears advisable to seek distinguishing characteristics among the various lesions as a basis for more adequately assessing their behavior.

In the soft tissues, a number of forms have been called fibromas, but in nearly all instances these include dermatofibroma, nodular fasciitis, nodular fibromatosis, and cicatrices, which doubtless are not true neoplasms. Occasional tumors of tendon sheath, neurofibromas, and leiomyomas may be completely overrun by fibrosis, which obscures their basic nature, so they may mimic fibromas to a remarkable degree. Certain terms, such as fibroma durum and fibroma molle, also are of an arbitrary nature but appear to have the sanction of usage. Usage also sanctions the terms nasopharyngeal fibroma (angiofibroma, p. 1216) and juvenile aponeurotic fibroma.

Juvenile aponeurotic fibroma

The term "juvenile aponeurotic fibroma" (calcifying fibroma) was suggested in 1953 to designate a distinctive fibroblastic tumor of the palms and soles of young children. Infrequently, however, analogous lesions suggesting cartilaginoid growths have been encountered in other superficial sites, chiefly the arms and legs and in the paravertebral region

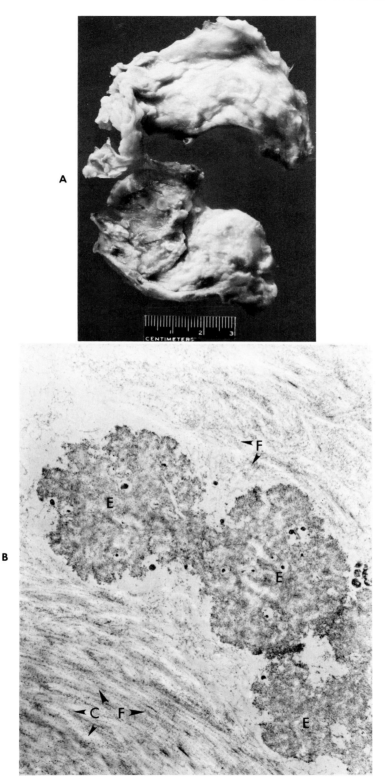

Fig. 43-1. A, Elastofibroma removed from subscapular area. Areas of degeneration are evident on cut surface. Margins are irregular and ill defined. **B,** Electron micrograph of elastofibroma shown in **A.** *E,* Elastic fibers; *C,* collagen fibrils; *F,* microfibrils. (28,500×.)

in adults as well as in children.[8] The precise nature and nosologic position of the lesion is still in question, but it appears to be clinically and morphologically related to fibromatosis. Unlike fibromatosis, however, it is a cellular and fibrillar growth, composed of parallel and circumferentially oriented strands and sheet-like masses of uniform, comparatively small rounded and spindle-shaped cells with minimal chondroid and osseous features and sometimes stippled with focal calcification. The lesion infiltrates and overgrows subcutaneous fat and voluntary muscle, often enveloping nerves and blood vessels, but not usually involving the aponeuroses or deep fascial structures. Apparently self-limiting, yet showing a disturbing tendency to invade locally and to recur postoperatively after limited excision, the growth usually is cured by re-excision.

Elastofibroma

Elastofibroma dorsi is a rare benign elasto-fibrous growth, usually occurring under the scapular muscles and frequently attached to the rib cage. It is a firm solid mass of fibrous and some adipose tissue. Fibrils that take elastic stains, elastinophilic masses, and a homogeneous matrix are the characteristic features. The mass has irregular margins that extend into adjacent fascia and muscle. It has been suggested that it is an elastodysplasia or degenerative pseudotumor, rather than a true neoplasm. (See Fig. 43-1.)

Congenital generalized fibromatosis and fibrous hamartoma of infancy

Congenital generalized fibromatosis (poly-fibromatosis, multicentric mesenchymal dysplasia, fibromatous hamartomatosis) is a rare systemic disturbance manifested by multiple, often widely scattered, nodular and locally infiltrative fibroblastic lesions in the superficial and deep soft tissues, viscera, and bone. Most observers regard the disorder as a generalized form of fibromatosis (polyfibromatosis) of infancy and childhood. Nevertheless, the occurrence of the lesions in other mesenchymal tissues and usually smooth muscle elements and vasoformative tissue, often in angiomatous arrangement, intermingled with the predominant fibrous component, suggests a developmental disturbance such as multicentric mesenchymal dysplasia or so-called fibromatous hamartomatosis. Undoubtedly, some of the reported cases of infantile neuro-fibromatosis and congenital fibrosarcoma with or without widespread metastases or what is sometimes referred to as aggressive infantile fibromatosis belong to this entity. Usually present at birth, or appearing shortly thereafter, the condition in its more florid form is incompatible with life. Apparently, milder forms of the disease also occur. A familial relationship has been described in which the condition occurred in four members of one family.

Fibromatosis hyalinica multiplex juvenilis is a recently described entity usually manifested in young children but not present at birth. It may represent a morphologically destructive form of multicentric fibromatosis, although its exact nature is uncertain. It is a slowly growing subcutaneous tumor, occurring in varying numbers throughout the body, but particularly on the scalp. It consists of spindle-shaped cells forming minute strands with an amorphous eosinophilic stroma. Although there may be some deformities of the head and trunk, physical and mental development of the children is usually normal. New single growths may appear throughout childhood, and some tumors recur after enucleation. Recurring digital fibrous tumors of infancy and childhood may be part of the spectrum of congenital fibromatoses.

Fibrous hamartoma of infancy (subdermal fibromatous tumor of infancy) appears to be an analagous, usually solitary, fibromatous tumor situated almost exclusively in the dermis and subcutaneous fat. It may be found on various parts of the body, but particularly in the axilla, shoulder, and upper arm of infants and young children. Grossly, the tumors average 3 to 4 cm in diameter but with wide deviations. Except for poorer circumscription, they resemble fibrolipomas. Histologically, the fibrous hamartoma of infancy may be difficult to differentiate from juvenile fibromatosis and certain neurogenic tumors. However, clusters of mature-appearing fat cells interposed between well-defined fibrous trabeculae, foci resembling primitive mesenchyme, or whorls and masses of spindle-shaped cells are distinguishing features.

Nodular fasciitis

The entity nodular fasciitis (fasciitis, infiltrative fasciitis, subcutaneous pseudosarcomatous fibromatosis) is a tumorlike fibroblastic proliferation that histologically may suggest sarcoma, although it is clinically benign. The pathogenesis of the lesion is uncertain, although it is probably a reactive or inflammatory process, possibly induced by a virus and related to the myxoma-fibroma group of lesions in animals. Usually developing in young adults, particularly on the extremities, neck, and trunk, it arises in the subcutaneous fascia or occasionally in the superficial portions of the deep fascia of the underlying muscle sheath. The overlying skin may be raised, with slight brownish discoloration, but is uninvolved by the growth. Parosteal fasciitis, a similar, self-limited benign lesion occurring in relation to bone, has also been described.

The nodule generally appears suddenly and is frequently characterized by rapid growth. It may reach its maximum size within a few days or weeks. At other times, it may grow more slowly, or it may show no appreciable growth over a period of many months. Appearing almost invariably as a single, discrete, slightly tender or asymptomatic nodule, varying from 4 mm to about 4 cm in diameter, it is circumscribed but unencapsulated and, on section, appears grayish white to tan in color, with mucoid and gelatinous areas.

Although the microscopic appearance is variable, there are certain uniform features:

1. A nodular proliferation of young, actively growing, large multipolar to spindle-shaped fibroblasts, with variable amounts of cytoplasm and plump, oval or round hyperchromatic nuclei with prominent nucleoli
2. A syncytial stromal meshwork of delicate fibrillary processes extending out in all directions from the parent fibroblasts, together with intercellular reticulin and collagen fibers and variable amounts of amorphous ground substance
3. A vascular component consisting of slitlike spaces, capillary buds, and occasional well-formed blood vessels of small caliber
4. A variable cellular component that may include multinucleated giant cells of various types; mesenchymal cells not readily distinguishable from fibroblasts; extravasations of red blood cells and infiltrates of inflammatory cells—predominantly lymphocytes, plasma cells, and macrophages
5. Involvement of superficial or deep fascia in all cases

The organization of the lesion varies from that of an exuberant granulation tissue to a fibroma-like appearance (Figs. 43-2 and 43-3). When the fibroblasts are large and hyperchromatic with frequent mitoses, the lesion

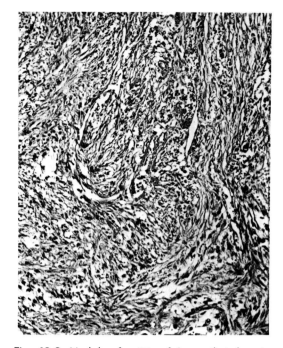

Fig. 43-2. Nodular fasciitis of 3 months' duration in subcutaneous deltoid region. Cells and fibers in compact arrangement with formation of bundles and whorls. (AFIP 60-4736.)

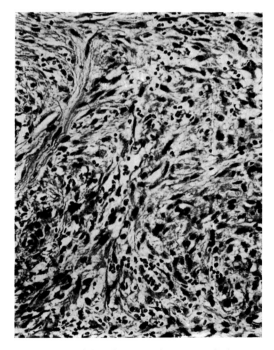

Fig. 43-3. Nodular fasciitis showing cellular area of haphazardly arranged oval and spindle cells with hyperchromatic nuclei, among which are slitlike spaces containing erythrocytes and mononuclear cells. (AFIP 60-4860.)

may resemble a fibrosarcoma (Fig. 43-3). The myxoid growths must be differentiated from myxoid liposarcoma, embryonal myxoid rhabdomyosarcoma, and edematous neurofibroma or neurilemoma. Evidence based on follow-up studies indicates that fasciitis is a benign condition, the treatment of which is simple local excision.

Palmar and plantar fibromatosis

The tumorlike proliferations that occur in the palmar and plantar aponeuroses are similar except that the flexion deformities associated with palmar fibromatosis (Dupuytren's contracture, p. 2040) are uncommonly observed in the feet. Involvement may be unilateral or bilateral, and concomitant involvement of both hands and feet occurs in about 5% to 10% of cases. The background appears to be hereditary, but·trauma may be a factor. The condition is found most frequently in middle-aged and older male adults. It is relatively uncommon in children. On the basis of ultrastructural studies, it has been suggested that the fibroblasts in Dupuytren's contracture have modulated into contractile cells (myofibroblasts) and that their contraction plays a role in the pathogenesis of the contracture.

The lesions grow slowly, appearing as localized nodular enlargements or occasionally diffuse thickenings, that develop in or infiltrate the fascia and sometimes involve the overlying skin and subcutaneous tissues. Dorsal extension with fixation to the deeper structures is uncommon, although recurrent nodules may become adherent to the underlying tendons. The tumors usually are circumscribed but unencapsulated and range in size from a few millimeters to 4 or 5 cm or more. They are firm and grayish white and have a whorled, fasciculated appearance.

The microscopic picture of the nodules is distinctive. It is characterized by a compact intertwining proliferation of uniform spindle-shaped to fusiform fibroblasts and by variable amounts of collagen interdigitated with the dense acellular bundles of normal fascia (Fig. 43-4). The number of mitotic figures in the more cellular areas may be as high as three to four per high-power field. The borders of the nodules are usually poorly defined and merge imperceptibly with surrounding fascia. Other nodules consist of dense, poorly cellular fasciculi of collagenous tissue scarcely distinguishable from normal preexisting fascia.

Although the lesions are almost invariably

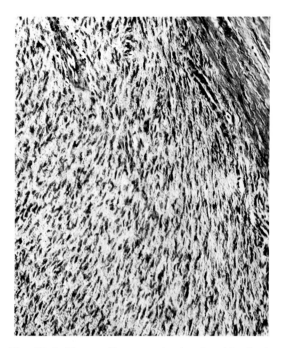

Fig. 43-4. Plantar fibromatosis showing histologic pattern. (AFIP 60-4877.)

benign, the recurrence rate is relatively high unless the palmar or plantar fascia is totally excised. Because of their tendency to recur after simple excision, small asymptomatic nodules are perhaps best left untreated. Occasionally, highly cellular tumors with large atypical fibroblasts and numerous mitotic figures are difficult to distinguish from fibrosarcoma, but this latter diagnosis should be considered only after repeated recurrences and with extensive involvement of the deeper structures.

Musculoaponeurotic fibromatosis (desmoid fibromatosis)

Arising primarily from fascial sheaths and musculoaponeurotic structures in various parts of the body are benign fibrous growths that differ from simple palmar and plantar fibromatoses in that characteristically they infiltrate or develop in skeletal muscle. Similar but less well-defined tumors, not necessarily involving muscle, occasionally occur in the periosteum (periosteal desmoid), orbit, mediastinum, and mesentery. The lesions are seen in all age groups but most commonly in young adults. They constitute the majority of fibrous tumors of the soft parts exclusive of skin.

The noncommittal term "desmoid tumors," or, more recently, "desmoid fibromatosis," is

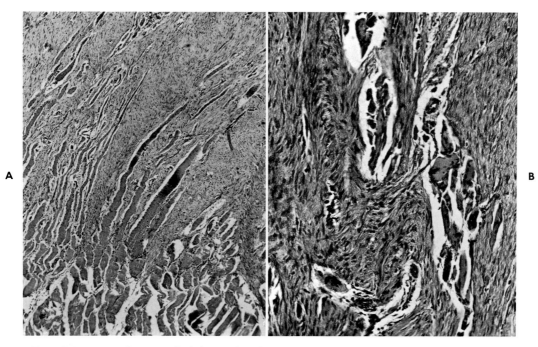

Fig. 43-5. Desmoid tumor of abdominal wall in 36-year-old multipara. **A,** Broad trabeculae of dense fibrous tissue infiltrate and destroy muscle bundles. **B,** Higher power showing wavy collagen bundles and muscle giant cells. (**A,** AFIP 52-1835; **B,** AFIP 52-1836.)

applied to the group as a whole. This is based on their fundamental similarity in origin and behavior to the distinctive tumors arising from the musculoaponeurotic structures of the abdominal wall that occur especially (but not exclusively) in parous women. In its classic form, the abdominal desmoid tumor is situated in the anterior sheath of the rectus abdominis muscle just below the umbilicus and is believed to be initiated by the trauma of delivery. It may occur at the site of operation or other injury. It may develop spontaneously, however, in any part of the abdominal wall in either sex. The extraabdominal tumors also show a predilection for certain regional areas, the most common sites being the upper and lower extremities, head, and neck. Experience has demonstrated that the behavior of any single lesion is unpredictable, recurrences frequently following attempts at local removal. In some areas, particularly about the shoulder girdle, inguinal region, and lower extremities, they possess aggressive infiltrative tendencies (aggressive fibromatosis, p. 1882) and may spread to involve contiguous soft parts and osseous structures, but they do not metastasize. Rarely, fibromatosis of the head and neck may cause death by encroaching upon vital structures.

Fibromatosis of childhood (juvenile fibromatosis) is also prone to aggressive behavior. However, *fibromatosis colli (congenital wryneck, torticollis),* which may be incidental to birth injury, has been known to undergo spontaneous regression or usually can be prevented by early excision before deformity becomes permanent. Age and regional considerations are of more importance in assessing the growth potential of the various lesions than is their morphologic appearance, which does not usually reflect their biologic behavior (p. 1270).

The lesions present initially as asymptomatic or slightly painful tumors, apparently arising within muscle, over which the skin is freely movable. With progressive growth or recurrences, they may infiltrate the skin, become fixed to deeper structures, and engulf nerve trunks, producing numbness, hyperesthesia or severe pain, and limitation of motion. On gross examination, they usually are solitary tumors, varying in size from 1 to 15 cm or more, with an average of 6 to 8 cm. They are well circumscribed and may give the appearance of encapsulation, but during removal it is apparent that there is fixation to surrounding muscle with infiltration of fascial planes. They have a firm, rubbery consistency and are a homogeneous grayish white color, with intersecting fibrous bands and occasional areas of cystic degeneration.

Histologically, the general pattern is that of cellular interlacing bands of fibroblasts and collagen fibers, with some included muscle fibers. The latter usually are represented peripherally by compressed or isolated muscle bundles and, toward the center of the lesion, by individual atrophied muscle fibers and degenerated muscle giant cells (Fig. 43-5). There is considerable variation from one lesion to another and in different areas within the same lesion. Some are relatively acellular and composed of dense eosinophilic bands of collagen resembling hypertrophic keloidlike scar tissue whereas others are more cellular and have a fasciculated appearance or occasionally interstitial mucoid material may be present in portions of the tumor. Generally, the fibroblastic proliferation shows considerable uniformity and maturity, in many instances producing a tendonlike appearance, but in occasional highly cellular growths the fibroblasts may be large, with prominent vesicular or hyperchromatic nuclei and a few mitotic figures. The tumors must be completely removed by wide local excision. Recurrences and inoperable cases are sometimes satisfactorily controlled over long periods by radiation therapy.

Fibrosarcoma

The term "fibrosarcoma" is applied to a diverse group of tumors, all of which are believed to represent malignant growths of fibroblasts. However, truly malignant fibroblastic tumors capable of metastasis are relatively uncommon and of limited distribution. A majority of so-called fibrosarcomatous growths, particularly in the soft parts, are intermediate or borderline malignancies clinically and pathologically indistiguishable from aggressive fibromatoses or extra-abdominal desmoid tumors. This borderline group includes tumors exhibiting variable rates of growth and degrees of structural differentiation, but it appears nonetheless to represent a distinct class. In addition, there are a number of clinicopathologic variants of uncertain nature and position, some of which exhibit regionally specific characteristics. The generic term "fibrosarcoma" will be retained for the entire group.

In order to correlate structure with behavior and because of the therapeutic and prognostic implications, it is advisable to divide these tumors into two main classes:

(1) the well-differentiated, low-grade nonmetastasizing fibrosarcomas (aggressive fibromatoses) and (2) the poorly differentiated, moderately anaplastic, malignant fibrosarcomas.

Although described in nearly all locations where fibrous connective tissue is found, about 80% to 90% of fibrosarcomatous growths arise in the soft tissues. They may occur at any age, but approximately 70% are seen between the ages of 20 and 50 years, with a slight preponderance in males. Most of these tumors develop spontaneously, but many are noted after repeated trauma, although an etiologic relationship is difficult to ascertain in any given case.

Differentiated fibrosarcoma

Nonmetastasizing fibrosarcoma (aggressive fibromatosis) arises in both superficial and deep structures. The superficial lesions originating in skin and subcutaneous tissues are, with few exceptions, of the well-differentiated type, and they rarely, if ever, metastasize. An unquestionable primary fibrosarcoma of the superficial tissues is very uncommon, although it is sometimes seen after radiation injury or within scars. The disproportionately large number of cases reported in some series are found, on critical evaluation, to consist mostly of nodular fasciitis and dermatofibrosarcoma protuberans. *Nodular fasciitis,* as previously indicated, is a benign lesion that microscopically may sometimes appear deceptively like fibrosarcoma.

A majority of **deep fibrosarcomas of the differentiated type (aggressive fibromatoses)** arising in soft tissues have an origin and distribution similar to that of the musculoaponeurotic fibromatoses, i.e., in musculofibrous septa, in aponeuroses, and occasionally in deep connective tissue structures about tendon sheaths. They occur most often in the extremities, particularly about the shoulder girdle, but are not uncommon in the abdominal wall, back, head, and neck. Internal growths of this type in the retroperitoneum and mediastinum are great rarities, but they are somewhat less rare in the mesentery and omentum or other intraabdominal sites. Parosteal fibrosarcomas are seen occasionally, the tumor being either a large, circumscribed, ovoid mass intimately attached to the periosteum or encircling bone and extensively invading adjacent soft tissues (p. 2005). Well-differentiated fibrosarcomas have also been described in the orbit, nasopharynx, central nervous system, and certain viscera and in nearly all areas of the body in which fibrous connective tissue is found.

Well-differentiated fibrosarcomas cannot always be distinguished from musculoaponeurotic fibromatoses. Diagnostic judgment must be based also on clinical and regional considerations. When fibromatous growths of questionable morphology are located other than in the abdominal wall and recur after excision, they often are indiscriminately diagnosed as fibrosarcomas. However, recurrence is not necessarily a criterion of malignancy, and it is well known that these lesions frequently occur in individuals with an inherent tendency to develop spontaneously exaggerated fibroblastic proliferation, a so-called desmoplastic diathesis. In any event, whether regarded as aggressive fibromatoses or as differentiated fibrosarcomas, they are characteristically unencapsulated, infiltrating, and locally destructive growths that may recur repeatedly over many years but without disposition to metastasize. Microscopically, the

fibroblasts are well differentiated, but with occasional mitotic figures, and tend to form obtuse or sinuously interlaced bundles, sometimes assuming a herringbone pattern (Fig. 43-6) an arrangement often believed to distinguish true fibrosarcoma from aggressive fibromatosis. However, in addition to such organized structure in which there are numerous collagen and reticulin fibers, the pattern may be variable, and in areas the tumor may show a dense keloidlike scar tissue with a relative paucity of fibrocytes. Recurrences are frequently more mature and more characteristic of desmoid tumors than is the primary growth.

Treatment of the early operable cases necessitates surgical excision well beyond the palpable margins of the tumor. In many instances, recurrences respond well to radiation therapy. In a survey of 35 cases of aggressive fibromatosis from the shoulder region, there was a recurrence rate of 74% and only one death as a result of the tumor growth penetrating the chest wall.

Poorly differentiated fibrosarcoma

Approximately 20% of soft-part fibrosarcomas are poorly differentiated, and it is necessary by the usual criteria to regard them as malignant tumors. However, although such fibrosarcomatous lesions are rapidly growing and locally aggressive, the majority do not metastasize. Five- and 10-year survival rates range from 60% to 80%. They usually exhibit increased cellularity with moderate to strong anaplasia, cell irregularity, and increased numbers of mitotic figures. Bizarre cells and small hyperchromatic spindle cells usually are present in profusion in the more malignant tumors, which produce comparatively little collagenous stroma. Giant cells are never a conspicuous feature in fibrosarcoma and, when present, should suggest a different type of sarcoma, such as leiomyosarcoma, liposarcoma, or malignant fibrous xanthomas.

An uncommon variety of fibrosarcoma, which is of high malignant potential showing a strong propensity to metastasize, is the so-called immature macrocellular spindle cell sarcoma of the older writers. It is well demarcated, usually of moderate size, and appears to arise in connection with tendons and periarticular structures as well as aponeuroses. It may represent a monophasic variant of synovial sarcoma. Histologically, it is composed of closely packed bands and bundles of large, elongated spindle cells of uniform type with abundant eosinophilic cyoplasm and hyper-

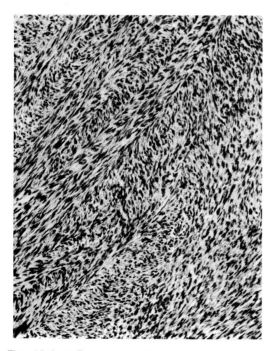

Fig. 43-6. Differentiated fibrosarcoma (aggressive fibromatosis) of shoulder region in 29-year-old man that recurred 2 years after primary excision. Section illustrated was selected from densely cellular area in order to demonstrate so-called fibrosarcoma pattern. Although locally aggressive, it is unlikely that such tumor will metastasize. (AFIP 60-4851.)

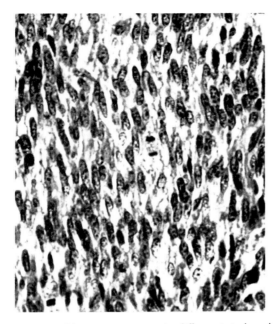

Fig. 43-7. Fibrosarcoma, poorly differentiated and of immature macrocellular spindle cell type. Highly cellular, and nuclei assume large vesicular form. Note mitotic figures and scarcity of intercellular collagen. (AFIP 53-10393.)

chromatic nuclei showing frequent mitotic activity. It lacks differentiation in that little or no collagenous matrix is elaborated, although reticulin (precollagen) is present in various amounts (Fig. 43-7). In this undifferentiated malignant type, radical extirpative surgery, either wide excision or amputation, affords the only possibility of cure.

BENIGN AND MALIGNANT TUMORS OF PROBABLE HISTIOCYTIC ORIGIN

In recent years, the terms "benign" and "malignant fibrous histiocytoma" have been used by pathologists to refer to a broad spectrum of benign and malignant tumors of probable histiocytic origin. More specific terms have been applied to different well-recognized morphologic subtypes. Fibrous histiocytomas arise in both superficial and deep soft-tissue structures of any part of the body, although the number of clinical and histologic variants often clouds their recognition as related entities. The benign lesions, most of which suggest nonneoplastic tumefactions are easily recognized histologically, but the obviously malignant lesions in many instances are mistaken for pleomorphic liposarcoma or pleomorphic rhabdomyosarcoma. Often, the differentiation may be dependent on the demonstration of a storiform stromal pattern, believed to be the histologic hallmark of these tumors. The concept of fibrous histiocytoma is based on classic but as yet unresolved studies, suggesting that the tumors are composed largely of cells with the characteristics of histiocytes by light microscopic, tissue culture, and ultrastructural studies. It is hypothesized that the proliferating histiocytes transform into fibroblast-like cells (facultative fibroblasts) with collagen-synthesizing ability and so are responsible for the more or less prominent fibroblastic component of these tumors. The admixtures of xanthomatous cells and giant cells, constituent elements of most fibrous histiocytomas, are also believed to be histiocytic derivatives. Despite the debatable histogenesis of this group of tumors, the terminology has gained wide acceptance and, therefore, tentatively is being adopted here.

With respect to their anatomic and regional location, morphology, and behavior characteristics, the fibrous histiocytomas may be classified as follows:

A. Benign fibrous histiocytoma (fibrous xanthoma)
  1. Dermatofibroma (histiocytoma, fibrous xanthoma, sclerosing hemangioma, nodular subepidermal fibrosis)
  2. Giant cell tumor of tendon sheath (fibrous xanthoma, localized nodular tenosynovitis)
  3. Pigmented villonodular synovitis and bursitis
  4. Juvenile xanthogranuloma (nevoxanthoendothelioma, nevoid histiocytoma)
  5. Reticulohistiocytoma (localized and generalized giant cell reticulohistiocytoma)
  6. Xanthofibromatous pseudotumor (postradiation pseudotumor, pseudotumor in association with squamous carcinoma, postinflammatory pseudotumor of lung)
  7. Retroperitoneal xanthogranuloma (Oberling)
B. Intermediate type of fibrous histiocytoma (intermediate type of fibrous xanthoma)
  1. Atypical fibroxanthoma (pseudosarcomatous dermatofibroma, atypical fibrous histiocytoma, paradoxical fibrosarcoma, pseudotumor)
  2. Dermatofibrosarcoma protuberans (progressive and recurring dermatofibroma, storiform fibrous xanthoma)
C. Malignant fibrous histiocytoma (malignant fibrous xanthoma, fibroxanthosarcoma)
  1. Malignant fibrous histiocytoma, pleomorphic and predominantly fibrous type
  2. Malignant retroperitoneal xanthogranuloma (malignant fibrous xanthoma)
  3. Malignant histiocytoma, questionable type
    a. Epithelioid sarcoma of soft tissues
    b. Malignant giant cell tumor of soft tissue
    c. Sclerosing reticulum cell sarcoma of soft tissue (extremely rare)

Benign fibrous histiocytoma (fibrous xanthoma)

Benign fibrous histiocytomas occur primarily as localized nodular lesions in the skin (dermatofibroma) and about tendon sheaths (giant cell tumor of tendon sheaths) or as composite nodular or diffuse masses in points and bursae (pigmented villonodular synovitis and bursitis). In addition, the term "fibrous histiocytoma" is also applied, often inconsistently, to a variety of different lesions found almost anywhere in the body, as seen in the classification. Although the majority of such lesions are generally considered reactive or proliferative processes, they cannot always be differentiated from true neoplastic conditions. Histologically, a composite picture of the lesions is impossible to describe. The typical nodules are composed predominantly of fibroblast-like cells showing variable degrees of fibrogenesis or, in addition, histiocytes and multinucleated giant cells. Lipid-filled histiocytes and tendon giant cells together with an intermingling of chronic inflammatory cells and variable amounts of hemosiderin pigment are additional features seen in some of the lesions. The xanthomatous or postinflammatory pseudotumor of the lung in particular may show a striking storiform pattern, otherwise uncommonly encountered in the benign fibrous xanthomas.

Intermediate type of fibrous histiocytoma
Atypical fibroxanthoma

Atypical fibroxanthoma (pseudosarcomatous dermatofibroma) has been singled out as a special form of fibrohistiocytic tumor with a number of characteristic clinical and pathologic features. The lesion usually occurs as a solitary, ulceronodular tumor on the exposed skin of the head and neck (chiefly the ears, cheeks, and nose) of elderly patients. A clinical variant has also been described in the skin of the trunk and limbs of younger individuals. Judged by their ominous histologic appearance, atypical fibroxanthoma may be incorrectly interpreted as highly malignant neoplasms, although they usually prove benign. Indeed, atypical fibroxanthoma may simulate malignant melanoma, pleomorphic sarcoma, or anaplastic spindle cell carcinoma, and the morphologic distinction between these lesions has been appreciated only during recent years. The majority of the nodules develop as circumscribed cellular proliferations within the dermis, but they frequently extend into the subcutaneous tissue. Histologically, there is considerable variation in the cellular pattern of the atypical fibroxanthomas, and they range from those resembling benign fibroxanthomas to highly pleomorphic forms. Briefly, the features that characterize the more pleomorphic lesions are the variable proportions of bizarre mononucleated and multinucleated giant cells, some resembling Touton type of giant cells, and others with grotesque hyperchromatic nuclei, dispersed in a stromal background of plumpish spindle-shaped and ovoid cells, sometimes arranged in interlacing fascicles. Mitotic figures, often abnormal, may be frequent in these cells. A storiform pattern is uncommon in atypical fibroxanthoma, although fibrillar collagenous substance may be abundant in some tumors.

As to the clinical behavior of the atypical fibroxanthomas, published reports suggest that the lesions are almost uniformly benign. However, personal experience indicates that their aggressiveness and malignant potential may be greatly underrated. From the standpoint of practical importance, it appears that tumors restricted to the dermis, or at most extending into the superficial subcutis, have a highly favorable prognosis and generally follow a benign course. However, deep subcutaneous infiltration may result in local recurrences and even metastasis, although the latter is uncommon. One should note that tumors with the histologic pattern of highly pleomorphic atypical fibroxanthoma may involve deeper soft-tissue structures either primarily or secondarily, but often they fungate and present initially as primary intracutaneous lesions. Such tumors have a malignant potential and should be regarded as malignant fibrous histiocytomas or fibroxanthosarcomas.

Dermatofibrosarcoma protuberans

Dermatofibrosarcoma protuberans (progressive and recurring dermatofibroma, storiform fibrous xanthoma) is a borderline sarcoma first accorded recognition as an entity by Darier and designated dermatofibrosarcoma protuberans by Hoffmann in 1925. Based on morphologic and tissue culture observations, a histogenetic relationship has been postulated between dermatofibroma and its questionable malignant counterpart dermatofibrosarcoma protuberans and benign and malignant fibrous histiocytomas or fibrous xanthomas. The matter of histogenesis has not been settled unequivocally, and the previously held view that the tumors are of fibroblastic origin, cannot be completely discarded.

Dermatofibrosarcoma protuberans is easily recognized by its distinctive, relatively pure,

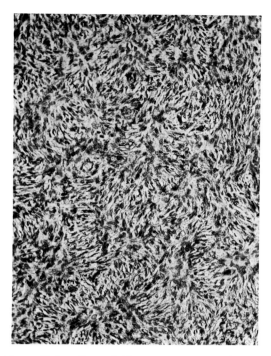

Fig. 43-8. Dermatofibrosarcoma protuberans. Spindle cells arranged in interwoven pattern and radiating from focal points of condensed collagen. (AFIP 60-1930.)

storiform pattern of growth, a feature now generally believed to be highly characteristic of the fibrous histiocytomas. The lesion is predominantly an intracutaneous growth, arising as a single or multiple, hard, coalescence of nodules or plaques that enlarge slowly and become fixed to the skin and subcutaneous tissues. A protruding mass is formed varying from a few centimeters to 20 cm or more in diameter, which after a variable period (ranging from 6 months to 25 years or more) may fungate and ulcerate. Microscopically the appearance is that of a uniform cellular growth with spindle cells arranged in an interwoven rhythmic pattern or radiating from central focal points of condensed collagen, giving the appearance of spiral galaxies or the so-called spoke wheel—the storiform pattern (Fig. 43-8). Occasional examples present a fasciculated pattern, with the cells lying in parallel rows. Sometimes, myxoid areas are prominent, usually in recurrent lesions. Collagen production is variable but usually scanty. Cellular morphology may vary widely sometimes approaching that of true fibrosarcoma, and mitotic figures may be fairly numerous in some areas. Frequently primary tumors are more cellular

than recurrent lesions. Giant cells and abnormal histiocytes are rarely found in these lesions. Occasionally, dermatofibrosarcoma protuberans presents a formidable appearance clinically, and about 30% recur after excision, although they can be controlled by reexcision. A few instances of metastases have been reported in the literature, but in a study of 115 cases at the Armed Forces Institute of Pathology, metastasis was not observed.

Malignant fibrous histiocytoma (malignant fibrous xanthoma)

Malignant pleomorphic fibrous histiocytomas (fibroxanthosarcomas) are preponderantly neoplasms of deep soft-tissue structures of middle-aged or older adults, although the age range is wide. The tumors occur principally in the extremities, particularly the thigh and leg, but less frequently they are encountered on the trunk and in the retroperitoneum, or in other parts of the body. They have a relatively poor prognosis and frequently metastasize to regional lymph nodes and lungs or more widely by the hematogenous route. Radiation may have a beneficial effect upon the primary tumor or its metastases.

On gross examination, the malignant fibrous histiocytomas vary greatly in appearance, size, and texture. Most are poorly delimited multinodular masses of soft or firm grayish yellow tissue with cystic and necrotic areas, and they may vary from 2 to 20 cm or more in diameter. The tumors usually invade adjacent tissues and tend to recur locally after limited surgical removal. Microscopically, the malignant pleomorphic fibrous histiocytomas show a highly variegated sarcomatous-appearing spindle-cell stroma and large numbers of pleomorphic histiocytes or xanthoma cells, with granular or foamy cytoplasm and bizarre histiocytic giant cells, often including fantastic forms with clumped nuclei or fragmented masses of nuclear material. Numerous normal and abnormal mitotic figures may be found throughout the tumor. There may be variable amounts of fibrillar collagen between the stromal cells, and almost always there is a recognizable, if only focal and abortive, storiform pattern in parts of the tumor, a distinguishing feature to be looked for. Otherwise, it may be impossible to distinguish the tumor from pleomorphic rhabdomyosarcoma or pleomorphic liposarcoma, tumors that bear remarkable histologic similarity to the malignant fibrous xanthomas.

Tumors developing in deep soft-tissue structures and exhibiting histologic features of atypical fibroxanthoma, should be included among the malignant pleomorphic fibrous histiocytomas. Also, the very exceptionally encountered infiltrating retroperitoneal tumors with an inflammatory xanthogranulomatous pattern and variable amounts of fibrous tissue, as first described by Oberling, appear to include both benign and malignant forms, but the usual histologic variant appears to follow a highly unpredictable course. Recently, there has been quite general agreement that such lesions, which are undoubtedly morphologic variants of fibrous xanthomas, should be regarded as potentially malignant, with an exceptionally poor prognosis when the histologic picture of malignancy is clear cut. Similar lesions may also occur in other sites. Many malignant fibrous xanthomas present a predominantly spindle-cell fibrogenic pattern with numerous or sparse mononuclear and multinuclear histiocytic or xanthomatous giant cells. These tumors, which may resemble dermatofibrosarcoma protuberans, fibrosarcoma, or even leiomyosarcoma, are locally aggressive neoplasms but probably of somewhat lower overall malignancy than the more pleomorphic types.

Juvenile aponeurotic fibroma

The term "juvenile aponeurotic fibroma" (calcifying fibroma) was suggested in 1953 to designate a distinctive fibroblastic tumor of the palms and soles of young children. From the relevant cases in the literature, the lesions apparently exhibit a predilection for the hand, most often the palm, although the wrist, metacarpal area, and fingers may be the site of involvement in adults as well as in children. Frequently, analogous lesions suggesting cartilaginoid fibrous growths have been encountered in the deep musculofascial and paraskeletal tissues, chiefly the arms and legs and in the paravertebral region. Aponeurotic fibroma has also been described in the superficial subcutaneous tissues without involvement of deeper structures. The precise nature and nosologic position of the lesion is still in question, but it appears to be clinically and morphologically related to fibromatosis. Unlike fibromatosis, however, it is a cellular fibroblastic growth, composed of irregularly arranged or whorled, parallel and circumferentially oriented strands and sheetlike masses of rounded and spindle-shaped cells with foci of stippled, or heavy amorphous calcification surrounding and within a zone of chondroid metaplasia. Ocasional osteoclast-like giant cells may be found adjacent to the calcium deposits, within the compact cellular rim of the chondroid focus. Although atypical histologic features are absent, the lesion infiltrates and overgrows subcutaneous fat and voluntary muscle often enveloping nerves and blood vessels, but not usually involving tendons, the aponeuroses, or deep fascial structures when located in the hands or feet. Although showing a disturbing tendency to invade locally and to recur, sometimes repeatedly, the growth is usually controlled by conservative surgical procedures.

TUMORS OF UNDIFFERENTIATED AND PLURIPOTENTIAL MESENCHYME
Myxoma

A peculiar form of mesenchymal tumor, myxoma reproduces the structure of primitive mesenchyme or of the mucoid connective tissue (Wharton's jelly) of the umbilical cord. Since this tissue does not exist in the adult but is widespread in the embryo, it has been postulated to arise from embryonic rests (Ewing) or to represent the reappearance of mucin in the intercellular matrix of some fibroblastic growths (Willis). Although the neoplasm is relatively uncommon, it occurs in the heart, skin, subcutaneous and aponeurotic tissues, muscle, certain bones, especially the jawbones (odontogenic myxoma, p. 1256), genitourinary tract, and other unusual sites. Except for the skin and subcutaneous tissue, a myxoma seldom develops in the soft parts other than in relationship to the large muscles and aponeuroses of the limbs, chiefly the thigh and shoulder. It may be found in any age group but more commonly in middle-aged adults, and there is no obvious preponderance in either sex.

The lesions range in size from small subcutaneous tumors to giant deep growths, sometimes weighing several kilograms but usually they do not attain a size of more than 6 to 7 cm in diameter. The deep tumors tend to infiltrate contiguous structures but recur infrequently after excision. Although typical myxomas sometimes are considered malignant, they do not metastasize or undergo true sarcomatous change. Grossly, they are solitary, unencapsulated, soft to slightly firm, mucoid or slimy, and, at times, cystic in appearance. Histologically, they are composed of large stellate or spindle-shaped cells, probably fibroblasts, with anastomosing processes separated by an abundant basophilic mucoid ground substance rich in acid mucopolysaccharides in which there are granular and fibrillary precipitates and thin collagen fibers (Fig. 43-9). The poor

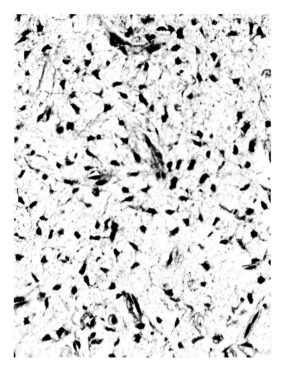

Fig. 43-9. Myxoma showing characteristic histologic pattern. Note sparse vascular supply consisting of occasional small-caliber blood vessels within delicate fibrous septa. (AFIP 60-4754.)

vascularization is important in differentiation from the highly-vascularized well-differentiated liposarcoma. Rarely, the tumor may show denser fibrous areas. The rarity of these tumors in deeper soft tissues should be appreciated, for they may be confused with a variety of malignant neoplasms susceptible to myxomatous change, such as myxoid liposarcoma, chondrosarcoma, embryonal rhabdomyosarcoma, mesenchymoma, and fibrosarcoma. The treatment of myxoma is complete local excision. Roentgenotherapy has uniformly proved to be ineffectual.

Mesenchymoma (hamartoma—mixed mesodermal tumor)

Mesenchymoma is a complex, supposedly dysontogenetic growth that displays the pluripotentialities and differential characteristics of the primitive mesenchyme from which it is derived. Composed of a variety of mesenchymal tissues (including fibrous, adipose, myxomatous, angiomatous, osseous, cartilaginous, muscle, and lymphoid) in various proportions and combinations, it has been appropriately designated mesenchymoma or

mixed mesodermal tumor. The diagnosis must be made with discrimination and is justified only in the presence of two or more mesenchymal elements other than ubiquitous benign or malignant fibroblastic tissue. Excluded from this category are those neoplasms known to undergo metaplastic change, such as liposarcoma, which may contain osseous and cartilaginous as well as fibrous tissue. It appears to be uncommon in the soft parts.

Although both benign and malignant mesenchymomas have been reported, evidence for a benign variety has not always been convincingly presented. The term "benign mesenchymoma" is sometimes applied to small, circumscribed, fatty, tumorlike masses associated with vascular and smooth muscle proliferations that occur in children and young adults. These are widely recognized, however, as congenital malformations and are either hamartomas or choristomas.

Malignant mesenchymoma may occur at any age and in any location, but the deeper structures of the extremities and retroperitoneum appear to be predilected sites. It consists of mature and immature tissues, including two or more sarcomatous elements of different histogenesis (such as leiomyosarcoma, liposarcoma, chondrosarcoma, osteogenic sarcoma, reticulum cell sarcoma) in various proportions and combinations. Inclusions of fibrosarcoma and undifferentiated primitive mesenchyme, although frequent, are not recognized as separate elements contributing to a diagnosis. Predominance of one tissue may result in what appears to be a homogeneous neoplasm, so that meticulous examination of many parts of the tumor is necessary. Malignant mesenchymoma is similar to mixed mesodermal tumor of the urogenital system (p. 1718), except that epithelial components never can be demonstrated. The tumors are not grossly distinctive except that they tend to be large and to infiltrate contiguous structures. They may recur locally and, in a few cases, have metastasized widely. In general, the prognosis is poor, the degree of malignancy corresponding to the most malignant element.

TUMORS OF ADIPOSE TISSUE
Lipoma and diffuse lipomatosis

Lipoma is one of the most common of all benign neoplasms and may arise almost anywhere in the body. The name is sometimes applied to any circumscribed nodular collection of fat. Characteristically, a lipoma consists of rounded, multilobulated masses of adipose tissue enclosed in a delicate fibrous capsule, although occasionally it may infiltrate. Usually solitary but sometimes multiple, these tumors vary in size from minute growths to huge masses weighing many kilograms. They may occur from early childhood to advanced age, but from 40% to 50% appear between the fourth and fifth decades, when the body begins to accumulate excess fat, at which time the incidence of these tumors is about twice as high in women as in men.

The majority of lipomas occur in the subcutaneous tissues, especially on the neck, back, shoulders, and abdominal wall, and only rarely on the face, scalp, hands, and feet. As a rule, the subcutaneous tumors appear as localized lumps and cause few symptoms, but in dependent areas, such as the perineum and inner surfaces of the thighs, they may form pendulous masses reaching to the ground. Lipomas may be found in connection with voluntary muscle, fascias, and articular capsules of the larger joints. Intramuscular and intermuscular lipomas usually encountered in the deeper soft tissues of the extremities and trunk often attain fairly large size, tend to be poorly circumscribed, and frequently infiltrate adjacent tissues. Such infiltrating intramuscular or intermuscular lipomas are distinguished from well-differentiated liposarcomas by the absence of cellular atypia. Lipomas described in tendon sheaths and in synovial membranes of joint cavities (lipoma arborescens) probably represent inflammatory proliferations of the lining structures. The retroperitoneum, mediastinum, and gastrointestinal tract are the predominant sites of the relatively uncommon internal lipomas, although even the central nervous system, larynx, and solid viscera may be involved. A prominent feature of the retroperitoneal tumors, which have a predilection for the perirenal area, and of the far less common mediastinal growths, is the gigantic proportions they sometimes attain— weights of more than 5 kg frequently have been recorded.

Multiple lipomatosis appears to be a condition of localized and diffuse adipose overgrowths that adopt a bewildering variety of forms and are not true tumors. Such lipomatous masses may be haphazardly or symmetrically distributed in various parts of the body. Frequently associated with other endocrine and neurologic disturbances, these overgrowths probably result from disordered fat metabolism. The occurrence of multicentric symmetric lipomas, sometimes in large numbers

and with a regional localization similar to that of multiple neurofibromas, has sometimes suggested a central nervous system defect or a connection with peripheral nerves. In congenital lipomatosis, diffuse or localized lipomatous masses sometimes are mingled with other heterotopic components, usually cavernous angiomas, and often are asociated with developmental anomalies and deformities of muscles and bones. Many lipomatoses resemble true tumors and are grouped with the lipomas for taxonomic purposes. Thus, in replacement lipomatosis of atrophying kidney, thymus, or lymph nodes, fatty growths of moderate to large dimensions may be produced, with partial or complete effacement of these structures.

Lipomas with an admixture of other mesenchymal elements may be designated fibrolipoma, angiolipoma, myolipoma, or benign mesenchymoma, although the majority are undoubtedly hamartomas. Lipomatous masses containing hemopoietic tissue are referred to as myelolipomas (p. 1675). They occur most often in the adrenal glands, but in the soft tissues they appear to have a predilection for the prevertebral position.

Microscopically, a typical lipoma is similar to normal adipose tissue, and differentiation may be impossible without gross evidence of circumscription or encapsulation. In addition, however, to adult fat cells, which may be fairly uniform in character or may vary greatly in size and shape, xanthoma-like cells with granular to foamy cytoplasm may be present and also variable amounts of irregularly distributed supporting stroma. Although mucoid and myxomatous components are sometimes encountered in a benign lipoma, such features are more common in liposarcoma and therefore demand a careful search for malignancy in other parts of the tumor.

The symptoms of a lipomatous tumor depend on the amount of compression it produces, and death may result from pressure on vital structures. Liposarcomatous transformation is exceedingly uncommon. Since most lipomas usually grow expansively without infiltrating adjacent structures, they are easily excised and seldom recur.

Hibernoma

The term "hibernoma" is applied to a special type of lipoma, infrequently encountered in man, which is considered to arise from vestiges of brown fat similar to the glandular brown adipose tissue occurring in the hiber-

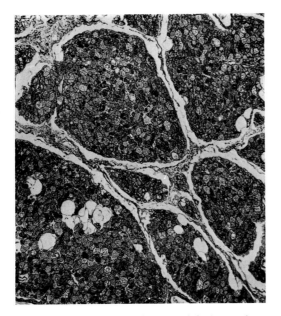

Fig. 43-10. Hibernoma showing lobular architecture. Note finely granular, multiloculated, and adult fat cells. (AFIP 53-7111.)

nating organs of certain animal species. The tumor is composed of lobular masses of multiloculated, coarsely granular, sudanophilic cells whose high lipochrome content and rich vascularity account for their light tan-brown color (Fig. 43-10). Most have occurred in young adults of either sex and in the neck, interscapular region, axilla, and mediastinum—areas in which brown fat has been identified in human beings. They are solitary, encapsulated, slow-growing neoplasms, do not recur after removal, and are not known to undergo malignant change.

Lipoblastomatosis (embryonic lipoma, fetal lipoma)

Lipoblastomatosis refers to another special form of immature lipomatous tumor different from hibernoma.[107] It is essentially benign and occurs predominantly in infants and children, usually during the first few years of life. The tumors usually present as circumscribed, grayish yellow lobulated masses separated by partitions of loose fibrous tissue. Occasionally there are more deeply situated infiltrating lesions. On section, there are lobulated masses of grayish yellow tissue with gelatinous and cystic areas. On histologic examination, differing parts of the lobules consist of continuous groups of multivacuolated fat cells closely re-

sembling those of fetal adipose tissue with interspersed unilocular fat cells of adult type. Progressive maturation toward a more common lipoma has been observed. Careful search almost always will disclose variable proportions, sometimes dominant areas, of stellate and spindle-shaped embryonal lipoblasts set in a myxomatous stroma with a richly developed network of blood capillaries in plexiform arrangement. These myxomatous and vascular features exclude hibernoma but understandably may erroneously suggest myxoid liposarcoma, a tumor of rare occurrence in infancy and childhood. Although the tumor may recur occasionally, radical therapy is not required, since complete local excision or reexcision appears to result in a cure.

Liposarcoma

Liposarcoma is the most common primary malignant neoplasm of the soft tissues, constituting about 20% of all soft-part sarcomas. Unlike lipoma, it arises primarily in deeper structures, with a recognized predilection for certain anatomic sites, particularly the thigh, leg, gluteal region, and retroperitoneum. Of 499 examples reviewed at the Armed Forces Institute of Pathology, 205 were in the lower extremities, 107 in the retroperitoneum, 61 in the upper extremities, including shoulder and axilla, 53 in the trunk, 10 in the neck, 5 in the mediastinum, and smaller numbers in widely scattered areas throughout the body. Although liposarcomas occur predominantly in middle and later life and are uncommon before 20 years of age, unequivocal examples have been recorded in children. The frequency in males and females is about equal.

The majority of liposarcomas arise spontaneously. Only rarely do the pathologic findings indicate a malignant transition in a preexisting lipoma. They are believed to take origin from undifferentiated perivascular mesenchyme, which is directly converted into malignant lipoblastic tissue, although retaining to some extent a capacity for more diverse differentiation. In the extremities, the growths usually occur about deep fascial structures, in intermuscular planes, and in periarticular regions. Beginning as inconspicuous swellings, they have usually attained appreciable size before they are first diagnosed and treated. Retroperitoneal tumors may reach enormous dimensions—weights of 5 to 10 kg or more frequently have been observed.

Grossly, liposarcomas form bulky multinodular masses varying from some firmness to a soft mucoid consistency. On section, they have a yellow to yellow-white color and usually show cystic areas with hemorrhage and necrosis. The myxoid tumors usually can be identified readily by their gelatinous appearance, although they often contain firmer fibrous nodules. Although primary tumors may appear sharply demarcated or give the false impression of encapsulation, they regularly infiltrate surrounding structures, producing satellite nodules, and precise boundaries are exceedingly difficult to define.

Microscopically, liposarcomas present a wide divergence of structural patterns, which may vary from specimen to specimen and even within different areas of the same tumor. Nonetheless, division into several more or less distinct varieties is possible and has therapeutic and prognostic usefulness.

Differentiated liposarcoma

Differentiated adult liposarcoma retains a fairly intact lobular architecture and is composed mostly of mature fat in which variable amounts of mucoid and myxomatous tissue are accompanied by fusiform and stellate cells and occasional bizarre lipoblasts. It is usually well circumscribed and a few centimeters in diameter. This relatively benign, borderline liposarcoma merges imperceptibly with the lipomas. It may recur locally after excision, and in the retroperitoneal area it may become aggressive and show true malignant transformation.

Myxoid liposarcoma

Myxoid liposarcoma, the most common form of liposarcoma, may be well differentiated or poorly differentiated. The former is of embryonal type (myxoliposarcoma) and composed of an intricate vascular meshwork of fusiform and stellate cells in a myxomatous and mucoid background, containing variable numbers of vacuolated lipoblasts (Figs. 43-11 and 43-12). Such tumors may resemble fetal fat, myxoma, or lymphangioma. The poorly differentiated myxoid liposarcoma contains, in addition to embryonal and adult fat cells, large numbers of anaplastic cells and bizarre giant lipoblasts, with interspersed lipid-laden foam cells resembling atypical mononucleated and multinucleated xanthoma cells or Touton giant cells (Fig. 43-12). It displays a strong tendency to undergo fibrosis, with the production of areas resembling fibrosarcoma, and sometimes shows osseous and cartilaginous

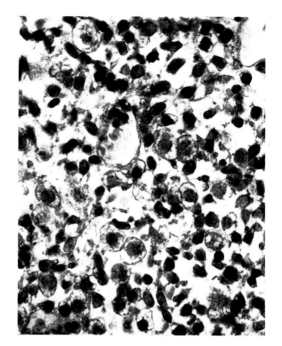

Fig. 43-11. Liposarcoma showing numerous embryonal fat cells. (AFIP 53-4683.)

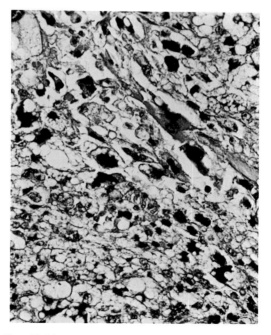

Fig. 43-12. Liposarcoma. Many bizarre giant lipoblasts with large pyknotic nuclei evident in this poorly differentiated myxoid liposarcoma. (AFIP 60-4858.)

metaplasia. The well-differentiated tumors (age group 25 to 50 years) regularly infiltrate surrounding structures. In a series of more than 100 cases personally reviewed, approximately 60% recurred from one to 10 times after radical local excision, although recurrences were sometimes delayed as much as 5, 10, or even 20 years. When located in the thigh, the tumor extends more cephalad with each recurrence, and ultimately there may be direct peritoneal extension, but no more than 5% metastasize to lungs, liver, and bone. The poorly differentiated myxoid tumors (age group 40 to 60 years) also are locally aggressive, infiltrating widely and metastasizing in from 25% to 40%. It has been emphasized repeatedly that the rare liposarcomas observed in children are characterized by more favorable clinical behavior and rarely, if ever, metastasize. Such tumors are mainly of the well-differentiated myxoid type, and their morphologic distinction from such benign lesions as lipomatosis and particularly lipoblastomatosis may prove difficult.

Undifferentiated liposarcoma

Pleomorphic liposarcoma, generally highly anaplastic, is difficult to distinguish from other highly undifferentiated mesenchymal tumors, and even from some of the epithelial neoplasms such as amelanotic malignant melanoma. Some of these tumors would now be considered malignant fibrous histiocytomas. However, recognizable bizarre lipoblastic cells usually can be demonstrated in parts of the tumor. Occurring particularly in the gluteal region in elderly patients, these tumors metastasize widely by the hematogenous route.

Treatment of a liposarcoma should take into consideration a number of factors, such as degree of malignancy, regional location, recurrent status, infiltration, and metastasis. Radical local excision or amputation usually is the treatment of choice, although radiation therapy is sometimes considered a valuable adjunct. The value of chemotherapy has not yet been established.

TUMORS OF SMOOTH MUSCLE
Leiomyoma

Although benign tumors of smooth muscle occur infrequently outside the uterus and gastrointestinal tract, they occasionally may be found almost anywhere in the body, including the kidney, urinary bladder, spermatic cord, round ligament, veins, bronchus, tongue, orbit, and eye. Leiomyomas of the soft parts largely are confined to the skin and subcutaneous tissues (p. 1861) and have only rarely been described in the deeper peripheral soft tissues, mediastinum, and retroperitoneum. It should be stressed that even well-differentiated large leiomyomatous masses, particularly in the retroperitoneal area, usually prove malignant. This does not apply, however, to intraligamentary growths of uterine origin or to extracapsular renal leiomyomas that, on thorough examination, usually show foci of other mesodermal elements and probably represent hamartomas. In the thorax, especially, leiomyomas are so rare as to be practically nonexistent, and when an intrathoracic tumor is called a leiomyoma, it often is a misdiagnosed neurilemoma. The differentiation between leiomyoma and neurilemoma or neurofibroma may be difficult.

Grossly, the leiomyomas in the deeper tissues show few distinctive characteristics. They are well circumscribed and rarely reach more than 3 to 5 cm in diameter. Microscopically, they consist of intertwining bundles of spindle cells of fairly uniform size, slightly larger than normal smooth muscle cells, with elongated, blunt-ended nuclei. Intracellular myofibrils can easily be demonstrated in appropriately stained sections. The amount of fibrous connective tissue is variable but usually scanty, although fine reticulin fibers encircle or run parallel to the long axes of the cells. Mitosis is very infrequent. The symptoms caused by these tumors depend on their size, vascularity, and location. Subcutaneous tumors, like the glomus tumors, may cause attacks of paroxysmal pain. Actually, some tumors may show both glomus and smooth muscle elements surrounding well-defined vascular spaces (glomangiomyoma).

Bizarre leiomyoma

Bizarre leiomyomas (epithelioid leiomyoma, leiomyoblastoma) are increasingly recognized as peculiar morphologic variants of smooth muscle tumors that usually are encountered in the gastrointestinal tract, especially in the gastric wall, but occasionally elsewhere. Rarely, the tumors arise in the superficial and deep soft tissues but, when they occur in these sites, are seldom structurally typical representations. Grossly, they have the characteristics of smooth muscle tumors, but their principal variables are size (they vary from small to enormous) and softness. Frequently, they are hemorrhagic and exhibit small cystic areas. Microscopically, the bizarre leiomyomas are composed predominantly or entirely of round or polygonal cells with faintly acidophilic cytoplasm, show no myofibrils, and often have a clear zone partially or completely surrounding the nucleus. Mitoses usually are scanty. A telltale feature is the frequent transitions toward elongated cells recognizable as smooth muscle elements. Occasional tumors have a full malignant potential, but their recognition may prove difficult because of poor correlation between histologic appearance and biologic behavior.

Leiomyosarcoma

Relatively few malignant smooth muscle tumors have been reported in the soft somatic tissues, but apparently their true incidence is much greater than most statistical data indicate. Stout listed 25 collected cases in various soft-tissue sites and in a later review[123] described 36 tumors in the skin and subcutaneous tissues. While at the Armed Forces Institute

of Pathology, I (R. S.) reviewed 462 leiomyosarcomas, 125 of which (27%) arose in soft-tissue sites. In order of frequency, their distribution was as follows: retroperitoneum, 76; extremities (deep tissues), 23; subcutaneous, 10; omentum and mesentery, 8; venous system, 3; abdominal wall, 2; orbit, 2; mediastinum, 1. The highest age incidence is between the fourth and sixth decades.

The typical soft-part leiomyosarcoma appears as a large rounded, nodular mass of firm, gray to grayish brown tissue with areas of hemorrhage and necrosis. In the retroperitoneum, the tumors are poorly delimited, acting as progressive growths that attain large size and extend by infiltration into adjacent tissues and organs. After a time, they metastasize most often to the liver and lungs. The deep peripheral tumors, usually situated in the extremities, may appear well circumscribed but nonetheless show a high incidence of local recurrence and often metastasize widely after attempts at local extirpation (Figs. 43-13 and 43-14). Primary leiomyosarcomas arising in the walls of large veins are nearly always intraluminal and metastasize readily to the lungs.

Microscopically, leiomyosarcomas consist mainly of long, spindle-shaped cells of more

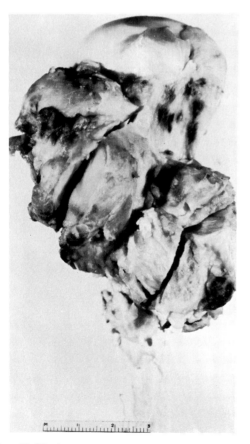

Fig. 43-13. Leiomyosarcoma. Gross specimen removed after disarticulation of arm. Bulky multinodular tumor with areas of hemorrhage surrounds neck of humerus. (AFIP 55-22183.)

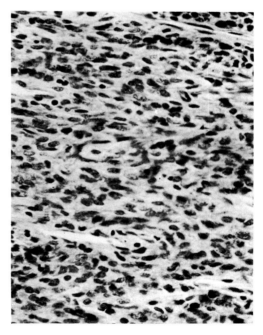

Fig. 43-14. Histologic appearance of tumor shown in Fig. 43-13. Note conspicuous cellularity, variations in size and appearance of cells, and mitotic figures. (AFIP 60-4745.)

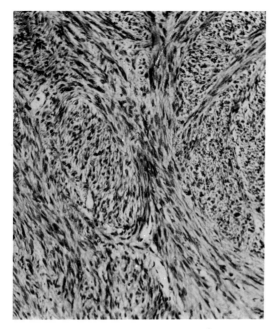

Fig. 43-15. Leiomyosarcoma showing well-differentiated histologic pattern. (AFIP 60-4723.)

or less uniform size arranged in interlacing fascicles. The nuclei are elongated, with blunt ends, and are sharply outlined by pink-staining cytoplasm in which myofibrils usually can be demonstrated (Fig. 43-15). Study of many sections, however, usually will disclose less well-differentiated areas with occasional giant cells, strap cells, ovoid to polygonal cells of varying size, and small round cells with hyperchromatic nuclei. Mitotic figures generally are scarce but when numerous indicate a high degree of malignancy. Frequently, there is a tendency for the nuclei in smooth muscle tumors to be aligned in parallel rows (palisading) so as to mimic neurogenic neoplasms. Actually, cytologic criteria for the distinction of benign from malignant leiomyomatous growths are not always reliable. When doubt exists, size and location are valuable diagnostic aids. Evidence obtained from analysis of a large series of cases appears to indicate that smooth muscle tumors over 5 cm in diameter in the deep soft tissues of adults are almost invariably malignant. Irradiation seems to have little effect upon these tumors, and radical surgical resection or amputation affords the only hope of cure. In children, many of the extremely rare growths of the superficial soft tissues diagnosed histologically as leiomyosarcoma are of low biologic malignancy and appear to have a favorable prognosis. Those

tumors of high malignant potential described in the prostate and bladder, sometimes listed as predilected sites in infants and children, are probably mainly botryoid rhabdomyosarcomas.

TUMORS OF STRIATED MUSCLE
Rhabdomyoma

It is doubtful whether benign striated muscle tumors occur in pure form other than in the heart, and even these are probably congenital malformations rather than true neoplasms (p. 839). However, a few highly differentiated rhabdomyomas have been described, most of which occurred in the orocervical region, particularly in the tongue of infants and children.

Rhabdomyosarcoma

Rhabdomyosarcomas are among the more common malignant tumors of soft parts, exceeded in frequency only by liposarcomas and possibly by fibrosarcomas. They form a complex group of tumors with various adult and embryonal forms. A recent classification includes three main types, with the designations of adult pleomorphic rhabdomyosarcoma, embryonal alveolar rhabdomyosarcoma, and embryonal botryoid rhabdomyosarcoma. Each is a distinct oncologic entity, delineated according to embryogenic, histologic, gross anatomic, and clinical characteristics. Among 162 cases studied at the Armed Forces Institute of Pathology prior to 1956, 21 (13%) were of adult pleomorphic type, 67 (41%) of embryonal alveolar type, and 74 (46%) of embryonal botryoid type. As of 1964, there were approximately 600 cases of rhabdomyosarcoma on file at the Armed Forces Institute of Pathology, and these lesions were second in frequency among all malignant soft-tissue tumors.

Embryonal botryoid rhabdomyosarcoma

Besides the so-called grapelike sarcomas (sarcoma botryoides) that occur predominantly in the genitourinary organs of infants and children (p. 996), related tumors with identical histologic appearance and behavior characteristics are observed in other soft-tissue sites in patients of this age group. The most controversial of the rhabdomyosarcomas, these neoplasms are widely believed to represent mixed tumors, or even teratomatous growths—in which various heterologous tissues besides striated muscle may be present. However, in 155 cases personally reviewed (R. S.), only three (associated with testicular and vaginal growths) contained components other than striated muscle. Most of such tumors, other than those in the genitourinary tract, occur in locations in which skeletal muscle arises directly in mesoderm or in its mesenchymal derivatives, and they recapitulate, sometimes strikingly, the ontogenetic development of striated muscle. The impression is gained that the stages in the development of skeletal muscle, which have not been well worked out in man, may be traced through botryoid and alveolar rhabdomyosarcoma.

Embryonal botryoid rhabdomyosarcomas are not uncommon tumors of the soft tissues, although until recently relatively few large series of cases have been recorded. In the 155 cases I (R. S.) reviewed, the majority of which were studied at the Armed Forces Institute of Pathology, 73% occurred in the first decade of life and 91% in the first two decades, the median age being 4 years. The condition is about twice as common in males as in females. The head and neck are the most common sites, the lesions involving the orbit and nasopharynx in most instances. Next in frequency are sites in the genitourinary tract, particularly the vagina, bladder, and spermatic cord. The tumors are not confined to these areas, however, for a relatively small number occur in the common bile duct, retroperitoneum, and extremities.

Botryoid rhabdomyosarcomas, particularly those in the abdomen and genitourinary system, characteristically grow as large polypoid tumors of edematous myxomatous tissue. Frequently attached by a broad base in the nasopharynx, they appear as flattened polypoid projections often mistaken for benign mucous polyps. Usually arising in association with mucous surfaces, the tumors involve muscle and other structures only secondarily, and a primary growth in muscle is very likely not a botryoid rhabdomyosarcoma.

Although botryoid rhabdomyosarcomas display considerable microscopic variability, most are sufficiently characteristic to be recognized with comparative ease. Usually, variable numbers of small round cells and stellate cells with pyknotic nuclei and scanty cytoplasm are scattered in a loose myxomatous matrix. The stellate cells are connected by long fibrillary processes in a fine reticular syncytium, sometimes resembling myxoid liposarcoma, without the definite vascular pattern of the latter. Occasionally sparsely cellular neoplasms are mistaken for simple myxoma. In addition to the indifferent mesenchymal cells, rhabdomyoblastic elements usually are recognizable, con-

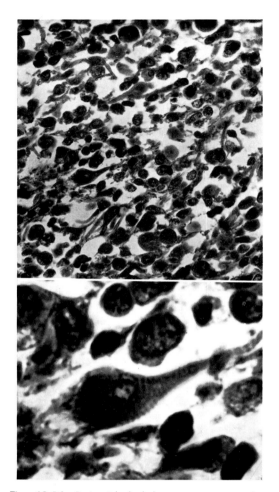

Fig. 43-16. Botryoid rhabdomyosarcoma, embryonal type, from nasopharynx in 7-year-old child. Highly cellular area showing various forms of rhabdomyoblasts with maturation. Note crossstriated tadpole-shaped cell in center of field. (AFIP 58-8885.)

sisting of large round cells with granular to homogeneous acidophilic cytoplasm, halo cells, and elongated spindle forms in which longitudinal and cross striations are sometimes discernible. Occasional strap cells, bizarre giant cells, and tadpole cells reminiscent of those in the pleomorphic and alveolar forms may be encountered. When the tumor is covered by a mucosal surface, a layering of cells usually occurs just beneath the epithelium, the so-called cambium layer of Nicholson, in which maturation is most advanced (Fig. 43-16). The tumor occasionally may mimic the pleomorphic or spindle adult form, although characteristic myxomatous areas always are present. Many of the neoplasms reach a high degree of maturation, approaching the appearance of adult muscle.

The prognosis of embryonal botryoid rhabdomyosarcomas is extremely poor. They tend strongly toward repeated local recurrences, and usually wide local extension proves fatal. In the later stages, blood and lymphatic metastases occur. Approximately 10% to 15% 5-year survivals are to be expected. Prompt aggressive surgery is indicated.

Embryonal alveolar rhabdomyosarcoma (juvenile rhabdomyosarcoma)

Defined as a clinicopathologic entity within recent years, this specific primary malignant tumor of skeletal muscle occurs with far greater frequency than generally suspected. In embryonal rhabdomyosarcomas, the cells frequently display the capacity to differentiate along rhabdomyoblastic lines, with the formation of striated muscle elements. The histogenesis is uncertain, although they appear to recapitulate in an abortive form the embryonic development of skeletal muscle from primitive myotomal segments or, less often, from mesenchyme derivatives.

The term "alveolar" has sometimes been encountered in the literature on rhabdomyosarcomas, but it is probable that most such tumors are confused with synovial sarcoma, neuroblastoma, reticulum cell sarcoma, hemangioendothelioma, and carcinoma—lesions that usually must be considered in the differential diagnosis. Alveolar rhabdomyosarcoma usually is observed in children and young adults. In a series of 67 cases, 36% were observed in the first decade of life and 58% in the first two decades. Only eight patients were 30 or more years of age. There were 48 males and 19 females. The presenting lesions were located chiefly in the extremities, 20 in the upper and 27 in the lower. Of the remainder, 10 occurred in the trunk, nine in the head and neck, and one in the perineum. In the extremities, the larger muscles of the thigh and forearm are the most common sites, but the tumor also may be found in the small muscles of the hands and feet. In the region of the head, the orbital and facial muscles are more likely to be involved.

Clinically, embryonal rhabdomyosarcomas may appear as small, symptomless swellings in the superficial muscles, but the typical patient complains of severe, intermittent or persistent pain in the affected area, sometimes for several months before a definite tumor mass is noted. Grossly, most of the tumors give the impression

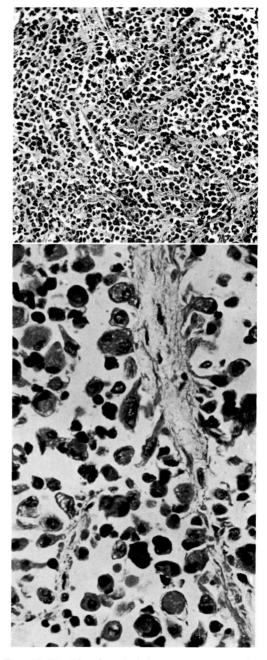

Fig. 43-17. Alveolar rhabdomyosarcoma, embryonal type, showing distinctive pattern. Embryonal muscle cells loosely attached to trabeculae and lying free in alveolar spaces.

of circumscription, although it is apparent during removal that adjacent tissues are infiltrated. On section, they are grayish white and of almost cartilaginous consistency, but cystic areas filled with jellylike material or turbid fluid may be present.

Microscopically, alveolar rhabdomyosarcomas show small nodular tumor masses, which usually give the impression of replacing individual primary and secondary muscle bundles, frequently leaving intervening bundles substantially intact. A variety of histologic patterns merging imperceptibly with each other are produced in different examples and in different areas of the same tumor. The prevailing pattern is alveolar but not infrequently the neoplastic cells are oriented about blood vessels, resembling pseudorosettes, or are aligned in papillary formation. Loosely adherent to the interstitial connective tissue or fibrovascular septa, the tumor cells tend to trail off and become freely floating in the alveolar spaces (Fig. 43-17). The characteristic cells are likely to be large, oval, or rounded, uninuclear forms with scanty cytoplasm, resembling reticulum cells, but among these cells are many with marginal highly chromatic nuclei and strongly acidophilic cytoplasm in which myofibrils are discernible. In addition, careful cytologic study reveals isolated polyhedral and giant cells, sometimes with marginal masses of dense nuclear chromatin, tadpole-shaped cells, and strap cells with multiple nuclei. Such cells may have vacuolated, granular, or homogeneous cytoplasm in which transverse striations often can be demonstrated. Some show a considerable degree of morphologic regularity and superficially resemble reticulum cell sarcoma of the soft parts, an entity that is still questionable.

Alveolar rhabdomyosarcoma has an extremely grave prognosis, with a high mortality even when definitive treatment is instituted early. Although 80% to 90% of the patients are dead of generalized metastases within 2 to 3 years of onset, the course is not necessarily run with such rapidity.

Undifferentiated adult pleomorphic rhabdomyosarcoma

Although uncommon, undifferentiated adult pleomorphic rhabdomyosarcoma is the familiar, supposedly classic form of rhabdomyosarcoma. It may arise in skeletal muscle in any part of the body, but the majority are situated in the extremities, about 50% occurring in the lower extremities, usually the thigh. Predilec-

tion for certain muscles frequently has been noted: in the lower extremities—the quadriceps, adductors, and semimembranosus; in the upper extremities—the biceps and brachialis internus. Nearly all patients with pleomorphic rhabdomyosarcoma are adults, with the greatest incidence being in the fourth to seventh decades. It is unlikely that the tumor occurs in infants and children. The clinical course and growth pattern of these tumors are quite variable. A few have a short but dramatic history of fulminating rapid growth with distant lymphatic and hematogenous metastases, but the usual case tends toward repeated local recurrences with ultimate metastasis. Occasional examples progress slowly or remain quiescent over long periods.

Adult pleomorphic rhabdomyosarcomas vary greatly in size and appearance. In superficial muscles, they may be relatively small, but in deep bulky muscles they usually attain large size (10 to 15 cm). Although most appear firm and well circumscribed, those growing rapidly are locally destructive and infiltrative. In rare instances, usually associated with a rapidly fatal course, they are hemorrhagic, cystic, and necrotic, resembling an old hematoma in which little viable tissue can be demonstrated.

Microscopically, most adult pleomorphic rhabdomyosarcomas are characterized by a high degree of cellular pleomorphism (Fig. 43-18). Large and small branching spindle-shaped cells predominate, sometimes almost exclusively, but usually are mingled with large and small cells that are oval or polygonal and have vesicular or pyknotic nuclei. There also are elongated straplike and ribbon cells, often with several nuclei arranged in tandem, and numerous giant cells of various types, often with bizarre hyperchromatic nuclei and vacuolated cytoplasm. Many of the cells have the tinctorial qualities of muscle cells, with strongly acidophilic cytoplasm varying from homogeneous to granular appearance. In carefully differentiated sections, the long, straplike cells with abundant cytoplasm almost invariably show longitudinal fibrils, but good cross striations can rarely, if ever, be demonstrated. In the hemorrhagic necrotic lesions, tumor cells may be sparse and diagnosis exceedingly difficult.

Because of the lack of cross striations, the evidence that such tumors are rhabdomyosarcomas is purely circumstantial. It is necessary, therefore, to restrict the diagnosis to those neoplasms occurring in skeletal muscle. In

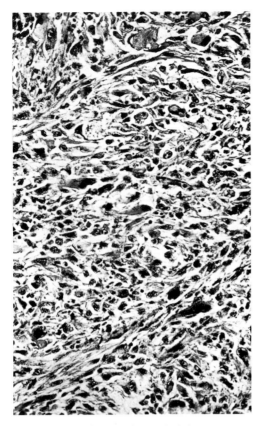

Fig. 43-18. Pleomorphic rhabdomyosarcoma, adult type, showing great variety of cells, mostly spindle shaped, with intermingling of bizarre giant cells. (AFIP 60-4750.)

other tissues, the cytologic pattern may be simulated by a variety of mesenchymal or epithelial neoplasms, both benign and malignant, and the pathologist must exercise considerable caution in interpretation.

TUMORS OF HETEROTOPIC BONE AND CARTILAGE
Chondroma, osteoma, and osteochondroma

Benign tumor masses of bone or cartilage, or mixtures of both, and properly referred to as chondromas, osteomas, or osteochondromas, are extremely rare in soft tissues. Criteria for soft-tissue origin are that they should be unattached to periosteum or periarticular structures, appear to be of spontaneous origin and not secondary to trauma or inflammation, and not be related to maldevelopment (e.g., a hamartoma of the branchial cleft area). Such neoplasms seldom attain more than a few centimeters in diameter and usually are of little clinical significance.

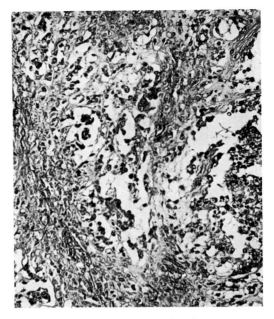

Fig. 43-19. Chondrosarcoma of soft tissues. Portions of two nodules with clusters of chondroblasts in fibrillary and mucoid matrix shown. (AFIP 60-4855.)

Chondrosarcoma (extraosseous)

Primary chondrosarcomatous tumors in the extraskeletal soft tissues are extremely rare. My (R. S.) experience with soft-tissue chondrosarcoma includes about 29 cases. The favored site is the extremities, especially the lower, mostly in young and middle-aged adults. The majority are situated in muscle, although they may develop in connection with fascia, tendon sheaths, and periarticular structures. Grossly, soft-tissue chondrosarcomas may vary from a few centimeters to 20 cm or more in diameter. Characteristically, they consist of a mass or masses of soft mucoid to moderately firm gray tissue in which there are nodular areas of cartilaginous consistency. Cyst formation, hemorrhage, necrosis, and focal calcification are not uncommon. Microscopically, they are comparable to chondrosarcomas in bone, but with larger areas of poorly organized mucoid or myxomatous matrix and relatively few foci of mature hyaline cartilage. Usually, they are composed of small, vaguely defined lobules separated by a loose fibrous stroma. Clusters and strands of rounded to stellate cells, with single and double nuclei, having the usual characteristics of chondroblasts, are irregularly disposed in the mucoid and myxomatous matrix and tend to be concentrated about the periphery of the individual lobules (Fig. 43-19). Anaplastic or undifferentiated variants rarely are seen. Apparently, the neoplasms arise anew and not in preexisting chondromatous growths, although their source of origin is still an enigma.

Extraskeletal chondrosarcomas are extremely variable in their growth potentialities. Some infiltrate widely but do not metastasize despite multiple recurrences. Others metastasize within a relatively short time. Small growths located in the hands and feet often are confused with mixed tumors of the skin and larger, more deeply situated lesions are confused with liposarcoma. The treatment of choice is radical removal of the affected area or amputation, depending on the site.

Osteogenic sarcoma

Although well recognized, malignant ossifying tumors originating in extraskeletal soft tissues and exhibiting clinical and pathologic features comparable to those of conventional osteogenic sarcomas primary in bone are extremely rare. Arising primarily in skeletal muscle and deep fascial structures of the extremities, particularly the lower, a few have been encountered in other soft-tissue sites, including the retroperitoneum and mediastinum. These are essentially tumors of middle and old age, but children and young adults are not always spared. Although the origin of these sarcomas is obscure, evidence suggests that they develop from neoplastic connective tissue with latent osteogenic potencies, under some unknown physiochemic influence of their environment. Usually, the growths arise anew and often have attained considerable size in patients with symptoms of only a few weeks' or months' duration. On the other hand, in some reported instances, they appear to have developed by malignant transformation of preexisting, benign, bone-forming lesions of long standing, such as myositis ossificans and calcifying hematomas. However, genuine malignant transformation in such lesions, most of which have followed a relatively benign course, is unquestionably extremely rare. Great caution, therefore, must be taken in interpreting these so-called pseudomalignant osseous tumors of the soft parts, which may closely mimic osteogenic sarcoma histologically (myositis ossificans, p. 2071). Radiographic appearance in conjunction with clinical and microscopic findings may be helpful in differential diagnosis.

Grossly, typical primary osteogenic sarcomas of the soft tissues may be well circumscribed.

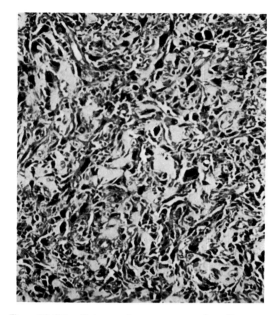

Fig. 43-20. Osteogenic sarcoma of soft parts. Formation of osteoid matrix by anaplastic tumor cells shown. (AFIP 54-7431.)

They are, however, notorious for recrudescence and extensive invasion of adjacent structures after attempts at local surgical procedures. On section, they are firm, grayish white, and gritty but usually have conspicuous areas of necrosis and hemorrhage. The histologic criteria for their recognition are similar to those for osteosarcomatous lesions of bone, and they appear to have a range equal to the latter tumors. Although most of them produce relatively little osteoid and osseous matrix and resemble osteolytic tumors of bone, others are densely sclerotic and highly ossified and resemble sclerosing osteogenic sarcomas of bone (Fig. 43-20). Occasionally, highly cellular transitional forms containing bizarre multinucleated tumor giant cells are encountered and are indistinguishable from giant cell tumors of bone. In contradistinction to pseudomalignant bone-forming lesions, which are condensed or circumscribed at their periphery by fibrous tissue or by a delimiting shell of well-formed bone, the advancing borders of soft-tissue osteogenic sarcomas, like those of their counterpart in bone, are usually their most cellular and least differentiated portion. The interiors of frankly malignant ossifying lesions also are far more atypical than those of the benign type. One should keep these facts in mind in dealing with these neoplasms. As might be expected, typical soft-tissue osteogenic sarcomas are highly malignant growths that metastasize early and consistently involve the lungs. Because the tumors are radioresistant, prompt ablative surgical treatment of the type used for osteogenic sarcoma of bone is required.

TUMORS OF UNDETERMINED TYPE
Alveolar soft-part sarcoma

A relatively uncommon soft-tissue neoplasm of uncertain histogenesis that occurs principally in voluntary muscle or musculofascial planes has been called by the descriptive term alveolar soft-part sarcoma. Previously, evidence linking these tumors with the vascular glomera or paraganglia had been presented and the term "malignant tumors of nonchromaffin paraganglia" was proposed. This hypothesis has found some favor but is not generally accepted. Others have considered these neoplasms to be malignant granular cell myoblastomas.

Alveolar soft-part sarcoma is prone to occur in adolescents and young adults, and females are affected more often than males. Its usual site is in an extremity, most often a lower, although it may arise in different situations. In 62 cases personally studied (R. S.), 41 arose in the lower extremities, nine in the upper extremities, and the remainder in such sites as the abdominal wall, para-anal region, tongue, floor of mouth, and orbit. The ages ranged from 1½ to 55 years.

Grossly, the tumor averages between 6 and 10 cm in diameter and usually is well circumscribed or partially encapsulated. Occasionally, there is invasion of surrounding structures at one or more sites. On section, the tumor is fairly firm and gray-yellow in color, but often it is mottled by necrotic and hemorrhagic areas. Fibrous trabeculae may divide it into lobules, producing a honeycombed effect. The microscopic features are characteristically uniform, and this uniformity is also preserved in metastatic lesions. There are rounded or cordlike aggregates of cells separated from similar groups of cells by delicate fibrous septa and thin-walled vascular spaces (Fig. 43-21). An organoid or endocrine-like arrangement often is suggested. The individual groups are composed of from five to 50 or more cells. The cell groups may be compact or centrally devoid of organized structure so that there is an alveolar or tubular appearance. The component cells resemble so-called granular cell myoblasts and contain diastase-resistant, PAS-positive, fine acidophilic granules and occasional vacuoles within the rather abundant cytoplasm. With special histochemical studies, the granules appear to represent lipid-protein-carbohydrate complexes sometimes recognizable as crystalline structures with the light microscope. On the basis of electron microscopic observations, the crystals have been interpreted as a possible secretory product formed in the Golgi complex. The occasional large pleomorphic cells with giant hyperchro-

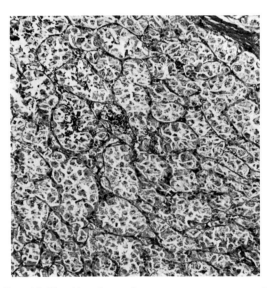

Fig. 43-21. Alveolar soft-part sarcoma—general architectural pattern. Thick fibrous septa divide tumor into irregular lobules. (AFIP 60-4735.)

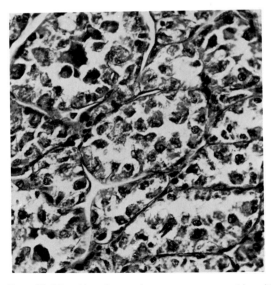

Fig. 43-22. Alveolar soft-part sarcoma. Alveoli composed of large granular cells with occasional bizarre giant forms. (AFIP 60-4739.)

matic nuclei are probably degenerating forms (Fig. 43-22).

Alveolar soft-part sarcoma is a slowly growing neoplasm that may recur locally after simple excision. Pulmonary, cerebral, and skeletal metastasis occurs in more than 50% of cases, and rarely a metastasis gives rise to the initial symptoms. Whether or not amputation is required depends on the accessibility of the tumor to radical excision.

REFERENCES
General

1 Evans, R. W.: Histological appearances of tumours, ed. 2, Baltimore, 1968, The Williams & Wilkins Co.
2 Enzinger, F. M.: Histological typing of soft tissue tumours, Geneva, 1969, World Health Organization.
3 Suit, H. D., Russell, W. O., and Martin, R. G.: Cancer 35:1478-1483, 1975 (histology and treatment).

Tumors of fibrous tissue
Fibroma
Juvenile aponeurotic fibroma

4 Allen, P. W., and Enzinger, F. M.: Cancer 26: 857-867, 1970.
5 Brown, A.: Proc. Roy. Soc. Med. 62:327, 1969.
6 Goldman, R. L.: Cancer, 26:1325-1331, 1970 (cartilage analog).
7 Keasby, L. E., and Fanselau, H. A.: Clin. Orthop. 19:115-131, 1961.
8 Lichtenstein, L., and Goldman, R. L.: Cancer 17:810-816, 1964 (cartilage analog).
9 Rios-Dalenz, J., Kim, J. S., and McDowell, F. W.: Am. J. Clin. Pathol. 44:632-635, 1965.
10 Shapiro, L.: Arch. Dermatol. 99:37-42, 1969 (infantile digital fibromatosis).

Elastofibroma

11 Barr, J. R.: Am. J. Clin. Pathol. 45:679-683, 1966.
12 Burdick, C. O.: New Eng. J. Med. 275:154-155, 1966.
13 Contanzi, G., and Evsebi, V.: Tumori 57:349-352, 1971.
14 Delvaux, T. C., and Lester, J. P.: Am. J. Clin. Pathol. 43:72-74, 1965.
15 Freilich, J. K., and Bendix, R. M.: Geriatrics 24:65-67, 1969.
16 Järvi, O. H., and Saxen, E.: Acta Pathol. Microbiol. Scand. (suppl.) 144:83-84, 1961.
17 Järvi, O. H., Saxen, A. E., Hopsu-Havu, V. K., Wartiovaara, J. J., and Vaissalo, V. T.: Cancer 23:42-63, 1969.
18 Lansing, A. J., Rosenthal, T. B., Alex, M., and Dempsey, E. W.: Anat. Rec. 114:555-575, 1952 (electron microscopy).
19 Marston, A., and Jones, E. W.: Br. J. Surg. 52:980-981, 1965.
20 Mirra, J. M., Straub, L. R., and Järvi, O. H.: Cancer 33:234-238, 1974.
21 Stemmermann, G. N., and Stout, A. P.: Am. J. Clin. Pathol. 37:499-506, 1962.
22 Winkelmann, R. K., and Sams, W. M., Jr.: Cancer 23:406-415, 1969.

Congenital generalized fibromatosis

23 Balsaver, A. M., Butler, J. J., and Martin, R. G.: Cancer 20:1607-1616, 1967 (congenital fibrosarcoma).
24 Beatty, E. C., Jr.: Am. J. Dis. Child. 103:620, 1962.
25 Drescher, E., Woyke, S., Markiewicz, C., and Tegi, S.: J. Pediatr. Surg. 2:427-430, 1967 (fibromatosis hyalinica multiplex juvenilis).
26 Enjoji, M., Kato, N., Kamikazuru, K., and Arima, E.: Acta Med. Univ. Kagoshima (suppl.) 10:145-151, 1968.
27 Enzinger, F. M.: Fibrous tumors of infancy. In Tumors of bone and soft tissue, Chicago, 1965, Year Book Medical Publishers, Inc., pp. 375-396.
28 Gonzalez-Crussi, F.: Cancer 26:1289-1299, 1970 (ultrastructure of congenital fibrosarcoma).
29 Goslee, L., Clermont, V., Bernstein, J., and Wooley, P. V., Jr.: J. Pediatr. 65:377-387, 1964 (superficial connective tissue tumors in early infancy).
30 Policard, A., Collet, A., Roussel, G., Martin, J. C., and Renet, C.: Pathol. Biol. (Paris) 12:32-38, 1963.
31 Mande, R., Hennequet, A., Loubry, P., Cloup, M., and Marie, J.: Ann. Pediatr. (Paris) 12:692, 1965.
32 Reye, R. D. K.: Arch. Pathol. 80:228-231, 1965 (recurring digital fibrous tumors of childhood).
33 Shnitka, T. K., Asp, D. M., and Horner, R. H.: Cancer 11:627, 1958.
34 Welsh, R. A., and Meyer, A. T.: Arch. Pathol. 84:354-362, 1967 (collagen fibers).
35 Woyke, S., Domagala, W., and Olszewski, W.: Cancer 26:1157-1168, 1970 (ultrastructure).

Nodular fasciitis

36 Allen, P. W.: Pathology 4:9-26, 1972.
37 Hutter, R. V. P., Stewart, F. W., and Foote, F. W., Jr.: Cancer 15:992-1003, 1962.
38 Hutter, R. V. P., Foote, F. W., Jr., Francis, K. C., and Higinbotham, N. L.: Am. J. Surg. 104:800-807, 1962 (parosteal).
39 Price, E. B., Jr., Silliphant, W. M., and Shuman, R.: Am. J. Clin. Pathol. 35:122-136, 1961.
40 Soule, E. H.: Arch. Pathol. (Chicago) 73:437-444, 1962.
41 Stout, A. P.: Cancer 14:1216-1222, 1961 (children).

Palmar and plantar fibromatosis

42 Allen, R. A., Woolner, L. B., and Ghormley, R. K.: J. Bone Joint Surg. (Am.) 37:14-26, 1955 (plantar fibromatosis).
43 Battifora, H., and Hines, J. R.: Cancer 27:1530-1536, 1971 (recurrent digital fibromas of childhood; an electron microscope study).
44 Dupuytren, G.: J. Univ. Med. Chir. (Paris) 5:352-355, 1831-1832 (Dupuytren's contracture).

45 Gabbiani, G., and Majno, G.: Am. J. Pathol. **66:**131-146, 1972 (fibroblast contraction).

46 Larsen, R. D., and Posch, J. L.: J. Bone Joint Surg. (Am.) **40:**773-792, 1958 (Dupuytren's contracture).

47 Majno, G., Gabbiani, G., Hirschel, B. J., Ryan, G. B., and Statkov, P. R.: Science **173:**548-549, 1971 (contraction of granulation tissue in vitro).

48 Pickren, J. W., Smith, A. G., Stevenson, T. W., Jr., and Stout, A. P.: Cancer **4:**846-856, 1951 (plantar fascia).

49 Ross, R.: The connective tissue fiber forming cells. In Ramachandran, G. N., and Gould, B. S., editors: Treatise on collagen, New York, 1968, Academic Press, Inc., vol. 2, part A, pp. 1-82.

Musculoaponeurotic fibromatosis

50 Chandler, F. A.: Bull. Hosp. Joint Dis. **14:**158-171, 1953 (congenital muscular torticollis).

51 Conley, J., Healey, W. V., and Stout, A. P.: Am. J. Surg. **112:**609-614, 1966 (head and neck).

52 Enzinger, F. M., and Shiraki, M.: Cancer **20:**1131-1140, 1967 (shoulder girdle).

53 Dahn, I., Jonsson, N., and Lundh, G.: Acta Chir. Scand. **126:**305-314, 1963 (desmoid tumors).

54 Hough, G. deN., Jr.: Surg. Gynecol. Obstet. **58:**972-981, 1934 (congenital torticollis—review).

55 Hunt, R. T. N., Morgan, H. C., and Ackerman, L. V.: Cancer **13:**825-836, 1960 (extra-abdominal).

56 Kern, W. H.: Arch. Pathol. (Chicago) **69:**209-216, 1960 (proliferative myositis; pseudosarcomatous reaction to injury).

57 Kim, Dong-Heup, Goldsmith, H. S., Quan, S. H., and Huvos, A. G.: Cancer **27:**1041-1045, 1971 (desmoid tumor).

58 Kimmelstiel, P., and Rapp, I. H.: Bull. Hosp. Joint Dis. **12:**286-297, 1951 (parosteal desmoids).

59 Masson, J. K., and Soule, E. H.: Am. J. Surg. **112:**615-622, 1966 (head and neck).

60 Musgrove, J. E., and McDonald, J. R.: Arch. Pathol. (Chicago) **45:**513-540, 1948 (extra-abdominal).

Fibrosarcoma

61 Pritchard, D. J., Soule, E. H., Taylor, W. F., and Ivins, J. C.: Cancer **33:**888-897, 1974.

62 van der Werf-Messing, B., and van Unnik, J. A. M.: Cancer **18:**1113-1123, 1965.

Benign and malignant tumors of possible histiocytic origin

63 Bednar, B.: Cancer **10:**368-376, 1957 (storiform neurofibromas).

64 Bourne, R. G.: Med. J. Aust. **1:**504-510, 1963 (pseudosarcoma).

65 Fisher, E. R., and Hellstrom, H. R.: Cancer **19:**1165-1171, 1966 (dermatofibrosarcoma).

66 Fretzin, D. F., and Helwig, E. B.: Cancer **31:**1541-1552, 1973 (atypical fibroxanthoma).

67 Fu, Y.-S., Gabbiani, G., Kaye, G. I., and Lattes, R.: Cancer **35:**176-198, 1975 (malignant fibrous histiocytomas).

68 Gentele, H.: Acta Dermatol. Venereol. (Suppl.) (Stockh.) **31:**1-180, 1951 (skin).

69 Gonzalez-Crussi, F., and Campbell, R. J.: Arch. Pathol. **89:**65-72, 1970 (juvenile xanthogranuloma—ultrastructural study).

70 Gordon, H. W.: Arch. Dermatol. **90:**319-325, 1964 (pseudosarcomatous reticulohistiocytoma).

71 Hudson, A. W., and Winkelmann, R. K.: Cancer **29:**413-422, 1972 (fibroxanthoma of skin).

72 Kahn, L. B.: Cancer **31:**411-422, 1973 (malignant fibrous xanthoma).

73 Kempson, R. L., and Kyriakos, M.: Cancer **29:**961-976, 1972 (fibroxanthosarcoma).

74 Kempson, R. L., and McGavran, M. H.: Cancer **17:**1463-1471, 1964 (atypical fibroxanthomas of the skin).

75 Levan, N. E., Hirsh, P., and Kwong, M. Q.: Arch. Dermatol. **88:**908-912, 1963 (pseudosarcomatous dermatofibroma).

76 McPeak, C. J., Cruz, T., and Nicastri, A. D.: Ann. Surg. **166:**803-816, 1966 (dermatofibrosarcoma protuberans).

77 Merkow, L. P., Frich, J. C., Slifkin, M., Kyreages, C. G., and Pardo, M.: Cancer **28:**372-383, 1971 (ultrastructure of fibroxanthosarcoma).

78 O'Brien, J. E., and Stout, A. P.: Cancer **17:**1445-1455, 1964 (malignant fibrous xanthomas).

79 Ozarda, A. T., and Naifeh, G.: Cancer **26:**1109-1111, 1970 (retroperitoneal xanthogranuloma).

80 Ozzello, L., Stout, A. P., and Murray, M. R.: Cancer **16:**331-344, 1963 (cultural characteristics).

81 Pack, G. T., and Tabah, E. J.: Arch. Surg. (Chicago) **62:**391-411, 1951 (dermatofibrosarcoma protuberans).

82 Papadimitriou, J. M., and Matz, L. R.: Arch. Pathol. **83:**535-542, 1967 (retroperitoneal xanthogranuloma).

83 Parker, P., and Odland, G. F.: Am. J. Pathol. **53:**537-565, 1968 (experimental xanthomas).

84 Parker, P., and Odland, G. F.: J. Invest. Dermatol. **52:**136-147, 1969 (ultrastructure).

85 Rosas-Uribe, A., Ring, A. M., and Rappaport, H.: Cancer **26:**827-831, 1970 (malignant fibroxanthoma).

86 Soule, E. H., and Enriquez, P.: Cancer **30:**128-143, 1972 (histiocytoma).

87 Sutton, J. S.: J. Cell Biol. **28:**303-332, 1966 (ultrastructure).

88 Waller, J. I., Hellwig, C. A., and Barbosa, E.: Cancer **10:**388-392, 1957 (retroperitoneal xanthogranuloma).

Tumors of undifferentiated and pluripotential mesenchyme
Myxoma

89 Enzinger, F.: Am. J. Clin. Pathol. **43:**104-113, 1965 (intramuscular myxoma).

90 Kindblom, L.-G., Stener, B., and Angervall, L.: Cancer **34:**1737-1744, 1974 (intramuscular myxoma).

91 Leung, T. K., Vauzelle, I. L., Patricot, L. M., Lejoune, E., and Queneau, P.: Ann. Anat. Pathol. (Paris) **16:**417-428, 1971 (ultrastructure).

92 Uehlinger, E.: Virchows Arch. (Pathol. Anat.) **306**:255-299, 1940 (osteofibrosis deformans juvenilis).
93 Wirth, W. A., Leavitt, D., and Enzinger, F. M.: Cancer **27**:1167-1173, 1971 (intramuscular myxomas).

Tumors of adipose tissue
Lipoma

94 Booher, R. J.: J. Bone Joint Surg. **47-A**:727-740, 1965 (hands and feet—literature review).
95 Dodge, O. G., and Evans, D. M. D.: J. Pathol. Bacteriol. **72**:313-317, 1956 (myelolipoma).
96 Greenberg, S. D., Isensee, C., Gonzalez-Angulo, A., and Wallace, S. A.: Am. J. Clin. Pathol. **39**:66-72, 1963 (thigh).
97 Howard, W. R., and Helwig, E. B.: Arch. Dermatol. (Chicago) **82**:924-931, 1960 (angiolipoma).
98 Keeley, J. L., and Vana, A. J.: Int. Abstr. Surg. **103**:313-322, 1956. In Surg. Gynecol. Obstet., October 1956 (mediastinum).
99 Kindblom, L.-G., Angervall, L., Stener, B., and Wickbom, I.: Cancer **33**:754-762, 1974 (muscle).
100 Stimpson, N.: Br. J. Surg. **58**:464-466, 1971 (angiolipomas of skeletal muscle).
101 Sullivan, C. R., Dahlin, D. C., and Bryan, R. S.: J. Bone Joint Surg. **38-A**:1275-1280, 1956 (tendon sheath).
102 Wells, H. G.: J.A.M.A. **114**:2177, 1940 (adipose tissue).

Hibernoma

103 Angervall, L., Nilsson, L., and Stener, B.: Cancer **17**:685-692, 1964 (microangiographic and histologic studies).
104 Brines, O. A., and Johnson, M. H.: Am. J. Pathol. **25**:467-479, 1949.
105 Cramer, W.: Br. J. Exp. Pathol. **1**:184-196, 1920 (relation to endocrine organs and vitamin problem).
106 Van Meurs, D. P.: Br. J. Surg. **34**:282-284, 1947 (embryonic lipoma; transformation to common lipoma).
107 Vellios, F., Baez, J. M., and Shumacker, H. B.: Am. J. Pathol. **34**:1149-1159, 1958 (lipoblastomatosis—fetal fat different from hibernoma).

Lipoblastomatosis

108 Chung, E. B., and Enzinger, F. M.: Cancer **32**:482-492, 1973.
109 Jaffe, R. H.: A.M.A. Arch. Pathol. **1**:381-387, 1926 (recurrent).
110 Shear, M.: Br. J. Oral Surg. **5**:173-179, 1967.
111 Tedeschi, C. G.: Arch. Pathol. **42**:320-337, 1946 (multicentric lipoblastosis).

Liposarcoma

112 Amador, E., and Danzig, L. S.: Dis. Chest **41**:95-101, 1962 (mediastinum).
113 DeWeerd, J. H., and Dockerty, M. B.: Am. J. Surg. **84**:397-407, 1952 (retroperitoneum).
114 Enterline, H. T., Culberson, J. D., Rochlin, D. B., and Brady, L. W.: Cancer **13**:932-950, 1960.
115 Enzinger, F. M., and Winslow, D. J.: Virchows

Arch. (Pathol. Anat.) **335**:367-388, 1962 (103 cases).
116 Kinne, D. W., Chu, F. C. H., Huvos, A. G., Yagoda, A., and Fortner, J. G.: Cancer **31**:53-64, 1973 (treatment).
117 Reszel, P. A., Soule, E. H., and Coventry, M. B.: J. Bone Joint Surg. **48-A**:229-244, 1966.
118 Spittle, M. F., Newton, K. A., and Mackenzie, D. H.: Br. J. Cancer **24**:696-704, 1970.

Tumors of smooth muscle
Leiomyoma

119 Fisher, W. C., and Helwig, E. B.: Arch. Dermatol. (Chicago) **88**:510-520, 1963 (skin).
120 Yannopoulos, K., and Stout, A. P.: Cancer **15**:958-971, 1962 (benign and malignant, in children).

Leiomyosarcoma

121 Botting, A. J., Soule, E. H., and Brown, A. L., Jr.: Cancer **18**:711-720, 1965 (benign and malignant, in children).
122 Penner, D. W.: Cancer **6**:776-779, 1953 (spontaneous regression).
123 Stout, A. P., and Hill, W. T.: Cancer **11**:844-854, 1958 (superficial soft tissues).
124 Thomas, M. A., and Fine, G.: Cancer **13**:96-101, 1960 (veins—literature review).

Tumors of striated muscle
Rhabdomyoma

125 Goldman, R. L.: Cancer **16**:1609-1613, 1963 (multicentric).
126 Moran, J. J., and Enterline, H. T.: Am. J. Clin. Pathol. **42**:174-181, 1964 (pharynx—literature review).
127 Ross, C. F.: J. Pathol. Bacteriol. **95**:556-558, 1968 (sternomastoid).

Rhabdomyosarcoma

128 Albores-Saavedra, J., Martin, R. G., and Smith, J. L., Jr.: Ann. Surg. **157**:186-197, 1963 (35 cases).
129 Cappell, D. F., and Montgomery, G. L.: J. Pathol. Bacteriol. **44**:517-548, 1937 (rhabdomyoma and myoblastoma).
130 Horn, R. C., and Enterline, H. T.: Cancer **11**:181-199, 1958.
131 Lawrence, W., Jr., Jegge, G., and Foote, F. W., Jr.: Cancer **17**:361-376, 1964 (clinicopathologic study).
132 Patton, R. B., and Horn, R. C., Jr.: Surgery **52**:572-584, 1962 (comparison with human fetal and embryonal skeletal muscle).
133 Porterfield, J. F., and Zimmerman, L. E.: Virchows Arch. (Pathol. Anat.) **335**:329-344, 1962 (orbit).
134 Potenza, A. D., and Winslow, D. J.: J. Bone Joint Surg. **43-A**:700-708, 1961 (hand).
135 Potter, G. D.: Cancer **19**:221-226, 1966 (embryonal, in middle ear, in children).
136 Soule, E. H., Geitz, M., and Henderson, E. D.: Cancer **23**:1336-1346, 1969 (embryonal, in limbs).
137 Stobbe, G. D., and Dargeon, H. W.: Cancer **3**:826-836, 1950.
138 Stout, A. P.: Ann. Surg. **123**:447-472, 1946.

Tumors of heterotopic bone and cartilage
Chondrosarcoma (extraosseous)

139 Kauffman, S. L., and Stout, A. P.: Cancer **16:**432-439, 1963 (osteogenic sarcomas and chondrosarcomas in children).

140 Stout, A. P., and Verner, E. W.: Cancer **6:**581-590, 1953.

Osteogenic sarcoma

141 Binkley, J. S., and Stewart, F. W.: Arch. Pathol. (Chicago) **29:**42-56, 1940 (osteogenic sarcoma and pseudo-osteosarcoma).

142 Butler, F. E., and Woolley, I. M.: Radiology **26:**236-237, 1936 (from a calcified hematoma).

143 Fine, G., and Stout, A. P.: Cancer **9:**1027-1043, 1956.

144 Jaffe, H. L.: Tumors and tumorous conditions of the bones and joints, Philadelphia, 1958, Lea & Febiger.

145 Pack, G. T., and Braund, R. R.: J.A.M.A. **119:**776-779, 1942 (myositis ossificans).

146 Salm, R.: Br. J. Cancer **13:**614-617, 1959.

Tumors of undetermined type
Alveolar soft-part sarcoma

147 Abrikossoff, A. I.: Virchows Arch. (Pathol. Anat.) **280:**723-740, 1931.

148 Christopherson, W. M., Foote, F. W., Jr., and Stewart, F. W.: Cancer **5:**100-111, 1952.

149 Fisher, E. R.: Am. J. Pathol. **32:**721-737, 1956 (histochemistry, reference to histogenesis).

150 Lieberman, P. H., Foote, F. W., Jr., Stewart, F. W., and Berg, J. W.: J.A.M.A. **198:**1047-1051, 1966.

151 Pearse, A. G. E.: J. Pathol. Bacteriol. **62:**351-362, 1950 (histogenesis, granular cell perineural fibroblastoma).

152 Ross, R. C., Miller, T. R., and Foote, F. W., Jr.: Cancer **5:**112-121, 1952 (malignant granular cell myoblastoma).

153 Shipkey, F. H., Lieberman, P. H., Foote, F. W., Jr., and Stewart, F. W.: Cancer **17:**821-830, 1964 (ultrastructure).

154 Unni, K. K., and Soule, E. H.: Mayo Clin. Proc. **50**(10):591-598, 1975 (electron microscopy).

44/Metabolic and other nontumorous disorders of the bone

STEVEN L. TEITELBAUM

Bone is a heterogenous tissue that is not only structurally important but plays the central role in mineral homeostasis. It may be functionally divided into its cortical (compact) and trabecular (cancellous) components. Structural stability is provided by cortical bone, which comprises approximately 80% of the skeleton. It contains haversian canals through which longitudinally oriented blood vessels pass and horizontally arranged Volkmann's canals containing vascular offshoots. Surrounding each haversian canal is a series of concentric, lamellar, mineralized collagen bundles forming an osteon, which is the remodeling unit of cortical bone. Separating osteons are basophilic, metachromatic markers known as cement lines (Fig. 44-1).

Trabecular bone consists of a meshwork of spicules between which are the marrow elements. The orientation of these spicules is generally along the lines of stress (Fig. 44-2). The surface area of trabecular bone is much greater than that of cortical bone and therefore its primary role is metabolic rather than structural. Its surface, the endosteum, is covered by a syncytium of cells, which probably functionally separates bone from marrow space (Fig. 44-3).

The three major cellular activities of bone are modeling, remodeling, and repair. Modeling is intimately associated with growth and includes those functions responsible for shaping the small bones of the newborn into the much larger, identically shaped bones of a fully grown adult. The factors initiating the resorptive and formative activities of bone that are responsible for the ever-changing shape during growth are unknown.

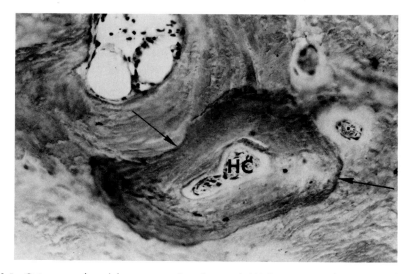

Fig. 44-1. Osteon enclosed by cement line *(arrows)*. Within center of osteon is haversian canal, **HC.** (Undecalcified, toluidine blue; 100×.)

Remodeling occurs in both the growing and fully grown skeleton. It is intimately related to mineral homeostasis. The histologic manifestations of remodeling such as osteoclasts and osteoblasts are probably reflections of long-term metabolic demands. Maintenance of minute-to-minute mineral homeostasis may not be reflected morphologically and is probably accomplished by changing ionic fluxes.

The most distinctive cellular activity of remodeling is the coupling of resorption and formation. In the normal adult these processes are inexorably linked. After bone cell activation, a selective focus of bone (activation site) undergoes osteoclastic resorption to be followed in the same location by osteoblastic bone deposition. The description of the linkage of precursor cell activation and bone resorption and formation by Frost[1] has laid the foundation for the quantitative evaluation of bone remodeling by morphologic techniques. Even in states of abnormal bone turnover, such as

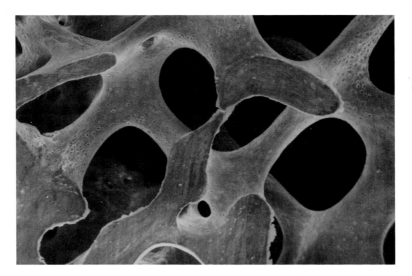

Fig. 44-2. Scanning electron micrograph of trabecular bone after removal of marrow. All trabeculae are joined in a complicated meshwork. Small holes on surface are osteocytic lacunae. (57×.)

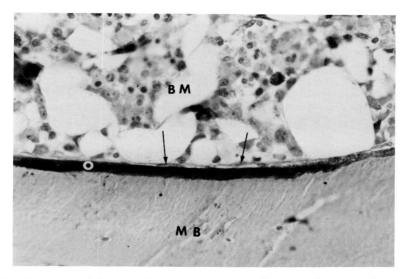

Fig. 44-3. Syncytium of flat, membranous-appearing cells *(arrows)* covering bone surface, which probably functionally separates bone from the general extracellular fluid. **BM,** Bone marrow; **MB,** mineralized bone; **O,** osteoid. (Undecalcified, Goldner stain; 250×.)

Paget's disease and hyperparathyroidism, this local tethering of formation and resorption persists, although, as is obvious by changing skeletal mass, the rates of each function may differ. This association may be temporarily disrupted when the skeletal system is perturbed by a new stimulus such as a therapeutic agent. It is therefore extremely important that the effects of a stimulus be evaluated at a point past the transient time, which may be determined morphologically.[2] Undoubtedly, many misconceptions of the effects of various drugs on the skeleton have arisen from evaluation of transient phenomena.

Repair is the third distinct functional activity of bone. Not only does this process occur in a gross manner, but microfractures are probably always undergoing repair somewhere in the skeleton.

The importance of recognizing the distinction between these three processes relates not only to appreciation of human skeletal dynamics, but also to the choice of laboratory animals. Much work related to bone remodeling is of limited value because the rat has been used as the experimental animal. As this animal continues to grow to death,[3] the processes of modeling and remodeling cannot be distinguished.

As demonstrated by Frost,[4] bone surfaces are covered by three cellular envelopes. These envelopes, which respectively cover the periosteum, haversian canals, and endosteum, function independently of each other. Hence,

it is possible, such as in corticosteroid excess, to have relative sparing of cortical bone and aggravated loss of cancellous bone.[5]

COMPOSITION AND STRUCTURE OF BONE
Cellular phase
Osteoblasts

Osteoblasts are the cells that synthesize bone matrix and probably play a role in its mineralization.[6] In nondecalcified sections they appear mononuclear with extremely basophilic cytoplasm containing a perinuclear clear zone. Osteoblasts are almost invariably found lining an osteoid seam, which is nonmineralized bone collagen (Fig. 44-4).

Flat, membranous-appearing cells actually line most osteoid seams (Fig. 44-3). The nature of these cells is controversial. Whereas some believe these are relatively "inactive" osteoblasts,[7] others see them as a part of a membranous system separating bone surfaces from its vascular supply[8] and taking an active part in calcium homeostasis.[9] In any event, these cells are associated with bone that is replacing itself relatively slowly, whereas a predominance of columnar osteoblasts is seen in states of stimulated bone metabolism.

Abundant endoplasmic reticulum lined by ribonuclear protein particles accounts for osteoblastic basophilia. These cells are almost never found in mitoses and therefore probably do not replicate themselves.[7] Although cytoplasmic processes extend from cell to cell, osteoblasts

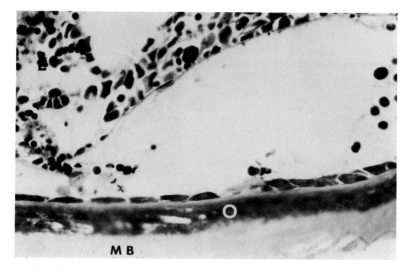

Fig. 44-4. Obsteoblasts lining osteoid seam, **O. MB,** Mineralized bone. (Undecalcified, Goldner; 250×.)

are not fused. Narrow spaces exist between these cells, which may function as channels of communication between the vascular supply and bone surfaces.[9] Pinocytotic vesicles, which are abundant, may have a similar function.

Osteoblasts are rich in enzymatic activity. Alkaline phosphatase is abundant.[10] Although the enzyme decreases in the matrix with progresssive bone mineralization, it persists in the osteocytes.[11]

Osteoblasts undergo morphologic alterations with varying humoral stimuli such as parathyroid hormone,[12] vitamin D,[13] or calcitonin.[14] After cessation of bone growth, these cells are rarely present on the periosteal surface except in pathologic states. In these circumstances they may reappear, resulting in periosteal new bone formation,[15] an important roentgenologic sign of bone disease.

The origin of osteoblasts is controversial. Whereas most investigators postulate a common progenitor cell of osteoblasts and osteoclasts[7] (as well as chondroblasts[16]), Rasmussen and Bordier[17] have offered a controversial hypothesis in which osteoclasts, by cell fission, are the source of osteoblasts. Recently however, Kahn and Simmons[18] have presented exciting new evidence indicating a hematogenous origin of osteoclasts and a skeletal origin of osteoblasts.

Osteocytes

After matrix deposition, the osteoblast is incorporated into osteoid, becoming an osteo-cyte. It retains contact with its fellows and overlying osteoblasts by canaliculae through which cell processes extend, meeting each other in tight junctions[8] (Fig. 44-5). It is likely that this cell system regulates the transfer of metabolites between the bone surface and extracellular fluid.[9]

Contrary to the long-accepted belief that osteocytes are relatively inert, they are capable of significant metabolic activity. They not only engage in bone resorption (osteocytic osteolysis) under the influence of such substances as parathyroid hormone[19] and vitamin D[20] but also are able to form and mineralize bone matrix.[21,22] It is therefore possible that as osteocytes and their processes cover much more bone surface than do any other cell types, their metabolic activity plays a significant role in calcium homeostasis. As hours are needed for osteoclast mobilization, osteocytic osteolysis may be responsible for meeting demands of immediate skeletal mobilization.[23] However others deny that this phenomenon plays a significant role in mineral homeostasis.[24]

The ratio of matrix volume to osteocyte number varies with the state of bone turnover. Woven bone contains many more of these cells than does lamellar bone. In addition, the osteocytic lacunae of woven bone are larger than their counterparts in lamellar bone (Fig. 44-6).

Ultrastructurally those osteocytes closest to the cell surface most resemble osteoblasts.[25] With progressive age they lose much of their cytoplasmic organelles. Whereas osteocytes en-

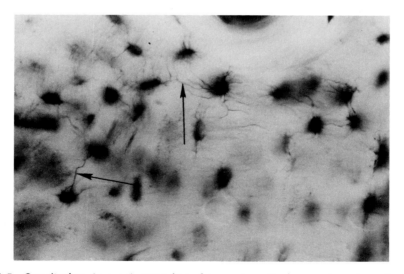

Fig. 44-5. Canaliculae *(arrows)* extending from osteocytic lacuna to osteocytic lacuna. (Fresh, unembedded ground section; Villanueva bone stain; 250×.)

gaging in bone formation and mineralization contain a prominent Golgi apparatus and rough endoplastic reticulum,[26] the cytoplasm of the resorbing cells is characterized by lysosomes.

Osteoclasts

Osteoclasts are the large, mobile, resorptive cells of bone that carry on osteolysis with dramatic physical activity.[27] Although usually multinuclear, they may contain only one nucleus. Their appearance differs from megokaryocytes in that osteoclast nuclei are separated whereas those of megokaryocytes are fused.

Osteoclasts engaged in resorptive activity are juxtaposed to the bone surface in scalloped areas known as Howship's lacunae or resorptive bays (Fig. 44-7). These resorptive bays, with or without osteoclasts, merely inform the observer that resorption has taken place at that location and offers no information about resorptive rate. On occasion, in nondecalcified thin sections, a striated border between osteoclast and adjacent bone is apparent. This probably represents the ruffled or brush border of the cell, easily visualized by electron microscopy, particularly when the cell is stimulated by parathyroid hormone (Fig. 44-8). This structure, consisting of complicated villuslike infoldings of the cell membrane, plays an intimate role in bone resorption.[28]

Similar to osteoblasts, osteoclasts are never seen in mitosis. Although their ultimate fate

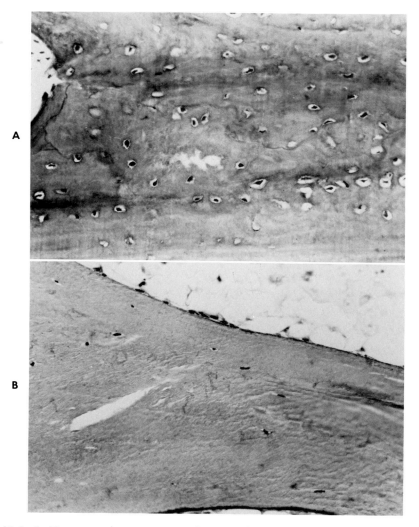

Fig. 44-6. A, Numerous, large osteocytic lacunae characterizing woven bone as compared to normal, lamellar bone, **B.** (Undecalcified, Goldner; 250×.)

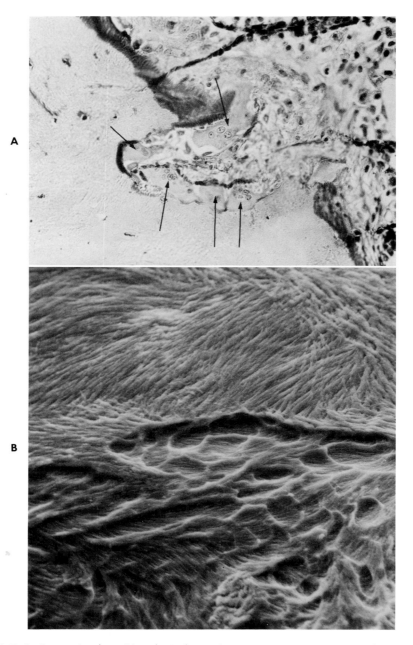

Fig. 44-7. A, Resorptive bay (Howship's lacuna) containing numerous osteoclasts *(arrows).* **B,** Scanning electron micrograph of large resorptive bay. **(A,** Undecalcified, Goldner, 250×; **B,** 750×.)

is unknown, there are suggestions that osteoclasts may eventually undergo amitotic fission.[17]

The known stimuli of osteoclast-remodeling activity are parathyroid hormone and vitamin D. Obviously in modeling and fracture repair, other stimuli are responsible for their activation. In addition, certain neoplastic tissues, particularly that from lymphoid tumors, elaborate a bone-resorbing substance that mediates its effect through osteoclast proliferation.[29] A similar substance is obtained from cultured normal human leukocytes stimulated by phytohemagglutinin.[30] Furthermore, prostaglandin E_2 may promote bone resorption.[31]

The process of bone resorption involves both

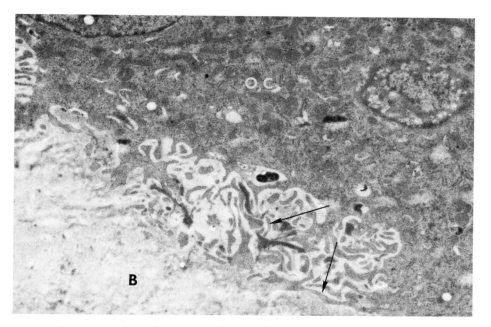

Fig. 44-8. Osteoclast, **OC,** with large ruffled border *(arrows)* resorbing bone, **B.** (13,000×; Courtesy Dr. Barbara Mills, San Marino, Cal.)

the organic and inorganic phases.[28] Hence osteoclasts are in general unable to digest osteoid.[32] Resorption also probably involves lysosomal activity because osteoclasts are rich in enzymes such as acid phosphatase, the release of which is stimulated by parathyroid hormone.[33] In addition, carbonic anhydrase[34] and local acidification[35] may play a role in bone resorption.

Organic phase

Bone may be functionally conceptualized as a variety of cells undergoing metabolic activity within an organic and inorganic matrix. The organic component, about 90% of which is collagen,[36] represents approximately 25% of the dry weight of bone.[37] Bone collagen as compared to that of other tissues is characterized by its relative insolubility.[36] Since the amino acid structures of bone and skin collagen are relatively similar, the insolubility of the former is probably related to the extent and nature of the intermolecular cross-links.[36] Lathyrogenic agents, which promote bone collagen solubility, do so by destroying these cross-links.[36]

Nonfetal bone collagen is normally deposited in a lamellar pattern, characterized by parallel, relatively uniform bundles. The architecture of fetal bone collagen is "woven." These bundles vary in size and are arranged in a random pattern. Woven bone also occurs in any state of accelerated bone synthesis such as fracture repair or hyperparathyroidism. In normal skeletal development or repair, woven bone serves as a scaffolding for lamellar bone deposition and eventually undergoes osteoclastic resorption (Fig. 44-9).

Hydroxyproline, an amino acid almost unique to collagen, is important in the evaluation of bone turnover. With significant collagen degradation, which in the majority of instances is of bone origin, increased quantities of this amino acid appear in the urine. In addition, hydroxyproline is released from newly formed bone. Whereas the amino acid released by bone degradation is unbound, hydroxyproline representing bone formation is excreted as an oligopeptide. These moieties may be distinguished by dialysis.[38]

The noncollagenous organic component of bone is the ground substance. This contains a variety of compounds of which glycosaminoglycans and proteoglycans are present in the greatest concentrations.[39] Both of these groups of compounds exist in greater quantities in cartilage than in bone.[39]

Glycosaminoglycans are the acid mucopolysaccharides of bone and are therefore metachromatic. They are characterized biochemically by their high hexosamine content.[40] As in cartilage, the major member of this group

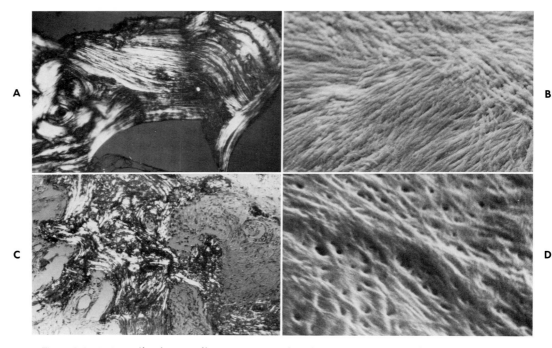

Fig. 44-9. A, Lamellar bone collagen as viewed under polarized light. Fibers are of uniform diameter and arranged in parallel fashion. **B,** Scanning electron micrograph of lamellar bone. **C,** Woven bone collagen viewed under polarized light. There is a random directionality of the fibers. **D,** Scanning electron micrograph of woven bone. The architectural arrangement and dimensions of the collagen bundles are varied. (**A,** Decalcified; **A** and **C,** hematoxylin and eosin; 100×; **B** and **D,** 1000×.)

is chondroitin sulfate.[39] This group of substances may not only play a role in mineralization, but also appears to aggregate with collagen fibrils, perhaps increasing their stability.[41]

Proteoglycans are protein polysaccharides in which chondroitin sulfate is bound to protein by covalent bonding.[39] Other components of ground substances include glycoproteins and phospholipids. The latter, which is demonstrable by sudan black staining, appears to play a role in mineral deposition.[42]

Mineral phase

The mineral component of bone, hydroxyapatite, $Ca_{10}(PO_4)_6(OH)_2$, exists in two phases.[36] It is initially deposited in a form that is amorphous when examined ultrastructurally[43] or by x-ray diffraction analysis.[44] Within a short period of time, amorphous calcium phosphtae is converted to crystalline hydroxyapatite, also having distinctive ultrastructural[43] and x-ray diffractive[44] appearances.

Although the mechanism by which mineralization occurs is in debate, there is little question that the relationship of the inorganic phase to its organic counterpart is of vital importance. Similar to any structure, the strength of bone is dependent not only on the absolute quantities of its various components, but on the way in which these components are related to each other. Hence, although Pagetic bone may contain normal quantities of organic and inorganic material, because of its composition, it is relatively weak.[36] Therefore abnormalities of bone must be evaluated in qualitative as well as quantitative terms.

Bone cells probably play an active role in mineralization. One popular theory holds that intracellular granules composed of amorphous calcium phosphate are important in mineralization.[6] These particles may be transiently stored in the mitochondria of osteoblasts and osteocytes from which they are passed into the the cytoplasm, packaged, and extruded into the osteoid as double membrane–bound matrix vesicles.[45]

Ultimately, mineral deposition parallels the distribution of collagen fibers (Fig. 44-10). Whether the collagen fibril serves as the initial locus of calcification, however, remains in question. Glimcher and Krane[36] propose that

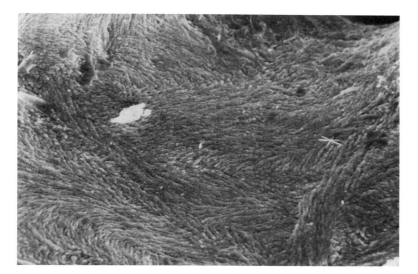

Fig. 44-10. Scanning electron micrograph of lamellar bone after extraction of all organic material. Arrangement of mineral phase of bone parallels that of bone collagen. (540×.)

tropocollagen molecules are arranged in a quarter-stagger pattern resulting in holes paralleling their 640 Å periodicity. They postulate that it is within these holes that mineralization initially occurs. Moreover, they propose that collagen, associated with inorganic phosphate, serves to nucleate bone crystals. Conversely, according to Bonnucci,[46] matrix mineralization is initiated within the ground substance. He believes crystallization initially parallels these fibrils.

The major unsolved question regarding calcification is why collagen such as that of bone and dentin mineralizes, whereas that of skin and muscle fails to do so. Differences in the biochemical structure of bone and skin collagen do exist. However, it is possible that subtle architectural distinctions in molecular packing, perhaps in association with ground substance deposition, may be responsible for the differences in propensity to mineralize.[47] An equally intriguing concept involves the role of mineralization inhibitors, particularly pyrophosphate. This compound is postulated to interfere with the deposition of amorphous calcium phosphate and slow its transformation to crystalline hydroxyapatite.[48] Perhaps alkaline phosphatase influences mineralization by catalyzing the hydrolysis of pyrophosphate.[48]

SKELETAL DEVELOPMENT

Prenatal bone development occurs by either endochondral or intramembranous ossification. The former entails partial replacement of a cartilaginous model by bone, with the residual cartilage serving as the epiphyseal plate and articular surface. Intramembranous ossification occurs by differentiation of primitive mesenchymal cells directly into osteoblasts, which produce bone in the absence of cartilage.

Endochondral ossification

Cartilage is of mesenchymal derivation and originates with primitive cells clustering together and differentiating into chondroblasts (Fig. 44-11). These cells secrete an intracellular, nonvascular substance rich in mucopolysaccharides and collagen. Like bone, cartilage can grow appositionally by perichondrial cells differentiating into chondrocytes. The ability of cartilage to grow interstitially however, enables it to serve as the skeletal growth plate. Interstitial growth implies duplication of chondrocytes within the substance of cartilage, which in turn produce additional intracellular matrix, and therefore the chondrocytes expand the cartilaginous mass.

Long bones develop within a cartilaginous model by differentiation of perichondrial cells into osteoblasts. Invasion by these cells and their blood supply results in mineralization and death of cartilage (Fig. 44-12). This focus, an ossification center, serves as a scaffold for the deposition of woven bone. With continued diaphyseal and metaphyseal replacement by bone, the growth plate differentiates into four distinct zones. The zone of resting cartilage is firmly adherent to the overlying epiphyseal bone. The proliferating zone of cartilage is characterized by vertical columns of chondro-

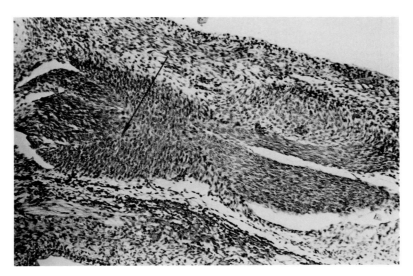

Fig. 44-11. Cluster of primitive mesenchymal cells *(arrow)* prior to differentiation into chondroblasts. (Hematoxylin and eosin; 80×.)

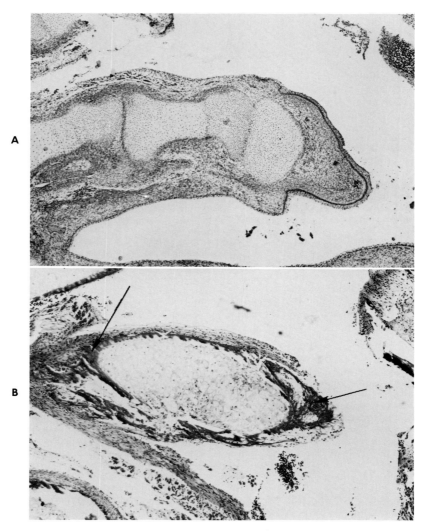

Fig. 44-12. A, Cartilaginous model of digit that will undergo endochondral ossification. **B,** Bone *(arrows)* forming in periphery of cartilaginous model in normal endochondral ossification. (**A** and **B,** Hematoxylin and eosin; **A,** 40×; **B,** 80×.)

cytes, which expand the plate interstitially until they enter the hypertrophic zone where they enlarge and become less polar. It is in this zone that P_{O_2} is lowest and the cellular metabolism entirely anaerobic.[49] Alkaline phosphatase is produced by the hypertrophic cells closest to the metaphysis, promoting formation of the zone of calcified cartilage and associated cell death. The calcified cartilage then functions as a lattice for the deposition of bone by osteoblasts that appear against the dead spicules, with the resultant formation of the metaphyseal trabeculae (Fig. 44-13). Therefore, while the epiphyseal plate is expanded by interstitial growth of the proliferative zone, it is attenuated by replacement by bone on the diaphyseal side, resulting in elongation of the shaft. As longitudinal bone growth occurs, it becomes necessary to expand and shape the bone to adult proportions. Structural model-

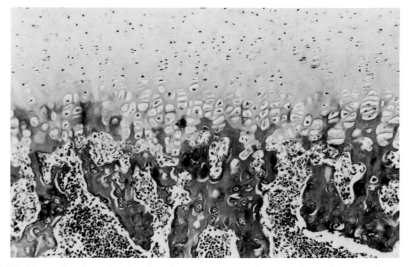

Fig. 44-13. Normal epiphysis. As chondrocytes approach metaphyseal bone, they enlarge. With increasing P_{O_2}, cartilage undergoes mineralization, dries, serves as a lattice for deposition of bone, and is eventually resorbed. (Hematoxylin and eosin; 40×.)

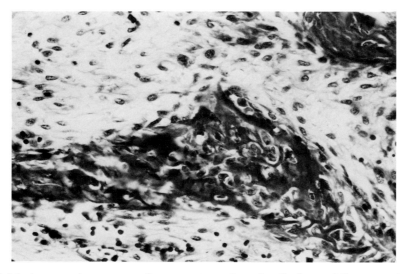

Fig. 44-14. Intramembranous ossification. Mesenchymal cells have differentiated directly into osteoblasts and are forming bone in absence of cartilaginous model. (Hematoxylin and eosin; 250×.)

ing is accomplished by apposition and resorption of bone at appropriate locations on the subperiosteal and endosteal surfaces.

Intramembranous ossification

Intramembranous ossification, which occurs only in flat bones, differs from endochondral ossification in that no cartilaginous model is formed. As bone cannot grow interstitially, intramembranous bone develops only by apposition. However, because this type of ossification does not occur in long bones, the absence

of epiphyseal growth is of no particular disadvantage.

The process originates with collection of mesenchymal cells, which cluster together in centers of ossification. These cells differentiate into large osteoblasts, which in turn secrete collagen matrix and ground substance. Coincidentally with secretion of alkaline phosphatase, mineralization occurs. This initial trabeculum lined by osteoblasts, branches into other trabeculae by apposition (Fig. 44-14). As the trabeculae expand in width, osteoblasts

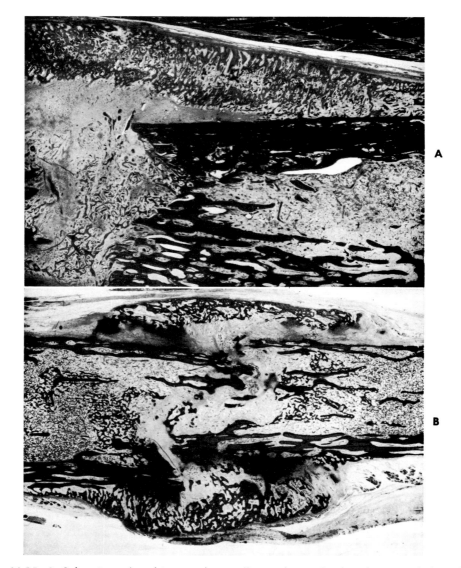

Fig. 44-15. A, Subperiosteal and intermediate callus evident in healing fracture of tibia of young child. **B,** Ten-month-old fracture site in rib of elderly woman. Interlocking ends of fractured bone encased in abundant external and internal callus, which is in part cartilaginous and in part bony. (**A** and **B,** 8×; from Bennett, G. A., and Bauer, W.: In Scudder, C. L., editor: The treatment of fractures, Philadelphia, 1938, W. B. Saunders Co.)

become incorporated in the matrix as osteo-cytes. The trabeculae destined to form compact bone continue to expand, incorporating blood vessels into haversian canals. As the ossification center expands and joins its neighbors, structural modeling begins in a manner similar to that occurring in endochondral ossification.

REPAIR

The prototype of bone repair is fracture healing. Repair is initiated after bone death as a result of tearing of the periosteal and haversian vessels. This dead bone either undergoes osteoclastic resorption or serves as a scaffolding for the deposition of callus.

Callus is tissue deposited during fracture

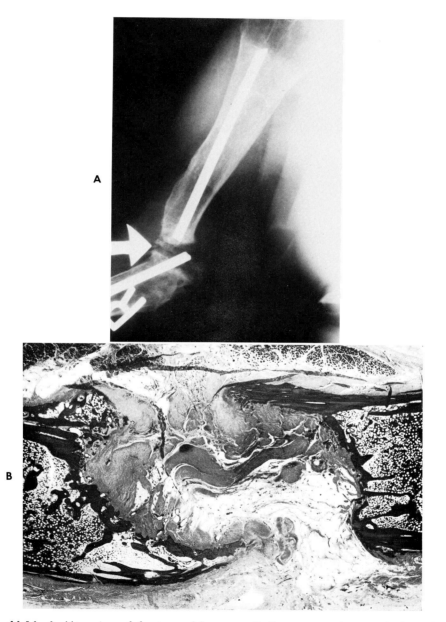

Fig. 44-16. A, Nonunion of fracture of humerus. **B,** Fracture site has resulted in fibrous union, and no evidence of reparative changes remains. Medulla of each fractured bone end closed by osseous plate into which dense connective tissue bundles insert. (**A,** Courtesy Dr. Jerome Gilden, St. Louis, Mo.; **B,** 9×.)

repair and eventually modeled into normal bone. Analogous to growing bone, it is dynamic tissue that undergoes structural change much faster than does mature bone. Shortly after fracture, proliferation of periosteal osteoprogenitor cells occurs close to the fracture site as well as along the entire shaft.[50] Locally these cells initiate formation of early external callus, collaring the ends of the fragments. Endosteal progenitor cell proliferation promotes internal callus formation, which appears first at the endosteal surface and grows into the interfragmentary space. The stimulatory effect of fracture on bone formation is manifested clinically by the propensity of a traumatized extremity of a child to grow longer than its contralateral partner[51] (Fig. 44-15).

Callus is composed primarily of fibrous tissue, woven bone, and cartilage.[52] Because of its rapid growth and relative lack of proximity to blood vessels, superficial callus is less vascular than deep callus. In relatively anoxic tissue, osteoprogenitor cells differentiate into chondroblasts rather than osteoblasts.[52] Hence early superficial callus is composed primarily of cartilage, whereas in the deep, more vascular location, woven bone is directly formed. With vascular encroachment, the cartilaginous portion of callus is mineralized, dies, and is replaced by woven bone, all of which is initially trabecular in type. Active modeling of the mature callus now occurs with replacement of woven bone by its lamellar counterpart. Similar to intramembranous ossification, com-

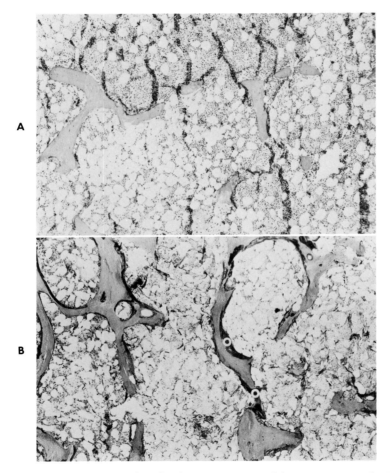

Fig. 44-17. A, Osteoporotic trabecular bone. Quantity of bone matrix is diminished but normally mineralized. **B,** Osteomalacic trabecular bone. Excess of osteoid, O, (unmineralized bone matrix) is present. Both **A** and **B** were taken from patients with skeletons roentgenographically exhibiting identical degree of osteopenia. (**A** and **B,** Undecalcified, Goldner; 40×.)

paction of trabecular bone into cortex occurs where appropriate.

Fractures that are in poor alignment form exuberant callus. Those that are well aligned, particularly if internally immobilized, form little if any external callus. Therefore, callus formation may be a response to stress upon fractured bone. In addition, fracture repair entails modeling of haversian systems, which eventually cross the interfragmentary space. The speed with which this occurs depends on the degree of alignment.[53]

It is apparent that the periosteum plays a central role in fracture repair. Because of its greater vascularity, when fracture occurs, an extent of periosteum less linear than that of bone dies. However, if there is extensive damage to the periosteal blood supply, failure of fracture healing (nonunion) may ensue.[53] Nonunion may also occur in osteomalacia, in which the matrix component of callus fails to mineralize and therefore remains relatively radiopaque (Fig. 44-16).

Electrical forces can stimulate osteogenesis and promote fracture healing.[54] Not only does the rate of repair increase with electrical stimulation, but the callus appears more highly organized.[54]

DISORDERS OF REMODELING
Morphologic methods of diagnosis

Metabolic bone diseases are generally disorders of remodeling. They are characterized by involvement of the entire bony skeleton. That is not to say that the morphologic manifestations of the disorder may not be more severe in one location than in another. However, as distinct from neoplastic or inflammatory processes, which are focal or multifocal, metabolic bone diseases are diffuse. Therefore, with the realization that various bones have different quantities of cortex and trabeculae and are subjected to different physical stresses, skeletal tissue from any site in a patient with a metabolic bone disease will exhibit some evidence of the disorder.

In the majority of patients with metabolic bone diseases it is impossible to radiologically distinguish diminished bone mass caused by decreased quantities of normally mineralized bone (osteoporosis) from that caused by defective mineralization (osteomalacia) (Fig. 44-17). More sophisticated techniques of delineating abnormalities of skeletal mass such as photon-absorption bone densitometry are also incapable of making this distinction. These various types of deficient skeletal mass, in-

distinguishable by noninvasive techniques should be classified under the generic term "osteopenia." To discriminate among the osteopenias, histologic examination of the skeleton is usually necessary. However, since many metabolic disorders of bone are associated with defective mineralization, bone processed by decalcification prior to paraffin embedding, as is performed in the routine histology laboratory, will obscure the differences between mineralized and nonmineralized bone collagen (osteoid). Therefore the distinction of osteomalacia from osteoporosis can only be made from nondecalcified bone sections (Fig. 44-18).

The structural characteristics of bone lend themselves to histologic quantitation. The

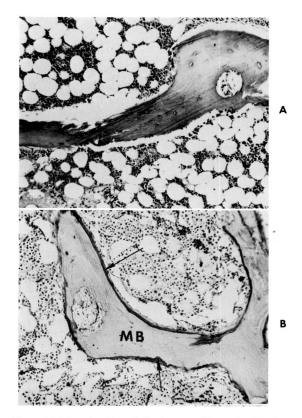

Fig. 44-18. A, Decalcified, paraffin-embedded bone biopsy. It is not possible to distinguish mineralized from nonmineralized bone matrix by this technique. **B,** Undecalcified, plastic-embedded section of bone taken simultaneously with **A.** Distinction between mineralized bone, *MB,* and nonmineralized bone matrix or osteoid *(arrows)* is easily made. In addition, there is superior preservation of bone architecture. (**A,** Hematoxylin and eosin; **B,** Goldner; **A** and **B,** 100×.)

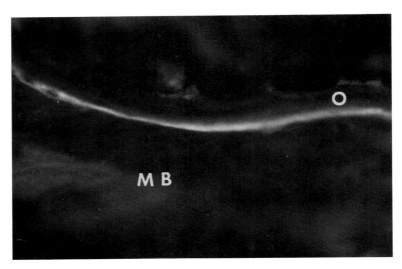

Fig. 44-19. Normal linear fluorescence of mineralization front after administration of tetracycline. Mineralization front is located at the interface between osteoid, **O,** and mineralized bone, **MB.** (Undecalcified, unstained; 250×).

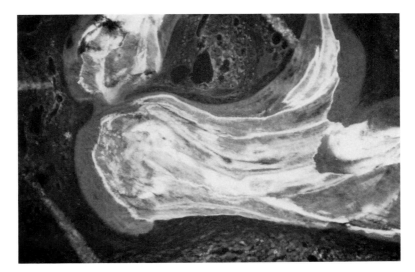

Fig. 44-20. Fluorescent micrograph of woven bone after administration of tetracycline. Bone diffusely fluoresces without distinct formation of calcification front. (Undecalcified, unstained; 100×).

amounts of mineralized and nonmineralized organic matrix are easily determined from nondecalcified sections. In addition, the cellular components of the skeleton may be quantitated with a high degree of precision (55-58).

It is important to appreciate that rates of bone turnover cannot be determined by examination of a histologic section representing one point in time. This is analogous to the impossibility of calculating the doubling time of the lung tumor from a single x-ray film. Although numerous osteoclasts and osteoblasts

are often associated with states of increased bone resorption and formation respectively, large numbers of these cells may exist where these activities are suppressed.[59,60] One must therefore distinguish between cellular level and tissue level rates of resorption and formation.[1] Cellular rates relate to the activity of the average osteoclast or osteoblast. Tissue rates reflect the total quantity of skeleton resorbed or formed per unit bone volume per unit period of time regardless of the number of cells. Therefore pathologic conditions exist in

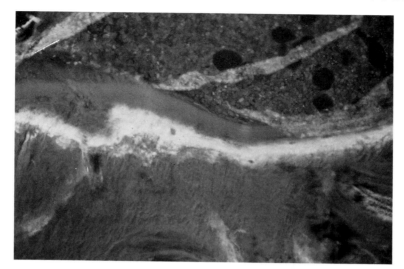

Fig. 44-21. Fluorescent micrograph of bone biopsy from patient with osteomalacia. Compare with Fig. 44-19 and note wide, diffuse appearance of fluorescent tables after administration of tetracycline. (Undecalcified, unstained; 250×).

which the cellular and tissue rates differ from normal in opposite directions.[61] For example, parathyroid hormone is a general activator of bone cells (i.e., stimulates formation of osteoblasts and osteoclasts from their precursors). However, in certain circumstances it may suppress the mean rate of osteoblastic bone formation. Hence, although tissue level formation may be increased in primary hyperparathyroidism, some patients with this disease may have suppressed cellular level formation.[61] Fortunately, the use of time-spaced tetracycline markers that fluoresce in bone enables one to measure these kinetic parameters in a single, nondecalcified section.[1]

Because of their fluorescent properties[1] and ability to combine with calcium,[62] tetracyclines are the most useful morphologic markers of mineralization. In normal lamellar bone, they are deposited exclusively at the calcification (mineralization) front located at the interface between osteoid and mineralized lamellar bone (Fig. 44-19).[63] The predisposition of these antibiotics for this location is attributable to their property of stochiometrically binding to amorphous calcium phosphate,[64] which is normally found only at the calcification front.[65] Woven bone, which contains no calcification front, diffusely fluoresces when labeled with tetracycline (Fig. 44-20).

Deficiencies of mineralization are often reflected by abnormalities of calcification front formation. Although states of severe vitamin D or phosphate deficiency are associated with a

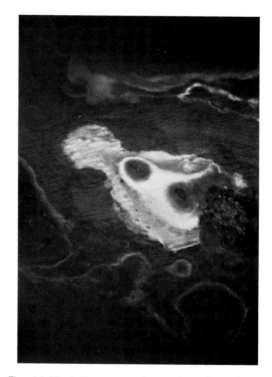

Fig. 44-22. Entire osteon fluorescing after administration of tetracycline to patient with chronic renal failure. (Undecalcified, unstained; 40×.)

decrease in the percentage of osteoid seams with a fluorescent label, more subtle abnormalities of mineralization are characterized by wider and more diffuse patterns of fluorescence[66] (Fig. 44-21). This commonly occurs

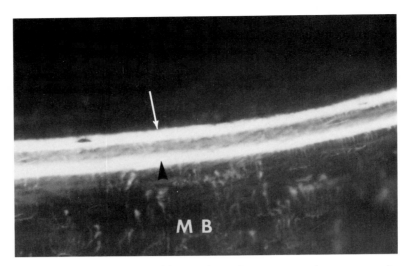

Fig. 44-23. Fluorescent micrograph of bone after administration of two tetracycline labels. Label *(arrowhead)* deepest in mineralized bone, **MB**, was administered first. Second label *(arrow)* was administered 2 weeks later. Appositional rate is determined by measurement of distance between these labels. (Undecalcified, unstained; 500×.)

in chronic renal disease,[67] Paget's disease, and hypophosphatemic rickets[66] and experimentally in early vitamin D deprivation[68] and probably reflects a delay in maturation of amorphous calcium phosphate to its crystalline phase.[69] In addition, fluorescent antibiotics usually diffuse through entire hypomineralized osteons in these diseases (Fig. 44-22). As mineral maturation is abnormal in experimental renal failure,[70] it is likely that this pattern of tetracycline fluorescence reflects the morphologic counterpart of this abnormality.

The fluorescent properties of tetracycline enable its use as a marker of bone kinetics. If two doses of the drug are administered, separated by a known period of time, one calculates the rate of bone formation at the cellular level (appositional rate) by determining the mean distance between the two labels and dividing this distance by the interim between doses.[1] One may then calculate the tissue-level bone formation rate by multiplying this factor by the total surface area participating in bone formation (Fig. 44-23).

Physiologic effects of hormones, vitamins, enzymes, and inorganic compounds on bone with attendant dysfunctions

Parathyroid hormone

Responding to circulating levels of ionized calcium, the parathyroid glands secrete the hormone that is most important in maintaining mineral homeostasis. Parathyroid hormone is a general stimulus of bone cell activity. The mechanism by which this phenomenon occurs involves activation of membrane-bound adenyl cyclase[71] to form intracellular cyclic AMP.[72] In the presence of adequate stores of vitamin D, hyperparathyroidism activates both osteoclastic and osteocytic osteolysis.[73] As hours are required for osteoclast mobilization, it has been postulated that the immediate, exquisitely sensitive mechanism whereby bone is mobilized in response to parathyroid hormone, is osteocytic resorption.[23]

The role of parathyroid hormone in collagen formation is not well defined. Ultrastructurally, this hormone induces synthesis of endoplasmic reticulum in osteoblasts and osteocytes,[73] a fact suggesting accelerated protein synthesis. This cytoplasmic change is followed by an increase in osteoid formation and bone alkaline phosphatase.[12] Paradoxically, collagen synthesis as measured by bone proline incorporation significantly decreases after parathyroid hormone administration.[74] However, after 3 days of hormonal stimulation, collagen production increases above control values.[74] Proline incorporation measured against DNA concentration[74] illustrates this phenomenon is the result of increased collagen production by individual cells as well as of formation of additional osteoblasts.

Primary hyperparathyroidism

Primary hyperparathyroidism is the state of parathyroid hormone excess in a relatively uncomplicated milieu. It therefore is the path-

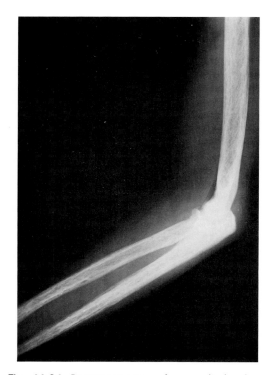

Fig. 44-24. Roentgenogram of upper limb of patient with primary hyperparathyroidism. There is advanced skeletal demineralization. (Courtesy Dr. James W. Debnam, Jr., Chesterfield, Mo.)

ologic condition that most accurately reflects experimental administration of the hormone.

The clinical manifestations of the disease are protean. In the past, patients usually presented with either renal or skeletal complications. With the advent of multiphasic screening, most are presently asymptomatic[75] and only 20% have skeletal changes on x-ray film.[76,77] Although these changes occur in asymptomatic individuals, they may represent a subpopulation of patients with larger parathyroid tumors.[76]

Skeletal disease when symptomatic may be striking. Not only do patients experience bone pain and fractures,[78] but skeletal deformities, particularly those produced by cystic lesions, may also be crippling (Fig. 44-24).

The cystic lesions of von Recklinghausen's disease of bone when present are easily diagnosed. More subtle radiographic changes particularly occur in the hands. The distal phalangeal tufts and the subperiosteal bone of the middle phalanges often show evidence of resorption. Intracortical striations are signs of early resorption (Fig. 44-25). The distal ends of the clavicles also are frequently resorbed. Resorption may also occur in the lamina dura of the jaw and at the sites of tendon insertion, resulting in their avulsion.[79]

osteitis Fibrosa cystica (handwritten margin note)

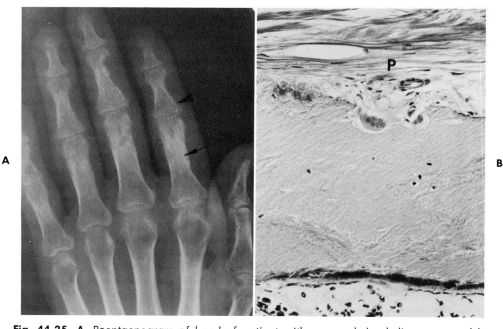

Fig. 44-25. A, Roentgenogram of hand of patient with severe skeletal disease caused by hyperparathyroidism. Intracortical striations *(arrow)* are present, as is subperiosteal resorption *(arrowhead).* **B,** Osteoclasts resorbing subperiosteal bone in hyperparathyroidism. **P,** Periosteum. (**A,** Courtesy Dr. James W. Debnam, Jr., Chesterfield, Mo.; **B,** undecalcified, Goldner; 100×.)

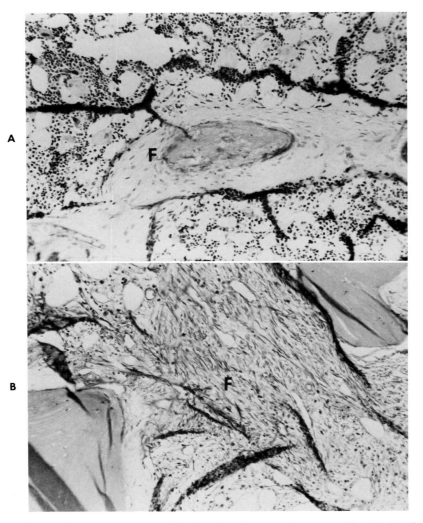

Fig. 44-26. A, Characteristic peritrabecular distribution of marrow fibrosis, *F,* of osteitis fibrosa. **B,** Distribution of fibrous tissue, *F,* in idiopathic myelofibrosis. Distribution of fibrous tissue is not peritrabecular. (**A** and **B,** Undecalcified, Goldner; 100×.)

Whereas most patients with primary hyperparathyroidism have no roentgenographic abnormalities, when evaluated by more sophisticated techniques such as bone densitometry, they usually are osteopenic.[80,81] On occasion, they may be osteosclerotic.[82] This virtual universality of abnormal bone morphology[78] reflects the widely variable bone dynamics accompanying primary hyperparathyroidism.[61]

As parathyroid hormone is a general activator of bone cells, not only are osteoclasts more numerous, but osteoblasts proliferate as well. Some investigators describe osteocytic osteolysis as universal in this disorder.[23] The disease is also associated with a general increase in osteoid volume,[78] probably because of accelerated collagen synthesis. However, as parathyroid hormone is a phosphaturic agent and may accelerate the rate of vitamin D metabolism, it has been postulated that a mineralization defect may also play a role in producing the hyperosteoidosis.[83]

Although the fibrous components of osteitis fibrosa may occasionally be extensive in primary hyperparathyroidism, it is rarely as prominent as that accompanying secondary hyperparathyroidism. The fibrosis first appears adjacent to trabeculae, particularly those areas undergoing active resorption of formation. Idiopathic myelofibrosis does not show this predilection (Fig. 44-26).

The cystic lesions of von Recklinghausen's

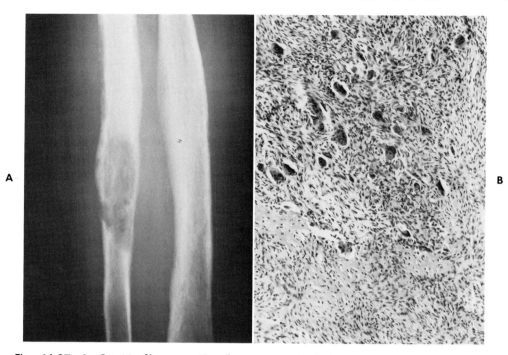

Fig. 44-27. A, Osteitis fibrosa cystica (brown tumor) of ulna. **B,** Osteitis fibrosa cystica (brown tumor). Numerous giant cells are present in cellular stroma. (**A,** Courtesy Dr. James W. Debnam, Jr., Chesterfield, Mo.; **B,** hematoxylin and eosin; 100×)

disease of bone histologically resemble giant cell tumors. There is osteoclast proliferation in a cellular, fibrous stroma, characteristically associated with hemosiderin deposition (brown tumor). These lesions are best distinguished from giant cell tumors by their predilection for the diaphyseal portion of long bones and the jaw and skull[84] (Fig. 44-27). If a giant cell tumor appears in a location other than the paraepiphyseal portion of a long bone, hyperparathyroidism should be considered. In addition, fibrous dysplasia occurs with increased frequency in primary hyperparathyroidism.[85]

After parathyroidectomy, osteoclasts begin to rapidly decrease in number and return to their normal population within a few hours.[86] For reasons unknown, osteoblasts proliferate after surgery reaching a peak in population within 2 weeks, after which they decline in number.[86] Within months, marrow fibrosis is sharply reduced or disappears (Fig. 44-28).

Ectopic hyperparathyroidism

Ectopic hyperparathyroidism is a state of parathyroid hormone excess attributable to production of parathormone or parathormone–like substances by neoplastic tissue. With the use of a sensitive immunoassay specific for the carboxyl terminal of the parathyroid hormone molecule, Benson and co-workers detected hyperparathyroidism in 95.3% of patients with hypercalcemia associated with malignant tumors.[87] Both patients with and without skeletal manifestations have increased circulating parathyroid hormone. This suggests that, in general, the hypercalcemia of malignancy is probably the result of ectopic hyperparathyroidism, rather than of direct invasion of bone by carcinoma.[87]

The most common source of ectopic parathyroid hormone is squamous cell carcinoma of the lung,[88] followed by tumors of the genitourinary system.[89] Characteristic roentgenographic and histologic changes of hyperparathyroidism occur in the skeleton. Neither they, nor the associated hypercalcemia, respond to parathyroidectomy.[90]

Hypoparathyroidism

Although the effects of parathyroid hormone deficiency on bone have been studied in experimental animals, less is known of its morphologic manifestations in man.[91] In the rat, thyroparathyroidectomy with thyroxin replacement results in decreased bone formation and mineralization as well as subnormal resorption.[91] Growth is also impaired.[92]

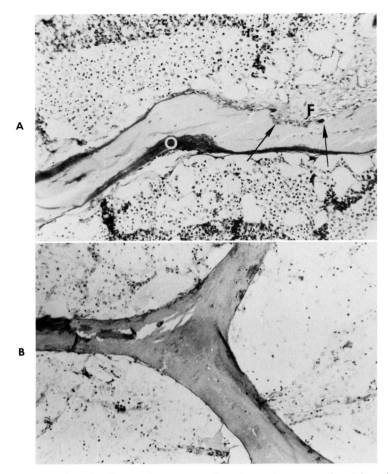

Fig. 44-28. A, Trabecular bone of patient with primary hyperparathyroidism biopsied at time of parathyroidectomy. Osteitis fibrosa is present as manifested by peritrabecular fibrosis, *F,* deep resorptive bays *(arrows)* containing osteoclasts, and wide osteoid seams, O, lined by columnar osteoblasts. **B,** Bone biopsy taken from same patient 1 year after parathyroidectomy. Histologic appearance of bone is now normal. (**A** and **B**, Undecalcified, Goldner; 100×.)

Most patients with surgical hypoparathyroidism, the most common form of the human parathyroprivic state, have some residual parathyroid function.[93] Therefore a situation analogous to the parathyroidectomized animal may not obtain. However, the appearance of the bones of these patients suggests a decreased rate of metabolic activity.[94] As expected, there is a paucity of osteoclasts.[94] Although some investigators report that vitamin D does not promote osteoclastosis in the human hypoparathyroid state,[94] others suggest that pharmacologic doses of this vitamin result in significant numbers of these cells in the parathyroid-deficient rat.[13]

Patients with idiopathic hypoparathyroidism are more likely to exhibit clinical musculoskeletal abnormalities than do their counterparts with iatrogenically induced abnormalities. However, the bones of those few individuals with idiopathic hypoparathyroidism that have been examined at autopsy have been reported as normal.[95] It is not uncommon to encounter clinical features usually associated with pseudohypoparathyroidism in these patients.[95,96] These features include soft-tissue calcification and ossification,[97] abnormal dentition,[95] and osteosclerosis.[95] Intracranial calcification[95] and ankylosing spondylitis[97] also occur. The etiology of extraskeletal calcification in idiopathic hypoparathyroidism is unknown. Its relationship to the often encountered variability of the response of bone to vitamin D in hypoparathyroidism[98] has also yet to be defined.

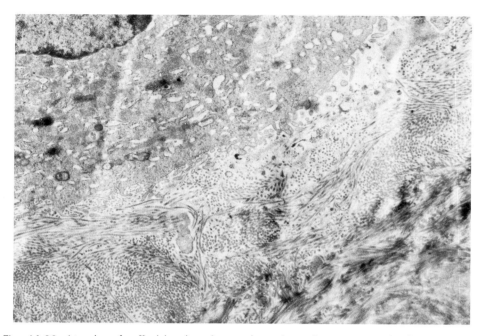

Fig. 44-29. Atrophy of ruffled border of osteoclast after administration of calcitonin. Compare with Fig. 44-8. (15,500×; courtesy Dr. Barbara Mills, San Marino, Cal.)

Calcitonin

Although thyrocalcitonin is a potent hypocalcemic agent, its physiologic function, if any in man, is yet to be determined. As secondary hyperparathyroidism frequently accompanies calcitonin administration,[99,100] only in vitro studies or those performed on parathyroidectomized animals enables one to distinguish the skeletal effects of this agent from those of parathyroid hormone.

There is little question that calcitonin acts directly on bone, since this tissue contains adenyl cyclase–receptor sites sensitive to the hormone.[101] The ionic mode of action may be related to stimulation of calcium uptake and inhibition of its release by bone cells.[102]

The ultrastructure of osteoclasts is the morphologic feature of bone most strikingly affected by calcitonin. Shortly after administration of the hormone, these cells leave the bone surface and lose their ruffled border[103,104] (Fig. 44-29). A layer of osteoblasts often becomes interposed between osteoclasts and the trabecular surface.[104] A decrease in osteoclast number precedes calcitonin-induced hypocalcemia and the magnitude of the two changes are directly related.[105] As manifested by changes in serum calcium and urinary hydroxyproline excretion, the hormone is most effective in states of osteoclastosis.[105]

Osteocytes are also rapidly altered by calcitonin.[106] The first change occurring in these cells is shrinkage by egress of intracellular fluid, probably related to phosphate loss. Particles of amorphous calcium phosphate then form in the periosteocytic osteoid matrix. Coincidental with cellular rehydration, mineralized granules appear within mitochondria. Histologically, these changes have been interpreted as decreased osteocytic osteolysis and numerous "dead" osteocytes.[99]

By morphometric analysis, calcitonin appears to suppress bone formation.[107] However, its morphologic effects on osteoblasts are less clear than on other bone cells. In vivo there is disruption of osteoblast orientation on bone surfaces[104] and biochemical evidence of decreased collagen formation.[108]

The net effect of decreased rates of resorption and formation induced by calcitonin are unclear. It not only promotes experimentally induced fracture healing[109] but also may be etiologically related to experimental osteopetrosis.[110,111] Moreover, chronically administered calcitonin has been reported to increase cortical bone mass in rats.[112] On the other hand, calcitonin administered to man results in osteoporosis, presumably because of parathyroid hormone–induced resorption.[100] Consequently, despite initial hopes for the use of calcitonin as an agent in the treatment of osteoporosis, little such success has been achieved. Paget's disease, in which the hormone suppresses both the accelerated rates of resorption and formation, is the only pathologic condition that responds favorably with some regularity to calcitonin therapy.[108]

The effect of calcitonin on bone mineralization is also a matter of controversy. Whereas some investigators note increased mineralization after hormonal administration,[113] firm evidence that calcitonin promotes calcium deposition is lacking. Indeed there are morphologic data that point to inhibition of mineralization by this agent.[99] Because calcitonin inhibits 1-hydroxylation of 25-hydroxycholecalciferol in vitro,[114] there is circumstantial evidence supporting the latter hypothesis.

Patients with medullary carcinoma of the thyroid and many of their relatives are the only individuals exposed to chronic, endogenous hypercalcitoninemia.[115] Associated hyperparathyroidism is unusual in these patients unless they have the familial form of the carcinoma.[99] Afflicted individuals are not osteosclerotic and may be osteopenic.[99] Histologically, the bones of patients with medullary carcinoma of the thyroid appear inactive.[99]

Growth hormone

Growth hormone is probably the factor most responsible for longitudinal skeletal development. Its growth-promoting properties appear to be effected through sulfation factor, a substance that, in conjunction with somatotropin, stimulates sulfate uptake and mitogenesis in epiphyseal cartilage.[116]

The influence of growth hormone on epiphyseal growth is best studied in the hypophysectomized state. In the absence of somatotropin, the epiphysis diminishes in width, chondrocyte columns decrease in number, and extracellular matrix becomes relatively more abundant.[117] Moreover, vascular invasion of the epiphysis from the marrow disappears and a transverse bone seal forms between the metaphysis and epiphysis.[117] In the hypophysectomized rat, metaphyseal bone may be resorbed without replacement, resulting in osteoporosis.[117]

Growth hormone administration to a hypophysectomized, growing animal results in epiphyseal widening as a result of chondrocyte proliferation and matrix synthesis.[117] Vascular invasion from the metaphysis reappears and the transverse bone seal is resorbed.[117] Continued somatotropin administration to a grow-

ing individual results in gigantism because of persistent endochondral growth. The rapid proliferation of the growth plate in growing patients administered this hormone can result in slipped epiphyses.[118]

The effects of growth hormone on the skeleton appear to be that of a general stimulus of bone progenitor cell proliferation. Ramser and co-workers[119] maintain that increased bone turnover induced by excess somatotropin is attributable to formation of additional bone remodeling sites, while the activity of individual cells remains unaltered. Regardless of the mechanism, the net result is acceleration of both formation and resorption with the magnitude of these processes directly related to the circulating levels of immunoreactive growth hormone.[120]

The relative predominance of these activities may differ on various bone surfaces.[121] Therefore in acromegaly, a net increase in bone formation obtains at the endosteal and periosteal surfaces, whereas resorption is dominant in the haversian envelope.[121] The resultant morphology is often increased cortical thickness and porosity.[121,122]

The bone-proliferating effects of growth hormone are related to its ability to stimulate collagen formation.[117] In addition, this hormone results in retention of phosphorus,[120] an ion also capable of stimulating bone formation. Of interest is the failure of circulating alkaline phosphatase to increase with growth hormone administration.[121]

Growth hormone stimulates calcium metabolism. This is associated not only with accelerated skeletal calcium accretion and resorption but also with increased intestinal absorption[123] and urinary excretion of this ion.[123,124] However, although some patients with acromegaly are in positive or negative calcium balance, absorption and excretion are usually equal.[124]

Although periosteal accretion is the rule in acromegaly,[125] osteosclerosis is an unusual complication. Despite some investigators[126] who report a relatively high incidence of osteopenia in acromegalic patients, others fail to substantiate this finding and morphologically note increased trabecular width[120] (Fig. 44-30).

Growth hormone deficiency in man occurs in hypopituitary midgets who may have an isolated defect in somatotropin synthesis. This deficiency may also be combined with that of other pituitary hormones. Since growth hormone is not necessary for in utero growth,[127] birth length is normal in infants with the

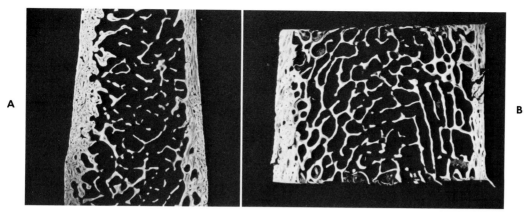

Fig. 44-30. Microroentgenograms of anterior iliac crest biopsies of normal 24-year-old male, **A**, and similarly aged acromegalic male, **B**. Note increased trabecular width in acromegalic bone. (Courtesy Dr. Jenifer Jowsey, Rochester, Minn.; from Aloia, J. F., et al.: J. Clin. Endocrinol. Metab. **35**:543, 1972.)

monotropic deficiency[128] and growth retardation is not apparent until 6 months to 1 year of age.[128] Although thyroid hormone affects bone maturation to a greater degree than does growth hormone, bone age is retarded in pituitary dwarfs.[117] With puberty, growth spurts are frequent.[128]

Because of its bone-forming properties, growth hormone has been proposed as a therapeutic agent in the treatment of senile osteopenia.[122] Perhaps related to loss of responsivity of the skeleton to sulfation factor with age[129] and because of the bone-resorbing properties of somatotropin,[120] little such success has been achieved.

Thyroid hormone

Thyroid hormone not only directly affects bone by accelerating turnover,[130] but probably also influences its maturation.[131] Intestinal absorption of calcium is suppressed,[132] and urinary excretion is increased by the hormone,[133] which when present in excessive quantities causes a negative calcium balance.[134]

Chronically untreated hyperthyroidism is frequently associated with osteopenia.[135] However, although the duration of the thyrotoxicosis is directly related to the incidence of bone disease, no such relationship exists between the skeletal lesion and the magnitude of hyperthyroidism.[133] Experimentally, physiologic quantities of this hormone is an influence in the induction of disuse osteoporosis.[136]

Hyperthyroidism may be associated with a lattice-like radiographic appearance of the phalanges and a "flaky" quality of cortical bone.[133] This latter phenomenon may be related to the predilection of osteoclastic activity for cortical bone in this disorder, and the attendant increase in cortical porosity.[133]

The osteopenic effects of thyroxin are related to its role as a general stimulus of bone cell activity, in which its osteolytic properties predominate over its ability to promote bone formation. Pathologically, thyroxin-stimulated bone often resembles that of hyperparathyroidism.[137] The trabeculae are thin and small, and osteoclasts and osteoblasts are numerous. As the disease is characterized by equal acceleration of both the rates of bone collagen synthesis and mineralization, osteoid is not increased in most patients but may be abundant.[133] Marrow fibrosis may also be encountered (Fig. 44-31).

Despite the association of hyperthyroidism with negative calcium balance,[134] circulating parathyroid hormone is generally not elevated in afflicted patients.[138] Some postulate that thyroxin exerts an osteolytic role by potentiating the action of vitamin D.[130] Both hyperthyroidism and hypothyroidism may be associated with increased sensitivity to vitamin D and nephrocalcinosis.[139]

Although hyperthyroid children may grow faster than normal,[140] a direct effect of thyroxin on growth is yet to be proved. Hypothyroidism results in growth retardation. However, because thyroxin may act synergistically with somatotropin to be growth promoting,[117] this phenomenon is possibly secondary to pituitary atrophy.

The growth-inhibiting effect of hypothyroidism is probably related to abnormal chondrogenesis.[141] In the hypoparathyroid state, the

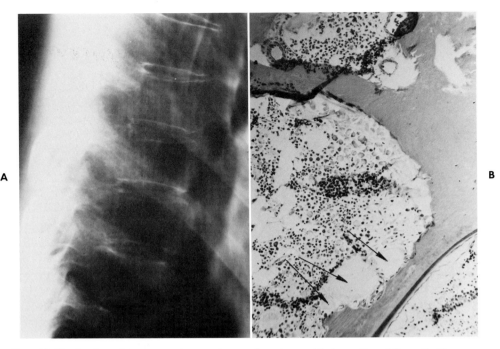

Fig. 44-31. A, Grossly osteopenic vertebrae of patient with hyperthyroidism. **B,** Numerous osteoclasts *(arrows)* and wide osteoid seams present in bone biopsy taken from patient in **A. (B,** Undecalcified, Goldner; 100×.)

maturation of epiphyseal cells is retarded and the matrix calcifies irregularly.[141] Roentgenologically the growth plates are fragmented and have a stippled appearance.[142] Vascular penetration of the epiphyseal plate occurs prematurely, and ultrastructurally there is an abnormal accumulation of glycogen in the chondrocytes.[141] The depth of the growth plate is reduced, and metaphyseal development is retarded.[141]

Despite the not infrequent association of hypothyroidism with increased circulating parathyroid hormone,[138] the bones of adults with this disease appear generally inactive.[137] Trabecular mass is either normal or increased and both osteoclasts and osteoblasts are rare. Although bone mass does not appear affected in these individuals, they may have abnormalities of calcium balance because of defective bone turnover.[143]

Adrenal corticosteroids

Since these agents are used therapeutically with increasing frequency, the skeletal effects of adrenal corticosteroids, particularly glucocorticoids, are commonly encountered. In addition, steroid-induced osteopenia of noniatrogenic etiology is perhaps more frequent than commonly appreciated. Young osteopenic adults may have hypercortisonism caused by micronodular hyperplasia of the adrenal glands.[144] I have also encountered a number of postmenopausal, osteopenic females and older osteopenic males with increased urinary corticoid excretion.

Adrenal corticosteroids have dramatic skeletal effects involving trabecular more than cortical bone[5] (Fig. 44-32). Patients treated chronically with these agents are usually osteopenic and have a high fracture rate. Moreover, because corticosteroids retard skeletal repair, these fractures are often slow to heal.[145]

At low as well as high doses, glucocorticoids directly inhibit formation and activity of osteoblasts resulting in suppression of cellular and tissue level bone formation.[146-148] The skeletal inactivity induced by glucocorticoids relates to their antianabolic effects.[149] These substances not only inhibit collagen synthesis but also protein formation in general.[149] Mucopolysaccharide synthesis by cartilage is suppressed,[150-152] and RNA content of isolated bone cells exposed to corticosteroids, declines.[149]

Corticosteroids suppress intestinal absorption[153] and renal tubular reabsorption[154] of calcium. They also antagonize the bone calcium–mobilizing effect of parathyroid hormone[155-157]

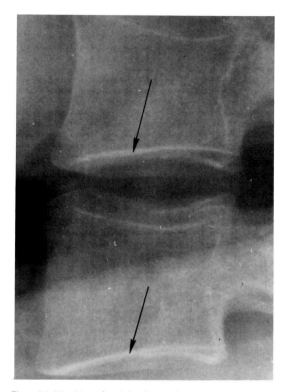

Fig. 44-32. Vertebral bodies of patient who had been treated with corticosteroids for years. There is severe trabecular osteopenia. Note relative spacing of cortical bone *(arrows)*. (Courtesy Dr. James W. Debnam, Jr., Chesterfield, Mo.)

and shorten the half-life of vitamin D.[158] All these factors promote secondary hyperparathyroidism, which commonly accompanies hypercortisonism. In addition, cortisone, perhaps through its induction of hyperparathyroidism, may promote synthesis of 1,25-dihydroxycholecalciferol, a potent bone resorber.[159] Therefore one may see numerous osteoclasts accompanied by a paucity of osteoblasts in patients treated with low doses of steroids (Fig. 44-33).

Although osteoclasts may be present in increased number, experimental evidence suggests that both the cellular and tissue levels of resorption are suppressed in hypercortisonism.[147] For example, despite abundant osteoclasts, the metaphysis of steroid-treated rats becomes sclerotic because of failure of resorption of the primary spongiosa.[152,160] Regardless of the exacerbation of secondary hyperparathyroidism with increasing doses of steroids, the suppressive influence of these agents on bone cell activation overrides the activating effects of parathyroid hormone, and a paucity of osteoclasts ensues.[146] The resultant histologic picture is one of osteoporosis with thin trabeculae and few osteoblasts or osteoclasts (Fig. 44-34, *A*). As the number of bone-remodeling units is sharply reduced, tetracycline uptake is minimal[161] (Fig. 44-34, *B*). It is of interest that tetracycline sequestration may increase dramatically with tapering of steroids from a therapeutic to a maintenance dose (Fig. 44-35). This may represent a rebound phenomenon resulting in excessive activation of osteoblasts.

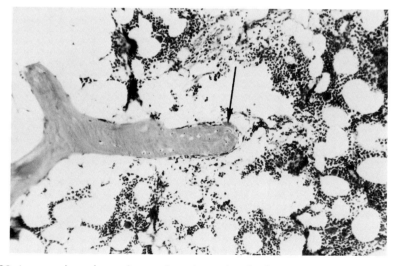

Fig. 44-33. Increased numbers of osteoclasts *(arrow)* with absence of osteoblasts in trabecular bone of patient treated with corticosteroids. (Undecalcified, Goldner; 100×.)

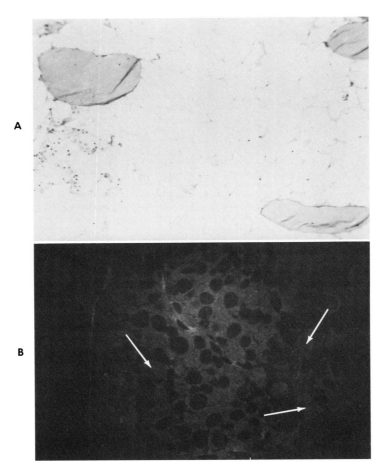

Fig. 44-34. A, Trabecular bone of patient on long-term corticosteroid therapy. There is severe osteoporosis and virtual absence of osteoblasts and osteoclasts. **B,** Fluorescent micrograph of specimen in **A.** There is virtually complete absence of trabecular tetracycline fluorescence *(arrows)* indicating suppression of bone formation. (**A** and **B,** Undecalcified; **A,** Goldner, 100×; **B,** unstained, 40×.)

While the skeletal sensitivity to corticosteroids exhibits interspecies variation, they virtually universally inhibit growth.[162] The growth-retarding effects of corticosteroids are probably largely related to direct skeletal inhibition.[163] However, it is of interest that these agents are inhibitors of growth hormone release as well.[164]

Children with adrenocortical hyperplasia[165] or iatrogenically induced hypercortisonism[166] fail to grow. Although the rate of growth may approach normal after cessation of the hypercorticoid state, normal height is often never achieved.[166] Moreover, demineralized portions of the skeleton often persist, to be surrounded by normally dense bone.[167] Radiographically this phenomenon appears in the vertebral body as a lucent core.[167] Histologically, cortico-

steroids result in thinning of the epiphyseal plate, atrophy of the proliferative zone, and disarray of the zones of hypertrophy and provisional calcification.[162]

Senile osteopenia

Loss of skeletal mass with age is the most common form of symptomatic osteopenia. Although the clinical manifestations of osteopenia often occur in white females after the menopause, bone loss in this population begins in the latter part of the fourth decade.[168] Blacks are relatively immune to clinically significant age-related bone loss, but white males are less so.[169] However, since the bone mass of white males decreases at a slower rate than that of white females[170] and since men have greater initial skeletal mass,[168] the clinical

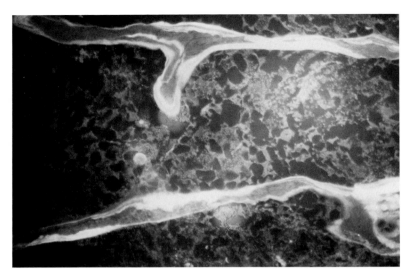

Fig. 44-35. Bone biopsy from patient undergoing tapering of corticosteroid dosage after long-term administration. Virtually every trabecular surface assumes a tetracycline label, indicating sharp increase in rate of bone formation. (Undecalcified, unstained, fluorescent micrograph; 40×.)

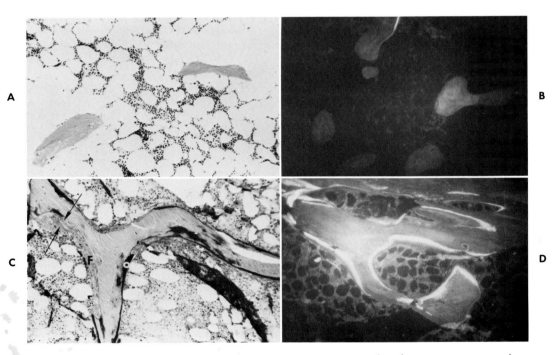

Fig. 44-36. Histologic spectrum of senile osteopenia. **A,** Biopsy taken from postmenopausal, osteopenic patient consisting of scattered trabeculae exhibiting virtually no osteoblasts or osteoclasts. **B,** Fluorescent micrograph of specimen in **A.** Most trabecular surfaces exhibit no tetracycline label, indicating a suppressed rate of bone formation. **C,** Osteitis fibrosa of elderly osteopenic female. Numerous osteoclasts *(arrows)*, peritrabecular fibrosis, *F,* and thick osteoid, *o,* seams are present. **D,** Fluorescent micrograph of specimen in **C.** There is significant increase in tetracycline uptake, indicating acceleration of bone formation. (**A** to **D,** Undecalcified, 100×; **A** and **C,** Goldner; **B** and **D** unstained.)

manifestations of this process in men are later to appear. In addition, females with systemic osteopenia are generally slighter of frame than their nonaffected counterparts and perhaps develop clinical bone disease as a consequence of a relative paucity of bone mass at maturity.[168]

Bone densitometric measurements indicate parallel loss of cortical and trabecular bone with senescence.[5] However, since approximately 80% of the skeleton is compact, haversian and endosteal resorption are essentially indefinitely progressive, whereas the absolute quantity of cancellous bone loss is self-limited by diminished mass.[171]

The syndrome of postmenopausal osteopenia probably represents a potpourri of pathogenetic mechanisms. Hence, the skeletal histologic features of afflicted patients are variable. Although a continuum of changes exists, the microscopic features may be divided into those that suggest slow skeletal turnover as contrasted to those in which bone metabolism appears accelerated (Fig. 44-36). The former group probably reflects the hypothesis posited by Albright[172] that postmenopausal osteoporosis is a disorder of osteoblast dysfunction. The bones of these individuals contain few osteoblasts, osteoclasts, or osteoid and have diminished bone formation rates as demonstrated by tetracycline labeling. On the other hand, the majority of patients with postmenopausal osteopenia have normal rates of bone formation.[173] They also frequently have increased numbers of osteoblasts and cortical osteoclasts, a fact suggesting that bone turnover may be accelerated.[174] On occasion, subperiosteal osteoclasts may appear. Therefore, not only does attenuation of compact bone occur, but also increased cortical porosity is a function of age.[175] The lack of osteoclasts in trabecular bone in advanced senile osteopenia despite striking intracortical resorption probably reflects the paucity of trabecular bone surface available to these cells.[174]

Collateral with morphologic evidence of accelerated bone resorption, a number of postmenopausal patients have increased circulating immunoreactive parathyroid hormone.[174] Parathormone appears to play a fundamental role in the development of osteopenia in calcium-deprived animals as parathyroidectomy protects against this form of bone loss.[176] Although some older patients with normocalcemic, primary hyperparathyroidism are undoubtedly diagnosed as having postmenopausal osteoporosis, the majority of hyperparathyroidism occurring in the elderly is undoubtedly second-

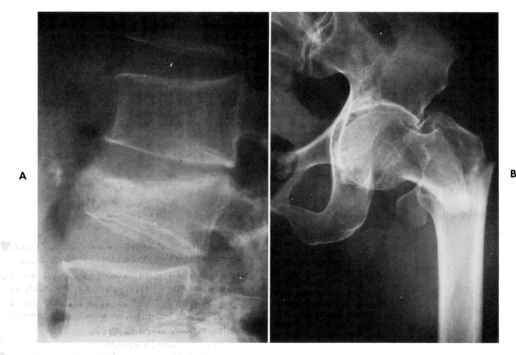

Fig. 44-37. A, Crush fracture of vertebral body of patient with senile osteopenia. **B,** Intertrochanteric hip fracture that occurred in elderly, osteopenic patient.

ary. These changes are probably related to negative calcium balance associated with deficient intestinal absorption,[177] decreasing renal function,[178] and hypercalciuria with age.[170] The high acid residue diet of Western man[179] and varying dietary calcium[180] and phosphorus contents[181,182] may also be factors. Moreover, geriatric patients may have suboptimal stores of vitamin D.[183] This may relate to the frequency with which osteomalacia is encountered in bone biopsies of elderly osteopenic patients.[184-186] Approximately one third of our untreated osteopenic, postmenopausal patients have increased quantities of osteoid.

The inhibitory effects that estrogens and androgens have on parathyroid hormone–induced bone resorption may relate to the development of senile osteopenia.[187] Diminished quantities of these substances with age may accelerate bone resorption. Indeed, the increased resorption of postmenopausal osteopenia may be a product not of excessive parathyroid hormone, but of normal quantities of this substance in a less inhibited milieu.[171] Attempts to demonstrate estrogenic receptors in bone, however, have to date been unrewarding.[188]

The morbid consequences of diminished bone mass are an increase in the incidence of fracture and its attendant dysfunctions.[189] Of approximately 1 million fractures occurring each year in the United States in women at least 45 years of age, it has been estimated that 700,000 are associated with osteopenia.[190] Although osteopenic females commonly sustain fractures of the distal radius and vertebral bodies,[191] it is intertrochanteric hip fractures that are responsible for the greatest attendant morbidity and mortality. Females with intertrochanteric hip fractures are significantly more osteopenic than age-matched controls, and the incidence of this fracture reflects the incidence of severe skeletal demineralization[192,193] (Fig. 44-37).

Ovarian dysgenesis

Turner's syndrome is commonly associated with skeletal abnormalities. Affected patients are short, and bone maturation is frequently arrested at age 12 to 13.[194] They often have hypoplasia of the first cervical vertebra[195] and fusion of adjacent bones throughout the skeleton.[194] In addition, similar to changes of pseudohypoparathyroidism, there is shortening of the fourth metacarpal, presumably attributable to generalized growth arrest.[194]

Osteoporosis is common in Turner's syndrome.[194,196] Although the severity increases with age,[195] even young dysgenetic females have significant bone loss. Although these patients may have accelerated rates of bone resorption,[196,197] controversy exists as to whether the rate of formation is normal[196] or depressed.[197]

Histologically the bone exhibits little evidence of cellular activity. Osteoid is sparse, and the general morphologic impression is one of suppressed turnover.

Vitamin D

Within the past few years, great advances have been made particularly by DeLuca's group[198,199] in defining the biochemistry of vitamin D. Although other metabolites have been described, the two major metabolic products of vitamin D are its 25-hydroxylated and 1,25-dihydroxylated compounds, which are synthesized in the liver[200] and kidney,[201] respectively. The concentrations of circulating 25-hydroxycholecalciferol, the major circulating metabolite of vitamin D, are directly related to dietary consumption of the vitamin and its synthesis in the skin.[202] The blood levels of this substance are highest in the summer months,[203] when the incidence of osteomalacia in hip fractures is lowest.[204] 1,25-Dihydroxycholecalciferol is the metabolite that acts on the intestine to promote calcium absorption.[198]

Vitamin D plays a critical role in bone mineralization. However, though circumstantial evidence suggests a direct physiologic action of the vitamin on bone mineralization,[205] this has yet to be experimentally proved.[198] The calcification accompanying the administration of this compound to osteomalacic patients may theoretically be attributable to an associated increase of calcium or phosphorus, or both, in the extracellular fluid because of stimulated intestinal absorption of calcium or bone resorption,[198] or to reduction of lysosomal activity in rachitic tissue.[206] In hypophosphatemic patients, normal calcification will not be induced by high doses of vitamin D unless phosphate is also administered.[66]

The well-defined, direct role of vitamin D on bone relates to its osteolytic properties.[207] Although the hypercalcemia that often attends administration of large doses of vitamin D is in part attributable to increased intestinal absorption of calcium,[208] it is also related to mobilization of bone. The bone-resorptive properties of pharmacologic doses of the vitamin do not depend on the presence of parathyroid hormone,[13] although the latter promotes 1-hydroxylation of 25-hydroxychole-calciferol.[209] In addition, the relative potencies of vitamin D and its metabolites differ greatly. Whereas the parent compound has no resorptive properties in vitro, 25-hydroxycholecalciferol has significant potency, only to be superseded one-hundredfold by 1,25-dihydroxy-cholecalciferol.[209]

The direct effects of vitamin D on bone are best studied experimentally on a person in the parathyroidectomized state. In these circumstances pharmacologic doses of cholecalciferol induce osteoclastic and osteoblastic hyperplasia and proliferation of epiphyseal chondrocytes.[13] Bone alkaline phosphatase also increases.[13] These changes accompany hydroxyprolinuria and a rise in serum calcium to within the normal range.[13] Physiologic doses of vitamin D

administered to these animals fail to induce these biochemical changes and produce no distinctive morphologic alterations.[13] It therefore appears that the physiologic effects of vitamin D upon the skeleton are synergistically dependent on parathyroid hormone. Similarly, the skeletal effects of parathyroid hormone are blunted in the vitamin D–deficient state.

Vitamin D deficiency

The major skeletal effect of vitamin D deficiency is failure of normal mineralization. Osteomalacia occurs in the vitamin D–deprived child and adult. Prior to epiphyseal closure, rickets also complicates vitamin D deficiency.[210] The rachitic state is characterized by osteoid, which fails to mineralize. Affected tion. The growth plate widens and its archi-

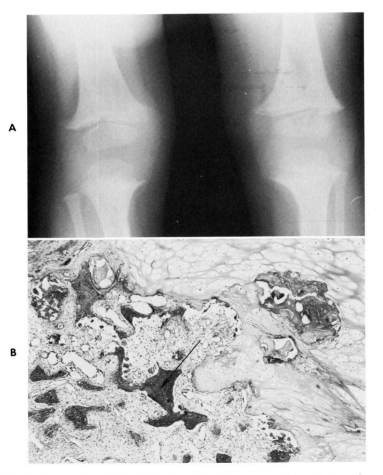

Fig. 44-38. A, Knees of rachitic child. Growth plates are wide and irregular. **B,** Rachitic epiphysis. Compare with Fig. 44-13. Note loss of columnar orientation of chondrocytes. Junction between growth plate and metaphysis is irregular, and large areas of osteoid (*arrow*) are evident. Metaphyseal marrow is fibrotic. (**B,** Hematoxylin and eosin; 40×; courtesy Dr. Ruth Silberberg, Jerusalem, Israel.)

tecture becomes disarrayed. The columnar arrangement of the distal chondrocytes is lost, and the zone of provisional calcification disappears. Cartilaginous cores extend deeply into the metaphysis where they become surrounded by osteoid, which fails to mineralize. Affected children usually develop bowed legs because of structural weakness of the widened epiphyses and osteomalacic bone. Radiographically, the junction between the growth plate and epiphyses is irregular. The cup-shaped curve of the growth plate is caused by indentation from metaphyseal pressure (Fig. 44-38).

Secondary hyperparathyroidism usually accompanies the vitamin D–deficient state.[211] As opposed to primary hyperparathyroidism, which is the disorder of autonomous, hyperfunctioning parathyroid glands, secondary hyperparathyroidism is a generic term encompassing the many conditions in which continuous parathyroid gland hyperactivity is stimulated by low circulating calcium. The most commonly diagnosed cause of secondary hyperparathyroidism in the United States is chronic renal failure. However, any cause of vitamin D deficiency results in parathyroid gland stimulation. This phenomenon almost universally accompanies severe malabsorption of vitamin D, such as associated with biliary cirrhosis or sprue. It occurs in the large numbers of Asian immigrants with vitamin D–deficient osteomalacia who inhabit Great Britain.[210] Secondary hyperparathyroidism may also accompany osteomalacia that frequently occurs after gastric resection.[212-214]

Regardless of etiology, the skeletal lesions of secondary hyperparathyroidism are qualitatively similar. As deficient mineralization is almost universal in this disorder, the osteoid seams are wide and tetracycline fluorescence is abnormal (Fig. 44-21). If the osteomalacia is severe, characteristic Looser's zones or pseudofractures appear, particularly in the pelvis. These linear, cortical interruptions represent callus that has failed to mineralize. It is one of the few roentgenographic signs diagnostic of a histologic skeletal lesion of a metabolic bone disorder (Fig. 44-39).

Because of attendant hyperparathyroidism, increased numbers of osteoclasts usually accompany osteomalacia. However, when osteoid seams, which are in general not resorbable,[215] cover the entire endosteum, there may be a paucity of these cells (Fig. 44-40). The quan-

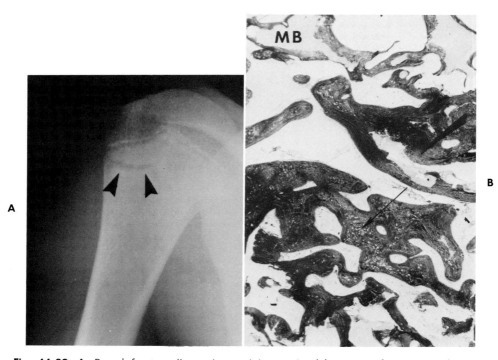

Fig. 44-39. A, Pseudofracture (Looser's zone) in proximal humerus of patient with osteomalacia. **B,** Biopsy of pseudofracture (Looser's zone). Lesion is characterized by trabeculae consisting entirely of osteoid *(arrow)*. *MB,* Mineralized bone. (**B,** Undecalcified, Goldner; 40×.)

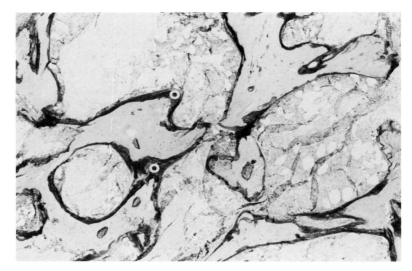

Fig. 44-40. Trabecular bone of patient with osteomalacia. Wide osteoid seams, **O,** cover virtually all trabecular surfaces without increased numbers of osteoclasts. (Undecalcified, Goldner; 40×.)

tities of osteoblasts and fibrosis usually parallel the number of osteoclasts. All histologic abnormalities return to normal after appropriate therapy.[216]

Vitamin D–dependent rickets

Vitamin D–dependent rickets (hereditary pseudo–vitamin D deficiency rickets) is an autosomal dominant disorder of vitamin D metabolism that may mimic X-linked familial hypophosphatemia. The metabolic abnormality of vitamin D dependency lies in deficient 1-hydroxylation of 25-hydroxycholecalciferol, resulting in abnormal calcium absorption and secondary hyperparathyroidism.[217] The biochemical and morphologic manifestations of the disease respond rapidly to administration of 1,25-dihydroxycholecalciferol.

Vitamin C

Clinical scurvy rarely occurs in Western society and therefore has become largely a disease of historic interest. Current histologic descriptions of the skeletal changes are therefore almost exclusively dependent on scorbutic animals.

The essential role of vitamin C in skeletal metabolism relates to collagen formation. The vitamin promotes hydroxylation of both proline[218] and lysine,[219] and in its absence, collagen synthesis ceases. Ascorbic acid induces ribosome aggregation on the endoplasmic reticulum of collagen-producing cells.[220] Consequently, in scurvy, osteoblasts lose their char-

acteristic ribonuclear protein-dependent basophilia.[221]

Vitamin C also plays a role in hexosamine metabolism as illustrated by defective uptake of labeled sulfate by cartilage exposed to a scorbutic environment.[220] Although some investigators report that ascorbic acid deprivation results in defective mineralization, this is probably a reflection of deficient bone matrix production.[222] From these observations, it is apparent that clinical effects of scurvy involve not only the skeleton but all connective tissues.

The uptake of ascorbic acid by cells declines with age,[223] and the manifestations of vitamin C deficiency are most dramatic in the growing animal. As the skeletal disease of scurvy primarily reflects defective collagen synthesis, hemorrhages, particularly in the periosteum, are common. These may go on to calcify[224] or, in the partially scorbutic animal, ossify.[225] This new periosteal bone, which is poorly vascularized, pushes beneath the cortex and the now easily elevated periosteum. There is failure of formation of cortex from the newly deposited bone, which, when associated with fracture, may extend along the entire shaft.[225]

In the totally scorbutic animal, complete failure of collagen synthesis results in cessation of periosteal apposition. As endosteal resorption continues, the cortex becomes greatly attenuated.[226] Osteoblasts decrease in number and become shriveled and spindle shaped.[227] Trabecular bone mass sharply decreases and a peculiar gelatinous area (*Gerüstmark*) con-

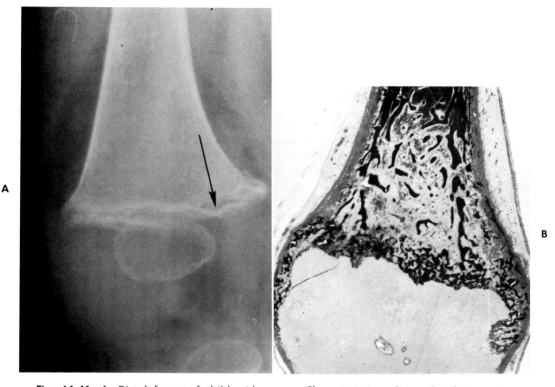

Fig. 44-41. A, Distal femur of child with scurvy. Characteristic radiographic features include relative sclerotic rimming of distal metaphyses. Area of radiolucency is present (arrow) immediate to metaphyseal sclerosis. **B,** Classic features of well-advanced scurvy in costochondral junction. Bone shows evidence of osteoporosis, and marrow spaces filled with loosely textured and edematous connective tissue in which some hemorrhage has occurred. Metaphyseal end of bone widened and made up of irregularly arranged spicules of heavily calcified matrix. (**A,** Courtesy Dr. William McAlister, St. Louis, Mo.; **B,** 10×.)

taining mesenchymal cells juxtaposed to skeletal detritis develops at the bone ends.[227] Since this area does not appear in immobilized limbs of scorbutic animals,[228] it probably represents the effects of trauma in poorly developing callus.[229]

Fracture repair is greatly impaired in hypovitaminosis C.[230] The initial clot is slow to resorb,[224] and callus formation by both endosteum and periosteum is arrested.[231] However, since lack of ascorbic acid does not affect already synthesized collagen, healed fractures do not break down in scurvy.[224] In addition, no evidence exists that additional vitamin C given to a nonscorbutic animal accelerates fracture repair.

Both collagen and ground substance synthesis by cartilage is impaired in scurvy. Hence epiphyseal growth stops, cellularity of the growth plate diminishes, and chondrocytes appear disoriented.[227,229] The epiphyseal trabeculae atrophy, and reflecting diminished

mucopolysaccharide concentrations, lose their metachromasia.[232] However, a peculiar peripheral deposition of mucopolysaccharides occurs in these trabecula.[232]

Because of disruption of collagen ground-substance synthesis, epiphyseal slippage is common in scurvy.[227] Moreover, the growth plate and metaphysis push into each other so that irregularity of the metaphyseo-epiphyseal line and expansion of the bone ends result.[226,227] Therefore the chest wall of a scorbutic child may contain features resembling a rachitic rosary (Fig. 44-41).

During the past few years, vitamin C has been ingested in large quantities in Western society. Little is known of the effects of hypervitaminosis C on the skeleton although it appears to stimulate bone turnover.[233]

Vitamin A

Both excesses and deficiencies of vitamin A are associated with skeletal pathologic conditions. Chronic hypervitaminosis A may be encountered in children ingesting large quantities of fish oil[234] or in Eskimos who eat polar bear liver.[235] The skeletal effects involve stimulation of modeling and remodeling, and inhibition of endochondral growth. The vitamin directly promotes osteoclastic[236] and osteocytic[237] resorption of bone and as such may result in osteopenia, with particular thinning of the long bones[238] and skull.[239] Since this acceleration of resorption in a growing animal is largely a manifestation of rapid modeling, only those portions of the bone involved in the modeling process are affected.[238] As such, the gross architecture of the bone may be significantly deformed.[238]

Osteoid proliferation may occur in apposition to accelerated resorptive activity in vitamin A toxicity.[238] Whether this represents stimulation of osteoblastic activity or a mineralization defect is unclear. However, abundant, well-mineralized callus commonly accompanies repair of the frequent fractures that occur in the vitamin A toxic rat.[238] Moreover, periosteal mineralization[240] and abnormal bone formation[237] are usual manifestations of the disorder.

Since this substance has degenerative effects on cartilaginous matrix and chondrocytes in vitro,[241] it is not surprising that endochondral growth is greatly affected by excess vitamin A.[242] Premature epiphyseal closure occurs because of endochondral calcification associated with penetration of the growth plate by metaphyseal vessels. Because of failure of growth and accelerated resorption of modeling sites, there is a decrease in the anteroposterior diameter of the long bones of the vitamin A–toxic rat.[238]

The skeletal manifestations of hypervitaminosis A differ somewhat in man from those in the experimental animal. Although resorption is accelerated and thinning of the cortex and long bones may occur, human osteopenia is not so frequent an accompaniment of the disorder.[239] Moreover, in contrast to the vitamin A–toxic rat, fractures are unusual in man.[243] The most common clinical manifestation of the toxicity is the proliferation of tender, moundlike, periosteal calcifications and exostoses, almost invariably involving the ulna.[234] Histologically, the periosteum is thickened and calcification of the tendons and ligaments may occur[244] (Fig. 44-42).

Childhood hypervitaminosis A has resulted in permanent skeletal deformities.[242] The epiphyses may be impressed into cup-shaped, wide metaphyses, particularly about the knees.

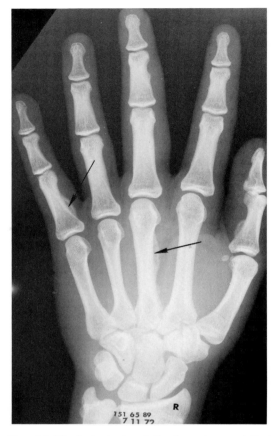

Fig. 44-42. Periosteal calcifications (arrows) that characterize hypervitaminosis A. (From Frame, B., Jackson, C. E., Reynolds, W. A., et al.: Ann. Intern. Med. **80:**44, 1974.)

Although premature epiphyseal closure has occurred in these children,[242] infants less than 6 months of age who are vitamin A toxic have wide epiphyses.[239] Unlike those of rickets, these growth plates are sharply demarcated from the adjacent metaphyses.[239]

In vitamin A deficiency, remodeling may virtually cease.[238] Osteoclastic activity disappears from the subperiosteal surface, and apposition of cancellous bone continues in that location resulting in overgrowth of the entire skeleton.[245] Because of failure of modeling of trabecular bone into cortex, the absolute quantity of cortical bone diminishes in hypovitaminosis A.[245] This proliferation of new bone may encroach on spaces containing neurologic tissues.[245] Consequently, symptoms such as loss of hearing are not unusual.[246] Gerlings[246] postulates that oxycephaly with associated narrowing of the internal auditory canal may be caused by a lack of this vitamin.

As a result of failure of proliferation of chondrocytes associated with continued vascular penetration, epiphyseal growth stops in hypovitaminosis A.[238] A bone plate develops across the face of the epiphyseal disc, isolating it from the underlying metaphysis.[238] Therefore, because of a combination of failure of both remodeling and growth, with continuous periosteal apposition, the bones of the vitamin A–deficient state are short and thick,[238] with a predominance of newly formed cancellous, periosteal bone.

Phosphorus

Inorganic phosphorus plays many roles in the metabolic activities of bone. It probably promotes bone collagen formation and mineralization.[247,248] Supplemental phosphorus increases the tensile strength[249] and accelerates the rate of healing[250] of fractures. There is a major intracellular requirement for this ion by osteocytes and osteoblasts[251] that relates to calcification.[6,252] In addition, the formation of collagen-orthophosphate bonds may be an important mechanism in the mineralization of osteoid.[253] This is illustrated clinically by the failure of normal calcification front formation in hypophosphatemic states despite adequate vitamin D stores.[66,69] Moreover, since phosphorus is intimately linked to the cellular uptake and intracellular distribution of calcium, its presence is necessary for the actions of the latter ion as a second messenger, enabling bone cells to respond to hormonal stimuli.[254]

Because of its reciprocal relationship with circulating calcium, administration of phosphorus leads to parathyroid hormone secretion.[255] Therefore it is important to individualize the effects of these agents on bone.

Phosphorus deficiency results in osteomalacia that is not responsive to vitamin D therapy.[66] Repletion of the euparathyroid, hypophosphatemic patient with phosphorus may lead to striking biochemical and morphologic evidence of skeletal synthesis, including extensive woven-bone proliferation.[66]

It is less clear if phosphorus exerts a direct influence on bone resorption. Baylink and co-workers[256] report accelerated resorptive activity in the hypophosphatemic rat independent of parathyroid hormone. In vitro studies however suggest a direct inhibitory effect of phosphorus on parathyroid hormone–induced osteoclastic activity.[257] However, other investigators find no suppression of resorptive activity by phosphorus[258] and note increased numbers of osteoclasts in the euparathyroid, hypophosphatemic patient after repletion with this ion.[66]

Hypophosphatemic (vitamin D–resistant) osteomalacia

Familial hypophosphatemic rickets is the most common form of rickets in western societies.[259] It is transmitted as an X-linked dominant[260] and characterized by hypophosphatemia,[260] hyperphosphaturia,[261] and abnormal vitamin D metabolism.[262] Probably related to defective phosphorus transport,[263] intestinal absorption of calcium is impaired. The renal phosphorus leak is attributable to loss of a parathyroid hormone–sensitive component of phosphate transport in the renal tubule.[261]

The clinical manifestations of the disease often appear within the second year of life. Affected patients fail to grow and have bowed legs.[259] As opposed to other forms of rickets, muscular weakness is uncommon.[259] Radiographically, typical rachitic epiphyses are present, particularly in the extremities. The axial skeleton is relatively spared. With age, bony protuberances often appear at the sites of tendon insertion. The resultant restriction of motion may be significant.

Histologically, the bone, although not osteopenic, contains extremely wide osteoid seams.[264] There is usually little evidence of parathyroid hormone effect. However, the bones of some patients have typical features of osteitis fibrosa, correlating with biochemical evidence of hyperparathyroidism (Fig. 44-43).[265] Although this is to be expected with phosphorus therapy, for unknown reasons it also appears in untreated patients. A peculiar "halo effect" about the osteocytic lacunae is present, particularly on thick hand-ground sections when stained with basic fuchsin[266] or examined microradiographically.[267] The phenomenon probably represents a delay of osteocyte-induced mineralization.[268] The "halo effect" has been documented by scanning electron microscopy to be hypomineralized zones characteristically polarized towards the nearest free bone surfaces[69] (Fig. 44-44).

The major efforts in treating vitamin D–resistant rickets have concentrated on vitamin D[269,270] and its metabolites[271] and inorganic phosphorus.[272] Since phosphorus alone heals the disease both biochemically and radiographically and since high doses of vitamin D, if used alone, are necessary to accomplish healing, the effects of the latter may be attributable to mobilization of bone stores of phosphorus to achieve mineralization of osteoid.[270]

A nonfamilial form of hypophosphatemic rickets usually appearing in the adolescent or young adult years differs from the X-linked variety by the presence of severe osteopenia.[259] It is also characterized by muscle weakness and glycinuria.[259] Both the muscle weakness and bones respond dramatically to vitamin D and phosphorus therapy.[66]

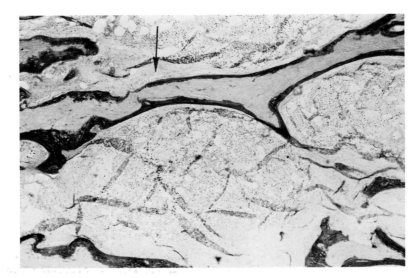

Fig. 44-43. Bone biopsy of a patient with hypophosphatemic (X-linked) osteomalacia. Wide osteoid seams cover virtually entire trabecular surface. Correlating with elevated circulating immunoreactive parathyroid hormone levels, biopsy exhibits peritrabecular fibrosis *(arrow)*. (Undecalcified, Goldner; 40×.)

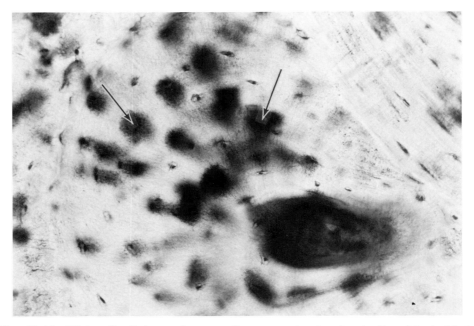

Fig. 44-44. "Halo effect" *(arrows)* surrounding osteocytes in vitamin D–resistant rickets. (Fresh, ground sections; Villanueva bone stain; 390×; courtesy Mr. Antonio R. Villanueva, Detroit, Mich.)

Alkaline phosphatase
Hypophosphatasia

Hypophosphatasia is a congenital disorder caused by deficient synthesis of skeletal alkaline phosphatase.[273] The attendant failure of normal bone mineralization offers convincing evidence of the fundamental role this enzyme must play in skeletal calcification.

Approximately half of the patients exhibit clinical evidence of the disorder at birth and usually die prior to 1 year of age.[274] Those infants in whom the disease becomes manifest past 6 months of age are less severely affected and may eventually undergo significant recovery. Occasionally, the diagnosis is made in adulthood.[275]

The cardinal features of the disease are a rickets-like radiographic picture with particular involvement of the calvaria. Wide sutures consisting of osteoid separate poorly mineralized bone. As a result of arrested calvarial growth, bulging fontanelles, often associated with craniostenosis, are present.[275] Endochondral growth is retarded, and the epiphyses are radiologically and histologically indistinguishable from those of vitamin D–deficient rickets. Osteoblasts, which retain their capability to synthesize collagen, appear normal. A morphologic feature distinguishing the disease from other rachitic lesions is the common occurrence of subperiosteal new bone formation in hypophosphatasia.[276]

Because of deficient alveolar bone synthesis or poor dental root development, early loss of anterior deciduous teeth is a frequent and important diagnostic feature of this disorder.[277] Patients with hypophosphatasia have low levels of circulating alkaline phosphatase, virtually all of which is of intestinal origin.[278] They also excrete increased quantities of urinary phosphoethanolamine.[279] Clinically unaffected heterozygotes frequently exhibit these biochemical abnormalities.[276] In vitro studies have demonstrated that hypophosphatasic serum is capable of mineralizing rachitic rat cartilage,[280] whereas costochondral tissue from affected patients fails to calcify in normal serum.[279] It therefore appears that the disorder is primary within the skeleton and is manifested by low levels of circulating alkaline phosphatase.

Fluoride

Fluoride, which first came to the attention of osteologists because of its toxic skeletal effects, has ironically become a major form of therapy for the most common of metabolic bone diseases—postmenopausal osteopenia. Industrial cryolite (Na_3AlF_6) workers often develop crippling skeletal fluorosis.[281] Endemic

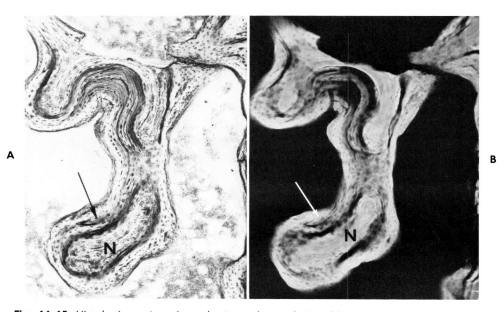

Fig. 44-45. Histologic section, **A,** and microradiograph, **B,** of bone of patient after 2 years of fluoride treatment. Abnormally calcified bone *(arrow)* has been deposited on normal trabeculae, *N.* (Basic fuchsin; 50×; from Jowsey, J., Schenk, R. K., and Reutter, F. W.: J. Clin. Endocrinol. **28:**869, 1968.)

areas of the disorder, because of high concentrations of the substance in the drinking water, exist in India[282] and Qatar.[283]

Patients with this disease have skeletal pains and restriction of spinal motion.[284] Radiologically there is severe osteosclerosis[282,284] with periosteal new bone formation.[284] There may be calcification of the interosseous membrane, ligaments, and tendons.[284] Grossly, the bones have a yellow-brown discoloration.[285]

The primary skeletal effect of fluoride is displacement of hydroxyl ions from apatite to form fluorapatite.[286] This crystal is larger than its normal analog and hence less soluble.[286] Moreover, because of direct inhibition of mineralization, osteomalacia and rickets may attend fluorosis.[287] These factors, associated with suppression of intestinal absorption of calcium,[288] are probably responsible for the secondary hyperparathyroidism commonly accompanying ingestion of large quantities of fluoride.[282] This may be reflected radiologically and grossly by cystic expansion of small bones[284] and subperiosteal bone resorption.[282, 284,289] Since parathyroid hormone stimulates bone formation as well as resorption, the osteosclerotic effect of fluoride may at least in part be the result of associated hyperparathyroidism in a state in which the skeleton is resistant to resorption.

Fluoritic bones histologically exhibit increased quantities of osteoid, osteoclasts, and Howship's lacunae, and on occasion marrow fibrosis.[282,284,289,290] Osteoblasts are numerous, correlating with elevated levels of circulating alkaline phosphatase.[283,284] Woven bone may be abundant[285,291,292] and microfractures have been reported as common.[285] The defective rate of mineralization is often reflected by a broad, irregular calcification front.[285] Although some investigators report numerous bone-remodeling sites[285,289,293] associated with increased cortical porosity,[289,293] others postulate a suppression of the rate of skeletal turnover[294] (Fig. 44-45).

The therapeutic uses of fluoride were prompted by studies demonstrating significantly less vertebral crush fractures and osteopenia among older adult women in areas with fluoridated as opposed to nonfluoridated water.[295] The results of clinical studies employing this agent in postmenopausal osteopenia are less than convincing that salutary symptomatic changes occur despite encouraging morphologic and densitometric data.[296,297] This disparity is perhaps attributable to abnormal structural features of fluoritic bone,[291,292] which, despite increased microhardness,[298] has not proved more resistant to fracture.[289,299,300]

Renal osteodystrophy

Chronic renal disease has a profound and varied effect upon bone metabolism and structure. Consequently, renal osteodystrophy is a generic term representing a number of bone and soft-tissue abnormalities that attend the chronic uremic state. With the advent of life-prolonging techniques, particularly maintenance hemodialysis, these complications assume increasing significance.

Prior to chronic dialysis, the osseous consequences of renal disease were overshadowed by its uremic manifestations.[301] More than 90% of patients on dialysis for at least 2 years have roentgenologic bone disease.[302] Despite suggestions to the contrary, there is no evidence that dialysis per se affects the natural history or pathologic pattern of uremic bone disease.

The principal metabolic abnormalities of uremia that affect bone structure are related to parathyroid hormone excess and altered vitamin D, calcium, and phosphorus metabolism. Essentially all uremic patients have parathyroid gland hyperplasia and evidence of resistance to the intestinal effects of vitamin D.[303] The latter is related to deficient 1-hydroxylation of 25-hydroxycholecalciferol, thereby resulting in a paucity of the vitamin D metabolite most potently affecting intestinal absorption of calcium.[198]

Reflecting these metabolic abnormalities, uremic osteodystrophy is usually combinations of osteitis fibrosa, osteosclerosis, and osteomalacia.[301] When compared to nonuremic, osteopenic patients, total bone mass correlates poorly with the incidence of fractures. The osseous defect of renal failure is therefore probably more qualitative than quantitative and relates to the abnormal maturation of bone mineral and collagen, which exists in experimental uremia.[70]

Uremic bones may be histologically indistinguishable from those of other types of secondary hyperparathyroidism. Marrow fibrosis and woven bone, two characteristics of increased bone turnover, are present in most cases of long-standing uremia. However, the calcemic effect of parathyroid hormone on bone is blunted in renal failure.[304] Therefore the number of osteoclasts per unit of circulating immunoreactive parathyroid hormone may not be so striking as in primary hyperparathyroidism.[304a] However, as circulating levels of immunoreactive parathyroid hormone are in general much higher in renal failure than in primary hyperparathyroidism, uremic bones usually contain a greater absolute number of osteoclasts. The resistance of uremic bone to parathyroid hormone is probably in part related to the inability of osteoclasts to resorb the thick osteoid seams covering much more trabecular surface than normal.[215] In addition, the rate of resorption per osteoclast is usually depressed in renal failure.[305]

Osteosclerosis, increased matrix volume per volume of whole bone, may be the most common form of renal osteodystrophy.[301] Since it does not commonly result in obvious deformities, the condition may escape clinical detection. Roentgenographically, the most severely affected patients have a "rugger-jersey spine," a pathognomonic feature attributable to alternating bands of increased and normal bone density (Fig. 44-46). Pathologically, there is loss of distinction between cortical and trabecular bone. The trabeculae are wide and

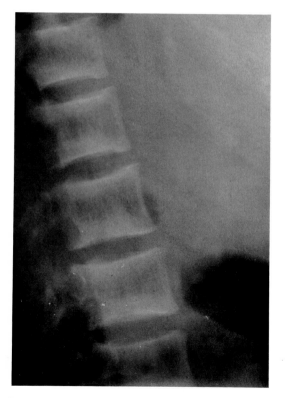

Fig. 44-46. Osteosclerosis of spine associated with long-standing renal failure. The rugger jersey appearance is attributable to alternating bands of sclerotic and normally dense bone.

usually covered by thick osteoid seams. Large quantities of woven bone are usually present and osteitis fibrosa progresses in tandem with osteosclerosis (Fig. 44-47).

Whether the kinetic mechanism involved in osteosclerosis is increased formation or decreased resorption is uncertain. However, decreased rates of bone formation[59] and resorption[60] commonly accompany chronic uremia. It is therefore this combination of events, with a decrease in resorption predominating, that is probably responsible for the development of osteosclerosis. Furthermore, since woven bone may mineralize where lamellar bone fails to do so,[306] the presence of large quantities of woven bone may also be responsible for the increased skeletal mass of renal disease.

Although osteomalacia occurs in some uremic patients, its incidence and severity in the United States are much less than in Europe.[307] This may be related to greater vitamin D stores in Americans than in Europeans.[307]

Probably related to active skeletal growth, clinical bone disease is much more common in uremic children than in adults.[308] The predominant changes are osteosclerosis and rickets. Children with renal disease are usually older than those with nutritional rickets and consequently heavier and more ambulant. Therefore the varus or valgus deformities of the lower extremities of uremic children tend to be more severe.[308]

As contrasted to other forms of therapy, renal transplantation may completely reverse the uremic state.[309] However, since involution of the glands may take years, evidence of increased parathyroid hormone effect on bone may persist for some time. Moreover, immunosuppressive agents administered to these patients inhibit bone cell activity and are responsible for the development of avascular necrosis.[310] In addition, posttransplantation patients frequently develop transient hypercalcemia.[311] This is presumably attributable to renewed synthesis of 1,25-dihydroxycholecalciferol and to newly mineralized bone that becomes available to osteoclastic activity in a non–parathyroid hormone resistant state.

Pseudohypoparathyroidism

A multitude of phenotypic expressions represent the syndrome of pseudohypoparathyroidism. Affected patients are usually short and obese with a characteristic moon facies. They have abnormal dentition and shortening of the bones of the hands and feet, particu-

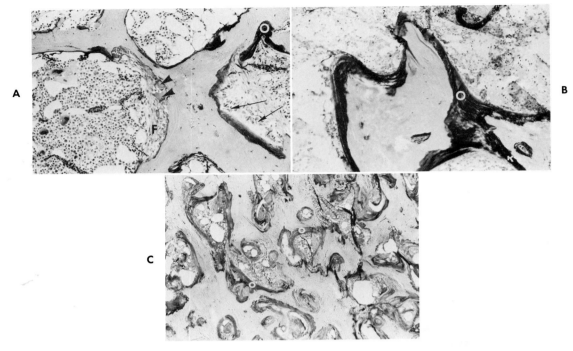

Fig. 44-47. Histologic spectrum of renal osteodystrophy. Combinations of three basic lesions are usually found. **A,** Osteitis fibrosa is characterized by peritrabecular fibrosis, F; numerous osteoclasts *(arrowheads)*; increased osteoid, O; and osteoblast proliferation *(arrows)*. **B,** Osteomalacia exhibits a predominance of wide osteoid, O. **C,** Osteosclerosis. Quantity of trabecular bone is greatly increased. Eventually one cannot distinguish trabecular from cortical bone. Osteoid, O, is also commonly increased. (Undecalcified, Goldner; 40×.)

larly the metacarpals and metatarsals (Fig. 44-48). The long bones often appear curved. Soft-tissue mineralization and ossification are common as are cataracts and basal ganglion calcification.[312] Although bone density is roentgenologically normal in most, these patients may be osteopenic or osteosclerotic. Although most investigators believe the mode of inheritance is X-linked dominant,[313,314] some suggest an autosomal dominant pattern.[315] Women with this condition outnumber men two to one.[95] The disease usually appears within the first decade and invariably by the end of the second.[95]

The major physiologic defect rests in resistance of the renal tubule to the effects of parathyroid hormone. This is characteristically manifest as an absence of phosphaturia in response to exogenous parathyroid hormone administration. However, the disease is best diagnosed by the failure of the patient to excrete urinary cyclic AMP under these circumstances.[316] A smaller group of patients with pseudohypoparathyroidism type II have the classic phenotypic changes.[317] These individuals however excrete cyclic AMP in response to parathyroid hormone while failing to excrete phosphorus.[317] Whereas the classical form of the disease is related to deficient cyclic AMP production by the kidney, pseudohypoparathyroidism type II is caused by defective responsivity of the renal tubule to the nucleotide.[317] In addition, the bones of patients with both forms of the disease are less responsive than normal to parathyroid hormone.[318,319]

Because of failure to excrete phosphorus, the characteristic biochemical features of pseudohypoparathyroidism are hyperphosphatemia and hypocalcemia, with attendant secondary hyperparathyroidism. The bones therefore show changes of osteitis fibrosa both radiologically and histologically. These changes may be reversed by a phosphorus-poor diet and supplemental vitamin D.[320]

The epiphyses of the short bones are histologically and histochemically abnormal.[321] The growth plates are narrow and the cells arranged in short columns. Premature closure

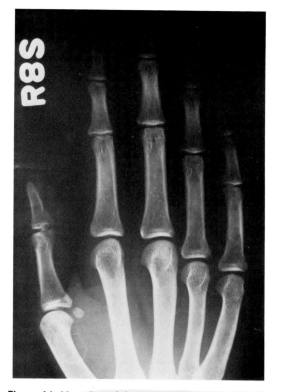

Fig. 44-48. Pseudohypoparathyroidism. Note shortening of fourth metacarpal. Although this phenomenon occurs frequently in pseudohypoparathyroidism, it is not pathognomonic and may be seen in a variety of congenital metabolic disorders. (Courtesy Dr. James W. Debnam, Jr., Chesterfield, Mo.)

of these epiphyses accounts for the retarded growth.[313]

A number of patients with pseudohypoparathyroidism are hypothyroid.[322] In addition, thyrocalcitonin content of the gland is extremely high,[323] a finding that suggests a role of the hypocalcemic agent in the etiology of the disease. However, total thyroidectomy fails to correct the biochemical abnormalities.[323]

Idiopathic hypoparathyroidism, pseudohypoparathyroidism, and pseudo-pseudohypoparathyroidism represent a spectrum of physical and biochemical abnormalities.[96,324,325] Patients with idiopathic hypoparathyroidism frequently have many physical features similar to those with pseudohypoparathyroidism,[316] whereas some patients with the hormone-resistant disease appear physically unremarkable.[325]

Osteitis deformans (Paget's disease)

In 1877 Sir James Paget[326] described a potentially deforming bone disease of unknown etiology affecting 3% to 4%[327,328] of the population. It is rarely encountered before the fourth decade,[329] is the most frequent accompaniment of primary malignant bone tumors in the adult,[330] may be familial,[331] and is usually undiagnosed prior to autopsy.[328] The cardinal feature of this disorder is focal acceleration of bone resorption and formation.[332] Although some view it as a form of idiopathic hyperplasia or benign neoplasia of skeletal mesenchymal cells,[94] the continued coupling of resorption and formation that characterizes Paget's disease suggests that it is a form of abnormal remodeling.

Although it may be monostotic,[328,329] the disease usually involves multiple portions of the skeleton with predilection for the skull, pelvis, tibia, and femur. Individually involved bones simultaneously contain many stages of the disease process. Therefore osteitis deformans is not a generalized bone disease and probably not of metabolic origin.[333] As the disease is nonuniform within the skeleton, histologic examination of a bone specimen is of no value in predicting changes in other bones or in following the effects of therapy in a single patient.

Reflecting the general phenomenon of bone remodeling, a focus of Paget's disease begins as active resorption. This lytic phase may progress rapidly and result in considerable softening of bone. Characteristic transverse fissure fractures, particularly of the tibia, femur, and humerus often occur.[334] These fractures when stressed, heal normally. However, since osteolysis is stimulated by immobilization, placing these limbs in a restrictive cast frequently accelerates the lytic process.[329]

When involving a long bone, the process invariably begins at one end. Osteoporosis circumscripta, characteristically occurring in the frontal or occipital poles of the skull, is a manifestation of osteolytic Paget's disease.[335] In addition, platybasia, bowed back, curvatures of the femur and tibia, erosion of the lamina dura, and protrusion deformities of the acetabulum are attributed to bone softening. On occasion, there is cord compression secondary to vertebral collapse.[336]

Histologically, the trabeculae of the osteolytic phase of Paget's disease are slender and extremely vascular. Because of osseous hyperperfusion, the skin over involved bone is warm and, in severe cases, cardiac output is greatly elevated.[337] Although the long hypothesized existence of arteriovenous shunts in pagetic bone has been disproved,[338] the existence of

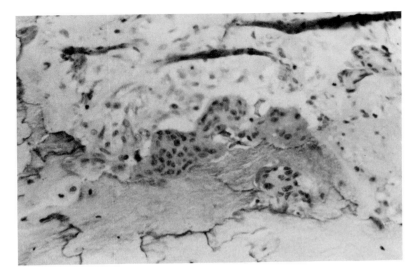

Fig. 44-49. Pagetic osteoclasts containing large numbers of nuclei distributed throughout cytoplasm. (Undecalcified, toluidine blue; 250×.)

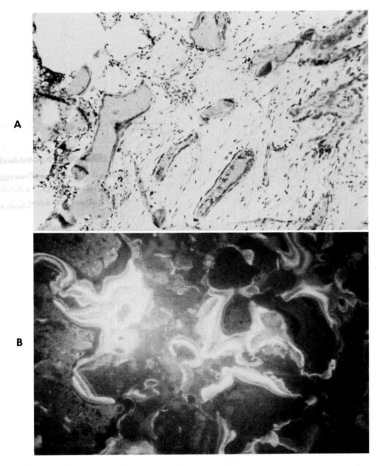

Fig. 44-50. A, Mixed phase of Paget's disease. There are numerous osteoclasts and osteoblasts. Marrow has a myxomatous appearance, and woven bone is present. **B,** Fluorescent micrograph of biopsy of site of active Paget's disease. As seen by exuberant uptake of tetracycline, there is noticeable acceleration of bone turnover. (**A,** Undecalcified, Goldner; 100×; **B,** undecalcified, unstained; 40×.)

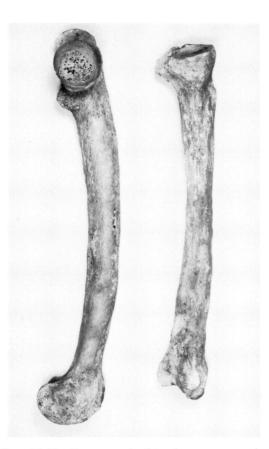

Fig. 44-51. Femur and tibia from a severely pagetic skeleton. Note anterior bowing of both bones and pronounced periosteal reaction. (Courtesy Dr. Stephen Molnar, St. Louis, Mo.; W.U. 76-2964.)

a decreased difference in arterial and venous oxygen saturations remains unexplained.

The hallmark of the lytic phase of osteitis deformans, and a pathognomonic feature of Paget's disease, is giant osteoclast, which may contain up to 100 nuclei. Whereas the nuclei of normal osteoclasts are located adjacent to the nonresorbing surface of the cell, those of pagetic osteoclasts are randomly distributed throughout the cytoplasm (Fig. 44-49).

The mixed phase of Paget's disease is characterized by accelerated formation as well as resorption. Radiologically this appears as a V-shaped advancing edge of osteolytic activity followed by a blastic zone. The proliferative region contains irregular, vascular trabeculae lined by thick osteoid seams. Numerous large, often bizarre osteoblasts appear and are responsible for the increased concentrations of blood alkaline phosphatase characterizing the disorder. The presence of thick osteoid seams likely reflects accelerated collagen production. Woven bone proliferates in abundance as does fibrous tissue in the marrow. These changes may be confused with hyperparathyroidism, particularly since on occasion the roentgenographic lesions appear similar[332] (Fig. 44-50).

Paradoxically, the areas most roentgenographically characteristic of Paget's disease are the ones that are no longer active or symptomatic.[339] The bone of the sclerotic or "burned-out" phase of the disorder is rock hard and difficult to cut. The sclerotic nature of the bone may lead to neurosensory deaf-

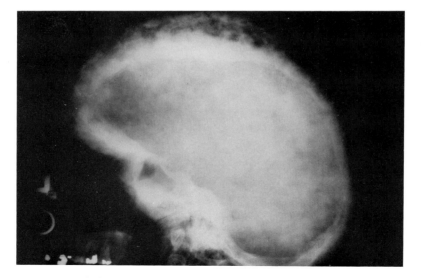

Fig. 44-52. Pagetic skull with characteristic cotton-ball appearance. (Courtesy Dr. James W. Debnam, Jr., Chesterfield, Mo.)

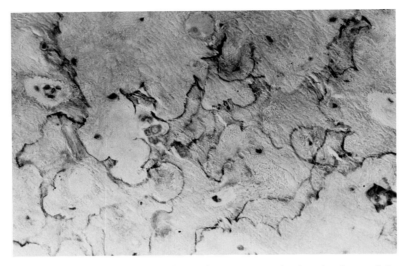

Fig. 44-53. Mosaic pattern of cement lines characteristic of sclerotic phase of Paget's disease. (Undecalcified, toluidine blue; 100×.)

ness as a result of degeneration of sensory receptors within the temporal bones.[340] Extremely active periosteal new bone formation results in a rough, uneven surface (Fig. 44-51). The bone width is increased and the anatomic structure distorted, resulting in a characteristic radiographic cotton-ball appearance of the skull and coarse trabecular striations (Fig. 44-52). The distinction between cortical and trabecular bone is lost and osteonal architecture distorted. Trabeculae are wide and disorganized and vascular sinusoids not so prominent as in the earlier stages of the process. Although osteoclasts and osteoblasts are much fewer in number, the striking histologic feature of this phase of the disease is a "mosaic" pattern of cement lines reflecting the previously active alternating processes of resorption and formation (Fig. 44-53).

Immobilization osteoporosis

Osteopenia in immobilized portions of the skeleton is a universal phenomenon. Not only does this occur with bed rest,[341] paralysis,[342] and plaster cast immobilization,[343] but, as observed with the advent of space travel, in a weightless environment.[344] In addition, since arrest of longitudinal bone growth frequently occurs in association with childhood poliomyelitis, it may occur with limb denervation.[345]

The pathogenesis of disuse osteopenia is not only controversial, but different patterns of bone loss appear as well in denervated as opposed to nondenervated immobilized limbs.[346] Compensation for loss of weight on the vertebral column does not prevent the negative calcium balance induced by horizontal immobilization.[347] Therefore the lack of direct mechanical stress on bone does not appear to be the primary inducer of immobilization osteoporosis.

The rate of trabecular bone formation falls off rapidly while periosteal bone accretion[348] may be increased at least in the early stages of immobilization.[348] However, endosteal resorption is accelerated to an even greater degree, resulting in net cortical bone loss.[347] The early rapid loss of immobilized bone may be followed by a new steady state of formation and resorption in which there is little further diminution of skeletal mass.[349]

Since thyroparathyroidectomy protects against loss of bone mass in nondenervated, immobilized limbs,[136] a humoral substance is perhaps responsible for this form of disuse osteopenia. The absence of osteoporosis in the contralateral, functional limb may be attributed to local factors that increase the sensitivity of immobilized bone to normal circulating levels of thyroid or parathyroid hormone, or both.[136]

CONGENITAL DISORDERS OF MODELING
Disorders of collagen formation
Osteogenesis imperfecta

Osteogenesis imperfecta, a heritable disorder of connective tissue, usually becomes clinically manifest by a predisposition toward multiple bone fractures. Although significant overlap occurs, there are two general pheno-

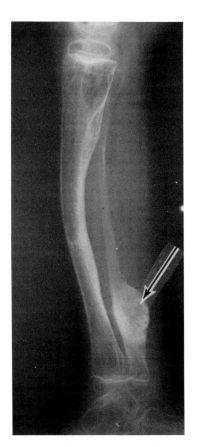

Fig. 44-54. Severely osteopenic and distorted tibia and fibula of child with osteogenesis imperfecta. A healing fracture exhibits abundant callus formation *(arrow)*. (Courtesy Dr. James W. Debnam, Jr., Chesterfield, Mo.)

typic expressions of the disorder. At birth, infants with osteogenesis imperfecta congenita, the more severe form of the disease, have multiple fractures and subsequently develop crippling deformities. Although the mode of inheritance is probably autosomal recessive,[350] few patients with this disease are capable of reproduction. Hence the genetic pattern remains uncertain.

Children with osteogenesis imperfecta tarda, the more latent form of the disease, usually transmitted as an autosomal dominant,[351] may be born with fractures. However, clinical evidence of bone disease often does not appear until after the perinatal period. Bowing of the extremities is of particular diagnostic significance.[352] Regardless of the phenotypic expression, the mass of cortical and trabecular bone is significantly reduced. The bones are often so distorted that the roentgenograph is diagnostic of the disease (Fig. 44-54).

Fractures, although frequent, heal normally with exuberant callus formation.[352] Histologically, the bone is characterized by a failure of normal modeling of trabecular into compact bone, resulting in poorly demarcated, thick trabeculae and a porous cortex. The replacement of woven bone is usually delayed past the second decade, correlating with the reduction in the fracture rate often occurring with puberty.[352] This delay in the morphologic maturation of bone is reflected biochemically by a lack of maturation of collagen cross-linkage.[353]

The bone surface lined by Howship's

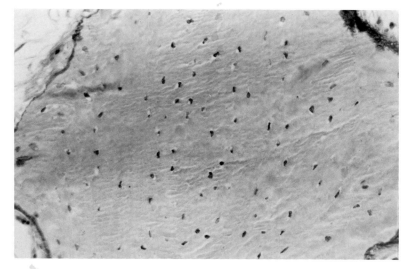

Fig. 44-55. Note the large increase in number of osteocytes in lamellar bone from patient with osteogenesis imperfecta as compared to Fig. 44-6, *B.* (Undecalcified, Goldner; 100×)

lacunae is increased in osteogenesis imperfecta, but there may be no excess of osteoclasts.[354] This is of particular significance as Villanueva and Frost[355] report essentially normal or increased bone formation rates and thereby conclude the associated osteopenia must be attributable to accelerated resorption.

A sharp increase in the osteocyte concentration per unit volume of bone is perhaps the histologic feature most diagnostic of the disease. This large number of osteocytes suggests a decrease in the volume of bone under the metabolic influence of each cell. Not only does woven bone, which normally has abundant osteocytes, display this feature, but lamellar bone as well.[354] Correlating with osteocyte dysfunction, Villanueva and Frost find decreased cellular and increased tissue level bone

formation rates, an indication of defective osteoblast function[355] (Fig. 44-55).

Osteogenesis imperfecta is not a disease confined to the skeleton. Clinical features such as blue scleras, thin translucent skin, hypermobile joints, and cardiac valve incompetence reflect a generalized disorder of mesenchyme and a relationship to the Marfan-like group of diseases. Fibroblast cultures of skin from patients with this disease are morphologically abnormal.[356] Although histochemical studies suggest a sulfation defect of glycosoaminoglycans,[357] Penttinen et al.[358] have recently described deficient skin procollagen I synthesis in this disease. Since there are convincing reports of abnormal bone collagen fiber structure, particularly of a striking defect of aggregation of thin into thick fibers,[359] a relationship between these morphologic defects and deficient procollagen synthesis appears likely (Fig. 44-56).

Fibrogenesis imperfecta ossium

Fibrogenesis imperfecta ossium is a rare disease that occurs in midadult life, clinically characterized by skeletal pain, tenderness, and a propensity toward fracture.[360,361] Radiographically, the cancellous bone of these patients with the disease is opaque.[360] Histologically, the cortex is thin, and the trabeculae are wide and irregular and contain patchy areas of granular calcification.[360] The increased skeletal radiopacity is apparent by microradiography in which these abnormally mineralized areas are accentuated.[360] Moreover, the hydroxyapatite content of bone is increased above normal.[360]

Reflecting defective collagen as the structural abnormality of the disorder, there is a paucity of doubly refractile bone fibers by polarizing microscopy.[360,361] In the earlier stages of the process, one may see normally polarizing skeletal tissue deep to recently deposited abnormal bone.[360] Moreover, as the disorder progresses, osteoclasts and osteoblasts, which may be abundant early in the disease,[360] virtually disappear.[361]

Osteomalacia is another component of fibrogenesis imperfecta ossium.[360,361] The abnormally shaped trabeculae are covered by wide osteoid seams, many of which fail to assume a tetracycline label.[361] As is commonly associated with stages of defective mineralization, the bone appositional rate is low.[361] The etiology of the osteomalacia in this disorder is unknown, although some postulate that it is secondary to abnormal collagen structure.[361]

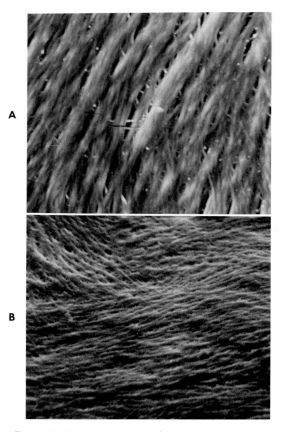

Fig. 44-56. A, Scanning electron micrograph of osteoid of normal 11-year-old patient. Note thick interweaving fiber bundles. **B,** Scanning electron micrograph of 11-year-old patient with osteogenesis imperfecta. Fibers fail to aggregate into bundles of normal width. (**A** and **B,** 2200×; from Teitelbaum, S. L., Kraft, W. J., Lang, R., et al.: Calcif. Tissue Res. **17**(1):75, 1974.)

Some symptomatic improvement may occur with vitamin D therapy.[360]

Disorders of ground substance and cartilage
Mucopolysaccharidoses

The mucopolysaccharidoses are a group of disorders of defective degradation of mucopolysaccharides. Identification of various specific enzyme defects has enabled McKusick[362] to classify these diseases into six categories. Cultured fibroblasts from patients of each group exhibit abnormal metachromasia correctible by the addition of normal serum or that of individuals with other forms of mucopolysaccharidoses.[363] Although significant bone disease may exist in patients with any of the mucopolysaccharidoses, those with Morquio's (MPS IV) and Maroteaux-Lamy (MPS VII) syndromes are the most strikingly affected.

Hurler's syndrome (MPS I H), the first of the mucopolysaccharidoses to be described, is caused by deficient α-L-iduronidase.[364] It is associated with increased tissue stores and excretion of dermatan and heparan sulfate.[365] "Gargoylism" describes the characteristic troll-like appearance of these patients. The gross skeletal defects that are also present in other mucopoysaccharidoses represent a spectrum of changes called "dysostoses multiplex."[366]

Patients with Hurler's syndrome are dwarfed, with saber-shaped, broad, flat ribs, clawed hands, and a characteristic shoe-shaped sella turcica.[366] Because of expansion of the marrow cavity, the tubular bones are swollen. The proximal one third of the femur however is narrow.[366] Focally decreased anteroposterior development and replacement of defective areas by radiolucent cartilage result in a hook-shaped radiologic appearance of some lumbar-vertebral bodies.[367] These defectively developed vertebrae may displace posteriorly, resulting in spinal cord compression.[368]

Histologically there is arrest of endochondral growth in Hurler's syndrome.[367,368] The resting zone of the epiphysis appears normal whereas the proliferative zone is attenuated.[368] The cells of the hypertrophic zone are severely disarrayed. The chondrocytes are enlarged, contain abundant intracellular glycoprotein, and completely fill their lacunae.[369] Moreover, an abnormal variant of mucopolysaccharides, which may appear focally fibrillar and birefringent,[369] is present in Hurler cartilaginous matrix.[370]

Ultrastructurally, the chondrocytes in Hurler cartilage contain numerous, often coalescing vacuoles, which push the endoplasmic reticulum to the periphery of the cells.[371] Since the mucopolysaccharidoses are diseases of enzyme deficiencies, these abnormal vacuoles may be derived from lysosomes. Presumably as a result of discharge of cytoplasmic contents into the matrix, normal chondrocytes have scalloped cell membranes. These crenations however are not present in chondrocytes of patients with Hurler's syndrome.[371] Silberberg and co-workers[371] believe that this absence of scalloping represents deficient release of intracellular contents by chondrocytes (Fig. 44-57).

The thin cortices of Hurler bone are essentially unremarkable histologically. A transverse bony plate commonly develops between the epiphysis and the metaphysis.[367] Little osteoblastic activity is present, and the osteocytes may be enlarged.[367] Whereas "gargoyle cells" are common in cartilage and periosteum in Hurler's syndrome,[367] there is little evidence that they infiltrate osseous tissue.[368] Therefore, the etiology of the osteopenia associated with this disease may be different from that of abnormality in endochondral growth.[368]

Hunter's syndrome (MPS II) is also associated with abnormal excretion of dermatan and heparan sulfate.[372] Patients with this affliction may have skeletal changes similar to, but less severe than those with Hurler's syndrome.[362,366]

Because of sulfamidase deficiency,[373] patients with Sanfilippo's syndrome (MPS III) have high urinary and tissue content of heparan sulfate.[374] Although often characterized by slight dwarfism, the gross skeletal abnormalities of this disorder tend to be the mildest of the mucopolysaccharidoses.[375] Ultrastructurally, chondrocytes of patients with Sanfilippo's syndrome are distended with distinct types of vacuoles, which, as in Hurler's syndrome, may represent altered lysosomes.[371] Moreover, similar to Hurler chondrocytes, these cells exhibit a lack of cell membrane scalloping, again suggesting a failure of egress of cytoplasmic contents (Fig. 44-58).

The skeletal changes of patients with Morquio's syndrome (MPS IV) are among the most severe of the mucopolysaccharidoses.[376] These patients excrete excessive amounts of keratan sulfate.[377] They appear normal at birth, and clinical manifestations usually develop between the first and second years. Because of severe dysplasia of epiphyseal growth centers, virtually all bones other than those of the skull are affected.[376] Generalized osteoporosis is present. The vertebral bodies are

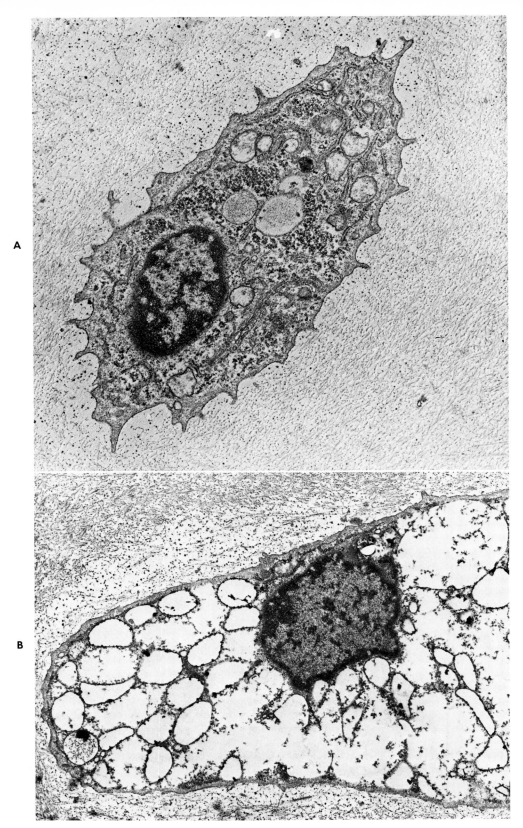

Fig. 44-57. A, Normal chondrocyte. Note scalloped cell membrane. **B,** Giant chondrocyte from patient with Hurler's syndrome. Note large, distended cytoplasmic vacuoles and absence of scalloping of cell membrane. (**A** and **B,** 19,900×; courtesy Dr. Ruth Silberberg, Jerusalem, Israel.)

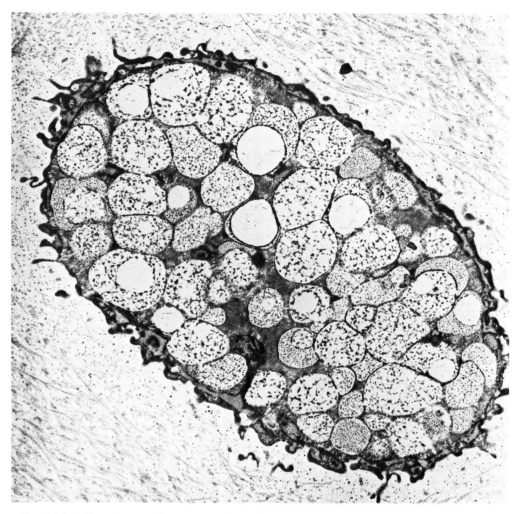

Fig. 44-58. Chondrocyte of patient with Sanfilippo's syndrome. Note distinctive cytoplasmic vacuoles. (19,900×; courtesy Dr. Ruth Silberberg, Jerusalem, Israel.)

characteristically flat (platyspondyly),[376] and because of hypoplasia of the first cervical vertebra, high spinal cord compression is one of the complications of the disorder.[378] The ribs resemble paddles and the epiphyses are misshapen.[376] The hips are enlarged and irregular.[376]

The characteristic histologic alterations in Morquio's syndrome are confined to the skeleton, particularly the cartilage.[376,379,380] There are several abnormalities of the epiphyses, with short, disorganized zones of proliferative and hypertropic cartilaginous cells. The chondrocytes are big and contain large amounts of metachromatic material.[380] These cells are generally sparse and clumped. Ultrastructurally they exhibit distended ergastoplasmic sacs.[381]

Distinct areas of clumped, metachromatic granules, juxtaposed to nonmetachromatic foci are common in Morquio cartilaginous matrix.[376] Not uncommonly, areas of this cartilage have the birefringent qualities of fibrillar connective tissues such as collagen.[376,379,380] Fibrous tissue strands containing areas of intramembranous bone formation may be interposed between cartilage and bone in the epiphyses.[380]

Although severe osteopenia is common in Morquio's syndrome, the bony abnormalities may be secondary to cartilage dysfunction.[376,379] As in Hurler's syndrome, a transverse osseous plate forms across the face of the metaphyseo-epiphyseal junction.[379] Although osteoblastic and osteoclastic activity appears normal, there is a disorderly array of sparse trabeculae.[380] Calcified cartilage persists in these trabeculae, but there are no foam cells in the bone.[376,379] It is therefore likely that deficient metaphyseal osteogenesis in this disease results from inadequate chondrocyte proliferation and maturation.[379]

Maroteaux-Lamy syndrome (MPS IV) is a rare form of the mucopolysaccharidoses. It is associated with excessive excretion of dermatan sulfate.[382] The skeletal changes of this disorder are severe. However no information regarding pathology in cases in which the diagnosis is certain is yet available.

Patients with Maroteaux-Lamy syndrome are strikingly dwarfed and have severe dysostosis multiplex. Radiolucencies suggesting residual islands of cartilage are present in the tibial and distal femoral metaphyses.[362] Irregular ossification of the femoral head, which may be confused with Legg-Calvé-Perthes disease, is also present.[362] Similar to Morquio's syndrome, there is often hypoplasia of the odontoid process.[362]

Achondroplasia

Achondroplasia is the most common of the chondrodystrophies and the most frequent etiology of disproportionate, short stature. It is inherited as an autosomal dominant.[383] However, because of physical and social difficulties of reproduction, 80% of cases are sporadic.[128] The characteristic appearance of these patients reflects failure of normal endochondral ossification. They are short limbed, and although spinal abnormalities are common, truncal length is relatively normal.[383] As a result of decreased interpedicular distance and a narrow foramen magnum, the most serious complications of the disorder are cord and nerve root compression.[383] Achondroplastics have a prominent lumbar lordosis and versus deformities of the knees. Wide spacing of the third and fourth fingers result in a "trident" appearance of the hand. A saddle-nose deformity exists. Because intramembranous ossification is not affected, there is disproportionate growth of the calveria resulting in prominent frontal bossing and mild macrocephaly. The base of the skull develops largely in cartilage and is therefore relatively hypoplastic (Fig. 44-59).

There is much debate concerning the histologic appearance of achondroplastic cartilage. Ponseti[384] and Stannescu and co-workers[385] report striking morphologic abnormalities of the epiphyses, including dis-

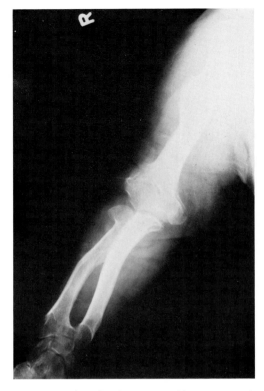

Fig. 44-59. Achondroplastic arm. Note attenuation of diaphyseal length with normal width. The metaphyses are characteristically flared. (Courtesy Dr. Hyman R. Senturia, St. Louis, Mo.)

array and paucity of chondrocytes, fibrosis of cartilaginous matrix, and attenuation of the hypertrophic zone with attendant failure of cell maturation. There is histochemical evidence of decreased quantities of mucopolysaccharides about the chondrocytes and an absence of glycogen in the superficial cells of the hypertrophic zone.[385] Furthermore, there may be deficiencies of lysosomal enzymes, including alkaline phosphatase, in the cartilaginous matrix.[385] Particularly in older achondroplastic children, the cartilaginous proteoglycans are less soluble than normal, and the glucosamine concentration is frequently increased.[386] These changes may be related to curvilinear inclusion bodies composed of rough endoplasmic reticulum present in chondrocytes of pseudoachondroplastic dwarfs, a disorder similar to, but less severe than achondroplasia.[387] Cooper and co-workers interpret these bodies as manifestations of failure and chondrocytes to transfer synthesized protein from ergastoplasm to the Golgi apparatus.[387]

Rimoin and co-workers view the chondrodystrophies as (1) those with histologically well-ordered endochondral ossification and (2) those in which endochondral ossification is histologically disordered.[388] They believe achondroplastic cartilage is morphologically well ordered, and the dysfunctions of growth are probably rate related rather than caused by gross cartilaginous abnormalities. They state that those reports of disordered cartilage in achondroplasia were actually observations of other chondrodystrophies, particularly thanatrophic and metatrophic dwarfism, as well as achondrogenesis. One should appreciate, however, that although investigators reporting morphologically abnormal achondroplastic cartilage were examining long bone epiphyses, the studies of Rimoin et al.[388] were confined to costochondral cartilage and iliac crest, which Ponseti[384] also finds morphologically normal.

Regardless of the controversial appearance of their cartilage, little question exists that the gross and roentgenographic appearances of epiphyses of patients with achondroplasia are abnormal. The plates are V shaped, with the apex pointing toward the metaphyses.[384] As a consequence of normal periosteal bone formation associated with retarded endochondral ossification, periosteal bone grows over and into the perichondrium resulting in cup-shaped costochondral junctions.[389]

Osteopetrosis

Osteopetrosis is a disease characterized by a densely radiopaque appearance of the entire skeleton. The sclerotic process usually starts in the diaphyses of the long bones and spreads to the metaphyses,[390] which assume a characteristic club-shaped appearance.[391] The progression of the disease may fluctuate, resulting in alternating bands of greater and lesser density[391] (Fig. 44-60).

Although each affects approximately 50% of patients,[390] the genetic patterns of the benign and malignant forms of the disorder differ. Benign osteopetrosis is characterized by relatively normal longevity and is inherited as an autosomal dominant. The malignant form, which because of anemia or secondary infection invariably results in death before the end of the second decade, is recessive and often associated with a history of consanguinity.[390] Radiographic distinction cannot be made between the two forms.

The diagnosis of benign osteopetrosis is often not made until the second or third decade.[390] Although patients not infrequently have only radiologic manifestations of the disease, a num-

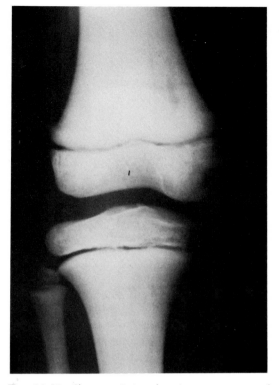

Fig. 44-60. Characteristic sclerotic appearance of osteopetrotic bones. Distinction between cortical and trabecular bone is lost. (Courtesy Dr. James W. Debnam, Jr., Chesterfield, Mo.)

ber sustain many fractures that heal normally.[390] Osteomyelitis, particularly of the mandible, is common in benign osteopetrosis,[390] as is cranial nerve palsy from progressive obliteration of the foramina of the skull.[391] Although the sex ratio of osteopetrotic patients is one, males, with a greater propensity to skeletal fractures, are more frequently symptomatic.[390]

Malignant osteopetrosis is characterized by high incidences of optic atrophy and hepatosplenomegaly.[390] Many afflicted children grow poorly, and mental retardation and deafness are common. The only frequently encountered biochemical abnormality in either form of this disease is elevation of the blood acid phosphatase.

Pathologically, the bone is dense and the medullary cavity absent.[390] Microfractures are common. Reflecting a failure of modeling, the fetal shape of a thick cortex is retained. The unique histologic feature of the disorder is hyaline bars of nonresorbed cartilage that intermingle with bone that is largely woven (Fig. 44-61). The disease is therefore a result

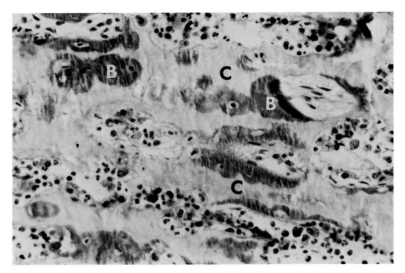

Fig. 44-61. Trabecular bone of osteopetrotic patient. Because the disorder is one of osteoclast dysfunction, bars of mineralized cartilage, **C,** persist among abnormal bone, **B.** (Undecalcified, Goldner; 100×.)

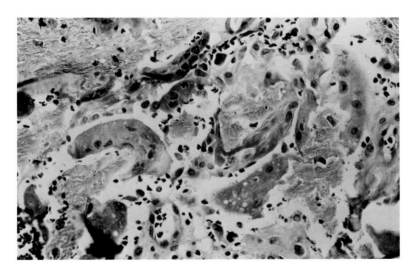

Fig. 44-62. Bizarre osteoclasts characteristic of osteopetrosis. (Undecalcified, Goldner; 200×.)

of deficient replacement of the growth plate by bone. There is also impairment of skeletal response to resorptive stimuli[392] such as parathyroid hormone or vitamin D.[393]

The cellular defect of the disease is failure of osteoclast function. These cells may be decreased or increased in number. When present in large concentrations, the osteoclasts appear extremely bizarre (Fig. 44-62).

Since osteopetrotic children have normal levels of circulating thyrocalcitonin, the disease does not appear to be attributable to a sup-

pressive effect of this hormone on osteoclast function.[394] Furthermore, there is commonly absence of epiphyseal invasion by metaphyseal vessels. The growth plate therefore fails to mature, and these patients may consequently have rachitic changes on x-ray films (Fig. 44-63).

There are numerous experimental models of osteopetrosis.[395-398] Osteoclasts of affected incisor-absent *(ia)* rats lack a ruffled border.[399] Although capable of synthesizing the enzyme, they are not able to normally release acid

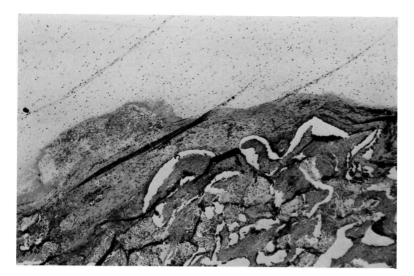

Fig. 44-63. Failure of growth plate maturation in osteopetrosis.

phosphatase.[397] These changes are of particular interest because hepatic lysosomal activity of osteopetrotic patients is normal.[400]

The studies of Walker[395, 396, 398] are undoubtedly the most important yet performed to delineate the pathogenesis of this disease. By parabiosis of osteopetrotic mice with their normal littermates, he has cured the abnormal animal without affecting its parabiotic partner. These studies indicate that lack of a humoral substance may be responsible for the development of this experimental form of the disease. The exacerbation of experimental osteopetrosis by parathyroid hormone suggests a pathogenetic role of this agent.[398] However, suppression of parathormone activity does not cure the human disorder.[398]

AVASCULAR NECROSIS

Avascular (aseptic) necrosis of bone is an infarctive process of debated etiology that most commonly involves the femoral head. Three times more males than females are affected,[401] usually within the fifth or sixth decades.[402] Since the etiology of the disorder is unknown, it is frequently referred to as idiopathic. However, it is often associated with alcoholism,[403] corticosteroid therapy,[404] and hyperuricemia.[405]

Subcapital fractures of the femoral neck most commonly precede avascular necrosis.[405] Traumatic dislocation is also a major predisposing factor.[401] Other conditions that are frequently attended by avascular necrosis are Gaucher's disease,[406] systemic lupus erythematosis,[407] and various hemoglobinopathies.[402, 408]

It is often associated with congenital hip dysplasias and slipped capital femoral epiphysis.[405] A large number of patients undergoing renal homotransplantation develop this complication within 2 years of surgery.[310] Perhaps related to intravascular nitrogen bubbles, it is also seen in caisson workers.[409]

There are three major hypotheses regarding the etiology of avascular necrosis. These include thrombotic or mechanical interference with arterial blood supply,[410] fat embolization to the subchondral vessels,[411, 412] and abnormal biomechanical structure of the hip joint.[413] The frequent association of the disorder with subcapital femoral neck fracture[405] suggests a vascular etiology. In addition, the arterial blood supply[410] and venous drainage of the femoral head are severely compromised in avascular necrosis.[414] However, this may represent the results rather than the etiology of the disorder. The vascular hypothesis has prompted the sobriquet "coronary disease of the hip" for idiopathic avascular necrosis.[415]

On the basis of the presence of lipid in the subchondral vessels of necrotic femoral heads, invesgtigators have postulated fat embolization as the etiologic factor of this disorder.[411, 412] Jones[411] believes the lipid particles are mobilized from fatty livers induced by alcoholism or corticosteroids. The presence of lipid emboli in necrotic and nonnecrotic femoral heads with similar frequencies[404] and the failure to produce aseptic necrosis in corticosteroid-treated rabbits, despite the occurrence of fat emboli,[416] places this hypothesis in question.

The incidence of avascular necrosis after femoral neck fracture is directly related to the degree of malreduction.[413] Hence biomechanical factors are likely to play a role in this constellation of events. This, of course, implies that the etiology of traumatic avascular necrosis differs from that of the idiopathic type, a not unlikely conclusion, particularly since the high incidence of bilaterality in the latter suggests a systemic cause.[402] The likelihood of a systemic etiology is further supported by observations of Laurent and co-workers that

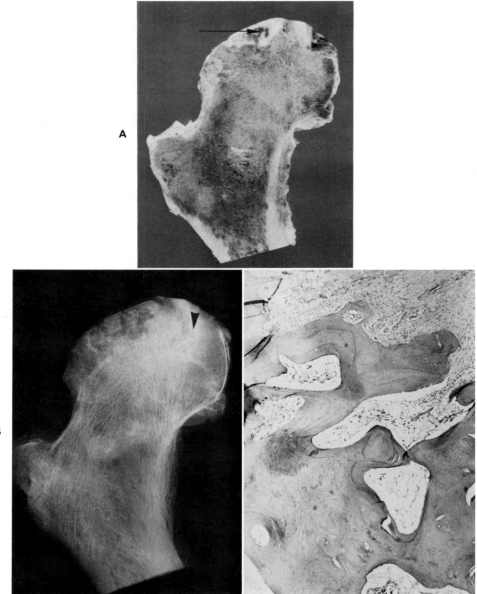

Fig. 44-64. A, Sagittal section of femoral head resected for avascular necrosis. Necrotic focus *(arrow)* is surrounded by articular cartilage that has collapsed into the bone. **B,** Roentgenogram of specimen **A.** Fractures of cortical bone over area of necrosis are apparent as is sclerotic area *(arrowhead)* surrounding lucent necrotic focus. **C,** Section taken from border of sclerotic bone and fibrous tissue. Necrotic bone, not shown, was adjacent to fibrous tissue. (Hematoxylin and eosin; 40×.)

most iliac crest biopsies of patients with idiopathic avascular necrosis are abnormal, with many exhibiting osteomalacia.[417] They therefore propose that idiopathic avascular necrosis is attributable to a subchondral fatigue fracture occurring on a pathologic background.

When epiphyseal bone undergoing avascular necrosis is encountered, it usually exhibits changes of a continuum of necrosis and repair. The first radiologic abnormality is a subchondral lucent line paralleling the articular cartilage.[418] This represents a fracture of the trabecular bone in that location surrounded by an area of necrosis. The articular cartilage overlying the necrotic bone initially appears normal. However, it eventually becomes irregular and fissured. This area of dead bone consists of a wedge-shaped, radiolucent zone, usually in the anterosuperior portion of the femoral head, which contains acellular trabeculae and, eventually, granulation tissue.

The radiologic hallmark of avascular necrosis is increased density of the reparative zone abutting on and replacing necrotic bone. It is therefore the healing stage that is most often diagnostic of the lesion. With progression of the process, collapse of the femoral head occurs, resulting in disruption of the normal weight-bearing relationships of the hip and subsequent degenerative arthritis. It is important to appreciate that the irregularity of the femoral head, and hence the destructive changes in the hip joint, are in a large part caused by the exuberant reparative process in response to bone death. Moreover, it is the reactive synovitis that commonly causes the limitation of motion and pain that are the first symptoms attending avascular necrosis (Fig. 44-64).

Although ischemic necrosis occurs in numerous locations in the growing skeleton, as in the adult, the femoral head is most commonly involved. This childhood disorder, Legg-Calvé-Perthes disease, has many pathologic and radiologic similarities to idiopathic avascular necrosis of the adult femoral head. However, since it involves growing bone, some differences do exist.[419] The femoral capital epiphyseal plate is open in patients with Legg-Calvé-Perthes disease and perhaps is the primary site of involvement.[420] Histologically, the cartilage appears irregular and fragmented.[421] Ponseti and Cotton[420] postulate that since Legg-Calvé-Perthes disease is ischemic necrosis of the proximal femoral head, the destroyed growth plate restricts the blood supply to this portion of the bone. The prognosis of this disorder is dependent on the percentage of femoral head involved, the presence of metaphyseal cysts, which probably reflect extension of the necrotic process, and the degree of subluxation.[422]

MYOSITIS OSSIFICANS PROGRESSIVA

Although myositis ossificans progressiva is histologically identical to its localized counterpart, each is a distinct pathologic entity. Appearance of lesions of the disseminated disorder is commonly unassociated with trauma[423] representing primary abnormalities of the tissue in which the mineral is deposited.

Myositis ossificans progressiva becomes clinically manifest before the age of 20 and usually in the first few years of life.[423] Less than 10% of patients have a familial history of the disease.[423] Associated congenital abnormalities, particularly microdactyly or adactyly of the thumbs or great toes, are common.[423] The disorder affects the voluntary musculature, with early predisposition for the paravertebral and sternocleidomastoid areas.[423] The initial stage represents fibroblast proliferation and fibrosis,[424] followed by calcification and extraosseous ossification.[425] Ankylosing spondylitis is among the first manifestations of restrictions of motion with ultimate impairment of virtually all joints.[426] Premature death usually results from respiratory embarrassment[423, 427] or inanition from involvement of the muscles of mastication.[423]

Whether myositis ossificans progressiva is a primary myofibril disease or a manifestation of muscle involvement secondary to changes in associated fibrous tissues is unresolved. Smith and co-workers[425] report abnormalities of myofibril structure and adenosine triphosphate content in areas histologically exhibiting no evidence of the disease. Moreover, electromyographic changes in these areas resemble those of a myopathy.[425] McKusick,[362] however, suggests that the disease is attributable to exuberant fibroblast proliferation within fibrous tissue, resulting in compression and regeneration of adjacent myofibrils, which subsequently ossify.[426] He therefore offers "fibrodysplasia ossificans progressiva" as a more pathophysiologic name.

Some biochemical studies suggest that abnormal alkaline phosphatase activity plays an etiologic role in myositis ossificans progressiva.[425] However, Lutwak[423] proposes that the absence of a normally circulating inhibitor of calcification may be responsible for initiating the extraskeletal mineralization. In this regard, it is of interest that significant therapeutic success with this disease has been achieved by use of diphosphonates, which inhibit hydroxyapatite formation.[428]

OSTEOMYELITIS
Pyogenic osteomyelitis

Osteomyelitis, the generic term for bone infections, may be divided into cases of hematogenous origin, those from direct extension of an associated infection, and those related to peripheral vascular disease.[429] Prior to epiphyseal closure, most osteomyelitis is of hematogenous origin.[430] However, increasing numbers of patients over 30 years of age develop this complication.[429] The organisms most frequently involved are *Staphylococcus aureus* and gram-negative bacilli.[431] Sickle-cell anemia is characterized by a high frequency

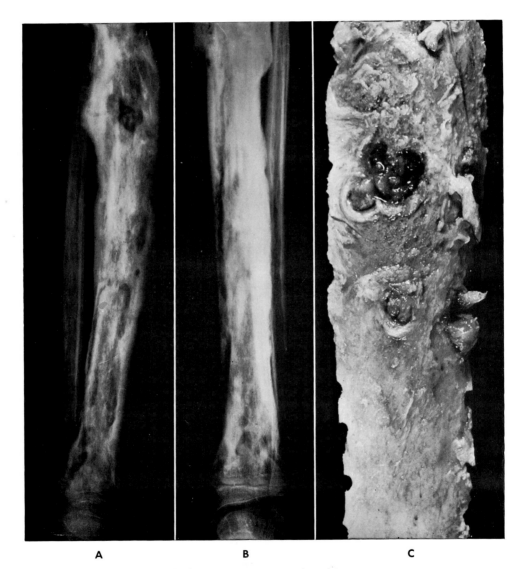

A   B   C

Fig. 44-65. Osteomyelitis of tibia. **A** and **B,** Lateral and anteroposterior roentgenograms showing destructive and proliferative changes of long-standing pyogenic osteomyelitis. Sequestrated segments of original tibial shaft visible through shadows cast by ossified granulation tissue (involucrum). **C,** Specimen of bone removed from tibia illustrated in **A** and **B.** Granulation tissue—filled sinus openings clearly evident on external surface of bone. These sinuses formed communications between skin surfaces and sequestrum enclosed in bony cavity.

of hematogenous osteomyelitis from *Salmonella*.[432] Although the lower extremities are the most common sites of osteomyelitis, there has recently been a significant increase in the incidence of vertebral disease, particularly complicating urinary tract infections or pelvic surgery.[429]

In adulthood, direct extension from soft-tissue infections, or more commonly, from operative intervention related to fracture repair, is responsible for the majority of skeletal infections.[429] Peripheral vascular disease, particularly among diabetics, is associated with osteomyelitis of the small bones of the hands and feet.[429]

The skeletal vascularity and its relation to the epiphyseal plate appear largely responsible for the varied locations of hematogenous osteomyelitis within a given bone.[433] In the first year of life, the metaphyseal branches of the nutrient artery penetrate the growth plate. Consequently, infantile osteomyelitis spreads to the epiphyseal bone, often with permanent growth plate damage. In childhood, these vessels turn back upon themselves proximal to the growth plate, whereupon they enter large vascular channels, resulting in relative stasis of blood flow. Since pooling of blood and the

presence of necrotic tissue are the common factors predisposing toward osteomyelitis,[430] it is in the metaphysis that childhood infections localize. After epiphyseal closure, the metaphyseal vessels cross into epiphyseal bone. Hence adult osteomyelitis localizes in a subchondral focus, often with extension into the joint space.

The rigid limits of the marrow cavity define the spread of purulent exudate. In the child, pus is forced through haversian and Volkmann's canals, breaking into the subperiosteal space at points of cortical attenuation. By dissecting between the periosteum and cortex, it tears the periosteal vessels, with the result of sequestration of the outer portion of the cortical bone. This focus of necrosis may persist as a nidus of reinfection. The separated periosteum exuberantly synthesizes new bone some distance from the cortex, forming the involucrum. It is the formation of sequestra and a large involucrum that largely distinguishes childhood from adult hematogenous osteomyelitis.

In the adult, pus may break through the epiphyseal cortical bone and enter the joint space. Because of pressure atrophy, focal trabecular osteoporosis occurs. Since the peri-

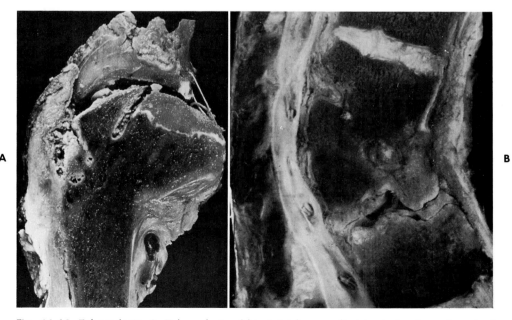

Fig. 44-66. Tuberculosis. **A,** Tuberculosis of hip joint has resulted in destruction of most of femoral caput and acetabular cup. Tuberculous osteomyelitis with extension of sinus tracts into adjacent articular capsule and soft tissues evident on left. **B,** Compression of vertebrae with angulation of spine has resulted from tuberculous osteomyelitis that affected three vertebral bodies and two intervertebral discs.

osteum is now rigidly attached, it is unusual for cortical sequestration and involucrum formation to occur in the mature skeleton. Repair is more likely to follow the classic pattern of removal of necrotic bone, new bone formation, and fibrosis. Hence the radiologic appearance of hematogenous osteomyelitis often exhibits both lytic and sclerotic features. Because of exuberant periosteal new bone formation, the process is frequently confused with malignant skeletal tumors, particularly Ewing's sarcoma.[434] In the many cases of osteomyelitis in which the x-ray films are not diagnostic, biopsy should be performed.

The clinical course and pathologic features of osteomyelitis have been drastically altered by the advent of antibiotics. Although one no longer encounters the gross deformities associated with the chronic process, persistent disease does exist, particularly when associated with sequestration.[430] Brodie's abscess, a lytic process surrounded by a sclerotic margin usually in metaphyseal bone, represents a persistent low-grade focus of chronic osteomyelitis that no longer contains purulent material[430,435] (Fig. 44-65).

Skeletal tuberculosis

After the virtual disappearance of transmission of bovine tuberculosis to man in Western society, the incidence of skeletal tuberculosis has sharply decreased.[429] However bone, now almost exclusively caused by *Mycobacterium tuberculosis*, remains the most common site of the extrapulmonary form of the disease.[436] Approximately 1% of patients with pulmonary tuberculosis develop skeletal complications.[436] Although half the patients with tuberculous osteomyelitis have, or have had, a pulmonary focus, an equal number give no such history.[429, 436]

The major sites of skeletal tuberculosis are the spine and hips.[429] The knees, ankles, and small bones of the hands and feet are also commonly involved.[429] Multiple skeletal sites are not unusual.[436] The basic lesion is often a combination of tuberculous osteomyelitis and arthritis.[436] The latter arises hematogenously or by extension from epiphyseal bone.[436] Tuberculous osteomyelitis usually does not produce the degree of bone destruction and repair common in its pyogenic counterpart.[436] Since the quantity of purulent exudate is not great, sequestration and involucrum formation are uncommon.[436] Histologically, the classic changes of tuberculosis are present, including caseation and granuloma formation (Fig. 44-66).

REFERENCES

1 Frost, H. M.: Tetracycline-based histological analysis of bone remodeling, Calcif. Tissue Res. **3**:211, 1969.
2 Frost, H. M.: Bone dynamics in metabolic bone disease, J. Bone Joint Surg. **48A**:1192, 1966.
3 Jowsey, J.: Age and species differences in bone, Cornell Vet. **58**(Suppl.):74, 1968.
4 Frost, H. M.: The bone dynamics of osteoporosis and osteomalacia, Springfield, Ill., 1966, Charles C Thomas, Publisher.
5 Hahn, T. J., Boisseau, V. C., and Avioli, L. V.: Effect of chronic corticosteroid administration on diaphyseal and metaphyseal bone mass, J. Clin. Endocrinol. Metab. **39**:274, 1974.

Composition and structure of bone
Cellular phase
 Osteoblasts

6 Martin, J. H., and Matthews, J. L.: Mitochondrial granules in chondrocytes, osteoblasts, and osteocytes. An ultrastructural and micro-incineration study, Clin. Orthop. **68**:273, 1970.
7 Pritchard, J. J.: The osteoblast. In Bourne, G. H., The biochemistry and physiology of bone. Vol. 1: Structure, ed. 2, New York, 1972, Academic Press, Inc., p. 191.
8 Holtrop, M. E., and Weinger, J. M.: Ultrastructural evidence for a transport system in bone. In Talmadge, R. V., and Munson, P. L., editors: Calcium, parathyroid hormone and the calcitonins, Int. Congr. Ser. No. 243, Amsterdam, 1972, Excerpta Medica Foundation, p. 365.
9 Matthews, J. L., and Martin, J. H.: Intracellular transport of calcium and its relationship to homeostasis and mineralization. An electron microscope study, Am. J. Med. **50:** 589, 1971.
10 Martin, B. F., and Jacoby, F.: Diffusion phenomenon complicating the histochemical reaction for alkaline phosphatase, J. Anat. **83:** 351, 1949.
11 Bevelander, G., and Johnson, P. L.: A histochemical study of the development of membrane bone, Anat. Rec. **108**:1, 1950.
12 Weisbrode, S. E., Capen, C. C., and Nagode, L. A.: Effects of parathyroid hormone on bone of thyroparathyroidectomized rats. An ultrastructural and enzymatic study, Am. J. Pathol. **75**:529, 1974.
13 Weisbrode, S. E., Capen, C. C., and Nagode, L. A.: Fine structural and enzymatic evaluation of bone in thyroparathyroidectomized rats receiving various levels of vitamin D, Lab. Invest. **28**:29, 1973.
14 Mills, B. G., Haroutinian, A. M., Holst, P., Bordier, P. J., and Tun-Chot, S.: Ultrastructural and cellular changes at the costochondral junction following in vivo treatment with calcitonin or calcium chloride in rabbits. In Taylor, S., editor: Endocrinology 1971. Proceedings of the third international symposium, London, 1972, Wm. Heinemann, p. 79.
15 Pritchard, J. J., and Ruzicka, A. J.: Comparison of fracture repair in the frog, lizard and rat, J. Anat. **84**:236, 1950.
16 Tonna, E. A., and Pentel, L.: Chondrogenic

cell formation via osteogenic cell progeny transformation, Lab. Invest. **27:**418, 1972.

17 Rasmussen, H., and Bordier, P.: The cellular basis of metabolic bone disease, New Eng. J. Med. **289:**25, 1973.

18 Kahn, A. J., and Simmons, D. J.: Investigation of cell lineage in bone using a chimera of chick and quail embryonic tissue, Nature **258:**325, 1975.

Osteocytes

19 Belanger, L. F.: Osteocytic osteolysis, Calcif. Tissue Res. **4:**1, 1969.

20 Remagen, W., Hohling, H. J., Hall, T., and Caesar, R.: Electron microscopical and microprobe observations on the cell sheath of stimulated osteocytes, Calcif. Tissue Res. **4:**60, 1969.

21 Young, R. W.: Cell proliferation and specialization during endochondral osteogenesis in young rats, J. Cell Biol. **14:**357, 1962.

22 Baylink, D., and Wergedal, J.: Bone formation and resorption by osteocytes. In Nichols, G. V., and Wasserman, R. H., editors: Cellular mechanisms for calcium transfer and homeostasis, New York, 1971, Academic Press, Inc., p. 257.

23 Bordier, P. J., Arnaud, C., Hawker, C., Tun-Chot, S., and Hioco, D.: Relationship between serum iPTH, osteoclastic and osteocytic bone resorptions and serum calcium in primary hyperparathyroidism and osteomalacia. In Frame, B., Parfitt, A. M., and Duncan, H., editors: Clinical aspects of metabolic bone diseases, Int. Congr. Ser. No. 270, Amsterdam, 1973, Excerpta Medica Foundation, p. 222.

24 Liu, C.-C., Baylink, D. J., and Wergedal, J.: Vitamin D–enhanced osteoclastic bone resorption at vascular canals, Endocrinology **95:**1011, 1974.

25 Doty, S. B., and Schofield, B. H.: Metabolic and structural changes within osteocytes of rat bone. In Talmadge, R. V., and Munson, P. L., editors: Calcium, parathyroid hormone and the calcitonins. Proceedings of the fourth parathyroid conference, Chapel Hill, N.C., 1971, Int. Congr. Ser. No. 243, Amsterdam, 1972, Excerpta Medica Foundation, p. 353.

26 Baud, C. A.: Structure et fonctions des ostéocytes dans les conditions normales et sous l'influence de l'extrait parathyroïdien, Schweiz. Med. Wochenschr. **98:**717, 1968.

Osteoclasts

27 Goldhaber, P.: Behavior of bone in tissue culture. In Sognnaes, R. F., editor: Calcification in biological systems, publ. 64, Washington, D.C., 1958, American Association for the Advancement of Science, p. 349.

28 Bonucci, E.: The organic-inorganic relationships in bone matrix undergoing osteoclastic resorption, Calcif. Tissue Res. **16:**13, 1974.

29 Mundy, G. R., Luben, R. A., Raisz, L. G., Oppenheim, J. J., and Buell, D. N.: Bone-resorbing activity in supernatants from lymphoid cell lines, New Eng. J. Med. **290:**867, 1974.

30 Horton, J. E., Raisz, L. G., Simmons, H. A., Oppenheim, J. J., and Mergenhagen, S. E.: Bone resorbing activity in supernatant fluid from cultured human peripheral blood leukocytes, Science **177:**793, 1972.

31 Tashjian, A. H., Jr., Voelkel, E. F., Levine, L., and Goldhaber, P.: Evidence that the bone resorption–stimulating factor produced by mouse fibrosarcoma cells is prostaglandin E$_2$. A A new model for the hypercalcemia of cancer, J. Exp. Med. **136:**1329, 1972.

32 Cameron, D. A.: The ultrastructure of bone. In Bourne, G. H., editor: The biochemistry and physiology of bone. Vol. 1: Structure, ed. 2, New York, 1972, Academic Press, Inc., p. 191.

33 Walker, D. G.: Enzymatic and electron microscopic analysis of isolated osteoclasts, Calcif. Tissue Res. **9:**296, 1972.

34 Minkin, C., and Jennings, J. M.: Carbonic anhydrase and bone remodeling: sulfonamide inhibition of bone resorption in organ culture, Science **176:**1031, 1972.

35 Nichols, G.: In vitro studies of bone resorptive mechanisms. In Mechanisms of hard tissue destruction, publ. 75, Washington, D.C., 1963, American Association for the Advancement of Science, p. 557.

Organic phase

36 Glimcher, M. J., and Krane, S. M.: The organization and structure of bone, and the mechanism of calcification. In Gould, B. S., editor: Treatise on collagen. Vol. 2, Biology of collagen, New York, 1968, Academic Press, Inc., p. 67.

37 Oldroyd, D., and Herring, G. M.: A method for the study of bone microsubstances by using collagenase, Biochem. J. **104:**20P, 1967.

38 Haddad, J. G., Couranz, S., and Avioli, L. V.: Nondialyzable urinary hydroxyproline as an index for bone collagen formation, J. Clin. Endocrinol. Metab. **30:**282, 1970.

39 Herring, G. M.: The organic matrix of bone. In Bourne, G. H., editor: The biochemistry and physiology of bone. Vol. 1: Structure, ed. 2, New York, 1972, Academic Press, Inc., p. 127.

40 Hjertquist, S. O., and Vejlens, L.: The glycosaminoglycans of dog compact bone and epiphyseal cartilage in the normal state and in experimental hyperparathyroidism, Calcif. Tissue Res. **2:**314, 1968.

41 Gelman, R. A., and Blackwell, J.: Interaction between collagen and chondroitin-6-sulfate, Connect. Tissue Res. **2:**31, 1973.

42 Irving, J. T., and Wuthier, R. E.: Histochemistry and biochemistry of calcification with special reference to the role of lipids, Clin. Orthop. **56:**237, 1968.

Mineral phase

43 Luben, R. A., Sherman, J. K., and Wadkins, C. L.: Studies of the mechanisms of biological calcification. IV. Ultrastructural analysis of calcifying tendon matrix, Calcif. Tissue Res. **11:**39, 1973.

44 Posner, A. S.: Bone mineral on the molecular level, Fed. Proc. **32:**1933, 1973.

45 Matthews, J. L., Martin, J. H., Kennedy, J. W., III, and Collins, E. J.: An ultrastructural study of calcium· and phosphate deposition

and exchange in tissues. Hard tissue growth and repair. Ciba Foundation Symposium II (new series), Amsterdam, 1973, Excerpta Medica Foundation, p. 187.

46 Bonnucci, E.: The locus of initial calcifications in cartilage and bone, Clin. Orthop. **78**:108, 1971.

47 Avioli, L. V.: Collagen metabolism, uremia and bone, Kidney Int. **4**:105, 1973.

48 Wuthier, R. E., Bisaz, S., Russell, R. G. G., and Fleisch, H.: Relationship between pyrophosphate amorphous calcium phosphate and other factors in the sequence of calcification in vivo, Calcif. Tissue Res. **10**:198, 1972.

Skeletal development
Endochondral ossification

49 Brighton, C. T., and Heppenstall, R. B.: Oxygen tension in zones of the epiphyseal plate, the metaphysis and diaphysis, J. Bone Joint Surg. **53A**:719, 1971.

Repair

50 Tomna, E. A., and Cronkite, E. P.: Changes in the skeletal cell proliferative response to trauma concomitant with aging, J. Bone Joint Surg. **44A**:1557, 1962.

51 Bisgard, J. D.: Longitudinal overgrowth of large bones with special reference to fractures, Surg. Gynecol. Obstet. **62**:823, 1936.

52 Bassett, C. A. L., and Hermann, I.: Influence of oxygen concentration and mechanical factors on differentiation of connective tissues in vitro, Nature **190**:460, 1961.

53 Ham, A. W., and Harris, W. R.: Repair and transplantation of bone. In Bourne, G. H., editor: The biochemistry and physiology of bone. Vol. III: Development and growth, ed. 2, New York, 1971, Academic Press, Inc., p. 337.

54 Bassett, C. A. L., Pawluk, R. J., and Pilla, A. A.: Augmentation of bone repair by indirectively coupled electromagnetic fields, Science **184**:575, 1974.

Disorders of remodeling
Morphologic methods of diagnosis

55 Merz, W. A., and Schenk, R. K.: Quantitative structural analysis of human cancellous bone, Acta Anat. **75**:54, 1970.

56 Courpron, P., Meunier, P., Vignon, G., Edouard, C., Bernard, J., and Thomas, J. D.: Données histologiques quantitatives sur le vieillissement osseux humain, Lyon Med. **226**:755, 1971.

57 Bordier, P. J., and Tun-Chot, S.: Quantitative histology of metabolic bone disease, Clin. Endocrinol. Metabol. **1**:197, 1972.

58 Teitelbaum, S. L., Bone, J. M., Stein, P. M., Gilden, J. J., Bates, M., Boisseau V. C., and Avioli, L. V.: Calcifediol in chronic renal insufficiency, J.A.M.A. **235**:164, 1976.

59 Hitt, O., Jaworski, Z. F., Shimizu, A. G., and Frost, H. M.: Tissue level bone formation rates in chronic renal failure measured by means of tetracycline bone labeling, Can. J. Physiol. Pharmacol. **48**:824, 1970.

60 Jaworski, Z. F. G., Lok, E., and Wellington, J. L.: Impaired osteoclastic function and linear bone erosion rate in secondary hyperparathyroidism associated with chronic renal failure, Clin. Orthop. **107**:298, 1975.

61 Wilde, C. D., Jaworski, Z. F., Villanueva, A. R., and Frost, H. M.: Quantitative histological measurements of bone turnover in primary hyperparathyroidism, Calcif. Tissue Res. **12**:137, 1973.

62 Ibsen, K. H., and Urist, M. R.: The biochemistry and the physiology of the tetracyclines, with special reference to mineralized tissue, Clin. Orthop. **32**:143, 1964.

63 Frost, H. M.: Tetracycline labeling of bone and the zone of demarcation of osteoid seams, Can. J. Biochem. Pharmacol. **40**:485, 1962.

64 Rolle, G. K.: The distribution of calcium in normal and tetracycline modified bones of developing chick embryo, Calcif. Tissue Res. **3**:142, 1966.

65 Wergedal, J. E., and Baylink, D. J.: Electron microprobe measurements of bone mineralization rate in vivo, Am. J. Physiol. **226**:345, 1974.

66 Teitelbaum, S. L., Rosenberg, E. M., Bates, M. S., and Avioli, L. V.: The effects of phosphate and vitamin D therapy on osteopenic, hypophosphatemic osteomalacia of childhood, Clin. Orthop. **116**:38, 1976.

67 Avioli, L. V., and Teitelbaum, S. L.: The renal osteodystrophies. In Brenner, B. M., and Rector, F. C., editors: The kidney, Philadelphia, W. B. Saunders Co. (In press.)

68 Baylink, D., Stouffer, M., Wergedal, J., and Rich, C.: Formation, mineralization and resorption of bone in vitamin D–deficient rats, J. Clin. Invest. **49**:1122, 1970.

69 Steendijk, R., and Boyde, A.: Scanning electron microscopic observations on bone from patients with hypophosphatemic (vitamin D resistant) rickets, Calcif. Tissue Res. **11**:242, 1973.

70 Russell, J. E., Termine, J. D., and Avioli, L. V.: Abnormal bone maturation in the chronic uremic state, J. Clin. Invest. **52**:2848, 1973.

Physiologic effects of hormones, vitamins, enzymes, and inorganic compounds on bone with attendant dysfunctions
Parathyroid hormone

71 Chase, L. R., Fedak, S. A., and Aurbach, G. D.: Activation of skeletal adenyl cyclase by parathyroid hormone in vitro, Endocrinology **84**:761, 1969.

72 Chase, L. R., and Aurbach, G. D.: The effect of parathyroid hormone on the concentration of adenosine $3',5'$-monophosphate in skeletal tissue in vitro, J. Biol. Chem. **245**:1520, 1970.

73 Weisbrode, S. E., Capen, C. C., and Nagode, L. A.: Influence of parathyroid hormone on ultrastructural and enzymatic changes induced by vitamin D in bone of thyroparathyroidectomized rats, Lab. Invest. **30**:786, 1974.

74 Nichols, G., Jr., Flanagan, B., and Woods, J. H.: Parathyroid influence on bone biosynthesis mechanisms. In Gaillard, P. J., Talmadge, R. V., and Budz, A. M., editors: The parathyroid glands: ultrastructure, secretion and

function, Chicago, 1965, University of Chicago Press, p. 243.

Primary hyperparathyroidism

75 Purnell, D. C., Scholz, D. A., Smith, L. H., Sizemore, G. H., Black, B. M., Goldsmith, R. S., and Arnaud, C. D.: Treatment of primary hyperparathyroidism, Am. J. Med. **56**:800, 1974.

76 Purnell, D. C., Smith, L. H., Scholz, D. A., Elveback, L. R., and Arnaud, C. D.: Primary hyperparathyroidism: a prospective clinical study, Am. J. Med. **50**:670, 1971.

77 Gordon, G. S., Eisenberg, E., Loken, H. F., Gardner, B., and Hayashido, T.: Clinical endocrinology of parathyroid hormone excess, Recent Progr. Horm. Res. **18**:297, 1962.

78 Byers, P. D., and Smith, R.: Quantitative histology of bone in hyperparathyroidism. Its relation to clinical features, x-ray and biochemistry, Q. J. Med. **40**:471, 1971.

79 Preston, E. T.: Avulsion of both quadriceps tendons in hyperparathyroidism, J.A.M.A. **221**: 406, 1972.

80 Dalén, N., and Hjern, B.: Bone mineral contents in patients with primary hyperparathyroidism without radiological evidence of skeletal changes, Acta Endocrinol. **75**:297, 1974.

81 Forland, M., Strandjord, N. M., Paloyan, E., and Cox, A.: Bone density studies in primary hyperparathyroidism, Arch. Intern. Med. **122**: 236, 1968.

82 Genant, H. K., Baron, J. M., Straus, F. H., Paloyan, E., and Jowsey, J.: Osteosclerosis in primary hyperparathyroidism, Am. J. Med. **59**:104, 1975.

83 Bordier, P. J., Woodhouse, N. J. Y., Sigurdsson, G., and Joplin, G. F.: Osteoid mineralization defect in primary hyperparathyroidism, Clin. Endocrinol. **2**:377, 1973.

84 Clark, O. H., and Taylor, S.: Osteoclastoma of the jaw and multiple parathyroid tumors, Surg. Gynecol. Obstet. **135**:188, 1972.

85 Ehrig, U., and Wilson, D. R.: Fibrous dysplasia of bone and primary hyperparathyroidism, Ann. Intern. Med. **77**:234, 1972.

86 Merz, W. A., Olah, A. J., Schenk, R. K., Dambacher, M. A., Gunaga, J., and Haas, H. G.: Bone remodeling in primary hyperparathyroidism. Preoperative and postoperative studies, Isr. J. Med. Sci. **7**:494, 1971.

Ectopic hyperparathyroidism

87 Benson, R. C., Riggs, B. L., Pickard, B. M., and Arnaud, C. D.: Radioimmunoassay of parathyroid hormone in hypercalcemic patients with malignant disease, Am. J. Med. **56**:821, 1974.

88 Bender, R. A., and Hensen, H.: Hypercalcemia in bronchogenic carcinoma. A prospective study of 200 patients, Ann. Intern. Med. **80**:205, 1974.

89 King, W. W., Cox, C. E., and Boyce, W. H.: Pseudohyperparathyroidism and seminoma, J. Urol. **107**:809, 1972.

90 Scholz, D. A., Riggs, B. L., Purnell, D. C., Goldsmith, R. C., and Arnaud, C. D.: Ectopic hyperparathyroidism with renal calculi and subperiosteal bone resorption. Report of a case, Mayo Clin. Proc. **48**:124, 1973.

Hypoparathyroidism

91 Wergedal, J., Stauffer, M., Baylink, D., and Rich, C.: Inhibition of bone matrix formation, mineralization and resorption in thyroparathyroidectomized rats, J. Clin. Invest. **52**:1052, 1973.

92 Keil, L. C., Evans, J. W., and Prinz, J. A.: Effect of parathyroidectomy on bone growth and composition in the young rat, Growth **38**: 519, 1974.

93 Parfitt, A. M.: The spectrum of hypoparathyroidism, J. Clin. Endocrinol. Metab. **34**:152, 1972.

94 Rasmussen, H., and Bordier, P.: The physiological and cellular bases of metabolic bone disease, Baltimore, 1974, The Williams & Wilkins Co., p. 157.

95 Bronsky, D., Kushner, D. S., Dubin, A., and Snapper, I.: Idiopathic hypoparathyroidism and pseudohypoparathyroidism: Case reports and review of the literature, Medicine **37**:317, 1958.

96 Moses, A. M., Rao, K. J., Coulson, R., and Miller, M.: Parathyroid hormone deficiency with Albright's hereditary osteodystrophy, J. Clin. Endocrinol. Metab. **39**:496, 1974.

97 Jimenea, C. V., Frame, B., Chaykin, L. B., and Sigler, J. W.: Spondylitis of hypoparathyroidism, Clin. Orthop. **74**:84, 1971.

98 Avioli, L. V.: The therapeutic approach to hypoparathyroidism, Am. J. Med. **57**:34, 1974.

Calcitonin

99 Melvin, K. E. W., Tashjian, A. H., and Bordier, P.: The metabolic significance of calcitonin-secreting thyroid carcinoma. In Frame, B., Parfitt, A. M., and Duncan, H., editors: Clinical aspects of metabolic bone disease, Int. Congr. Ser. No. 270, Amsterdam, 1973, Excerpta Medica Foundation, p. 193.

100 Jowsey, J., Riggs, B. L., Goldsmith, R. S., Kelly, P. J., and Arnaud, C. D.: Effects of prolonged administration of porcine calcitonin in post-menopausal osteoporosis, J. Clin. Endocrinol. **33**:752, 1971.

101 Marx, S. J., Woodard, C. J., and Aurbach, G. D.: Calcitonin receptors of kidney and bone, Science **178**:999, 1972.

102 Harell, A., Binderman, I., and Rodan, G. A.: The effect of calcium concentration on calcium uptake of bone cells treated with thyrocalcitonin (TCT) hormone, Endocrinology **92**: 550, 1973.

103 Kallio, D. M., Garant, R. R., and Minkin, C.: Ultrastructural effects of calcitonin on osteoclasts in tissue culture, J. Ultrastruct. Res. **39**: 205, 1972.

104 Zichner, L.: The effect of calcitonin on bone cells in young rats. An electron microscopic study, Isr. J. Med. Sci. **7**:359, 1971.

105 Bordier, P., Hioco, D., and Tun-Chot, S.: Calcitonin: acute effects upon serum calcium, urinary hydroxyproline excretion and osteoclasts in man. In Taylor, S., and Foster, G.,

editors: Calcitonin, 1969, New York, 1970, James H. Heineman, Inc., p. 339.

106 Matthews, J. L., Martin, J. H., Collins, E. J., Kennedy, J. W., and Powell, E. L.: Immediate changes in the ultrastructure of bone cells following thyrocalcitonin administration. In Talmadge, R. V., and Munson, P. L., editors: Calcium, parathyroid hormone and the calcitonins, Int. Congr. Ser. No. 243, Amsterdam, 1972, Excerpta Medica Foundation, p. 375.

107 Baylink, D., Morey, E., and Rich, C.: Effect of calcitonin on the rates of bone formation and resorption in the rat, Endocrinology **84:** 261, 1969.

108 Krane, S. M., Harris, E. D., Singer, F. R., and Potts, J. T.: Acute effects of calcitonin on bone formation in man, Metabolism **22:**51, 1973.

109 Delling, G., Schafer, A., and Ziegler, R.: The effect of calcitonin on fracture healing and ectopic bone formation in the rat. In Taylor, S., and Foster, G., editors: Calcitonin 1969, New York, 1970, James H. Heineman, Inc., p. 175.

110 Marks, S. C., and Walker, D. G.: The role of the parafollicular cell of the thyroid gland in the pathogenesis of congenital osteopetrosis in mice, Am. J. Anat. **126:**299, 1969.

111 Krook, L., Lutwak, L., and McEntee, K.: Dietary calcium, ultimobronchial tumors and osteopetrosis in the bull. Syndrome of calcitonin excess? Am. J. Clin. Nutr. **22:**115, 1969.

112 Wase, A. W., Solewski, J., Rickes, E., and Seidenberg, J.: Action of thyrocalcitonin bone, Nature **214:**388, 1967.

113 Baud, C. A., DeSiebenthal, J., Langer, B., Tupling, M. R., and Mach, R. S.: The effects of prolonged administration of thyrocalcitonin in human senile osteoporosis. In Taylor, S., and Foster, G., editors: Calcitonin 1969, New York, 1970, James H. Heineman, Inc., p. 540.

114 Rasmussen, H., Wong, M., Bikle, D., and Goodman, D. B. P.: Hormonal control of the renal conversion of 25-hydroxycholecalciferol to 1,25-dihydroxycholecalciferol, J. Clin. Invest. **51:**2502, 1972.

115 Tashjian, A. H., Howland, B. G., Melvin, K. E. W., and Hill, C. S.: Immunoassay of human calcitonin. Clinical measurement, relation to serum calcium and studies in patients with medullary carcinoma, New Eng. J. Med. **283:** 890, 1970.

Growth hormone

116 Daughaday, W. H., and Kipnis, D. M.: The growth-promoting and anti-insulin actions of somatotropin, Recent Progr. Horm. Res. **22:** 49, 1966.

117 Urist, M. R.: Growth hormone and skeletal tissue metabolism. In Bourne, G. H., editor: The biochemistry and physiology of bone. Vol. II: Physiology and pathology, ed. 2, New York, 1972, Academic Press, Inc., p. 155.

118 Fidler, M. W., and Brook, C. G. D.: Slipped upper femoral epiphyses following treatment with human growth hormone, J. Bone Joint Surg. **56A:**1719, 1974.

119 Ramser, J. R., Frost, H., and Smith, R.: Tetracycline-based measurement of the tissue and cell dynamics in rib of a 25-year-old man with active acromegaly, Clin. Orthop. **49:**169, 1966.

120 Riggs, B. L., Randall, R. V., Wahner, H. W., Jowsey, J., Kelley, P. J., and Singh, M.: The nature of the metabolic bone disorder in acromegaly, J. Clin. Endocrinol. Metab. **34:** 911, 1972.

121 Harris, W. H., Heaney, R. P., Jowsey, J., Cockin, J., Akins, C., Graham, J., and Weinberg, E. H.: Growth hormone: the effect on skeletal renewal in the adult dog. I. Morphometric studies, Calcif. Tissue Res. **10:**1, 1972.

122 Harris, W. H., and Heaney, R. P.: Effect of growth hormone on skeletal mass in adult dogs, Nature **223:**403, 1969.

123 Henneman, P. H., Forbes, A. P., Moldawer, M., Dempsey, E. F., and Carroll, E. L.: Effects of human growth hormone in man, J. Clin. Invest. **39:**1223, 1960.

124 Bell, N. H., and Bartter, F. C.: Studies of ^{47}Ca metabolism in acromegaly, J. Clin. Endocrinol. **27:**178, 1967.

125 Doyle, F. H.: Radiology of the skeleton in endocrine disease, Proc. Roy. Soc. Med. **60:** 1131, 1967.

126 Eisenberg, E., and Gordon, G. S.: Skeletal dynamics in man measured by non-radioactive strontium, J. Clin. Invest. **40:**1809, 1961.

127 Grunt, G. A., and Reynolds, D. W.: Insulin, blood sugar and growth hormone levels in an anencephalic infant before and after intravenous administration of glucose, J. Pediatr. **76A:**112, 1970.

128 Scott, C. I.: The genetics of short stature. In Steinberg, A. G., and Bearn, A. B., editors: Progress in medical genetics, New York, 1972, Grune & Stratton, Inc., p. 243.

129 Heins, J. N., Garland, J. T., and Daughaday, W. H.: Incorporation of ^{35}S-sulfate into rat cartilage explants in vitro: effects of aging on responsiveness to stimulation by sulfation factor, Endocrinology **87:**688, 1970.

Thyroid hormone

130 Parfitt, A. M., and Dent, C. E.: Hyperthyroidism and hypercalcemia, Q. J. Med. **39:** 171, 1970.

131 Ray, R. D., Asling, C. W., Walker, D. G., Simpson, M. E., Li, C. H., and Evans, H. M.: Growth and differentiation of the skeleton in thyroidectomized-hypophysectomized rats treated with thyroxine, growth hormone, and the combination, J. Bone Joint Surg. **36A:**94, 1954.

132 Lekkerkerker, J. F. F., and Doorenbos, H.: The influence of thyroid hormone on calcium absorption from the gut in relation to urinary calcium excretion, Acta Endocrinol. **73:**672, 1973.

133 Meunier, P. J., Bianchi, G. S., Edouard, C. M., Bernard, J. C., Courpron, P., and Vignon, G. E.: Bony manifestations of thyrotoxicosis, Orthop. Clin. North Am. **3:**745, 1972.

134 Clerkin, E. P., Haas, H. G., Mintz, D. H., Meloni, C. R., and Canary, J. J.: Osteomalacia in thyrotoxicosis, Metabolism **13:**161, 1964.

135 Adams, P. H., Jowsey, J., Kelley, P. J., Riggs,

B. L., Kinney, V. R., and Jones, J. D.: Effects of hyperthyroidism on bone and mineral metabolism in man, Q. J. Med. 36:1, 1967.

136 Burkhart, J. M., and Jowsey, J.: Parathyroid and thyroid hormone in the development of immobilization osteoporosis, Endocrinology 81: 1053, 1967.

137 Bordier, P., Miravet, L., Matrajt, H., Hioco, D., and Ryckewaert, A.: Bone changes in adult patients with abnormal thyroid function (with special reference to ⁴⁵Ca kinetics and quantitative histology), Proc. Roy. Soc. Med. 60:1132, 1967.

138 Bouillon, R., and DeMoor, P.: Parathyroid function in patients with hyper- or hypothyroidism, J. Clin. Endocrinol. Metab. 38: 999, 1974.

139 Newman, R. J.: The effects of thyroid hormone on vitamin D–induced nephrocalcinosis, J. Pathol. 111:13, 1973.

140 Wilkins, L.: The diagnosis and treatment of endocrine disorders in childhood and adolescence, Springfield, Ill., 1950, Charles C Thomas, Publisher, p. 137.

141 Dearden, L. C., and Mosier, H. D.: Growth retardation and subsequent recovery of rat tibia, a histochemical, light and electron microscopic study. I. After propylthiouracil treatment, Growth 38:253, 1974.

142 Wilkin, L.: Epiphyseal dysgenesis associated with hypothyroidism, Am. J. Dis. Child. 61: 13, 1941.

143 Jowsey, J., and Detenbeck, L. C.: Importance of thyroid hormones in bone metabolism and calcium homeostasis, Endocrinology 85:87, 1969.

Adrenal corticosteroids

144 Ruder, H. J., Loriaux, D. L., and Lipsett, M. B.: Severe osteopenia in young adults associated with Cushing's syndrome due to micronodular adrenal disease, J. Clin. Endocrinol. Metab. 39:1138, 1974.

145 Sissons, H. A.: The osteoporosis of Cushing's syndrome, J. Bone Joint Surg. 38B:418, 1956.

146 Jee, W. S. S., Roberts, W. E., Park, H. Z., Julian, G., and Kramer, M.: Interrelated effects of glucocorticoid and parathyroid hormone upon bone remodeling. In Talmadge, R. V., and Munson, P. L., editors: Calcium, parathyroid hormone and the calcitonins, Amsterdam, 1972, Excerpta Medica Foundation, p. 430.

147 Klein, M., Villanueva, A. R., and Frost, H. M.: A quantitative histological study of rib from eighteen patients treated with adrenal cortical steroids, Acta Orthop. Scand. 35:171, 1965.

148 Epker, B. N.: Studies on bone turnover and balance in the rabbit. I. Effects of hydrocortisone, Clin. Orthop. 72:315, 1970.

149 Peck, W. A., Brandt, J., Miller, I.: Hydrocortisone-induced inhibition of protein synthesis and uridine incorporation in isolated bone cells in vitro, Proc. Natl. Acad. Sci. U.S.A. 57:1599, 1967.

150 Whitehouse, M. W., and Lash, J. W.: Effect of cortisone and related compounds on the biogenesis of cartilage, Nature 189:37, 1961.

151 Sisson, J. C., Kirchick, H., and Kothary, P.: Inhibition of glycosaminoglycans production

in retrobulbar fibroblast cultures by ethacrynic acid and hydrocortisone, J. Clin. Endocrinol. Metab. 38:777, 1974.

152 Hulth, A., and Westerborn, O.: Effect of cortisone on epiphyseal cartilage. A histologic and autoradiographic study, Virchows Arch. (Pathol. Anat.) 336:209, 1963.

153 Kimberg, D. V., Baerg, R. D., Gershon, E., and Graudusius, R. T.: Effect of cortisone treatment on the active transport of calcium by the small intestine, J. Clin. Invest. 50: 1309, 1971.

154 Laake, H.: The action of corticosteroids on the renal reabsorption of calcium, Acta Endocrinol. 34:60, 1960.

155 Eliel, L. P., Thomsen, C., and Chames, R.: Antagonism between parathyroid extract and adrenal cortical steroids in man, J. Clin. Endocrinol. 25:457, 1965.

156 Talmage, R. V., Park, H., and Jee, W.: Parathyroid hormone and thyrocalcitonin function in cortisol-treated rats, Endocrinology 86: 1080, 1970.

157 Raisz, L. G., Trummel, C. L., Wener, J. A., and Simmons, H.: Effect of glucocorticoids on bone resorption in tissue culture, Endocrinology 90:961, 1972.

158 Avioli, L. V., Berger, S. J., and Lee, S. W.: Effects of prednisone on vitamin D metabolism in man, J. Clin. Endocrinol. 28:1341, 1968.

159 Lukert, B. P., Stanbury, S. W., and Mawer, E. B.: Vitamin D and intestinal transport of calcium: effects of prednisone, Endocrinology 93:718, 1973.

160 Bernick, S., and Ershoff, B. H.: Histochemical study of bone in cortisone treated rats, J. Clin. Endocrinol. Metab. 72:231, 1963.

161 Duncan, H.: Bone histodynamic changes in the rheumatic diseases, Clin. Orthop. 49:124, 1966.

162 Sissons, H. A., and Hadfield, G. J.: The influence of cortisone on the structure and growth of bone, J. Anat. 89:69, 1955.

163 Maassen, A. P.: The effect of desoxycorticosterone acetate (Doca) on body-growth and ossification, Acta Endocrinol. 9:291, 1952.

164 Frantz, A. G., and Rabkin, M. T.: Human growth hormone. Clinical measurement, response to hypoglycemia and suppression by corticosteroids, New Eng. J. Med. 271:1375, 1964.

165 Bailey, C. C., and Komrowen, G. M.: Growth and skeletal maturation in congenital adrenal hyperplasia. Review of 20 cases, Arch. Dis. Child. 49:4, 1974.

166 Friedman, M., and Strang, L. B.: Effect of long-term corticosteroids and corticotrophin on the growth of children, Lancet 1:568, 1966.

167 Iammaccone, A., Gabrilove, J. L., Brahms, S. A., and Soffer, L. J.: Osteoporosis in Cushing's syndrome, Ann. Intern. Med. 52:570, 1960.

Senile osteopenia

168 Garn, S. M., Rohmann, C. G., and Wagner, B.: Bone loss as a general phenomenon in man, Fed. Proc. 6:1729, 1967.

169 Trotter, M., Bromar, G. E., and Peterson, R. R.: Densities of bones of white and Negro skeletons, J. Bone Joint Surg. 42A:50, 1960.

170 Nordin, B. E. C.: Clinical significance and pathogenesis of osteoporosis, Br. Med. J. 1: 571, 1971.

171 Nordin, B. E. C., Young, M. M., Bulusu, L., and Horsman, A.: Osteoporosis reexamined. In Barzel, U. S., editor: Osteoporosis, New York, 1970, Grune & Stratton, Inc., p. 47.

172 Albright, F., Bloomberg, E., and Smith, P. H.: Post-menopausal osteoporosis, Trans. Assoc. Am. Physicians 55:298, 1940.

173 Heaney, R. P., and Whedon, G. D.: Radiocalcium studies of bone formation rate in human metabolic bone disease, J. Clin. Endocrinol. 18:1246, 1958.

174 Teitelbaum, S. L., Rosenberg, E. M., Richardson, C. A., and Avioli, L. V.: Histological studies of bone from normocalcemic postmenopausal osteoporotic patients with increased circulating parathyroid hormone, J. Clin. Endocrinol. Metab. 42:537, 1976.

175 Jowsey, J.: Age changes in human bone, Clin. Orthop. 17:210, 1960.

176 Jowsey, J., and Raisz, L. G.: Experimental osteoporosis and parathyroid activity, Endocrinology 82:384, 1968.

177 Avioli, L. V., McDonald, J. E., and Lee, S. W.: The influence of age on the intestinal absorption of ^{47}Ca in women and its relation to ^{47}Ca absorption in post-menopausal osteoporosis, J. Clin. Invest. 44:1960, 1965.

178 Davies, D. F., and Shock, N. W.: Age related changes in glomerular filtration rate, effective renal plasma flow, and tubular excretory capacity in adult males, J. Clin. Invest. 29: 496, 1950.

179 Barzel, U. S.: The effect of excessive acid feeding on bone, Calcif. Tissue Res. 4:94, 1969.

180 Gershon-Cohen, J., and Jowsey, J.: The relationship of dietary calcium to osteoporosis, Metabolism 13:221, 1964.

181 Jowsey, J., and Balasubramaniam, P.: Effect of phosphate supplements on soft tissue calcification and bone turnover, Clin. Sci. 42:289, 1972.

182 Kelly, P. J., Jowsey, J., Riggs, B. L., and Elveback, L. R.: Relationship between serum phosphate concentration and bone resorption in osteoporosis, J. Lab. Clin. Med. 69:110, 1967.

183 Corless, D., Beer, M., Boucher, B. J., Gupta, S. P., and Cohen, R. D.: Vitamin D status in long stay geriatric patients, Lancet 2:1404, 1975.

184 Johnson, K. A., Riggs, B. L., Kelly, P. J., and Jowsey, J.: Osteoid tissue in normal and osteoporotic individuals, J. Clin. Endocrinol. Metab. 33:745, 1971.

185 Jenkins, D. H. R., Roberts, J. G., Webster, D., and Williams, E. O.: Osteomalacia in elderly patients with fracture of the femoral neck, J. Bone Joint Surg. 55B:575, 1973.

186 Aaron, J. E., Gallagher, J. C., Anderson, J., Stasiak, L., Longton, E. B., Nordin, B. E. C., and Nicholson, M.: Frequency of osteomalacia and osteoporosis in fractures of the proximal femur, Lancet 1:785, 1974.

187 Riggs, B. L., Jowsey, J., Goldsmith, R. S., Kelly, P. J., Hoffman, D. L., and Arnaud, C. D.: Short and long term effects of estrogen and synthetic anabolic hormone in post-menopausal osteoporosis, J. Clin. Invest. 51: 1659, 1972.

188 Nutik, G., and Cruess, R. L.: Estrogen receptors in bone. An evaluation of the uptake of estrogen into bone cells, Proc. Soc. Exp. Biol. Med. 146:265, 1974.

189 Smith, D. M., Khairi, M. R. A., and Johnston, C. C.: The loss of bone mineral with aging and its relationship to risk of fracture, J. Clin. Invest. 56:311, 1975.

190 Iskrant, A. P., and Smith, R. W., Jr.: Osteoporosis in women 45 years and over related to subsequent fracture, Public Health Rep. 84:33, 1969.

191 Newton-John, H. F., and Morgan, D. B.: The loss of bone with age, osteoporosis and fractures, Clin. Orthop. 71:229, 1970.

192 Stevens, J., Freeman, P. A., Nordin, B. E. C., and Barnett, E.: The incidence of osteoporosis in patients with femoral neck fracture, J. Bone Joint Surg. 44B:520, 1962.

193 Alhava, E. M., and Puittinen, S.: Fractures of the upper end of the femur as an index of senile osteoporosis in Finland, Ann. Clin. Res. 5:398, 1973.

Ovarian dysgenesis

194 Preger, L., Steinbach, H. L., Moskowitz, P., Scully, A. L., and Goldberg, M. B.: Roentgenographic abnormalities in phenotypic females with gonadal dysgenesis, Am. J. Roentgenol. 104:899, 1968.

195 Finby, N., and Archibald, R. M.: Skeletal abnormalities associated with gonadal dysgenesis, Am. J. Roentgenol. 89:1222, 1963.

196 Brown, D. M., Jowsey, J., and Bradford, D. S.: Osteoporosis in ovarian dysgenesis, J. Pediatr. 84:816, 1974.

197 Garn, S. M., Poznanski, A. K., and Nagy, J. M.: Bone measurement in the differential diagnosis of osteopenia and osteoporosis, Radiology 100:509, 1971.

Vitamin D

198 DeLuca, H. F.: Vitamin D—1973, Am. J. Med. 57:1, 1974.

199 DeLuca, H. F.: The kidney as an endocrine organ involved in the function of vitamin D, Am. J. Med. 58:39, 1975.

200 Bhattacharyya, M. H., and DeLuca, H. F.: The regulation of rat liver calciferol-25-hydroxylase, J. Biol. Chem. 268:2969, 1973.

201 Fraser, D. R., and Kodicek, E.: Unique biosynthesis by kidney of a biologically active vitamin D metabolite, Nature 228:764, 1970.

202 Haddad, J. G., and Chyu, K. J.: Competitive protein-binding radioassay for 25-hydroxycholecalciferol, J. Clin. Endocrinol. 33:992, 1972.

203 Haddad, J. G., and Stamp, T. C. B.: Circulating 25-hydroxyvitamin D in man, Am. J. Med. 57:57, 1974.

204 Aaron, J. E., Gallagher, J. C., and Nordin, B. E. C.: Seasonal variation of histological osteomalacia in femoral neck fractures, Lancet 2:84, 1974.

205 Teitelbaum, S. L.: Histological effects of vitamin D and its analogs on bone, Am. J. Clin. Nutr. 29:1300, 1976.

206 Eisenstein, R., Sorgente, N., Arsenis, C., and Kuettner, K. E.: Vitamin D effects on tissue and serum lysozyme, Arch. Pathol. **94**:479, 1972.

207 Carlsson, A.: Tracer experiments on the effect of vitamin D on the skeletal metabolism of calcium and phosphorus, Acta Physiol. Scand. **26**:212, 1952.

208 Omdahl, J. L., and DeLuca, H. F.: Regulation of vitamin D metabolism and function, Physiol. Rev. **53**:327, 1973.

209 Reynolds, J. J., Holnick, M. F., and DeLuca, H. F.: The role of vitamin D metabolites in bone resorption, Calcif. Tissue Res. **12**:295, 1973.

Vitamin D deficiency

210 Holmes, A. M., Enoch, B. A., Taylor, J. L., and Jones, M. E.: Occult rickets and osteomalacia amongst the Asian immigrant population, Q. J. Med. **42**:125, 1973.

211 Jaffe, B. I., Hocking, W. H. L., Seftel, H. C., and Hartdegen, R. G.: Parathyroid-hormone concentrations in nutritional rickets, Clin. Sci. Mol. Med. **42**:113, 1972.

212 Bordier, Ph., Matrajt, H., Hioco, D., Hepner, G. W., Thompson, G. R., and Booth, C. C.: Subclinical vitamin D deficiency following gastric surgery, Lancet **1**:437, 1968.

213 Garrick, R., Ireland, A. W., and Posen, S.: Bone abnormalities after gastric surgery, Ann. Intern. Med. **75**:221, 1971.

214 Eddy, R. L.: Metabolic bone disease after gastric surgery, Am. J. Med. **50**:442, 1971.

215 Jowsey, J., Massry, S. G., Coburn, J. W., and Kleeman, C. R.: Microradiographic studies of bone in renal osteodystrophy, Arch. Intern. Med. **124**:539, 1969.

216 Melvin, K. E. W., Hepner, G. W., Bordier, P., Neale, G., and Joplin, G. F.: Calcium metabolism and bone pathology in adult coeliac disease, Q. J. Med. **39**:83, 1970.

Vitamin D–dependent rickets

217 Fraser, D., Kooh, S. W., King, H. P., Holick, M. F., Tanaka, Y., and DeLuca, H. F.: Pathogenesis of hereditary vitamin D–dependent rickets. An inborn error of vitamin D metabolism involving defective conversion of 25-hydroxyvitamin D to 1α,25-dihydroxyvitamin D, New Eng. J. Med. **289**:817, 1973.

Vitamin C

218 Peck, W. A., Birge, S. J., and Brandt, J.: Collagen synthesis by isolated bone cells: stimulation by ascorbic acid in vitro, Biochim. Biophys. Acta **142**:512, 1967.

219 Kivirikko, K. I., and Prockop, D. J.: Parietal purification and characterization of protocollagen lysine hydroxylase from chick embryos, Biochim. Biophys. Acta **258**:366, 1972.

220 Fernández-Madrid, F.: Collagen biosynthesis. A review, Clin. Orthop. **68**:163, 1970.

221 Follis, R. H.: Histochemical studies on cartilage and bone. II. Ascorbic acid deficiency, Bull. Johns Hopkins Hosp., **89**:9, 1951.

222 Bourne, G. H.: Some experiments on the possible relationship between vitamin C and calcification, J. Physiol. **102**:319, 1943.

223 Patnaik, B. K.: Age related studies on ascorbic acid metabolism, Gerontologia **17**:122, 1971.

224 Hertz, J.: Studies on the healing of fractures, with special references to the significance of the vitamin content of the diet, Acta Pathol. Microbiol. Scand. (Suppl.) **28**:134, 1936.

225 Murray, P. D. F., and Kodicek, E.: Bones, muscles and vitamin C. II. Partial deficiencies of vitamin C and mid-diaphyseal thickenings of the tibia and fibula in guinea pigs, J. Anat. **83**:205, 1949.

226 Murray, P. D. F., and Kodicek, E.: Bones, muscles and vitamin C. III. Repair of the effects of total deprivation of vitamin C at the proximal ends of tibia and fibula in guinea-pigs, J. Anat. **83**:285, 1949.

227 Hess, A. F.: Scurvy past and present, Philadelphia, 1920, J. B. Lippincott, p. 94.

228 Follis, R. H.: The pathology of nutritional diseases, Oxford, 1948, Blackwell Scientific Publications, Ltd.

229 Wolbach, S. B., and Maddock, C. L.: Cortisone and matrix formation in experimental scorbutus and repair therefrom, with contributions to the pathology of experimental scorbutus, Arch. Pathol. **53**:54, 1952.

230 Murray, P. D. F., and Kodicek, E.: Bones, muscles and vitamin C. I. The effects of a partial deficiency of vitamin C on the repair of bone and muscle in guinea-pigs, J. Anat. **83**:158, 1949.

231 Bourne, G. H.: The relative importance of periosteum and endosteum in bone healing and the relationship of vitamin C to their activities, Proc. Roy. Soc. Med. **37**:275, 1944.

232 Hill, C. R., and Bourne, G. H.: Histochemical changes in organs and tissues on scorbutic guinea-pigs, Br. J. Nutr. **12**:237, 1958.

233 Thornton, P. A.: Influence of exogenous ascorbic acid on calcium and phosphorus metabolism in the chick, J. Nutr. **100**:1479, 1970.

Vitamin A

234 Caffey, J.: Chronic poisoning due to excess of vitamin A. Description of the clinical and roentgen manifestations in seven infants and young children, Am. J. Roentgenol. **65**:12, 1951.

235 Rodahl, K.: Toxicity of polar bear liver, Nature **164**:530, 1949.

236 Barnicot, N. A.: The local action of vitamin A on bone, J. Anat. **84**:374, 1950.

237 Bélanger, L. F., and Clark, I.: Alpharadiographic and histological observations on the skeletal effects of hypervitaminosis A and D in the rat, Anat. Rec. **158**:443, 1967.

238 Wolbach, S. B.: Vitamin A deficiency and excess in relation to skeletal growth, J. Bone Joint Surg. **29**:171, 1947.

239 Persson, B., Tunell, R., and Ekengren, K.: Chronic vitamin A intoxication during the first half year of life. Description of 5 cases, Acta Paediatr. Scand. **54**:49, 1965.

240 Frame, B., Jackson, C. E., Reynolds, W. A., and Umphrey, J. E.: Hypercalcemia and skeletal effects in chronic hypervitaminosis A, Ann. Intern. Med. **80**:44, 1974.

241 Fell, H. B., and Thomas, L.: Comparison of the effects of papain and vitamin A on carti-

lage. I. The effects on organ cultures of embryonic skeletal tissue, J. Exp. Med. **111**:719, 1960.

242 Pease, C. N.: Focal retardation and arrestment of growth of bones due to vitamin A intoxication, J.A.M.A. **182**:980, 1962.

243 Ruby, L. K., and Mital, M. A.: Skeletal deformities following chronic hypervitaminosis A. A case report, J. Bone Joint Surg. **56**:1283, 1974.

244 Gerber, A., Raab, A. P., and Sobel, A. E.: Vitamin A poisoning in adults with description of a case, Am. J. Med. **16**:729, 1954.

245 Mellanby, E.: Nutrition in relation to bone growth and the nervous system, Proc. Roy. Soc. London (Biol.) **132**:28, 1944.

246 Gerlings, P. G.: Clinical and histopathological investigations of the labyrinth in oxycephaly, Acta Otolaryngol. **35**:91, 1947.

Phosphorus

247 Feinblatt, J., Bélanger, L. F., and Rasmussen, H.: Effect of phosphate infusion on bone metabolism and parathyroid hormone action, Am. J. Physiol. **28**:1624, 1970.

248 Haddad, J. G., and Avioli, L. V.: Comparative effects of phosphate and thyrocalcitonin on skeletal turnover, Endocrinology **87**:1245, 1970.

249 Goldsmith, R. S., Woodhouse, C. F., Ingbar, S. H., and Segal, D.: Effect of phosphate supplements in patients with fractures, Lancet **1**:688, 1967.

250 Nollen, A., and Bijvuet, O.: The effect of phosphate on fracture healing in rabbits, Isr. J. Med. Sci. **7**:508, 1971.

251 Matthews, J. L., and Martin, J. H.: Intracellular calcium in connective tissue cells, Int. Congr. Ser. No. 229, Amsterdam, 1970, Excerpta Medica Foundation, p. 216.

252 Matthews, J. L.: Ultrastructure of calcifying tissues, Am. J. Anat. **129**:451, 1970.

253 Glimcher, M. J., and Krane, S. M.: The incorporation of radioactive inorganic orthophosphate as organic phosphate by collagen fibrils in vitro, Biochemistry **3**:195, 1964.

254 Rasmussen, H.: Ionic and hormonal control of calcium homeostasis, Am. J. Med. **50**:567, 1971.

255 Reiss, E., Canterbury, J. M., Bercovitz, M. A., and Kaplan, E. L.: The role of phosphate in the secretion of parathyroid hormone in man, J. Clin. Invest. **49**:2146, 1970.

256 Baylink, D., Wergedal, J., and Stouffer, M.: Formation, mineralization and resorption of bone in hypophosphatemic rats, J. Clin. Invest. **50**:2519, 1971.

257 Bingham, P. J., and Raisz, L. G.: Bone growth in organ culture: effects of phosphate and other nutrients on bone and cartilage, Calcif. Tissue Res. **14**:31, 1974.

258 Rasmussen, H., Feinblatt, J., Nagata, N., and Pechet, M.: Effect of ions on bone cell function, Fed. Proc. **29**:1170, 1970.

Hypophosphatemic (vitamin D–resistant) osteomalacia

259 Dent, C. E., and Harris, H.: Hereditary forms of rickets and osteomalacia, J. Bone Joint Surg. **38B**:204, 1956.

260 Williams, T. F., and Winters, R. W.: Familial (hereditary) vitamin D–resistant rickets with hypophosphatemia. In Stanbury, J. B., Wyngaarden, J. B., and Frederickson, D. S., editors: The metabolic basis of inherited disease, ed. 3, New York, 1972, McGraw-Hill Book Co., p. 1465.

261 Glorieux, F., and Scriver, C. R.: Loss of a parathyroid hormone–sensitive component of phosphate transport in X-linked hypophosphatemia, Science **175**:997, 1972.

262 Avioli, L. V., Williams, T. F., Lund, J., and DeLuca, H. F.: Metabolism of vitamin D_3-^3H in vitamin D–resistant rickets and familial hypophosphatemia, J. Clin. Invest. **46**:1907, 1967.

263 Short, E. M., Binder, H. J., and Rosenberg, L. E.: Familial hypophosphatemic rickets: defective transport of inorganic phosphate by intestinal mucosa, Science **179**:700-702, 1973.

264 Villanueva, A. R., Ilnicki, L., Frost, H. M., and Arnstein, R.: Measurement of bone formation rate in a case of familial hypophosphatemic vitamin D–resistant rickets, J. Lab. Clin. Med. **67**:973, 1966.

265 Hahn, T. J., Scharp, C. R., Halstead, L. R., Haddad, J. G., Karl, D. M., and Avioli, L. V.: Parathyroid hormone status and renal responsiveness in familial hypophosphatemic rickets, J. Clin. Endocrinol. Metab. **41**:926, 1975.

266 Frost, H. M.: A unique histological feature of vitamin D resistant rickets observed in four cases, Acta Orthop. Scand. **33**:220, 1963.

267 Engfeldt, B., Zetterström, R., and Winberg, T.: Primary vitamin-D resistant rickets. III. Biophysical studies of skeletal tissue, J. Bone Joint Surg. **38A**:1323, 1956.

268 Buss, R. O., and Frost, H. M.: The prevalence of halo volumes in familial vitamin D–resistant rickets, Calcif. Tissue Res. **7**:76, 1971.

269 Nagant de Deuxchaisnes, C., and Krane, S. M.: The treatment of adult phosphate diabetes and Fanconi syndrome with neutral sodium phosphate, Am. J. Med. **43**:508, 1967.

270 Steendijk, R., Nielsen, H. K. L., and Kraii, A.: Osteotomy, vitamin D and the metabolism of calcium and inorganic phosphate in vitamin D–resistant rickets and osteomalacia, Helv. Paediatr. Acta **6**:627, 1968.

271 Brickman, A. S., Coburn, J. W., Kurokowa, K., Bethune, J. E., Harrison, H. E., and Norman, A. W.: Actions of 1,25-hydroxycholecalciferol in patients with hypophosphatemic vitamin D–resistant rickets, New Eng. J. Med. **289**:495, 1973.

272 Wilson, D. R., York, S. E., Jaworski, Z. F., and Yendt, E. R.: Studies in hypophosphatemic vitamin D–refractory osteomalacia in adults. Oral phosphate supplements as an adjunct to therapy, Medicine **44**:99, 1965.

Alkaline phosphatase
Hypophosphatasia

273 Rathburn, J. C.: Hypophosphatasia. A new developmental abnormality, Am. J. Dis. Child. **75**:822, 1948.

274 Fraser, D.: Hypophosphatasia, Am. J. Med. **22**:730, 1957.

275 Bethune, J. E., and Dent, C. E.: Hypophos-

phatasia in the adult, Am. J. Med. 28:615, 1960.

276 McCance, R. A., Fairweather, D. V. I., Barrett, A. M., and Morrison, A. B.: Genetic, clinical, biochemical and pathological features of hypophosphatasia, Q. J. Med. 25:523, 1956.

277 Pimstone, B., Eisenberg, E., and Silverman, S.: Hypophosphatasia: genetic and dental studies, Ann. Intern. Med. 65:722, 1966.

278 Warshaw, J. B., Littlefield, J. W., Fishman, W. H., Inglis, N. R., and Stolback, L. L.: Serum alkaline phosphatase in hypophosphatasia, J. Clin. Invest. 50:2137, 1971.

279 Fraser, D., and Yendt, E. R.: Metabolic abnormalities in hypophosphatasia, Am. J. Dis. Child. 90:552, 1955.

280 Fraser, D., Yendt, E. R., and Christie, F. H. E.: Metabolic abnormalities in hypophosphatasia, Lancet 1:286, 1955.

Fluoride

281 Faccini, J. M.: Fluoride and bone, Calcif. Tissue Res. 3:1, 1969.

282 Teotia, S. P. S., and Teotia, M.: Secondary hyperparathyroidism in patients with endemic skeletal fluorosis, Br. Med. J. 1:637, 1973.

283 Azar, H. A., Nucho, C. K., Bayyuk, S. Z., and Bayyuk, W. B.: Skeletal fluorosis due to chronic fluoride intoxication. Cases from an endemic area of fluorosis in the region of the Persian Gulf, Ann. Intern. Med. 55:193, 1961.

284 Faccini, J. M., and Teotia, S. P. S.: Histopathological assessment of endemic skeletal fluorosis, Calcif. Tissue Res. 16:45, 1974.

285 Baylink, D. J., and Bernstein, D. S.: The effects of fluoride therapy on metabolic bone disease, Clin. Orthop. 55:51, 1967.

286 Eanes, E. D., Zipkin, I., Harper, R. A., and Posner, A. S.: Small-angle x-ray diffraction analysis of the effect of fluoride on human bone apatite, Arch. Oral Biol. 10:161, 1965.

287 Bélanger, L. F., Visek, W. J., Lotz, W. E., and Commar, C. L.: Rachitomimetic effects of fluoride feeding on the skeletal tissue of growing pigs, Am. J. Pathol. 34:25, 1958.

288 Ramberg, C. F., Phang, J. M., Mayer, G. P., Norberg, A. I., and Kornfeld, D. S.: Inhibition of calcium absorption and elevation of calcium removal rate from bone in fluoride treated calves, J. Nutr. 100:981, 1970.

289 Weatherell, J. A., and Weidmann, S. M.: The skeletal changes of chronic experimental fluorosis, J. Pathol. Bacteriol. 78:233, 1959.

290 Jowsey, J., Schenk, R. K., and Reutter, F. W.: Some results of the effect of fluoride on bone tissue in osteoporosis, J. Clin. Endocrinol. 28:869, 1968.

291 Spencer, G. R., Cohen, A. L., and Garner, G. E.: Effect of fluoride, calcium and phosphorus on periosteal surface, Calcif. Tissue Res. 15:111, 1974.

292 Cass, R. M., Croft, J. D., Perkins, P., Nye, W., Waterhouse, C., and Terry, R.: New bone formation in osteoporosis following treatment with sodium fluoride, Arch. Intern. Med. 118:111, 1966.

293 Epker, B. N.: A quantitative microscopic study of bone-remodeling and balance in a human with skeletal fluorosis, Clin. Orthop. 55:87, 1967.

294 Singer, L., Armstrong, W. D., Zipkin, I., and Frazier, P. D.: Chemical composition and structure of fluoritic bone, Clin. Orthop. 99:303, 1974.

295 Bernstein, D. S., Sadowsy, N., Hegsied, D. M., Guri, C. D., and Stare, F. J.: Prevalance of osteoporosis in high and low fluoride areas in North Dakota, J.A.M.A. 198:499, 1966.

296 Jowsey, J., Riggs, B. L., Kelly, P. J., and Hoffman, D. L.: Effect of combined therapy with sodium fluoride, vitamin D and calcium in osteoporosis, Am. J. Med. 53:43, 1972.

297 Franke, J., Rempel, H., and Franke, M.: Thirty years' experience with sodium fluoride therapy of osteoporosis, Acta. Orthop. Scand. 45:1, 1974.

298 Yamamoto, K., Wergedal, J. E., and Baylink, D. J.: Increased bone microhardness in fluoride treated rats, Calcif. Tissue Res. 15:45, 1974.

299 Riggins, R. S., Zeman, F., and Moon, D.: The effects of sodium fluoride on bone breaking strength, Calcif. Tissue Res. 14:283, 1974.

300 Weidmann, S. M., and Weatherell, J. A.: The uptake and distribution of fluoride in bones, P. Pathol. Bacteriol. 78:243, 1959.

Renal osteodystrophy

301 Ellis, H. A., and Peart, K. M.: Azotaemic renal osteodystrophy: a quantitative study on iliac bone, J. Clin. Pathol. 26:83, 1973.

302 Massry, S., Coburn, J. W., Popovitzer, M. M., Shinaberger, J. H., Maxwell, M. M., and Kleeman, C. R.: Secondary hyperparathyroidism in chronic renal failure. The clinical spectrum in uremia during hemodialysis and after renal transplantation, Arch. Intern. Med. 124:431, 1969.

303 Potts, J. J., Reitz, R. E., Deftos, L. J., Kaye, M. M., Richardson, J. A., Buckle, R. M., and Aurbach, G. D.: Secondary hyperparathyroidism in chronic renal disease, Arch. Intern. Med. 124:408, 1969.

304 Massry, S. G., Coburn, J. W., Lee, D. D. N., Jowsey, J., and Kleeman, C. R.: Skeletal resistance to parathyroid hormone in renal failure. Studies in 105 human subjects, Ann. Intern. Med. 78:357, 1973.

304a Bordier, P. J., Marie, P. J., and Arnaud, C. D.: Evolution of renal osteodystrophy: correlation of bone histomorphometry and serum mineral and immunoreactive parathyroid hormone values before and after treatment with calcium carbonate or 25-hydroxycholecalciferol, Kidney Int. 7:S102, 1975.

305 Villanueva, A. R., Jaworski, Z. F., Hitt, O., Sarnsethsiri, P., and Frost, H. M.: Cellular level bone resorption in chronic renal failure and primary hyperparathyroidism. A tetracycline-based evaluation, Calcif. Tissue Res. 20:288, 1970.

306 Ball, J., and Garner, A.: Mineralization of woven bone in osteomalacia, J. Pathol. Bacteriol. 91:563, 1966.

307 Lumb, G. A., Mawer, E. B., and Stanbury, S. W.: The apparent vitamin D resistance of chronic renal failure. A study of the physiology of vitamin D in man, Am. J. Med. 50:421, 1971.

308 Stanbury, S. W.: Bony complications of renal disease. In Black, D. A. K., editor: Renal disease, ed. 2, Philadelphia, 1967, F. A. Davis Co., p. 665.

309 Katz, A. I., Hampers, C. L., and Merrill, J. P.: Secondary hyperparathyroidism and renal osteodystrophy in chronic renal failure. Analysis of 195 patients with observations on the effects of chronic dialysis, kidney transplantation and sub-total parathyroidectomy, Medicine 48:333, 1969.

310 Pierides, A. M., Simpson, W., Stainsky, D., Alvarez-Ude, F., and Udall, P. R.: Avascular necrosis of bone following renal transplantation, Q. J. Med. 46:459, 1975.

311 Alfred, A. C., Jenkins, D., Groth, C. D., Schorr, W. S., Gecelter, L., and Ogden, D. A.: Resolution of hyperparathyroidism, renal osteodystrophy, and metastatic calcifications after renal homotransplantation, New Eng. J. Med. 279:1349, 1968.

Pseudohypoparathyroidism

312 Steinbach, H. L., and Young, D. A.: The roentgen appearance of pseudohypoparathyroidism (PH) and pseudo-pseudohypoparathyroidism (PPH). Differentiation from other syndromes associated with short metacarpals, metatarsals and phalanges, Am. J. Roentgenol. 97:49, 1966.

313 Mann, J. B., Alterman, S., and Hills, A. G.: Albright's hereditary osteodystrophy comprising pseudohypoparathyroidism and pseudo-pseudohypoparathyroidism, with a report of two cases representing the complete syndrome occurring in successive generations, Ann. Intern. Med. 56:315, 1962.

314 Lee, J. B., Tashjian, A. H., Streeto, J. M., and Frantz, A. G.: Familial pseudohypoparathyroidism. Role of parathyroid hormone and thyrocalcitonin, New Eng. J. Med. 279:1179, 1968.

315 Reinhart, R., Brickman, A. S., Kurokawa, K., Coburn, J. W., and Massry, S. G.: Studies in three generations of a kindred with pseudohypoparathyroidism, Clin. Res. 21:255, 1973.

316 Chase, L. R., Melson, G. L., and Aurbach, G. D.: Pseudohypoparathyroidism: defective excretion of 3'5'-AMP in response to parathyroid hormone, J. Clin. Invest. 48:1832, 1969.

317 Drezner, M., Neelon, F. A., and Lebovitz, H. E.: Pseudohypoparathyroidism type II: a possible defect in the reception of the cyclic AMP signal, New Eng. J. Med. 289:1056, 1973.

318 McDonald, K. M.: Responsiveness of bone to parathyroid extract in siblings with pseudohypoparathyroidism, Metabolism 21:521, 1972.

319 Rodriguez, H. J., Villarreal, H., Klahr, S., and Slatopolsky, E.: Pseudohypoparathyroidism type II. Restoration of normal renal responsiveness to parathyroid hormone by calcium administration, J. Clin. Endocrinol. Metab. 39:693, 1974.

320 Kolb, F. O., and Steinbach, H. L.: Pseudohypoparathyroidism with secondary hyperparathyroidism and osteitis fibrosa, J. Clin. Endocrinol. Metab. 22:59, 1962.

321 Stanescu, V., Bona, C., and Ionescu, U.: Histochemical and histoenzymological investigations of growing cartilage in pseudohypoparathyroidism, Acta Endocrinol. 60:433, 1969.

322 Marx, S. J., Hershman, J. M., and Aurbach, G. D.: Thyroid dysfunction in pseudohypoparathyroidism, J. Clin. Endocrinol. Metab. 33:822, 1971.

323 Suh, S. M., Kooh, S. W., Chan, A. M., and Fraser, D.: Pseudohypoparathyroidism: no improvement following total thyroidectomy, J. Clin. Endocrinol. Metab. 29:429, 1969.

324 Nusjnowitz, M. L., and Klein, M. H.: Pseudo-idiopathic hypoparathyroidism. Hypoparathyroidism with ineffective parathyroid hormone, Am. J. Med. 55:677, 1973.

325 Frame, B., Hanson, C. A., Frost, H. M., Block, M., and Arnstein, A. R.: Renal resistance to parathyroid hormone with osteitis fibrosa: "pseudohypohyperparathyroidism," Am. J. Med. 52:311, 1972.

Osteitis deformans (Paget's disease)

326 Paget, J.: On a form of chronic inflammation of bones (osteitis deformans), Trans. Med. Chir. Soc. London 60:37, 1877.

327 Schmorl, G.: Ueber Osteitis deformans Paget, Virchows Arch. (Pathol. Anat.) 283:694, 1932.

328 Collins, D. H.: Paget's disease of bone. Incidence and subclinical forms, Lancet 2:51, 1956.

329 Edeiken, J., DePalma, A. F., and Hodes, P. J.: Paget's disease: osteitis deformans, Clin. Orthop. 46:141, 1966.

330 Price, C. H. G.: The incidence of osteogenic sarcoma in south-west England, and its relationship to Paget's disease of bone, J. Bone Joint Surg. 44B:366, 1962.

331 Galbraith, H. J. B.: Familial Paget's disease of bone, Br. Med. J. 2:29, 1954.

332 Nagant de Deuxchaisnes, C., and Krane, S. M.: Paget's disease of bone: clinical and metabolic observations, Medicine 43:233, 1964.

333 Albright, F., Aub, J. C., and Bauer, W.: Hyperparathyroidism, a common and polymorphic condition, as illustrated by seventeen proven cases from one clinic, J.A.M.A. 102:1276, 1934.

334 Allen, M. L., and John, R. L.: Osteitis deformans (Paget's disease). Fissure fractures—their etiology and clinical significance, Am. J. Roentgenol. 38:109, 1937.

335 Harris, E. D., and Krane, S. M.: Paget's disease of bone, Bull. Rheum. Dis. 18:506, 1968.

336 Franck, W. A., Bress, N. M., Singer, E. R., and Krane, S. M.: Rheumatic manifestations of Paget's disease of bone, Am. J. Med. 56:592, 1974.

337 Edholm, O. G., Howarth, S., and McMichael, J.: Heart failure and bone blood flow in osteitis deformans, Clin. Sci. 5:249, 1945.

338 Rhodes, B. A., Greyson, N. D., Hamilton, C. R., White, R. I., Giargina, F. A., and Wagner, H. N.: Absence of anatomic arteriovenous shunts in Paget's disease of bone, New Eng. J. Med. 287:686, 1972.

339 Khairi, M. R. A., Wellman, H. N., Robb, J. A., and Johnston, C. C.: Paget's disease of bone (osteitis deformans): symptomatic lesions and bone scan, Ann. Intern. Med. 79:348, 1973.

340 Lindsay, J. R., and Lehman, R. H.: Histopathology of the temporal bone in advanced Paget's disease, Laryngoscope 79:213, 1969.

Immobilization osteoporosis

341 Hulley, S. B., Vogel, J. M., Donaldson, C. L., Bayers, J. H., Friedman, R. J., and Rosen, S. N.: The effect of supplemental oral phosphate on the bone mineral changes during prolonged bed rest, J. Clin. Invest. 50:2506, 1971.

342 Heaney, R. P.: Radiocalcium metabolism in disuse osteoporosis in man, Am. J. Med. 33: 188, 1962.

343 Nilsson, B. E. R.: Post-traumatic osteopenia. A quantitative study of the bone mineral mass in the femur following fracture of the tibia in man using americium-241 as a photon source, Acta. Orthop. Scand. 37:Suppl. 91:1, 1966.

344 Lutwak, L., Whedon, G. D., and LaChance, P. A.: Mineral electrolyte and nitrogen balance studies of the Gemini-VII fourteen-dog orbital space flight, J. Clin. Endocrinol. Metab. 29: 1140, 1969.

345 Stinchfield, A. J., Reidy, J. A., and Barr, J. S.: Prediction of unequal growth of lower extremities in anterior poliomyelitis, J. Bone Joint Surg. 31A:478, 1949.

346 Pennock, J. M., Kalu, D. N., Clark, M. B., Foster, G. V., and Doyle, F. H.: Hypoplasia of bone induced by immobilization, Br. J. Radiol. 45:641, 1972.

347 Hantman, D. A., Vogel, J. M., Donaldson, C. L., Friedman, R., Goldsmith, R. S., and Hulley, S. B.: Attempts to prevent disuse osteoporosis by treatment with calcitonin, longitudinal compression and supplementary calcium and phosphate, J. Clin. Endocrinol. Metab. 36:845, 1973.

348 Dequeker, J.: Periosteal and endosteal surface remodeling in pathologic conditions, Invest. Radiol. 6:260, 1971.

349 Minaire, P., Meunier, P., Edouard, C., Bernard, J., Courpron, P., and Bourret, J.: Quantitative histological data on disuse osteoporosis, Calcif. Tissue Res. 17:57, 1974.

Congenital disorders of modeling
Disorders of collagen formation
Osteogenesis imperfecta

350 Goldfarb, A. A., and Ford, D.: Osteogenesis imperfecta in consecutive siblings, J. Pediatr. 44:264, 1954.

351 Rieseman, R. F., and Yates, W. M.: Osteogenesis imperfecta: its incidence and manifestations in seven families, Arch. Intern. Med. 67:950, 1941.

352 Falvo, K. A., Root, L., and Bullough, P. G.: Osteogenesis imperfecta: clinical evaluation and management, J. Bone Joint Surg. 56A:783, 1974.

353 Francis, M. J. O., Smith, R., and MacMillan, D. C.: Polymeric collagen of skin in normal subjects and in patients with inherited connective tissue disorders, Clin. Sci. 44:429, 1973.

354 Falvo, K. A., and Bullough, P. G.: Osteogenesis imperfecta: a histometric analysis, J. Bone Joint Surg. 55A:275, 1973.

355 Villanueva, A. R., and Frost, H. M.: Bone formation in human osteogenesis imperfecta measured by tetracycline bone labeling, Acta. Orthop. Scand. 41:531, 1970.

356 Lancaster, G., Goldman, H., Scriver, C. R., Gold, R. J. M., and Wong, I.: Dominantly inherited osteogenesis imperfecta in man: an examination of collagen biosynthesis, Pediatr. Res. 9:83, 1975.

357 Blümcke, S., Niedorff, H. R., Thiel, H. J., and Langness, U.: Histochemical and fine structural studies on the cornea with osteogenesis imperfecta congenita, Virchows Arch. (Zellpathol.) 11:124, 1972.

358 Pettinen, R. P., Lichtenstein, J. R., Martin, G. R., and McKusick, V. A.: Abnormal collagen metabolism in cultured cells in osteogenesis imperfecta, Proc. Natl. Acad. Sci. U.S.A. 72:586, 1975.

359 Teitelbaum, S. L., Kraft, W. J., Lang, R., and Avioli, L. V.: Bone collagen aggregation abnormalities in osteogenesis imperfecta, Calcif. Tissue Res. 17:75, 1974.

Fibrogenesis imperfecta ossium

360 Baker, S. L., Dent, C. E., Friedman, M., and Watson, L.: Fibrogenesis imperfecta ossium, J. Bone Joint Surg. 48B:804, 1966.

361 Frame, B., Frost, H. M., Pak, C. Y. C., Reynolds, W., and Argen, R. J.: Fibrogenesis imperfecta ossium. A collagen defect causing osteomalacia, New Eng. J. Med. 285:769, 1971.

Disorders of ground substance and cartilage
Mucopolysaccharidoses

362 McKusick, V. A.: Heritable disorders of connective tissue, ed. 4, St. Louis, 1972, The C. V. Mosby Co., p. 521.

363 Fratantoni, J. C., Hall, C. W., and Heufeld, E. F.: Hurler and Hunter syndromes: mutual correction of the defect in cultured fibroblasts, Science 162:570, 1968.

364 Bach, G., Friedman, R., Weissmann, B., and Neufeld, E. F.: The defect in Hurler and Scheie syndromes: deficiency of α-L-iduronidase, Proc. Natl. Acad. Sci. 69:2048, 1972.

365 Dorfman, A., and Lorincz, A. E.: Occurrence of urinary acid mucopolysaccharides in the Hurler syndrome, Proc. Natl. Acad. Sci. U.S.A. 43:443, 1957.

366 Caffey, J.: Gargoylism (Hunter-Hurler disease, dysostosis multiplex, lipochondrodystrophy); prenatal and neonatal bone lesions and their early postnatal evolution, Am. J. Roentgenol. 67:715, 1952.

367 Lindsay, S., Reilly, W. A., Gotham, T. J., and Skahen, R.: Gargoylism: study of pathologic lesions and clinical review of twelve cases, Am. J. Dis. Child. 76:239, 1948.

368 Dawson, I. M. P.: The histology and histochemistry of gargoylism, J. Pathol. Bacteriol. 67:587, 1954.

369 Bona, C., Stanescu, V., Streja, D., and Ionescu, V.: Histochemical and histoenzymological study of tibial growing cartilage in Hurler's syndrome, Acta Histochem. 23:231, 1966.

370 Bona, C., Stanescu, V., and Streja, D.: Differential regional distribution of mucopolysaccharides in the human epiphyseal cartilage matrix in normal and pathological conditions, Virchows Arch. (Pathol. Anat.) 342:274, 1967.

371 Silberberg, R., Rimoin, D. L., Rosenthal, R. E., and Hasler, M. B.: Ultrastructure of cartilage in the Hurler and Sanfilippo syndromes, Arch. Pathol. 94:500, 1972.

372 Kaplan, D.: Classification of the mucopoly-

saccharidoses based on the pattern of mucopolysacchariduria, Am. J. Med. **47**:721, 1969.

373 Matalon, R., and Dorfman, A.: Sanfilippo A syndrome. Sulfamidase deficiency in cultured skin fibroblasts and liver, J. Clin. Invest. **54**: 907, 1974.

374 Kresse, H., and Neufeld, E. F.: The Sanfilippo A corrective factor, purification and mode of action, J. Biol. Chem. **247**:2164, 1972.

375 Sanfilippo, S. J., Yunis, J., and Worthen, H. G.: An unusual storage disease resembling the Hurler-Hunter syndrome, Am. J. Dis. Child. **104**:553 (abstr. no. 81), 1962.

376 Schenk, E. A., and Haggerty, J.: Morquio's disease. A radiologic and morphologic study, Pediatrics **34**:839, 1964.

377 Pedrini, V., Lenuzzi, L., and Zambotti, V.: Isolation and identification of keratosulfate in urine of patients affected by Morquio-Ullrich disease, Proc. Soc. Exp. Biol. Med. **110**:847, 1962.

378 Einhorn, N. H., Moore, J. R., and Rowntree, L. G.: Osteochondrodystrophia deformans (Morquio's disease). Observations at autopsy in one case, Am. J. Dis. Child. **72**:536, 1946.

379 Anderson, C. E., Crane, J. T., Harper, H. A., and Hunter, T. W.: Morquio's disease and dysplasia epiphysalis multiplex. A study of epiphyseal cartilage in seven cases, J. Bone Joint Surg. **44A**:295, 1962.

380 Zellwager, H., Ponseti, I. V., Pedrini, F. S., and von Noorden, G. K.: Morquio-Ullrich's disease. Report of two cases, J. Pediatr. **59**:549, 1961.

381 Sengel, A., Stoebner, P., and Juif, J.: Les chondrocytes de la maladie de Morquio. Vacuoles ergastoplasmiques à inclusions spécifiques, J. Microsc. **10**:33, 1971.

382 Maroteaux, P., Lévêque, B., Marie, J., and Lamy, M.: Une nouvelle dysostose avec élimination urinaire de chondroitine-sulfate B, Press. Méd. **71**:1848, 1963.

Achondroplasia

383 Nelson, M. A.: Spinal stenosis in achondroplasia, Proc. Roy. Soc. Med. **65**:1028, 1972.

384 Ponseti, I. V.: Skeletal growth in achondroplasia, J. Bone Joint Surg. **52A**:701, 1970.

385 Stanescu, V., Bona, C., and Ionescu, V.: The tibial growing cartilage biopsy in the study of growth disturbances, Acta Endocrinol. **64**:577, 1970.

386 Pedrini-Mille, A., and Pedrini, V.: Studies of human iliac crest cartilage. III. Protein polysaccharides in human achondroplasia, Calcif. Tissue Res. **8**:106, 1971.

387 Cooper, R. R., Ponseti, I. V., and Maynard, J. A.: Pseudoachondroplastic dwarfism. A rough-surfaced endoplasmic reticulum storage disorder, J. Bone Joint Surg. **55A**:475, 1973.

388 Rimoin, D. L., Hughs, G. N., Kaufman, R. L., Rosenthal, R. E., McAlister, W. H., and Silberberg, R.: Endochondral ossification in achondroplastic dwarfism, New Eng. J. Med. **283**: 728, 1970.

389 Rimoin, D. L., McAlister, W. A., Salidino, R. M., and Hall, J. G.: Histologic appearances of some types of congenital dwarfism, Progr. Pediatr. Radiol. **4**:68, 1973.

Osteopetrosis

390 Johnston, C. C., Lavy, N., Lord, T., Vellios, F., Merritt, A. D., and Deiss, W. P.: Osteopetrosis. A clinical, genetic, metabolic and morphologic study of the dominantly inherited, benign form, Medicine **47**:149, 1968.

391 Dent, C. E., Smellie, J. M., and Watson, L.: Studies in osteopetrosis, Arch. Dis. Child. **40**:7, 1965.

392 Frost, H. M., Villanueva, A. R., Jett, S., and Eyring, E.: Tetracycline-based analysis of bone remodeling osteopetrosis, Clin. Orthop. **65**:203, 1969.

393 Fraser, D., Kooh, S. W., Chan, A. M., Cherian, A. G.: Congenital osteopetrosis—a failure of normal resorptive mechanisms of bone, Calcif. Tissue Res. **2**(suppl.):52, 1968.

394 Verdy, M., Beaulieu, R., Demers, L., Sturtridge, W. C., Thomas, P., and Ashwini-Kumar, M.: Plasma calcitonin activity in a patient with thyroid medullary carcinoma and her children with osteopetrosis, J. Clin. Endocrinol. Metab. **32**:216, 1971.

395 Walker, D. G.: Osteopetrosis cured by temporary parabiosis, Science **180**:875, 1973.

396 Walker, D. G.: Congenital osteopetrosis in mice cured by parabiotic union with normal siblings, Endocrinology **91**:916, 1972.

397 Marks, S. C.: Pathogenesis of osteopetrosis in the ia rat: reduced bone resorption due to reduced osteoclast function, Am. J. Anat. **138**: 165, 1974.

398 Walker, D. G.: Experimental osteopetrosis, Clin. Orthop. **97**:158, 1973.

399 Schofield, B. H., Levin, L. S., and Doty, S. B.: Ultrastructure and lysosomal histochemistry of ia rat osteoclasts, Calcif. Tissue Res. **14**:153, 1974.

400 Rosen, J. F., and Haymovits, A.: Liver lysosomes in congenital osteopetrosis. A study of lysosomal function, calcitonin, parathyroid hormone and 3′,5′-adenosine monophosphate, J. Pediatr. **81**:518, 1972.

Avascular necrosis

401 Thompson, V. P., and Epstein, H. C.: Traumatic dislocation of the hip. A survey of two hundred and four cases covering a period of twenty-one years, J. Bone Joint Surg. **33A**:746, 1951.

402 Malka, S.: Idiopathic aseptic necrosis of the head of the femur in adults, Surg. Gynecol. Obstet. **123**:1057, 1966.

403 Boettcher, W. G., Bonfiglio, M., Hamilton, H. H., Sheets, R. F., and Smith, K.: Nontraumatic necrosis of the femoral head. Part I. Relation of altered hemostasis to etiology, J. Bone Joint Surg. **52A**:312, 1970.

404 Solomon, L.: Drug-induced arthropathy and necrosis of the femoral head, J. Bone Joint Surg. **55B**:246, 1973.

405 Herndon, J. H., and Aufranc, O. E.: Avascular necrosis of the femoral head in the adult. A review of its incidence in a variety of conditions, Clin. Orthop. **86**:43, 1972.

406 Amstutz, H. C., and Carey, E. J.: Skeletal manifestations and treatment of Gaucher's disease, J. Bone Joint Surg. **48A**:670, 1966.

407 Bergstein, J. M., Wiens, C., Fish, A. J.,

Vernier, R. L., and Michael, A.: Avascular necrosis of bone in systemic lupus erythematosis, J. Pediatr. 85:31, 1974.

408 Nachamie, B. A., and Dorfman, H. D.: Ischemic necrosis of bone in sickle cell trait, Mt. Sinai J. Med. N.Y. 41:527, 1974.

409 McCallum, R. I., and Walder, D. N.: Bone lesions in compressed air workers, J. Bone Joint Surg. 48B:207, 1966.

410 Hayashi, M., Murata, T., Ohki, I., and Inoue, S.: Assessment of the ischemia of the femoral head in idiopathic avascular necrosis. A preliminary report, Clin. Orthop. 110:317, 1975.

411 Jones, J. P., and Engleman, E. P.: Avascular necrosis of bone in alcoholism, Arthritis Rheum. 10:287, 1967.

412 Fisher, D. E., and Bickel, W. H.: Corticosteroid-induced avascular necrosis. A clinical study of seventy-seven patients, J. Bone Joint Surg. 53A:859, 1971.

413 Garden, R. S.: Malreduction and avascular necrosis in sub-capital fractures of the femur, J. Bone Joint Surg. 53B:183, 1971.

414 Suramo, I., Puranen, J., Heikkinen, E., and Vuorinen, P.: Disturbed patterns of venous drainage of the femoral neck in Perthes disease, J. Bone Joint Surg. 56B:448, 1974.

415 Chandler, F. A:. Coronary disease of the hip, J. Int. Coll. Surg. 11:34, 1948.

416 Jaffe, W. L., Epstein, M., Heyman, N., and Mankin, H. J.: The effect of cortisone on femoral and humeral heads in rabbits. An experimental study, Clin. Orthop. 82:221, 1972.

417 Laurent, J., Meunier, P., Courpron, P., Edouard, C., Bernard, J., and Vignon, G.: Recherches sur la pathogénie des necroses aseptiques de la tête fémorale, La Nouvelle Presse Médicale 2:1755, 1973.

418 Norman, A., and Bullough, P.: The radiolucent crescent line—an early diagnostic sign of avascular necrosis of the femoral head, Bull. Hosp. Joint Dis. 24:99, 1963.

419 Ferguson, A. B.: The pathology of Legg-Perthes disease and its comparison with aseptic necrosis, Clin. Orthop. 106:7, 1975.

420 Ponseti, I. V., and Cotton, R. L.: Legg-Calvé-Perthes disease—pathogenesis and evolution, J. Bone Joint Surg. 43A:261, 1961.

421 McKibben, B., and Ralis, Z.: Pathological changes in a case of Perthes disease, J. Bone Joint Surg. 56B:438, 1974.

422 Katz, J. F., and Siffert, R. S.: Capital necrosis, metaphyseal cyst and subluxation in coxa plana, Clin. Orthop. 106:75, 1975.

Myositis ossificans progressiva

423 Lutwak, L.: Myositis ossificans progressiva. Mineral, metabolic and radioactive calcium studies of the effects of hormones, Am. J. Med. 37:269, 1964.

424 Frame, B., Azad, N., Reynolds, W. A., and Saeed, S. M.: Polyostotic fibrous dysplasia and myositis ossificans progressiva. A report of coexistence, Am. J. Dis. Child. 124:120, 1972.

425 Smith, D. M., Zeman, W., Johnston, C. C., and Deiss, W. P.: Myositis ossificans progressiva. Case report with metabolic and histochemical studies, Metabolism 15:521, 1966.

426 Lockhart, J. D., and Burke, F. G.: Myositis ossificans progressiva. Report of a case treated with corticotropin (ACTH), Am. J. Dis. Child. 86:626, 1954.

427 Buhain, W. J., Rammohan, G., and Berger, H. W.: Pulmonary function in myositis ossificans progressiva, Am. Rev. Respir. Dis. 110:333, 1974.

428 Russell, R. G. G., Smith, R., Bishop, M. C., and Price, D. A.: Treatment of myositis ossificans progressiva with a diphosphonate, Lancet 1:10, 1972.

Osteomyelitis
Pyogenic osteomyelitis

429 Waldvogel, F. A., Medoff, G., and Swartz, M. W.: Osteomyelitis: a review of clinical features, therapeutic considerations and unusual aspects, New Eng. J. Med. 282:198, 260, 316, 1970.

430 Kahn, D. S., and Pritzker, K. P. H.: The pathophysiology of bone infection, Clin. Orthop. 96:12, 1973.

431 Kelley, P. J., Wilkowske, C. J., and Washington, J. A.: Comparison of gram-negative bacillary and staphylococcal osteomyelitis of the femur and tibia, Clin. Orthop. 96:70, 1973.

432 Curtiss, P. H.: Some uncommon forms of osteomyelitis, Clin. Orthop. 96:84, 1973.

433 Trueta, J.: The three types of acute haematogenous osteomyelitis, J. Bone Joint Surg. 41B:671, 1959.

434 Harris, N. H., and Kirkaldy-Willis, W. H.: Primary subacute pyogenic osteomyelitis, J. Bone Joint Surg. 47B:526, 1965.

435 Kandel, S. N., and Mankin, H. J.: Pyogenic abscess of the long bones in children, Clin. Orthop. 96:108, 1973.

Skeletal tuberculosis

436 Davidson, P. T., and Horowitz, I.: Skeletal tuberculosis. A review with patient presentations and discussion, Am. J. Med. 48:77, 1970.

45/Tumors and tumorlike conditions of bone

JUAN ROSAI

ETIOLOGY AND PREDISPOSING FACTORS

There are various circumstances and diseases that are seen associated with the appearance of bone neoplasms in a significant fashion. However, they account for only a minority of the cases even when considered as a group.

The possibility of *trauma* predisposing to the development of bone sarcoma has been suggested many times but never proved. Major trauma to the bone, such as fracture, surgery (particularly amputation), and exodontia, has no statistical relation with bone sarcoma. It is therefore difficult to believe that the relatively insignificant trauma that patients with bone tumors often cite could have possibly been the cause of the neoplasm.

It has been known for many years that various modalities of *ionizing radiation* can result in the appearance of bone sarcomas. One of the first demonstrations of this occurrence was the production by Lacassagne[63] of fibrosarcoma of the tibia in a rabbit 36 months after administration of radiations to an abscess near the bone. Osteosarcomas in laboratory animals can be induced with intraperitoneal injections of ^{45}Ca or ^{89}Sr.[49] It is interesting that the radioactive calcium produces sarcomas chiefly in the spine and pelvis, whereas the strontium induces sarcomas in the bones of the limb.[4] A large number of osteosarcomas have been seen after the use of thorium in the treatment of tuberculosis and ankylosing spondylitis.[100] Cases of bone sarcomas developing in apparent connection with the local administration of radiations for therapeutic purposes have been reported from several centers.[18,45] All bones in the skeletal system are susceptible to this complication. The average interval between the time of irradiation and the clinical appearance of the tumor is 9 years.[5]

In most reported cases, the dosis of radia-tion has been very high and the patient has received repeated courses. The practical hazard of radiation-induced osteosarcoma appears to be very remote and should not be a consideration in the selection of the best mode of treatment for a given lesion. The most spectacular series of radiation-induced bone sarcomas was the one reported by Martland and Humphries[70] (Fig. 45-1). The victims were young women employed in the painting of clock dials with luminous paint made of zinc sulfide and 1 part in 40,000 of radium, mesothorium (an isotope of radium), and radiothorium. It was the custom of the workers to moisten the bristles of the brush between their lips, and this led to the ingestion of a certain amount of radioactive material. Eighteen patients died of radium poisoning, five of whom had developed osteosarcoma.

It has been well documented that *Paget's disease* predisposes to the development of bone tumors, considerably more in men than in women. Osteosarcomas predominate, but chondrosarcomas, fibrosarcomas, and giant cell tumors have also been reported. The osteosarcoma developing in Paget's disease usually occurs in the areas in which the process is most advanced. In order of descending frequency, the bones involved by sarcoma are femur, humerus, pelvis, tibia, skull and facial bones, and scapula.[51] The prognosis for sarcoma arising in Paget's disease is extremely poor.

Fibrous dysplasia may also be complicated with bone sarcoma, although the incidence is very low. Most of the cases are of the polyostotic type.[97] The tumor is usually an osteosarcoma, although chondrosarcoma can also occur.[53]

Recently, an increasing number of malignant bone tumors has been reported at the site of bone infarcts, such as those seen in *caisson* workers. The microscopic types were malignant fibrous histiocytoma, fibrosarcoma, and osteosarcoma.[38,74]

Two polyostotic bone disorders, of either a

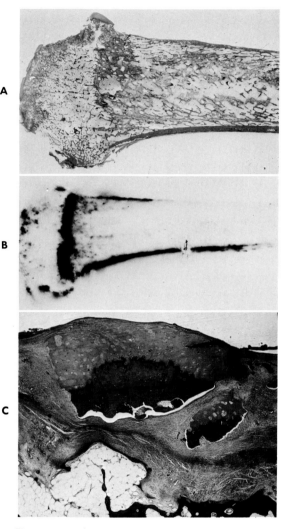

Fig. 45-1. Photographic representation of bone and cartilage changes caused by irradiation. Patient, 46-year-old woman, had worked as watch- and clock-dial painter for 3½ months when 16 years of age. Lower extremity was amputated because of sarcomatous change originating in diseased femur. Tumor was classified as fibrosarcoma. **A,** Large section of lower segment of femur showing necrosis. **B,** Autoradiogram made from section similar to specimen shown in **A.** Note evidence of intense radioactivity in region of metaphyseal end of diaphysis, which marks growth zone at time patient was exposed to radioactive material. **C,** As result of radiation injury, articular cartilage and subchondral bone have undergone necrosis and fragmentation.

neoplastic or developmental nature, are associated with an increased occurrence of chondrosarcoma; these are known as enchondromatosis and osteochondromatosis and are discussed in the section of chondroblastic (cartilage-forming) tumors.

Fraumeni[36] made the intriguing observation that youngsters under 18 years of age with osteosarcomas were significantly taller than those in a control group with nonosseous malignant tumors.

Osteosarcomas have been produced by viral inoculations into the chicken and mouse[34] and by local implantation of beryllium salts into rabbits.[108] There are several clinical and laboratory observations suggesting the possibility of a viral etiology for human osteosarcoma. The concurrent development of tumors in members of the same family implicates either genetic or infectious factors. This has been documented for osteosarcoma, chondrosarcoma, and Ewing's sarcoma.[44,92] Also in favor of this hypothesis is the observation of unusual clustering of sarcomas in a small community.[111] The possibility that human osteosarcomas may be produced by viruses is being seriously considered after the demonstration by immunofluorescence techniques of a high incidence of antibodies to osteosarcomas in the sera of patients with this disease and their close associates, which reacted with a common antigen or antigens in osteosarcomas.[76] This observation obviously suggests the association of an infectious agent with this neoplasm, which appears capable of infecting close associates of the patients.

Another experiment suggesting a viral etiology for human osteosarcoma is the one performed by Finkel and collaborators.[33] They were able to produce osteosarcomas, fibrosarcomas, and benign bone tumors in neonatal hamsters by injecting them with cell-free extracts of human osteosarcomas. These authors also demonstrated cross-reactivity between human osteosarcoma sera and hamster sarcomas.

Electron microscopy also lends some support to the viral hypothesis. Thin sections of human bone tumors and of pelleted extracts of these tumors have shown particles that could possibly be associated with viral DNA.[41]

The above-mentioned studies strongly suggest a relation between a viral infectious agent and human osteosarcoma. However, the fundamental question as to whether this agent is directly related to the tumor etiology or is an incidental passenger remains largely unanswered.

Table 45-1. Usual age and sex of patient and location and behavior of most common primary bone tumors and tumorlike lesions*†

Tumor or tumorlike lesion	Age (yr)	Sex M:F	Bones more commonly affected (in order of frequency)	Usual location within long bone	Behavior
Osteoma	40-50	2:1	Skull and facial bones	—	Benign
Osteoid osteoma	10-30	2:1	Femur, tibia, humerus, hands and feet, vertebrae, fibula	Cortex of metaphysis	Benign
Osteoblastoma	10-30	2:1	Vertebrae, tibia, femur, humerus, pelvis, ribs	Medulla of metaphysis	Benign
Osteosarcoma	10-25	3:2	Femur, tibia, humerus, pelvis, jaw, fibula	Medulla of metaphysis	Malignant; 20% 5-year survival rate
Juxtacortical (parosteal) osteosarcoma	30-60	1:1	Femur, tibia, humerus	Juxtacortical area of metaphysis	Malignant; 80% 5-year survival rate
Chondroma	10-40	1:1	Hands and feet, ribs, femur, humerus	Medulla of diaphysis	Benign
Osteochondroma	10-30	1:1	Femur, tibia, humerus, pelvis	Cortex of metaphysis	Benign
Chondroblastoma	10-25	2:1	Femur, humerus, tibia, feet, pelvis, scapula	Epiphysis, adjacent to cartilage plate	Practically always benign
Chondromyxoid fibroma	10-25	1:1	Tibia, femur, feet, pelvis	Metaphysis	Benign
Chondrosarcoma	30-60	3:1	Pelvis, ribs, femur, humerus, vertebrae	Central—medulla of diaphysis Peripheral—cortex or periosteum of metaphysis	Malignant; 5-year survival rate—low grade, 78%; moderate grade, 53%; high grade, 22%
Mesenchymal chondrosarcoma	20-60	1:1	Ribs, skull and jaw, vertebrae, pelvis, soft tissues	Medulla or cortex of diaphysis	Malignant; extremely poor prognosis
Giant cell tumor	20-40	4:5	Femur, tibia, radius	Epiphysis and metaphysis	Potentially malignant; 50% recur; 10% metastasize
Ewing's sarcoma	5-20	1:2	Femur, pelvis, tibia, humerus, ribs, fibula	Medulla of diaphysis or metaphysis	Highly malignant; 20%-30% 5-year survival rate in recent series
Malignant lymphoma, histiocytic (reticulum cell sarcoma) and mixed cell types	30-60	1:1	Femur, pelvis, vertebrae, tibia, humerus, jaw, skull, ribs	Medulla of diaphysis or metaphysis	Malignant; 22%-50% 5-year survival rate
Plasma cell myeloma	40-60	2:1	Vertebrae, pelvis, ribs, sternum, skull	Medulla of diaphysis, metaphysis, or epiphysis	Malignant; diffuse form uniformly fatal; localized form often controlled with radiation therapy
Hemangioma	20-50	1:1	Skull, vertebrae, jaw	Medulla	Benign
Desmoplastic fibroma	20-30	1:1	Humerus, tibia, pelvis, jaw, femur, scapula	Metaphysis	Benign
Fibrosarcoma	20-60	1:1	Femur, tibia, jaw, humerus	Medulla of metaphysis	Malignant; 28% 5-year survival rate

Chordoma	40-60	2 : 1	Sacrococcygeal, spheno-occipital, cervical vertebrae	—	Malignant; slow course; locally invasive; 48% distant metastases
Solitary bone cyst	10-20	3 : 1	Humerus, femur	Medulla of metaphysis	Benign
Aneurysmal bone cyst	10-20	1 : 1	Vertebrae, flat bones, femur, tibia	Metaphysis	Benign; sometimes secondary to another bone lesion
Metaphyseal fibrous defect	10-20	1 : 1	Tibia, femur, fibula	Metaphysis	Benign
Fibrous dysplasia	10-30	3 : 2	Ribs, femur, tibia, jaw, skull	Medulla of diaphysis or metaphysis	Locally aggressive; rarely complicated by sarcoma
Eosinophilic granuloma	5-15	3 : 2	Skull, jaw, humerus, rib, femur	Metaphysis or diaphysis	Benign

*It should be emphasized that these data correspond to the typical case and that they should not be taken in an absolute sense. Isolated exceptions to practically every one of these statements have occurred.

†From Ackerman, L. V., and Rosai, J.: Surgical pathology, ed. 5, St. Louis, 1974, The C. V. Mosby Co.

CLASSIFICATION AND DISTRIBUTION

The presence of a large variety of tissues within the skeletal system, the rarity of bone neoplasms and the uncertainty that still exists regarding their histogenesis have all contributed to the confusion in terminology and classifications that for many years have plagued this field of tumor pathology. Fortunately, a satisfactory degree of uniformity in the nomenclature has now been reached. The main contributions for these achievements have been the pioneering work of H. L. Jaffe,[55] the fascicle called "Tumors of Bone and Cartilage" of the *Atlas of Tumor Pathology* series (now in its second series)[101] and the manual by Schajowicz, Ackerman, and Sissons, published under the auspices of the World Health Organization as part of their *International Histological Classification of Tumours* series.[91]

The classification presented in this chapter is largely based on the latter work and is of histogenetic character. Tumors are classified according to the tissue or cell type from which they are presumed to arise, which in turn is mainly deduced from the tissue that the tumor cells are able to manufacture. Thus a bone tumor composed of cells that produce osteoid or bone is presumed to originate from osteoblasts, a tumor composed of cells that produce cartilage (and only cartilage) is presumed to originate from chondroblasts, and so on. In other instances, the histogenetic presumption of origin is derived not from the identification of a manufactured product of the tumor cell but rather from the morphologic similarity of this cell to a given normal cell by light microscopy, histochemistry, and electron microscopy. For instance, a malignant bone tumor composed of small round cells that morphologically resemble normal lymphocytes is presumed to arise from these cells and is therefore designated as malignant lymphoma. Some terms that have very little histogenetic meaning have remained either to honor the scientist who first recognized them (e.g., Ewing's sarcoma) or for no other reason than tradition (e.g., myeloma).

The reader who first scans a classification of bone neoplasms such as the one presented below is likely to wonder what its real practical significance is. This is understandable because there have been in the past (and it is possible that there still are) classifications of tumors that describe minimal morphologic variations of a basic tumor pattern that have no clinical, surgical, or prognostic significance whatsoever. The reader may be assured that this is not the case with the present classification of bone tumors. Each one of the entities below listed has a personality of its own: its preference for a given bone, site within the bone, age of the patient, radiographic appearance, and behavior are distinctive and allow the clinician to suggest a specific diagnosis, plan therapy, and predict the evolution with a high degree of accuracy.

The basic information regarding these parameters is included in Table 45-1. The data concerning age, sex, bone, and bone site most commonly involved will generally not be repeated in the text. For a proper understanding of this table, a brief recapitulation of some terms of normal bone anatomy might be helpful. *Medulla* (medullary cavity or marrow cavity) refers to the inner or central portion of the bone, composed of network of cancellous (spongy, reticular) bone trabeculae that enclose bone-marrow hematopoietic elements, adipose tissue, blood and lymph vessels, and nerves. The *cortex,* composed of compact (dense) bone and essentially devoid of bone marrow and other soft-tissue components, surrounds the medulla in a circumferential fashion. The *periosteum,* which covers the external surface of the bone, consists of a thick external layer of fibrous connective tissue and a thin osteoblastic layer. Bone tumors located in the region of the periosteum, and possibly arising from it, are designated as periosteal, parosteal, or juxtacortical.

A typical adult long bone is composed of a *diaphysis,* which is the central cylindric shaft; the *epiphyses,* which are two roughly spheric terminal regions covered by the articular cartilage; and the *metaphyses,* two intermediate conelike regions connecting the shaft and the articular ends (Fig. 45-2). The metaphysis is particularly important in bone pathology because in the growing individual it is adjacent to a cartilaginous *epiphyseal plate.* The latter represents the area of most active bone growth and, perhaps as a result, it is the most common site of occurrence of many bone neoplasms.

Definitions of normal bone histologic features that are important to remember in the context of the subject of this chapter include the following. *Osteoid* (preosseous tissue) is the extracellular material produced by the osteoblasts and composed of collagen fibers and an amorphous protein-poysaccharide matrix. *Bone* refers to the same tissue after calcium salts have been deposited on it. *Woven (membrane) bone* is the type of bone produced nor-

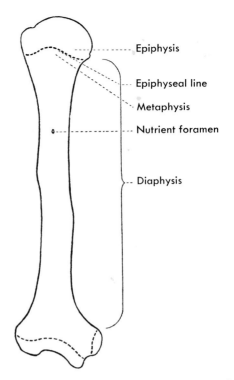

Fig. 45-2. Sketch of long bone (humerus) identifying different anatomic landmarks important for localization of bone neoplasms.

mally in the course of intramembranous ossification and abnormally in a fracture callus, fibrous dysplasia, and a variety of bone neoplasms; it is characterized by the fact that the collagen fibers run in an haphazard fashion throughout the osteoid matrix. One can observe this particularly well with polarizing lenses. *Lamellar bone,* on the other hand, is laid down in lamellae containing collagen in ordered parallel arrays.

The classification listed below also includes a group of nonneoplastic conditions, most of them of obscure pathogenesis, that can closely resemble a bone neoplasm on radiographic and morphologic grounds.

*Classification of bone tumors**
  OSTEOBLASTIC (BONE-FORMING) TUMORS
    Benign
      Osteoma
      Osteoid osteoma and osteoblastoma
    Malignant
      Osteosarcoma
      Juxtacortical (parosteal) osteosarcoma

*Modified from Schajowicz, F., Ackerman, L. V., and Sissons, H. A.: Histological typing of bone tumours, International Histological Classification of Tumours, No. 6, Geneva, 1972, World Health Organization.

CHONDROBLASTIC (CARTILAGE-FORMING) TUMORS
   Benign
      Chondroma
      Osteochondroma
      Chondroblastoma
      Chondromyxoid fibroma
   Malignant
      Chondrosarcoma
      Mesenchymal chondrosarcoma
GIANT CELL TUMOR
MARROW TUMORS
   Ewing's sarcoma
   Malignant lymphoma
   Plasma cell myeloma
VASCULAR TUMORS
   Benign
      Hemangioma
      Lymphangioma
      Glomus tumor
   Malignant
      Angiosarcoma, low grade
      Angiosarcoma, high grade
FIBROUS TISSUE TUMORS
   Benign
      Desmoplastic fibroma
   Malignant
      Fibrosarcoma
OTHER PRIMARY TUMORS
   Chordoma
   "Adamantinoma" of long bones
   Tumors of peripheral nerves
   Tumors of adipose tissue
   Tumors of probable histiocytic origin
METASTATIC TUMORS
UNCLASSIFIED TUMORS
TUMORLIKE LESIONS
   Solitary bone cyst
   Aneurysmal bone cyst
   Ganglion cyst of bone
   Metaphyseal fibrous defect (nonossifying
      fibroma)
   Fibrous dysplasia
   Myositis ossificans
   Histiocytosis X (eosinophilic granuloma,
      Hand-Schüller-Christian disease, and
      Letterer-Siwe disease)

DIAGNOSIS, TREATMENT, AND PROGNOSIS

The diagnosis of bone tumors should always be made on the basis of a combined clinical, radiographic, and pathologic evaluation. In some specific instances, biochemical and hematologic information is also of crucial importance. Laboratory data that are particularly important in this regard include serum levels of calcium, phosphorus, alkaline phosphatase, and acid phosphatase. The tumors and tumorlike conditions in which the knowledge of these data is essential are hyperparathyroidism, Paget's disease, plasma cell myeloma, and metastatic carcinoma. Bone marrow cytology and serum and urinary immunoglobulin determinations are important for the diagnosis of plasma cell myeloma; a thorough hematologic

investigation is essential in the evaluation of malignant lymphoma and leukemia of bone; and urinary catecholamine determination is a useful adjunct for the diagnosis of metastatic neuroblastoma.

The most important clinical parameter is the patient's age. Most bone neoplasms show a definite preference for a given age range and are distinctly unusual in another. For instance, a diagnosis of giant cell tumor in a child or that of Ewing's sarcoma in an octogenarian should be viewed with great skepticism. Along the same line, a malignant bone tumor of uniform small round cells in an infant is likely to be a metastatic neuroblastoma, that in a child a Ewing's sarcoma, and that in an adult a malignant lymphoma. The sex of the patient, on the other hand, is of little importance in the differential diagnosis of bone tumors, except for some types of metastases. Symptoms are also of only minor relevance in this field, and on occasions they may be misleading. For instance, a bone tumefaction associated with local pain and redness, fever, and leukocytosis may lead the physician to a diagnosis of osteomyelitis, yet Ewing's sarcoma can result in an identical picture. In general, the larger the tumor is, the more likely that it will be malignant. However, one of the largest and more spectacular masses that one can encounter is an aneurysmal bone cyst, which is probably not even neoplastic in nature.

The other information of importance regarding the clinical evaluation pertains to the existence of any of the conditions that are known to predispose to a greater or lesser degree to the appearance of bone tumors, such as Paget's disease, irradiation, bone infarcts, enchondromatosis (Ollier's disease), osteochondromatosis, and fibrous dysplasia.

Radiologic investigation is always of extreme importance. Routine roentgenograms in different views usually provide most of the necessary data for a proper evaluation, but in selected cases tomographs and arteriograms provide useful additional information.[116] The radiographic data important for the diagnosis of a bone tumor are the bone involved, precise localization of the lesion (whether medullary, cortical, or juxtacortical and whether diaphyseal, metaphyseal, or epiphyseal if located in a long bone), indication as to whether the lesion has originated in bone or has extended to it from soft tissues, size and shape, margins (whether sharply or ill-defined), nature of any changes in the surrounding bone, and the presence and type of calcification in the lesion.

On some occasions, a tumor that is extensively involving a given bone can hardly be detected by radiographic examination. The explanation is that the tumor diffusely permeates the bone marrow spaces without destroying the bone trabeculae.

Despite the fact that a good degree of diagnostic accuracy can be reached on the basis of the radiographic examination of the lesion, the final diagnosis on which all prognostic and therapeutic considerations will be made should always remain in a careful pathologic study. I must also emphasize that the relevant clinical and radiographic information should always be available to the pathologist before a final diagnosis is made. This is important because lesions that have a totally different clinical and radiographic presentation and are therefore easily separable on this basis can have a very similar appearance under the microscope.

Histologic study of a bone tumor usually involves examination of a biopsy specimen, a procedure that should never be omitted whenever radical surgery, radiation therapy, or chemotherapy are contemplated. The specimen is obtained by either open surgical biopsy (incisional or excisional biopsy) or needle biopsy (aspiration or trochar biopsy).[93] Performance of an open surgical biopsy entails a small risk of tumor implantation in the soft tissue, especially in the case of cartilaginous tumors. However, the information obtained by the use of the biopsy far outweighs this potential risk and should never be omitted.

The majority of pathologic diagnoses are based on the examination of routinely processed material, i.e., tissue that has been subjected to formalin fixation, decalcification if needed, paraffin embedding, and hematoxylin-eosin staining. On occasions, histochemical stains provide additional information of diagnostic significance, such as glycogen identification in Ewing's sarcoma, pyroninophilia of the cytoplasm in plasma cell myeloma and intense alkaline phosphatase activity in osteosarcoma. Electron microscopic examination, in selected instances, has given diagnostic support for a given diagnosis or has proved of value in elucidating the histogenesis of a neoplasm, as in the case of so-called adamantinoma of long bones.

The therapeutic approach to bone tumors varies a great deal according to their nature. The three main modalities are surgery, radiation therapy, and chemotherapy. The surgical approach, which is used for most neoplasms, generally consists of curettage and packing for benign lesions (such as chondroblastoma), block excision for more aggressive but not fully malignant tumors, and radical operations (amputation or disarticulation) for highly malignant neoplasms. Radiation therapy is particularly important for Ewing's sarcoma and malignant lymphoma.[106]

From the point of view of behavior, most classifications (including the present one) divide bone neoplasms into a benign and a malignant category. This is done for orientation purposes, but it represents a gross oversimplification of the problem. As is often the case in real life as compared to western movies, bone neoplasms cannot be sharply segregated into the "bad guys" and the "good guys." There is instead a whole range of intermediate characters between the perfectly innocuous tumor and the highly invasive and metastasizing neoplasm.

As a general rule, the most benign tumors are well circumscribed, with well-defined outlines and often sclerotic borders (indicative of slow growth), located either within the medulla or the cortex, with no evidence of soft-tissue extension or periosteal reaction. The most malignant bone tumors tend to be large and poorly circumscribed, often permeate the medullary cavity, extend into the soft tissues, elicit prominent new bone formation from the periosteum, and have the capacity to give distant metastases. The latter property is the main basis by which a bone tumor has been included in the "malignant" category in the classification presented in this chapter. The majority of distant metastases of bone tumors are blood-borne and appear in the lungs. Some bone sarcomas, such as Ewing's sarcoma and osteosarcoma, initially located within a single bone, have a tendency to show up later in other bones. Whether these foci represent metastases from the original lesion or multicentric foci of involvement is a moot point.[2] The rarest form of distant metastasis in bone sarcoma is the lymph-borne type. Although instances of lymph node metastases in osteosarcoma and other bone tumors have been reported, the incidence is so low that it can be disregarded when one plans therapy.

One should understand well that the fact that a tumor recurs locally after conservative surgical therapy is not necessarily an indication that it is of a malignant nature. The reason for this should be obvious. The most common surgical approach to benign bone tumors consists of unroofing the lesion and removing it in bits with a sharp curette; the space thus formed is then packed with bone chips. The fact is that no matter how thorough the curettage is, the possibility always exists that a small portion of tumor will remain in situ and provide the nidus for a recurrence.

OSTEOBLASTIC (BONE-FORMING) TUMORS

The common property of this group of bone tumors is the capacity of their constituent cells to produce osteoid or bone, or both, thus fulfilling the criterion of functional osteoblasts.

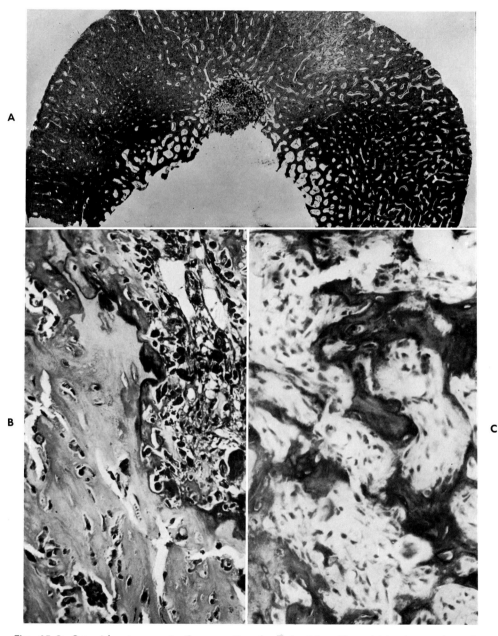

Fig. 45-3. Osteoid osteoma. **A,** Cross section through nidus. Note thickening and condensation of surrounding cortical bone. In **B** and **C,** note composition of osteoid osteoma. **B,** Abundant osteoid. **C,** Irregular well-calcified osseous spicules encased by highly vascular and moderately cellular connective tissue. Osteoclasts present in moderate numbers. (**B,** 180×; **C,** 250×.)

Understand that for osteoid or bone formation to be significative in this regard, it must be the direct product of the tumor cells. The occurrence of reactive bone formation by non-neoplastic osteoblasts at the periphery of a tumor, or the endochondral ossification that neoplastic cartilage can undergo in the same fashion as normal cartilage, does not qualify a tumor as being of osteoblastic derivation.

Benign tumors

Osteoma. This lesion is composed of well-differentiated compact bone of lamellar structure. It has an extremely slow rate of growth. It is almost entirely restricted to the skull and facial bones, from which it may grow into the paranasal sinuses.[42] The radiographic appearance is that of a dense ivorylike mass. Osteomas can be seen as a component of Gardner's syndrome (intestinal polyposis and soft-tissue tumors).[14] The behavior of osteomas is perfectly benign.

It seems likely that the bone lesion we call osteoma is not a true neoplasm and perhaps

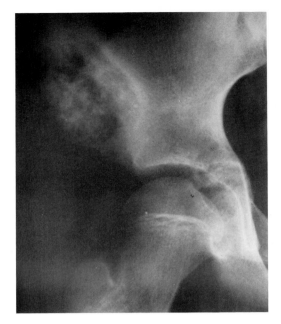

Fig. 45-5. Osteoblastoma of iliac bone. Lesion is well circumscribed, has sclerotic borders, and shows diffuse ossification.

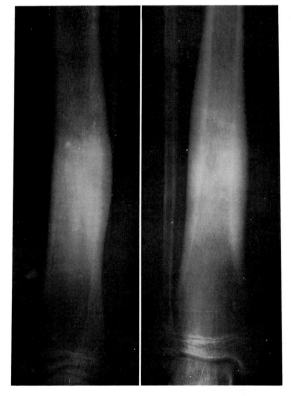

Fig. 45-4. Osteoid osteoma. Lateral and anteroposterior roentgenograms showing typical osteosclerosis associated with osteoid osteoma.

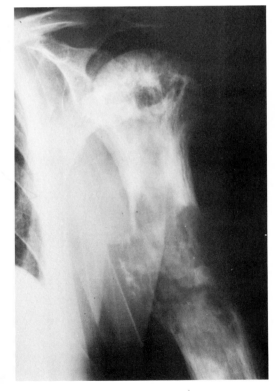

Fig. 45-6. Paget's disease complicated by osteosarcoma and pathologic fracture. Note thickening of bone resulting from Paget's disease and destructive lytic process in center of figure, corresponding to poorly differentiated osteosarcoma with scanty osteoid formation.

not even a uniform entity. Some cases seem to represent the site of a former traumatic injury, such as a subperiosteal hematoma or a localized inflammatory process; others appear to be hamartomas, i.e., a type of malformation; still others probably represent the end result of osteochondroma or fibrous dysplasia.

Osteoid osteoma and osteoblastoma. These two types of benign bone tumors are so closely related that it is better to discuss them together.[96] Their common features include a benign behavior, a preference for children and young adults, and a microscopic appearance characterized by an extremely active formation of osteoid and immature bone by plump osteoblasts situated in a highly vascularized stroma

(Fig. 45-3). The differences between the two, which are not always clear cut in an individual case, refer to size, presence of pain, location, and radiographic appearance. *Osteoid osteoma* is small (usually less than 1 cm), often located in the cortex of a long bone, painful, clearly demarcated, and surrounded by a zone of sclerotic reactive bone[69] (Fig. 45-4). Thus it appears radiographically as a small radiolucent area (the nidus) with or without a minute dense center, in an otherwise sclerotic mass. In the past, it was often confused with a chronic bone abscess or sclerosing osteomyelitis. *Osteoblastoma* is larger (usually more than 1 cm), painless, located in the vertebrae, in the medulla of long bones, or in the iliac

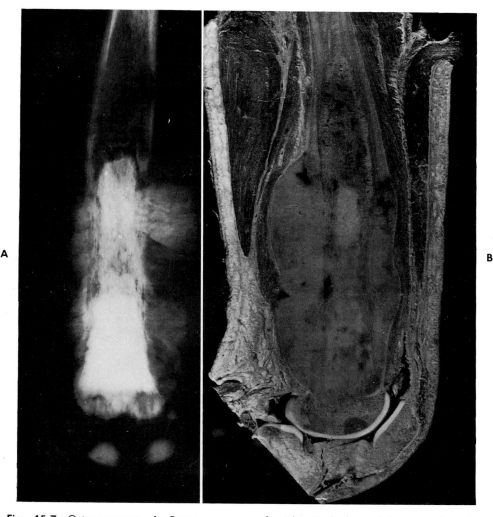

Fig. 45-7. Osteosarcoma. **A,** Roentgenogram of midsagittal slice of femur undergoing replacement by sclerosing osteosarcoma. Note condensation and loss of architectural design of affected segment of femur and pronounced osseous tissue growth subperiosteally. **B,** Gross appearance of sectioned surface of sarcoma illustrated in **A.**

bone, and usually accompanied by little or no reactive bone formation (Fig. 45-5). It is possible that many of these differences are simply related to the respective sites of the two lesions when they involve a long bone: cortical for osteoid osteoma and medullary for osteoblastoma.[10,27]

Malignant tumors

Osteosarcoma. Osteosarcoma is the primary malignant tumor of osteoblasts and is identified microscopically by the *direct* formation of osteoid or bone, or both, by the neoplastic cells. It is the most common primary malignant tumor of bone, and it is also known as osteogenic sarcoma.[23] Most cases appear in adolescents and young adults. Males are affected more often than females. A good proportion of osteosarcomas presenting after middle age represent a complication of Paget's disease or irradiation therapy to the area[5] (Fig. 45-6). The classic site of occurrence is the medulla of the metaphysis of long bones, particularly the lower end of the femur, the upper end of the tibia, and the upper end of the humerus. It is a highly invasive neoplasm. On the one hand, it permeates the medullary cavity and can extend for a long distance from its site of inception (this being the cause for the stump recurrences that often occur after amputations done too close to the tumor mass)[65]; on the other hand, it breaks through the cortex, elevates the periosteum, and grows relentlessly into the soft tissues (Fig. 45-7). There is only one tissue that is able to stop, at least temporarily, the advance of this tumor; it is the cartilage of the epiphyseal plate (Fig. 45-8). Because of this, it is very uncommon for osteosarcomas occurring in young individuals (when the epiphyseal plate is present) to extend into the epiphyses; once the cartilage from the epiphyseal plate has disappeared, the tumor freely extends into the articular end of the bone and may even penetrate the joint cavity. Distant metastases are common and the reason for the present high rate of failures in the treatment of this neoplasm. They are generally blood-borne, and the lungs are the most common site of involvement (Fig. 45-9).

The roentgenographic appearance depends a great deal on the relative amount of bone produced in a particular tumor. A tumor that produces a large amount of osteoid matrix that calcifies will appear as a highly sclerotic lesion; a less differentiated tumor that produces little or no recognizable bone will present as a lytic lesion (Figs. 45-7 and 45-10).

The gross appearance of an osteosarcoma depends a great deal on the relative amount of osteoid, bone, and cartilage being produced

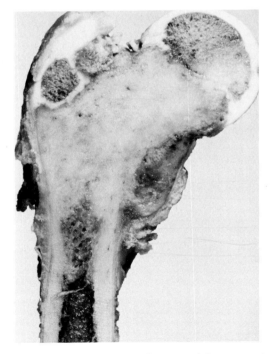

Fig. 45-8. Osteosarcoma of proximal femur in 10-year-old boy. There is massive involvement of medullary cavity, invasion of cortex and soft tissues, and periosteal elevation. Note how tumor growth is restrained by epiphyseal cartilage.

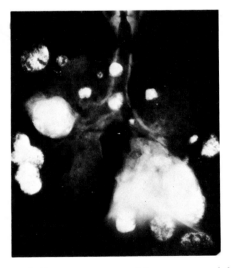

Fig. 45-9. Roentgenogram of lungs removed from patient who died of osteosarcoma. Metastases consist of bone that is heavily mineralized.

(Fig. 45-11). Tumors with an abundance of this material have a hard, partially calcified appearance, whereas more undifferentiated tumors are softer, whitish or pink, with frequent areas of necrosis and hemorrhage. Foci of cartilage formation present as white, glistening, somewhat mucoid areas. Some osteosarcomas are accompanied by telangiectatic blood vessels that result in a multicystic appearance not dissimilar from that of aneurysmal bone cyst.[30]

Osteosarcomas show a considerable variation in microscopic pattern. The tumor cells may be small and more or less uniform in size and shape or highly pleomorphic, with bizarre nuclear and cytoplasmic shapes and numerous mitoses (Figs. 45-10 and 45-12). In addition to osteoid and bone, the tumor cells may produce cartilage, fibrous tissue, or myxoid tissue. As a matter of fact, in some osteosarcomas the production of cartilage or fibrous tissue is even greater than that of osteoid or bone (Fig. 45-13). Other areas may have a totally undifferentiated appearance, without any type of intercellular material being deposited. However, I should emphasize that as long as a malignant bone tumor is producing osteoid or bone directly from the neoplastic cells, it should

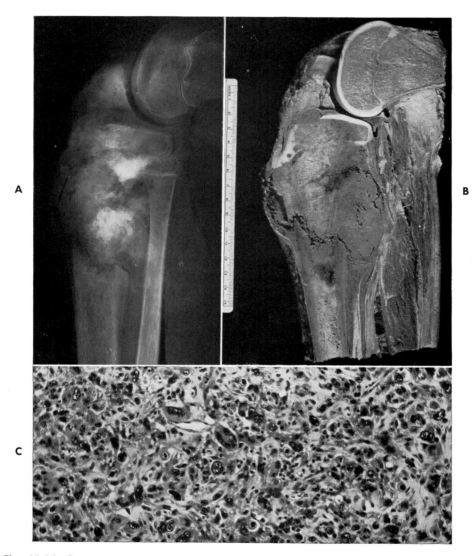

Fig. 45-10. Osteosarcoma. **A** and **B,** Destructive and rapidly growing sarcoma of tibia that has resulted in pathologic fracture. **C,** Variation in size and shape of cells, bizarre mitoses, and little or no evidence of bone matrix formation are noteworthy features in this lytic form of osteosarcoma. (165×; AFIP 73613.)

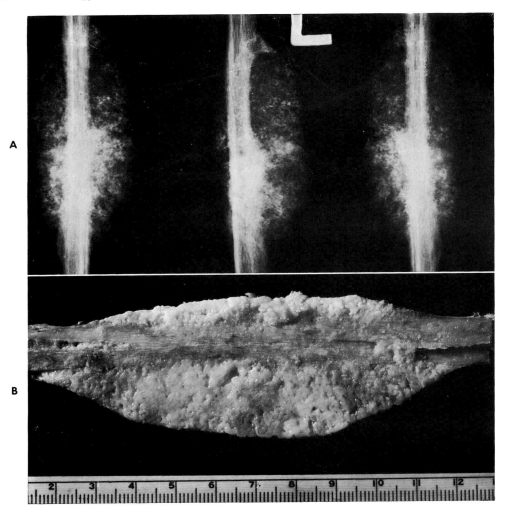

Fig. 45-11. A, Sclerosing osteosarcoma of fibula. Tumor was slowly growing. It was made up of both osseous and cartilaginous tissues (see Fig. 45-13). **B,** Specimen illustrated in **A.**

be designated as osteosarcoma regardless of how focal this production may be and regardless of how many other materials (cartilage, fibrous tissue) are being produced elsewhere by the tumor. Histochemically, the cells of osteosarcoma are seen to contain large amounts of enzymes of the alkaline phosphatase group. At a fine structural level, the cytoplasm of the tumor cells resembles that of a normal osteoblast by virtue of a prominent development of the granular endoplasmic reticulum.

As previously mentioned, most osteosarcomas arise within the medullary cavity. There is, on the other hand, a type of osteosarcoma that originates in a location extrinsic to the cortex, i.e., in the periosteal or parosteal region. It is designated as *juxtacortical* or *parosteal osteosarcoma*[114] (Fig. 45-14). It is an osteosarcoma

in the true sense of the word, in that it produces neoplastic osteoid and bone. However, it deserves to be separated from the more common medullary variety because of its distinct form of presentation and different prognosis.[29] It occurs in an older age group, shows no sex predilection, grows relatively slowly, and is circumscribed and sometimes lobulated. Roentgenologic examination usually reveals a dense bony mass that, although firmly attached to the bone cortex over a wide base, tends to encircle the shaft as a bulky and heavily calcified growth (Fig. 45-15, *A*). Microscopically, it usually shows a high degree of structural differentiation. It is composed of a mass of bone trabeculae, often mature and lamellar, which are seen merging with the adjacent cortical bone (Fig. 45-15, *B*). As in the case

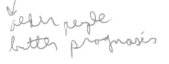

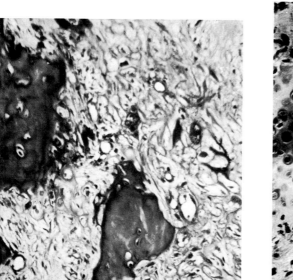

Fig. 45-12. Osteosarcoma. Bizarre cellular pattern and irregular ossification of sclerosing osteogenic sarcoma. (230×; AFIP 63769.)

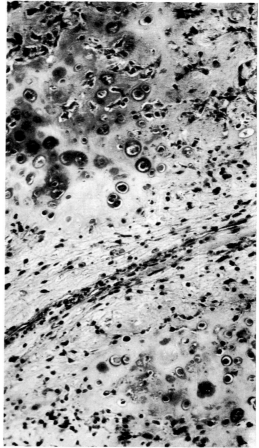

Fig. 45-13. Imperfectly formed bone and cartilage make up this malignant tumor. Histologic features portrayed here similar to those seen in tumor illustrated in Fig. 40-56. (170×; AFIP 66706.)

of the medullary osteosarcoma, fibrous tissue and cartilage may also be present. The tumor cells are often well differentiated, with few mitoses and very little pleomorphism. The diagnosis is often difficult and usually requires a combined evaluation of radiographic and microscopic findings. Many of the cases are misdiagnosed as atypical osteochondromas or myositis ossificans. The prognosis is much better than that of the usual osteosarcoma.

CARTILAGINOUS (CARTILAGE-FORMING) TUMORS

Benign tumors

Chondroma. The chondroma is a relatively common tumor, composed of the elements of mature hyaline cartilage. It typically involves the short tubular bones of the hands and feet and, less commonly, the ribs (particularly at the costochondral junction) and long bones.[107]

Chondroma may be solitary or multiple; the latter condition, which is not familial, is referred to as *multiple enchondromatosis*. Cases of multiple enchondromatosis with an exclusive or predominant unilateral distribution are known as *Ollier's disease,* or *dyschondroplasia*. When multiple chondromas are accompanied by multiple soft-tissue hemangiomas, the term *Maffucci's syndrome* is used.[3]

Most chondromas are located in the medullary portion of the diaphysis and are therefore referred to as enchondromas. They result radiographically in a well-circumscribed lytic lesion, which often has small foci of calcification. A less common variant of chondroma is seen outside the cortex and is referred to as *juxtacortical* or *parosteal chondroma*.[67]

Grossly and microscopically, chondromas recapitulate the appearance of normal adult

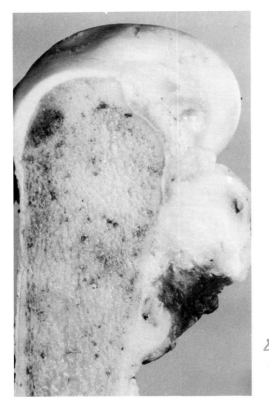

Fig. 45-14. Classic juxtacortical osteosarcoma occurring in 57-year-old man. Patient remains well over 10 years after amputation.

hyaline cartilage, although their pattern of orientation is abnormal. They have a characteristic lobulated appearance and may undergo necrosis, calcification, endochondral ossification and myxoid degeneration (Fig. 45-16). The nuclei of the cartilaginous cells are small, single, and irregular; mitotic figures are absent. The behavior of both solitary and multiple chondromas is benign. However, a small percentage of patients with multiple enchondromatosis develop chondrosarcomas.[17] Keep in mind that benign cartilaginous tumors of long and flat bones are very rare; any cartilaginous tumor in these locations should be viewed with suspicion even if the microscopic features are those of a well-differentiated neoplasm.

Osteochondroma. The term "osteochondroma" refers to an exophytic mass protruding from the metaphyseal area of a long bone and invariably pointing in a direction opposite to the articular cavity (Fig. 45-15, A). It is also referred to as an *exostosis* or *osteocartilaginous exostosis* in the orthopedic literature. It is probably the most common bone tumor. As in the case of the osteoma, it is doubtful whether

osteochondroma is a true neoplasm. It may well represent instead a disorder of growth. It is usually solitary although it may appear as part of a generalized condition known as *multiple hereditary exostoses* (diaphyseal aclasis, hereditary deforming chondrodysplasia) (Fig. 45-17).

Grossly, osteochondromas may have either a broad or a narrow base that is continuous with the cortical bone (Fig. 45-18). Microscopically, they are composed of a center of mature lamellar bone covered by a cartilaginous cap (Fig. 45-19). Active endochondral ossification is seen at the interphase between the two tissues. Eventually, all the cartilage is replaced by bone that contains bone marrow elements between its trabeculae. It is not clear whether *subungual exostosis* is a type of osteochondroma or an independent entity; it is often painful and forms beneath the nail of the finger or toe, especially the great toe.

Malignant transformation, usually in the form of chondrosarcoma, is exceptional with the solitary osteochondroma but is seen with some frequency in patients with multiple hereditary exostoses.

Chondroblastoma. This rare benign cartilaginous tumor occurs almost exclusively in the epiphyseal ends of long bones, adjacent to the epiphyseal cartilage plate.[94] Occasionally, it extends into the adjacent metaphysis. The majority of the patients are under 25 years of age. The radiographic appearance is that of a well-circumscribed lytic lesion with multiple small foci of calcification.[54] The gross appearance is not distinctive. It has a granular texture and a gray to whitish color (Fig. 45-20). Microscopically, the first impression is not that of a cartilaginous tumor. What one sees is a polymorphic, highly cellular lesion, in which scattered multinucleated cells with the appearance of osteoclasts alternate with much more numerous, small, polygonal, or round mononuclear cells. Because of the numerous multinucleated giant cells, this lesion was originally misinterpreted as a variant of giant cell tumor. In this regard, it is important to remember that the mere presence of multinucleated giant cells in a bone tumor is by no means justification to label this tumor as a giant cell tumor. One should realize, instead, that giant cells are a common nonspecific accompaniment of a variety of benign and malignant bone tumors and tumorlike nonneoplastic conditions. The important cells are the smaller and more numerous mononuclear elements. These are chondroblasts, as evi-

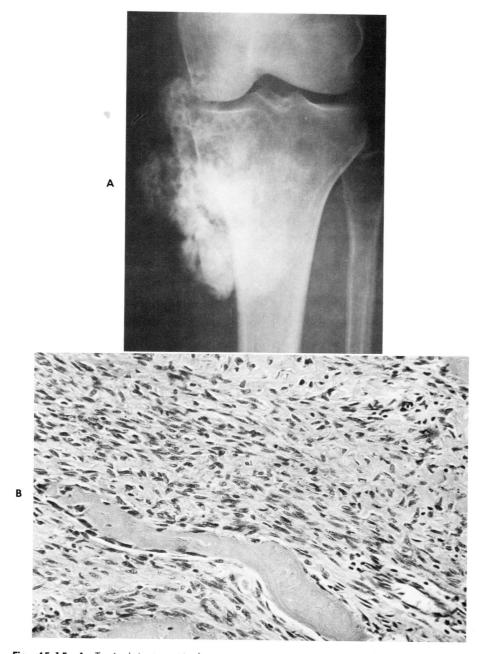

Fig. 45-15. A, Typical juxtacortical osteosarcoma occurring in 40-year-old woman. Note large extracortical component. **B,** Same lesion shown in **A** demonstrating well-differentiated character of sarcomatous stroma. This lesion had been present for several years. (250×.)

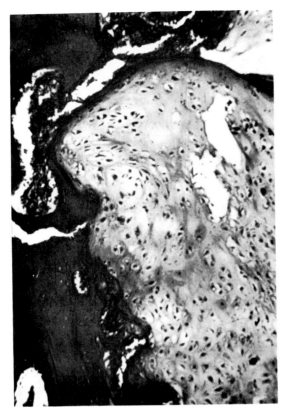

Fig. 45-16. Structural and cytologic features of typical enchondroma. (130×; AFIP 90709.)

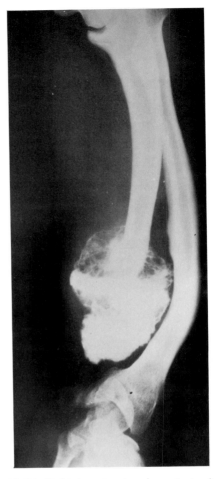

Fig. 45-17. Multiple osteochondromatosis. A large osteochondroma is seen involving distal end of ulna and deforming radius by compression.

denced by their electron microscopic appearance and the fact that a careful search under the light microscope will invariably reveal the presence of small amounts of cartilaginous intercellular matrix with areas of focal calcification.[64] In some instances, typical areas of chondroblastoma alternate with large blood-filled vascular spaces reminiscent of aneurysmal bone cysts. These are referred to as "cystic chondroblastomas."

The behavior of chondroblastoma is generally benign. Some cases recur after curettage, and on occasions they extend into the articular space or the soft tissue.[16] Exceptionally, a tumor that has all the microscopic appearance of chondroblastoma has been seen to give rise to distant metastases.[60] This occurrence is so uncommon that for purposes of therapy, chondroblastoma should be regarded and treated as a benign neoplasm.

Chondromyxoid fibroma. A chondromyxoid fibroma is also a benign tumor of cartilaginous origin, despite its name, which suggests a primarily fibrous derivation.[58] It often presents

in the metaphysis of long bones, and the upper end of the tibia is the single most common area of involvement.[85] The bones of the feet are another site of preferential involvement by this tumor. Radiographically, it appears at an eccentric, sharply outlined, radiolucent area that often causes expansion of the bone[95] (Fig. 45-21). Calcification within the lesion is not so common as with other cartilaginous tumors. A thin sclerotic inner border is usually present, as in most benign bone tumors. Grossly, it is solid, often lobulated, and of a yellowish white or tan color. Usually, there is a quality of translucency, suggesting cartilaginous derivation. Microscopically, a lobulated architecture can be readily observed under low-power examination. The lobules are separated by bands of fibrous tissue lined on the sides by a variable number of multinucleated giant cells with the

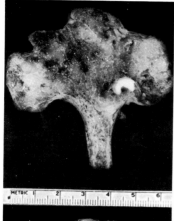

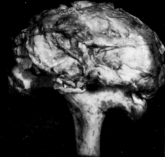

Fig. 45-18. Typical mushroom-shaped osteochondroma.

appearance of osteoclasts (Fig. 45-22). The lobules themselves are composed of immature cartilage with a prominent myxoid pattern. Easily identifiable chondroblasts alternate with stellate myxoid cells and scattered large pleomorphic cells. The latter may result in an erroneous diagnosis of malignancy. Mitoses are exceptional. Rarely, tumors representing hybrids between chondromyxoid fibroma and chondroblastoma are encountered.[22] This is not surprising in view of the close histogenetic relationship of these neoplasms.

Chondromyxoid fibroma is essentially a benign tumor, yet it may manifest a certain degree of aggressive behavior. The recurrence rate after curettage approaches 25%, and because of this some orthopedic surgeons prefer to treat it with an en bloc excision. Extension into soft tissues has also been seen, but distant metastases have not been encountered so far.

Malignant tumors

Chondrosarcoma. As the name indicates, chondrosarcoma represents a malignant tumor of chondroblasts.[8] It usually presents in the

middle age or later. Two distinct varieties exists.[25] The *central* chondrosarcoma originates in the medullary cavity of the diaphysis or metaphysis, presumably anew. It results in a very typical radiographic appearance of an osteolytic lesion with splotchy calcification, ill-defined margins, fusiform thickening of the shaft, and perforation of the cortex[71] (Fig. 45-23). The *peripheral* form, which may be either cortical or parosteal, can arise anew or represent a malignant degeneration in the cartilage of an osteochondroma. Radiographically, it presents as a large tumor, with a heavily calcified center surrounded by a less dense periphery with splotchy calcification.

The gross appearance of chondrosarcoma betrays its cartilaginous composition. The tumor is often extremely large and has a lobulated outline (especially in the peripheral variety), firm consistency, and a glistening white or bluish, translucent cut surface (Fig. 45-24). A gelatinous or myxoid quality is often evident. Calcification is often present and may be extreme. Foci of ossification may be encountered. The central chondrosarcoma may be seen pushing into the cortex and eventually reaching the periosteum and surrounding soft tissues.[80]

Microscopically, the hallmark of chondrosarcoma is the presence of chondroblasts having atypical cytologic features, situated in a more or less organized cartilaginous matrix (Fig. 45-25). The cytologic signs of malignancy can be very obvious or quite subtle. In the well-differentiated examples, the pathologist has to rely on minimal morphologic deviations, such as plump nuclei, multinucleated chondroblasts, presence of multiple chondroblasts in a single lacuna, and strikingly accelerated growth activity at the margins of the individual lobules or nodules. In these cases, evaluation of the clinical and radiographic features is of paramount importance. The above-mentioned minor microscopic characteristics, if present in an invasive tumor of the medullary cavity of a long bone, are diagnostic of chondrosarcoma but, if present in a small cartilaginous tumor of the hand, are probably of no significance.

Neoplastic cartilage, like its normal counterpart, may be replaced by bone by a mechanism of endochondral ossification. In this process, the cartilage is reabsorbed and new bone is laid down in its place by osteoblasts, i.e., different cells from those that produced the cartilage. Presence of endochondral ossification in a neoplastic cartilage is not an indication that the tumor is an osteosarcoma or a reason

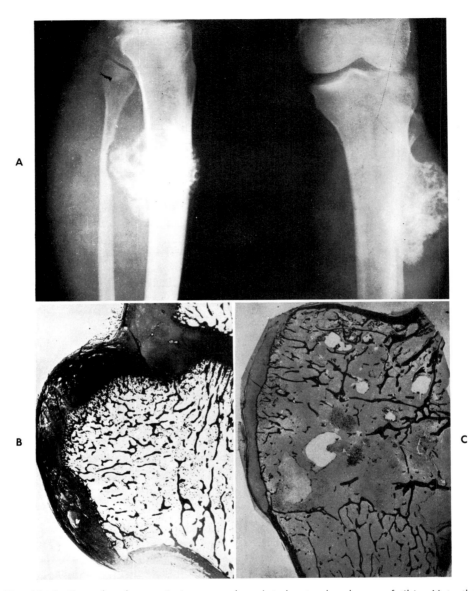

Fig. 45-19. Osteochondroma. **A,** Large, pedunculated osteochondroma of tibia. Note that direction of growth has been away from epiphyseal end of shaft. Pressure atrophy of fibula from contact with tumor apparent in lateral view. **B,** Osteochondroma in early stage of development in young child. Section through junction of metaphyseal end of tibia (lower three fourths) and epiphysis (upper right). Relation of tumor to perichondrium apparent. **C,** Flat osteochondroma of upper end of femur. Note perichondrial layer, growing cartilage, and irregular trabecular bone that has resulted from imperfect endochondrial ossification. (**A,** AFIP 77515.)

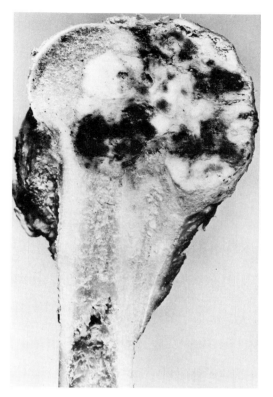

Fig. 45-20. Well-outlined chondroblastoma involving epiphysis of humerus in young adult.

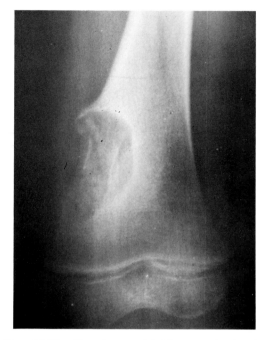

Fig. 45-21. Chondromyxoid fibroma. As is the rule with this tumor, lower femoral metaphysis is involved, borders are sharp and sclerotic, and lesion is eccentrically located.

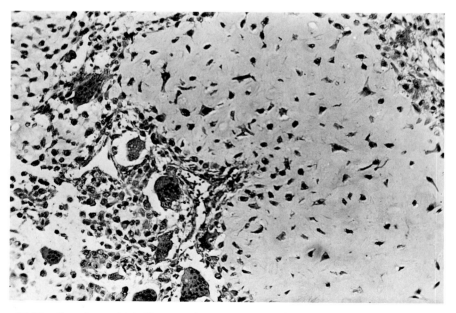

Fig. 45-22. Chondromyxoid fibroma showing giant cells, cartilage, and cellular zones. (200×.)

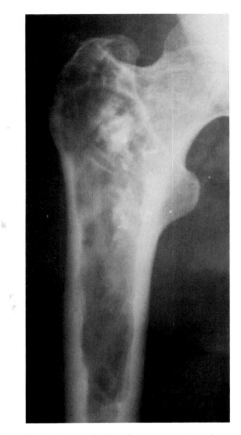

Fig. 45-23. Central chondrosarcoma involving upper metaphysis of femur. Note splotchy calcification, lobulated contour, and cortical destruction.

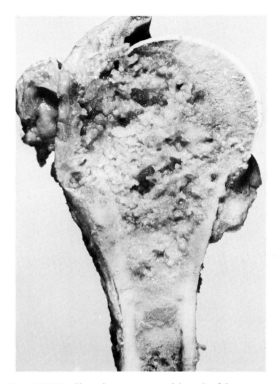

Fig. 45-24. Chondrosarcoma of head of humerus.

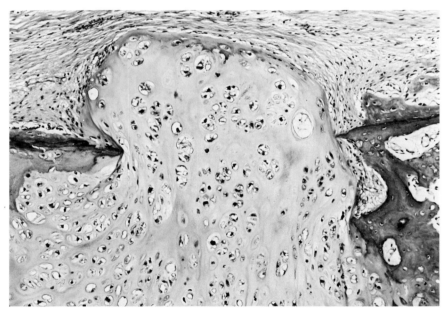

Fig. 45-25. Bizarre and "plump" nuclei in rather well-differentiated chondrosarcoma from pelvis. This histologic section also shows tumor protruding through cortical bone into surrounding soft tissues. This feature and lobular pattern seen grossly illustrate danger of enucleating these tumors. Persistent tumor is almost inevitable. (125×.)

to call the tumor an osteochondrosarcoma. It is only when the bone or osteoid is produced directly by the neoplastic cells, i.e., without the interposition of a cartilaginous phase, that the term "osteosarcoma" should be used. Although both chondromas and osteochondromas (especially the generalized forms) can lead to chondrosarcoma development, it seems likely that the majority of chondrosarcomas arise anew.

The behavior of chondrosarcoma varies a great deal according to the degree of microscopic differentiation. Well-differentiated ("low grade") neoplasms grow slowly and rarely metastasize. Poorly differentiated ("high grade") tumors invade quickly and are prone to distant metastases, particularly to the lungs. A peculiar feature of chondrosarcoma is its capacity to implant in soft tissues as a result of surgical manipulation, with this property being probably attributable to the relatively low need for oxygen that cartilaginous tissue is known to have. In some instances, autopsy reveals a continuous intravascular growth of tumor, which may extend to the right side of the heart or even into the pulmonary arteries.

A variant of chondrosarcoma that deserves to be treated separately is the *mesenchymal chondrosarcoma*.[88] It is more malignant than the conventional variety and more often multicentric. A significant percentage of cases arises primarily in the soft tissues.[40] Their distinctive microscopic appearance is provided by the alternate arangements of two greatly different patterns—one of relatively well-differentiated cartilage and one of highly cellular and vascularized spindle-celled elements. Although the latter have some morphologic resemblance to pericytes at a light microscopic level, their fine structural appearance and relationship with the other component of the tumor suggest that they are instead poorly differentiated chondroblasts.

GIANT CELL TUMOR (OSTEOCLASTOMA)

The giant cell tumor belongs to a category by itself in most classifications of bone tumors, mainly because of the uncertainty that still exists regarding its histogenesis. Some investigators even doubt whether it constitutes a valid entity. However, the elimination from the category of giant cell tumor of many neoplasms and tumorlike conditions that simulated it because of their high content of giant cells has resulted in the delineation of a lesion with quite definite clinicopathologic features.[24,79]

Giant cell tumor is, by and large, a tumor of adults. Although well-documented cases have been recorded in children, one should always keep in mind that if a giant cell–containing lesion is found in a patient of less than the age of 20 years, the chances are overwhelming that it will prove to be something other than a true giant cell tumor.

This neoplasm shares with chondroblastoma a predilection for epiphyseal involvement, although in the case of the former there is often also some extension to the metaphysis. It may be significant in this regard that the overwhelming number of giant cell tumors occurs after the epiphyses have closed. The lower end of the femur, upper end of the tibia, and lower end of the radius are the most common sites of involvement, in that order of frequency. Pain that is especially severe on weight bearing and motion is usually the first symptom. Later, there may be noticeable swelling. A pathologic fracture may supervene. Radiographically, it appears as a somewhat lobulated lytic lesion, without sclerosis of the borders and usually located eccentrically within the epiphysis, in a

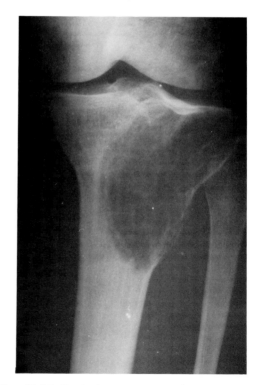

Fig. 45-26. Typical roentgenographic appearance of giant cell tumor of bone. Tumor involves upper tibial epiphysis and diaphysis. It is eccentrically located and shows little if any sclerosis of margins.

condyle (Fig. 45-26). On gross inspection, it is well circumscribed and often has a granular hemorrhagic appearance (Fig. 45-27). The expanded portion is partially or completely encased in a thin shell of bone. The neoplastic tissue is firm and friable. It is often grayish, with either a pinkish or a brownish tint. Focal areas of degeneration, of yellow-brown color, and hemorrhagic areas of red or dark brown color, depending on the age of the hemorrhage, are usually present.

The microscopic hallmark of this neoplasm is the presence of a large number of multinucleated giant cells that are *regularly scattered* throughout the tumor mass (Fig. 45-28). This spatial relationship between giant cells and stromal cells is important in the differential diagnosis with the diseases that simu-

late giant cell tumors because in the latter the giant cells are irregularly distributed, often in clumps or surrounding blood vessels, with large tumor areas being devoid of them.

The giant cells of giant cell tumor of bone have an abundant acidophilic cytoplasm and as many as 100 nuclei. Their light microscopic, enzyme, histochemical, and fine structural features are extremely similar to those of normal osteoclasts.[90] As in osteoclasts, acid phosphatase activity is very high and a large number of mitochondria is present in the cytoplasm.[104] Because of these similarities, giant cell tumor of bone is also known as osteoclastoma.

The second microscopic component of the giant cell tumor is often designated with the unassuming name of "stromal cell." Although far less spectacular than the giant cell when examined under the microscope, it probably represents the basic tumor element. It is certainly more important numerically than the giant cell. It is their relative number and appearance that correlates with the clinical

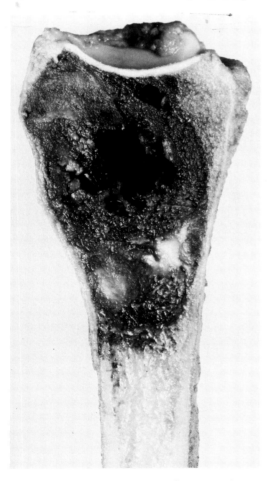

Fig. 45-27. Gross appearance of giant cell tumor involving upper epiphysis and metaphysis of tibia. Note poor circumscription, granular hemorrhagic appearance, and central cystic degeneration. Articular cartilage is intact.

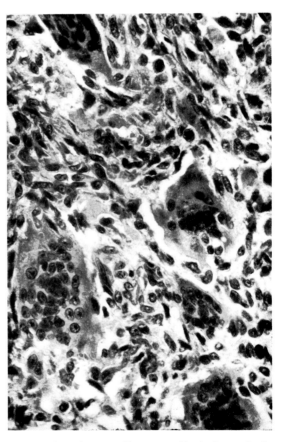

Fig. 45-28. Giant cell tumor. Typical cytologic and structural features. (765×; AFIP 63505.)

evolution. In locally aggressive and metastasizing lesions, one often gets the impression that the stromal cell component has "taken over" the neoplasm. The stromal cells of a typical giant cell tumor are medium-sized, oval or spindle, and with rather plump nuclei and ill-defined acidophilic cytoplasm (Fig. 45-28). The stroma is richly vascularized and contains a small amount of collagen. In about a third of the cases, foci of osteoid or bone formation of reactive appearance are found. Under the electron microscope, the stromal cells are seen to contain a well-developed granular endoplasmic reticulum. Their appearance is reminiscent of either a fibroblast or an osteoblast.[43]

Giant cell tumors are aggressive lesions. As many as 60% will recur after curettage, and about 10% will result in distant metastases, usually to the lungs. The latter occurrence is almost always preceded by a history of repeated curettages and recurrences. Because of

this, many authors recommend en bloc excision as the treatment of choice for this neoplasm.

In microscopy the grading systems proposed in order to allow prediction of the clinical behavior of this tumor have not proved satisfactory, and there is today no agreement on specific histologic features that dependably indicate the likelihood of malignant behavior.

MARROW TUMORS

Ewing's sarcoma. Ewing's sarcoma, a highly malignant neoplasm first described by James Ewing in 1921, usually occurs in patients between the ages of 5 and 20. In the usual case, the patient complains of pain in the affected area. Swelling may be present. The patient may have slight fever, and the leukocyte count and erythrosedimentation rate may be slightly or moderately elevated. These signs and symptoms may lead to an erroneous diagnosis of osteomyelitis. Radiographically, it is predomi-

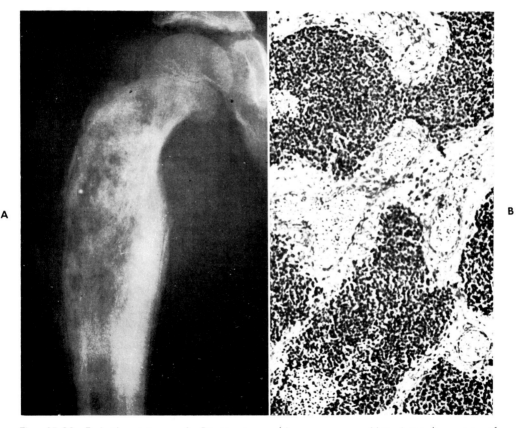

Fig. 45-29. Ewing's sarcoma. **A,** Roentgenographic appearance. Note irregular areas of osteoporosis and osteosclerosis, loss of bone architecture, and multilayered periosteal new bone formation. **B,** Closely packed small round cells make up substance of this tumor. Note loosely textured connective tissue containing numerous blood vessels, which forms partitions between masses of tumor cells. (160×; AFIP 73775.)

nantly osteolytic. However, the bone destruction is often associated with patchy reactive periosteal bone formation, which may result in the pattern that radiologists call onion-skin appearance (Fig. 45-29). Grossly, the tumor is white and exceedingly soft and friable; large areas of necrosis and hemorrhage are often encountered. The side of origin is the medullary canal of the diaphysis or metaphysis, from which it permeates the cortex and invades the soft tissues. The bone marrow permeation can be quite extensive and still leave the bone trabeculae relatively undisturbed so that the tumor may be missed on radiographic examination. Distant metastases are common, particularly to lung, liver, other bones, and the central nervous system.[72]

Microscopically, the tumor tissue has a rather uniform appearance. It is made up of densely packed small cells with round nuclei, frequent mitoses, scanty cytoplasm, and ill-defined cytoplasmic outlines (Fig. 45-29). The cytoplasm contains a moderate to large amount of glycogen granules, a feature of importance in the differential diagnosis.[89] Fibrous septa divide the tumor tissue into irregular lobules. Areas of necrosis are frequent; these may be secondarily infiltrated with acute inflammatory cells. Vascularization is usually well developed. The tumor cells may be grouped around blood vessels, producing a false rosette. The fine structural appearance is that of primitive cells without signs of differentiation.[37] New bone formation is usually encountered; this is invariably of reactive nature.

The histogenesis is still disputed, although most investigators favor an origin from primitive bone marrow elements.[59] If this turns out to be the case, Ewing's sarcoma may then be regarded as a type of malignant lymphoma, although still one that needs to be individualized from other lymphomas because of its distinct features.

The microscopic differential diagnosis has to be made primarily with two other "small round cell tumors" of bone—malignant lymphoma and metastatic neuroblastoma. Malignant lymphoma affects an older age group, the cells are larger, the nuclei often have a vesicular or indented configuration, glycogen is absent, and reticulin is more prominent. In metastatic neuroblastoma the bone lesions are often multiple and the predilection is for patients under 3 years of age. Glycogen is absent and rosettes may be present. When grown in tissue culture, neurites will form in 24 to 48 hours; urinary catecholamine derivatives are almost always elevated.

The prognosis of Ewing's sarcoma used to be dismal. Most series quoted a 5-year survival rate of less than 5%. This has been dramatically changed in the last few years with the institution of an aggressive combined therapeutic regime consisting of radiation therapy to the entire bone affected and systemic (and sometimes intrathecal) chemotherapy.[87]

Malignant lymphoma. All types of malignant lymphoma and leukemia can involve the skeletal system, either as an expression of systemic involvement or as the first manifestation of the disease.[13] *Hodgkin's disease* produces radiographically visible bone lesions in 15% of the cases.[48] The involvement is multifocal in 60%, and the bones most often involved are the vertebrae, pelvis, and ribs. In the vertebrae, the lesions often have a striking osteoblastic appearance. Of the four microscopic types of Hodgkin's disease, mixed cellularity and lymphocyte depletion have a greater tendency to involve bones.

Malignant lymphoma primarily involving bones tends to occur in patients over the age of 30 years.[98] It involves the shaft or metaphysis of the bone, producing a radiographically ill-defined cortical and medullary destruction

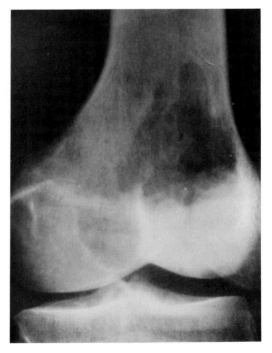

Fig. 45-30. Malignant lymphoma of distal femur. Note lytic nature of lesion, irregular outlines, lack of calcification, and absence of periosteal reaction.

(Fig. 45-30). It has been observed that the affected patients may remain in good health, even when the tumor has reached a large size, and that metastases are slow to occur.[9] Grossly, it is pinkish gray and granular. It frequently extends into the soft tissues and invades the muscle. Microscopically, most bone lymphomas are composed of round cells with relatively large vesicular nuclei, often indented or horseshoe-shaped and with prominent nucleoli. Cytoplasmic outlines tend to be well defined, and the cytoplasm is abundant and eosinophilic. A rich reticulin framework surrounds individual cells. In the traditional classification of malignant lymphoma, this tumor would be classified as a reticulum cell sarcoma; in Rappaport's classification, most cases would probably be included in the "histiocytic" category. In the light of recent immunologic and immunohistochemical observations, it is likely instead that, in the bone as well as in the lymphoid organs, it represents a tumor of "transformed" or blastic cells of the lymphocytic line.[1] A combination of radiation therapy and surgery is the treatment of choice.[115]

Plasma cell myeloma. This malignant tumor of plasma cells offers a variety of clinicopatho-logic expressions.[6] The most common form is usually known as multiple myeloma. It usually occurs between 40 and 60 years of age and presents with symptoms of pain, weakness, weight loss, and osteolytic lesions in the vertebrae, pelvis, rib, sternum, and skull (Fig. 45-31). Signs and symptoms referable to pressure upon the spinal cord or the spinal nerves may occur. Another complication of the disease is represented by compression fractures of vertebrae or pathologic fractures of other involved bones. Some degree of anemia is usually noted, and examination of the blood often reveals excessive *rouleau* formation. Roentgenologic examination reveals multiple small and large areas of bone destruction. These have sharp borders ("punched-out areas") and are unaccompanied by proliferative reactions at the margins, unless a fracture has occurred. In advanced cases, extraskeletal spread may be seen, either in the soft tissues adjacent to involved bones or as distant metastases to lymph nodes, spleen, liver, and other organs.[83] Immunoglobulin abnormalities are very common (87% of the cases) and express the functional capability of the neoplastic plasma cells. In a series of 112 patients, increased serum IgG was

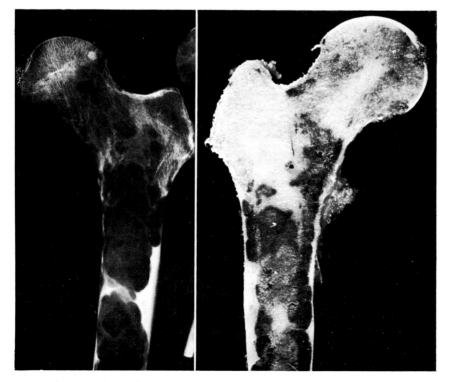

Fig. 45-31. Plasma cell myeloma of femur. Roentgenogram and gross photograph of hemisection showing extensive bone destruction caused by tumor. Note absence of any reactive bone formation.

found in 61%, IgA in 18%, and light chains only (Bence Jones protein) in 9%.[12] The most common finding in the urine of myeloma patients is the presence of Bence Jones protein, which represents the light chain of the immunoglobulin molecule. Rarely, neoplastic plasma cells are detected in the peripheral circulation. The name "plasma cell leukemia" is sometimes used to designate this phase of plasma cell myeloma. (See also p. 1568.)

The other major clinicopathologic form of plasma cell myeloma is represented by the appearance of a solitary tumor mass, either in a bone or in the soft tissues (nasopharynx, nose, tonsil).[62,73] These are usually not accompanied by immunoglobulin abnormalities. Many of these localized lesions eventually become disseminated in bone, although this may occur many years later and even then run a more prolonged course than the form that is generalized from the beginning.

The gross and microscopic features of the disease are similar in the generalized and localized forms. Grossly, the tissue is soft, friable, and hemorrhagic (Fig. 45-31). The focal, slowly growing tumor may have a fairly well-defined border.

Microscopically, there is a wide range of differentiation that the neoplastic cells may exhibit (Fig. 45-32). On one extreme, there is the tumor that is composed of plasma cells so well differentiated that a confusion with an inflammatory condition may arise; on the other, one sees a highly undifferentiated tumor with formation of tumor giant cells, in which the plasmacytic nature may be missed altogether. The characteristic features of plasma cells, which persist in all but the more undifferentiated neoplasms, include oval cytoplasm, eccentric nucleus with cartwheel distribution of the chromatin and a distinct perinuclear clear halo. The high ribosomal content of the cytoplasm can be made evident with the methyl green–pyronine stain, which stains cytoplasmic and nucleolar RNA red (pyroninophilic) and nuclear DNA green. By electron microscopy, the most distinctive features are the presence of a highly developed granular endoplasmic reticulum, usually arranged in the form of parallel cisternae, and a prominent Golgi apparatus, which corresponds to the perinuclear clear halo of light microscopy.[35]

Osteomyelitis rich in plasma cells (so-called plasma cell osteomyelitis) can be differentiated from plasma cell myeloma by the absence of atypical nuclear forms; no or few binucleated plasma cells; presence of abundant Russell's

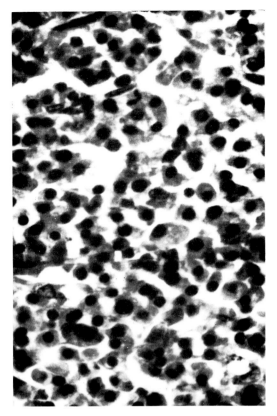

Fig. 45-32. Plasma cell myeloma. Closely packed tumor cells resembling plasma cells.

bodies (intracytoplasmic round eosinophilic bodies that represent inspissated immunoglobulin and are of very rare ocurrence in myeloma); presence of other inflammatory components, such as lymphocytes, eosinophils, and neutrophils; and a richer reticular and collagenous background.

In a certain percentage of myeloma cases, a deposition of amyloid is observed in the tumor tissue or in other organs.

Vascular tumors. The most common vascular tumor is the benign tumor of the blood vessel, i.e., *hemangioma*.[113] It is usually of the cavernous variety, in the sense that it is composed of capillaries and venules with thin walls and greatly dilated lumens packed with red blood cells. The vascular spaces permeate the bone marrow and, if large enough, expand the bone and elicit periosteal new bone formation. In flat bones, particularly the skull, this results in a typical "sunburst" effect on radiographic examination. The most common locations of clinically significant hemangiomas are the skull, vertebrae, and jawbones. Collections of dilated blood-filled vessels are commonly encountered in the vertebrae at autopsy, but they probably represent malformations rather than true neoplasms.

Bone hemangiomas can be multiple, especially in children; half of the cases are associated with cutaneous, visceral, or soft-tissue hemangiomas.[102]

Massive osteolysis (Gorham's disease) is a disease characterized by a progressive replacement of the bone structures by heavily vascularized fibrous tissue. This may lead eventually to resorption of a whole bone or several bones.[39]

Two benign vascular tumors that are exceptional in bones are *lymphangioma* and *glomus tumor (glomangioma)*. The former is usually multiple and associated with similar lesions in soft tissues. The latter is invariably located in a terminal phalanx.[68] Benign and malignant *hemangiopericytomas* primary in bone have been described.

Most malignant vascular tumors of bone arise from endothelial cells of blood vessels and are better designated as *angiosarcomas*. Grossly, these tumors may be cellular, friable, and gray or, because of the high degree of vascularity, may be red and ooze blood when sectioned. Two distinct varieties are recognized, both of which tend to be multicentric.[28] Low-grade angiosarcoma (also known as hemangioendothelioma) is characterized by the formation of anastomosing cell cords, some with a central lumen. The endothelial cells lining the spaces are plump but without bizarre cytologic or nuclear features. The clinical course is prolonged, with frequent local recurrence but a very low incidence of distant metastases.[81] High-grade osteosarcoma has a similar architecture, but it also has obvious atypia of the endothelial cells, together with the formation of solid areas and the appearance of necrosis. Distant metastases are common, particularly to the lungs.

Well-vascularized osteosarcoma and metastatic carcinoma to bone (particularly from the kidney) can closely simulate the microscopic pattern of angiosarcoma.

FIBROUS TISSUE TUMORS

Desmoplastic fibroma. Desmoplastic fibroma is a nonmetastasizing but locally aggressive neoplasm that is characterized microscopically by the presence of mature fibroblasts separated by abundant collagen.[84] The absence of pleomorphism, necrosis, and mitotic activity differentiate this tumor from fibrosarcoma. Local recurrences are common. It is likely that des-

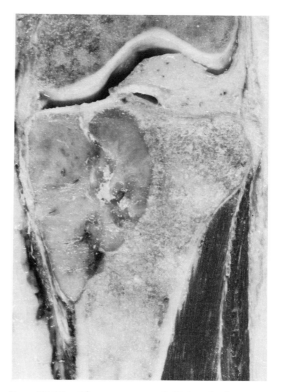

Fig. 45-33. Fibrosarcoma of tibia. Lesion produced osteolytic defect and was confused radiographically with giant cell tumor.

moplastic fibroma represents the osseous counterpart of soft-tissue fibromatosis (so-called desmoid tumor).

Fibrosarcoma is the malignant counterpart of desmoplastic fibroma.[26] It usually involves the metaphysis of long bones in adult individuals. It appears radiographically as an osteolytic lesion with frequent extension into soft tissues.[52] Most cases arise within the medullary canal (endosteal or medullary fibrosarcomas),[20] but indubitable periosteal examples have also been reported. Grossly, the tumor is whitish, firm, and homogeneous (Fig. 45-33). The microscopic appearance is similar to that of the more common fibrosarcoma of soft tissue and characterized by atypical spindle cells that form interlacing bundles of collagen fibers *but no cartilage or bone.* The latter feature is important in the differential diagnosis because both osteosarcoma and chondrosarcoma can have similar spindle cell areas.

Fibrosarcomas are less malignant as a group than are osteosarcomas, especially the better differentiated variants.

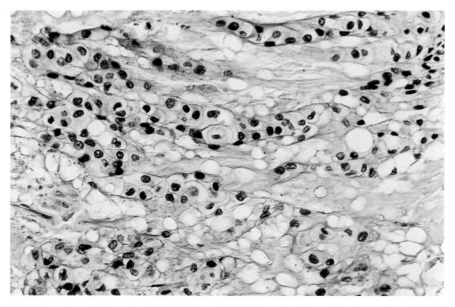

Fig. 45-34. Chordoma of spheno-occipital region. Cuboid and polyhedral cells of central nucleus form rows and nests among abundant myxoid matrix. (350×.)

OTHER PRIMARY TUMORS

Chordoma. Malignant chordoma is believed to arise from developmental remnants of the notochord. The notochord is the original axial skeleton that is subsequently replaced by the spine; its remnants are represented by the nucleus pulposus of the intervertebral discs and small clumps of notochordal cells within the vertebral bodies. Because of their highly vacuolated cytoplasm, these cells are also known as physaliphorous (*physalis,* 'bubble'; *phoros,* 'bearing').

Naturally, all chordomas arise in the axial skeleton. The sacral and spheno-occipital regions are the commonest sites,[46] with the intervening vertebrae being involved only rarely. Chordomas are slowly growing tumors. They infiltrate adjacent structures and stubbornly recur after excision. However, distant metastases are quite rare. Radiographically, chordomas appear as an osteolytic or rarely an osteoblastic process. The tumor may encroach upon the spine and give rise to symptoms of spinal cord compression.[47] Grossly, they are gelatinous and soft and often contain areas of hemorrhage. Microscopically, the tumor is formed by cell cords and lobules separated by a variable but usually abundant amount of myxoid intercellular tissue (Fig. 45-34). The tumor cells are quite large, with vacuolated cytoplasm and prominent vesicular nucleus. The cytoplasm contains glycogen and muco-substances, but no fat. Areas of cartilage and bone may be present.

"Adamantinoma" of long bones. This mysterious neoplasm, rarely seen in long bones (predominantly the tibia), is so designated because of its microscopic resemblance to the adamantinoma (ameloblastoma) of jaw-bones.[7,75] The origin of the latter tumor is the odontogenic tissue, but this can hardly be the case for its long-bone counterpart. Three major hypotheses have been put forward to explain it—tumor of epithelial cells, vascular tumor, and tumor of intraosseous synovial tissues. The weight of the evidence favors the first interpretation. The typical tumor has an obvious epithelial architecture, being formed by lobules with peripheral palisading and a central looser arrangement (Fig. 45-35). By electron microscopy, the tumor cells contain tonofibrils and complex desmosomes, two well-known markers of epithelial cells.[86] Naturally, the question arises as to what an epithelial tumor is doing inside a long bone. Significative in this regard is that the most common location is the tibia, which is closer to the skin than any other long bone. It is conceivable that epithelial cells from the epidermis or its adnexa find their way beneath the periosteum, either as a result of traumatic inclusion or as an abnormality of development, and later undergo a neoplastic transformation. In support of this interpretation, there is a close morphologic

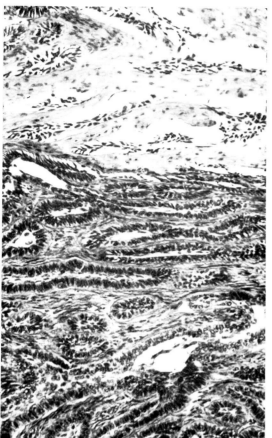

Fig. 45-35. "Adamantinoma" of tibia. Alveolar arrangement of tall cylindric cells with centrally placed fusiform and oval cells. Invasion of bone evident at left margin. Section prepared from tumor shown in Fig. 45-36. (145×.)

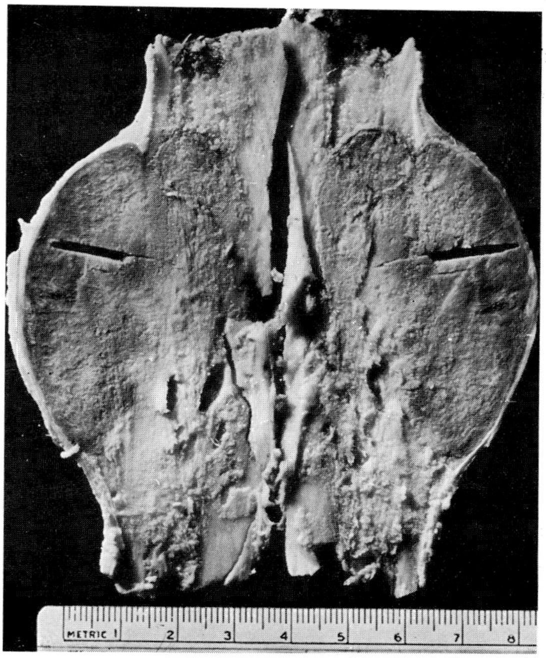

Fig. 45-36. "Adamantinoma" of long bones. Large solitary tumor mass in midportion of tibia has led to sharply defined bone destruction. Neoplasm was dense but moderately cellular and friable and, on section, revealed features similar to those of adamantinoma (ameloblastoma) of jawbones (see Fig. 45-35).

similarity between "adamantinoma" of long bones and sweat gland carcinoma of the skin.

Long-bone "adamantinoma" produces rounded or oval, sometimes loculated, areas of bone destruction to be seen in roentgenograms and on gross examination (Fig. 45-36). Occasionally, it is seen in association with a lesion of fibrous dysplasia in the same bone[15]; it is a malignant neoplasm, prone to local recurrence and even distant metastases.[112]

Tumors of peripheral nerves. Peripheral nerve tumors are exceptional and mainly represented by the *neurilemoma*.[31] Although von Recklinghausen's disease is often accompanied by skeletal deformities, the occurrence of intraosseous neurofibromas is virtually nonexistent.[50]

Tumors of adipose tissue. Adipose tissue tumors are exceptional and basically represented by the benign *lipoma*. This presents as a small to medium-sized nodule of fat tissue fairly demarcated from bone marrow. Whether a primary liposarcoma of bone exists is debatable; most cases so designated are presently regarded as examples of other tumors, such as malignant fibrous histiocytoma.

Tumors of probable histiocytic origin. It is now accepted that a relatively large number of soft-tissue neoplasms arise from "fixed" histiocytes (as distinguished from the "mobile" histiocytes of lymphoid and hematopoietic organs).[61] They are designated as histiocytomas and fibrous histiocytomas, the latter having in addition to the histiocytic elements a fibroblastic component, perhaps originated from the histiocytes by virtue of a metaplastic process.[82] Each category can be divided into a benign and a malignant type. It is becoming evident that similar tumors exist within the bone, although their frequency is certainly less than in the soft tissue.[32] *Benign histiocytomas* often have a prominent component of fat-containing foamy macrophages (xanthoma cells) and are also referred to as xanthomas. The rib is the most common location. *Malignant fibrous histiocytomas*, also known as fibroxanthosarcomas and xanthosarcomas, predominate in long bones, where they tend to involve the medullary portion in the metaphyseal area. Radiographically, they appear as large lytic destructive lesions. The gross appearance is that of a variegated tumor with yellow foci alternating with areas of hemorrhage. Microscopically, spindle cells predominate. They are often arranged about a central point, producing radiating spokes grouped at right angles to each other, a pattern referred to as *storiform*. Foamy cells, hemosiderin-laden macrophages and bizarre giant tumor cells are common.

Some cases of malignant fibrous histiocytomas have been reported as a late complication of bone infarcts.[74]

The clinical behavior is unpredictable, although the degree of malignancy is less than that of osteosarcoma. Metastases to regional lymph nodes can occur.

Metastatic tumors. Metastases to the skeletal system of neoplasms arising in other organs are the most frequent of all malignant neoplasms of bone. Carcinomas greatly predominate over sarcomas. The most common types of cancer resulting in bone metastases are tumors of breast, prostate, lung, kidney, stomach, thyroid, and adrenal medulla. Cancers arising in other organs, such as the body and cervix of the uterus, bladder, and testicle, also may spread to bone. Melanomas sometimes give rise to extensive skeletal involvement. The metastatic foci can be multiple or single. The latter are particularly common with thyroid and renal cancers. In order of frequency, the bones most commonly involved are as follows: spine, pelvis, femur, skull, ribs, and humerus. Metastases to distal bones, such as the bones of forearm, wrist, hand, leg, ankle, and foot are quite unusual. Radiographically, most metastases appear as destructive lytic lesions (Fig. 45-37). Others may be seen as a mixture of lytic and sclerotic changes, and still others elicit such an exuberant osteoblastic reaction as to produce a radiographic osteoblastic appearance. Tumors with a particular tendency to produce osteoblastic bone metastases are prostate, carcinoid tumor, oat cell tumor of lung, and, rarely, breast and stomach cancer.[78,109] The mechanism for the osteoblastic stimulation is not known. Metastases from renal and thyroid cancers may pulsate and give rise to an audible bruit because of their pronounced vascularity. Pathologic fracture is often the first evidence that metastasis to a bone has taken place.

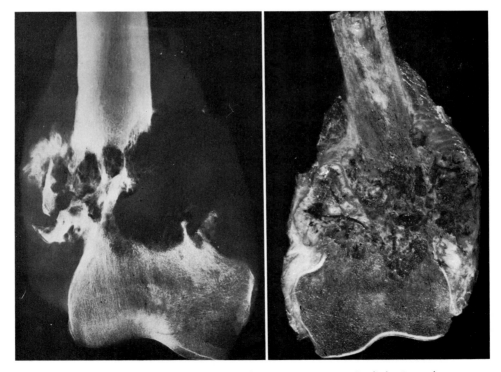

Fig. 45-37. Carcinoma of kidney (hypernephroma) metastasis. Radiologic and gross appearances of slice of femur showing large destructive lesion with pathologic fracture.

The area of a long bone most commonly involved by a metastatic process is the metaphysis, presumably by virtue of its greater vascularity.

As mentioned above, sarcomas metastasize to the skeletal system only rarely. The outstanding exception is *embryonal rhabdomyosarcoma* of soft tissues, which is complicated by blood-borne osseous metastases in a large percentage of cases.[11]

Skeletal metastases, when demonstrated in any given patient, are obviously of great importance in determining prognosis and in guiding treatment. In general, the consequence of such lesions to the patient are pain that is frequently intolerable and disability to the point of complete invalidism until the disease has terminated fatally.

TUMORLIKE LESIONS

Solitary bone cyst. This benign condition, also known as simple or unicameral bone cyst, presents as a cavity filled with clear or blood-tinged fluid in the metaphysis of a long bone, particularly the upper end of the humerus and femur[57] (Fig. 45-38). Most cases occur in

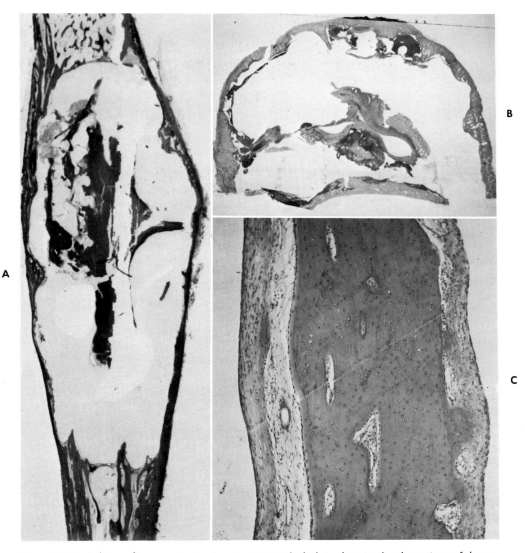

Fig. 45-38. Solitary bone cyst. **A,** Intact cyst included in longitudinal section of bone. Cortex greatly reduced in thickness and bone shaft widened. **B,** Cross section illustrating fibrous tissue septa that partially divide such cysts. **C,** Thin bony wall of cyst with fibrous connective tissue lining on left and proliferative changes in subperiosteal layer on exterior surface of expanded bone on right.

children and adolescents.[105] The pathogenesis is unknown. Microscopically, the cavity is lined by a membrane of variable thickness that is formed by loose connective tissue with a scattering of osteoclasts (Fig. 45-38). A layer of fibrin or hyalinized fibrous tissue is commonly present in the wall, together with newly formed bone trabeculae of reactive nature. Areas of recent or old hemorrhage and cholesterol clefts can sometimes be found, particularly after a fracture of the cyst. The latter is a common event. The treatment consists of curettage followed by packing of the cavity with bone chips.

Aneurysmal bone cyst. The aneurysmal bone cyst, which was often confused in the past with the giant cell tumor, presents as an expansile mass formed by blood-filled spaces of variable but often large size. Most cases occur in patients under 30 years of age and involve either the shaft of metaphysis of long bones or the vertebral column.[66] Pain and swelling are the predominant symptoms. The radiographic appearance is quite distinctive by virtue of the expansile nature of the mass, resulting in a ballooned-out distention of the periosteum[110] (Fig. 45-39). Grossly, it forms a spongy hemorrhagic mass that may extend into the soft tissue and be covered by a thin shell of reactive bone. Microscopically, the cyst cavity is not lined by endothelial cells but rather by fibrous septa containing osteoid and numerous osteoclast-like multineucleated giant cells. The pathogenesis is not clear. Lichtenstein[66] postulated a persistent local alteration in hemodynamics leading to increased venous pressure and the subsequent development of a dilated and vascular bed within the transformed bone area.

Cystic changes, apparently secondary and closely resembling those of aneurysmal bone cyst, are occasionally found in chondroblastoma, fibrous dysplasia, giant cell tumor, osteosarcoma, and other lesions.[21] Therefore it is important to rule out these conditions by examining carefully the entire material when confronted with this situation.

Ganglion cyst of bone. Ganglion cyst is a common lesion of soft tissue, where it appears as a mucus-filled cystic mass in a periarticular location. Sometimes a lesion of similar appearance and pathogenesis is found within a bone, usually the lower end of the tibia or humerus.[99] Radiographically, it appears as a well-defined osteolytic area with a surrounding zone of osteosclerosis. Microscopically, it lacks synovial lining. It has instead a flat fibrous lining, like its soft-tissue counterpart.

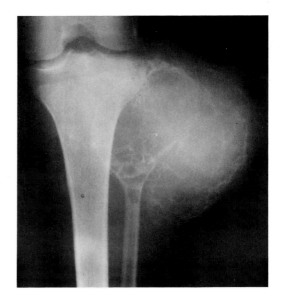

Fig. 45-39. Aneurysmal bone cyst of upper fibula. Lesion started in metaphysis but is now involving entire end of bone. Note classic ballooned-out appearance.

Metaphyseal fibrous defect. The metaphyseal fibrous defect is a radiographically distinctive benign lesion occurring in the diaphyseal cortex of long bones in children[19] (Fig. 45-40). It is usually solitary but may appear as multiple or even bilaterally symmetric defects. The upper or lower tibia and the lower femur are the sites of predilection. Radiographically, the lesion is eccentric, has sharply delimited borders, and is centered in the metaphysis. More extensive lesions, involving the medullary canal and resulting in a fusiform expansion of the bone, are sometimes referred to as *nonossifying* or *nonosteogenic fibromas*[56] (Fig. 45-41). The morphologic appearance of the two lesions is very similar, suggesting that they are examples of the same entity.[103] Grossly, the lesion is granular and brown or dark. Dense bone can be seen around it.[77] Microscopically, it consists of cellular masses of fibrous tissue with a storiform pattern of growth, with scattered osteoclast-like giant cells, hemosiderin-laden macrophages, and foamy cells. The lesion is often asymptomatic and is usually discovered incidentally in a roentgenogram taken for another reason.

The pathogenesis is unknown. The designation "defect" implies that the lesion arises as the result of some developmental aberration at the epiphyseal plate. Another possibility is that it belongs to the group of tumors de-

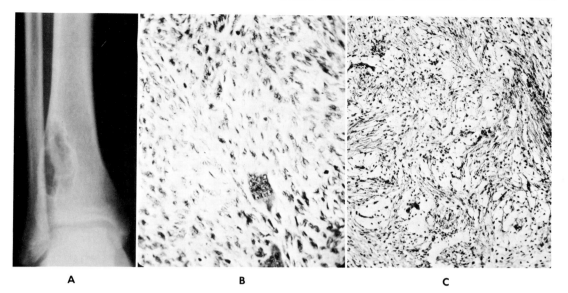

Fig. 45-40. Metaphyseal fibrous defect. **A,** Eccentric lytic area with sharply delimited sclerotic borders in the metaphysis. **B,** Cellular lesion, composed of plump fibroblasts and scattered giant cells. **C,** Clusters of lipid-laden histiocytes among spindle cells.

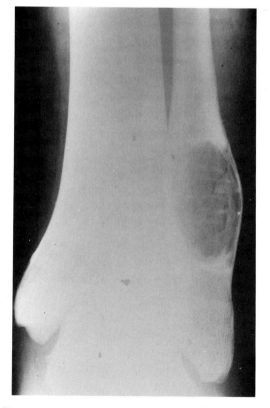

Fig. 45-41. Nonossifying fibroma with superimposed fracture. Lesion, which involves lower metaphysis of tibia, is distinguished from metaphyseal fibrous defect by virture of its large size and presence of medullary involvement and bone expansion.

scribed above in the discussion of tumors of probably histiocytic origin. The histologic resemblance with them is certainly pronounced.

REFERENCES

1 Aisenberg, A. C., and Bloch, K. J.: Immunoglobulins on the surface of neoplastic lymphocytes, New Eng. J. Med. 287:271-276, 1972.

2 Amstutz, H. C.: Multiple osteogenic sarcomata —metastatic or multicentric? Report of two cases and review of literature, Cancer 24:923-931, 1969.

3 Anderson, I. F.: Maffucci's syndrome; report of a case with a review of the literature, S. Afr. Med. J. 39:1066-1070, 1965.

4 Anderson, W. A. D., Zander, G. E., and Kuzma, J. F.: Cancerogenic effects of Ca^{45} and Sr^{89} on bones of CF_1 mice, Arch. Pathol. 62:262-271, 1956.

5 Arlen, M., Higinbotham, N. L., Huvos, A. G., Marcove, R. C., Miller, T., and Shah, I. C.: Radiation-induced sarcoma of bone, Cancer 28:1087-1099, 1971.

6 Azar, H. A.: Plasma cell myelomatosis and other monoclonal gammopathies, Pathol. Annu. 7:1-17, 1972.

7 Baker, P. L., Dockerty, M. B., and Coventry, M. B.: Adamantinoma (so-called) of the long bones, J. Bone Joint Surg. (Am.) 36:704-720, 1954.

8 Barnes, R., and Catto, M.: Chondrosarcoma of bone, J. Bone Joint Surg. (Br.) 48:729-764, 1966.

9 Boston, H. C., Jr., Dahlin, D. C., Ivins, J. C., and Cupps, R. E.: Malignant lymphoma (so-called reticulum cell sarcoma) of bone, Cancer 34:1131-1137, 1974.

10 Byers, P. D.: Solitary benign osteoblastic lesions of bone—osteoid osteoma and benign osteoblastoma, Cancer 22:43-57, 1968.

11 Caffey, J., and Andersen, D. H.: Metastatic

embryonal rhabdomyosarcoma in the growing skeleton: clinical, radiographic, and microscopic features, Am. J. Dis. Child. 95:581-600, 1958.

12 Carbone, P. P., Kellerhouse, L. E., and Gehan, E. A.: Plasmacytic myeloma; a study of the relationship of survival to various clinical manifestations and anomalous protein type in 112 patients, Am. J. Med. 42:937-948, 1967.

13 Chabner, B. A., Haskell, C. M., and Canellos, G. P.: Destructive bone lesions in chronic granulocytic leukemia, Medicine (Baltimore) 48:401-410, 1969.

14 Chang, C. H. J., Piatt, E. D., Thomas, K. E., and Watne, A. L.: Bone abnormalities in Gardner's syndrome, Am. J. Roentgenol. Radium Ther. Nucl. Med. 103:645-652, 1968.

15 Cohen, D. M., Dahlin, D. C., and Pugh, D. G.: Fibrous dysplasia associated with adamantinoma of the long bones, Cancer 15:515-521, 1961.

16 Coleman, S. S.: Benign chondroblastoma with recurrent soft-tissue and intra-articular lesions, J. Bone Joint Surg. (Am.) 48:1554-1560, 1966.

17 Cowan, W. K.: Malignant change and multiple metastases in Ollier's disease, J. Clin. Pathol. 18:650-653, 1965.

18 Cruz, M., Coley B. C., and Stewart, F. W.: Postradiation bone sarcoma, Cancer 10:72-88, 1957.

19 Cunningham, J. B., and Ackerman, L. V.: Metaphyseal fibrous defects, J. Bone Joint Surg. (Am.) 38:797-808, 1956.

20 Cunningham, M. P., and Arlen, M.: Medullary fibrosarcoma of bone, Cancer 21:31-37, 1968.

21 Dabska, M., and Buraczewski, J.: Aneurysmal bone cyst; pathology, clinical course and radiologic appearances, Cancer 23:371-389, 1969.

22 Dahlin, D. C.: Chondromyxoid fibroma of bone, with emphasis on its morphological relationship to benign chondroblastoma, Cancer 9:195-203, 1956.

23 Dahlin, D. C., and Coventry, M. B.: Osteogenic sarcoma; a study of 600 cases, J. Bone Joint Surg. (Am.) 49:101-110, 1967.

24 Dahlin, D. C., Cupps, R. E., and Johnson, E. W., Jr.: Giant-cell tumor; a study of 195 cases, Cancer 25:1061-1070, 1970.

25 Dahlin, D. C., and Henderson, E. D.: Chondrosarcoma, a surgical and pathological problem, J. Bone Joint Surg. (Am.) 38:1025-1038, 1956.

26 Dahlin, D. C., and Ivins, J. C.: Fibrosarcoma of bone; a study of 114 cases, Cancer 23:35-41, 1969.

27 de Souza Dias, L., and Frost, H. M.: Osteoid osteoma—osteoblastoma, Cancer 33:1075-1081, 1974.

28 Dorfman, H. D., Steiner, G. C., and Jaffe, H. L.: Vascular tumors of bone, Hum. Pathol. 2:349-376, 1971.

29 Edeiken, J., Farrell, C., Ackerman, L. V., and Spjut, H.: Parosteal sarcoma, Am. J. Roentgenol. Radium Ther. Nucl. Med. 111:579-583, 1971.

30 Farr, G. H., Huvos, A. G., Marcove, R. C., Higinbotham, N. L., and Foote, F. W., Jr.: Telangiectatic osteogenic sarcoma; a review of twenty-eight cases, Cancer 34:1150-1158, 1974.

31 Fawcett, K. J., and Dahlin, D. C.: Neurilemoma of bone, Am. J. Clin. Pathol. 47:759-776, 1967.

32 Feldman, F., and Norman, D.: Intra- and extraosseous malignant histiocytoma (malignant fibrous xanthoma), Radiology 104:497-508, 1972.

33 Finkel, M. P., Biskis, B. O., and Farrell, C.: Osteosarcomas appearing in Syrian hamsters after treatment with extracts of human osteosarcomas, Proc. Natl. Acad. Sci. 60:1223-1230, 1968.

34 Finkel, M. P., Biskis, B. O., and Jinkins, P. B.: Virus induction of osteosarcoma in mice, Science 151:698-701, 1966.

35 Fisher, E. R., and Zawadski, A.: Ultrastructural features of plasma cells in patients with paraproteinemias, Am. J. Clin. Pathol. 54:779-789, 1970.

36 Fraumeni, J. F., Jr.: Stature and malignant tumors of bone in childhood and adolescence, Cancer 20:967-973, 1967.

37 Friedman, B., and Gold, H.: Ultrastructure of Ewing's sarcoma of bone, Cancer 22:307-322, 1968.

38 Furey, J. G., Ferrer-Torells, M., and Reagan, J. W.: Fibrosarcoma arising at the site of bone infarcts; a report of two cases, J. Bone Joint Surg. (Am.) 42:802-810, 1960.

39 Gorham, L. W., and Stout, A. P.: Massive osteolysis (acute spontaneous absorption of bone, phantom bone, disappearing bone); its relation to hemangiomatosis, J. Bone Joint Surg. (Am.) 37:985-1004, 1955.

40 Guccion, J. G., Font, R. L., Enzinger, F. M., and Zimmerman, L. E.: Extraskeletal mesenchymal chondrosarcoma, Arch. Pathol. 95:336-340, 1973.

41 Gyorkey, F., Sinkovics, J. G., and Gyorkey, P.: Electron microscopic observations on structures resembling myxovirus in human sarcomas, Cancer 27:1449-1454, 1971.

42 Hallberg, O. E., and Begley, J. W., Jr.: Origin and treatment of osteomas of the paranasal sinuses, Arch. Otolaryngol. 51:750-760, 1950.

43 Hanaoka, H., Friedman, B., and Mack, R. P.: Ultrastructure and histogenesis of giant cell tumor of bone, Cancer 25:1408-1423, 1970.

44 Harmon, T. P., and Morton, K. S.: Osteogenic sarcoma in four siblings, J. Bone Joint Surg. 48B:493-498, 1966.

45 Hatcher, C. H.: The development of sarcoma in bone subjected to roentgen or radium irradiation, J. Bone Joint Surg. 27:179-195, 1945.

46 Heffelfinger, M. J., Dahlin, D. C., MacCarty, C. S., and Beabout, J. W.: Chordomas and cartilaginous tumors at the skull base, Cancer 32:410-420, 1973.

47 Higinbotham, N. L., Phillips, R. F., Farr, H. W., and Hustu, O.: Chordoma; thirty-five-year study at Memorial Hospital, Cancer 20:1841-1850, 1967.

48 Horan, F. T.: Bone involvement in Hodgkin's disease, Br. J. Surg. 56:277-281, 1969.

49 Howard, E. B., Clarke, W. J., Karagianes, M. T., and Palmer, R. F.: Strontium-90–induced bone tumors in miniature swine, Radiat. Res. 39:594-607, 1969.

50 Hunt, J. C., and Pugh, D. G.: Skeletal lesions in neurofibromatosis, Radiology 76:1-19, 1961.

51 Hutter, R. V. P., Foote, F. W., Jr., Frazell, E. L., and Francis, K. C.: Giant cell tumors

complicating Paget's disease of bone, Cancer 16:1044-1056, 1963.

52 Huvos, A. G., and Higinbotham, N. L.: Primary fibrosarcoma of bone; a clinicopathologic study of 130 patients, Cancer 35:837-847, 1975.

53 Huvos, A. G., Higinbotham, N. L., and Miller, T. R.: Bone sarcomas arising in fibrous dysplasia, J. Bone Joint Surg. 54A:1047-1056, 1972.

54 Huvos, A. G., Marcove, R. C., Erlandson, R. A., and Mike, V.: Chondroblastoma of bone; a clinico-pathologic and electron microscopic study, Cancer 29:760-771, 1972.

55 Jaffe, H. L.: Tumors and tumorous conditions of the bones and joint, Philadelphia, 1958, Lea & Febiger.

56 Jaffe, H. L., and Lichtenstein, L.: Nonosteogenic fibroma of bone, Am. J. Pathol. 18:205-221, 1942.

57 Jaffe, H. L., and Lichtenstein, L.: Solitary unicameral bone cyst, Arch. Surg. 44:1004-1025, 1942.

58 Jaffe, H. L., and Lichtenstein, L.: Chondromyxoid fibroma of bone; a distinctive benign tumor likely to be mistaken especially for chondrosarcoma, Arch. Pathol. 45:541-551, 1948.

59 Kadin, M. E., and Bensch, K. G.: On the origin of Ewing's tumor, Cancer 27:257-273, 1971.

60 Kahn, L. B., Wood, F. M., and Ackerman, L. V.: Malignant chondroblastoma; report of two cases and review of the literature, Arch. Pathol. 88:371-376, 1969.

61 Kempson, R. L., and Kyriakos, M.: Fibroxanthosarcoma of the soft tissues; a type of malignant fibrous histiocytoma, Cancer 29:961-976, 1972.

62 Kotner, L. M., and Wang, C. C.: Plasmacytoma of the upper air and food passages, Cancer 30:414-418, 1972.

63 Lacassagne, A.: Conditions dans lesquelles ont été obtenus, chez le lapin, des cancers par action des rayons x sur des foyers inflammatoires, C. R. Soc. Biol. (Paris) 112:562-564, 1933.

64 Levine, G. D., and Bensch, K. G.: Chondroblastoma—the nature of the basic cell; a study by means of histochemistry, tissue culture, electron microcopy, and autoradiography, Cancer 29:1546-1562, 1972.

65 Lewis, R. J., and Lotz, M. J.: Medullary extension of osteosarcoma: implications for rational therapy, Cancer 33:371-375, 1974.

66 Lichtenstein, L.: Aneurysmal bone cyst; observations on fifty cases, J. Bone Joint Surg. (Am). 39:873-882, 1957.

67 Lichtenstein, L., and Hall, J. E.: Periosteal chondroma; a distinctive benign cartilage tumor, J. Bone Joint Surg. 34:691-697, 1952.

68 Mackenzie, D. H.: Intraosseous glomus; report of two cases, J. Bone Joint Surg. (Br). 44:648-651, 1962.

69 MacLennan, D. I., and Wilson, F. C., Jr.: Osteoid osteoma of the spine; a review of the literature and report of six new cases, J. Bone Joint Surg. (Am.) 49:111-121, 1967.

70 Martland, H. S., and Humphries, R. E.: Osteogenic sarcoma in dial painters using luminous Joint Surg. (Am.) 49:111-121, 1967.

71 McKenna, R. J., Schwinn, C. P., Soong, K. Y., and Higinbotham, N. L.: Sarcomata of the osteogenic series (osteosarcoma, fibrosarcoma, chondrosarcoma, parosteal osteogenic sarcoma, and sarcomata arising in abnormal bone), J. Bone Joint Surg. (Am.) 48:1-26, 1966.

72 Mehta, Y., and Hendrickson, F. R.: CNS involvement in Ewing's sarcoma, Cancer 33:859-862, 1974.

73 Meyer, J. E., and Schulz, M. D.: "Solitary" myeloma of bone: a review of 12 cases, Cancer 34:438-440, 1974.

74 Mirra, J. M., Bullough, P. G., Marcove, R. C., Jacobs, B., and Huvos, A. G.: Malignant fibrous histiocytoma and osteosarcoma in association with bone infarcts, J. Bone Joint Surg. 56A:932-940, 1974.

75 Moon, N. F.: Adamantinoma of the appendicular skeleton; a statistical review of reported cases and inclusion of 10 new cases, Clin. Orthop. 43:189-213, 1965.

76 Morton, D. L., and Malmgren, R. A.: Human osteosarcomas: immunologic evidence suggesting an associated infectious agent, Science 162:1279-1281, 1968.

77 Mubarak, S., Saltzstein, S. L., and Daniel, D. M.: Non-ossifying fibroma; report of an intact lesion, Am. J. Clin. Pathol. 61:697-701, 1974.

78 Muggia, F. M., and Hansen, H. H.: Osteoblastic metastases in small-cell (oat-cell) carcinoma of the lung, Cancer 30:801-805, 1972.

79 Murphy, W. R., and Ackerman, L. V.: Benign and malignant giant-cell tumors of bone, Cancer 9:317-339, 1956.

80 O'Neal, L. W., and Ackerman, L. V.: Chondrosarcoma of bone, Cancer 5:551-557, 1952.

81 Otis, J., Hutter, R. V. P., Foote, F. W., Jr., Marcove, R. C., and Stewart, F. W.: Hemangioendothelioma of bone, Surg. Gynecol. Obstet. 127:295-305, 1968.

82 Ozzello, L., Stout, A. P., and Murray, M. R.: Cultural characteristics of malignant histiocytomas and fibrous xanthomas, Cancer 16:331-344, 1963.

83 Pasmantier, M. W., and Azar, H. A.: Extraskeletal spread in multiple plasma cell myeloma; a review of 57 autopsied cases, Cancer 23:167-174, 1969.

84 Rabhan, W. N., and Rosai, J.: Desmoplastic fibroma; report of ten cases and review of the literature, J. Bone Joint Surg. (Am.) 50:487-502, 1968.

85 Rahimi, A., Beabout, J. W., Ivins, J. C., and Dahlin, D. C.: Chondromyxoid fibroma; a clinicopathologic study of 76 cases, Cancer 30:726-736, 1972.

86 Rosai, J.: Adamantinoma of the tibia; electron microscopic evidence of its epithelial origin, Am. J. Clin. Pathol. 51:786-792, 1969.

87 Rosen, G., Wollner, N., Tan, C., Wu, S. J., Hajdu, S. I., Cham, W., D'Angio, G. J., and Murphy, M. L.: Disease-free survival in children with Ewing's sarcoma treated with radiation therapy and adjuvant four-drug sequential chemotherapy, Cancer 33:384-393, 1974.

88 Salvador, A. H., Beabout, J. W., and Dahlin, D. C.: Mesenchymal chondrosarcoma; observations on 30 new cases, Cancer 28:605-615, 1971.

89 Schajowicz, F.: Ewing's sarcoma and reticu-

lum-cell sarcoma of bone; with special reference to the histochemical demonstration of glycogen as an aid to differential diagnosis, J. Bone Joint Surg. (Am.) 41:349-356, 1959.

90 Schajowicz, F.: Giant-cell tumors of bone (osteoclastoma); a pathological and histochemical study, J. Bone Joint Surg. (Am.) 43: 1-29, 1961.

91 Schajowicz, F., Ackerman, L. V., and Sissons, H. A.: Histologic typing of bone tumours, International Histological Classification of Tumours, No. 6, Geneva, 1972, World Health Organization.

92 Schajowicz, F., and Bessone, J. E.: Chondrosarcoma in three brothers, J. Bone Joint Surg. 43A:1-29, 1961.

93 Schajowicz, F., and Derqui, J. C.: Puncture biopsy in lesions of the locomotor system: review of results in 4,050 cases, including 941 vertebral punctures, Cancer 21:531-548, 1968.

94 Schajowicz, F., and Gallardo, H.: Epiphysial chondroblastoma of bone; a clinico-pathological study of sixty-nine cases, J. Bone Joint Surg. (Br.) 52:205-226, 1970.

95 Schajowicz, F., and Gallardo, H.: Chondromyxoid fibroma (fibromyxoid chondroma) of bone; a clinico-pathological study of thirty-two cases, J. Bone Joint Surg. (Br.) 53:198-216, 1971.

96 Schajowicz, F., and Lemos, C.: Osteoid osteoma and osteoblastoma, Acta Orthop. Scand. 41: 272-291, 1970.

97 Schwartz, D. T., and Alpert, M.: The malignant transformation of fibrous dysplasia, Am. J. Med. Sci. 247: 1-20, 1964.

98 Shoji, H., and Miller, T. R.: Primary reticulum cell sarcoma of bone; significance of clinical features upon the prognosis, Cancer 28:1234-1244, 1971.

99 Sim, H., and Dahlin, D. C.: Ganglion cysts of bone, Mayo Clin. Proc. 46:484-488, 1971.

100 Spiess, H., Poppe, H., and Schoen, H.: Strahleninduzierte Knochentumoren nach Thorium X-Behandlung, Monatsschr. Kinderheilkd. 110: 198-201, 1962.

101 Spjut, H. J., Dorfman, H. D., Fechner, R. E., and Ackerman, L. V.: Tumors of bone and cartilage. In Atlas of tumor pathology, Sect. II, Fasc. 5, Washington, D. C., 1971, Armed Forces Institute of Pathology.

102 Spjut, H. J., and Lindbom, A.: Skeletal angiomatosis; report of two cases, Acta Pathol. Microbiol. Scand. 55:49-58, 1962.

103 Steiner, G. C.: Fibrous cortical defect and nonossifying fibroma of bone, Arch. Pathol. 97:205-210, 1974.

104 Steiner, G. C., Ghosh, L., and Dorfman, H. D.: Ultrastructure of giant cell tumors of bone, Hum. Pathol. 3:569-586, 1972.

105 Stewart, M. J., and Hamel, H. A.: Solitary bone cyst, South. Med. J. 43:926-936, 1950.

106 Suit, H. D.: Role of therapeutic radiology in cancer of bone, Cancer 35:930-935, 1975.

107 Takigawa, K.: Chondroma of the bones of the hand, J. Bone Joint Surg. (Am.) 53:1591-1600, 1971.

108 Tapp, E.: Osteogenic sarcoma in rabbits following subperiosteal implantation of beryllium, Arch. Pathol. 88:89-95, 1969.

109 Thomas, B. M.: Three unusual carcinoid tumours, with particular reference to osteoblastic bone metastases, Clin. Radiol. 19:221-225, 1968.

110 Tillman, B. P., Dahlin, D. C., Lipscomb, P. R., and Stewart, J. R.: Aneurysmal bone cyst, an analysis of 95 cases, Mayo Clin. Proc. 43: 478-495, 1968.

111 Turner, R. C.: Unusual group of tumours among schoolgirls, Br. J. Cancer 21:17-26, 1966.

112 Unni, K. K., Dahlin, D. C., Beabout, J. W., and Ivins, J. C.: Adamantinomas of long bones, Cancer 34:1796-1805, 1974.

113 Unni, K. K., Ivins, J. C., Beabout, J. W., and Dahlin, D. C.: Hemangioma, hemangiopericytoma, and hemangioendothelioma (angiosarcoma) of bone, Cancer 27:1403-1414, 1971.

114 Van der Heul, R. O., and Von Ronnen, J. R.: Juxtacortical osteosarcoma; diagnosis, differential diagnosis, treatment, and an analysis of eighty cases, J. Bone Joint Surg. (Am.) 49: 415-439, 1967.

115 Wang, C. C., and Fleischli, D. J.: Primary reticulum cell sarcoma of bone, with emphasis on radiation therapy, Cancer 22:994-998, 1968.

116 Yaghniai, I., Zia, A., Shariat, S., and Afshari, R.: Value of arteriography in the diagnosis of benign and malignant bone lesions, Cancer 27: 1134-1147, 1971.

46/Diseases of joints

RUTH SILBERBERG

NORMAL JOINT STRUCTURE AND FUNCTION
Diarthrodial joints

The joints most commonly affected by disease are the diarthrodial or synovial joints. Unlike the serosal cavities of pleurae and peritoneum, joint spaces are not closed or lined by a continuous layer of mesothelial cells. Instead, they are open tissue spaces, communicating directly with the periarticular tissues.

The articulating ends of two bones are held together by the joint capsule, a tubular structure of dense connective tissue inserting at the outer surfaces of the bony shafts. The capsule has an abundant supply of sensory nerve fibers that are highly sensitive to stretching and twisting and that are primarily responsible for the intense pain accompanying many joint lesions. Ligaments and tendons insert at the outer surface of the capsule. The capsule is lined by the synovial membrane, or synovium, which also covers the soft structures within the joints, fat pads, and ligaments and which forms outpouchings (bursae). The bursae communicate with the joint space and are therefore likely to become involved in pathologic processes affecting the joints and vice versa. The articulating surfaces of the bones are covered by bluish, glistening hyaline cartilage, which varies in thickness not only in different joints but also within one and the same joint, with weight-bearing areas usually having a thicker cartilage cover than non–weight-bearing areas. The cartilage is supported by a layer of cancellous bone.

A small amount of free viscid fluid is present in the joint space and, by forming a thin layer over the cartilage, acts as a lubricant during joint motion.

Histologically and by electron microscopy, the surface of the articular cartilage is not smooth, but shows innumerable roundish pits 20 to 30 μm in diameter,[43] which correspond to the underlying most superficially located cartilage cells. The articular surface proper is entirely composed of matrix without cells. This architecture is of importance to the nutrition of the avascular articular cartilage, since it facilitates the flow of the synovial fluid into the cartilage. The chondrocytes vary in size, shape, and distribution; three zones are usually distinguishable—a superficial zone characterized by spindle-shaped cells with their long axis oriented circumferentially; an intermediate or midzone of groups or small columns of polygonal cells, which are capable of multiplying and which are highly active metabolically[187]; and the deepest, the pressure zone, possessing the largest cells, often in perpendicular orientation in relation to the joint surface and separated from the underlying bone by a narrow layer of calcified matrix. By electron microscopy, articular chondrocytes have been shown to possess all the subcellular organelles of cells engaged in active synthesis and secretion—rough endoplasmic reticulum, free ribosomes, a Golgi apparatus, mitochondria, etc. They produce the intercellular matrix and have been shown to respond readily to changes in the internal environment.[187]

The matrix of the articular cartilage is composed of an amorphous phase (the ground substance) and a fibrillar phase (collagen fibrils). The ground substance consists of a variety of protein-polysaccharides (glycosaminoglycans), chiefly chondroitin sulfates A and C and keratan sulfate,[167] responsible for the physical properties of the cartilage, especially its elasticity. The collagen fibrils vary in thickness and distribution. Near the surface, they are oriented in a circumferential direction, an arrangement that enables the cartilage to resist shearing forces; in the midzone they are mesh-like in distribution, and in the deep zone, where they are thicker and more densely packed than elsewhere, they are often found in perpendicular orientation in relation to the joint surface. "Arcades," formed by fibers, presumably in

2015

conformity with mechanical stresses[18] and visualized at the tissue level, are not apparent in electron micrographs.

The synovial membrane is composed of an outer layer of loose vascular connective tissue and an inner discontinuous layer of specialized cells, the synoviocytes.[71] Synoviocytes synthesize and secrete hyaluronate, which is given off into the joint space. Two morphologic types of synoviocytes have been described, one rich in endoplasmic reticulum (B cells), the other with a prominent Golgi apparatus (A cells). It is likely that these two types represent different functional states of one and the same cell.

The articular cartilage is constantly exposed to mechanical stresses occurring during joint motion as well as a result of static loading. The mechanical forces acting on a joint are those of tangential shear and of static pressure, forces that may act with sudden impact or in a protracted fashion. Static forces are brought about by weight and, more importantly, by the action of muscles and ligaments. A number of mechanisms protect the joints from damage by such forces: the elasticity and the surface architecture of the cartilage permit it to absorb some force; the synovial fluid provides lubrication that is ideally adapted to maintain joint function.[159,197,227]

The synovial fluid or "synovia," a term used first by Paracelsus, is a dialysate of plasma, which becomes viscid because of the discharge into it of protein hyaluronate, secreted by the synoviocytes. Under normal conditions, the synovial fluid forms a thin film on the cartilaginous surfaces[227]; the total amount of synovial fluid is small, amounting to about 3 ml in the adult knee joint. Its lubricating effect is enhanced by changes in viscosity with joint motion: at rest or at slow motion it is more viscid than at high rates of motion.[24] Normal synovial fluid contains about 3.5 mg/gm of hyaluronate bound to protein, plasma components, polymorphonuclear and mononuclear leukocytes, and some sloughed-off synoviocytes. The fluid acts not only as a lubricant but also as the main source of nutrients for the articular cartilage into which it penetrates because of a pumping effect created by joint motion.[169]

The biomechanical mechanisms by which joint lubrication is accomplished are still under discussion. The original concept of simple hydrodynamic action[128] has been supplemented by the concepts of boundary lubrication[40] and of weeping lubrication.[122] The former stresses the interaction of small irregularities in the articulating surfaces (as shown by scanning electron microscopy) with extremely thin layers of lubricating fluid in the lubricating process; the second concept is based on the fact that cartilage acts like a sponge, from which tissue fluid is expressed during stresses on the joint and into which fluid is sucked after release of the stress.[233] Whatever the mechanisms of lubrication, a decrease in lubrication will result in increasing friction between the articulating surfaces and lead to tissue damage.

Vertebral joints

Vertebrae possess two kinds of joints. (1) The small apophyseal joints linking the spinal processes are typically diarthrodial in architecture. Thus anatomic, physiologic, and pathologic principles governing these joints are the same as those applying to all other diarthrodial joints. (2) The articulations between the vertebral bodies are unique in that the free joint space is replaced by the intervertebral discs, which cushion the impact of mechanical forces on the vertebrae by virtue of their elasticity and their intrinsic pressure. The discs have a jelly-like center, the nucleus pulposus, containing much water and a variety of mucopolysaccharides, and an outer coat of dense connective tissue, the annulus fibrosus. The annulus restrains the nucleus within its boundaries during motion; it inserts at the opposing "end plates" of the vertebral bodies. These end plates are the actual articulating surfaces of the vertebral bodies and are composed of stratified cartilage structured similar to that of the diarthrodial joints. In the course of time, this cartilage may be partly replaced by bone, so that the annulus is inserted in bone rather than in cartilage.

CONGENITAL MALFORMATIONS AND DEVELOPMENTAL DEFECTS OF JOINTS

Disregarding traumatic dislocation of joints during birth, congenital deformities occur in about 6% of newborns.[19] Such lesions may be secondary to abnormalities in muscles or capsular connective tissue, or they may be primary to the osseous system.

Generalized joint rigidity, a rare condition, is seen in *arthrogryphosis multiplex* characterized by clubfeet, clubhands, and contractures of the large joints. The etiology of the disorder is unknown.

The opposite condition, joint flaccidity is generalized in the *Ehlers-Danlos syndrome*, which is associated with hyperextensibility of joints; it results in loosening of the joint capsule. This abnormality is often the cause for congenital subluxation of the hip.[38] The condition is hereditary, is transmitted as an autosomal recessive, and results from inadequate cross-linking of the collagen molecule. The basic defect is one of inadequate hydroxylation of lysine.[158a]

Clubfoot, a positional abnormality involving flexion of the ankle, inversion of the foot, and medial rotation of the tibia, has been attributed to intrauterine compression, a widely held, but poorly substantiated point of view. The increased concordance of the lesion in monozygotic twins (32%) as compared to 2.9% in fraternal twins suggests the presence of a genetic factor.[91]

Defective development, *dysplasia, of the acetabulum of the hip* is difficult to diagnose in the newborn but becomes more distinct with increasing age. Inadequate ossification of the roof of the acetabulum prevents the formation of a close-fitting socket for the femoral head. Consequently, the latter becomes dislocated cranially, posteriorly or laterally, with resulting complete luxation of the hip.[82]

NONINFLAMMATORY JOINT DISEASES
Joint disorders caused by physical injury

The term "traumatic arthritis," under which these disorders are usually classified, is a misnomer. Although physical injury may cause inflammatory changes, as implied in the term, the sequelae of physical injury are most often noninflammatory. All tissue components of the joints may be affected, and most repair processes correspond to those seen in other locations. However, those involving the articular cartilage have special significance. Although articular chondrocytes retain some growth potential into old age, the healing tendency of the cartilage is poor. Once the continuity of the surface has been disrupted, it is only rarely, if ever, restored to normal, despite active proliferation and synthetic activity of many of the chondrocytes in the middle and deep layers of the articular covering. Defects that reach as deep as the subchondral bone are repaired by fibrous tissue growing into the defect from the bone marrow. Under the effect of friction and pressure during motion, this "scar" may be transformed into fibrocartilage.[36,126]

Injuries of the joints resulting from physical forces are of two main types: (1) acute injuries, which are usually produced by the action of a single violent force, and (2) chronic injuries, which occur after minor and frequently repeated inflictive forces.

1. Any one of the component parts of a joint may be injured by physical force, particularly if the stress is applied suddenly. If a joint is twisted, hyperextended, hyperflexed, or otherwise forced to move beyond the limits permitted by the elasticity of its ligaments, a sprain, subluxation, or dislocation occurs. Such injuries represent varying degrees of a single type of damage. Thus, as the result of a twist, blow, or fall, the synovial tissues, the ligaments, or the capsule may be stretched, lacerated, or ruptured. In the knee, menisci may be displaced, detached, or torn. The articular cartilage may be compressed, split, or detached from the underlying bone.

Injuries that include severe lacerations of ligaments and articular capsules may be associated with dislocation of the bone ends. In these more severely damaged joints, there may be permanent weakening and instability, as well as predisposition to recurrent dislocation. With greater violence, the joint may be dislocated or the bones may be fractured, and there may be a bloody effusion into the joint space.

Usually, the extravasated blood is completely absorbed. In some instances, however, the blood clot organizes, with the production of fibrous adhesions across the joint space. Portions of bone that are completely detached by the fracture become necrotic, though the cartilage survives. These detached fragments of cartilage and bone remain in the joint as loose bodies ("joint mice") and may cause pain or recurrent locking of the joint. Malalignment of the fracture fragments may cause an uneven joint surface and thus excessive friction. The relation of these factors to secondary osteoarthrosis is discussed in a later section of this chapter.

Open laceration of a joint capsule may lead to secondary infection. In addition, physical injury may trigger recurrence of, or reactivate, old quiescent lesions, such as tuberculosis, gouty arthritis, or pyogenic infections.

2. Injuries from minor repeated forces are of many kinds and grades of severity. They include injuries incurred in daily activities, those sustained in recreational or occupational pursuits, and mechanical dysfunction induced by abnormal posture, disturbed locomotion, and skeletal deformities.

The articular changes produced are varied both in kind and in extent of involvement. In some instances, the lesions are found in the periarticular structures, including ligaments, tendon sheaths, or bursae. More frequently, the joint proper is the site of involvement. Effusions of fluid into the bursae, tendon sheaths, or articular cavities occasionally occur. Loose bodies may be present within distended bursal or synovial cavities. Occasionally, calcification will be found in tendons or bursal walls. Such changes are especially common in the region of the shoulder.[139]

Neuropathic joint disease (Charcot's joint)

The lesions, usually monoarticular, are seen in patients suffering from a variety of neurologic disorders. Originally described by Charcot in 1868, they were attributed chiefly to tabes or syringomyelia; they are now known to be associated with spina bifida, with amyloid infiltration in the course of multiple myeloma,[178] with diabetes mellitus,[163,190] and chronic alcoholism.[215] The site of the neurologic lesion determines which joint is affected; with tabes, it is commonly a knee, with syringomyelia the shoulder, with spina bifida the hip, and with diabetes the small joints of the feet and the ankles.

An initial nonspecific noninflammatory effusion within the joint space may subside without further damage. Subsequently, there is increasing deterioration and erosion of the articular cartilage and sclerosis of the adjacent bone. Eventually the bone also undergoes necrosis and disintegrates, a condition leading to gross disfiguration or even disappearance of the involved epiphysis.

Anesthetization of the joint caused by the disrupted nerve supply has been incriminated as a main contributor to the lesion. The patient suffering no pain is not aware of a disease process and continues to traumatize the joint. This mechanism is also responsible for the massive necrosis of joints seen after treatment with large doses of cortisone.[210] However, factors other than purely neurologic dysfunction may be involved in the pathogenesis of some forms of Charcot's joints; diabetic neuropathy especially may be complicated by simultaneous vascular disease, and the disturbed glucose metabolism may directly alter the protein-polysaccharide composition of the cartilage matrix.

Amyloid arthropathy

Generalized amyloidosis may affect multiple joints with deposition of amyloid in the synovium, in cartilage, and in the joint cavity. The shoulder is a site of predilection, but elbows, hands, knees, and temporomandibular and sternoclavicular joints are commonly in-

volved. Large quantities of amyloid may be free in the joint cavity or deposited in the tissues.[143] Cartilage containing amyloid is whitish opaque, and infiltrated synovium is stiffened. By electron microscopy, typical amyloid fibrils with a 75 to 100 Å diameter and a periodicity of 2 or 3 per 100 Å length are found extracellularly in the synovium. With special stains, amyloid may be identified as a thin layer on and slightly below the surface of the cartilage. The surface may be smooth or frayed, depending on whether there is associated degradation of the matrix. No amyloid is found within the chondrocytes.[32] The problem as to how the amyloid reaches the joint cavity—whether by precipitation from the synovial fluid, or by discharge of synovial deposits into the free joint space—is unresolved.

Arthropathy associated with ochronosis

The joint disease associated with ochronosis is caused by the intra-articular deposition of polymerized homogentisic acid, a black pigment. The latter is the product of incomplete degradation of tyrosine and phenylalanine, occurring because of an inborn absence of the enzyme homogentisic acid oxidase. The joints involved are primarily those of the vertebral column, although later in the course of the disorder, hips, knees, and shoulder joints may become affected. Grossly, the large joints may be distended by effusion, which is usually noninflammatory. The cartilage is stained a deep black to various shades of gray and is fragmented and brittle (Plate 6, A and B). The synovium has hypertrophic folds, which contain small fragments of detached deteriorated cartilage.

Microscopically, granular pigment is seen within chondrocytes, and the matrix is stained diffusely.[150] The synovium may show evidence of acute or chronic inflammation. By electron microscopy, amorphous pigment particles have been demonstrated both in chrondrocytes and in the surrounding matrix.[111]

Arthropathy associated with hemochromatosis

Joint involvement is seen in about one half the cases of primary hemochromatosis, and frequently there is associated chondrocalcinosis. The small joints of the hands are most conspicuously affected, but knees, hips, and the vertebral column also become involved.[33,181]

Grossly, the synovium is of brownish-red color, and, in the presence of chondrocalcinosis, multiple, whitish, chalk-like deposits are

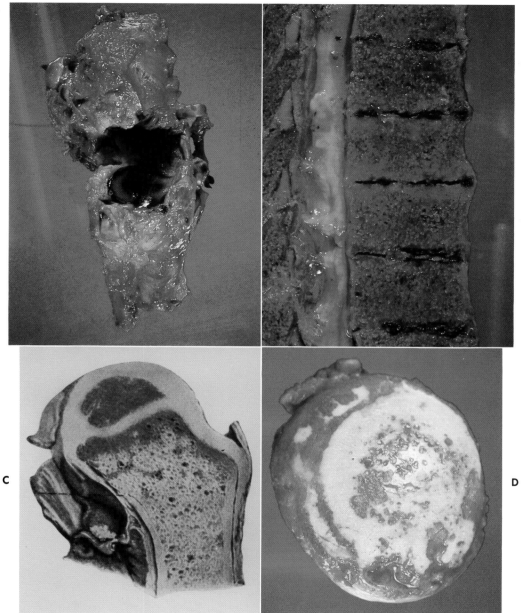

Plate 6

A, Ochronosis of knee joint. Intensely black stain of articular cartilage.

B, Ochronosis of intervertebral discs. Discs are stained deep black.

C, Purulent arthritis developing in course of staphylococcic osteomyelitis. Purulent exudate in both joint capsule *(E)* and bone marrow. *P,* Communication between bone marrow and joint space.

D, Osteoarthrosis of femoral head. Pronounced ulceration of articular cartilage and some marginal lipping.

(**A** and **B,** Courtesy Dr. Steven L. Teitelbaum, St. Louis, Mo.; **C,** from Henke, F., and Lubarsch, O., editors: Handbuch der pathologischen Anatomie und Histologie, New York, 1934, Springer-Verlag, vol. 9, chap. 2; **D,** B.H. 75-1635.)

present in the cartilage, especially in fissures and erosions, which appear during the course of the disease.

Microscopically, the synovium shows slight hyperplasia with proliferation of fibroblasts, perivascular deposits of hemosiderin in the deep layers, thickening of the vessel walls, occasional microaneurysms and medial calcification. By electron microscopy, the pigment can be demonstrated mainly in B cells.[175] Inflammatory changes are negligible. The cartilage does not contain pigment, but calcium pyrophosphate crystals can be demonstrated together with the fibrillation and erosion characteristic of chondrocalcinosis.

The pathogenetic mechanism leading to the joint changes is unknown. The deposition of hemosiderin as such is apparently not injurious, since the lesions do not occur in other conditions associated with iron deposition in joints. This raises the question as to a possible role of the abnormal glucose metabolism of hemochromatosis.

Arthropathy associated with hemophilia

Of hemophiliacs, 80% to 90% will sooner or later develop adverse joint manifestations because of hemorrhage into the articular cavities. A single hemorrhagic episode may be followed by complete resorption and restoration of normal conditions. Repeated hemorrhage, however, sets off a sequela of changes resulting in severe disfiguration and functional impairment of the involved joints.

Grossly, the synovium takes on a reddish-brown color, it becomes hypertrophic with polypous folds or diffuse, mosslike thickening. With increasing duration of the condition, there is increasing fibrous thickening of the synovium, as well as of the subsynovial connective tissue, and development of fibrous adhesions between the opposing surfaces of the joint. The cartilage becomes eroded and cystic because of focal necrosis. The subchondral bone responds with early sclerosis, which may give way to atrophy and breakdown with formation of cysts in the epiphyses. Such cysts enclose organizing blood clot; they may communicate with the articular cavity.

Microscopically, the synovium contains numerous hemosiderin-laden macrophages, especially in the near-surface layers. The lining cells, particularly B cells, are hyperplastic, as are the fibroblasts of the deep layers. Especially near the insertion of ligaments, ingrowth of synovium into degenerating cartilage may be seen. In advanced cases, the cartilage resembles that found in osteoarthrosis.[106,155]

Osteochondroses

Osteochondroses result from aseptic necrosis of the bone underlying the articular cartilage. Since the articular cartilage does not depend on blood vessels for its nutritional supply, the injury to the cartilage is not attributable to nutritional failure. Rather, it is the loss of mechanical support from the underlying bone that causes the cartilage to break down. The ensuing defects may initially be small, but there may be further deterioration of the articular covering and reactive chondrocyte proliferation, resulting in lesions similar to those of osteoarthrosis. Many syndromes associated with osteochondrosis have been described in various skeletal sites. (See Chapter 44.)

Osteochondrosis dissecans

The formerly used term "osteochondritis" is a misnomer, which should be abandoned. The lesion has no inflammatory component whatsoever, and therefore the suffix "-itis" is inappropriate. The characteristic gross findings in the joints are single or multiple loose or lightly attached bodies composed of cartilage and underlying bone. These bodies, termed "joint mice," are ovoid or roundish in shape and measure 0.5 to 1.5 cm in diameter and several millimeters in thickness (Fig. 46-1). Often, a groove in the articular surface indicates the site from which a body has been detached. Microscopically, the grooves are covered with fibrous tissue. The cartilage of the fragments may be intact or show various degrees of fibrillation and foci of calcification. The attached bone is usually sclerotic with thickened trabeculae.

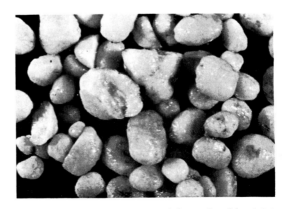

Fig. 46-1. Joint mice removed from shoulder joint. Synovial membrane was studded with small nodules composed of dense fibrous tissue and cartilage. Detachment of these tissue excrescences was apparent source of loose bodies.

The lesions are commonly found in children and adolescents, in boys more often than in girls, and involve most often the knee joint, especially the medial condyle of the femur. However, hip, shoulder, and elbow may also be affected.[160] Mechanical forces, acting on normal joint tissue or on local developmental defects, have been considered as a major cause of the changes; the lesions also develop as a result of aseptic necrosis of subchondral bone and secondary disruption of the cartilage overlying the necrotic bone.[192]

Arthropathy associated with sickle-cell disease

Sickling and thrombosis occur in small vessels of the articular tissues as in non skeletal locations. Thrombi composed of dead cells, platelets, and red blood corpuscles occlude vascular lumens; as a result, microinfarcts may develop in the synovium. The vascular basement membranes are thickened, and perivascular fibrosis is present.[175] The synovium shows low-grade infiltration by mononuclear leukocytes. The cartilage becomes involved secondarily, because of avascular necrosis of the subchondral bone. Tissue destruction, which may become extensive, thus resembles that seen in aseptic avascular necrosis, and, in advanced cases, in osteochondrosis dissecans. The joints most commonly involved are hip, shoulder, and knee in the order mentioned.

Hypertrophic osteoarthropathy

The clubbing of fingers and toes characteristic of the disorder is primarily attributable to periarticular and periosteal hyperemia and fibroblastic proliferation and to overgrowth of bone; joints may become involved with an increase of synovial fluid, which is rich in mucins but has fewer cells than would be present in an inflammatory lesion. The condition is found in association with circulatory failure as occurring in congenital heart disease, with a variety of digestive disorders, but chiefly with malignant or chronic benign pulmonary disease.

In addition to this secondary type of clubbing, there is a primary form of the disease, pachydermatoperiostosis, which is inherited as a sex-linked dominant trait.[162]

Aging of articular cartilage

The articular cartilage changes with age in regard to its morphologic, biochemical, and physical properties. These changes are important pathogenetically because they render the cartilage more susceptible to the action of injurious factors.

The growth potential and the cellularity of the articular cartilage decrease progressively from birth to the end of the growth period, but some growth potential persists throughout life.[185] This fact is responsible for lifelong cell renewal, the gradual remodeling of the articular contour,[96] and the resumption of cell proliferation under pathologic conditions, such as osteoarthrosis of old age or of hyperpituitarism. During adulthood, the decline in cellularity slows down, and in old age, a slight increase in the number of cells may occur.[206] Associated with this increase in cell number, is an increase in cellular activity as indicated by increased uptake of radiosulfate by the articular chondrocytes.[46] An age-linked increase in intracellular lipid apparently does not interfere with the functioning of the chondrocytes.

The matrix likewise changes with advancing age.[207] During growth, the ratio of chondroitin sulfate A to chondroitin sulfate C decreases, and keratan sulfate is deposited in increasing quantities. The latter process continues into midlife, whereas from early adulthood on, there is a net loss of total mucopolysaccharides from the matrix. In many joints, mucopoly-

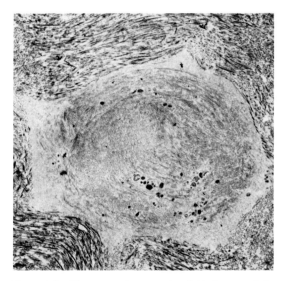

Fig. 46-2. Electron micrograph of "microscar" in aging human articular cartilage of hip joint. Whorls of collagen fibrils with intermingled electron-dense fat globules have replaced disintegrated chondrocytes. Scar is still surrounded by halo of relatively electron-lucent matrix, which surrounded the former chondrocyte. Regular matrix with collagen fibrils at periphery. (Courtesy Dr. Max Spycher, Zurich.)

saccharide content becomes stabilized thereafter, and no further changes occur, unless additional pathogenic factors become active.

As mucopolysaccharides decrease, the collagen fibrils increase in thickness and become packed more tightly than in the young individual.[202] Focal whorl-like aggregations of collagen fibrils develop at the sites of disintegrated cells (Fig. 46-2). All these changes, together with loss of water, lead to impairment of elasticity, increase the stiffness of the articular cartilage,[233] inhibit the flow of nutrient fluid, and thus cause attrition of many chondrocytes. The remaining cells, in an apparent attempt at compensation, become temporarily overactive and, after this, are prematurely exhausted and die; thus a vicious cycle is initiated resulting ultimately in osteoarthrosis. The age-linked progressive accumulation of lipid in the matrix[69] results from distintegration of cell components but does not seem to influence subsequent disease processes.

Age changes in capsule, ligaments, and synovial membrane presumably are the same as those in connective tissue in other locations.[76,221]

Osteoarthrosis

Osteoarthrosis is a noninflammatory disorder of synovial joints, characterized by regressive changes and proliferation of the articular cartilage and by overgrowth of subchondral and juxta-articular bone and of intra-articular soft tissues. The disease is, so far as is known, a strictly skeletal disorder without accompanying changes in the biochemistry of body fluids or in nonskeletal tissues.

SYNONYMS. In view of the absence of inflammatory changes, synonyms like osteoarthritis, hypertrophic arthritis, or arthritis deformans are misnomers. The term "degenerative joint disease" is correct only insofar as it denotes general deterioration of the joints; it does not take into account the prominent processes of growth occurring in the course of the disease; moreover, the term disregards the fact that "degeneration" of articular tissues occurs in many other joint disorders.

Prevalence and distribution

Osteoarthrosis is one of the oldest and most widespread diseases known. The characteristic alterations have been observed in the skeletons of prehistoric animals, in many nonmammalian and mammalian species of present-day animals,[196] and in modern man. The disease is age linked, starting as subtle microscopic changes at the beginning of the third decade, becoming radiographically noticeable at the end of the fourth decade, and giving rise to clinical symptoms some time thereafter. Practically no aging human individual is spared, osteoarthrosis developing sooner or later in one or several locations. Particularly severe or early involvement of one joint may be so prominent as to make the clinical disease appear monoarticular, though commonly mutliple joints will be affected to some lesser degree. Pathologic involvement is thus more widespread than clinical symptomatology would suggest, and localized monoarticular osteoarthrosis should be considered as a special occurrence rather than as the rule. The higher incidence of clinical disease in women as compared to man is not borne out by autoptic and radiographic observations. Men develop the disease at least as often and even at earlier ages than do women; however, the advanced lesions of later ages seem to be more common in women than in men.[84,101,102,217]

Osteoarthrosis is most conspicuous in the large joints of the lower extremity, knees, and hips, but the interphalangeal, shoulder, metacarpophalangeal, and sternoclavicular joints are commonly involved. The temporomandibular joints may also be affected by the disease.

Histogenesis

The early stages of the disease merge imperceptibly with the late aging changes.[16] Because of loss of mucopolysaccharides, which normally invest the collagen fibrils, the latter are unmasked and the cartilage appears fibrillated; the fibrils are held together less tightly than normal, and, if this process involves the surface layer, they change from the circumferential to a radial orientation as the articular surface becomes frayed and fissured (Fig. 46-3). The chondrocytes respond with proliferation and hypertrophy, followed by accelerated disintegration (Fig. 46-4). Once the surface continuity has been disrupted, the conditions for smooth joint motion and normal lubrication no longer exist, and mechanical forces contribute to further erosion of the articular surface; the cartilage may show increased calcification, invasion by blood vessels, and progressive ulceration (Fig. 46-5 and Plate 6, *D*). The underlying bone is bared and reacts with osteosclerosis; the epiphyseal bone marrow often becomes fibrotic and occasionally cystic. The intra-articular soft tissues, synovial villi, and fat pads become hypertrophic, but unlike conditions in inflammatory joint disease, pan-

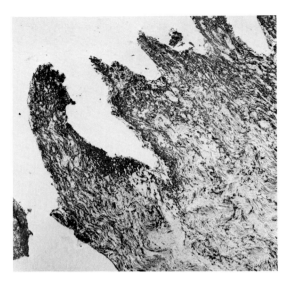

Fig. 46-3. Electron micrograph from osteoarthrotic ulcer at femoral head. Surface of lesion is frayed, and villous projections are composed of short, irregularly clustered collagen fibrils, mainly in radial orientation to joint surface. (Courtesy Dr. Max Spycher, Zurich.)

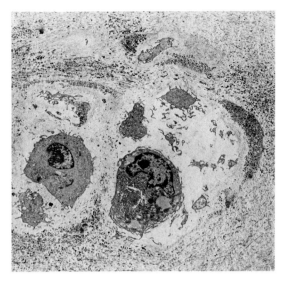

Fig. 46-4. Electron micrograph from osteoarthrotic femoral head. Cluster of chondrocytes indicating proliferation. Two chondrocytes are shown completely; others are sectioned tangentially and only partly shown. Numerous electron-dense granules —some scattered diffusely and others aggregated in crescents—represent lipid derived from disintegrated cells. (Courtesy Dr. Max Spycher, Zurich.)

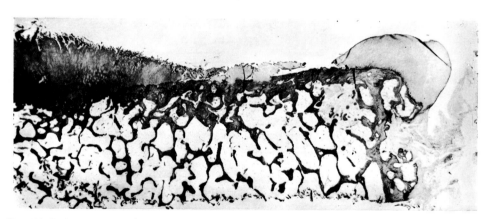

Fig. 46-5. Low-power photomicrograph of cartilage of patellar surface of femur. Osteoarthrosis. Fibrillation and splitting of matrix present. Fragmentation and detachment of cartilage evident toward *right*, where subchondral bone has been denuded. (10×; AFIP 67996.)

nus does not develop. Fragments of cartilage may be detached into the joint cavity and persist and move about as free bodies. Although destructive processes are prominent in the center regions of the joints, the cartilage and bone at the joint margins proliferate, forming large, elevated and overhanging outgrowths (Figs. 46-6 and 46-7). This process described as "lipping" results in further distortion of the articular surface, with considerable functional impairment. However, even in severely altered osteoarthrotic joints, complete immobilization hardly ever occurs.

Etiology and pathogenesis

Osteoarthrosis is now recognized as being of multifactorial origin, and the earlier simplistic concept of a "wear and tear disease" is outdated. From an etiologic point of view, primary and secondary osteoarthrosis may be distinguished, although morphologically the two types are indistinguishable. Secondary

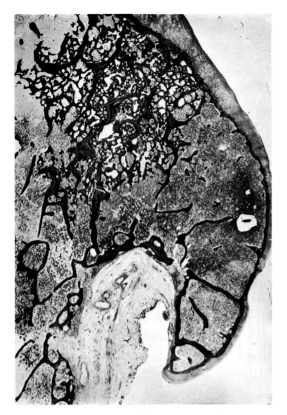

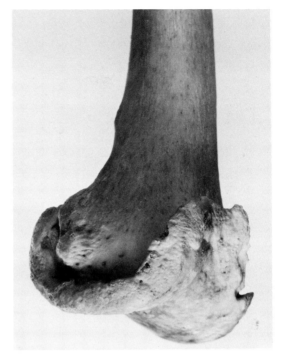

Fig. 46-7. Macerated specimen of lower femur. Pronounced osteoarthrosis of femoral aspect of knee joint with extensive marginal lipping.

Fig. 46-6. Low-power photomicrograph of joint, showing extensive marginal lipping. "Lip" is extension of epiphyseal end of tubular bone. (AFIP 67998.)

osteoarthrosis is posttraumatic in the widest sense of the term, with trauma being related to (1) action of mechanical force on a joint, either by single impact or, more commonly, by repeated, occupational insults as seen in shoulder and elbow joints of men working with pneumatic drills, (2) malalignment of joints attributable to congenital malformations, to metabolic or circulatory bone disease, or to superimposition on previous inflammatory disease associated with fibrosis and scarring of the joint capsule, (3) deposition of injurious material within the articular tissues.

Osteoarthrosis is considered as primary, if none of the above conditions apply. In the absence of unequivocal evidence as to the etiology of the disorder, a number of hypotheses have been advanced in the past, among which the "wear and tear" hypothesis was the most widely held. This concept maintained that the "microtrauma" of daily wear and tear was the basic etiologic factor in the disorder; accordingly, it was postulated that the greater the mechanical stress of weight bearing, the greater the propensity of a particular joint to become diseased. This concept does not clearly distinguish between the traumatic and the primary forms of the disease; it does not account for the facts that osteoarthrosis commonly involves non–weight bearing joints[186] and that particularly severe forms of the disease occur in such locations as the interphalangeal joints regardless of the amount of use these joints have been put to before the onset of the disease. The problem may be overcome by introduction of the concept of tissue susceptibility. In the presence of high tissue susceptibility, a comparatively low grade extraneous influence suffices to produce a lesion; whereas more powerful stimuli are required as triggers of disease if the tissue is comparatively resistant. The following factors have been shown to determine the susceptibility of the articular cartilage to become arthrotic:

1. *Genetic factors,* demonstrated by increased familial incidence of a special type of osteoarthrosis of the interphalangeal joints, Heberden's nodes,[203] and of polyarticular osteoarthrosis.[103]

2. *Hormonal factors,* as indicated by the hastened onset and increased severity of osteoarthrosis associated with acromegaly and with diabetes.[186,226]

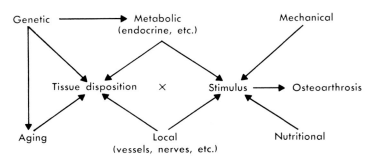

Fig. 46-8. Diagram illustrating the multifactorial etiology of osteoarthrosis. (From Silberberg, R., and Silberberg, M.: Pathol. Microbiol. [Basel] **27**:447, 1964.)

3. *Nutritional factors,* as shown by the frequent coexistence of osteoarthrosis and obesity. This coexistence is neither fortuitous, nor is osteoarthrosis the consequence of the increased weight bearing associated with obesity.[170] This is demonstrated by the finding that Heberden's nodes are as common in obese as in nonobese men. It appears more likely that both obesity and osteoarthrosis are related to a metabolic disorder involving lipid metabolism.

4. *Biologic age.* The articular changes occurring at a relatively early age are pacemakers for the disease. The rate at which these age changes proceed are decisive for the subsequent pathologic events into which they gradually merge.

5. *Local factors,* i.e., blood and nerve supply.

The concept of multiple etiologic factors acting on the joints to produce osteoarthrosis may be illustrated in a diagrammatic fashion (Fig. 46-8).

Osteoarthrosis associated with acromegaly

Patients suffering from acromegaly develop joint lesions that are grossly indistinguishable from those of the usual type of osteoarthrosis.[4, 23,225] Microscopically, proliferation of chondrocytes may be more pronounced than that in senile osteoarthrosis, especially in the young acromegalic person,[59,184] a quantitative difference not sufficient to prove a specific nature of the arthropathy. The changes that distinguish the arthropathy of acromegaly from the age-linked disorder are associated with extra-articular skeletal manifestations of hyper-pituitarism, particularly the resumption of osteogenesis at periosteal surfaces.

Kashin-Beck disease

Kashin-Beck disease is a special form of severe osteoarthrosis endemic to certain areas of Siberia. It occurs in young children and is associated with pronounced disturbances of skeletal growth. The joint lesions, typically those of osteoarthrosis, have been attributed to the presence of a fungus, *Fusarium sporotrichiella,* in grain used in the diet and to toxic effects of the fungus on cartilage.[145]

INFLAMMATORY JOINT DISEASES
Arthritis caused by infectious agents

Infectious arthritis is one of the possible complications of any infectious disease. Although the incidence of infectious joint lesions has decreased with the advent of antibiotic therapy, the disorders still are of considerable clinical importance.

The histogenetic mechanisms active in the development of infectious arthritides are the same as those prevailing in other connective-tissue spaces, modified by the special anatomic and physiologic conditions prevailing in joints. The infection may be attributable to direct contamination as in open wounds, to extension from the adjacent tissue, or to lymphatic spread, or it may be blood borne (Plate 6, *C*). The process begins acutely with hyperemia and swelling of the synovium, infiltration by polymorphonuclear and mononuclear leukocytes, and development of an effusion in the joint cavity. The exudate may be predominantly serous, or fibrinous, or purulent, depending on the severity of the infection, the resistance of the host, and the duration of the process. The synovium may be involved diffusely, or focally. A predominantly serous effusion or comparatively small amounts of fibrin may disappear completely, the latter after fibrinolysis has occurred. With increasing amounts of fibrin and increasing duration of the infection, however, granulation tissue develops with formation of adhesions between the soft tissues of the joints and between opposing articular surfaces; synovium and subsynovial tissues become thickened and fibrotic. In pyogenic infections, this is accompanied by abscess formation, which may involve the entire joint space or more or less isolated pockets. Even after successful surgical intervention, which usually is required to remove the exudate, the increase in fibrous tissue and the subsequent collagenization may result in permanent impairment of joint motion.

The characteristic feature of inflammatory arthritis is the involvement of the articular cartilage. The changes are degenerative rather than inflammatory, which is consistent with the fact that the cartilage contains no blood vessels. With the development of the exudate in the joint cavity and the granulation tissue in the synovium, the cartilage becomes frayed and eroded. In advanced cases it may disappear completely, and the underlying bones undergo osteosclerosis, or it may be thinned out and eroded by granulation tissue. This tissue may then invade the epiphyseal marrow cavity.

The injury to the cartilage is presumably brought about by lysosomal enzymes, such as cathepsins, collagenase, and hyaluronidase, which attack both the protein and the nonprotein moieties of the matrix. Since chondrocytes contain few lysosomes, it has to be surmised that the degradative enzymes are chiefly derived from leukocytes of the exudate and the synovium.[112,119,228,229]

The pathogenic organisms most commonly found in bacterial arthritis of adults are *Staphylococcus aureus,* hemolytic streptococci,[45,105] *Neisseria gonorrhoeae*[90,157] and *Haemophilus influenzae.* In infants and children, *Haemophilus influenzae* arthritis and, in adults, *Serratia* arthritis are seen with increasing frequency.[53a,144] Pneumococci,[216] *Pseudomonas, Proteus, Salmonella, Enterobacter, Bacteroides,* and *Escherichia* are among the rarer organisms causing bacterial arthritis[105] (Plate 6, *C*).

Joint involvement is monoarticular more often than polyarticular. The large joints of the lower limbs, knee, and hip are most commonly affected. In the most instances, predisposing factors are demonstrable, such as oral or local corticosteroid administration, diabetes, or preexisting rheumatoid arthritis.[98]

Viral arthritis

Rubella, mumps, infectious mononucleosis, lymphogranuloma venereum, variola, and other generalized viral infections may be ac-companied by episodes of acute arthritis,[65] yet reports of tissue changes are scanty. The findings in mumps-associated arthritis are probably characteristic of viral joint inflammations in general; synovial biopsies show edema, lymphocytic infiltration, and hyperplasia of synoviocytes. A patchy fibrinous exudate completes the picture of a nonspecific synovitis.[236]

With the use of immunohistochemical methods evidence for the presence of virus in synovial tissue can be obtained in arthritis after smallpox or rubella vaccination.[188]

Tuberculous arthritis

Approximately 1% of subjects with tuberculosis have skeletal involvement; in 30%, hips or knees are involved, and in 20%, various other joints are affected. Not uncommonly, the skeletal infection may remain dormant and without clinical symptoms for many years.[57] Almost invariably, tuberculous arthritis results from hematogenous dissemination of the organisms. These may reach the synovial membrane directly, or they may involve the joint secondarily, spreading from a focus of tuberculous osteomyelitis close to the articulation. Thus, in the knee of adults, the synovial membrane is frequently the primary site, whereas in children, the secondary spread from a focus in the adjacent metaphyseal or epiphyseal bone is the more common occurrence. Regardless of the point of origin, the end result of the infection is likely to be the same. The synovial membrane becomes hyperemic and edematous. A grayish yellow exudate is deposited on its surface, and occasionally tubercles may be recognized on gross inspection. In some cases, the synovium is transformed into a necrotic mass mixed with a shaggy fibrinous exudate; the joint space contains grayish white bodies, the size and shape of melon seeds, and varying amounts of turbid or clear exudate. Occasionally an excessive amount of fluid distends the joint (tuberculous hydrops). The changes in the articular cartilage depend to a considerable extent on the duration of the infection. In early stages, the cartilage may merely lose its glistening appearance, a change sometimes accompanied by the extension of tuberculous granulation tissue from the synovium over the cartilaginous surfaces. In more severely affected joints, fragments of cartilage are loosened and detached from the underlying bone, leaving an uneven granular ulcerated base of necrotic bone and exudate.

Microscopically, the loosened fragments consist of necrotic cartilage with faintly staining matrix and devoid of cells. The involved areas of bone show caseous necrosis surrounded by tuberculous granulation tissue. The necrotic trabeculae undergo gradual resorption (caries). The synovial membrane contains numerous solitary or conglomerate tubercles.

Healing may occur, with the end result depending on the extent of the lesion. If the lesion was confined to the synovial membrane, functional impairment may be limited; advanced involvement of cartilage and bone may result in total destruction of the articulation, with either fibrous or bony union of the articulating bones (ankylosis).

Syphilitic arthritis

The frequency with which joints are involved in syphilis is declining. Arthritis may, however, occur in congenital as well as in acquired forms of the disease.

In congenital syphilis, varying degrees of involvement of the joint capsules and epiphyses may accompany the characteristic changes of osteochondritis and periostitis. Microscopically, these joints show hyperemia, edema, lymphoid and plasma cell infiltration, and proliferation of fibroblasts. In addition, there may be small areas of necrosis in cartilage, bone, and capsular tissues.

In older children showing manifestations of congenital syphilis, a peculiar form of arthritis, known as Clutton's joint,[44] may develop. One or both knees, and occasionally other joints, are swollen and lax and contain an excessive amount of fluid. The synovial membrane is thickened and appears gelatinous. Microscopically, there is edema, diffuse infiltration with lymphocytes and plasma cells, and occasional gummas.[3]

Acquired syphilis

Pathologic investigations of joint tissues in secondary syphilis are notably lacking; however, inflammatory and vascular lesions resembling those found in skin and mucous membranes may produce an acute synovitis, sometimes associated with a transitory effusion. The knee joint is more often affected than other articulations, and the involvement is often bilateral.

In later stages of acquired syphilis, the joints may be the site of gumma formation or of a diffuse chronic nonspecific synovitis with more or less pronounced effusion. Gummas may also be found in ligaments, cartilage, and adjacent bone. Conversely, gummas may spread by direct extension from the bone marrow and bone to neighboring joints.

As a nonspecific sequela of tabes dorsalis, neuropathic joint disease may ensue.

Arthritis of brucellosis

Arthritis occurs as a complication of *Brucella bovis* or *B. suis* infection in about 10% of affected individuals. Hips, sacroiliac, and the small joints of hands and feet may be the site of acute suppurative synovitis or of chronic synovitis and bursitis.[201] Involvement of the spine is prominent. Subacute osteomyelitis of the vertebral bodies with destruction of cancellous bone and microabscesses are associated with destruction of the end plates, separating the vertebral body from the intervertebral disc, and with breakdown of the discs. There is a tendency to repair, with production of granulomas. Although blood-borne infection of the intervertebral discs has been considered as a primary event in the evolution of the lesion, it appears more logical, in the absence of clear-cut evidence, to assume that the process starts as an osteomyelitis and involves the discs secondarily as seen in other chronic infections.[124]

Fungal arthritis

A variety of fungal organisms may lodge in the synovium and give rise to suppurative or granulomatous lesions. The synovium may be the primary site of joint involvement, or the infection may spread from the marrow cavity to the subchondral bone and from there into the articular tissues.[65]

Whipple's disease

For reasons discussed on p. 1300, the disease is no longer considered to be metabolic but one caused by an infectious agent. The arthritis associated with the disorder is a transient, migratory, nonspecific synovitis that subsides without residual changes.[39,104] The rodlike particles seen in large numbers in the intestinal laminae propriae have not been demonstrated in articular tissues.

Arthritis associated with rheumatic fever

The arthritis that occurs in most patients with acute rheumatic fever is characteristically an acute, transient, migratory disorder, involving most commonly the large articulations such as knees, ankles, and wrists. A nonspecific synovitis involves the joint cavity proper as well as bursae and tendon sheaths. The effusion present in the joint cavity is always sterile; initially, the inflammatory cells are predominantly polymorphonuclear leukocytes, with varying numbers of eosinophils; at later stages, mononuclear cells may predominate. If the occlusive vasculitis, characteristic of rheumatic fever, is present in synovium or periarticularly, the diagnosis of rheumatic arthritis can be made. The arthritis usually subsides after a few weeks without residual changes.[141]

Rheumatic arthritis is often accompanied by the appearance of subcutaneous nodules, developing in the vicinity of joints. These nodules resemble in some ways the subcutaneous nodules of rheumatoid arthritis on the one hand and the Aschoff bodies of the myocardium on the other. The nodules usually measure several millimeters in diameter; microscopically, they have an acellular center of eosinophilic material; much of the latter can be identified as swollen or disintegrated collagen, with an admixture of mucopolysaccharides and, more rarely, necrotic tissue elements. This center is surrounded by a rim of lymphocytes, large and small monocytes, multinucleated giant cells, and occasionally eosinophils. Typical rheumatic vasculitis is usually found in the immediate vicinity of the nodules.[15] The nodules may be completely resorbed after a few weeks of existence. Some of the features that distinguish the rheumatic from the rheumatoid nodules seem related to the time factor involved in their pathogenesis: nodules of rheumatic fever come and go quickly and fail to show the extensive necrosis and the granulomatous character of the rheumatoid nodules, which develop and regress in a more chronic fashion.[17]

The pathogenesis of the arthritis of rheumatic fever is unknown although it has been shown experimentally that streptolysin, injected into the joint cavity, will produce arthritis, probably by disrupting lysosomes and thus liberating enzymes.[228] The possibility that streptococcal debris might also call forth the synovial inflammation has not been ruled out.

Repeated attacks of rheumatic arthritis of the hands or feet may be followed by flexion deformities, particularly striking in metacarpophalangeal joints. The condition, described first by Jaccoud in 1869,[42] and therefore termed Jaccoud's arthritis, is associated with pronounced ulnar deviation of the digits. However the deformities seem to be attributable to fibrosis of fasciae and tendons rather than to synovitis.[31]

Rheumatoid arthritis

Rheumatoid arthritis (RA) is a chronic progressive inflammatory arthritis of unknown origin involving multiple joints and characterized by a tendency to spontaneous remissions and subsequent relapses.

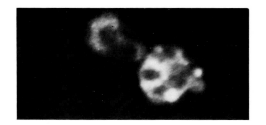

Fig. 46-9. Cell from synovial fluid from patient with rheumatoid arthritis. Cell was treated with serum containing antigammaglobulin. Brightly fluorescent globular inclusion suggests presence of rheumatoid factor (RF). (From Zucker-Franklin, D.: Arthritis Rheum. **9**:24, 1966.)

Arthritis is the most prominent manifestation of rheumatoid disease, a generalized connective tissue disorder that may involve para-articular structures such as bursae, the tendon sheath, and tendons, and extra-articular tissues such as the subcutis,[198] the cardiovascular system,[120,195] lungs,[57,171,189] spleen, lymph nodes, skeletal muscle,[48] peripheral nervous system, and eyes.

Rheumatoid disease is often accompanied by the presence of characteristic immunoglobulins, called "rheumatoid factors" (RF), in the affected persons' serum. These factors are of considerable complexity; they are capable of acting as antigammaglobulins and of forming complexes with abnormal antigenic gamma globulins in vivo and in vitro. With appropriate techniques, such antigens or antibodies or their complexes can be demonstrated in serum, in synovial fluid, in leukocytes of blood and articular exudates, and in the synovial tissues (Fig. 46-9). Several tests have been developed to detect these immune bodies, utilizing the agglutination of antibody on antigen-coated particles, such as red blood corpuscles,[223] bacteria,[114] or inert latex or bentonite particles.[27,220]

Rheumatoid factor is present in only 85% to 95% of subjects suffering from rheumatoid arthritis, and a distinction is therefore made between "seropositive" and "seronegative" forms of the disease. On the other hand, RF may be found in 2% to 7% of patients suffering from connective tissue diseases other than rheumatoid arthritis. Yet, the tests are considered useful for diagnostic and prognostic purposes, since there is a positive correlation between the level of the serum titers of RF and the severity of the clinical disease.

Distribution and prevalence

Young adults are frequently affected, but with increasing age an increase in prevalence has been reported.[218] Depending on the criteria used for diagnosis, women are 2½ to 5 times more often affected than are males.[154,218] Familial aggregation seems safely established for the severe forms of seropositive disease, whereas no such aggregation is seen in seronegative or low-grade seropositive forms.[21,116] Geographic distribution, considered significant at one time, has recently been shown to be random.[29,116] A slightly increased incidence is seen in males engaged in occupations requiring physical work as compared to males in professional or managerial positions.[218] The small joints of hands and feet are usually the first and the most common to be involved, with lesions of the large joints appearing later in the course of the disease.

Pathologic anatomy

The basic tissue changes of rheumatoid disease are similar, regardless of site. In different locations they are modified in accordance with the properties peculiar to the tissue in which they take place. None of the changes is by itself specific, but in combination, they give a fairly typical and diagnostically suggestive picture. It is of interest that similar uncertainties exist in regard to the clinical diagnosis of rheumatoid arthritis.[166]

The rheumatoid lesion is characterized by

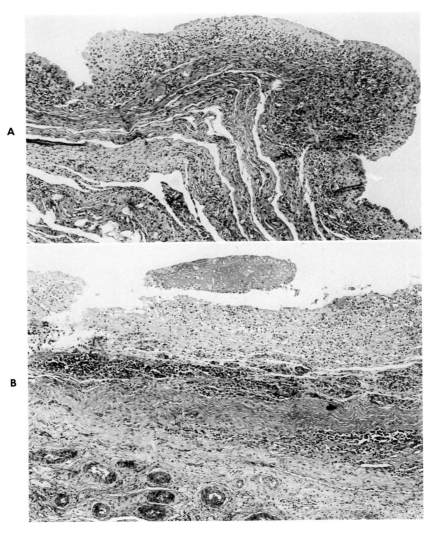

Fig. 46-10. Rheumatoid synovitis. **A,** Infiltration of synovium by lymphocytes. **B,** Fibrinous exudate superimposed on inflamed synovium. Necrosis of superficial layer of synovium. Thickening and fibrosis of subsynovial tissue.

(1) diffuse or focal infiltration of the tissue by lymphocytes or plasma cells, or both, and by development of lymphoid centers; (2) vasculitis with endothelial proliferation, narrowing or occlusion of the lumen, "fibrinoid" change or necrosis of the wall, and perivascular aggregation of lymphocytes and plasma cells; (3) the rheumatoid granuloma, a focal lesion with an amorphous center composed of necrotic tissue, fibrin, and immune complexes surrounded by a band of oblong histiocytes often in palisade-like radial orientation, and an outer zone of granulation tissue containing a variety of mononuclear leukocytes, capillaries, and fibroblasts. With time, the granuloma may undergo resorption or increasing fibrosis and collagenization.

In the joints, the early changes involve the synovium, which becomes congested, edematous, and infiltrated by lymphocytes (Fig. 46-10). There often are small areas of superficial necrosis of synovial lining cells with formation of superficial erosions, covered by "fibrinoid" deposits; these deposits are composed of fibrin and small amounts of gamma globulin and complement components.[146] An exudate containing polymorphonuclear leukocytes accumulates in the joint cavity. At later stages, the synovitis is characterized by plasma cells, lymphoid centers, occasional multinucleated giant cells, and vasculitis. Granulation tissue composed of synovial fibroblasts and capillaries causes grossly recognizable villous thickening of the synovium, whose lining cells become hypertrophic and hyperplastic. In some of these lining cells as well as in lymphocytes and plasma cells of the synovium and in leukocytes of the synovial fluid, rheumatoid factor, gamma globulins, and antigen-antibody complexes can be demonstrated after incubation of smears or of tissue sections with the proper fluorescein-conjugated antigens.[25,28,89,135] The granulation tissue does not remain localized to the synovium but spreads over the surface of the articular cartilage and produces adhesions between the opposing joint surfaces (Figs. 46-11 to 46-13). This "pannus," comes to be interposed between the cartilage and the lumen of the joint cavity; it may interfere with the flow of synovial fluid into the cartilage. Thus malnutrition of the cartilage may contribute to its destruction, although most of the destruction is attributed to the action of hydrolytic enzymes released from lysosomes of neutrophils and cells of the pannus.[228] As the pannus ages, increasing fibrosis and collagenization lead to shrinkage of the capsule, progressive narrowing of the joint space, and displacement or increasing approximation of the ends of the opposing bones. Closely opposing bones may

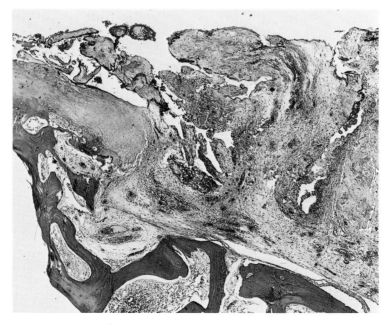

Fig. 46-11. Rheumatoid pannus. Exuberant granulation tissue replacing most of articular cartilage and forming hypertrophic villi projecting into joint space. Some preserved articular cartilage is seen at *left side.*

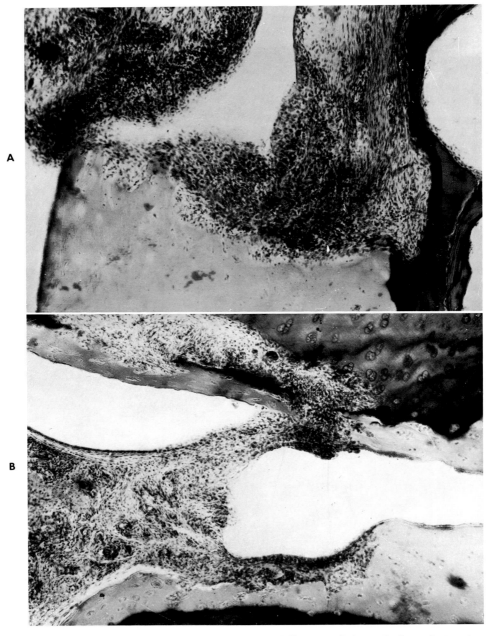

Fig. 46-12. Rheumatoid arthritis. **A,** Early stage of fibrous ankylosis. **B,** Granulation tissue projecting inward from margin of interphalangeal joint has formed adhesion across joint space. Nearly all articular cartilage has disappeared beneath pannus, which is clearly shown in lower half.

become fused by bony bridges developing in the scar tissue, or they may be telescoped into each other, with complete elimination of the joint (Fig. 46-14 to 46-16). Disuse osteoporosis develops locally in the immobilized bones and becomes generalized in patients totally crippled by the disease and bedridden for long periods of time. The osteopenia may be compounded by prolonged corticosteroid therapy given to alleviate the arthritic symptoms.

Rheumatoid arthritis occurring before the age of 16 has been termed *juvenile rheumatoid arthritis* (JRA), or Still's disease.[205] Morphologically, the lesions are identical with those of the adult disorder, but clinically the disease differs from the former. Three clinical forms are distinguished, depending on the presence of systemic involvement with fever, lymphadenopathy, skin rash, pleurisy, pericarditis, or iridocyclitis. Joint involvement may be polyarticular; lesions are found predominantly in the joints of the hand, or a few of the large joints (knees, ankles, and elbows) may be affected. This variability in the distribution of the lesions, in the clinical course, and in the results of immunologic tests for rheumatoid and antinuclear factors have suggested to some

investigators that JRA is not a single disease entity but a group of heterogeneic disorders.[173]

Extra-articular rheumatoid disease and syndromes associated with rheumatoid arthritis

The most common extra-articular lesion is the subcutaneous nodule, a granuloma, a few millimeters to several centimeters in size and developing usually in areas close to the joints and subject to minor mechanical insults (Fig. 46-17 to 46-19). An arteritis is often found nearby[198] and may contribute to the gradual expansion of the necrotic center of the granuloma. Nodules may also be found in bursae and tendon sheaths. In contradistinction to the similar but smaller nodules of rheumatic fever, the rheumatoid nodules develop and regress slowly and are less rich in hydroxyproline than are the former nodules.[238]

Vasculitis, wherever it occurs, may result in ischemia and microinfarcts, characteristically seen along the nail beds; occlusive involvement of larger vessels may cause gangrene of terminal phalanges of fingers and toes.

Visceral involvement has been observed in 16% of patients with rheumatoid arthritis.[189]

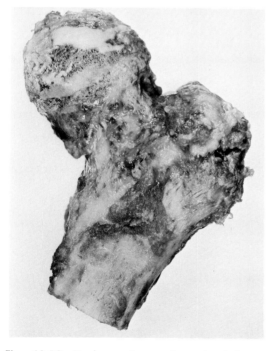

Fig. 46-13. Fresh specimen of proximal femur. Rheumatoid arthritis with destruction of joint surface by pannus. (W.U. 49-5578.)

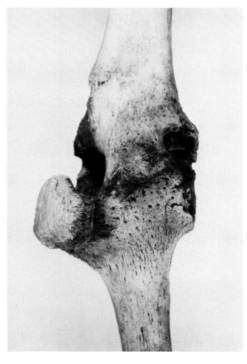

Fig. 46-14. Macerated specimen of knee joint. Advanced rheumatoid arthritis with bony fusion (ankylosis) of patella, femur, and tibia.

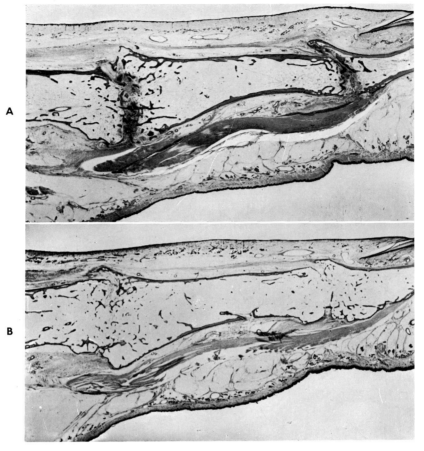

Fig. 46-15. Midline longitudinal sections of second and fourth digits. Atrophy of osseous and dermal tissues evident in both **A** and **B**. Active chronic inflammation shown in middle and terminal interphalangeal joints in **A**. All other joints have been destroyed and bony ankylosis is evident.

Pulmonary lesions may be focal and granulomatous or diffuse, interstitial, or intra-alveolar.[57,171,213] The end result is focal or diffuse fibrosis. In association with pneumoconiosis, especially of coal miners, "rheumatoid pneumoconiosis" develops[37] (see Chapter 26). Rheumatoid factor has been demonstrated in such lungs.[224]

Pericardium, myocardium, and valvular endocardium may be involved with vasculitis, granulomas, fibrous scarring, and amyloidosis.[42,120,189,198]

Lymph nodes, especially those draining the areas of involved joints show hyperplasia and, less commonly, granulomas (Fig. 46-20).

Several types of scleritis have been described in about 1% of patients with rheumatoid disease.[95]

Of patients with rheumatoid arthritis, 10% to 15% develop Sjögren's syndrome, an

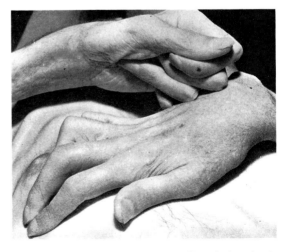

Fig. 46-16. Deformed and stiffened hands in chronic rheumatoid arthritis. Note evidence of muscular atrophy and smooth glossy skin.

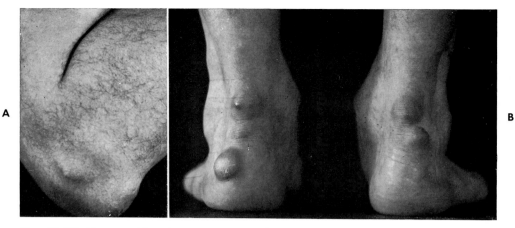

Fig. 46-17. Rheumatoid arthritis. **A,** Large subcutaneous nodule over olecranon process. **B,** Subcutaneous nodules of tendo Achillis areas having typical morphologic features of nodule of rheumatoid arthritis. (Courtesy Dr. F. A. Chandler.)

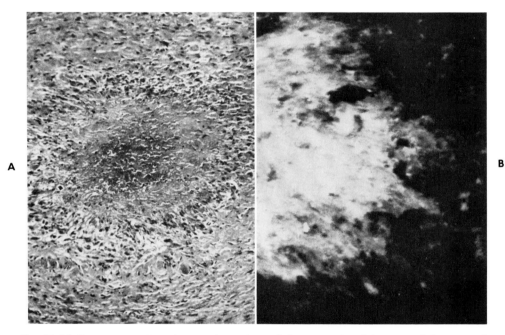

Fig. 46-18. Two consecutive microscopic sections of rheumatoid nodule. **A,** With hematoxylin and eosin stain, showing center of fibrinoid necrosis and a rim of macrophages with some palisading. **B,** Unstained, treated with fluorescein-conjugated antigammaglobulin. Large fluorescing area indicates presence of gamma globulin in nodule. (From Vazquez, J. J., and Dixon, F. J.: Lab. Invest. **6:**205, 1957.)

association of typical, but relatively mild, nondestructive rheumatoid arthritis with keratoconjunctivitis sicca, iridocyclitis, and parotitis.[182,191]

The association of rheumatoid arthritis with splenomegaly and leukopenia is known as Felty's syndrome.[7,61]

Amyloidosis is a late complication of rheu-matoid arthritis, with data on the frequency varying widely, from 25% to 60%.[36,214]

Etiology and pathogenesis

Of the factors once believed to play a role in the etiology or pathogenesis of rheumatoid arthritis, several, such as allergy, endocrine imbalance, climate, or "collagen disease," have

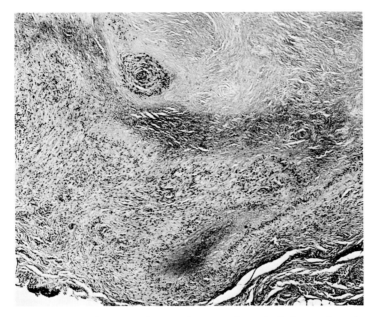

Fig. 46-19. Subcutaneous rheumatoid granuloma with occluded vessel at its periphery.

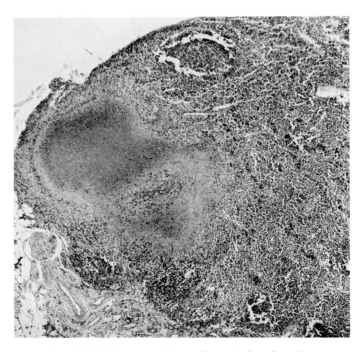

Fig. 46-20. Rheumatoid granuloma in lymph node.

not stood tests by strict standards; others, especially *infections, postinfectious immunopathology, autoimmunity,* and *heredity* are still being actively investigated, as are the effects of psychophysiologic disorders that seem to be related to the onset of attacks.[62,136]

No living organism has consistently been found in rheumatoid joints despite widespread search, which in years past was directed mainly against streptococci.[5] The significance of diphtheroids,[11,204] of *Mycoplasma,*[121] which has been demonstrated occasionally, or of viruses[172,193] remains controversial. Yet infection, often observed clinically some time prior to an attack[88,133] may be responsible for initiating a sequence of immune processes, which in turn seem involved in the pathogenesis of articular and extra-articular lesions.

The pathogenic role of immune processes in the development of rheumatoid lesions is suggested by the following observations made in subjects suffering from rheumatoid disease:

1. The presence of gammaglobulins, in particular, IgG and IgM in synovial fluid,[156] in synovial plasma cells,[135,219] in synovial lymphoid centers,[129] in leukocytes of the synovial fluid,[89] and in subcutaneous nodules.[135] These gammaglobulins are, however, not a direct cause of rheumatoid disease, since the disorder occurs in persons with agammaglobulinemia.[74]

2. The presence of rheumatoid factor in synovial plasma cells.[135]

3. The presence of antigen-antibody complexes (RF and gamma globulin) in synovial plasma cells[25] and in synoviocytes.[107]

4. The presence in synovial leukocytes of complement components,[28] associated with decreased complement titers in the synovial fluid.[83]

5. The presence of antinuclear factors (ANF) in the serum of patients with advanced disease suggests a role of autoimmunity if not as the ultimate cause, but perhaps in the chronicity of the process.[8]

6. The common association of rheumatoid arthritis with amyloidosis.[35,214]

A role of heredity in rheumatoid arthritis is not inconsistent with that of abnormal immune mechanisms. The propensity to formation of abnormal gamma globulins or to abnormal tissue reactivity to all kinds of challenges may well be under genetic control.[72] The first mentioned possibility is strongly supported by clinical observations: some rheumatoid factors show familial aggregation regardless of the presence or absence of joint disease.[117]

Results of investigations into the role of heredity in rheumatoid arthritis differ with the methods of sampling. On the basis of criteria established by the American Rheumatism Association, the existence of familial aggregation has been questioned.[149] With the use of strict criteria, i.e., inclusion into the surveys of only those patients with severe erosive involvement of multiple joints, familial aggregation was demonstrated.[116] This familial aggregation is apparently not attributable to the common environment shared by members of the same family: in pairs of monozygotic twins, rheumatoid arthritis occurred 33 times more often than in pairs of dizygotic twins. The latter show no higher propensity to develop the disease than expected from a sample of the general population.

On the basis of available histologic and immunologic data a concept of the pathogenesis of rheumatoid arthritis has evolved. An antigen, which could be extraneous (related to infection) or endogenous (related to abnormal gamma globulins), forms a complex with rheumatoid factor; the complex activates the complement sequence, which in turn stimulates leukotaxis and phagocytosis. The immune complex to which complement may have been added is taken up by the lysosomes of the polymorphonuclear leukocytes, which are termed "RA cells," or rhagocytes.[239] In the process, lysosomal membranes are presumed to be damaged, and hydrolytic enzymes released from the lysosomes act on the surrounding material. They participate in fibrinolysis and removal of cellular debris of the exudate, but they also degrade the protein-polysaccharide of the cartilage matrix[232] and thus have a major part in the destruction of the joint.

No plausible concept has as yet been developed to explain the chronicity of the disease. There is no spontaneous animal analog of the disorder, and numerous attempts to create an animal model with consistent chronicity without the need for repeated challenge have failed.[67] This has reinforced the hypothesis that autoimmunity may be involved in this as well as in other aspects of RA.[2]

Arthritis associated with immune complex disease

These arthritides are characterized by a transitory monoarticular or polyarticular synovitis, often with effusion, often relapsing, sometimes subsiding without residual damage, and in other instances leading to permanent morphologic alterations and functional impairment of the joints. As a result of the problems arising from surgical interference, reports on tissue changes are scanty at best.

Arthritis associated with viral hepatitis

The disorder occurs in the presence of high serum titers of hepatitis-associated antigen (HAA) and decreased serum levels of the C_4 component of complement.[1,152] Although no immune complexes have as yet been demonstrated in the articular tissues, it is believed that complexes of HAA antigen, homologous antibody, and early components of complement are causes of the joint lesions.

Arthritis of familial Mediterranean fever (FMF)

A genetic background has been demonstrated for this form of arthritis, which occurs commonly in Sephardic Jews. The acute, subacute, or chronic synovitis may be accompanied by an effusion, which is sterile on culture. After repeated attacks, changes of early osteoarthrosis may develop. One joint is usually involved at a time, but in the course of years, multiple joints may be affected.[85]

Arthritis associated with sarcoidosis

Acute or chronic nonspecific, often symmetric synovitis may develop in the course of the disease.[200] Formation of granulomas in the synovium may be followed by erosion of the cartilage, advanced joint destruction, and osteophytic outgrowth at the joint margins. Ankle and knee joints are most commonly affected, but, as a rule, joint involvement is less conspicuous than that of adjacent or distant bones.

Behçet's syndrome

Behçet's disease, a multisystem disease causing ulceration of skin, eyes, and mucous membranes, involves large and small joints of about 90% of diseased persons, with a nonspecific self-limiting synovitis. The resulting changes are similar to those of rheumatoid arthritis.[134,151]

Enteropathic arthritis

The existence of this type of arthritis has been doubted; however a number of facts argue strongly in favor of arthritides related to such disorders as regional ileitis and ulcerative colitis. First, as well as recurring, episodes of acute joint inflammation always follow, never precede, bowel involvement, and after surgical removal of the diseased segment of the intestine, there are no further attacks of arthritis.[234]

The disease is usually monoarticular, with the knee being most commonly involved and the ankle next in order of frequency. Ankylosing spondylitis is also seen in association with ulcerative colitis. However, causal relationship between these two disorders appears more doubtful than that between the intestinal disease and arthritis. The latter relationship has been explained as an immune response to an antigen from the large bowel.[234]

Reiter's syndrome

Reiter's syndrome was originally described as a combination of conjunctivitis, urethritis, and arthritis. More recently, keratodermia, oral ulcerations, and cardiovascular abnormalities have been added to the list of characteristic lesions. The arthritis is polyarticular and asymmetric, involving the knee and ankles and often starting at the heel. The usual subacute stage is characterized by a fibrinopurulent exudate. The synovium is hyperemic and infiltrated by polymorphonuclear leukocytes, lymphocytes, and a few plasma cells. Some extravasation of red blood corpuscles may occur and lead to deposition of small amounts of hemosiderin. Commonly, there is no major residual change; a few lymphocytic foci in the synovium may be the only evidence of the earlier involvement.

More rarely, the subacute process progresses with development of synovial hypertrophy and with proliferation of synovial lining cells and fibroblasts. This pannus spreads over the cartilage and erodes it as well as the subchondral bone. Ultimately, the appearance of the joints may be similar to that found in rheumatoid arthritis.[110] However, a para-articular ossifying periostitis distinguishes these lesions of Reiter's syndrome from rheumatoid arthritis.

The spondylitis of Reiter's syndrome resembles radiologically that of psoriasis in the random distribution of osteophytic outgrowths.[130]

The etiology of Reiter's syndrome is unknown; a genetic background has been demonstrated, but its role in the pathogenesis of the disease has not been clarified.

Arthritis associated with psoriasis

The association of arthritis and psoriasis is more than coincidental but occurs probably in only 5% to 7% of patients suffering from psoriasis. The chronic destructive lesions involve mainly the distal interphalangeal joints in an asymmetric fashion. Histologically, the chronic fibrosing synovitis and subsequent destruction of the joint resemble rheumatoid arthritis. In advanced stages, osteolysis of the tips (acra) of the phalanges occurs.[12,138] A characteristic finding is terminal convolutions of the nail capillaries in the vicinity of the affected joints, suggesting a role of decreased vascular supply in the necrotizing process involving the epiphyses of the phalanges. A triggering role has been attributed to mechanical injury. Spondylitis also occurs as a complication of psoriasis; the lesions resemble those of Reiter's syndrome.

Arthritis associated with "connective tissue diseases"

Acute transitory arthritides may be a more or less prominent occurrence in serum sickness, lupus erythematosus, erythema nodosum, and various forms of vasculitis.[13] Usually, no permanent lesions ensue. An exception are the changes seen in progressive systemic sclerosis. In this disorder, progressive resorption of the tufts of the terminal phalanges eventually involves the distal interphalangeal joints; because of occlusive disease of the afferent vessels, the subchondral bone and the overlying cartilage undergo avascular necrosis accompanied by fibrinous synovitis and progressive synovial fibrosis.[164,230]

Gout (crystal deposition disease, type I)

Gout is a disorder of purine metabolism directly related to serum levels of uric acid and characterized by deposition of monosodium urate monohydrate crystals in various connective tissues. A distinction is usually made between primary or idiopathic gout, developing on the basis of a primary abnormality of purine metabolism, and secondary gout, associated with diseases conducive to "secondary" hyperuricemia. There is no known difference in the tissue changes seen in the two forms of gout.

Historic background

Gout belongs to that group of diseases known to and discussed by men through the ages.[75,81,165] From Hippocrates to Galen and to the Renaissance the disease was considered to be caused by bad humors, poisoning the body in association with excessive eating, drinking, and generally lecherous living. Paracelsus was the first to attribute the disease to the deposition of an abnormal substance, tartar, derived from food and subsequently altered to form stony material, especially when mixed with "synovia," an egg white–like substance contained in the joints. Sydenham still held onto the concept of ill humors but elaborated specifically on the connection between gout and stone formation and gave a classic description of the disease.

Modern thinking about gout seems to have originated in 1769 with the discovery by Scheele that kidney stones found in patients with gout were made up of an acid, which was also present in the urine. The identification of urates in tophi by Wollaston in 1797[231] and the discovery of hyperuricemia in patients suffering from gout by Garrod in 1848[68] created new directives for all subsequent work dealing with this disorder. Gout is distinctly familial in distribution, with both hereditary and environmental factors having been shown to be involved in the pathogenesis.[26,153,177,180]

Distribution and prevalence

The disease usually begins in the third decade. Males are affected more often and at an earlier age than females. The higher the serum level of uric acid, the greater the likelihood that an individual will develop the disease. Yet, the number of persons with hyperuricemia, who actually develop gouty arthritis is small, probably not exceeding 2% or 3%.[115,118] The mere presence of hyperuricemia at one time or another is a prerequisite for local manifestations of gout to appear, regardless of the cause of hyperuricemia. Hyperuricemia may be primary or secondary; one form of primary hyperuricemia is the result of an enzyme defect that inhibits reconversion of hypoxanthine to inosinic acid, a step in purine resynthesis. Consequently, hypoxanthine is further degraded to produce excessive quantities of uric acid.[14,78,86,100,235] Secondary hyperuricemia is seen under conditions when excessive amounts of nuclear material are being degraded as in leukemia or polycythemia, or when renal excretion is impaired as in lead poisoning or renal calcification. Characteristically, in secondary hyperuricemia, the pathways of purine degradation are normal.

The joint most commonly involved is the metatarsophalangeal joint of the big toe, but knees and ankles, elbows and fingers, and spinal and sternoclavicular joints are commonly affected. Not all patients suffering from gout develop arthritis; lesions may be confined to periarticular tissues and extraskeletal sites, such as the outer ear, the eyelids, scleras, kidneys, heart valves, blood vessels, and cartilages of the respiratory system.

Pathologic anatomy

The acute lesion is triggered by precipitation of needle-shaped crystals of monosodium urate from serum or synovial fluid. In the joints, the crystals produce an acute synovitis accompanied by an effusion, with numerous polymorphonuclear leukocytes. These leukocytes

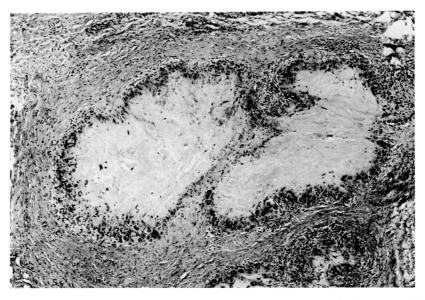

Fig. 46-21. Photomicrograph of portion of gouty tophus in periarticular tissue. Two of several aggregates of which tophus is composed. Urate crystals originally present have been dissolved in processing of tissue and only proteinaceous matrix is preserved in centers. Latter are surrounded by corona of granulation tissue with numerous multinucleated giant cells. (B.H. 69-1754.)

may take up as much as 95% of the urates either into their cytoplasm or into phagosomes.[161,183] There is hyperplasia of synoviocytes, some of which are being sloughed off into the effusion. Urates are also found interstitially in the synovial membrane, where they tend to form clusters.[237]

With recurring attacks, the lesions become chronic. The deposits enlarge, and urate crystals, disposed radially around an amorphous proteinaceous matrix, become the center of a foreign body granuloma with a rim of fibroblasts and multinucleated giant cells (Fig. 46-21). The granuloma is spoken of as "tophus" (Latin *tophus* or *tofus,* 'porous stone'). Tophi vary in size from a few millimeters to several centimeters in diameter; if located subcutaneously, they present as prominent nodules; if located on the hands or feet, they may cause conspicuous disfiguration. More or less diffuse fibrosis may develop around tophi as the lesions age. Synovial granulomas may erode the articular cartilage, but crystals are also directly precipitated in the cartilage. Since articular cartilage is avascular, there is no inflammatory reaction to such deposits; urates at first occupy the superficial layers of the cartilage, which undergo necrosis and assume an opaque, whitish, chalky appearance. Incrustation of the deeper layers of the cartilage is seen in association with advanced regression, resembling the changes of early osteoarthrosis (Fig. 46-22).

Pathogenesis

The mechanism that causes deposition of urates in tissues is complex and is discussed in Chapter 3. Rapid fluctuations in uric acid serum levels as occurring after excessive consumption of alcohol, after fasting, and initially after administration of uricosuric drugs[132] are likely to trigger and acute attack in persons predisposed to gout.

Tissues with low oxygen tension are particularly prone to be the site of urate precipitation. Moreover, the peak incidence of gouty arthritis coincides with the age at which age-linked loss of mucopolysaccharide from the cartilaginous matrix is maximal.

The irritating effect of urate crystals is attributable to their physical configuration and not to their chemical composition: a minor inflammatory response is observed after introduction of dissolved sodium urate into tissues, in contradistinction to the intense reaction to crystalline monosodium urate. Agents differing from sodium urate chemically, but similar in crystallinity, evoke an inflammatory reaction resembling that produced by crystalline sodium urate.[60]

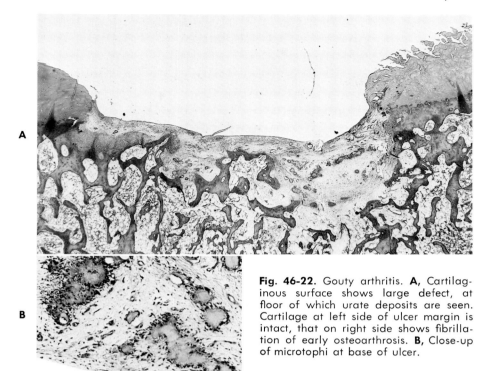

Fig. 46-22. Gouty arthritis. **A,** Cartilaginous surface shows large defect, at floor of which urate deposits are seen. Cartilage at left side of ulcer margin is intact, that on right side shows fibrillation of early osteoarthrosis. **B,** Close-up of microtophi at base of ulcer.

Decrease in pH as occurring in acute inflammation promotes crystal deposition,[180] and thus a vicious cycle may be initiated responsible for self-perpetuation of the lesion.

Activation of Hageman factor by the crystals[99] suggests an action mediated by the kallikrein-kininogen-kallidin system and promoting an inflammatory response. Likewise unexplained is the role of polymorphonuclear leukocytes: in the absence of polymorphonuclear leukocytes in experimentally produced aleukocytosis no attack develops.[180]

Pyrophosphate arthropathy

SYNONYMS. Articular calcinosis, pseudogout, crystal deposition disease type II, and others.

This abnormality was recognized after demonstration of calcium pyrophosphate in the synovial fluid of certain inflamed joints.[109] It constitutes an example of crystal deposition disease characterized by the presence of calcium pyrophosphate dihydrate crystals in articular cartilage, synovium, articular ligaments, and intervertebral discs. The crystals can be demonstrated by polarized light or by x-ray diffraction.[20,113] The disorder differs from true gout not only by the chemical nature of the crystals, but also in distribution; in pseudogout, the large joints such as knees, hips, and shoulders are preferably involved rather than the small joints of hand and feet.

Pyrophosphate arthropathy occurs by itself or, more rarely, in association with other metabolic aberrations such as hyperparathyroidism, true gout, diabetes, or acromegaly.[50] The joints show an acute synovitis, often with a large effusion—changes that may subside without residual damage. With repeated recurrences, or insidiously without acute phase, changes typical of osteoarthrosis develop, and deposits of calcium pyrophosphate are found in the articular cartilage. These deposits are composed of crystals or microspheroliths[20]; they are confined to the midzone of the cartilage and have no apparent relationship to chondrocytes.

Neither the etiology nor the pathogenetic mechanism by which the lesions evolve is known. Occasional familial aggregation of persons with the disorder point to a genetic background.[222] No basic biochemical abnormalities have been found.

Relapsing polychondritis (chronic atrophic polychondritis)

Relapsing polychondritis, which occurs in both men and women, is characterized by degeneration and inflammation of any of the cartilages of the body.[53] The disintegration of the cartilage leads to gross deformities, such as floppy ears, saddlenose, or collapse of the trachea. Involvement of intervertebral discs may lead to spondylitis and, at late stages, to deformities of the spine. In the joints, a picture resembling rheumatoid arthritis is seen. The synovium is infiltrated by lymphocytes and plasma cells, and there is an increase in both A and B cells. The cartilage matrix loses some of the acid mucopolysaccharides, resulting in decreased staining with alcian blue and other cationic dyes. The cartilage is infiltrated by lymphocytes, and many chondrocytes disappear from their capsules. By electron microscopy chondrocytes have peculiar bulbous bodies attached to or within the elongated cytoplasmic processes; the cells contain an unusual number of lysosomes and dense bodies, both signs of degeneration. In the cell vicinity, aggregates of granular material appear from which long spacing bodies are formed.[137] The nature of this material is unknown, but it seems related to degenerative processes in both cells and matrix. The etiology of the disorder is likewise unknown.

Diseases of bursae, tendons, and fasciae
Bursitis

Since bursae are synovial membrane–lined sacs, their reaction to injury may be expected to resemble that of the synovial lining of joints (Fig. 46-23). The common lesions are those resulting from mechanical insults or infection.

Traumatic bursitis may result from a single injury, such as a blow upon the elbow (olecranon bursa) or the knee (prepatellar bursa). More commonly, however, it is the repeated injuries from excessive pressure or bruises that initiate the inflammatory changes. This is well exemplified by "housemaid's knee," in which the prepatellar bursa becomes enlarged and painful as the result of crawling on floors and closing drawers and doors with the knee.

Purulent inflammation of bursal cavities may result from the localization of pathogenic microorganisms. This may follow penetrating injuries, be an extension of infection from an adjacent cellulitis or abscess, or result from embolization of blood-borne organisms.

Tendinitis and tenovaginitis

Inflammation of tendons and tendon sheaths may result from chronic mechanical insults or from direct or blood-borne infection. The lesions may assume any form of acute or chronic inflammation with or without effusion, with or without suppuration, or with development of

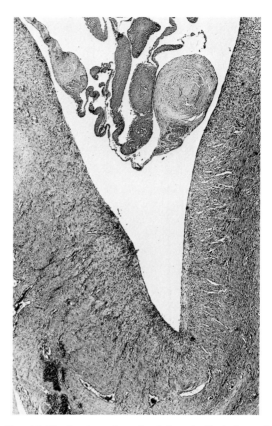

Fig. 46-23. Portion of wall of chronically inflamed bursa. Synovial lining has been replaced by layer of vascular fibrous tissue infiltrated by lymphocytes. Inspissated old exudate is present in bursal lumen.

diffuse granulation tissue or granulomas. A special type of tenovaginitis is stenosing tenovaginitis. This lesion develops preferably in places where tendons pass over bony prominences, especially at the wrist. The tendon sheath is narrowed because of annular fibrosis of the wall, which inhibits the free motion of the tendon. The tendon distal to the stenosis becomes thickened and at times locked in a certain position, from which it has to be unlocked before normal motion is restored.

Dupuytren's contracture

Contracture of the digits of the hand first observed by Plater in 1614 was recognized as an affection of the palmar aponeurosis by Dupuytren[54] and more recently reported as also occurring in the plantar aponeurosis. The lesion results in permanent flexion contracture, with the fifth, fourth, and third digits being usually involved in this order of frequency. Males are more commonly affected than females, and in about half of the patients the lesion is bilateral.

Grossly, the involvement may be diffuse or nodular. Microscopically, three developmental phases have been described[125]: (1) proliferation of fibroblasts, (2) decreasing cellularity and increasing collagenization, and (3) a residual stage, characterized by regression of the nodules, atrophy of the fibrous cords, and almost complete acellularity. The lesions extend into the adjacent subcutaneous fat tissue and into the corium, thus causing attachment of the aponeurosis to the skin. In the past, contraction of the excessive collagen has been considered as the principal pathogenic mechanism involved. However, electron microscopic investigations have disclosed a cytoplasmic fibrillar system and other evidence of contractility in the cells of the lesion. The involved cells thus appear to be myofibroblasts, which have the ability to contract.[64] This property is believed to play a role in the clinical contracture.

The etiology of the lesion is unknown. A more than coincidental association with diabetes has been observed,[52] and heredity may be involved in some cases.[208]

CYSTS OF JOINTS AND PARA-ARTICULAR TISSUES
Cysts of ganglion

These round or ovoid, movable subcutaneous lesions are cystic or semicystic, occurring most commonly on the wrist, but also on the dorsal surface of the foot, close to the ankle, or about the knee. They may or may not have a pedicle attachment to or communicate with a tendon sheath or a joint cavity. The cysts are filled with a clear mucinous fluid, which by electron microscopy contains flakes or delicate filaments and distintegrated collagen. In some instances the cysts have a more or less continuous lining of cells resembling synovial cells; in others, the lining is discontinuous or lacking altogether; the cyst wall then consists of dense connective tissue lined by necrotic cells, cell debris, and disintegrated collagen.[70] Other ganglia contain fragments of tissue resembling synovium incorporated in a loose edematous connective tissue mass.

The histogenesis of the lesion is disputed. Herniation of the synovium into the surrounding tissue, displacement of synovial tissue during embryogenesis, or posttraumatic degeneration of connective tissue have been incriminated as causes.[199] More recently demonstrated aggregates of cytoplasmic filaments suggest a relationship to smooth-muscle fibrils. It was therefore suggested that the lesions are the result of proliferation of pluripotential mesenchymal cells.

Cysts of semilunar cartilage

Cysts of the semilunar cartilages are usually located in the lateral meniscus near its anterior insertion. They contain a number of indistinct locules filled with mucinous or gelatinous fluid. Microscopic sections may reveal bits of synovial lining and diffuse fraying of the fibrocartilage of the meniscus. The fraying probably results from the extravasation of mucin-containing fluid into the interstices of the dense and relatively accellular connective tissue of the pre-existing semilunar cartilage. These lesions have much in common with ganglia of tendon sheath origin and are probably formed in a similar manner.

Bursal cysts that are connected with the knee joint are not uncommon. In some instances, the openings connecting the cysts with the articular cavity are long and tortuous. Not infrequently, the opening becomes obliterated by cicatrization. These examples of bursal cysts usually are referred to as Baker's cysts, although Baker's original papers described cystic lesions in association with a variety of pathologic conditions of dissimilar causation.[6,108]

Bursal cysts have a dense fibrous wall of variable thickness. The enclosed cavity often is divided partially or completely into two or more chambers by fibrous septa that project inwardly from the cyst wall. The cavity contains fluid that may be either clear or turbid, and either watery or mucinous. At times, the fluid is stained with blood pigments. Not frequently, the cavities contain "melon seed" bodies originating from detached small excrescences or tips of villi projecting into the cavity.

Microscopically, apparent synovial membrane may be present, but more frequently the cyst space is lined by dense fibrous connective tissue that contains focal and diffuse infiltrations of lymphocytes and hemosiderin-laden phagocytes. Baker's cysts are not infrequent in patients with rheumatoid arthritis.

TUMORS AND TUMORLIKE LESIONS OF JOINTS, BURSAE, TENDONS, AND TENDON SHEATHS

Any of the tissue components of the articulations, including bursae, tendons, and tendon sheaths, may give rise to benign or malignant neoplasms. Among the benign tumors, chondromas, osteochondromas, myxomas, angiomas, fibromas, and lipomas occasionally are encountered. These neoplasms and the malignant tumors derived from corresponding cell types are no different from tumors of the same histologic composition seen elsewhere in the body. Neoplasms whose origin and behavior are determined by the presence of specialized synovial-lining cells, and which are thus peculiar to structures normally lined by such cells, may be benign or malignant.

Xanthofibroma

SYNONYMS. Giant cell tumor of tendon sheaths, benign synovioma.

These lesions occur most commonly on fingers, wrists, ankles, feet, and knees. They grow slowly, with compression and displacement of the adjacent tissues. Where the tendons and other tissues are firmly anchored in bone, the tumors may cause surface erosions or deep rounded depressions in the bone from pressure atrophy.

The gross appearance of these tumors varies within wide limits. They measure from a few millimeters to several centimeters in greatest diameter. They have a dense fibrous covering formed by the compressed surrounding tissues. They are firm and only slightly elastic. Cut surfaces show a gray, dense, inelastic tissue and, in many instances, yellowish flecks or streaks, proportional to the amount of lipid contained within histiocytes. Because of the yellow color, these lesions have been named "xanthomas" or "xanthofibromas."

Microscopically the tumors are characteristic; they are composed of small oval or spindle-shaped cells, multinucleated giant cells, lipid-laden macrophages, and irregularly placed bundles of connective tissue. The ratio of these elements is exceedingly variable, both within the same and in different tumors. Some neoplasms are highly cellular and show active cell proliferation. Others are dense and fibrous with few cellular elements. Giant cells may be numerous or few. They contain many small oval nuclei that are usually crowded together in one portion of the cell. The cytoplasm may be scant or abundant, and the shape of the cells is equally variable. The number of lipid-laden phagocytes ("foam cells") is also varia-

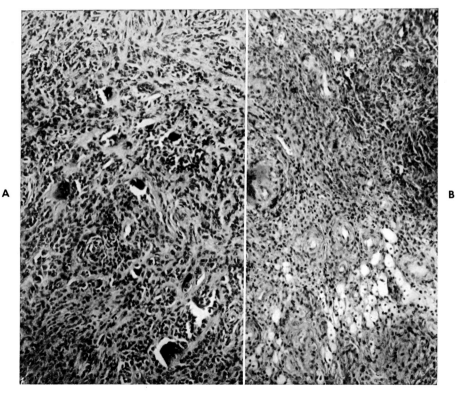

Fig. 46-24. Xanthofibromas of tendon sheath. **A,** Tumor composed of spindle-shaped fibroblasts and giant cells. **B,** Tumor containing many lipid-laden cells. (**A** and **B,** 130×; **A,** AFIP 90662; **B,** AFIP 82251.)

ble. Some tumors are composed chiefly of foam cells, whereas others contain only small aggregates or scattered single such cells (Fig. 46-24).

Some tumors show irregular slitlike cavities lined by oval or flattened cells. Small tufts of these cells may project into the cavities. Cellular tumors with many clefts and tufts may be difficult to distinguish from synovial sarcoma.

The origin and histogenesis of xanthofibroma has been traced to the proliferation of synovial cells resembling histiocytes. These cells are transformed into multinucleated giant cells and macrophages laden with hemosiderin or lipid. The underlying tissue is infiltrated by lymphocytes, a finding of basic significance in support of the view that the nodules are of inflammatory rather than of neoplastic origin. As the nodules age, collagenous and often hyalinized matrix is laid down between the cells. Doubt has been cast on the neoplastic character of the lesions especially because similar changes may involve the synovium of joints, bursae, and tendon sheaths multifocally or diffusely. The term "villonodular synovitis" is being used to describe the diffuse lesion; benign giant cell tumor of the tendon sheath and villonodular synovitis have been considered as manifestations of the same underlying process: a chronic granulomatous inflammation, of as yet unknown etiology.[93]

Osteochondromatosis

Osteochondromatosis may occur as an isolated lesion or in conjunction with other forms of joint disease. It is characterized by the development, in the synovial tissues, of cartilaginous nodules that tend to undergo secondary ossification. The synovial lining contains translucent masses of cartilage projecting from the surface or hanging from narrow pedicles into the joint space (Fig. 46-25). Many of the nodules become detached and dozens or even hundreds of them float free in the joint fluid, where they may continue to grow. By electron microscopy, transition from regular synovial cells to chondrocytes producing cartilaginous matrix, and deposition of crystals along the collagen fibrils of the matrix can be demonstrated.[47]

The etiology of the disorder is unknown. Although mechanical injury and inflammation have vaguely been implicated, the lesions may occur in the absence of either. Histogenetically, two mechanisms have to be considered: metaplasia from regular elements of the synovium, or development from undifferentiated chondrogenic cells. Such cells are to be expected, especially at the reflection of the synovium, where during embryogenesis cells develop either into synoviocytes or into chondrocytes.[158]

An uncommon variant of osteochondromatosis has been described as "osteomatosis." In this disorder, multiple osseous bodies develop in the synovial tissue without previous formation of cartilage.[55,142]

Synovioma (synovial sarcoma)

The term "synovioma" was suggested to designate a group of rare malignant tumors involving the regions of diarthrodial joints and once believed to arise from the synovium.[193] However, only 10% of the tumors develop within the joint cavities; the rest arise in tissues close to the articulations and seem to involve the synovium secondarily.[209] The tumor is most often seen in young adults, and the sex ratio is 3 : 2, with males predominating. The knee joint is the most common site. The survival rate is poor,[79,131] and metastases spread more often by the bloodstream than by lymphatics.

Grossly, the tumors usually are single, roughly ovoid in shape, often lobulated, and vary in size from 1 to 18 cm in diameter.[34]

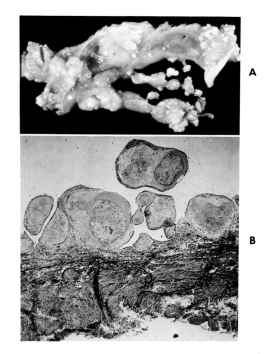

Fig. 46-25. Osteochondromatosis. **A,** Portions of synovial membrane showing numerous attached and superimposed cartilaginous nodules. **B,** Photomicrograph of synovial membrane showing ectopic cartilage forming numerous nodules projecting into joint cavity.

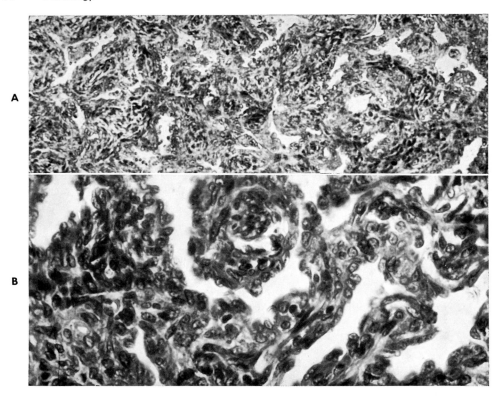

Fig. 46-26. Synovial sarcoma. **A,** Low-power view. **B,** High-power view. (**A** and **B,** AFIP 90623.)

They may be sharply delimited but may extend along fascial planes. Growing expansively, they are partially or completely surrounded by a pseudocapsule formed by the compressed or attenuated adjacent nontumorous tissue. On the cut surface, the tumors may be firm, focally gritty, or spongy and friable. Homogeneous areas alternate with those of fibrous, even whorl-like appearance, and hemorrhage, necrosis, or cysts may be present, the cysts containing gelatinous or mucinous material.

Microscopically, the tumors are characterized by a biphasic cell pattern: (1) areas resembling fibrosarcoma, composed of fairly uniform spindle-shaped cells with hyperchromatic nuclei and densely packed in bands or sheets, and (2) cells resembling epithelium ("synovioblastic" cells), arranged in pseudoglandular structures, lining clefts in the fibrosarcomatous stroma, or forming papillae (Figs. 46-26 and 46-27). These cells vary in shape from cuboid to tall columnar; they may secrete a mucopolysaccharide, probably hyaluronic acid, which is also found in the occasional cysts. The cell sheets are surrounded by abundant masses of reticulin, but no fibrils are found between the cells. In addition, there is nonfibrillar eosinophilic material that resembles osteoid and sometimes contains deposits of calcium. In the presence of an old hemorrhage, hemosiderin-laden macrophages or, more rarely, foreign body giant cells may be found. The number of mitosis varies from moderate to large. The tumor may invade adjacent tissues and blood vessels.

The biphasic pattern of the tumors has been confirmed by electron microscopy.[63,127] Stromal cells have folded nuclei with clumped chromatin at the membrane and prominent nucleoli; the cytoplasm is vesiculated. Endoplasmic reticulum, both rough or smooth, and microfilaments are more prominent than Golgi apparatus or mitochondria. The epithelium-like cells, by contrast, contain many mitochondria. The cells are always in contact with one another. The plasmalemma has characteristic desmosomes and other special junctional zones. A basement membrane may but need not be present at the junction of stromal and epithelium-like cells.

The histogenesis of the tumors is obscure. The similarity of the cells to the two types of

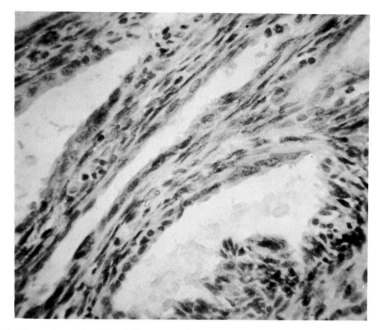

Fig. 46-27. Example of highly differentiated synovial sarcoma illustrating epithelium-like cells forming surface lining of tissue clefts.

cells found in normal synovium has been suggestive of synovial origin. However, the extra-articular origin of the majority of the tumors, the presence of transitional cell types, and the behavior of the tumor cells in tissue culture are not consistent with this hypothesis; it seems more justified to consider a pluripotential undifferentiated mesenchymal cell as the true precursor of the neoplasm.

Clear-cell sarcoma of tendon sheaths and aponeuroses

This neoplasm has been recognized only recently.[22,58] It occurs preferably in the region of the feet or hands. The spheric smooth or nodular tumors are attached to tendons or aponeuroses; on cut surface they are grayish white, solid, and sometimes gritty, with occasional foci of necrosis or cysts. Microscopically, they are not biphasic as the synoviomas, but consist of nests of pale, fusiform "epithelioid" cells surrounded by delicate fibrous septa. The tumor cell have light-staining nuclei with contrasting prominent nucleoli and do not contain lipid. Multinucleated giant cells are common. By electron microscopy, melanosomes were found in such a tumor.[87]

Miscellaneous malignant lesions

Malignant giant cell tumor of the tendon sheath combines features of clear-cell sar-

coma and benign giant cell tumor of tendon sheaths. It differs from the former in that there are transitions between the clear cells and foam cells, and multinucleated giant cells of osteoclastic or Touton type. The intercellular substance, which can be removed with bovine hyaluronidase, is closely related to the plasma membrane of the tumor cells, a finding that suggests secretion of the substance by the membrane.[97,148]

Chondrosarcoma of the joint is a rare and highly malignant neoplasm.[73] It involves the joints diffusely, simulating benign chondromatosis at the early stages. The tumor may arise from the synovium directly or from previously present chondromatosis.[140] Histologically, the neoplasm is characterized by large atypical cells with hyperchromatic nuclei and by large binucleated or multinucleated cells.

Multicentric histiocytic reticulosis may involve multiple or simple joints by development of granulomatous tissue in the synovium. As elsewhere in this disorder, the granulation tissue is characterized by the presence of numerous histiocytes, of multinucleated giant cells, and of forms transitional between the two. All these cells may characteristically have a foamy cytoplasm and, with special stains, can be shown to contain neutral fats and phospholipids.[10] More rarely, lipid may be absent from the cells.[56] The granulation tissue spreads aggressively, and with time, there is extensive destruction of the articular cartilage and the adjacent bone, leading to partial or complete loss of joint function.

DISEASES OF VERTEBRAL COLUMN
Deformities

The significance of spinal deformities lies in their effects on motor activity, on the integrity of peripheral joints, and on viscera, which depend on normal spatial relations for their proper functioning, such as heart and lungs.

Deformities of the spine may be caused by changes in the vertebral bodies (a topic outside the scope of this chapter) or by changes in the intervertebral discs. Three types of deformities involving large segments of the spine exist: kyphosis, characterized by increased convexity of the spine in the anteroposterior direction; lordosis, increased concavity in the anteroposterior direction; and scoliosis, lateral deviation from the normal orientation. One of the most common deformities, kyphosis of old age, or senile kyphosis, is caused by uneven distribution of degenerative processes in the discs, which cause them to collapse anteriorly and to tilt the anterior portions of the vertebral bodies towards each other.

Disc disease

Starting in late adolescence and progressing with increasing age the intervertebral discs deteriorate (Sylvén et al., 1957). Water is lost from the nucleus, and there are loss of chondroitin sulfate, increase of keratan sulfate and of collagen, and calcification. These changes lead to a decrease in intranuclear pressure and to loss of elasticity. The annulus fibrosus likewise loses water, becomes fibrillated and fissured, and loses its tight attachment to the vertebral bone. It thus exerts less than normal restraints on the nucleus during mechanical stress. Sudden, or, more commonly, chronic stretching and bending that produces mechanical strain may then force the nucleus out of the confines of the annulus into neighboring structures. If the prolapse occurs into the spinal canal, pressure on and potential damage to neural tissues ensue. Another site of predilection for prolapses are the terminal plates of the vertebrae; disc tissue may penetrate into the bone marrow space of the vertebral body and there form globular masses. These structures are termed "Schmorl's nodules"; radiologically they have a superficial resemblance to metastatic tumors. Prolapsed nuclei undergo further

degeneration, such as hyalinization and sclerosis.

Spondylosis

Degenerating discs, even if they do not prolapse, may yet assume a role in the initiation of spondylosis deformans. Spondylosis deformans, or hypertrophic spondylosis, is a disease peculiar to vertebral bodies and their articulating surfaces. It does not involve the small joints of the spinal processes, which are subject to develop osteoarthrosis like other, large diarthrodial joints. Spondylosis deformans is an age-linked disorder, having its steepest rise in incidence during the fourth to sixth decades, after which age the number of affected individuals is practically 100%.[174] Men seem to be affected somewhat more severely and at an earlier age than are women.[84] The increased incidence of the disorder in miners as compared to that found in factory workers or craftsmen, suggested to some investigators an etiologic role of extraneous mechanical stresses.

The fully developed lesions of spondylosis are characterized by fraying, fibrillation, and chondrocyte proliferation of the cartilage of the terminal plates and by chondro-osseous outgrowths (osteophytes) at the vertebral margins. Osteophytes may bridge the narrowed intervertebral space and overlap the adjacent vertebral edge (Fig. 46-28). Two opposing osteophytes may fuse, thus causing immobilization of the joint. The origin of the osteophytes is disputed, but one should keep in mind that during development, the edge of the vertebral body consists of a cartilaginous ring. Although this ring ossifies in due course of time, the adjacent fibrous tissues still contain cells with a chondrogenic or osteogenic potential that is activated under the effect of stimulating factors. The age-linked loosening of the annulus fibrosus in association with the narrowing of the intervertebral space gives rise to friction, which has long been recognized as one of the causes of spondylosis. The frequent association with diabetes mellitus[80] indicates that metabolic factors may enter into the etiology of the disorder, either by acting on the vertebral end plates directly, or by first causing abnormalities in the intervertebral discs.

In ochronosis, the intervertebral discs are discolored a deep black; they are softened or calcified and brittle, shrunken, and often prolapsed posteriorly into the spinal canal or anteriorly through the retaining ligaments. With

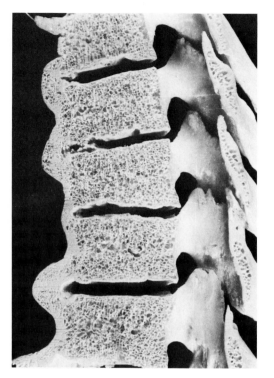

Fig. 46-28. Hyperostotic spondylosis. Anterior fusion of vertebral bodies by osseous bridges. (Courtesy Dr. Max Aufdermaur, Lucerne.)

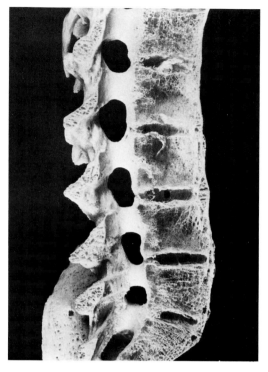

Fig. 46-29. Ankylosing spondylitis. Bony fusion of vertebral processes and narrow bony bridges between vertebral bodies. Note advanced osteopenia of vertebral bodies. (Courtesy Dr. Max Aufdermaur, Lucerne.)

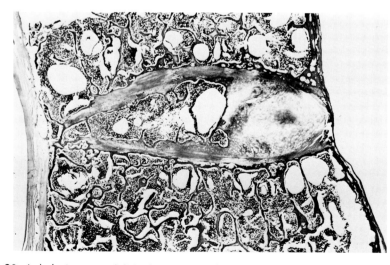

Fig. 46-30. Ankylosing spondylitis, low-power photomicrograph. Two vertebral bodies are fused, and part of intervertebral disc is replaced by bone. (Courtesy Dr. Max Aufdermaur, Lucerne.)

shrinkage of the discs, the intervertebral spaces are narrowed, and eventually the vertebral bodies touch and become fused by osseous links (Plate 6, *B*).

Ankylosing spondylitis (Marie-Strümpell-Bekhterev disease)

Ankylosing spondylitis is a chronic progressive inflammation of unknown origin, involving primarily the small apophyseal and costovertebral joints of the spine as well as the sacroiliac joints. The overall incidence of the disorder in a general population is less than 1%; males are affected nine times more frequently than females; the disease usually starts late in the second or in the third decade, progresses to involve several segments or the entire length of the spine, and terminates in ankylosis of individual joints and in immobilization of the involved segments of the spine. The histologic changes are basically similar to those seen in rheumatoid arthritis: a nonspecific chronic synovitis with destruction of the cartilage by pannus, adhesions between the opposing surfaces of the joint, and thickening and fibrosis of the joint capsule. In contradistinction to spondylosis, the intervertebral spaces are not narrowed, but the discs may be partially or completely destroyed by granulation tissue, which undergoes fibrosis, calcification, and ossification.[49] Consequently, adjacent vertebrae become fused by osseous bridges, which often protrude from under the longitudinal ligament and give rise to the gross appearance of the "bamboo" spine (Figs. 46-29 and 46-30).

Etiology

Earlier claims relating the disease to infection of the male genitourinary system have not been adequately supported, and despite the morphologic similarity of the lesions to those of rheumatoid arthritis, the two disorders differ in distribution and in immunologic respects: the sex ratio is reversed, and tests for rheumatoid fatcors are almost always negative in ankylosing spondylitis.

REFERENCES

1 Alpert, E., Isselbacher, K. J., and Schur, P. H.: The pathogenesis of arthritis associated with viral hepatitis, New Eng. J. Med. **285**:185-189, 1971.
2 Anderson, J. R., and Watson-Buchanan, W.: Autoimmunity and the rheumatic diseases. In Hill, A. G. S., editor: Modern trends in rheumatology, London, 1966, Butterworth & Co. (Publishers), vol. 1, pp. 70-209.
3 Argen, R. J., and Dixon, A. St. J.: Clutton's joint with keratitis and periostitis, Arthritis Rheum. **6**:341-348, 1963.
4 Arnold, J.: Acromegalie, Pachyacrie oder Ostitis, Beitr. Pathol. Anat. **10**:1-79, 1891.
5 Aronoff, A., Bywaters, E. G. L., and Fearnley, G. R.: Lung lesions in rheumatoid arthritis, Br. J. Med. **2**:228-232, 1955.
6 Baker, W. M.: On the formation of synovial cysts in the leg in connection with disease of the knee joint, St. Bartholomew's Hosp. Rep. **13**:245-261, 1877.
7 Barnes, C. G., Turnbull, A. L., and Vernon-Roberts, B.: Felty's syndrome, Ann. Rheum. Dis. **30**:359-374, 1971.
8 Barnett, C. H.: Maintenance of articular surfaces, Fed. Proc. **25**:1077-1078, 1966.
9 Barnett, E. V., North A. F., Jr., Condemi, J., Jacox, R. F., and Vaughn, J. H.: Antinuclear factors in systemic lupus erythematosus and rheumatoid arthritis, Ann. Intern. Med. **63**:100-108, 1965.
10 Barrow, M. V., Sunderman, F. W., Jr., Hackett, R. L., and Coloni, W. S.: Identification of tissue lipids in lipid dermatoarthritis (multicentric reticulohistiocytosis), Am. J. Clin. Pathol. **47**:312-315, 1967.
11 Bartholomew, H. E., and Nelson, F. R.: *Corynebacterium* acnes in rheumatoid arthritis. Isolation and antibody studies, Ann. Rheum. Dis. **31**:22-27, 1972.
12 Bauer, W., Bennett, G. A., and Zeller, J. W.: The pathology of joint lesions in patients with psoriasis and arthritis, Trans. Assoc. Am. Phys. **56**:349-352, 1941.
13 Bauer, W., Giansiracusa, J. E., and Kulka, J. P.: The protein nature of connective tissue disease. In Rheumatic diseases, postgraduate medicine and surgery, Philadelphia, 1952, W. B. Saunders Co., pp. 349-400.
14 Becker, M. A., Meyer, L. J., Wood, A. W., and Seegmiller, J. E.: Purine overproduction in man associated with increased phosphoribosylpyrophosphate synthetase activity, Science **179**:1123-1126, 1973.
15 Bennett, G. A.: Comparison of the pathology of rheumatic fever and rheumatoid arthritis, Ann. Intern. Med. **19**:111-113, 1943.
16 Bennett, G. A., Waine, H., and Bauer, W.: Changes in the knee joints at various ages with particular reference to the nature and development of degenerative joint disease, New York, 1942, Commonwealth Fund.
17 Bennett, G. A., Zeller, J. W., and Bauer, W.: Subcutaneous nodules of rheumatoid arthritis and rheumatic fever, Arch. Pathol. **30**:70-89, 1940.
18 Benninghoff, A.: Form und Bau der Gelenkknorpel in ihren Beziehungen zur Funktion, Z. Zellforsch. **2**:783-862, 1925.
19 Bick, E. M.: Congenital deformities of the musculoskeletal system noted in the newborn, Am. J. Dis. Child. **100**:861-868, 1960.
20 Bjelle, A. O.: Morphological study of articular cartilage in pyrophosphate arthropathy, Ann. Rheum. Dis. **31**:449-456, 1972.
21 de Blécourt, J. J.: Hereditary factors in rheumatoid arthritis and ankylosing spondylitis. In Kellgren, J. H., Jeffrey, M. R., and Ball, J., editors: The epidemiology of chronic rheuma-

tism, Philadelphia, 1963, F. A. Davis Co., pp. 258-266.

22 Bliss, B. O., and Reed, R. J.: Large cell sarcomas of tendon sheath, Am. J. Clin. Pathol. **49:**776-781, 1968.

23 Bluestone, R., Bywaters, E. G. L., Hartog, M., Holt, P. J. L., and Hyde, S.: Acromegalic arthropathy, Ann. Rheum. Dis. **30:**243-268, 1971.

24 Blumberg, B. S., and Ogston, A. G.: Physicochemical studies on hyaluronic acids. In Wolstenholme, E. W., and O'Connor, M., editors: Ciba Foundation Symposium on the chemistry of mucopolysaccharides, Boston, 1958, Little, Brown & Co., pp. 22-41.

25 Bonomo, H., Tursi, A., Trizio, D., Gillardi, V., and Dammaco, F.: Immune complexes in rheumatoid synovitis: a mixed staining immunofluorescence study, Immunology **18:**557-563, 1970.

26 Boyle, J. A., Greig, W. R., Jasani, M. K., Duncan, A., Diver, M., and Watson-Buchanan, W.: Relative roles of genetic and environmental factors in the control of serum uric acid levels in normouricemic subjects, Ann. Rheum. Dis. **26:**234-238, 1967.

27 Bozicevich, J., Bunim, J. J., Freund, J., and Ward, S. B.: Bentonite flocculation test for rheumatoid arthritis, Proc. Soc. Exp. Biol. Med. **97:**180-183, 1958.

28 Britton, M. C., and Schur, P. H.: The complement system in rheumatoid synovitis. II. Intracytoplasmic inclusions of immunoglobulins and complement, Arthritis Rheum. **14:**87-95, 1971.

29 Bunim, J. J., Burch, T. A., and O'Brien, W. M.: Influence of genetic and environmental factors on the occurrence of rheumatoid arthritis and rheumatoid factors in American Indians, Bull. Rheum. Dis. **15:**349-350, 1964.

30 Byers, P. D., Contepomi, C. A., and Farkas, T. A.: A postmortem study of the hip joint including the prevalence of the features of the right side, Ann. Rheum. Dis. **29:**15-31, 1970.

31 Bywaters, E. G. L.: The relation between heart and joint disease including "rheumatoid heart disease" and chronic postrheumatic arthritis (type Jaccoud), Br. Heart. J. **12:**101-131, 1950.

32 Bywaters, E. G. L., and Dorling, J.: Amyloid deposits in articular cartilage, Ann. Rheum. Dis. **30:**294-306, 1971.

33 Bywaters, E. G. L., and Hamilton, E. B. D.: The spine in idiopathic hemochromatosis, Ann. Rheum. Dis. **30:**457-465, 1971.

34 Cadman, N. L., Soule, E. H., and Kelly, P. J.: Synovial sarcoma: an analysis of 134 tumors, Cancer **18:**613-627, 1965.

35 Calkins, E., and Cohen, A. S.: Diagnosis of amyloidosis, Bull. Rheum. Dis. **10:**215-218, 1960.

36 Cambell, C. J.: The healing of cartilage defects Clin. Orthop. **64:**45-63, 1969.

37 Caplan, A., Payne, R. B., and Withey, J. L.: A broader concept of Caplan's syndrome related to rheumatoid factors, Thorax **17:**205-212, 1962.

38 Carter, C., and Wilkinson, J.: Persistent joint laxity and congenital dislocation of the hip, J. Bone Joint Surg. **46B:**40-45, 1964.

39 Caughey, D. E., and Bywaters, E. G. L.: The arthritis of Whipple's disease, Ann. Rheum. Dis. **22:**327-335, 1963.

40 Charnley, J.: The lubrication of animal joints in relation to surgical reconstruction by arthroplasty, Ann. Rheum. Dis. **19:**10-19, 1960.

41 Chung, S. M. K., and Ralston, E. L.: Necrosis of femoral head associated with sickle cell anemia and its genetic variant, J. Bone Joint Surg. **51A:**33-58, 1969.

42 Clark, W. S., Kulka, P., and Bauer, W.: Rheumatoid arthritis with aortic regurgitation, Am. J. Med. **22:**580-592, 1957.

43 Clarke, J. C.: Surface characteristics of human articular cartilage—a scanning electron microscope study, J. Anat. **108:**23-30, 1971.

44 Clutton, H. H.: Symmetrical synovitis of the knee in hereditary syphilis, Lancet **1:**391-393, 1866.

45 Cohen, A. S., and Kim, I. C.: Acute suppurative arthritis. In Hill, A. G. S., editor: Modern trends in rheumatology, London, 1966, Butterworth & Co. (Publishers), vol. 1, pp. 347-361.

46 Collins, D. H., and McElligott, T. F.: Sulphate ($^{35}SO_4$) uptake by chondrocytes in relation to histological changes in osteoarthritic human cartilage, Ann. Rheum. Dis. **19:**318-330, 1960.

47 Cotta, H., Rauterberg, K., Binsus, G., and Dettmer, U.: Electronenoptische und biochemische Untersuchungen an der Gelenkchondromatose, Arch. Orthop. Unfallchir. **63:** 73-91, 1968.

48 Cruickshank, B.: Focal lesions in skeletal muscles and peripheral nerves in rheumatoid arthritis and other conditions, J. Pathol. Bacteriol. **64:**21-32, 1952.

49 Cruickshank, B.: Lesions of cartilaginous joints in ankylosing spondylitis, J. Pathol. Bacteriol. **71:**73-84, 1956.

50 Currey, H. L. F.: Pyrophosphate arthropathy and calcific periarthritis, Clin. Orthop. **71:** 70-80, 1970.

51 Davidson, P. T., and Horowitz, J.: Skeletal tuberculosis, Am. J. Med. **48:**77-84, 1970.

52 Devach, M., and Cabilli, C.: Dupuytren's contracture and diabetes mellitus, Isr. J. Med. Sci. **8:**774-775, 1972.

53 Dolan, D. L., Lemmon, J. B., Jr., and Teitelbaum, S. L.: Relapsing polychondritis, Am. J. Med. **41:**285-299, 1966.

53a Donovan, T. L., Chapman, M. W., Harrington, K. D., and Nagel, D. A.: *Serratia* arthritis, J. Bone Joint Surg. **58A:**1009-1011, 1976.

54 Dupuytren, G.: Permanent retraction of the fingers produced by an affection of the palmar fascia. (Translation from French: Leçons Orales 1:1, 1832.) Med. Classics **4:**142-150, 1939.

55 Ehalt, W., Ratzenhofer, M., and Gergen, M.: Die synoviale Osteochondromatose kombiniert mit paraartikulärer cartilaginärer Exostose und die Beziehungen zu einem seltenen Fall primärer synovialer Osteomatose, Chirurg **40:** 464-468, 1969.

56 Ehrlich, G. E., Young, J., Nosheny, S. Z., and Katz, W. A.: Multicentric reticulohistiocytosis

(lipid dermatoarthritis). A multisystem disorder, Am. J. Med. **52**:830-840, 1972.

57 Ellman, P., and Ball, R. E.: Rheumatoid disease with joint and pulmonary manifestations, Br. Med. J. **2**:816-820, 1948.

58 Enzinger, F. M.: Clear cell sarcoma of tendons and aponeuroses, Cancer **18**:1163-1174, 1965.

59 Erdheim, J.: Die Lebensvorgänge im normalen Knorpel und seine Wucherung bei Akromegalie. Pathologie und Klinik in Einzeldarstellungen, Berlin, 1931, Springer Verlag.

60 Faires, J. S., and McCarty, D. J., Jr.: Acute synovitis in normal joints of man and dog produced by injections of microcrystalline sodium urate, calcium oxalate and corticosteroid esters, Arthritis Rheum. **5**:295-296, 1962.

61 Felty, A. R.: Chronic arthritis in the adult associated with splenomegaly and leucopenia, Bull. Johns Hopkins Hosp. **35**:16-20, 1924.

62 Friedman, H.: Aspects psychosomatiques de la polyarthrite chronique évolutive (PCE) ou polyarthrite rhumatoïde, Acta Psychiatr. Belg. **72**:117-141, 1972.

63 Gabbiani, G., Kaye, G. I., Lattes, R., and Majno, G.: Synovial sarcoma. Electron microscopic study of a typical case, Cancer **28**:1031-1039, 1971.

64 Gabbiani, G., and Majno, G.: Dupuytren's contracture: fibroblast contraction? An ultrastructural study, Am. J. Pathol. **66**:131-146, 1972.

65 Gardner, D. L.: Pathology of connective tissue diseases, Baltimore, 1965, The Williams & Wilkins Co.

66 Gardner, D. L.: The experimental production of arthritis, Am. Rheum. Dis. **19**:297-317, 1960.

67 Gardner, E.: The nerve supply of muscles, joints and other deep structures, Bull. Hosp. Joint Dis. **21**:153-161, 1960.

68 Garrod, A. B.: The nature and treatment of gout, London, 1859, Walton & Maberly.

69 Ghadially, F. N., Meachim, G., and Collins, D. H.: Extracellular lipid in the matrix of articular cartilage, Ann. Rheum. Dis. **24**:136-146, 1965.

70 Ghadially, F. N., and Mehta, P. N.: Multifunctional mesenchymal cells resembling smooth muscle cells in ganglia of the wrist, Ann. Rheum. Dis. **30**:31-42, 1971.

71 Ghadially, F. N., and Roy, S.: Ultrastructure of synovial joints in health and disease, New York, 1969, Appleton-Century-Crofts.

72 Glynn, L. E.: Pathogenesis and etiology of rheumatoid arthritis, Ann. Rheum. Dis. **31**:412-420, 1972.

73 Goldman, R. L., and Lichtenstein, L.: Synovial chondrosarcoma, Cancer **17**:1233-1240, 1964.

74 Good, R. A., and Rotstein, J.: Rheumatoid arthritis and agammaglobulinemia, Bull. Rheum. Dis. **10**:203-207, 1960.

75 Graham, W., and Graham, K. M.: Martyrs to the gout, Metabolism **6**:209-217, 1966.

76 Gross, J.: Ageing of connective tissue. In Bourne, G. H., editor: Structural aspects of ageing, London, 1961, Pitman Medical Publishing Co., pp. 177-195.

77 Gutman, A. B.: Renal mechanisms for regulation of uric acid excretion with special reference to normal and gouty man, Sem. Arthritis Rheum. **2**:1-46, 1972.

78 Gutman, A. B., and Yü, T. F.: Hyperglutamatemia in primary gout, Am. J. Med. **54**:713-724, 1973.

79 Haagensen, C. D., and Stout, A. P.: Synovial sarcoma, Ann. Surg. **120**:826-842, 1942.

80 Hajkova, Z., Streda, A., and Skrha, F.: Hyperostotic spondylosis and diabetes mellitus, Ann. Rheum. Dis. **24**:536-543, 1965.

81 Hartung, E. F.: Historical considerations, Metabolism **6**:196-208, 1957.

82 Hass, J.: Congenital dislocation of the hip, Springfield, Ill., 1957, Charles C Thomas, Publisher.

83 Hedberg, H.: Studies on the depressed hemolytic complement activity of synovial fluid in adult rheumatoid arthritis, Acta Rheum. Scand. **9**:165-170, 1963.

84 Heine, J.: Ueber die Arthritis deformans, Virchows Arch. (Pathol. Anat.) **260**:521-663, 1926.

85 Heller, H., Gafni, J., Michael, D., Shahin, N., Sohar, E., Ehrlich, G., Karten, J., and Sokoloff, L.: The arthritis of familial Mediterranean fever, Arthritis Rheum. **9**:1-17, 1966.

86 Henderson, J. F., Rosenbloom, F. M., Kelley, W. N., and Seegmiller, J. E.: Variations in purine metabolism of cultured skin fibroblasts from patients with gout, J. Clin. Invest. **47**:1511-1516, 1968.

87 Hoffman, G. J., and Carter, D.: Clear cell sarcoma of tendons and aponeuroses with melanin, Arch. Pathol. **95**:22-25, 1973.

88 Hollander, J. L., Brown, E. M., Jr., Jessar, R. A., Hummeler, K., and Henle, W.: Studies on the relationship of virus infections to early or acute rheumatoid arthritis, Arch. Interamer. Rheum. **5**:137-148, 1962.

89 Hollander, J. L., McCarty, D. J., Jr., Astorga, G., and Castro-Murillo, G.: Studies on the pathogenesis of rheumatoid joint inflammation. I. The RA cell and a working hypothesis, Ann. Intern. Med. **62**:271-280, 1965.

90 Holmes, K. K., Counts, G. W., and Beatty, H. N.: Disseminated gonococcal infection, Ann. Intern. Med. **74**:979-993, 1971.

91 Idelberger, K.: Die Ergebnisse der Zwillingsforschung beim angeborenen Klumpfuss, Verh. Dtsch. Ges. Orthop. **33**:272, 1939.

92 Jaccoud, F. S.: Leçons de clinique médicale faites à l'Hôpital de la Charité, 23. leçon, ed. 2, Paris, 1869, Delahaye.

93 Jaffe, H. L., Lichtenstein, L., and Sutro, C. J.: Pigmented nodular synovitis, bursitis and tenosynovitis, Arch. Pathol. **31**:731-765, 1941.

94 Jansson, E.: Isolation of fastidious mycoplasma from human sources, J. Clin. Pathol. **24**:53-56, 1971.

95 Jayson, M. I. V., and Jones, D. E. P.: Scleritis and rheumatoid arthritis, Ann. Rheum. Dis. **30**:343-347, 1971.

96 Johnson, L. C.: Morphologic analysis in pathology. In Frost, H. M., editor: Bone dynamics, 1964, Little, Brown & Co., Boston, pp. 543-654.

97 Kahn, L. B.: Malignant giant cell tumor of the tendon sheath. Ultrastructural study and re-

view of the literature, Arch. Pathol. **95**:203-208, 1973.

98 Karten, I.: Septic arthritis complicating rheumatoid arthritis, Ann. Intern. Med. **70**:1147-1158, 1969.

99 Kellermeyer, R. W.: Hageman factor and acute gouty arthritis, Arthritis Rheum. **11**:452-459, 1958.

100 Kelley, W. N., Greene, M. L., Rosenbloom, F. M., Henderson, J. F., and Seegmiller, J. E.: Hypoxanthine-guanine-phosphoribosyltransferase deficiency in gout, Ann. Intern. Med. **70**:155-206, 1969.

101 Kellgren, J. H.: Osteoarthrosis in patients and populations, Br. Med. J. **1**:1-6, 1961.

102 Kellgren, J. H., in discussion of Lawrence, J. L., and Bier, F.: Nodal and non-nodal forms of generalized osteoarthrosis, Ann. Rheum. Dis. **23**:205, 1964.

103 Kellgren, J. H., Lawrence, J. S., and Bier, F.: Genetic factors in generalized osteoarthrosis, Ann. Rheum. Dis. **22**:237-255, 1963.

104 Kelly, J. J., III, and Weisiger, B. B.: The arthritis of Whipple's disease, Arthritis Rheum. **6**:615-832, 1963.

105 Kelly, P. J., Martin, W. J., and Coventry, M. B.: Bacterial (suppurative) arthritis in the adult, J. Bone Joint Surg. **52A:** 1595-1602, 1970.

106 Key, J. A.: Hemophilic arthritis, Ann. Surg. **95**:198-225, 1932.

107 Kinsella, T. D., Baum, J., and Ziff, M.: Immunofluorescent demonstration of an IgG-B₁C complex in synovial lining cells of rheumatoid synovial membrane, Clin. Exp. Immunol. **4:** 265-271, 1969.

108 Kogstad, O.: Baker's cyst, Acta Rheum. Scand. **11**:194-204, 1965.

109 Kohn, N. N., Hughes, R. E., McCarty, D. J., Jr., and Faires, J. S.: The significance of calcium phosphate crystals in the synovial fluid of arthritic patients: the pseudogout syndrome, Ann. Intern. Med. **56**:738-745, 1962.

110 Kulka, J. P.: The lesions of Reiter's syndrome, Arthritis Rheum. **5**:195-201, 1962.

111 Kutty, M. K., Iqbal, Q. M., and Teh, E.-C.: Ochronotic arthropathy, Arch. Pathol. **96**:100-103, 1973.

112 Lack, C. H.: Lysosomes in relation to arthritis. In Dingle, J. T., and Fell, H. B., editors: The lysosomes, New York, 1968, John Wiley & Sons, Inc., vol. I, pp. 493-508.

113 Lagier, R., Baud, C. A., and Buchs, M.: Crystallographic identification of calcium deposits as regards their pathological nature with special reference to chondrocalcinosis. In Fleisch, H., Blackwood, H. J. J., and Owen, M., editors: New York, 1966, Springer Publishing Co., pp. 158-162.

114 Lamont-Havers, R. W.: Nature of serum factors causing agglutination of sensitized sheep cells and group A hemolytic streptococci, Proc. Soc. Exp. Biol. Med. **88**:35-38, 1955.

115 Lawee, D.: Uric acid: the clinical application of 1000 unsolicited determinations, Can. Med. Assoc. J. **100**:838-841, 1969.

116 Lawrence, J. S.: Heberden oration: Rheumatoid arthritis—nature or nurture? Ann. Rheum. Dis. **29**:357-379, 1970.

117 Lawrence, J. S.: Rheumatoid factors in families, Sem. Arthritis Rheum. **3**:177-188, 1973.

118 Lawrence, J. S., Hewitt, J. V., and Popert, A. J.: Gout and hyperuricemia in the United Kingdom. In Kellgren, J. H., Jeffrey, M. R., and Ball, J., editors: The epidemiology of chronic rheumatism Philadelphia, 1963, F. A. Davis Co., pp. 176-181.

119 Lazarus, G. S., Brown, R. S., Daniels, J. R., and Fullmer, H. M.: Human granulocyte collagenase, Science **159**:1483-1485, 1968.

120 Lebowitz, W. B.: The heart in rheumatoid disease, Ann. Intern. Med. **58**:102-123, 1963.

121 Letters. Mycoplasma and rheumatoid arthritis, Arthritis Rheum. **15**:648-651, 1972.

122 Lewis, P. R., and McCutchen, C. W.: Experimental evidence for weeping lubrication in mammalian joints, Nature **184**:1285, 1959.

123 Ling, R. S. M.: The genetic factor in Dupuytren's disease, J. Bone Joint Surg. **45B:**709-718, 1963.

124 Lowbeer, L.: Brucellosis osteomyelitis in man and animals, Am. J. Pathol. **24**:723-724, 1948.

125 Luck, V.: Dupuytren's contracture, J. Bone Joint Surg. **41A**:635-664, 1959.

126 Luck, V.: Articular cartilage: responses to destructive influence. In Basset, C. E., editor: Cartilage, degradation and repair, Washington, D.C., 1967, Nat. Res. Council, pp. 143-164.

127 Luse, S. A.: A synovial sarcoma—studies by electron microscopy, Cancer **13**:321-322, 1960.

128 MacConnaill, M. A.: The function of intra-articular fibrocartilage, with special reference to the knee and inferior radio-ulnar joint, J. Anat. **60**:210-227, 1931.

129 McCormick, J. N.: An immunofluorescence study of rheumatoid factor, Ann. Rheum. Dis. **22**:1-10, 1963.

130 McEwen, C., diTata, D., Lingg, C., Porini, A., Good, A., and Rankin, T.: Ankylosing spondylitis accompanying ulcerative colitis, regional ileitis and Reiter's disease, Arthritis Rheum. **14**:291-318, 1971.

131 Mackenzie, D. H.: Synovial sarcoma, Cancer **19**:169-180, 1966.

132 MacLachlan, M. D., and Rodnan, G. P.: Effects of food, fast and alcohol on serum uric acid and acute attacks of gout, Am. J. Med. **42:** 38-57, 1967.

133 Martenis, T. W., Bland, J. H., and Phillips, C. A.: Rheumatoid arthritis after rubella, Arthritis Rheum. **11**:683-687, 1968.

134 Mason, R. M., and Barnes, C. G.: Behçet's syndrome with arthritis, Ann. Rheum. Dis. **28:** 95-103, 1969.

135 Mellors, R. C., Heimer, R., Corcos, J., and Korngold, L.: Cellular origin of rheumatoid factor, J. Exp. Med. **110**:875-886, 1959.

136 Meyerowitz, S.: The continuing investigation of psychosocial variables in rheumatoid arthritis. In Hill, A. G. S., editor: Modern trends in rheumatology, London, 1971, Butterworth & Co. (Publishers), vol. 2, pp. 92-105.

137 Mitchell, N., and Shepard, N.: Relapsing polychondritis. An electron microscopic study of synovium and articular cartilage, J. Bone Joint Surg. **54A**:1235-1245, 1972.

138 Moll, J. M. H., and Wright, V.: Psoriatic arthritis, Sem. Arthritis Rheum. **3:**55-78, 1973.

139 Moseley, H. F.: Shoulder lesions, ed. 3, Baltimore, 1969, The Williams & Wilkins Co.

140 Mullins, F., Berard, C. W., and Eisenberg, S. H.: Chondrosarcoma following synovial chondromatosis, Cancer **18:**1180-1188, 1965.

141 Murphy, E. G.: The histopathology of rheumatic fever: a critical review. In Lewis, L. T., editor: Rheumatic fever, Minneapolis, 1952, University of Minnesota Press, pp. 28-51.

142 Murphy, F. P., Dahlin, D. C., and Sullivan, C. R.: Articular synovial chondromatosis, J. Bone Joint Surg. **44A:**77-86, 1962.

143 Nashel, D. J., Widerlite, L. W., and Pekin, T. J.: IgD myeloma with amyloid arthropathy, Am. J. Med. **55:**426-430, 1973.

144 Nelson, J. A., and Koontz, W. C.: Septic arthritis in infants and children, Pediatrics **38:**966-971, 1966.

145 Nesterov, A. I.: The clinical course of Kashin-Beck disease, Arthritis Rheum. **7:**29-40, 1964.

146 Nowoslawski, A.: Immunopathological features of rheumatoid arthritis. In Mueller, W., Harwerth, H. G., and Fehr, K., editors: Rheumatoid arthritis, New York, 1971, Academic Press, Inc., pp. 325-338.

147 Nugent, C. A.: Renal urate excretion in gout studied by feeding ribonucleic acid, Arthritis Rheum. **8:**671-685, 1965.

148 O'Brien, J. E., and Stout, A. P.: Malignant fibrous xanthomas, Cancer **17:**1445-1455, 1964.

149 O'Brien, W. W.: Twin studies in rheumatic diseases, Arthritis Rheum. **11:**81-86, 1968.

150 O'Brien, W. M., Banfield, W. C., and Sokoloff, L.: Studies on the pathogenesis of ochronotic arthropathy, Arthritis Rheum. **4:**137-152, 1961.

151 O'Duffy, J. D., Carney, J. A., and Deodhar, S.: Behçet's disease: a report of 10 cases, three with new manifestations, Ann. Intern. Med. **75:**561-570, 1971.

152 Onion, D. K., Crumpacker, C. S., and Gilliland, B. C.: Arthritis of hepatitis associated with Australia antigen, Ann. Intern. Med. **75:**29-33, 1971.

153 O'Sullivan, J. B.: Gout in a New England town. A prevalence study in Subdury, Mass., Ann. Rheum. Dis. **31:**166-169, 1972.

154 O'Sullivan, J. B., and Cathcart, E. S.: The prevalence of rheumatoid arthritis, Ann. Intern. Med. **76:**573-577, 1972.

155 DePalma, A. F.: Hemophilic arthropathy, Clin. Orthop. **52:**145-165, 1967.

156 Panush, R. S., Bianco, N. E., and Schur, P. H.: Serum and synovial fluid IgG, IgA and IgM antigammaglobulins in rheumatoid arthritis, Arthritis Rheum. **14:**737-747, 1971.

157 Partain, J. O., Cathcart, E. S., and Cohen, A. S.: Arthritis associated with gonorrhea, Ann. Rheum. Dis. **27:**156-162, 1968.

158 Paul, G. R., and Leach, R. E.: Synovial chondromatosis of the shoulder joint, Clin. Orthop. **68:**130-135, 1970.

158a Pinnell, S. R., Krane, S. M., Kenzora, J. E., and Glimcher, M. J.: A heritable disorder of connective tissue. Hydroxylysine-deficient collagen disease, New Eng. J. Med. **286:**1013-1020, 1972.

159 Radin, E. L., and Paul, I. L.: A consolidated concept of joint lubrication, J. Bone Joint Surg. **54A:**607-616, 1972.

160 Reichelt, A.: Beiträge zur Ätiologie der Osteochondrosis dissecans des Hüftgelenkes, Arch. Orthop. Unfallchir. **65:**220-235, 1969.

161 Riddle, J. M., Bluhm, G. B., and Barnhart, M. J.: Ultrastructural study of leucocytes and urates in gouty arthritis, Ann. Rheum. Dis. **26:**389-401, 1967.

162 Rimoin, D. L.: Pachydermoperiostosis; genetic and physiologic considerations, New Eng. J. Med. **222:**923-931, 1965.

163 Robillard, R., Gagnon, P. A., and Alarie, R.: Diabetic neuropathy: report of four cases, Can. Med. Assoc. J. **91:**795-804, 1964.

164 Rodnan, G. P.: The nature of joint involvement in progressive systemic sclerosis (diffuse scleroderma); clinical study and pathologic examination of synovium in twenty-nine patients, Ann. Intern. Med. **56:**422-439, 1962.

165 Rodnan, G. P.: Early theories concerning etiology and pathogenesis of gout, Arthritis Rheum. **8:**599-609, 1965.

166 Ropes, M. W., Bennett, G. A., and Cobb, S.: Revision of diagnostic criteria for rheumatoid arthritis, Ann. Rheum. Dis. **18:**49-53, 1958.

167 Rosenberg, L., Johnson, B., and Schubert, M.: Proteinpolysaccharides from human articular and costal cartilage, J. Clin. Invest. **44:**1647-1656, 1956.

168 Ruettner, J., and Spycher, M.: Electron microscopic investigations on aging and osteoarthrotic human cartilage, Pathol. Microbiol. **31:**14-24, 1968.

169 Sääf, J.: Effect of exercise on adult articular cartilage, Acta Orthop. Scand., Suppl. 7, 1950.

170 Saville, P. D.: Age and weight in osteoarthritis of the hip, Arthritis Rheum. **11:**635-644, 1968.

171 Scadding, J. G.: The lungs in rheumatoid arthritis, Proc. Roy. Soc. Med. **62:**227-238, 1969.

172 Schachter, J.: Isolation of *Bedsonia* from human arthritis and abortion tissue, Am. J. Ophthalmol. **63:**1082-1086, 1967.

173 Schaller, J., and Wedgwood, R. J.: Juvenile rheumatoid arthritis: a review, Pediatrics **50:**940-953, 1972.

174 Schmorl, G., and Junghanns, H.: The human spine in health and disease. (English translation by S. P. Wilkins and L. S. Coin.) New York, 1959, Grune and Stratton, Inc.

175 Schumacher, H. R., Jr.: Ultrastructure of the synovial membrane in idiopathic hemochromatosis, Ann. Rheum. Dis. **31:**465-473, 1972.

176 Schumacher, H. R., Andrews, R., and McLaughlin, G.: Arthropathy in sickle cell disease, Ann. Intern. Med. **78:**203-211, 1973.

177 Scott, J. T., and Pollard, A. C.: Uric acid excretion in the relatives of patients with gout, Ann. Rheum. Dis. **29:**397-400, 1970.

178 Scott, R. B., Elmore, S. McD., Brackett, N. C., Harris, W. O., and Still, W. J. S.: Neuropathic joint disease (Charcot joints) in Waldenström's macroglobulinemia with amyloidosis, Am. J. Med. **54:**535-543, 1973.

179 Seegmiller, J. E., Howell, R. R., and Malawista, S. E.: The inflammatory reaction to sodium urate, J.A.M.A. **180:**469-475, 1962.

180 Seegmiller, J. E., Laster, L., and Howell, R. R.: Biochemistry of uric acid and its relation to gout. III. New Eng. J. Med. **268:**821-827, 1963.

181 de Sèze, S., Solnica, J., Mitrovic, D., Miravet, L., and Dorfman, H.: Joint and bone disorders and hyperparathyroidism in hemochromatosis, Sem. Arthritis Rheum. 2:71-94, 1972.

182 Shearn, M. A.: Sjögren's syndrome, Philadelphia, 1971, W. B. Saunders Co.

183 Shirahama, T., and Cohen, A. S.: Ultrastructural evidence for leakage of lysosomal contents after phagocytosis of monosodium urate crystals, Am. J. Pathol. 76:501-520, 1974.

184 Silberberg, M., and Silberberg, R.: The effects of endocrine secretions on articular tissues and their relation to the aging process. In Slocum, C. H., editor: Rheumatic diseases, Philadelphia, 1952, W. B. Saunders Co., pp. 151-163.

185 Silberberg, M., and Silberberg, R.: Aging changes in cartilage and bone. In Bourne, G. H., editor: Structural aspects of ageing, London, 1961, Pitman Medical Publishing Co., Ltd., pp. 87-108.

186 Silberberg, M., Frank, E. L., Jarrett, S. R., and Silberberg, R.: Aging and osteoarthrosis of the human sternoclavicular joint, Am. J. Pathol. 35:831-865, 1959.

187 Silberberg, R.: Ultrastructure of articular cartilage in health and disease, Clin. Orthop. 57:233-257, 1968.

188 Silby, H. M., Farber, R., O'Connell, C. J., Acher, J., and Marme, E. J.: Acute monoarticular arthritis after vaccination, Ann. Intern. Med. 62:347-350, 1965.

189 Sinclair, R. J. G., and Cruickshank, B.: A clinical and pathologic study of rheumatoid arthritis with extensive visceral involvement "rheumatoid disease," Q. J. Med. (N.S.) 25: 312-332, 1956.

190 Sinha, S., Munichovdappa, C. L., and Kozak, G. P.: Neuro-arthropathy (Charcot joints) in diabetes mellitus, Medicine 51:191-200, 1966.

191 Sjögren, H.: Keratoconjunctivitis sicca and chronic polyarthritis, Acta Med. Scand. 130: 484-488, 1948.

192 Smillie, J. L.: Osteochondritis dissecans: loose bodies in joints; etiology, pathology, treatment. Edinburgh, 1960, E. & S. Livingstone.

193 Smith, L. W.: Synoviomata, Am. J. Pathol. 3:355-364, 1927.

194 Smith, C. B.: A synovial culture model for the study of the possible infectious etiology of rheumatoid arthritis. In Christian, C. L., Phillips, P. E., and Williams, R. C., editors: Atypical virus infections, The Arthritis Foundation Conference, Ser. No. 15, New York, 1971, The Arthritis Foundation, pp. 54-58.

195 Sokoloff, L.: The heart in rheumatoid arthritis, Am. Heart J. 45:635-643, 1954.

196 Sokoloff, L.: Comparative pathology of arthritis, Adv. Vet. Sci. Comp. Med. 6:193-250, 1960.

197 Sokoloff, L.: The biology of degenerative joint disease, Chicago, 1969, University of Chicago Press.

198 Sokoloff, L., McCluskey, R. T., and Bunim, J. J.: Vascularity of the early subcutaneous

199 Soren, A.: Pathogenesis and treatment of ganglion, Clin. Orthop. 48:173-179, 1966.

200 Spilberg, J., Silzbach, L. E., and McEwen, C.: The arthritis of sarcoidosis, Arthritis Rheum. 12:126-137, 1969.

201 Spink, W. W.: The nature of brucellosis, Minneapolis, 1956, University of Minnesota Press, pp. 175-180.

202 Spycher, M., Moor, H., and Ruettner, J.: Electron microscopic investigations on aging and osteoarthrotic human articular cartilage, Z. Zellforsch. Mikrosk. Anat. 98:512-524, 1969.

203 Stecher, R. M.: Heberden oration: Heberden's nodes. A clinical description of osteoarthritis of the finger joints, Ann. Rheum. Dis. 14:1-10, 1955.

203a Stein, C.: The interrelationship of synovium and articular cartilage, doctoral thesis, University of Oxford, 1976.

204 Stewart, S. M., Alexander, W. R. M., and Duthie, J. J. R.: Diphtheroid organisms and rheumatoid arthritis, Lancet 1:678-679, 1970.

205 Still, G. F.: On a form of chronic joint disease in children, Med. Chir. Trans. (London) 80: 47-59, 1897.

206 Stockwell, R. A.: The cell density of human articular and costal cartilage, J. Anat. 101: 753-763, 1967.

207 Stockwell, R. A.: Changes in the acid glycosaminoglycan content of the matrix of aging human articular cartilage, Ann. Rheum. Dis. 29:509-515, 1970.

208 Stougaard, J.: Familial occurrence of osteochrondritis dissecans, J. Bone Joint Surg. 46B: 542-543, 1964.

209 Stout, A. P., and Lattes, R.: Tumors of soft tissues. In Atlas of tumor pathology, Ser. 2, Fasc. 1, Bethesda, Md., 1967, Armed Forces Institute of Pathology, pp. 164-171.

210 Sutton, R. D., Benedek, T. G., and Edwards, G. A.: Aseptic bone necrosis and corticosteroid therapy, Arch. Intern. Med. 112:594-602, 1963.

211 Swinyard, C. A., and Mayer, V.: Multiple congenital contractures (arthrogryphosis), J.A.M.A. 183:23-27, 1963.

212 Sylven, B., Paulson, S., Hirsch, C., and Snellman, O.: Biophysical and physiological investigations on cartilage and other mesenchymal tissues. II. The ultrastructure of bovine and human nuclei pulposi, J. Bone Joint Surg. 33A: 333-340, 1951.

213 Talbott, J. A., and Calkins, E.: Pulmonary involvement of rheumatoid arthritis, J.A.M.A. 189:911-913, 1964.

214 Teilum, G., and Lindahl, A.: Frequency and significance of amyloid changes in rheumatoid arthritis, Acta Med. Scand. 149:449-455, 1954.

215 Thornhill, H. L., Richter, R. W., Shelton, M. L., and Johnson, C. A.: Neuropathic arthropathy (Charcot forefeet) in alcoholics, Orthop. Clin. North Am. 4:7-20, 1973.

216 Torres, J., Rathbun, H. K., and Greenough, W. B., III: Pneumococcal arthritis: report of a case and review of the literature, Johns Hopkins Med. J. 132:234-241, 1973.

217 U.S. National Center of Health Statistics:

nodule of rheumatoid arthritis, Arch. Pathol. 55:475-495, 1955.

Prevalence of osteoarthritis in adults, Ser. 11, No. 15, 1961/1962.

218 U.S. National Health Service: Rheumatoid arthritis in adults, Public Health Service Publications, Ser. 11, No. 17, 1966.

219 Vaughn, J. H., Barnett, E. V., Sobel, M. V., and Jacox, R. F.: Intracytoplasmic inclusions of immunoglobulins in rheumatoid arthritis and other disorders, Arthritis Rheum. **11:**125-134, 1968.

220 Vaughn, J. H., and Butler, V. P., Jr.: Current status of rheumatoid factor, Ann. Intern. Med. **56:**1-11, 1962.

221 Verzár, F.: Aging of connective tissue, J. Gerontol. **12:**915-921, 1964.

222 Vlasik, J., Zitman, D., and Sitaj, S.: Articular chondrocalcinosis. II. Genetic study, Ann. Rheum. Dis. **22:**153-157, 1963.

223 Waaler, E.: The occurrence of a factor in human serum activating the specific agglutination of sheep blood corpuscles, Acta Pathol. Scand. **17:**173-188, 1940.

224 Wagner, J. C., and McCormick, J. N.: Immunological investigations of coalworkers disease, J. Roy. Coll. Phys. **2:**49-56, 1967.

225 Waine, H., Bennett, G. A., and Bauer, W.: Joint disease associated with acromegaly, Am. J. Med. Sci. **209:**671-678, 1947.

226 Waine, H., Nevinny, D., Rosenthal, J., and Joffe, I. B.: Association of osteoarthritis and diabetes, Tufts Folia Med. **7:**13-19, 1961.

227 Walker, P. S., Dowson, D., Longfield, M. D., and Wright, V.: Boosted lubrication in synovial joint by fluid entrapment and enrichment, Ann. Rheum. Dis. **27:**512-520, 1968.

228 Weissmann, G.: Lysosomes and joint disease, Arthritis Rheum. **9:**834-840, 1966.

229 Weissmann, G.: Studies on lysosomes. VII. Acute and chronic arthritis produced by intra-articular injections of streptolysin S in rabbits, Am. J. Pathol. **46:**129-247, 1968.

230 Wilde, A., Mankin, H. J., and Rodnan, G. P.: Avascular necrosis of the femoral head in scleroderma, Arthritis Rheum. **13:**445-447, 1970.

231 Wollaston, W. H.: On gouty and urinary concretions, Philosoph. Trans. Roy. Soc. London **87:**388-400, 1797.

232 Wood, G. C., Pryce-Jones, R. H., and White, D. D.: Chondromucoprotein-degrading neutral protease activity in rheumatoid fluid, Ann. Rheum. Dis. **30:**73-77, 1971.

233 Wright, V., Dowson, D., and Unsworth, A.: The lubrication and stiffness of joints. In Hill, A. G. S., editor: Modern trends in rheumatology, London, 1971, Butterworth & Co. (Publishers), vol. 1, pp. 30-45.

234 Wright, V., and Watkinson, G.: The arthritis of ulcerative colitis, Medicine **38:**243-262, 1959.

235 Wyngaarden, J. B.: The overproduction of uric acid in primary gout, Arthritis Rheum. **8:**648-658, 1965.

236 Yanez, J. E., Thompson, G. R., Mikkelsen, W. M., and Bartholomew, L. E.: Rubella arthritis, Ann. Intern. Med. **64:**772-777, 1966.

237 Zevely, H. A., French, A. J., Mikkelsen, W. M., and Duff, I. F.: Synovial specimens obtained by knee joint punch biopsy, Am. J. Med. **20:**510-520, 1956.

238 Ziff, M., Kantor, T., Bien, E., and Smith, A.: Studies on the composition of the fibrinoid material in the subcutaneous nodule of rheumatoid arthritis, J. Clin. Invest. **32:**1253-1259, 1953.

239 Zucker-Franklin, D.: The phagosomes in rheumatoid synovial fluid leukocytes: a light, fluorescence and electron microscope study, Arthritis Rheum. **9:**24-36, 1966.

47/Diseases of skeletal muscle

A. R. W. CLIMIE
JACOB L. CHASON

EMBRYOGENESIS AND STRUCTURE[1,3,4,6]

An understanding of the embryogenesis of muscle is of value in the interpretation of histopathologic changes in certain diseases, since damaged or regenerating muscle fibers frequently resemble embryonic fibers at various stages of development. Myoblasts develop in the myotomes of the embryonic somites, in the limb buds, and in the mesenchyme of the branchial arches. Initially myoblasts multiply by mitotic division, but later elongate and become multinucleated myocytes either by amitotic nuclear division or by fusion of adjacent cells. By the ninth week of fetal life each cell forms a long myotube with a row of central nuclei and scanty peripheral cytoplasm in which fine fibrils are randomly dispersed. Filaments of actin, 6 to 7 nm in diameter, are the first to form. Shortly thereafter thicker 10 nm filaments composed of myosin appear, and these are immediately surrounded by actin filaments forming a hexagonal pattern that is retained throughout adult life. The myosin-actin complexes initially become oriented in a linear fashion to form a nonstriated myofibril, but by the eleventh week cross striations can be detected; these become more apparent in subsequent weeks. Concurrent with these changes, the nuclei move to their definitive position and the myofibrils toward the center. Longitudinal splitting of muscle fibers occurs during the twelfth to fourteenth weeks of embryogenesis, but thereafter no additional new fibers are formed. A gradual increase in the length and width of the fibers follows. Connective tissue develops simultaneously with the formation of myoblasts but does not penetrate between individual fibers until late in fetal life. Nerve fibers, present earlier in the connective tissue, reach the muscle fibers by the eleventh week of embryogenesis, and by the thirteenth week motor nerve endings are recognized.

In the adult, skeletal muscle fibers are long multinucleated cells enclosed by an inner plasma membrane (sarcolemma) separated by a uniform space from the external basement membrane. The cytoplasm consists of myofibrils paralleling the long axis of the fiber and of sarcoplasm containing mitochondria, glycogen particles, lipid bodies, lysosomes, and an intermyofibrillary tubular complex composed of the sarcoplasmic (endoplasmic) reticulum and a transverse (T) tubular system. The latter is formed by periodic invaginations of the plasma membrane. The T system, the ends of which open on the surface of the fiber, is believed to conduct the depolarizing electrical impulse into the fiber, releasing calcium from the sarcoplasmic reticulum. The calcium then activates myosin adenosine triphosphatase to hydrolyze ATP with release of energy; thus contraction is initiated by a sliding interaction of myosin and actin. The cross striations, which are perpendicular to the long axis of the muscle fiber, are caused by the alignment of corresponding parts of adjacent myofibrils that have differing indices of refraction. With light microscopy, two bands are clearly visible—a darker, anisotropic (A) band and a lighter, isotropic (I) band. In the middle of the I band is a thin, darker zone, the Z* band or disc. With electron microscopy, an additional light zone, the H band, can be discerned in the center of the A band and this in turn contains a central, darker M band. The structural unit of the muscle fiber, the sarcomere, extends between two anchoring Z bands (Fig. 47-1). The banded appearance of muscle fibers results from the intracellular arrangement of the two major proteins of muscle, actin and myosin. Thin actin fibrils are attached at right angles to the Z disc and interdigitate with thicker

---

*Other abbreviations are from German: Z = *Zwischenscheibe* (intermediate disc), H = *heller* (lighter, brighter), M = *Mittelscheibe* (middle disc).

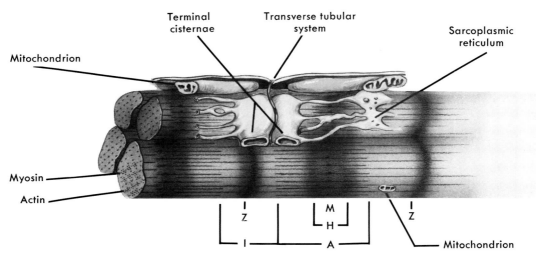

Fig. 47-1. Skeletal muscle fiber. Important components of sarcomere.

myosin fibers which occupy the central portion of the sarcomere. The light I band is composed only of actin filaments on both sides of the Z disc. The darker A band consists of overlapping actin and myosin filaments, the intermediate H band of myosin filaments, and their central M band of so-called M substance. The width of all the bands, except the Z disc, varies with the state of contraction of the muscle. In normal muscle virtually all the nuclei are in a subsarcolemmal location, but internal nuclei may be seen near myotendinous junctions. A few nuclei are located between the plasma membrane and basement membrane. These belong to satellite cells or persisting myoblasts that have the capacity to proliferate with fiber injury and that are a source of regenerative activity. The supporting connective tissue of the muscle is the endomysium, a thin sheath of fine reticulin fibers, surrounding the basement membrane of each fiber. The endomysium extends into the perimysium, which surrounds varying numbers of fibers arranged in fascicles. The whole muscle, composed of numbers of fascicles, is enclosed by the epimysium, which forms the attachments to fascia and tendons. The arrangement of this supporting tissue is such as to permit normal contraction and relaxation and to prevent overstretching.

Each muscle is supplied by one or more motor nerves originating from alpha motoneurons at one or more levels of the spinal cord or brainstem. In the extraocular muscles each neuron supplies only one fiber, but in other muscles each axon divides into multiple branches thereby innervating scattered fibers through motor end plates located on the surface of each fiber. In the motor end plate the axon, devoid of myelin and covered by a Schwann cell coat, lies in contact with synaptic folds of the sarcolemma. Terminal dilatations of the axon contain synaptic vesicles of acetylcholine, which is released in hundreds of quanta when reached by a nervous impulse. The acetylcholine attaches to the postsynaptic membrane rendering it more permeable to sodium, potassium, and calcium ions and so initiating depolarization of the cell. Cholinesterase from the postsynaptic and presynaptic membranes and Schwann cells then hydrolyzes the acetylcholine, and repolarization occurs as the muscle fiber relaxes. An anterior horn cell, its axon, and the muscle fibers supplied by its branches form a motor unit. The muscular nerves contain 30% to 50% of sensory fibers, many from muscle spindles located in the perimysium between fascicles. Each spindle consists of small, central muscle fibers surrounded by a thick connective-tissue capsule. The central (intrafusal) fibers penetrate the ends of the capsule, thereby becoming partially extrafusal in location. Specialized sensory nerve endings surround the intrafusal fibers and are responsible for measuring the tension of muscle.

The range of cross-sectional diameters of normal skeletal muscle fibers in the adult varies from 20 μm for the extraocular muscles up to 100 μm for the gluteus maximus. In commonly biopsied muscles from the limbs, the average diameter in men is 60 to 70 μm and in women 50 to 60 μm.[14,16] In children, the average diameter shortly after birth is 15 μm,

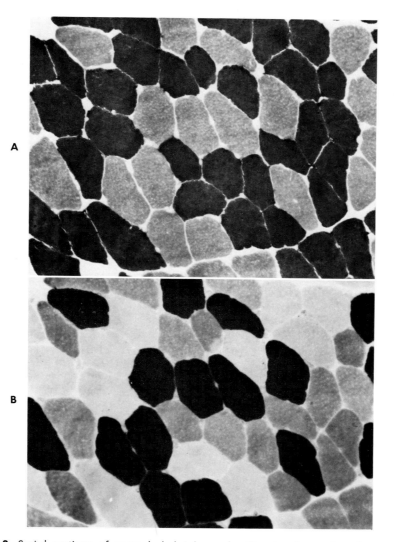

Fig. 47-2. Serial sections of normal skeletal muscle. Mosaic of type I and type II fibers. **A,** Myosin ATPase, pH 9.4: type I fibers light, type II fibers dark. **B,** Myosin ATPase, preincubated at pH 4.6: type I fibers dark, type IIA light, type IIB intermediate. (175×.)

and there is a steady increment of 2 to 4 μm annually until adult size is reached about 15 years of age.[15]

Human skeletal muscle is composed of a mixture of two major types of fibers identified by histochemical reactions.[16,38,59] Type I fibers contain numerous mitochondria and lipid droplets and are rich in oxidative enzymatic activity (e.g., nicotinamide adenine dinucleotide dehydrogenase, succinic dehydrogenase) and low in glycogen and in myophosphorylase and myofibrillar adenosine triphosphatase (myosin ATPase) activities. Type II fibers have fewer mitochondria, depend more on glycolysis for energy, and have reciprocal histochemical

properties. Type I fibers correspond roughly to the slow-twitch, red muscles, and type II fibers correspond to the fast-twitch, white muscles of certain animals. In man, however, all muscles are mixed, with the two types of fibers randomly distributed in an approximate ratio of one third type I to two thirds type II. A cross section of muscle appropriately prepared appears as a mosaic of light and dark fibers (Fig. 47-2). In women the diameter of type II fibers is generally smaller than that of type I fibers, whereas the converse is true in men.[14,58] In general, there is more variability in the size of type II than of type I fibers, a factor of some importance in the diagnosis of certain types of atrophy. The myosin ATP-ase reaction is probably the most reliable for fiber typing and has the added advantage of being technically simple.[23] With this reaction at pH 9.4, type I fibers stain light and type II dark. Preincubation of sections at pH 4.6 reverses these staining qualities, revealing subtype fibers IIA and IIB in approximately equal numbers.[16] Type I fibers under these conditions stain dark, type IIA are almost unstained, and type IIB are of intermediate intensity.

It is clear from cross-innervation experiments in animals and from studying the results of reinnervation of previously denervated muscles in humans that the histochemical reactivity of a muscle fiber is not an intrinsic property of the fiber but is determined by the specific type of alpha motoneuron from which its nerve supply is derived.[38] It has been proposed that each motoneuron supplies four "factors" to muscle cells to which it is connected.[41] The first, acetylcholine, is excitatory to the muscle. A second (trophic) factor maintains the health and size of the myofiber. The third factor is similar to the trophic factor and is responsible for establishing the histochemical type of the fiber. The fourth factor is inhibitory in action, preventing the myofiber from discharging spontaneously and so causing fibrillation and myotonia. Deficiency of these factors, alone or in combination, may be the pathogenetic mechanism for a variety of congenital and acquired diseases, some of which have heretofore been considered to be primarily myopathic rather than neurogenic in origin.

MUSCLE BIOPSY[2,22,23,37]

Muscle biopsy is valuable in diagnosis when properly performed. Care must be taken to select a muscle actively involved by the disease. It is important to obtain in advance a baseline estimation of serum creatine phosphokinase, since its elevation may occur after the trauma of biopsy. Sites of prior intramuscular injection or electromyographic needling must be avoided because of the associated focal necrosis and reactive inflammation. Local anesthetic should not be injected into the specimen of muscle, which should measure approximately 2 cm in length and 1 cm in diameter with the muscle fibers oriented longitudinally. The contractile nature of muscle is such that formalin-fixed sections show many retraction and contraction artifacts that obscure minor pathologic changes. This difficulty is best avoided by flash-freezing of blocks of muscle in isopentane cooled to $-160°$ C by liquid nitrogen and then by preparation

of frozen sections for both routine stains and histochemical reactions. Tissue frozen at customary cryostat temperatures of $-20°$ to $-30°$ C contains artifacts because of the formation of ice crystals. Frozen tissue remaining after sectioning should be retained for possible biochemical analysis. Longitudinally oriented fresh fragments of muscle, 3×1 mm, may be fixed in glutaraldehyde for electron microscopic studies. Formalin-fixed, paraffin-embedded tissue is useful for identification of inflammatory cell types and for a permanent record. If material is limited, preference should be given to transverse sections of muscle from which more information can usually be obtained. As a minimum, serial, flash-frozen, transverse sections should be stained with hematoxylin and eosin, with a trichrome method, and for myosin ATPase activity. Phosphotungstic acid–hematoxylin and stains for glycogen and lipid are of value in selected cases. In specific instances, or for investigative purposes, other histochemical reactions may be indicated. Examination of muscle at autopsy has the advantage of offering widespread sampling. Although not always so well defined as in biopsy specimens during life, most histochemical reactions are of value for 48 hours after death.

PATHOLOGIC REACTIONS OF MUSCLE[5,13,87,88]

The histopathologic reactions of muscle fibers are limited. Those related to loss of motor nerve supply are considered in the section on denervation atrophy. An increase in lipid bodies may be noted in certain atrophic fibers; in the aged a slight increase in lipochrome pigment may develop in the sarcoplasm at the ends of the nuclei. Injury to muscle is followed by a relatively constant series of histopathologic changes. First to be noticed is cloudy swelling of the fiber with blurring of the striations. Ultrastructurally this is attributable to swelling and disruption of Z discs, increase in the number and size of mitochondria, and formation of membranous structures derived from the sarcoplasmic reticulum or mitochondria. Zenker's hyaline or waxy degeneration, classically associated with typhoid fever, is indicative of more severe damage and is characterized by a homogeneous, brightly eosinophilic appearance with loss of cross striations. Affected fibers seem peculiarly prone to rupture. (Fibers showing "Zenker's degeneration" frequently occur at the edges of muscle biopsy specimens, presumably from surgical trauma;

this should not be interpreted as preexisting intrinsic disease.) Granular or floccular degeneration is a form of fiber necrosis that follows more prolonged or severe injury. The cytoplasm breaks up into small granules or larger, eosinophilic, flocculent masses, while the nuclei become pyknotic and may migrate centrally into the necrotic area. The plasma membrane and sarcoplasmic tubules rupture, as do the enlarged mitochondria. Z disc substance is the first to be lost, followed by the I bands and finally the entire myofibrillar substructure. The basement membrane may remain intact, thus forming a supporting structure for subsequent regenerative attempts by the satellite cells.

Inflammatory cells appear in the muscle within a few hours of injury. Neutrophils may be present transiently, but more striking is the perivascular accumulation of lymphocytes and the invasion of necrotic fibers by larger mononuclear macrophages, which phagocytize and remove cellular debris. Fragments of sarcoplasm that contain nuclei, or the remaining intact portion of a fiber only segmentally necrotic, frequently undergo attempts at regeneration. Complete regeneration of muscle occurs only under certain circumstances. When the basement membrane remains intact and the necrotic segment is not too large, complete reconstitution of the original structure is possible. If the fiber has been completely sectioned and the distance between two regenerating ends is short continuity may be reestablished but not necessarily with the original fiber. If the distance is greater or fibrous tissue intervenes, regeneration remains incomplete. With a focally necrotic fiber, regenerative activity is indicated when the adjacent sarcoplasm becomes deeply basophilic and the nuclei enlarge, become vesicular, develop prominent nucleoli, and migrate centrally into the fiber. Portions of fragmented fibers may develop into spindle-shaped cells or myoblasts in which the nuclei are believed to undergo at least one mitotic division. Adjacent myoblasts may then fuse to form multinucleated sarcoblasts in which further nuclear division is amitotic. Genesis of myofibrils and other subcellular components proceeds in sarcoblasts much as in embryonic life, but the resulting cell is functionally deficient, for regeneration is limited and continuity of fibers usually is not achieved. The role of the nerve supply in regeneration of muscle is not well defined, but it is unlikely that complete functional reconstitution can occur in the absence of innervation.

Hypertrophy of muscle results from increased activity or work load and is frequently seen as a compensatory mechanism in cells adjacent to atrophic fibers. After birth, individual fibers increase in diameter and length but not in numbers. This principle also applies in hypertrophy, but it is less clear whether the bulk of individual fibers is caused by an increase in the amount of sarcoplasm and the size of myofibrils or whether there may be neogenesis of myofibrils.

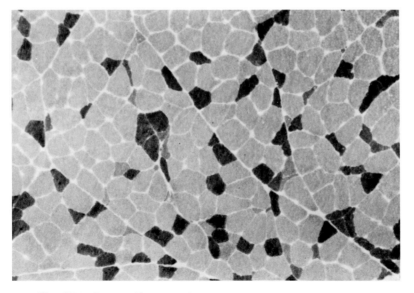

Fig. 47-3. Type II fiber atrophy. (Myosin ATPase, pH 9.4; 80×.)

ATROPHY OF DISUSE AND STEROID THERAPY[38,62,72,86]

Prolonged disuse of normally innervated muscle causes a preponderant or exclusive atrophy of type II fibers. Similar changes may be seen in cachetic patients and in those on long-term steroid therapy or with Cushing's syndrome. Except in cases of long duration, type I fibers remain of normal size whereas type II fibers are reduced in size, are angular in cross section and often have concave rather than the normal, slightly convex borders (Fig. 47-3). In some patients type IIB fibers are predominantly affected. Sarcolemmal nuclei retain their peripheral location while fiber necrosis and inflammatory changes are absent. Electron microscopic studies in type II atrophy show a preponderant loss of myofilaments from the peripheral portion of the fiber, with glycogen granules filling the empty spaces.[72] Mitochondria are decreased in number, and the sarcoplasmic reticulum is dilated. The plasma and basement membranes are widely separated, but the nuclei are normal. The findings are similar to those in denervation atrophy, possibly suggesting an alteration of the trophic neural influence on the fibers, particularly of type II. Type II fiber atrophy is reversible with appropriate exercise or discontinuation of steroid therapy. It should be stressed that a diagnosis of type II fiber atrophy cannot be made in the absence of fiber typing. At best, routine sections will demonstrate scattered atrophic fibers indistinguishable from the pattern in many patients with early denervation. Care should be taken not to overdiagnose type II atrophy, since normal type II fibers vary considerably in size. This is especially important in biopsies from women in whom type II fibers are smaller than those of type I.

DENERVATION ATROPHY[13,25,38]

Denervation (neurogenic) atrophy of muscle results from interruption of the motor nerve supply at any point from the motor nerve cell to its terminal axonal sprouts, which reach the motor end plates. Among the more common neurologic diseases causing denervation are the peripheral neuropathies and motoneuron disease. It is not usually possible to determine the cause of denervation from an examination of the histopathology of the muscle as this is similar in almost all diseases. The gross appearance of the muscle is not remarkable until very late in the course of the disease when the atrophic muscle is largely replaced by fat and fibrous tissue. It is convenient to divide the changes from denervation into early, advanced, and terminal stages. The first detectable change in cross-section is the presence of scattered, small, angular fibers with concave margins (Fig. 47-4). The atrophic fibers sometimes occur in small groups surrounded by fibers of normal size and shape. Type I and

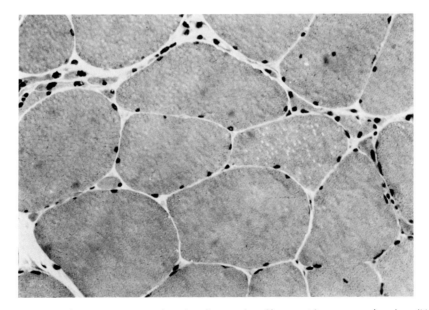

Fig. 47-4. Early denervation atrophy. Small angular fibers with concave border. (Hematoxylin and eosin; 260×.)

type II fibers are usually equally affected. Sarcolemmal nuclei remain peripherally located and cross striations are retained. A diagnostic feature not always present is the appearance of target fibers, which may represent either recently denervated[64] or recently reinnervated fibers.[13] This change is usually restricted to type I fibers, which on myosin ATPase stains have a central zone devoid of reactivity, surrounded first by a zone of increased activity and then by a zone of normal activity. Fiber necrosis, regenerative changes, and interstitial inflammation are rarely seen and probably indicate an abnormal susceptibility of denervated fibers to minor trauma. At a more advanced state of denervation, type grouping of fibers is common. The normal mosaic of type I and type II fibers is replaced

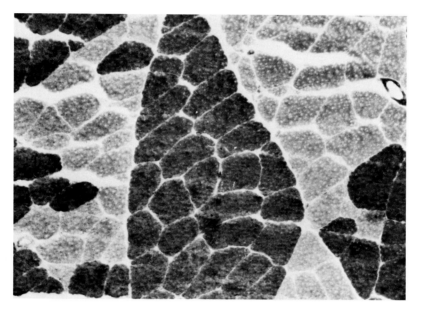

Fig. 47-5. Denervation atrophy with reinnervation showing grouping of fiber types. (Myosin ATPase, pH 9.4; 150×.)

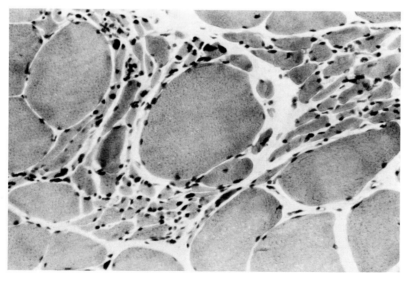

Fig. 47-6. Advanced denervation atrophy. Fascicular atrophy of muscle fibers. (Hematoxylin and eosin; 260×.)

by large clusters of fibers, all with like histochemical reactivity (Fig. 47-5). Type grouping is the result of reinnervation of fibers within a restricted zone by axonal sprouts from healthy motoneurons. It is probably most common in the recovery phase of an acute polyneuropathy. If these reinnervated fibers become denervated, the classic picture of denervation atrophy results (Fig. 47-6). There will then be large groups or fascicles in which the fibers are all atrophic and of approximately the same size, except for a rare normal fiber, which derives its nerve supply from an intact motoneuron. In longitudinal sections the loss of sarcoplasm results in a relative increase in the subsarcolemmal nuclei, which become pyknotic and are arranged in chains or clusters. In terminal stages many fibers have vanished, and those remaining measure only 10 to 15 μm in diameter and consist of little more than a sarcolemmal sheath containing clumped nuclei. Fat and fibrous tissue replace the muscle, but it is important to emphasize that this is a late occurrence when compared with similar changes in muscular dystrophy and severe polymyositis. Muscle spindles remain unaffected throughout and thus appear unusually prominent in the end stage of denervation atrophy. The alterations in fine structure in denervation atrophy are similar to those described for type II fiber atrophy in disuse. Infantile spinal muscular atrophy (Werdnig-Hoffmann disease) differs in appearance from the other denervation processes in two ways: the atrophic fibers remain rounded rather than angular, and there is a selective hypertrophy of type I fibers in certain fascicles.[25]

MUSCULAR DYSTROPHY[93-95]

The muscular dystrophies represent a group of hereditary and progressive disorders of skeletal muscle of unknown etiology. Myosin from normal and dystrophic muscle is identical when examined chemically and electrophoretically.[83] Recent electromyographic studies in Duchenne, limb-girdle, and myotonic dystrophies have suggested that there is a selective loss of motor units in affected muscles, an indication that lack of trophic influence from a "sick" motoneuron may be a significant etiologic factor.[70,71] Accepting loss of trophic influence for myotonic dystrophy, Engel and associates have proposed an alternative etiologic hypothesis in Duchenne dystrophy based on the similarity between the histopathologic changes in that disease and those produced experimentally by arterial embolization of rab-

bit muscle.[39,54,73] Further study is necessary to determine if the arterial narrowing commonly present in dystrophic muscle is a primary or secondary phenomenon. Neither theory for the etiology of muscular dystrophy can be considered established.

Numerous classifications of muscular dystrophy have been proposed, of which the most practical is that of Walton.[93] Based on the mode of inheritance and clinical features, it is presented here in slightly modified form.

Muscular dystrophy
  Sex-linked inheritance
    Severe (Duchenne type)
    Benign (Becker type)
  Autosomal recessive inheritance
    Limb-girdle type
  Autosomal dominant inheritance
    Facioscapulohumeral type
    Myotonic dystrophy
  Miscellaneous dystrophies (distal, ocular, oculopharyngeal)

Clinical features

Duchenne muscular dystrophy is transmitted by a sex-linked recessive gene although spontaneous mutations are relatively common. Only boys are affected; females are carriers. Symptoms begin in childhood usually before the age of 4. The muscles of the pelvis are the first to be affected; so the initial symptoms are difficulty in walking, running, and rising from a sitting position. Other muscles, especially those of the shoulder girdle, are affected in relentless progression until the patient is confined to a wheelchair or bed when contractures rapidly supervene. At some stage of the disease hypertrophy of muscles is usually noted, particularly in the calves. This change is probably attributable in part to true hypertrophy of muscle fibers and in part to a pseudohypertrophy produced by fatty infiltration of the muscle. Involvement of the heart muscle is virtually constant. Death is caused by either respiratory or cardiac failure and usually occurs before the age of 20. Serum enzymes, especially the serum creatine phosphokinase (CPK), are invariably elevated early, but the CPK level drops rapidly after the age of 10.[74] Abnormal electromyographic findings are constant. Approximately 70% of female carriers also show elevation of the serum CPK although this is not constant and may only be detected after repeated measurement.[85] Carriers also show electromyographic abnormalities, and fiber necrosis may be found on muscle biopsy. By the combined use of the serum CPK, electromyography, and biopsy, approximately 80% of carriers can be identified; thus genetic counseling is greatly aided.

The Becker variety of sex-linked dystrophy comes to attention between the ages of 5 and 25 years. Similar in other respects to the Duchenne variety, it has a much slower clinical course and is usually without cardiac involvement. These individuals frequently survive to sexual maturity, and so transmission of the trait from affected males becomes possible.

Limb-girdle dystrophy, transmitted as an autosomal recessive trait, affects both sexes. Spontaneous mutations are not uncommon. Initial symptoms begin in early adult life and first affect muscles of the shoulder or pelvic girdle. Pseudohypertrophy of the calves occurs, but cardiac involvement is rare. The progress of the disease is variable, but few patients live a normal life-span. Longevity is, however, considerably greater than that in Duchenne dystrophy.

Facioscapulohumeral dystrophy bears many resemblances to the limb-girdle variety. Major differences include autosomal dominant inheritance in most, the occurrence of weakness of facial muscles, the rarity of pseudohypertrophy, the occurrence of incomplete forms of the disease, and a normal life expectancy in all but the most rapidly progressive cases.

Myotonic dystrophy (dystrophia myotonica, myotonia atrophica) is transmitted by an autosomal dominant gene, and its manifestations are not confined to skeletal muscle. Other lesions include cardiac involvement, frontal baldness, cataracts, gonadal atrophy, and mental deficiency. Symptoms usually begin in early adult life, and the muscles most commonly affected include those of the face, forearm, and lower legs. This distal pattern of involvement, together with the phenomenon of myotonia (inability to relax the muscles after contraction), distinguishes the disease from most of the other dystrophies, which predominantly affect proximal muscles.

The miscellaneous dystrophies (distal, ocular, oculopharyngeal) are too rare to justify separate attention. Some may have been confused with various rare familial denervation diseases.

Elevation of the serum CPK activity is a common finding in all varieties of dystrophy except the myotonic, in which it is variable. Levels are highest in Duchenne dystrophy and may even be normal at times in other varieties during quiescent periods. The elevation of the enzyme in the serum is probably related to the number of actively necrotic muscle fibers from which it leaks. The CPK can therefore be expected to be highest in the acute phases of muscle destruction and when the disease is rapidly progressive.

Pathologic features

Gross pathologic changes in muscular dystrophy are nonspecific. They consist of an early replacement by fat and fibrous tissue so that the muscle appears yellow or white and floats in the fixative solution. It is this infiltration that gives rise to the pseudohypertrophic appearance of certain muscles although transient compensatory hypertrophy of individual fibers may occur. Except for myotonic dystrophy, the histopathologic aspect of the various forms of muscular dystrophy varies only in minor respects. The earliest change is the appearance of focally necrotic fibers infiltrated by macrophages but generally without an associated interstitial inflammatory infiltrate. Adjacent to the zone of necrosis there is basophilia of sarcoplasm and internal migration of enlarged nuclei characteristic of regeneration. Continuity of necrotic fibers may be reestablished in the early stages of the disease, but regenerative activity decreases later as the destructive process predominates. In dystrophy, atrophic fibers tend to retain a rounded cross-sectional appearance, differing in this respect from the angular, atrophic fibers of denervation (Fig. 47-7). Uninvolved fibers commonly are hypertrophied so that a transverse section of muscle appears as a haphazard mosaic of small, normal-sized, and enlarged fibers. Internal migration of nuclei, longitudinal splitting[57] of fibers and ring fibers may all be prominent. Ring fibers, which may be seen in other diseases and occasionally in normal muscle, consist of a peripheral layer of myofibrils running at right angles to, or in spiral fashion about, a central core of longitudinally oriented myofibrils. Electron microscopic changes in fibers with early necrosis are nonspecific; they consist of streaming or fragmentation of the Z discs, shredding of myofibrils, dilatation of the sarcoplasmic reticulum, swelling and disruption of mitochondria, and accumulation of lipid vacuoles and myelin-like figures. As the dystrophic process advances, individual fibers are separated by ever-increasing amounts of endomysial fibrous tissue (Fig. 47-8). Histochemical typing is less reliable in dystrophic than in normal muscle. However, with care, one can demonstrate that both fiber types are

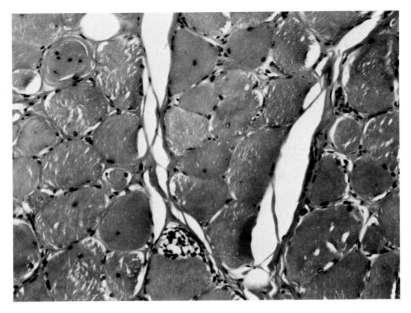

Fig. 47-7. Early muscular dystrophy. Variation in fiber size, necrotic fiber infiltrated by macrophages, and ring fiber in *upper left*. (Hematoxylin and eosin; 200×.)

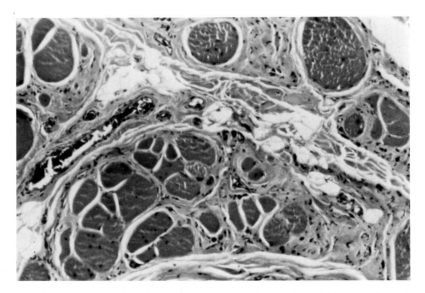

Fig. 47-8. Advanced muscular dystrophy. Haphazard atrophy of fibers with replacement by fat and fibrous tissue. (Hematoxylin and eosin; 175×.)

affected, though the normal orderly relationship may be lacking.[9] In the terminal stages the muscle is replaced by fat and fibrous tissue in which rare surviving fibers can be seen together with muscle spindles, which are seldom affected. At this point histologic differentiation from end-stage denervation atrophy or polymyositis is not possible. The histopathologic aspect of myotonic dystrophy differs from the other diseases in this group in several respects. Early changes include atrophy of type I fibers but relatively little necrosis or phagocytosis. Later, chains of central nuclei, ring fibers, and sarcoplasmic masses are common.

MYOSITIS

Inflammatory diseases of muscles are divisible into two major groups, those with known and those of unknown etiology. A practical classification is as follows:

Myositis

1. Known etiology
   a. Bacterial
   b. Fungal
   c. Parasitic
   d. Viral
   e. Mechanical, physical, and chemical agents
2. Unknown etiology
   a. Polymyositis (dermatomyositis)
      (1) Acute
      (2) Chronic
   b. Acute rhabdomyolysis
   c. Interstitial myositis
      (1) Collagen diseases
          Polyarteritis nodosa
      (2) Sarcoidosis

Bacterial myositis is uncommon and is almost always caused by direct implantation of the causative organism. The course of localized inflammation, necrosis, and abscess formation differs little from that seen in other tissues. The effectiveness of repair and regeneration after resolution of the inflammatory process depends on the extent of the destruction. In most cases regeneration will be incomplete and a fibrous scar will remain. Specific diseases such as gas gangrene, fungal and viral infections, and parasitic infestations have been considered previously under their appropriate designations. Heat, cold, and trauma result in nonspecific necrosis, degeneration, and regeneration of muscle.

Polymyositis[79,80]

Polymyositis is a disease of unknown etiology, but the frequent elevation of serum globulins, the association with "autoimmune" diseases of the collagen group, and the response to therapy with steroids have all suggested a relationship to an autoimmune phenomenon. Support for such a hypothesis comes from a demonstration that rat lymphocytes sensitized to rabbit muscle are cytopathic to tissue cultures of fetal rat skeletal muscle.[61] It is therefore proposed that the infiltrating lymphocytes in polymyositis, heretofore considered reactive in nature, may have previously been sensitized to muscle in some manner and so are directly responsible for initiating necrosis of fibers.

Polymyositis may occur at any age, but the peak incidence is in the fourth through sixth decades. It is twice as common in women as in men.[67] A cutaneous rash is associated with approximately 50% of patients with polymyositis (then known as dermatomyositis). The histopathologic changes in the muscles are identical in both groups. Dermal lesions are particularly common in the 15 to 20% of cases of polymyositis with an associated internal malignancy, usually a carcinoma. The incidence of concomitant malignancy is much greater in patients whose disease begins after age 50. Polymyositis may be associated with other collagen diseases such as rheumatoid arthritis, lupus erythematosus, and scleroderma. Raynaud's phenomenon is not uncommon, and there is also an association with Sjögren's syndrome. The onset of polymyositis may be acute or gradual. When it is acute, the patient experiences severe muscular weakness, fever, malaise, and other constitutional symptoms. Death may occur from failure of the respiratory muscles. More often, the onset of polymyositis is gradual, with the development of muscular weakness first affecting proximal limb muscles and then progressing to others. There may be muscular pain and tenderness. When the dermal component of the disease is present, it typically takes the form of an erythematous rash seen especially on the face but also on the trunk and proximal limbs. Serum enzymes, especially CPK, are elevated in proportion to the amount of muscle necrosis. Serial estimations of CPK are useful in following the activity of the disease and its response to treatment.

In acute polymyositis there is atrophy, degeneration, and necrosis of muscle fibers. Both fiber types and muscle spindles are affected. The peripheral fibers of fascicles are often predominantly affected early whereas the central fibers are spared, but later in the course this selective pattern of involvement is lost (Fig. 47-9). Muscle fibers show a complete spectrum of degeneration from vacuolar changes to frank necrosis. Segmental involvement of fibers is frequent. Regenerative attempts are prominent both in the form of isolated myoblasts as well as of muscle giant cells and proliferating buds at the disrupted ends of fibers. Electron microscopic findings are nonspecific and generally are indistinguishable from those described under muscular dystrophy. The endomysium and perimysium are infiltrated by variable numbers of lymphocytes, plasma cells, macrophages and lesser numbers of neutrophils. There is little relationship between the amount of inflammatory exudate and the degree of muscle damage. As the necrotic muscle is removed, it is replaced by connective tissue and fat, until

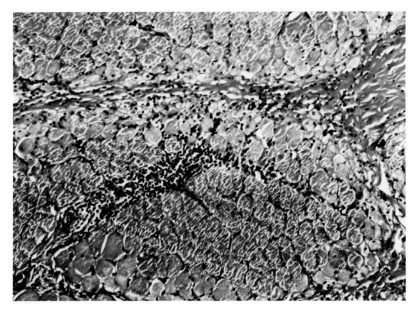

Fig. 47-9. Polymyositis. Selective atrophy of fibers at periphery of fascicles. Infiltrate of lymphocytes. (Hematoxylin and eosin; 80×.)

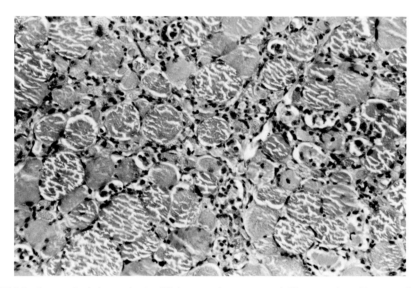

Fig. 47-10. Acute rhabdomyolysis. Widespread necrosis of fibers with infiltration by macrophages. Little interstitial inflammation. (Hematoxylin and eosin; 120×.)

in the terminal stage the appearance is nonspecific.

In chronic cases the histopathologic changes may be limited to isolated necrotic fibers and an associated minor inflammatory infiltrate. Since there is also variation in fiber size, the findings may be remarkably similar to those in early muscular dystrophy; thus they pose a problem in differential diagnosis.[27]

Acute rhabdomyolysis[1,69]

Acute rhabdomyolysis or paroxysmal myoglobinuria is characterized by attacks of muscle pain and cramps associated with severe weakness and, on occasion, with systemic symptoms. Half the cases occur after an episode of unaccustomed physical exertion,[47] and the remainder are related to trauma, viral infections,[12] excessive alcohol intake,[60] potassium deficiency,[21,63] or exposure to certain drugs and toxins.[28,56,68] Shortly after the onset of an attack, dark urine containing myoglobin is passed. In severe cases renal tubular necrosis may develop and be followed by oliguria and azotemia. It is important to analyze both serum and urine for myoglobin during the acute attack because plasma clearance is rapid and later specimens may be normal. Differentiation of myoglobinuria from hemoglobinuria is difficult.[42] Histologically there is a striking segmental necrosis of muscle fibers with concomitant attempts at regeneration from adjacent unaffected zones. Necrotic segments are infiltrated by macrophages, but there is little interstitial inflammatory infiltrate in relation to the amount of muscular damage (Fig. 47-10). Regeneration is usually complete because the basement membrane and endomysium remain intact. If repeated attacks occur, there may be permanent muscular damage and weakness.

Interstitial myositis

Focal interstitial collections of inflammatory cells, especially lymphocytes, are found in a variety of diseases. Scattered necrosis of muscle fibers may also be noted but is not usually prominent. Lesions of this type are most common in the collagen group of diseases, especially rheumatoid arthritis, lupus erythematosus, scleroderma, and polymyalgia rheumatica.[17] The findings are nonspecific and should not be misinterpreted as polymyositis. Type II fiber atrophy may coexist on the basis of disuse, steroid therapy, or both.

Polyarteritis nodosa[81]

Polyarteritis nodosa affects skeletal muscle in over 50% of cases although clinically it is not always apparent. It may also involve peripheral nerves with secondary denervation atrophy of muscles. In selection of a muscle for biopsy the chance of success in demonstrating the lesion is proportional to the local severity of pain or weakness. Most commonly the affected arteries lie in the perimysium and the perivascular inflammatory infiltrate frequently extends into the peripheral zones of adjacent muscle fascicles. Necrosis and degeneration of muscle may be present, and should sections lack a typical arterial lesion, it may be impossible to distinguish the disease from polymyositis.

Sarcoidosis[26]

Sarcoidosis may affect skeletal muscle more commonly than is generally realized. Clinical evidence of muscular pain or weakness is uncommon, but biopsies have revealed typical noncaseating epithelioid cell granulomas in over 50% of patients. The granulomas are usually located in the perimysium, often adjacent to an artery or vein. More rarely a granuloma may develop in the endomysium often associated with focal atrophy or necrosis of the adjacent muscle fibers. In the differential diagnosis it is important to consider that a granulomatous response can be seen adjacent to each *Trichinella* larva. Sarcoidosis involving peripheral motor nerves results in secondary denervation atrophy of muscle.

MYASTHENIA GRAVIS[44,55,77,89]

Myasthenia gravis is believed to be caused by a deficiency in the production, storage, release or premature degradation of acetylcholine at the motor end plate. This results in excessive weakness and fatigue after repetitive movements or with sustained muscular contraction. Its prevalence approximates 1 per 20,000 population. Age at onset reaches a peak in the third decade for women and the sixth decade for men. The overall incidence is greater in women than in men in a ratio of 3 : 2. Although familial cases have been reported, there is no heritable pattern.[20] Onset is usually gradual, with manifestations restricted to ocular muscles in 20%; in another 50% ocular symptoms and mild or moderate generalized myasthenia are concomitant. In 10% weakness is severe, progressive, and generalized with involvement of the "bulbar" and respiratory muscles. Remissions occur in the early stages but become less common and of shorter duration as the disease progresses. Death is usually attributable to respiratory failure and aspiration pneumonia that results from the severe dysphagia.

Myasthenia gravis has been associated with hyperthyroidism, diabetes mellitus, pernicious anemia, rheumatoid arthritis, lupus erythematosus, polymyositis and neoplasia, especially carcinoma of the breast. Thymomas are present in 10% of patients, with the incidence increasing with age at onset. In two thirds of the patients, the thymus is of normal size and weight but contains germinal centers and increased numbers of lymphocytes and plasma cells in its medulla.[48] Similar changes of "thymitis" may be present in the thymus surrounding a thymoma.

The classic, but inconstant, lesion in muscle is a focal lymphocytic infiltrate ("lymphorrhage"), usually perivascular but less often located in the endomysium where it displaces adjacent muscle fibers. Although muscle atrophy is constant in the later stage, necrosis is rare. The usual pattern of atrophy is that of denervation, but type II fiber atrophy may predominate as a result of disuse or treatment with steroids. Electron microscopic studies have disclosed shortening and simplification of the postsynaptic membrane at the motor end plate.[36] Investigations with the use of microelectrodes have shown that the quanta of acetylcholine released from the presynaptic vesicles are normal in number but only one fifth normal in size.[29]

Considerable evidence has accumulated to suggest that myasthenia gravis may be an autoimmune disease.[89] Serum complement levels are depressed in proportion to the severity of the disease. In 30% to 40% of patients serum antibodies to skeletal muscle antigens can be recognized by indirect immunofluorescence and antibodies are detectable in more than 50% when multiple methods are utilized. The reactive antigens are common to cardiac muscle and the spindle-shaped "myoid" cells of the thymus. With polarizing microscopy the antibodies appear to attach especially to the A bands, which contain both actin and myosin, but microcomplement-fixation studies of isolated muscle components have demonstrated that myosin is the active antigen and that actin is nonantigenic. It has been proposed that the antibodies are to ATPase or to ATP- or calcium-binding myosin chains, thus leading to interference with energy sources for muscle contraction. Additional immunologic evidence is the finding of antinuclear antibodies in 20% of patients with uncomplicated myasthenia gravis and in all patients with a concomitant "autoimmune" disease.

A cell-mediated immunologic process has also been related etiologically to myasthenia gravis. Migratory inhibition techniques have shown that extracts of myosin produce significant lymphocytic inhibition in two thirds of myasthenic patients. No patient has humoral antibody who does not also have a cell-mediated immunologic response suggesting that the cellular component may be the more important. It is, however, possible that both types of immunologic response are required for production of the disease. Evidence for a thymic cellular role is twofold. There is a relationship between the number of medullary germinal centers and the severity of the disease, and improvement or remission is seen in 75% of patients after thymectomy. This beneficial re-

sponse may be delayed, often for 2 to 5 years or longer, possibly as a result of the presence of an extrathymic pool of long-lived immunocompetent T lymphocytes.[78]

The thymus secretes a hormone (thymin) that acts by inhibiting neuromuscular transmission[49-51] and in excess may cause myasthenia. "Thymitis" produced in animals by injection of extracts of thymus or striated muscle resembles that seen in many patients with myasthenia gravis, and the affected animals develop a partial neuromuscular block curable by thymectomy. Excess thymin may therefore be significant etiologically in the 75% of patients who have either "thymitis" or a thymoma. Regardless of the nature of the initiating etiologic factor, other evidence suggests that it may act on the alpha motoneuron rather than directly on muscle; thus it causes first a decrease in axonal acetylcholine.[40,41] The neuronal trophic factor decreases later, first affecting type II fibers but eventually both types with a resulting denervation atrophy. This theory and the morphologic changes are not incompatible with an autoimmune concept although the target organ is shifted from muscle to neuron (see also p. 1588).

GLYCOGEN-STORAGE DISEASE[8,91,92]

The glycogen-storage diseases are inborn, heritable errors of metabolism characterized by an abnormal accumulation of glycogen in the tissues. The classification (Table 47-1) now includes at least 10 types in which a specific enzymatic defect has been established. Additional isolated cases have been reported in which the defect has not as yet been defined. Abnormal deposition of glycogen in skeletal muscle is found in all but types I, VI, and IX although the amount present varies considerably with the different enzymatic defects. Diagnosis depends on biochemical identification of the enzymatic abnormality, except for type II in which the histologic appearance is characteristic and type V in which a reliable histochemical method is available. The less rare glycogenoses of muscle are types II, III, and V.

Type II glycogenosis (Pompe's disease) is transmitted by an autosomal recessive gene and becomes manifest at 3 to 4 months of age with muscular weakness, cyanosis, and cardiac and lingual enlargement. The muscular weakness correlates poorly with the firm, apparently well-developed muscles. Death usually occurs within the first year of life because of cardiac failure or pneumonia. The enzymatic defect

Table 47-1. The glycogenoses

Type		Enzymatic defect	Organ affected
I	(von Gierke's disease)	Glucose-6-phosphatase	Liver, kidney
II	(Pompe's disease)	α-1,4-Glucosidase	Generalized; liver, muscle
III	(Cori's disease) (Forbes' disease)	Amylo-1,6-glucosidase or oligo-1,4$\rightarrow$ 1,4-glucan transferase, or both	Generalized; liver, muscle
IV	(Andersen's disease)	Amylo-1,4$\rightarrow$1,6-transglucosylase	Generalized; liver
V	(McArdle's syndrome)	Muscle phosphorylase	Muscle
VI	(Hers' disease)	Hepatic phosphorylase	Liver, leukocytes
VII		Phosphofructokinase or phosphoglucomutase	Muscle, erythrocytes
VIII		Inhibitor of phosphohexoisomerase	Muscle
IX		Hepatic phosphorylase kinase	Liver
X		Cyclic AMP–dependent phosphorylase kinase	Liver, muscle
—		UDPG-glycogen transglucosylase	Decreased hepatic and muscle glycogen

is a deficiency in lysosomal α-1,4-glucosidase (acid maltase). At autopsy, massive accumulations of glycogen are found in a variety of organs including skeletal, cardiac, and smooth muscle, liver, kidneys, and central nervous system. In muscle the glycogen appears as large vacuoles which are PAS-positive. Islands of myofibrillar substance remain as condensed masses often in a subsarcolemmal location. With electron microscopy the excess glycogen is seen to lie free, in membrane-bound structures and in autophagic vacuoles.[31] Glycogen in normal muscle is probably ingested by lysosomes and later digested by the lysomal acid maltase. In the absence of the enzyme, glycogen accumulates and distends the lysomes to such an extent that myofibrils are mechanically disrupted. The onset of symptoms in type II glycogenosis has occasionally been delayed until later childhood or adulthood.[35] Cardiac involvement has then been absent, and the disease may mimic muscular dystrophy. Heterozygous carriers can be detected by assay of muscle enzyme content.[33]

Type III glycogenosis (limit dextrinosis, debrancher enzyme defect, Forbe's disease, Cori's disease) is caused by a deficiency of one or both of amylo-1,6-glucosidase or oligo-1,4$\rightarrow$1,4-glucan transferase. These enzymes are responsible for hydrolysis at the α-1,6 linkage and hence for the continuation of glycogenolysis after the initial breakdown of the straight outer chains of the molecule by phosphorylase. In their absence an abnormal glycogen with short outer chains accumulates in the affected organs. Four subtypes are now recognized depending on whether one or both of the enzymes are absent from liver, muscle, or both. The mode of inheritance has not been established. Symptoms begin in the neonatal period and

may decrease with age. They are related more to involvement of the liver than to muscle, with hypoglycemia, hyperlipidemia, hepatomegaly, infections, and ketoacidosis. Muscle weakness when present may be mistaken for muscular dystrophy and in some patients may not become apparent until adult life. The excessive glycogen is subsarcolemmal, often in a semilunar vacuole. Electron microscopy reveals the glycogen to be free and membrane bound both in intermyofibrillar spaces as well as beneath the sarcolemma. The extremely rare type IV glycogenosis (Andersen's disease) is caused by a deficiency of amylo-1,4$\rightarrow$1,6-transglucosylase. Its mode of inheritance is not established. Excess glycogen resembling amylopectin is found in many organs including skeletal muscle. Symptomatology is primarily related to hepatic damage.

Type V glycogenosis (McArdle's disease) is an autosomal recessive disease characterized by an absence of phosphorylase from muscle but not from liver.[69] The enzymatic lack blocks the breakdown of glycogen to glucose-1-phosphate, and hence excess glycogen collects in the muscle. Muscular stiffness, weakness, and pain upon exertion usually begin in childhood but may be delayed until adult life. Exercise with ischemia results in contracture of the muscles, with inability to relax and electrical silence on electromyography. Failure of blood lactate to rise after a period of ischemic exercise should suggest the diagnosis. Histochemical examination of muscle reveals the complete absence of phosphorylase. Excess glycogen may or may not be detectable in muscle. When present, it is likely to be in subsarcolemmal blebs or in the intermyofibrillar spaces. Excess glycogen has also been described in enlarged mitochondria. Myopathic changes characterized by isolated fiber necrosis may be seen and thus simulate an early stage of muscular dystrophy.

The remaining types of glycogen-storage diseases are even more rare. In all there may be an excess of glycogen in skeletal muscle while symptoms and laboratory findings resemble those of type V glycogenosis. Type VII is caused by a deficiency of phosphofructokinase or phosphoglucomutase. Type VIII may be caused by the action of an inhibitor of phosphohexoisomerase rather than deficiency of a specific enzyme, and in type X there is an absence of phosphorylase kinase from muscle. A form of glycogenosis that results in decreased glycogen in both liver and muscle has also been described.[66] The disease is caused by a deficiency of UDGP-glycogen transglucosylase, probably transmitted by an autosomal recessive gene. Symptoms begin shortly after birth and are characterized by hypoglycemic convulsions. Mild ketonuria may be present. The fasting hypoglycemia is unresponsive to glucagon given intramuscularly.

PERIODIC PARALYSES[82]

The several forms of periodic paralyses are all characterized by episodic attacks of flaccid paralysis. The primary or familial periodic paralyses can be divided into hypokalemic, normokalemic, and hyperkalemic varieties. Secondary periodic paralyses are associated with thyrotoxicosis, primary aldosteronism, and abnormalities of potassium metabolism in diabetic acidosis and renal tubular acidosis.

The most common primary periodic paralysis is the hypokalemic form, which is transmitted by an autosomal recessive gene but is three times more frequent in males than in females. Attacks of paralysis are characteristically nocturnal and occur after a period of vigorous exercise. Symptoms usually appear first in the second decade and tend to become less severe with age. The attack, which may last from a few hours to several days, affects the musculature of the limbs and trunk but spares the facial and respiratory muscles. Although associated with low levels of serum potassium, weakness may begin at potassium levels higher than those that would induce paralysis in a normal individual.

Histologic examination of muscle fibers reveals single or multiple, centrally located, intracellular vacuoles with displacement of the myofibrils to the periphery. Type I and type II fibers are equally affected. The vacuoles appear to begin as dilatations of the sarcoplasmic

reticulum that are later surrounded by a membrane derived from the T-tubular system, which connects the vacuoles with the extracellular fluid.[30] This form of periodic paralysis is believed to be related to an alteration in cellular polarization attributable either to defects in the sarcolemma or sarcoplasmic reticulum or to abnormal intracellular carbohydrate metabolism. Attacks may be aborted by the administration of oral or intravenous potassium.

Hyperkalemic and normokalemic periodic paralyses are more rare. In the former, paralysis occurs typically by day during rest after a period of exercise and is often associated with myotonia. In the latter, the characteristic attacks are nocturnal and prolonged, often lasting for days or weeks. Vacuolar changes occur in the muscle fibers in both the hyperkalemic and hypokalemic types of periodic paralyses but are less constant and severe than in the hypokalemic form.

MISCELLANEOUS DISEASES

Myopathic changes have been described in association with a number of endocrinopathies. Among them may be included the muscular weakness experienced by certain patients with hyperthyroidism, hypothyroidism, hyperparathyroidism, hyperaldosteronism, Addison's disease, Cushing's syndrome, and diabetes mellitus. Although electromyographic findings may be abnormal at some time in all, demonstrable abnormalities in muscle are either absent or nonspecific though type II atrophy from disuse may be seen.

Myopathy is an uncommon complication of chronic alcoholism. When it does occur, proximal muscle weakness is usual, with isolated fiber necrosis, a vacuolar myopathy, and rarely rhabdomyolysis.[60,84] Recently it has been suggested that these lesions may be secondary to chronic hypokalemia, but since denervation atrophy has also been reported, it is possible that the mucular weakness is the result of a concomitant peripheral neuropathy with secondary myopathic changes.[43]

Congenital myotonia (Thomsen's disease) is characterized by a delay in relaxation of muscle resulting in a tonic cramp and immobility. Patients with Thomsen's disease have difficulty initiating movement after a period of rest, but persistent and repetitive attempts usually result in normal freedom of response. Twenty-five percent of cases are transmitted as an autosomal dominant trait, whereas the remainder appear to arise spontaneously. Symptoms usually begin in childhood but may be delayed until early adult life. No pathologic lesions are recognized in muscle other than striking hypertrophy of muscle fibers from an increase in the number of myofibrils.

A number of congenital myopathies have been described and classified primarily on the basis of particular morphologic abnormalities within muscle fibers. The names given to these diseases (nemaline [rod],[76] centronuclear or myotubular,[11,19,75] central core,[52] multicore,[34] mitochondrial,[45] tubular aggregate,[38] reducing body,[18] fingerprint body[32] myopathies) reflect the most prominent histologic findings, but the rarity of the conditions precludes detailed discussion here.

Myositis (fibroplasia) ossificans progressiva is a rare disease characterized by the development of extraosseous connective tissue masses that eventually become ossified. The disease usually begins in childhood with the appearance of rubbery masses in the connective tissues of the neck or back and later in the limbs. The lesions may form in connective tissue or muscle and initially consist of proliferating fibroblasts devoid of inflammatory reaction. When muscle is affected, the fibers are fragmented and destroyed and contractures develop as the nodule matures into collagen. Finally osteoid is formed either directly in the collagen or through an intermediate cartilaginous step. The end result is progressive immobility because of ossification of many muscle groups. Pneumonia, the commonest cause of death, follows involvement of the respiratory muscles. Although this has not been established with certainty, the disease is probably hereditary in nature and may be transmitted by an autosomal dominant gene. Congenital abnormalities may occur, particularly microdactyly of the great toe or thumb. Cases have also been associated with polyostotic fibrous dysplasia, a finding that suggests that the basic defect is a disseminated dysplasia of connective tissue.[46] Recurrence is usually rapid if the ectopic bone is surgically removed, but administration of the diphosphonate disodium ethidronate prior to operation has been successful in preventing reossification.[90]

Arthrogryposis multiplex congenita[10,24] is a rare congenital condition characterized by deformities of the limbs and trunk. Mental retardation coexists in about half the cases. It appears there may be multiple causes. Some cases are the result of maldevelopment of anterior horn cells in the spinal cord with resultant failure of innervation of specific mus-

cles. Others represent a failure to recruit myoblasts from the primitive mesenchyme during fetal life or are examples of a congenital muscular dystrophy. In neurogenic arthrogryposis muscle fibers are extremely small, whereas in the myopathic forms there is variation in fiber size and increase in endomysial fibrous tissue.

The stiff-man syndrome[53,65] begins with intermittent pain and tightness of the muscles of the neck and trunk and later progresses to involve the limbs so that all voluntary movement becomes increasingly difficult. Severe, painful spasms or cramps then develop and may be triggered by both physical or emotional stimuli. It is likely that other conditions with spasticity or rigidity have been confused with the stiff-man syndrome. The diagnosis should be restricted to those in whom electromyography shows constant tonic muscle contractions associated with continuous firing of nerve impulses. The abnormal electrical and contractile state is abolished by sleep, myoneural blocking agents, nerve block, and general anesthesia. The pathophysiology of the stiff-man syndrome is uncertain but probably involves a central mechanism. There are many similarities to tetanus, and there is probably more than one cause. Necrosis and other nonspecific changes accounted for by trauma induced by the spasms are all that are found on muscle biopsy.

TUMORS OF SKELETAL MUSCLE

Tumors and tumorlike lesions of skeletal muscle have been considered elsewhere (p. 1894).

REFERENCES
General
1 Adams, R. D.: Diseases of muscle. A study in pathology, ed. 3, Hagerstown, Md., 1975, Harper & Row, Publishers.
2 Dubowitz, V., and Brooke, M. H.: Muscle biopsy: a modern approach, Philadelphia, 1973, W. B. Saunders Co.
3 Pearson, C. M., editor: The striated muscle, Baltimore, 1973, The Williams & Williams Co.
4 Walton, J. N., editor: Disorders of voluntary muscle, ed. 2, London, 1969, J. & A. Churchill, Ltd.

Specific
5 Adams, R. D.: In Walton, J. N.: See reference 4, pp. 143-202 (pathologic reactions).
6 Allen, E. R.: In Pearson, C. M.: See reference 3, pp. 40-57 (myogenesis).
7 Alpert, L. I., Rule, A. H., Nonio, M., Kott, E., Komfeld, P., and Osserman, K. E.: Am. J. Clin. Pathol. 58:647-653, 1972 (myasthenia gravis).
8 Aponte, G. E., and Mancall, E. L.: In Sunderman, F. W., and Sunderman, F. W., Jr., editors:

The clinical pathology of infancy, Springfield, Ill., 1967, Charles C Thomas, Publisher, pp. 72-102 (glycogenoses).

9 Baloh, R., and Cancilla, P. A.: Neurology (Minneapolis) **22:**1243-1252, 1972 (fiber types in dystrophy).

10 Bharucha, E. P., Pandya, S. S., and Dastur, D. K.: J. Neurol. Neurosurg. Psychiatry **35:** 425-434, 1972 (arthrogryposis).

11 Bethlem, J., Van Wijngaarden, G., Mumenthaler, M., and Meijer, A. E. F. H.: Arch. Neurol. **23:**70-73, 1970 (centrotubular myopathy).

12 Berkin, B. S., Simon, N. M., and Bovner, R. N.: J.A.M.A. **227:**1414-1415, 1974 (myoglobinuria).

13 Brooke, M. H.: In Pearson, C. M.: See reference 3, pp. 86-122 (histochemistry).

14 Brooke, M. H., and Engel, W. K.: Neurology (Minneapolis) **19:**221-233, 1969 (muscle fiber size in adults).

15 Brooke, M. H., and Engel, W. K.: Neurology (Minneapolis) **19:**591-605, 1969 (muscle fiber size in children).

16 Brooke, M. H., and Kaiser, K. K.: Arch. Neurol. **23:**369-379, 1970 (muscle fiber types).

17 Brooke, M. H., and Kaplan, H.: Arch. Pathol. **94:**101-118, 1972 (muscle in rheumatoid arthritis, polymyalgia, and polymyositis).

18 Brooke, M. H., and Neville, H. E.: Neurology (Minneapolis) **22:**829-840, 1972 (reducing body myopathy).

19 Bradley, W. G., Price, D. L., and Watanabe, C. K.: J. Neurol. Neurosurg. Psychiatry **33:**687-693, 1970 (centronuclear myopathy).

20 Bundey, S.: J. Neurol. Neurosurg. Psychiatry **35:**41-51, 1972 (genetics of myasthenia gravis).

21 Campion, D. S., Arias, J. M., and Carter, N. W.: J.A.M.A. **220:**967-969, 1972 (rhabdomyolysis and hypokalemia).

22 Cancilla, P. A.: In Pearson, C. M.: See reference 3, pp. 19-27 (muscle biopsy, stains, and artifacts).

23 Climie, A. R. W.: Am. J. Clin. Pathol. **60:**753-770, 1973 (muscle biopsy).

24 Dastur, D. K., Razzak, Z. A., and Bharucha, E. P.: J. Neurol. Neurosurg. Psychiatry **35:**435-450, 1972 (arthrogryposis).

25 Dorman, J. D.: In Pearson, C. M.: See reference 3, pp. 249-262 (denervation atrophy).

26 Douglas, A. C., MacLeod, J. G., and Matthews, J. D.: J. Neurol. Neurosurg. Psychiatry **36:**1034-1040, 1973 (sarcoidosis).

27 Dowben, R. M., Vawter, G. F., Brandfonbrenner, A., Sniderman, S. P., and Kaegy, R. D.: Arch. Intern. Med. **115:**584-594, 1965 (polymyositis).

28 Duane, D. D., and Engel, A. G.: Neurology (Minneapolis) **20:**733-739, 1970 (emetine myopathy).

29 Elmqvist, D., Hofmann, W. W., Kugelberg, J., and Quastel, D. M. J.: J. Physiol. **174:**417-434, 1964 (myasthenia gravis).

30 Engel, A. G.: Mayo Clin. Proc. **45:**774-814, 1970 (hypokalemic periodic paralysis).

31 Engel, A. G.: In Pearson, C. M.: See reference 3, pp. 301-341 (vascular myopathies).

32 Engel, A. G., Angelini, C., and Gomez, M. R.: Mayo Clin. Proc. **47:**377-388, 1972 (fingerprint myopathy).

33 Engel, A. G., and Gomez, M. R.: J. Neurol. Neurosurg. Psychiatry **33:**801-804, 1970 (type II glycogenosis).

34 Engel, A. G., Gomez, M. R., and Groover, R. V.: Mayo Clin. Proc. **46:**666-681, 1971 (multicore disease).

35 Engel, A. G., Gomez, M. R., Seybold, M. E., and Lambert, E. H.: Neurology (Minneapolis) **23:**95-106, 1973 (type II glycogenosis).

36 Engel, A. G., and Santa, T.: Ann. N.Y. Acad. Sci. **183:**46-63, 1971 (myasthenia gravis).

37 Engel, W. K.: Pediatr. Clin. North Am. **14:**963-995, 1967 (muscle biopsy).

38 Engel, W. K.: Arch. Neurol. **22:**97-117, 1970 (muscle fiber types and reactions).

39 Engel, W. K.: In Pearson, C. M.: See reference 3, pp. 453-472 (Duchenne dystrophy).

40 Engel, W. K., and Warmolts, J. R.: Ann. N.Y. Acad. Sci. **183:**72-87, 1971 (myasthenia gravis).

41 Engel, W. K., and Warmolts, J. R.: Muscle Biol. **1:**229-253, 1972 (muscle pathology related to motoneuron abnormalities).

42 Farmer, T. A., Hammack, W. J., and Frommeyer, W. B.: New Eng. J. Med. **264:**60-66, 1961 (rhabdomyolysis).

43 Faris, A. A., and Reyes, M. G.: J. Neurol. Neurosurg. Psychiatry **34:**86-92, 1971 (alcoholic myopathy).

44 Fields, W. S., editor: Myasthenia gravis (symposium), Ann. N.Y. Acad. Sci. **183:**3-386, 1971.

45 Fisher, E. R., and Danowski, T. S.: Am. J. Clin. Pathol. **51:**619-630, 1969 (mitochondrial myopathy).

46 Frame, B., Azad, N., Reynolds, W. A., and Sneed, S. M.: Am. J. Dis. Child. **124:**120-122, 1972 (myositis ossificans progressiva).

47 Geller, S. A.: Hum. Pathol. **4:**241-250, 1973 (rhabdomyolysis).

48 Goldstein, G.: Annu. Rev. Med. **22:**119-124, 1971 (myasthenia gravis).

49 Goldstein, G.: Triangle **11:**7-14, 1972 (myasthenia gravis).

50 Goldstein, G.: In Pearson, C. M.: See reference 3, pp. 498-512 (myasthenia gravis).

51 Goldstein, G., and Hofmann, W. W.: In Rowland, L. P., editor: Immunological disorders of the nervous system, Baltimore, 1971, The Williams & Williams Co., pp. 241-259 (myasthenia gravis).

52 Gonatas, N. K., Percy, M. C., Shy, G. M., and Evangelista, I.: Am. J. Pathol. **47:**503-524, 1965 (central core disease).

53 Gordon, E. G., Januszko, D. M., and Kaufman, L.: Am. J. Med. **42:**528-599, 1967 (stiff-man syndrome).

54 Hathaway, P. W., Engel, W. K., and Zellwego, H.: Arch. Neurol. **22:**365-378, 1970 (muscular dystrophy).

55 Howard, C. W. H.: Br. Med. J. **3:**437-440, 1973 (myasthenia gravis).

56 Itabashi, H. H., and Kokmen, E.: Arch. Pathol. **93:**209-218, 1972 (chloroquine neuromyopathy).

57 Isaacs, E. R., Bradley, W. G., and Henderson, G.: J. Neurol. Neurosurg. Psychiatry **36:**813-819, 1973 (muscular dystrophy).

58 Jennekens, F. G. I., Tomlinson, B. E., and Walton, J. N.: J. Neurol. Sci. **13:**281-292, 1971 (muscle fiber sizes).

59 Jennekens, F. G. I., Tomlinson, B. E., and

Walton, J. N.: J. Neurol. Sci. **14**:245-257, 1971 (muscle fiber sizes).

60 Kahn, L. B., and Meyer, J. S.: Am. J. Clin. Pathol. **53**:516-530, 1970 (alcoholic myopathy).

61 Kakulas, B. A.: In Pearson, C. M.: See reference 3, pp. 485-497 (polymyositis).

62 Klinkerfuss, G. H., and Haugh, M. J.: Arch. Neurol. **22**:309-320, 1970 (disuse atrophy).

63 Knochel, J. P.: New Eng. J. Med. **287**:927-928, 1972 (rhabdomyolysis).

64 Kovarcky, J., Schochet, S. S., Jr., and Mc-Cormick, W. F.: Am. J. Clin. Pathol. **59**:790-797, 1973 (denervation atrophy).

65 Layzer, R. B., and Rowland, L. P.: New Eng. J. Med. **285**:31-40, 1971 (stiff-man syndrome).

66 Lewis, G. M., Spencer-Peet, J., and Stewart, K. M.: Arch. Dis. Child. **38**:40-48, 1963 (glycogenoses).

67 Logan, R. G., Bandera, J. M., Mikkelson, W. M., and Duff, I. F.: Ann. Intern. Med. **65**:996-1007, 1966 (polymyositis).

68 Macdonald, R. D., and Engel, A. G.: J. Neuropathol. Exp. Neurol. **29**:479-499, 1970 (chloroquine myopathy).

69 McArdle, B.: In Walton, J. N.: See reference 4, pp. 607-638 (type V glycogenosis).

70 McComas, A. J., Sica, R. E. P., and Campbell, M. J.: Lancet **1**:321-325, 1971 (motoneurons and muscle disease).

71 McComas, A. J., Sica, R. E. P., and Upton, A. R. M.: Arch. Neurol. **30**:249-254, 1974 (motoneurons and muscle disease).

72 Mendell, J. R., and Engel, W. K.: Neurology (Minneapolis) **21**:358-365, 1971 (type II fiber atrophy).

73 Mendell, J. R., Engel, W. K., and Derrer, E. C.: Science **172**:1143-1145, 1971 (Duchenne dystrophy).

74 Munsat, T. L., Baloh, R., Pearson, C. M., and Fowler, W., Jr.: J.A.M.A. **226**:1536-1543, 1973 (serum enzymes in neuromuscular disorders).

75 Munsat, T. L., Thompson, L. R., and Coleman, R. F.: Arch. Neurol. **20**:120-131, 1969 (centronuclear myopathy).

76 Neustein, H. B.: Arch. Pathol. **96**:192-195, 1973 (nemaline myopathy).

77 Osserman, K. E., and Genkins, G.: Mt. Sinai J. Med. N.Y. **38**:497-537, 1971 (myasthenia gravis).

78 Papatestas, A. E., Alpert, L. I., Osserman, K. E., Osserman, R. S., and Kark, A. E.: Am. J. Med. **50**:465-474, 1971 (myasthenia gravis).

79 Pearson, C. M.: Annu. Rev. Med. **17**:63-82, 1966 (polymyositis).

80 Pearson, C. M.: In Walton, J. N.: See reference 4, pp. 501-539 (polymyositis).

81 Pearson, C. M.: In Walton, J. N.: See reference 4, pp. 532-533 (polyarteritis nodosa).

82 Pearson, C. M.: In Pearson, C. M.: See reference 3, pp. 427-441 (periodic paralyses).

83 Penn, A. S., Clark, R. A., and Rowland, L. P.: Arch. Neurol. **27**:159-173, 1972 (muscular dystrophy).

84 Perkoff, G. T., Hardy, P., and Velez-Garcia, E.: New Eng. J. Med. **274**:1277-1285, 1966 (alcoholic myopathy).

85 Perry, T. B., and Frazer, F. C.: Neurology (Minneapolis) **23**:1316-1323, 1973 (serum enzymes in Duchenne dystrophy).

86 Pleasure, D. E., Walsh, G. O., and Engel, W. K.: Arch. Pathol. **22**:118-125, 1970 (steroid-induced atrophy).

87 Price, H. M.: In Pearson, C. M.: See reference 3, pp. 144-184 (ultrastructural pathology).

88 Reznik, M.: In Pearson, C. M.: See reference 3, pp. 185-225 (muscle regeneration).

89 Rule, A. H., and Kornfeld, P.: Mt. Sinai J. Med. N.Y. **38**:538-572, 1971 (myasthenia gravis).

90 Russell, R. G. G., Bishop, M. C., Smith, R., Price, D. A., and Squire, C. M.: Lancet **1**:10-11, 1972 (myositis ossificans progressiva).

91 Schotland, D. L.: In Pearson, C. M.: See reference 3, pp. 410-426 (glycogenoses).

92 Sidbury, J. B., Jr.: The glycogenoses. In Gardner, L. I., editor: Endocrine and genetic disease of childhood, Philadelphia, 1969, W. B. Saunders Co., pp. 853-866 (glycogenoses).

93 Walton, J. N., and Gardner-Medwin, D.: In Walton, J. N.: See reference 4, pp. 455-499, (muscular dystrophy).

94 Walton, J. N.: In Pearson, C. M.: See reference 3, pp. 263-291 (muscular dystrophy).

95 Zundel, W. S., and Tyler, F. H.: New Eng. J. Med. **273**:537-543, 596-601, 1965 (muscular dystrophy).

48/Nervous system

JACOB L. CHASON

Central nervous system

The diseased nervous system offers an exceptional opportunity for the correlation of structure with function. Although the pathologic processes that affect the nervous system differ little from those occurring elsewhere in the body, the functional changes that result have both greater variability and uniformity. The variability of the effects upon neurologic function is related to the anatomic localization of the disease. The uniformity of neurologic response, on the other hand, is dependent on several factors, among which are the following:

1. Fixed size of space enclosing the central nervous system (after fusion of the sutures of the skull)
2. Limited mobility of the nervous system within the space
3. Immobility of the dura and dural folds
4. The uniformity of structural change and progression of most lesions, i.e., "the biologic behavior of the lesion" (essential to the correlation of structure and function is an understanding of the reactions of the components of the nervous system to injury)

CELL STRUCTURE: FUNCTION AND REACTION TO INJURY
Neuron

The nerve cell consists of a nucleus and a cell body, the perikaryon, with one or more processes known as dentrites and a single larger process, an axon. The perikaryon of the cell ranges in diameter from 5 μm in internal granular cells of the cerebellum to 80 μm or more in the Betz cells of the motor cortex.

The larger cells have a single, large, round to oval, usually vesicular nucleus with a well-defined nuclear membrane and a large nucleolus. With the exception of some cells of the hypothalamus, brainstem, and Clarke's column of the spinal cord, the nucleus is in a central portion in the perikaryon. The cytoplasm, except at the base of the axon, contains basophilic, granular to blocklike material called Nissl substance. This material, as identified by electron microscopy, represents the ribosomes and the rough endoplasmic reticulum, which are the sites of protein metabolism. Nissl substance has the staining characteristics of the nucleolus, where it is believed to be formed and from which it spreads throughout the cytoplasm, appearing initially as a nuclear cap. In most large cells, the Nissl substance is relatively evenly divided throughout the cytoplasm. In the cells normally having an eccentric nucleus, it is characteristic for the Nissl substance to be concentrated at the peripheral margins of the cell cytoplasm.

Many of the larger cells contain a brown, granular, intracytoplasmic lipochrome or lipofuscin pigment that increases with age.[4,7] This pigment has the same staining characteristics and significance as the lipofuscin in parenchymal cells elsewhere. A neuromelanin pigment, morphologically similar to that of melanin, is normally present in the cytoplasm of the perikaryon of the cells of the substantia nigra, the locus ceruleus, and some cells of the motor nuclei along the floor of the fourth ventricle[61] and in melanophores in the posterior lobe of the pituitary gland. This pigment first appears in the cells of the locus ceruleus, microscopically visible at about the eighth intrauterine month and grossly visible by the eighth postnatal month. In the substantia nigra, the pigment appears microscopically visible at approximately 1½ years of age and grossly visible at 3 years of age. Adult pigment levels are reached by the end of adolescence.[61]

Dendrites and axons of variable lengths are cytoplasmic extensions of the neurons. The longest, the axons of the Betz cells, extend for almost 1 meter. Coursing from a dendrite to the axon through the perikaryon are microtubules and neurofilaments (both types individually visible only with electron microscopy). It is believed that these structures help maintain the shape of the cell and are the pathways for the orderly transfer of materials from one part of the cell to the other. Aggregates of the neurofilaments or neurotubules characteristic of certain diseased states can usually be seen only with special silver stains.

Other components of the nerve cells generally cannot be adequately demonstrated or studied either individually or in groups by light microscopy. Their presence and actual or potential activities sometimes can be demonstrated from the enzyme content. The acid phosphatase reaction is a marker for, and represents one of, the enzymatic actions of the lysosomes. Some of the oxidative enzyme reactions are used as markers for mitochondria and to demonstrate the type and relative amounts of the enzymes.

The specialized sites, being forms of the contact of the nerve cells, called the synapses, require electron microscopy for study. The presynaptic terminally expanded axon contains mitochondria and vesicles with acetycholine or, in some, norepinephrine. Release of the chemical at the synapse results in the transmission of the impulse to the receptor, usually the dendrite, or to the end button (synaptic knob, end foot, *bouton terminal*), cell body, or even axon, of the succeeding cell.

The recognition and separation of antemortem and postmortem changes in nerve cells are essential. Because minor degrees of structural variation within the cells may be associated with abnormalities of function, constant use of control sections is necessary for separation of the normal appearance from fixation artifacts, structural variations caused by disease, and autolytic change.

Shrinkage and increased staining of the entire cell with tortuosity of the cell processes constitute one of the commonest of nerve cell changes (chronic neuronal disease). Although it has been described as an aging process in some cells and is a form of reaction to a variety of acute and chronic diseases, it is also commonly found in the second and third cortical layers, where it is attributable to the effects of fixation. Low-grade chronic injury to nerve cells is believed to result in an abnormal increase in the intracytoplasmic lipofuscin (lipochrome) pigment. This is known as pigmentary atrophy and more recently has been associated with the disease lipofuscinosis. The abnormal increase in this pigment, which is sudanophilic and sometimes acid-fast, is believed to interfere with the normal cellular metabolic activity, perhaps by causing coating of the cell organelles. Cloudy swelling or, as it is known in the central nervous system, acute nerve cell change is characterized by cellular swelling and staining pallor of the perikaryon with loss of Nissl substance. This condition is considered to be reversible up to the point at which the cell processes are fragmented and separated from the cell body. It is a nonspecific response to a variety of injurious agents and is a well-known postmortem change. Ischemic change in the cell results from hypoxia, anoxia, and hypoglycemia or occurs after the ingestion of poisons that block the utilization of oxygen or glucose. With ischemia, there is early pronounced cytoplasmic eosinophilia accompanying the rapid destruction of the Nissl substance. The cell soon begins to swell, the cytoplasm becomes finely granular, and the nucleus becomes pyknotic. Shortly thereafter the eosinophilia begins to fade, the perikaryon shrinks, and the nucleus undergoes karyorrhexis with total cell disintegration. Central chromatolysis, (retrograde or axonal degeneration) occurs after injury to the cell axon (only when near the perikaryon). In the affected cell, the nucleus is displaced to one side of the swollen and rounded perikaryon, and the Nissl substance is lost first about the nucleus and later toward the periphery. With recovery, the nucleolus enlarges, the Nissl substance reappears initially as a nuclear cap, later filling the perikaryon and dendrites, while the nucleus gradually resumes its normally central position. Complete structural recovery may take several months. By light microscopy, this entire series of changes can be adequately studied only with the Nissl stain. Because cells with eccentrically placed nuclei and peripheral Nissl substance are normally present in certain portions of the sections, adequate control must be utilized. Degeneration with swelling and fragmentation of the axon distal to the site of injury (wallerian degeneration) resembles that of the peripheral nervous system (p. 2140). The covering myelin formed by the oligodendrogliocytes simultaneously degenerate. Mononuclear inflammatory cells, attracted to the area, phagocytize the axonal fragments and the altered myelin, converting the myelin to neutral fats. The portion of the axon attached to the perikaryon may swell and have one or more fine silver positive sprigs extend from it, but effective regeneration of the axon as in the peripheral nervous system does not occur. Since oligodendroglial cells may be the source of myelin for more than one axon, they degenerate only with loss of significant numbers of axons. Wallerian degeneration is grossly recognizable only after several months and only when a large and relatively compact tract is affected. The affected tract may gradually become more white and sharply demarcated from the surrounding tissue, especially when it is the result of a rapid and massive destruction of the axons. If the cause results in gradual axonal destruction, the affected tract may barely be discerned and then only by a decrease in its cross-sectional size. Other specific nerve cell changes are described with the diseases with which they are associated.

One should recognize that an oligodendroglial cell can be destroyed without structural damage to the surrounded axon. Conversely, destruction of the axon, either directly or indirectly (because of injury to the nerve cell), always results in destruction of the covering myelin sheath and sometimes of the oligodendrocyte. With the hematoxylin and eosin stain, one of the earliest reliable indications of myelin damage is the presence of myelin-containing or lipid-containing macrophages, first within the area of damage and later about adjacent blood vessels. Occasionally, one is able to recognize swelling of the axon and surrounding myelin by the presence of 20 to 25 μm, circular or cylindric, eosinophilic masses in the white matter of the brain or spinal cord. The darker core of these eosinophilic structures indicates the swollen axon, and the lighter outer zone represents the altered myelin. Simultaneously, but difficult to recognize, are shrinkage and further hyperchromatism of the oligodendroglial nucleus. These changes are more easily and adequately recognized with special stains for myelin and axons that demonstrate irregular swelling, pallor, and fragmentation of both structures well before the routine stains appear abnormal. Although slight staining pallor of the area may be recognizable with the routine stains after the loss or removal of myelin, the state is more easily appreciated with any of the variety of stains for myelin. The interfascicular oligodendrocytes of the white matter cover a single segment of one or more axons. The junction between the two cell membranes covering an axon is known as a node of Ranvier. With brain edema or swelling, the nonstaining halo of the interfascicular oligodendrocyte may be-

come filled with a pink mucoid material (mucinous degeneration). The nonstaining halo seen about almost all of the oligodendroglial nuclei may increase in size as a part of the postmortem autolytic change. Oligodendrocytes also are found in the gray matter of the central nervous system, where they form satellite cells about the larger nerve cells. The satellite type of oligodendroglial cell has been considered by some to act both as a protector of the perikaryon and as a part of the route for the transport of nutrients to the cells. With the routine stains and at the usual 6 to 7 μm thickness of the sectioned tissue, one and occasionally two satellite cells may be found around one nerve cell body.

Neuroglia: neuroectodermally derived supporting cells of central nervous system

The astrocytes are the principal supporting cells of the central nervous system. Astrocytes supply structural support to the central nervous system, their foot processes form an important part of the blood-brain barrier, and they may be the transport route for nutrients to nerve cells from blood vessels and of the reverse transport of metabolites. Astrocytic processes surround and isolate synapses. Finally, much like fibroblasts, they function as a reparative response to injury. With the routine hematoxylin and eosin stain, the only component of a normal astrocyte that ordinarily can be seen is the nucleus. It is 8 to 10 μm in diameter, round to oval, and vesicular with finely granular chromatin and has a definite nuclear membrane of uniform thickness. A nucleolus ordinarily is not visible with light microscopy.

Astrocytes of two basic structural forms differing in their processes have been described. The more common fibrous astrocyte located predominantly in the white matter and on the cortical surface has long, thin, and usually nonbranching fibrillary processes, one of which extends to the wall of a blood vessel, whereas another may extend to the pial membrane. Protoplasmic astrocytes, present in the gray matter, have shorter, wider, and branching processes. Some astrocytes with both types of processes as well as with the ability to convert from one to the other have been described. The structural distinction does not appear to indicate an essential functional or biologic difference. The reactive astrocyte, whatever the source type, regularly assumes a fibrous appearance. The Fanana cell of the cerebellar cortex has some similarity with the protoplasmic astrocyte, whereas the Bergmann cell of the internal granular layer of the cerebellum has greater resemblance to the fibrous form.

The response of the astrocyte to injury can be recognized in a variety of ways. The presence of a slightly eosinophilic halo about the nucleus is one form of early reactive change visible with the hematoxylin and eosin stain. It is, however, also characteristic of many normal astrocytes present in newborn infants and young children. When there is an abundant amount of eosinophilic cytoplasm, the astrocyte is of the gemistocytic type. This structural change can be seen within hours of injury. It is associated with the rapid formation of mitochondria and their enzymes. Another form of reactive change is indicated by the presence of nuclear pairs and sometimes tetrads. This, of course, is interpreted as representing cell multiplication supposedly by amitosis, because a reactive astrocyte in mitosis is seen very rarely. The increase in astrocytes is known as astrocytosis. In astrocytic gliosis, another type of response to injury, there is an increase in the fibrillar processes of the astrocytes. When the gliotic pattern follows the preexisting normal structure, it is called isomorphic gliosis; in anisomorphic gliosis the proliferation of processes has a haphazard arrangement. These are best seen with special stains, although they usually can be recognized with the routine stains. In chronic toxic states, either endogenous, as in uremia, in liver disease with jaundice, and in Wilson's disease, or exogenous, with a variety of toxins, some astrocytic nuclei may enlarge as a result of swelling and become more vesicular. The nucleus maintains a definite nuclear membrane with several infoldings, and one or more nucleoli may become evident. These are the Alzheimer's type II cells. In Wilson's disease, also known as hepatolenticular or hepatocerebral degeneration, transitions from type II cells to the Alzheimer type I cell have been described. The type I cell has a large, darkly basophilic nucleus with a single darker nucleolus and a lighter basophilic, sometimes granular, cytoplasm. Processes are not found extending from the bodies of these cells. Among the poorly understood changes occurring in astroytes are the corpora amylacea. There are slightly eosinophilic to basophilic, sometimes concentrically laminated, PAS-positive, 10 to 15 μm spheric bodies. They are present in astrocytic processes in both the gray and white matter of the central nervous system in larger numbers in the aged and when there has been preexisting disease.

Myelin is a complex proteolipid formed by the winding of double layers of the cell membrane of the oligodendrocytes about the axons of most nerve cells of the central nervous system. Each layer (seen only by electron microscopy) is composed of the double plasma membranes—the inner membrane surfaces have come together, displacing the cytoplasmic contents toward the nucleus of the cell. The sandwich of double plasma membrane, by differential growth of these approximated cell membranes, is believed to result in the spiral coating about the axon. The oligodendrocyte nulceus and cytoplasm are gradually displaced ahead of their newly formed plasma membrane in its spiral about the axon. Only the 5 to 7 μm, round, hyperchromatic nucleus of the oligodendrocytes stains with hematoxylin and eosin. The cytoplasm and plasma membrane remain as a clear unstained halo about the nucleus.

Cuboid to columnar cells, the *ependymal* cells, line the ventricles, the choroid plexuses, and the central canal of the spinal cord. Microscopic remnants of detached portions of ventricles, predominantly at the occipital and, to a lesser extent, the frontal poles of the lateral ventricles, and the ventriculus terminalis of the filum terminale also are lined. Some cells are ciliated, presumably to help propel the cerebrospinal fluid. The presence of blepharoplasts (best seen with the Mallory phosphotungstic acid–hematoxylin stain), which are small cytoplasmic hematoxylinophilic granules surrounded by a clear halo, can be of great help in the identification of cells of ependymal origin. These granules are believed to be remnants of the cilia whose portions outside the cell have disappeared. Reactions of the ependyma to injury are few. Ulceration of the ventricular lining may be seen with and after local inflammations and when there is pronounced dilatation of the ventricular system. The underlying reactive subependymal astrocytes may produce nodules of astrocytic fibers that occasionally surround trapped ependymal cells. This produces an irregularity of the ventricular surface and is known as granular ependymitis or ependymal granulations.

Microglia (mesodermal glia)

During the period of vascularization early in the development of the central nervous system, another type of "glial" cell makes its appearance. Of mesodermal origin, the microglial cells represent a portion of the reticulo-endothelial system. These cells are scattered irregularly in both gray and white matter and among the astrocytes and oligodendrocytes. In the resting phase, only the short, oval to kidney-shaped hyperchromatic nuclei of these cells are stained with hematoxylin and eosin. Their scant cytoplasm and their relatively few processes (as compared with the astrocytes) are best demonstrated with the Hortega silver stain. Microglial cells react in response to injury with a great variety of structural change. Initially, they may proliferate locally about a small area of necrosis with the formation of a small group of cells, forming a so-called glial nodule. Their occurrence in a group phagocytizing a dead nerve cell is known as neuronophagia. Because of chemotactic influences, the cells may move toward the area damaged. In the process of movement, there is enlargement and elongation of their nuclei. Because of the shape of the cells during such movement, they are known as rod cells. A microglial cell also may be transformed into a mononuclear (less often multinuclear) macrophage, during which its processes are lost and its cytoplasm becomes evident, in part, because of the phagocytized content of myelin, lipid, etc. They are then known as scavenger cells, gitter cells, compound granular corpuscles, lipophages, myelinophages, etc. Many of the cells so named, however, may have their origin from lymphocytes and monocytes that reach the central nervous system through the bloodstream.

Vasculature

The blood vessels of the central nervous system, in addition to their usual functions, help through their contribution to the blood-brain barrier to maintain hemostasis and to aid in the return of interstitial fluid to the veins across the perivascular (Virchow-Robin) space. The blood-brain barrier is a physiologic phenomenon with which several structural features have been associated.[37] Although the movement of water and lipid-soluble substances across this barrier is relatively unrestricted, the transfer of other substances such as glucose, amino acids, and inorganic ions is inhibited to varying degrees. It has been stated that the large size of some molecules and the nonutilization by the nervous system of many smaller molecules determine the degree of their exclusion by the blood-brain barrier. However, the mechanism for this barrier effect is not known. It has been related to the properties of the capillary endothelium, the basement membrane, and the pericytes; to the astrocytic foot processes that almost completely surround the capillaries; and to the relative absence of an extracellular space (from early electron microscopic studies). Except in the absence of endothelial pores, the structure of the capillaries of the central nervous system does not differ significantly from that of the capillaries in many parts of the body. Only approximately 85% of their circumference is covered by the astrocytic glial sheath. Moreover, the size of the extracellular space has not been settled.[72,121] Although no agreement has been reached between the estimates derived from chemical studies and those derived from electron microscopy, the size of the space is now believed to be approximately 10% to 15% of the volume of the brain.

The perivascular or Virchow-Robin space lies between the adventitia and the pial membrane and is continuous with the subarachnoid space. Extending only as far as the capillaries, it is believed to form a route for the return of subarachnoid fluids and of cells through the subarachnoid space to the vascular system.

DEVELOPMENTAL DISORDERS

The nervous system begins as a longitudinal, mid-dorsal, ectodermal thickening. Cellular proliferation with ventral grooving and dorsal fusion of the freed lateral margins results in the formation of the neural tube, which is separated from the adjacent neural crest and the overlying skin. Continued orderly development with cell proliferation, peripheral migration, growth, and maturation are paralleled by growth, closure, and fusion of surrounding bones.[14,39,161]

The long period of maturation of the central nervous system is an important factor in its involvement in approximately half of all congenital defects. The known or suspected causes of these defects include the following:

1. Genetic disturbances
2. Maternal infections (i.e., rubella)
3. Fetal infection
4. Fetal hypoxia
5. Irradiation
6. Nutritional deficiencies and excesses
7. Chemical agents
8. Mechanical forces

Each of these factors appears to be capable of producing its effect only at a particular time in the course of development of the embryo.[34,42,51,73,152,153] Since the continued normal development is dependent on the preceding stage, the earlier the injury, the more serious the malformation.

Agenesis is the term applied to the condition in which there is absence of the anlage of a structure. In anencephaly,[152] the most severe form of agenesis, most of the brain is absent and sometimes also the spinal cord (amyelia). There are usually associated failures of closure of the skull and vertebral arches (rachischisis). All of these changes appear to begin with early defective closure of the neural tube (dysrhaphia). In those instances in which the calvaria remain intact with the skull of normal size and with the brain replaced by fluid (hydranencephaly), one should suspect paranatal injury rather than dysrhaphia and agenesis. Agenesia of specific portions of the brain, though not common, is well known. Many such defects are compatible with life and may be first recognized as incidental findings at postmortem examination. Among these are agenesis of the cerebellum and agenesis of all or only the caudal portion of the corpus callosum.[20,105,132,142] Absence of the cerebral pallium with failure of separation of the cerebral tissue (telencephalon impar) is accompanied by absence of the calvaria. Cyclencephaly is caused by failure of separation of the cerebral hemispheres. When accompanied by a single median eye (cyclopia) and by a supraorbital nasal trunk with arrhinencephaly, it is usually compatible with survival for only a few hours. Agenesis of a portion of the brain usually is bilateral and most often affects the parietal lobes. The underlying lateral ventricles at these sites are dilated and communicate with the subarachnoid space (porencephaly) (p. 2083). Similar ventricular dilatation may be seen after occlusion of the arteries or veins supplying or draining these areas or after trauma or infection, all occurring early in embryonic development with failure of development of the affected portion of one or both cerebral hemispheres.

Errors of closure of the neural tube and fusion of the surrounding bony structures are common, particularly at the lumbosacral level of the spinal cord. When the defect is complete, the dorsal portion of the spinal cord is not formed and its lateral margins remain attached to the modified ectoderm (amyelocele). The most frequent developmental defect of the neural tube, however, is that of failure of complete closure of the vertebral arches (spina bifida). Herniation of only the meninges through this defect is known as a meningocele. When a portion of the cord also is included, the defect is called a meningomyelocele. A meningomyelocystocele includes the meninges, a portion of the cord, and a portion of the central canal. With spina bifida occulta, the failure of fusion of the affected vertebral arches may result in dimpling of the overlying skin and separating fibrous tissue, but with no herniation of the cord or its coverings. Herniations of a portion of the brain and its covering during closure of the skull bones are far less frequent. These occur in the region of the glabella, the occipital bone, and at the roof of the mouth.[15] Like those of the spinal cord, they are known as meningocele, meningoencephalocele, and meningoencephalocystocele.

In the Arnold-Chiari malformation, there is caudal displacement of the medulla and vermis of the cerebellum below the level of the foramen magnum into the spinal canal.[125] A notch frequently develops on the anterior surface of the cervical cord where it is overridden by the displaced medulla. The malformation is associated with a small posterior fossa and flattening of the base of the skull (platybasia) and sometimes with internal hydrocephalus and a meningomyelocele. The association of internal hydrocephalus with the platybasia has suggested to some that the brain has been forced downward during development. Fixation of the spinal cord in the patients with a meningomyelocele, on the other hand, may have displaced the brainstem and spinal cord downward because of the greater growth of the vertebra as compared with the spinal cord. Both hypotheses have been refuted by evidence suggesting the initial

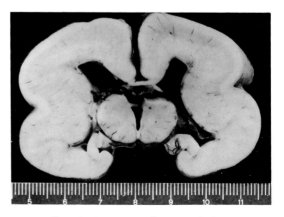

Fig. 48-1. Agyria (lissencephaly).

defect to be failure of formation of the pontine flexure.

Defective cell migration and maturation result in faulty cell position (heterotopia) and abnormalities in the formation of the gyri. The absence of gyrus formation is known as lissencephaly (agyria).[38] (Fig. 48-1). It is often, but not always, associated with generalized hypoplasia of the brain (microcephaly) and with developmental hydrocephalus. Focal hypoplasias are uncommon. They usually involve the related nuclei of the pons, medulla, and cerebellum.

Conversely, an overly large brain, macrocephaly (megalocephaly), is due in part to hyperplasia and often in part to dysplastic development.[154]

Tuberous sclerosis

Tuberous sclerosis is a heredofamilial, autosomally dominant disease caused by dysplastic development and heterotopia of the ectodermal cells of the central nervous system.[98] Often associated are a variety of developmental abnormalities of other organs of the body, including the skin—the "adenoma sebaceum" at the nasolabial folds and the subungual nodules, both of which are fibrovascular overgrowths, and shagreen skin *(peau de chagrin)* of the midlumbar skin of the back. Accompanying renal tumors, often bilateral, are either mixtures of blood vessels, fibrous tissue, fat, and smooth muscle (the angiomyolipofibromas) or tubular adenomas.[81] Nodular, gray-yellow, glycogen-filled myocardial tumors incorrectly diagnosed as rhabdomyomas may be found in some patients who die early with the disease. Pulmonary fibrosis, cysts, and bronchial hamartomas also have been seen.

The brain is usually of normal size or small. Affected gyri are slightly to greatly enlarged, white, and hard, with poor demarcation between the cortex and the white matter. The first layer of a cortical tuber may have foci of thick astrocytic fibrillae in a characteristic sheaflike arrangement (Fig. 48-2). The normal laminar arrangement of the cortical cells is considerably disturbed. In addition to an astrocytic gliosis, there are large globoid to spidery cells with both neuronal and astrocytic characteristics. Hard nodular areas, more easily felt than seen, may be found in the white matter and are composed of foci of astrocytic gliosis. Periventricular gray to white, hard, often mineralized, tumors project into the lateral ventricles. The periventricular nodules are formed by partly mineralized clusters of large bizarre

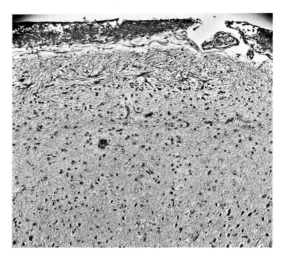

Fig. 48-2. Tuberous sclerosis with characteristic sheaflike astrocytic gliosis in first cortical layer. (Hematoxylin and eosin; 90×.)

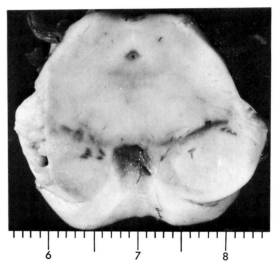

Fig. 48-3. Congenital aqueductal gliotic stenosis after intrauterine infection.

cells of astrocytic appearance. Retinal lesions, referred to as phakomas, are related tumors formed by the abnormally developed glial cells.

Aqueductal stenosis

Abnormal formation of the cerebral aqueduct in fetal life may be attributable either to an intrauterine inflammation with periaqueductal gliosis or to a disturbance in development. On rare occasions, the aqueduct is developmentally small and may be double, the so-called forking of the aqueduct. The two channels are too small for adequate cere-

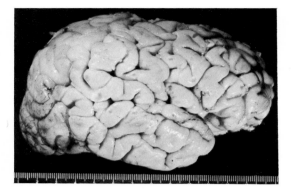

Fig. 48-4. Mongolism. Small superior temporal gyrus and blunted occipital lobe.

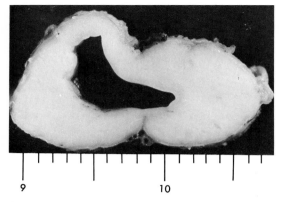

Fig. 48-5. Syringomyelia—cervical portion of spinal cord.

brospinal fluid flow. Hydrocephalus resulting from any of the causes may be first manifest either at birth (congenital) or during infancy or early childhood, depending on the degree of stenosis. Accurate recognition of its cause (Fig. 48-3) requires a good history, multiple sections of the aqueduct taken at close intervals and at right angles to its path, and comparison with normal controls.

Mongolism (Down's syndrome)[87]

At least two karyotypes of mongolism have been reported. The more common form, characterized by an extra 21 chromosome, is the result of the failure of separation of one pair of these chromosomes in oogenesis and is more likely to occur in infants of older mothers. In the other type, not related to maternal age, the extra 21 chromosome is believed to have been translocated to the end of another large chromosome. Translocation mongolism may be familial. One of the parents may be found to have the translocation (usually to chromosome 15) and with only 45 chromosomes, or it may have arisen during gamete formation in normal parents.

A variety of structural abnormalities has been reported in the brains of these patients. The more characteristic is the blunting of the occipital portion of the brain and a small superior temporal gyrus (Fig. 48-4). The cerebellum may be small as well. No uniform microscopic changes have been described although senile plaques have been seen. Diagnosis, however, is based upon the characteristic mongol facies with rounded head, prominent epicanthal folds, oblique palpebral fissures, dysplastic ears, high-arched palate, palm-print abnormalities, a palm with four finger lines, a curved fifth finger, large space between the first and second toes, other nonspecific body changes, and occasional cardiac malformations.

Syringomyelia and syringobulbia[117]

Named for its irregular tubular cavity, syringomyelia is a disorder of the spinal cord ascribed to multiple causes. One form, sometimes associated with neurofibromatosis, is believed to be caused by a defect in closure of the alar plates of the spinal cord. On the other hand, the cavity or cavities may be the residual of a previous inflammation, infarct, or hemorrhage or a component of a glial neoplasm. The cervical portion of the spinal cord is the most frequently affected and, when the lesions are multiple, usually contains the largest of the cavities. Each syrinx is filled with a watery to slightly xanthochromatic fluid. The lesion may begin anywhere within the cord; in the developmental form it is most often in the cervical cord, extending both longitudinally and laterally to involve the gray and white matter (Fig. 48-5). Its lining is formed by astrocytic processes (Fig. 48-6) except in those areas in which there is residual ependyma of an included central canal. The cavity may extend for only a few segments or involve the entire cord or, as noted previously, there may be multiple cavities. The lateral extent of the cavity or cavities determines the site and degree of ascending and descending wallerian degeneration. Involvement of the medulla (syringobulbia) may occur separately or as an extension of a lesion in the cervical portion of the cord. In the medulla, the cavity is a slit in a dorsolateral winglike position. It may be bilateral and roughly symmetric. Similar cavities have been described as occurring in the pons and even more rarely in the cerebral

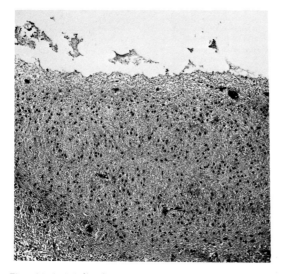

Fig. 48-6. Wall of syrinx with astrocytic proliferation. (Hematoxylin and eosin; 90×.)

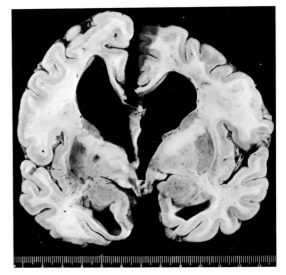

Fig. 48-7. Internal hydrocephalus of lateral and third ventricles caused by obstructive lesion in fourth ventricle (not illustrated).

hemispheres, where they end in the head portion of either or both caudate nuclei.

Dilatation of the central canal (hydromyelia) is a frequent and asymptomatic finding seen at all levels of the spinal cord examined routinely post mortem. Some consider it the mildest form of spinal dysrhaphia, i.e., the mildest form of syringomyelia.

Hydrocephalus[138]

The descriptive term "hydrocephalus" is used to indicate an increased amount of cerebrospinal fluid in the ventricles, in the subarachnoid space about the brain, or in both. In practice, this is recognized from enlargement of these spaces rather than by measurement of the fluid. The condition is classified in several different ways. When the increased fluid accumulation is limited to the dilated ventricular system, the hydrocephalus is called internal (Fig. 48-7). External hydrocephalus, on the other hand, is the presence of excess fluid in the enlarged subarachnoid space over the brain. Separation of hydrocephalus into communicating and noncommunicating types is useful for the clinician. In the communicating type, there is normal free flow of fluid between the ventricles and the subarachnoid space about the cauda equina. Obstruction or block of this free flow is considered to be a noncommunicating hydrocephalus. Varying degrees, sites, and causes of flow impedance are causes for limitation of the value of this classification.

The most useful classification is that described by Russell[138] and slightly modified here. To understand this classification, a limited knowledge of formation, flow, and removal of spinal fluid is essential. Cerebrospinal fluid is formed, in the main, by the choroid plexuses of the lateral, third, and fourth ventricles. From the lateral ventricles, flow is directed into the third ventricle through the two foramina of Monro. The fluid then follows the cerebral aqueduct into the fourth ventricle, from which it exits into the subarachnoid spaces through the two lateral recesses and the foramina of Luschka and through the middle foramen of Magendi. Most of the fluid finally is returned to the venous system through the arachnoid villi that lie in several of the venous sinuses. With this brief description as a background, hydrocephalus can then be considered to have arisen from an imbalance or derangement of one or more of these factors.

Hydrocephalus from the overproduction of cerebrospinal fluid is the least common. Proved instances of overproduction (i.e., caused by hypertrophy or neoplasms of choroid plexuses) are medical curiosities. Obstruction of the great vein of Galen, previously considered a cause of fluid overproduction, has not been confirmed.

Decreased outflow (or absorption) of fluid through the arachnoidal lining cells or through narrowed or closed pores in the arachnoid villi offers another possible mechanism.[52] Di-

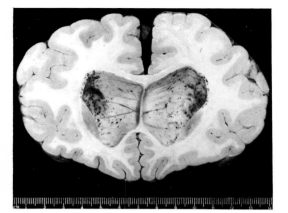

Fig. 48-8. Acute internal hydrocephalus with numerous subependymal petechiae caused by obstructive lesion in fourth ventricle (not illustrated).

rect and adequate examination of these pores is possible only by means of electron microscopy, and such has not been described. Moreover, there is some question whether such pores actually exist. The mechanism of decreased outflow, however, has been utilized, probably correctly, to explain the hydrocephalus seen with fibrosis covering the arachnoid granulations and with thrombosis of the superior sagittal sinus.

Obstruction to the flow of fluid is a common cause of internal hydrocephalus. The obstructing lesion may be developmental, inflammatory, mechanical, or neoplastic and may be almost anywhere in the flow tract. The pattern of ventricular enlargement frequently can be used as a guide to determine the site of the obstructing lesion. Ventricular dilatation is limited to that portion proximal to the obstruction (Fig. 48-7). Dilated ventricles with subependymal petechial hemorrhages are diagnostic of an acute obstructive hydrocephalus (Fig. 48-8).

Two other mechanisms also should be considered in the production of hydrocephalus. Once the fontanels are closed and growth has ceased, the skull encloses an intracranial space of fixed size. Loss of brain tissue for any reason must, therefore, be accompanied by increase in fluid and enlargement of the subarachnoid or ventricular spaces. This is known as compensatory hydrocephalus (hydrocephalus ex vacuo). It is the most common form of hydrocephalus although, in most instances, it is not clinically symptomatic. Among the less frequent causes of hydrocephalus and one that often is not considered is that caused by failure

in development of all or a portion of the brain. Although the ventricles, in such instances, are small, they are relatively large when compared with the overall size of the brain. This is developmental hydrocephalus.

Porencephaly,[112] is a related condition. The term originally was meant to designate an abnormal cavity that connected the ventricular and subarachnoid spaces through a defect in the cerebrum. With this definition, the cause was attributable to the failure of development of a portion of the primitive ependymal lining in the line of the primary fissure. The defect was usually bilateral and symmetric. Much of this meaning has been lost, for most observers now use the term to describe any large intracerebral cavity usually with an opening into an adjacent ventricle.

VASCULAR DISEASES
Hypoxic encephalopathy (anoxic encephalopathy)

Despite the many variables that could be expected to alter the pattern of damage to the central nervous system subjected to hypoxia, there is an unusual degree of uniformity of histologic change. The increased susceptibility of the central nervous system to oxygen deprivation is the result of a combination of factors each of which is of critical importance. Almost all of the central nervous system function is subserved by energy derived from aerobic metabolism of carbohydrates. This 2% of the body utilizes 20% of the oxygen and 20% of the cardiac output in the resting state. Because of the lack of significant oxygen and carbohydrate reserves within the central nervous system, a constant resupply of both is required. The structural changes are dependent on the degree and duration of the hypoxia, on length of survival, and, when present, on a preceding period of a lesser degree of hypoxia. Antecedent asymptomatic or mild hypoxia[104] depletes the affected cells of enzymes that promote individual cell destruction. Lindenberg[104] believes that a preceding mild hypoxia is therefore desirable in that structural and functional recovery are then more likely to occur. Gross structural changes generally are not striking with hypoxia except when associated with severe venous engorgement that produces duskiness of the entire central nervous system and petechial hemorrhages. When the cause is ischemia, there is mild to pronounced pallor. The brain is slightly to greatly swollen with some blurring of the margins between the cortex and the underlying white matter; occasionally, there are petechiae about the third ventricle and in the floor of the fourth ventricle.

Although the first microscopic changes may be seen after survival of only 4 hours, they usually are not discernible until after survival of at least 8 to 12 hours. With general hypoxia (as with cardiac failure, respiratory disease, and anemia, or to thromboemboli), the most susceptible cells, including their processes, are those in Sommer's sector in the hippocampal portion of the temporal lobe, the Purkinje cells of the cerebellum, and the cells of the third and fourth cortical layers of the cerebral hemispheres. The earliest microscopic changes consist of slight cell enlargement and cytoplasmic eosinophilia with loss of the Nissl substance. Affected cells occur singly or in clusters and may be separated by cells with a normal appearance. The hypoxic cells and adjoining blood vessels are surrounded by edematous zones that stain less intensely than the normal.

Later, the affected cells become irregularly shrunken and their nuclei eccentric, small, and hyperchromatic. Eventually, the cells and their processes that are injured beyond recovery disappear. Petechiae that occur without other tissue damage disappear without remnants; with necrosis, the area becomes organized and recognizable because of residual macrophages with hemosiderin.

Infarcts

A localized area of necrosis caused by circulatory insufficiency is known as an infarct. Large infarcts may be associated with atherosclerosis with or without thrombosis, with emboli in large arteries, with venous occlusive disease, and rarely with a dissecting hematoma that compresses the lumen of the affected artery.[11,23,41,53,111] Small infarcts occur with disease of small arteries and arterioles (usually related to hypertension) and sometimes because of emboli in these vessels. With adequate collateral channels, particularly through the circle of Willis and leptomeningeal vessels, gradual occlusion of even a large artery may not result in an infarct. Conversely, the gradual narrowing of a small artery can, in the absence of an adequate collateral, cause infarction. Infarcts are classified as pale (anemic) or red (hemorrhagic), depending on the amount of blood present in the necrotic area (Fig. 48-9). They also are divided into those that are recent (usually under 3 weeks), old (3 to 6 weeks), and remote (over 6 weeks).

Anemic infarcts most frequently are asso-

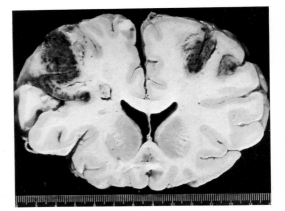

Fig. 48-9. Recent mixed hemorrhagic and anemic infarcts secondary to emboli in middle cerebral arteries.

ciated with atherosclerosis with or without thrombosis. In the absence of a thrombus, there is often a preceding episode of hypotension or hypoxia or both. Anemic infarcts are more likely to occur in normotensive or hypotensive states and in the presence of disseminated vascular disease that impairs the limited collateral circulation. Initially, an anemic infarct is dusky because of continued deoxygenation of the retained intravascular blood. Shortly afterward, the infarct begins to enlarge in volume because of the influx of fluid from adjacent functioning blood vessels and tissues. The increasing volume of the infarct within the fixed intracranial space compresses the contained vessels. By forcing the sludged intravascular blood away into the draining venous channels, the infarct becomes pale. There is a simultaneous and progressive decrease in size of the adjacent spaces (subarachnoid and ventricular). In some, the rapid increase in volume of a large infarct may produce brain displacement, with herniations and even secondary pressure hemorrhages in the brainstem. The initial microscopic changes are similar to those described under hypoxic encephalopathy but with more diffuse and severe involvement.

An infarct of the third and usually also the fourth and fifth layers of the cerebral cortex, regularly in the depth of a convolution, is known as a laminar (or pseudolaminar) infarct. When more severe, the infarct extends to involve the cortex toward the crest of the gyri and the second and deeper cortical layers and may even extend into the underlying white matter. The first cortical layer regularly demonstrates only a reactive astrocytosis. The

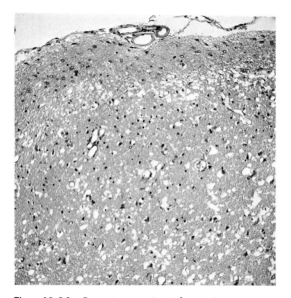

Fig. 48-10. Recent anemic infarct. Intact outer cortical layer with reactive astrocytosis. Pallor, cellular pyknosis, and microcavitation secondary to edema in deeper cortical layers. (Hematoxylin and eosin; 90×.)

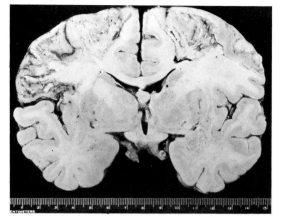

Fig. 48-11. Liquefaction of recent anemic infarcts with beginning gross cavitation (end of second week), secondary to emboli in branches of middle cerebral arteries.

laminar infarct occurs more frequently in the so-called watershed zones of the parieto-occipital convexities but may be found in all parts of the cerebral cortex and even in the cerebellum. This type of infarct frequently is found in a patient after a period of prolonged shock as may occur with gastrointestinal bleeding, hypoglycemia, myocardial infarction, temporary cardiac arrest, etc.

In the following description of the natural history of infarcts, one should recognize that the time sequences are approximations. The rates and degrees of reaction are dependent on many variables existing among individuals and in the same patient with differing conditions. These variations may be present even in different portions of a single large infarct.

In all anemic infarcts, the cytoplasm of the nerve cell initially becomes eosinophilic and its nucleus shrunken and hyperchromatic. With the influx of fluid, the infarcted tissue progressively becomes more pale staining (Fig. 48-10) except the intact first cortical layer, in which only a reactive astrocytosis occurs. The first reactive cells, seen between the eighteenth and twenty-fourth hour of the infarct, are neutrophils. These cells, usually in small numbers, are found in the walls of blood vessels within the infarct and the immediately adjacent necrotic tissue near the periphery of the infarct. They may reach the adjacent subarach-

noid space. Activation of the surrounding microglial cells and the appearance of perivascular lymphocytes and monocytes at the edges of the infarct may begin by the second day but most frequently are not found until the third day. During the following two weeks, the infarct continues to enlarge and soften, with evidence of liquefaction (Fig. 48-11). Beginning by the fourth day and increasing thereafter, it is progressively filled by the mononuclear cells, many of which have become lipophages. The blood vessels within the infarct are gradually reopened by the flow of blood from the collateral channels. Reactive astrocytes in the brain immediately surrounding the infarct, first seen during the third day, become easily evident by the fifth day. The volume of the anemic infarct is greatest during the second week. Thereafter, its gradually decreasing volume is associated with the disappearance of the lipophages and loss of fluid. At the end of the third week, its volume approximates that of the original tissue. Continued removal of the necrotic material and of fluid gradually transforms the infarct by the sixth week into a pale spongelike cavity traversed by a network of small blood vessels, some of which are newly formed (Fig. 48-12). A few lipophages within the infarct and a narrow wall of reactive and often gemistocytic astrocytes remain for the life of the individual. The presence of an intact first cortical layer aids in the separation of an infarct from a contusion or laceration (Fig. 48-11). The adjacent spaces, first narrowed and compressed, have enlarged (compensatory hydrocephalus) as the infarct volume decreases.

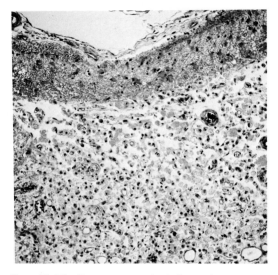

Fig. 48-12. Remote anemic infarct. Intact outer cortical layer with reactive astrocytosis. Scattered macrophages and newly formed capillaries in cavity. (Hematoxylin and eosin; 135×.)

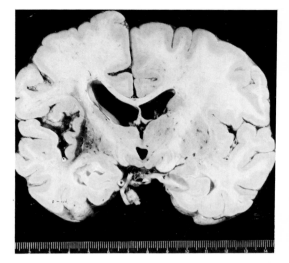

Fig. 48-13. Remote anemic and hemorrhagic infarcts in putamina and caudate nuclei. Patient with long-standing hypertension. Compensatory internal hydrocephalus. Segmental atherosclerosis, severe.

Hemorrhagic infarcts are associated with hypertension, with emboli, with those who have a tendency toward bleeding, and with venous occlusion. The duskiness of the early infarct becomes dark red because of the inflow of blood into the necrotic tissue from reopening of the occluded vessel or from collateral channels, or because the initial lesion was the result of a venous occlusion. In comparison with the anemic infarct, the hemorrhagic infarct enlarges more rapidly and to a greater degree and retains its increased volume for a longer period. Hemosiderophages, found with extreme difficulty before the third or fourth day, become progressively more prominent thereafter and, like the lipophages, some remain locally for the life of the individual. Reactive astrocytes forming the infarct wall sometimes contain hemosiderin granules. The brown color of the remote lesion (over 6 weeks), attributable to hemosiderin and hematoidin, distinguishes it from an anemic infarct, and the bridging blood vessels separate it from a massive hemorrhage. Compensatory hydrocephalus, external or internal, may also be associated with the larger hemorrhagic infarcts.

Mixed anemic and hemorrhagic infarcts (Fig. 48-9) are not rare. The hemorrhagic component is always in the gray whereas the anemic component can involve both white and gray matter.

Infarcts, anemic and hemorrhagic, from 1 mm to 1 cm in size are common in the putam-

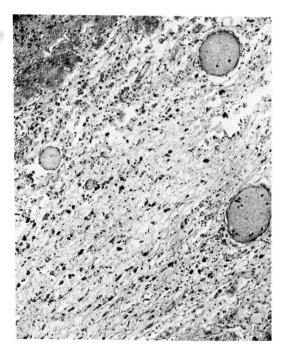

Fig. 48-14. Remote hemorrhagic infarct containing newly formed capillaries, hemosiderin-laden macrophages, and fibrous tissue. Hypertensive patient. (Hematoxylin and eosin; 90×.)

ina and thalami (Fig. 48-13) and, to a lesser degree, in the base of the pons and in the other central gray masses of the cerebral hemispheres in patients with a long history of hypertension.[59,78] Bilateral lesions are almost limited to patients with long-standing hypertension. Slightly larger infarcts in the central white matter of the cerebral hemispheres are equally characteristic of long-standing hypertension, especially when the infarcts are hemorrhagic or have more than the expected amount of connective tissue about the blood vessels within them (Fig. 48-14). Small, subcortical areas of necrosis usually have been considered as infarcts resulting from severe arteriolosclerosis in patients with hypertension.[122] Recently, however, these have been described as the end stages of recurrent or severe local edema associated with hypertensive encephalopathy.[55] The associated clinical state is known as Binswanger's disease.[55,122]

Hemorrhage

Hemorrhage into the central nervous system may result from any of the diseases that destroy the integrity of the blood vessels or decrease the coagulability of the blood.[27,115,123] Petechial hemorrhages, especially those in the floor and walls of the third ventricle and floor of the fourth ventricle, are most often the result of hypoxia from respiratory failure in which the heart has continued to beat for a short time. They may be seen with mechanical trauma to the head, with fat embolism, with chemical toxins such as the arsenical compounds, with intrinsic disorders of the hematopoietic system that have a tendency toward bleeding, after anticoagulant therapy, in endogenous toxic conditions such as uremia, and with diseases of the blood vessels. In most instances, there are multiple causative agents that act synergistically. A recent petechial hemorrhage, often confused with an engorged blood vessel, may be recognized because it is usually significantly larger than the otherwise normal but dilated vessels in the area, is slightly irregular, has a less sharp margin than that seen with an engorged blood vessel, and, with semitangential lighting, has a convex meniscus rather than the concave meniscus of blood within a vessel. When not completely resorbed, the petechial hemorhages are brown to yellow and slightly depressed. This is the result of the conversion of the hemoglobin to hemosiderin and hematoidin by the macrophages accompanied by some tissue loss and a mild reactive astrocytosis. Massive hemorrhages (3 cm or more in the cerebrum, 1.5 cm or more in the brainstem and cerebellum) may be ascribed to any of the aforementioned causes. Under these circumstances (not associated with hypertension), the hemorrhages are frequently multiple,

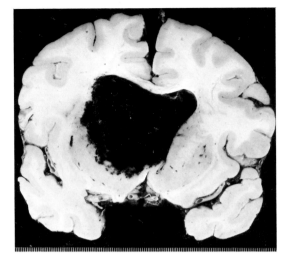

Fig. 48-15. Recent massive hemorrhage, inner striate area, with rupture into lateral ventricle in patient with hypertension. Remote lacunar infarcts in putamina.

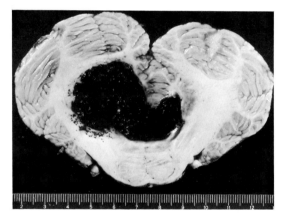

Fig. 48-16. Recent massive cerebellar hemorrhage with petechiae in wall and rupture into fourth ventricle in patient with hypertension.

sharply demarcated, with petechiae peripherally, and usually with no swelling or edema of the adjacent brain. Although these hemorrhages may sometimes extend through the cortex into the subarachnoid space, these nonhypertensive hemorrhages rarely rupture into an adjoining ventricle.

Massive brain hemorrhages are a common cause of death in patients with inadequately treated and uncontrolled hypertension.[47,62] About 70% of the hemorrhages are in the lateral or medial ganglionic regions of the cerebral hemispheres (lenticular nuclei, thalami, and internal capsules [Fig. 48-15]).[21,49]

From these regions, the hemorrhages may track downward along the nerve tracts to the midbrain and even to the pons or into the adjacent frontal or parietal lobes. The cerebral hemispheres are equally affected. About 20% of the hemorrhages begin initially in the midbrain, pons, or white matter of the cerebellum (Fig. 48-16). The remaining 10% begin in any of the remaining portions of the cerebral hemispheres. The medulla is never the primary site of this type of hemorrhage and is rarely involved by extension. The hemorrhages in fatal cases almost always have ruptured into the adjacent ventricle and from there have followed the cerebrospinal flow to reach the subarachnoid space. Relatively few rupture directly into the overlying subarachnoid space, and very rarely have the hemorrhages ruptured simultaneously or successively into both. Less than 1% of these massive hemorrhages are multiple. Death occurs in over 90% of these patients and usually within 96 hours (except in those patients maintained by respirator for longer periods). On examination, the brain is pale and swollen and asymmetric, usually with a symmetric subarachnoid hemorrhage at the base (Fig. 48-17). With this asymmetrically swollen brain, the larger hemisphere contains

the hemorrhage. It usually is covered by a lesser degree of subarachnoid blood because of greater compression of the space by the more swollen gyri. Brain displacement with herniations and secondary brainstem hemorrhage are common. The occurrence and localization of these secondary changes are dependent on the site and size of the massive hemorrhage.

The brain immediately surrounding the hemorrhage is greatly swollen and edematous and often has many petechiae in one or more areas immediately about the hemorrhage. The absence of brain tissue within the hemorrhage and the presence of blood beyond the region supplied by an artery or drained by a vein serves to distinguish macroscopically the hemorrhage from a hemorrhagic infarct. On microscopic examination, a characteristic structural pattern usually can be recognized. Within the hemorrhage, only a rare remnant of nerve tissue is found among the blood cells. The immediately surrounding swollen and edematous brain contains numerous severely sclerotic small arteries and arterioles as well as capillaries and venules. In the regions with petechial hemorrhages, there usually are necrotic arterioles, venules, and capillaries infiltrated and surrounded by red blood cells and sometimes some neutrophils. When the routine

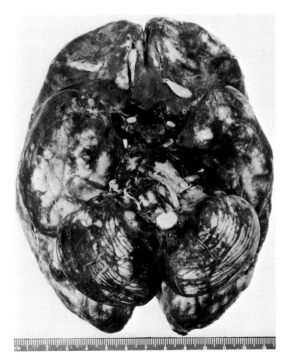

Fig. 48-17. Recent diffuse subarachnoid hemorrhage in patient with massive intracerebral hemorrhage.

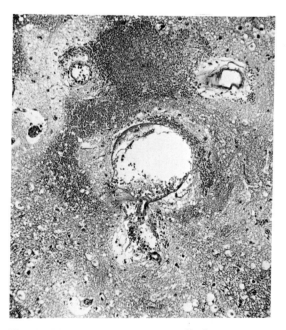

Fig. 48-18. Microaneurysm in wall of massive recent hypertensive hemorrhage. (Hematoxylin and eosin; 90×.)

examination includes only a single or, at most, several sections through this region, infrequent recognizable aneurysmally dilated arterioles and small arteries are to be found (Fig. 48-18). Serial sections through these zones often result in a significant increase in their yield, but they are never frequent. The zone immediately peripheral to the petechial hemorrhages contains hyalinized thick-walled blood vessels surrounded by large lakes of fluid high in protein content. There is a moderate degree of brain swelling and edema in this area, but this is less than that seen in the portion of the brain immediately adjacent to the hemorrhage. In the remainder of the brain, there are arterioles and small arteries that exhibit varying degrees of arteriolosclerosis. Frequently, many of the infarcts previously described as occurring in patients with hypertension are also present. In those hypertensive patients in whom no petechial hemorrhages are to be found in the walls of the massive hemorrhage, there is a different structural stratification. At one edge of the hemorrhage, one may, on occasion, find evidences of a preexisting or simultaneously occurring anemic or hemorrhagic infarct. The other portions of its wall are similar to those seen in the other hemorrhages with brain swelling, edema, and arteriolosclerosis of moderate to pronounced degrees.

These findings have stimulated at least three hypotheses as to the pathogenesis of the massive hemorrhages[27,32,33]:

1. Necrotizing arteriolitis with rupture of many arterioles
2. Arteriolosclerosis with a few or many arterioles undergoing necrosis, microaneurysm formation, and rupture (Fig. 48-18)
3. Massive hemorrhage in an area of earlier infarct

In 5% to 10% of the hypertensive patients with a massive hemorrhage, the lesion is not fatal. Although this may occur with the larger cerebral hemorrhage that has not ruptured into a ventricle, it is more frequently seen with the smaller ganglionic hemorrhages that have neither extended nor ruptured into the ventricular or subarachnoid spaces. In these, only the outer 1 to 2 mm of the hemorrhage is organized, with conversion of the hemoglobin to hemosiderin and hematoidin. A mild reactive astrocytic proliferation is present in the immediately surrounding brain. The blood in the interior of the hemorrhage becomes dark (chocolate red) and remains semiliquid and unorganized. When the blood is manually evacuated, a brown smooth-walled cavity not traversed by blood vessels remains.

Hypertensive encephalopathy characterized by recurrent attacks of sudden and severe headaches with vomiting, mental confusion, and visual, sensory, or motor disturbances is common in patients with untreated or inadequately treated hypertension.[165] Although one of these attacks may precede the appearance of a massive hemorrhage, death during an uncomplicated attack is rare. The mechanism of the syndrome is not known, though arteriolar spasm and arteriolar and capillary thrombi have been suggested. The changes in the brain are neither characteristic nor uniform. Brain swelling with pallor and scattered petechiae has been described. There are others, however, in whom no gross abnormalities have been recognized. On microscopic examination, there are usually varying degree of arteriolosclerosis. In some, there is arteriolar necrosis with surrounding petechiae. Identical changes also may be seen in hypertensive patients dying in chronic uremia. The relationship of hypertensive encephalopathy to the small and larger hemorrhages and to the areas of necrosis in patients with hypertension is not known, although there has been much speculation.

Aneurysms

Aneurysms of the arteries of the circle of Willis have been classified as berry (so-called congenital), atherosclerotic, inflammatory (mycotic), traumatic, and developmental. Of this group, only the first is of frequent clinical importance. The traumatic lesion usually is an arteriovenous fistula rather than an aneurysm. True developmental aneurysms are exceptionally rare.

Berry aneurysms.[25,68] The most common of this group of blood vessel lesions, berry aneurysms are found in 5% to 6% of all adults at postmortem examination.[25] Most occur in the bifurcation pockets of the arteries forming (Fig. 48-19) or extending from the circle of Willis (Fig. 48-20). The initial defect is considered by many to be a developmental deficiency to absence of the medial smooth muscle in the crotch of the bifurcation. Similar aneurysms not in these pockets are said to occur after incomplete resorption of unused embryonic arteries. The aneurysms form later after damage of the internal elastic lamina, probably because of a preceding focal atherosclerotic change. Some, however, have incorrectly considered this damage to be caused by disease of the vasa vasorum of these vessels.

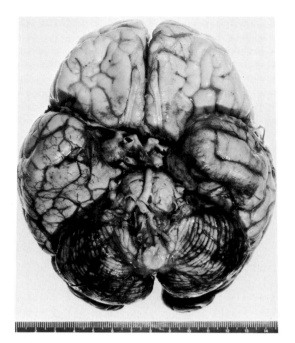

Fig. 48-19. Berry aneurysm at junction of right internal carotid and posterior communicating arteries. Pons is slightly widened and fore-shortened, and there is cerebellomedullary herniation—both caused by rupture of aneurysm with intracerebral and intraventricular extension of hemorrhage that has reached cerebellar subarachnoid space through the ventricular system.

The normal thin adventitia of the arteries of the circle of Willis contributes significantly to the lack of adequate resistance to the intravascular pressure.

The aneurysms are, for reasons not known, twice as common in women as in men. Only about 40% found at necropsy show evidence of bleeding or of rupture. About 30% are multiple and, of these, two thirds are bilateral. Association with polycystic renal disease and with coarctation of the aorta can usually be related to the coexistent hypertension. Hypertension is present in 80% of those who have these aneurysms (with and without bleeding). The average mean age at the time of fatal rupture is between 50 and 55 years. The mortality of the first rupture is between 25% and 50%, and it is believed to be even higher with each succeeding rupture. In those with fatal ruptures, death occurs within 24 hours in almost half, many within the first hour, and in 95% within 2 weeks. The arteries forming the anterior half of the

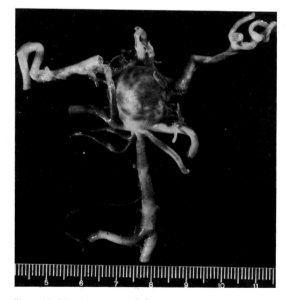

Fig. 48-20. Unruptured berry aneurysms. Larger aneurysm at terminal portion of basilar artery. Smaller aneurysm in bifurcation angle of middle cerebral artery on right.

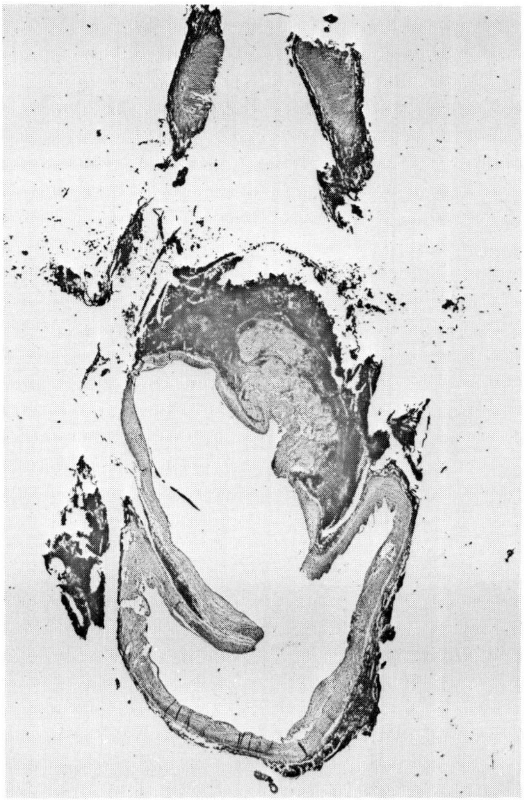

Fig. 48-21. Recently ruptured berry aneurysm. Thrombus in fundus at site of rupture. (Hematoxylin and eosin; 8×.)

circle are involved about six times more frequently than those of the posterior half.[25] The sides of the circle are affected equally.

Although some aneurysms are cylindric, most are berry shaped. They have narrowed necks of variable lengths. The mouth of the aneurysm internally often is constricted by an encircling endothelial fibrous cushion covering the frayed ends of the internal elastic lamina[139] (Fig. 48-21). The wall of the aneurysm is formed by a few layers of connective tissue devoid of the elastic lamina. It progressively become more thin toward the fundus, where rupture is most likely to occur (Fig. 48-21).[106] A recent electron microscopic study of these aneurysms has suggested the presence of smooth muscle cells within the wall of the aneurysm.[100] The occasional presence of a few neutrophils in the wall immediately adjacent to sites of leakage or rupture has led some to suggest incorrectly that these lesions are basically inflammatory.

In over two thirds of the patients with fatal rupture, the asymmetric subarachnoid hemorrhage is but one of the complications.[25] Extension of the hemorrhage into the adjacent brain and often into a ventricle is common. Subdural hemorrhage occurs but is infrequent. Cerebral infarcts occurring with or after rupture are frequent. Some are caused by emboli and some by severe and prolonged local vasospasm. Brain displacement, herniation, and brainstem hemorrhage also are frequent secondary complications.

Atherosclerotic aneurysms. Atherosclerotic aneurysms are usually manifest as elongated cylindric dilatations affecting the terminal portions of the internal carotid arteries and the basilar artery. Although rupture is very rare, the carotid aneurysms often compress either or both optic nerves, sometimes with recognizable and characteristic narrowing of the visual fields. The wall of the atherosclerotic aneurysm is characterized by a thickening of the intima by fibrous tissue with a few lipophages and occasional cholesterol-crystal clefts. The internal elastic lamina is represented by only a few residual fragments of elastic tissue and the media by a few layers of fibrous tissue almost devoid of smooth muscle. There is a thin fibrous adventitia.

Inflammatory aneurysms. An inflammatory (mycotic) aneurysm occurs at the site of attachment to an infected embolus whose usual source is a vegetation from a left-sided heart valve or pulmonary infection. The aneurysms are more frequent in the first and second major bifurcations of either middle cerebral artery. They are sometimes associated with a purulent leptomeningitis, a brain abscess, or a cerebral infarct. The aneurysm infrequently ruptures into the subarachnoid space.

Arteriovenous fistula (internal carotid artery–cavernous sinus fistula). Before entering the intracranial cavity, the internal carotid arteries pass through the lumens of the cavernous sinus. Disruption of the internal carotid artery at this level often is associated with a blow to the frontal area of the head, sometimes with fracture of one of the bones of the paranasal sinus. In some, a history of antecedent injury is not obtained. The presence of significant concomitant degenerative disease of the carotid artery has not received adequate attention, since this region has not been routinely examined at necropsy. Rupture of the artery results in severe distention of the cavernous sinus and of the veins draining into it.

Developmental (true congenital) aneurysms.[149] Developmental aneurysms are exceedingly rare lesions. In a recent summary, only 16 had been recorded, all occurring in children under the age of 2 years. The aneurysms differ structurally from the berry aneurysms. Our material contains a single previously unrecorded case of an aneurysm of the left posterior inferior cerebellar artery in a 6-week-old infant. There were no endothelial changes. The wall was completely devoid of elastic tissue, and the tunica media contained a thin layer of loosely arranged plump spindle cells suggesting smooth muscle. The adventitia was thin and loose. The aneurysm did not occur at a bifurcation, and there was no endothelial cushion.

TRAUMA

The effects of mechanical forces, either direct or indirect, upon the central nervous system, atlhough varied, are frequently predictable. A systematic approach to the structural changes resulting from mechanical forces causing injury, usually begins with lesions of the dura, followed by the lesions that are produced at successively deeper levels.

Epidural hematoma

The dura mater covering the brain is represented by a fusion of dura and periosteum of the skull. Below the level of the foramen magnum, the two layers are separated by adipose tissue, blood vessels, and nodular accumulation of lymphocytes, sometimes with follicle formation. Epidural hematomas from

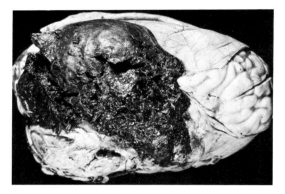

Fig. 48-22. Acute epidural hematoma secondary to skull fracture with tear of middle meningeal artery and vein.

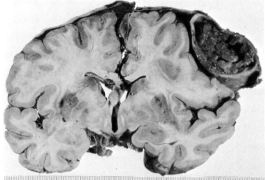

Fig. 48-23. Chronic subdural hematoma with compression of underlying brain and lateral ventricle. Bone formation in falx. Uncal herniation on side of hematoma.

blunt traumatic forces are almost limited to the region of the skull[115] (Fig. 48-22). They usually are associated with a recent skull fracture that, in crossing the groove of the middle meningeal artery, tears that artery and often the accompanying vein as well. Rarely, the hematoma may be attributable to a tear of the anterior or posterior meningeal artery or to a tear of a vein between the skull and dura. Because of its position, the lesion also can be considered as a subperiosteal hematoma.

These hematomas rarely, if ever, organize or resolve without surgical intervention. The usual amount of blood found at autopsy in untreated patients varies between 75 and 125 gm. This amount is in the same range found in fatal acute subdural hematomas and intracerebral hypertensive hemorrhages. Death is caused by the effects of brain compression, with brain displacement, herniation, and secondary brainstem hemorrhages associated with neurogenic pulmonary edema.

Subdural hematoma

Subdural hematomas usually result from blunt injury to the skull without fracture. They can, however, occur without direct injury to the skull. This is particularly true in older individuals with brain atrophy in whom sudden anterior or posterior movement of the head, as from stumbling, may easily tear one of the bridging veins. On rare occasions, arterial bleeding may be the cause of the hematoma.

With the acute subdural hematoma, blood accumulates rapidly after a tear of a bridging vein at the point where the vessel leaves the subdural space (a potential space) to enter the dura. Because most veins cross the subdural space in the vicinity of the superior sagittal sinus, most hematomas begin parasagittally. The reason they remain as tumorous collections in this region rather than form a diffuse hematoma is not known. Some believe that it is caused by the pressure exerted by the brain at the rim of the hematoma. There is little or no evidence of early organization of the acute subdural hematoma on its dural surface or at its margins, nor is there ever any evidence of organization of the hematoma from the arachnoid membrane except when this membrane is torn.

Organization of subdural blood in the formation of a chronic subdural hematoma begins within the first week and is quite evident after 2 weeks. The hematoma is encapsulated by highly vascular granulation tissue originating from the overlying dura, with the dura at the edges of the hematoma contributing to the formation of the granulation tissue that separates the blood from the underlying arachnoid membrane (Fig. 48-23). The granulation tissue on the dural surface is known as the outer membrane, that on the undersurface, the inner membrane (Fig. 48-24).

Others believe that some chronic subdural hematomas result from the tearing of a bridging vein as it crosses between the outer and inner layers of the meningeal dura.

Whatever the original site of the hemorrhage, the granulation tissue that surrounds the hematoma contains large thin-walled vessels that act as semipermeable membranes (Fig. 48-24). With destruction of the blood cells, the hematoma becomes hypertonic and attracts fluid from the surrounding dilated

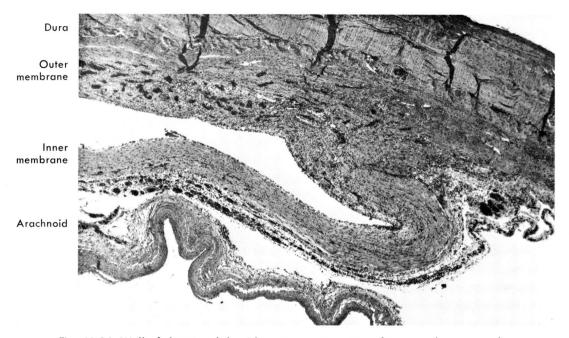

Dura

Outer
membrane

Inner
membrane

Arachnoid

Fig. 48-24. Wall of chronic subdural hematoma at junction of inner and outer membranes. (Hematoxylin and eosin; 30×.)

thin-walled vessels. This results in enlargement of the hematoma, with stretching, tearing, and hemorrhage from the vessels at the margins. Repetition of these processes leads to continued gradual and steplike enlargement of the hematoma. This theory, however, has recently been challenged in that no evidence of increased osmolarity was found. These hematomas regularly are associated with brain displacement, herniations, and, when fatal, brainstem hemorrhages and neurogenic pulmonary edema. Clinical classification of subdural hematomas with acute, subacute, and chronic types are more related to the time of development of signs and symptoms and their duration than to the structural characteristics.

A history of trauma is not obtained in every patient with a chronic subdural hematoma, even those capable of giving reliable histories. This is attributable, in part, to the occasional long interval between the causative event and the first signs and symptoms. In some, the episode may have been ignored or forgotten, since the trauma appeared to be trivial or was to another part of the body (such as a fall on the buttocks or a jerking of the entire body on stumbling). Individuals on anticoagulant therapy, particularly those who are older and have vascular disease, are more susceptible.

Organized subdural hemorrhages recognized grossly as rusty discoloration of the inner dural layer are frequent when the autopsy population has a high proportion of alcoholics and other adult groups with an unusual incidence of minor head trauma. In these, the hemoglobin has been converted to hemosiderin and hematoidin. Occasionally, a small recent hemorrhage is found, suggesting a new injury or the beginning of the cycle toward the formation of a hematoma.

A localized subdural collection of a yellow fluid with a high protein content is known as a subdural hygroma. It is an uncommon lesion believed to occur after a valvelike tear of the arachnoid, permitting only the outward flow of subarachnoid fluid into the subdural space. Origin from a chronic subdural hematoma has been suggested for the encapsulated hygroma whose wall has a rusty brown discoloration. In these, organization has resulted in the gradual removal of the cellular blood elements but with the retention of fluid stained to variable degrees by residual hemosiderin and hematoidin.

Subarachnoid hemorrhage

Bleeding into the subarachnoid space has many causes, one of the more common of which is blunt trauma to the skull with or without fracture. Although bleeding can be the sole result of trauma (at least clinically), at postmortem examination the hemorrhages often are associated with other lesions (i.e., contusions and lacerations). With small hemorrhages, the blood may be completely removed by following the cerebrospinal fluid flow into the draining sinuses. In some individuals, particularly those with other traumatic brain lesions, the blood may be trapped by adhesions and then converted to hemosiderin and hematoidin.

Contusion

Contusions of the brain are caused by blunt head trauma. The effects are transmitted to the brain by the deformation of the skull and by the inertia of the brain. Coup lesions occur at the point of impact and the contrecoup lesion at a point away from the impact site. The latter is generally at or near the diametrically opposite side of the skull from the impact. The exact point depends on the skull curvature, direction of impact, etc. The energy transferred to the brain—either positive (coup) or negative (contrecoup)—is accentuated by the inertia of the brain and the inbending at the point of impact and outbending of the deformed skull at the contrecoup site, combined with shearing rotational movements of this lacerated brain. Damage is diminished by the shape of the skull and the falx and tentorium.

Most contusions are sustained by the impact of the moving head against a fixed or relatively stationary object. The contrecoup lesion with these deceleration injuries is usually larger than the coup lesion and is the result of the negative pressure. The coup and contrecoup lesions are roughly conic, with the base of the cone directed toward the arachnoid surface at the apex of one or more convolutions (Fig. 48-25). All tissues, including the surface cortical layer (therefore, all contusions are lacerations as well), are destroyed or damaged for varying depths. Initially, the lesions are filled with necrotic cells and focal or diffuse collections of fresh blood from torn blood vessels. There is a variable degree of edema and swelling of the adjacent tissue. Early and transiently, a few neutrophils may be found in the walls of an occasional vessel at the margin of a contusion. Perivascular mononuclear cells appear during the second and third days, and reactive astrocytes are seen in the adjoining brain at about the same time. Organization proceeds with the formation of lipophages and the conversion of the blood

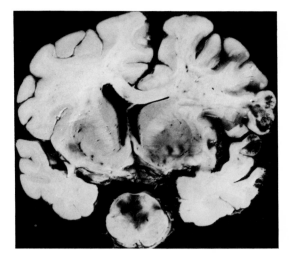

Fig. 48-25. Recent contusions of frontal and temporal lobes. Displacement of cingulate gyrus and lateral ventricles. Secondary hemorrhages in lower midbrain—upper pons.

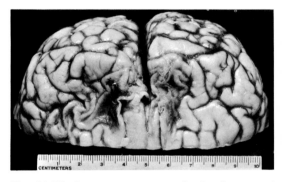

Fig. 48-26. Remote contusions of orbital gyri and olfactory bulbs.

to hemosiderin and hematoidin, much of which remains within the lesion. Thereafter, the contusion-laceration is represented by an orange-brown, depressed, wedge-shaped region with a flattened apex (Fig. 48-26). The lesion, widest at the crest of a gyrus or gyri, often is covered by a leptomeningeal-cortical scar.

Contusion-lacerations are most frequent at the tips and orbital portions of the frontal lobes and tips and lateral portions of the temporal lobes. Other areas of involvement are the tips of the occipital lobes, the corpus callosum (from damage by the free margin of the falx), the cerebellum, and base of the pons.

Intracerebral hematoma

Intracerebral hematomas occurring after nonpenetrating trauma to the skull are pre-

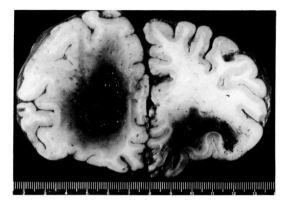

Fig. 48-27. Recent hematomas in frontal lobes, posttraumatic.

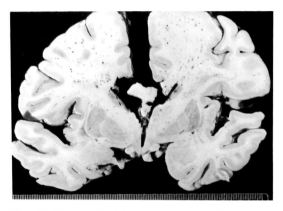

Fig. 48-28. Petechial hemorrhages in white matter in posttraumatic fat embolism.

sumably the result of shearing stresses upon intracerebral vessels. The rupture of one or more large vessels may lead to a large hematoma or to several (Fig. 48-27). They are more likely to occur in the frontal lobes but may be found in other portions of the brain, including cerebellum. The midbrain, pons, and medulla rarely contain a large traumatic hemorrhage.

Multiple small hemorrhages, primarily in the white matter of the brain after nonpenetrating skull trauma, are more likely the result of hypoxia or of fat embolism. Although the hemorrhages of fat embolism are far more frequent in the white matter (Fig. 48-28), fat emboli are found more frequently in the adjoining gray matter. Although fat emboli may be found in the central nervous system in patients with injuries to long bones with or without fractures, they also are seen after burns or mechanical damage to large areas of subcutaneous fat, in sickle-cell crises, in

patients with severe fatty change in the liver, and in patients with active pancreatitis. Fat emboli need not be accompanied by petechial hemorrhages. The fat obstructs many arterioles and capillaries throughout the brain. The vascular stasis with anoxia and the endothelial damage produce the petechiae.

Concussion

Concussion is the sudden loss of neurologic function immediately upon blunt injury, usually to the head. Much has been written concerning the definition of this entity, the mechanism of injury, and the physical principles involved in the transmission of force, as well as the structural changes, if any.

Uncomplicated concussion in the human being is rarely, if ever, fatal. Among those who have reported experimental observations, there is agreement that structural changes at the light microscopic level do occur. These changes consist of central chromatolysis of variable numbers of cells in the reticular substance of the brainstem with similar but lesser involvement of cells in the cerebral cortex.[29,30] Some believe that these changes are secondary to damage to axons in the ventral portion of the upper cervical portion of the spinal cord, whereas others are of the opinion that the changes are caused by shear stresses directly upon the affected cells.

Penetrating injuries to brain

The brain and spinal cord may be penetrated by bullets and fragments of metal and bone sometimes covered by scalp, hair, and other contaminated foreign material. The damage in the high-velocity bullet injuries is generalized as well as local. Its effects are caused by the sudden increase in intracranial pressure, the shearing and tearing of the tissue, and the intense local heat. There is extensive necrosis and hemorrhage in and about the tract of the missile. In low-velocity injuries, the damage is limited to the penetrated area.

Posttraumatic brain swelling and edema

Occasionally in children (rarely in adults), a minor degree of head trauma is associated with generalized and progressive swelling and edema of the brain. Other traumatic lesions are usually absent. The brain is enlarged and symmetric. The convolutions are flattened, the sulci narrowed, and the ventricles small. The white matter is prominent—bulging and dry in the swollen areas, depressed and wet in the

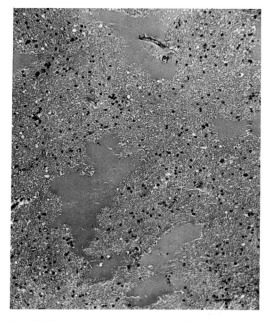

Fig. 48-29. Brain edema. Intercellular lakes of high protein content fluid. (Hematoxylin and eosin; 90×.)

edematous sites. Edema fluid high in protein content may be found about the blood vessels and in the Virchow-Robin space and tissue in brain edema (Fig. 48-29). The myelin sheaths are irregularly swollen and pale with enlarged clear spaces about the oligodendroglial nuclei in the areas of swelling. Increasing amounts of eosinophilic cytoplasm of the involved astrocytes become visible by the end of the first day. Death usually is associated with hypoxia and neurogenic pulmonary edema.

Trauma of spinal cord

The spinal cord of the newborn infant can be injured in breech deliveries by the exertion of too great an extractile force with the hyperextended head. The overstretched cord, usually at the cervico-thoracic level, has an hourglass narrowing (Fig. 48-30).

Hematomyelia with necrosis of the cord is usually caused by fractures or dislocations of the vertebrae with compression of the cord. In some, the lesion appears to follow extreme degrees of hyperextension (Fig. 48-30) and hyperflexion at the cervical level with fracture or dislocation. The cord appears to be slightly to moderately narrowed at the level of compression, with bulging and softening above and below caused by necrosis with hemorrhage into the gray matter (Fig. 48-31). This may extend for several levels to either side of the point of initial injury.

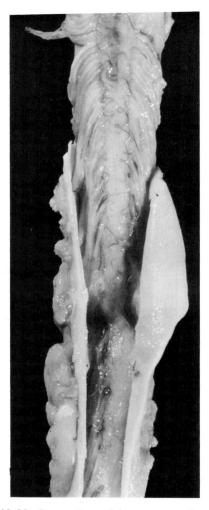

Fig. 48-30. Destruction of lower cervical portion of spinal cord of infant attributed to stretching during breech delivery.

The spinal cord may be compressed on its ventral surface by a herniated intervertebral disc (Fig. 48-32) or by osteophytic lipping of the vertebral bodies.[77,86,110,148] The former is more likely to affect the lumbar portion and the latter the cervical portion of the cord. There are, however, many exceptions. The spinal cord, stabilized by the denticulate ligaments, is injured by direct compression locally. Less often, the changes are from compression of the anterior spinal artery.

CEREBRAL BIRTH INJURY[5,151]

Cerebral birth injury (cerebral palsy, Little's disease, spastic diplegia) is a disorder of paranatal origin characterized clinically by disturbances of movement, sometimes associated with mental retardation. The disorder may be hereditary or caused by mechanical forces,

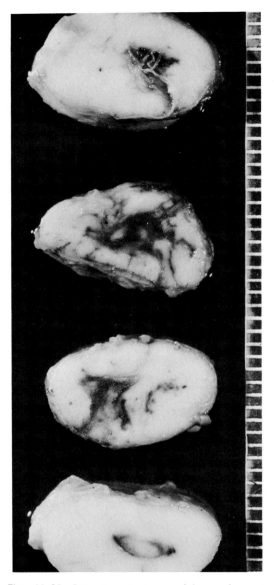

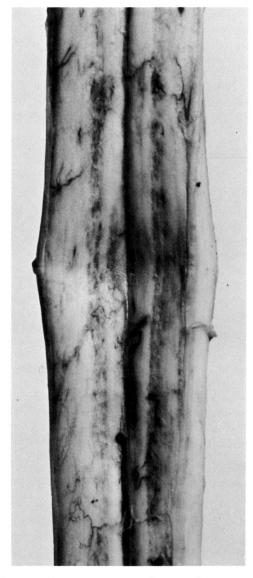

Fig. 48-31. Recent contusion and hemorrhage in cervical portion of spinal cord (hematomyelia) after dislocation of cervical vertebra.

Fig. 48-32. Compression of cervical portion of spinal cord by ruptured disc. Patient was asymptomatic.

anoxia, maternal infection, metabolic disease, or vascular disease, with the morphologic lesions spanning almost the entire range of neuropathic forms. Each of the lesions should be evaluated separately.

DEGENERATIVE DISEASES
Brain atrophies[113,120]

Continuous loss of nerve cells and their processes and of the surrounding myelin and intercellular fluid regularly accompanies aging. The cell and fluid loss results in a compensatory hydrocephalus. There may also be slight

focal fibrotic thickening of the leptomeninges.

On microscopic examination, the nerve cell loss may be recognizable within the cortex and the central gray matter by the presence of patchy areas devoid of cells. Many of the remaining, often shrunken, nerve cells contain excessive amounts of intracytoplasmic lipofuscin pigment. A mild to moderate reactive astrocytic gliosis is present and is most easily recognized in the outermost layers of the cortex. Hyaline congophilic thickening of the capillary walls in the occipital cortex frequently accompanies the aging process. Corpora amylacea are often prominent.

In the aging brain, the loss of nerve cells and their processes results in a temporary condensation of interfascicular oligodendrocytes and eventual loss of white matter. In some individuals, the process of aging is so severe as to produce varying degrees of dementia.

Alzheimer's disease

Formerly considered to be a disease whose clinical onset preceded the sixth decade, Alzheimer's disease is now recognized as a pathologic entity whose cause is unknown and whose clinical onset, though most frequent in the fourth to sixth decades, may occur even before the age of 15 years.

The brain is diffusely atrophic with a compensatory hydrocephalus. All the microscopic characteristics of the aging brain are present in great profusion. In addition there are senile plaques, Alzheimer's neurofibrillary tangles, and granulovascular changes in certain of the nerve cells. Senile plaques (Fig. 48-33) are to be found irregularly distributed in all parts of the cerebral cortex in the region of the neuropil, in the mammillary bodies, uncommonly in other gray matter, and rarely in white matter and in the brainstem. With the hematoxylin and eosin stain, plaques are eosinophilic fibrillar spheres 15 to 125 μm in diameter. The fibrils are either haphazardly arranged or radi-

ate from a central hyaline eosinophilic core; at the periphery of the latter plaque there may be a deeply eosinophilic rim. Plaques are, however, more easily seen with silver stains (Fig. 48-34); the central cores stain as amyloid and with electron microscopy have the characteristics of amyloid. Variable numbers of reactive astrocytes surround the plaques. Alzheimer's neurofibrillary tangles occur in the perikaryon of many of the larger cortical nerve cells and are recognizable only with special silver stains or by electron microscopy. These argyrophilic fibrillar tangles are formed by the condensation and twisting of the neurotubules with simultaneous displacement of the other cytoplasmic contents (Fig. 48-34). Granulovascular changes occur primarily in the larger cells of the hippocampus; the cells contain hematoxylinophilic and argyrophilic cytoplasmic granules each within a nonstaining vacuole.

Pick's disease (lobar sclerosis, circumscribed cortical atrophy)

Pick's disease[159] is an uncommon, sometimes familial disease of unknown cause. Although

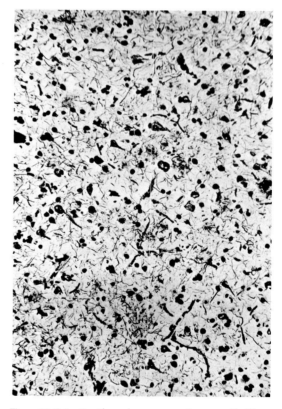

Fig. 48-34. Senile plaques and neurofibrillary tangles in Alzheimer's disease. (Hortega silver carbonate; 135×.)

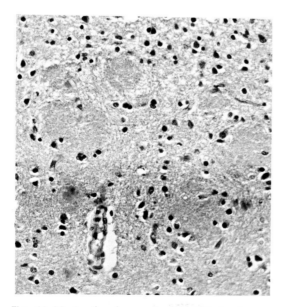

Fig. 48-33. Senile plaques in Alzheimer's disease. (Hematoxylin and eosin; 280×.)

patients usually become symptomatic during the sixth and seventh decades, onset in the third decade and in the tenth decade has been recorded. Women are affected more often than men. The disease characteristically is fatal in 5 to 10 years.

The lobar atrophy, from which one of the names of the disease is derived, is most noticeable in the temporal and frontal lobes with the formation of the "saber gyri" (Fig. 48-35). The atrophy is usually symmetric and may extend to involve the insular cortex. Compensatory hydrocephalus is pronounced. The atrophy is primarily the result of the severe loss of nerve cells in the outer three cortical layers, frequently leaving a vacuolated appearance. Some of the residual degenerating nerve cells are swollen with peripheral displacement of their nuclei. These abnormal cells, Pick's cells, contain intracytoplasmic, amphophilic (with hematoxylin and eosin), argyrophilic, and granular material. An astrocytic gliosis, sometimes very pronounced, in the outer cortical layers of the atrophic gyri is regularly present.

Spinocerebellar degenerations

The spinocerebellar degenerations are an overlapping group of related diseases that

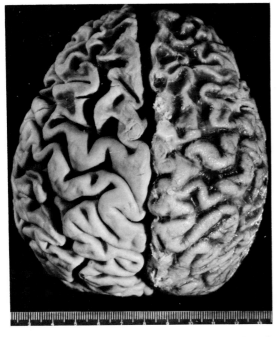

Fig. 48-35. Pick's disease. Pronounced atrophy of rostral frontal lobes with compensatory external hydrocephalus.

affect the portions of the central nervous system that control coordination. The systems of cells involved are developmentally, functionally, and anatomically related. Although many of the diseases are hereditary (either dominant or recessive), previous infections, alcoholism, and the remote effects of cancer also have been implicated.

The disorders are first apparent clinically and structurally in the most peripheral portion of the processes of the affected cells, with retrograde progression toward the perikaryon. For ease of understanding, these disorders have been divided into (1) primarily spinal, (2) primarily cerebellar, and (3) mixed types.

Primarily spinal atrophies

The more common of the degenerations that are primarily spinal are Friedreich's ataxia and peroneal muscular atrophy.

Friedreich's ataxia. Friedreich's ataxia (hereditary spinal ataxia) is a rare progressive disease whose usual onset occurs during the first two decades of life. The sexes are affected equally, and the average life-span after clinical onset is approximately 15 years. The cerebrum, brainstem, and cerebellum are normal. On the other hand, the spinal cord, its posterior roots, and the spinal ganglia are small at the time of death. This is attributed at first to demyelination and later to loss of axons in the posterior half of the cord.

Initially, the fasciculi graciles are affected. With progression, the disease in turn affects the fasciculi cuneati, the posterior roots, and the dorsal and then the ventral spinocerebellar tracts. In far-advanced disease, the lateral and later the anterior corticospinal tracts also may be involved. The cells of Clarke's columns, with loss of Nissl substance become small, and finally many cells may disappear. At the time of death, about half the patients have myocardial lesions: hypertrophy, fatty infiltration, focal myocarditis, and fibrosis, in any combination.

Peroneal muscular atrophy. Peroneal muscular atrophy (Charcot-Marie-Tooth disease; progressive neural muscular atrophy) is a hereditary disease. It may occur in families in which other members have Friedreich's ataxia. The lesions are characterized by demyelination followed by axon loss beginning in the most distal portions of the peroneal nerves, initially involving the fibers supplying the small muscles of the feet. With progression, the lesions ascend the nerves to involve the anterior horn cells and the cells of the spinal ganglions. In some patients, the posterior columns of the spinal cord exhibit degeneration. Reactive proliferation of the Schwann cells around some residual axons in the peripheral nerves produce an onionskin appearance.

The rare primary spinal atrophies include hereditary areflexic dystaxia (Roussy-Levy syndrome) and heredopathia atactica polyneuritiformis (Refsum's disease).

Primarily cerebellar atrophies

The degenerations that are primarily cerebellar include lamellar atrophy of Purkinje cells, degeneration of the internal granular layer, focal cerebellar sclerosis, and olivopontocerebellar atrophy. In this group of disorders, in contrast with the spinal forms, there is a later clinical onset, more common involvement of the extrapyramidal tracts, and, less commonly, extraneural signs.

Lamellar atrophy of Purkinje cells. Lamellar atrophy of Purkinje cells is a disorder of adults, more often past the age of 40 years. It usually is not hereditary. Some instances have been associated with alcoholism. Other suggested causes have included a variety of toxins, infections, and premature aging.

The cerebellum grossly appears normal or is only slightly decreased in size. Microscopically, there is a sharp loss of Purkinje cells (Fig. 48-36) that may be complete in the superior and anterior portions of the cerebellar vermis. There is a lesser loss of cells in the hemispheres. The molecular layer of the cerebellum is unaltered. A mild loss of the internal granular cells is sometimes noted.

Subacute cerebellar degeneration. Diffuse loss of Purkinje cells (subacute cerebellar degeneration) has been ascribed to the remote effects of cancer. The great sensitivity of these cells to hypoxia, hyperthermia, a variety of chemical toxins, heavy metals and possibly alcohol, obscures the significance of cancer as the cause of this change.

Degeneration of internal granular layer. Degeneration of the internal granular layer with either partial or complete loss of the cells is a common postmortem finding. It is regular as an autolytic change in the so-called

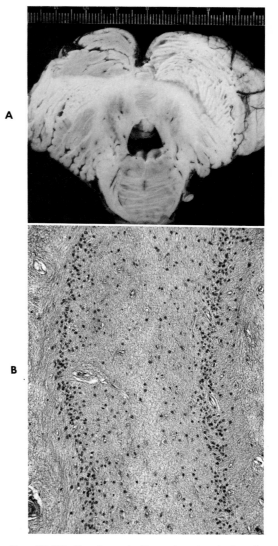

Fig. 48-37. Focal cerebellar sclerosis. **A,** Involvement of several cerebellar folia. **B,** Focus of loss of Purkinje and most internal granular cells. Reactive astrocytic gliosis. (Hematoxylin and eosin; 90×.)

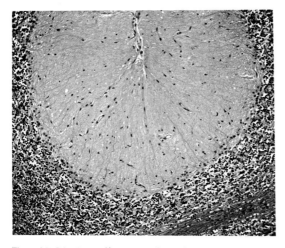

Fig. 48-36. Lamellar atrophy of Purkinje's cells. (Hematoxylin and eosin; 90×.)

respirator brain and is seen in a great variety of disorders frequently associated with hyperthermia, as well as in alcoholism. Familial cases with onset in the first year of life associated with mental deficiency and ataxia also have been described. The cerebellum may be normal in size or slightly smaller than normal. The degree of internal granular cell loss is variable. Purkinje cells are far less involved and occasionally may be displaced into the molecular or granular layers. The presence of a mild to moderate reactive astrocytosis, in some, suggests an extrinsic cause rather than a developmental lesion.

Focal cerebellar sclerosis (circumscribed atrophy of the cerebellar cortex). In focal cerebellar sclerosis, there is a focal and severe degeneration of all three cerebellar layers and a strong reactive proliferation of Bergmann cells (Fig. 48-37). The superior and inferior semilunar and simplex lobules are most frequently involved. The cause of this usually clinically silent disease is not known.

Olivopontocerebellar atrophies[97]

This is a group of related disorders characterized by the loss of nerve cells in the cerebellar cortex, the base of the pons, and the inferior olives (Fig. 48-38). Separation into five types has been based upon their hereditary background, their clinical and pathologic characteristics, and involvement of other portions of the central nervous system. All but one are dominantly inherited. The life-span after clinical onset is usually less than 10 years.

The great atrophy of the cerebellum (usually sparing the vermis), base of pons, and inferior olives is diagnostic and basic to all five types. This is caused by the loss of internal granular and Purkinje cells with an astrocytosis in the cerebellum and loss of neurons in the base of the pons and inferior olives. Type 1 additionally exhibits degeneration of the middle cerebellar peduncles and the spinocerebellar tracts and posterior columns of the spinal cord with a decrease in cells in the anterior and posterior horns. Type 2 is recessively inherited with loss of cells of the substantia nigra in addition to the basic disorder. In type 3, the changes are those of the type 1 with added retinal degeneration. Degeneration of cells of the vagus and hypoglossal nuclei superimposed upon the basic changes is seen in type 4. In the type 5 there is also loss of cells in the cerebral cortex, caudate and lenticular nuclei, and the second and third cranial nerves.

Parkinson's disease

Formerly considered as a disease, parkinsonism is now regarded as a symptom-complex most frequently of idiopathic or viral origin.[43,50] Other causes are local vascular disease with infarction, anoxia caused by carbon monoxide, toxins, and drugs (manganese and the phenothiazines), metastatic lesions, and injury from mechanical forces. The term paralysis agitans usually is reserved for the idiopathic variety.

In most patients, the recognizable lesions are confined to the cells of the substantia nigra, locus ceruleus, and other pigmented

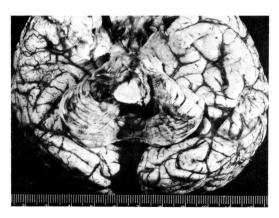

Fig. 48-38. Olivopontocerebellar atrophy. Pronounced atrophy of cerebellum, pons, and inferior olives.

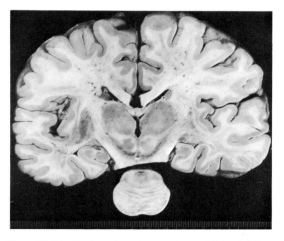

Fig. 48-39. Brain of patient who exhibited idiopathic parkinsonism shows partial loss of pigment in substantia nigra and complete loss in locus ceruleus, both bilaterally.

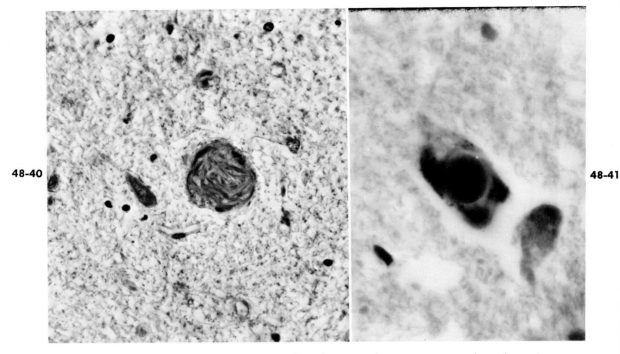

Fig. 48-40. Neurofibrillary change in cell of locus ceruleus in patient with parkinsonism. (Hematoxylin and eosin; 600×.)

Fig. 48-41. Lewy body in cell of substantia nigra in patient with parkinsonism. (Hematoxylin and eosin; 1100×.)

cells of the brainstem (i.e., dorsal nucleus of the vagus). The grossly visible loss of pigment in these areas (Fig. 48-39) is the result of destruction of the cells with phagocytosis and removal of the cell products and specific pigment—neuromelanin. Many of the remaining cells are shrunken, and some are vacuolated. In others cells of these nuclei, a coarse thickening of the neurofibrils (neurofibrillary tangles) may be visible even with routine hematoxylin and eosin stain (Fig. 48-40) and with Congo red and polarized light. Some cells may contain single or multiple cytoplasmic, spheric, hyaline, eosinophilic inclusions with dark centers; these are Lewy bodies (Fig. 48-41). Mild to moderate degrees of focal reactive astrocytosis often are present in the affected regions. In patients younger than 60 years, the presence if general brain atrophy and Lewy bodies is more characteristic of the idiopathic type (paralysis agitans), whereas Alzheimer's neurofibrillary changes and disseminated focal astrocytic scars are more suggestive of the inflammatory variety. These distinctions are far less secure in older patients.[50]

Other lesions, not generally accepted, have been described in patients with either type

of parkinsonism.[43] These include loss of the large cells of the caudate nuclei and putamina and "perivascular degeneration" of the outer segments of the globus pallidus with pallor from loss of myelinated fibers.

In patients with parkinsonism from other causes, the lesions are generally widespread with the additional involvement of the substantia nigra.

Among the Chamorros in the Mariana islands, parkinsonism often is associated with dementia or amyotrophic lateral sclerosis, or both. In these patients, there is a loss of pigmented cells, no Lewy bodies, many neurofibrillary tangles, frontal and temporal lobe atrophy, and, in some, microscopic changes characteristic of motor neuron disease. The disease may be the result of a "slow virus" infection.

Motor neuron disease (amyotrophic lateral sclerosis)[21,101]

Motor neuron disease is a disease that primarily if not exclusively affects the pyramidal (motor) system. Its clinical and structural variants are dependent on the motor level predominantly affected. Although amyotrophic lateral sclerosis denotes the entire group, it also has been used to describe that variant in which the principal level of involvement is in the cells of the motor cortex and in their processes. In progressive bulbar palsy, the most significant lesions are in the motor cranial nuclei. The anterior horn cells are primarily affected in the type known as progressive (spinal) muscular atrophy. When the lesions are confined to the lateral and anterior corticospinal tracts with little or no recognizable change in the motor cortex, the disease is considered by some to represent primary lateral sclerosis. One of the many causes of the "floppy infant" is infantile progressive spinal muscular atrophy (Werdnig-Hoffmann disease, amyotonia congenita, Oppenheim's disease). It has the microscopic appearance of progressive (spinal) muscular atrophy and progressive bulbar palsy.

The unitarian concept of this group of diseases is suggested by the simultaneous involvement, often clinically and regularly at microscopy, of two or more levels of the motor system. Motor neuron disease has been classified among the abiotrophic conditions of the central nervous system. These are diseases in which genetic factors are considered to result in the gradual and premature death of the cells ordinarily destined to live many more years. This may account for the approximately 6% to 10% familial incidents in the adult form of this disease and the generally accepted autosomal recessive heredity of the infantile form. The initial degenerative change occurs in the most peripheral part of the longest cell process. With progression, there is retrograde deterioration toward the cell body. It recently has been suggested that the disease may be caused by a slow virus, i.e., one with an incubation period of years.[63,64] It is assumed that the effect of the as yet unidentified virus is to gradually produce a change in the cell identical with that of the abiotrophic state. Previous suggestions of a host of other causes of motor neuron disease such as toxins, syphilis, and trauma have not been substantiated.

The gross appearance of the brain and spinal cord is usually not helpful for diagnosis. In a few, there may be a slight to moderate degree of atrophy of the motor cortex, gray-white change in the lateral corticospinal tracts, or a decrease in size of the ventral roots at the lumbar and cervical levels of the spinal cord. The latter is difficult to evaluate because of the normally great variation in size of these roots. Amyotrophic lateral sclerosis, the most common of the motor neuron diseases, is usually most easily recognized on microscopic examina-

tion (with special stains for axons and myelin) by the presence of axonal and myelin degeneration affecting the motor tracts. This change is seen at all levels of the spinal cord and may be traced upward in the pyramidal system, usually easily as far as the pons, and sometimes as far as the internal capsule. At the latter level, degeneration of the myelin and axons is recognizable in less than one third of the patients. Only an occasional lipid-containing macrophage and a few perivascular lymphocytes are found at any level. This suggests more the very gradual progression of the disease rather than its inactivity. Neuronophagia of the cells of the motor cortex usually is not prominent and often may go unnoticed.

With progressive bulbar palsy, there is degeneration, neuronophagia, and loss of the cells of the cranial motor nuclei with a reactive astrocytosis in these areas. The nuclei most frequently and severely affected, in descending order, are the hypoglossal nucleus, the nucleus ambiguus, and the motor nuclei of the seventh and fifth nerves.

In spinal muscular atrophy, there is severe loss of anterior horn cells and usually much reactive astrocytosis. Neuronophagia is not prominent probably because the disease at this level is most prolonged. Axonal degeneration, evident in the ventral rootlets, corresponds to the anterior horn cells involved. Neurogenic atrophy is seen in the muscles innervated by the affected anterior horn cells.

The lesions in infantile progressive muscular atrophy involve loss or absence of the cells of the anterior horns of the spinal cord and the cranial motor nerve nuclei. The affected muscles have small fibers of the "fetal" or atrophic types.

Huntington's chorea

Huntington's chorea is an autosomal, dominantly inherited disease. Its late clinical onset, rare before the end of the second decade, allows the patient to have a family (often large) before there is significant mental deterioration or choreiform movements. The disease is slowly progressive with a long period of dementia.

The brain is moderately to greatly atrophic, particularly the frontal and temporal gyri. There is a sharp decrease in size of the caudate nuclei and the putamina and some decrease in size of the corpus callosum (Fig. 48-42). Compensatory internal and external hydrocephalus is characteristic. The changes in the caudate nuclei and putamina are caused by a

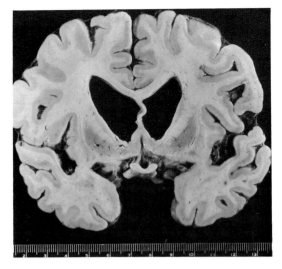

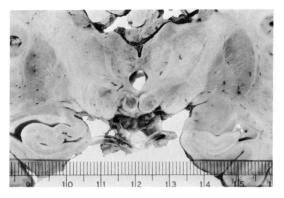

Fig. 48-43. Acute Wernicke's disease with involvement of mammillary bodies, hypothalami, and thalami.

Fig. 48-42. Huntington's chorea. Diagnostic atrophy of caudate nuclei and putamina. Moderate cortical atrophy. Compensatory internal and external hydrocephalus.

great loss of their small nerve cells with a pronounced reactive astrocytosis. In the atrophic cerebral cortex, the nerve cell loss and the reactive astrocytosis are more prominent in the outer layers.

DEFICIENCY DISEASES
Wernicke's polioencephalopathy[136]

Like beriberi, Wernicke's syndrome is caused by a deficiency of vitamin B_1. Characteristically occurring in chronic alcoholics, it also has been found in persons with a variety of debilitating diseases in whom the diet consists primarily of carbohydrates. The principal lesions, in decreasing order of frequency, involve the mammillary bodies, the gray matter of the hypothalami and thalami immediately surrounding the third ventricle (Fig. 48-43), the periaqueductal gray matter, and the floor and sometimes the roof of the fourth ventricle. Petechial hemorrhages in these regions, and from which the disease derived its original name (polioencephalitis hemorrhagica superior and inferior), may be absent or insignificant and are more likely the result rather than the cause of the initial lesions.

The early lesion is accompanied by decreased eosinophilia and granularity of the intercellular substance with loss of oligodendroglia and myelin in the affected sites. There is activation of the microglia with the formation of some lipophages. The resultant vascular dilatation leads to engorgement, some endothelial hypertrophy and hyperplasia, and variable numbers

of petechiae. A mild reactive astrocytosis is seen in the older lesions. Neurons in the affected regions are surprisingly little altered. A few may be shrunken, and a few may show eosinophilic homogenization. If death does not occur, and with adequate therapy, the lesions become inactive. The areas affected, particularly the mammillary bodies, collapse and become more brown than normal. At this stage, which is associated with the clinical state known as Korsakoff's syndrome, there is staining pallor, loosening of the tissues, increased lipofuscin in the nerve cells, and occasionally a few hemosiderophages.

Subacute necrotizing encephalomyelopathy (Leigh's disease)[54,56,67,130]

First described as limited to infants, subacute necrotizing encephalomyelopathy has also been reported in children and adults.[42,43,76,145] The necrotic lesions with a pronounced infiltration of lipophages are characteristically bilaterally symmetric. They involve the hypothalamus, the periaqueductal gray matter, the tegmental portion of the pons, and infrequently the mammillary bodies. The medulla and spinal cord sometimes are also involved.

The disease is presumed to be a metabolic defect that is genetically controlled. Because of the structural similarity to Wernicke's encephalopathy, it has been suggested that this defect involves the utilization of thiamine or of its derivatives.

Pellagra

Inadequate amounts of nicotinic acid in the diet can result in pellagra. The characteristic light-sensitive dermatitis and diarrhea may be accompanied or, as is more usual, followed by disorders of mentation and even of movement.

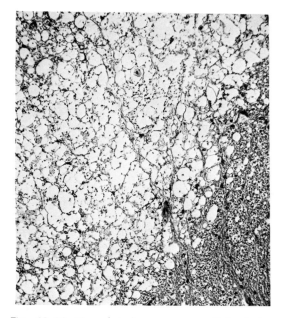

Fig. 48-44. Vacuolated appearance of fasciculus gracilis in patient with vitamin B$_{12}$ deficiency. (Hematoxylin and eosin; 90×.)

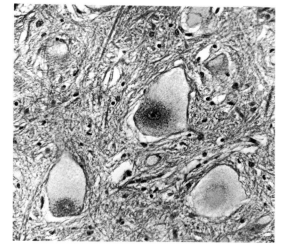

Fig. 48-45. Tay-Sachs disease. Anterior horn cells. Displacement of nucleus and Nissl substance attributed to accumulation of ganglioside. (Hematoxylin and eosin; 280×.)

There are usually no gross changes in the central nervous system. Microscopically, many neurons at all levels of the central nervous system have the appearance characteristic of central chromatolysis with some increase in lipofuscin. There is little recognizable degeneration of the axons.

Posterolateral sclerosis (subacute combined degeneration of spinal cord)[136,151]

Because of a deficiency of vitamin B$_{12}$, posterolateral sclerosis is associated with addisonian (pernicious) anemia. It may be seen in patients with sprue, with gastric cancer, after gastrectomy, or with folate deficiency. The spinal cord may be of normal size or slightly small in circumference, with pallor and softening of the posterior columns. On microscopic examination of the spinal cord, there is loss of myelin and oligodendroglia and of axons in the posterior and lateral columns. The early lesions may contain many lipophages. The later lesions are characteristically spongy, with almost complete absence of a reactive astrocytosis (Fig. 48-44). Moderate loss of nerve cells of the cerebral cortex with areas of degeneration of the white matter have been described.[58]

NEURONAL LIPID-STORAGE DISEASES[17]

The neuronal lipid-storage diseases are a group of rare enzymatic disturbances of lipid metabolism that sometimes can be diagnosed ante mortem because of nerve cell involvement seen on brain, rectal, jejunal, or muscle biopsy and by enzyme assays of circulating leukocytes, serum, cultured fibroblasts, or amniotic cells. The group includes Tay-Sachs disease and its variants, Gaucher's disease, Niemann-Pick disease, Fabry's disease, etc.

Amaurotic familial idiocy[140]

Because of slight enzymatic differences there are several variations of amaurotic familial idiocy. Most instances are of the infantile form (Tay-Sachs disease), with congenital, late infantile, juvenile, and adult forms having been described.

Early enlargement of the brain is followed by a decrease in size as the disease progresses. The larger nerve cells at all levels, including the Purkinje cells and the anterior horn cells of the spinal cord, are distended with a complex lipid containing sphingosine, hexoses, chondrosamine, and neuraminic acid. It is classified as a ganglioside and is oil-red positive. As the intracytoplasmic material accumulates, the Nissl substance is gradually displaced to a small zone about the nucleus (Fig. 48-45). The material also is to be found enlarging the cell processes. Lipid-containing macrophages can be found in the affected central nervous system and in the leptomeninges. There is a moderate reactive astrocytosis in the older lesions.

Niemann-Pick disease

In Niemann-Pick disease, nerve cells and the cells of the reticuloendothelial system and liver are distended with sphingomyelin. The similarity of nerve cells bloated with this stored material with those of amaurotic idiocy makes it exceedingly difficult to structurally separate the diseases. Involvement of the liver and of the reticuloendothelial system is helpful in differentiating the two (p. 1508).

Gaucher's disease

The accumulation of a cerebroside (protein-bound glycolipid) is regularly seen in the perikaryon of nerve cells in patients with *Gaucher's disease*. The enzymatic defect is glucosyl ceramide-β-glucosyl hydrolase. The material is periodic acid–Schiff positive. With routine stains, the nerve cells appear vacuolated. Involvement of the reticuloendothelial system is described elsewhere (p. 1507).

Gargoylism (Hurler-Pfaundler disease, Hunter-Hurler disease, lipochondro-dystrophy)

In gargoylism the material that accumulates in many nerve cells and in reticuloendothelial macrophages and in bone and cartilage cells is a mucopolysaccharide. A sphingolipid is sometimes also found. The disease is recessively inherited, either sex linked (Hunter's) or autosomally (Hurler's), and is apparently attributable to the absence of one or more of a group of enzymes that degrade mucopolysaccharides (p. 1395).

METABOLIC DISTURBANCES
Wilson's disease, hepatolenticular degeneration[13]

Wilson's disease is believed to be caused by, at least in part, an absence or insufficiency of the serum alpha globulin ceruloplasmin, which binds the serum copper. As a result, the bound and total serum copper is low and free copper is deposited in the putamina and striate bodies, in Descemet's membrane of the eye, and in the liver. There is often an aminoaciduria, presumably as a result of renal tubular disease. In over one half the patients, the disease is apparently inherited through a rare recessive gene (p. 1375).

The brain is usually atrophic. There may be no grossly visible changes. In some, there is softening with brown discoloration of the striate areas. On microscopic examination, there is often a pronounced astrocytosis with type I and type II Alzheimer's astrocytes in the central gray matter of the cerebral hemispheres. Large oval cells with small nuclei, the Opalski cells, sometimes are found in these same areas. The patients have a nodular cirrhosis and the brown Kayser-Fleischer rings of deposited copper at the margins of the corneas.

Amino acid disturbances

Several rare disorders of amino acid metabolism have been described. Among these is *phenylketonuria* (phenylpyruvic oligophrenia) caused by the lack of phenylalanine hydrolase, an enzyme that converts phenylalanine to tyrosine. Consequently phenylalanine accumulates in the tissues, blood, and cerebrospinal fluid while phenylpyruvic acid, the deaminated by-product of phenylalanine is excreted in the urine. Characteristic structural changes in the central nervous system have not been described in this recessively inherited condition. *Hartnup disease*[83] is ascribed to a defect in the conversion of tryptophan to nicotinic acid. The central nervous system changes in this familial disease resemble those of pellagra (p. 631). Large amounts of 3-indolylacetic acid and indolylacetyl glutamine are excreted in the urine. The affected children have a pellagra-like skin rash, cerebellar ataxia, nystagmus, and sometimes dementia. *Maple syrup urine disease* is ascribed to an enzymatic deficiency that results in the accumulation in the tissues of the branched-chain α-keto acid derivatives of isoleucine, leucine, and valine; their excretion in the urine imparts the characteristic odor. The disease is familial; structural changes in the nervous system have not been recorded.

KERNICTERUS (NUCLEAR JAUNDICE)[69]

Abnormally high concentrations of lipid-soluble, indirect-reacting bile pigments may discolor the globi pallidi, subthalamic nuclei, hippocampi, dentate nuclei, and inferior olivary nuclei in the newborn, especially when premature. The cerebral and cerebellar cortices and cochlear nuclei are less regularly affected. The high concentrations of bile pigment are most frequently attributed to severe hemolytic disease of the infant resulting from the presence of maternal antibodies, usually anti-D, but sometimes to an ABO incompatibility or to structural defects in erythrocytes leading to increased hemolysis. A further increase in the blood of the indirect-reacting bile pigment in the immature infant is attributed, in part, to an initial liver deficiency of glucuronyl transferase. The presence of a low serum albumin to which the indirect-reacting pigment ordinarily forms a loose attachment permits the pigment to enter the tissues more easily. Although a level of indirect-reacting bile pigment of 18 to 20 mg per 100 ml is considered critical, all factors must be considered. Nuclear jaundice has also been recorded in congenital familial nonhemolytic jaundice of the Crigler-Najjar type.[35] Localizations of the pigment deposits in the nuclear areas have been ascribed to focal immaturity of the blood-brain barrier and to previous hypoxic damage to the nerve cells in these areas; structural changes are variable. In many of the pigmented areas (subthalamic nucleus, globus pallidus, and hippocampus), the affected nerve cells have undergone severe ischemic changes and mineralization of their Golgi apparatus; the stained cells of the dentate nuclei and inferior olives may show little change.

Some surviving children, although actively treated, later manifest signs and symptoms resulting from damage, destruction and loss of many cells in the affected nuclei (see also p. 1389).

EPILEPSY

Epilepsy is an abnormal functional state of the central nervous system that is characterized by uncontrolled outbursts of nerve cell activity and clinically by convulsive seizures with or without loss of consciousness or by their equivalents. In the idiopathic (primary, or essential) form, the only structural changes are those related to hypoxia, which accompanies the attacks. The secondary (symptomatic) form of epilepsy has been associated with a great variety of diseases that affect the central nervous system. Loss of cells in Sommer's sector of the hippocampus with a reactive astrocytosis may be seen in both forms and in patients without epilepsy. In severe epilepsy with repeated and frequent attacks, there are usually other evidences of anoxic changes, including laminar cell loss in the cerebral cortex (third through fifth layers), especially in the cortex that lies in the depths of the sulci. Loss of Purkinje cells, especially in the depths of the folia, is a common structural evidence of any hypoxic state, including that which accompanies epileptic seizures.

A special form of epilepsy, *myoclonus* (inclusion body) *epilepsy,* is a rare disease of unknown cause in which spheric intracytoplasmic basophilic inclusions (Lafora's bodies) are found in the larger nerve cells of the cerebral cortex and the subcortical gray matter, the brainstem, and the subcortical gray areas of the cerebellum, as well as in myocardial fibers and liver cells (particularly those at the periphery of the lobules).

INFLAMMATION

Inflammations of the brain and spinal cord generally are complications of similar inflammations elsewhere in the body. Normally there is great protection afforded the central nervous system by the surrounding covering structures and by the actions of the blood-brain barrier. Once these defenses are breached, the resistance to infection is less than that of most of the other organs of the body. There are four general routes by which pathogenic organisms may reach the central nervous system.

1. The most frequently utilized route is that of the blood vessels. Most intravascular spread to the central nervous system is by way of the arteries, the organisms usually having first produced disease of the lungs or heart valves. Less often, organisms reach the central nervous system through emissary or diploic veins as a component of a retrograde thrombophlebitis or embolus draining adjacent infections, or from distant structures.[71] The paravertebral venous system is rarely implicated.

2. Infections of the mastoid sinuses, middle ears, paranasal sinuses, skull, and vertebra may extend directly to involve the brain or spinal cord or their coverings.

3. Organisms, chemical toxins, or even particulate materials may be directly implanted upon the coverings or within the central nervous system as a result of gunshot wounds, mechanical trauma, or medical procedures, including surgery and lumbar puncture.

4. Certain viruses, including rabies and possibly herpes simplex and zoster, once implanted within the axoplasm of a peripheral nerve, can, by centripetal movement within the cell cytoplasm and perhaps through the neurotubules, reach the perikaryon within the spinal ganglia, spinal cord, or brain.

Once within the central nervous system, further dissemination of the infection may proceed by direct continuity or by way of the fluid within the ventricular, subarachnoid, or Virchow-Robin spaces in the usual direction of flow, retrograde, or both.

• • •

Inflammations of the central nervous system are classified according to the site of involvement and to the type of exudate.

Meningeal infections

Meningeal infections may be separated into those affecting the dura mater and those affecting the pia-arachnoid.

Pachymeningitis. Purulent infections of the

dura are most frequently from *Diplococcus pneumoniae, Staphylococcus aureus,* and β-hemolytic streptococci. These infections are characterized as external (epidural, or extradural) when the inflammation involves the outer surface and internal (subdural) when the inner surface is affected.

In the skull, most instances of epidural infection are the result of extension from an adjacent infection of the paranasal or mastoid sinuses with the formation of a small epidural (subperiosteal) abscess. Over the spinal cord, these abscesses are usually secondary to infections of the vertebra. Less frequently, they may follow retroperitoneal or retropleural infections with extension to the epidural space through an intervertebral foramen. The epidural abscess of the spinal cord tends to become larger than that of the skull because the spinal dura is separate from the periosteum and the intervening tissues offer little mechanical resistance to spread. The prognosis is good in either of the abscesses only if the lesion is treated early and adequately.

Purulent subdural infections (subdural empyema, subdural abscess) (Fig. 48-46), like their epidural counterparts, are most often complications of adjacent infections and occur with or without epidural infections.[75] The organisms may bypass the external dura by extending through a dural sinus and bridging vein into the subdural space or may be spread there by eroding the dura locally. Once in the subdural space, continued spread over the brain unilaterally is rapid, and it frequently becomes bilateral. The rare purulent spinal subdural infection is most likely to lie over the lower portion of the spinal cord and cauda equina. Reaction to the infection at both levels, at least initially, is from the vascular inner portion of the dura. There is no contribution from the arachnoid. Attempts to localize the infection by the formation of vascular pyogenic granulation tissue is late and generally inadequate. The tendency of the exudate and organisms to disseminate widely through the subdural space, to compress the underlying nervous system, and to spread to the subarachnoid space contributes to the high mortality in this condition.

Leptomeningitis. Purulent infections of the leptomeninges (leptomeningitis, meningitis) are seen with an ever-increasing variety of bacteria. At present, the most common in adults are from *Streptococcus pneumoniae, Staphylococcus aureus,* β-hemolytic streptococci, meningococcus *(Neisseria meningitidis),* whereas in children the most common causative organisms are *Haemophilus influenzae* and *Escherichia coli.* Almost all the routes of invasion described earlier are utilized. The bac-

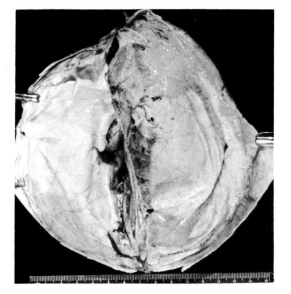

Fig. 48-46. Unilateral acute subdural empyema. Secondary to frontal sinusitis.

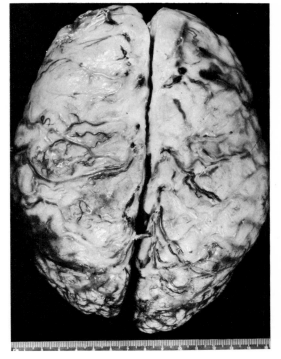

Fig. 48-47. Severe acute purulent leptomeningitis with thrombophlebitis.

teria that reach the subarachnoid space through the arteries may do so by exiting from the small thin-walled arteries in the subarachnoid space or may reach the subarachnoid space indirectly after exiting from the choroid plexuses into the ventricles. Contiguous paranasal and sinus infections are frequent sources. In any leptomeningitis, the source should be identified and that lesion treated as well as the infection of the central nervous system.

Early, the brain is variably swollen and its vessels engorged. When the patient has succumbed very quickly, as some do with a fulminant meningococcemia, little or no exudate may be visible macroscopically. The earliest exudate that can be seen is recognizable first as thin gray streaks that parallel the lateral margins of superficial veins that lie over the sulci. The exudate soon becomes more diffuse, thick, gray, and often slightly green. Initially, it fills the sulci and later overlays and obscures the gyri (Fig. 48-47) and finally the cisterns become filled. Later the exudate tends to concentrate in the subarachnoid space to either side of the superior sagittal sinus, with lesser amounts toward the base of the brain. Over the spinal cord, the exudate covers the posterior aspect greatest in amount at the thoracic level, probably because of gravity in the relatively immobile patient lying in the recumbent position.

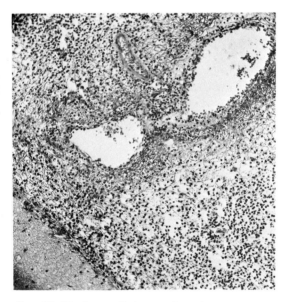

Fig. 48-48. Acute fibrinopurulent leptomeningitis with numerous neutrophils and some fibrin. (Hematoxylin and eosin; 90×.)

When there has been little or no visible exudate macroscopically, sections from multiple areas or of rolls of leptomeninges covering all or portions of a hemisphere may contain only a few neutrophils, usually in small clusters. In the usual fatal case in which the infection had been present for 24 hours or more, the exudate initially is characterized by an extensive neutrophilic infiltration most concentrated about the blood vessels (Fig. 48-48). The exudate later becomes more diffuse and is accompanied by increasing amounts of fibrin. With a gram stain, both free and phagocytized organisms may be found. As the disease progresses and there is evidence of response to therapy, the exudate gradually changes to one in which the predominant cell types are lymphocytes, monocytes, and, finally, mononuclear macrophages. In the fatal cases and, presumably to a lesser extent, in patients who recover, toxic effects of the leptomeningeal disease result in a reactive astrocytosis seen in the molecular layer (first layer) of the cortex with shrinkage and hyperchromatism of some of the superficial nerve cells in the second and third cortical layers. With uncomplicated recovery, the exudate disappears apparently by exiting into the dural venous sinuses through the arachnoid villi and, possibly, by entering some of the thinner-walled leptomeningeal veins. No structural residua may be seen in patients treated early and adequately.

Thrombophlebitis involving several or many veins, particularly those draining the parasagittal portions of the cerebral hemispheres, occurs in some patients. The occurrence of an arteritis or thromboarteritis is less common. Small cortical and subcortical hemorrhagic or anemic infarcts are the usual sequelae of these vascular complications. When the infarcts are of significant numbers and sizes and are situated at functionally important sites, they are manifest by a variety of clinical complications. In some patients, the subarachnoid infection may extend into the brain along the Virchow-Robin spaces or in veins as a retrograde thrombophlebitis and result in the formation of one or more brain abscesses. Retrograde extension from the subarachnoid space through the lateral recesses of the fourth ventricle reaching the ventricular system then produces an ependymitis and choroid plexitis, initially of the fourth and later of the other ventricles. In these, the fibrinopurulent exudate covers the surfaces with areas of ependymal ulceration. Perivascular lymphocytic cuffs in the subependymal cell plate is evidence of further reaction to the inflammation. Not infrequently in children, rarely in adults, a unilateral or bilateral serous subdural effusion may overlie the purulent meningitis.

Small patches of leptomeningeal fibrosis frequently have been attributed to preexisting infections of the leptomeninges in which the exudate has been organized with the formation of a fibrous scar. These scars are significant when they are extensive or occur at critical areas in the path of cerebrospinal flow. An adhesive or constrictive band of scar tissue (adhesive or constrictive arachnoiditis) may be formed. Contraction of the scar can irritate the adjoining cells or destroy the encircled nervous system, including cranial nerves and spinal cord. A saclike leptomeningeal scar, by permitting the ingress of fluid and impeding its egress, can form the pocket for an enlarging subarachnoid cystic collection of fluid that compresses the underlying brain or spinal cord.

Brain abscess

As with the purulent leptomeningitides, the organisms producing an abscess can reach the brain through any of the routes previously described (p. 2107) or as a complication of a purulent meningitis. Abscesses occurring after septic emboli are usually multiple and occur most frequently in the distribution areas of the middle cerebral arteries. When in the white matter, early there is sparing of the subcortical U fibers. Both cerebral hemispheres are affected equally. An abscess whose source is a contiguous infection is usually single and more often involves the adjacent portion of the brain. Extension from the middle ear is to the ventrocaudal portion of the homolateral temporal lobe, whereas the abscess of mastoid origin is usually in the homolateral cerebellar hemisphere. Rarely, any of these infections may extend as a thrombophlebitis of a dural sinus to enter the brain at some point other than that adjacent to the original infection.

In its earliest stages, before abscess formation, the area is congested, edematous, soft and with numerous petechiae; it is diffusely infiltrated with neutrophils. This is the stage known to clinicians as "cerebritis." More intense neutrophilic infiltration with liquefaction necrosis rapidly ensues. Variable numbers of bacteria may lie free in the abscess or in neutrophils or in both. Without adequate therapy, there is continued enlargement and coalescence of abscesses, often with extension into the subarachnoid or ventricular cavities.

Adequate medical therapy decreases the

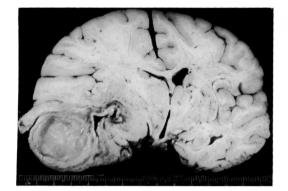

Fig. 48-49. Chronic brain abscesses in temporal lobe and insula. Surrounding brain swelling and edema. Compression and displacement of lateral and third ventricles. Cingulate gyrus and uncal herniations.

local spread and the surrounding edema and swelling. Usually, inadequate amounts of vascular granulation tissue form about the abscess. The source of the granulation tissue is the mesenchymal cells in the walls of the blood vessels within the brain and adjoining leptomeninges and possibly the microglia. With treatment, the neutrophils within the abscess gradually are replaced by lymphocytes, monocytes, and macrophages. The surrounding granulation and fibrous tissue remains thin and is surrounded by a narrow zone of reactive astrocytes and more peripherally by a moderately edematous and swollen brain in which there are perivascular lymphocytic cuffs. Although specific and intensive antibiotic therapy may have been given, a portion of the wall of almost every abscess, however chronic, shows evidence of continued enlargement with necrosis and often with the formation of satellite lesions (Fig. 48-49).

Granulomatous infections

Tuberculosis. The decreasing incidence of pulmonary tuberculosis, coupled with more adequate therapy, has made tuberculosis of the central nervous system relatively uncommon. Extension of a tuberculous infection from a vertebra to the epidural and subdural spaces is rare. A tuberculous leptomeningitis in children is most often a part of a generalized miliary infection. In adults, the usual association is with pulmonary tuberculosis. The early report of Rich and McCordock, that a tuberculous leptomeningitis represents extension from an adjacent focus in the brain in at least 90% of the patients, has not been substanti-

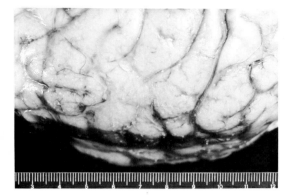

Fig. 48-50. Tuberculous leptomeningitis with numerous leptomeningeal tubercles.

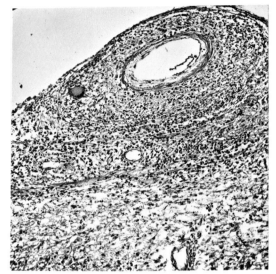

Fig. 48-51. Tuberculous leptomeningitis. Presence of Langhans' type of giant cell is unusual. (Hematoxylin and eosin; 90×.)

ated. As with purulent inflammations, many now believe that the organisms enter the central nervous system from other infections elsewhere in the body by way of the choroid plexuses or through the walls of the leptomeningeal vessels.

Early in tuberculous leptomeningitis, the exudate is usually scant, diffuse, and gray-white, sometimes with a faint green tinge. Later, 1 to 3 mm, discrete, gray nodules may be found, particularly along the course of the leptomeningeal blood vessels (Fig. 48-50). In patients with a relatively long history of tuberculous leptomeningitis, as with most granulomatous infections of the meninges, the exudate is more prominent at the base of the brain. The initial diffuse exudate is formed by lymphocytes, large mononuclear cells, serum and fibrin with small foci of caseation, and occasional neutrophils at sites of recent extension. The discrete nodules seen macroscopically consist of foci of caseation necrosis with fibrin surrounded by varying numbers of lymphocytes, plasmocytoid cells, and large mononuclear cells. Giant cells of Langhans' type are less frequent here than in other tissues (Fig. 48-51). Acid-fast bacilli may be numerous or rare. As with pyogenic infections, there may be spread along the ventricular system, and into the brain along the Virchow-Robin spaces. Blood vessels within the leptomeningeal exudate have lymphocytes in their walls. They may exhibit a reactive, endothelial hypertrophy and hyperplasia, sometimes with thrombosis, leading to small anemic infarcts in the adjacent brain and spinal cord.

Early chemotherapy modifies the response and decreases the degree of fibrous tissue scarring. Because the exudate and the scars are more abundant at the base of the brain, they may significantly impede the flow of cerebrospinal fluid and thereby produce an obstructive internal hydrocephalus, and constriction of the scar may impair the function of one or more cranial nerves.

A tuberculous encephalitis usually presents in one of two structural forms. In one there may be multiple granulomas all of about the same size (usually up to 1 cm). In the other there are one or a few that may reach a diameter of 5 to 6 cm, are solid, and have "growth rings" formed by the successive addition of layers of granulation tissue. The larger lesions are more common in the cerebellum.

Cryptococcosis. Cryptococcosis (*Cryptococcus neoformans,* formerly *C. hominis*) of the central nervous system is a worldwide disease of increasing incidence. It is seen in patients with diabetes, in those who have undergone cardiac surgery, and in those after having immunosuppressive treatment for a variety of diseases. The central nervous system disease is associated with infection of other organs, particularly the lungs, spleen, bone marrow, liver, and kidneys (p. 505).

The leptomeninges and brain usually are involved simultaneously. The leptomeningeal exudate is variable in amount, clear to turbid, watery to gelatinous, and usually more prominent at the base of the brain and over the dorsal aspect of the thoracic portion of the

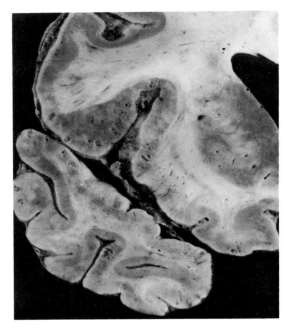

Fig. 48-52. Cryptococcosis with thin watery leptomeningeal exudate and many cortical cavities.

spinal cord. Within the brain, especially in the gray matter, there may be many smooth-walled cavities from less than 1 mm to as much as 1 cm in diameter (Fig. 48-52). These are filled with fluid identical to that seen in the subarachnoid space. The ventricular system, particularly in the region of the choroid plexuses, may contain the same type of exudate. The degree of cellular response is variable. In some areas, organisms may be present free in the subarachnoid and ventricular spaces or in the cystic cavities with almost no cell response. In other areas, particularly when the lesions have been present for a long time, there may be many lymphocytes, large mononuclear macrophages, some neutrophils and fibrin, and giant cells of both foreign body and Langhans' types. Characteristic organisms are usually easily found in all areas and in the lumbar cerebrospinal fluid. Mixed infections are sometimes seen.[95]

Coccidioidomycosis. Coccidioidomycosis (*Coccidioides immitis*) is an endemic disease of the southwestern portion of the United States. The central nervous system infection is always a complication of a disseminated disease, particularly that originating from an initial pulmonary infection (p. 504).

The leptomeningeal exudate, although similar in many respects to that of tuberculosis, is usually more diffuse, more tenacious, and more abundant. The granulomas have a greater degree of central liquefaction. The infiltrates consist of mixtures of lymphocytes, neutrophils, plasma cells, large mononuclear cells, and giant cells of Langhans' type. Typical organisms are found in these cells as well as in the tissues.

Histoplasmosis and blastomycosis. Histoplasmosis (*Histoplasma capsulatum*) and blastomycosis (*Blastomyces dermatitidis*) are similar in that their involvement in the brain and spinal cord resembles tuberculosis. Both are associated with primary infection elsewhere in the body, most frequently of the respiratory tract.

With histoplasmosis, there is usually diffuse involvement of the reticuloendothelial system. In blastomycosis, the skin and bones also are involved. In both, the leptomeningeal exudate may be diffuse and gray with or without well-defined, firm, gray nodules. Similar nodules often are seen within the brain. The diffuse exudate consists of lymphocytes, large mononuclear cells, some plasma cells, and neutrophils embedded in a moderate amount of fibrin. The nodules are formed by lymphocytes and epithelioid and giant cells of both Langhans' and foreign body types, all surrounding a central core of necrotic debris. The organisms are found both free and in the large mononuclear and giant cells. Distinction between the two is sometimes difficult unless cultural studies are done (see also p. 502).

Actinomycosis. Actinomycotic infections of the central nervous system are rare. When they do occur, they are more likely caused by the acid-fast aerobe than by the non–acid fast anaerobe. As with the other fungi, the central nervous system infection (usually abscess) is most frequently a complication of pulmonary disease and less frequently an extension from an adjacent infection. The cellular response is identical with that seen elsewhere in the body.

Neurosyphilis

The decreased incidence of syphilis of the central nervous system is the consequence of better control and of more adequate treatment during the early stages of the disease. Involvement of the central nervous system by the spirochete occurs during the secondary or the latent stage of the disease, always within the first 2 or 3 years of the infection.

Since syphilis may become inactive even without treatment (i.e., "burned out"), both before and after meningeal spread and because early meningeal involvement may be

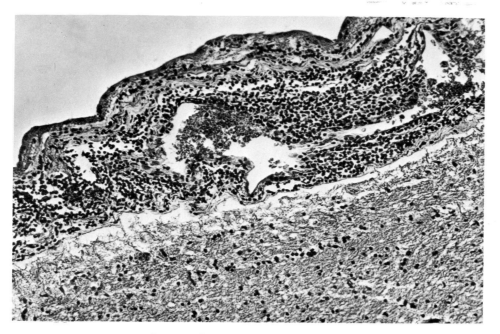

Fig. 48-53. Meningovascular syphilis. Lymphocytes and plasma cells in leptomeninges. (Hematoxylin and eosin; 180×.)

asymptomatic, the spinal fluid must be repeatedly examined for cells (lymphocytes), increase in proteins (globulin), and the presence of a positive serology. The symptomatic phase may resolve spontaneously or with treatment or progress to a more advanced stage of neurosyphilis (see also p. 441).

Meningovascular syphilis. In the early stages of meningovascular syphilis, there may be a cloudy gray exudate within the leptomeninges, usually more prominent at the base of the brain and, to a lesser extent, along the blood vessels over the cerebral convexities. Occasionally, the cloudiness may be in patches or more diffuse. The characteristic exudate is one composed primarily of lymphocytes, plasma cells, and large mononuclear cells, all with a tendency toward adventitial and perivascular concentration (Fig. 48-53). It is said that in about 5% of the patients, the disease may begin as a severe acute meningitis. In these, the exudate is more abundant and, in addition, the characteristic cellular infiltrate also contains neutrophils and fibrin. After adequate therapy and possibly spontaneously, the exudate becomes organized with patches or even extensive areas of fibrosis.

A significant part of the leptomeningeal infection is the accompanying involvement of the smaller arteries. In the more severe infections, the inflammatory cells migrate into the media, separate the muscle fibers, split the internal elastic lamina, and stimulate a reactive intimal hyperplasia and endothelial hypertrophy (Heubner's endarteritis and panarteritis). These vascular changes, depending on their numbers, degree, and rapidity of involvement, can produce numerous small or large anemic infarcts.

General paresis (paretic dementia, etc.). General paresis is a form of progressive syphilitic meningoencephalitis. Adequate therapy only halts its progression. With the early or minimal lesion, no gross abnormalities may be recognized. In the usual patient, however, there is patchy or diffuse thickening of the leptomeninges and cortical atrophy, often more noticeable over the frontal lobes. There may be a characteristic but nondiagnostic granularity of the ependyma lining the moderately enlarged ventricles. The floor of the fourth ventricle may have a thickened, gray appearance because of a highly characteristic, diffuse astrocytic glial proliferation.

The meningeal exudate is identical with that seen in syphilitic meningitis and usually is accompanied by the typical vasculitis. Within the brain, the lesions are more concentrated in the cerebral cortex and in the central gray matter than in the white matter. The intensity of the reactions roughly parallels the degree of overlying leptomeningeal involvement. The vessels within these areas and, to a lesser degree, those of the underlying white matter are surrounded by lymphocytes, plasma cells, and a few large mononuclear cells. Their walls are greatly thickened, and their lumens narrowed because of endothelial hyperplasia and hypertrophy. As a result, many nerve cells are lost or in varying stages of ischemic change, and there is proliferation and rodlike elongation of the surrounding microglial cells. As the lesions undergo resolution and organization, they resemble microscopic infarcts with loss of cells, leading to focal collapse of the cortex, and distortion of the normal layering of the residual cells. There is a pronounced reactive astrocytosis. Iron-containing pigment in macrophages and in the walls of cortical blood vessels is highly characteristic of general paresis. In Lissauer's type of general paresis, there is an associated spongy destruction of the upper cortical layers and chromatolytic changes in some nerve cells of the fifth and sixth layers. In the untreated patient, spirochetes may be found singly and in clusters about the blood vessels and in the cortex.

With treatment, demonstrable spirochetes rapidly disappear. The cellular exudate and the vascular changes decrease far more slowly. Leptomeningeal scars, the disseminated focal cortical atrophy and characteristic cortical disorganization, the ependymal granularity, the gliosis of the floor of the fourth ventricle, and the iron granules in macrophages and walls of the cortical blood vessels are the unalterable structural remnants of the disease.

Tabes dorsalis. The spinal cord in the patient with syphilis may be involved separately or in combination with the brain. Of the several patterns of spinal cord involvement, tabes dorsalis has been the most frequent. The exact site of syphilitic inflammation that results in degeneration of the fasciculi graciles and sometimes of the fasciculi cuneati and of the dorsal roots is not known. One hypothesis suggests localization of the toxic effects of the spirochetes on the dorsal rootlets as they pass through the Obersteiner-Redlich area. The second assumes that there is involvement of the cells of the spinal ganglia and the fibers from these cells entering the spinal cord. In both hypotheses, the caudalmost portion of the spinal cord is affected earliest and to the greatest degree.

The gross appearance of the spinal cord is characteristic but not diagnostic. The posterior columns are smaller than normal, often with dorsal concavity rather than convexity. Spe-

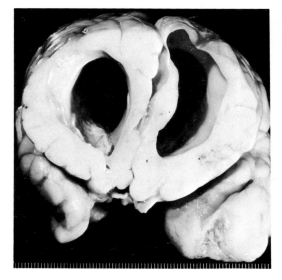

Fig. 48-54. Toxoplasmosis. Conspicuous internal hydrocephalus, obstructive, with numerous subependymal calcifications, in 2-year-old child.

cial stains reveal the absence of axons and myelin sheaths in the affected tracts. With tabes dorsalis, the optic nerves are often similarly involved. The exact site of the lesion that produces the Argyll Robertson pupil seen in this disease is not known.

The spinal cord may be affected in a variety of patterns that are less frequent and less characteristic of syphilis. These are attributed to differing localizations of lesions that extend into the cord from the leptomeninges and from variations in the sites of the vasculitis.

Toxoplasmosis[57,144]

A disease with worldwide distribution, toxoplasmosis is most often recognized in infants. It may, however, be the cause of a febrile or unsuspected disease in adults. The causative agent is the protozoan *Toxoplasma gondii*. The infant is infected in utero during the short period of parasitemia in the early stages of the disease in the mother who may be asymptomatic. Fetal infection and damage are highest when maternal infection occurs during the first and second trimesters of pregnancy. Serologic tests become positive after the period of infectivity. Infections and clinical disease are increasing in incidence in adults treated with immunosuppressive drugs. Cats are considered to be the animal host.

The inflammatory aqueductal stenosis in the infant results in an obstructive hydrocephalus (Fig. 48-54); microcephaly has been described

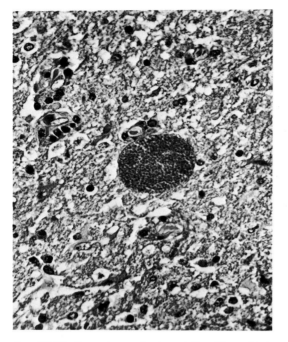

Fig. 48-55. Toxoplasmosis, in adult with multiple myeloma. "Cyst" formation containing many organisms. (Hematoxylin and eosin; 370×.)

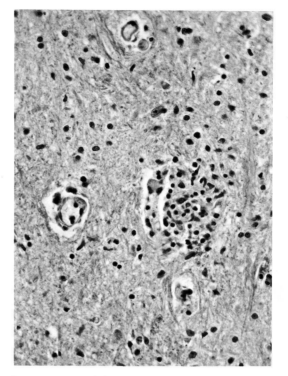

Fig. 48-56. Nodule of lymphocytes and mononuclear cells about wall of a capillary in patient with scrub typhus. (Hematoxylin and eosin; 280×.)

in some newborns. There may be necrotic paraventricular basal ganglionic lesions that lead to mineralization often visible by x-ray examination. In the adult there are multiple small areas of necrosis within the central portions of the brain. Involvement of the surface of the brain is associated with a focal chronic (lymphocytic) leptomeningitis. The ovoid organisms, which are 4 to 6 μm long and 2 μm wide, usually are found in clusters in the cytoplasm of a mononuclear macrophage. This is known as the pseudocyst (Fig. 48-55). The areas of necrosis in which the organisms are found and from which they may be cultured are surrounded by varying degrees of mononuclear cells and reactive astrocytosis.

In infants, other organs such as the eye or the myocardium often are affected as well. In adults, the lungs and lymph nodes usually are involved (see also p. 536).

Rickettsial encephalitides

Focal collections of a few neutrophils with lymphocytes and mononuclear macrophages in and about the walls of the smaller blood vessels in the brain are known as typhus nodules and are the characteristic but not diagnostic lesions in the rickettsial diseases (Fig. 48-56). Hypertrophy and hyperplasia of the endo-

thelial cells result from the intraendothelial multiplication of the rickettsias. These are the lesions characteristic of typhus fever caused by *Rickettsia prowazekii* (see also p. 454).

In Rocky Mountain spotted fever caused by *Rickettsia rickettsii*,[162] the inflammatory and vascular changes are usually more severe, whereas in scrub typhus caused by *Rickettsia orientalis,* the vascular lesions are fewer and less severe.

Viral infections[48,84]

Human viral infections were expected to almost disappear with the use of the poliomyelitis vaccines. This has not occurred. Increased numbers of mild, severe, and fatal viral encephalitides are now recognized. The basic similarities of the structural changes in the central nervous system in all viral diseases are ascribed to the obligate intracellular position of the viruses.

When the injury is recent or mild, the infected nerve cells become slightly swollen, later to undergo shrinkage and neuronophagia by surrounding mononuclear cells. The later changes are accompanied by a perivascular

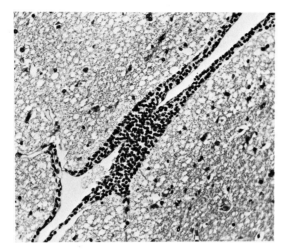

Fig. 48-57. Chronic encephalitis, viral type. (Hematoxylin and eosin; 90×.)

inflammatory cell infiltrate, which initially and transiently may be neutrophilic. Later and more characteristically, the cellular infiltrates are composed of lymphocytes, some plasmacytoid cells, and large mononuclear cells and macrophages (Fig. 48-57). Variations in this pattern are dependent on the locations of the cells, including glial as well as nerve cells, that are affected and the degree of necrosis of cells and surrounding tissues. In some of the viral infections, intranuclear or intracytoplasmic inclusion bodies may be formed within nerve and glial cells. Cowdry type A intranuclear inclusions (Fig. 48-67) may be found in the encephalitides caused by the measles virus, herpes simplex, cytomegalic inclusion disease, and herpes zoster. The relationship of Cowdry type B inclusion bodies to viral diseases is not certain.

When the infection is limited to nerve cells, the central nervous system grossly may appear unchanged or, at most, focally or diffusely engorged. With a necrotizing encephalitis that includes destruction of white and gray matter, the nervous system early is enlarged, swollen, and engorged. The areas of necrosis that follow may be small and scattered or large, extending beyond the boundaries of an area supplied by a single or several blood vessels. In addition to the usual cellular infiltrate, there may be a pronounced reactive astrocytosis and a lesser gliosis.

Acute poliomyelitis (infantile paralysis). The sharp decrease in incidence of acute poliomyelitis in the past several years is one of the triumphs of medicine. Poliomyelitis is consid-

ered here because it is a prototype of the viral diseases. Formerly, it occurred both sporadically and more frequently in epidemics during the summer and autumn. The enterovirus enters the body through the gastrointestinal tract, from which, by way of the bloodstream, it spreads to involve the central nervous system. There is an incubation period of 7 to 10 days (see also p. 467).

Alterations in the central nervous system vary with the intensity and duration of the illness. The nerve cells characteristically affected are the large anterior horn cells of the spinal cord, particularly those at the cervical and lumbar enlargements. With a more severe and usually fatal disease, the large nerve cells of the brainstem motor nuclei are affected (bulbar poliomyelitis), and in the most severe forms the large nerve cells of the motor cortex are involved, as well as cells in the thalamus and hypothalamus and brainstem. It has never been clear why only some cells in each area may be affected. Because of the similarity of change at all levels, it has been assumed that the cells were infected at one time.

The gross and microscopic appearances are those previously described for the nonnecrotizing encephalomyelitis. In the early and rapidly fatal disease, there is vascular engorgement of the affected areas. There may be a few neutrophils in the leptomeninges and about some vessels within the affected areas. These are soon replaced by a considerable amount of perivascular lymphocytic infiltrates. The early swollen nerve cells rapidly undergo neuronophagia by large mononuclear cells. Loss of nerve cells is followed by degeneration of the axons and their sheaths with neurogenic atrophy of the muscles they innervate. The healed lesion is represented by a selective loss of nerve cells, collapse of the area, and focal astrocytic gliosis.

Other enteroviral encephalomyelitides. Other enteroviruses are often the cause of infections of the central nervous system. These include a large group of coxsackieviruses and the echovirus. One, the coxsackievirus type A7, is known to produce a disease that is structurally inseparable from that produced by the poliomyelitis viruses. The usual illness, however, is nonparalytic and generalized, sometimes with a myalgia or encephalalgia.

Epidemic encephalitides. The epidemic encephalitides are a group of diseases that occur in epidemics and are presumed to be of viral origin. Among these is the lethargic encephalitis of von Economo, which may be ascribed to several different viruses. Others included in this group are St. Louis encephalitis and equine encephalitis (see also p. 470).

The localization of the pathologic changes varies greatly. In the von Economo type, the lesions characteristically affect the brainstem most severely; the parkinsonian state may occur after an interval of weeks to years. The microscopic changes include nerve cell degeneration and adventitial infiltrates composed of lymphocytes, plasmacytoid cells, and large mononuclear cells; a few may persist for years after the onset of the disease.

Necrotizing and sclerosing encephalitides. The necrotizing encephalitides have been reported under a variety of names, including Dawson's inclusion body encephalitis, von Bogaert's subacute sclerosing leukoencephalitis, and Pette-Döring panencephalitis. One of these diseases is currently designated as subacute sclerosing panencephalitis. Formerly considered to be caused by the herpes simplex virus, recent evidence is strongly suggestive that the measles virus is the cause.[19,71,82,89,124,133,141,164] The virus is believed to lay dormant in the individual, usually a child, for a period, sometimes years, after which it is reactivated. It characteristically destroys cortical nerve cells and supporting glia and may even involve the cells of the central gray matter, pons, and cerebellum. The disease is gradually progressive, with death in months to a few years. Cowdry type A intranuclear inclusions may be found in affected nerve cells and glia with a perivascular, usually mononuclear infiltration containing macrophages. A reactive astrocytosis in the affected areas is prominent.

The necrotizing encephalitis caused by the herpes simplex virus is characterized by extensive necrosis with some hemorrhage in the limbic lobe of the brain[80] (Fig. 48-58). The active portions of the disease exhibit the usual mixed mononuclear perivascular infiltrates. Cowdry type A inclusion bodies may be seen and are more likely to be found in oligodendrocytes than in the rapidly destroyed neurons (Fig. 48-59). There is a moderate, loose reactive astrocytosis. Cytomegalic inclusion disease[70,159] is caused by the cytomegalic virus, a large DNA virus of the herpes subgroup. In the brain, there are areas of necrosis that are predominantly periventricular, frequently with mineralization (calcification). There is little cellular response. The Cowdry type A intranuclear inclusions are exceedingly large and prominent; intracytoplasmic inclusions are also to be found. The disease may be generalized

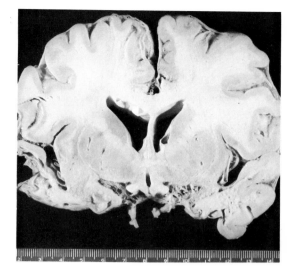

Fig. 48-58. Chronic necrotizing encephalitis caused by herpes simplex. Necrosis of temporal lobes, insula, and cingulate gyri.

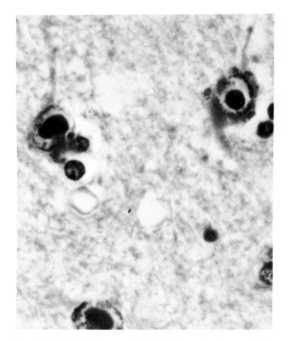

Fig. 48-59. Viral encephalitis. Cowdry type A intranuclear inclusions in nerve cells. (Hematoxylin and eosin; 1100×.)

and present acutely and in a fulminant fashion. Although the infection occurs most frequently in newborn infants infected by their asymptomatic mothers, it has been recognized in adults in whom there is an impaired immune response.

Lymphocytic choriomeningitis. The virus of lymphocytic choriomeningitis produces moderate lymphocytic infiltrations in the leptomeninges, choroid plexuses, and vessels beneath the ependyma. It appears to be transmitted to man through the urine of infected mice that act as the host reservoir. The disease, rarely fatal in man, also has been called benign lymphocytic meningitis. Diagnosis usually is made by the presence of a rising titer of specific neutralizing antibodies.

Progressive multifocal leukoencephalopathy.[6,163] Progressive multifocal leukoencephalopathy is a recently recognized and as yet uncommon disease. Initially described as occurring particularly in patients with neoplastic diseases of the reticuloendothelial system, especially chronic lymphatic leukemia, and in sarcoidosis, it has now been seen in association with a variety of diseases, including "senility." Further reports have suggested that the etiologic agent is a slow (SV40) virus that is able to produce disease only in a patient with a greatly depressed immune response.

In the fixed specimen, the islandlike multiple lesions affecting the brain and spinal cord have a granular gray appearance. In only half of the reported cases are there perivascular cellular infiltrates consisting of lymphocytes and plasmacytoid cells. The viruses destroy the oligodendrocytes within the lesion while some at the periphery may contain an eosinophilic intranuclear inclusion. The nuclei of many of the surrounding astrocytes are enlarged, bizarre, irregular, and hyperchromatic, highly suggestive of an early stage of neoplastic transformation.

DISEASES OF MYELIN

Myelin diseases are a group of disorders of the oligodendrocytes in which the effects are more apparent upon myelin, the cell membrane. The surrounded axons are completely or relatively spared; when they are affected, it follows involvement of the myelin. Neither clinical nor etiologic classifications have been satisfactory because of overlapping clinical appearances and because the causes are either unknown or in dispute. The diseases have been categorized as demyelinating (i.e., myelinoclastic) or dysmyelinating (leukodystrophy, i.e., disorders of myelin formation).[129]

Demyelinating diseases

Multiple sclerosis (disseminated sclerosis, insular sclerosis). Multiple sclerosis is the most common of the demyelinating diseases and is among the most common primary diseases of the central nervous system. It is characteristically chronic and relapsing, although acute and unremitting forms occur.[147,166] Of the innumerable theories concerning its cause, those associated with disorders of blood vessels, with developmental defects of the glia, and with a great variety of toxic agents are no longer seriously considered. Currently, the theories most supported are those related to autoimmunity and to viral infection. The increased prevalence in the colder latitudes, in families one of whose members has the disease, and the exacerbations and remissions, often years apart, have defied explanation. Seen at all ages after childhood, onset is more common between the ages of 20 and 40 years. Both sexes are affected, women more frequently and at an earlier age. The mean duration of the disease is over 20 years.

In the chronic relapsing form, the gross appearance of the central nervous system is usually diagnostic. The brain is either normal in size or slightly atrophic, and the spinal cord is variably small. Lesions in the white matter are, on the cut surface, slightly depressed, gray to gray-pink, and sharply demarcated. Although these lesions (plaques) are more easily seen in the white matter, they

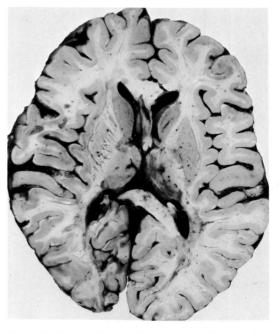

Fig. 48-60. Multiple sclerosis, chronic relapsing type with numerous plaques. Plaques in all characteristic areas. Cortex and U fibers involved in several areas.

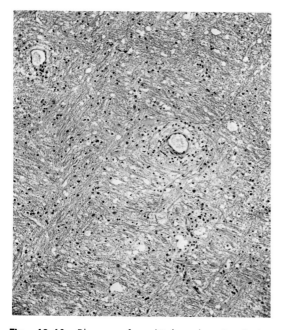

Fig. 48-61. Plaque of multiple sclerosis. Active lesion with perivascular lymphocytes. Slightly lighter staining area in lower half of section is plaque. (Hematoxylin and eosin; 90×.)

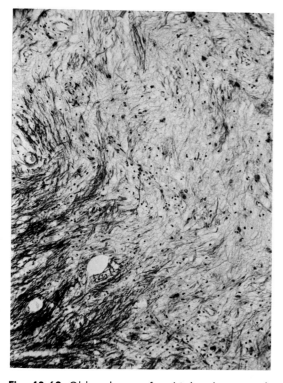

Fig. 48-62. Older plaque of multiple sclerosis with loss of myelin and retention of some axons in lighter-staining area. (Luxol-fast blue–silver nitrate; 135×.)

extend into the gray matter in almost every patient (Fig. 48-60). Plaques vary in size, shape, number, and position. In almost all patients, however, some plaques are seen with their bases at the angles of the lateral ventricles and with their apices toward the cortex. Plaques are frequently in the central and convolutional white matter of the brain and in the brainstem, cerebellum, and spinal cord.

All stages of the plaque development may be found in the patient in relapse. Perivascular lymphocytes and plasmacytoid cells (Fig. 48-61) characterize the acute lesions, with spillover of the cells into the leptomeninges in some instances. The degree and stages of oligodendroglial injury with myelin destruction and loss are seen with routine as well as with special stains (Fig. 48-62). In the slightly older and active lesions, there is a decrease in the myelin staining with swollen myelin. Here, in addition to the usual inflammatory cells, are macrophages with fragments of myelin, metachromatic granules, or neutral fat. The older and inactive lesions are sharply demarcated regions of myelin loss without inflammatory cells. Although the plaques are devoid of oligodendroglia, variable number of axons remain and are surrounded by a mild to moderate increase in astrocytes whose fibrillary processes follow the original axonal pattern (isomorphic gliosis).

Diffuse sclerosis (Schilder's disease, cerebral sclerosis, encephalitis periaxialis diffusa). In contrast with multiple sclerosis, in almost half

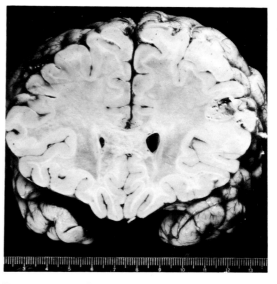

Fig. 48-63. Diffuse sclerosis. Extensive loss of myelin in both frontal lobes.

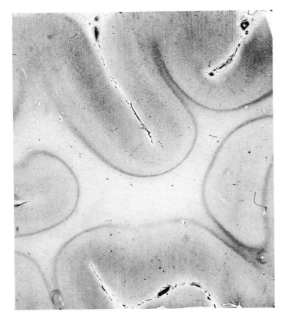

Fig. 48-64. Diffuse sclerosis. Partial retention of U fibers. (Mahon stain; 8×.)

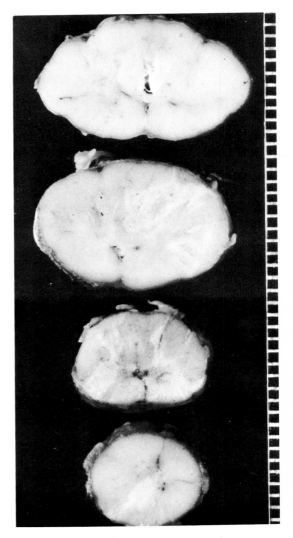

Fig. 48-65. Spinal cord in neuromyelitis optica.

of the patients with diffuse sclerosis the onset of disease occurs before the age of 10 years, with the mean duration of life being 6 years. The disease has been described in older adults. There is usually bilateral but not necessarily symmetric involvement of the white matter of the cerebral hemispheres (Fig. 48-63), especially that of the occipital lobes. The lesions are sharply demarcated, often spare the subcortical U fibers (Fig. 48-64), and unite with each other across the corpus callosum. The older lesions frequently have areas of cavitation.

The cellular response and destruction of myelin follow the same pattern as that seen in multiple sclerosis. Many axons are swollen, fragmented, and destroyed, whereas others are preserved. Reactive astrocytes are usually fibrillary, but many are gemistocytic and some are multinucleate. Axonal degeneration secondary to severe injury to the axons may be seen.

Intermediate or transitional form. In *neuromyelitis optica* (Devic's disease, neuro-ophthalmomyelitis), the spinal cord (Fig. 48-65) and the optic nerves and chiasm are the principal sites of clinical and anatomic involvement. Like diffuse sclerosis, the disease is more common in the young (under 10 years of age) but is also seen in older individuals. Although the disease is usually unremitting and progressive, it may become stationary or have

relapses. The anatomic findings support an intermediate position of this disease between diffuse sclerosis on the one hand and multiple sclerosis on the other.

Many segments of the spinal cord usually are involved at one or more levels. Early, the affected white matter is swollen, soft, and slightly pink. Older lesions are depressed and gray, and some that are large may be cavitated. The optic nerves and chiasm are similarly affected. Both portions of the nervous system may be at the same stage or in different stages of involvement and may be affected equally, or, as is more usual, unequally. In some patients there may be lesions in other parts of the brain identical with those of multiple sclerosis.

The microscopic changes in the typical patient vary from the characteristic plaques of multiple sclerosis in all of its stages to those of diffuse sclerosis with areas of necrosis and with axonal degeneration.

Acute perivenous encephalomyelitis (postvaccinal encephalomyelitis, postexanthematous encephalomyelitis). A disseminated infectious or postvaccinal encephalomyelitis may appear during the course of or shortly after recovery from several exanthems, such as chickenpox, German measles, or smallpox and, rarely, after inoculations against smallpox, rabies, and typhoid. Although most of these illnesses are caused by viruses, none has, as yet, been identified in patients with postvaccinal encephalomyelitis.

The clinical and pathologic similarities of the involvement of the central nervous system and the uniform structural change have suggested an autoimmune response on the part of the central nervous system or the activation of a latent virus. In the fatal case, the central nervous system is hyperemic, slightly swollen, and with an occasional petechial hemorrhage. Micoscopically the lesions appear to be mainly confined to the white matter. Early, the congested vessels are surrounded by a few neutrophils that are soon replaced by lymphocytes and plasmacytoid cells. Macrophages, some containing lipid, occur during the later stages of the disease. The loss of myelin about the veins and the relatively undamaged axons are usually only to be recognized with special stains. The disease is not progressive.

Acute necrotizing hemorrhagic encephalitis (acute hemorrhagic leukoencephalitis, acute hemorrhagic leukoencephalopathy).[79] This is a rare, usually rapidly fatal disorder that is often preceded by a nondescript infection, characteristically respiratory, from which the patient is recovering or has recovered. The brain is congested and swollen, with many isolated and confluent petechiae in the white matter. The lesions often involve one portion of the brain to a greater degree than another (Fig. 48-66).

On microscopic examination, the walls of the small vessels are necrotic, with edema of the surrounding brain. Early, there are variable numbers of neutrophils and fibrin in the necrotic vessel walls. Lymphocytes and plasma cells later replace the neutrophils because the surrounding edematous and hemorrhagic brain also undergoes necrosis. Death usually supervenes before macrophages are to be found. This condition may represent a severe form of perivenous encephalomyelitis.

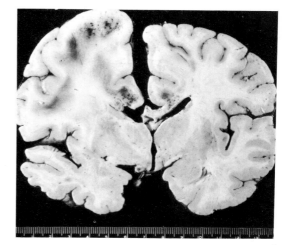

Fig. 48-66. Acute hemorrhagic leukoencephalitis, predominantly unilateral. (Courtesy Dr. J. Langston; from Chason, J. L.: In Saphir, O., editor: A text on systemic pathology, vol. 2, New York, 1958, Grune & Stratton, Inc.; by permission.)

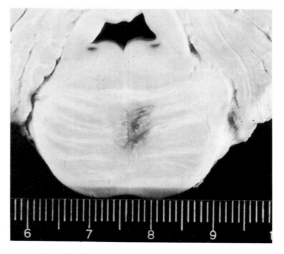

Fig. 48-67. Central pontine myelinolysis.

Central pontine myelinolysis.[26,99] Described first in 1959, it has been associated with alcoholism, malnutrition, disturbances of electrolytes and water, extraneural infections, local venous obstruction, and unidentified agents. The lesion occurs in the central portion of the base of the pons, with its greatest transverse diameter at the level of the external origins of the trigeminal nerves (Fig. 48-67). Rostrally, the plaque may reach almost into the midbrain. Its caudal extent generally spares the lowermost pons. The well-formed lesion is granular, gray, well demarcated, and depressed.

On coronal section, it is diamond shaped, triangular with its base dorsal, or cylindric. In some, only a poorly defined gray change is noted at the appropriate level. The area is pale with the routine hematoxylin and eosin stain and with occasional lipophages in the early and active lesions. Special stains disclose loss of myelin and retention of most, if not all, of the axons. Metachromatic granular material may be seen early. In some plaques, the myelin going in one direction may be lost, with sparing of the myelin sheathing fibers running in another direction. Oligodendrocytes are decreased to absent in the lesion. Reactive astrocytosis and gliosis are usually minimal.

Leukodystrophies

The leukodystrophies are metabolic diseases characterized by a disturbance in the formation of myelin (dysmyelinating diseases). They have been considered to be genetically determined and are often familial. There is a similarity in some to the lipidoses. The leukodystrophies differ from the demyelinating diseases in that the lesions are likely to be bilateral and symmetric, involve more of the nervous system, and occur in younger individuals. The subcortical U fibers are regularly spared, and the axons usually are destroyed. The biochemical criterion for this group of diseases is an increase in hexosamine content of the affected area. Whereas the leukodystrophies are similar in appearance grossly, they have characteristic microscopic features that permit their separation into subgroups. Only those that are generally accepted and are less rare are described below.

Metachromatic leukodystrophy (sulfatide lipidosis).[12,66,85,127,140] Metachromatic leukodystrophy is a disease of both children and adults. The basic defect in myelin metabolism is a deficiency of the enzyme arylsulfatase A. The involved areas of the white matter contain large amounts of a sulfatide that exhibits gamma metachromasia with the von Hirsch–Pfeiffer cresyl violet–acetic acid stain. A relationship to the lipidosis has been suggested because the abnormal material also has been found in tissues other than the central nervous system, including the cells of the liver and kidneys, the white blood cells, and cells of the gallbladder. Schwann cells of the peripheral nerves and the cells of nerve plexuses also are involved. The anatomic diagnosis often can be made by biopsy examination of a peripheral nerve (usually sural) or of the nerve plexuses (rectum). The specific stain done on frozen

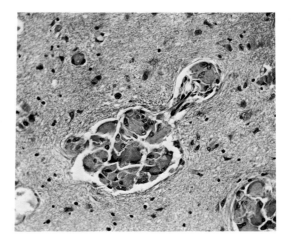

Fig. 48-68. Globoid sclerosis (Krabbe's disease). (Hematoxylin and eosin; 135×.)

sections with the presence of gamma metachromasia as described is diagnostic. Analysis of the more easily available urine, leukocytes, or fibroblasts in tissue cultures for the enzyme deficiency is a safer and more reasonable approach for diagnosis.

Globoid cell leukodystrophy (Krabbe's disease, globoid sclerosis). Globoid cell leukodystrophy is a disease that affects only the central nervous system of children. The accumulation of an abnormal PAS-positive material, possibly a cerebroside of the kerasin type, leads to the formation of large epithelioid and multinucleated giant cells (the globoid cells) (Fig. 48-68). The mononuclear cells are found in clusters of varying sizes about blood vessels, whereas the multinucleated cells occur more frequently in the affected white matter. Galactosyl ceramide-β-galactosyl hydrolase and other enzyme deficiencies have been described.[3]

Neutral fat leukodystrophy (sudanophilic leukodystrophy). Although neutral fat leukodystrophy resembles diffuse sclerosis, significant differences have suggested its inclusion with the dysmyelinating diseases. These include genetic background with a family history and increase in hexosamine in the affected area.

NEOPLASMS

No accurate statistics reporting the frequency of neoplasms of the central nervous system are available. Estimates based upon a variety of observations often include granulomas and are biased by the character of the hospital or clinic and by the interests of the clinician and pathologist. The estimate that 9.2% of all neoplasms (excluding those of the skin) are primary in the central nervous system is, at present, most reasonable.

Theories concerning the development of neoplasms elsewhere in the body have their counterparts in the nervous system. Early tumor classifications were based upon the cell rest theory of Cohnheim, in which neoplasms were believed to originate from activation of aberrant immature cells.[8,10] Cytologic similarities of neoplastic cells to those at different stages of maturation reinforced the opinions. Later classifications were based upon the belief that fully mature cells could be stimulated to reproduce and to dedifferentiate.[94] Experimental production of central nervous system lesions has not resolved these differences. The issues have become even more debatable by evidence that the structure of these neoplasms may be related to their position within the nervous system and that there is often a mixture of glial elements. Most modern classifications make use of both theories.

Gliomas

Tumors classified as gliomas should be limited only to those neoplasms whose origin is from the ectodermal supporting tissues (neuroglia) of the central nervous system. It has been customary, however, to include among these the medulloblastomas and the pineal neoplasms. The classification proposed in 1926 by Bailey and Cushing[10] was based upon the then current theories of histogenesis of the nervous system. The more recent classification proposed by Kernohan et al.[94] and, for the most part, adopted here includes interpretations of the suggestions of Willis and of Sherer. It is based upon the assumption that some gliomas arise by dedifferentiation of adult cells.

Astrocytic series

Astrocytoma, grade I. Among the grade I astrocytomas, which constitute about 15% of all gliomas, are the fibrillary, protoplasmic, and pilocytic types. Although these types differ as to the amount of visible cytoplasm and degree of production of neuroglial fibers, they have, in general, the same biologic behavior. They are relatively slow growing, with an average survival in excess of 3 years after the onset of symptoms. They may be found in any part of the central nervous system.

In adults, those neoplasms are usually in one of the cerebral hemispheres. In young adults and in children, the tumors are more frequent in the pons and cerebellum.[2,18,108] Those oc-

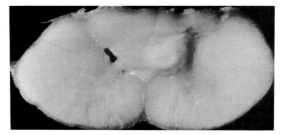

Fig. 48-69. Grade I astrocytoma (cytic) in cervical cord.

curring in the cerebrum and pons are solid, gray, and firm, with very poorly defined borders. Small cystic areas sometimes may be found in the tumors of the cerebrum. The cerebellar neoplasms more often are cystic. The cyst walls are surrounded by neoplastic cells in 60%, whereas in 40% only a mural nodule composed of neoplastic astrocytes is found.[18,108] The cavity contains a clear amber fluid high in protein. Similar but smaller lesions also occur in the spinal cord (Fig. 48-69).

The microscopic recognition of these neoplasms may be exceedingly difficult particularly at biopsy because of the following:

1. Astrocytes forming the tumors are within the cytologic limits of normality.
2. Mitoses are not found.
3. There is no area of necrosis or hemorrhage (except operative).
4. In the diffuse forms, normal-appearing nerve cells often are included within the lesion.
5. There are no changes of the blood vessels (see following) except an occasional perivascular scant lymphocytic cuff.

Diagnosis by biopsy is dependent on an evaluation of the history and the presence of increased numbers of astrocytes in the absence of an apparent cause for their numerical increase.

The boundaries of the neoplasms that are solid or diffuse are difficult to demarcate by microscopic study. The reasons are the very gradual centrifugal decrease in numbers of astrocytes and the absence of evidence of compression or destruction of the surrounding brain. In occasional neoplasms examined in detail, there are nests of enlarged and sometimes pleomorphic astrocytes and recognizable increases in blood vessels, some with proliferation of the endothelial and adventitial layers. These are interpreted as evidence of increased dedifferentiation and biologic activity.

Occasionally, a tumor of the cerebral hemispheres may be composed either entirely (less commonly) or in part by well-differentiated astrocytes with abundant eosinophilic cytoplasm. These are gemistocytic astrocytes. The biologic behavior of gemistocytic astrocytomas usually differs from those just described. These neoplasms rapidly undergo malignant dedifferentiation usually to grade III astrocytoma (glioblastoma multiforme). Because of this, it has been our practice to empirically add one cytologic grade to the neoplasm when clusters of these cells are found.

Astrocytoma grade II. This neoplasm has also been called astroblastoma because of the resemblance of many of its constitutent cells to astroblasts. It forms approximately 1% of all gliomas. More common in young adults than in children, these neoplasms are solid and gray-white to white. The macroscopically discernible apparent borders sometimes give rise to a false impression of sharp demarcation because of compression of the surrounding brain.

Microscopically, the tumor is more cellular than the lower grade astrocytoma. The cells are generally larger, and in many there are cells with one or more plump cell processes that radiate about the walls of the moderately increased numbers of blood vessels. Mitoses and areas of necrosis are rare. When the lesions are examined to include the gross line of demarcation, neoplastic cells singly and in groups can be found to extend well beyond this point.

The average postoperative survival of patients with grade II astrocytomas is approximately 2 years.

Astrocytoma grade III and grade IV. This group includes glioblastoma multiforme, spongioblastoma multiforme, polar spongioblastoma, monstrocellular or gigantocellular glioblastoma, etc. These highly malignant and uniformly fatal neoplasms constitute 50% to 60% of all gliomas. They are more common in adults and in the cerebral hemispheres. Beginning more often in white matter, they often appear to be well demarcated because the surrounding brain is compressed, swollen, and edematous. The neoplasm is usually slightly more firm than the adjacent tissue. Its surface has a variegated gray, white, yellow (necrotic), and reddish brown (hemorrhagic) appearance (Fig. 48-70). The tumors frequently extend into and across the corpus callosum into the opposite hemisphere. Multicentric origin (i.e., two or more separate neoplasms) has been described in 15%. However, on microscopic study, I have frequently found neoplastic cells connecting the grossly separate

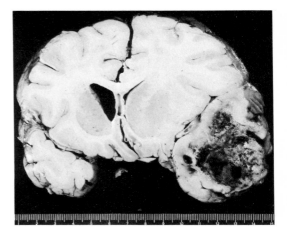

Fig. 48-70. Grade III astrocytoma in temporal lobe. Brain displacement with cingulate gyrus herniation and compression of lateral ventricle.

tumors. It is my experience that multicentric origin does not exceed 5%.

The microscopic appearance of these lesions usually is characterized by profuse numbers of pleomorphic and frequently bizarre cells (Fig. 48-71). Among these are many cells with enlarged and irregular nuclei. Some cells can be identified by their processes as being of astrocytic origin. Other cells may be small with oval, hyperchromatic nuclei resembling the undifferentiated small cells of a bronchogenic carcinoma. In other areas, there may be large cells with irregular large, vesicular nuclei and with an abundant eosinophilic cytoplasm suggesting an origin from gemistocytic astrocytes. In many areas within the neoplasm, one may find bizarre, multinucleate cells with abundant cytoplasm resembling strap cells of rhabdomyosarcomas. Mitoses, often abnormal, are usually easily found either in clusters or spread fairly regularly throughout the neoplasm. In many regions within the neoplasm, there are large and small areas of necrosis often with a garland of small cell nuclei at the periphery (Fig. 48-72). Blood vessels are greatly increased in numbers and usually with endothelial or adventitial hypertrophy and hyperplasia. Occasionally, vessels with these changes are found well beyond the apparent microscopic limits of the neoplasm.

Despite the apparent sharp gross demarcation, neoplastic cells extend far beyond these borders because of the infiltration from the tumor and perhaps also because of the continued dedifferentiation of the surrounding cells. A sudden increase in signs and symptoms in patients with these neoplasms usually can

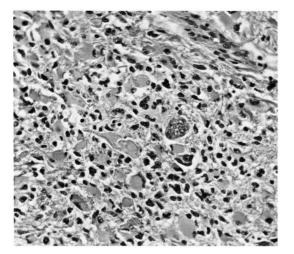

Fig. 48-71. Grade III astrocytoma. Gemistocytic astrocytes and multinucleate cells. (Hematoxylin and eosin; 280×.)

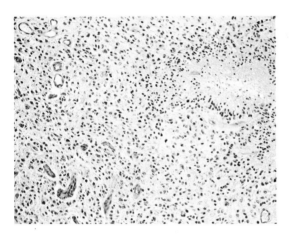

Fig. 48-72. Grade III astrocytoma. Area of necrosis with garland formation. Vascular proliferation. (Hematoxylin and eosin; 135×.)

be correlated with the occurrence of large areas of necrosis caused by the vascular changes, often with superimposed thromboses. Massive hemorrhages within the neoplasms less frequently cause rapid tumor enlargement and clinical deterioration.

Cells of any of the astrocytic neoplasms, but particularly those that are more malignant, may reach the subarachnoid or the ventricular spaces. From this point, they may spread by way of the ventricular and cerebrospinal fluid and implant in other portions of the central nervous system. The presence of free neoplastic cells recognized on cytologic examination of cerebrospinal fluid does not necessarily indicate

metastasis. Extracranial metastasis, though rare, is more apt to occur after operative removal of a portion of the neoplasm.

Most of the patients with a grade III astrocytoma live fewer than 18 months after diagnosis. More extensive surgical therapy has increased only the survival time—not the rate of cure.

In the rare cerebrospinal glioblastomatosis (gliomatosis cerebri), there may be no grossly visibly neoplasm or at most one or two poorly defined areas of enlargement usually within the brain, less often in the spinal cord. On microscopic examination there are multiple areas in the brain and spinal cord composed of bizarre, neoplastic astrocytes of the type seen in the grade III (and grade IV) astrocytomas. Most are so remote from possible implantation sites as to suggest that the lesions are multicentric in origin.

Ependymoma[60,91]

Approximately 5% of the intracranial gliomas are ependymomas, with 60% of the latter arising in the posterior fossa. In the spinal cord, 60% of the gliomas are of the ependymal group. Intracranial ependymomas have their origins from cells lining the ventricles, the choroid plexuses, and the cells of ependymal streaks that represent obliterated portions of the ventricles. In the spinal cord, they arise from the ependymal cells lining the central canal or its remnants and from the cells of the ventriculus terminalis in the filum terminale. It is also possible that these neoplasms may arise (usually mixed with other glial cells) from the cells of the subependymal plate.

These neoplasms are gray, moderately firm, and well demarcated from the adjoining compressed tissues (Fig. 48-73). Those in the fourth ventricle are usually solid, whereas those in the cerebral hemispheres and in the spinal cord are frequently cystic. Neoplasms of the choroid plexuses are gray-pink, fungating, and papillary. Ependymomas of the filum terminale are thinly encapsulated and cystic. The capsule may be breached in the larger lesions.

The microscopic appearances of these neoplasms are exceedingly variable among the tumors as a group and in different areas of the same tumor. Except for the choroid plexus papilloma, the most characteristic pattern of growth is the epithelial type whose cells line large tubular or ventricle-like spaces called "rosettes" (Fig. 48-74). The lining cells are cuboid to columnar, with the appearance of ependymal cells. In some areas, the cells line

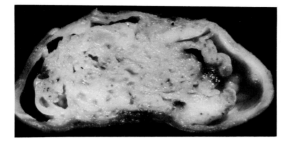

Fig. 48-73. Ependymoma of cervical portion of spinal cord. Residual spinal cord represented by peripheral rim of tissue.

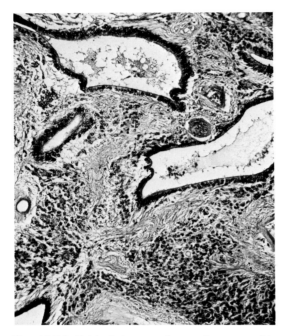

Fig. 48-74. Epithelial type of ependymoma with many rosettes. Tissue from that in Fig. 48-73. (Hematoxylin and eosin; 90×.)

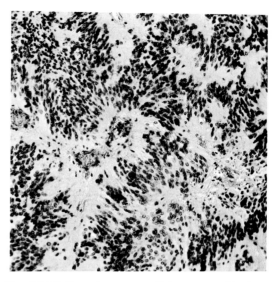

Fig. 48-75. Ependymoma, cellular type, with characteristic perivascular arrangement. (Hematoxylin and eosin; 90×.)

pattern, except for occasional cells whose processes radiate about a blood vessel[91] (Fig. 48-75).

There are two varieties of papillary ependymomas: choroid plexus type and myxopapillary type. These tumors are formed by cuboid to columnar cells lining a central core of connective tissue containing a capillary. In the *choroid plexus papilloma,* the structure is very similar to that of a normal choroid plexus with the exception that the epithelial cells are taller and larger than those of the normal plexus (Fig. 48-76). The *myxopapillary type* can occur throughout the cerebrospinal axis and even in the hollow of the sacrum, but it is far more frequent at the level of the cauda equina. The vascular and connective tissue cores of the papillae have undergone a great degree of myxoid change.

In approximately one third of the ependymomas, there are nests of cells with the appearance of oligodendrocytes.

Histologic grading of this group of neoplasms was developed by Kernohan and Uihlein[92] using the same general criteria described with the astrocytoma group. The prognosis, however, is more dependent on the site of origin than on the histologic dedifferentiation, and therefore these neoplasms are usually not graded.

Medulloepitheliomas are neoplasms that are believed to originate from residual cells of the embryonic medullary canal. These tumors are exceedingly rare. Their structural similarities

what has been interpreted as representative of a small portion of a poorly formed space, a partial rosette. Blepharoplasts are structures that represent the cytoplasmic residua of cilia. They may be found in some cells when stained with Mallory's phosphotungstic acid–hematoxylin and examined under high magnification (oil). Blepharoplasts are small, circular, or rod-shaped structures surrounded by a narrow unstained halo. They lie in that portion of the cell cytoplasm that is directed toward the lumen of the rosette. In other areas of the neoplasm and in other ependymomas, the tumors are formed by a diffuse proliferation of polygonal cells without a characteristic

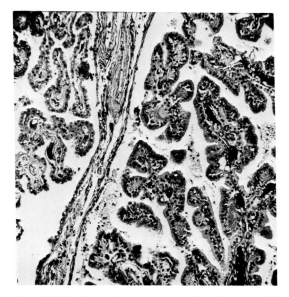

Fig. 48-76. Ependymoma, choroid plexus papilloma type. Larger papillary projections to the right of the lining represent the neoplasm. Lesion was in left cerebellopontine angle. (Hematoxylin and eosin; 90×.)

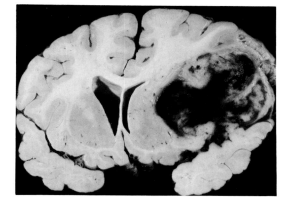

Fig. 48-77. Oligodendroglioma with operative hemorrhage. Brain and ventricular displacement with cingulate gyrus herniation.

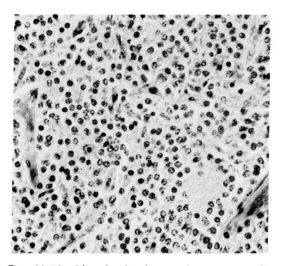

Fig. 48-78. Oligodendroglioma. Compartmentalization of cells by blood vessels. Some cells have nonstaining halos. (Hematoxylin and eosin; 280×.)

to the ependymomas makes their separation difficult, if not impossible.

Oligodendrogliomas[9,158]

Like the ependymomas, the oligodendrogliomas constitute about 5% of all gliomas. They are slow-growing tumors that are found in the white matter of a cerebral hemisphere of an adult, most frequently during the fourth or fifth decade of life. The tumors are gray-pink, well demarcated, and soft and frequently extend into the leptomeninges locally. About 20% are cystic, and in most the neoplastic tissue entirely surrounds the cyst. Areas of necrosis, hemorrhage, and mineralization are common in the larger lesions (Fig. 48-77). Mineralization (calcification) in the walls of the blood vessels and in larger confluent masses is visible on x-ray films in some 40% and is found on microscopic examination in 70%.

The usually described neoplastic cell has a lymphocyte-like nucleus surrounded by a clear, nonstaining halo with a definite cell membrane (Fig. 48-78). Groups of these cells produce the characteristic honeycombing. However, this appearance may be obscured in the better preserved areas of the neoplasm by the staining of the finely granular, slightly hematoxylinophilic cytoplasm. Compartmentalization of groups of tumors cells by blood vessels is commonly present and is characteristic. The border

zones of the neoplasms are relatively narrow but less well defined than the gross demarcation would suggest. Mitoses are rare. Their presence, sometimes in large numbers, in neoplasms containing cells with large pleomorphic nuclei has led some to classify the latter group as oligodendroblastomas.

Prognosis is related neither to the degree of mineralization nor to the cytologic appearance. Most patients live more than 4 years after clinical onset. Evidence of leptomeningeal spread is commonly found at necropsy and may be related to previous operative treatment.

Astrocytes frequently are found within these neoplasms, predominantly about blood vessels, perhaps serving as stromal support. In almost one third, there are nests of ependyma-like cells.

Medulloblastoma (neuroblastoma, granuloblastoma)[31,87,137]

Medulloblastomas are highly malignant and uniformly fatal neoplasms whose origin is restricted to the cerebellum. Representing approximately 8% of all neuroglial neoplasms, they occur predominantly in children. The greatest incidence is in those 5 to 9 years of age; with another increase in incidence occurring between the ages of 20 to 24 years. Males are affected more than twice as frequently as females. Familial occurrences, including tumors in identical twins, have been described. In children, most of the tumors originate in the region of the cerebellar vermis, possibly from microscopic remnants of the external granular layer of the cerebellum. In the older patients, the tumors may arise from one of the hemispheres.

Medulloblastomas are gray-pink to red, soft, friable, and often hemorrhagic and necrotic. Demarcation from the adjacent cerebellum is usually sharp. Because of the sites of origin, the fourth ventricle is almost regularly filled by the rapidly growing neoplasm, often with extensions of the tissue into and through the lateral recesses, the posterior roof of the fourth ventricle, the cerebral aqueduct, and the tissues of the floor and walls of the fourth ventricle. Nodules and sheets of implanted neoplastic cells are frequent in the lateral and third ven-

tricles and in the subarachnoid space, particularly in the regions of the cauda equina because of spread via the cerebrospinal fluid (Fig. 48-80). These highly cellular neoplasms are composed of cells with small, round to oval, usually hyperchromatic nuclei. There is little visible cytoplasm (Fig. 48-79). The number of mitoses are variable. Although the neoplastic cells tend to grow about the blood vessels with necrosis at a distance, in most there is no special histologic pattern. Rosettes and a perivascular arrangement (pseudorosette) have been described, and evidences of continued maturation of some cells toward nerve cells and glial cells, though rare, may be seen.

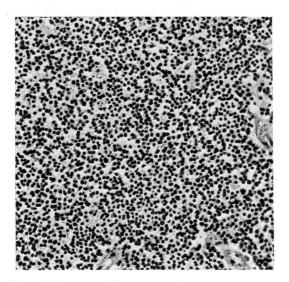

Fig. 48-79. Medulloblastoma originating in vermis of cerebellum. (Hematoxylin and eosin; 280×.)

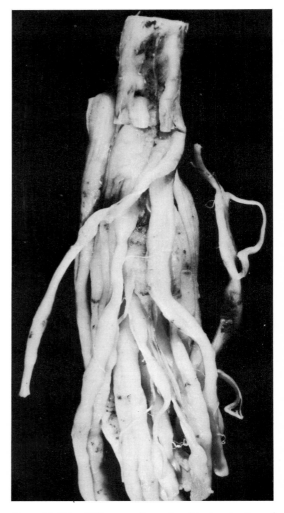

Fig. 48-80. Diffuse subarachnoid implants of medulloblastoma onto filaments of cauda equina. Every filament is covered with the implants; they are 5 to 20 times thicker than they should be.

Differences in the cytologic appearance and the histogenic pattern led some to the opinion that the group of neoplasms that lie predominantly in the leptomeninges are cerebellar sarcomas. Others have concluded that the atypical features are attributable to spread and growth of cells of a medulloblastoma in the confines of the subarachnoid space.[114]

Pinealoma (germinoma, teratoma, pineoblastoma, pineocytoma, pineal neuroblastoma, etc.)[40]

There are many classifications and interpretations of the 0.5% of all primary intracranial neoplasms that originate in and about the pineal gland. The cysts (dermoid) and the gliomas should be so identified and designated. The very small group of neoplasms remaining are the pinealomas (germinomas) (Fig. 48-81). The component cells are of two types. There are large, pale polyhedral to spheroid cells separated into lobules by vascular connective tissue trabeculae, next to which are small nests of cells with the appearance of lymphocytes. Those observers who recognize cells in transition between the two types diagnose them as pinealomas; others consider them as germinomas since the neoplasms are indistinguishable from seminomas (Fig. 48-82). When other structural components characteristic of teratomas are found, the interrelationship is apparent.

Mixed gliomas

Gliomas of more than one cell type are common. However, the predominance of one cell type usually permits classification into one of the groups previously described. There are other gliomas that arise from cells of the subependymal cell plate.[16,22] These neoplasms are

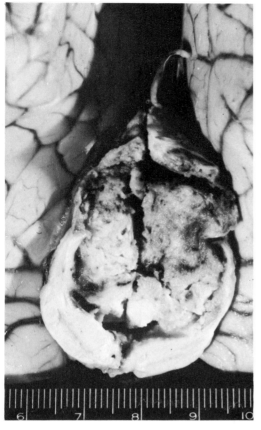

Fig. 48-81. Germinoma of pineal gland. Gross compression of midbrain.

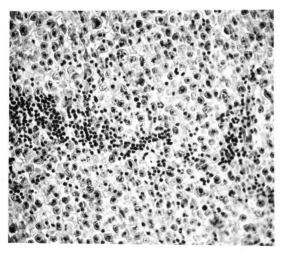

Fig. 48-82. Germinoma of pineal gland (pinealoma). (Hematoxylin and eosin; 135×.)

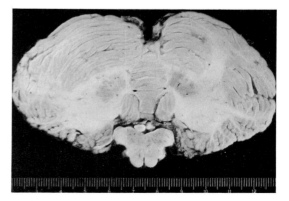

Fig. 48-83. Subependymal mixed gliomas arising in roof of fourth ventricle.

usually small, frequently multiple, and asymptomatic unless so strategically placed as to impede or obstruct the flow of cerebrospinal fluid. Although more common in the fourth ventricle (Fig. 48-83), identical neoplasms have been found in all parts of the ventricular system and about the central canal of the spinal cord. The tumors are solid, gray-white, well demarcated, firm, and sometimes mineralized. The larger neoplasms appear to be formed by the coalescence of smaller nodules of similar appearance. They are formed by plump spindle cells, some of which are in small clusters. Blepharoplasts have been demonstrated in some of the cells within the clusters. Though rosettes have been described, the usual arrangement is more like that of the obliterated central canal of the spinal cord. Surrounding these cell clusters, but also separately, are tight nodules of astrocytes with many fibrillary processes. These neoplasms have been classified as subependymal glomerate astrocytomas, as mixed subependymal gliomas, and as subependymomas. It is unexplained why most have occurred in adult males.

Ganglioglioma

Gangliogliomas are rare, usually slow-growing neoplasms that are usually composed of a mixture of neoplastic nerve cells and astrocytes. The structural criteria necessary for their diagnosis require the definite identification of neoplastic nerve cells rather than included normal cells. For this, it is generally required that binucleate and multinucleate nerve cells be present in addition to the neoplastic astrocytes and, less commonly, oligodendrocytes.

Craniopharyngioma (Rathke's pouch tumor, supracellular or epidermoid cyst, etc.)

Craniopharyngiomas form approximately 3% of all intracranial neoplasms. They appear to arise from squamous cell remnants of Rathke's pouch (Erdheim cell rests). These are cell nests that can be found at any level from the nasopharynx to the arachnoid covering the mammillary bodies. Although craniopharyngiomas may be seen at most ages, there are two peaks of incidence—one in late childhood and early adulthood and the other in the fifth decade.

The encapsulated tumor has a smooth, usually lobulated, gray surface. The sectioned surface is pale gray in the solid portions with one or more cysts filled with an amber to brown fluid containing cholesterol or grumous, yellow-gray material, or both (Fig. 48-84).

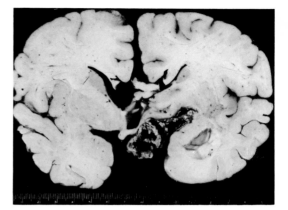

Fig. 48-84. Craniopharyngioma displacing floor of third ventricle and hypothalamus.

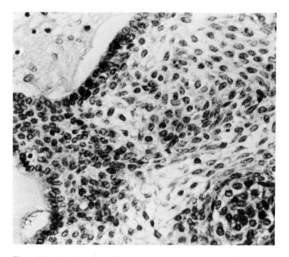

Fig. 48-85. Craniopharyngioma. Interior of islands with stellate cells and cuboid to columnar cells adjacent to stroma.

In almost two thirds, areas of mineralization or ossification can be found scattered throughout the solid portions of the tumor. Compression of the pituitary, optic chiasm, nerves, and tracts and elevation of the floor of the third ventricle are common.

The solid portions of the neoplasm are formed by a thin layer of dense connective tissue containing a mosaic of anastomosing sheets and cords of squamous cells. The inner portions of the epithelial structures are often loose and vacuolated, whereas the outer layers of cells are usually cuboid to cylindric. Liquefaction of the epithelial structure leads to the formation of the cystic spaces lined by stratified squamous epithelium (Fig. 48-85).

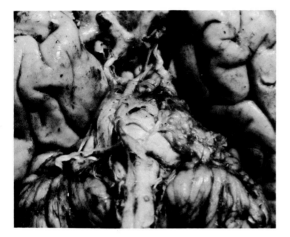

Fig. 48-86. Dermoid cyst. "Pearly" tumor is on left side of the ventral surface of pons near the cerebellopontine angle.

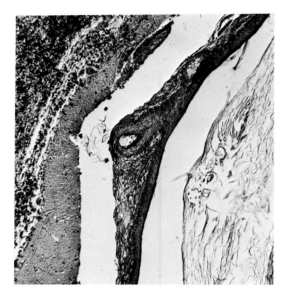

Fig. 48-87. Dermoid cyst. Stratified squamous epithelial lining of cyst contains hair follicle. Cyst lumen filled with keratin. (Hematoxylin and eosin; 90×.)

Dermoid and epidermoid cysts

It is generally conceded that the midline cysts of the dermoid and epidermoid varieties result from defects of closure of the neural tube with the heterotopic inclusion of the skin, sometimes with accessory skin structures. The cysts usually are found at or near the midline of the posterior fossa (Fig. 48-86), near the vermis, or even in the fourth ventricle. The small group of epidermoid cysts usually in the lateral positions at the base of the brain are

believed to represent portions of the linings of the sinuses trapped during closure of the bones of the skull.

The cysts are rounded and circumscribed, with an outer thin connective tissue wall and with an inner cavity filled with a thick, sticky, yellow material. A stratified squamous layer with keratohyaline granules and intercellular bridges lines the cavities of the epidermoid cyst. In the dermoid cyst (Fig. 48-87), the walls, in addition, contain sweat glands, sebaceous glands, hair follicles, or all three. Spread of the contents, usually postoperative, leads to the formation of multiple small nodules formed by keratin-containing foreign body giant cells.

This entire group of cysts comprises less than 1% of all primary intracranial neoplasms.

Colloid cyst (paraphyseal cyst)[74,143]

According to a recent study, there are two types of ependyma-lined cysts. Both are limited to the roof of the third ventricle. The more frequent type arises after closure of an ependymal pouch whose cuboid to columnar cells contain blepharoplasts or cilia. The second type, also lined by cuboid or columnar cells without blepharoplasts or cilia, is believed to arise because of persistence of the embryonic paraphyseal pouch. The cysts are spheric masses attached to the most rostral portion of the roof of the third ventricle midway between the interventricular foramina (Fig. 48-88).

Whatever their origin, the content of these cysts is usually gray and gelatinous. When brown, the color is the result of preceding hemorrhage. The inner lining of either type of cyst wall is formed by a single layer of cuboid to columnar cells. These cells are the source of the amorphous, eosinophilic, PAS-positive contents in which a few desquamated cells may be present. The outer cyst wall is formed by a thin fibrous connective tissue capsule that extends to the tela choroidea of the third ventricle. The autopsy incidence of about 2% of all intracranial tumors exceeds the clinical incidence of 0.5%, since only about one fourth of these neoplasms reach the clinically significant size of 1 cm.

Meningioma

Among all symptom-producing intracranial neoplasms, approximately 15% are classified as belonging to the meningiomas. This is a broad group of miscellaneous neoplasms with a variety of cells of origin.[36] Most have a dural

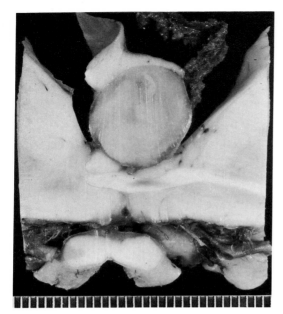

Fig. 48-88. Colloid cyst of third ventricle. Narrowed foramina of Monro are to either side of cyst.

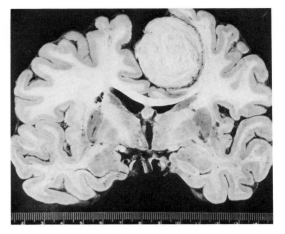

Fig. 48-89. Parasagittal meningioma, fibrous type. Small, remote anemic infarcts in internal capsules and left putamen.

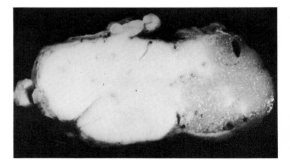

Fig. 48-90. Lipoma in leptomeninges of lumbar spinal cord. Lack of capsule on side of spinal cord is evident.

attachment and are relatively slow growing. They are slightly more common in women and in the fifth decade. In decreasing order of frequency, the meningiomas occur parasagittally (Fig. 48-89) over the cerebral convexities, laterally over the sphenoid ridges, medially in the olfactory grooves, and in the posterior fossa (cerebellopontine angle).

Based, as the classification has been, upon the anatomic site of origin of the tumor rather than upon its cytologic origin, it is surprising that reasonably accurate generalizations as to biologic behavior are possible.[27,75] Only one cell type, the arachnoid cap cell (meningocyte or meningothelial cell) is found solely in the leptomeninges. The remaining cells are those associated with the supporting tissues and blood vessels. Tumors arising from these cells have the appearance, both gross and microscopic, of similar tumors occurring elsewhere—i.e., fibroma, hemangioma, osteoma, chondroma, lipoma (Fig. 48-90), etc.—and therefore need no further description. The unencapsulated lipoma may represent a maldevelopment. About 90% to 95% of the meningiomas encountered are meningothelial, fibromatous, or inseparable mixtures of the two.

The meningothelial (meningocytic) meningioma is a thinly encapsulated, flat to spheric, moderately firm, yellow-gray, solid neoplasm usually firmly adherent at some point to the dura. The cell forming this type of neoplasm is polygonal, with poorly defined cell boundaries. Its centrally placed nucleus is relatively large and round and contains finely divided chromatin without an evident nucleolus. In some tumors, the cells are arranged in onionskin-like whorls or in sheets of varying sizes (Fig. 48-91). In the centers of many of the whorls and at the edges or within the sheets are capillaries or slightly larger blood vessels. Connective and elastic tissue and reticulin are confined to the blood vessel walls and act as a stroma supporting the neoplasm. Calcospheres (psammoma bodies) in varying numbers may be found in these neoplasms. They apparently represent a degenerative change with mineralization within the walls of blood vessels or tumor cells. When they predominate, the meningothelial meningioma is considered by some to be of the psammo-

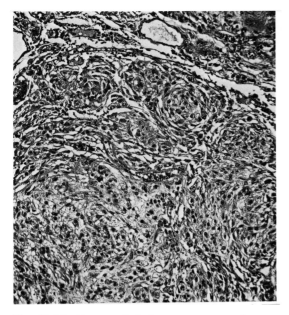

Fig. 48-91. Meningothelial meningioma with typical whorls. (Hematoxylin and eosin; 90×.)

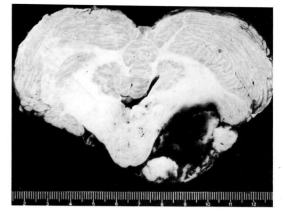

Fig. 48-92. Right cerebellopontine-angle schwannoma with recent operative hemorrhage. Compression and displacement of pons, cerebellum, and fourth ventricle.

matous type. This is a common occurrence at the spinal level, where it is associated with a long history and very slow progression of signs and symptoms.

Although these neoplasms are classified as benign, there may be recurrence even after the entire tumor appears to have been removed. Multiple tumors are infrequent. In addition, they have the propensity for growing into adjacent dura, dural sinus, and skull, just as do arachnoid granulations. Metastasis, on the other hand, is extremely rare. Cytologic and histologic criteria suggesting malignancy such as nuclear enlargement, irregularity, and hyperchromatism and growth beyond the capsule occur in about 10% of the surgically removed meningothelial meningiomas. This is, however, far in excess of any malignant biologic activity.

Extension of the neoplasm through the dura with reaction of the overlying bone may be helpful in determining the rate of growth of the tumor. Benign and slow-growing meningiomas often are associated with destruction of the inner table of the skull with a "sunburst" type of bone production of the outer table. More rapidly growing tumors destroy both tables without reactive bone formation.

"Incidental" asymptomatic, small meningiomas, usually of the meningothelial and fibromatous types, are a frequent finding at postmortem examination. Their numbers exceed those that have produced clinical symptoms and signs.

Schwannoma (neurilemoma, neurofibroma, etc.)

Schwannomas, neoplasms arising from the Schwann cells of peripheral nerves, comprise 8% of all intracranial neoplasms. They originate most commonly from the vestibular portion of the eighth nerve in the region of the internal acoustic meatus (Fig. 48-92) and grow into the cerebellopontine angle. They may arise from any of the cranial nerves having a Schwann sheath; the nerves of origin in decreasing order of frequency are the ninth, seventh, eleventh, fifth, and fourth.

The intracranial tumors are most frequently clinically apparent during the fourth through sixth decades and are two to three times more common in women than in men. The neoplasms are usually single; when multiple, they may be a manifestation of von Recklinghausen's disease (Fig. 48-93).

The intracranial tumors are encapsulated, firm, and gray-white and are attached to or appear as part of the cranial nerve, which is then stretched about or within the mass. The larger lesions often have an irregular lobulated surface with yellow, softened, and sometimes hemorrhagic areas internally. Among the several characteristic microscopic features of these neoplasms are the following:

1. The capsule is relatively thick (as compared with the meningioma).
2. The larger lesions are divided into compact, solid areas that are relatively highly cellular (Antoni type A) and areas that

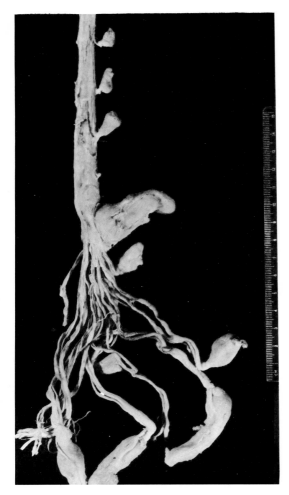

Fig. 48-93. Neurofibromatosis involving cauda equina and spinal ganglia in patient with von Recklinghausen's disease.

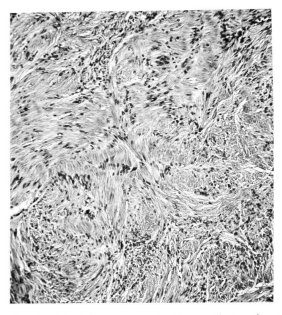

Fig. 48-94. Schwannoma. Portion with interlacing fascicular pattern. (Hematoxylin and eosin; 90×.)

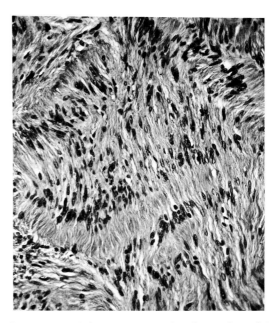

Fig. 48-95. Schwannoma. Palisading of nuclei. (Hematoxylin and eosin; 185×.)

are loose, reticular, and less cellular (Antoni type B).

3. The cells of the more cellular areas are spindle shaped with long processes and nuclei that are long and narrow with finely granular chromatin.

4. A portion of the tumor regularly has cells with an interlacing fascicular pattern (Fig. 48-94).

5. In some areas, the nuclei tend to align as palisades (Fig. 48-95).

6. An occasional whorl-like arrangement is believed to simulate a tactile end organ (Verocay body).

7. In the Antoni type B areas, the neoplastic cells are more plump and more varied in appearance.

8. Pronounced hyalinization with thickening of the walls of the blood vessels is characteristic; it often leads to necrosis and hemorrhage, sometimes with thrombosis.

9. The cystic areas containing numerous lipid and hemosiderin-laden macrophages may be organized, with the formation of granulation tissue.

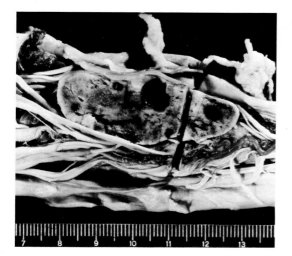

Fig. 48-96. Schwannoma originating in filament of cauda equina.

The intracranial schwannomas are histologically benign lesions, although they frequently recur if incompletely removed. Rarely do they undergo malignant transformation.

Almost one third of spinal tumors are schwannomas. They are always attached to a nerve root and occur at all levels, including the cauda equina (Fig. 48-96). In most, the nerve root that is involved lies between the spinal cord and the dura. Of the remaining, an equal number involve the nerve root as it traverses the dura or lie outside the dura. The spinal schwannomas are smaller than those of the eighth cranial nerve and, though they have the usual gross and microscopic features, the Antoni type A appearance is by far the more frequent.

Vascular malformations and neoplasms

Vascular malformations in the central nervous system are frequent. During a 5-year period when the brain at postmortem examination was routinely sectioned at 2 to 3 mm intervals, vascular malformations were found in over 5%. In the majority, the lesions were incidental. There is no classification that satisfactorily encompasses the range of their structural appearances.[106] When thorough analyses are made of the lesions, frequently portions are found to have features of more than one type of lesion.

Telangiectasia (capillary telangiectasis, capillary angioma). Telangiectasia is the most frequent of the vascular malformations. They are found in adults of both sexes and in all portions of the brain. Because of their usual small size (usually less than 1 cm) and because they are usually single, they often are missed on the routine sectioning of the brain. They appear as well-circumscribed but nonencapsulated dark red areas in which there is a fine stippling caused by the engorged blood vessels. One portion or the entire area on occasion may have an orange-brown appearance because of remote bleeding.

Microscopically, the lesion is composed of capillaries with some variation in size. In the usual small lesion, intervening brain tissue separates the capillaries. In the larger lesions, this is noted only at the periphery, since the center contains larger capillary vessels with no intervening nerve tissue. These lesions occasionally lead to a small local hemorrhage. Their recognition in the wall of a massive hemorrhage, sometimes extending into the ventricular or subarachnoid spaces, is difficult.[94] To adequately investigate such an instance, one should strain the blood obtained from the lesion through several layers of gauze as it is being washed, with the residual tissue retained by the gauze being examined for the presence of the vascular lesion.

Arteriovenous malformations. Although less frequent than the telangiectasia, arteriovenous malformations involve the brain (Fig. 48-97) and spinal cord. From the appearance of the vessel wall, traditional divisions of these lesions have been made to include arteriovenous and venous types.

The arteriovenous malformation is composed of a complex tangle of enlarged dilated arteries and veins without intervening identifiable capillaries. The lesions appear to be more common in men and are often in the area of the middle cerebral artery. On microscopic examination, there is irregular fibrous thickening of the arterial intima, often with fraying, reduplication or the destruction of the internal elastic lamina, and variable thickening of the media. The thinner-walled veins usually have undergone varying degrees of hyalinization of their media and intimal fibrosis so that they resemble arteries. Although these lesions may be in the brain or in the leptomeninges, the malformation often enlarges sufficiently to involve both. Occasionally only venous types of vessels are recognized. These lesions may be asymptomatic or, with rupture, be associated with the signs and symptoms of intraventricular or subarachnoid hemorrhage. In most, with their continued enlargement and some with minor bleeding as well, there is a surrounding astrocytic gliosis and gray-matter

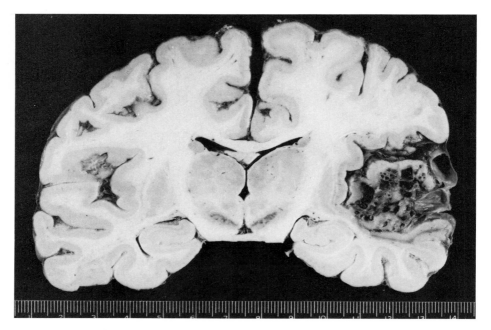

Fig. 48-97. Vascular malformation in superior temporal gyrus with large draining vein.

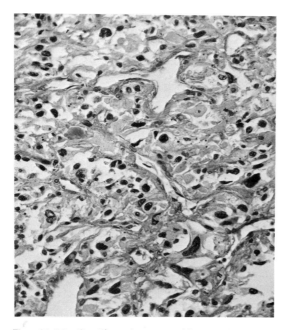

Fig. 48-98. Capillary hemangioblastoma in cerebellum. (Hematoxylin and eosin; 135×.)

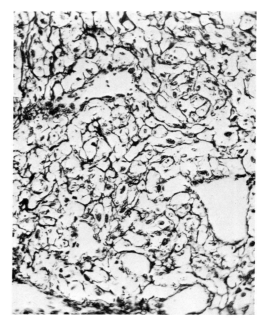

Fig. 48-99. Capillary hemangioblastoma in cerebellum. (Reticulum stain; 90×.)

atrophy; the resulting symptoms depend on the site of the malformation.

Sturge-Weber-Dimitri disease (cephalic neurocutaneous angiomatosis). Sturge-Weber-Dimitri disease is a rare developmental disturbance of blood vessels involving both the skin and the brain. It has been found in families and has been associated in some with mental retardation.

In this disease occurring in the leptomeninges and in atrophic portions of the brain (mainly the occipital and parietal lobes) including the cortex and white matter, there is a striking increase in blood vessels with collagenization of many. Mineralization is generally limited to those vessels in the cortex and, when pronounced, produces a characteristic x-ray pattern. Cortical atrophy is accompanied by a reactive astrocytic gliosis and focal compensatory hydrocephalus. The associated skin lesion is a homolateral facial nevus flammeus (port-wine stain) in the distribution of one or more branches of the trigeminal nerve. Other developmental lesions have been associated in a few instances.

Capillary hemangioblastomas (hemangioendothelioma, angioblastic meningioma).[90,118,134] Hemangioblastomas are red to yellow-gray firm neoplasms of varying size. Although found in all portions of the central nervous system, they are more common in the cerebellum. In the posterior fossa, they form 7% of all primary tumors. They may be solid, as is usual in the cerebral lesions. The cerebellar lesion is more characteristically cystic with a mural nodule. The neoplasm may be single or multiple but always with a leptomeningeal attachment.

The tumor is composed of well-formed capillaries with prominent endothelial cells (Fig. 48-98) in an abundant reticulin network extending radially from or concentrically about the capillaries (Fig. 48-99). Large lipid-containing macrophages are found scattered throughout the tumor, often imparting a yellow background to the usual red-gray gross appearance. The nuclei of the cells are usually large and uniform. Although variation in nuclear size may be found (Fig. 48-98), this is not indicative of malignant transformation.

The cerebellar lesion is usually single and near the midline, but exceptions to both have been described. In less than 10% of the cerebellar lesions, there may be a similar tumor in the retina, vascular malformation of the spinal cord, cysts of the pancreas and liver, and cysts or tumors of the kidney (adenocarcinoma). This combination, known as von Hippel–Lindau disease, is more likely to occur with multiple cerebellar tumors. Familial occurrences and associations with polycythemia and pheochromocytomas have been reported.

Sarcomas[92,126]

Sarcomas of the central nervous system originate from the multipotential cells in the walls of the blood vessels and from the microglial cells within the substance of the brain and spinal cord. Although almost any type of

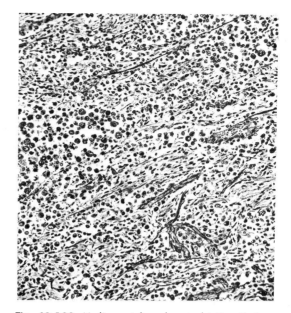

Fig. 48-100. Malignant lymphoma, histiocytic type (reticulum cell sarcoma) in brain. (Hematoxylin and eosin; 90×.)

mesodermal tumor could develop from these cells, the most common are those that resemble one of the malignant lymphomas (Fig. 48-100). Similar lesions may be found in lymph nodes, spleen, and bone marrow. The position of the "cerebellar sarcoma" as previously described is under active debate. At the present time, the evidence suggests that this is a form of medulloblastoma with extension into the leptomeninges.

Metastatic neoplasms[28]

It has been suggested that metastatic neoplasms form up to 30% of all intracranial tumors. The great variation in the estimated frequency is ascribed to inadequate and biased sampling. Metastatic tumors are well demarcated and multiple in over 80% of cases (Fig. 48-101). Those under 1 cm in size are usually solid. Larger lesions are cystic because of central necrosis, often with a 1 to 2 mm rim of neoplasm. Extension of the neoplasm into the subarachnoid space is common. Smaller metastases are often found in the white matter just beneath the U-shaped fibers.

The primary sources, in decreasing order of frequency, are the lungs, breasts, kidneys, skin (melanoma), gastrointestinal tract, and prostate. Neoplastic cell emboli reach the nervous system almost exclusively by way of the arteries with preceding involvement of the lungs.

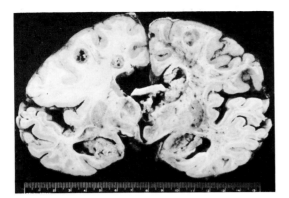

Fig. 48-101. Multiple metastases to brain and ependyma from carcinoma of lung.

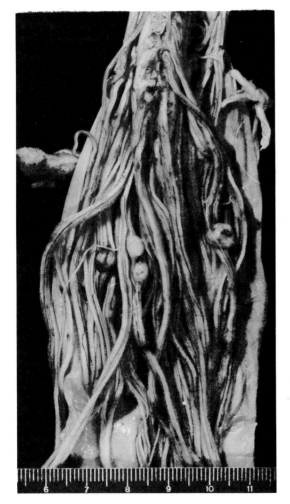

Fig. 48-102. Metastatic carcinoma onto filaments of cauda equina.

Sole localization within the leptomeninges (primary meningeal carcinomatosis, carcinomatous meningitis) is rare. In 2% of those with brain metastases, the spinal cord or cauda equina, or both (Fig. 48-102) are also involved.

BRAIN SWELLING AND EDEMA[155]

Enlargement of the brain from the intracellular accumulation of colloidally bound fluid is known as brain swelling, or dry brain. Enlargement from the presence of an increased amount of intercellular fluid is known as brain edema or wet brain. Both have been related to many causes, including trauma, neoplasms, toxic states, hypoxia, inflammations, etc. The mechanism of production of swelling and edema is not known. Brain swelling is much more common and usually precedes brain edema. The enlarged and swollen brain is heavy, with a decrease in size of the subarachnoid and ventricular spaces. The cerebral convolutions are large, and their crests are flat with compression of the sulci. The sectioned surface of the brain is pale and dry and bulges slightly. The increase in size is attributable entirely to the increase in size of the central white matter. Despite the obvious gross changes, with routine stains the microscopic changes are minimal.

An accompanying edema can be recognized by depression and wetness of the cut surface. This is the result of the separation of the cell processes and myelin sheaths by the accumulation of fluid between them and about the blood vessels. When the fluid is high in protein content and is eosinophilic, recognition is obvious. Separation of the microscopic changes from postmortem and processing artifacts is difficult when the fluid is low in protein and only enlargement of the spaces is to be seen.

Persistence of the edematous state is accompanied by a reactive astrocytosis characterized by cytoplasmic eosinophilia, focal enlargement and fragmentation of axons, loss of myelin, and occasional macrophages.

BRAIN DISPLACEMENT AND HERNIATION[93,95,104]

An expanding intracranial mass often combined with brain swelling and edema is frequently associated with brain displacement and herniation. The more slowly the expansion occurs, the greater the changes that may follow. When the lesion is in the midline and frontal or if both hemispheres are generally and equally affected, the cerebral hemispheres and portions of the midbrain are displaced downward through the incisura of the tentorium. As a result, the midbrain is elongated and the unci become notched by the free margins of the tentorium. The structures occupying the posterior fossa may simultaneously be displaced downward, with impaction of the medulla and cerebellar tonsils into the funnel-shaped foramen magnum (Fig. 48-103). With this downward displacement, the cerebellar tonsils become elongated and notched and the ventral surface of the medulla becomes flattened, sometimes even notched. The displaced pons simultaneously becomes foreshortened and widened. Each downward displacement produces a degree of obstruction of the flow of cerebrospinal fluid.

An expanding lateral or eccentrically placed cerebral mass may produce asymmetric brain displacement and herniation. When the displacement is toward the opposite hemisphere, the cingulate gyrus is forced across the midline beneath the free margin of the falx. Downward displacement to the side homolateral to the mass produces a hemolateral uncal groove (Fig. 48-104) compression of the homolateral third nerve, and sometimes a notching of the homolateral cerebral peduncle by the free margin of the tentorium. With this caudal displacement, the free margin of the tentorium compresses the overriding homolateral posterior cerebral artery. The occlusion can, in turn, result in the production of an anemic and, on release, a hemorrhagic infarct in the area supplied (Fig. 48-104). The combination of downward and contralateral displacement produces another combination of herniations. More frequently, there is compression of the uncus on the homolateral side, and contralateral compression of the cerebral peduncle[93] and posterior cerebral artery occur.

Tumors of the posterior fossa are associated with downward displacement and notching of the medulla and cerebellar tonsils. There may be notching of the superior surface of the cerebellum should either or both hemispheres of the cerebellum be displaced upward.

Downward displacements can be accentuated by the injudicious use of the lumbar puncture.

The brain also may herniate through dural defects and irregularities such as the points of entrance or exits of the blood vessels. A large dural defect such as may be produced after operation can permit a large local herniation, fungus cerebri.

The microscopic appearances with each of

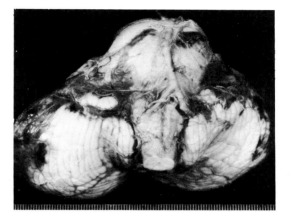

Fig. 48-103. Foreshortening and widening of pons with cerebellomedullary herniation. Secondary to cerebral mass lesion with brain swelling, edema, and displacement.

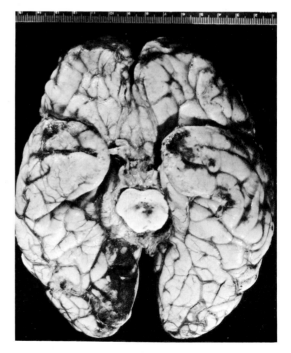

Fig. 48-104. Brain displacement with large right uncal herniation. Compression of right posterior cerebral artery with hemorrhagic infarct of medial portion of occipital lobe and with overlying subarachnoid hemorrhage. Secondary hemorrhages in lower midbrain.

the herniations are characteristic of focal ischemia and sometimes with small areas of necrosis.

Midbrain, pontine, and sometimes thalamic hemorrhages are common fatal secondary effects produced by supratentorial expanding masses. The mechanism producing these hemorrhages is not known.[95] They appear to be related to the downward displacement of the brain without the simultaneous displacement of the basilar artery and its branches. This produces a compression or angulation of the vessels within the brainstem that is believed to result in the hemorrhages of the brainstem.[144]

Peripheral nervous system
Structure and function

Because much of the peripheral nervous system has been covered in the description of diseases of the various organs, this discussion is limited to that supplying the limbs. This portion of the nervous system includes the sensory fibers whose unipolar cell bodies are in the spinal ganglia and whose dendritic processes extend from the limbs and whose axons reach to the spinal cord or brainstem. The motor fibers begin as peripheral nerves in the motor nerve root area of the spinal cord and brainstem. At the nerve root, the myelin sheath, both on the sensory and motor sides, is abruptly changed from that formed by oligodendrocytes centrally to that formed by Schwann cells peripherally. This occurs at a node of Ranvier, and the portion of the nerve in the subarachnoid area proximal to this change is called the Obersteiner-Redlich space or area. The site of change is easily recognizable with the hematoxylin and eosin stain because of the lighter staining of the central portion and the darker staining of the peripheral nervous system portion. Sensory, motor, and mixed nerves have the same general organizational pattern. Individual axons are surrounded by Schwann cells in a linear series separated at the junctions of Schwann cells. These are called the nodes of Ranvier. A thin, fibrous layer, the endoneurium, surrounds each axon and its covering Schwann cells. Fascicular groups of fibers are surrounded by a more easily seen and thicker layer of connective tissue, the perineurium. The epineurium surrounds the entire nerve and extends to the surrounding connective tissues. The perikaryons of the cells of the spinal ganglia are large and spheric. They are surrounded by a single layer of flattened cuboid cap cells. These cells are considered to be the counterpart of Schwann cell peripherally and of the oligodendrocytes centrally.

Degenerations

Degenerative changes of the spinal ganglia cells and their reactions are similar to those of the large nerve cells elsewhere. Aging is associated with the progressive accumulation of lipofuscin, a yellow to brown granular pigment, either about or to one side of the nucleus. Shrinkage of the cell is associated with irregularities of shape, pyknosis of the nucleus, and proliferation of the surrounding cap cells. The changes of central and peripheral chromatolysis are identical with those of the cells of the central nervous system. Cell death is accompanied initially by proliferation of and, later, phagocytosis by the cap cells. Nageotte clusters represent a residual whorled arrangement of cap cells after the loss of a ganglion cell. Cell counts have demonstrated that there is a gradual and continuous loss of spinal ganglion cells with increasing age.

Disintegration of the axons may follow damage to the cell body or may be the result of local injury. With the latter, the change progresses centrally only as far as the next node of Ranvier. They may become focally swollen with varicosities or generally swollen and fragmented and later demonstrate increasing granularity. Myelin beading, swelling, and fragmentation accompany the changes in the axons. Chemical changes in the myelin sheath, demonstrable by special stains, first appear 8 to 10 days after the initial injury and probably are related to the formation of cholesterol esters. Stainable neutral fats appear soon afterward and are slowly removed by macrophages and, according to some, by Schwann cells. Regeneration is possible when the damage to the nerve cells of the spinal ganglia is minimal or is limited to the peripheral axon. Concurrently with the degenerative changes, Schwann cells begin to proliferate, primarily from their distal end toward the central stump, forming the so-called neurolemmal tubules. Multiple fibrillary outgrowths from the central end of the damaged axon make their initial appearance at the end of the first week in myelinated nerves and after the second week in the unmyelinated fibers. The down-growing fibers enter the proximal ends of the neurolemmal tubules, sometimes before there is complete degeneration and removal of the injured tissues. It is assumed that there is an influence that governs the pattern of regeneration. There is, however, always some degree of loss of the normal relationships so that not all fibers reach and grow into the correct neurolemmal tubule. The degree of disorganization is more pronounced in the presence of foreign material and with the formation of scar tissue. The factor that determines which of the fiber branches continues to grow downward into the tubule and which disappears is not known. It is believed that those fibers that have entered improper tubules (i.e., sensory fibers in a motor area) do not achieve function and eventually degenerate. Initially, all regenerated fibers are nonmyelinated. Myelination about some fibers proceeds from the central end distalward, making its proximal appearance about 1 month after injury.

When these structures are examined routinely at autopsy, it can be seen that the spinal ganglia and peripheral nerves participate in many so-called nonneurologic diseases that affect the individual.

The causes of damage to a peripheral nerve are many, and the initial locus of damage is equally varied. Nerve biopsy is not common in these conditions, and the early changes usually are inferred from those found at autopsy or are found in the course of examination for other diseases. The limited response on the part of the peripheral nerve, however, places many disorders in relatively uniform categories of structural change. In all of these nonneoplastic disorders, the changes in the axons and myelin sheaths are those of swelling and fragmentation and eventual loss of the myelin sheath at that level. A mild to moderate reactive fibrosis is part of the response about the affected fibers. With continued injury, the degenerative changes may progress toward the perikaryon. Early, one may find a mononuclear response with lipid-containing phagocytes in the areas of damage. With the most severe states of sensory nerve involvement, axonal degeneration may be seen in the cells of the spinal ganglia (central chromatolysis) and with accompanying satellitosis and even neuronophagia.

Cysts of spinal ganglia[46]

Although of frequent occurrence, cysts of the spinal ganglia are only rarely symptomatic. It has been assumed that they result from the cerebrospinal fluid pressure exerted upon the sleeves of pia-arachnoid that accompany the nerves as they exit toward the intervertebral spaces. When the fine porous openings in the pia-arachnoid through which the nerve fibers course become narrowed, perhaps as a result of scarring, the cerebrospinal fluid pressure, increased by the long periods of upright position in man, becomes more effective in bulging the walls of this funnel-like space. This results in the formation of a cyst whose distal outer wall often is in the proximal portion of the spinal ganglion. When clinically symptomatic, it is believed to be attributable to the effect of the pressure upon the included nerve fibers.

Metastatic cancer to spinal ganglia and peripheral nerves

The spinal ganglia, like all living tissue of the body, can be expected to be the site for metastatic disease (Fig. 48-105). In the only prospective postmortem study, the spinal ganglia were involved in 2% of all patients with carcinoma that had separately metastasized to the central nervous system as well.[28] It was recognized that this must have represented a minimal involvement since usually one ganglion and rarely more than two ganglia were examined in this study.

Involvement of the peripheral nerve by metastatic cancer has been reported on many occasions. This is particularly true in certain cancers, such as those of the prostate, urinary bladder, and cervix, where their mode of spread is believed to be through the perineural lymphatic spaces.

Spinal ganglia and peripheral nerves frequently are involved in patients with a lymphoma, leukemia (Fig. 48-106), or multiple

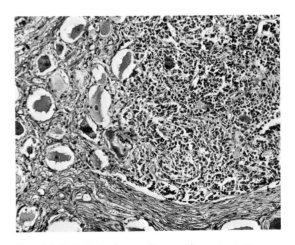

Fig. 48-105. Spinal ganglion with metastatic carcinoma from prostate. (Hematoxylin and eosin; 135×.)

myeloma.[45] The lack of clinical recognition, as with the carcinoma, is probably related to the more pressing and more symptomatic involvement of other tissues.

Amyloidosis

Amyloidosis, with the exception of familial cases, is a late and uncommon complication

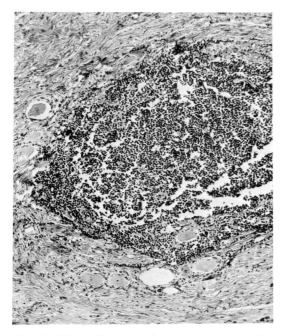

Fig. 48-106. Infiltrate of chronic granulocytic leukemia in spinal ganglion. (Hematoxylin and eosin; 90×.)

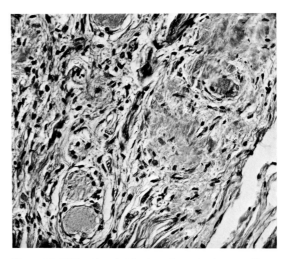

Fig. 48-107. Amyloidosis of spinal ganglion. (Hematoxylin and eosin, 280×.)

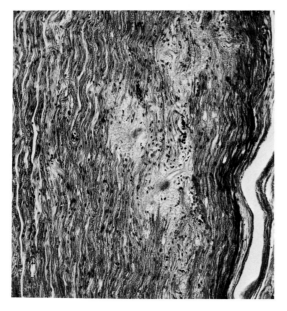

Fig. 48-108. Amyloidosis of peripheral nerve. (Hematoxylin and eosin; 90×.)

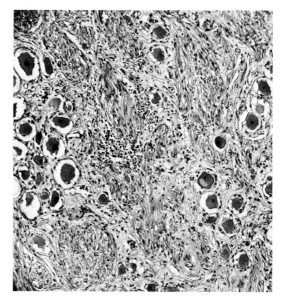

Fig. 48-109. Lumbar spinal ganglion with nonspecific focal chronic inflammation. (Hematoxylin and eosin; 90×.)

of those diseases with which generalized amyloid deposition is to be expected. It is characterized by hyaline eosinophilic balls between nerve fibers in the spinal ganglia (Fig. 48-107) and in the peripheral nerves (Fig. 48-108). A relation to blood vessel walls is not always apparent. Typical deposition in the walls of smaller blood vessels also is seen. Familial cases of amyloidosis have been described as occurring in certain Portuguese families, possibly from genetic causes.

Hemorrhage

Hemorrhage into the proximal half of the dorsal root ganglion is not uncommon. Most frequently, it represents extension of subarachnoid hemorrhage in the pia-arachnoid sleeve that surrounds the peripheral rootlets. In most instances, the blood appears to finally escape along the usual channels of cerebrospinal fluid flow. In some, the blood becomes locally organized. The hemoglobin is converted to hemosiderin and hematoidin, and there is a moderate degree of reactive fibrosis. In our material, none of the hemorrhages were recognized as clinically symptomatic.

Inflammation

Nonspecific inflammatory changes in the spinal ganglia and peripheral nerves are not uncommon (Fig. 48-109). These changes are characterized by cellular infiltrates, predominantly lymphocytic, and sometimes by degenerative changes in the axons and in the myelin sheaths. Abnormalities of this type were seen in approximately 5% of routine autopsies in a general city hospital. The lesions appear to be nonspecific and related more to a general state of the body than to a disease specifically affecting the nervous system. In most instances, there was no clinical recognition of such involvement. When severe and limited to the rootlets, sometimes with involvement of the spinal cord, the Landry-Guillain-Barré syndrome results.

In herpes zoster infection, the changes and the inflammatory responses are striking. The affected spinal ganglia may be swollen and red because of the considerable necrosis with hemorrhage, which simulates a hemorrhagic infarct (Figs. 48-110 and 48-111). Changes in the motor component result in damage to the motoneurons with satellitosis and neuronophagia of the anterior horn cells at that level.

The peripheral nervous system is, of course, involved in all varieties of inflammatory disease, including the purulent, granulomatous, and viral diseases, the collagen diseases, and sometimes after chemotherapy[65,116] (Fig. 48-112).

Vascular disease

Degenerative vascular disease such as seen in patients with atherosclerosis and with diabetes frequently affects the peripheral nervous system. Infarction of the spinal ganglia must

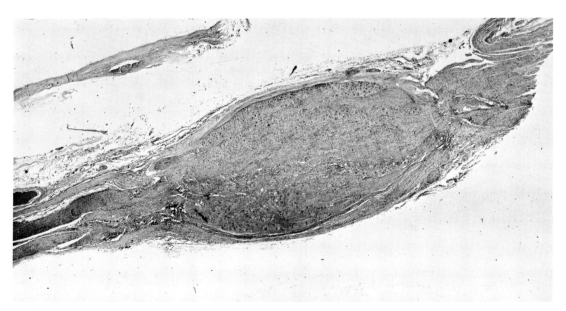

Fig. 48-110. Herpes zoster. Necrosis of upper half of spinal ganglion. (Hematoxylin and eosin; 8×.)

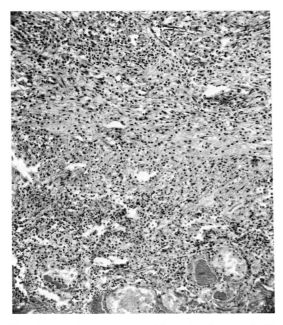

Fig. 48-111. Herpes zoster. Necrosis of upper half of spinal ganglion. (Hematoxylin and eosin; 90×.)

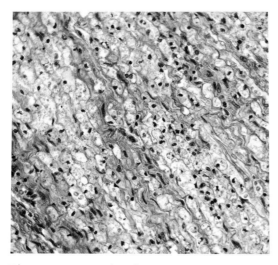

Fig. 48-112. Peripheral neuritis occurring after vincristine therapy. Fragmentation and loss of axons and destruction of myelin. (Hematoxylin and eosin; 280×.)

be exceedingly rare, never having been recognized in our series of over 10,000 ganglia. Involvement of both sensory and motor nerves is, however, very common, particularly in the lower limbs of diabetic patients.[131]

A neuropathy from focal areas of degeneration in the peripheral nervous system has been seen in 16% of patients with diabetes mellitus in the fifth decade of life and in 37% of those in the seventh decade. The clinical and structural appearance of pseudotabes from wallerian degeneration secondary to changes in the peripheral nervous system also has been described in diabetic patients. Involvement of the peripheral nerves and perhaps also the intermediolateral columns of the spinal cord is probably an important factor in the development of the Charcot joints in patients with diabetes.

Pressure

Constant and prolonged pressure upon the peripheral nerve can lead to structural as well as functional changes. The larger fibers are the most susceptible. The myelin sheaths are damaged first, followed by changes in the axon. Initially, there is fragmentation of the myelin sheaths, followed by the chemical changes characteristic of myelin destruction. When the axons are damaged, they become swollen and fragmented. Both are removed by macrophages. Wallerian degeneration follows. Recovery is related to the reconstitution of the axons followed by the formation of the surrounding myelin. Dependent on the degree of damage and the degree of fibrosis, recovery may take weeks or months.

Nutritional deficiencies

A peripheral neuropathy related to vitamin B_1 deficiency has been described frequently. The changes affect the distalmost portion of the fibers first, with a progressive dying back of the central portion of the neuron. The nerve cells appear to remain intact. The axons and myelin sheaths undergo swelling and fragmentation, followed by phagocytosis and removal. Recovery takes the pattern previously described for nerve fiber regeneration.

Toxic disorders

Segmental demyelination involving both sensory and motor nerves has been described in the peripheral nervous system in patients with diphtheria, with heavy metal poisoning (lead and arsenic), and with porphyria.

Peroneal muscular atrophy (Charcot-Marie-Tooth disease)

Peroneal muscular atrophy is a heredofamilial disease with degenerative changes beginning in the distalmost portion of the peroneal nerve. The fibers that lead to the small muscles of the foot are affected first. As the disease progresses, the lesions affect more and

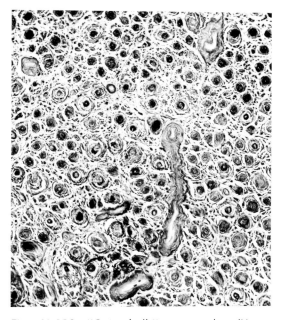

Fig. 48-113. "Onion-bulb" neuropathy. (Hematoxylin and eosin; 90×.)

more of the peripheral nerve to structurally include the cells of the spinal ganglia and anterior horn cells of the spinal cord. In some instances, the posterior columns also demonstrate secondary axonal degeneration. Proliferation of the connective tissue around the residual axons of the peripheral nerve can produce an appearance structurally similar to that seen in hypertrophic interstitial neuropathy (Dejerine-Sottas disease).

In some of the patients with peroneal muscular atrophy, other members of the family have exhibited diseases suggestive of Friedreich's ataxia as well as peroneal muscular atrophy, whereas in others, only a few muscles of the lower leg may be affected.

"Onion-bulb" neuropathies (Dejerine-Sottas disease, hypertrophic interstitial radiculoneuropathy, Refsum's disease, etc.)[119,128,130,156]

The "onion-bulb" neuropathies are a group of conditions related only in that they are represented by a concentric-ring proliferation of Schwann cells and connective tissue about a peripheral axon. This reactive change can occur in almost any chronic peripheral neuropathy that is characterized by recurrent episodes of demyelination and remyelination.

Hypertrophic interstitial neuropathy of Dejerine-Sottas is a rare disorder resulting in enlargement of the sensory and motor nerves.

It is characterized microscopically by the presence of concentric rings of connective tissue forming an onionskin-like layering about the peripheral axon (Fig. 48-113). Formerly considered to be a specific reaction, at the present time it is not known if the proliferation of the connective tissue represents a genetic response or is evidence of excessive regeneration.

Neoplasms

Neoplasms of the peripheral nervous system, except those of the eighth cranial nerve, are unusual. They are seen more commonly in patients with von Recklinghausen's disease, in whom neurilemomas or neurofibromas or diffuse hyperplasias of a portion of the peripheral nervous system (usually confined to a limb) are seen. The appearances of these tumors are identical with those described for the peripheral nerves attached to the brain and spinal cord.

REFERENCES

1 Adams, R. D., and Richardson, E. P., Jr.: In Folch-Pi, J., editor: Chemical pathology of the nervous system, New York, 1961, Pergamon Press, Inc., pp. 163-194 (demyelinating diseases).

2 Alpers, B. J., and Yaskin, J. C.: Arch. Neurol. Psychiatry (Chicago) 41:435-459, 1939 (gliomas of pons).

3 Andrews, J. M., Cancilla, P. A., Grippo, J., and Menkes, J. H.: Neurology (Minneapolis) 21: 337-352, 1971 (globoid cell leukodystrophy).

4 Andrew, W.: J. Chronic Dis. 3:575-596, 1956 (aging).

5 Arey, J. B.: J. Pediatr. 40:621-625, 1952 (cerebral palsy).

6 Astrom, K. E., Mancall, E. L., and Richardson, E. P., Jr.: Brain 81:93-111, 1958 (leukoencephalopathy).

7 Bailey, A. A.: Arch. Neurol. Psychiatry (Chicago) 70:299-309, 1953 (aging in spinal cord).

8 Bailey, P.: In Penfield, W., editor: Cytology and cellular pathology of the nervous system, New York, 1932, Paul B. Hoeber, Inc., vol. 2, p. 903 (cellular types in primary tumors of brain).

9 Bailey, P., and Bucy, P. C.: J. Pathol. Bacteriol. 32:735-751, 1929 (oligodendroglioma).

10 Bailey, P., and Cushing, H.: A classification of the tumors of the glioma group on a histogenetic basis with a correlated study of prognosis, Philadelphia, 1926, J. B. Lippincott Co.

11 Barnett, H. J. M., and Hyland, H. H.: Brain 76:36-49, 1953 (intracranial venous thrombosis).

12 Bass, N. H., and Hirose, G.: Neurology (Minneapolis) 22:312-320, 1972 (adult metachromatic leukodystrophy).

13 Bearn, A. G., and Kunkel, A. G.: J. Clin. Invest. 33:400-409, 1954 (Wilson's disease).

14 Benda, C. E.: Developmental disorders of mentation and cerebral palsies, New York, 1952, Grune & Stratton, Inc.

15 Black, B. K., and Smith, D. E.: Arch. Neurol. Psychiatry (Chicago) **64:**614-630, 1950 (nasal glioma).

16 Boykin, F. C., Cowen, D., Iannucci, C. A. J., and Wolf, A.: J. Neuropathol. Exp. Neurol. **13:** 30-49, 1954 (astrocytoma).

17 Brady, R. O.: In Albers, R. W., Siegel, G. J., Katzman, R., and Agranoff, B. W., editors: Basic neurochemistry, Boston, 1972, Little, Brown & Co., pp. 485-495 (sphingolipidoses).

18 Bucy, P. C., and Thieman, P. W.: Arch. Neurol. (Chicago) **18:**14-19, 1968 (astrocytomas of cerebellum).

19 Cape, C. C., Martinez, A. J., Robertson, J. T., Hamilton, R., and Jabbour, J. T.: Arch. Neurol. **28:**124-127, 1973 (subacute sclerosing panencephalitis in adult).

20 Carpenter, M. B., and Druckemiller, W. H.: Arch. Neurol. Psychiatry (Chicago) **69:**305-322, 1953 (agenesis of corpus callosum).

21 Carpenter, S.: Neurology (Minneapolis) **18:** 841-851, 1968 (motor neuron disease).

22 Chason, J. L.: J. Neuropathol. Exp. Neurol. **15:** 461-470, 1956 (subependymal mixed gliomas).

23 Chason, J. L.: Radiology **70:**811-814, 1958 (cerebral infarction).

24 Chason, J. L., and Dickenman, R. C.: Unpublished data, 1959 (inflammations of spinal ganglia).

25 Chason, J. L., and Hindman, W. M.: Neurology (Minneapolis) **8:**41-44, 1958 (berry aneuysms).

26 Chason, J. L., Landers, J. W., and Gonzalez, J. E.: J. Neurol. Neurosurg. Psychiatry **27:** 317-325, 1964 (pontine myelinolysis).

27 Chason, J. L., Mahoney, W. F., and Landers, J. W.: Minn. Med. **49:**27-31, 1966 (intracerebral hemorrhage).

28 Chason, J. L., Walker, F. B., and Landers, J. W.: Cancer **16:**781-787, 1963 (metastatic carcinoma).

29 Chason, J. L., Hardy, W. G., Webster, J. E., and Gurdjian, E. S.: J. Neurosurg. **15:**135-139, 1958 (concussion).

30 Chason, J. L., Fernando, O. U., Hodgson, V. R., Thomas, L. M., and Gurdjian, E. S.: J. Trauma **6:**767-769, 1966 (concussion).

31 Chatty, E. M., and Earle, K. M.: Cancer **28:** 927-983, 1971 (medulloblastoma).

32 Cole, F. M., and Yates, P.: Brain **90:**759-768, 1967 (microaneurysms).

33 Cole, F. M., and Yates, P. O.: J. Neurol. Neurosurg. Psychiatry **30:**61-66, 1967 (cerebral hemorrhage).

34 Cowen, D., and Geller, L. M.: J. Neuropathol. Exp. Neurol. **19:**488-527, 1960 (prenatal x irradiation).

35 Crigler, J. F., Jr., and Najjar, V. A.: Pediatrics **10:**169-179, 1952 (kernicterus).

36 Cushing, H., and Eisenhardt, L.: Meningiomas; their classification, regional behaviour, life history and surgical end results, Springfield, Ill., 1938, Charles C Thomas, Publisher.

37 Dal Santo, G.: In Harmel, M. H., editor: Clinical anesthesia; neurologic considerations, Philadelphia, 1967, F. A. Davis Co. ("blood-brain barrier": pathology and importance in anesthesia).

38 Daube, J. R., and Chou, S. M.: Neurology (Minneapolis) **16:**179-191, 1966 (lissencephaly).

39 Davies, J.: Human developmental anatomy, New York, 1963, The Ronald Press Co.

40 Dayan, A. D., Marshall, A. H. E., Miller, A. A., Pick, F. J., and Ramkin, N. E.: J. Pathol. Bacteriol. **92:**1-29, 1966 (pinealomas).

41 DeReuck, J., Chattha, A. S., and Richardson, E. P.: Arch. Neurol. **27:**229-236, 1972 (periventricular leukomalacia).

42 DeMyer, W.: Neurology (Minneapolis) **14:**806-808, 1964 (vinblastine-induced malformations).

43 Denny-Brown, D.: The basal ganglia and their relation to disorders of movements, London, 1962, Oxford University Press.

44 Desnick, R. J., Dawson, G., Desnick, S. J., Sweeley, C. C., and Krivit, W.: New Eng. J. Med. **284:**739-744, 1971 (glycosphingolipoidoses).

45 Dickenman, R. C., and Chason, J. L.: Am. J. Pathol. **34:**349-361, 1958 (dorsal root ganglia).

46 Dickenman, R. C., and Chason, J. L.: Arch. Pathol. (Chicago) **77:**366-369, 1964 (cysts of dorsal root ganglia).

47 Dinsdale, H.: Arch. Neurol. (Chicago) **10:**200-217, 1964 (hemorrhage in posterior fossa).

48 Dorfman, L. J.: Neurology (Minneapolis) **23:** 136-144, 1973 (cytomegalovirus encephalitis in adults).

49 Dyck, P. J., and Gomez, M. R.: Mayo Clin. Proc. **43:**280-296, 1968 (Dejerine-Sottas disease).

50 Earle, K. M.: J. Neuropathol. Exp. Neurol. **27:** 1-14, 1968 (Parkinson's disease).

51 Elizan, T. S., Ajero-Froehlich, L., Fabiyi, A., Ley, A., and Sever, J. L.: Arch. Neurol. (Chicago) **20:**115-119, 1969 (malformations of central nervous system).

52 Ellington, E., and Margolis, G.: J. Neurosurg. **30:**651-657, 1969 (subarachnoid hemorrhage).

53 Fawcett, F. J., and Smith, W. T.: Postgrad. Med. J. **42:**5-15, 1966 (strokes).

54 Feigin, I., and Goebel, H.: Neurology (Minneapolis) **19:**749-759, 1969 (necrotizing encephalopathy).

55 Feigin, I., and Popoff, N.: J. Neuropath. Exp. Neurol. **22:**500-511, 1963 (cerebral edema).

56 Feigin, I., and Wolf, A.: J. Pediatr. **45:**243-263, 1954 (Wernicke's encephalopathy).

57 Feldman, H. A.: New Eng. J. Med. **279:**1431-1437, 1968 (toxoplasmosis).

58 Ferraro, A., Arieti, S., and English, W. H.: J. Neuropath. Exp. Neurol. **4:**217-239, 1945 (cerebral changes in pernicious anemia).

59 Fisher, C. M.: Neurology (Minneapolis) **15:** 774-784, 1965 (cerebral infarcts).

60 Fokes, E. C., Jr., and Earle, K. M.: J. Neurosurg. **30:**585-594, 1969 (ependymoma).

61 Foley, J. M., and Baxter, D.: J. Neuropathol. Exp. Neurol. **17:**586-598, 1958 (pigment granules).

62 Freytag, E.: J. Neurol. Neurosurg. Psychiatry **31:**616-620, 1968 (intracerebral hematoma).

63 Gibbs, C. J., Jr.: Curr. Top. Microbiol. Immunol. **40:**44-58, 1967 (search for infectious etiology in chronic and subacute degenerative diseases of central nervous system).

64 Gibbs, C. J., Jr., Gajdusek, D. C., Asher, D. M., Alpers, M. P., Beck, E., and Daniel, P. M.: Science **161:**388-389, 1968 (Creutzfeldt-Jakob disease).

65 Gottschalk, P. G., Dyck, P. J., and Kiely, J. M.: Neurology (Minneapolis) 18:875-882, 1968 (alkaloid neuropathy).

66 Greene, H. L., Hug, G., and Schubert, W. K.: Arch. Neurol. (Chicago) 20:147-153, 1969 (leukodystrophy).

67 Greenhouse, A. H., and Schneck, S. A.: Neurology (Minneapolis) 18:1-8, 1968 (necrotizing encephalomyelopathy).

68 Hamby, W. B.: Intracranial aneurysms, Springfield, Ill., 1952, Charles C Thomas, Publisher.

69 Haymaker, W., Margolis, C., Pentschew, A., Jacob, H., Lindenberg, R., Arroyo, L. S., Stockdorph, O., and Stowens, D.: Kernicterus and its importance in cerebral palsy, Springfield, Ill., 1961, Charles C Thomas, Publisher.

70 Heard, B. E., Hassan, A. M., and Wilson, S.: J. Clin. Pathol. 15:17-20, 1962 (cytomegalic inclusion disease).

71 Herndon, R. M., and Rubinstein, L. J.: Neurology (Minneapolis) 18:8-20, 1968 (Dawson's encephalitis).

72 Hess, A.: J. Comp. Neurol. 98:69-91, 1953 (ground substance of central nervous system).

73 Hicks, S. P.: Arch. Pathol. (Chicago) 57:363-378, 1954 (radiation anencephaly).

74 Hirano, A., and Ghatak, N. R.: J. Neuropathol. Exp. Neurol. 33:333-341, 1974 (colloid cysts).

75 Hitchcock, E., and Andreadis, A.: J. Neurol. Neurosurg. Psychiatry 27:422-434, 1964 (subdural empyema).

76 Hsieh, H.: Neurology (Minneapolis) 17:752-762, 1967 (cerebrovascular disease).

77 Hughes, J. T., and Brownell, B.: Neurology (Minneapolis) 14:1073-1077, 1964 (cervical spondylosis).

78 Hughes, W.: Lancet 2:19-21, 1965 (origin of lacunes).

79 Hurst, E. W.: Med. J. Aust. 2:1-6, 1941 (hemorrhagic leukoencephalitis).

80 Illis, L. S., and Gostling, J. V. T.: Herpes simplex encephalitis, Bristol, 1972, Scientechnica (Publishers) Ltd.

81 Inglis, K.: Am. J. Pathol. 30:739-755, 1954 (tuberous sclerosis).

82 Jenis, E. H., Knieser, M. R., Rothouse, P. A., Jensen, G. E., and Scott, R. M.: Arch. Pathol. 95:81-89, 1973 (subacute sclerosing panencephalitis).

83 Jervis, S. A.: In Folch-Pi, J., editor: Chemical pathology of the nervous system, New York, 1961, Pergamon Press, Inc.

84 Johnson, R. T., and Mims, C. A.: New Eng. J. Med. 278:23-30, 84-92, 1968 (viral infections).

85 Julius, R., Buehler, B., Aylsworth, A., St. Petry, L., Rennert, O., and Greer, M.: Neurology (Minneapolis) 21:15-18, 1971 (metachromatic leukodystrophy).

86 Kahn, E. A.: Neurosurg. 4:191-199, 1947 (lateral sclerosis).

87 Kallen, B., and Levan, A.: In Tedeschi, C. G., editor: Neuropathology methods and diagnosis, Boston, 1970, Little, Brown & Co., pp. 558-559 (mongolism).

88 Kane, W., and Aronson, S. M.: Acta Neuropathol. (Berlin) 9:273-279, 1967 (cerebellar medulloblastoma).

89 Katz, M., Rorke, L. B., Masland, W. S., Koprowski, H., and Tucker, S. H.: New Eng. J. Med. 279:793-798, 1968 (sclerosing panencephalitis).

90 Kawamura, J., Garcia, J. H., and Kamijyo, Y.: Cancer 31:1528-1540, 1973 (cerebellar hemangioblastoma).

91 Kernohan, J. W., and Fletcher-Kernohan, E. M.: Assoc. Res. Nerv. Ment. Dis. Proc. 16: 182-209, 1935 (ependymoma).

92 Kernohan, J. W., and Uihlein, A.: Sarcomas of the brain, Springfield, Ill., 1962, Charles C Thomas, Publisher.

93 Kernohan, J. W., and Woltman, H. W.: Arch. Neurol. Psychiatry (Chicago) 24:274-287, 1929 (brain tumor).

94 Kernohan, J. W., Mabon, R. F., Svien, H. J., and Adson, A. W.: Proc. Staff Meet. Mayo Clin. 24:71-75, 1949 (gliomas).

95 Klintworth, G. K.: Am. J. Pathol. 53:391-408, 1968 (secondary brainstem hemorrhages).

96 Kolodny, E. H., Brady, R. O., and Volk, B. W.: Biochem. Biophys. Res. Commun. 37:526-531, 1969 (Tay-Sachs disease).

97 Konigsmark, B. W., and Weiner, L. P.: Medicine 49:227-242, 1970 (olivopontocerebellar atrophies).

98 Lagos, J. C., and Gomez, M. R.: Mayo Clin. Proc. 42:26-49, 1967 (tuberous sclerosis).

99 Landers, J. W., Chason, J. L., and Samuel, V. N.: Neurology (Minneapolis) 15:968-971, 1965 (pontine myelinolysis).

100 Lang, E. R., and Kidd, M.: J. Neurosurg. 22: 554-562, 1965 (cerebral aneurysms).

101 Lawyer, T., Jr., and Netzky, M. G.: Arch. Neurol. Psychiatry (Chicago) 69:171-192, 1953 (amyotrophic lateral sclerosis).

102 Leary, T.: J.A.M.A. 103:897-903, 1934 (subdural hemorrhage).

103 Leigh, D.: J. Neurol. Neurosurg. Psychiatry 14:216-221, 1951 (necrotizing encephalomyelopathy).

104 Lindenberg, R.: J. Neuropathol. Exp. Neurol. 14:223-243, 1955 (compression of brain arteries).

105 Loeser, J. B., and Alvord, E. C., Jr.: Brain 91: 553-570, 1968 (agenesis of corpus callosum).

106 McCormick, W. F., Hardman, J. M., and Boulter, T. R.: J. Neurosurg. 28:241-251, 1968 (vascular malformations).

107 Macdonald, R. D., Rewcastle, N. B., and Humphrey, J. G.: Arch. Neurol. (Chicago) 20: 565-585, 1969 (periodic paralysis).

108 Mabon, R. F., Svien, H. J., Adson, A. W., and Kernohan, J. W.: Arch. Neurol. Psychiatry (Chicago) 64:74-88, 1950 (astrocytoma of cerebellum).

109 Mabon, R. F., Svien, H. J., Kernohan, J. W., and Craig, W. M.: Proc. Staff Meet. Mayo Clin. 24:65-71, 1949 (ependymomas).

110 Mair, W. G. P., and Druckman, R.: Brain 76: 70-91, 1953 (cervical disk protrusion).

111 Mannen, T.: Geriatrics 21:151-160, 1966 (vascular lesions in spinal cord).

112 Marburg, O.: Arch. Neurol. Psychiatry (Chicago) 53:248, 1945 (porencephaly).

113 Margolis, G.: Lab. Invest. 8:335-370, 1959 (senile cerebral disease).

114 Margolis, G., Odom, G. L., Woodhall, B., and Bloor, B. M.: J. Neurosurg. 8:564-575, 1951 (intracerebral hematoma).

115 Markham, J. W., Lynge, H. N., and Stahlman,

G. E. B.: J. Neurosurg. **26**:334-342, 1967 (spinal epidural hematoma).

116 Moress, G. R., D'Agostino, A. N., and Jarcho, L. W.: Arch. Neurol. (Chicago) **16**:377-384, 1967 (leukemia treated with vincristine).

117 Netzky, M. G.: Arch. Neurol. Psychiatry (Chicago) **70**:741-777, 1953 (syringomyelia).

118 Nibbelink, D. W., Peters, B. H., and McCormick, W. F.: Neurology (Minneapolis) **19**:455-460, 1968 (pheochromocytoma and cerebellar hemangioblastoma).

119 Nichols, P. C., Dyck, P. J., and Miller, D. R.: Mayo Clin. Proc. **43**:297-305, 1968 (hypertrophic neuropathy).

120 Nikaido, T., Austin, J., Trueb, L., and Rinehart, R.: Arch. Neurol. **27**:549-554, 1972 (aging of the brain).

121 Oldendorf, W. H., and Davson, H.: Arch. Neurol. (Chicago) **17**:196-205, 1967 (cerebrospinal fluid).

122 Olszewski, J.: World Neurol. **3**:359-375, 1962 (Binswanger's disease).

123 Paulson, O. B.: Stroke **2**:327-360, 1971 (cerebral apoplexy).

124 Payne, F. E., Baublis, J. V., and Itabashi, H. H.: New Eng. J. Med. **281**:585-589, 1969 (sclerosing panencephalitis).

125 Peach, B.: Arch. Neurol. **12**:527-536, 1965 (Arnold-Chiari malformation).

126 Peison, B.: Cancer **20**:983-990, 1967 (microglial glioma).

127 Pilz, H.: Arch. Neurol. **27**:87-90, 1972 (adult metachromatic leukodystrophy).

128 Pleasure, D. E., and Towfighi, J.: Arch. Neurol. **26**:289-301, 1972 (onion-bulb neuropathies).

129 Poser, C. M.: In Minckler, J., editor: Pathology of nervous system, New York, 1968, Blakiston Division, McGraw-Hill Book Co., p. 767 (diseases of myelin).

130 Prineas, J. W.: Acta Neuropathol. **18**:34-57, 1971 (recurrent idiopathic polyneuropathy).

131 Raff, M. C., Sangalang, V., and Asbury, A. K.: Arch. Neurol. (Chicago) **18**:478-499, 1968 (ischemic mononeuropathy).

132 Rakic, P., and Yakovlev, P. I.: J. Dairy Sci. **132**:45-72, 1968 (corpus callosum).

133 Resnick, J. S., Engel, W. K., and Sever, J. L.: New Eng. J. Med. **279**:126-129, 1968 (sclerosing panencephalitis).

134 Rivera, E., and Chason, J. L.: J. Neurosurg. **25**:452-454, 1966 (cerebral hemangioblastoma).

135 Robertson, D. M., Dinsdale, H. B., and Campbell, R. J.: Arch. Neurol. **24**:203-209, 1971 (subacute combined degeneration).

136 Rosenblum, W. I., and Feigin, I.: Arch. Neurol. (Chicago) **13**:627-632, 1965 (Wernicke's encephalopathy).

137 Rubinstein, L. J., and Northfield, D. W. C.: Brain **87**:379-412, 1964 (medulloblastoma).

138 Russell, D. S.: Observations on the pathology of hydrocephalus, Med. Res. Counc. Spec. Rep. Ser. (London) No. 265 (third impression with appendix), 1966.

139 Sahs, A. L.: J. Neurosurg. **24**:792-806, 1966 (aneurysms).

140 Schneck, L., Volk, B. W., and Saifer, A.: Am. J. Med. **46**:245-263, 1969 (gangliosidoses).

141 Schneck, S. A.: Neurology (Minneapolis) **18** (no. 1, pt. 2):79-82, 1968 (measles vaccination).

142 Shaw, C.-M., and Alvord, E. C., Jr.: Brain **92**:213-224, 1969 (cava septi pellucidi).

143 Shuangshoti, S., Roberts, M. P., and Netzky, M. G.: Arch. Pathol. (Chicago) **80**:214-224, 1965 (colloid cysts).

144 Siim, J. C., editor: Human toxoplasmosis, Baltimore, 1960, The Williams & Wilkins Co.

145 Sipe, J. C.: Neurology (Minneapolis) **23**:1030-1038, 1973 (Leigh's syndrome in adult).

146 Snyder, R. O., and Brady, R. O.: Clin. Chem. Acta **25**:331-338, 1969 (lipid-storage diseases and white blood cells).

147 Steiner, G.: J. Neuropathol. Exp. Neurol. **11**:343-372, 1952 (multiple sclerosis).

148 Stoltmann, H. F., and Blackwood, W.: Brain **87**:45-50, 1964 (myelopathy in cervical spondylosis).

149 Thompson, R. A., and Pribram, H. F. W.: Neurology (Minneapolis) **19**:785-789, 1969 (aneurysm).

150 Towbin, A.: Pathology of cerebral palsy, Springfield, Ill., 1960, Charles C Thomas, Publisher.

151 Ungley, C. C.: Brain **72**:382-427, 1949 (subacute combined degeneration).

152 Vogel, F. S., and McClenahan, J. L.: Am. J. Pathol. **28**:701-723, 1952 (anencephaly).

153 Warkany, J.: J. Cell. Comp. Physiol. **43**(suppl. 1):207-236, 1954 (vitamin deficiencies).

154 Warner, F. J.: J. Nerv. Ment. Dis. **118**:1-18, 1953 (macrogyria).

155 Wasterlain, C. G., and Torack, R. M.: Arch. Neurol. (Chicago) **19**:79-87, 1968 (cerebral edema).

156 Webster, G. H., et al.: J. Neuropathol. Exp. Neurol. **26**:276-289, 1967 (role of Schwann cells in onion-bulb formation).

157 Weir, B., and Elvidge, A. R.: J. Neurosurg. **29**:500-505, 1968 (oligodendroglioma).

158 Weller, T. H.: New Eng. J. Med. **285**:203-214, 267-274, 1971 (cytomegalic inclusion disease).

159 Wisniewski, H., Coblentz, J. M., and Terry, R. T.: Arch. Neurol. **26**:97-108, 1972 (Pick's disease).

160 Wisniewski, H., Terry, R. D., and Hirano, A.: J. Neuropathol. Exp. Neurol. **29**:163-176, 1970 (neurofibrillary pathology).

161 Wolstenholme, G. E. W., and O'Connor, C. M., editors: Ciba Foundation Symposium on Congenital Malformations, Boston, 1960, Little, Brown & Co.

162 Woodard, T. E., and Jackson, E. B.: In Horsfall, F. L., Jr., and Tamm, I., editors: Viral and rickettsial infections in man, ed. 4, Philadelphia, 1965, J. B. Lippincott Co., p. 1095.

163 Woolsey, R. M., and Nelsen, J. S.: Neurology (Minneapolis) **15**:662-666, 1965 (leukoencephalopathy).

164 Zeman, W., and Kolar, O.: Neurology (Minneapolis) **18**:1-7, 1968 (sclerosing panencephalitis).

165 Ziegler, D. K., Zosa, A., and Zileli, T.: Arch. Neurol. (Chicago) **12**:472-478, 1965 (hypertensive encephalopathy).

166 Zimmerman, H. M., and Netzky, M. G.: Assoc. Res. Nerv. Ment. Dis. Proc. **28**:271-312, 1950 (multiple sclerosis).

Index